Nammalwar's Principles and Practice of
PEDIATRIC NEPHROLOGY

Nammalwar's Principles and Practice of PEDIATRIC NEPHROLOGY

THIRD EDITION

Editors

Arpana A Iyengar
MD DNB FPN FRCP
Professor
Department of Pediatric Nephrology
St John's National Academy of Health Sciences
Bengaluru, Karnataka, India

Susan Uthup
MD DNB (Ped) DM (Nephro) DNB (Nephro) FISN
Professor and Head
Department of Pediatric Nephrology
SAT Hospital, Government Medical College
Thiruvananthapuram, Kerala, India

Sudha Ekambaram
DNB (Peds) FPN FISN (Singapore)
Head
Department of Pediatric Nephrology
Mehta Multispeciality Hospitals India Pvt Ltd
Chennai, Tamil Nadu, India

Foreword
Kumud Pravin Mehta

JAYPEE

JAYPEE BROTHERS MEDICAL PUBLISHERS
The Health Sciences Publisher
New Delhi | London

Jaypee Brothers Medical Publishers (P) Ltd.

Headquarters

Jaypee Brothers Medical Publishers (P) Ltd
EMCA House, 23/23-B
Ansari Road, Daryaganj
New Delhi 110 002, India
Landline: +91-11-23272143, +91-11-23272703
+91-11-23282021, +91-11-23245672
Email: jaypee@jaypeebrothers.com

Corporate Office

Jaypee Brothers Medical Publishers (P) Ltd
4838/24, Ansari Road, Daryaganj
New Delhi 110 002, India
Phone: +91-11-43574357
Fax: +91-11-43574314
Email: jaypee@jaypeebrothers.com

EU GPSR Authorised Representative
Logos Europe, 9 rue Nicolas Poussin
17000, La Rochelle, France
Phone: +33 (0) 6 67 93 73 78
E-mail: Contact@logoseurope.eu

Website: www.jaypeebrothers.com
Website: www.jaypeedigital.com

Inquiries for bulk sales may be solicited at: jaypee@jaypeebrothers.com

Nammalwar's Principles and Practice of Pediatric Nephrology

First Edition: 2004

Second Edition: 2013

Third Edition: **2023, Reprint: 2025**

ISBN: 978-93-5465-490-9

Printed in India

Dedicated to

Late Dr M Vijayakumar

Contributors

Abhijeet Saha
Professor
Division of Pediatric Nephrology
Department of Pediatrics
Lady Hardinge Medical College and
Kalawati Saran Children's Hospital
New Delhi, India

Aditi Das
Senior Resident
Department of Pediatrics
Lady Hardinge Medical College and
Kalawati Saran Children's Hospital
New Delhi, India

Aditi Sinha
Associate Professor
Division of Nephrology
Department of Pediatrics
All India Institute of Medical Sciences
New Delhi, India

Alpana Ohri
Associate Professor, Pediatrics
In-Charge, Pediatric Nephrology
Bai Jerbai Wadia Hospital for Children
Consultant Pediatric Nephrology
Jaslok Hospital
Mumbai, Maharashtra, India

Amish Udani
Consultant
Department of Pediatric Nephrology
Bai Jerbai Wadia Hospital for Children
Lokmanya Tilak Municipal General
Hospital and Lokmanya Tilak Municipal
Medical College
Mumbai, Maharashtra, India

Anil Vasudevan
Professor and Head
Department of Pediatric Nephrology
St. John's Medical College Hospital
Bengaluru, Karnataka, India

Anila Abraham Kurien
Pathologist
Renopath, Center for Renal and Urological
Pathology
Chennai, Tamil Nadu, India

Anoop Subash
Pediatric Surgeon
Shishoo—The Children's Hospital
Mysuru, Karnataka, India

Anshuman Saha
Assistant Professor
Department of Pediatric Nephrology
Institute of Kidney Disease and Research
Centre
Gujarat Institute of Transplantation
Sciences
Ahmedabad, Gujarat, India

Arpana A Iyengar
Professor
Department of Pediatric Nephrology
St John's National Academy of Health
Sciences
Bengaluru, Karnataka, India

Arvind Bagga
Professor and Chief
Division of Nephrology
Department of Pediatrics
All India Institute of Medical Sciences
New Delhi, India

Asok Kumar GM
Professor
Department of Pediatric Surgery
Government Medical College
Thiruvananthapuram, Kerala, India

Banigallapati Vijay Kiran
Assistant Professor
Department of Nephrology
Nizam's Institute of Medical Sciences
Hyderabad, Telangana, India

Beena SV
Professor
Department of Pediatric Surgery
Government Medical College
Thiruvananthapuram, Kerala, India

Binu MK
Assistant Professor
Department of Pediatric Surgery
Government Medical College
Thiruvananthapuram, Kerala, India

BR Nammalwar
Consultant
Department of Pediatric Nephrology
Mehta Multispecialty Hospital
Chennai, Tamil Nadu, India

Brinda Panchal Jain
Consultant Pediatric Nephrologist
Thunga Hospital
Former Specialty Medical Consultant
Hinduhrudaysamrat Balasaheb Thackarey
Medical College and Dr Rustom Narsi
Cooper Municipal General Hospital
Mumbai, Maharashtra, India

Christy Cathreen Thomas
Assistant Professor
Pediatric Nephrology
Department of Pediatrics
SAT Hospital, Government Medical
College
Alappuzha, Kerala, India

CS Aravind
Associate Professor
Department of Pediatric Surgery
SAT Hospital, Government Medical
College
Thiruvananthapuram, Kerala, India

CV Kanimozhi
Consultant Pediatric Radiologist
Kanchi Kamakoti CHILDS Trust Hospital
Chennai, Tamil Nadu, India

Deepthi RV
Assistant Professor
Division of Pediatric Nephrology
Child Health Unit 2, Department of Child
Health
Christian Medical College
Vellore, Tamil Nadu, India

Devi S Sruthi
Assistant Professor
Department of Nephrology
TD Medical College
Thiruvananthapuram, Kerala, India

Dimpy Waghela
Fellow, Pediatric Nephrology
Division of Pediatric Nephrology and
Renal Transplantation
Institute of Child Health
Sir Ganga Ram Hospital
New Delhi, India

Edwin Fernando M
Professor and Head
Department of Nephrology
Government Stanley Medical College,
Chennai
Senior Consultant Nephrologist and
Transplant Physician
Mehta Multispecialty Hospital
Chennai, Tamil Nadu, India

G Nandhini
Pediatric Surgeon and Urologist
Mehta Children's Hospital
Chennai, Tamil Nadu, India

G Sangeetha
Assistant Professor
Department of Pediatric Medicine and
Division of Pediatric Nephrology
Sri Ramachandra Institute of Higher
Education and Research
Chennai, Tamil Nadu, India

Geetika Singh
Professor
Department of Pathology
All India Institute of Medical Sciences
New Delhi, India

Girish C Bhatt
Associate Professor
Department of Pediatrics
All India Institute of Medical Sciences
Bhopal, Madhya Pradesh, India

Gurdeep Dhooria
Associate Professor
Department of Pediatrics
Dayanand Medical College and Hospital
Ludhiana, Punjab, India

Gurinder Kumar
Past fellow
Department of Pediatric Nephrology
St John's Medical College Hospital,
Bengaluru
Metrohealth Medical Center
Cleveland, Ohio, USA

Hamsa V Reddy
Assistant Professor
Division of Pediatric Nephrology
Department of Pediatrics
Ramaiah Medical College and Teaching
Hospital
Bengaluru, Karnataka, India

Indira Agarwal
Professor and Head
Subdivision of Pediatric Nephrology
Head, Division of Pediatrics
Christian Medical College Hospital
Vellore, Tamil Nadu, India

Jayati Sengupta
Consultant
Department of Pediatrics
AMRI Hospitals and
Department of Pediatric Nephrology
Institute of Child Health
Kolkata, West Bengal, India

Jitendra Meena
Assistant Professor
Department of Pediatrics
Postgraduate Institute of Medical
Education and Research
Chandigarh, India

Jyoti Sharma
Consultant Pediatric Nephrologist
King Edward Memorial Hospital
Pune, Maharashtra, India

Jyoti Singhal
Junior Consultant Pediatric Nephrologist
King Edward Memorial Hospital
Pune, Maharashtra, India

Kalaivani Ganesan
Senior Consultant
Department of Pediatric Nephrology
Mehta Multispecialty Hospital
Chennai, Tamil Nadu, India

Kanav Anand
Consultant Pediatric Nephrologist
Division of Pediatric Nephrology and
Renal Transplantation
Institute of Child Health
Sir Ganga Ram Hospital
New Delhi, India

Kanika Kapoor
Associate Professor
Department of Pediatrics
Vardhman Mahavir Medical College and
Safdarjung Hospital
New Delhi, India

Karalanglin Tiewsoh
Associate Professor
Department of Pediatric Nephrology
In-Charge, Pediatric Nephrology Unit
Postgraduate Institute of Medical
Education and Research
Chandigarh, India

Kiran Sathe
Consultant Pediatric Nephrologist
Department of Pediatrics
Sir HN Reliance Foundation Hospital and
Research Centre
Mumbai, Maharashtra, India

Kirtisudha Mishra
Associate Professor
Department of Pediatrics
Chacha Nehru Bal Chikitsalaya
New Delhi, India

Leema George
Scientist
MV Hospital for Diabetes and
Prof M Viswanathan Diabetes Research
Centre
Chennai, Tamil Nadu, India

Liji R
Senior Consultant
Department of Nephrology
Government General Hospital
Thiruvananthapuram, Kerala, India

Madhuri Kanitkar
Vice Chancellor
Maharashtra University of Health Sciences
(MUHS)
Nashik, Maharashtra, India

Mahantesh V Patil
Professor and Head
Department of Pediatrics
In-Charge, Pediatric Nephrology Division
Consultant Pediatric Nephrologist
KLES Dr Prabhakar Kore Hospital and
Medical Research Centre
Belagavi, Karnataka, India

Manish Kumar
Professor
Department of Pediatrics
Chacha Nehru Bal Chikitsalaya
New Delhi, India

Manoj G Matnani
Pediatric Nephrologist
Department of Pediatrics
KEM Hospital
Pune, Maharashtra, India

Mehul A Shah
Consultant Pediatric Nephrologist
Apollo Health City and
Little Stars Children's Hospital
Hyderabad, Telangana, India

Menka Yadav
Assistant Professor
Division of Pediatric Nephrology
Department of Pediatrics
Lady Hardinge Medical College and
Kalawati Saran Children's Hospital
New Delhi, India

MS Yasmeen
Registrar
Department of Pediatric Nephrology
Little Stars Children Hospital
Hyderabad, Telangana, India

Mukta Mantan
Professor
Department of Pediatrics
Maulana Azad Medical College
New Delhi, India

N Prahlad
Senior Consultant Pediatric Nephrologist
Rainbow Children hospital
Chennai, Tamil Nadu, India

N Prasad
Former Head
Department of Pediatrics Surgery
Institute of Child Health
Chennai, Tamil Nadu, India

Nachiket Shankar
Professor
Department of Anatomy and Medical Education
St John's Medical College
Bengaluru, Karnataka, India

Neha Bandari
Pediatric Nephrologist
Akash Healthcare Superspecialty Hospital
New Delhi, India

Nisha Krishnamurthy
Associate Consultant
Pediatric Nephrology
SRCC Children Hospital
Mumbai, Maharashtra, India

Nivedita Kamath
Associate Professor
Department of Pediatric Nephrology
St. John's Medical College Hospital
Bengaluru, Karnataka, India

OP Mishra
Professor
Division of Pediatric Nephrology
Department of Pediatrics
Banaras Hindu University
Varanasi, Uttar Pradesh, India

Pankaj Hari
Professor
ICMR Center for Advanced Research in Nephrology
Department of Pediatrics
All India Institute of Medical Sciences
New Delhi, India

Pankaj Pandurang Bhansali
Orchid Pediatric Superspecialty Clinic
Mahatma Gandhi Missions Medical College
Kamalnayan Bajaj Hospital
Aurangabad, Maharashtra, India

Prajnya Ranganath
Additional Professor and Head
Department of Medical Genetics
Nizam's Institute of Medical Sciences, Hyderabad
Adjunct Scientist, Diagnostics Division
Centre for DNA Fingerprinting and Diagnostics
Hyderabad, Telangana, India

Priya Pais
Associate Professor
Pediatric Nephrology
St John's Medical College Hospital
Bengaluru, Karnataka, India

Priyanka Khandelwal
Assistant Professor (Adhoc)
Division of Pediatric Nephrology
Department of Pediatrics
All India Institute of Medical Sciences
New Delhi, India

Radhika C Radhakrishnan
Assistant Professor
Department of Pediatric Nephrology
SAT Hospital, Government Medical College
Thiruvananthapuram, Kerala, India

Raji RP
Senior Consultant
Department of Pediatric Nephrology
GG Hospital
Thiruvananthapuram, Kerala, India

Rajiv Sinha
Head
Department of Pediatric Nephrology
Institute of Child Health
Kolkata, West Bengal, India

Ranjeet W Thergaonkar
Professor
Department of Pediatrics
INHS Ashwini
Mumbai, Maharashtra, India

Rehna Rahman
Pediatric Nephrologist
Aster MIMS Hospital
Kozhikode, Kerala, India

Reshma Mirshad
Research Associate
MV Hospital for Diabetes and Prof M Viswanathan Diabetes Research Centre
Chennai, Tamil Nadu, India

Richa Prakash
Assistant Professor
Pediatric Nephrology Division
Kalawati Saran Children's Hospital
New Delhi, India

RW Thergaonkar
Professor
Department of Pediatrics
INHS Asvini
Mumbai, Maharashtra, India

S Muralinath
Consultant Pediatric Radiologist
Chennai, Tamil Nadu, India

S Prabha
Former Head and Senior Consultant
Department of Pediatric Nephrology
Mehta Multispecialty Hospital
Chennai, Tamil Nadu, India

S Thangavelu
Pediatric Consultant and Director of Pediatrics
Mehta Multispecialty Hospital
Chennai, Tamil Nadu, India

Saravanan M
Consultant Nephrologist
Apollo Children's Hospital
Chennai, Tamil Nadu, India

Saroj Kumar Patnaik
Professor and Head
Senior Advisor Pediatrics and Pediatric Nephrologist
Command Hospital Air Force
Bengaluru, Karnataka, India

Sasidaran Kandaswamy
Head
Advanced Pediatric Critical Care Center
Mehta Multispecialty Hospital
Chennai, Tamil Nadu, India

Sethunath S
Professor and Head
Department of Pediatric Surgery
SAT Hospital, Government Medical College
Thiruvananthapuram, Kerala, India

Sheeja Sugunan
Pediatric Intensivist and Associate Professor
Department of Pediatrics
SAT Hospital, Government Medical College
Thiruvananthapuram, Kerala, India

Shinaz Sadiq
Assistant Professor
Department of Pediatric Surgery
SAT Hospital, Government Medical College
Thiruvananthapuram, Kerala, India

Shubha AM
Professor and Head
Department of Pediatric Surgery
St Johns National Academy of Health Sciences
Bengaluru, Karnataka, India

Shweta Priyadarshini
Consultant Pediatric Nephrologist
Apollo Hospital, Hyderabad
Associate Professor
Department of Pediatric Nephrology
Apollo Health Education and Research Foundation
Hyderabad, Telangana, India

Soumya Reddy
Senior Resident
Department of Pediatric Nephrology
St John's Medical College Hospital
Bengaluru, Karnataka, India

Sripathi V
Senior Consultant Pediatric Urologist and Director Fellowship Program
Pediatric Urology Unit
Apollo Children's Hospital
Chennai, Tamil Nadu, India

Sriram Krishnamurthy
Additional Professor
Department of Pediatrics
Jawaharlal Institute of Postgraduate Medical Education and Research
Puducherry, India

Subhankar Sarkar
Consultant
Institute of Child Health
Kolkata, West Bengal, India

Subhasis Saha
Consultant
Department of Pediatric Surgery
Calcutta Medical Research Institute
Kolkata, West Bengal, India

Sudha Ekambaram
Head
Department of Pediatric Nephrology
Mehta Multispeciality Hospitals India Pvt Ltd
Chennai, Tamil Nadu, India

Sukanya Govindan
Consultant
Department of Pediatric Nephrology
Mehta Multispecialty Hospital
Chennai, Tamil Nadu, India

Suprita Kalra
Pediatric Nephrologist
Department of Pediatrics
Army Hospital Research and Referral
New Delhi, India

Suresh M
Assistant Professor
Department of Pediatrics
KMCH Institute of Health Sciences and Research
Coimbatore, Tamil Nadu, India

Susan Uthup
Professor and Head
Department of Pediatric Nephrology
SAT Hospital, Government Medical College
Thiruvananthapuram, Kerala, India

Sushmita Banerjee
Consultant Pediatrician
Calcutta Medical Research Institute
Kolkata, West Bengal, India

Swathi Shiri
Senior Resident
Department of Pediatric Nephrology
St John's Medical College Hospital
Bengaluru, Karnataka, India

Thirumurthi K
Chief of Nuclear Medicine
Madras Medical Mission
Chennai, Tamil Nadu, India

Uma S Ali
Senior Consultant
Department of Pediatric Nephrology
SRCC Children's Hospital, Lilavati Hospital, Jupiter Hospital
Mumbai, Maharashtra, India

Urmila Anandh
Senior Consultant and Head
Department of Nephrology
Yashoda Hospital
Secunderabad, Telangana, India

Vaishali More
Consultant Pediatric Nephrologist
Tara Children's Kidney Care
SRCC Children's Hospital, SL Raheja Hospital, Wockardt Hospital
Mumbai, Maharashtra, India

Vaishnavi Raman
Senior Resident
Department of Pediatrics
ESI Hospital
Chennai, Tamil Nadu, India

Vidhya T
Pediatric Urology Unit
Apollo Children's Hospital

Vijay Viswanathan
Head and Chief Diabetologist
MV Hospital for Diabetes and Prof M Viswanathan Diabetes Research Centre
Chennai, Tamil Nadu, India

Vinod Choudhary
Consultant Pediatric Nephrologist
Radiant Children's Hospital
Jodhpur, Rajasthan, India

Vivek Parameswara Sarma
Associate Professor
Department of Pediatric Surgery
SAT Hospital, Government Medical College
Thiruvananthapuram, Kerala, India

Message

A Dream in 1989 Comes True

Dr Arpana A Iyengar invited me to write on the birth and growth of the *Principles and Practice of Pediatric Nephrology*. A poor resemblance to the present book was released on January 7, 1989, at an annual CME of the then Indian Pediatric Nephrology Group (IPNG). It was titled Pediatric Nephrology—Selected Topics. It all began as a *potpourri* of 15 articles contributed by senior nephrologists in adult medicine and pediatricians who were striking in the field of pediatric nephrology. At that time, I had a dream. Here in is an extract from my Editor's column of that book.

"There has been a long felt need for a small book on renal medicine which would be of use to the postgraduates and practicing pediatricians. This book is born out of such a need. It is designed to be easy, simple to read, helpful to plan management and yet its scientific qualities not diluted. This is a collection of lecture notes and articles on Nephrology from many Senior Nephrologists and Pediatricians. *It is hoped that in the future this small nucleus will grow into a standard textbook of Pediatric Nephrology of Indian origin."*

The second book titled Handbook of Glomerular Diseases was released in 1991. This book consisted of 14 chapters photocopied from different journals and books and was spiral bound.

Encouraged by pediatric colleagues and appreciative reception from postgraduates for these two attempts, I was encouraged to venture out for a comprehensive textbook in pediatric nephrology to cater to the needs of postgraduates in pediatric medicine and practicing pediatricians. Fortunately, Dr M Vijayakumar, with all his dynamism, supported the proposal. This book, published in 1993, included articles by authors of Indian origin in the United States and their department heads and was printed by M/s Alamu Printers from Chennai, Tamil Nadu. The copies were carried by us to various conferences and meets. We were happy with the acceptance by the students.

After a long break, we set out for the next edition in 2004. This time, two policy decisions were made. First, the book should also meet the needs of DM Nephrology students of Internal Medicine. Second, the book should be published by a prominent publisher to increase its publicity and visibility. Thanks to M/s Jaypee Brothers Medical Publishers (P) Ltd, New Delhi, India who accepted to print and publish. The Foreword was by Dr HPS Sachdev, Editor of Indian Pediatrics at that time. The publishers were strong in terming it the First Edition.

In 2013, the second edition was published. Dr M Vijayakumar took over the Chief Editorship. In keeping with his farsightedness, he added new topics on Genetics in Kidney Diseases, Molecular Basis of Inherited Kidney Diseases, and Pediatric Urology. The book was contributed by 61 authors, of which 59 were Indian authors—an astonishing mammoth and rapid growth of pediatric nephrology in India. We were honored by a Foreword by Dr Gokulnath, President of the Indian Society of Nephrology, Southern Chapter and Peritoneal Dialysis Society of India.

Dr M Vijayakumar is no longer with us and I was lost as to the future growth of the book. Drs Arpana A Iyengar, Susan Uthup, and Sudha Ekambaram with their magnanimity accepted the editorship and carried it forward. The third edition of the *Nammalwar's Principles and Practice of Pediatric Nephrology* is in the offing and in safe hands. Now I can rest in peace.

BR Nammalwar
Consultant
Department of Pediatric Nephrology
Mehta Multispecialty Hospital
Chennai, Tamil Nadu, India

Foreword

I am greatly honored and privileged to write the foreword for the 3rd edition of the book *Nammalwar's Principles and Practice of Pediatric Nephrology* edited by Dr Arpana A Iyengar, Dr Susan Uthup and Dr Sudha Ekambaram under the able guidance of Professor BR Nammalwar, Mehta Children's Hospital, Chennai, Tamil Nadu, India.

The book has 100 chapters divided into 15 sections. Each section includes 3–12 topics. The presentation is simple, lucid, and gives current information as well as recent advances on the evaluation and management of diseases affecting the kidneys and urinary tract. Simple bedside tests and sophisticated investigations, especially in the field of immunology and genetics have been incorporated.

Professor Nammalwar is known for promoting the younger generation to come to the forefront of academic activities. It is encouraging to see names of the younger generation of Pediatric Nephrologists in the list of authors.

Highlights of this book include a comprehensive in-depth review of all recent aspects in the field using flowcharts, illustrations, and algorithms. Authors from all major centers across the country have contributed to the making of this book. Every chapter includes a conclusion and key points. In addition, references have been cited. Emphasis has been given to IPNA (International Pediatric Nephrology Association) guidelines and Indian Society of Pediatric Nephrology guidelines. A dedicated chapter on the current pandemic of COVID-19 and its effect on the kidney is timely and appropriate. Inclusion of current topics like nephro-pharmacology, bio-ethics, registries, database, nomograms, and transition to adult nephrology are special additions to this edition.

My sincere congratulation to Professor BR Nammalwar and his entire team for launching this 3rd edition of *Nammalwar's Principles and Practice of Pediatric Nephrology*. I am sure that this 3rd edition will be a valuable reference guide for all pediatric postgraduates, nephrology fellows and residents across India.

Kumud Pravin Mehta
Senior Consultant
Pediatric Nephrologist
Jaslok Hospital and Research Center
Mumbai, Maharashtra, India

Preface to the Third Edition

The *Nammalwar's Principles and Practice of Pediatric Nephrology*, introduced by Professor BR Nammalwar, has successfully fulfilled the need for a reference book providing concise, practical information to pediatricians and fellows in training for two decades. We are pleased to introduce a new generation of learners to the 3rd edition of this book, completely updated and written in a new format.

This textbook had a modest beginning in the year 2000 as a compilation of teaching materials from the Pediatric Nephrology National conference held in Chennai by Dr BR Nammalwar, the doyen of Pediatric Nephrology in South India. This new edition is a tribute to the late Dr M Vijayakumar, who supported Dr Nammalwar's quest to make the knowledge of children's kidney diseases accessible to all. Dr M Vijayakumar was a great clinician, a teacher par excellence, and the editor of previous two editions of this book.

This 3rd edition reflects the immense advances that pediatric nephrology has seen in recent times and has many new features to enhance learning. The entire spectrum of pediatric kidney disease is presented comprehensively, yet in an easy-to-read format with colorful illustrations, tables and flowcharts. Each of the 15 sections has been written to provide the necessary theoretical concepts to understand a disease, yet focuses on the practical approach to a patient. For the first time, each chapter includes references. We have introduced new chapters on genetics of kidney disease, COVID-19-related kidney disease, nephro-pharmacology, AKI to CKD progression, bio-ethics, and transition of care from pediatric to adult nephrology. In keeping with today's practice, the book contains online links to disease registries and databases. The appendices contain easy to reference normative data charts and algorithms.

In this edition, many senior authors in India who are experts in the field have collaborated with younger colleagues and members of the Indian Society of Pediatric Nephrology in writing these chapters. We are confident that this will foster the growth of pediatric nephrology as a specialty and also encourages the feeling of community amongst pediatric nephrologists in India. We acknowledge the efforts and timely contributions of all the authors.

Words are not enough to express our gratitude to Professor Dr BR Nammalwar, for his timely advice, unfailing support and above all the encouragement to accomplish our goal of editing this edition. We are grateful to Dr Rajul Jain (Development Editor) and the entire team of M/s Jaypee Brothers Medical Publishers (P) Ltd, New Delhi, India for their efforts in publishing this book. We are thankful to Mr Suresh for his sincere secretarial assistance and for coordinating communication with all contributors.

We take immense pride in bringing out this new 3rd edition. We hope that it maintains the spirit and fulfils the goal of the earlier editions of the book as a comprehensive reference book of Pediatric Nephrology for medical students, fellows in training and any physician caring for children with kidney diseases.

Arpana A Iyengar
Susan Uthup
Sudha Ekambaram

Preface to the First Edition

The third edition of *Principles and Practice of Pediatric Nephrology* is being published after 10 years. The second edition was published in 1993. Since then, there has been constant request from the postgraduates and colleagues for the next edition. The outcome of this encouragement and support is the printing of this third edition. We have attempted to make this textbook as comprehensive as possible and at the same time to keep the presentation in simple language. Newer chapters such as Inherited Diseases of the Kidney, Genetic Basis of Renal Diseases, Renal Replacement Therapy and Newer Investigation Modalities have been included in this book.

Our friends Drs N Somu, L Subramanyam, A Balachandran, K Nedunchelian, NC Gowrishankar, S Lakshmi and So Shivbalan, have contributed extensively in every respect in the production of this book as in the earlier edition.

We are thankful to our colleagues and senior pediatric nephrologist, for their contribution to this book. We cannot forget our friends and colleagues from India and abroad, who have contributed their experience to the book. If this book is good and useful, it is because of contributions from these Authors.

We are grateful to Dr Radhakrishna Baliga, the center pin, for the success in obtaining contributions from senior and respected faculty from abroad. We are fortunate to have the unstinted support of our former colleagues Dr Vivek Narendran, Dr Aravind Kasaragode, for their own contribution and also from their colleagues.

We are thankful to Dr HPS Sachdev, our friend and guide as well as a senior pediatrician of India, for his 'Foreword' to this book.

We are sincerely thankful and grateful to our friends, Mr G Suresh and Mr S Rajkumar, for their sincere and unconditional secretarial assistance.

We are thankful to our wives, children and our family members, for their patience and mental support to bring out this book.

We are grateful to M/s Jaypee Brothers Medical Publishers (P) Ltd, New Delhi, India, for their willingness to support our cause by accepting to print and publish this book, *Principles and Practice of Pediatric Nephrology*.

We request our readers, the postgraduates, teachers and colleagues, for their critical review, suggestions and comments to improve in the next edition.

Nammalwar BR
Vijayakumar M

Contents

Section 1: Basics of Developmental Nephrology

Section 2: Investigating a Child with Kidney Disease

Section 3: Symptoms and Signs of Kidney Disease

Section 4: Approach to Management of Fluid, Electrolyte and Acid-base Disorders

Section 5: Neonatal Nephrology

Section 6: Glomerular Diseases

Section 7: Kidney Manifestation of Systemic Diseases

Section 8: Tubular Disorders

Section 9: Ciliopathies and Hereditary Tubulointerstitial Diseases

Section 13: Pediatric Urology

Section 14: Assorted Themes

Section 15: Clinical Practice Resources

SECTION

1

Basics of Developmental Nephrology

CHAPTER

1.1

Embryology of the Kidney and Urinary Tract

Nachiket Shankar

INTRODUCTION

The three germ layers from which all the tissues of the body develop are the ectoderm, endoderm, and mesoderm. The mesoderm is further subdivided into the paraxial, intermediate, and lateral plate components. The kidney and urinary tract develop from the *intermediate mesoderm* **(Fig. 1)**.

The intermediate mesoderm lies between the paraxial mesoderm medially and the lateral plate mesoderm laterally.[1] It extends craniocaudally on each side of the primitive dorsal aorta, projects into the dorsal wall of the coelomic cavity, and is covered by coelomic epithelium. It extends from the cervical region to the sacral region of the embryo. In the cervical and upper thoracic regions, the intermediate mesoderm shows segmentation and each segment is known as a *nephrotome*. The rest of the intermediate mesoderm forms an unsegmented column on either side of the dorsal aorta, known as the *urogenital ridge*.[2] The urogenital ridge is divided into the *gonadal ridge* that forms the gonads and the *nephrogenic cord* that contributes to the development of the excretory system. Several important structures are formed in relation to the urogenital ridge on each side as follows **(Fig. 2)**:

- Gonad (testis or ovary), which develops from the coelomic epithelium lining the medial side of the urogenital ridge
- Excretory tubules associated with the development of the kidney
- Nephric duct or primary excretory duct
- Paramesonephric duct or Mullerian duct

The other structure that contributes to the development of the urinary tract is the *primitive urogenital sinus* **(Figs. 3A to C)**.

The *cloaca* is the dilated post-allantoic part of the hindgut. It is subdivided by the urorectal septum into the primitive urogenital sinus ventrally and the primitive rectum dorsally. The primitive urogenital sinus is subdivided into a cranial part called the *vesicourethral canal* and a caudal part called the *definitive urogenital sinus*. The openings of the mesonephric ducts lie at the junction of these two subdivisions. Later, the definitive urogenital sinus shows a division into a cranial pelvic part and a caudal phallic part. The urogenital system is derived from structures that develop from the intermediate mesoderm and subdivisions of the primitive urogenital sinus.[3]

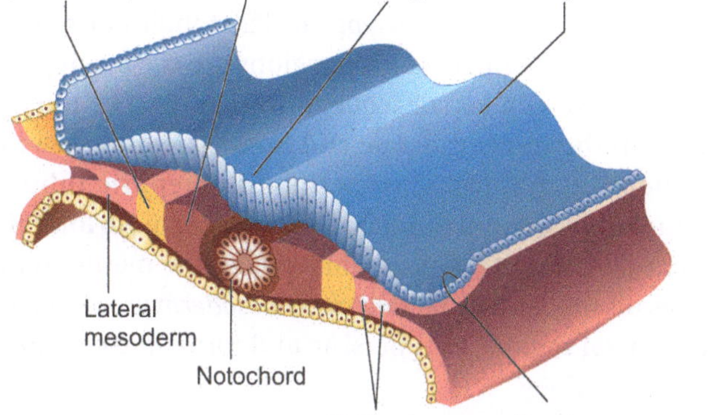

Fig. 1: Transverse section of an embryo in the third week of development showing the location of the intermediate mesoderm.
Source: With permission from Moore KL, Persaud TVN, Torchia MG. The Developing Human, 10th edition. Amsterdam: Elsevier; 2017.

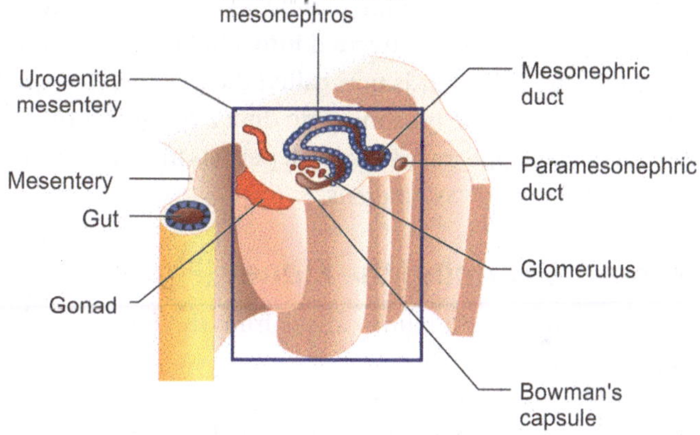

Fig. 2: Transverse section of an embryo in the fifth week of development showing the components of the urogenital ridge enclosed within the blue box.
Source: With permission from Sadler TW. Langman's Medical Embryology, 12th edition. Amsterdam: Wolters Kluwer; 2011.

DEVELOPMENT OF THE KIDNEYS

Formation of the Excretory Tubules (Fig. 4)

Excretory tubules arise in a craniocaudal direction from the cervical region to the sacral region.[1] As more caudal tubules

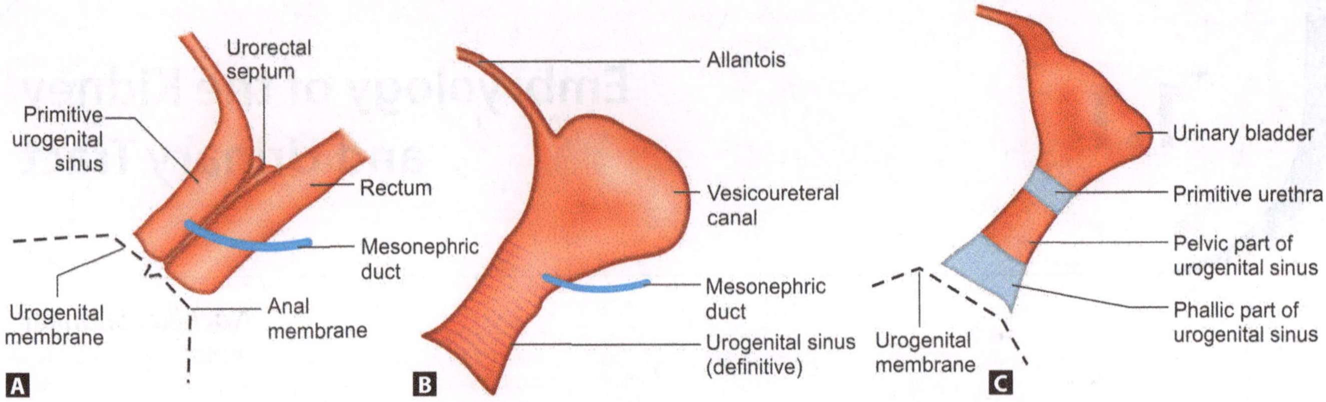

Figs. 3A to C: The formation and parts of the primitive urogenital sinus.
Source: With permission from Subhadra Devi V. Inderbir Singh's Human Embryology, 11th edition. New Delhi: Jaypee Brothers Medical Publishers; 2018.

form, the cranial tubules disappear. The tubules formed in the cervical and upper thoracic regions are the pronephric tubules. These tubules subsequently disappear. The tubules formed in the lower thoracic and lumbar regions are the mesonephric tubules. Most of the mesonephric tubules disappear, but some of the caudal tubules persist to form the efferent ductules of the testes. In females, the mesonephric tubules disappear. The *metanephric mesoderm* is seen in the lumbosacral region. This persists and forms the excretory part of the kidney.

Nephric Duct (Fig. 4)

The nephric duct or the primary excretory duct is initially situated dorsally in the nephrogenic cord as a solid rod of cells.[1] It differentiates before the nephric tubules. As it lengthens, its caudal end separates from the nephrogenic cord and passes anteriorly to approach the cloaca. This solid rod of cells is progressively converted into a hollow duct, which opens into the cloaca. It is now called the *mesonephric duct* or Wolffian duct. The mesonephric duct after giving off the ureteric bud disappears in females. It persists in males to form the epididymis and vas deferens.

Primordia Forming the Kidney (Fig. 5)

The definitive human kidney arises from the following two distinct sources:[2]

1. The excretory tubules or nephrons are derived from the metanephric mesoderm, also called the *metanephric blastema.*
2. The collecting part, which is derived from a diverticulum of the mesonephric duct called the *ureteric bud.*

Collecting System (Figs. 6A to D)

The *ureteric bud* gives rise to the collecting ducts of the permanent kidney.[2] The bud penetrates the metanephric tissue, which forms a cap over its distal end. The primitive renal pelvis develops from a dilatation of the bud. It then

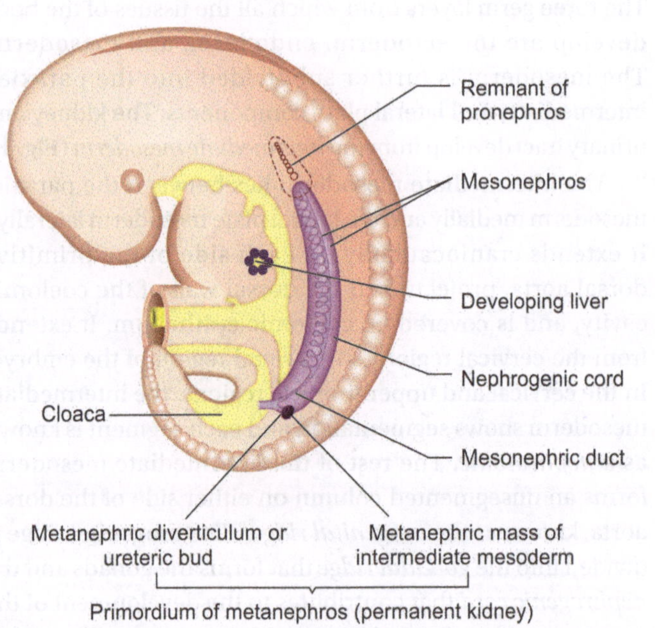

Fig. 4: Formation of the three sets of excretory tubules and the mesonephric duct. Primordium of metanephros (permanent kidney)
Source: With permission from Moore KL, Persaud TVN, Torchia MG. The Developing Human, 10th edition. Amsterdam: Elsevier; 2017.

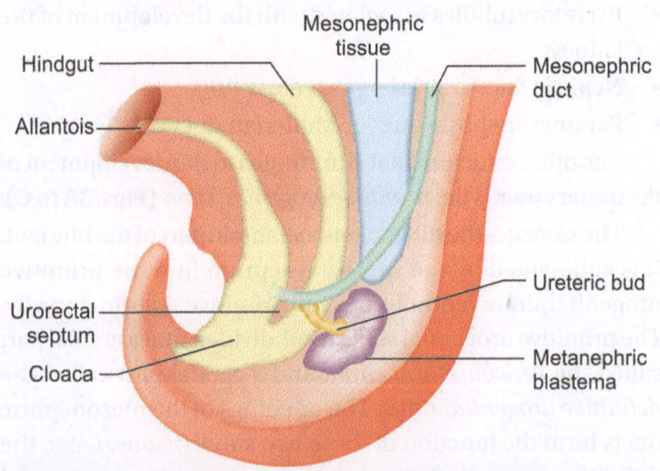

Fig. 5: The two primordia that form the kidney, namely the ureteric bud and the metanephric blastema.
Source: With permission from Sadler TW. Langman's Medical Embryology, 12th edition. Amsterdam: Wolters Kluwer; 2011.

divides into cranial and caudal parts which give rise to the future major calyces. As each calyx penetrates the metanephric tissue, it divides into two new buds. Two further subdivisions of these buds occur. The minor calyces are formed by an enlargement of the second-order tubules which absorb those of the third and fourth orders. The renal pyramid is formed by a substantial lengthening of the collecting tubules of the fifth and subsequent orders and their convergence upon the minor calyces. Thus, the ureteric bud gives rise to the following structures:

- Ureter
- Renal pelvis
- Major and minor calyces
- Approximately one to three million collecting tubules

Excretory System (Figs. 7A to F)

A *metanephric tissue cap* covers the distal ends of each of the subdivisions of the ureteric bud.[2] *Renal vesicles* are formed from these metanephric caps after induction by the ureteric bud. These vesicles are converted into small S-shaped tubules. The ends of these tubules become indented by capillaries which form glomeruli. The glomeruli and tubules together constitute the *nephrons* or excretory units. The portion of the nephron which is in close proximity to the glomerulus develops into Bowman's capsule. The distal end of each nephron establishes continuity with a collecting tubule. The other parts of the nephron, namely the proximal convoluted tubule, loop of Henle, and distal convoluted tubule, develop as the nephron continues to elongate.

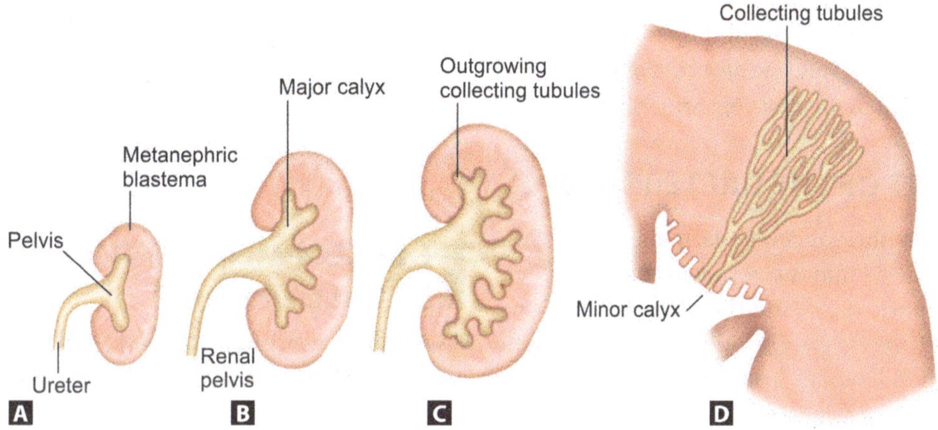

Figs. 6A to D: Developments of the renal pelvis, calyces, and collecting tubules from the ureteric bud.
Source: With permission from Sadler TW. Langman's Medical Embryology, 12th edition. Amsterdam: Wolters Kluwer; 2011.

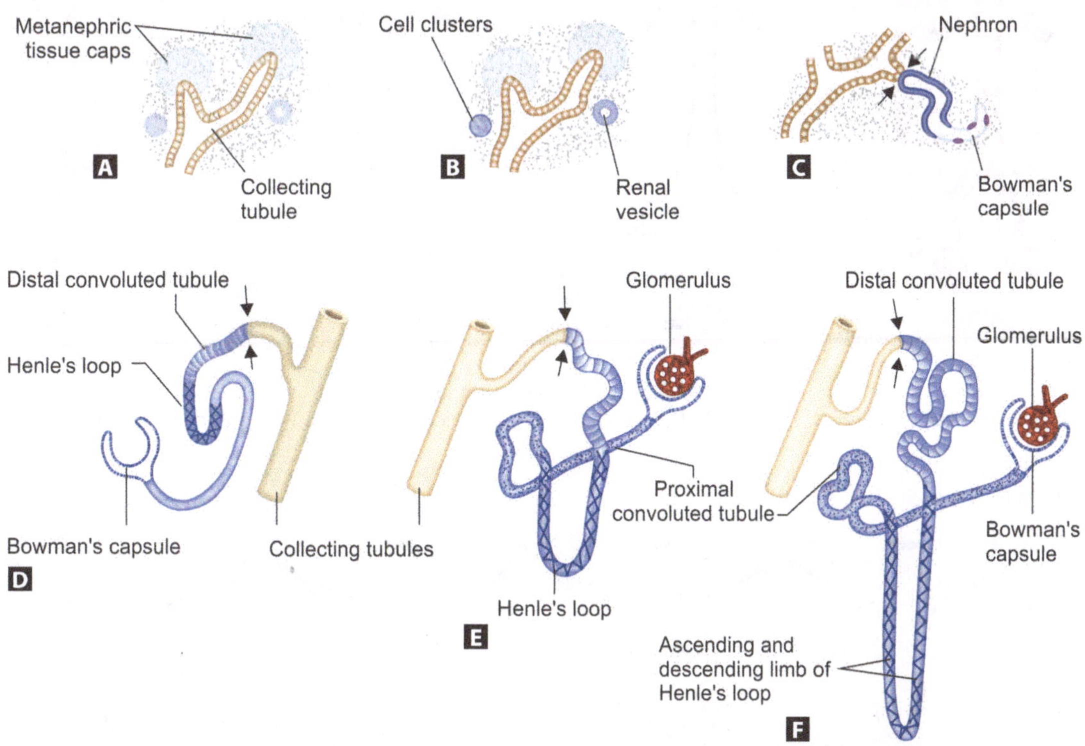

Figs. 7A to F: Stages in the development of nephrons and their communication with the collecting tubules.
Source: With permission from Sadler TW. Langman's Medical Embryology, 12th edition. Amsterdam: Wolters Kluwer; 2011.

Ascent and Rotation of the Kidneys (Figs. 8A to D)

The kidneys are initially situated in the pelvic region. They progressively ascend to reach their final location in the abdomen. Ascent of the kidneys to the lumbar region occurs because of differential growth of the body wall.[1] The kidneys receive their arterial supply from the lateral splanchnic branches of the abdominal aorta. Unlike the gonads which retain their initial arterial supply, the arteries that supply the kidney change with their ascent. The lateral sacral arteries initially supply the kidneys. The superior branches of the aorta take over the supply as they ascend. The definitive renal artery is a lateral splanchnic branch of the aorta that arises at the level of the second lumbar vertebra. As the kidneys ascend, their hila face anteriorly. The kidneys rotate medially as they reach their final location in the abdomen, so their hila eventually face the midline[1]. Fetal kidneys are lobulated, and this condition persists up to the first year after birth.

DEVELOPMENT OF THE URETERS (FIG. 9)

The parts of the mesonephric ducts caudal to the origin of the *ureteric buds* are absorbed into the vesicourethral canal.[4] As a result, the mesonephric ducts and the ureteric buds have separate openings into the cloaca. The openings of the ureteric bud move cranially and laterally. The triangular area on the dorsal wall of the vesicourethral canal between the openings of the ureteric buds and those of the mesonephric ducts is therefore of mesodermal origin. The ureter is derived from the part of the *ureteric bud* that lies between the pelvis of the kidney and the vesicourethral canal.

DEVELOPMENT OF THE URINARY BLADDER (FIGS. 3 AND 9)

The entire mucosa of the bladder, except the internal trigone, is developed from the endoderm of the *vesicourethral part* of the *primitive urogenital sinus.* The apex of the bladder is derived from absorption of the proximal part of the allantoic diverticulum. The *internal trigone* of the bladder is developed from *mesoderm* by incorporation of the caudal parts of the *mesonephric ducts.* The musculature and serous walls of the bladder are developed from the splanchnic layer of *lateral plate mesoderm,* which surrounds the cloaca. The distal part of the allantoic diverticulum is obliterated and persists as the *urachus,* which extends from the apex of the bladder to the umbilicus. It is known as the median umbilical ligament in the adult.[4]

DEVELOPMENT OF THE FEMALE URETHRA

The female urethra is derived from the caudal part of the *vesicourethral canal* (endoderm). The posterior wall of

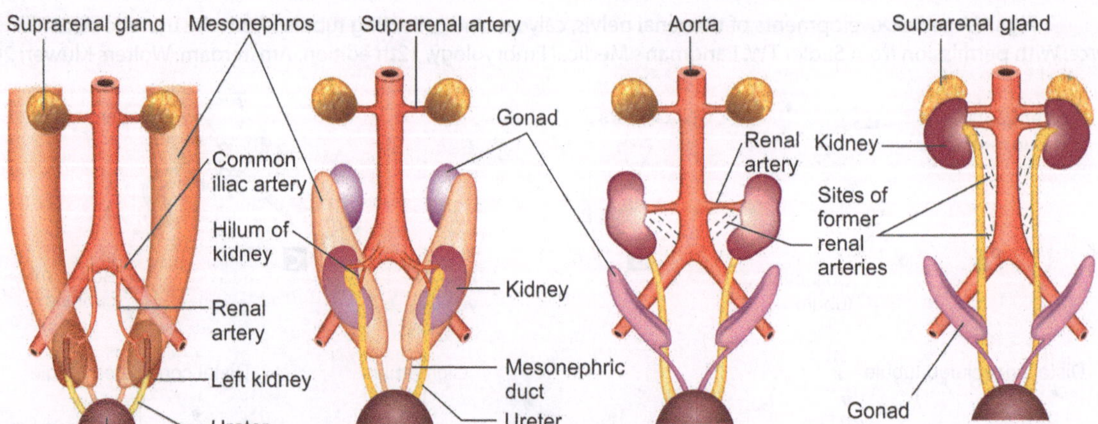

Figs. 8A to D: Ascent and rotation of the kidneys.
Source: With permission from Moore KL, Persaud TVN, Torchia MG. The Developing Human, 10th edition. Amsterdam: Elsevier; 2017.

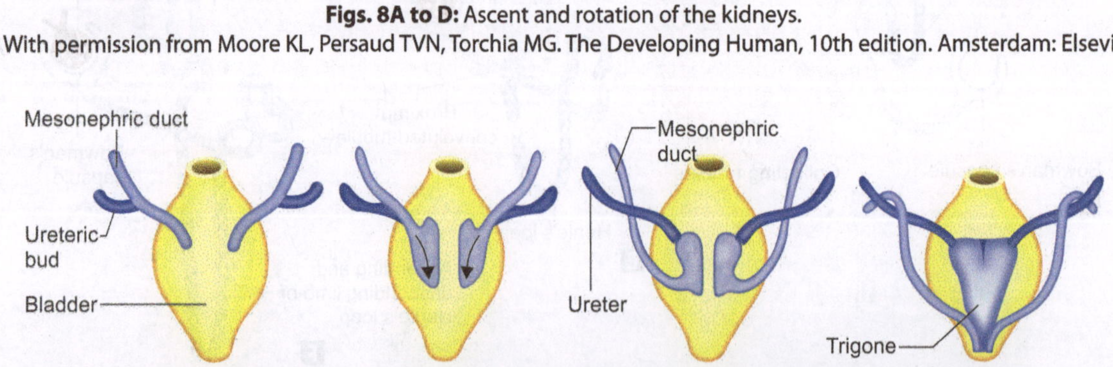

Fig. 9: Development of the trigone of the urinary bladder from the absorbed mesonephric ducts.
Source: With permission from Schoenwolf G, Bleyl S, Brauer P, Francis-West P. Larsen's Human Embryology, 5th edition. Amsterdam: Elsevier; 2014.

the urethra is derived from the mesonephric ducts and is mesodermal in origin. The female urethra may receive a slight contribution from the pelvic part of the urogenital sinus.[2]

DEVELOPMENT OF THE MALE URETHRA (FIGS. 10A TO D)

The caudal portion of the *vesicourethral canal* (endoderm) gives rise to the proximal part of the *prostatic urethra* up to the openings of the ejaculatory ducts. The absorbed mesonephric ducts (mesoderm) form the posterior wall of this part of the urethra. The *pelvic part* of the *definitive urogenital sinus* develops into the rest of the prostatic urethra and *membranous urethra*. The *phallic part* of the *definitive urogenital sinus* gives rise to the *penile urethra* with the exception of its most distal portion. The female urethra is developmentally analogous to the prostatic part of the male urethra.[2]

To understand the development of the *penile urethra*, it is essential to review the development of the external genitalia.[2] The *cloacal folds* are paired, elevated structures derived from mesenchymal cells that migrate from the primitive streak to a region around the cloacal membrane. The genital tubercle is formed by fusion of the cranial ends of the cloacal folds. The caudal portions of the cloacal folds become subdivided into the ventral *urethral folds* and dorsal anal folds. The genital swellings are elevations that develop immediately lateral to the urethral folds on each side. Up to this stage, development is common to both males and females. Testosterone secreted by the fetal testes influences the development of the male external genitalia. The genital tubercle elongates rapidly and is now called the phallus, which is the precursor of the penis. The urethral folds are drawn anteriorly by the growth of the phallus resulting in the formation of a *urethral groove*. The urethral groove is seen to occupy the ventral aspect of the enlarging phallus except for its terminal portion, the glans. The epithelial lining of the groove, which is endodermal, forms the *urethral plate*. The two urethral folds close over the urethral plate, forming the penile urethra. The most distal part of the penile urethra is formed by the canalization of a short cord of *ectodermal cells* which penetrate inwards from the tip of the glans.

MOLECULAR REGULATION AND FUNCTION (FIG. 11)

Differentiation of the kidney involves interactions between the epithelial and the mesenchymal primordia from which it develops. The epithelium of the ureteric bud induces the metanephric cap mesenchyme to differentiate into nephrons. The definitive kidneys developed from the metanephros start functioning around the 12th week. **Figure 11** summarizes the four stages in the development of the uriniferous tubules and the molecular mechanisms that regulate them.[5]

CONCLUSION

Kidneys develop from two sources. The metanephros gives rise to excretory tubules and the ureteric bud forms the collecting system. Nephron formation is a critical event that stems from the interaction between the metanephric blastema and the ampulla of the ureteric bud. The urinary bladder, female urethra, and prostatic proximal urethra are derived from the vesicourethral canal, whereas the rest of the male urethra develops from the urogenital sinus. **Flowcharts 1 and 2** illustrate key events in the development of the kidney and urinary tract, respectively.

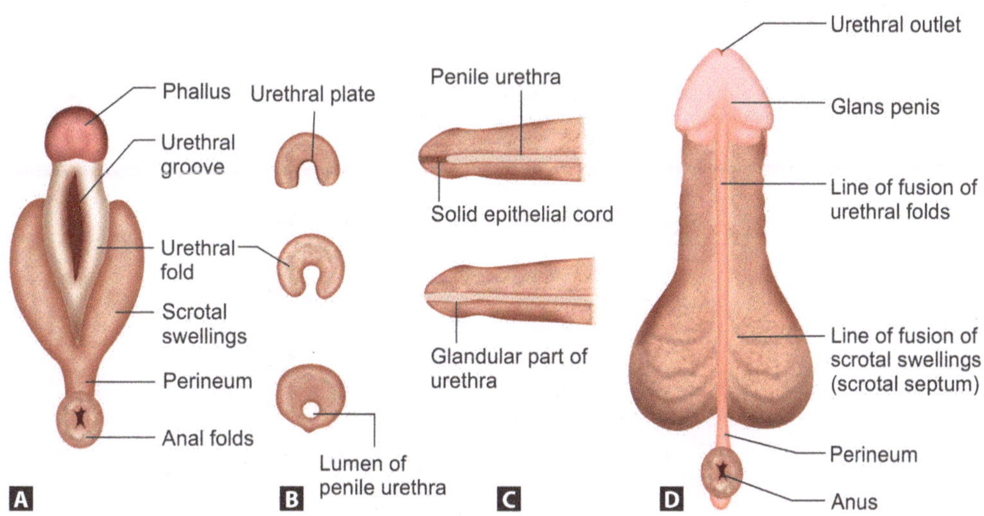

Figs. 10A to D: Development of the penile urethra. (A) Ventral view of the developing urethra; (B) Cross section through the shaft of the developing penis showing the stages in the development of the urethra; (C) Formation of the terminal portion of the urethra from ectoderm; (D) Ventral view of the external genitalia in a neonate.
Source: With permission from Sadler TW. Langman's Medical Embryology, 12th edition. Amsterdam: Wolters Kluwer; 2011.

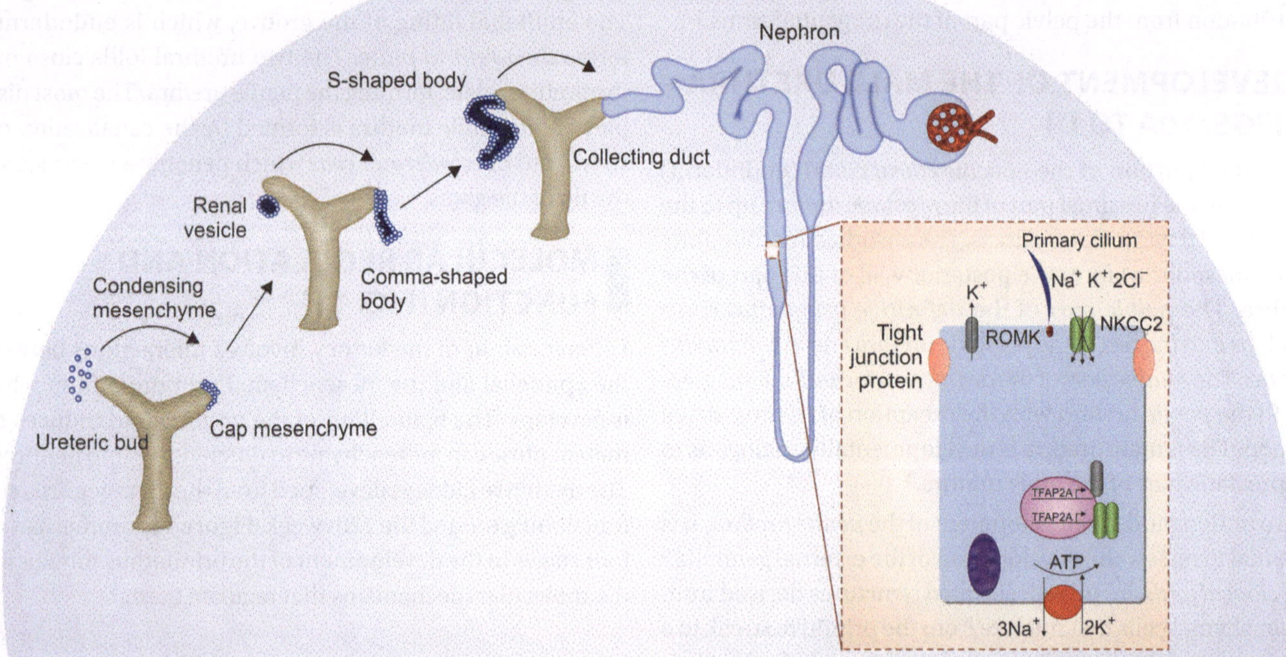

Metanephric mesenchyme	Nephron epithelialization and outgrowth	Nephron regionalization	Terminal differentiation
• Ureteric epithelium invades metanephric mesenchyme and branching begins • Nephron progenitor cells are contained in the cap mesenchyme and are regulated by many factors	• Formation of RV, CSB, SSB resulting in nephron • Changes from cell adhesion molecules to epithelial markers • Changes in polarity • Lumen formation	Molecular factors regulate regionalized signaling pathways	• Cells express genes specific to their roles • Expression of functional proteins, tight junction proteins, and soluble transporter proteins

Fig. 11: A summary of the molecular regulation of the development of the kidney. The details of molecular changes are listed in the table. (CSB: comma-shaped body; NPC: nephron progenitor cells; RV: renal vesicle; SSB: s-shaped body).
Source: With permission from Chambers JM, Wingert RA. Tissue Barriers. 2020;8(4). https://doi.org/10.1080/21688370.2020.1832844.

Flowchart 1: Development of the kidney.

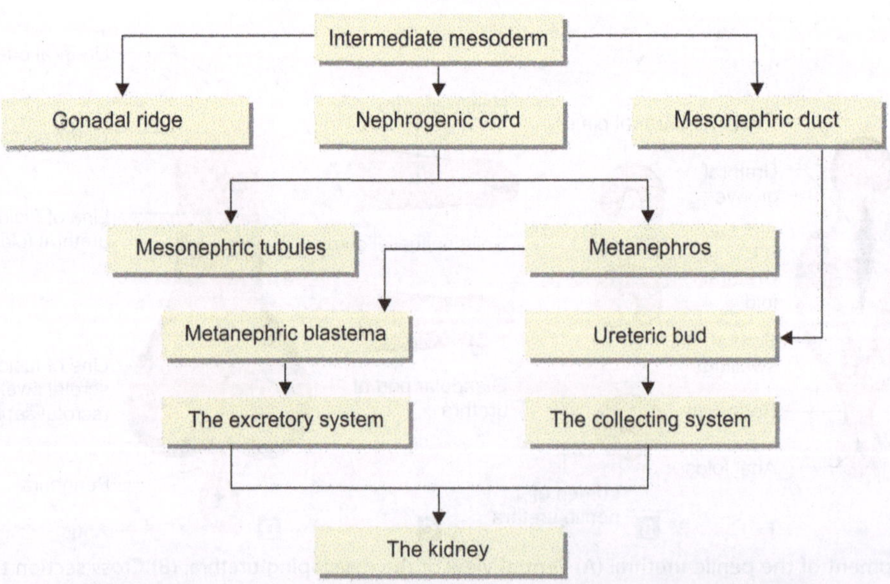

Flowchart 2: Development of the urinary bladder and urethra.

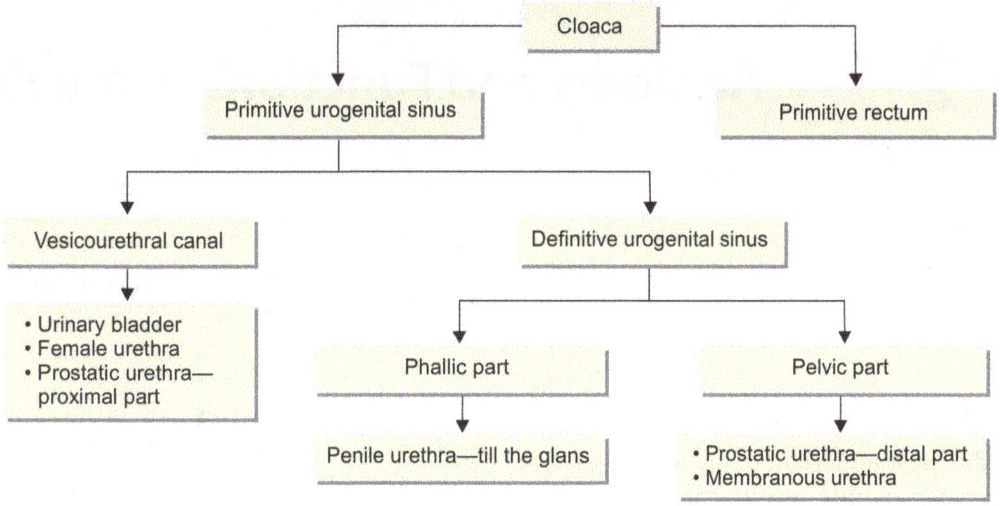

KEY POINTS

- Excretory system develops from the intermediate mesoderm.
- Kidneys form from the ureteric bud and metanephric blastema.
- Nephrons arise from the metanephric blastema.
- Collecting ducts develop from the ureteric bud.
- Ascent of kidneys takes place from the pelvic to the lumbar region.
- Ureters develop from ureteric buds.
- Urinary bladder forms from the vesicourethral canal, absorbed mesonephric ducts, and lateral plate mesoderm.
- Male urethra develops from primitive urethra and pelvic and phallic parts of definitive urogenital sinus.
- Female urethra forms from primitive urethra and pelvic part of definitive urogenital sinus.
- Molecular regulation involves epithelial-mesenchymal interactions between the ureteric bud and the metanephric mesenchyme.

REFERENCES

1. Moore KL, Persaud TVN, Torchia MG. The Developing Human, 10th edition. Amsterdam: Elsevier; 2017.
2. Sadler TW. Langman's Medical Embryology, 12th edition. Amsterdam: Wolters Kluwer; 2011.
3. Subhadra Devi V. Inderbir Singh's Human Embryology, 11th edition. New Delhi: Jaypee Brothers Medical Publishers; 2018.
4. Schoenwolf G, Bleyl S, Brauer P, Francis-West P. Larsen's Human Embryology, 5th edition. Amsterdam: Elsevier; 2014.
5. Chambers JM, Wingert RA. Tissue Barriers. 2020;8(4). https://doi.org/10.1080/21688370.2020.1832844

CHAPTER

1.2 Anatomy and Functions of the Kidneys

Sudha Ekambaram, BR Nammalwar

INTRODUCTION

The kidneys are the most important of the four regulatory systems and have a dynamic role in maintaining the homeostasis of the human body. The others are lungs, gastrointestinal tract, and the skin. The kidneys, in addition to maintaining homeostasis, have multiple metabolic functions: detoxify and remove toxins, regulate blood pressure through production of angiotensin and humoral factors, activate vitamin D production for bone metabolism, and release erythropoietin for red blood cell production in the bone marrow and gluconeogenesis. This chapter presents at first an introduction to the anatomy and function of the fetal kidney (FK) followed by that in children.

DEVELOPING ANATOMY OF FETAL KIDNEYS

Morphogenesis of the human kidney starts at the 5th week of gestation and extends up to the end of the last trimester of pregnancy. In premature neonates, functional maturation extends up to 2 weeks after birth.

The metanephros develops by about 5th week of embryonic life and represents the final adult kidney. The zone of transition between cortex and medulla appears at the start of the 14th week. An arcade system along with well-defined pyramids appears at 16–18 weeks. The kidney pelvis is very small and undifferentiated at 10 weeks and only fully differentiated at 18 weeks. The FK is made up of lobes. The number of lobes is about three to four at 8th week and increases to 40 to 50 in the 34th week. Each lobe is self-contained and is made up of a group of papillary ducts, their branches accompanied by nephrons and vessels.[1] The lobules start fusing with each other at 15 weeks of gestation. The number of lobes decreases to form the normal smooth surface of adult kidney at term.[2]

DEVELOPING FUNCTIONS OF FETAL KIDNEY

Metanephros forms nephrons at about 10 weeks. The fetal glomerular ultrafiltration process starts at 10–11 weeks of gestation. The important factor that determines the volume of glomerular ultrafiltrate depends on the number of functional nephron units or total renal mass. The FK filtrates the blood and makes a hypotonic urine. Urine output increases from 2.2 mL/h at 22 weeks to 12.2 mL/h at 32 weeks and 28 mL/h at term. The urine sodium and chloride content is lower than that in fetal plasma. The average pH is 6.0, slightly acidic. Fetal urine has more urea and creatinine than fetal plasma but contains little protein and glucose.[3] The urine forms two third of the amniotic fluid (AF). The amount of AF depends on the integrity of FK function. The swallowed AF is absorbed from the intestines and transported through circulation back to the kidneys where it is filtrated. The cycle goes on and on. However, this filtration is not sufficient to eliminate the waste materials. The waste materials are eliminated by the maternal kidneys when they are transported into the mother's blood through the placental membrane. In short, homeostasis of the fetus is primarily the responsibility of the placenta. The FK helps in synthesis of vitamin D, angiotensin, prostaglandin, and kallikrein–kinin system, which are active in the second half of the gestational period.[1]

Blood Supply

In the early gestational period, only about 2% of cardiac output goes to the kidneys. Systemic blood pressure is around 40–60 mm Hg, and kidney blood flow is low. Low renal blood flow (RBF) is due to elevated renal vascular resistances (RVRs). The FK blood flow increases with the increase of gestational age, kidney volume, and cardiac output, whereas the RVRs to blood flow decrease. During fetal hypoxia, there is redistribution of the fetal blood flow with an increase of the perfusion of brain, heart, liver, and adrenals and a decrease of the perfusion of the kidney. The humoral response of the kidney increases the fetal arterial pressure which maintains the hemodynamic compensation to hypoxia for some period of time. Ultimately, in hypoxic ischemic FK, the urine production is diminished.[4]

Glomerular Function

During fetal life, the glomerular filtration rate (GFR) is low due to low kidney blood flow associated with elevated RVRs. With the active development of FK, the GFR increases progressively although RVRs remain elevated. This state is due to a subtle equilibrium between vasoconstrictive factors, namely the renin-angiotensin system (RAS), renal sympathetic nervous system, and vasodilating factors such the prostaglandins and nitric oxide (NO). In the FK, the RAS is the principal vasoconstrictive factor. Angiotensin II increases the glomerular efferent tone while the renal sympathetic nervous system increases both afferent and efferent arteriole tone. The RAS is upregulated during active nephrogenesis and downregulated at the end of this process. The RAS maintains RBF and renal perfusion pressure. The FK releases renin circulation, which does not cross the placenta and remains higher than maternal serum levels.[5] Use of angiotensin-converting enzyme inhibitors and angiotensin II receptor blockers has been associated with adverse fetal effects.[6] Vasoconstrictive forces are counterbalanced by vasodilating factors that principally act on the glomerular afferent arteriole to maintain a sufficient RBF. Prostaglandins, NO, and kallikrein-kinin system are the principal factors. Prostaglandins are produced by both the placental membranes and the fetus, from the action of two enzyme isoforms, the cyclooxygenase types 1 and 2 (COX-1 and COX-2), and their production is stimulated by angiotensin II.[5] COX-2 is constitutively expressed in FK and appears essential for the development and function of the kidney.[7] Administration of COX inhibitors during pregnancy decreases kidney blood flow, impairs kidney function, and induces oligohydramnios. Other factors such as endothelin and atrial natriuretic factors modulate kidney hemodynamics.

Tubular Function

Individual tubular segments of the FK have different secretion and reabsorption activities. The individual tubular transporters mature at different periods during the development of the nephrons. In general, as in adult kidneys, the proximal tubule (PT) is principally involved in reabsorption of fluid, electrolytes, amino acids, and glucose, and the distal tubules (DTs) and collecting ducts are involved in fluid and tonicity regulation. The functions of the renal tubules of the FK are influenced by various hormones: RAS, aldosterone, prostaglandins, atrial natriuretic peptide, and cortisol.

The FK produces hypotonic urine at about 300 mL/kg fetal weight/day. The low concentration capacity and the hypotonic urine are due to (1) structural immaturity of the loop of Henle (LOH), (2) preferential distribution of blood flow to the inner cortex, (3) a low osmotic gradient concentration in the medulla due to low amounts of urea generated, (4) a low expression of aquaporin 2 (AQP2), and (5) low arginine vasopressin synthesized. The final result is hypotonic urine of about 100–250 mOsm. If the mother becomes dehydrated, some renal conservation of water occurs in the fetus. The very immature fetus copes less well than the mature, as both the release of arginine vasopressin and the renal effectiveness of this hormone increase significantly only over the last third of gestation.[8] The immaturity of tubular functions in the early pregnancy causes the high rate of AF production and, with its maturation, decreases AF production at the end stage of gestation. Filtration in FK is not necessary for the elimination of the waste materials as they are transported into the mother's blood through the placental membrane. That is why, the blood urea and serum creatinine levels reflect the maternal values.

In FK, the urinary sodium is reabsorbed by the sodium/hydrogen exchangers (NHEs), located at the luminal membrane of tubular cells. Unlike, as in postnatal life, in the FK the urinary sodium is mainly reabsorbed in the immature DTs. In the immature PT, the expression of NHE is downregulated as its activity is dependent on the expression of the tubular sodium-potassium pump (Na^+, K^+-ATPase) which is downregulated in immature kidney.

The tubular potassium and phosphorus channels mature early in the DT to meet the needs for growth and cellular functions. The fetal serum potassium levels are higher than those in the mother due to active transplacental transfer and renal immaturity. Urinary potassium excretion increases toward term with increase in glomerular and tubular surface area, with maturation of tubular Na^+, K^+-ATPase activity, and with the progressive tubular sensitivity to aldosterone.

During fetal development, the placenta regulates the fetal acid-base balance. The fetal tubular NHE mediates the exchange of one sodium for one hydrogen and contributes to the acidification of urine. The reabsorption of bicarbonates and chloride in the PT increases with gestational age and at term the fetus fully participates in acid-base homeostasis. This function is mainly related to the maturation of the carbonic anhydrase activity.

The fetus has a positive phosphorus balance resulting from a transplacental transport against a concentration gradient, a high rate of tubular reabsorption via a sodium-phosphorus cotransporter, and a relative parathyroid insufficiency.

Calcium is important for the adequate mineralization, growth, and fetal skeleton. Vitamin D-dependent calcium-binding proteins, involved in transepithelial calcium transfer, are present in FK. The major role of the kidney in fetal calcium homeostasis is the production of $1,25(OH)_2D_3$ rather than renal regulation of calcium excretion.

Anatomical Position

During early development, the kidneys lie close together in the sacral region of the embryo. However, as the abdomen enlarges, the kidneys are drawn apart and ascend to their final position in the lumbar region between 6 and 9 weeks. During their pelvic position, the kidneys are vascularized by the branches of the common iliac artery. When the kidneys migrate upward, the renal arteries develop from the corresponding segments of the aorta while the more caudal branches disappear. Due to the position change of the kidneys, 25% of the population may have two or more renal arteries.[9]

ANATOMY OF THE KIDNEYS IN CHILDREN

The kidneys are paired organs that lie on the posterior wall of the abdomen behind the peritoneum on either side of the vertebral column. The kidneys grow rapidly in the first year of life, from 4.5 cm in length at birth to 6.5 cm in childhood and to 11 cm in adulthood. The weight of both kidneys at birth is about 23 g and increases to 150–200 g in adults. The renal artery and vein, nerves, and pelvis enter the kidney on the medial side **(Fig. 1)**. The renal tissue is divided into the outer region, the cortex, and the inner medulla and is composed of nephrons, blood vessels, lymphatics, and nerves. The medulla in the human kidney is divided into conical masses called renal pyramids with the intervening renal columns. The base of the pyramids originates at the corticomedullary border and the apices are the papillae, which project into the minor calyces, wherein urine is collected from the papillae. The minor calyces are cup-like structures joining within the kidney to form three or four major calyces. The major calyces in turn unite to form the pelvis, the upper expanded region of the ureter, which carries urine to the urinary bladder **(Fig. 2)**.

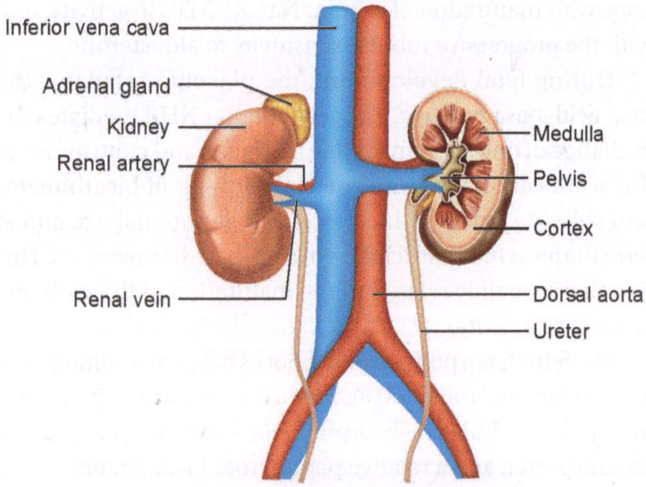

Fig. 1: Anatomy of the kidney and ureters in relation to the vascular system.

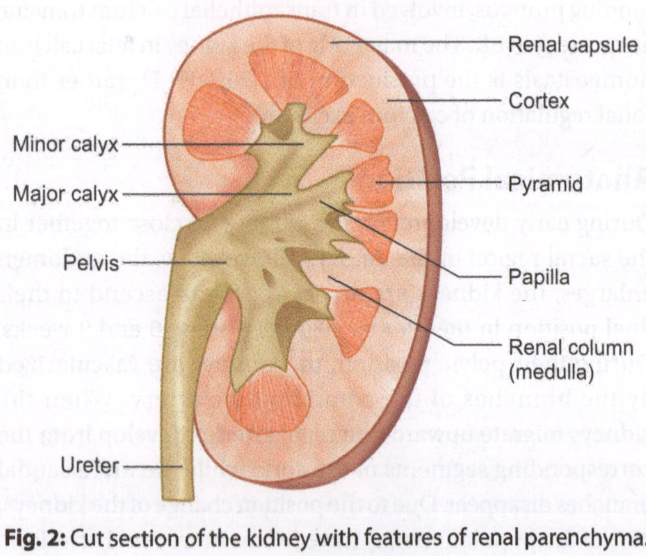

Fig. 2: Cut section of the kidney with features of renal parenchyma.

The walls of the calyces, pelvis, and ureters contain smooth muscle that contracts to propel the urine toward the urinary bladder.

Renal Vascular System

The renal arteries branch off from the abdominal aorta and supply the kidneys with blood. There may be one or more renal arteries supplying each kidney. The renal artery divides into five segments, which subsequently branches up the sides of the pyramids to form the interlobar artery, the arcuate artery, the interlobular artery, and the afferent arteriole which leads to glomerular capillaries **(Fig. 3)**. The glomerular capillaries come together to form the efferent arteriole, which leads into a second capillary network, the peritubular capillaries, which supply blood to the nephron. The vessels of the venous system run parallel to the arterial vessels and progressively form the interlobular, arcuate, interlobar, and renal veins.

Renal Nervous System

Sympathetic fibers originate in the lower splanchnic nerves and travel through the lumbar ganglion to the kidney. Stimulation of the sympathetic nervous system reduces RBF by causing intrarenal vasoconstriction. It also stimulates the local renin–angiotensin aldosterone system and enhances sodium reabsorption. The kidney also receives input from the parasympathetic nervous system, by way of the renal branches of the vagus nerve (cranial nerve X), which causes vasodilation and increased blood flow of the afferent arterioles. Due to this mechanism, sympathetic nervous stimulation will decrease urine production, while parasympathetic nervous stimulation will increase urine production.

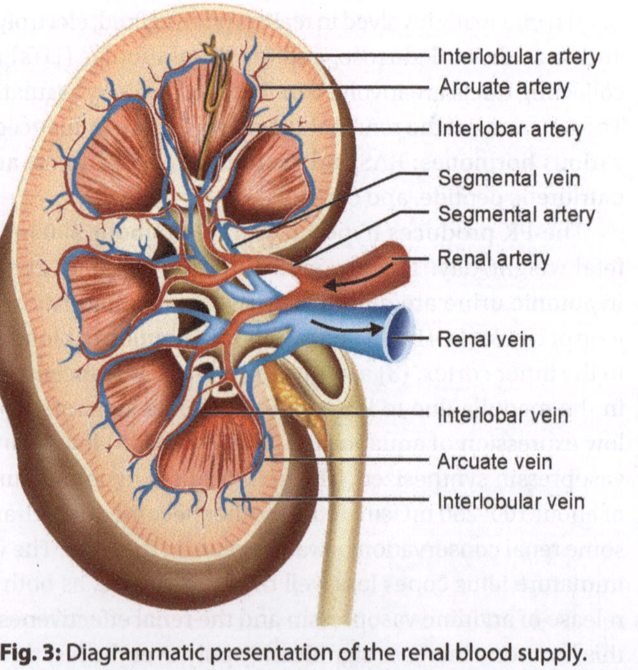

Fig. 3: Diagrammatic presentation of the renal blood supply.

FUNCTIONS OF THE KIDNEY

- *Regulation of the volume and composition of the body fluids:*
  - Osmotic pressure (osmolality) of the body fluids by excreting osmotically dilute or concentrated urine
  - Volume of the extracellular fluid by controlling sodium and water excretion
  - Concentrations of numerous ions in blood plasma, including Na^+, K^+, Ca^{2+}, Mg^{2+}, Cl^-, HCO^{3-}, $PO4^{3-}$, and $SO4^{2-}$.
  - Acid-base balance by excreting H ions when there is excess acid or HCO_3 when there is excess base
- *Regulation of arterial blood pressure:*
  - Arterial blood pressure by modulating the intraglomerular hemodynamics, adjusting sodium excretion, and producing various substances (e.g., renin) that can affect blood pressure.
- *Excretory function:*
  - Eliminates the waste products of metabolism, such as urea, the main nitrogen-containing end product of protein metabolism; uric acid, the end product of purine metabolism; and creatinine, the end product of muscle degradation.
  - Eliminates drugs and toxic compounds
- *Endocrine function:*
  - Kidneys are the sites of production of hormones: Erythropoietin, calcitriol, renin, and important producer of prostaglandins, endothelins, adrenomedullin, autocrine, and paracrine molecules.[10]
- *Degradation function:*
  - Degrade several polypeptide hormones, such as insulin, glucagon, and parathyroid hormone (PTH).
- *Production function:*
  - Synthesize ammonia, which plays a role in acid-base balance
  - Synthesize substances that affect RBF and sodium excretion, viz arachidonic acid derivatives, prostaglandins, thromboxane A2, and kallikrein, a proteolytic enzyme, that results in the production of kinins.
  - Gluconeogenesis

STRUCTURE AND FUNCTIONS OF THE NEPHRON

Nephron

The nephron is a unit of the kidney. Each human kidney contains approximately 1.2 million nephrons. The nephron consists of a glomerulus, PT, LOH, juxtaglomerular apparatus (JGA), DT, and collecting duct system (CDS). There are two types of nephrons: (1) cortical nephrons (85%), which are superficial in the renal cortex, and (2) juxtamedullary nephrons (15%), which lie in the renal cortex close to the renal medulla (**Fig. 4A**). Let us see their functional importance. The glomerulus of each superficial nephron is located in the outer region of the cortex. Its thin LOH and the thick ascending limb (TAL) are primarily confined to the cortical region. The efferent arteriole branches into peritubular capillaries that surround the nephron segments of its own and adjacent nephrons. This capillary network serves as a pathway to deliver substances to the nephron for secretion and return of reabsorbed water and solutes to the circulatory system. The glomerulus of the juxtamedullary nephron is located at the corticomedullary junction and has long LOH. The TAL is primarily within the medullary region, and its loop extends deep into the inner medulla. The efferent arteriole of the juxtamedullary nephron forms both a network of peritubular capillaries and a number of vascular loops called the vasa recta, deep in the medulla. The long LOH and its vasa recta form the countercurrent system, which serves in concentrating and diluting the urine (**Fig. 4B**).

Glomerulus

The glomerulus consists of a network of capillaries supplied by the afferent arteriole and drained by the efferent arteriole. The glomerular meningeal cells provide a structural support for the capillary network. The glomerular capillaries press into the closed end of the PTs, forming the Bowman capsule of the glomerulus. The capillaries are covered by epithelial cells, called podocytes, which form the visceral layer of the capsule of Bowman. The visceral cells continue at the vascular pole to form the parietal layer of the Bowman capsule. The space between the visceral and the parietal layers is the Bowman space, which at the urinary pole of the glomerulus becomes the lumen of the PT (**Fig. 5**). The endothelial cells of the glomerular capillaries are covered by the glomerular basement membrane (GBM) which is surrounded by foot processes of the podocytes on the other side. In other words, the GBM interposes between the endothelial cells of the capillaries and the foot processes of the podocytes. The capillary endothelium, GBM, and foot process of podocytes form the filtration barrier. The endothelium is fenestrated with pores. The pores are on average 60–100 nm wide and are freely permeable to water, small solutes, and most proteins but not permeable to cellular components. The endothelial cells have negatively charged glycoproteins on their surface, which retard the filtration of negatively charged proteins into Bowman space. The endothelial cells synthesize a number of vasoactive substances, angiotensin, prostaglandins, nitric acid, endothelin-1, bradykinins, and glucocorticoids that are important in controlling renal flow. The GBM has a thick, dense central layer, the lamina densa, which is covered by thinner, more electron-lucent inner and outer layers and the lamina rara interna and lamina rara externa. The GBM is a porous matrix of negatively charged proteins including type IV collagen, laminin 521, the proteoglycans agrin and perlecan, and fibronectin. The GBM acts as a permselective

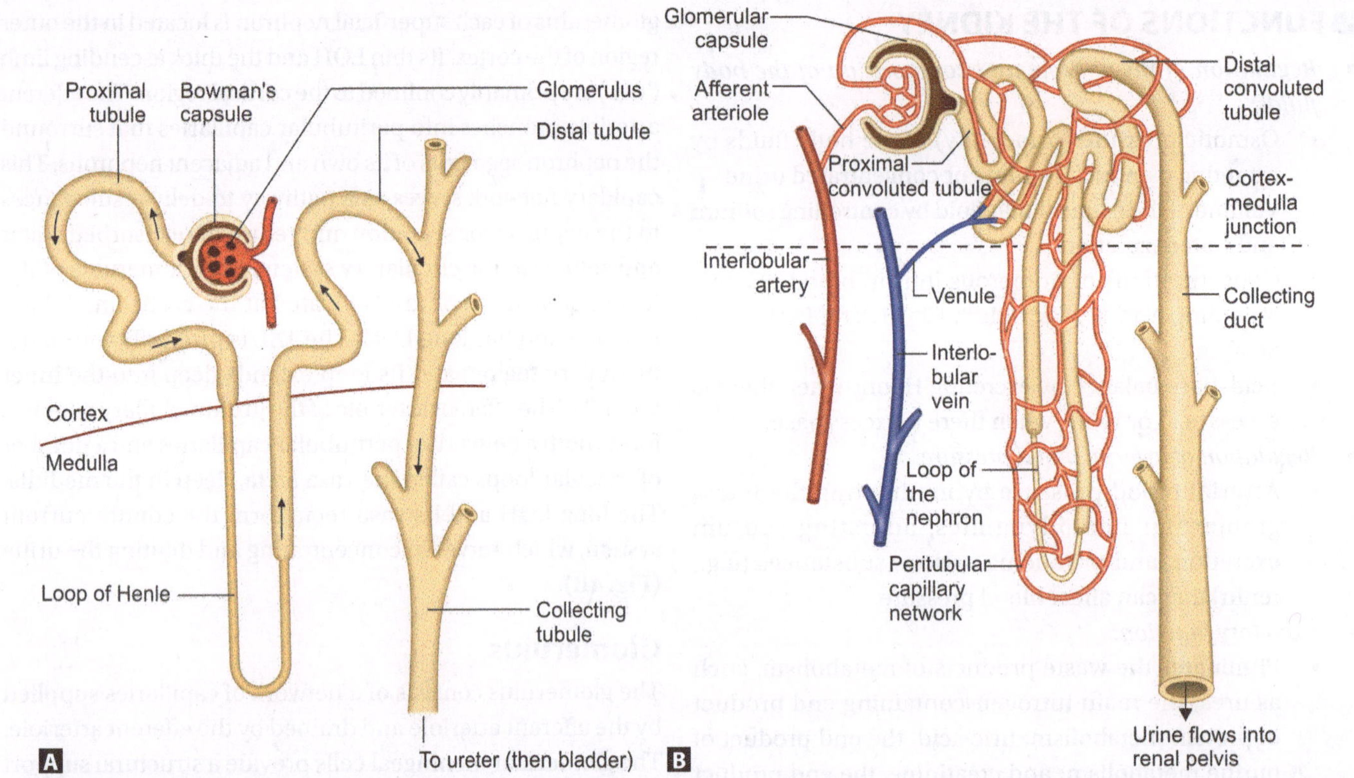

Figs. 4A and B: (A) Diagram of a short-looped cortical nephron and a long-looped juxtaglomerular nephron together with the collecting system; (B) Vascular supply to the cortical glomeruli is short and loops off at the corticomedullary junction. Vascular supply to the juxtamedullary junction glomeruli is long and extends deep into the medulla forming the vasa recta.

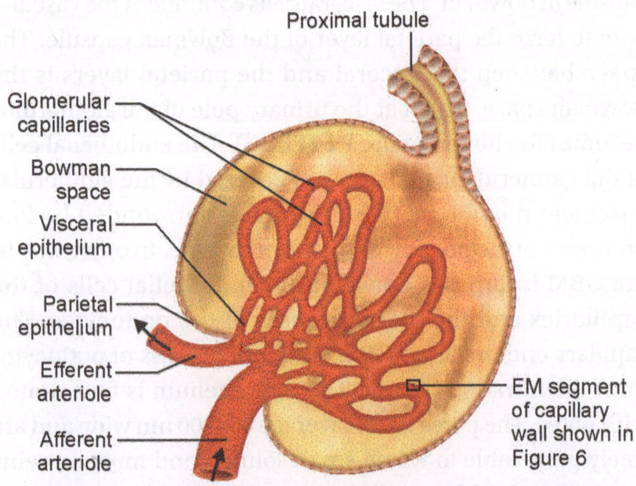

Fig. 5: Diagrammatic presentation of the structure of the glomerulus. (EM: electron microscopy).

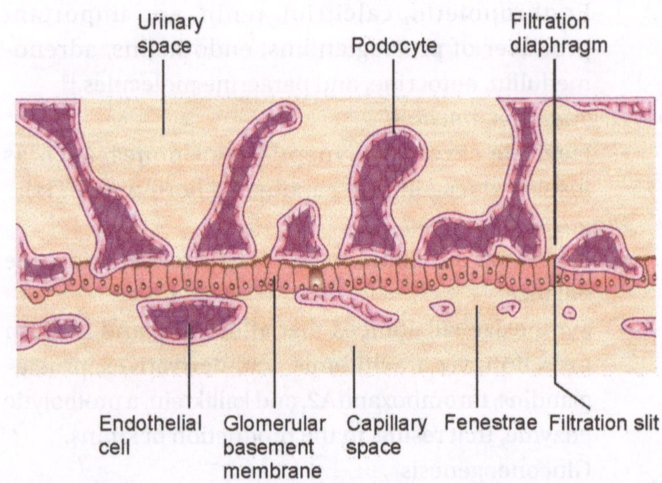

Fig. 6: Electron microscopic presentation of the glomerular capillary wall showing the components of the filtration barrier.

filter and restricts the permeability to macromolecules. The GBM filtration process is primarily based on size (70 kDa) and electrical charge. The more cationic the protein, the more permeable it is. The podocytes have long, finger-like tentacles, called foot processes, that interlace to cover the basement membrane and are separated by apparent gaps called filtration slits. Each filtration slit is bridged by a thin diaphragm, about 40 nm wide, and contains pores (**Fig. 6**). The pores in the filtration slit diaphragm are around 7 nm wide and function primarily as the size-selective filter. They retard the filtration of proteins and macromolecules that tend to cross the basement membrane from entering the Bowman space. The filtration slit diaphragm is composed of several proteins including nephrin, podocin, alpha-actinin 4, and CD2-associated protein (CD2AP) (**Fig. 7**).

Podocytes maintain the GBM with reciprocal crosstalk between glomerular podocytes and endothelial cells.[11] The foot processes also provide the mechanical resistance

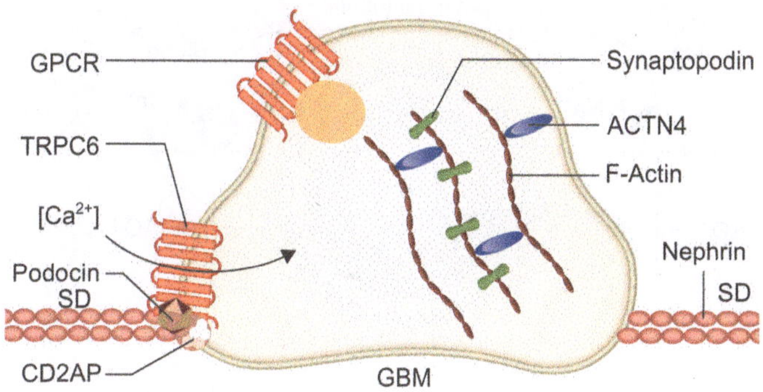

Fig. 7: Gene products in the podocytes and slit diaphragm. Podocyte foot process. (ACTN4: actinin 4; CD2AP: CD2-associated protein; GBM: glomerular basement membrane; GPCR: G protein-coupled receptor; SD: slit diaphragm; TRPC6: transient receptor potential cation channel)

against blood pressure that compresses the GBM, preserving permselectivity and preventing loss of albumin and other macromolecules.[12] Podocytes prevent clogging of the GBM filter by constant phagocytosis of the immunoglobulins, immune complexes, and proteins.

The glomerular mesangial cells provide a structural support to the glomerular tuft and play a role in the functions of renal glomerulus. Through its modified smooth muscle cell activity, the mesangial cell contracts or relaxes in response to a number of vasoactive agents and modifies glomerular filtration locally. The glomerular mesangial cells constantly remodel the basement membrane structure, generate prostaglandins, mediate inflammation, synthesize cytokines, and uptake of macromolecules, including immune complexes.[13]

The glomerulus is responsible for filtering the blood and providing a barrier to the passage of protein and cells into the urine. It is a passive process in which hydrostatic pressure pushes fluid and solute through a membrane with no energy requirement. The outward and inward force from the capillaries determines how much water and solutes cross the filtration membrane. Hydrostatic pressure from the glomerular capillaries is the major filtration force with a pressure of 60 mm Hg. The other potential filtration force is Bowman's capsular space colloid osmotic pressure, but it is zero because proteins are not usually present within the capsular space. The hydrostatic pressure within the capsular space and the colloid osmotic pressure in glomerular capillaries negate the filtration force of the glomerular capillaries resulting in a net filtration pressure which plays a big role in the glomerular filtration. The sum of all of the influences, both osmotic and hydrostatic, results in an effective net filtration pressure of 10–20 mm Hg: blood hydrostatic pressure (60 mm Hg), colloid osmotic pressure within capillaries (30 mm Hg), and hydrostatic pressure within the Bowman space (15 mm Hg).

Proximal Tubule

The proximal tubule (PT) initially forms several coils, followed by a straight piece that descends toward the medulla. The PT is the first segment of the renal tubule, which is divided into three morphologically distinct segments. The cells at the proximal convoluted segment of the tubule (S1 segment) have an apical membrane with a brush border, which increases the surface area for absorption compared with the straight portions (S2 and S3 segments) and late proximal convoluted tubule. The wide brush border contains greater numbers of microvilli, an extensive network of mitochondria, Golgi apparatuses, and more invaginations of the basolateral membrane and therefore possesses a larger capacity for reabsorption. Almost all the cells in the nephron have a single nonmotile primary cilium, which protrudes into tubule fluid. Primary cilia are mechanosensors, which sense changes in the flow rate of tubular fluid, and chemosensors, which respond to compounds in the surrounding fluids and calcium-dependent signaling pathways including those that control kidney cell function, proliferation, differentiation, and apoptosis.

The PT fulfills most of the reabsorptive role for sodium chloride and sodium bicarbonate, leaving the fine-tuning to the distal nephron. The PT also completes the reabsorption of glucose, amino acids, and important anions, including phosphate and citrate. The process of movement (reabsorption) of solutes, electrolytes, and water from the tubular fluid, across the renal tubular cell membrane, to the peritubular capillary blood and its reversal (secretion) from the peritubular capillary blood to tubular fluid is the result of specialized membrane carrier proteins called transporters, channels, or by passive diffusion. Active transporters are H^+/K^+-ATPase and H^+-ATPase. The passive transporters are $Na^+/K^+/Cl^-$ and Na^+/glucose cotransporters and Ca^{2+}/Na^+, NHE^+ exchangers and finally the AQPs.[14]

The PT also plays a basic role in regulating acid–base balance through absorption of approximately 80% of filtered bicarbonate. Dysfunction of the PT results in proximal renal tubular acidosis. The PT secretes acid (H^+ ions) into the tubule lumen, thereby reabsorbing approximately 80% of the filtered base (HCO_3). In addition, the PT generates HCO_3^- for regulating blood pH.[15] The PT cells deaminate glutamine to glutamic acid and then form α-ketoglutaric acid, liberating one ammonia (NH_3) group. During chronic acidosis, there is an increased rate of deamination of glutamine. The NH_3 in the tubule fluid liberated from these reactions binds to H^+ ions secreted by the cells. Once it binds to H^+ to form ammonium (NH_4), it can no longer easily penetrate the apical membrane and is excreted. Thus, there is a gain of one base equivalent.

The PT reabsorbs 70% of the filtered water. The driving force for water reabsorption is a transtubular osmotic gradient established by solute reabsorption (e.g., NaCl and glucose). However, water re-absorption by the kidney requires the presence of water channels in the nephron epithelium. The water channels, AQPs1, are present in the apical and basolateral membranes of the tubule cells and are responsible for the "obligatory" water re-absorption of the PT, while the

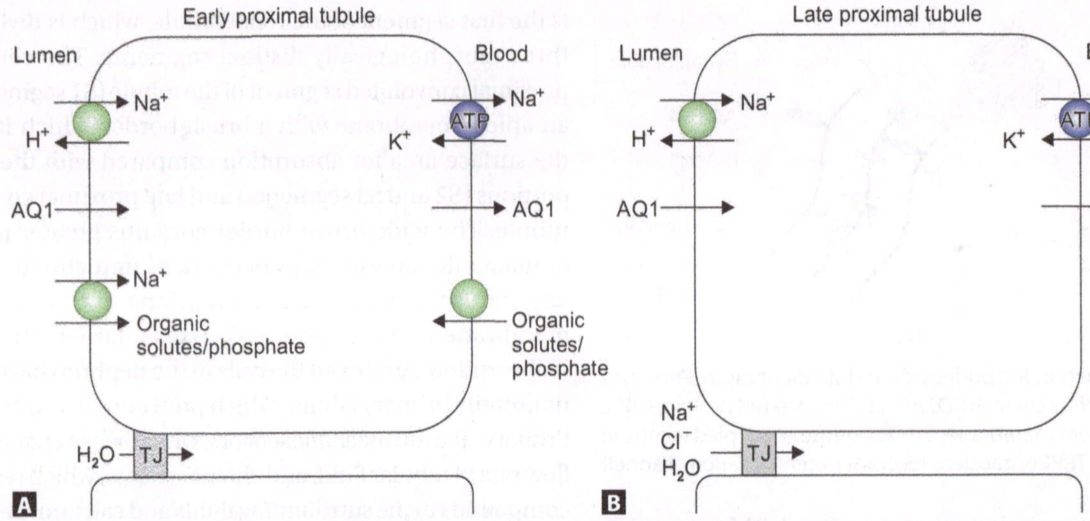

Figs. 8A and B: Two segments of the proximal tubule with their transcellular transporters. Note paracellular transport via claudin of sodium, chloride, and water. See the text for details. (ATP: adenosine triphosphate)

"facultative absorption" is under the control of vasopressin in the distal nephron. In the kidney, AQP1 is extremely abundant in the PT and descending thin limb and is essential for urinary concentration with no significant expression at other nephron sites. It is present in both apical and basal membranes.[16] AQPs 3, 7, 8, and 9 appear to affect the membrane's permeability to larger solutes, such as glycerol. These AQPs have been termed "aquaglyceroporins"[17] **(Figs. 8A and B)**.

The PT is a metabolic organ. It is where the 24-hydroxylase reaction converts 25-hydroxyvitamin D and 1,25-dihydroxy-vitamin D to their inactive forms and produces the active form erythropoietin. It is the site of gluconeogenesis that parallels the liver.

Loop of Henle

The next segment, LOH, has a hairpin configuration with a thin descending limb and both a thin and a TAL. The thin descending and ascending segments have thin epithelial membranes with no brush borders and minimal metabolic activity. The thin descending limb is highly permeable to water, with reabsorption occurring passively via AQP1 channels. Very low amounts of urea, sodium, and other ions are reabsorbed into the tubule. The water reabsorption is driven by the hyperosmotic environment created by active reabsorption of sodium in the TAL. This increases tubular fluid osmolarity to about 1,200 mOsm/L. The thin ascending limb is impermeable to water but permeable to sodium and chloride. As the liquid returns through the thin ascending limb, the sodium and chloride diffuse paracellularly out of the tubule into the surrounding tissue. This is due to the difference in osmolarity between the tubule and the interstitium where the sodium chloride concentration is lower.

However, the primary site of sodium reabsorption in the LOH is the thick ascending limb. The TAL is impermeable to water. The Na^+/K^+ ATPase on the basolateral membrane actively pumps three sodium ions out of the cell into the interstitium and two potassium ions into the cell. By creating a low intracellular concentration of sodium ions, the inside of the cell becomes negatively charged, creating an electrochemical gradient. Sodium ions then move into the cell (from the tubular lumen) down the electrical and chemical gradients, through the NKCC2 transporter on the apical membrane. This transporter moves one sodium ion, one K^+ ion, and two Cl^- ions across the apical membrane. Potassium ions are transported back into the tubule by renal outer medullary potassium (ROMK) channels on the apical membrane to prevent toxic build-up within the cell. Chloride ions are transported into the tissue fluid via ClC-Kb channels. The LOH contributes to the absorption of approximately 25% of filtered sodium and can be targeted by furosemide diuretic therapy. This leads to a drop in the osmolarity of fluid from 1,200 to 100 mOsm/L and a hypotonic solution arrives at the DT. In addition to the above urine concentrating mechanisms, there is significant paracellular reabsorption of magnesium, calcium, sodium, and potassium and uromodulin synthesis **(Fig. 9)**.

Juxtaglomerular Apparatus

At the end of the ascending limb of LOH and the beginning of DT, where the nephron passes between the afferent and the efferent arterioles of the same nephron, is the JGA. This is made up of an area of thickened epithelial cells of the afferent arteriole, the granular cells. They manufacture, store, and release renin. Renin is involved in the formation of angiotensin-II and ultimately aldosterone. The area of specialized cells lining the wall of the tubule is the macula densa and the extraglomerular mesangial cells **(Fig. 10)**. The JGA activates the RAS, aldosterone secretion, sodium conservation, and the blood volume.

Distal Tubule

The DT starts shortly after the macula densa. The DT is comprised of the distal convoluted tubule (DCT) and the

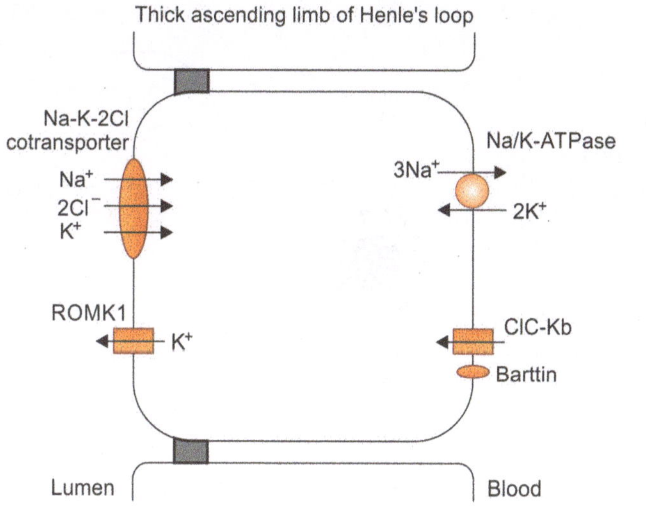

Fig. 9: Thick ascending limb of loop of Henle with their transcellular transporters. See text for details. (ROMK: renal outer medullary potassium)

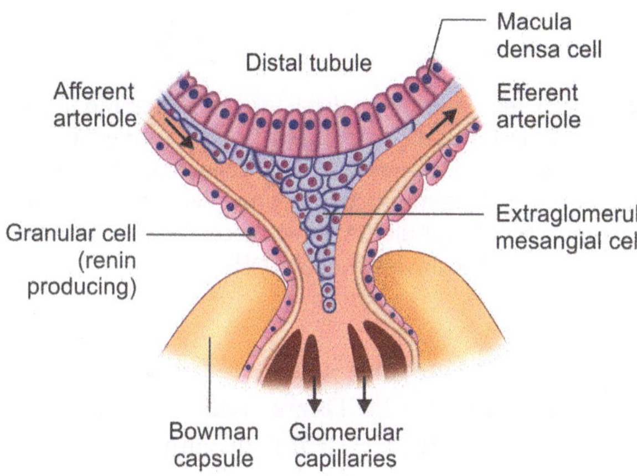

Fig. 10: Diagrammatic presentation of the juxtaglomerular apparatus.

connecting tubule (CNT). The DCT is the shortest segment of the nephron, of about 5 mm in length. The DCT consists of two distinct subsegments, DCT1 and DCT2. The DCT1 and DCT2 together reabsorb roughly 5–10% of the filtered sodium load. In addition to sodium chloride reabsorption, it has a role in potassium secretion and in calcium and magnesium handling.

Sodium

Sodium absorption from the tubular lumen in DCT1 is by thiazide-sensitive NaCl cotransporter (NCC). In addition to NCC, the DCT2 segment expresses the amiloride-sensitive Epithelial sodium channel (ENaC) on the apical side. In other words, in DCT2, both NCC and ENaC sodium channels are present. In both DCT1 and DCT2, sodium is moved through the basolateral membrane to the peritubular interstitium by the Na^+–K^+-ATP supported by the potassium channel (Kir4.1), a potassium leak channel. Note that unlike NCC, aldosterone activates ENaC. In DCT2, sodium is reabsorbed and drives potassium secretion through the ROMK and Maxi-K channels[18] **(Fig. 11)**.

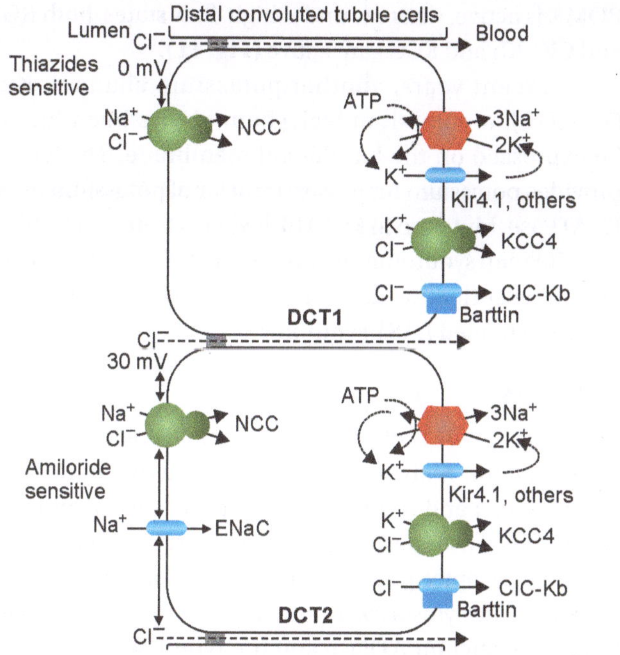

Fig. 11: Distal convoluted tubules 1 and 2 with their transporters. See text for details. *Note:* Paracellular transport of chloride. (ATP: adenosine triphosphate; DCT: distal convoluted tubule; KCC4: potassium chloride cotransporter 4; NCC: NaCl cotransporter)

Chloride

Intracellular transport of chloride is through the NCC. Extracellular transport is carried out by the chloride channel (ClC-Kb) and potassium chloride cotransporter 4 (KCC4). Both these transporters move the intracellularly accumulated potassium and chloride to peritubular interstitium and maintain lumen to cell-negative transepithelial voltage. The cell-negative transepithelial voltage is augmented in the later part of DCT by the paracellular chloride transport **(Fig. 11)**.

Potassium

Approximately 10% of filtered potassium reaches the DCT and downstream. The luminal potassium concentration progressively increases, indicating that net potassium secretion occurs along the DT. The potassium secretion is mediated by the ROMK channel. At the same time, the basolateral potassium efflux into peritubular interstitium in the DCT is by potassium transporters, ClC-Kb and KCC4. The potassium secretion does not stop here but occurs more distally in the CNT and cortical collecting duct by ROMK. Increased plasma potassium concentration decreases NCC activity and increases sodium delivery to the downstream aldosterone-sensitive DCT2, CNT, and where the CDS begins. Herein, increased aldosterone-mediated ENaC intracellular sodium transport generates a driving force for ROMK-mediated potassium secretion into the tubular fluid. A reduction in plasma potassium concentration activates NCC activity. This effect causes salt retention and reduces sodium delivery and flow to downstream segments resulting in decreased potassium secretion.[17] Under low-flow conditions,

ROMK is active, whereas under high-flow states, both ROMK and ClC-Kb and KCC4 are active **(Fig. 11)**.

In recent years, another potassium channel, Kir4.1 (KCNJ10), a potassium leak channel, has been found to be expressed on the basolateral membrane. This channel provides potassium for inward transfer of potassium by Na^+–K^+-ATPase. Mutation in KCNJ10 develops features resembling the Gitelman syndrome and presents in infancy with epilepsy, ataxia, sensorineural deafness, and salt wasting. The disease has been named EAST syndrome.[19]

Calcium

In the DCT, 7–10% of filtered calcium is reabsorbed. In the DCT, calcium reabsorption occurs by active transcellular mechanisms and not through the paracellular route as in other segments. Apical calcium transport is mediated by the transient receptor potential channel subfamily V member 5 (TRPV5). The cytosol calcium is extruded into the peritubular fluid by a calcium ATPase and the type 1 sodium-calcium exchanger (NCX1).

Magnesium

The DCT reclaims some 5–10% of the filtered magnesium. Yet this amount is large for it represents 60–70% of the magnesium delivered to the DCT from LOH. Transepithelial magnesium absorption is active in the DCT as transport is against luminal-to-interstitial electrical and concentration gradients. The magnesium channel transient TRPM6 activity is stimulated by the magnesiotropic hormone, epithelial growth factor receptor (EGFR), which triggers an intracellular signaling cascade in the DCT. After transluminal entry, cytosolic Mg^{2+} transport out through the basolateral membrane of the DCT into the interstitium is unknown but suspected to be an active process.[20]

Connecting Tubule

The CNT lies between the DCT and the initial portion of the CDS **(Fig. 12)** and functionally simulates both segments. The CNT (1) is impermeable to water even with antidiuretic hormone (ADH); (2) participates in active calcium reabsorption, in response to PTH and calcitriol; (3) partially reabsorbs sodium by a thiazide-sensitive NCC; (4) reabsorbs sodium in exchange for potassium secretion in principal cells; and (5) reabsorbs sodium via ENaC and potassium excretion in response to aldosterone. Aldosterone stimulates uptake of sodium by the ENaC and potassium secretion by the luminal potassium channels that are accumulated in the cell by the apical potassium transporter Na^+-K^+-ATPase.[21]

Collecting Duct System

The CNT from different adjacent nephrons merge together to form the arcade of initial collecting tubules (ICTs). The ICTs merge together to form cortical collecting ducts (CCDs). The CCDs receive filtrate from multiple cortical collecting tubules

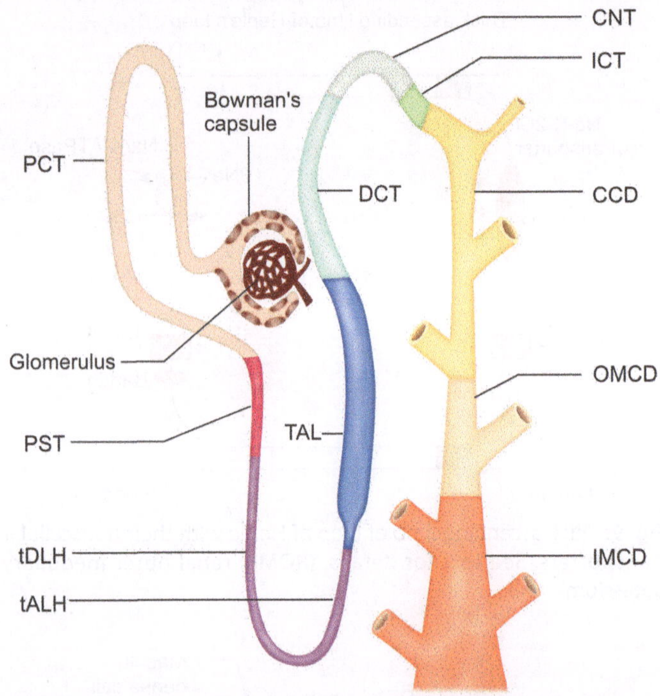

Fig. 12: Various segments of the distal tubule. *Source:* Modified from reference 7. (CCD: cortical collecting duct; CNT: connecting tubule; DCT: distal convoluted tubule; ICT: initial collecting tubules; OMCD: outer medullary collecting duct; PCT: proximal convoluted tubule; PST: proximal straight tubule; TAL: thick ascending limb; tALH: thin ascending LOH; tDLH: thin descending LOH).

(CCTs) and descend into the renal medulla to form medullary collecting ducts (MCDs). MCDs are divided into outer MCDs (OMCDs) and inner MCDs (IMCDs), the latter reaching more deeply into the medulla which leads to papillary duct that empties into a minor calyx via the duct of Bellini **(Fig. 4A)**. Anatomically the CDS is not considered as a part of the nephron because embryologically it arises from the ureteric bud. The CDS performs the final adjustment of the products of renal excretion **(Fig. 12)**.[22]

The CDS consists of different cell types and plays an important role in maintaining homeostasis. The CDS epithelium consists of principal cells and intercalated cells (ICs); the latter are subdivided into type A (or alpha), type B (or beta), and non-A, non-B cells.

Principal Cells

The principal cells of the CCDs form a part of the aldosterone-sensitive distal nephron, where the urinary excretion of sodium, potassium, and chloride is fine-tuned so as to match dietary intake. Principal cells express the ENaC and the ROMK channel at the apical membrane and Na^+-K^+-ATPase pump at the basolateral membrane. CCD reabsorbs sodium and chloride and secretes potassium in response to sodium depletion or aldosterone treatment, whereas little transport occurs under basal conditions.[23] AQP2 is the sensitive water channel in the apical membranes of the principal cells of the collecting tubules and ducts. There is little AQP2 in the basal membrane. The ability of the CCDs to reabsorb water is controlled by ADH or arginine vasopressin. In the presence of ADH, AQP2-containing vesicles fuse with the apical membrane allowing water to enter the cell. Water exits from the basolateral aspect via AQP3 and AQP4 channels. Between them, AQP4 is thought to be the primary exit pathway for water to leave the cells. The action of ADH on the CCD allows for the production of concentrated urine and protects against dehydration[24] **(Fig. 13)**.

Intercalated Cells

There are three main types of ICs, types A, B, and "non-A, non-B", each with a distinct morphology. They express different transport proteins on the apical and basolateral membranes with different roles in homeostasis. ICs are present in the late DCTs, CNTs, CCDs, and OMCDs and are an early part of the IMCDs. ICs maintain acid–base status of the organism: (1) ICs reabsorb a small amount of residual bicarbonate, (2) ICs dispose acid that is generated by dietary intake and cannot be eliminated via the lungs, called fixed or nonvolatile acid, and thus produce new bicarbonate. The primary mechanism of new bicarbonate generation involves renal ammonia metabolism. Renal ammoniagenesis, utilizing glutamine as the primary metabolic substrate, generates equivalent amounts of ammonium and bicarbonate. The bicarbonate produced is preferentially transported across the basolateral plasma membrane, absorbed into peritubular capillaries, and returned to the systemic circulation, (3) participates in NaCl transport-mediated intravascular volume regulation along with principal cells, (4) takes part in potassium uptake, and (5) plays a role in the innate immune system. It is to be remembered that ICs have one common pathway to generate new bicarbonate. All three types of ICs express carbonic anhydrase in their cytoplasm. It is by the hydration of CO_2 by the intracellular carbonic anhydrase II (CAII). This reaction generates H_2CO_3 that disassociates into H ion and base HCO_3 **(Fig. 13)**.

Type A ICs express H^+–ATPase and H^+/K^+-ATPase at their apical membrane and Cl/HCO_3 which is encoded by anion exchanger (AE) at their basolateral membrane and lack pendrin expression. Type A ICs secrete H ion into urine via H^+-ATPase or H^+/K^+-ATPase at their apical membrane. The latter pump exchanges one potassium ion for each extruded H ion. The secretion of an H ion into the tubular lumen, whether it is in exchange for potassium reabsorption or not, results in the generation of intracellular bicarbonate via CAII, which is reabsorbed into the interstitium in exchange for chloride by the Cl/HCO_3 exchanger. A chloride channel transporter (Cl) is also expressed at the apical membrane. These pumps are stimulated by acidemia and aldosterone.[25]

Type B ICs have an inverse orientation of pumps and channels as compared to type A ICs. Type B ICs are responsible for secretion of bicarbonate via a specialized Cl/HCO_3 exchanger known as pendrin located on the apical membrane of B-ICs. The H^+–ATPase at the basolateral membrane moves hydrogen ions from the interstitium into the intracellular cytoplasm. The presence of a H ion in the cytoplasm results in the generation of intracellular bicarbonate via CAII, which is secreted into the tubular lumen in exchange for chloride by pendrin, the Cl/HCO_3 exchanger. Given its dual function of bicarbonate secretion and chloride reabsorption, pendrin has an important role in systemic acid–base balance and electrolyte and vascular volume homeostasis in physiological conditions. Type B IC has a sodium-driven Cl^-/HCO_3^- exchanger (NDCBE) at their apical membrane. The reabsorption of sodium chloride from the lumen by NDCBE is energized by the basolateral H^+–ATPase. The transepithelial transport of sodium and chloride into the interstitium, the peritubular capillaries, and ends in the systemic circulation. Thus, type B ICs contribute to the protection of intravascular volume in addition to principal cells.[25] These pumps are stimulated by acidemia and aldosterone. Experimentally induced metabolic acidosis results in the conversion of type B ICs to type A ICs giving the kidney a greater ability to secrete protons and return pH to the normal range **(Fig. 13)**. The non-A, non-B ICs express both the H^+-ATPase and pendrin at their apical membrane.

In essence, in acidemic conditions the CCD secretes hydrogen ions, and in alkalemic conditions the CCD secretes

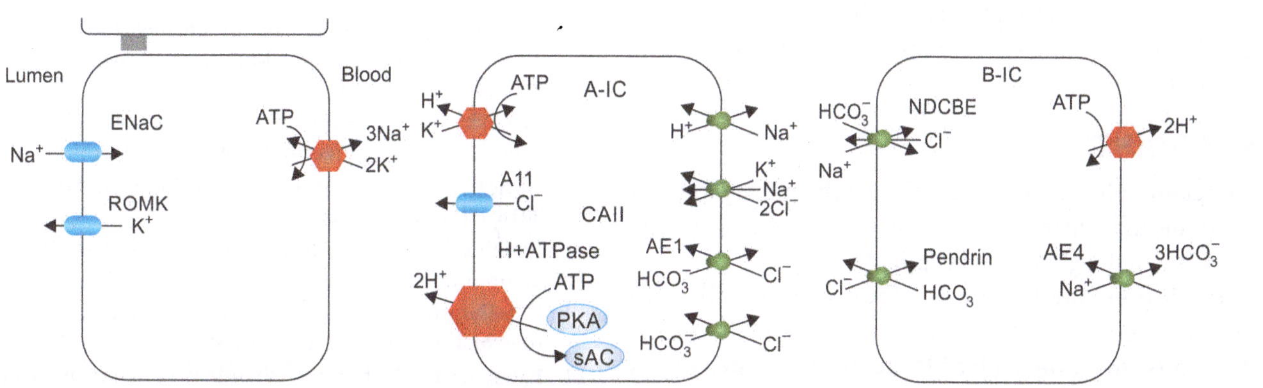

Fig. 13: Cortical collecting ducts and their transporters. (AE: anion exchanger; ATP: adenosine triphosphate; IC: intercalated cells; PKA: protein kinase A; NDCBE: sodium-driven Cl^-/HCO_3^- exchanger; ROMK: renal outer medullary potassium; sAC: soluble adenylyl cyclase).

bicarbonate. Furthermore, these segments are involved in the regulation of calcium and magnesium homeostasis and water and urea transport.

The paracellular route has long been recognized as an important chloride transport pathway in the CCD. Paracellular chloride reabsorption is driven by the lumen-negative transepithelial potential difference that is established by ENaC. The permeability of the paracellular pathway is imparted by tight junction proteins, claudins, that form selective channels.[25]

Water Absorption in the Collecting Duct System

Water reabsorption and concentration of urine occur at the IMCDs. The osmotic gradient created by the countercurrent multiplier system in the LOH provides the force responsible for water reabsorption through the CCDs. Urea is not reabsorbed in the earlier segments. This results in a high urea concentration in the terminal IMCD. There, the urea is rapidly reabsorbed mediated by specific urea transporters UT-A1 and UT-A3 in the basolateral and the apical membranes, respectively, where it accounts for about one half of the interstitial solute. This process is regulated by ADH. The high urea concentration in the inner medullary interstitium sets up the intrarenal osmotic gradient. It is this hypertonic interstitium that facilitates urine concentration. The rate of osmotic movement is determined by the permeability to water which is proportional to the number of AQPs in the epithelial cells of both segments. The ADH facilitates transportation of AQP2 from storage vesicles in the cytoplasm to the apical cells in plasma membrane. Water exits from the basolateral aspect via constitutively present AQP3 and AQP4 channels. After passage through the collecting duct and the duct of Bellini, the fluid leaves the kidney as urine and brought into the ureter and bladder.

CONCLUSION

The function of the kidneys is to maintain the physiological state of extracellular and intracellular environment for efficient function of other organ cells in spite of daily variations in food and water intake, nonrenal losses of fluid and electrolytes, onslaught of toxins, and the ongoing generation of metabolic waste products.

KEY POINTS

- The glomerulus is a passive mechanical filter that produces a glomerular filtrate effected by a positive hydrostatic pressure in the glomerular capillaries.
- The glomerular filtrate is blood minus cells and macromolecules.
- In adults, the glomerular filtrate produced per day is about 180 L/day, but the average urine produced is only about 1.5 L/day. The reabsorption of 99% of the glomerular filtrate with its dissolved components is due to a sophisticated tubular network.
- The PT reabsorbs ions, water, and nutrients from the filtrate into the interstitial fluid and actively transports toxins and drugs from the interstitial fluid into the filtrate and contributes toward maintaining acid-base balance. It is the site of production of 1,25$(OH)_2$ vitamin D_3 and erythropoietin.
- In the thin and thick parts of the LOH, sodium and chloride shift into the interstitial fluid, and the filtrate becomes hypotonic as it travels up the limb.
- In the DCT, potassium and hydrogen ions are selectively secreted into the filtrate, whereas sodium, chloride, and bicarbonate ions are reabsorbed to maintain pH and electrolyte balance in the blood.
- The CDS is the last part of nephron and participates in fine-tuning of electrolyte, fluid balance, and concentration of urine.

REFERENCES

1. Cukuranovic R, Vlajkovic S. Age related anatomical and functional characteristics of human kidney. Med Biol. 2005;12:61-9.
2. Sharma S, Raina S. Study of human fetal kidney. Int J Anat Res. 2014;2:785-90.
3. Caruthers B. Kidney development and function in the fetus. Surg Technol. 1999;1:16-20.
4. Luzi G, Bori S, Lammarino G, Taddei F, Martines G, Piatti P, et al. Functional aspects of the fetal urinary apparatus in relation to growth. Arch Ital Urol Androl. 1996;68(5 Suppl):9-12. (English abstract).
5. Boubred F, Simeoni U. Pathophysiology of fetal and neonatal kidneys. In: Buonocore G, Bracci R, Weindling M (Eds). Neonatology. Cham: Springer; 2018. Available from https://doi.org/10.1007/978-3-319-18159-2_261-2 [Last accessed May, 2021].
6. Magee LA, Ornstein MP, Von Dadelszen P. Management of hypertension in pregnancy. BMJ. 1999;318:1332-6.
7. Khan KNM, Stanfield KM, Dannenberg A, Seshan SV, Baergen RN, Baron DA, et al. Cyclooxygenase-2 expression in the developing human kidney. Pediatr Dev Pathol. 2001;4:461-6.
8. Lumbers E. Renal function during intrauterine life. Physiology. 1987;2:220-3.
9. Zweyer M. Embryology of the kidney. In: Quaia E (Ed). Radiological Imaging of the Kidney. Medical Radiology. Berlin, Heidelberg: Springer; 2010. pp. 3-16.
10. Sahay M, Kalra S, Bandgar T. Renal endocrinology: the new frontier. Indian J Endocrinol Metab. 2012;16:154-5.
11. Garg P. A review of the podocyte biology. Am J Nephrol. 2018;47(Suppl 1):3-13.
12. Benzing T, Salant D. Insights into glomerular filtration and albuminuria. N Engl J Med. 2021;384:1437-46.
13. Schlondorff D. The glomerular mesangial cell: an expanding role for a specialized pericyte. FASEB J. 1987;1:272-81.
14. Lawrence EA, Doherty D, Dhanda R. Function of the nephron and the formation of urine. Anaesth Intensive Care Med. 2018;19:249-53.

15. Boron WF. Acid-base transport by the renal proximal tubule. J Am Soc Nephrol. 2006;17:2368-82.
16. Nielsen S, Frøkiaer J, Marples D, Kwon TH, Agre P, Knepper MA. Aquaporins in the kidney: from molecules to medicine. Physiol Rev. 2002;82:205-44.
17. Lote CJ. Applied physiology: the renal tubule. Curr Paediatr. 2006;16:453-7.
18. Palmer BF, Clegg DJ. Physiology and pathophysiology of potassium homeostasis: core curriculum. Am J Kidney Dis. 2019;74:682-95.
19. Bockenhauer D, Feather S, Stanescu HC, Bandulik S, Zdebik AA, Reichold M, et al. Epilepsy, ataxia, sensorineural deafness, tubulopathy, and KCNJ10 mutations. N Engl J Med. 2009;360: 1960-70.
20. Subramanya AR, Ellison DH. Distal convoluted tubule. Clin J Am Soc Nephrol. 2014;9:2147-63.
21. Staruschenko A. Regulation of transport in the connecting tubule and cortical collecting duct. Compr Physiol. 2012;2:1541-84.
22. Kriz W, Bankir LA. Standard nomenclature for structures of the kidney. Kidney Int. 1988;33:1-7.
23. Edwards A, Gilles Crambert G. Versatility of NaCl transport mechanisms in the cortical collecting duct. Am J Physiol Renal Physiol. 2017;313:F1254-63.
24. Lote CJ. Applied physiology: the renal tubule. Curr Paediatr. 2011;11:207-11.
25. Roy A, Al-bataineh MM, Pastor-Soler NM. Collecting duct intercalated cell function and regulation. Clin J Am Soc Nephrol. 2015;10:305-24.

CHAPTER

1.3 Nephron Endowment: Hypertension and Chronic Kidney Disease

Sudha Ekambaram, Arpana A Iyengar

INTRODUCTION

Chronic kidney disease (CKD) is one of the major causes of mortality and poses a great risk to human health. "Developmental programming" has given rise to the concept that CKD can begin in early life. This refers to the process in which any insult during the critical window of development can lead to long-term effects on the structure or function of an organism.[1]

Nephrogenesis is completed at 36 weeks of gestation except in extreme preterm infants in whom nephrogenesis is observed until day 40 of birth.[2] Kidney development in utero is vulnerable to various adverse events that can lead to permanent morphological and functional changes, termed renal programming. This forms an important link to the development of CKD in later life. The basis for this form of CKD is mainly due to reduction in nephron numbers formed in utero.[1] Early life environmental insults, such as undernutrition, uteroplacental insufficiency, gestational diabetes, glucocorticoid exposure, drug exposure, and molecular mechanisms, such as oxidative stress and epigenetic regulation, lead to low nephron endowment.[1] Let us see in detail the programming mechanism of kidney development and the strategies of reprogramming that could potentially help us address the growing burden of CKD.

NEPHRON NUMBERS IN HUMANS

The nephron number varies in human kidneys. Counting nephrons is feasible only during postmortem, and it is a tedious task. Studies show that the average nephron number in each kidney is approximately 9,00,000 to 1 million and varies between 2 and 2.5 million.[3] The nephron number declines with age and has been estimated to reduce by 4,500 glomeruli/kidney/year between 18 and 70 years. The lowest and highest estimated glomerular count is 3,31,000 and 14,24,000, respectively. These variations are attributed to a combination of nephron loss during nephrogenesis and postnatal life.[4] The glomerular filtration rate (GFR) helps to assess the function of all nephrons, whereas single-nephron GFR (SNGFR) assesses the function of individual nephrons. A higher SNGFR is associated with nephromegaly, glomerulosclerosis, and arteriosclerosis favoring CKD development.[5]

METHODS TO ESTIMATE NEPHRON NUMBER

Autopsy study is the current technique used for counting nephron numbers. Noninvasive methods for counting nephron numbers have not been established yet. Glomerular hypertrophy is a consequence of oligonephronia. This potentially limits the utility of kidney size as a surrogate marker of nephron number by ultrasound. Other limitations are interobserver variation and difficulty in measurement in obese individuals.[6] A recent study has attempted to estimate the nephron number by magnetic resonance imaging (MRI) and labeling glomeruli through cationic ferritin. This method has the potential to measure the actual nephron number in living subjects but needs further validation.[7]

DETERMINANTS OF NEPHRON NUMBER

There is individual variation of nephron number with variability of up to 10-fold within select population. Despite this variation, each individual possesses an average of 9,00,000 nephrons in each kidney. The final nephron number that is determined at birth is termed nephron endowment. This results in a complex interplay of genetic and environmental factors on renal function with a potential risk for hypertension (HTN) and kidney disease in later life.[2] With regard to developing strategies to preserve nephron number, it becomes important to first understand the determinants of nephron number during kidney development. Various prenatal and postnatal factors affecting the nephron number during one's lifetime are listed in **Table 1**.[6] We will briefly discuss a few important factors affecting the nephron number.

Antenatal Factors

Genetics

Nephrogenesis is a finely orchestrated process requiring signals from the ureteric bud to initiate condensation of the metanephric mesenchyme into nephrons (via pretubular aggregate, renal vesicle, and S-shaped body transitions), while the metanephric mesenchyme reciprocally induces growth and branching of the ureteric bud. Genetic and environmental factors can disrupt this delicate balance leading to alteration

TABLE 1: Factors determining reduced nephron number.[6]

Antenatal	*Postnatal*
• Genetic factors – *RET* – *PAX 2* – *FGF* – *EYA 1* – *SIX 2* • Maternal dietary deficiencies – Iron deficiency – Vitamin A and D deficiency – Maternal undernutrition • Uterine ischemia • Gestational exposure – Angiotensin-converting enzyme inhibitors – Nonsteroidal anti-inflammatory drug – Aminoglycoside – Cyclosporine – Alcohol – Tobacco • Maternal hyperglycemia	• Intrauterine growth retardation • Low birth weight • Prematurity • Acute kidney injury • Hypertension • Obesity • Nephrotoxic medication exposure • Acquired renal scars • Partial nephrectomy
Fetal	
• Urinary tract obstruction • Renal hypodysplasia	

(*EYA 1*: eyes absent homolog 1; *FGF*: fibroblast growth factor; *PAX 2*: paired box gene; *RET*: ret proto-oncogene; *SIX 2*: SIX homeobox 2)

in nephrogenesis. Mutations affecting the nephron number either affect the ureteric bud or the metanephric mesenchyme. Some of the important genes involved in the pathway of nephrogenesis are glial cell line-derived neurotrophic factor (*GDNF*)/rearranged during transfection (*RET*), fibroblast growth factor (*FGF*), paired box protein (*PAX 2*), SIX homeobox 2 (*SIX 2*), and Hedgehog (*HH*). For example, *SIX 2*, a renal-specific transcription factor, is involved in nephrogenesis and its mutation leads to renal hypoplasia.[6] *PAX 2* has a wide range of functions in kidney development and *RET* is required for branching nephrogenesis. Variants in both these genes cause renal hypoplasia. Mutations in other common genes include *EYA 1*, *SaLL 1*, and *TCF 2*, resulting in reduced nephron number and smaller kidney size.[8] Understanding the role of genetic control on nephrogenesis will help us to identify those individuals who are at a greater risk for lower nephron number.

Low Birth Weight

It is defined as a birth weight of <2,500 g. The known risk factors for low birth weight (LBW) and intrauterine growth restriction (IUGR) are maternal HTN, maternal smoking, poor maternal weight gain during pregnancy, shorter maternal height, poor antenatal care, and lower socioeconomic status. A reduction in birth weight either due to IUGR or due to premature birth has an impact on nephrogenesis. It has been reported that every 1 kg increase in birth weight leads to an average increase of 2,60,000 additional nephrons.[9] LBW is most strongly associated with lower nephron number with an increased long-term risk of CKD.[10,11]

Preterm Birth

Preterm birth is associated with interruption of normal organogenesis of the kidney and the vascular tree, leading to low nephron endowment, HTN, endothelial dysfunction, and proteinuria in some individuals. Individuals are born with incompletely formed kidneys, and the degree of immaturity is inversely proportional to the gestational age. Nephrogenesis stops at 40 days after birth. Preterm newborns surviving ≥40 days without renal dysfunction develop glomerulomegaly, whereas the same has not been documented in long-term survivors with renal dysfunction. This is because individuals surviving without renal dysfunction develop a compensatory mechanism through hyperfiltration that probably helps kidneys to maintain glomerular function.[12] Preterm birth is an important risk factor for renal disease later in life.[10,13] This phenomenon is a multihit one that includes race, ethnicity, fetal–parental genome, and environmental and socioeconomic profile of the individual.[14]

Postnatal Factors

Nutrition and Catch-up Growth

Among preterm infants, protein–energy malnutrition in the early postnatal period is associated with reduction in estimated GFR (eGFR) at the age of 7 years.[15] On the contrary, there is evidence to suggest that rapid "catch-up" growth (i.e., upward crossing of weight centiles) leads to the development of high blood pressure, insulin resistance, cardiovascular and renal risks later in life. Catch-up growth is necessary as it improves child survival, stunting, and malnutrition but not to an extent of overweight or obesity. Adverse effects are most marked among those who had been LBW or preterm and became overweight or obese.[16] A follow-up study of obese preterm children showed that these children are more prone to kidney injury compared to their term counterparts.[17]

The other clinical markers associated with nephron number reduction in humans include gender, adult height, age, and ethnicity. Female gender has 12% lower nephron number than males. There is an increase in 28,000 glomeruli per centimeter increase in height. After the age of 18 years, a total of 3,676 glomeruli reduce per kidney per year. Aboriginal Australians have lower nephron number when compared to the US Whites and Blacks.[16]

RENAL PATHOLOGICAL CHANGES ASSOCIATED WITH LOW NEPHRON NUMBER

Glomerular Size

The nephron number does not increase after birth, but the kidney matches its filtration capacity to the body's demands through glomerular hypertrophy. Most studies have reported a strong inverse correlation between the glomerular numbers and the mean glomerular volume (Vglom). These findings suggest that larger glomeruli may be a sign of compensatory hyperfiltration and hypertrophy in subjects with a fewer number of nephrons. These hypertrophied glomeruli may be more susceptible to hyperfiltration and glomerulosclerosis.[7] Glomerular hypertrophy is an integral feature of hypertensive nephropathy and appears to precede rather than compensate for glomerulosclerosis.[18] Thus, an increase in the glomerular size may be an additional risk factor for HTN and CKD.

Glomerulosclerosis

Young et al. observed an inverse relation between the total nephron number and glomerulosclerosis in adults.[19] Glomerular hyperfiltration damage, as a result of low nephron number, may lead to arteriolosclerosis in the periglomerular arteries as well as glomerulosclerosis due to ischemia.[7]

Glomerular Density

Glomerular density is the glomerular number per renal cortical area that correlates with weight of the neonate. Kidneys of LBW neonates contain fewer glomeruli per unit area of cortex than neonates with a normal birth weight.[20] Glomerular density has been hypothesized to reflect the unique nephron number of every individual and is inversely correlated with the mean glomerular volume.[7]

BARKER AND BRENNER HYPOTHESIS

In 1980s, David J Barker, a British physician and epidemiologist, said, "Womb may be more important than Home." He discovered that the mortality rate of coronary heart disease correlated with birth weight. This strongly contributed to the concept "fetal origin of adult disease."[21] Brenner et al. hypothesized that the developmental programming in the kidney leads to reduction in nephron number, which may be due to a congenital or an acquired nephron deficit, and these individuals were at a risk for adult HTN and chronic nephropathy.[22]

LONG-TERM CLINICAL CONSEQUENCES OF LOW NEPHRON NUMBER

Both LBW and preterm birth are associated with an increased risk of elevated blood pressure and CKD in later life. The fact that only one risk factor is present may not increase the risk of CKD, but the presence of multiple factors could lead to the development of HTN and CKD in later life. **Figure 1** illustrates the key clinical consequences of low nephron number, which include glomerular hyperfiltration, glomerulosclerosis, proteinuria, HTN, and CKD.

Low Nephron Number and Hypertension

Low birth weight with reduced nephron number is a risk factor for HTN in adulthood. It has been estimated through large epidemiological studies that blood pressure levels increase by an average of 1-4 mm Hg/kg decrease in birth weight.[23] The risk of HTN may correlate with the severity of the nephron deficit. The lower the nephron number, the higher the blood pressure. When the nephron number is markedly reduced (>50%), as observed in patients with severe congenital renal hypoplasia and in experimental studies in which the nephron number is dramatically reduced down to 70% or more, early HTN is more likely to occur.[24,25] It has also been shown that children with solitary kidney are prone to developing HTN and early CKD compared to general population.[26,27]

Low birth weight and preterm birth lead to an interruption in angiogenesis, which includes endothelial dysfunction, impaired endothelial-dependent arterial relaxation, reduction in microvascular density, reduced arterial dimensions, and arterial elasticity. These characteristics of the vascular system in LBW and preterm neonates are the cause for predisposition to HTN independent of genetic or environmental factors.[28] Apart from arterial factors, endocrine mechanisms involved in the programming of HTN comprise increased hypothalamic-pituitary-adrenal axis activity and overexpression of the renin-angiotensin-aldosterone system. Recent work has identified the key role of neonatal oxidative stress in programming both renal and vascular dysfunctions.[29] In LBW infants apart from

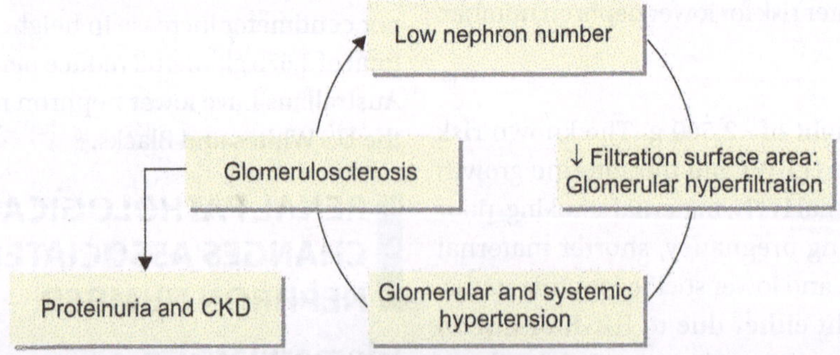

Fig. 1: Clinical consequences of low nephron number. (CKD: chronic kidney disease)
Source: Adapted from Luyckx VA, Shukha K, Brenner BM. Low nephron number and its clinical consequences. Rambam Maimonides Med J. 2011;2(4):e0061.

reduced nephron number, salt sensitivity has been shown to be the cause of HTN. The reduction in the filtration surface area limits the sodium excretion.[2] Programmed alteration in sodium handling in LBW children with reduced renal mass leads to increased salt sensitivity and HTN in later life.[30]

Low Nephron Number and Chronic Kidney Disease

Low birth weight and preterm birth are risk factors for CKD. Renal function measurements showed that the urinary microalbumin/creatinine ratio and plasma creatinine levels in adulthood were inversely proportional to birth weight in this population. In addition, increased microalbuminuria and decreased GFR were observed in those patients who were born small for gestational age.[31] Many studies have shown that LBW, when compared to normal birth weight, has a higher risk of albuminuria and kidney failure.[32] Infants born prematurely with extreme LBW have a significantly smaller kidney volume, and their renal functions are also affected with significant elevation in serum cystatin C levels. A detailed longitudinal study of LBW children gives us the evidence that kidney dysfunction may already be evident by childhood based on laboratory markers or imaging evident by smaller kidneys which reflects reduced nephron number.[33] In the Norwegian kidney biopsy registry, those with immunoglobulin A (IgA) nephropathy and LBW were associated with an increased risk of CKD.[34] The large nationwide Swedish cohort study showed that preterm and early term births were strong risk factors for the development of CKD from childhood into mid-adulthood.[35]

FOLLOW-UP

Neonatologists and pediatricians caring for premature and LBW infants should have a high suspicion for kidney dysfunction as they are at an increased risk due to reduced nephron number. It is imperative to review the birth history, neonatal intensive care unit (NICU) admissions, and childhood status for a proper management. Early identification of renal dysfunction through blood pressure measurement and urinalysis is important as HTN and albuminuria may be the early markers of CKD. Hence, long-term follow-up of these children is mandatory for high-risk neonates as shown in **Flowchart 1** though we do not have robust guidelines.

PREVENTION

With advances in neonatal care and better survival of preterm neonates, a conscious approach to preserve kidney function and protect injured kidneys is critical. Strategies to maximize nephron endowment at birth are not available at present. Hence, it is important that we follow certain preventive measures to overcome this burden.

Preconception Preventive Strategy

The optimum time to intervene is perhaps before mothers even realize that they are pregnant. Women need to be

Flowchart 1: Recommended follow-up of high-risk infants.

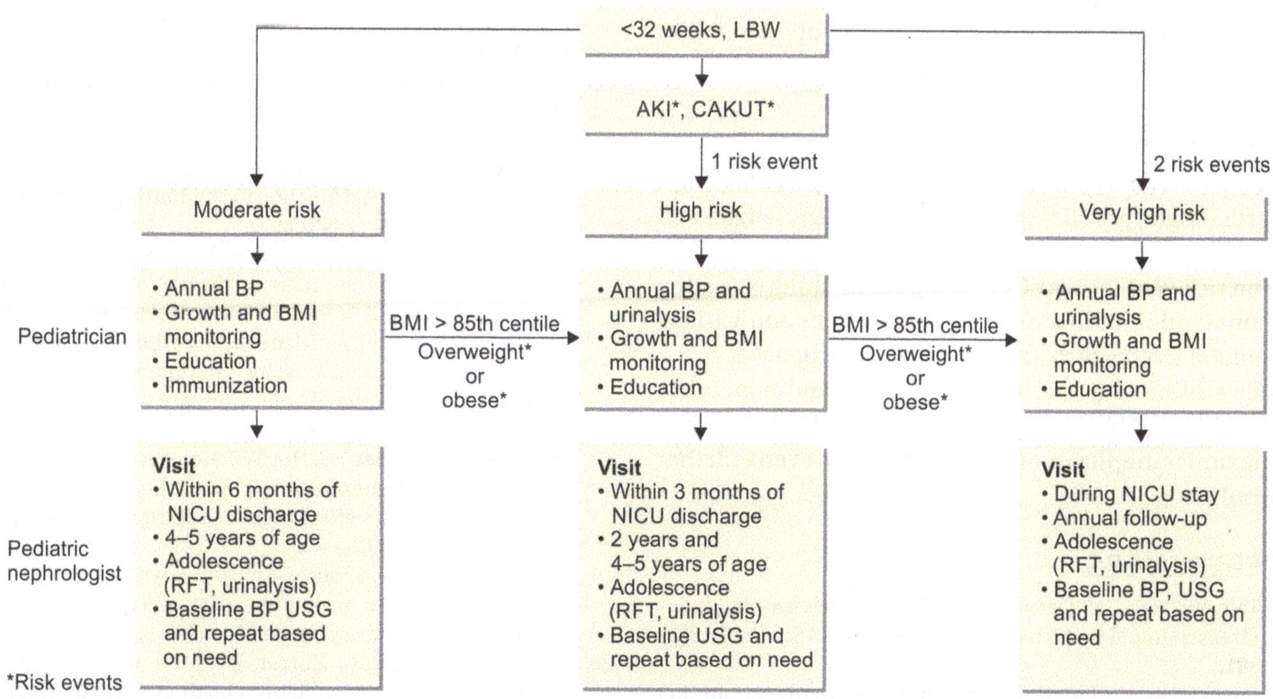

(AKI: acute kidney injury; BMI: body mass index; BP: blood pressure; CAKUT: congenital anomalies of kidney and urinary tract; LBW: low birth weight; NICU: neonatal intensive care unit; RFT: renal function test; USG: ultrasound).

educated on healthy lifestyle habits even before marriage. As genetics also play a role in congenital anomalies of kidney and urinary tract (CAKUT), we need to discourage a consanguineous marriage. In those with a family history of CAKUT, it would be ideal to provide genetic counseling before conception.

Intranatal Preventive Strategy

Regular screening during pregnancy with importance to nutrition and treatment of infections is advisable. Routine antenatal ultrasound is imperative for diagnosing early CAKUT, and an early follow-up with a pediatric nephrologist should be advised.

Postnatal Preventive Strategy

Exclusive breastfeeding for the initial 6 months should be encouraged. Parents need to be educated about healthy lifestyle choices and avoidance of rapid catch-up growth and obesity in high-risk infants. Growth and blood pressure monitoring, early identification of acute kidney injury (AKI), and avoidance of nephrotoxic medications will be helpful in these infants. Prompt referral to a pediatric nephrologist for those at high risk as shown in **Flowchart 1** is warranted.[10]

CONCLUSION

Addressing the long-term consequences of prematurity, IUGR, and LBW in the context of potential risk for CKD in later life needs focus. A coordinated effort by neonatologist, pediatrician, and pediatric nephrologist is required not only to identify the infants at high risk of CKD but also to advocate for early evaluation and appropriate referral. This may allow for future avoidance of modifiable risk factors that might accelerate CKD progression.

KEY POINTS

- Nephron number varies in humans with gestational age, birth weight, genetics, gender, nutrition, age, height, and ethnicity.
- The risk of HTN and CKD is higher in children with a combination of low nephron endowment and various multihit factors such as obesity, AKI, and diabetes.
- High-risk neonates need regular follow-up and monitoring.
- Appropriate preventive strategies are to be followed to maximize nephron endowment and prevent further insults.

REFERENCES

1. Tain YL, Hsu CN. Developmental origins of chronic kidney disease: should we focus on early life? Int J Mol Sci. 2017:18(2): 381.
2. Luyckx VA, Shukha K, Brenner BM. Low nephron number and its clinical consequences. Rambam Maimonides Med J. 2011;2(4):e0061.
3. Bertram JF, Douglas-Denton RN, Diouf B, Hughson MD, Hoy WE. Human nephron number: implications for health and disease. Pediatr Nephrol. 2011;26(9):1529-33.
4. Nyengaard JR, Bendtsen TF. Glomerular number and size in relation to age, kidney weight, and body surface in normal man. Anat Rec. 1992;232(2):194-201.
5. Denic A, Mathew J, Lerman LO, Lieske JC, Larson JJ, Alexander MP, et al. Single-nephron glomerular filtration rate in healthy adults. N Engl J Med. 2017;376(24):2349-57.
6. Charlton JR, Springsteen CH, Carmody JB. Nephron number and its determinants in early life: a primer. Pediatr Nephrol. 2014;29(12):2299-308.
7. Kanzaki G, Tsuboi N, Haruhara K, Koike K, Ogura M, Shimizu A, et al. Factors associated with a vicious cycle involving a low nephron number, hypertension and chronic kidney disease. Hypertens Res. 2015;38(10):633-41.
8. Cain J, Di Giovanni V, Smeeton J, Rosenblum ND. Genetics of renal hypoplasia: insights into the mechanisms controlling nephron endowment. Pediatr Res. 2010;68:91-8.
9. Hughson M, Farris AB 3rd, Douglas-Denton R, Hoy WE, Bertram JF. Glomerular number and size in autopsy kidneys: the relationship to birth weight. Kidney Int. 2003;63(6):2113-22.
10. Hirano D, Ishikura K, Uemura O, Ito S, Wada N, Hattori M, et al.; Pediatric CKD Study Group in Japan in conjunction with the Committee of Measures for Pediatric CKD of the Japanese Society of Pediatric Nephrology. Association between low birth weight and childhood-onset chronic kidney disease in Japan: a combined analysis of a nationwide survey for paediatric chronic kidney disease and the National Vital Statistics Report. Nephrol Dial Transplant. 2016;31(11):1895-900.
11. Kanda T, Murai-Takeda A, Kawabe H, Itoh H. Low birth weight trends: possible impacts on the prevalences of hypertension and chronic kidney disease. Hypertens Res. 2020;43(9):859-68.
12. Rodríguez MM, Gómez AH, Abitbol CL, Chandar JJ, Duara S, Zilleruelo GE. Histomorphometric analysis of postnatal glomerulogenesis in extremely preterm infants. Pediatr Dev Pathol. 2004;7(1):17-25.
13. Chehade H, Simeoni U, Guignard JP, Boubred F. Preterm birth: long term cardiovascular and renal consequences. Curr Pediatr Rev. 2018;14(4):219-26.
14. Abitbol CL, Ingelfinger JR. Nephron mass and cardiovascular and renal disease risks. Semin Nephrol. 2009;29(4):445-54.
15. Bacchetta J, Harambat J, Dubourg L, Guy B, Liutkus A, Canterino I, et al. Both extrauterine and intrauterine growth restriction impair renal function in children born very preterm. Kidney Int. 2009;76(4):445-52.
16. Low Birth Weight and Nephron Number Working Group. The impact of kidney development on the life course: a consensus document for action. Nephron. 2017;136(1):3-49.
17. Abitbol CL, Chandar J, Rodríguez MM, Berho M, Seeherunvong W, Freundlich M, et al. Obesity and preterm birth: additive risks in the progression of kidney disease in children. Pediatr Nephrol. 2009;24(7):1363-70.
18. Hughson MD, Puelles VG, Hoy WE, Douglas-Denton RN, Mott SA, Bertram JF. Hypertension, glomerular hypertrophy and nephrosclerosis: the effect of race. Nephrol Dial Transplant. 2014;29(7):1399-409.
19. Young RJ, Hoy WE, Kincaid-Smith P, Seymour AE, Bertram JF. Glomerular size and glomerulosclerosis in Australian aborigines. Am J Kidney Dis. 2000;36:481-9.
20. Manalich R, Reyes L, Herrera M, Melendi C, Fundora I. Relationship between weight at birth and the number and size of renal glomeruli in humans: a histomorphometric study. Kidney Int. 2000;58:770-3.

21. Barker DJ. The fetal and infant origins of adult disease. BMJ. 1990;301(6761):1111.
22. Brenner BM, Garcia DL, Anderson S. Glomeruli and blood pressure. Less of one, more the other? Am J Hypertens. 1988; 1:335-47.
23. Huxley RR, Shiell AW, Law CM. The role of size at birth and postnatal catch-up growth in determining systolic blood pressure: a systematic review of the literature. J Hypertens. 2000;18:815-31.
24. Singh RR, Denton KM, Bertram JF, Jefferies AJ, Head GA, Lombardo P, et al. Development of cardiovascular disease due to renal insufficiency in male sheep following fetal unilateral nephrectomy. J Hypertens. 2009;27:386-96.
25. Keller G, Zimmer G, Mall G, Ritz E, Amann K. Nephron number in patients with primary hypertension. N Engl J Med. 2003;348:101-8.
26. Thorner PS, Arbus GS, Celermajer DS, Baumal R. Focal segmental glomerulosclerosis and progressive renal failure associated with a unilateral kidney. Pediatrics. 1984;73(6): 806-10.
27. Mei-Zahav M, Korzets Z, Cohen I, Kessler O, Rathaus V, Wolach B, et al. Ambulatory blood pressure monitoring in children with a solitary kidney—a comparison between unilateral renal agenesis and uninephrectomy. Blood Press Monit. 2001;6(5): 263-7.
28. Abitbol CL, Rodriguez MM. The long-term renal and cardiovascular consequences of prematurity. Nat Rev Nephrol. 2012; 8(5):265-74.
29. Simeoni U, Ligi I, Buffat C, Boubred F. Adverse consequences of accelerated neonatal growth: cardiovascular and renal issues. Pediatr Nephrol. 2011;26(4):493-508.
30. Simonetti GD, Raio L, Surbek D, Nelle M, Frey FJ, Mohaupt MG. Salt sensitivity of children with low birth weight. Hypertension. 2008;52(4):625-30.
31. Keijzer-Veen MG, Finken MJ, Nauta J, Dekker FW, Hille ET, Frolich M, et al. Microalbuminuria and lower glomerular filtration rate at young adult age in subjects born very premature and after intrauterine growth retardation. J Am Soc Nephrol. 2005;16:2762-8.
32. White SL, Perkovic V, Cass A, Chang CL, Poulter NR, Spector T, et al. Is low birth weight an antecedent of CKD in later life? A systematic review of observational studies. Am J Kidney Dis. 2009;54(2):248-61.
33. Starzec K, Klimek M, Grudzień A, Jagła M, Kwinta P. Longitudinal assessment of renal size and function in extremely low birth weight children at 7 and 11 years of age. Pediatr Nephrol. 2016;31(11):2119-26.
34. Ruggajo P, Svarstad E, Leh S, Marti H-P, Reisæther AV, Vikse BE. Low birth weight and risk of progression to end stage renal disease in IgA nephropathy—a retrospective registry-based cohort study. PLoS One. 2016;11(4):e0153819.
35. Crump C, Sundquist J, Winkleby MA, Sundquist K. Preterm birth and risk of chronic kidney disease from childhood into mid-adulthood: national cohort study. BMJ. 2019;365:l1346.

SECTION

2

Investigating a Child with Kidney Disease

CHAPTER

2.1 Urinalysis

Nivedita Kamath, Arpana A Iyengar

INTRODUCTION

Urinalysis is a basic but important tool for the diagnosis of a wide range of renal diseases. Microscopic examination of the urine is considered a bedside tool, an important adjunct to arrive at a clinical diagnosis. Urinalysis has its unique role in the diagnosis of glomerular diseases, tubulointerstitial diseases, and infections. In this chapter, we discuss the collection of urine sample for analysis, processing the urine sample, and the evaluation of urine for physical and chemical parameters and microscopic examination and its relevance to clinical practice. The details of evaluation of electrolytes, acidification, concentrating ability of urine, etc., are discussed in relevant chapters.

COLLECTION OF URINE FOR ANALYSIS

Single Urine Sample/Spot Sample

A single sample of urine can be collected by one of these techniques:

- *Bag collection:* This is useful in infants and toddlers who are not able to void on command. After cleaning the genital area, a self-adhesive bag is attached around it. The child is given an adequate amount of fluids and the voided urine is collected. This technique is cumbersome to use in female infants. Given the high risk of contamination, this method of collection is also not suitable in a child with a suspected urinary tract infection (UTI).[1]
- *Clean catch sample:* This is a simple method of obtaining a urine sample in a child who is toilet trained. After cleaning the genital area, the collection of the sample begins midstream after the first few milliliters of urine have been voided. This is a fairly reliable method of collection of urine for all tests including testing for UTI.
- *Catheter sample:* A suitable sample for urine culture can be obtained by inserting an infant feeding tube by a one-time catheterization with aseptic precautions. This is used only in infants and toddlers when UTI is being evaluated.[1]
- *Suprapubic aspiration:* This is a sparingly used procedure, reserved only when collection by other methods is not feasible in an infant with a suspected UTI. The procedure is performed after maintaining thorough asepsis. The child should be fed at least 30 minutes prior to the procedure. The suprapubic aspiration is performed by inserting a 22-gauge needle attached to a 5 cm^3 syringe. The needle is inserted in the midline 1–2 cm above the pubic symphysis at an angle of 30° toward the pelvis. At a depth of 1.5–2 cm, urine can be aspirated after which the needle is withdrawn. This procedure can be performed under ultrasound guidance to improve the yield.

Timed Collection of Urine

Twenty-four-hour Collection of Urine

A 24-hour sample of urine is required for the estimation of creatinine clearance, urinary protein estimation, and measurement of urinary excretion of electrolytes. This method, however, is cumbersome, prone to error, and may not be feasible in young children. The time point of collection starts from the second voided sample of the first day and includes all voided samples of the day and night and ends with the collection of the next day's first voided sample. The urine should be collected in a designated jar and stored in a cool place. In partially toilet-trained children, timed samples can be collected, i.e., a 6–12-hour collection, and the results extrapolated to a 24-hour sample.[1]

Timing of Urine Sample Collection

The first voided sample is ideally suited for biochemical evaluation. However, the second voided sample may be more feasible to obtain in office practice.

PROCESSING THE URINE SAMPLE

Urine should be collected in a sterile, transparent, wide-mouthed container. The collected sample of urine must be processed within 2–4 hours of collection to avoid lysis of particles. Alternately, the urine sample can be stored at 2–8°C for up to 24 hours. However, this may result in precipitation of phosphates and urates and makes the examination of urine inaccurate. Preservatives such as formaldehyde and glutaraldehyde can be used with caution as they may alter the findings of urine microscopy.[2]

EXAMINATION OF URINE

The examination of urine consists of examination of physical parameters, chemical parameters, and microscopic examination.

Physical Parameters

- *Color:* The color of the urine should be examined in natural light against a white background. The normal color of the urine ranges from pale yellow to amber colored based on the state of hydration. The abnormal color of urine may give a clue to various conditions. Reddish/pink urine may suggest the presence of blood, hemoglobin, myoglobin, porphyrin, or nonpathological pigments (beets, food-coloring agents). Cola-colored urine is typically seen in glomerular hematuria. Blue-green appearance of urine may be seen in the presence of biliverdin or in infection with *Pseudomonas*. Drugs such as rifampicin (orange color) and nitrofurantoin (brownish color) may also result in the abnormal color of the urine. The various conditions that result in a change in the color of urine are discussed in **Table 1**.[2]
- *Turbidity:* Normal urine is usually transparent. Turbid urine is most often seen in concentrated urine, or increased number of cells such as erythrocytes, leukocytes, or bacteria, or increased concentration of phosphate or rarely in chyluria.
- *Odor:* Infection is the most common cause of foul-smelling urine. The odor of the urine is an important clue to several metabolic conditions. The most common conditions are maple syrup urine disease (maple syrup odor), phenylketonuria (musty odor), and hypermethioninemia (fishy odor). The various conditions resulting in a change in the odor of urine are discussed in **Table 1**.

TABLE 1: Altered color and odor of urine.

Altered color	*Clinical relevance*
White	Chyle, pus, phosphate crystals
Red/brown	Blood, hemoglobin, myoglobin, methemoglobin Cola-colored glomerulonephritis *Drugs:* Methyldopa, metronidazole
Yellow/orange	Bilirubin *Drugs:* Rifampicin, phenazopyridine
Blue/green	Biliverdin, *Pseudomonas* UTI, dyes *Drugs:* Triamterene, amitriptyline
Altered odor	***Clinical relevance***
Fruity	Ketones
Ammoniacal	Urease-splitting organisms
Maple syrup	Maple syrup urine disease
Musty	Phenylketonuria
Sweaty feet	Isovaleric acidemia
Rancid	Tyrosinemia

- *Relative density:* The relative density of urine can be assessed in different ways.
  - *Specific gravity:* The specific gravity of the urine is a measure of the number and weight of dissolved particles. It is measured with a urinometer. Though simple and quick to use, it requires a fairly large amount of urine. The urinometer is now obsolete and rarely used in clinical settings. A dipstick test is commonly used to assess specific gravity. The normal specific gravity of urine ranges from 1.005 to 1.030.
  - *Osmolality:* This is the gold standard for measurement of relative density. It is measured using an osmometer. Osmolality is measured on a fresh sample of urine using freezing point depression osmometry. The normal osmolality of urine varies from 50 to 1,200 mOsm/kg.
  - *Refractrometry:* This is measured using the refractive index. It is a commonly used measure and the advantage is that it can be measured with a single drop of urine.
  - *Dipstick:* The dipstick is a rapid and simple test and is commonly used in office practice.[2]

Chemical Parameters

Several substances in the urine can be detected using chemical reactions. However, with the advent of the dipstick, it has become a commonly used tool at the bedside and in the laboratory for the detection of several substances alone or in combination. The dipstick with the various parameters that can be measured are shown in **Figure 1**.

- *Urine pH:* The urine pH should be ideally measured on a freshly passed sample of urine using a pH meter. However, in routine practice, pH is often measured using dipsticks.
- *Blood:* The dipstick detects hemoglobin in the urine. The pseudoperoxidase activity of heme catalyzes the

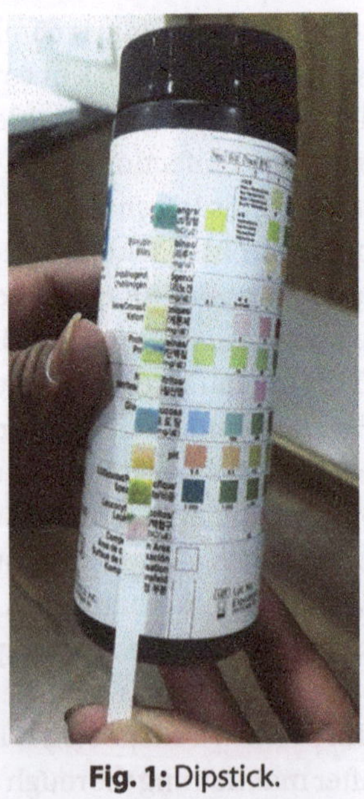

Fig. 1: Dipstick.

reaction of peroxide with a chromogen resulting in a color change. When the hemoglobin is sequestered in the intact erythrocytes, it produces green spots, whereas free hemoglobin produces a diffuse green color. However, in massive hematuria, a large number of intact red blood cells (RBCs) also could give a diffuse green color. Hence, dipstick cannot differentiate between hemoglobinuria and hematuria. A microscopic examination of the urine will support the diagnosis of hematuria. Myoglobin, which is chemically similar to hemoglobin, can result in a false-positive test. Myoglobinuria can be differentiated from hemoglobin using the rapid ammonium sulfate precipitation test. To 5 mL of urine, 2.8 g of ammonium sulfate is added and the sample is centrifuged. Hemoglobin precipitates resulting in a clear supernatant, while the supernatant remains reddish in the presence of myoglobin.[3]

The other important false positives are from the heavy growth of pseudoperoxidase-producing bacteria (enterococci, staphylococci, streptococci). Ascorbic acid causes a false-negative reaction.

- *Protein:* There are several methods of estimation of protein. The tests may be quantitative, semiquantitative, or qualitative. Quantitative tests are 24-hour urinary estimation of proteinuria and protein-creatinine ratio. Most commonly used tests such as dipstick assessment and turbidimetric tests are semiquantitative. Qualitative assessment of proteins could be done using radioimmunoassays or high-performance liquid chromatography to detect specific proteins.
  - *Dipstick:* The dipstick uses the protein error of estimation—the presence of protein causes a change in the pH that is proportional to the concentration of the protein. This change in pH results in a change in the color of the chromogen tetrabromophenol blue. The dipstick has a high sensitivity for the detection of albumin and low sensitivity for other proteins. The sensitivity of the dipstick for the measurement of albumin is 15–30 mg/dL. Microalbuminuria which is defined as urine albumin excretion between 30 and 300 mg/day or 30 and 300 µg/mg creatinine may not be detected by dipsticks. The dipstick offers a semiquantitative estimation of the protein content in the urine which is expressed on a scale from 0 to 4+.
  - *Urine protein to creatinine estimation:* This is a quantitative estimation of protein in the random spot sample of urine, preferably the first morning sample. The protein-creatinine ratio correlates well with the 24-hour estimation of protein. This is a simple, easy-to-perform test, which is useful in measuring proteinuria in children and is a useful test to use during follow-up for assessing the response to treatment. A protein to creatinine ratio of <0.2 is considered normal, 0.2–2 as non-nephrotic range proteinuria, and >2 as nephrotic range proteinuria.
  - *24-hour estimation of proteinuria:* The 24-hour estimation of proteinuria is considered the gold standard. However, it is difficult to get an accurate collection of the sample in children, time consuming, and not practical for follow-up assessment of response to therapy. To assess the accuracy of sample collection, the 24-hour urinary creatinine should be measured and reported within the normal range (20 mg/kg in girls and 30 mg/kg in boys).
  - *Turbidimetric tests:* Tests such as the heat coagulation tests and the sulfosalicylic acid tests which are semiquantitative tests based on the assessment of turbidity of urine are simple bedside tests. However, they are cumbersome and prone to error.

    In the heat coagulation test, 10 mL of urine is taken in a test tube and the upper part of the test tube is heated to boiling point. The precipitate formed does not disappear when three drops of acetic acid are added.

    In the sulfosalicylic acid test, five to eight drops of 20% sulfosalicylic acid are added to 5 mL of urine. The turbidity is measured as 1+ (15–30 mg/dL)—turbidity without granule formation, 2+ (30–100 mg/dL)—turbidity with granule formation, 3+ (150–300 mg/dL) turbidity with flocculation, and 4+ (>500 mg/dL)—flocculent precipitation.
  - *Microalbuminuria:* It refers to urinary albumin excretion in the range of 30–300 mg/day. It is measured using the radioimmunoassay technique. It can also be expressed as 30–300 µg/mg creatinine or 20–200 µg/min.[2,4]
- *Glucose:* The dipstick is commonly used to measure glucose in the urine. Glucose in the urine is oxidized to gluconic acid and hydrogen peroxide. Using the catalyzing activity of a peroxidase, hydrogen peroxide reacts with a chromogen to form a colored product. A false-positive test can occur in the presence of oxidizing agents and hydrochloric acid. False-negative results occur in the presence of ascorbic acid and bacteria. Nonglucose-reducing sugars cannot be detected by a dipstick test.
- *Leukocyte esterase and nitrite:* The dipstick uses indoxyl esterase activity from lysed neutrophils to detect leukocyturia. In alkaline or dilute urine, the leukocytes lyse giving a false-positive result. Conversely, in concentrated urine, a false-negative result may be obtained. False-negative results are also seen in the presence of high glucose or protein concentration and in the presence of drugs such as tetracyclines and cephalosporins.
- *Nitrite:* The dipstick is able to detect the presence of bacteria with the ability of reducing nitrates to nitrites using nitrate reductase. Most gram-negative organisms, which are the common uropathogens, have this enzyme

and produce a positive result. A false positive may be seen in a diet rich in nitrates.

- *Others:* Ketones and bile pigments are tested in specific clinical situations using a dipstick.

Microscopic Examination of Urine

Microscopic examination of the urine is an integral part of the overall clinical assessment of a child with a renal disease. The second morning sample is generally preferred for the microscopic evaluation. The first morning sample is not preferred as it is usually concentrated and has been collected in the bladder for a long time which could cause lysis of cells in the urine.

Procedure for the Preparation of a Sample for Microscopy

The second morning sample is generally preferred; however, any available sample could be used. The midstream sample must be collected in a wide-mouthed container. The sample must be processed within 2–3 hours of collection. A 10-mL sample of urine is centrifuged at 2,000 rpm for 10 minutes. The supernatant is discarded, and the sediment is resuspended in 0.5-mL urine. About 50 µL of urine is transferred on to a slide and covered with a coverslip. A phase-contrast microscope is ideal, but a traditional bright light microscope could be used. The phase-contrast microscope allows better visualization of the details of cells and has a greater sensitivity for hyaline and RBC casts. The addition of polarized light is useful in the identification of crystals. The examination of the slide is done under low power (×10) and then under high power (×40). A minimum of 20 high-power fields should be examined. Casts tend to move toward the edges of the coverslip, and this part of the slide must be included in the examination. Casts are better visualized under low power and are expressed as number per low-power field. The cells are expressed as number per high-power field.

The microscopic examination of the urine should always be preceded by the physical examination and dipstick assessment of urine. Alkaline pH and low specific gravity can result in lysis of cells and should be interpreted with caution. The pH of the urine is also important for the visualization of various crystals.[2]

Examination

Cells

Cells in the urine can be derived from the circulation—erythrocytes and leukocytes—or from the epithelium—renal tubular cells and urothelial cells.

- *Erythrocytes (RBC):* They have a translucent biconcave appearance (4–7 µm) with no nucleus. They may be normal in shape (isomorphic) or appear to have irregular shape and contour. Though the guidelines for the evaluation of hematuria by the Indian Society of Pediatric Nephrology define hematuria as the presence ≥5 RBCs/hpf,[5] the more recent guidelines recommend that the presence of >3 RBC/hpf is considered significant.[4] Isomorphic hematuria is suggestive of nonglomerular hematuria **(Fig. 2)**. Dysmorphic cells are typically seen in glomerular hematuria **(Fig. 3)**. RBCs appear dysmorphic due to changes in pH and osmolality as they traverse the various parts of the tubule. Acanthocytes are a type of dysmorphic erythrocytes, which are ring shaped with one or more protrusions. Though there is no standard cutoff for the number of dysmorphic RBCs, the presence of >40% dysmorphic RBCs or >5% acanthocytes is considered significant.[4]
- *Leukocytes [white blood cell (WBC)]:* Neutrophils are the most commonly found leukocytes in the urine **(Fig. 2)**. They are larger (7–13 µm) than the erythrocytes and are identified by the presence of a granular cytoplasm and lobulated nucleus. The presence of >5 WBC/hpf in a

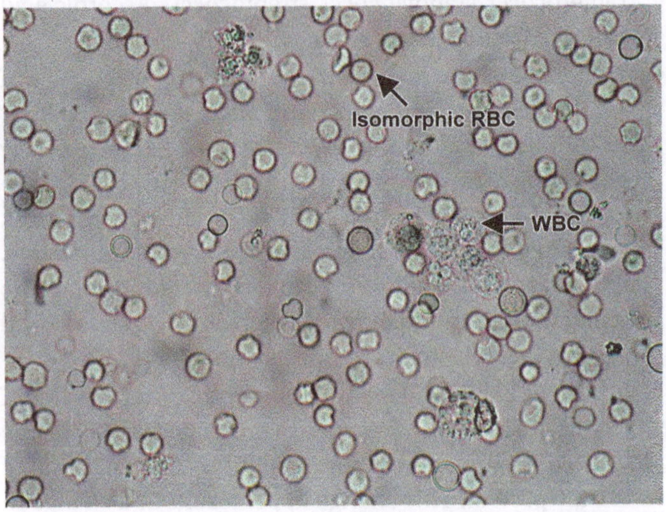

Fig. 2: A cluster of WBCs seen in a field with numerous isomorphic RBCs in the background. (RBC: red blood cell; WBC: white blood cell)

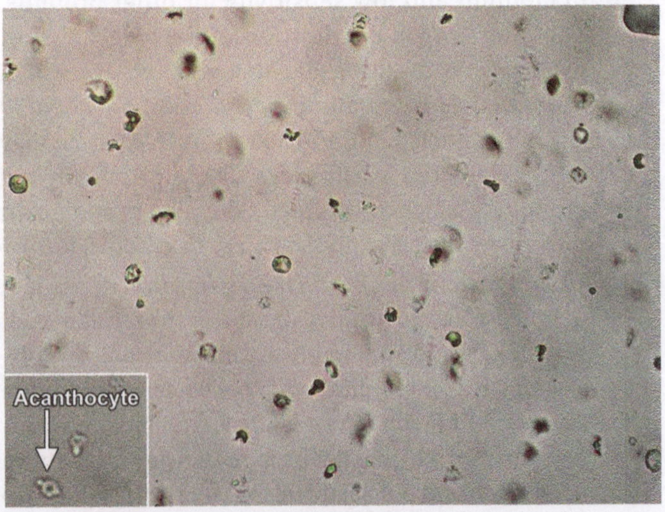

Fig. 3: Dysmorphic red blood cells (RBCs) seen in the microscopic examination of urine.

centrifuged sample of urine is considered significant.[6] Neutrophils are commonly seen in UTIs but may also be found in tubulointerstitial nephritis and acute glomerulonephritis. Eosinophils are found in conditions such as drug-induced tubulointerstitial nephritis. Eosinophils can be identified by using the Wright stain or Hansel stain. Lymphocytes are rarely seen in the urine. Macrophages appear as large cells and may contain phagocytosed lipid particles giving the appearance of oval fat bodies.

- *Renal tubular epithelial cells:* Tubular epithelial cells vary in size and shape depending on the segment of the tubule they are shed from. They have a distinct nucleus with prominent nucleoli. Tubular cells indicated tubular damage, commonly seen in acute tubular necrosis, acute interstitial nephritis, and acute cellular rejection.[2]
- *Urothelial cells:* These cells are derived from the urothelial lining from the renal calyces to the proximal urethra. These cells are large, oval, or club shaped and are commonly seen in UTIs and ureteric calculi.[2,4]
- *Decoy cells:* These are desquamated urothelial cells with intranuclear inclusions. They are seen in polyoma virus infection following renal transplantation.

Casts

Casts are cylindrical structures of renal origin where cells of different kinds are enmeshed in a matrix of Tamm–Horsfall (TH) protein. TH proteins are secreted by the thick ascending limb of the loop of Henle. The presence of casts in the urine is called cylindruria. The most common types of casts are hyaline, epithelial, granular, fatty, broad, waxy, RBC, and WBC casts. The common casts seen in urine **(Fig. 4)** and their clinical relevance are discussed in **Table 2.** "Telescopic urine" is a term used to describe a urine sample that has a variety of cells and casts. It is usually seen in proliferative glomerulonephritis such as lupus nephritis.

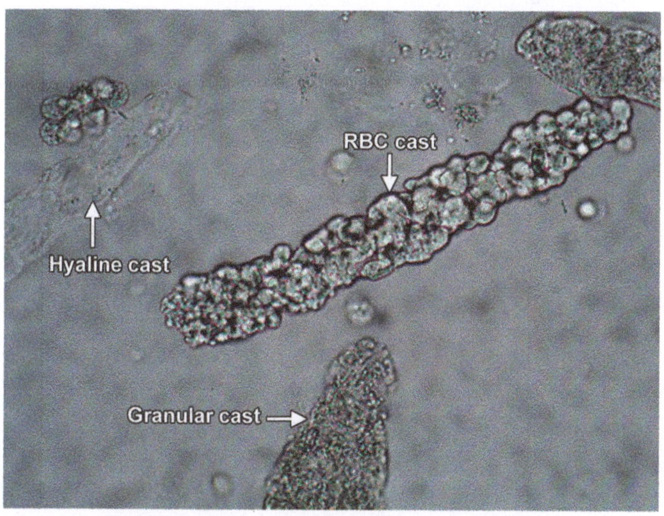

Fig. 4: Casts in the urine. (RBC: red blood cell).

Crystals

Crystals are commonly seen in urine. They may consist of normal constituents of urine, pathological constituents, or drug-related crystals. Some crystals such as calcium oxalate or calcium phosphate are present normally in the urine and may be transiently supersaturated and precipitated in the presence of dehydration. Some crystals such as cystine and dihydroxyadenine are always pathological. Variations in temperature and pH can be associated with precipitation of crystals. Acid urine is associated with calcium oxalate, uric acid, and amorphous urate crystals. Alkaline urine is associated with calcium phosphate, triple phosphate, and amorphous phosphates. The various crystals found in urine **(Figs. 5A to C)** and their clinical significance are given in **Table 3.**

Organisms

- *Bacteria:* These are commonly found in the urine as a contaminant from an improperly collected sample or from growth in a sample that has not been processed within 2–3 hours.
- *Candida: Candida* in the urine is usually seen from contamination with genital secretions.
- *Schistosoma haematobium:* Urine microscopy is an important tool in the diagnosis of urinary schistosomiasis.

Clinical relevance: The urine analysis is a key investigation in the diagnosis of common renal diseases. The findings on urine analysis in common renal diseases such as acute glomerulonephritis, nephrotic syndrome, UTI, and acute kidney injury are described in **Table 4.**

ADVANCES IN THE EVALUATION OF URINE

With improvement in technology, automated urine analysis including automated microscopy is being increasingly used

TABLE 2: Common casts and their clinical relevance.

Casts	*Clinical relevance*
Hyaline: Tamm–Horsfall proteins	Dehydration, congestive heart failure, diuretics
Epithelial: Renal epithelial cells	Acute tubular necrosis, glomerulonephritis
Granular: Degenerated epithelial cells	Acute tubular necrosis
Fatty: Granular or hyaline with lipid droplets	Fabry disease (Maltese cross on polarized light), nephrotic syndrome
RBC casts: RBC enmeshed in TH protein	Glomerular hematuria (100% sensitivity)
WBC cast: WBC enmeshed in TH protein	Pyelonephritis, interstitial nephritis

(RBC: red blood cell; TH: Tamm–Horsfall; WBC: white blood cell)

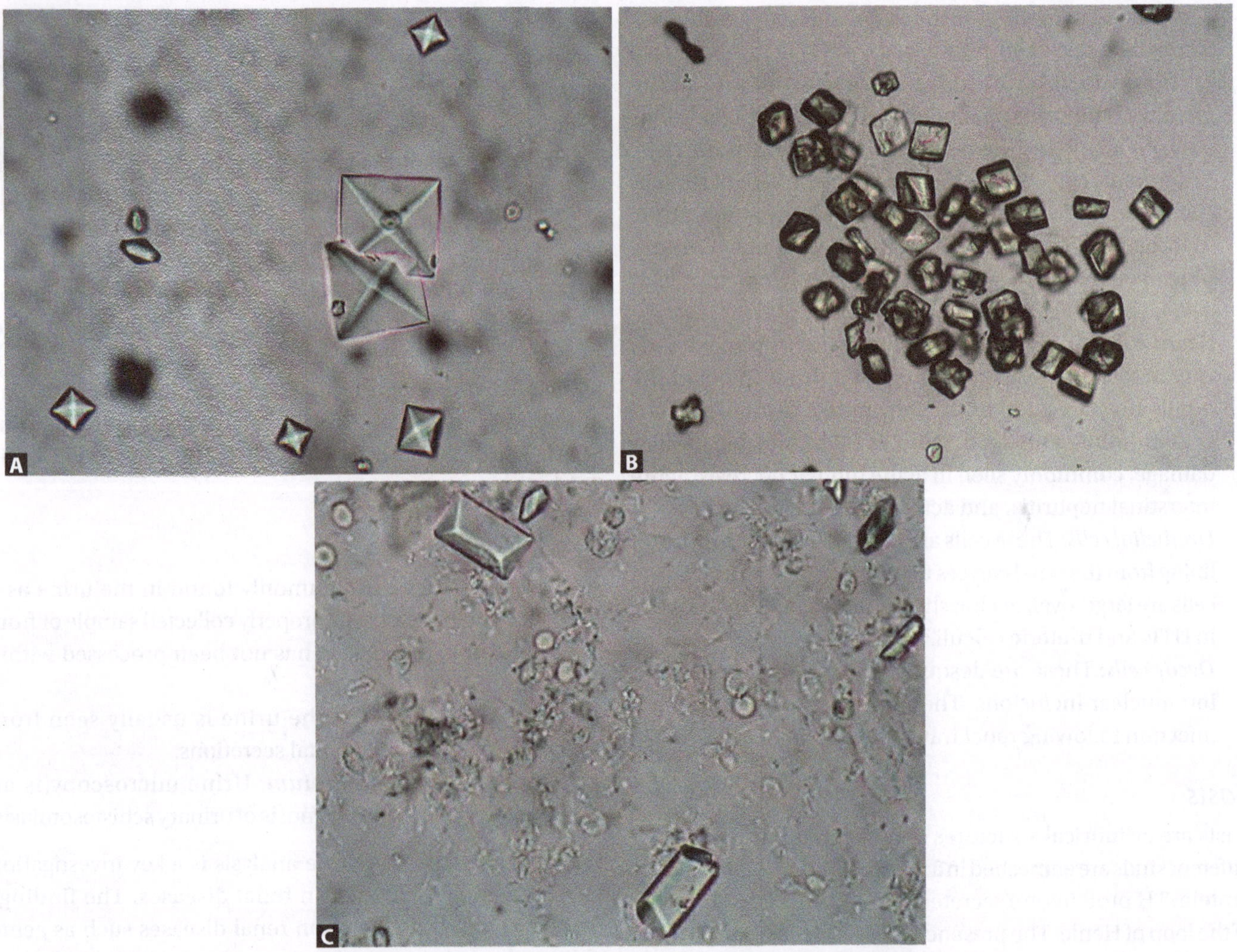

Figs. 5A to C: Crystals in the urine: (A) Calcium oxalate; (B) Uric acid; (C) Triple phosphate.

Courtesy: Photographs of urine microscopy by Dr. Anila Abraham, Nephropathologist, Renopath Laboratory Private Limited, Chennai.

TABLE 3: Common crystals and their clinical relevance.

Crystals	*Clinical relevance*
• *Calcium oxalate monohydrate:* Dumbbell shaped • *Calcium oxalate dihydrate:* Envelope-shaped crystals	High oxalate diet, primary hyperoxaluria, ethylene glycol poisoning
Uric acid: Diamond-shaped, multicolor birefringence on polarized light	Uric acid calculi, hyperuricosuria, tumor lysis
Phosphate: • *Calcium phosphate:* Coffin lid appearance • *Triple phosphate:* Rectangular prism	Associated with recurrent UTI
Cystine: Hexagonal	Cystinuria
Drugs: • *Acyclovir:* Needle shaped • *Indinavir:* Plates and stars • *Amoxicillin:* Broom/brush shaped	

(UTI: urinary tract infection)

TABLE 4: Urinary findings in common renal diseases.

Urinary parameters	*Acute glomerulonephritis*	*Nephrotic syndrome*	*Urinary tract infection*	*Acute kidney injury*
Gross appearance	Cola color	Dark yellow, amber, turbid	Turbid, may be foul smelling	Dark yellow
Protein	+ to ++	+++ to ++++	+ to ++	+ to ++
Blood	Present	Absent	Absent	Absent
Leukocyte esterase, nitrite	Negative	Negative	Likely to be positive	Negative
Microscopy cells	Several RBC dysmorphic	Occasional RBC, WBC	WBC	WBC (interstitial nephritis), eosinophils (drug-induced interstitial nephritis)
Casts	RBC casts	Hyaline casts, fatty casts	WBC casts	Epithelial cell casts, granular casts

(RBC: red blood cell; WBC: white blood cell)

in modern-day laboratories. Laser-based flow cytometry and digitalized microscopy are the two common techniques used for automated microscopic examination of the urine. These methods require small amounts of urine (2–3 mL), can process several samples at once, and correlate fairly well with the manual method.[7]

CONCLUSION

Urine analysis is a simple, easily available bedside tool in the diagnosis and follow-up of renal disease in children and is a useful adjunct to the clinical assessment in patients with renal disease.

KEY POINTS

- Urine analysis, especially the dipstick test, and microscopic evaluation of urine are important tools for the diagnosis of kidney diseases in children.
- The physical evaluation examines the color, odor, and specific gravity of urine.
- The chemical analysis is performed most often with a dipstick and examines the pH, presence of protein, glucose, blood, and other substances.
- The microscopic examination is often done on a centrifuged sample of urine and examines the presence of cells (erythrocytes, leukocytes, epithelial cells), casts (RBC, white blood cell, hyaline, granular, etc.), and crystals (calcium oxalate, urate, phosphate, etc.).

Note: For a comprehensive and interactive review on urine analysis, the reader is referred to "Urine—A window to diagnose kidney disease—A pediatric perspective" On ISN Academy. (https://academy.theisn.org/isn/2017/elearning_modules/193117/arpana.iyengar.urine.analysis.a.window.to.diagnose.kidney.disease.)

REFERENCES

1. Utsch B, Klaus G. Urinalysis in children and adolescents. Dtsch Arztebl Int. 2014;111(37):617-25.
2. Fogazzi GB, Verdesca S, Garigali G. Urinalysis: core curriculum 2008. Am J Kidney Dis. 2008;51(6):1052-67.
3. Trivedi DJ, Kulkarni SP, Mudaraddi R. Primary myoglobinuria: differentiate myoglobinuria from hemoglobinuria. Indian J Clin Biochem. 2017;32(3):367-9.
4. Mutter WP. Urinalysis. In: Turner N, Lameire N, Goldsmith DJ, Winearls CG, Himmelfarb J, Remuzzi G (Eds). Oxford Textbook of Clinical Nephrology, 4th edition. Oxford: Oxford University Press; 2015. pp. 35-43.
5. Phadke KD, Vijayakumar M, Sharma J, Iyengar A; Indian Pediatric Nephrology Group. Consensus statement on evaluation of hematuria. Indian Pediatr. 2006;43(11):965-73.
6. Mishra OP, Abhinay A, Prasad R. Urinary infections in children. Indian J Pediatr. 2013;80(10):838-43.
7. Becker GJ, Garigali G, Fogazzi GB. Advances in urine microscopy. Am J Kidney Dis. 2016;67(6):954-64.

CHAPTER

2.2 Glomerular and Tubular Functions

Liji R, Susan Uthup

ASSESSMENT OF GLOMERULAR AND TUBULAR FUNCTIONS

The kidneys play an important role in the excretion of nitrogenous waste products and regulation of acid–base, electrolyte, and water balance in our body. Assessment of glomerular and tubular functions is important for the early detection and management of renal disease, to monitor the response to treatment, and to assess the progression of the disease.

Assessment of Glomerular Function

Renal glomerulus is a semipermeable filter which filters water and solutes and sieves macromolecules of size greater than or equal to albumin. Glomerular function can be assessed by evaluation of glomerular filtration rate (GFR); assessment of proteinuria; and measurement of serum concentrations of markers such as urea, creatinine, and cystatin C.

Glomerular Filtration Rate

Glomerular filtration is the process of producing an ultrafiltrate of blood as it flows through the glomerular capillaries. GFR is the volume of fluid filtered by the glomerulus in unit time. Assessment of GFR plays a crucial role in the diagnosis of acute kidney injury (AKI) and chronic kidney disease, early intervention to prevent the progression of chronic kidney disease, modification of the dose of drugs cleared by the kidney, and monitoring for side effects of the drugs.

Glomerular filtration rate can be assessed by measuring the clearance of substances that are eliminated predominantly by glomerular filtration. Clearance of a substance is defined as the volume of plasma cleared of that substance in unit time and can be calculated by the formula:

$$\text{Clearance of a substance (mL/min)} = UV/P$$

where U and P are the urine concentration and plasma concentration of that substance, respectively, and V is the volume of urine in unit time.

For accurate assessment of GFR using any substance, the following criteria should be met by that substance as defined by Smith et al.[1] These criteria include the following:

- The substance is freely filtered by the glomerulus.
- It is neither secreted nor reabsorbed by the tubules.
- It is physiologically inert and nontoxic.
- It is neither cleared nor metabolized in extrarenal organs or tissues.
- It is not synthesized, stored, or metabolized by the kidney.
- It is not bound to plasma proteins and its level remains reasonably constant.
- Its clearance is at a constant rate regardless of the amount that is in the solution in the plasma.

Clearance of both exogenous and endogenous solutes is used for the determination of GFR. Exogenous markers include iohexol, inulin, iodoacetate, and diethylenetriaminepentaacetic acid (DTPA). GFR estimation using these exogenous markers, though more accurate, is time consuming and cumbersome. Endogenous markers used for assessment of GFR include plasma creatinine, beta-trace protein, and cystatin C.

Inulin: The inulin clearance is the time-tested gold standard method for GFR estimation.[2] It is a fructose polymer that is completely filtered at the glomerulus and is not reabsorbed or secreted by the tubules. Urinary clearance of inulin during its continuous infusion is used as a reference method to measure GFR.

Blood urea: Urea, the major end product of protein catabolism, is filtered by the glomerulus and reabsorbed by the tubules. Reabsorption of urea mainly occurs at the proximal tubule and also through urea transporters present in the collecting duct. Apart from renal failure, blood urea levels are affected by protein intake, liver disease, and catabolic states. The rate of urea production is so variable in infants that it is only a crude reflection of GFR and can only be used to detect gross changes.

Plasma creatinine: Creatinine is the most commonly used marker for assessing renal function in clinical practice. It is freely filtered at the glomerulus due to its small size and lack of protein binding. It is also actively secreted by the proximal tubules. The fraction of tubular secretion increases with decreasing GFR leading to an overestimation by 10–40% when compared to inulin clearance. Estimation of creatinine to assess renal function is difficult in children, as there is a steady increase in plasma creatinine after 2 years of life due to an increase in muscle mass. Excessive dietary intake of meat increases plasma creatinine while the levels may be erroneously low in anorectic adolescents and malnourished children. Only when kidney function is reduced by >50% do creatinine concentrations in serum or plasma increase beyond the reference levels. A measured creatinine clearance may provide more diagnostic information in such situations.[3]

Creatinine can be determined by using various modifications of the Jaffe principle (alkaline picrate reaction) by enzymatic dry chemistry or enzymatic colorimetric methods. Creatinine estimation by the Jaffe method can be affected by pseudochromogens such as acetone. Bilirubin is also a negative interferent in creatinine estimation by both Jaffe's and enzymatic methods resulting in the underestimation of serum creatinine in hyperbilirubinemia.[4] To overcome this negative interference, several modifications in the assay methods have been used.

Cystatin C: Cystatin C is produced endogenously at a constant rate by all nucleated cells. It is freely filtered by the glomerulus, completely reabsorbed, and metabolized by the tubular cells.[5] Cystatin C level in blood is independent of age, height, or muscle mass. Obesity or malnutrition will not affect cystatin C levels and is not influenced by dietary protein. Thus, serum cystatin C is more accurate than serum creatinine. When GFR is <75 mL/min, tubular secretion of creatinine will affect GFR assessment while cystatin C levels in the blood will be more accurate.[5,6] However, cystatin C has not yet replaced creatinine in clinical practice due to its high cost, difficult assay methods, and standardization. Cystatin C reference values[7] are given in **Table 1**.

Estimated GFR: Estimated GFR (eGFR) is GFR calculated using creatinine and/or cystatin C taking into consideration both height and muscle mass. Schwartz formula, the most commonly used one for calculating creatinine clearance in children, is already corrected for body surface area.

$$\text{Creatinine clearance (mL/min/1.73 m}^2) = k \times \text{length (in cm)/serum creatinine (mg/dL)}$$

where *k* is an empirical constant and is determined by length/serum creatinine ratio against measured GFR.

In malnourished children, the low muscle mass may affect the value of constant *k*, thus leading to overestimation of GFR. Also, the value of *k* is different depending on the method of serum creatinine estimation. Creatinine estimation by enzymatic methods that use isotope dilution mass spectroscopy (IDMS)-based reference standards are more accurate and specific compared to Jaffe method.

If *Jaffe method* is used *for creatinine estimation,* the value of "*k*" is directly proportional to the muscle mass and varies with age. In adolescents, the value of *k* varies with the sex of the patient as well.[7-10] When the Jaffe method is used for creatinine estimation and is expressed as mg/dL, the value for *k* is as follows.

- Preterm infants up to 1 year—0.33
- Term infants up to 1 year—0.45
- Children above 2 years—0.55
- Adolescent females—0.55
- Adolescent males—0.77

When serum creatinine is estimated by enzymatic methods and expressed as mg/dL, a modified Schwartz formula is used. Here the value of "*k*" is equal to 0.413 for all children aged 1–16 years with CKD.[11] However, it has been validated only for a GFR range of 15–75 mL/min/1.73 m² in children below 18 years. Further work is needed to assess the accuracy of this calculation in children with higher levels of GFR. The Schwartz equation is currently the most accurate and least complex formula in clinical practice for calculating eGFR in children. As the value of *k* will vary depending on height and muscle mass, local population characteristics must be considered for improving the accuracy and reducing the bias of GFR estimation. The constant *k* should be locally derived based on the method of creatinine estimation and the reference used. In Indian children, Hari et al. found the value of *k* to be 0.42 when creatinine was estimated by the kinetic Jaffe method. GFR estimation by ^{99}mTc-DTPA was the reference used by Hari et al.[12,13]

Cystatin C-based equations: Compared to the creatinine-based equations, cystatin C-based equations are more accurate in eGFR calculation. Equations for eGFR using both creatinine and cystatin C, also combining demographic variables such as height, weight, age, and sex, have been derived recently like the CKiD equation. The current Kidney Disease Improving Global Outcomes (KDIGO) guidelines recommend the use of the CKiD equation in children. The CKiD equation is :

$$\text{GFR (mL/min/1.73 m}^2\text{) CKiD equation} = 39.1[(\text{height (m)/creatinine (mg/dL)})]^{0.516} \times [1.8/\text{cystatin C (mg/L)}]^{0.294} [30/\text{BUN (mg/dL)}]^{0.169} [1.099]^{(\text{male})} [\text{height (m)}/1.4]^{0.188}$$

This equation, though more complex, is in better agreement with the measured GFR compared to the updated Schwartz equation. This formula is valid in combination with enzymatic methods of creatinine estimation and calibration traceable to the IDMS reference procedure. The Lund-Malmö equation developed in 2011 for adults was later revised and validated for both children and adults.[14] It can be used with similar accuracy to dedicated pediatric equations in children with normal renal function, but yields marked overestimations in children with CKD. Thus, Lund-Malmö revised (LMR) equation is presently not an equation for the full spectrum of age and renal function.[15]

TABLE 1: Cystatin C reference values.[7]

Age group	*mg/L*
<1 month	1.37–1.89
1–12 months	0.73–1.17
Adult men	0.50–0.96
Adult women	0.57–0.96

British Columbia Children's Formulas 1 and 2: Of late, a new height-independent estimation of eGFR has been developed.

Some of them are given below.[16] GFR estimation based on serum creatinine and age is developed by Zapitelli et al., i.e., British Columbia Children's Formulas 1 and 2 (BCCH1 and 2). These equations are given below:

British Columbia Children's Hospital Formula 1 (BCCH1)

$$\text{inverse ln (eGFR - BCCH) (mL/min/1.73 m}^2) = 8.067 + \{1.034 \times \ln [0.011/(\text{serum creatinine (mg/dL)})]\} + \{0.305 \times \ln [\text{age (years)}]\} + 0.064 \text{ if male.}$$

British Columbia Children's Hospital Formula 2 (BCCH2):

$$\text{eGFR} = [43.82 \times \exp (0.003 \times \text{Ht})]/(\text{CysC}^{0.635} \times \text{Scr}^{0.547}) \times 1.165 \text{ if renal transplant} \times 1.57\ \text{Scr}^{0.925} \text{ if spina bifida}$$

Chehade formula: The Chehade formula may replace the combined Schwartz formula for children with moderate chronic kidney disease:

$\text{eGFR} = 0.42 \times (\text{Ht/Scr}) - 0.04 \times (\text{Ht/Scr})^2 - 14.5 \times \text{CysC} + 0.69 \times \text{Age} + (18.25 \text{ if female, or } 21.88 \text{ if male})$, with Scr in mg/dL, height in cm, cystatin C in mg/L, age in years.

eGFR by pottel: Median serum creatinine reference values are used in the eGFR formula by Pottel et al.[17]

$$\text{eGFR - Pottel (mL/min/1.73 m}^2) = 107.3/\left|\frac{\text{serum creatinine (mg/dL)}}{Q}\right|$$

Q is the median serum creatinine in children based on age and sex.[16]

Glomerular filtration rate using radioisotopes: A radioisotope handled by the kidney in the same manner as inulin can be used to assess GFR. The renal concentration of the radioisotope can be determined by measuring the activity using a scintillation camera or monitoring of timed blood samples. The relative uptake of isotopes by each kidney is proportional to the blood flow and thus the contribution of each kidney to the overall renal function can be estimated. Radioisotopes used for estimating GFR include chromium-51 ethylenediaminetetraacetic acid (^{51}Cr-EDTA), ^{99}TcDTPA, ^{125}I-iothalamate, and iohexol.[18] GFR assessment by urinary clearance of ^{51}Cr-EDTA shows underestimation by 5–15% compared to inulin clearance as there is a degree of tubular reabsorption. ^{99}TcDTPA is an analog of EDTA and is labeled with technetium 99m (^{99}mTc). Advantages include a short half-life of 6 hours, minimum radiation exposure, and a high counting efficiency of ^{99}TcDTPA. The major disadvantage is underestimation of GFR as ^{99}Tc from DTPA binds plasma proteins. Iohexol and iothalamate are radiocontrast agents that can be used as exogenous GFR markers comparable to inulin and ^{51}Cr-EDTA. The limitations of iohexol are protein binding, tubular reabsorption, high cost, and iodine allergy in some patients. Iothalamate has some tubular secretion also apart from all the above limitations.

Newer methods to estimate GFR: A promising potential marker, especially in neonates, is beta-trace protein, a circulating endogenous low-molecular-weight protein. As the blood levels of this protein are independent of size, gender, and muscle mass, it is considered as a promising surrogate marker for eGFR estimation.[19] Fluorescein-based assays using fluorescein isothiocyanate inulin (FITC) are also upcoming.

Renal plasma flow (RPF): RPF can be measured using a substance in plasma that is cleared completely on a single passage through the kidneys. Para-aminohippuric acid (PAH), an organic acid, is commonly used as the marker to measure RPF. It is given intravenously to achieve a low concentration and its clearance is calculated to estimate RPF. PAH clearance in neonates is 65% at birth. It increases after birth and by 5 months reaches 90% of the adult value. Normal adult RPF is 625 mL/min. At 8 days of life in a full-term infant, RPF is 140 mL/min/1.73 m^2. By 5 months of age, it becomes 580 mL/min/1.73 m^2.[20]

Proteinuria: This is defined as urine protein levels of >4 mg/m^2/h or 100 mg/m^2/day. In neonates, protein excretion can be as high as up to 300 mg/m^2/day, due to the reduced reabsorption of filtered proteins reflecting the immaturity of their tubular function. Proteinuria can be assessed by qualitative tests such as dipstick or quantitative tests such as 24-hour urine protein or a spot urine protein–creatinine (PC) ratio. 24-hour urine protein estimation, though technically difficult, in children is the gold standard test for quantitative evaluation of proteinuria. Urine PC ratio by spot urine analysis is preferred in children because of greater convenience. PR ratio is preferably calculated in the first morning urine. This avoids the possible variation caused by the circadian rhythm of protein excretion, which is maximal in the day and minimum in the night compared to urinary excretion of creatinine which is fairly constant over the day. In children older than 2 years of age, a urine PR ratio < 0.2 on a spot sample is considered normal. From 6 months to 2 years, the upper limit of normal urine PC ratio is 0.5.[21]

Nephrotic proteinuria is urine protein of >40 mg/m^2/h in an overnight specimen or >50 mg/kg/day or urine PR ratio of >2. Glomerular proteinuria caused by increased glomerular permeability is an indicator of glomerular dysfunction. It can be selective or nonselective. Selective proteinuria is characterized by the presence of predominantly anionic proteins with a molecular weight of 50–80 kDa (e.g., albumin). In nonselective proteinuria, larger proteins with molecular weight >50–80 kDa [e.g., immunoglobulin G (IgG)] are found, which is indicative of more severe damage to glomeruli. The selectivity of glomerular proteinuria can be assessed by selectivity index which is the ratio of clearance of IgG (molecular weight 150 kDa) to clearance of transferrin (molecular weight 80 kDa).

$$\text{Selectivity index} = (\text{urinary IgG/plasma IgG})/(\text{urinary transferrin/plasma transferrin})$$

When the ratio is <0.1, proteinuria is highly selective and strongly suggests steroid-responsive minimal change disease in children with nephrotic syndrome. The response to treatment is moderate if the ratio is between 0.11 and 0.20

and anything >0.21 is nonselective proteinuria and indicates pathology such as focal segmental glomerulosclerosis.[22]

Assessment of Tubular Function

Evaluation of proximal and distal tubule is important in the diagnosis of tubular disorders. Proximal tubular functions include reabsorption of bicarbonate, glucose, amino acids, phosphate, and calcium whereas distal tubular functions include potassium secretion, urinary acidification, and concentration.

Assessment of Proximal Tubular Functions

Glucose: Detectable amount of glucose in the urine is termed glycosuria. Normally <1.5 mmol (300 mg)/day/1.73 m^2 of glucose is excreted.[23] Dipsticks can only pick up a glucose concentration of >5 mmol/L. Hence, glycosuria in the presence of dilute urine may be missed. A formal biochemical measurement is preferable.[24] Glycosuria can be due to increased filtered load as in diabetes mellitus or due to incomplete reabsorption of normal filtered loads as in renal glycosuria. So concomitant blood glucose measurement is needed.

Phosphate: Fractional excretion of phosphate is determined on a timed urine specimen. Tubular reabsorption of phosphate (%) is calculated from the fractional excretion of phosphate obtained from a timed urine sample (6-, 12-, or 24-hours):[24]

$$\text{Fractional excretion of } PO_4(\%) = \frac{\text{Urine } PO_4 \times \text{plasma creatinine}}{\text{Plasma } PO_4 \times \text{urine creatinine}} \times 100$$

$$\text{Tubular reabsorption of } PO_4(\%) = 100 - \text{Fractional excretion of } PO_4$$

Tubular reabsorption of PO_4 is not a satisfactory indicator of tubular PO_4 handling as it depends on plasma phosphate and GFR.[25] Tubular maximum for PO_4 corrected for GFR (TMP/GFR) is independent of plasma PO_4 and renal functions. It can be used as an index of renal handling for PO_4 and is determined as follows.

$$\text{TMP/GFR (mg/dL)} = \text{Plasma phosphate} - \frac{\text{Urine phosphate} \times \text{plasma creatinine}}{\text{Urine creatinine}}$$

Normal values of TMP/GFR are age dependent and should be compared with age-appropriate reference levels. The typical reference range in children aged 2–15 years is 3.6–7.6 mg/dL (1.15–2.44 mmol/L). Normal age-specific values of TMP/GFR[24] are given in **Table 2**.

Calcium: In children, hypercalciuria is diagnosed when urine calcium exceeds 4 mg/kg/day. Urine calcium-creatinine ratio in a spot sample collected from the second void in the morning after overnight fast correlates with 24-hour urine collection. Normal urine calcium-creatinine ratio values vary with age. In infants with age up to 6 months, it is 0.8 mg/mg; for 6–12 months, it is 0.6 mg/mg; for 1–2 years, it is 0.5 mg/mg; and for older children, it is 0.2.[25]

TABLE 2: Normal age-specific values of tubular maximum for PO_4 corrected for glomerular filtration rate.[23]

Age	*mmol/L*
<1 month	1.48–3.43
1–3 months	1.48–3.30
4–6 months	1.15–2.60
7 months to 2 years	1.10–2.70
2–4 years	1.04–2.79
4–6 years	1.05–2.60
6–8 years	1.26–2.35
8–10 years	1.10–2.31
10–12 years	1.15–2.58
12–15 years	1.18–2.09
>15 years	0.8–1.35

Distal Tubular Functions

Tests for urinary acidification:

Plasma anion gap

The difference between unmeasured anions and cations in the plasma is the anion gap (AG) and is calculated as follows:

$$AG = Na^+ - (Cl^- + HCO_3^-)$$

The normal AG is 10–12 mEq/L. Metabolic acidosis may be associated with normal or increased AG. Calculation of AG helps to differentiate between normal and high AG metabolic acidosis.[26]

Urine pH

pH meter or reagent strips are used to measure urine pH. A freshly voided, preferably morning sample of urine should be used for urine pH assessment. It is collected under mineral oil to prevent loss of CO_2 and promptly taken up into a syringe. Urine pH ranges from 4.5 to 8 depending on systemic acid-base status. Urine pH reflects the concentration of free H^+ ions. This accounts for <1% of the total H^+ ions excreted in urine. The remaining 99% is excreted as titratable acid with HPO_4^- and as ammonium. There are two important factors that need to be considered when analyzing urine pH:

1. Evaluation of urine pH should be in conjunction with net acid secretion, especially the ammonium concentration in urine. Ammonium production is increased in chronic metabolic acidosis or hypokalemia and urine pH will be high even with normal acidification mechanisms. Ammonia in urine will bind to more H^+ ions, decreasing the free H^+ concentration, thereby increasing the pH. On the other hand in type IV renal tubular acidosis (RTA),

there is decreased ammonia generation and less ammonia is available to buffer free H^+ ions. So the urine pH will be maximally acidic.[25]

2. Another important factor affecting urine pH is distal sodium delivery. Volume depletion as occurs with diarrhea and vomiting decreases the distal sodium delivery. This causes reduction in lumen-negative transepithelial potential difference which is the major driving force for free H^+ secretion. The reduced H^+ secretion leads to high urine pH despite an intact distal acidification process.[25]

Conditions associated with high urine pH:

- Inadequately collected sample or delayed examination of urine
- With normal distal acidification mechanisms:
  - Chronic metabolic acidosis of any etiology
  - Hypokalemia
  - Severe volume depletion
  - Infection with urea-splitting organisms, e.g., *Proteus*
- With impaired distal acidification mechanisms:
  - Distal RTA

Urine anion gap

Urine AG is the difference between cations and anions in urine. Normally, the sum of cations in urine (Na^+, K^+, NH_4^+, Ca^{2+}, and Mg^{2+}) is equal to the sum of anions in urine (Cl^-, HCO_3^-, SO_4^{2-}, PO_4^{2-}, and organic anions). HCO_3^- concentration in acid urine is negligible. Urine AG provides an estimation of urine ammonium (NH_4^+) concentration which is an unmeasured cation. If the small amount of Ca^{2+} and Mg^{2+} ions in the urine is ignored and other anions together are taken as "unmeasured anions," then we get the equation: $(Na^+) + (K^+) + (NH_4^+) = (Cl^-) + (\text{unmeasured anions})$.[26] Usually, in metabolic acidosis ammonium accompanies chloride when the kidney attempts to excrete more H^+ ions. Since ammonium is not included in calculating AG, the concentration of urinary chloride will be greater than the sum of urine Na and K in this situation (i.e., urine Cl^- > urine Na^+ + urine K^+). Here, the AG is negative as seen in clinical situations such as diarrhea where the renal acidification is intact.

Conversely, if the urine sodium and potassium are more than urine chloride, it may be assumed that urine NH_4 excretion is low. Here the urine AG is positive and indicates a distal acidification defect. However, a positive urinary AG does not always indicate ammonium deficiency. Ammonium may be excreted with other anions such as ketones, hippurate, penicillin, and lithium. Urine osmolal gap calculation helps in the assessment of this situation.[25,26] The acidification of the urine requires adequate distal delivery of sodium and urinary AG is unreliable if the urinary sodium level is <20 mmol/L.

If the kidney function remains normal, normal AG or hyperchloremic acidosis should lead to increased excretion of ammonium in urine. The measurement of urinary ammonium may be used to differentiate between renal and extrarenal causes of normal AG acidosis. Urinary ammonium is not measured routinely; the urinary AG ($[Na^+] + [K^+] - [Cl^-]$) and urinary osmolal gap ($[Na^+] + [K^+]$ + glucose + BUN − $[Cl^-]$ in mmol/L) may be used to measure ammonium excretion in urine.

The normal urine AG is positive (about +20 to +90 mmol/L) in healthy individuals. Ammonium is excreted as NH_4Cl. The excretion of chloride must be high in metabolic acidosis. The urine AG become negative in diarrhea (about −30 to −50 mEq/L). In distal RTA, urine AG will be positive. Low chloride excretion due to impaired urinary ammonium (NH_4^+) excretion as ammonium chloride (NH_4Cl) is the underlying cause. In proximal RTA, bicarbonate reabsorption is defective, but the ammonium excretion remains intact, and, therefore, a negative urinary AG will be found in RTA type 2.[27-29]

Urine osmolal gap

The urinary osmolal gap determines the difference between measured and calculated urinary osmolality. Urine osmolality is measured by the freezing point depression method from the laboratory. Urine osmolality is calculated from urine sodium, potassium, urea nitrogen, and urine glucose levels (if the dipstick for urine glucose is positive). If urine AG is positive and it is unclear whether it is due to an increased level of unmeasured anions other than chloride in urine, calculation of the urine osmolal gap helps in estimating urinary ammonium.

Urine osmolal gap = Measured urine osmolality − calculated urine osmolality

The urinary osmolality is calculated as follows:

$(2\,[Na^+] + 2\,[K^+])$ + (urine urea nitrogen in mg/dL/2.8) + (urine glucose in mg/dL/18) or $(2\,[Na^+] + 2\,[K^+])$ + (urine urea nitrogen in mmol/L) + (urine glucose in mmol/L).

The multiple of two accounts for the anions accompanying sodium and potassium. The denominators 2.8 and 18 are for converting the units from mg/dL to mOsm/kg. A normal urine osmolal gap is approximately 10–100 mOsm/kg, with urinary ammonium excretion being approximately one half of this value (5–50 mmol/L) due to accompanying anions.

The urinary osmolal gap better reflects the level of ammonium, except in the presence of large quantities of a nondissociated acid, such as β-hydroxybutyric acid in ketoacidosis and hippurate in toluene intoxication. A high urine osmolal gap >200 mEq/L suggests a high urine ammonium concentration, and a nonrenal cause for the acidosis such as diarrhea (often >300–400 mEq/L) is more likely than RTA.[29,30] If the urine osmolal gap is 160 mOsm/kg, ammonium excretion should be approximately one half of this value due to accompanying anions, i.e., 80 mEq/L which is appropriate in a patient with metabolic acidosis if renal acid excretion is normal.[25,26] A urinary osmolal gap <40 mmol/L in normal AG acidosis indicates impairment in urinary ammonium excretion.[28]

Acid-load test

The purpose of this test is to evaluate renal acidification by inducing metabolic acidosis. Ammonium chloride (at 0.15 mg/kg) is given orally to induce marked systemic acidemia (blood pH < 7.20, plasma HCO_3^- < 15 mEq/L). Urine is collected for the next 4–8 hours. If the urine pH is >5.5 in spite of significant systemic acidemia suggests the diagnosis of distal RTA.[26]

Urine to blood CO_2 difference

Secretion of H^+ ions into alkaline urine in the distal tubule leads to the formation of H_2CO_3, which dissociates into H_2O and CO_2. The CO_2 thus generated is retained in the medulla as the urothelium prevents the diffusion of luminal CO_2 into the blood. Urine carbon dioxide excretion is thus an indicator of H^+ secretion and urine to blood CO_2 difference is taken as an index of distal renal acidification.

In patients with urine pH of >7.6 (either spontaneous or induced by administration of alkali), a urine minus blood pCO_2 <10 implies a distal acidification defect. In patients with proximal RTA where there is increased distal delivery of bicarbonate and an intact distal H^+ secretory mechanism, $UpCO_2$ will be high and hence, the difference between urine minus blood pCO_2 is >20 mm Hg.[25,26]

Furosemide test

Furosemide blocks the $Na^+/K^+/2Cl^-$ pump in the loop of Henle. Administration of furosemide increases the distal delivery of sodium with augmented sodium reabsorption in the distal tubule. This induces voltage-mediated increase in H^+ ion and K^+ secretion. A normal response is an increase in net acid secretion leading to lowering of urine pH to <5.6 and kaliuresis. An abnormal furosemide test indicates a secretory or voltage-dependent distal acidification defect.[26]

Fractional excretion of bicarbonate

Fractional excretion of bicarbonate is a marker of proximal tubular bicarbonate handling. Normally, proximal tubule reabsorbs 85–90% of the filtered bicarbonate. Distal tubular reabsorption of bicarbonate accounts for 10–15%. Normal FE_{HCO_3} is < 5%. Bicarbonaturia >15% suggests proximal RTA. Before the test, it is required that the patient's serum bicarbonate level should be restored to normal before collecting blood and urine:[25]

$$\text{Fractional excretion of } HCO_3 = \frac{\text{Urine } HCO_3 \times \text{plasma creatinine}}{\text{Plasma } HCO_3 \times \text{Urine creatinine}} \times 100$$

Tests for Urinary Concentration

Kidneys play an important role in water homeostasis. Water reabsorption takes place in proximal convoluted tubule, thin descending limb of loop of Henle, and collecting duct.[31] The concentrating ability of kidneys can be assessed by the following tests.

Urine-specific gravity

Urine-specific gravity is the measure of dissolved solute particles in urine. It is measured by a urinometer or total solids refractometer. Reagent strips use polyelectrolyte reagent and measure specific gravity from 1.000 to 1.030. An amount of 50–100 mL of urine is needed in the urinometer, whereas two to three drops of urine are adequate to measure specific gravity using total solids refractometer and reagent strips. If proteins or glucose are present, specific gravity should be corrected for them. Specific gravity increases by 0.001 for each 0.4 g/dL increase of protein and each 0.27 g/dL increase of glucose. Early morning urine-specific gravity of >1.010 is indicative of good concentration. A fixed specific gravity of 1.010 is isosthenuria whereas a specific gravity of 1.007 or less is termed hyposthenuria.[31,32]

URINE OSMOLALITY AND PLASMA OSMOLALITY

Osmolality reflects the amount of osmotically active molecules of solutes in a unit solution and is expressed as mOsm/kg of water. In general, urine osmolality of 50 mOsm/kg is approximately equal to a specific gravity of 1.000; 350 mOsm/kg, a specific gravity of 1.010; and 800 mOsm/kg, a specific gravity of 1.020. Under normal circumstances, 0.010 unit change in specific gravity causes 350 mOsm/kg change in urine osmolality approximately.

Plasma osmolality and urine osmolality must be measured simultaneously for better results. This is done by depression of the freezing point method. Normal plasma osmolality is 280–295 mOsm/kg and urine osmolality is variable and may be as low as 40 mOsm/kg in water-excess states and as high as 1,400 mOsm/kg in water-restricted states.[31]

In hyponatremia, low urine osmolality indicates water intoxication and high urine osmolality indicates dehydration with excess urinary sodium loss. In hypernatremia, low urine osmolality indicates polyuria as in diabetes insipidus (DI) and high urine osmolality indicates excessive salt ingestion. In oliguric states, a urine osmolality of >500 mOsm/kg indicates preserved renal function.[31]

Water-deprivation Test

This test is used to assess the renal concentrating ability. The prerequisite for performing the test is that the baseline plasma osmolality and serum sodium are within the normal range and urine osmolality is <300 mOsm/kg. The child is deprived of fluids for 6–8 hours (4 hours for infants) or until 2–5% of weight loss occurs or upper limits of serum sodium and osmolality are reached or urine osmolality rises >800 mOsm/kg. If at the end of the test, urine osmolality is >800 mOsm/kg primary polydipsia is likely. Urine osmolality persisting <300 mOsm/kg after the water-deprivation test suggests the possibility of central or nephrogenic DI. For further evaluation, vasopressin is administered intranasally (10–20 μg) or subcutaneously (1–3 μg). Urine osmolality is then assessed at 1–2 hours' interval and an increase in urine osmolality by >50% from baseline, 1 hour after vasopressin is diagnostic of central DI. In nephrogenic DI, the increase in urine osmolality is minimal or nil. If urine osmolality is between 300 and 800 mOsm/kg after water deprivation further evaluation is needed to differentiate partial DI and polydipsia.[25,31]

Urinary Dilution

The capacity to produce dilute urine depends on the reabsorption of solutes without water in the thick ascending limb of loop of Henle. A simple water loading test is used to assess the diluting capacity of the kidney. 20 mL/kg of water is administered over 30 minutes and half hourly urine volumes are collected for the next 5 hours. >75% of the administered water load should be excreted in the next 3 hours. Urine osmolality should fall below 100 mOsm/kg (specific gravity < 1.003). The ability of kidneys to dilute urine can be assessed also by free water clearance (C_{H_2O}). The free water clearance is based on the concept that urine volume can be divided into two components. The first component is urine volume needed to excrete solutes at a concentration equal to that of plasma (isotonic). This is termed osmolar clearance (C_{osm}). The second component is free water clearance (C_{H_2O}), which is the volume of solute-free water that has been reabsorbed or added to the isotonic component (C_{osm}) to create hypertonic or hypotonic urine, respectively, i.e., it is the amount of water that must be added to or taken away from urine to make it isotonic with plasma. It is calculated as follows:

$$V = C_{osm} + C_{H_2O}$$
$$C_{H_2O} = V - C_{osm}$$
$$C_{H_2O} = V - (U_{osm}/U_{osm})V$$

$$C_{H_2O} = \frac{1 - U_{Osm}}{P_{Osm}} V$$

where C_{H_2O} is the free water clearance, U_{osm} is the urine osmolality, P_{osm} is the plasma osmolality, and V is the urine flow rate.

A positive free water clearance means that urine is more dilute than plasma and a negative free water clearance means urine is more concentrated.[31]

TESTS FOR POTASSIUM HANDLING

Renal potassium handling can be assessed by a 24-hour urine K or a spot urine K/creatinine ratio. 24-hour urine K < 15 mEq/L or a urine spot K (mEq)/creatinine (mg) ratio <13 in hypokalemia suggests an extrarenal cause. The influence of renal water handling on urine potassium concentration is the major limitation of urine spot potassium. Two patients with the same potassium excretion can have significantly different potassium concentration in urine depending on whether the urine is dilute or concentrated. To overcome this problem, transtubular K^+ gradient (TTKG) is used. It is calculated as follows:

$$\text{TTKG} = (\text{urine K} \times \text{plasma osmolality})/(\text{plasma K} \times \text{urine osmolality})$$

Transtubular K^+ gradient evaluates the gradient between the K concentration in the luminal fluid of the distal tubule and peritubular capillaries, which is a reflection of aldosterone activity. It is based on the assumptions that only water reabsorption and no potassium reabsorption or secretion takes place below this level and peritubular capillary potassium concentration is equal to systemic venous potassium concentration. TTKG can be used only in the presence of sufficient distal sodium delivery (urine Na > 25 mmol/L) so that sodium delivery is not rate limiting for potassium secretion and also the urine osmolality should be more than or equal to serum osmolality.[25] In children with hyperkalemia, a TTKG < 4.1 (<4.9 in infants) indicates reduced mineralocorticoid activity. With hypokalemia, TTKG > 2 is indicative of ongoing aldosterone activity in the distal tubule.

FRACTIONAL EXCRETION OF SODIUM

Fractional excretion of sodium (FE_{Na}) is the percentage of filtered sodium that is excreted in urine. It is a measure of the kidney's ability for sodium reabsorption as well as the effect of endogenous and exogenous factors on tubular reabsorption. A spot urine sample can be used for the assessment of FE_{Na}. It does not require timed urine collections and is calculated as follows:

$$\text{Fractional excretion of Na}(\%) = \frac{\text{Urine Na} \times \text{plasma creatinine}}{\text{Plasma Na} \times \text{urine creatinine}} \times 100$$

FeNa is useful in the differentiation of prerenal AKI from acute tubular necrosis. FE_{Na} is usually <1% (<3% in neonates) in prerenal AKI suggesting avid tubular sodium reabsorption as a result of the decrease in effective circulatory volume. A value of >2% is indicative of acute tubular necrosis.[24] But in early acute glomerulonephritis, when the tubular function is intact, a low FE_{Na} is seen despite volume expansion because of the decrease in surface area available for filtration in the glomerulus. FE_{Na} may not accurately reflect effective circulatory volume while on diuretics. In such situations, fractional excretion of urea can be used. A low FE_{urea} < 35% indicates low effective circulatory volume.[25,31,32]

CONCLUSION

Assessment of glomerular and tubular function is important for the early detection and management of renal disease. These tests have utility in identifying the presence of renal disease, determining the progression of the disease, and monitoring the response to treatment. Assessment of glomerular functions involves estimation of GFR, RPF, and measurement of proteinuria. The modified Schwartz formula still remains the commonly used formula for GFR estimation in children, though height-independent formulas are developed recently. Tubular function tests involve the evaluation of proximal tubular functions such as reabsorption of glucose and phosphate, and distal tubular functions include urinary acidification, concentration, and potassium secretion.

KEY POINTS

- Glomerular function can be assessed by the evaluation of GFR, measurement of markers such as urea, creatinine, and assessment of proteinuria.
- Clearance of exogenous markers such as inulin or endogenous markers such as creatinine can be used for GFR estimation.
- eGFR estimates GFR using creatinine and/or cystatin C-based formulae which also include height and muscle mass.
- Assessment of tubular functions involves evaluation of proximal tubular functions such as reabsorption of glucose and phosphate, and distal tubular functions include urinary acidification, concentration, and potassium secretion.
- Urine AG and urine osmolal gap are useful in differentiating various causes of metabolic acidosis and reflect urine ammonium excretion.

REFERENCES

1. Smith HW. The Kidney: Structure and Function in Health and Disease. New York: Oxford University Press; 1951. pp. 271-2.
2. Rahn KH, Heidenreich S, Brückner D. How to assess glomerular function and damage in humans. J Hypertension. 1999;17(3):309.
3. Tufro A, Gulati A. Development of glomerular circulation and function. In: Avner ED, Harmon WE, Niaudet P, Yoshikawa N, Emma F, Goldstein SL (Eds). Pediatric Nephrology, 7th edition. Berlin: Springer-Verlag; 2016. pp. 37-60.
4. Shemesh O, Golbetz H, Kriss JP, Myers BD. Limitations of creatinine as a filtration marker in glomerulopathic patients. Kidney Int. 1985;28(5):830.
5. Dharnidharka VR, Kwon C, Stevens G. Serum cystatin C is superior to serum creatinine as a marker of kidney function: a meta-analysis. Am J Kidney Dis. 2002;40(2):221-6.
6. Roos JF, Doust J, Tett SE, Kirkpatrick CMJ. Diagnostic accuracy of cystatin C compared to serum creatinine for the estimation of renal dysfunction in adults and children—a meta-analysis. Clin Biochem. 2007;40(5-6):383-91.
7. Finney H, Newman DJ, Thakkar H, Fell JM, Price CP. Reference ranges for plasma cystatin C and creatinine measurements in premature infants, neonates, and older children. Arch Dis Child. 2000;82:71-5.
8. Schwartz GJ, Work DF. Measurement and estimation of GFR in children and adolescents. Clin J Am Soc Nephrol. 2009;4:1832-43.
9. Schwartz GJ, Haycock GB, Edelmann CM Jr, Spitzer A. A simple estimate of glomerular filtration rate in children derived from body length and plasma creatinine. Pediatrics. 1976;58(2):25.
10. Schwartz GJ, Feld LG, Langford DJ. A simple estimate of glomerular filtration rate in full-term infants during the first year of life. J Pediatr. 1984;104(6):849.
11. Schwartz GJ, Munoz A, Schneider MF, Mak RH, Kaskel F, Warady BA, et al. New equations to estimate GFR in children with CKD. J Am Soc Nephrol. 2009;20:629-37.
12. Sethi SK. Estimating accurate glomerular filtration rate in children. Indian Pediatr. 2014;51:263-4.
13. Hari P, Biswas B, Pandey R, Kalaivani M, Kumar R, Bagga A. Updated height- and creatinine-based equation and its validation for estimation of glomerular filtration rate in children from developing countries. Clin Exp Nephrol. 2012;16:697-705.
14. Nyman U, Bjork J, Lindstrom V, Grubb, A. The Lund-Malmö creatinine-based glomerular filtration rate prediction equation for adults also performs well in children. Scand J Clin Lab Invest. 2008;68:568-76.
15. Björk J, Nyman U, Berg U, Delanaye P, Dubourg L, Goffin K, et al. Validation of standardized creatinine and cystatin C GFR estimating equations in a large multicentre European cohort of children. Pediatr Nephrol. 2019;34:1087-98.
16. Blufpand HN, Westland R, van Wijk JAE, Roelandse-Koop EA, Kaspers GJL, Bokenkamp A. Height-independent estimation of glomerular filtration rate in children: an alternative to the Schwartz equation. J Pediatr. 2013;163:1722-7.
17. Pottel H. Measuring and estimating glomerular filtration rate in children. Pediatr Nephrol. 2017;32(2):249-63.
18. Stevens LA, Levey AS. Measured GFR as a confirmatory test for estimated GFR. J Am Soc Nephrol. 2009;20, 2305-13.
19. Filler G, Kusserow C, Lopes L, Kobrzyński M. Beta-trace protein as a marker of GFR–history, indications, and future research. Clin Biochem. 2014;47(13-14):1188-94.
20. Calcagno PL, Rubin MI. Renal extraction of para amino hippurate in infants and children. J Clin Invest. 1963;42:1632-9.
21. Koopman MG, Krediet RT, Koomen GC, Strackee J, Arisz L. Circadian rhythm of proteinuria: consequences of the use of urinary protein: creatinine ratios. Nephrol Dial Transplant. 1989;4:9-14.
22. Cameron JS, Blandford G. The simple assessment of selectivity in heavy proteinuria. Lancet. 1966;2(7457):242-7.
23. Elsas LJ, Rosenberg LE. Familial renal glycosuria: a genetic reappraisal of hexose transport by kidney and intestine. J Clin Invest. 1969;48(10):1845-54.
24. Bockenhauer D, Kleta R. Approach to the patient with renal Fanconi syndrome, glycosuria or aminoaciduria. In: Turner N, Lamieire N, Goldsmith DJ, Winearls CG, Himmelfarb J, Remuzzi G (Eds). Oxford Text Book of Clinical Nephrology, 4th edition. Oxford: Oxford University Press; 2016. pp. 412-21.
25. Bagga A, Bajpai A, Menon S. Approach to renal tubular disorders. Indian J Pediatr. 2005;72:771-76.
26. Speeckaert M, Delanghe J. Assessment of renal function. In: Turner N, Lamieire N, Goldsmith DJ, Winearls CG, Himmelfarb J, Remuzzi G (Eds). Oxford Textbook of Clinical Nephrology, 4th edition. Oxford, UK: Oxford University Press; 2016. pp. 44-65.
27. Reddy P, Mooradian AD. Clinical utility of anion gap in deciphering acid-base disorders. Int J Clin Pract. 2009;63:1516-25.
28. Rodriguez Soriano J. Renal tubular acidosis: the clinical entity. J Am Soc Nephrol. 2002;13:2160-70.
29. Berend K. Review of the diagnostic evaluation of normal anion gap metabolic acidosis. Kidney Dis (Basel). 2017;3(4):149-59.
30. Rastegar M, Nagami GT. Non-anion gap metabolic acidosis: a clinical approach to evaluation. Am J Kidney Dis. 2017;69: 296-301.
31. Madden N, Trachtman H. Physiology of developing kidney: sodium and water disorders and its homeostasis. In: Avner ED, Harmon WE, Niaudet P, Yoshikawa N, Emma F, Goldstein SL (Eds). Pediatric Nephrology, 7th edition. Berlin: Springer-Verlag; 2016. pp. 37-60.
32. Schrier RW. Renal sodium excretion, oedematous disorders and diuretic use. In: Renal and Electrolyte Disorders, 8th edition. Philadelphia, PA: Wolters Kluwer; 2018. pp. 98-174.

CHAPTER

2.3 Imaging Studies

S Muralinath, CV Kanimozhi

INTRODUCTION

Arguably, the most important step that follows clinical evaluation and the acquisition of laboratory data is the process of imaging. Imaging offers a wealth of information in a simple and straightforward manner while sorting out diagnostic and therapeutic dilemmas. Basically, everyone is a physician. A radiologist is a "physician" who utilizes technology to look inside and seek additional information. This is to augment the information garnered already through clinical and laboratory means. Hopefully, this trio will help in the diagnosis and management of the disease. When it comes to imaging, one has an array of imaging modalities and procedures to choose from, such as plain X-ray, computed tomography (CT), magnetic resonance imaging (MRI), and micturating cystourethrogram (MCU). This implies that all of them have limitations. For this, one has to have a comprehensive idea of the issue at hand, so as to choose an optimum modality or procedure or modalities or procedures in combination, to arrive at a conclusion. This makes it imperative that the physician (clinician) and the radiologist act in conformity to establish a decisive imaging protocol.

This essentially is an overview of the role of radiology and imaging in the practice of nephrology and urology. The focus is on the essentials with an emphasis on a practical approach that leads to decision-making from a problem-solving perspective.

X-RAY

Plain X-ray is a ubiquitous study that provides a unique planar perspective of the regional anatomy. The advantage of this modality is that it is inexpensive, imparts a relatively low radiation dose, and is widely available. Plain films serve as a guide to determine the need and type of further imaging needed for a particular problem. The common indications for a plain radiograph in nephrology and urology include evaluation of urinary tract stones, evaluation of ureteric stent position **(Figs. 1A and B)**, and assessment of osseous structures. These are discussed here.

- Plain X-ray of kidney, ureter, and bladder (KUB) is useful in the evaluation of a child with suspected renal colic.

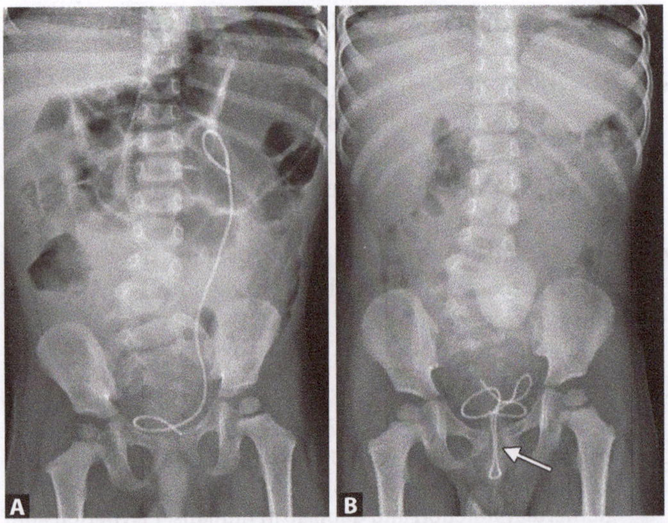

Figs. 1A and B: Plain radiographs in a 2-year-old child following left pyeloplasty. (A) Initial radiograph shows a well-positioned double-J (DJ) stent with upper end projected over the left renal shadow and distal end projected over the bladder; (B) Follow-up radiograph shows a displaced stent coiled in the bladder and extending into the urethra (arrow).

Radiopaque calculi (calcium phosphate and calcium oxalate deposits) can be readily seen on the plain film **(Figs. 2A to D)**. However, cystine and struvite stones are poorly demonstrated on plain films; uric and matrix stones are not apparent on radiographs.[1] Renal calcification, when evident may suggest a certain pathology by its nature and distribution, as in, acute cortical necrosis, medullary nephrocalcinosis, or medullary sponge kidney; a global nephrocalcinosis could suggest hyperoxalosis.

When urolithiasis is multiple and bilateral, an underlying metabolic cause would need to be considered.

- Retroperitoneal tumors having characteristic calcific and ossific inclusions can be identified as teratoma, fetus-in-fetu, or dermoid **(Fig. 3)**.
- The evaluation of osseous structures is paramount. The study of the vertebrae is of value in the evaluation of VACTERL (vertebral defects, anal atresia, cardiac defects, tracheoesophageal fistula, renal anomalies, and limb abnormalities) associations. A dysgenic, agenic, or scimitar sacrum (anterior meningocele) could be the pointer

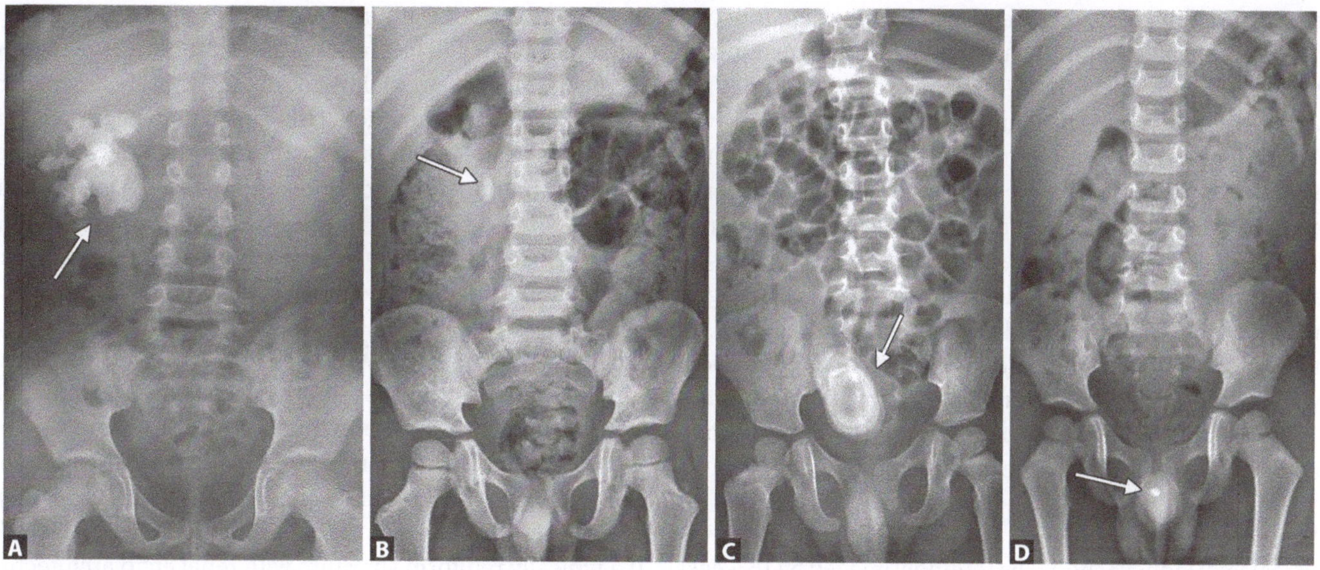

Figs. 2A to D: A series of plain radiographs in different children demonstrating various types of urolithiasis. (A) Staghorn calculus (arrow) projected over the right kidney; (B) Right upper ureteric calculus (arrow). Note the typical longitudinal lie of the calculus in the ureter; (C) A large bladder calculus (arrow) having the characteristic lamellated appearance; (D) An impacted urethral calculus (arrow) in a male child.

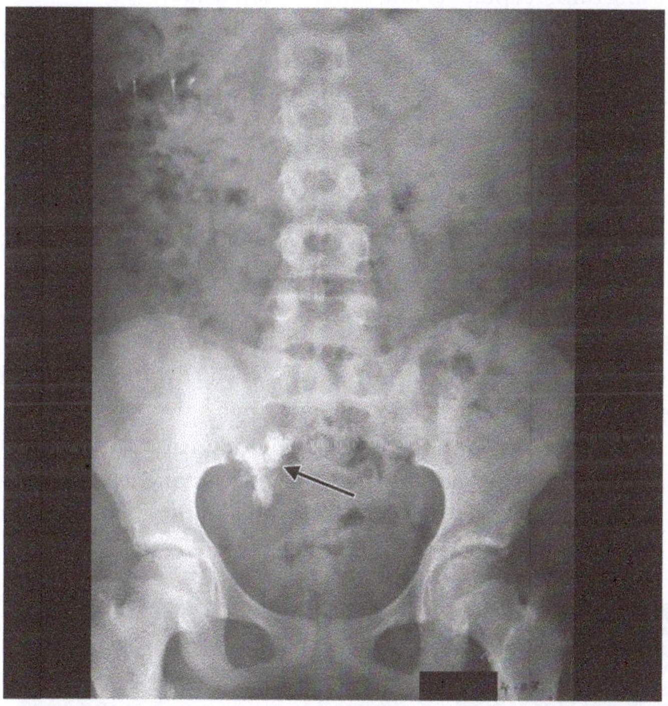

Fig. 3: Pelvic teratoma. Abdominal radiograph shows a heterogeneous lesion in the right side of the pelvis containing teeth-like calcifications (arrow).

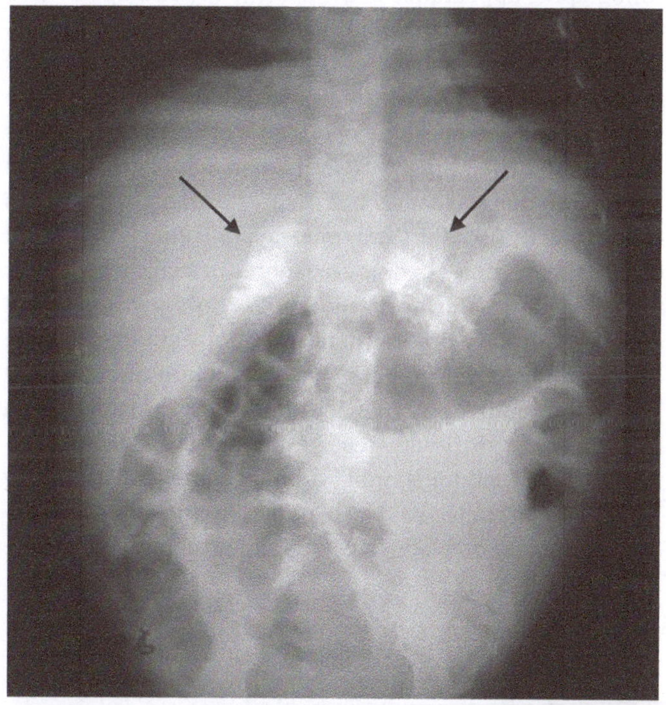

Fig. 4: Plain X-ray abdomen of a 6-month-old infant with diarrhea and failure to thrive. Both adrenals are enlarged with diffuse punctate calcifications (arrows). Though enlarged, the adrenals retain their normal shape.

toward a neurogenic uropathy. Lumbosacral dysgenesis/agenesis can be seen in caudal regression syndrome, particularly in type 1 where the conus medullaris has a high and abrupt termination. Widely separated pubic bones (pubic diastasis) are seen in patients with ectopia vesicae. A rugger jersey spine and rachitic changes would imply a chronic renal disease.

An example of a disease where the diagnosis can be confidently made using plain radiographs is Wolman's disease. This is a familial lipoidosis, which has the characteristic radiographic finding of dense calcification in enlarged adrenal glands **(Fig. 4)**.

Thus, as discussed earlier plain X-ray KUB is an ideal starting, for it offers a wealth of information to the discerning eye.

ULTRASONOGRAPHY

With the sole exception of antenatal ultrasound, nowhere else is the impact of the ultrasound profoundly felt than in pediatric urology. It has superseded intravenous urography in the assessment of structure and to a certain extent function of the urological system. It can be easily performed and is noninvasive with no risk to the patient or operator and is not dependent on the biological function of the organ. However, it is an operator-dependent investigation and requires the service of a skilled pediatric radiologist. A full bladder is needed to visualize the lower ureter as well as to adequately visualize the gonads in a female child. Restraining a child from voiding may not be practical. Hence, advise the parents to give the child plenty of fluids while awaiting the ultrasound. In this section, we will discuss the basics of renal measurement by sonography, the importance of renal size in pediatric nephrology and urology, and the application of the ultrasound in the most common pediatric renal scenarios.

Fetal Urinary Tract

Normal fetal kidneys should be routinely imaged by 16 weeks of gestational age as paired, hypoechoic, ovoid, and paraspinal structures in the posterior mid abdomen.[2] Identification and sonographic appearance of the kidneys depend upon when the study is performed. In the early to mid-second trimester, the hypoechoic renal cortex is poorly delineated from the renal sinus and perinephric tissues. By the middle to late second trimester, the kidneys are more readily visualized, as echogenic perinephric fat accumulation delineates the renal outline.[2] At this stage, the central sinus region also becomes echogenic. By the mid-third trimester, the renal borders and central sinus echoes become even more distinctly hyperechoic with the identification of the hypoechoic pyramids and corticomedullary differentiation. Various standards have been established for renal size as a function of menstrual age. A commonly used rule of thumb is that renal length in millimeters approximates fetal gestational age in weeks.

The fetal bladder should also be routinely identified by 16 weeks. Normally, the fetal bladder fills and empties every 30–45 minutes and bladder volume should change during the sonographic examination. The fetal bladder is thin walled, and nondilated and fetal ureters are not routinely visualized.

Assessment of amniotic fluid volume is a critical step in the evaluation of renal function. Urine formation begins early in the second trimester. Prior to 16 weeks, the kidneys contribute little to amniotic fluid formation and thus a normal amount of fluid may be present in the absence of renal function. However, in the second half of the pregnancy fetal urine production is the source of most of the amniotic fluid.

Postnatal Renal Ultrasound

Locating the kidneys is not always easy, particularly in patients with spinal deformity. Do not assume that an atypical structure in the renal bed is a kidney; it could be a bowel loop. Remember, thickened/compressed bowel loops or bowel lesions give rise to the "pseudokidney appearance". If a typically reniform structure with renal echo architecture is not seen in the renal bed, search for ectopic kidneys **(Figs. 5A and B)**. When in doubt, do a radionuclide study using dimercaptosuccinic acid (DMSA) scan.

When the kidney is located, assess the position, mobility, size, contour, parenchymal echo pattern, central echo complex/collecting system, and adjacent structures including the renal artery, vein, pelvis, and perinephric space.

The normal ureter is small in caliber and is not usually visualized. When the ureter is dilated, assess the extent and degree of dilatation, course, peristaltic activity, thickening of the wall and tortuosity, and intraluminal lesion or extra-luminal compression.

In the bladder, assess the following: contour, morphology of the wall, V-U junction, and area of the trigone and intraluminal lesion if any and contents.

The posterior urethra is imaged through the transperineal approach and posterior urethral dilatation characteristic of the posterior urethral valve (PUV) can be identified or a hidden calculus in the posterior urethra be revealed.

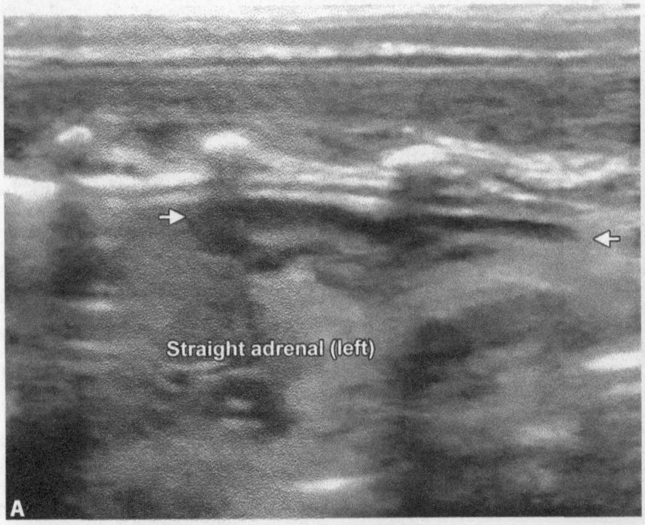

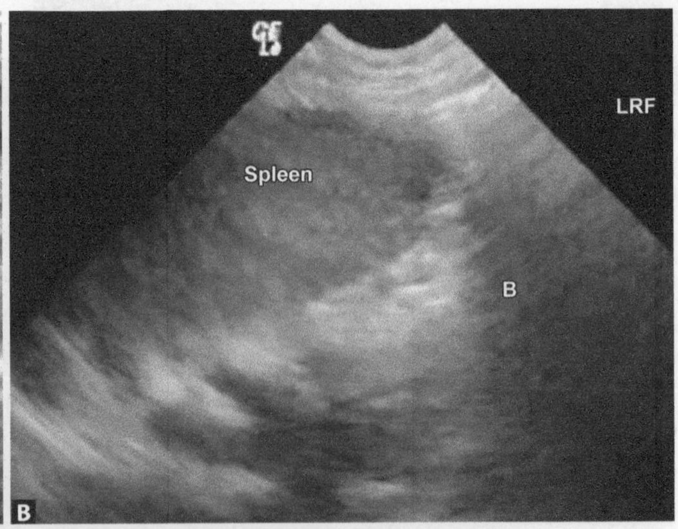

Figs. 5A and B: (A) Straight adrenal is seen (between calipers); (B) Empty left renal fossa (LRF) occupied by bowel loops. This suggests ectopic or absent left kidney.

Normal Renal Sonographic Anatomy

Older Infants and Children

The echoanatomy is essentially that of the adults. The renal parenchymal echo pattern is compared with adjacent organs.[3] The renal cortex is normally less echogenic than hepatic or splenic parenchyma. The medullary pyramids are hypoechoic relative to the cortex. The corticomedullary junction is demarcated by the arcuate arteries, which are seen as small echogenic foci. The central sinus echoes formed by the collecting system, vessels, and connective tissue at the center of the kidney are the most echogenic part of the kidney.

Newborns and Infants

Normal kidneys in newborn and young infants have several distinct sonographic features that differentiate them from the kidneys of older children and adults **(Table 1)**.

These differences from the adult are attributable to the immature structure of the still developing kidney. Although the full complement of nephrons is present by 36 weeks of gestation, their histology refinement and structural realignment are still taking place. In neonates, the renal cortex is more echogenic with echogenicity equal to the liver and spleen. The renal cortex of the right kidney and adjacent liver are equally echogenic in 65% of neonates; the cortex of the left kidney and spleen are equally echogenic in 50% of the neonates. In the remaining neonates, the cortex is slightly less echogenic than the liver or spleen. The renal cortex becomes less echogenic than the liver or spleen in the majority of the infants by 2 or 3 months of age, and by 6 months of age almost 100% of infants demonstrate an adult echo pattern.[4] Although the echogenicity of the renal cortex can be equal to that of the liver or spleen, it is usually not more echogenic than these structures in term infants. In contrast, in premature infants, the normal renal cortex can be hyperechoic relative to the adjacent liver. The more premature the infant is, the higher is the likelihood that the renal cortex will be hyperechoic.

TABLE 1: Differentiating features between neonatal and adult kidneys.

Features	*Neonatal*	*Adult*
Contour	Lobed	Smooth usually
Cortex reflectivity	+++	+
Medulla size	+ (relatively)	–
Sinus	Echo-poor	Echogenic
Pelvicalyceal system	Often apparent	Usually inapparent

In neonates and young infants, the medullary pyramids are hypoechoic and prominent, the result of a large medullary and smaller cortical volume in neonates relative to that of older children and adults **(Figs. 6A and B)**. The ratio of the cortex to the medulla is 1.64:1 in the neonate compared with 2.59:1 in the adult kidney. By 6 months of age, the pyramids demonstrate an adult pattern. The prominent and hypoechoic pyramids in the neonate should not be mistaken for hydronephrosis or cysts. The central sinus echoes in the neonate and young infants are not as echogenic as they are in older children because of the paucity of fat in this area. Adolescent kidneys have echogenic central sinus, which is typical of adults. The infant kidney contour is frequently lobulated resulting from residual fetal lobulation.

Renal Size

The importance of the assessment of renal size can never be overestimated. Its significance and practical application are all too obvious. Ultrasound has made renal size assessment a fairly simple, nonhazardous, and bedside job. The parameters to measure the growth of the kidneys include the use of two dimensions, namely renal length and breadth, use of pole to pole length (PPL), and renal volume. With advances in 3D ultrasound, accurate assessment of renal volume is possible. However, acquiring an acceptable 3D sweep in young children may not always be possible as it requires some cooperation on the part of the patient. 3D technology in infants and

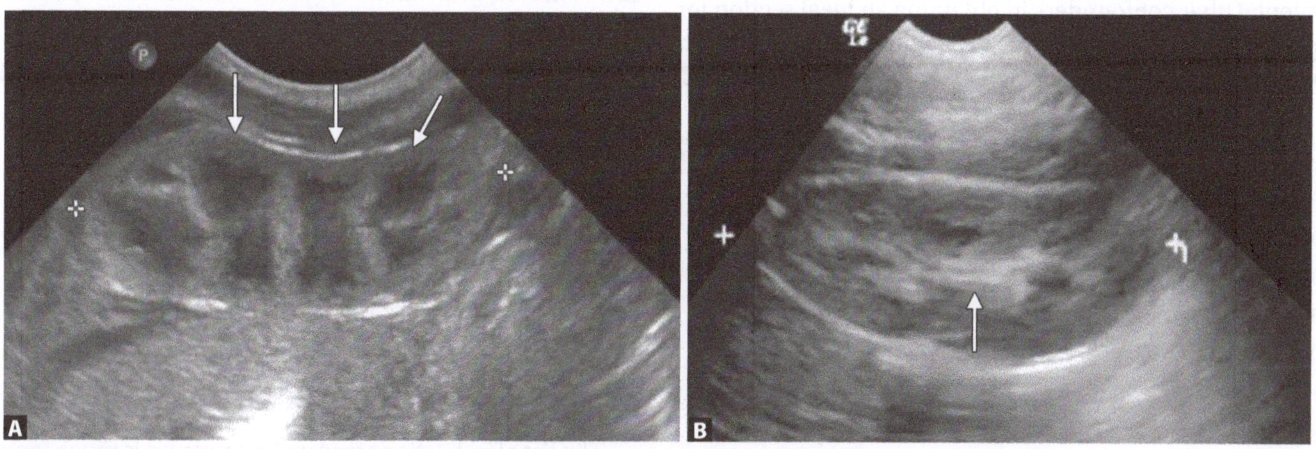

Figs. 6A and B: (A) Normal neonatal kidney. Ultrasound image of the kidney in a neonate shows large hypoechoic renal pyramids (arrows) and relatively smaller cortical volume; (B) Normal adolescent kidney. Ultrasound image shows an echogenic renal sinus (arrow). The hypoechoic renal pyramids appear relatively smaller compared to the neonate.

toddlers still remains in the fetal stage. Many studies have shown that using two dimensions in measuring the kidney offers precious little additional information. Hence, the focus remains on measuring renal length in the best section. The renal size varies according to age, height, weight, and body surface area. Interestingly, the average length of the kidneys in male children did not differ much from that of the age-matched female children. In growing children, height is the most important factor associated with kidney growth; renal size correlates best with the child's height.[5,6] However, measurement of height and height centiles may be cumbersome in the ultrasound room. Hence, age will remain the most practical parameter for the comparison of renal size. However, when the renal size is at the extremes of the age-appropriate limits, it is always prudent to judge the size with regard to the patient's build and height. Renal size varies with age and in neonates, it also varies with maturity. A number of age-appropriate standards have been established including studies in healthy Indian children. **Table 2** is once such age-corrected renal length table.[3]

Various studies of the renal size in children have brought out some interesting observations. Unlike adults, where asymmetry in renal size is often reported as a common phenomenon, the right and left renal lengths are more or less equal, especially in younger children, and the size difference does not usually exceed 2 or 3 mm in older children. Hence, it is prudent to view with suspicion any disparity in size of >10% between the two kidneys. Exceptions to this rule include kidneys with bifid collecting system and minor rotational anomalies of the kidney. The right kidney is usually slightly smaller than the left in adults. This is because of the space occupied by the liver, which makes less space available for the kidney and pushes it into a more rotated configuration. This decreases the PPL. However, the fact remains that *there is no well-defined threshold to classify pathological asymmetry* in children.

The renal length may also be altered by a few nonbiological variables. The most common one is the position of the patient. Other confounders in obtaining an ideal section for measuring renal length include the equipment used (both the transducer and the software used), overlying bowel gas, tubes and dressings (especially a sick child in the critical care unit as well as children on peritoneal dialysis), superficially located kidneys (failure to change depth may obscure the margins and interfere with renal length measurement), and, more importantly, a frightened child. Hence, the measurement of renal size requires a great degree of patience and perseverance. The importance of this measurement in determining management, however, makes it worth the effort many times over.

The rate of growth of the kidney is the fastest in the first year of life, especially the first 6 months. The renal size increases from 4 cm at birth to 5 cm in the first 2 months of life. A commonly used rule of thumb in assessing renal size in preterm infants is that renal length in millimeters approximates gestational age in weeks.

In conditions with just one functioning kidney, such as solitary kidney and multicystic dysplastic kidney, the normal kidney should show a compensatory phenomenon, a greater renal size than that is normal for age. A single kidney is compatible with normal life and ultrasound may help in detecting deficiencies in renal compensation. It is worthwhile mentioning that prolonged follow-up in children with multicystic dysplastic kidney (MCDK) has failed to show an increased risk of malignant transformation or hypertension and that involution depends on the renal size by ultrasound at birth.

Despite its well-documented usefulness and simplicity, the renal length continues to be an often-overlooked entity. This is because of its interobserver variability and the high degree of operator skill required for an accurate measurement. Hence, it is often superseded by other characteristics such as the corticomedullary differentiation in chronic renal disorders. In the hands of an experienced pediatric radiologist, the renal size will be the most useful sonological renal parameter, a fact, which pediatric nephrologists the world over, will vouch for.

TABLE 2: Age-related renal length.[3]

Age	Length (mm)	Range (mm)
0–3 months	45	35–60
3–6 months	50	50–60
6–9 months	55	52–60
9–12 months	58	54–64
1–3 years	65	54–72
3–6 years	75	64–88
6–9 years	80	73–86
9–12 years	86	73–100

Common Indications for Renal Ultrasound

The common indications for renal ultrasound in pediatric practice include the following:

- Postnatal evaluation of antenatally detected hydronephrosis/anomalies
- Evaluation of urinary tract infection (UTI)
- Evaluation of pyrexia of undetermined origin
- Hematuria
- Suspected urolithiasis/ureteric colic
- Acute renal failure
- Unexplained chronic kidney disease
- Nephrotic syndrome
- Renal mass.

The list of indications for renal ultrasound is much longer and it suffices to say that this chapter may not be adequate for the purpose.

Diagnostic Approach

A brief and introductory approach utilizing size and echo pattern is given as an example in **Table 3**.[7]

A patient study of the kidneys for the size, structure, parenchymal changes, and corticomedullary differentiation can indicate the underlying disease and chronicity of the disease.

In the following section, we will discuss the common clinical situations in pediatric nephrology and the importance of ultrasound in these situations.

Evaluation of Urinary Tract Infection

The evaluation of UTI is probably the most common indication for renal ultrasound in pediatric practice. The importance of diagnosis and optimal treatment of UTIs and its implications in preventing chronic kidney disease in adulthood is well known to all pediatricians. The three most important causes of recurrent UTIs are renal structure abnormalities, vesicoureteric reflux (VUR), and voiding dysfunction. Imaging is used to diagnose the first two conditions. The third is diagnosed purely by obtaining a proper voiding history from the patient and his/her parents. Imaging only helps in quantifying the degree of renal damage.

The ultrasound is usually done as soon as the diagnosis of UTI is made or suspected. Ultrasound is cost-effective and useful in the detection of complications such as focal lobar nephronia, abscess formation, pyonephrosis, perinephric extension of disease, etc. It is a sensitive tool to distinguish pyelonephritis from simple UTI. Pyelonephritis causes edema of the renal parenchyma, and this manifests as increased renal size on ultrasound. However, increased size is not specific for pyelonephritis and can occur in any disorder associated with renal inflammation. Common causes include enteric fever, leptospirosis, acute leukemia, and Kawasaki disease. The association of sterile pyuria in Kawasaki disease further complicates differentiation from UTI. The increase in renal size may not always be due to inflammation of that kidney (refer case scenario further).

Ultrasound is not very sensitive in the evaluation of reflux. Criteria for suspected VUR on sonogram are unexplained transient fullness of the collecting system, prominent lower ureters that exhibit frequent peristalsis, focal renal scarring, parenchymal thinning, thickening of the renal pelvis (pyelitis), and renal size discrepancy. Careful and meticulous scanning techniques may prove rewarding. One must remember that ultrasound evaluation of the bladder is done at rest and hence high-pressure refluxes that occur during the act of voiding are beyond its ambit. Ultrasound usually suggests high-grade refluxes that result in upper tract dilatation and/or significant renal parenchymal damage. It is very likely to miss low-grade refluxes that do not result in upper tract dilatation. Ultrasound is also not very sensitive in picking up mild-to-moderate reflux-induced renal parenchymal damage. The most sensitive modality for picking up renal parenchymal damage is the cortical imaging agent DMSA. IVU is of intermediate sensitivity, not as good as DMSA scan but better than ultrasonography.

The diagnosis of voiding dysfunction is usually achieved by a careful voiding history. Guidelines exist for suspicion of voiding dysfunction in a child. Imaging observations, which may suggest the same, include bladder wall thickening **(Fig. 7)**, significant post-void residual urine, persistent high-grade reflux, and a spinning top urethra on MCU. Thickening of the bladder wall may be erroneously diagnosed as cystitis. This again underscores the importance of a proper voiding history, which alone can differentiate the two without the

TABLE 3: Ultrasonographic approach to renal disorders.[7]

Kidney size	*Corticomedullary differentiation preserved*	*Corticomedullary differentiation lost*	*Corticomedullary differentiation inverted*
Large kidneys	Acute glomerulonephritis*	ARPKD (babies)*	ARPKD (older child)
	Congenital nephrotic syndrome* (renal size can be normal)	Renal vein thrombosis*	
	Hemolytic uremic syndrome (glomerular form)	Storage disease (e.g., amyloidosis)*	
		Infiltration by tumor	
Small kidneys	Organoid hypoplasia	Terminal renal failure whatever the cause*	
		Hypoplasia with dysplasia*	
Normal size kidneys	Acute tubulointerstitial nephritis	Juvenile nephronophthisis*	Medullary nephrocalcinosis
	Hemolytic uremic syndrome (arterial form)	Chronic tubulointerstitial nephritis*	Transient anuria in neonates
	Acute renal artery thrombosis		

*Increased cortical echogenicity is seen in these conditions.
(ARPKD: autosomal recessive polycystic kidney disease)
Source: Adapted from Garel L, Pariente D. Ultrasound in pediatric nephrology. In: Kalifa G (Ed). Pediatric Ultrasonography. Berlin: Springer; 1986.

need for investigations. One should first rule out neurogenic causes such as spinal dysraphism.

Case Scenario

A 6-month-old boy was admitted with a history of high-grade fever and vomiting. Clinical examination did not localize the fever. Investigations showed neutrophilic leukocytosis, high C-reactive protein (CRP), and plenty of pus cells. Ultrasound showed a large right kidney and the impression was right pyelonephritis **(Figs. 8A to C)**. DMSA, however, showed multiple photopenic areas and mild scarring of the left kidney.

This discrepancy is because the left kidney was actually a previously scarred kidney and there was hence compensatory overgrowth of the right kidney. The current episode had increased the size of the left kidney to a normal for age value, but much less than the noninfected right kidney with compensatory hypertrophy. This example illustrates the deficiencies of ultrasound in the diagnosis of pyelonephritis and reflux nephropathy as it shows only structural changes and not functional implications. DMSA is the gold standard in the diagnosis of pyelonephritis. However, ultrasound is a

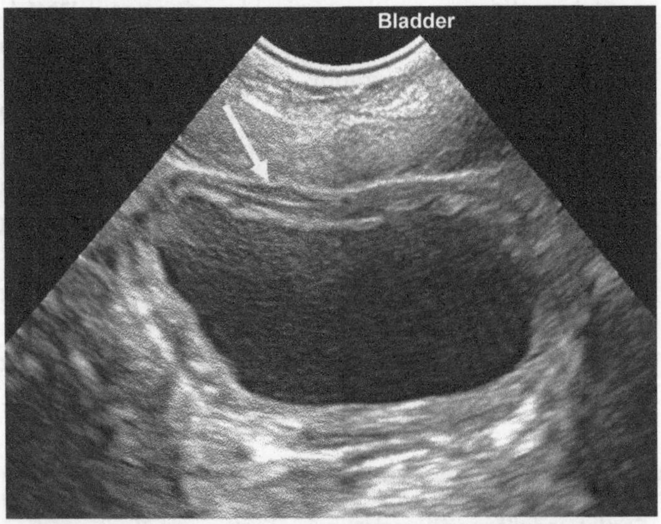

Fig. 7: Ultrasound image showing thickening of the bladder wall (arrow) in a child with voiding dysfunction.

much simpler option and remains the primary modality of investigating UTI.

Evaluation of Upper Urinary Tract Dilatation

Ultrasonography is the primary imaging modality of choice. In the majority of cases, sonography can reliably establish the degree and level of obstruction **(Flowchart 1)**. But it is not always possible to establish the cause for dilatation through sonographic examination alone.

Those who wish to be wise before the fact should realize that dilatation is not synonymous with obstruction.

Points to Remember

- Not all dilated systems are always obstructed and not all obstructed systems are always dilated.
- Situations leading to oliguria or anuria can mask dilatation/obstruction and will become manifest when the situation is relieved/corrected and when normal or near normal physiology is restored.
- A dilated system could be due to:
  - Obstruction—organic, functional
  - Reflux
  - Idiopathic
  - High outflow states (e.g., diabetes insipidus).

There are variable urodynamic parameters that have a role in causing a dilated urinary tract. They are urine flow rate; drainage rate; renal size; distensibility of calyces, pelvis, and ureter; and functional variations of bladder or urethra. Each one of them can possibly lead to variable dilatation of the upper urinary tract. Pure morphologic variants, whether physiologic or pathologic (e.g., megacalyces), compound the diversity of the phenomenon of hydronephrosis/hydroureter.[8]

The most common form of obstructive uropathy is a proximal stenosis of the ureter at the ureteropelvic junction. A "relative" ureteropelvic stenosis exists in patients with a large or very distensible extrarenal pelvis and in patients with high-grade VUR. Once the ureterovesical junction obstruction is cleared or reflux has resolved, the ureteropelvic junction is found to be normal. An unusual form of proximal "ureteral

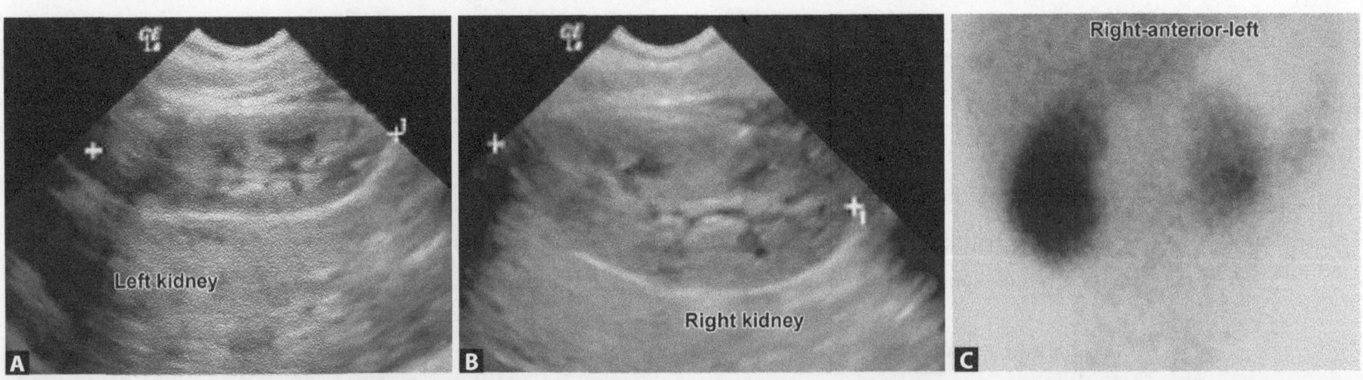

Figs. 8A to C: Ultrasound images in a 6-month-old infant with fever demonstrate a (A) Normal-sized left kidney; (B) Large right kidney. The impression was right pyelonephritis; and (C) Dimercaptosuccinic acid (DMSA) in the same infant shows a small left kidney with extensive photopenic areas indicating left pyelonephritis. The right kidney has normal appearances on DMSA.

Flowchart 1: Upper urinary tract dilatation: Diagnostic flowchart.

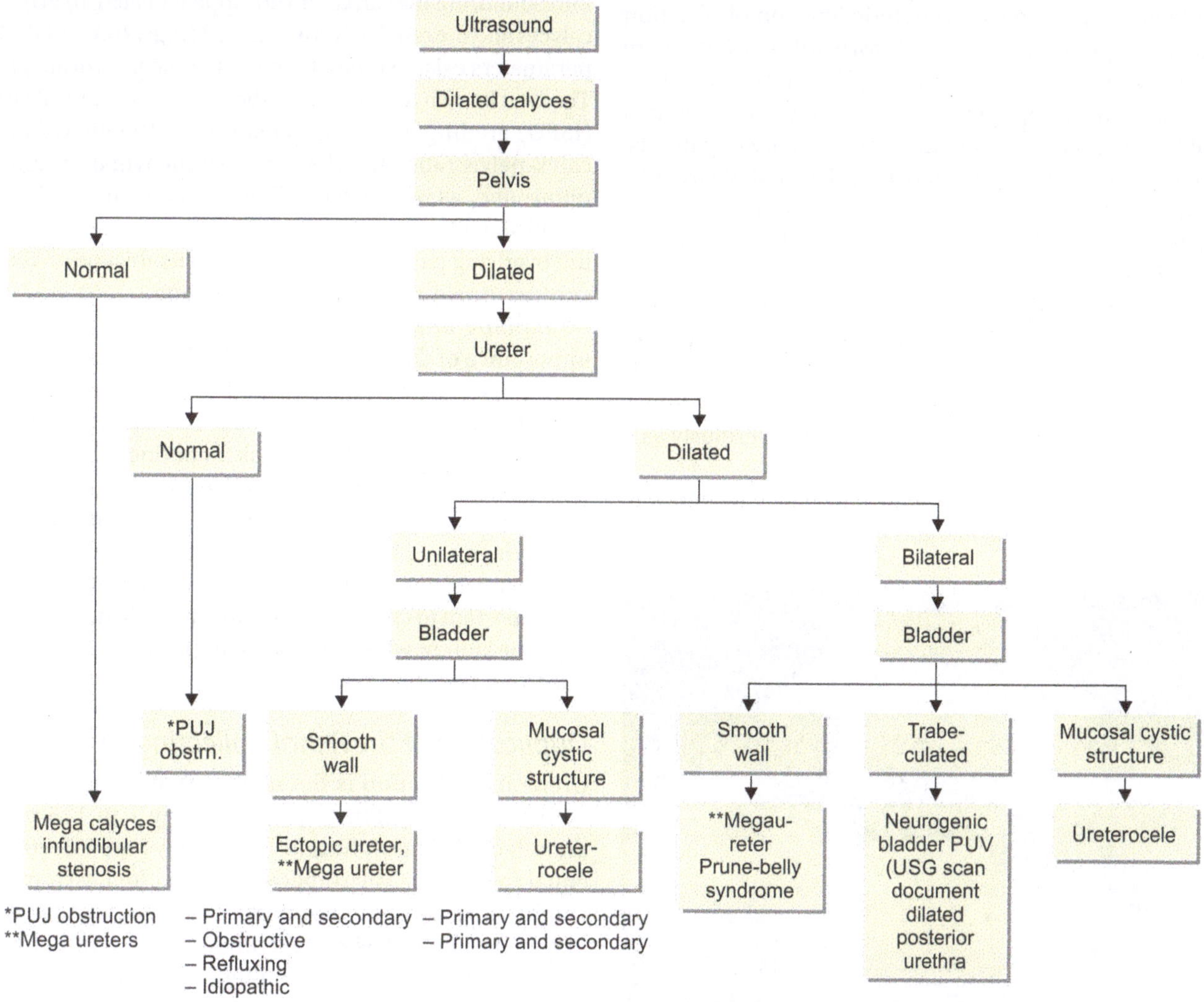

(PUJ: pelviureteric junction; PUV: posterior urethral valve; USG: ultrasonography)

obstruction" exists in conjunction with pelvoinfundibular hypoplasia, i.e., absence of the renal pelvis.

Obstruction may occur at various levels of the ureter and may be due to various etiologies. A common intrinsic form is fibrotic ureteral stenosis while a common extrinsic form is due to vascular ureteral compression (e.g., proximally by an aberrant renal artery and at mid ureter by a "retrocaval ureter"). More common than both etiologies mentioned is intraluminal ureteral obstruction of the ureter by a calculus. Often, little or no ectasia of the collecting system proximal to the obstruction is seen initially for a period of several days.

Primary obstructive megaureter is a common cause to compromise the urinary drainage at the ureterovesical junction. It may be associated with V–U reflux. Occasionally, there is hyperperistaltic activity of such a ureter. Both primary obstructive megaureter and primary refluxing megaureter may present with wall thickening due to hypertrophy resulting from hyperactivity. There is inadequate morphological ultrasonographic criteria to identify these complex forms of obstructive uropathy associated with severe reflux at the ureterovesical junction.

From the above discussion, it is evident that sonography alone cannot diagnose the etiology of the upper tract dilatation. It should be stressed that the morphodynamic examination of the urinary tract by micturition cystogram and IVU or radionuclide study [diethylenetriaminepentaacetic acid (DTPA)] is essential for the adequate evaluation of a dilated upper urinary tract. Nevertheless, ultrasound is the primary imaging modality of choice in the evaluation of the upper tract dilatation **(Fig. 9)**. One should attempt to define the morphology and the extent of the upper urinary tract ectasia as outlined below:

- Unilateral or bilateral
- Affecting the calyces, pelvis, and/or ureter
- Being part of a solitary system or segmental
- With or without an associated nephrourologic or other malformation
- Constant or intermittent.

Further diagnostic evaluation will require MCU and radionuclide studies, single or in combination to establish the diagnosis.

Pelviureteric Junction Obstruction

A couple of decades ago, pelviureteric junction obstruction (PUJO) management was straightforward. Patients were usually symptomatic and after imaging for confirmation of the diagnosis, the next step was pyeloplasty. However, advances in fetal imaging have resulted in a new category of patients: the infant for evaluation of antenatally detected obstructive uropathy. In such cases, ultrasound is best performed at the end of the first week of life. However, it can be done at any time after the first 3 days of life when the phase of physiological oliguria is completed. The ultrasound examination should look for the renal size, dilatation of the pelvis, and calyces as well as the renal parenchyma thickness.[9] The pelvis is a normally compliant structure unlike the calyces. Hence, any dilatation of the calyces should be viewed seriously as it usually implies a high-pressure obstruction.

In a normal anatomical variation, the renal pelvis tends to bulge medially outside the margins of the kidney. It is termed extrarenal pelvis. In this condition, the pelvis appears dilated on ultrasound, but the calyces do not appear dilated. In PUJO, both calyces and the renal pelvis are dilated **(Figs. 10A and B)**. Many parameters exist to predict renal outcome in hydronephrosis. The best known are the International Society of Fetal Urology (ISFU) grading, the anteroposterior (AP) pelvic diameter, calyx-pelvis ratio, and the renal parenchymal thickness on ultrasound, as well as the split renal function on DTPA. Any significant dilatation of the collecting system is likely to stretch the overlying parenchyma decreasing its thickness. Very thin cortices usually mean poor renal function.

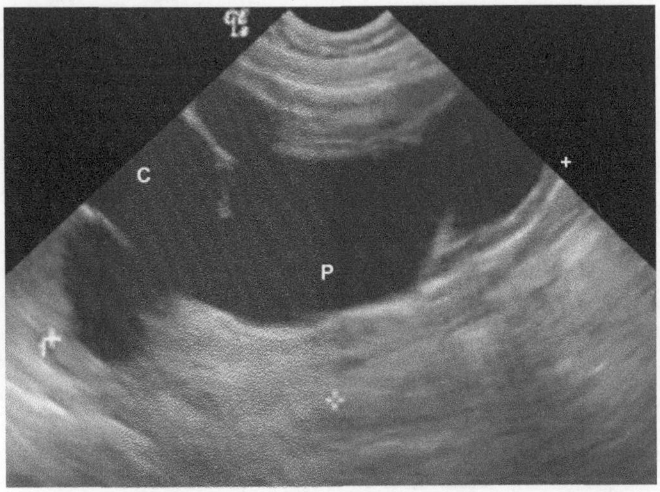

Fig. 9: Ultrasound image of a 1-year-old child showing a moderately dilated pelvis (P) and dilated calyces (C).

Equally important but frequently overlooked is the importance of the ultrasound in the follow-up of PUJO after pyeloplasty. Ultrasound in the immediate postoperative period shows an increase in renal size due to edema, and ultrasound is done mainly to look for perinephric collections. It is repeated 1 month postoperatively for checking the stent position. In the third month, the pelvis would have collapsed and a decrease in renal size is usually evident. Structural normality is seldom restored and residual dilatation is the rule. It is important to check for no undue increase in the size of the opposite kidney, which may be a compensatory phenomenon due to a failed surgery.

Duplication of the Renal Collecting System

Ureteral duplication is the most common anomaly of the genitourinary system. Approximately 1 in 125 patients are affected. The right and left kidneys are affected with equal frequency. The duplications are often asymmetrical. Duplication represents a spectrum of changes. A bifid pelvis may be thought of as representing the most minimal form of duplication, while in complete duplication the ureters enter the bladder separately. The ureters may join together within the bladder wall and have a common opening. The portion of the kidney drained by the lower pole system is usually larger than the upper pole segment.

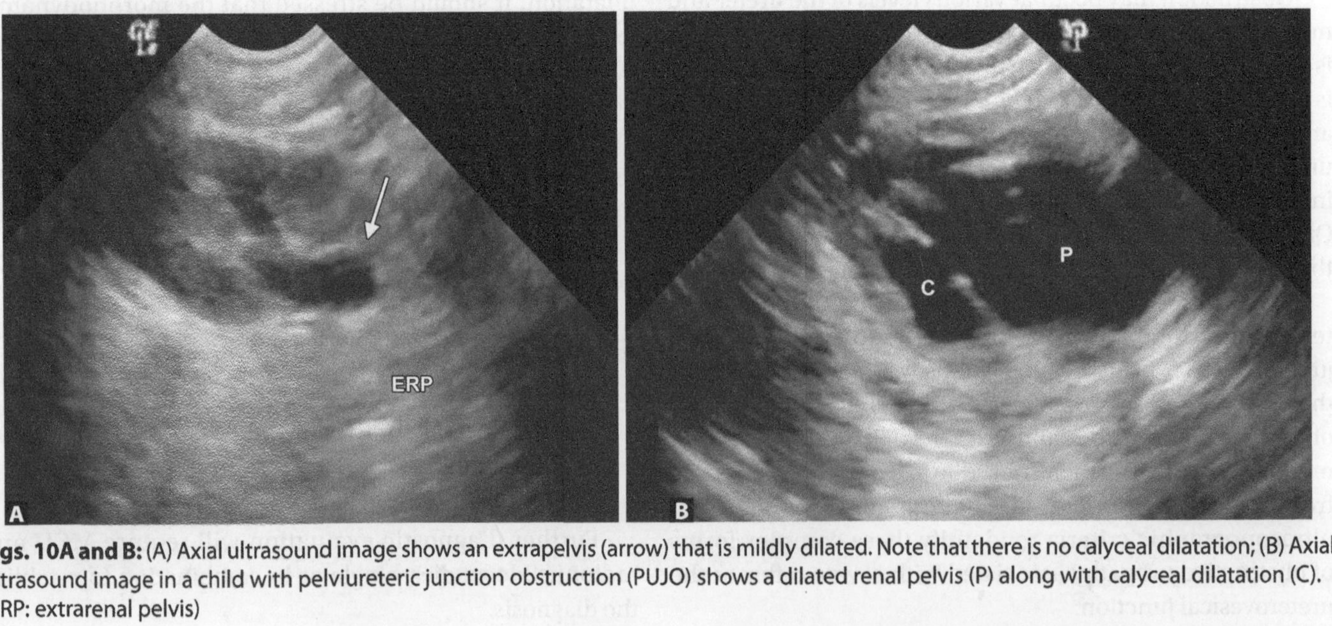

Figs. 10A and B: (A) Axial ultrasound image shows an extrapelvis (arrow) that is mildly dilated. Note that there is no calyceal dilatation; (B) Axial ultrasound image in a child with pelviureteric junction obstruction (PUJO) shows a dilated renal pelvis (P) along with calyceal dilatation (C). (ERP: extrarenal pelvis)

When the kidney is completely duplicated, two separate pelvicalyceal systems drain into two separate ureters, each having its own insertion into the bladder. The two openings generally are in one common sheath. The relationship of the insertion sites of the distal ureters is constant. The ureter from the upper pole moiety typically enters the bladder more caudally and more medially than the ureter draining the lower pole segment. This is known as the Weigert-Meyer rule. Ureteral ectopia is a common consequence of duplications. In either sex, the upper pole ureter may enter the bladder inferomedial to the trigone or at the level of the bladder neck **(Figs. 11A and B)**. In girls, it may also end ectopically in the vestibule, vagina, or urethra. In boys, the ectopic termination may be in the posterior urethra or seminal vesicles. In girls, the ureter may end distal to the external sphincter and in such cases the patient presents with dribbling. Patients with obstruction present with signs of infection. The upper pole ureter commonly ends in a ureterocele, resulting in various degrees of obstruction. Congenital ureteropelvic junction obstruction may occur in the setting of renal duplications. They are most likely to involve the lower pole. Reflux is a common occurrence, predominantly but not exclusively involving the lower pole moiety due to the distortion of tunneling through the bladder wall.

Reflux may result in scarring in the lower pole segment. Obstruction of the upper pole may result in severe thinning of the upper pole parenchyma. A markedly dilated upper pole ureter can cause secondary obstruction of the lower pole ureter. Obstruction of the upper pole system may result in a nonfunctioning upper pole. When the upper pole is nonfunctioning, renal scans and intravenous urograms give a classic appearance of the "drooping lily". The functioning lower pole is deviated laterally away from the spine by the large hydronephrotic upper pole. Ultrasound is useful in confirming the presence of the cystic nonfunctioning upper pole as the cause of the mass effect.

The ultrasonographic appearance of duplication varies, reflecting the type of duplication. In nonobstructed partial or complete duplications, the kidneys are slightly large in size and may show a separation of the renal sinus fat. These kidneys are difficult to differentiate from kidneys with prominent columns of Bertin.

When upper pole obstruction is present, the appearance of the kidney again varies, from mild hydronephrosis involving the upper third of the kidney with a rim of the normal-appearing kidney, to hydronephrosis with thinning of the upper pole rim parenchyma, to complete replacement of the upper third of the kidney by a large cystic mass. If the presenting problem is a UTI or sepsis, the upper pole collecting system may contain pus and appear echogenic. The lower pole may appear displaced from the psoas muscle by a large ectatic upper pole ureter. The ureter can often be followed to the level of the bladder. Ultrasound of the bladder is an excellent way of determining the presence of a ureterocele. Hydronephrosis of the lower pole may be present with or without renal scarring. Voiding cystourethrography is generally used to see if the lower pole dilatation is due to reflux. This may be suggested by ultrasonography if a change in distention of the renal pelvis is noted during patient voiding. Exposure of a baby to cold gel will often result in involuntary voiding. The bladder should therefore be evaluated early in the course of the examination.

Nephrotic Syndrome

Ultrasound examination is frequently done during evaluation of nephrotic syndrome. The kidneys are usually normal in size and echotexture in children with minimal change disease (MCD). An increase in size and echogenicity is usually

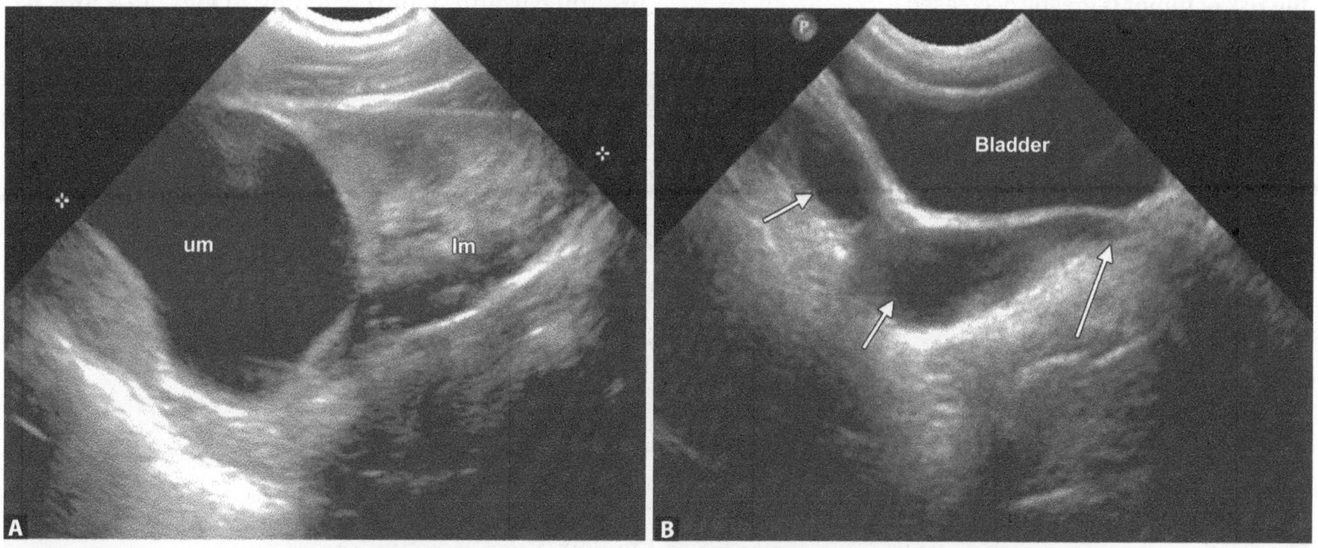

Figs. 11A and B: Ultrasound image in a 3-month-old infant with the first episode of urinary tract infection shows a duplex kidney. (A) Longitudinal ultrasound image of the kidney shows marked hydronephrosis in the upper moiety (um) with a thin rim of parenchyma. The lower moiety (lm) has normal appearances; (B) Longitudinal ultrasound image at the level of the bladder shows a dilated um ureter (short arrows) which has an ectopic insertion at the level of bladder neck (long arrow).

associated with a steroid-resistant phenotype such as focal segmental glomerulosclerosis (FSGS). An increased size with normal echotexture may be associated with frequent relapses, although the association has not been consistently proven to be statistically significant.

Renal Tumors

In pediatric practice, ultrasound has proven to be an adequate imaging modality in tumor evaluation and is the investigation of choice for tumor detection, localization, characterization, assessing extent and staging, guiding biopsy, and follow-up. In Wilms' tumor, the most common pediatric renal malignancy, it does all the above and also evaluates vascular extension with a great deal of accuracy. This provides vital preoperative knowledge in planning for therapy; for example, if the tumor thrombus is confined to renal vein or abdominal inferior vena cava (IVC) an abdominal surgical approach would suffice; to the contrary if the tumor thrombus has extended to the right atrium, a combined thoracoabdominal team approach becomes essential. The surveillance renal ultrasound to look for Wilms' tumor is periodically performed in patients with Beckwith-Wiedemann syndrome (BWS), Denys-Drash syndrome (DDS), and WAGR [Wilms tumor, aniridia, genitourinary anomalies, and intellectual disability (formerly referred to as mental retardation)] syndrome. It is equally important to look for foci of nephroblastomatosis. These may be intralobar nephrogenic rests (ILNRs) or perilobar nephrogenic rests (PLNRs). ILNRs are associated with early tumors in WAGR and DDS while PLNRs are associated with later onset of Wilms' tumor in BWS. In BWS, as per the consensus guidelines, the first scan is usually done at 1 month of age and bimonthly thereafter till 6 months of age. It is then done every 3 months till the age of 7 years. After 7 years, clinical examination of the abdomen biannually will suffice as the risk of tumor is greatly decreased.

RENAL DOPPLER

The following are the indications for "renal Doppler" studies in children:

- Renal transplant assessment
- Renal artery stenosis
- Renal vein thrombosis
- Complications after renal biopsy
- Evaluation of blood flow in acute and chronic kidney inflammation
- Distinction of obstructive and nonobstructive collecting system dilatation
- Evaluation of renal vascular resistance in various parenchymal renal diseases.

Umbilical artery catheter-associated thromboembolism affecting the aorta, the renal arteries, or both probably is the most common cause of hypertension observed in the typical newborn intensive care unit (NICU). The parameters normally studied in the renal Doppler include the resistivity index (RI), pulsatility index (PI), and acceleration time (AT). However, it should be kept in mind that the Doppler study is a technically difficult procedure. No study has established normative data in children. The continued use of adult normal values may result in wrong diagnosis. The cutoff for resistive index in adults is >0.70. Studies in younger children have shown that the same value could be used for children older than 10 years. However, in normal children younger than 6 years, the RI is usually higher. Studies have failed to consistently arrive at normal values for this age group. While renal Doppler has a good positive predictive value, it has a poor negative predictive value and hence a normal Doppler in the presence of clinical suspicion should always be confirmed by an angiogram.

Urolithiasis

Ultrasound is the primary modality for the diagnosis of urolithiasis and nephrocalcinosis **(Figs. 12A and B)** in

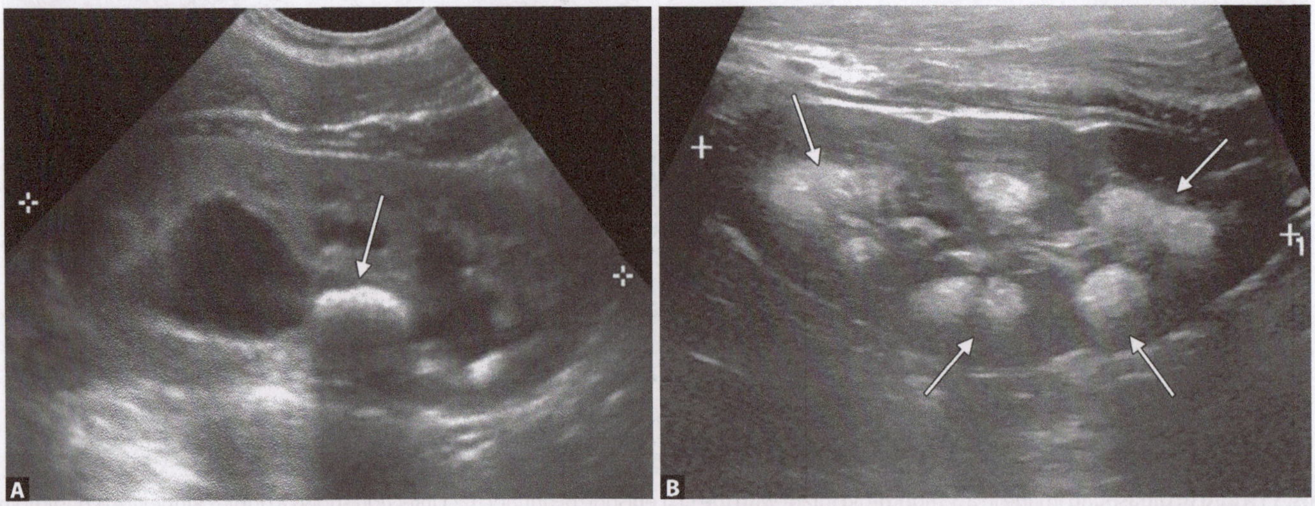

Figs. 12A and B: Urolithiasis. (A) Ultrasound image in a 6-year-old child with renal colic. Longitudinal ultrasound image of the left kidney shows a large calculus (arrow) in the renal pelvis causing hydronephrosis; (B) Ultrasound image of an infant with failure to thrive shows echogenic renal pyramids (arrows) consistent with medullary nephrocalcinosis.

children. A plain X-ray of the abdomen may aid in the diagnosis of a few calculi. Most renal and vesical calculi may be easily diagnosed by ultrasound. Ureteric calculi may be difficult to pick up on ultrasound. It is important to see the patient repeatedly. Secondary effects of the calculi, such as ureteric dilatation and urinary stasis, may aid in making the diagnosis. The use of CT abdomen in urolithiasis is discussed in this chapter (in CT section). The hazards of radiation in children are being increasingly recognized leading to an "Image Gently" campaign in pediatric urolithiasis. The ease of access, absence of harmful radiation, and high sensitivity in the hands of an experienced radiologist will mean that ultrasound will continue to remain the imaging modality of choice in urolithiasis.

VOIDING UROSONOGRAPHY

Voiding urosonography (VUS) is not technically a recent advance in uroradiology. Ultrasound evaluation of reflux has been in existence since the 1970s. Earlier studies used normal saline and the use of contrast became popular in the 1990s. Advances in ultrasound resolution have made accurate visualization of microbubbles possible and the emergence of safer second-generation contrast agents is a step in the right direction. However, it must be cautioned that VUS is still an invasive procedure requiring catheterization. It is more time consuming than MCU and is a more messy procedure. There is a lack of adequate validation data with respect to use in pediatrics.

The utility of ultrasound in pediatric nephrology does not end with the above-discussed conditions. The diagnosis of renal vein thrombosis in the newborn, polycystic kidney disease, and anorectal malformations, to mention a few, are not uncommon indications for a renal ultrasound. With a good clinicosonological correlation, it remains the premium investigation to make an accurate nephrological diagnosis. In conclusion, the assessment of the renal size, parenchymal echo pattern, and the status of the collecting system is the key to diagnostic decision-making in renal sonography. It has to be stressed that even basic clinical information will substantially help in reducing the number of possible differential diagnoses when dealing with a particular patient. Always evaluate the radiologic or imaging findings in the given clinical context. Radiology and imaging without clinical correlation is like clapping with one hand, an exercise in futility.

MICTURATING CYSTOURETHROGRAM

Micturating cystourethrogram is a commonly performed examination in pediatric radiology. When performed properly, it can provide anatomical and functional information about the lower urinary tract. MCU is the gold standard radiographic test to diagnose VUR. However, there are a few risks associated with this test. There is the risk of emotional trauma—MCU can be a distressing investigation for the child due to its invasive nature. A significant radiation exposure does occur during this test, and it is important to consider the risk of such radiation exposure versus the benefit of doing the test. MCU also carries with it the risk of iatrogenic UTI due to catheterization.

Indications

The common indications for MCU in children are for the assessment of recurrent UTI, for evaluation of VUR, and for suspected PUVs.[10]

There is considerable variation among pediatricians regarding the referral criteria for an MCU following UTI. One of the commonly used guidelines are those issued by the American Academy of Pediatrics (AAP). As per the AAP guidelines, MCU should not be routinely performed after the first episode of uncomplicated UTI. The AAP recommends MCU in young children with recurrent UTI, atypical UTI, or if the ultrasound shows significant hydronephrosis.[11] Minor renal pelvic dilatation and ureteric distension are nonspecific findings; on its own, such findings do not warrant an MCU. The guidelines issued by the Indian Society of Pediatric Nephrology (ISPN) are also widely used in our country. As per the revised guidelines of the ISPN,[12] the use of ultrasound, MCU, and DMSA is recommended in children younger than 1 year with the first episode of UTI. In older children between the ages of 1 and 5 years, evaluation includes the use of ultrasound and DMSA, with MCU being performed if either of those two tests shows an abnormality. In children older than 5 years, they suggest the use of a screening ultrasound, with further investigations only if the ultrasound is abnormal.

One must bear in mind that guidelines such as those discussed above, although useful, may not be applicable in every situation. Every institution has its preferences. It is crucial to take into account the age of the child when deciding the management. This is because infants and young children are at the highest risk for renal injury. The decision-making should be based on potential risks and benefits of performing a test and a thorough understanding of how such a test will, if at all, alter the patient's management.

Micturating cystourethrogram should not be done during an episode of acute infection. Clinical practice varies widely across institutions regarding the ideal timing of MCU following a UTI. Conventionally, MCU has been deferred for 4–6 weeks following a UTI as it was believed that edema at the ureteric mucosal orifice may lead to false-negative or false-positive study. Studies have disproved this line of reasoning. A recent review article states that early MCU can be performed after adequate antibiotic treatment of the acute episode of UTI.[13] They found that the timing of the MCU does not affect the detection rate of VUR. It is recommended that the procedure is done under antibiotic cover.[14] Sepsis and death following the procedure have been reported.[15]

Procedure

An appropriate-size feeding tube is inserted into the bladder. As a general guide, a 5 Fr feeding tube is used in infants and an 8 Fr feeding tube in older children; however, the ground reality will determine the exact size of the tube to be used in each patient. Once catheterized and the urine is drained, diluted contrast is instilled into the bladder. The bladder may be filled by the gravity dip method or by slow hand injection.[16] Low osmolar (nonionic) contrast media are ideal in neonates, infants, and high-risk groups, as they are less injurious than the high osmolar (ionic) contrast media. The contrast solution should be warmed to the body temperature as cold liquids initiate increased detrusor tone. Contrast is slowly infused, as quick injection will cause a sudden increase in bladder pressure. The following formula is used to calculate bladder volume in children. Volume infused in mL = wt. of the child × 7 (for a child <2 years); in a child 2–14 years: volume in mL = (age × 30) + 30.

However, this is not set in stone and should only serve as a guide. The volumes can differ from patient to patient even in the same age group. For example, a neurogenic bladder may need a greater volume to be infused, whereas a hyperactive bladder can accommodate only a small volume of fluid.

Practice varies from institution to institution—at some centers double cycle is performed,[16] where the bladder is filled and voided in two cycles; at others the bladder is filled only once. The images to be obtained include an AP plain film at the start of the study prior to catheterization. Following contrast instillation into the bladder, intermittent fluoroscopic screening may be done to visualize intermittent reflux. During voiding, a steep oblique view film and an AP view film are obtained in boys to visualize the entire course of the male urethra; in girls, only an AP view is obtained due to the short course of the urethra **(Figs. 13A and B)**. In cases of anorectal anomaly, along with the AP and oblique views, a lateral view is useful to assess the presence of a rectourethral fistula. A routine post-void image is generally not necessary. One must remember that an MCU is not a truly physiological test as the child is placed under considerable stress during the study. Thus, using this test to determine post-void residue is inaccurate and should be discouraged. The need for a post-void image is considered on a case-to-case basis. For example, in cases of reflux with suspected secondary PUJO a post-void film is useful **(Figs. 14A and B)**.

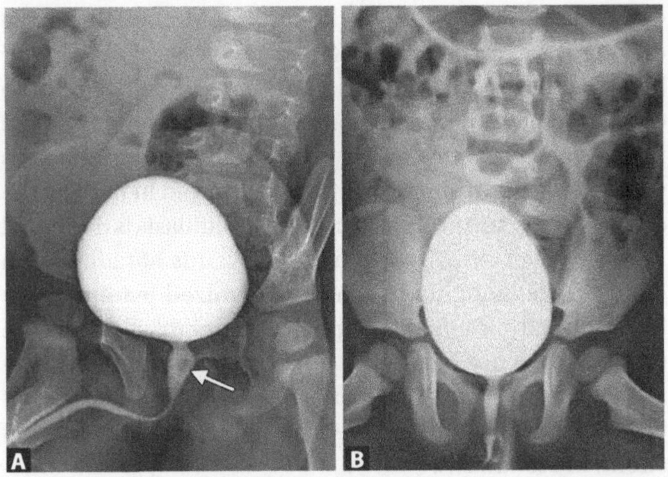

Figs. 13A and B: Micturating cystourethrogram—normal voiding images. (A) Steep oblique view in a boy showing the normal course of the entire male urethra. The small lucency (arrow) in the posterior urethra represents the normal verumontanum and should not be mistaken for pathology; (B) Anteroposterior voiding image in a girl demonstrates the short course of the female urethra.

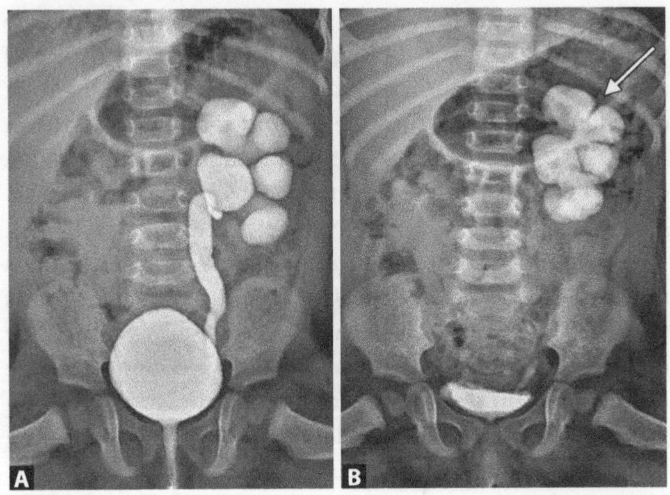

Figs. 14A and B: Micturating cystourethrogram—utility of postvoid image. (A) Voiding image shows left-sided reflux. Here, the calyces are dilated to a much greater degree compared to the ureters. This is abnormal. In such instances, it is useful to obtain a postvoid image; (B) Postvoid image shows that contrast in the ureter has drained whereas the contrast in the left renal collecting system is retained indicating a secondary left pelviureteric junction obstruction.

Pathology

Vesicoureteric Reflux

Vesicoureteric reflux is the retrograde flow of urine from the bladder into the ureter **(Figs. 15A and B)**. The reflux may be primary or secondary.

Primary VUR is due to abnormal tunneling of the distal ureter. The normal ureter has an oblique course through the bladder wall, which creates a valve-like mechanism. As the bladder fills, it compresses the submucosal part of the distal ureter and prevents reflux. When this submucosal tunnel is abnormal, the valvular mechanism becomes deficient and leads to reflux. In secondary VUR, the ureteric tunneling and valvular mechanism are normal to start with but are then overcome due to various factors, and this leads to reflux. Secondary causes of VUR include bladder outlet obstruction, voiding dysfunction **(Fig. 16)**, neurogenic bladder, and paraureteric diverticulum **(Figs. 17A and B)**. VUR also occurs if there is an abnormal site of ureteric insertion **(Figs. 18A and B)**. According to The International Reflux Grading System, there are five grades of reflux **(Table 4)**.

Posterior Urethral Valves

Posterior urethral valves are the most common congenital obstructive lesions in the urethra. The abnormality is a

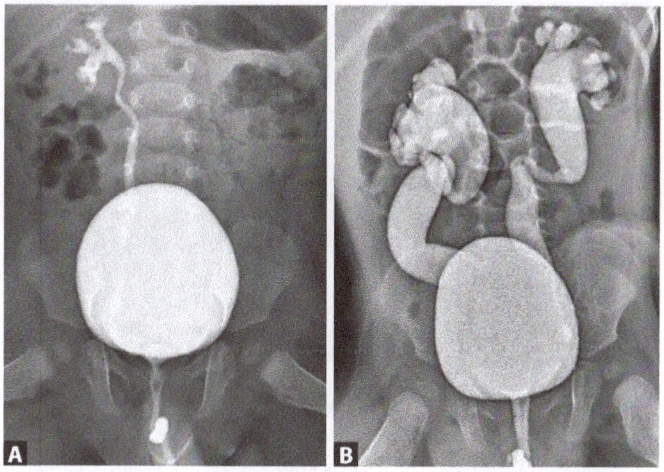
A
B

Figs. 15A and B: Micturating cystourethrogram—voiding images demonstrating vesicoureteric reflux (VUR). (A) Grade 2 VUR is seen on the right; (B) There is bilateral grade 5 VUR. There is dilatation and tortuosity of the ureters with loss of papillary impressions in the calyces.

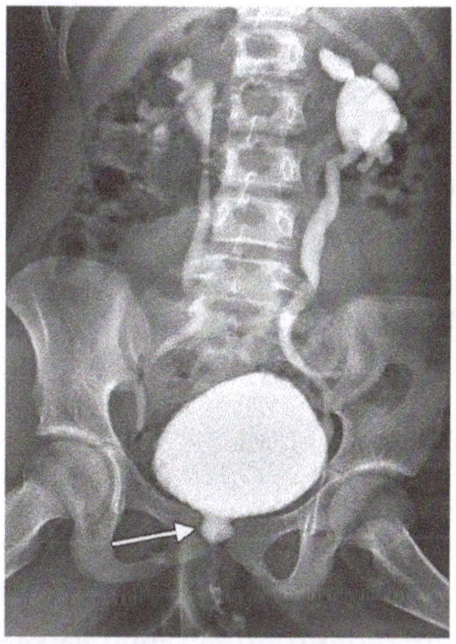

Fig. 16: Micturating cystourethrogram—voiding dysfunction. Anteroposterior voiding image in a girl child shows "spinning top" appearance (arrow) of the urethra indicating dysfunctional voiding. The high pressure bladder has led to bilateral vesicoureteric reflux.

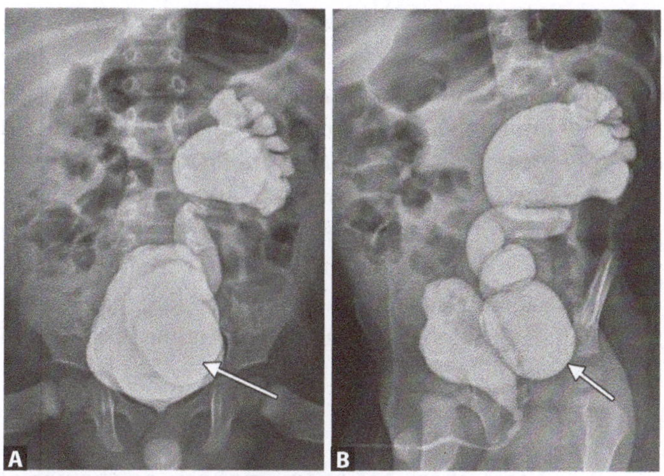
A
B

Figs. 17A and B: (A) Anteroposterior; and (B) Oblique voiding images in a male child showing left grade 5 vesicoureteric reflux secondary to a large paraureteric diverticulum (arrows).

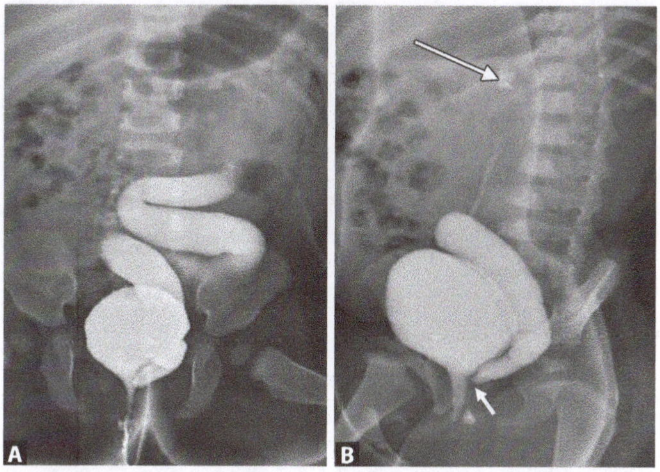
A
B

Figs. 18A and B: Micturating cystourethrogram—ectopic ureteric insertion. (A) Anteroposterior voiding image in a girl child shows reflux into a dilated tortuous left ureter; (B) This oblique image clearly shows ectopic insertion of the left ureter (short arrow) at the level of the bladder neck. Ectopic insertion can occur in single or in duplicated systems. Grade 2 reflux is also seen on the right (long arrow).

TABLE 4: Vesicoureteric reflux grading system.

Grade of VUR	Description
Grade 1	Reflux into ureter without any dilatation
Grade 2	Reflux into the ureter and pelvicalyceal system. There is no dilatation
Grade 3	Mild dilatation of the ureter and collecting system. Fornices are sharp
Grade 4	Calyces are blunted. Mild dilatation and tortuosity of the ureter
Grade 5	Ballooned out calyces with loss of papillary impressions. Markedly dilated and tortuous ureter

(VUR: vesicoureteric reflux)

thick valve-like membrane that courses obliquely from the verumontanum to the distal prostatic urethra. On an MCU, the essential finding is a dilated posterior urethra with a thin anterior urethral stream. There is associated bladder wall thickening and trabeculations. Unilateral or bilateral secondary VUR may be present.

On an MCU, the demonstration of the actual valve depends on the contrast density and angle of incidence of the X-ray beam. When seen, the valves appear as filling defects in the posterior urethra (**Figs. 19A and B**).

COMPUTED TOMOGRAPHY

In pediatrics, imaging modalities that do not use ionizing radiation are preferred. Thus, a dedicated pediatric ultrasound should be the first investigation of choice to evaluate the urinary tract in children. CT of the urinary tract should be considered in instances when an ultrasound is inconclusive and/or access to MRI is limited or where it may not be feasible to do an MRI. It is vital that pediatric settings are used when doing the CT and the number of CT phases should be kept to a minimum.

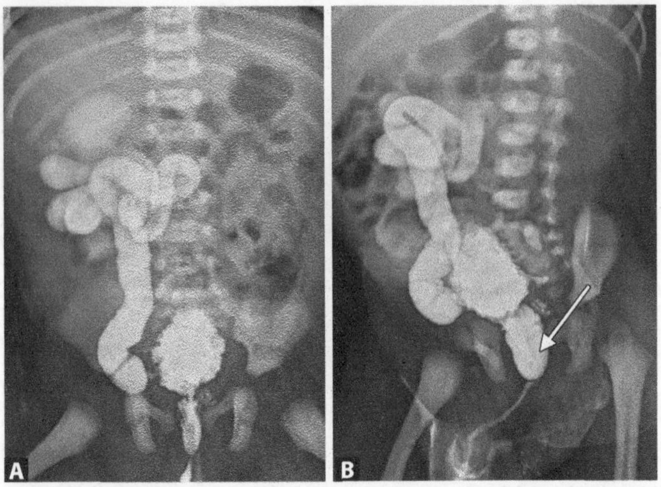

Figs. 19A and B: Micturating cystourethrogram—posterior urethral valves. (A) Anteroposterior; and (B) Oblique voiding images in a male neonate show a trabeculated bladder with a markedly dilated posterior urethra and thin anterior urethral stream. Linear filling defect (arrow) is seen in the posterior urethra representing valves. Right grade 5 VUR is present.

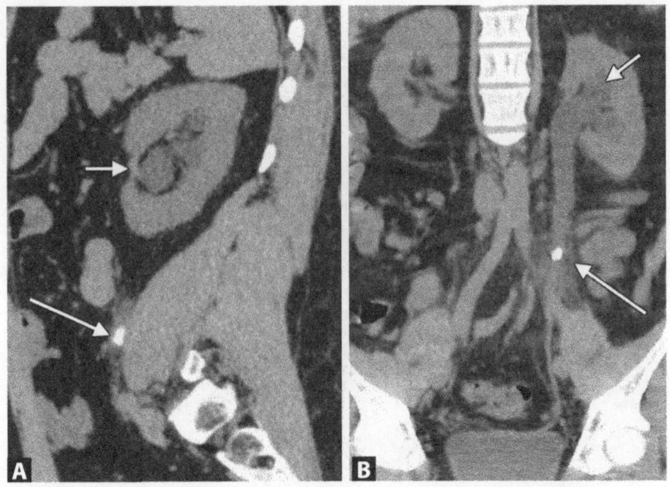

Figs. 20A and B: Computed tomography (CT) scan images of the kidney, ureter, and bladder: Ureteric calculus. (A) Sagittal; and (B) Coronal CT images in two different patients show an obstructing mid-ureteric calculus on the left (long arrows) with ureteric dilatation and dilated renal collecting system (short arrows).

The various indications for the use of CT in urology include urolithiasis, renal tumors, evaluation of renal artery stenosis, and renal trauma.

Urolithiasis

Computed tomography of KUB is a noncontrast, low-dose study that allows precise identification of calculi in the urinary tract. CT is considered as the gold standard for the assessment of urolithiasis in adults. However, in children one must be mindful of radiation dose as children are more sensitive to the deleterious effects of ionizing radiation.[17] If the CT parameters are not adjusted to suit the smaller body size in children, they may receive a larger radiation dose. Although CT of KUB is a relatively low-dose study (compared to other CT examinations), it is best to avoid unnecessary radiation exposures in children if possible.

Ultrasound is the primary imaging modality in a child with suspected urinary tract calculi.[18] Ultrasound is highly reliable for the demonstration of stones in the kidney, in the upper ureter, and in the distal ureter. However, it has a low sensitivity for the detection of calculi in the mid ureter due to bowel gas interference. Also, in children with obesity visualization of the ureter becomes difficult. In such cases, noncontrast CT KUB is useful for the assessment of ureteric calculi **(Figs. 20A and B)**. In recent years, there has been an increased use of CT in children and unfortunately CT is being used as the first line of investigation in suspected urinary tract calculi. This is concerning. In the majority of instances, an ultrasound is sufficient to make the diagnosis of urolithiasis.[19]

Renal Artery Stenosis

Computed tomography angiography is an important technique in the evaluation of renal artery stenosis. It allows high-resolution 2D and 3D reconstruction of the renal vessels. CT is ideal for depicting lesions involving the main renal artery and second-order branch vessels.[20] However, the sensitivity is lower for stenoses involving smaller intrarenal arteries. Despite this, CT angiography plays a valuable role in children with hypertension and it guides planning for further invasive procedures such as digital subtraction angiography and possible intervention.

Trauma

Multiphase contrast-enhanced CT of the abdomen is indicated in cases of polytrauma to detect intra-abdominal injury including renal trauma (such as vascular pedicle injury, urinary leak).[21] Indicators of possible renal injury include flank bruising, lower rib fractures, hematuria, and abdominal tenderness. In children, the degree of hematuria does not correlate with the severity of renal injury. Therefore, the current recommendation is to investigate any hematuria (microscopic or macroscopic) in a child with blunt injury abdomen.[22,23] The objective of imaging is to accurately grade the renal injury; this may be done using an ultrasound (in cases of mild trauma) or a contrast-enhanced CT.

Computed tomography provides precise demonstration of the presence and location of renal injuries **(Fig. 21)**. Delayed phase CT scans demonstrate collecting system injuries, if any. The most widely used grading system for renal trauma is the American Association for the Surgery of Trauma (AAST) renal injury scale **(Table 5)**.[24]

Tumors

In recent years. there has been emphasis on the use of magnetic resonance imaging (MRI) for the staging and preoperative evaluation of renal masses.[25] However, contrast-

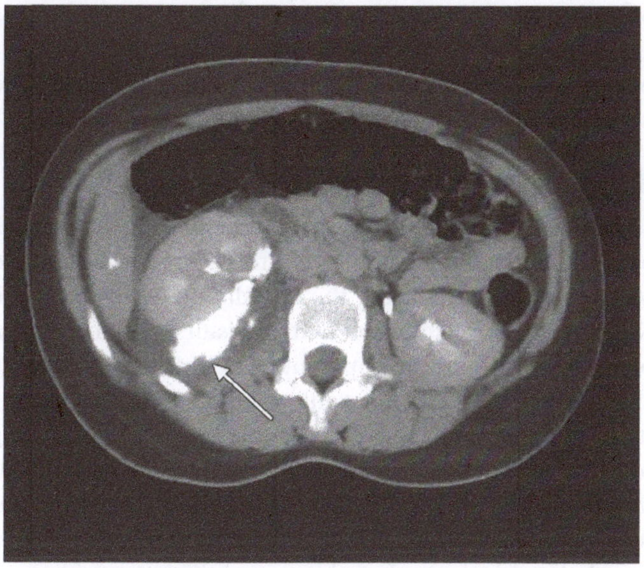

Fig. 21: Computed tomography (CT) scan in renal trauma. Postcontrast excretory phase CT scan of abdomen in a 9-year-old child with history of blunt trauma abdomen. Axial image at the level of the renal hilum shows a right pelviureteric junction injury leading to extravasation of contrast into the right perinephric space (arrow).

TABLE 5: American Association for the Surgery of Trauma (AAST) grading of renal injury.[24]

Grade	Description
Grade 1	• Subcapsular hematoma • Contusion
Grade 2	• Perirenal hematoma confined to Gerota fascia • Superficial laceration <1 cm depth not involving the collecting system (without urine extravasation)
Grade 3	• Laceration >1 cm without collecting system rupture or urinary extravasation • Vascular injury or active bleeding confined within perirenal fascia
Grade 4	• Laceration involving collecting system with urinary extravasation • Renal pelvis laceration and/or complete disruption of PUJ • Segmental vascular injury • Bleeding beyond Gerota's fascia into retroperitoneum or peritoneum
Grade 5	• Shattered kidney • Avulsion of renal hilum

(PUJ: pelviureteric junction)

enhanced multidetector CT is still widely used for this purpose due to greater availability, lower cost, and shorter scan times **(Fig. 22)**.

In children with malignancy, multiple follow-up imaging studies will be required. The cumulative radiation dose from such studies is significant. Hence, whenever possible MRI should be used in these children.

MAGNETIC RESONANCE IMAGING

In pediatrics, MRI is preferred over CT due to lack of ionizing radiation and inherent superior soft-tissue contrast.

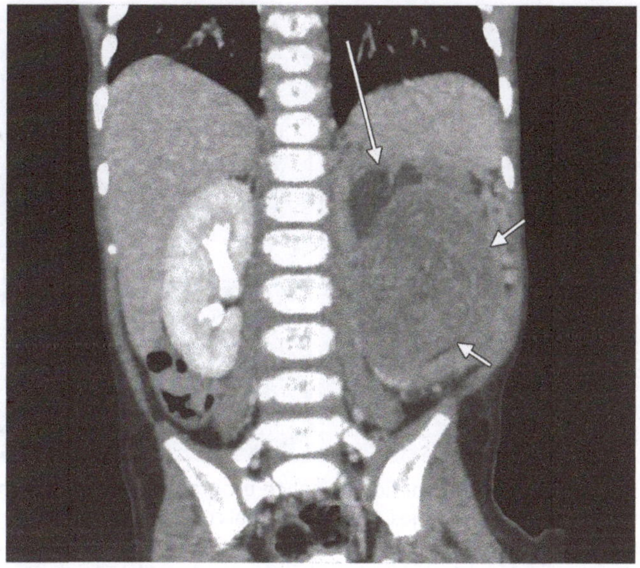

Fig. 22: Postcontrast computed tomography (CT) scan of abdomen in a 4-year-old child with palpable abdominal mass. Coronal CT image shows a large mass (short arrows) arising from the left kidney with pressure effect on the left collecting system (long arrow). This was a large Wilms' tumor.

Magnetic Resonance Urography

Magnetic resonance urography (MRU) permits anatomical and functional assessment of the urinary tract and kidneys.[26] In children, MRU is useful for the evaluation of suspected urinary tract obstruction, complex congenital anomalies of the urinary system, and preoperative planning **(Figs. 23A and B)**.

Magnetic resonance urography includes anatomic imaging of the abdomen and pelvis which permits morphological assessment of the renal parenchyma and urinary tracts. This is followed by functional imaging obtained after injection of IV contrast.[27]

In patients with suspected renal impairment, prior to administration of gadolinium-based contrast agents, glomerular filtration rate (GFR) needs to estimated. Although there are no pediatric-specific guidelines,[28] it is recommended that as per adult guidelines gadolinium should not be administered in those with estimated GFR (eGFR) < 30 mL/min,[29] and high-risk gadolinium agents should be avoided in children.

Postcontrast dynamic images allow determination of differential renal function. Using postprocessing techniques, renal parenchymal contrast uptake and excretion can be quantified. However, this entire set of anatomical and functional images need not be obtained in every patient. The MRU study needs to be tailored on a patient-to-patient basis depending on the specific clinical question to be answered.

Most often, MRU is used in problematic cases where other imaging modalities such as ultrasound and MCU have failed to provide sufficient information needed for treatment planning.

Magnetic Resonance Imaging in Oncology

Magnetic resonance imaging is increasingly being used in pediatric oncology due to lack of ionizing radiation, excellent

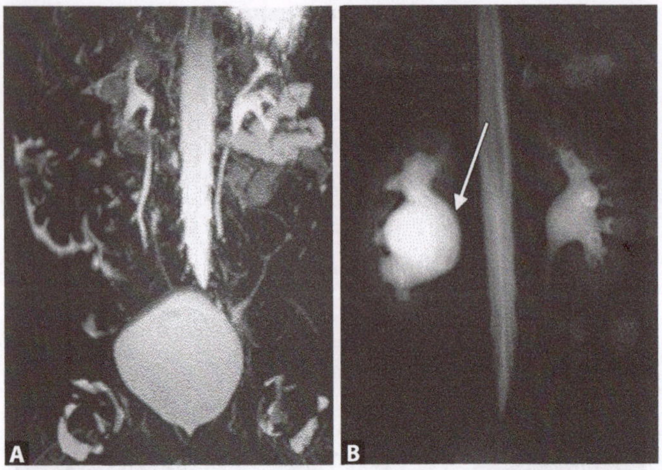

Figs. 23A and B: Magnetic resonance urography—3D maximum intensity projection images. (A) Normal renal collecting system, ureter, and bladder are demonstrated on both sides; (B) There is marked dilatation of the right pelvicalyceal system with a dilated extrarenal pelvis (arrow) suggestive of a right pelviureteric junction obstruction. Normal left collecting system and left ureter are seen.

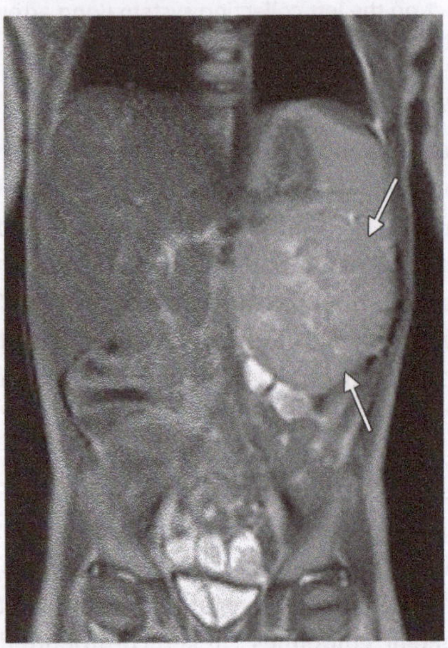

Fig. 24: Magnetic resonance imaging in oncology. Coronal T2-weighted image in a 2-year-old child shows a large heterogeneous mass (arrows) in the left upper quadrant. This was an extra-adrenal neuroblastoma.

soft-tissue resolution, and multiplanar capabilities[30] **(Fig. 24)**. The disadvantages of MRI include high cost, relatively long examination time, and image degradation due to motion artifact. Sedation/general anesthesia is usually needed in young children undergoing MRI studies.[31] Patients older than 8 years generally cooperate and tolerate MRI.

Magnetic resonance imaging is a valuable tool in the assessment of benign and malignant pediatric renal masses. It is useful for the characterization of renal lesions, to detect extracapsular spread, to demonstrate presence of metastatic lesions, and to assess for vascular invasion.

Magnetic resonance imaging of the abdomen may also be performed as part of whole-body MRI for the management of pediatric malignancies.[32] MRI offers a radiation-free alternative to CT for diagnosis, staging, and monitoring; this is particularly relevant in young children with malignancies who need to undergo serial long-term follow-up examinations.

CONCLUSION

The clinical history and physical examination are the bedrock over which the edifice of imaging rests. For the building to be strong and purposeful, the foundation has to be good. Never ever let go of the fact that one is first and foremost a physician. Nothing can supplant clinical analysis. Imaging and laboratory data are there only to supplement that process. It is imperative that the clinician decides on the imaging protocol in consultation with the radiologist to sort out the issue at hand. Remember, it is the clinical presentation that necessitates the imaging protocol and it is the clinical correlation that determines the diagnostic outcome.

In the realm of pediatrics, an aphorism that has been stated ad nauseam is this "children are not little adults". This basic self-evident truth seldom sinks in. If you wish to comprehend imaging and make astute judgments based on it, then one has to be conversant with the pathology and pathophysiology of the disease processes that are peculiar to that group. This is a sine qua non for success in clinical imaging.

KEY POINTS

- Ultrasound is the primary imaging modality in the evaluation of urinary tract in children.
- Use of appropriate ultrasound technique and accurate assessment of renal size is of utmost importance.
- In neonates, the renal cortex can be of increased echogenicity (compared to the liver or spleen), particularly in premature infants.
- MCU is indicated in children for the assessment of recurrent UTI, evaluation of VUR, and suspected PUVs.
- MCU is a morphodynamic study. One must remember that it is not a physiological test and it is not advisable to use this test to determine post-void residue.
- In pediatric urology, indications for CT include urolithiasis, renal trauma, renal artery stenosis, and renal tumors.
- Children are more sensitive to the deleterious effects of ionizing radiation; hence, caution is to be exercised when performing a CT. Wherever possible, radiation-free alternative imaging modalities are to be used.
- MRI is being increasingly used in pediatrics due to the lack of ionizing radiation and excellent soft-tissue resolution

REFERENCES

1. Culligan J. Renal stones permeable to the X-ray. Radiology. 1924;2:411-3.
2. Hindryckx A, De Catte L. Prenatal diagnosis of congenital renal and urinary tract malformations. Facts Views Vis Obgyn. 2011;3(3):165-74.

3. Cremin BJ. Real time ultrasonic evaluation of the paediatric abdomen: technique and anatomical variations. A personal view. BJR. 1985;58:859-68.
4. Fernbach SK, Feinstein KA. Normal findings and anatomical variants of kidney. In: Kuhn JP, Slovis TL, Haller JO (Eds). Caffey's Pediatric Diagnostic Imaging, 10th edition. Philadelphia, PA: Mosby Publications; 2004.
5. Kim BW, Song MK, Chung S, Kim KS. Evaluation of kidney size in children: a pilot study of renal length as a surrogate of organ growth. Korean J Pediatr. 2012;55(2):54-7.
6. Kim JH, Kim MJ, Lim SH, Kim J, Lee MJ. Length and volume of morphologically normal kidneys in Korean children: ultrasound measurement and estimation using body size. Korean J Radiol. 2013;14(4):677-82.
7. Garel L, Pariente D. Ultrasound in pediatric nephrology. In: Kalifa G (Ed). Pediatric Ultrasonography. Springer, Berlin, Heidelberg; 1986.
8. Willi UV. Hydronephrosis and hydroureter in a child, In: Nash DCH, Pettersson H (Eds). NICER Series on Diagnostic Imaging. Pediatric Radiology. Merit Communications; 1992.
9. Ruzal-Shapiro C. Neonatal hydronephrosis. In: Haller JO (Ed). Textbook of Neonatal Ultrasound, 1st edition. New York: Parthenon Publishing Group; 1998.
10. Riccabona M, Avni FE, Blickman JG, Dacher J-N, Darge K, Lobo ML, et al. Imaging recommendations in paediatric uroradiology: minutes of the ESPR workgroup session on urinary tract infection, fetal hydronephrosis, urinary tract ultrasonography and voiding cystourethrography, Barcelona, Spain, June 2007. Pediatr Radiol. 2008;38:138-45.
11. Subcommittee on Urinary Tract Infection. Reaffirmation of AAP clinical practice guideline: the diagnosis and management of the initial urinary tract infection in febrile infants and young children 2–24 months of age. Pediatrics. 2016;138(6):e20163026.
12. Vijaykumar M. Indian Society of Pediatric Nephrology revised statement on management of urinary tract infections. Indian Pediatr. 2011;48:709-17.
13. Mazzi S, Rohner K, Hayes W, Weitz M. Timing of voiding cystourethrography after febrile urinary tract infection in children: a systematic review. Arch Dis Child. 2020;105(3): 264-9.
14. Maskell R, Pead L, Vinnicombe J. Urinary infection after micturating cystography. Lancet. 1978;2:1191-2.
15. McAlister WH, Cacciarelli A, Shackelford GD. Complications associated with cystography in children. Radiology. 1974;111: 167-72.
16. Al-Imam OA, Al-Nsour NM, Al-Khulaifat S. Which is the best way of performing a micturating cystourethrogram in children? Saudi J Kidney Dis Transpl. 2008;19(1):20-5.
17. Brody AS, Frush DP, Huda W, Brent RL, American Academy of Pediatrics Section on Radiology. Radiation risk to children from computed tomography. Pediatrics. 2007;120:677-82.
18. Strohmaier WL. Imaging in pediatric urolithiasis—what's the best choice? Transl Pediatr. 2015;4(1):36-40.
19. Gupta A, Castellan M. Use of computed tomography (CT) for urolithiasis in pediatric patients. Transl Pediatr. 2015;4(1):33-5.
20. Orman G, Masand PM, Kukreja KU, Acosta AA, Guillerman RP, Jadhav SP. Diagnostic sensitivity and specificity of CT angiography for renal artery stenosis in children. Pediatr Radiol. 2021;51:419-26.
21. Kawashima A, Sandler C, Corl F, Clark West O, Tamm E, Fishman E, et al. Imaging of renal trauma: a comprehensive review. Radiographics. 2001;21:557-74.
22. Szmigielski W, Kumar R, Al Hilli S, Ismail M. Renal trauma imaging: diagnosis and management. A pictorial review. Pol J Radiol. 2013;78:27-35.
23. Fernandez-Ibieta M. Renal trauma in pediatrics: a current review. Urology. 2018;113:171-8.
24. Kozar RA, Crandall M, Shanmuganathan K, Zarzaur BL, Coburn M, Cribari C, et al. Organ injury scaling 2018 update: spleen, liver, and kidney. J Trauma Acute Care Surg. 2018;85(6):1119-22.
25. Smith EA, Dillman JR. Current role of body MRI in pediatric oncology. Pediatr Radiol. 2016;46(6):873-80.
26. Darge K, Anupindi S, Jaramillo D. MR imaging of the abdomen and pelvis in infants, children and adolescents. Radiology. 2011;261(1):12-29.
27. Morin CE, Mcbee MP, Trout AT, Reddy PP, Dillman JR. Use of MR urography in pediatric patients. Curr Urol Rep. 2018;19(11):93.
28. Weller A, Barber JL, Olsen ØE. Gadolinium and nephrogenic systemic fibrosis: an update. Pediatr Nephrol. 2014;29:1927-37.
29. Schlaudecker JD, Bernheisel CR. Gadolinium-associated nephrogenic systemic fibrosis. Am Fam Physician. 2009;80(7): 711-4.
30. Canale S, Vilcot L, Ammari S, Lemery M, Bidault F, Dalleyguier C, et al. Whole body MRI in paediatric oncology. Diag Interv Imaging. 2014;95(6):541-50.
31. Slovis TL. Sedation and anesthesia issues in pediatric imaging. Pediatr Radiol. 2011;41(Suppl. 2):514-6.
32. Goo HW. Regional and whole-body imaging in pediatric oncology. Pediatr Radiol. 2011;41:186-94.

CHAPTER

2.4

Radioisotope Imaging

Thirumurthi K

INTRODUCTION

Nuclear medicine techniques have now become one of the main modalities in the early diagnosis and follow-up of renal diseases in children.[1,2] They are sensitive in early detection of disease before anatomical changes are seen. Radioisotope studies provide functional and to a certain extent anatomic information with acceptable radiation exposure as compared to conventional radiology. They can be used in all pediatric age groups, in severely ill children, and also in patients with renal insufficiency. The radiopharmaceuticals are not toxic nor do they cause any allergic reaction and are isotonic. They do not cause or aggravate renal dysfunction.[2,3]

In nuclear imaging, usually a gamma ray emitting isotope is administered orally or parenterally. The radioactive substance is administered as such or it is tagged to a particular vehicle or transporting agent and administered into the body. It is carried to the organ of interest by the bloodstream. It gets distributed in the organ and emits gamma rays. The distribution of isotope (thereby its radioactivity) in an organ of interest is then mapped out by a gamma camera.

Similar to X-ray tomography (CT scan), the gamma camera can also be rotated around the patient and sectional images can be obtained. This procedure, known as SPECT (single-photon emission tomography), is particularly useful in studying renal scars, myocardial perfusion, cerebral perfusion, etc.

Technetium-99m (^{99m}Tc) is the radioisotope used widely.[4] It is combined with pharmaceuticals to study renal perfusion, filtration rate, and drainage pattern. It is very useful to detect acute pyelonephritis and scars if any.

RADIOPHARMACEUTICALS

- *DTPA (diethylenetriaminepentaacetic acid):* This chelating agent is solely filtered by the glomerulus and has similar properties to inulin. It has high extraction efficiency. Hence, it is the common choice for dynamic renal study (also called renogram).
- *MAG3 (mercaptoacetylglycylglycylglycine):* It is filtered by the glomerulus and also excreted by the tubules and is similar to iodohippurate. It has higher extraction efficiency than DTPA and is ideally suited for immature infant kidney evaluation and for poor-functioning kidneys. It is the ideal choice for a renogram.
- *EC (ethylene dicysteine):* It has all the properties of MAG3 and has the same very high extraction efficiency from the blood by the kidneys. It is produced in the country and less expensive than MAG3.
- *GHA (glucoheptonate):* It is both filtered and secreted by the tubules. There is retention of trace by the tubules. It is useful as a pelvicalyceal imaging agent (renogram), and the late images delineate cortical lesions.
- *DMSA (dimercaptosuccinic acid):* It is concentrated in the renal tubules and late image gives excellent images of the cortex. It is highly useful to determine relative function and define areas of inflammation and the scars.[5,6]

IMAGING TECHNIQUE

Preparation of Patient

No special preparation is required. Good hydration is essential for error-free renogram. Sedation may be necessary, especially in small children, to make them sleep to avoid movement. It is better to delay radioisotope studies for at least 24 hours after intravenous contrast administration by radiological procedures. Intravenous contrast administration will result in reduced renal uptake and prolonged transit time, and hence at least 24 hours should elapse between intravenous urogram (IVU) and dynamic nuclear scan. Hydration is important before the procedures. Either oral fluids or intravenous fluids can be given.

TECHNIQUES: RENOGRAM (DYNAMIC STUDY)

Dynamic imaging is performed most often with ^{99m}Tc-DTPA, ^{99m}Tc-MAG3, or ^{99m}Tc-EC. The tracers are rapidly cleared, and hence a continuous dynamic imaging (data acquisition) is carried out. Following a bolus intravenous injection of the radiopharmaceutical, continuous imaging is carried out for at least 20 minutes. The images that are obtained provide information relating to renal vascularity, renal function, and excretion. The first 30–60 seconds provide a vascular information of the major blood vessels and perfusion to kidneys, liver, and spleen. The amount of radioactivity at each kidney shows the relative vascularity. The tracer concentration in each kidney for about 2–4 minutes determines the function of the kidneys. Thereafter, cortical activity rapidly diminishes as the tracer is excreted by glomerular filtration or tubular secretion into the pelvis and ureters. To evaluate a dilated drainage system from an obstructed system, furosemide is administered to increase the hydrostatic pressure to determine drainage. There are three recognized protocols:

1. *F-15:* Furosemide is injected 15 minutes before the start of the study.
2. *F-0:* Furosemide is injected at the beginning of the study.
3. *F+15:* Furosemide is injected 15 minutes after the start of the study.

Postvoid images when possible are always acquired. Delayed images (1 hour to sometimes longer) are done to visualize poor-functioning kidneys and also to define the level and degree of obstruction.

Hydration

Good hydration before the study is essential to evaluate the excretory phase of renogram. Dehydration prolongs the excretory phase of renogram and may appear falsely as obstruction.

Bladder Drainage

Continuous bladder drainage in routine renogram is a controversy. Most centers avoid bladder drainage as good hydration and faster excreting traces such as MGG3 and EC are available. Bladder drainage is not required in cases in which simple upper tract obstruction is suspected, particularly when the ultrasound examination does not identify ureteric dilation. It is mandatory that children who can void on command should void before the commencement of the study. Bladder drainage may be necessary in evaluation of lower urinary tract dilation/obstruction.

ECTOPIC KIDNEY

In the presence of an ectopic kidney, the total and relative function estimation will be underestimating the function of the ectopic kidney in renogram. A ^{99m}Tc-DMSA scan with both posterior and anterior views is useful in such cases. Drainage may be difficult to assess in the dynamic study if the kidney lies close to the bladder. Postvoid images are useful.

STATIC IMAGING

Renal images are usually obtained 2–3 hours following intravenous injection of ^{99m}Tc-DMSA. Since rapid loss of tracer does not occur, several views of the kidneys can be obtained, including SPECT imaging. The static renal images obtained provide good definition of the cortical outline and, in addition, show the relative distribution of functional tissue. The ratio of tracer uptake between kidneys provides a measure of relative renal function.

RENOGRAM CURVE

The renogram curve is a time-activity curve depicting the blood flow, tracer concentration, intrarenal transit, and excretion from the kidney. The curve is obtained by drawing region of interest (ROI) over the whole kidneys or only cortex and/or only pelvis. The radioactivity or the counts in the ROI for each period of data acquisition and plotting these counts as a function of time. The renogram curve typically shows three phases: (1) *Vascular phase:* 0–1 minute shows the rapid tracer arrival in kidney and its exit through vascular channels. (2) *Uptake phase:* 2–4 minutes denote the tracer concentration in the glomerulus and tubules. The peak of the curve is a point where the excretion exceeds the input to the kidneys. (3) *Excretory phase:* This shows the drainage pattern in front of the kidney/pelvis. Normally, the intrarenal transit time is measured from the tracer entering the kidney till the tracer arrives in the pelvis. This is a useful parameter to decide the function and drainage. It is less than 5 minutes with DTPA and 2–4 minutes with faster clearing agents such as MAG3 or EC. Normal differential or relative function is usually defined as a relative uptake from 50 to 56/44 as normal and ≥60/40 as abnormal.

The excretory part of the curve depicts drainage from the kidney/pelvis. One of the simplest quantitative parameters to measure drainage is measuring the halftime (T1/2) of excretion. A T1/2 < 10 minutes is considered normal, a T1/2 between 10 and 20 minutes is considered indeterminate, and a T1/2 of >20 minutes is likely caused by an obstruction. Interpretation of T1/2 should be done with evaluation of the dynamic images, hydration, and other quantitative factors.

The relative function, excretory T1/2, and the intrarenal transit time of tracers are ideal in following pelviureteric junction (PUJ) obstructed kidneys.

CLINICAL APPLICATIONS

The glomerular filtration rate (GFR) is low in newborn period and preterm babies. The tracer concentration is low in the early period of life due to immature nephrons. Radionuclide studies done after 6 weeks of postnatal life give better results. Renal uptake of radioisotope will be lower, intrarenal transit time longer, and excretion slower in the newborn compared to older children. Measurement of total GFR is accurate with blood sampling methods using ^{99m}Tc-DTPA or Cr-EDTA.

URINARY TRACT INFECTIONS

To assess renal involvement in urinary tract infection (UTI), all young children should have a DMSA scan for assessing acute renal injury or renal scars and if necessary a micturating cystourethrogram (MCU) and direct radionuclide cystogram (DRCG) done to rule out vesicoureteral reflux (VUR). DMSA scan will show focal cold or photopenic areas **(Figs. 1 and 2)** with or without enlarged kidneys in acute pyelonephritis. Sensitivity and specificity of the test is >95%. The defects may be single or multiple. The upper and lower poles are usually affected. Rarely there may be diffuse decreased uptake in the affected kidney. All defects should be followed for at least 6 months to determine if the inflammation is healed with no significant scarring. Scarring reduces renal function; scars are permanent defects associated with loss of cortical volume appearing as cortical thinning, flattening, or a

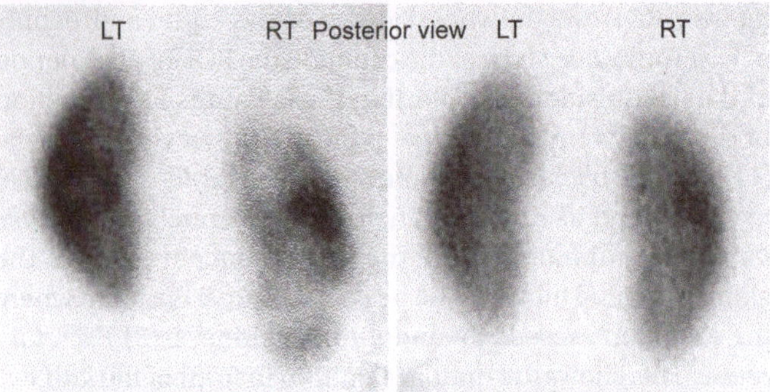

Fig. 1: Dimercaptosuccinic acid (DMSA) showing right pyelonephritis and resolution after treatment. (LT: left; RT: right)

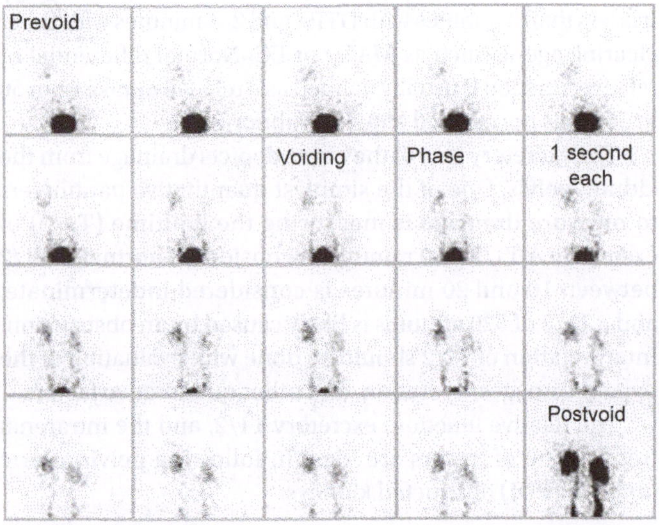

Fig. 2: Voiding direct cystogram with bilateral vesicoureteral reflux (VUR).

wedge-shaped defect. Transient photopenic areas due to acute infection resolve with treatment but untreated/unhealed areas appear as scars. Fetal lobulations, cysts, and splenic impression cause contour alterations. MCU is the gold standard for detecting VUR. DRCG is more sensitive than MCU. DRCG is carried out after bladder catheterization and filling bladder with radiotracer. Images are obtained continuously during filling and, if possible, during voiding. VUR can be detected both during filling and voiding or only in one phase. The disadvantage in DRCG is accurate grading, and delineation of urinary tract anatomy is not possible. A simpler method is to inject the isotope by suprapubic bladder puncture, which is the procedure, followed in most centers and avoids bladder catheterization.

HYDRONEPHROSIS AND OBSTRUCTION

Scintigraphy images vary depending on the type and severity of disease—site of obstruction and unilateral or bilateral pathology. PUJ and VUJ obstruction can be unilateral or bilateral. In bladder outlet obstruction such as posterior urethral valves (PUVs), there will be bilateral involvement. The hydronephrotic kidney in early images shows uptake in compressed or thinned-out cortex (directly related to functioning renal parenchyma) with pelvis appearing cold. The intrarenal transit is delayed. The pelvis later fills and drainage is delayed, and the degree of drainage depends upon the severity of obstruction. Detection of the severity and level of obstruction depends on adequate renal function. Diuretic renogram **(Fig. 3)** using furosemide (1 mg/kg) by one of the above-mentioned protocols is used for assessing PUJ obstruction. The F-15 method produces a good diuresis with fewer equivocal results. In functional obstruction, the radioactivity in the kidneys/pelvis is cleared after diuretic administration whereas in true obstruction it persists.

Output efficiency measured as a percentage of tracer excretion over 20 minutes from the input can also be used to measure obstruction. Normally, 80% tracer (MAG3 or EC) is cleared in 20 minutes. It is reduced in obstruction and in renal insufficiency. Antenatal diagnosed hydronephrosis may resolve over time. Serial measurements with sonography and renogram are required in follow-up of equivocal obstruction.

Indirect radionuclide voiding cystogram can also be done after DTPA or MAG3 renogram when the bladder is full and the child is ready to void, images being taken during voiding.

RENAL VASCULAR DISEASE

The prevalence of renovascular disease in selected groups of young hypertensive patients is at least 30%.

The baseline renogram may show that the affected kidney is small and has decreased perfusion and function. Renogram carried out post captopril administration is a useful screening test. A decrease in the function/GFR on the affected side of >10% post captopril is significant. A normal study rules out renovascular disease. It is also useful in assessment after intervention. In several centers, to avoid repetitive tests and reduce costs, the captopril test is done first and baseline study later only if the captopril study is abnormal. Parameters such as decreased renal uptake, increased cortical transit time, and retention in renal parenchyma are studied.

CONGENITAL ANOMALIES

Ectopic kidneys, fused kidneys, and horseshoe kidneys **(Fig. 4)** can be picked up easily with static DMSA scans, and their relative function of both kidneys including isthmus can be estimated. It should be noted that dilated mega ureters can be diagnosed; however, isotope studies are not useful in delineating other ureteral abnormalities such as double ureter and ectopic ureter.

ACUTE RENAL FAILURE

Renal scintigraphy has been used to predict recovery from acute tubular necrosis. Usually, appearance of renal uptake and excretion of isotope precede improvement in renal function.

ASSESSMENT OF GLOMERULAR FILTRATION RATE

^{51}Cr-EDTA has been used for estimation of GFR. It involves the use of a single dose of intravenous injection of the tracer

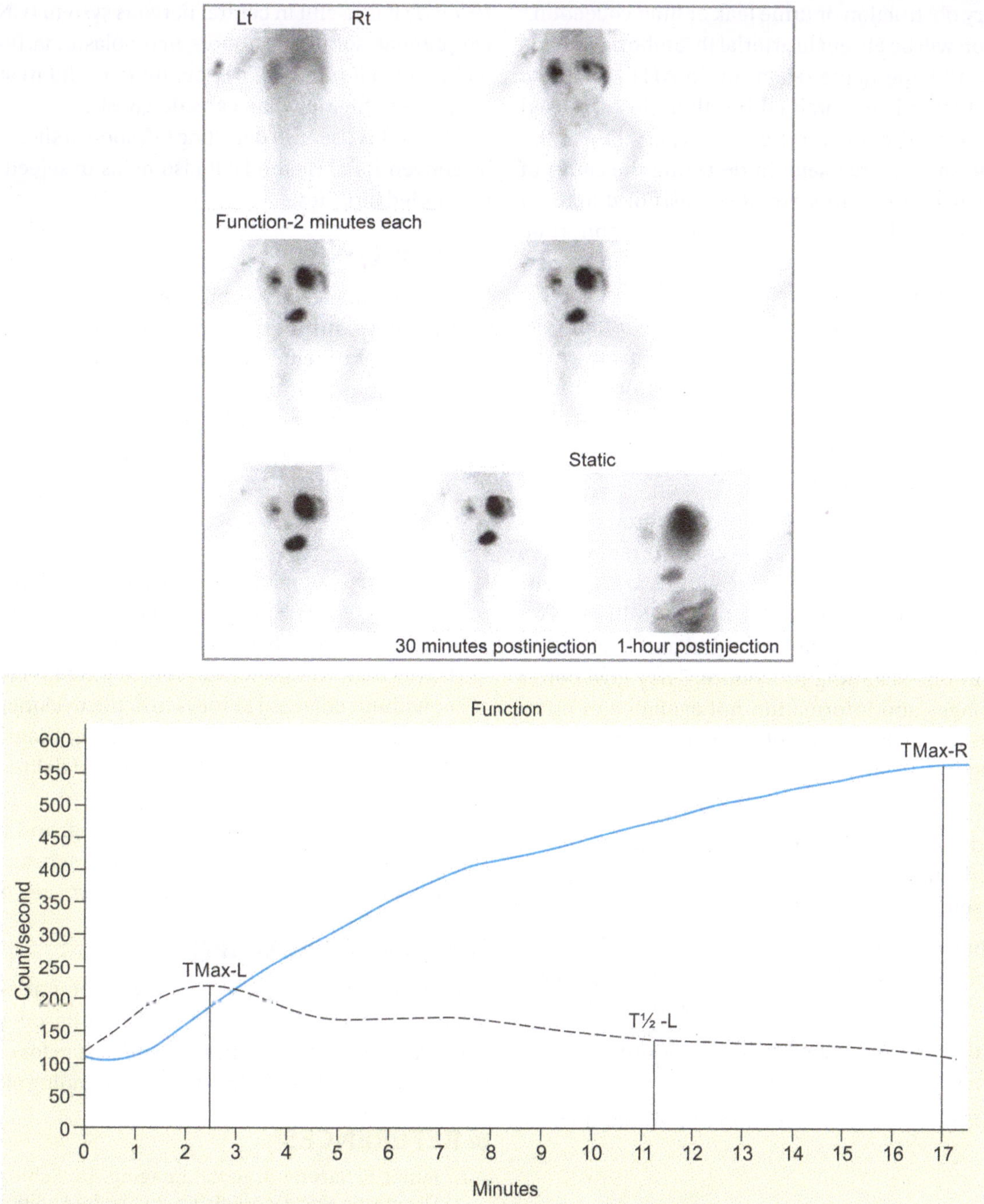

Fig. 3: Diuretic renogram showing right pelviureteric junction (PUJ) obstruction; renogram curve of same patient.

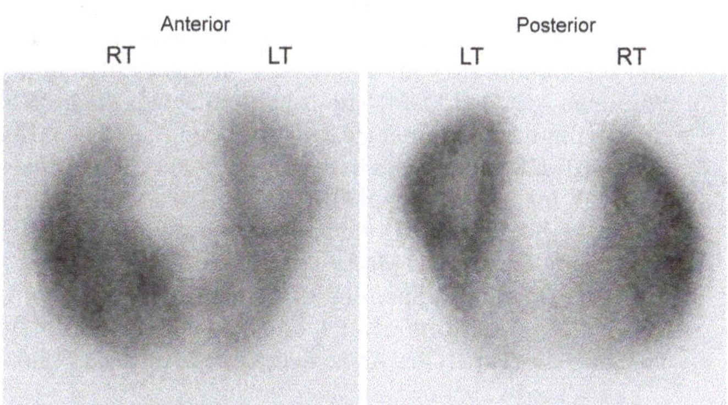

Fig. 4: Horseshoe kidney. (RT: right; LT: left)

followed by taking at least two blood samples at 2, 3, or 4 hours. External counting methods using ^{99m}Tc DTPA renogram images are not useful in children

EVALUATION OF RENAL TRANSPLANT (RENAL TX)

Radionuclide scans have a potential in evaluation of renal donors. In renal transplant recipients, it can be used to assess renal perfusion, assess the cause of renal dysfunction like acute tubular necrosis (ATN), rejection, damage due to immunosuppressive drugs, etc., and detect complications such as urinary obstruction or urine leak or fluid collection.[6] Renal perfusion will be absent in arterial thrombosis, venous thrombosis, and hyperacute rejection. In ATN and acute rejection, perfusion is maintained but there is decreased uptake and reduced concentration and excretion of the tracer. Isotope studies are useful in detecting the cause of obstruction, whether due to ureteral stenosis or due to an extraneous lymphocele. Urinary leak appears as abnormal tracer accumulation of tracer outside the transplant kidney, ureter, and bladder **(Fig. 5)**.

Isotope imaging methods have taken an important role, second only to ultrasonography, in pediatric renal practice. Isotope studies can identify parenchymal injury much before an anatomical abnormality sets in. Its availability and judicious usage help in prevention of renal damage, renal failure, dialysis, and transplant.

Positron emission tomography (PET) uses positron emitters resulting in dual photons. The positron emitting radiotracers are used as such or labeled to pharmaceuticals and used for imaging in a PET scanner which has a CT or MRI scanner in built with it. This gives both functional and anatomical information in one scanning procedure. They give better resolution images and information not available in other imaging modalities. The commonly used positron emitters are F-18, Ga-68, etc.

F-18: Fluorine 18 is a natural bone-seeking tracer and gives better resolution images than conventional bone scan with ^{99m}Tc methylene diphosphonate (MDP) and combining with CT it is more sensitive and specific.

FDG: F-18 labeled to glucose maps out regions of abnormal glucose utilizations. It is highly valuable in detecting primary tumors, detecting secondaries, and in evaluation of infection.

Fluorodopa: It is used in neuropsychiatric disorders and in detection of neuroendocrine tumors.

Ga-DOTANOC: It is used in detection of neuroendocrine tumors.

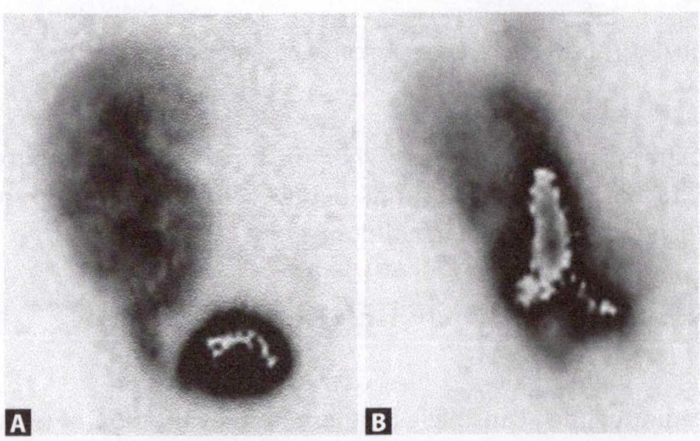

Figs. 5A and B: Normal Tx kidney, ureter, and bladder (A) and Tx kidney with urine leak (B).

PET/CT: It is useful in central nervous system (CNS) tumors, lymphomas, soft-tissue tumors, neuroblastoma, bone tumors, and germ cell tumors. They are more useful in staging, and response to therapy than early diagnosis.[7]

PET/CT is useful in detecting infection in sites not revealed by conventional methods. It also helps in selecting sites for CT-guided biopsies.

CONCLUSION

Nuclear medicine studies are noninvasive, not nephrotoxic, and provide subjective and objective information in management of renal disorders. They provide quantitative functional information making decisions easier in managing renal disease in the pediatric population. It is always advisable to correlate with clinical, biochemical, and anatomical studies for better understanding of nuclear imaging data.

KEY POINTS

- The relative function, excretory T1/2, and the intra renal transit time of tracers are ideal in following PUJ obstructed kidneys through dynamic renogram.
- DMSA scan will show focal cold or photopenic areas with or without enlarged kidneys in acute pyelonephritis.
- DRCG is more sensitive than MCU in diagnosing VUR but is not accurate in grading VUR and delineation of the urinary tract anatomy.
- PET/CT is useful in diagnosis, staging, and response to therapy in CNS tumors, lymphomas, soft-tissue tumors, neuroblastoma, bone tumors, and germ cell tumors.

ACKNOWLEDGMENTS

The author sincerely acknowledges the patients, all the scientific workers in the field, and web-based articles and teaching sites such as *www.auntMinnie.com* for contributing to enhancing the knowledge and understanding of the subject.

REFERENCES

1. Jamar F, Barone R. Renal imaging. In: Schiepers C (Ed). Diagnostic Nuclear Medicine, 2nd revised edition. New York: Springer; 2006.
2. Treves ST (Ed). Pediatric Nuclear Medicine/PET, 3rd edition. New York: Springer; 2007.
3. Bernier Donald R, Christian PE, Langan JK (Eds). Radioactive tracers: specific applications. In: Nuclear Medicine: Technology and Techniques, 3rd edition. St. Louis: Mosby; 1994.
4. Woolfson RG, Neild GM. The true clinical significance of renography in nephrourology. Eur J Nucl Med. 1997;24;557-70.
5. Hilson AJW. Radionuclides in the investigation of the urinary tract. BJU Int. 2000;86(Suppl 1):18-24.
6. Dubovsky EV, Russell CD. Radionuclide evaluation of renal transplants. Semin Nucl Med. 1988;18(3):181-98.
7. Kumar R, Shandal V, Shamim SA, Halanaik D, Malhotra A. Clinical applications of PET and PET/CT in pediatric malignancies. Expert Rev Anticancer Ther. 2010;10(5):755-68.

CHAPTER

2.5 Bladder Function Tests in Children

Vidhya T, Sripathi V

INTRODUCTION

The normal bladder functions as a reservoir to store urine at optimal pressure and when capacity is reached, voiding is initiated. Detrusor contraction with relaxation of urethral sphincter results in complete bladder emptying.

Normal bladder and urethral sphincter development and neural, volitional control over bladder-sphincter functions are essential for regulating lower urinary tract (LUT) function.[1] These maturation sequences are clinically evident by 5 years of age. In 17–22% of children, symptoms persist beyond 5 years of age resulting in LUT dysfunction. When LUT dysfunction (or LUTD) is associated with constipation, it is called bowel-bladder dysfunction (BBD). LUTD may lead to vesicoureteric reflux (VUR) and recurrent urinary tract infections (UTIs), thereby increasing the risk of renal scarring.

According to the International Children's Continence Society (ICCS), LUTD comprises overactive bladder, voiding postponement, underactive bladder, infrequent voiding, daytime-only urinary frequency, vaginal reflux, bladder neck dysfunction, and giggle incontinence.[2]

ASSESSMENT OF BLADDER FUNCTION

This includes a detailed clinical history, physical examination, bladder bowel diary, noninvasive investigations such as renal bladder ultrasound (RBUS) with postvoid measurement and uroflowmetry. Urodynamic study is invasive and a dynamic assessment of bladder function.

Clinical History

In children with bladder dysfunction, detailed history of symptoms and duration is vital. These include wetting, daytime voiding frequency, urgency, enuresis, holding maneuvers, stool frequency and consistency, and amount of water intake.

Physical Examination

The child is examined for distended bladder, palpable feculomas in the sigmoid, midline stigmata on the lumbosacral spine indicating occult spinal dysraphism, gluteal cleft asymmetry, anal canal laxity and a thorough lower limb neurological assessment.

Bladder Diary or Voiding Diary

Bladder diary is an objective record over a 7-day period of voided volume, voiding frequency, wetting, water intake, and stooling. In many instances, a review of the bladder diary will indicate the type and nature of the problem and will indicate appropriate and targeted investigations.[3]

Renal Bladder Ultrasound

RBUS is a noninvasive and readily available outpatient test, which plays an important role in determining upper tract status.

Renal Assessment

Imaging of kidney helps in identifying the following:

- Renal length and growth (5 cm at birth to 12 cm in adulthood)
- Corticomedullary differentiation, parenchymal thickness, cysts, and scarring
- Pelvicalyceal system and ureter (whether dilated or not)

Bladder Assessment

Transverse and longitudinal bladder scans will indicate turbidity of urine, wall thickness, postvoid residue, juxtavesical ureteral dilatation, and rectal diameter.

The normal bladder has a smooth contour. An irregular contour with a pear-shaped appearance is pathognomonic of a neurogenic bladder. The presence of sacculations and diverticulae is an indirect evidence of high bladder pressure.

Volume

Measurement of volume should be done in a full bladder. Length, transverse width, and anteroposterior depth are measured in centimeters and multiplied using a standard formula for measuring volume in an ellipsoid.

$$L \times D \times W \text{ (in cm)} \times 0.523$$

There are several formulae for bladder volume measurement. The simplest and easiest to remember is $(30 + 30X)$, where X is the age in years. This formula is applicable in children older than 2 years of age. In infants, the bladder capacity is calculated by the formula: (Age in months × 2.5 + 38).

As a rough rule, bladder capacity increases by 30 mL every year till 8 years of age.[4]

Wall Thickness

A thickened bladder wall indicates that the detrusor is working against resistance. This can be an anatomical obstruction like posterior urethral valve or a functional obstruction like a nonrelaxing external sphincter. The wall thickness can be accurately assessed only when the bladder is full. A normal bladder is <3 mm in thickness when full and <5 mm in thickness when empty.[5] This measurement of bladder wall thickness is very useful when assessing dysfunctional elimination.

Rectal Diameter

When imaged through a full bladder window (at the level of the ureteric orifices), a transverse rectal measurement of >3 cm indicates abnormal stool retention. This measurement is very important when assessing dysfunctional elimination.

Postvoid Residue

According to the ICCS[6] guidelines, any volume of urine remaining in the bladder is abnormal. However, on a practical basis, a residue of >10% of the expected bladder capacity for age is taken as abnormal. However, residue measurement should consider the following rules:

- It should be repeated as children are very capricious during voiding in a new environment.
- Residual assessment should be made within 5 minutes after voiding. At any time beyond this interval, 1–2 mL/min should be subtracted from the residual volume measurement to account for new urine production.

As a general rule in children 5 years or older, a residual volume of 20 mL or less is within normal limits.[5]

Micturating Cystourethrogram

Micturating cystourethrogram (MCU) is not routinely performed during assessment of bladder function. It is indicated in children in whom the posterior urethral valve or neurogenic bladder is suspected. It is also used to assess VUR in those with recurrent UTI and a scarred kidney (especially in those with BBD).

In a normal MCU, bladder has a smooth contour, normal urethral configuration, and no VUR **(Fig. 1)**.

Posterior urethral valve: Bladder contour is irregular with trabeculations or sacculations, dilated posterior urethra, narrow anterior urethral stream with or without VUR, and a hypertrophied bladder neck **(Fig. 2)**.

Neurogenic bladder: Bladder has an elongated irregular contour ("fir tree" appearance), with or without VUR. Voiding is incomplete (large residue). Vertebral anomalies are usually evident **(Fig. 3)**.

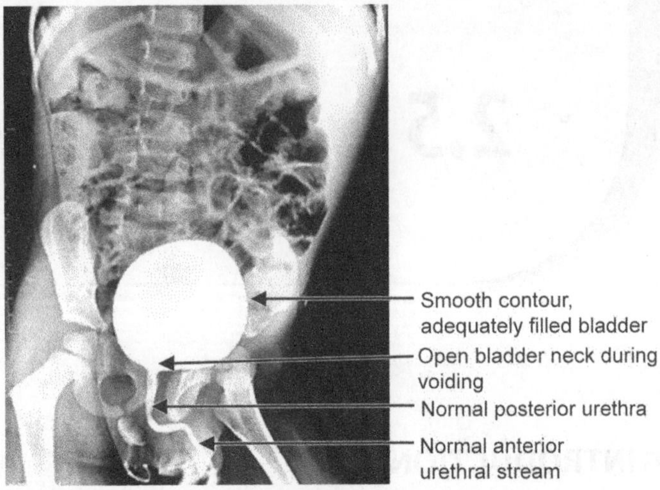

Fig. 1: Normal MCU showing smooth bladder contour, open bladder neck, normal urethral configuration, and urine stream. (MCU: micturating cystourethrogram)

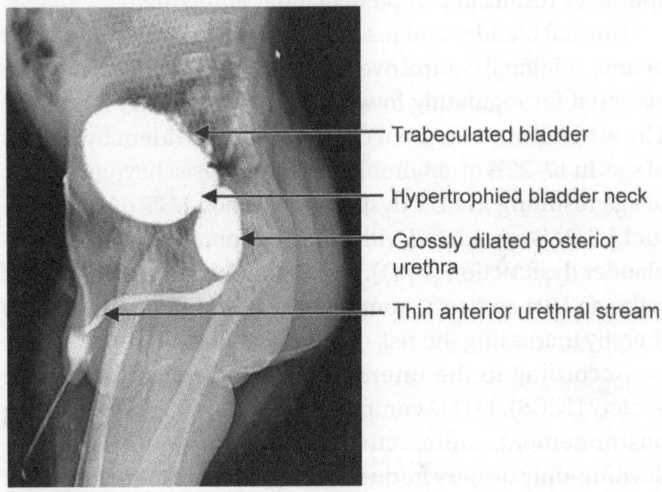

Fig. 2: MCU of a 3-month-old male child with PUV with bladder trabeculations, hypertrophied bladder neck, grossly dilated posterior urethra, thin anterior urethral stream, and no VUR. (MCU: micturating cystourethrogram; PUV: posterior urethral valve; VUR: vesicoureteric reflux)

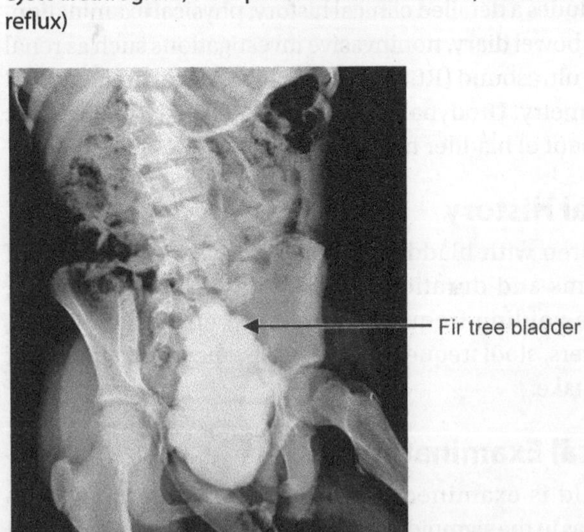

Fig. 3: Neurogenic bladder in a 12-year-old girl with lumbosacral vertebral segmentation errors MCU showing classic "fir tree" appearance. (MCU: micturating cystourethrogram)

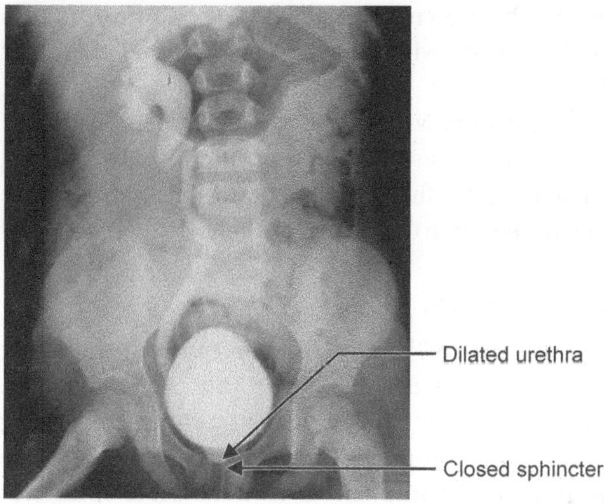

Fig. 4: MCU of a 6-year-old girl with voiding dysfunction showing the "spinning top bladder" indicating detrusor contraction against a closed external sphincter during voiding. Right-sided VUR grade 4 is seen. (MCU: micturating cystourethrogram; VUR: vesicoureteric reflux)

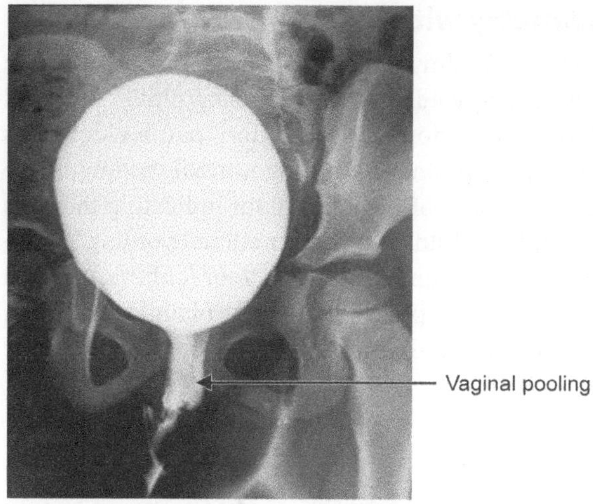

Fig. 5: MCU of a 7-year-old girl with voiding dysfunction. It shows normal bladder and urethra with vaginal pooling and left-sided grade 2 VUR. (MCU: micturating cystourethrogram; VUR: vesicoureteric reflux)

Voiding dysfunction: MCU in voiding dysfunction **(Figs. 4 and 5)** shows a near-normal bladder contour and dilated posterior urethra with closed external sphincter during voiding (spinning top configuration). As in neurogenic bladder disease, emptying is incomplete.

Uroflowmetry

Uroflowmetry is an outpatient procedure which assesses the rate of urine flow over time and the pattern of voiding. After voiding, ultrasound assessment of residual volume is an integral part of this study.

To perform uroflowmetry, the child should be above 5 years of age with the ability to hold and void urine on command. There are no defined indications for uroflowmetry. It can be used as an outpatient tool for any child whose stream is poor or who has dribbling (due to postvoid residue). It is used in the assessment and follow-up in bladder dysfunction and neurogenic bladder, for postoperative evaluation in PUV and hypospadias.

Procedure

A toilet-trained child with full bladder is asked to void in the uroflow commode and encouraged to relax. Older children are given privacy so that voiding is not inhibited. The voided volume, maximum rate of urine flow, time taken to void, and a graphical representation of all these values is obtained. Prevoid estimate of bladder fullness and postvoid estimate of bladder-emptying ability are mandatory. For meaningful results, a voided volume of more than 100 mL is essential.

The parameters of uroflowmetry are described here:

- Flow rate is defined as the volume of fluid expelled via the urethra per unit time (mL/sec).
- Voided volume is the total volume expelled via the urethra.
- Maximum flow rate (Q_{max}) is the maximum measured value of the flow rate after correction for artifacts.
- Average flow rate (Q_{ave}) is voided volume divided by the flow time. The average flow should be interpreted with caution if flow is interrupted or if there is a terminal dribble.
- Voiding time is the total duration of micturition (i.e., including interruptions). If voiding is completed without interruption, voiding time is equal to flow time.
- Flow time is the time over which measurable flow actually occurs.
- Time to maximum flow is the elapsed time from onset of flow to maximum flow.

According to ICCS recommendation, uroflowmetry curves are classified into five types: Bell, tower, plateau, staccato, and interrupted and they are described below:

- *Normal curve:* A normal void shows a "bell-shaped curve," as it gradually rises to a peak and then declines to reach the baseline. There are no "normal" numerical values for the "peak flow." If the square root of the "peak flow" value exceeds voided volume, then it is deemed normal for that child **(Fig. 6)**.
- *Tower curve:* The voiding curve reaches the peak instantly (named as supervoider). This is typically seen in children (especially girls) with severe urgency who are habituated to hold urine for prolonged periods of time.
- *Interrupted:* Voiding is accomplished by contraction of abdominal muscles. Small voids with a large postvoid residue characterizes "bladder atony" **(Fig. 7)**.
- *Staccato:* Voiding is interrupted by pelvic floor contraction causing dips in the uroflow curve.
- *Plateau curve:* This indicates voiding against resistance which can be organic (stricture) or functional (overactive sphincter). Void times are prolonged, peak uroflows are low, and postvoid residues are high.

Uroflowmetry with Electromyography

Uroflow with electromyography (EMG) recording of pelvic floor activity during voiding is called "uroflow EMG." To record pelvic floor contraction and relaxation, patch electrodes are placed on the perineum. During normal voiding, there is "complete silence" of the pelvic floor indicating that it is fully relaxed. In a child with "dysfunctional voiding," there is abnormal contraction of the pelvic floor (either sustained or intermittent) which prevents complete bladder emptying, thus creating a postvoid residual. This is called "dyssynergic voiding." Such dyssynergy is also pathognomonic of a neurogenic bladder with a denervated external sphincter (**Fig. 8**).

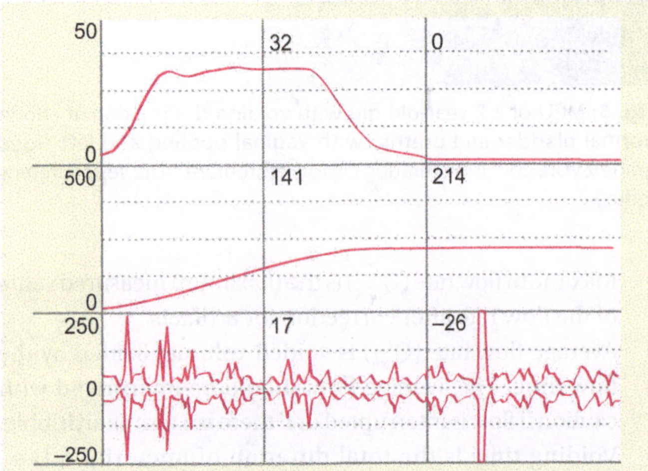

Fig. 6: A 14-year-old female child with recurrent urinary infections. Uroflow shows a "bell-shaped curve," good voided volume, good peak flow, nonactive external sphincter, and no postvoid residue.

The value of uroflow EMG is to graphically demonstrate to the parents and child as how voiding is inhibited by perineal muscle activity. Once this is understood, biofeedback can be instituted to overcome this abnormal behavior.[7]

Cystometrogram

Cystometrogram (CMG) is the study of pressure during filling and emptying phases of the bladder. In a normal bladder, pressure remains low during filling to capacity. During voiding, a detrusor contraction causes a sharp pressure rise and emptying is accomplished with complete sphincter relaxation (**Fig. 4**).

In any child with upper tract changes caused by a bladder abnormality, a cystometrogram study will be useful to find out the exact problem and treat it with either drugs or surgery. The usual conditions in which a CMG will be deemed useful include:

- Neurogenic bladder disease (caused by a myelomeningocele or occult tethering of the cord)
- Posterior urethral valve disease
- Prior to and following surgery for anorectal anomalies, Hirschsprung's disease, following surgery for cloacal anomaly, bladder exstrophy—epispadias
- Non-neurogenic bladder (with no obvious spinal cord abnormality)

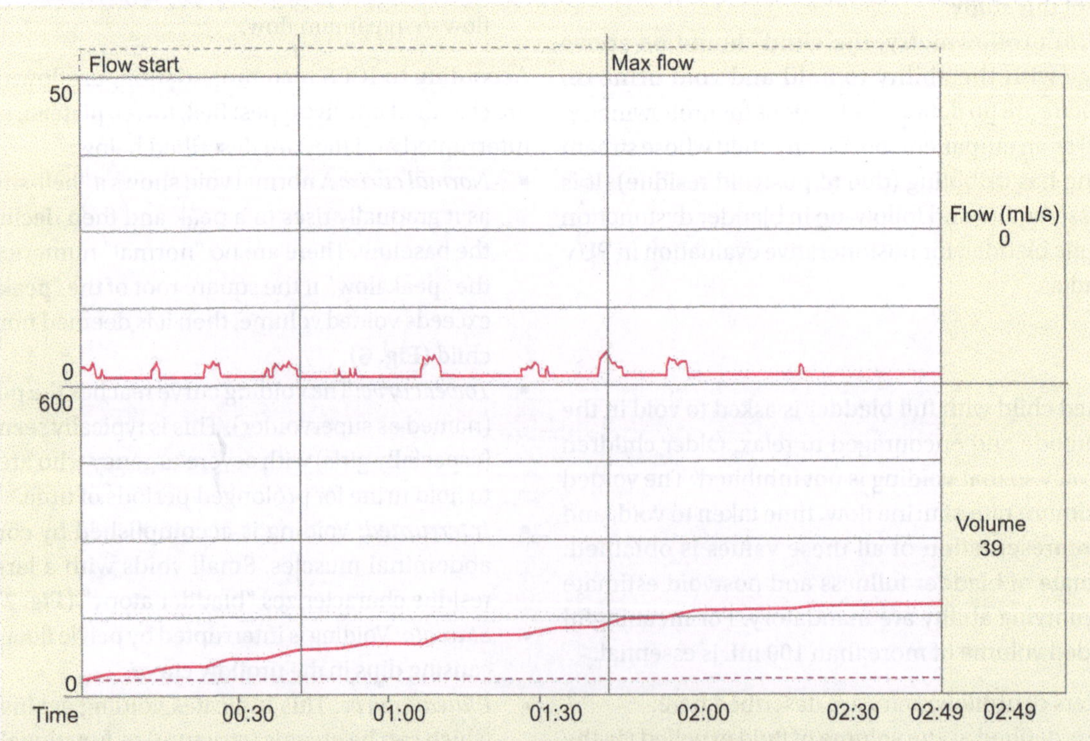

Fig. 7: A 10-year-old male child with urethra stricture showing an "interrupted flow pattern. Voiding by Valsalva results in small voids with intervals of no urine flow.

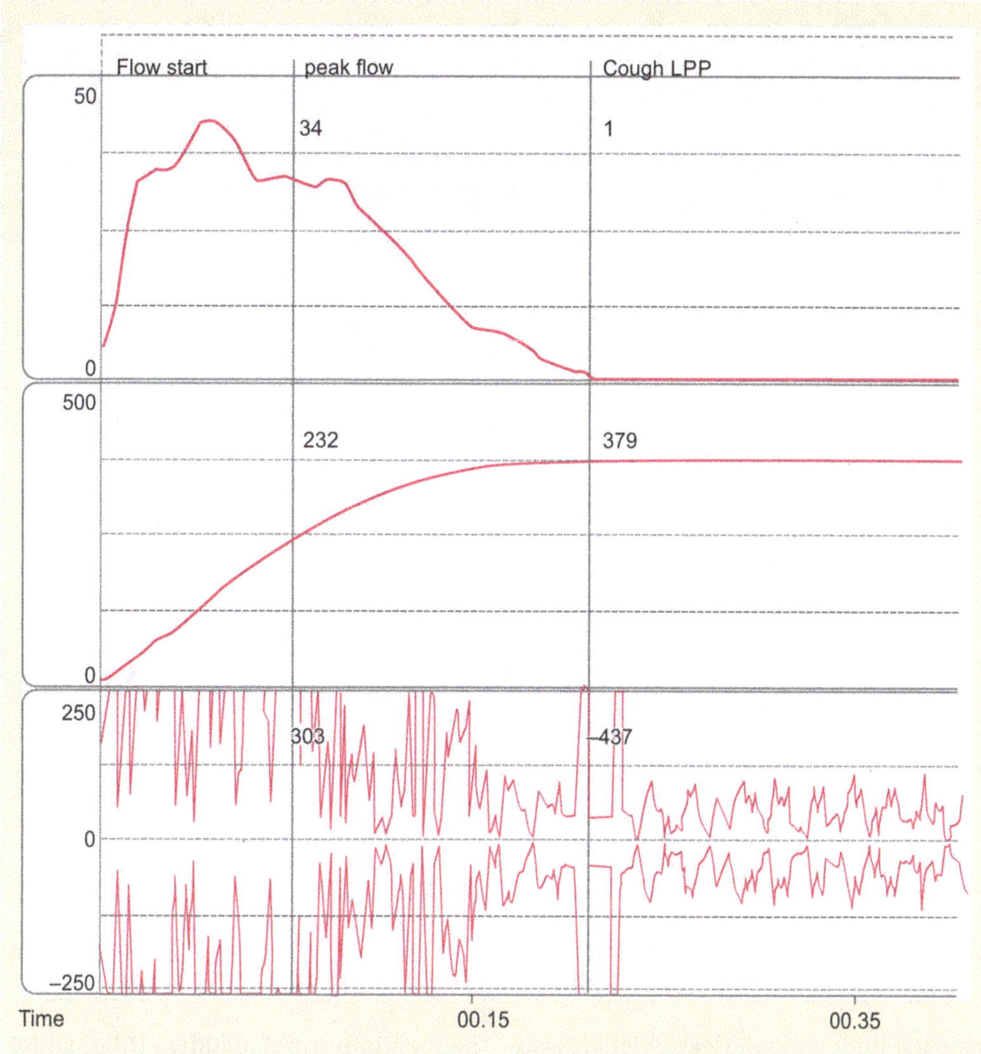

Fig. 8: Uroflow EMG in a 10-year-old female child presenting with recurrent urinary infections and wetting. EMG recording has picked up the pronounced sphincter activity during voiding contributing to a postvoid residue with wetting.

- Dysfunctional voiding
- Evaluation of the bladder prior to renal transplant

A complete clinical history and physical examination, sterile urine culture, RBUS with postvoid residual volume (PVR), MCU (to assess reflux status and grade) are the prerequisites prior to ordering urodynamic study.

Cystometrogram is an invasive test. Therefore, it should be not lightly ordered. Before requesting a CMG, it is useful to frame a clear question and then see if the test can provide the answer. For example, in a child with neurogenic bladder with sudden-onset wetting, the question should be: Have bladder pressures changed or is there dyssynergy between detrusor and sphincter? In a child with posterior urethral valves with worsening upper tracts, the question should be: is the bladder compliant?

Procedure

Under aseptic precaution, the bladder is catheterized with a double-lumen catheter of size 6 Fr/8 Fr (pressure, inflow). One lumen is used for filling the bladder and one for measuring pressure. A especially made catheter is inserted into the rectum to measure abdominal pressure. Normal saline is infused at a slow rate (5% of expected bladder capacity for age). The normal detrusor pressure should be <20 cmH_2O during filling phase. Once the child reports that he can no longer hold urine, he is instructed to void into the uroflow and voiding pressure is measured. After this, postvoid residue is estimated by ultrasound. If there is a leak during filling, the pressure at which it happens is noted.

Cystometrogram is a sophisticated real-time study and requires bedside monitoring by a knowledgeable physician. The study cannot be delegated to a technician as crucial events may be missed.

The following parameters are used when interpreting a CMG trace:

P_{ves} is the intravesical pressure measured by the bladder catheter, P_{abd} is the intra-abdominal pressure measured by the rectal catheter, and P_{det} is the mathematical value obtained

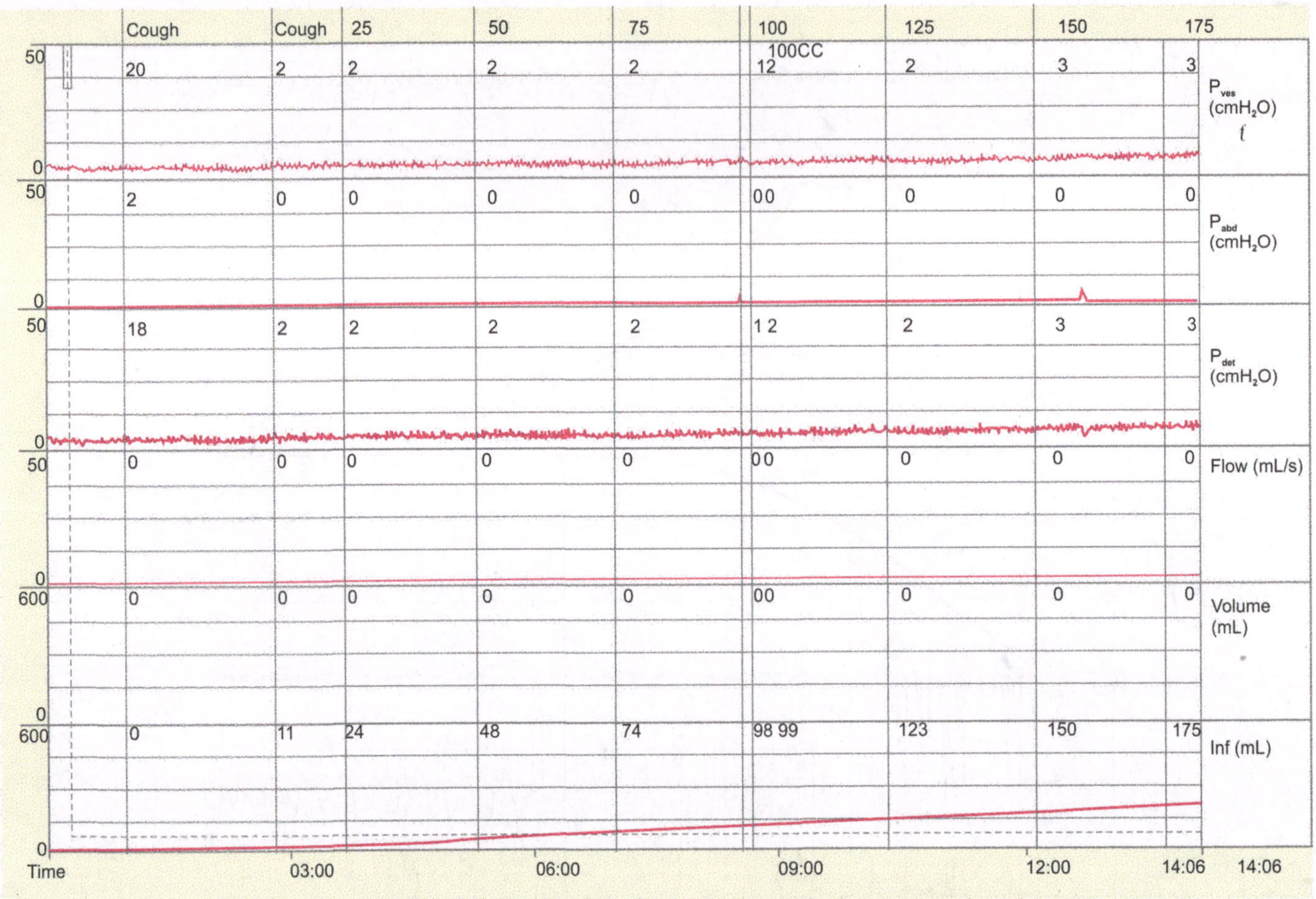

Fig. 9: Cystometrogram during bladder filling in a 3-year-old male child. Bladder pressure (P_{ves}), rectal pressure (P_{abd}), and detrusor pressure (P_{det}) are all within normal limits till bladder capacity is reached.

when P_{abd} is subtracted from P_{ves} and the leak point pressure is the bladder pressure at which pericatheter leak is noted

- *Normal urodynamic curve:* During the filling phase of bladder, detrusor pressure remains stable without undue pressure elevation or overactive contractions. The child is able to tolerate filling up to the expected bladder capacity for age **(Fig. 9)**.
- *Video CMG:* This is a urodynamic study performed after filling the bladder with contrast saline and with intermittent screening with a C-arm machine. This test is used in children with VUR. Fill volume and pressure are noted at the time of reflux. The information so obtained (low-pressure vs. high-pressure reflux) is used for decision-making.

COMMON URODYNAMIC ABNORMALITIES OBSERVED IN CHILDREN

Detrusor Overactivity

The detrusor contracts during filling leading to urgency. If the pressure generated by these detrusor contractions exceed 25 cmH_2O, the external sphincter undergoes a reflex relaxation (or is overcome) and wetting occurs. Overactivity can happen in normal bladders (idiopathic) or in those with neurogenic bladder disease. After urinary tract infections or in the presence of severe constipation, the bladder can exhibit irritability **(Fig. 10)**.

DETRUSOR SPHINCTER DYSSYNERGIA

This denotes failure of external sphincter relaxation during a strong detrusor contraction. This discordance does not allow complete bladder emptying and results in urinary residue (postvoid residue) which can be a cause of repeated UTI.

POOR COMPLIANCE

Compliance refers to the ability of the bladder to store urine at low pressures <15 cmH_2O during the filling phase. A bladder that shows progressive pressure rise with increase in fill volume is called a poorly compliant bladder. Filling pressures exceeding 25–30 cmH_2O are deleterious to the kidneys **(Fig. 11)**.

LEAK POINT PRESSURE

During filling, the external sphincter should be tightly closed. If there is leak (in the absence of detrusor overactivity), it means that either the sphincter is weak or the bladder

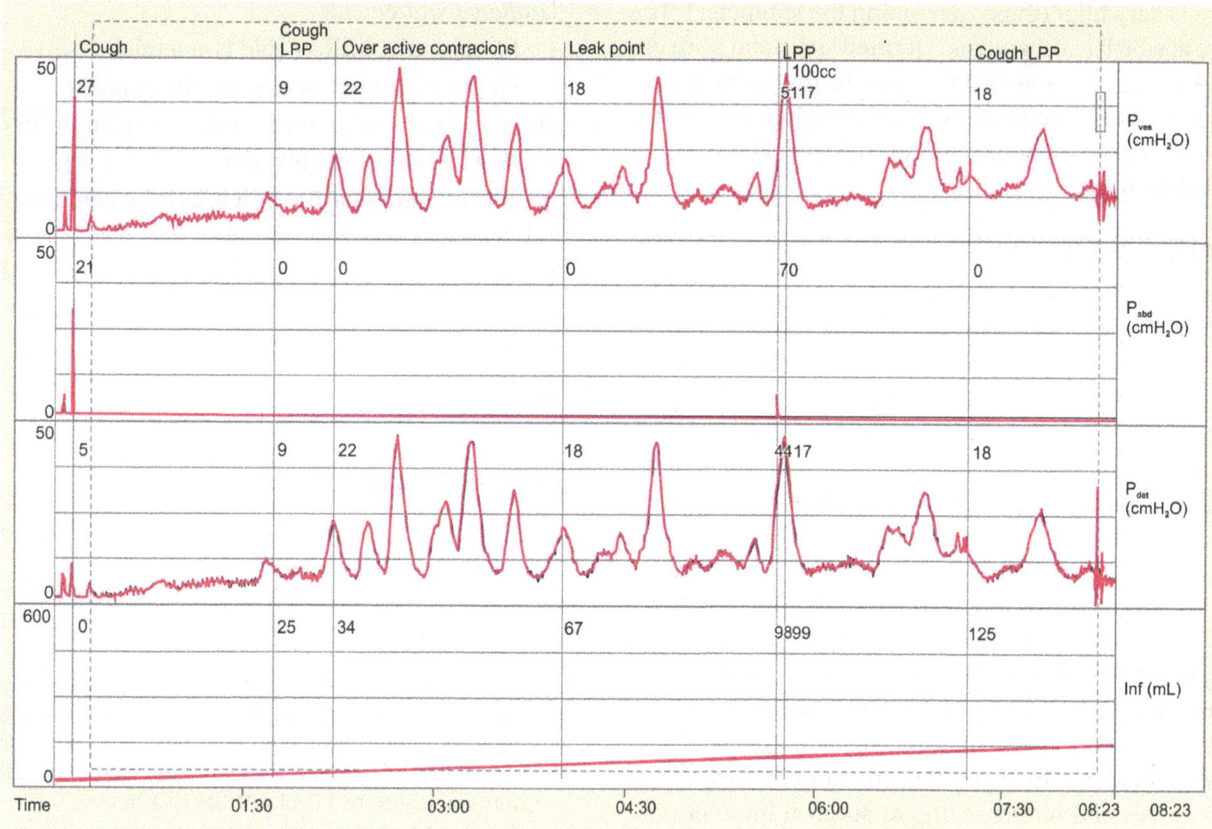

Fig. 10: Cystometrogram in an 11-year-old female presenting with wetting and urgency. The study shows pronounced detrusor overactivity (spikes in P_{ves} and P_{det}) warranting anticholinergic therapy.

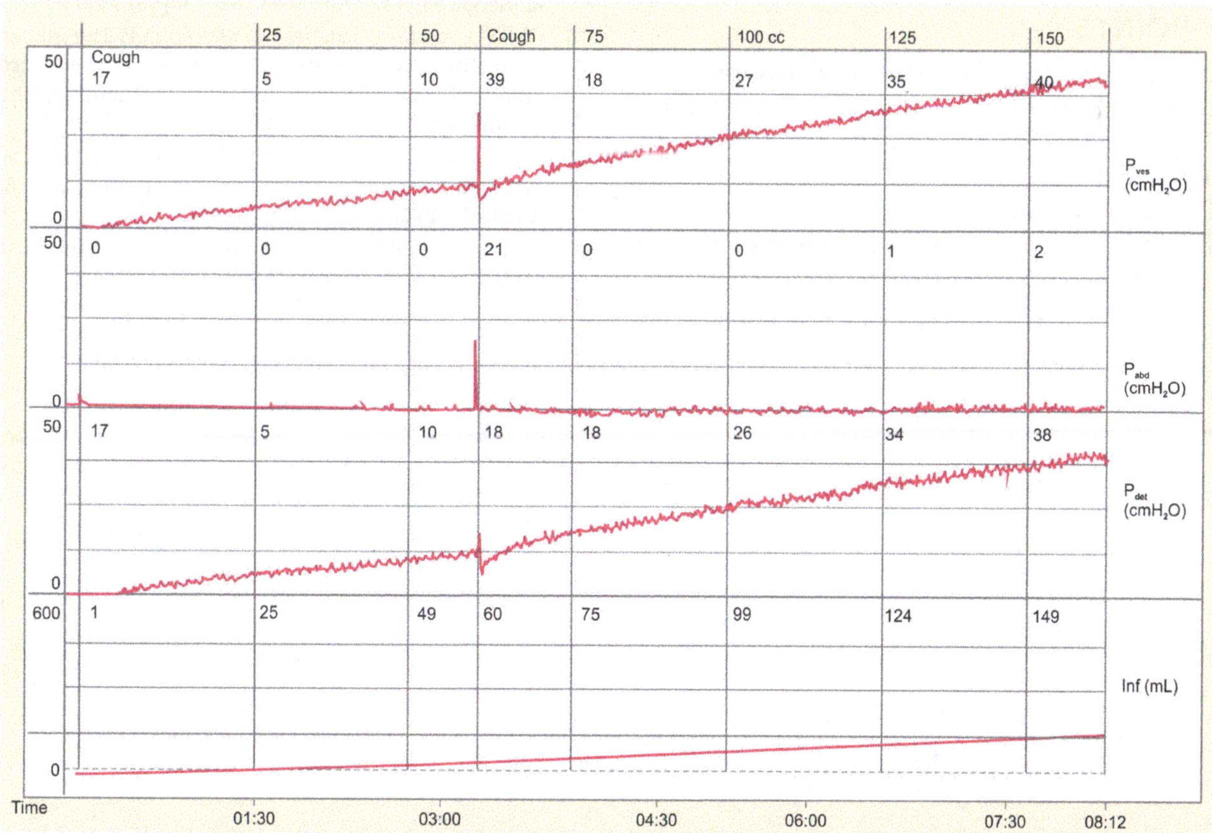

Fig. 11: Cystometrogram in a 9-year-old male child with neurogenic bladder. The P_{ves} and P_{det} traces show a linear pressure rise with filling indicating a severely "noncompliant bladder" needing augmentation cystoplasty.

pressure is very high (thus overcoming the sphincter). The pressure at which leak happens is termed leak point pressure (LPP). A high LPP is very damaging to the kidneys and usually mandates immediate surgical attention. Low LPP is an indication of an incompetent external sphincter or wide-open bladder neck.[8]

CONCLUSION

Functional assessment forms an integral part of bladder evaluation and is imperative before starting medication or planning surgery. A good clinical history and bladder diary give vital clues while RBUS, uroflowmetry, and urodynamics provide real-time data of bladder function. Uroflow is preferable in children over 5 years of age who are toilet trained and will hold and void on command. The pattern of flow and maximal flow can be evaluated provided that at least 100 mL is voided (this constitutes valid study). Detrusor sphincter dyssynergy (sphincter contracts when bladder empties) is identified in a uroflow EMG and is an important test in a dysfunctional voider. In every study, detrusor pressure and bladder compliance are measured during the filling phase and voiding pressure (and postvoid residue) is measured during the voiding phase. Poorly compliant bladders with high filling pressures are deleterious to the kidneys and mandate urgent surgical intervention. Before a urodynamic study is undertaken, a clear question to be answered should be formulated and the clinician should be present during the study.

KEY POINTS

- Bladder diary is an integral part of bladder assessment.
- Bladder wall thickness is a good indicator of dysfunctional voiding <3 mm full bladder and <5 mm empty bladder.
- Postvoid estimation gives a good idea about fecal loading and cause of dribbling.
- Uroflow studies can be done in co-operative children >5 years of age.
- *Uroflow requirement:*
    - Minimum 100 mL of void is essential.
    - Shape of curve indicates the abnormality.
- Filling phase urodynamic study is crucial for decision-making in neurogenic bladder.
- Bladder pressures have to be low till the capacity is reached (<15 cmH_2O).
- Voiding pressures are variable depending on the age (infant voiding pressures are higher than the older children).
- Overactive contractions >15 cmH_2O indicate bladder irritability and are a cause of wetting.

REFERENCES

1. de Groat WC, Griffiths D, Yoshimura N. Neural control of the lower urinary tract. Compr Physiol. 2011;5(1):327-96.
2. Rakowska-Silska M, Jobs K, Paturej A, Kalicki B. Voiding disorders in pediatrician's practice. Clin Med Insights Pediatr. 2020;14:1179556520975035.
3. Austin PF, Bauer SB, Bower W, Chase J, Franco I, Hoebeke P, et al. The standardization of terminology of lower urinary tract function in children and adolescents: update report from the Standardization Committee of the International Children's Continence Society. J Urol. 2014;191(6):1863-5.
4. Paliwalla M, Park K. A practical guide to urinary tract ultrasound in a child: Pearls and pitfalls. Ultrasound. 2014;22(4):213-22.
5. Chang SJ, Yang SS. Variability, related factors and normal reference value of post-void residual urine in healthy kindergarteners. J Urol. 2009;182(4 Suppl):1933-8.
6. Chase J, Austin P, Hoebeke P, McKenna P. The management of dysfunctional voiding in children: a report from the Standardisation Committee of the International Children's Continence Society. J Urol. 2010;183(4):1296-302.
7. Vijayakumar M, Nammalwar BR. Principles and Practice of Pediatric Nephrology, 2nd edition. New Delhi: Jaypee Brothers Medical Publishers; 2013. pp. 158-68.
8. De Jong TP, Klijn AJ. Urodynamic studies in pediatric urology. Nature Rev Urol. 2009;6(11):585.

CHAPTER

2.6 Kidney Biopsy

N Prahlad, BR Nammalwar

INTRODUCTION

Kidney biopsy (KB) has a crucial role in kidney diseases. The outcome of histological diagnosis after percutaneous kidney biopsy (PKB) can be utilized not only for diagnosis, prognosis, and program treatment for the specific illness but also as a research tool. Iversen and Brun introduced PKB of native kidneys in 1951 after localizing the kidney with intravenous pyelography and the patient in sitting position.[1] The tissue yield was inadequate, and hence there was a need to look for other percutaneous methods with tissue yields up to 95–99%. Iversen and Brun's PKB technique underwent several modifications by Kark and Muehrcke in 1954.[2] Subsequently, PKB has become a clinical tool for understanding the intrinsic aspects of childhood kidney diseases in children.

METHODS FOR KIDNEY BIOPSY

- *Percutaneous blind biopsy:* This technique is not practiced in small children.[3] The lower pole of the kidney of the child to be biopsied is localized using the anatomic landmark, which is usually posterior at the tip of the 12th rib. The left kidney is the preferred choice as it is further away from the main vessels.
- *Percutaneous blind biopsy after localizing by ultrasonogram:* It is performed blind after localizing the kidney with an ultrasound probe by the ultrasonologist in the sonogram room and then the child is moved to the procedure room.
- *Percutaneous real-time ultrasound-guided biopsy:* This technique is performed with real-time ultrasound guidance. This is the most popular method in pediatric nephrology and is done under sedation, both general and local.
- *Percutaneous CT-guided biopsy:* It is indicated in obese patients, patients with complex kidney anatomy such as vascular anomaly, horseshoe kidney (HSK), or focal lesions as in renal tumors. Interventional nephrologists or radiologists perform this procedure in the CT room.
- *Transjugular biopsy:* It is performed in a radiology room by either an interventional nephrologist or a radiologist with fluoroscopy guidance. The transjugular technique is preferred for combined liver and KB.
- *Laparoscopic biopsy:* It is performed by a urologist via the retroperitoneal approach or transperitoneal approach.
- *Open biopsy:* It is performed in patients with contraindication to PKB or during open abdominal surgeries for other renal indications.

Biopsy Needles Used for Kidney Biopsy

Over the years, there has been a modification in the biopsy needles, the main concerns being safety of the child, rapidity with which the tissue is cut, higher specimen tissue yield, and comfort of the performer[3] **(Figs. 1A to D)**.

INDICATIONS FOR KIDNEY BIOPSY

- *Idiopathic nephrotic syndrome (INS):* KB is not commonly performed in children between 1 and 8 years of age due to the high prevalence of minimal change disease and responsiveness to corticosteroids. Common indications for KB are given in the following text:
  - *Steroid-resistant nephrotic syndrome (SRNS):* Once a child is identified with SRNS, a KB should be performed except in a confirmed monogenic form of congenital and infantile SRNS. KB is justifiable where access to genetic testing is not available.[4] KB allows the confirmation of a primary podocytopathy, i.e., minimal change disease, focal segmental glomerulosclerosis (FSGS), diffuse mesangial sclerosis, membranous nephropathy, exclusion of secondary podocytopathy, lupus nephritis, membranoproliferative glomerulonephritis, and adaptive FSGS. Additionally, it permits grading of tubular atrophy, assessment of interstitial fibrosis, and glomerulosclerosis as prognostic markers. In inflammatory glomerular disease, as in lupus nephritis, the presence of inflammatory cells, proliferation of endothelial and mesangial cells, and cellular crescents mark the activity of the disease On the contrary, the presence of glomerular sclerosis, fibrous crescents, and tubular atrophy indicates the chronicity of the disease.
  - *INS on prolonged immunosuppressive:* Cyclosporine and tacrolimus can cause acute and chronic nephrotoxicity due to their renal vasoconstrictive effects and tubular structural injury. A study of KB specimens

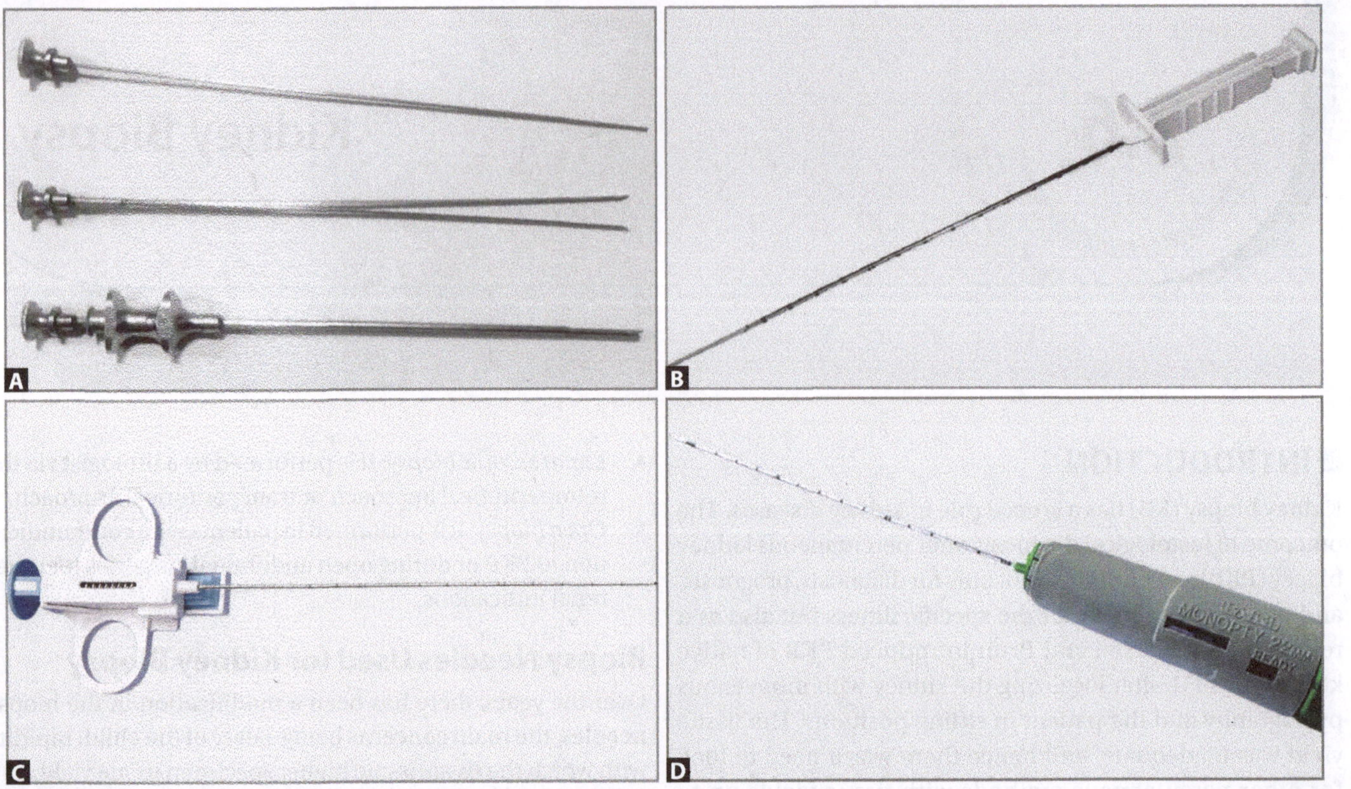

Figs 1A to D: The evolution of the biopsy needle over years. (A) Franklin modification of Vim Silverman liver biopsy needle in the year 1980; (B) Tru-Cut biopsy needle used in the year 1990; (C) Semiautomated biopsy needle used in the year 2000; (D) Automated spring-loaded biopsy device (the gun) currently in use.

from patients treated for 2 years or longer showed glomerulosclerosis.[5]
- INS with acute kidney injury (AKI) if the cause is not definite and is progressive.
- INS associated with suspected malignancies such as lymphoma or leukemia.

- *Nephritic syndrome:*
  - Acute nephritic syndrome with or without nephrotic proteinuria, persistent hypertension, rapidly increasing AKI, rapidly progressive glomerulonephritis (RPGN), presence of positive serum biomarkers, anti-glomerular basement membrane (anti-GBM) antibodies, antineutrophil cytoplasmic autoantibody (ANCA) and dsDNA, and persistent hypocomplementemia for more than 8 weeks. KB is considered as an urgent procedure in patients with RPGN to avoid severe chronic renal damage, as biopsy findings are vital to initiate appropriate treatment.
  - Nephritic syndrome and the presence of systemic symptoms such as fever, drowsiness, arthralgia, preceding dysentery, recurrent abdominal pain, nonitchy skin rashes, hepatosplenomegaly, rapidly falling platelet count, and hemoglobin which could indicate a primary systemic disease process such as Henoch-Schonlein purpura vascular nephritis, lupus nephritis, hemolytic uremic syndrome, and thrombotic thrombocytopenic microangiopathy.

- *Isolated glomerular hematuria:* Biopsy is not recommended unless there are strong indications for diseases such as Alport syndrome, thin basement membrane nephropathy, and immunoglobulin A nephropathy and after ruling out hypercalciuria.
- *AKI:* When prerenal and postrenal causes of AKI have been excluded and the cause of intrinsic AKI is unclear.[6]
- *Acute interstitial nephritis:* It is an important cause of AKI resulting from immune-mediated tubulointerstitial injury, initiated by medications and infection or direct toxic injury. Clinical features are those of AKI, and classic findings of fever, rash, and arthralgia are rarely present. KB remains the gold standard for diagnosis and will be required when there is no clinical improvement or increase in the severity of AKI even after removal of an offending agent or medication.
- In unexplained chronic kidney disease (CKD) with or without nephrotic range of proteinuria and a normal renal size
- *Post-transplant graft dysfunction:* Kidney allograft biopsy remains the gold standard to assess the cause. In acute graft dysfunction, the histology confirms acute rejection and the pathological mechanism. In chronic graft dysfunction, the histology assists in finding causes of chronic allograft nephropathy.
- Currently, "protocol" kidney biopsies are preferred for early diagnosis of kidney pathology before an increase in

serum creatinine levels could be seen. Common clinical conditions are post-transplant patients and in patients with systemic vasculitis on immunosuppressive therapy as in lupus nephritis. Such biopsies assist in early treatment modifications and predict long-term kidney outcomes.[7]

- In recent years, molecular pathology has made its presence. MicroRNAs are endogenous, short, noncoding lengths of RNA that control the expression of many genes. The study of microRNAs serve as biomarkers, a new way of examining KB tissues, to measure early and rapid changes in disease processes before pathological and clinical expression of the disease.[8]

CONTRAINDICATIONS FOR KIDNEY BIOPSY

Absolute contraindications for PKB are bleeding diathesis, unwilling parent, single functioning kidney, kidney with anatomic abnormalities, and bilateral small kidneys. HSK is considered a major contraindication owing to the anomalous and unpredictable location of internal renal structures and as the isthmus of the HSK often sits over the aorta. Relative contraindications are severe anemia, azotemia, on anticoagulation, skin infection at the biopsy site, acute pyelonephritis and hydronephrosis, or a large cyst in the kidney.[9]

PERCUTANEOUS KIDNEY BIOPSY PROCEDURE

Prebiopsy Evaluation

- Clinical evaluation includes a thorough history and physical examination with special emphasis on personal or family history of bleeding diathesis and blood pressure control.
- Laboratory evaluation includes:
  - Complete blood count which includes platelet count
  - Biochemical profile, especially renal function tests
  - Bleeding time, activated partial thromboplastin time (APTT), and prothrombin time (PT)
  - Urinalysis for presence of infection
  - Blood and Rh grouping
  - Serology for hepatitis B virus (HBV), human immunodeficiency virus 1 (HIV1), and HIV2
  - Ultrasound evaluation of kidney to assess the presence of anatomic abnormalities and to confirm the presence of both the kidneys.

Patient Preparation and Procedure

An informed preprocedure consent is obtained for the procedure and for administration of anesthesia. Early morning light breakfast is allowed if the procedure is performed late in the morning or afternoon. In children, PKB is preferentially done under general anesthesia in the minor operation theater (OT). The child lies in prone position with sandbag or rolled sheet under the abdomen. The lower pole of the kidney is localized using the ultrasound probe placed around the renal angle posteriorly. The area of skin overlying the lower pole can be marked and the probe removed (blind) or the probe is used to guide the biopsy needle throughout the procedure (real-time). The biopsy site is prepared, draped, and locally anesthetized. Additionally, a 20G spinal needle is used to localize the depth from the surface of the skin, as it moves with respiration upon penetrating the capsule of the lower pole. The spring-loaded biopsy needle is then inserted through a nick made on the anesthetized skin and advanced toward the renal capsule under real-time ultrasound guidance while the patient breaths gently. When the needle just pierces the renal capsule signified by a "give in feeling" and swinging of the biopsy needle with respiratory excursions, the patient breath is held if under general anesthesia or instructed to hold the breath, and the biopsy cut is taken. Usually, two cores of tissue are necessary for optimum evaluation, one for light microscopy and another for immunofluorescent study. If an electron microscopic study is contemplated, a third bit is taken.

Collection of Specimen

The biopsy specimen is to be removed from the biopsy needle with care not to stretch or crush the tissue with an 18G needle or a thin wooden stick, like a toothpick. Normal saline can also be used to wash the sample off the needle. The tissue is placed on a glass slide with normal saline and examined with or without a cover slip on a wet mount. The sample adequacy is assessed by the use of a dissecting microscope or hand lens. The glomeruli are visualized as small, red dots and can be recognized from fat, skeletal muscle and other nonkidney tissue. A renal sample is considered adequate for opinion if the yield of glomeruli is between 10 and 20. The minimum sample size for diagnosis varies greatly with the specific diagnosis. For example, MGN can be diagnosed even from a single glomerulus while focal FSGS can be missed if less than 10 glomeruli are obtained. Once it is determined that suitable cortical tissue is obtained, the first core is placed in formalin for LM study. The second is placed for immunofluorescence study in a vial containing Michel transport media (Zeus solution). For electron microscopy (EM), the third specimen is placed in 1–3% glutaraldehyde that acts as a fixative. Post biopsy, a firm dressing is applied and the child is observed in the minor OT until complete recovery from sedation and fairly oriented to recognize his parent. Then the child is moved to his bed and monitored for heart rate, blood pressure, and hematuria at least for 12 hours with minimum physical activity.

COMPLICATIONS OF KIDNEY BIOPSY

Microscopic hematuria is seen in almost 100% of patients and resolves spontaneously within 48 hours. If needed, 24 hours' postbiopsy hematocrit is done prior to discharge. The second most common risks are a silent hematoma at the puncture site and mild and transient hematuria. These complications are termed serious when there is a need for blood transfusion, surgical intervention, angiography, and embolization to control bleeding. Very rarely, there could be an arteriovenous fistula (AVF) formation or tear in the kidney needing nephrectomy of the injured kidney and loss of life. The AVF is generally asymptomatic. Patients with large or symptomatic AVF may require superselective transcatheter embolization or surgery. Serious complications are more likely in small children, in children with severe kidney failure, deranged coagulation profile, or on hemodialysis with heparinization and lack of experience of the performer.[10] The number of passes is more than three in children (five in adults) and the gauge of the biopsy needle bore size less than 16G correlates with increased bleeding risk. Automated needles 16G or 18G with larger bore and shorter bevel have been associated with larger fragment of tissue and fewer complications.[11] Complications become evident in the first 8–24 hours after biopsy. A 24-hour period of observation and a postbiopsy hematocrit on discharge ensure safety.

In children with prolonged BT and moderately elevated serum creatinine, desmopressin acetate 0.3 µg/kg IV 30 minutes or DDAVP 2–4 µg/kg intranasal is administered 2 hours before the procedure. This is associated with reduced bleeding complications but in children with kidney impairment, there is an increased possibility for hyponatremia.[12,13]

CONCLUSION

Renal biopsy is an integral procedure in the diagnosis and management of kidney disease. The current standard procedure for KB involves the use of real-time ultrasound to guide an automated spring-loaded biopsy device. Together, these two techniques have been shown to reduce complications of the procedure. Epidemiologically, the indications for KB over different nations and periods of time are variable and hence there is heterogeneity in observations and inferences based on them. However, the diagnostic value of a KB is undeniable in glomerular diseases, systemic diseases, CKD, unexplained AKI, and transplant kidney dysfunction.

KEY POINTS

- KB has redefined the diagnosis, prognostication, and therapy of glomerular and tubulointerstitial diseases.
- Primary indications of KB are glomerular hematuria and proteinuria with or without renal dysfunction and unexplained AKI and CKD.
- Biopsy needles have changed with times from Vim-Silverman needle to Tru-Cut needle to spring-loaded automatic gun.
- The procedure has developed from blind bedside biopsy to ultrasound marking to real-time ultrasound guidance and rarely to computerized tomography guidance, open biopsy, and transjugular KB.
- For gainful interpretation of KB, adequate sample and clinical information are mandatory.
- The most frequent complications of KB are microscopic hematuria and a silent hematoma.
- Complications are rare with increasing skill and availability of real-time ultrosonogram-guided KB.
- KB has come to stay as an investigatory tool of immense value in nephrology practice.

REFERENCES

1. Iversen P, Brun C. Aspiration biopsy of the kidney. Am J Med. 1951;11:324-30.
2. Cameron JS, Hicks J. The introduction of renal biopsy into nephrology from 1901 to 1961: a paradigm of the forming of nephrology by technology. Am J Nephrol. 1997;17:347-58.
3. Okoye O. (2019). Renal biopsy: Appraisal of the methods. In Renal Diseases. Tech Open. [online] Available from: http://dx.doi.org/10.5772/intechopen.86755 [Last accessed May, 2022].
4. Trautmann A, Vivarelli M, Samuel S, Gipson D, Sinha A, Schaefer F, et al; International Pediatric Nephrology Association. IPNA clinical practice recommendations for the diagnosis and management of children with steroid-resistant nephrotic syndrome. Pediatr Nephrol. 2020;35:1529-61.
5. Zachariae H, Kragballe K, Hansen HE, Marcussen N, Olsen S. Renal biopsy findings in long-term cyclosporin treatment of psoriasis. Br J Dermatol. 1997;136:531-5.
6. Waikar SS, McMahon GM. Expanding the role for kidney biopsies in acute kidney injury. Semin Nephrol. 2018;38:12-20.
7. Parikh SV, Alvarado A, Malvar A, Rovin BH. The kidney biopsy in lupus nephritis: past, present, and future. Semin Nephrol. 2015;35(5):465-77.
8. Halloran PF, de Freitas DG, Einecke G, Famulski KS, Hidalgo LG, MengeL M, et al. An integrated view of molecular changes, histopathology and outcomes in kidney transplants. Am J Transplant. 2010;10:2223-30.
9. Bandari J, Fuller TW, Turner RM II, D'Agostino LA. Renal biopsy for medical renal disease: indications and contraindications. Can J Urol. 2016;23:8121-6.
10. Manno C, Strippoli GF, Arnesano L, Bonifati C, Campobasso N, Gesualdo L, et al. Predictors of bleeding complications in percutaneous ultrasound-guided renal biopsy. Kidney Int. 2004;66:1570-77.
11. Roth R, Parekh S, Makey D, Foster J, Rozenblit G, Satoskar A, et al. When size matters: diagnostic value of kidney biopsy according to the gauge of the biopsy needle. Am J Nephrol. 2013;37:249-54.
12. Manno C, Bonifati C, Torres DD, Campobasso N, Schena FP. Desmopressin acetate in percutaneous ultrasound-guided kidney biopsy: a randomized controlled trial. Am J Kidney Dis. 2011;57:850-5.
13. Leclerc S, Nadeau-Fredette AC, Elftouh N, Lafrance JP, Pichette V, Laurin LP. Use of desmopressin prior to kidney biopsy in patients with high bleeding risk. Kidney Int Rep. 2020;5:1180-7.

CHAPTER

2.7 Histopathology of Renal Diseases

Anila Abraham Kurien

INTRODUCTION

Importance of renal biopsy:

- Establish a tissue diagnosis
- Exclude other diagnostic possibilities that could have a similar clinical presentation
- Assess the activity and severity of the disease
- Guide treatment
- Predict prognosis
- Help in understanding the pathogenesis.

The interpretation of renal biopsy can be challenging as the kidneys react both clinically and morphologically in only a limited fashion to a multitude of injurious agents. A particular disease can have different morphological patterns of renal involvement as in the case of lupus nephritis. Also, a particular morphologic pattern can be associated with different disease processes such as the focal and segmental glomerulosclerosis pattern, which may be a primary glomerular disease or a segmental scarring due to a wide variety of causes. Each of these has diverse etiologies, treatment, and prognoses. Obtaining clinically relevant information from a renal biopsy requires close cooperation between the clinician and the pathologist.[1-4]

HANDLING OF RENAL TISSUE

Renal tissue samples can be obtained by percutaneous needle biopsy or open wedge biopsy. An adequate assessment of a renal biopsy includes light microscopy (LM), immunofluorescence (IF) microscopy, and electron microscopy (EM). The biopsy should always be accompanied by relevant clinical information. A complete clinical history, physical examination, list of medications, radiological findings, and laboratory evaluation including relevant serological markers are required to evaluate a renal biopsy.

A minimum of two cores of tissue, each measuring 1-2 cm in length, are recommended.

The tissue should be handled with great care in order to avoid artifact. Forceps should not be used to remove the tissue from the needle as it can cause crush artifacts. A small wooden stick such as a toothpick can be used for manipulation of the tissue. Stretching or drying of the tissue should also be avoided.

Sample adequacy should be assessed with a hand magnifying glass or a dissecting microscope immediately after removal. The specimen is placed on a glass slide with normal saline and examined for the presence of glomeruli. The minimum number of glomeruli for diagnosis varies greatly with the specific diagnosis. As the percentage of glomerular involvement in a biopsy is used to estimate the severity of a focal glomerular lesion, a small biopsy sample size will cause considerable misclassification of disease severity. Also, a small sample size will make the exclusion of focal diseases difficult. For most biopsies, 15–20 glomeruli are considered to be adequate. However, larger numbers of glomeruli may be needed for focal lesions. For example, if only 10% of the glomeruli are affected, 30 glomeruli should be available in the biopsy tissue to have a >95% chance of sampling at least one affected glomerulus.[4]

Light Microscopy

The largest portion of the cortex should be placed in the 10% neutral-buffered formalin for LM.

Immunofluorescence Microscopy

Immunofluorescence tissue should include a piece of the cortex. Tissue for IF can be directly frozen or placed in tissue transport media such as Michel's medium. The tissue in Michel's medium is stable at room temperature for up to a week.

Electron Microscopy

Small, 1-mm bits of the cortex are allocated for EM and should be immediately placed in formalin or 2.5% glutaraldehyde.[1-4]

PROCESSING OF SPECIMENS

Light Microscopy

Because of the types of diseases and the various renal compartments that are involved, renal biopsy tissue processing mandates a variety of histochemical stains, which includes hematoxylin and eosin, periodic acid–Schiff (PAS), methenamine silver, and trichrome stains as given in **Table 1**. Each stain is complementary to the other and has its unique staining characteristics for both normal and abnormal structures and, as a rule, all these four stains are used in evaluating renal biopsies.

- Formalin-fixed, paraffin-embedded tissue cut as serial sections of 2–3 µm thickness is used for light microscopic evaluation. It is important to ensure that the sections are no more than 3 µm thick, because the definition of

TABLE 1: Histochemical stains identifying renal tissue.

Compartment	*Structure highlighted*
Hematoxylin and eosin stain	
Glomerular	Architecture, cellularity, characterize inflammatory infiltrate
Tubular	Epithelial cell damage, RBC casts, pigment casts, crystals
Interstitial	Edema, inflammation
Vascular	Fibrin thrombi, inflammation (vasculitis)
Periodic acid–Schiff stain	
Glomerular	Mesangial matrix, GBM thickening, hyalinosis, sclerosis
Tubular	Tubulitis, brush borders, tubular basement membrane thickening
Interstitial	IFTA
Vascular	Hyalinosis, arteriosclerosis
Jones methenamine silver stain	
Glomerular	Collagen, basement membrane spikes, pinholes, double contours, breaks in GBM, Bowman's capsule
Tubular	Tubular atrophy
Interstitial	Fibrosis
Vascular	Internal elastic lamina
Masson's trichrome stain	
Glomerular	Immune deposits, fibrin thrombi, fibrinoid necrosis, sclerosis
Tubular	Atrophy
Interstitial	Fibrosis
Vascular	Fibrinoid necrosis, fibrin thrombi

(GBM: glomerular basement membrane; IFTA: interstitial fibrosis and tubular atrophy; RBC: red blood cell)

glomerular cellularity is based on sections of this thickness **(Fig. 1)**.

- Hematoxylin and eosin, PAS, Jones methenamine silver, and Masson's trichrome are routinely performed on all biopsies.
- Congo red for amyloid, iron stains, special stains for fungus and acid-fast bacilli, etc., are the other stains performed to recognize specific features.

Immunofluorescence Microscopy

Immunofluorescence microscopy is required to identify and localize immunoglobulins, complement, fibrin, and light chains within the renal tissue using fluorescein-labeled antibodies.

- Fresh-frozen renal cortical tissue, with sections of 3–4 μm cut in a cryostat, is used.
- The antigens routinely examined include immunoglobulin G (IgG), IgM, IgA, complement components (C3, C1q), fibrin, and kappa and lambda light chains.
- C4d immunostain is performed on transplant biopsies.
- When frozen tissue is not available or glomeruli are not present on frozen sections, immunoperoxidase (IP) staining of the various antigens can be performed on paraffin-embedded sections.

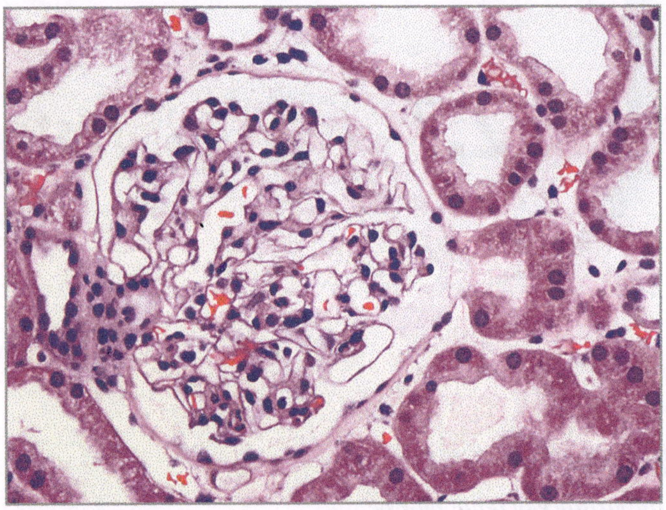

Fig. 1: Normal glomerulus. Glomerulus with normal cellularity, scanty mesangial matrix, and patent capillary loops. Hematoxylin and eosin stain, 2 μm section.

- IF on paraffin tissue sections can be done as a salvage method when frozen tissue is insufficient or not available. It is also used to unmask immunoglobulins or light chains when they are not detected in frozen tissue.[5]

Electron Microscopy

Electron microscopy helps to localize deposits, detect extremely small deposits, identify organized deposits, and recognize abnormalities in cellular and basement membrane structure.

- Tissue is fixed in 2.5% glutaraldehyde or 10% neutral-buffered formalin.
- Toluidine blue-stained, 1-μm "thick" sections are examined and structures for thin sectioning are identified.
- Glomeruli, the tubulointerstitium, and blood vessels are examined at low, medium, and high magnification.[1-4]

INTERPRETATION OF THE RENAL BIOPSY

The renal biopsy has to be evaluated by LM, IF, and EM in order to obtain maximum information.

All the compartments of the renal cortex have to be systematically assessed to provide the maximum clinically relevant information to the treating clinician.

Light Microscopy

Glomeruli

The biopsy tissue is evaluated for its adequacy using the low power objective of the microscope. The total number of glomeruli available is documented. The percentage or number of glomeruli showing sclerosis or disease is calculated. The term "*diffuse*" is applied when >50% of the glomeruli are involved and "*focal*" when changes occur only in a few glomeruli. The involvement is said to be "*global*" when the whole glomerulus is involved and "*segmental*" when only a part of the glomerulus is involved **(Fig. 2)**.

The first step in evaluating the glomerulus is to assess the cellularity, which is best done using the H&E or PAS-

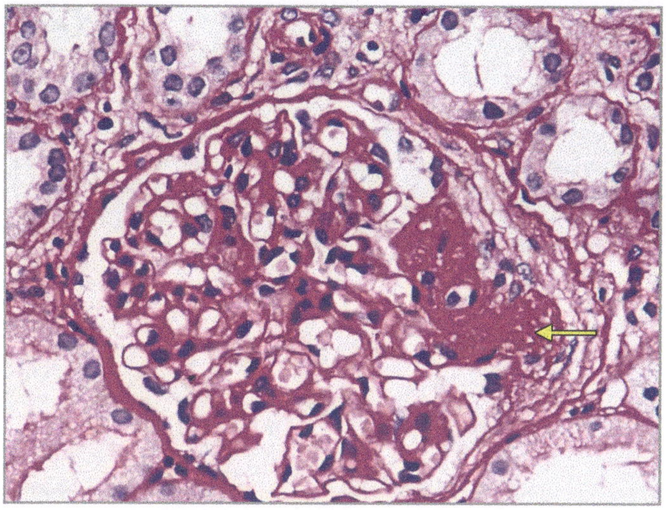

Fig. 2: Focal and segmental glomerulosclerosis. Arrow indicates segmental sclerosis of the capillary tuft (periodic acid–Schiff stain).

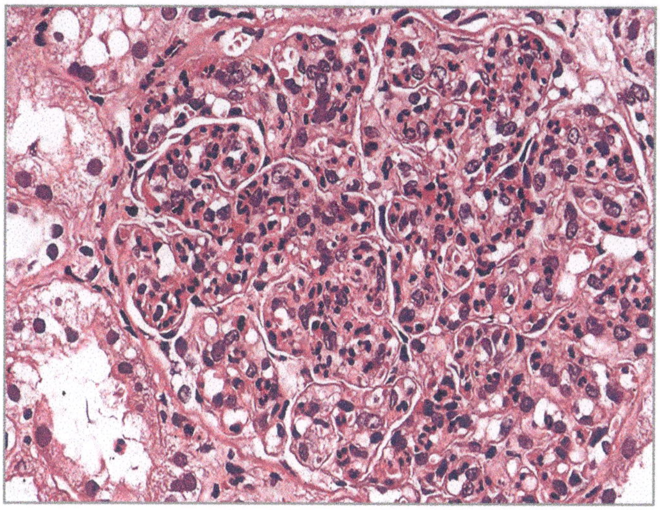

Fig. 3: Endocapillary hypercellularity. Enlarged and hypercellular glomerulus with marked acute inflammatory cell influx in a case of infection-related glomerulonephritis (hematoxylin and eosin stain).

stained sections. An increase in cellularity could be due to the proliferation of endothelial cells, mesangial cells, and by the infiltration of inflammatory cells. Endocapillary hypercellularity is defined as an increase in cellularity within the confines of the glomerular basement membrane composed of endothelial cells, mesangial cells, and/or inflammatory cells, resulting in narrowing or occlusion of the capillary lumen **(Fig. 3)**. Other features of proliferation are lobular accentuation, fibrinoid necrosis, karyorrhexis, and crescent formation. They indicate the severity of the lesion.

Mesangial changes include increase in the mesangial cells and/or matrix. Mesangial hypercellularity is defined as three or more cells per mesangial area, away from the vascular pole, in a 2–3-μm thick tissue section. The mesangial matrix may be expanded due to the accumulation of immune complex deposits, amyloid, collagen, or other abnormal proteins. It can have a diffuse or a nodular pattern of expansion.

Capillary wall/glomerular basement membranes are evaluated for their thickness, contours, and integrity. Although EM is the best way to study the structure of the basement membranes, a combination of the special stains that are routinely performed can provide reliable information. The thickness, irregularity, wrinkling, double contours, and spike formation can be observed by silver stains on LM **(Figs. 4A and B)**.

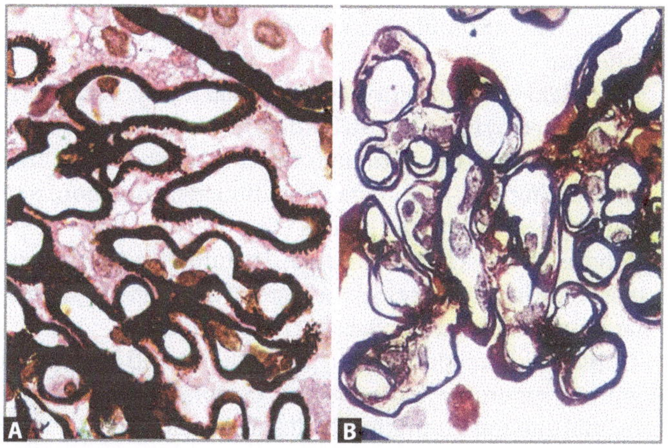

Figs. 4A and B: Glomerular basement membrane (GBM) changes. (A) Spike formation on the GBM; (B) The duplication of GBM (Jones silver stain).

Bowman's space or urinary space is studied for the presence of crescents, which are the build-up of more than two layers of cells caused by the proliferation of parietal epithelial cells, infiltrating inflammatory cells, and fibrin in the initial stages and collagen in the later stages within Bowman's space **(Fig. 5)**. Crescents are classified as cellular, fibrocellular, or fibrous depending on the predominant component.[4,6,7]

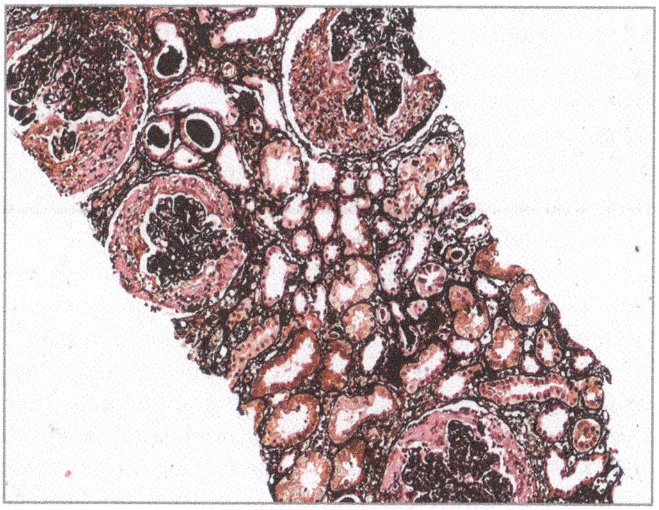

Fig. 5: Cellular crescent occupying the entire Bowman's space in all the glomeruli (Jones silver stain).

Tubules

Normal renal cortex has tubules packed close together with little intervening interstitium. In the medulla, the tubules are separated by varying amounts of interstitial tissue. The interpretation of tubular disease involves identifying tubular epithelial cell changes, tubular atrophy, tubular basement membrane changes, tubular casts and crystals in the lumen,

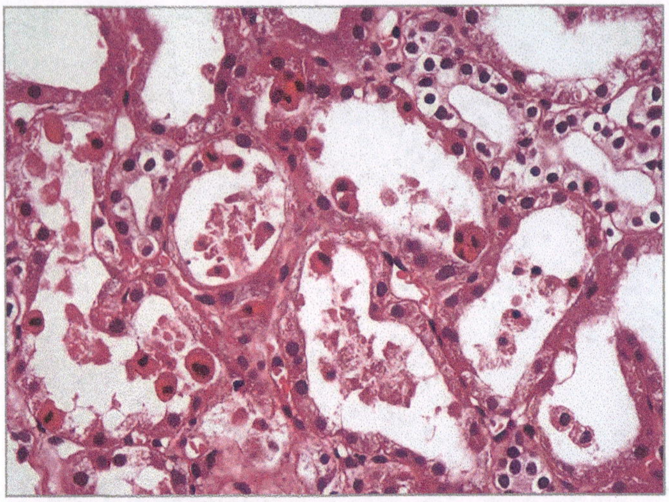

Fig. 6: Acute tubular injury. Many of the tubular epithelial cells have sloughed off and cell debris is seen in the lumen of the tubules (hematoxylin and eosin stain).

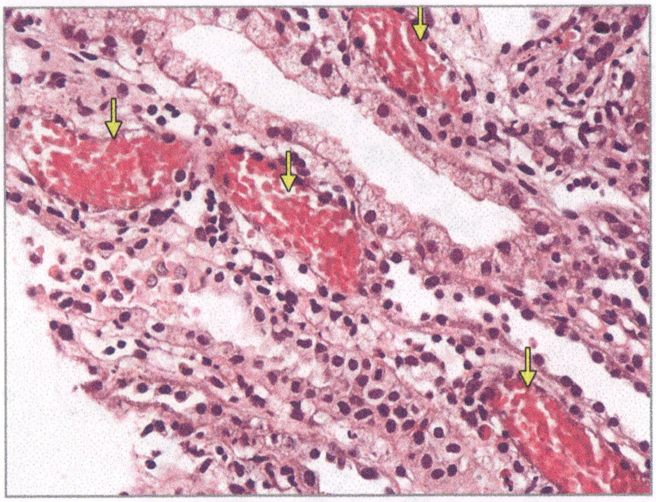

Fig. 7: Red blood cell (RBC) casts fill up some of the tubules in a patient with immunoglobulin A (IgA) nephropathy (hematoxylin and eosin stain).

and pigment accumulation or viral inclusions in the lining epithelium.

Tubular epithelial injury (acute tubular injury/necrosis) is characterized by loss of brush borders in the proximal tubular cells, cytoplasmic vacuolization, flattening of the epithelium with resulting tubular luminal dilatation, degeneration, and sloughing of cells into the lumina **(Fig. 6)**. Tubular epithelial cells have the capacity to regenerate. Features of regeneration/repair following an injury include increased nucleocytoplasmic ratio, cytoplasmic basophilia, and mitotic figures.

Lipid accumulation from hyperlipidemia and lipiduria in nephrotic syndrome may be seen as cytoplasmic vacuoles in proximal and less commonly in distal tubular cells.

The morphologic features of tubular atrophy include reduction in the caliber of the tubules and thickening and wrinkling of the tubular basement membrane.

The tubular basement membrane abnormalities include thickening and wrinkling which are seen in tubular atrophy, immune deposits in lupus nephritis, and deposition of abnormal proteins in amyloidosis.

The tubular lumen may contain various types of casts with different morphologic and staining characteristics. They may be a part of normal renal physiology, as a result of glomerulonephritis or a systemic disease. Hyaline casts are eosinophilic, homogeneous, strongly PAS positive and are seen in the lumina of the loop of Henle and the distal tubules. Red blood cell (RBC) casts, defined as compacted erythrocytes (intact or degenerated) within a tubular lumen, are formed due to the disruption of the glomerular filtration barrier and occur most commonly due to glomerulonephritis **(Fig. 7)**. Structural aberrations to the glomerular basement membrane can also give rise to RBC casts. Granular (necrotic cellular debris) casts are indicative of previous tubular cell necrosis. Neutrophilic or pus cell casts, which are associated with acute pyelonephritis, are a mixture of predominantly neutrophils accompanied by karyorrhectic debris and tubular epithelial cell debris. Myoglobin and hemoglobin casts are morphologically indistinguishable by LM and require immunohistochemistry for identification. They appear as reddish-brown granules and globules that may form rope-like or bead-like structures. They are associated with rhabdomyolysis and intravascular hemolysis, respectively.[4,6-8]

Intratubular crystal deposition of calcium salts, medications, or other chemicals may be seen on the renal biopsy. In children, congenital metabolic disorders, collectively known as primary hyperoxaluria, can induce the formation of oxalate crystals in the tubules.[9]

Interstitium

The interstitium has only limited structural manifestations of injury which include edema, inflammatory cell infiltration, and fibrosis.

Interstitial edema is identified by the separation of cortical tubules that are normally closely apposed. The tubular basement membranes are of normal thickness and contour.

Interstitial fibrosis is characterized by the separation of tubules by fibrous tissue. The tubules are atrophied, and their basement membrane is thickened and irregularly contoured **(Fig. 8)**.

Inflammation of the interstitium is classified as acute or chronic interstitial nephritis. The distinction between the two is made based on the presence of edema (acute interstitial nephritis) or fibrosis (chronic interstitial nephritis) in the area of inflammation, regardless of the type of infiltrating inflammatory cells.

The interstitium may be infiltrated by immune complexes (in autoimmune diseases such as lupus nephritis), amyloid, or foam cells (Alport syndrome).[4,6,7]

Blood Vessels

On the basis of LM, renal vascular lesions can be divided as inflammatory lesions and noninflammatory lesions.

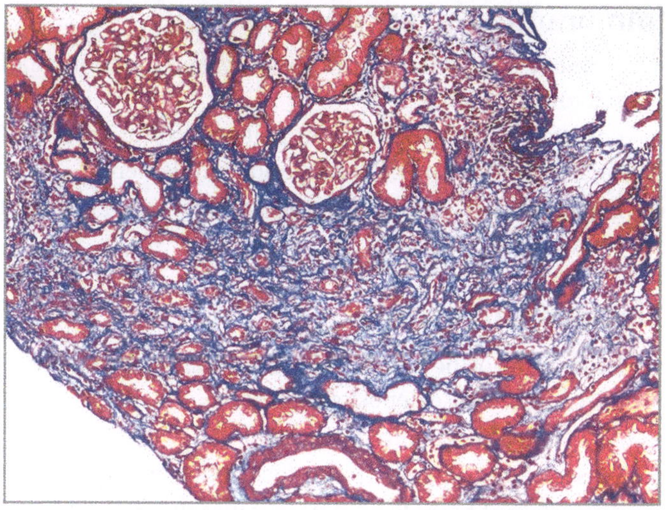

Fig. 8: Interstitial fibrosis and tubular atrophy. Interstitial fibrosis is seen as blue areas (Masson's trichrome stain).

Inflammation of the vessel wall is called vasculitis and it can affect vessels of all sizes, with different clinical and pathologic manifestations. Vasculitis is characterized by leukocytic infiltration, karyorrhexis, and fibrinoid necrosis of the vessel wall.

Narrowing of the vascular lumen, the thickness of the intima media, the integrity of the internal elastic lamina, and the presence of hyaline are features of noninflammatory vascular lesions.[4,6,7]

Activity and Chronicity Indices on Light Microscopy (Table 2)

After assessing all four compartments of the kidney, it is important to identify features that can predict the prognosis of the disease and thereby help in planning optimal treatment. The following are the histopathological features given in **Table 2**.

Immunofluorescence microscopy: Most primary glomerulonephritis and many secondary glomerular diseases are immunologic in nature. IF microscopy is a method to detect the presence of immunoglobulins and complements, their type, and their location. The slides are evaluated both qualitatively and semiquantitatively. The first and most important step in IF microscopy is to recognize if the positive staining is specific or not. With specific staining, the pattern can be linear, smudgy, or granular **(Fig. 9)**. It is important to identify the location(s) of the staining which could be on the glomerular capillary wall, mesangium **(Fig. 10)**, tubular basement membrane, tubular epithelium, tubular cast, or blood vessel wall. The final step is the semiquantification of staining intensity (scale 0 to +3 or 0 to +4).[1-4]

Electron microscopy: Electron microscopy can assess changes in cell structure such as effacement of podocyte foot processes and podocyte vacuolization and changes in the glomerular basement membrane structure such as thickening, thinning, irregularities, and duplication. EM helps identify and localize immune deposits **(Figs. 11 and 12)** and organized deposits.

Transmission electron microscope is used to evaluate the ultrastructure. One or two glomeruli are examined and a series of low, medium, and high magnification and photomicrographs are captured. This should include representative areas of capillary loops and mesangial regions. Tubulointerstitial and vascular structures are also examined for any pathological abnormality and images are captured. Interpretation of electron microscopic findings should be correlated with the findings in LM and IF microscopy.

Though it may not be necessary to perform EM on every renal biopsy, it is advisable to keep aside a small amount of material so that it may be used if required after studying the light and IF microscopic sections.[1-4]

TABLE 2: Activity and chronicity indices on light microscopy.

Activity indices	*Chronicity indices*
Cellular proliferation	Glomerular sclerosis
Crescent formation	Tubular atrophy
Fibrinoid necrosis	Interstitial fibrosis
Inflammation	Vascular sclerosis

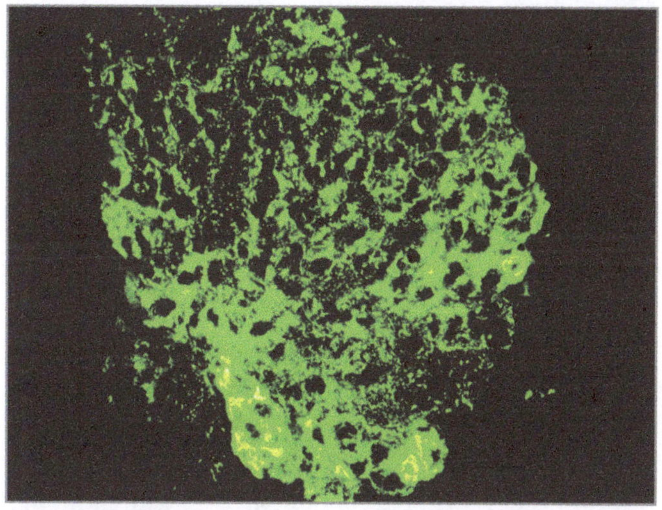

Fig. 9: Coarse granular deposits of C3 along the glomerular basement membrane (GBM) in a patient with infection-related glomerulonephritis.

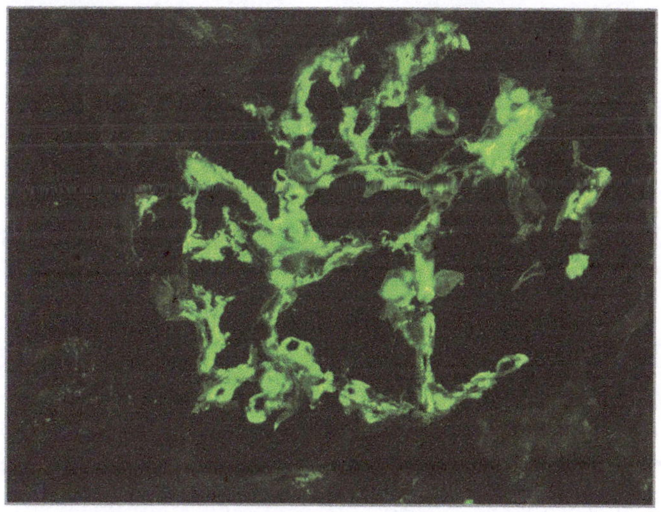

Fig. 10: Mesangial deposits of immunoglobulin A (IgA) in a patient with IgA nephropathy.

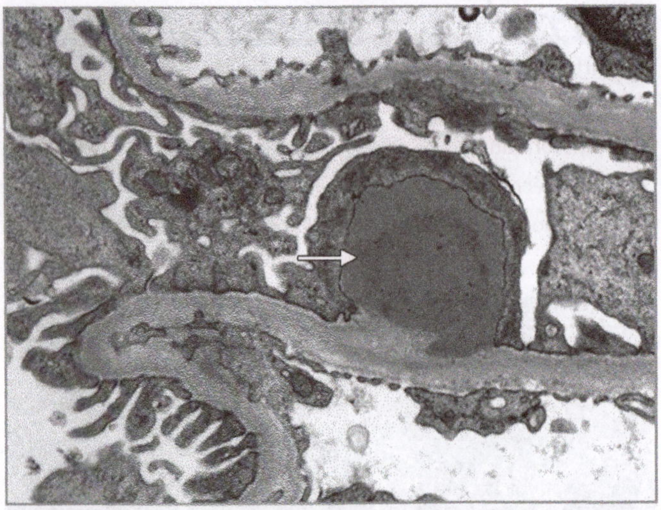

Fig. 11: Subepithelial "humps." Characteristic "hump"-like electron-dense deposits in the subepithelial region of glomerular basement membrane (GBM) in a patient with infection-related glomerulonephritis.

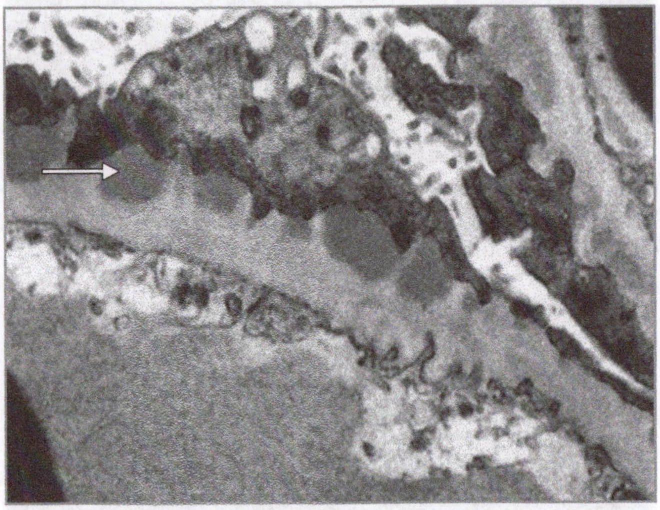

Fig. 12: Segment of a glomerular capillary loop shows subepithelial electron-dense deposits with spikes of glomerular basement membrane (GBM) between them.

CONCLUSION

Accurate interpretation of the biopsy sample requires the examination of all histological compartments of the kidney in multiple serial sections. The final diagnosis of the kidney biopsy requires the integration of histopathological features with the clinical information and other laboratory parameters of the patient.

KEY POINTS

Light Microscopy

- Presence of renal cortex and medulla and their relative proportion
- Number of glomeruli and the number/percentage of sclerotic or diseased glomeruli
- Detailed description of the morphology of the glomeruli, tubules, interstitium, and blood vessels
- Any significant negative finding should also be mentioned.

Immunofluorescence Microscopy

- Number of glomeruli and the number/percentage of sclerotic glomeruli
- Location, staining pattern, and intensity (scale of 0–3) of each of the immunoglobulins and complements
- Presence of staining in the tubulointerstitium or blood vessels.

Electron Microscopy

- Description of the location, size, appearance, and structure of electron-dense deposits, if present
- Any other abnormality, if present
- Presence and degree of foot process effacement
- Any relevant pathology of the tubules, interstitium, and blood vessels.

Diagnosis

- Morphologic pattern and the clinicopathologic category of the disease.

Comment

- List of differential diagnoses
- Histological prognostic indicators
- Clinicopathologic correlation.

REFERENCES

1. Walker, PD, Cavallo T, Bonsib SM. Practice guidelines for the renal biopsy. Mod Pathol. 2004;17:1555-63.
2. Walker PD. The renal biopsy. Archives Pathol Lab Med. 2009;133(2):181-8.
3. Kitterer D, Gürzing K, Segerer S, Dominik Alscher M, Amann K, Braun N, et al. Diagnostic impact of percutaneous renal biopsy. Clin Nephrol. 2015;84(6):311-22.
4. Jennette JC, Silva FG, Olson JL, D'Agati VD. Primer on the pathologic classification and diagnosis of kidney disease. In: Jennette JC, Olson JL, Silva FG, D'Agati VD (Eds). Heptinstall's Pathology of the Kidney, 7th edition.Philadelphia, PA: Wolters Kluwer; 2015. pp. 91-118.
5. Nasr HS, Fidler ME, Said SM. Paraffin immunofluorescence: a valuable ancillary technique in renal pathology. Kidney Int Rep. 2018;3(6):1260-6.
6. Johnson RJ, Floege J, Rennke HG, et al. Introduction to glomerular disease: pathogenesis and classification. In: Feehally J, Floege J, Johnson RJ (Eds). Comprehensive Clinical Nephrology, 3rd edition. Edinburgh: Mosby; 2007. pp. 181-91.
7. Colvin RB. Normal kidney structure. In: Colvin RB, Chang A (Eds). Diagnostic Pathology: Kidney Diseases, 3rd edition. Philadelphia, PA: Elsevier; 2019. pp. 24-36.
8. Dvanajscak Z, Cossey LN, Larsen CP. A practical approach to the pathology of renal intratubular casts. Semin Diagn Pathol. 2020;37(3):127-34.
9. Cossey LN, Dvanajscak Z, Larsen CP. A diagnostician's field guide to crystalline nephropathies. Semin Diagn Pathol. 2020;37(3):135-42.

CHAPTER

2.8 Genetic Analysis

Prajnya Ranganath

INTRODUCTION

Genetic factors play an important role in the causation of chronic kidney disease (CKD). Monogenic causes together account for around 30% of CKD in pediatric patients and around 5–30% of CKD in adult patients.[1,2] Till date around 450 monogenic disorders are known to be associated with various forms of renal involvement, and many of them have childhood onset, but some may manifest in adult life.[1,2] Recent technological advances, especially the development of next-generation sequencing (NGS) strategies, are helping to identify the genetic basis of an increasing number of conditions encountered in pediatric nephrology practice and also greatly facilitating the diagnosis of these disorders in the clinical setting.

Genetic tests can be broadly categorized into clinical diagnostic tests and research-based tests.[3]

- Clinical diagnostic tests are used for diagnosis, to aid in the treatment of an individual patient, or for prenatal genetic testing, presymptomatic detection, or carrier testing of family members.
- Research-based tests are performed to obtain a better understanding of the disease pathogenesis or to develop and validate a specific test for clinical application.

This chapter provides an overview of the various genetic testing modalities that are used in the clinical setting, with particular emphasis on their utility and applications in pediatric nephrology.

INDICATIONS FOR GENETIC TESTING

Over the past one or two decades, genetic tests have not only become more advanced, but also far more accessible and affordable. It is important to know when genetic testing needs to be offered to a particular individual. These are the various scenarios where genetic testing is usually offered in the setting of pediatric nephrology:

- *For the identification and/or confirmation of the genetic etiological diagnosis in the proband (index patient) in the following clinical scenarios:*
  - Clinical, laboratory, renal imaging, and/or renal histopathology features suggestive of a monogenic condition, e.g., autosomal recessive polycystic kidney disease (ARPKD), autosomal dominant polycystic kidney disease (ADPKD), Alport syndrome, primary hyperoxaluria, etc.
  - Clinical features suggestive of an etiologically heterogeneous condition where a proportion of cases are known to be due to genetic causes, e.g., steroid-resistant nephrotic syndrome (SRNS), medullary nephrocalcinosis, congenital anomalies of the kidney and urinary tract (CAKUT), etc.
  - In a patient with CKD, without an identified autoimmune or other acquired etiology
  - History of similar pattern of renal involvement in one or more family members.
- *For testing of family members of the proband:* This is usually done through targeted testing of the family member for the specific genetic mutation(s) already identified in the proband.
  - Prenatal genetic testing is done to diagnose the recurrence of a debilitating condition in the subsequent offspring, in the early antenatal period. The fetal sample is obtained through chorionic villus sampling (at 11–13 weeks of gestation) or amniocentesis (after 16 completed weeks of gestation), or less often through cordocentesis (after 18–20 weeks of gestation), and targeted testing of the mutation(s), already identified in the proband and/or carrier parents, is done in the fetal DNA. If the fetus is found to be affected, the option of termination of pregnancy, within the legally and medically permissible gestational age limit, could be considered. Fetal therapy is presently available only for a very few conditions and is not an option for most cases; however, there are likely to be developments in fetal therapeutics in the future.
  - Carrier testing of other family members in the reproductive age group is done to ascertain the risk of recurrence of the disorder in their offspring. It helps couples to make informed reproductive choices. Carrier testing is ideally done through targeted mutation testing of the family members, after prior identification of the genetic mutation(s) in the proband. However, if the proband is no longer alive and his/her genetic evaluation was not done prior to demise, the parents or sibling of the proband can be

directly evaluated and screened for mutations in the genes related to the deceased proband's phenotype. Carrier testing does not have any utility in childhood and should not be done in children.[4]

- Presymptomatic testing for late-onset genetic disorders is done in asymptomatic at-risk relatives of the proband, to identify or rule out their affected status. Presymptomatic testing helps individuals to make informed reproductive and lifestyle choices and enables early institution of therapy, intervention, and/or surveillance, if available. However, it is not recommended in children, unless some definitely beneficial course-altering therapy or intervention is available for the condition.[4]

- *For pharmacogenetic testing:* This is performed to optimize the choice of drug and the dosage for each individual patient, e.g., in the context of immunosuppressive therapy for renal transplantation.

GENETIC TESTS USED FOR CLINICAL DIAGNOSIS

Genetic tests that are used in the clinical diagnostic setting can be broadly classified as cytogenetic tests that are used for the diagnosis of chromosomal anomalies, and molecular genetic tests that are used to detect genetic mutations associated with monogenic disorders (also known as single-gene disorders or Mendelian disorders).

Most of the genetic renal disorders, such as the genetic glomerulopathies/podocytopathies, inherited renal tubulopathies, and primary ciliopathies, are monogenic disorders. A proportion of CAKUT cases, especially the ones associated with dysmorphic syndromes and multiple malformation disorders, may be caused by chromosomal abnormalities, though even monogenic causes account for some isolated as well as syndromic CAKUT cases.

Molecular Genetic Tests

Molecular genetic tests are performed in the deoxyribonucleic acid (DNA) sample [and less often in the ribonucleic acid (RNA) sample] of an individual to detect variants in genes. Genetic variants are alterations in the nucleotide sequence of a gene. A genetic variant that significantly alters the structure and/or function of the protein encoded by the gene, and thereby causes disease, is known as a "pathogenic variant" (conventionally referred to as a "mutation"). However, not all genetic variants are disease causing. Benign polymorphic genetic variants are present in normal individuals in the general population and do not have any significant effects on gene function.[5]

The main types of genetic variants are "single-nucleotide variants" (SNVs) (conventionally referred to as "point mutations", where one nucleotide is replaced by another), insertion or deletion of a few nucleotides, and deletion or duplication of one or more exons of the gene. SNVs may be "missense variants" (where substitution of one nucleotide by another results in replacement of the amino acid at that position by a different amino acid), "nonsense variants" (where nucleotide substitution results in an amino acid-coding codon being replaced by a stop codon, resulting in premature cessation of translation and production of a truncated protein), or "synonymous variants" (where there is no alteration of the amino acid, as the codon resulting from the nucleotide substitution codes for the same amino acid as the original codon).

Insertion or deletion of one or a few nucleotides (that are not in multiples of 3) alters the "reading frame" and are therefore referred to as "frameshifting" mutations. The reading frame refers to the fixed pattern in which the gene sequence is translated, with each group of three nucleotides, called a "codon", coding for one amino acid. Genetic variants that alter the normal splicing of a gene are called "splice variants". Splicing refers to the process by which the noncoding regions (i.e., introns) are removed from the precursor messenger RNA (pre-mRNA), and the coding regions (i.e., exons) are joined together to produce the mature mRNA, which is thereafter translated to synthesize the corresponding protein. Majority of the disease-causing genetic variants are located within the exons or the splice sites (exon–intron junctions) of genes, and only a small number of variants (usually <2–5%) are located in the deep intronic or promoter regions of genes.[5]

Based on the testing strategy used, molecular genetic tests done in the clinical setting can be broadly categorized as follows:

- Targeted testing of a specific genetic variant
- Sequence analysis of a specific gene
- Simultaneous sequence analysis of multiple genes related to a particular phenotype
- Dosage analysis for large deletions and duplications involving one or more exons
- Broad-spectrum testing.

Targeted Testing of a Specific Genetic Variant

This is done to look for a common genetic mutation known to be associated with the clinically diagnosed genetic disease (e.g., the p.Glu6Val missense variant in the *HBB* gene, which is the only mutation known to cause sickle cell disease). Targeted variant testing is also done when one has to look for a specific, already identified, genetic variant. This is usually done for the validation of a variant identified through NGS-based testing and for testing of family members for the variant identified in the proband. Family members are tested to study the familial segregation pattern of the variant, to check whether the pattern is consistent with what is expected for the mode of inheritance. Testing of the family members is also done for carrier testing, presymptomatic testing, and prenatal genetic testing (as illustrated in **Figs. 1A and B**). Sanger sequencing, which involves prior amplification of genomic regions of interest through polymerase chain reaction (PCR) followed by DNA sequencing, based on the method of in vitro DNA

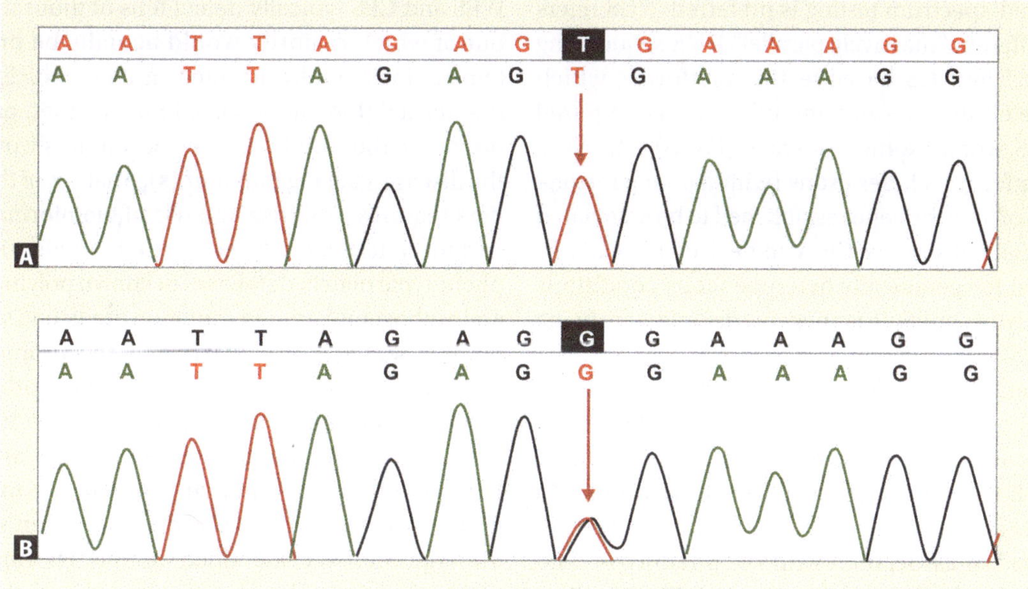

Figs. 1A and B: (A) Sanger sequence chromatogram of a child with Joubert syndrome (an autosomal recessive monogenic disorder) showing a homozygous pathogenic variant c.5668G>T (p.G1890Ter) in exon 41 of the *CEP290* gene (RefSeq sequence ENST00000552810; targeted Sanger sequencing was performed to validate the presence of the *CEP290* gene variant identified through clinical exome sequencing); (B) Sanger sequence chromatogram of the fetal DNA (obtained through chorionic villus sampling in the mother's next pregnancy) showing the presence of the same pathogenic variant c.5668G>T in a heterozygous state, indicating that the fetus (to-be-sibling of the proband) is only a carrier and not affected with the disease.

replication with selective incorporation of chain-terminating dideoxynucleotides, is the preferred technique for targeted variant testing of SNVs, few-nucleotide insertions, and few-nucleotide deletions.[6] Other methods such as restriction fragment length polymorphism (RFLP) analysis and amplification refractory mutation system-PCR (ARMS-PCR) may also be used for targeted testing of specific SNVs.

Sequence Analysis of a Specific Gene

When the clinical phenotype of a patient is clearly suggestive of a specific monogenic disorder known to be associated with only one gene, mutation analysis can be done for that gene alone [e.g., *GLA* (alpha-galactosidase) gene for Fabry disease, *VHL* gene for von Hippel-Lindau syndrome, and *PKHD1* gene for ARPKD]. As, in most cases, the mutation(s) can involve any nucleotide position of the gene, mutation identification in the proband requires sequence analysis of the entire gene. If the gene is relatively small (e.g., the *VHL* gene which has only three exons), the Sanger sequencing technique described above is preferred for sequence analysis of the gene. However, for sequence analysis of a large gene (e.g., the *PKHD1* gene which has 86 exons), Sanger sequencing is not a cost-effective method, and NGS is preferred.

Simultaneous Sequence Analysis of Multiple Genes/Multigene Panel Testing

This method is used for genetically heterogeneous conditions, where the phenotype can be caused by mutation(s) in any one of many different genes [e.g., *SRNS*, which can be caused by mutation(s) in any one of >20 different genes including *NPHS1*, *NPHS2*, *PLCE1*, *WT1*, *LAMB2*, etc.]. Testing of multiple genes in one single panel is done using the NGS technique. A broad-spectrum test such as clinical exome sequencing (CES) can also be used in this scenario.

Gene Dosage Analysis

This refers to testing for large deletions and duplications, which may involve one or more exons of a gene, and sometimes the whole gene. Sanger sequencing is not a suitable method for detecting these mutations. Different types of gene dosage analysis methods are available for molecular diagnosis, of which the most preferred is the multiplex ligation-dependent probe amplification (MLPA) technique, which can be used to look for deletions or duplications of all exons of a gene. MLPA is a modified multiplex PCR assay, wherein up to 40 probes can be used in each assay, to evaluate the relative copy number of different target genomic sequences.[7] Targeted testing for specific exonic deletions and duplications can also be done through quantitative real-time PCR (qPCR) or the less commonly used customized fluorescence in situ hybridization (FISH) technique. The recently developed exon-level genome-wide array method as well as whole genome sequencing (WGS) can be used to look for exonic deletions and duplications in any gene in the entire genome.

Broad-spectrum Testing

When multiple genes known to be associated with a specific phenotype (e.g., SRNS) have to be analyzed, or when the clinical features are not definitively suggestive of any specific syndrome or disorder (e.g., unexplained familial CKD),

NGS-based broad-spectrum testing is preferred. NGS refers to any one of different "massively parallel" DNA sequencing methodologies. The NGS-based testing platforms, which are used in the clinical setting, include multigene panel sequencing, CES, whole exome sequencing (WES), and WGS.

The CES platform includes exons (with flanking intron-exon junctions) of only the genes established to be associated with human genetic disorders. CES can be used instead of a multigene panel for genetically heterogeneous conditions such as SRNS or when multiple monogenic disorders are being considered as possible differential diagnoses.

The WES platform includes exons (with flanking intron-exon junctions) of all the genes in the genome. WES helps to identify causal variants in genes already known to be associated with the phenotype (the ones included in a multigene panel and/or CES), as well as in other genes not hitherto reported in association with the phenotype (and hence not included in the multigene panel/CES). WES is preferred in the evaluation of patients with conditions such as intellectual disability, congenital malformations such as CAKUT, etc., where the underlying etiology remains unknown in a significant proportion of cases. Trio-WES, i.e., simultaneous WES of the proband and of both parents, is the ideal test to be done in this scenario, as it allows for comparison of the variant data of the proband with that of the parents, which helps to corroborate the pathogenicity of the identified variants.

The WGS platform covers the entire genome; therefore, not just the exons, but also the introns and promoter regions of genes as well as the intergenic regions are covered in WGS. It can therefore detect deep intronic variants and promoter region variants not detected through CES or WES. Until recently, WGS was being used only in research settings, but over the past few years it is being increasingly used as a second-tier or third-tier diagnostic test for the evaluation of patients in whom a genetic etiology is strongly suspected, but where first- and second-tier tests such as CES and WES fail to identify any significant genetic variants.

Next-generation sequencing overcomes many of the limitations of Sanger sequencing. It is much more cost-effective and much less time consuming than Sanger sequencing, when larger genomic regions and multiple genes have to be sequenced. It also ensures a much higher depth of coverage and can detect even variants present at a low level of mosaicism.[8-10]

One of the biggest challenges faced with the high-throughput NGS-based tests is the detection of large numbers of genetic variants which one has to analyze and sift through, to identify the actual causal mutation(s). Variants are essentially nucleotide differences between the tested genomic sequences and the corresponding sequences in the reference genome, against which they are aligned and compared. The larger the genomic regions covered through NGS, the larger would be the number of variants detected. WES and CES typically detect tens of thousands of variants, out of which majority would actually be polymorphic or benign, incidentally detected variants, which are present in the normal population also. In most cases, only one or two out of the thousands of detected variants would actually be the disease-causing mutation(s). Analysis of the huge variant data requires expertise and use of bioinformatics tools. The variant data are analyzed through an algorithm based on phenotypic match, databases of known polymorphic variants and pathogenic variants, mutation prediction software results, familial segregation pattern, etc., to sort and filter out the exact disease-causing variant(s) from the other incidentally detected, thousands of variants, as shown in **Flowchart 1**. Detailed clinical phenotyping is an important prerequisite, because phenotypic match is one of the most important parameters taken into consideration when sifting through the large number of identified variants. The American College of Medical Genetics and Genomics and the Association for Molecular Pathology (ACMG/AMP) have formulated guidelines for the classification of gene variants, using criteria based on population data, computational data, functional data, and segregation data. Based on these guidelines, variants are categorized as "pathogenic", "likely pathogenic", "variant of uncertain significance" (VUS), "likely benign", and "benign."[11] Usually, in the clinical setting, identification of a pathogenic or likely pathogenic gene variant(s) which matches the clinical phenotype and follows the expected familial segregation pattern is considered to be confirmatory for the diagnosis of the particular genetic disorder associated with that gene. Benign and likely benign variants are usually not of clinical significance. Variants classified as VUSs may sometimes, but not always, be the disease-causing variants. Interpretation of VUSs is tricky, difficult, and often inconclusive. Apart from studying the clinical correlation, familial segregation pattern, and in silico prediction, additional evidences could be looked for, to corroborate the pathogenicity of a VUS identified in a gene. For example, if WES identifies a VUS in the *GLA* gene in a patient with unexplained CKD, alpha-galactosidase enzyme assay can be done for corroboration of the diagnosis of Fabry disease. Deficient enzyme activity in addition to the other aforementioned levels of evidence would confirm that the identified VUS in the *GLA* gene is the disease-causing variant in the patient. If sufficient evidence regarding the pathogenicity of a VUS is not obtained, it should not be assumed to be the disease-causing variant, and definitive actions such as prenatal or preimplantation genetic testing (PGT) should not be performed based on such a presumptive, unconfirmed diagnosis.

Cytogenetic Tests

Cytogenetic tests refer to the tests used for detecting chromosomal anomalies. These can be broadly categorized as "conventional cytogenetic tests" and "molecular cytogenetic tests".

Flowchart 1: Algorithm used for filtering and sorting of the large number of genetic variants identified through NGS-based testing platforms, to identify the actual disease-causing variant(s).

Genetic variants identified through NGS

↓

Polymorphic variants (variants with MAF >1% in population databases such as 1000 Genomes and gnomAD) filtered out

↓

Intergenic and deep intronic variants and synonymous SNVs filtered out

↓ ↓

Disease-variant databases such as HGMD and ClinVar checked to identify if any of the detected variants are previously reported as pathogenic variants

Mutation prediction software (such as MutationTaster, SIFT, Polyphen 2, CADD, Human splicing finder, etc.) Checked to filter out variants with in silico analysis scores not consistent with pathogenicity

↓ ↓

Genetic variant(s) with best match to patient's phenotype selected as potentially pathogenic

↓

Potential variant(s) tested in parents (and if possible, in affected and unaffected siblings, and in other affected family members) to confirm whether the familial segregation pattern is consistent with the pattern expected for the mode of inheritance

Databases and software mentioned in the flowchart:

- *1000 Genomes:* https://www.internationalgenome.org/1000-genomes-browsers/
- *gnomAD:* https://gnomad.broadinstitute.org
- *ClinVar:* https://www.ncbi.nlm.nih.gov/clinvar/
- *HGMD:* "Human Gene Mutation Database"; http://www.hgmd.cf.ac.uk/ac/index.php
- *PolyPhen-2:* http://genetics.bwh.harvard.edu/pph2/
- *SIFT:* "Sorting Intolerant From Tolerant"; https://sift.bii.a-star.edu.sg/
- *MutationTaster2:* http://www.mutationtaster.org/
- *CADD:* "Combined Annotation-Dependent Depletion"; https://cadd.gs.washington.edu/
- *Human Splicing Finder:* http://www.umd.be/HSF/

(MAF: minor allele frequency; NGS: next-generation sequencing; SNV: single-nucleotide variant)

Conventional Cytogenetic Tests

The most commonly used conventional cytogenetic test is karyotyping with G (Giemsa)-banding. Karyotyping can identify gross chromosomal anomalies such as chromosomal aneuploidies (e.g., trisomy 21, trisomy 13, trisomy 18, monosomy X, etc.) and structural rearrangements that are larger than around 5 Mb in size. Karyotyping is also used in the evaluation of disorders of sex development (DSDs), for ascertaining the chromosomal sex and for diagnosing sex chromosome aneuploidies.

Molecular Cytogenetic Tests

These tests are used for the detection of the smaller, submicroscopic, chromosomal copy number variations (CNVs), also referred to as microdeletions or microduplications. CNVs are defined as either the gain or loss of a stretch of DNA, as compared to the reference human genome, and may range in size from one kilobase to several megabases or even an entire chromosome. Different types of molecular cytogenetic tests are available.

If a specific microdeletion syndrome is suspected clinically, e.g., Williams–Beuren syndrome (chromosome 7q11.23 deletion) or DiGeorge syndrome (chromosome 22q11.21 deletion), targeted evaluation for the same can be done through techniques such as FISH or MLPA which use locus-specific probes.

If, however, a definite syndrome is not identifiable clinically, a broad-spectrum molecular cytogenetic test such as chromosomal microarray (CMA) is preferred. As CMA can detect CNVs throughout the genome, it is recommended as the first-line genetic test for the evaluation of patients with unexplained global development delay, intellectual disability, multiple malformations, and/or autism spectrum disorder.[12] CMA is also recommended as the first-tier test for prenatal genetic evaluation of fetal structural anomalies detected through antenatal scans. WGS is emerging as a better modality for detection of CNVs, as it can detect the chromosomal breakpoints down to the single nucleotide level.

GENETIC TESTING FOR SPECIFIC RENAL DISORDERS

The main categories of monogenic renal disorders are the renal ciliopathies, hereditary glomerulopathies, inherited renal tubulopathies, and monogenic nephrolithiasis conditions. In addition, around 20–30% of patients with CAKUT are identified to be associated with a syndromic or nonsyndromic monogenic cause or chromosomal anomaly.

Primary Ciliopathies

These disorders are caused by mutations in genes involved in determining the structure and function of the primary cilia. They are usually multisystemic disorders, with majority of them involving the kidneys. Primary ciliopathies with significant renal involvement include ADPKD, ARPKD, nephronophthisis, Bardet-Biedl syndrome (BBS), Joubert syndrome, Meckel-Gruber syndrome, and Senior-Loken syndrome. Cystic renal changes are a typical feature of these renal ciliopathies. Except ADPKD, which has an autosomal dominant pattern of inheritance, most of the other primary ciliopathies have an autosomal recessive inheritance pattern; in addition, digenic inheritance is reported in around 10% of the patients with BBS. As these disorders are genetically heterogeneous (e.g., ADPKD can be caused by heterozygous mutation in *PKD1* or *PKD2* gene, or in a few cases in *GANAB*, or *DNAJB11*; BBS can be caused by mutations in any one of around 25 different genes), or they are associated with a large gene (e.g., *PKHD1* which is associated with ARPKD has 67 exons), or they have significant phenotypic overlap (e.g., Joubert syndrome and Meckel-Gruber syndrome), NGS-based platforms are the preferred testing modality. A multigene panel or WES may be done as the first-line test, and if that does not yield the genetic etiology, WGS could be considered as the next line of testing.[13]

Hereditary Glomerulopathies

These include the early onset congenital nephrotic syndrome (CNS), the SRNS group, and Alport syndrome. CNS and SRNS may be nonsyndromic or they may be associated with syndromes such as Denys-Drash syndrome, Pierson syndrome, Galloway-Mowat syndrome, or Schimke immuno-osseous dysplasia. Causative pathogenic gene variants are identified in around 10–15% of young adults and 30% of children with SRNS, and approximately two-thirds of congenital and infantile onset nephrotic syndrome. Till date, around 60 monogenic causes of SRNS have been reported, of which *NPHS1* and *NPHS2* (1q25.2) are the two most commonly implicated genes in autosomal recessive SRNS, and *INF2* and *WT1* are the two most common causes of autosomal dominant SRNS.[14,15] Therefore, NGS-based multigene panel testing or WES would be the preferred first-line genetic test in these cases. However, if there is a strong clinical suspicion of a particular syndrome known to be caused by mutations in a specific gene, e.g., *WT1* gene for Denys-Drash syndrome (combination of SRNS with diffuse mesangial sclerosis on renal biopsy, Wilms tumor, and 46,XY DSD), sequence analysis of that particular gene may be considered first.

Approximately 85% of cases of Alport syndrome are X-linked (caused by *COL4A5* gene mutation), around 15% are autosomal recessive (caused by mutations in *COL4A3* or *COL4A4*), and a few cases caused by heterozygous *COL4A3* gene mutation have autosomal dominant inheritance.[16] NGS-based multigene panel testing or CES would be the preferred testing modality in a patient with suspected Alport syndrome.

Inherited Renal Tubulopathies

Currently, >50 genes are recognized to be associated with renal tubulopathies. Genetic disorders involving the proximal renal tubule include the monogenic forms of Fanconi renotubular syndrome, Fanconi-Bickel syndrome, Dent disease, hypophosphatemic rickets (X-linked and autosomal recessive forms), cystinuria, lysinuric protein intolerance, and Hartnup disease. Those that disrupt the function of the thick ascending limb include Bartter syndrome (types 1, 2, 3, 4a, 4b, and 5), familial hypomagnesemia with hypercalciuria and nephrocalcinosis, and autosomal dominant hypocalcemia. Genetic disorders involving the distal convoluted tubule include pseudohypoaldosteronism type 2, Gitelman syndrome, and autosomal dominant and autosomal recessive forms of familial hypomagnesemia. Monogenic disorders that impair the function of the collecting duct include pseudohypoaldosteronism type 1, Liddle syndrome, nephrogenic diabetes insipidus (X-linked, autosomal recessive, and autosomal dominant forms), and monogenic forms of distal renal tubular acidosis.[17] The preferred modality for genetic evaluation for these disorders is again NGS-based multigene panel testing or WES.

Congenital Anomalies of the Kidney and Urinary Tract

The CAKUTs may occur sporadically or may show a familial pattern. They may occur in isolation or as a part of a syndrome. To date, approximately 40 different genes have been identified to be associated with monogenic forms of CAKUT, but these together account for only around 10–20% of patients with CAKUTs.[18] In addition, around 10–15% of CAKUTs are found to be associated with chromosomal CNVs.[19] WES is the preferred modality to look for the monogenic causes and CMA is the recommended test to look for the chromosomal anomalies associated with CAKUT.

Metabolic Disorders Affecting the Kidneys

Renal involvement can be a component of certain inborn errors of metabolism (IEMs). For example, primary hyperoxaluria type 1 is caused by deficiency of the liver peroxisomal enzyme alanine-glyoxylate aminotransferase (due to mutations in the *AGXT* gene) and primary hyperoxaluria type 2 (PH2) is caused by deficiency of the enzyme glyoxylate reductase/hydroxypyruvate reductase (due to mutations in the *GRHPR* gene). Deficiency of these enzymes impairs the normal metabolism of glyoxylate and results in its conversion to oxalate, which in turn forms insoluble calcium oxalate crystals that result in severe nephrolithiasis. Glutaric acidemia II is associated with polycystic kidneys. Renomegaly, renal stones, and focal segmental glomerulosclerosis (FSGS) occur in glycogen storage disorder type I. Fabry disease and nephropathic cystinosis are the two main lysosomal storage disorders associated with renal impairment. Fabry disease (due to *GLA* gene-associated alpha-galactosidase deficiency) causes progressive glycosphingolipid accumulation in the kidney, which leads to proteinuria, isosthenuria, gradual deterioration of tubular reabsorption and secretion, azotemia, and finally end-stage kidney disease (ESKD). Nephropathic cystinosis (caused by mutations in the *CTNS* gene) is characterized by renal Fanconi syndrome and progressive impairment of glomerular functions. Peroxisomal disorders such as Zellweger syndrome may be associated with hydronephrosis and renal cortical microcysts. Whenever such IEMs are suspected clinically, the relevant metabolic testing, if available, can be performed, e.g., enzyme assay or metabolite assay, and further molecular confirmation can be done through sequencing of the associated gene(s).

Monogenic Causes of Renal Neoplasia/Malignancy

Around 1–2% of renal cell carcinomas occur due to inherited germline mutations. Around 10 syndromes have been identified to be associated with an increased risk of different types of kidney cancer. Increased risk for clear cell kidney cancer is seen with von Hippel–Lindau disease (caused by mutation in *VHL* gene), *PTEN* hamartoma tumor syndrome, germline mutations in the *BAP1* gene, and germline mutations in genes encoding proteins of the succinate dehydrogenase complex (*SDHB/SDHC/SDHD*). Germline mutations in the *MET* gene cause type 1 papillary kidney cancers, while type 2 papillary renal cancers are associated with the hereditary leiomyomatosis and renal cell cancer syndrome (HLRCC) due to *FH* gene (fumarate hydratase) mutations. Birt–Hogg–Dubé syndrome, caused by mutation in *FLCN* gene, is characterized by cutaneous lesions, pulmonary cysts, and various types of renal tumors especially chromophobe and oncocytic hybrid tumors.[20] Tuberous sclerosis complex, caused by mutation in *TSC1* or *TSC2* gene, is associated with renal angiomyolipomas. For patients with clinical suspicion of these disorders, sequence analysis of the relevant genes can be done through Sanger sequencing (if the gene is small, e.g., *VHL*) or NGS (if the gene is large or more than one gene is involved, e.g., *TSC1* and *TSC2*).

In all of the above scenarios, if sequencing of the exons and splice sites does not reveal the mutation(s), MLPA, exon-level microarray, or WGS may be required to look for large exonic deletion and duplication type of mutations. WGS additionally helps to look for deep intronic variants.

UTILITY OF GENETIC TESTING

Genetic testing helps to identify the exact etiology and obtain a precise diagnosis in individuals affected with monogenic disorders or chromosomal anomalies. This helps in accurate prognostication, appropriate management, and surveillance for anticipated manifestations and complications known to be associated with the condition. Disease-specific therapies, e.g., enzyme replacement therapy for Fabry disease, are now available for certain disorders and even mutation-specific therapies such as antisense oligonucleotide (ASO)-based exon-skipping therapy, etc., are being developed for certain others. In monogenic forms of CKD, identification of the underlying basis through genetic testing obviates the need for kidney biopsy, which is invasive and painful. Apart from these obvious benefits in terms of the clinical management of the affected individual per se, genetic testing helps the families as well. Identification of the exact genetic basis helps in accurate genetic counseling of the family. Based on the identified and confirmed genetic diagnosis, one can accurately ascertain the pattern of inheritance and thereby the risk of recurrence in the subsequent offspring of the parents, and perform prenatal genetic testing or preimplantation genetic testing (PGT) for their future pregnancies, to prevent this recurrence. It can also be used for carrier testing and presymptomatic testing of other at-risk family members, as discussed above. If kidney transplant is planned and the potential donor is a biological relative of the patient, presymptomatic genetic testing can be done to confirm the absence of the disease-causing mutations in the prospective donor.[1,2]

ETHICAL ISSUES RELATED TO GENETIC TESTING

Though genetic testing has significant utility and many potential benefits as listed above, there are important ethical considerations as well as legal and social concerns related to genetic testing. Privacy, confidentiality, and autonomy of the patient are very important considerations. In the case of a child, the parents or legal guardian are usually authorized to exercise these rights on behalf of the child. However, as children do not have autonomy over their genetic information and are not able to make informed decisions on the risks and benefits of this information, genetic tests that are not of clear medical benefit should not be done in children. Therefore, presymptomatic testing for a late-onset disorder without any standard disease-altering therapy or intervention, and carrier testing are not recommended in the pediatric age group.[3,4]

GENETIC COUNSELING

Before proceeding with a genetic test, the patient (or in the case of a child, the parents/legal guardian) should be counseled about the utility, diagnostic yield, cost, turnaround time (TAT), and limitations of the test. Implications of the test for clinical management, the procedure for sample collection and any associated risks, and the availability of alternative diagnostic methods and their comparative accuracy should also be discussed. Informed consent should be taken for the genetic test to be performed after completion of the pretest counseling process. Pretest counseling and informed consent are particularly essential for scenarios where there are special ethical, legal, and social issues (ELSI) such as prenatal genetic testing, PGT, carrier testing, or presymptomatic testing; in these situations, a trained genetic counselor and/or a clinical geneticist should be involved for appropriate counseling.[3]

Following confirmation of a monogenic or chromosomal disorder through genetic testing, genetic counseling is provided regarding the underlying basis of the condition, course and prognosis of the disorder, available management options, follow-up and surveillance plan, risk of recurrence in future offspring, reproductive options to prevent this recurrence (including prenatal genetic testing or PGT), newer therapeutic developments and ongoing clinical trials related to the disorder, and availability of patient support groups. Presymptomatic testing and/or carrier screening of other at-risk family members, as relevant, may also be suggested.

CONCLUSION

Many chronic renal disorders, especially the ones manifesting in childhood, have a genetic etiology. Thorough clinical evaluation, a detailed family history, and relevant laboratory investigations are essential to delineate the phenotype of a clinically suspected genetic condition and to choose the apt genetic testing strategy. Confirmation of the genetic etiology through appropriate genetic testing and identification of the underlying genetic basis helps in appropriate management and accurate prognostication of affected individuals, as well as in presymptomatic testing, prenatal genetic testing or PGT, and carrier testing of family members.

KEY POINTS

- Genetic testing has a very important role in the evaluation of chronic renal disorders, especially the ones manifesting in childhood.
- The main categories of monogenic renal disorders are the renal ciliopathies, hereditary glomerulopathies, and inherited renal tubulopathies. In addition, around 20–30% of CAKUTs are found to have a chromosomal anomaly or a monogenic defect.
- There are different testing modalities, ranging from targeted mutation testing and sequence analysis of one gene, to sequencing of a panel of multiple genes, or of the entire exome or genome, and the appropriate test to be chosen depends on the clinical scenario and the suspected clinical diagnosis.
- As majority of the genetic disorders affecting the kidneys are genetically heterogeneous monogenic conditions with overlapping phenotypes, NGS-based testing platforms such as multigene panel tests, CES or WES are the preferred first-line testing modality.
- Detailed phenotypic delineation, through thorough clinical evaluation and ancillary laboratory testing, is essential for choosing the apt genetic test(s) as well as for accurate interpretation and analysis of the test results.
- Pretest and post-test counseling have to be offered for any genetic test that is ordered. Appropriate genetic counseling by a clinical geneticist or a trained genetic counselor is necessary, to help the patient and the family cope with the disorder in the best possible manner.

REFERENCES

1. Arora V, Anand K, Verma IC. Genetic testing in pediatric kidney disease. Indian J Pediatr. 2020;87:706-15.
2. Connaughton DM, Hildebrandt F. Personalized medicine in chronic kidney disease by detection of monogenic mutations. Nephrol Dial Transplant. 2020;35:390-7.
3. Guay-Woodford LM, Knoers NVAM. Genetic testing: considerations for pediatric nephrologists. Semin Nephrol. 2009;29:338-48.
4. Phadke S, Gowda M. Genetic testing in children. Indian Pediatr. 2013;50:823-7.
5. Nussbaum RL, McInnes RR, Willard HF. Human genetic diversity: mutation and polymorphism. In: Nussbaum R, McInnes R, Willard H (Eds). Thompson & Thompson Genetics in Medicine, 8th edition. Philadelphia, PA: Elsevier Inc; 2016. pp. 43-56.
6. McCombie WR, McPherson JD, Mardis ER. Next-generation sequencing technologies. Cold Spring Harb Perspect Med. 2019;9:a036798.
7. Stuppia L, Antonucci I, Palka G, Gatta V. Use of the MLPA assay in the molecular diagnosis of gene copy number alterations in human genetic diseases. Int J Mol Sci. 2012;13:3245-76.
8. Mardis ER. Next-generation sequencing platforms. Annu Rev Anal Chem. 2013;6:287-303.
9. Metzker ML. Sequencing technologies: the next generation. Nat Rev Genet. 2010;11:31-46.
10. Behjati S, Tarpey PS. What is next-generation sequencing? Arch Dis Child Educ Pract Ed. 2013;98:236-8.
11. Richards S, Aziz N, Bale S, Bick D, Das S, Gastier-Foster J, et al. Standards and guidelines for the interpretation of sequence variants: a joint consensus recommendation of the American College of Medical Genetics and Genomics and the Association for Molecular Pathology. Genet Med. 2015;17:405-24.
12. Miller DT, Adam MP, Aradhya S, Biesecker LG, Brothman AR, Carter NP, et al. Consensus statement: chromosomal microarray is a first-tier clinical diagnostic test for individuals with developmental disabilities or congenital anomalies. Am J Hum Genet. 2010;86:749-64.
13. McConnachie DJ, Stow JL, Mallett AJ. Ciliopathies and the kidney: a review. Am J Kidney Dis. 2021;77:410-19.
14. Lipska-Ziętkiewicz BS, Ozaltin BS, Hölttä T, Bockenhauer D, Bérody S, Levtchenko E, et al. Genetic aspects of congenital nephrotic syndrome: a consensus statement from the ERKNet–ESPN inherited glomerulopathy working group. Eur J Hum Genet. 2020;28:1368-78.
15. Trautmann A, Vivarelli M, Samuel S, Gipson D, Sinha A, Schaefer F, et al. IPNA clinical practice recommendations for the diagnosis and management of children with steroid-resistant nephrotic syndrome. Pediatr Nephrol. 2020;35:1529-61.
16. Savige J, Gregory M, Gross O, Kashtan C, Ding J, Flinter F. Expert guidelines for the management of Alport syndrome and thin basement membrane nephropathy. J Am Soc Nephrol. 2013;24:364-75.
17. Downie ML, Lopez Garcia SC, Kleta R, Bockenhauer D. Inherited tubulopathies of the kidney: insights from genetics. Clin J Am Soc Nephrol. 2021;16:620-30.
18. van der Ven AT, Vivante A, Hildebrandt F. Novel insights into the pathogenesis of monogenic congenital anomalies of the kidney and urinary tract. J Am Soc Nephrol. 2018;29:36-50.
19. Sanna-Cherchi S, Kiryluk K, Burgess KE, Bodria M, Sampson MG, Hadley D, et al. Copy-number disorders are a common cause of congenital kidney malformations. Am J Hum Genet. 2012;91:987-97.
20. Haas NB, Nathanson KL. Hereditary kidney cancer syndromes. Adv Chronic Kidney Dis. 2014;21:81-90.

SECTION

3

Symptoms and Signs of Kidney Disease

CHAPTER

3.1

Oligoanuria

Shweta Priyadarshini, Vinod Choudhary

INTRODUCTION

Oligoanuria is a commonly encountered situation in a critical care setting. Oliguria as a condition has been historically mentioned by Hippocrates. It was first described by Ephesus and Galen as early as 100–200 AD.[1,2] Thereafter, an association of oliguria and renal failure was described by Heberden, an English physician, which he termed "ischuria renalis."[3] Oliguria is described as one of the early biomarkers of acute kidney injury (AKI).[4] The various causes of oligoanuria can be clinically apparent or may be subclinical. It is important to know the underlying pathophysiological mechanism of oligoanuria in various clinical settings, as in some situations it may be fully reversible. Oligoanuria is a very sensitive indicator of low-volume status and a consequent impaired end-organ perfusion. Hence, immediate attention is mandatory for a favorable clinical outcome. The importance of oligoanuria and its clinical impact is highlighted by the fact that it is an important criterion included in the classification of AKI, be it the RIFLE [Risk, Injury, Failure, Loss, end-stage kidney disease (ESKD)], pRIFLE (Pediatric RIFLE), AKIN (Acute Kidney Injury Network), or the KDIGO (Kidney Disease Improved Global Outcomes) classification.

DEFINITION

Oliguria is defined as a urine output <0.5 mL/kg/h or <300 mL/m²/day.[5] In infants, urine output <1 mL/kg/h is defined as oliguria. The terms oliguria and anuria are used interchangeably as their underlying pathophysiological mechanism and management remain the same. However, the term "anuria" implies complete cessation of urine flow and oliguria reduction in urine output enough to have an adverse effect on homeostasis.

These definitions just help to guide us with the management of the patients. In general, any urine output that is insufficient to maintain the fluid balance homeostasis and prevent volume overload can be deemed to be oligoanuria.[5]

The definition of oliguria aims to define a urine output threshold below which AKI, as reflected by elevation in serum creatinine, sets in. The longer the duration of collection of urine to define this urine threshold, the more the chances to include the pathological process causing oliguria that culminates in AKI.[6] A 12-hour observation period for oliguria has been found to significantly improve the prediction for worsening AKI.[7]

It is clinically relevant to note that using a weight-related urine output criterion for diagnosing AKI in obese individuals may lead to overdiagnosis of AKI. Hence, it is optimal to use ideal body weight for such calculations.[8]

Newborn babies, as per the above definition, are anuric for the first 24 hours of life and may continue to be oligoanuric till postnatal diuresis sets in by day 3 of life. However, this early neonatal oligoanuria is absolutely physiological and only warrants a wait-and-watch approach.

EPIDEMIOLOGY

The occurrence of oliguria is very common amongst hospitalized patients and mandates a close monitoring. Oliguria is more commonly seen in extremes of age groups, the newborn and the elderly, by the virtue of spectrum of disease and also the propensity to develop dehydration. Oligoanuria is common in the setting of intensive care unit (ICU).[9,10] However, patients who are in advanced stages of AKI, as per both the urine output and the serum creatinine criteria, have a greater adverse outcome than either of the criteria fulfilment alone.[11] Oliguria further has been found to be associated with lower rates of resolution of AKI.[12,13]

ETIOPATHOGENESIS

In the initial stages of oliguria, which cause decreased renal perfusion, various compensatory mechanisms to preserve the glomerular filtration rate (GFR) are activated. The activated myogenic autoregulation and the increase in vasodilatory prostaglandins lead to afferent dilatation; on the other hand, activation of renin–angiotensin–aldosterone system (RAAS) leads to efferent arterial constriction. These mechanisms lead to the maintenance of GFR. When these compensatory mechanisms are overwhelmed, decrease in GFR and ultimately oliguric AKI set in. The common causes of oliguria are listed in **Table 1**.

APPROACH TO OLIGURIA

It is important to evaluate the oliguric patients promptly and accurately to tailor the therapy for the same. Prompt

TABLE 1: Etiology of oliguria.

Prerenal	
Hypovolemia	• Gastrointestinal—diarrhea, vomiting • Renal loss—tubulopathies, diuretics, diabetes insipidus • Blood loss—trauma, surgery • Third spacing • Burns, sepsis, decreased intake
Cardiogenic	Cardiac tamponade, congestive cardiac failure, pulmonary embolism, myocardial failure causing myocardial infarction, congenital heart disease
Vascular	Renal vein or renal artery thrombosis, thromboembolism, capillary leak, neurogenic shock, anaphylactic shock
Intrinsic—Renal	• Vasculitis, glomerulonephritis, interstitial nephritis, malignant hypertension • Acute tubular necrosis due to nephrotoxins and radiocontrast agents • Transplant rejection • ATN due to prolonged prerenal failure
Postrenal	• Renal calculi • Lower urinary tract obstruction—bladder outlet obstruction, posterior urethral valve, tumors, meatal stenosis, neurogenic bladder, urethral trauma

(ATN: acute tubular necrosis)

diagnosis and management may help to reverse oliguria and prevent AKI, especially if prerenal or postrenal mechanisms are involved.

HISTORY

Hypovolemia

It is important to elicit the history of fluid losses such as diarrhea and vomiting. Causes of fluid loss, such as hemorrhage and burns, may be clinically apparent. History of surgery, shock, and nephrotic syndrome that can cause third spacing into interstitial space should be elicited. Causes of polyuria such as diabetes insipidus, diabetes mellitus, and renal tubular acidosis, which can cause volume depletion and consequent oliguria, should be evaluated for. Children often have weight loss with dehydration.

Drugs

Certain drugs such as cyclosporine, tacrolimus, and contrast agents impair myogenic renal autoregulation in face of early dehydration and precipitate oliguric AKI. Nonsteroidal anti-inflammatory drugs (NSAIDs), which inhibit renal production of vasodilatory prostaglandin, are the common drugs precipitating renal failure in a febrile dehydrated child.

Acute tubular necrosis can result due to administration of various drugs including aminoglycoside, amphotericin B, methotrexate, and contrast agents. Drugs such as penicillin, cephalosporins, ciprofloxacin, NSAIDs, and sulfonamides are the commonly used drugs known to cause interstitial nephritis. Hence, it is very important to elicit the detailed history of medications in a patient with oliguria and withdraw the use of the drug suspected to cause oliguria. Once the AKI sets in, care should be taken to modify the dosage of the medications based on GFR.

Glomerular Disease

Symptoms suggestive of glomerular etiology such as gross hematuria, edema, hypertension, pallor, sore throat, pyoderma preceding poststreptococcal glomerulonephritis (PSGN) and dysentery preceding hemolytic uremic syndrome (HUS) should be looked for. Children, commonly adolescents with lupus nephritis or other vasculitis with renal insult, may present with rash, joint involvement, and fever.

Infective Causes

A history of recent travel is also important to point toward prevalent infectious diseases, which can cause renal injuries, such as leptospirosis, malaria, dengue fever, and scrub typhus.

Bladder Outlet Obstruction

Urinary tract obstruction presents with poor urinary stream, difficulty in passing urine, dysuria, frequent urinary tract infections, and at times complete absence of urine output.

Chronic Kidney Disease

Chronic kidney disease (CKD) can also present as oliguria. Underlying causes of CKD may manifest as edema, hypertension, poor growth of the child, fatigue, pallor, hematuria, proteinuria, bone pains, and bony deformities.

PHYSICAL EXAMINATION

Keeping the various etiologies of oliguria, physical examination should be carried out meticulously.

A thorough physical examination should be carried out to assess the hydration status of the patient (skin turgor, mucous membranes, blood pressure). Evaluation of hemodynamic status can help in the identification of prerenal causes of oliguria. Patients with intravascular fluid depletion will have tachycardia, reduced skin turgor, and dry mucous membrane along with hypotension. Children with AKI may present with edema and hypertension as is seen in children with acute glomerulonephritis. Signs of volume overload, such as congestive cardiac failure (CCF) and hepatomegaly, should be looked for. Children with lupus nephritis, Henoch-Schönlein purpura (HSP) nephritis, interstitial nephritis, and various other diseases impacting the kidneys will have specific clinical signs and symptoms pertaining to the underlying disease. For example, children with lupus nephritis may have other signs of lupus such as butterfly rash and malar rash. Palpation of the urinary bladder may reveal a distended bladder secondary to urinary retention in acute cases. Besides oliguria, children with oliguric CKD will have stunted growth, anemia, hypertension, renal osteodystrophy, and edema.

INVESTIGATIONS

After a detailed history is obtained and thorough physical examination is performed, baseline investigative workup should be done.

Basic Laboratory Evaluation

Basic laboratory evaluation in any child with oliguria should include urinalysis and blood workup. Blood workup should include complete blood picture, serum creatinine, blood urea, serum electrolytes, and acid-base status. Depending on the clinical situation, serum complement levels, antinuclear antibody (ANA) profile, anti-double stranded DNA (anti-dsDNA), and other clinically relevant tests should also be done. Urinalysis should be done to look for protein, red blood cell (RBC), and casts in urine.

Urinary Indices

Simultaneous serum and urinary measurement of sodium, creatinine, and osmolality can help to differentiate between prerenal and intrinsic renal causes of oliguria.

The urinary indices for prerenal and intrinsic renal failure are detailed in **Table 2.**[14]

Imaging

Various imaging studies are helpful in evaluating oliguria. Renal ultrasound is a simple, noninvasive test that can give a lot of information with regard to renal size, which can be increased in AKI and reduced in CKD, both of which can present with oliguria. Bedside urinary bladder ultrasound may also be helpful and can instantaneously determine if there is retention of urine.

Renal Biopsy

Renal biopsy is not one of the initial evaluations. It may be required in occasional cases of oliguria secondary to glomerular cause. It is reserved for specific conditions such as suspected lupus nephritis, HSP nephritis, and rapidly progressing glomerulonephritis.[14,15]

Biomarkers

Biomarkers are increasingly being used to identify the risk of AKI and the underlying cause for oliguria, thereby helping to strategize appropriate intervention. One such biomarker is neutrophil gelatinase-associated lipocalin (NGAL), which has been found to predict the oliguria that can culminate in AKI, thus differentiating between reversible and nonreversible forms of oliguria.[4] However, more studies are required before biomarkers can be routinely proposed for use in evaluation of oliguria. Other biomarkers that have been studied are tissue inhibitor of metalloproteinases 2 (TIMP-2) and insulin-like growth factor-binding protein 7 (IGFBP-7).[4]

TABLE 2: Urinary indices for prerenal and intrinsic renal failure.

Urinary indices	*Prerenal failure*	*Intrinsic renal failure*
%FENa	<1%	>2%
Urinary sodium	<20 mEq/L	>40 mEq/L
Urine/plasma osmolality	>1.5	<1.1
Urine/plasma creatinine	>40	<20
Urinary specific gravity	>1.020	<1.010

(FENa: fractional excretion of sodium)

TREATMENT

A stepwise approach is recommended in the diagnosis and treatment of patients with oliguria as shown in **Flowchart 1**. Treatment depends mainly on the underlying etiology.

Initially, hypovolemia must be excluded in an oliguric patient and corrected to obtain adequate renal perfusion, although care should be taken to avoid volume overload.[16] A child with clinical evidence of hypovolemia and oliguria should be administered intravenous fluid challenge in the form of crystalloids at 20 mL/kg over 20–30 minutes to restore intravascular volume. Fluid boluses can be repeated depending on the response of the patient, with close monitoring for fluid overload. Restoration of adequate urine output after fluid replacement is consistent with diagnosis of the prerenal cause for oliguria. If oliguria persists despite adequate fluid replacement, a trial of intravenous furosemide at 1–5 mg/kg/dose or infusion of 0.05–0.4 mg/kg/h may be given. In a background of hypovolemia, if the child is not responding to fluid and diuretic challenge, it indicates acute tubular necrosis (intrinsic renal failure). The decision to initiate kidney replacement therapy (KRT) can be considered at this stage based on the clinical condition of the child.[14]

A pediatric surgeon/urologist should be involved in the postrenal cause of oliguria. Those with bladder outlet obstruction should undergo catheterization or surgical intervention depending on the cause.

PREVENTION

Once oliguria is identified, immediate attention should be directed to identify the cause. Dehydration, if identified and corrected early, has the potential to prevent oliguric AKI. Children with oliguria have reduced drug clearance and are at a higher risk for additional nephrotoxic medication-associated injury. Thus, daily evaluation of patient medication lists and dosages is required to optimize medication management and prevent progression of the underlying pathology.

CONCLUSION

Oliguria is an important sign for volume status and renal injury. Many causes of oliguria are reversible with timely evaluation and intervention. All children with oligoanuria should be assessed based on prerenal, renal, and postrenal etiologies to plan further management.

Flowchart 1: Management of oligoanuria.

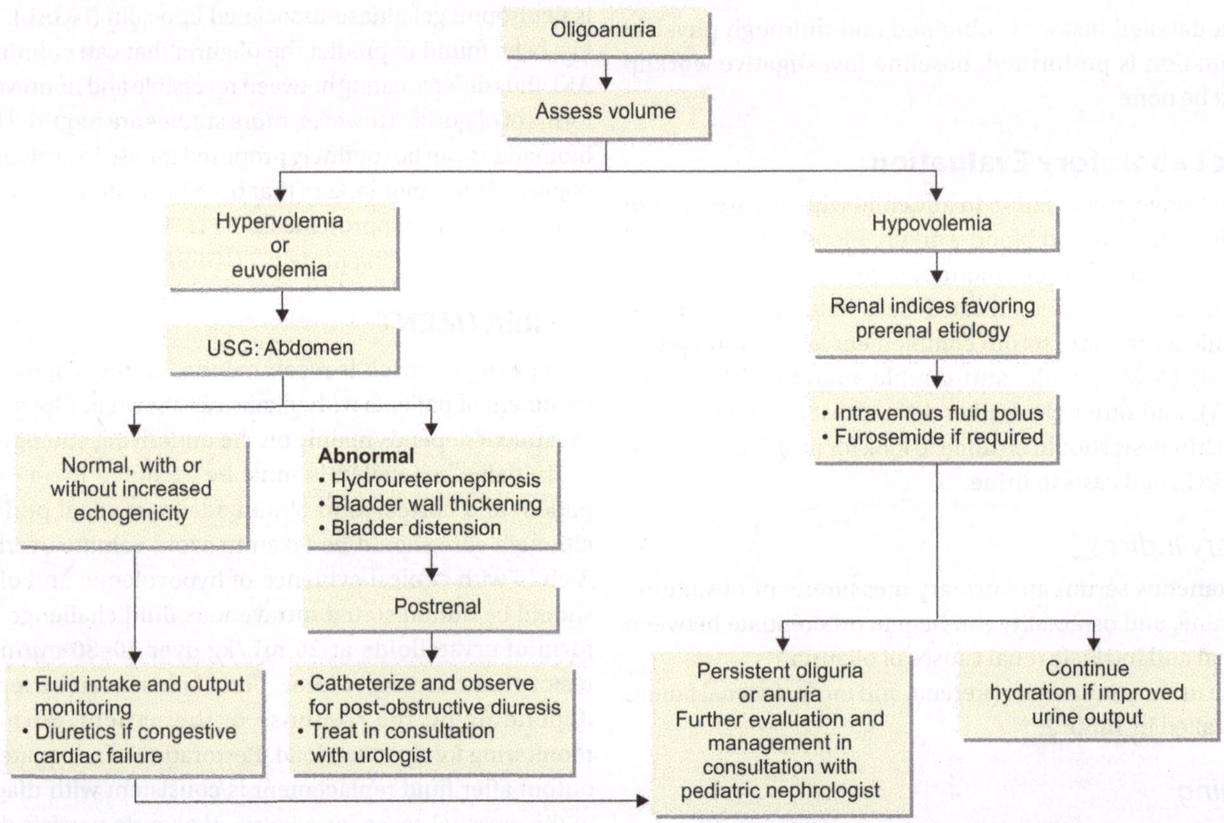

KEY POINTS

- Oliguria is defined as a urine output <0.5 mL/kg/h or <300 mL/m^2/day.
- Oliguria is commonly a result of prerenal causes and responds to fluid management.
- Oliguria is an important criterion to diagnose AKI and acute glomerulonephritis.
- Oliguria associated with hypervolemia needs diuretics and fluid/salt restriction.

REFERENCES

1. Eknoyan G. Rufus of Ephesus and his "Diseases of the Kidneys". Nephron. 2002;91(3):383-90.
2. Eknoyan G. The origins of nephrology—Galen, the founding father of experimental renal physiology. Am J Nephrol. 1989; 9(1):66-82.
3. Heberden W. Commentaries on the History and Cure of Diseases, 4th edition. London: Payne and Foss, Pall-Mall; 1816.
4. Klein SJ, Lehner GF, Forni LG, Joannidis M. Oliguria in critically ill patients: a narrative review. J Nephrol. 2018;31(6):855-62.
5. Goldstein SL. Oliguria in children. In: Vincent JL, Hall JB (Eds). Encyclopedia of Intensive Care Medicine. Berlin, Heidelberg: Springer; 2012. [online] Available from https://doi.org/10.1007/978-3-642-00418-6. [Last accessed June, 2022]
6. Md Ralib A, Pickering JW, Shaw GM, Endre ZH. The urine output definition of acute kidney injury is too liberal. Crit Care. 2013;17(3):R112.
7. Prowle JR, Liu YL, Licari E, Bagshaw SM, Egi M, Haase M, et al. Oliguria as predictive biomarker of acute kidney injury in critically ill patients. Crit Care. 2011;15(4):R172.
8. Ostermann M, Joannidis M. Acute kidney injury 2016: diagnosis and diagnostic workup. Crit Care. 2016;20(1):299.
9. Bailey D, Phan V, Litalien C, Ducruet T, Mérouani A, Lacroix J, et al. Risk factors of acute renal failure in critically ill children: a prospective descriptive epidemiological study. Pediatr Crit Care Med. 2007;8(1):29-35.
10. Macedo E, Malhotra R, Bouchard J, Wynn SK, Mehta RL. Oliguria is an early predictor of higher mortality in critically ill patients. Kidney Int. 2011;80(7):760-7.
11. Kellum JA, Sileanu FE, Murugan R, Lucko N, Shaw AD, Clermont G. Classifying AKI by urine output versus serum creatinine level. J Am Soc Nephrol. 2015;26(9):2231-8.
12. Federspiel CK, Itenov TS, Mehta K, Hsu RK, Bestle MH, Liu KD. Duration of acute kidney injury in critically ill patients. Ann Intensive Care. 2018;8(1):30.
13. Pistolesi V, Di Napoli A, Fiaccadori E, Zeppilli L, Polistena F, Sacco MI. Severe acute kidney injury following cardiac surgery: short-term outcomes in patients undergoing continuous renal replacement therapy (CRRT). J Nephrol. 2016;29(2):229-39.
14. Sharma J. Approach to oliguria. In: Vijayakumar M, Nammalwar BR (Eds). Principle and Practice of Pediatric Nephrology, 2nd edition. New Delhi: Jaypee Brothers Medical Publishers; 2013. pp. 185-90.
15. Stuart L, Zappitelli M. Evaluation and management of acute kidney injury in children. In: Avner ED, Harmon WE, Niaudet P, Yoshikawa N (Eds). Pediatric Nephrology, 7th edition. Heidelberg, Berlin: Springer-Verlag; 2016. pp. 2140-61.
16. Joannidis M, Druml W, Forni LG, Groeneveld ABJ, Honore PM, Hoste E, et al. Prevention of acute kidney injury and protection of renal function in intensive care unit: update 2017: Expert Opinion of the Working Group on Prevention, AKI section, European Society of Intensive Care Medicine. Intensive Care Med. 2017;43(6):730-49.

CHAPTER

3.2 Polyuria

MS Yasmeen, G Sangeetha

INTRODUCTION

Excessive urine output in a child is always a concern for the parents. Polyuria should be differentiated from the common complaints such as frequency or pollakiuria, in which urine output may not be increased. Polyuria is defined as consistent urine output of >4 mL/kg/h (or >2 L/m²/day) in infants and children and >6 mL/kg/h in neonates.[1]

WATER BALANCE

Water homeostasis in a healthy human being is principally achieved by three factors: (1) thirst, (2) vasopressin, and (3) renal function. All three determinants are closely inter-related. The release of vasopressin from the pituitary is principally regulated by any alterations in plasma osmolality. Water loss from the extracellular fluid of any causes increases plasma osmolality, and in turn, it stimulates vasopressin/antidiuretic hormone (ADH) release from the pituitary into the systemic circulation, whereas any reduction in plasma osmolality inhibits the secretion of vasopressin. As the osmoregulatory process is extremely sensitive, even 1% change in serum osmolality may alter the secretion of vasopressin. The released vasopressin acts on the kidney and increases free water reabsorption from the tubules, consequently increasing urine osmolality. Vasopressin V2 receptors (AVPR2)/antidiuretic receptors are situated on the basal aspect of the renal collecting tubular cells. Vasopressin binds to these receptors and allows the insertion of water channel proteins, aquaporin-2 (AQ2), into the cell membrane.[1] These channels transport water from the lumen of the nephron into the collecting duct cells along the osmotic gradient, thereby concentrating the urine. The subsequent passage of water from the cell into the renal interstitium and finally into the circulation is regulated principally by aquaporin-3 and -4 channels.

ETIOLOGY

Polyuria can result from the intake of a large quantity of fluids, solute (or osmotic) diuresis, and water diuresis:[2]

- *Increased fluid intake*: Primary polydipsia
- *Increased solute load (osmotic diuresis):*
    - Diabetes mellitus (DM) and other hyperglycemic conditions
    - The recovery phase of acute kidney injury
    - Mannitol infusion
- Water diuresis

Deficient ADH Secretion: Central Diabetes Insipidus

- *Development defects:* Septo-optic dysplasia, holoprosencephaly, agenesis of the corpus callosum, familial pituitary hypoplasia.
- *Genetic causes:* DIDMOAD [diabetes insipidus (DI), DM, optic atrophy, and deafness] syndrome, familial autosomal dominant/recessive [arginine vasopressin-neurophysin II (AVP-NPII) gene defect].
- Head injury, cerebral hemorrhage, thrombosis, or aneurysm.
- Intracranial tumors (craniopharyngioma, glioma, pinealoma).
- *Central nervous system infections:* Encephalitis, meningitis, and tuberculosis.

Impaired Renal ADH Responsiveness: Nephrogenic Diabetes Insipidus

Congenital:

- X-linked recessive *AVPR2* mutations
- Autosomal dominant and recessive (AQP2 mutations)

Diseases associated with secondary nephrogenic diabetes insipidus:

- Renal tubular acidosis (RTA)
- Salt-losing tubulopathies (Bartter syndrome and Gitelman syndrome)
- Ciliopathies (nephronophthisis and polycystic kidneys)
- Chronic tubulointerstitial nephritis, obstructive uropathy
- Chronic pyelonephritis
- Reflux nephropathy
- Sickle cell disease nephropathy, sarcoidosis, and analgesic nephropathy

DIAGNOSIS

Essential history-taking in polyuria includes polyhydramnios in antenatal scans, preterm delivery, failure to thrive,

Flowchart 1: A general approach to polyuria.

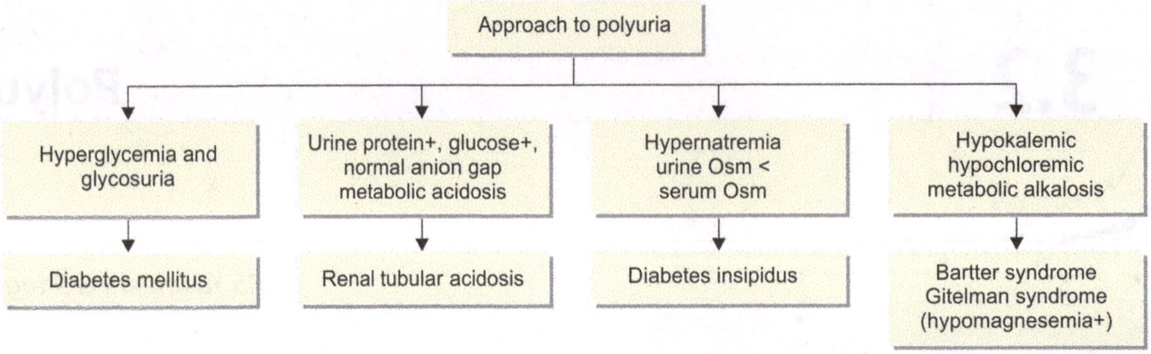

polydipsia, dehydration with no obvious gastrointestinal fluid loss, constipation, episodes of hypotonia, recurrent urinary tract infection, and the presence of bony deformities. An early morning urine sample will look very clear and dilute. Salt craving is an important finding observed in children with polyuria. A positive family history is usually present among other siblings. Psychogenic primary polydipsia that results in excessive intake of water is rare in children but needs to be kept in mind, especially while interpreting the water deprivation test. Parents are advised to maintain a record of fluid intake (frequency, quantity) and urine output record (frequency, quantity) of each day for at least 3–5 days to confirm excessive urine output and to rule out habitual polydipsia. **Flowchart 1** shows the general approach to a child with polyuria.

TABLE 1: Interpretation of fluid deprivation and desmopressin tests in patients with polyuria.

Urine osmolality (mOsm/kg)		
After fluid deprivation	***After desmopressin***	***Diagnosis***
<300	>750	Central DI
<300	<300	Nephrogenic DI
>750	–	Primary polydipsia
300–750	<750	Partial central DI/partial nephrogenic DI/primary polydipsia

(DI: diabetes insipidus)

Laboratory Investigations

- Urine-specific gravity (preferably first-morning sample) to look for renal concentrating ability.
- Urinalysis for proteinuria and glucosuria. Urine electrolytes to find out increased excretion of chloride and potassium in case of tubular disorders.
- Serum and urine osmolality in suspected DI
- Blood glucose levels in hyperglycemia conditions
- Arterial blood gas analysis, renal function test, serum electrolytes, serum calcium, serum phosphorous, serum alkaline phosphatase, and serum uric acid in suspected tubular disorders.
- Ultrasound of kidneys and bladder to look for kidney sizes, hydroureteronephrosis, and bladder status.
- MRI of the brain in suspected central DI
- Genetic testing to confirm congenital nephrogenic diabetes insipidus (NDI), RTA, and Bartter syndrome.

Water Deprivation Test

The water deprivation test is used to establish the diagnosis of partial or acquired conditions with polyuria and an initial serum osmolality value of <290 mOsm/kg. The main aim of the water deprivation test is to induce mild dehydration by stopping fluid intake and challenge the kidneys to preserve water by serial monitoring of urine and serum osmolality hourly for 4 hours in infants and 8 hours in children.[1,2] The test should be started after the void. Measure the body weight, serum sodium, and osmolality as a baseline. Measure the urine volume and urine osmolality with each void. Weight and vitals are monitored hourly. Serum sodium and osmolality are measured at 4 hours and then every 2 hours till the termination of the test. Measure ADH levels at the end of the test. The test must be stopped if the serum sodium is >145 mEq/L or serum osmolality >295 mOsm/kg or >3% loss of body weight or any symptoms of hypovolemia present. If the urine osmolality is >750 mOsm/kg, it indicates intact ADH release and its effect on the renal tubules. The test should be stopped as the patient does not have DI. If the patient has serum osmolality >295 mOsm/kg and urine osmolality <750 mOsm/kg, then DI is confirmed. To differentiate between central diabetes insipidus (CDI) and NDI, the vasopressin challenge test should be done.

Vasopressin Challenge Test

Vasopressin 5–10 μg (intranasally) or 2–4 μg (intravenously or subcutaneously) should be administered. The inability to concentrate urine >300 mOsm/kg in serial urine osmolality measurements performed once every 30 minutes for 2 hours favors NDI. The water deprivation test is not performed in newborns and in very young infants with suspected nephrogenic DI.[3,4] **Table 1** shows the interpretation of fluid deprivation and desmopressin (DDAVP) tests in patients with polyuria.

CONCLUSION

Polyuria in children can be missed unless specific pointers are identified. A general approach to a child with polyuria is described in this chapter and the detailed approach to evaluation and management of specific tubular disorders is mentioned in the respective chapters.

KEY POINTS

- Polyuria should be suspected in any child with failure to thrive with dehydration disproportionate to fluid losses.
- Polyuria is a manifestation of most tubular disorders and commonly presents in infancy.
- The approach to evaluating a child with polyuria and establishing a diagnosis is critical as the management is specific to the underlying tubular disorder.

REFERENCES

1. Van der Watt G, Omar F, Brink A, McCulloch M. Laboratory investigation of the child with suspected renal disease. In: Avner ED, Harmon WE, Niaudet P, Yoshikawa N, Emma F, Goldstein SL (Eds). Pediatric Nephrology, 7th edition. Heidelberg: Springer; 2016. pp. 631-2.
2. Mishra G, Chandrasekhar SR. Management of diabetes insipidus in children. Indian J Endocr Metab. 2011;15(Suppl S3):180-7.
3. Bagga A, Sinha A, Gulati A. Polyuria. Protocols in pediatric nephrology. New Delhi: CBS Publishers & Distributors; 2015. pp. 73-7.
4. Goodyer P. An approach to polyuria. In: Phadke K, Goodyer P, Bitzan M (Eds). Manual of Pediatric Nephrology. New York: Springer; 2014. pp. 232-3.

CHAPTER

3.3 Edema

Vaishnavi Raman, Sudha Ekambaram

INTRODUCTION

Edema, a cardinal sign of renal disease, is an abnormal collection of fluid within the interstitial tissue. It is often associated with effusion—fluid collection in the third space, namely pleural (hydrothorax/pleural effusion), abdominal (ascites), and pericardial space (hydropericardium/pericardial effusion). Massive severe edema is termed anasarca.[1]

Edema can be inflammatory or noninflammatory. Inflammatory edema is usually exudative, localized, and is associated with rubor, dolor, and calor. Noninflammatory edema is usually generalized and transudative. Noninflammatory edema can occur in renal, hepatic, and cardiac diseases or as a manifestation of angioedema, hypoproteinemia, and lymphatic obstruction.[2] The renal causes of edema are nephrotic syndrome (NS), acute glomerulonephritis (AGN), acute kidney injury (AKI), and end-stage kidney disease (ESKD).[3]

PHYSIOLOGY AND PATHOPHYSIOLOGY OF EDEMA

The concept of edema is still under evolution from the Hippocratic time as a general sign of disease to Richard Bright's anatomicopathological correlation linking edema to renal disease then to the Starling forces explaining the pathophysiology of edema and finally to the current modern molecular concepts of sodium retention.[4]

Modified Starling's Law

Factors preventing edema formation under a normal physiological state include the following:

- The tight balance of hemodynamic forces (Starling forces) along the capillary wall (capillary hydrostatic pressure favoring and colloid oncotic pressure preventing fluid movement into the interstitium).
- The permeability of capillaries determining fluid filtration and preventing protein leak across capillaries.
- The intact function of the lymphatic system returning retained interstitial fluid to the venous system.

Imbalance in these factors can lead to edema formation.[4-6]

Figure 1 shows an illustrative diagram of Starling forces.

Sodium and water retention, either leading to or as a consequence of imbalance of Starling forces, is the prime reason for edema in renal disease. The mechanism for the retention is different in different renal diseases. Let us see in detail the different mechanisms of edema formation in renal disease.

NEPHROTIC SYNDROME

Many mechanistic theories have been proposed with points for and against each of them.

Decreased Plasma Oncotic Pressure: The Underfill Hypothesis

In NS, the edema formation was considered to be secondary to increased sodium retention from transient intravascular

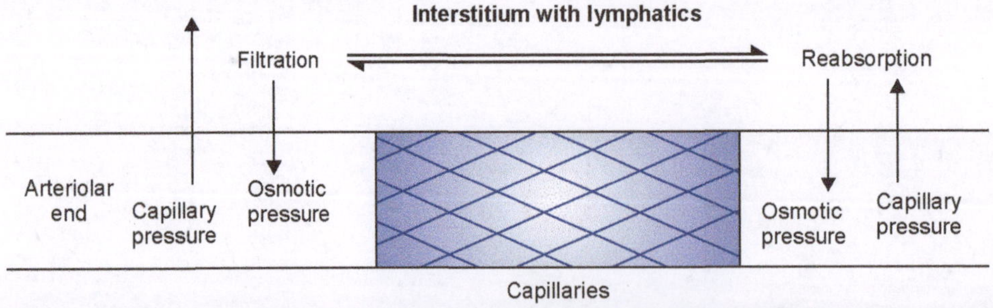

Note: Capillary pressure > osmotic pressure at arteriolar end favoring filtration and osmotic pressure > capillary pressure at venular end favoring reabsorption. Filtration at arteriolar end is balanced by reabsorption at venular end along with lymphatic reabsorption. Edema occurs when capillary pressure is high or osmotic pressure is low or lymphatic reabsorption is impaired.

Fig. 1: Illustrative diagram of Starling forces.

volume depletion from low plasma oncotic pressure referred to as the "underfill" hypothesis. Proteinuria → hypoproteinemia → reduced plasma oncotic pressure → accumulation of interstitial edema and transient *underfilling* of the circulation → reactive renal sodium retention through activation of the sympathetic nervous system, the renin-angiotensin-aldosterone axis, promotion of vasopressin secretion, and suppression of atrial natriuretic peptide (ANP) is the proposed sequence of event.[7,8] Hypoalbuminemia buffers the hemodynamic effects of acute increase in blood volume as it causes preferential interstitial sequestration of fluid. Hence, children with NS do not show a steep relationship between weight gain and hypertension unlike children with AGN.[9]

Pointers against Underfill Hypothesis

Contrary to belief of the underfill theory, reduced plasma oncotic pressure due to hypoalbuminemia does not directly lead to sodium retention and edema as accumulating evidences reveal.[5,10]

- It has been observed in acute NS that sodium retention commences before albumin levels fall substantially. Similarly, during remission, sodium excretion occurs (natriuresis and diuresis with partial resolution of edema) before serum albumin levels have shown a rise.
- With reduced plasma oncotic pressure due to hypoalbuminemia, there is a parallel fall in the interstitial oncotic pressure. Initial fluid shift from the intravascular space to the interstitium increases the interstitial fluid pressure and washes down the interstitial protein concentration. Thus, a parallel decrease in interstitial fluid albumin and an increase in interstitial fluid pressure serve to maintain edema driving forces constant, suggesting that hypoalbuminemia per say may not be the cause of edema.

Increased Plasma Hydrostatic Pressure: The Overfill Hypothesis

In the past two decades, many studies have supported the conceptually opposite idea of the "overfill" hypothesis of primary sodium retention.

- Induction and coordinated *overactivity of Na^+–K^+-ATPase and epithelial sodium channel (ENaC) in NS* leads to sodium and water retention. The principal cells in the cortical collecting duct are responsible for sodium and water reabsorption and potassium excretion, which are carried out by Na^+–K^+-ATPase on the basolateral membrane and ENaC on the apical membrane. In NS, aberrantly filtered plasminogen gets converted to its active form plasmin by tubular urokinase. Plasmin (the serine protease) causes increased proteolytic cleavage of the gamma subunit of ENaC at the cell surface and converts ENaC to its highly active form. The activated ENaC causes urinary sodium retention.[11]
- Proximal tubular sodium reabsorption is also enhanced by filtered albumin by directly stimulating *sodium-hydrogen exchanger* (NHE3), the major apical sodium transporter.[12,13]
- In patients with NS, *tubular resistance to ANP* caused by increased cyclic guanosine monophosphate (cGMP) phosphodiesterase activity leads to sodium retention.[14]
- There is also strong evidence that *tubulointerstitial inflammation and glomerulo-interstitial cross-talks* are involved in sodium retention and nephrotic edema formation. In acute phase, proteinuria → infiltration of the interstitium by inflammatory cells → reduction in glomerular co-efficient (Kf) and single-nephron glomerular filtration rate (GFR) → decline in sodium filtration. In longstanding NS, interstitial inflammation stimulates tubulointerstitial fibrosis leading to a more permanent decrease in GFR and thus sodium retention.[15]

However, not all children with NS present with features of increased circulatory volume (like hypertension). Hence, on review of literature, it appears that the underfill phase is common in acute conditions such as noninflammatory NS (minimal change disease), whereas the overfill phase is seen in the chronic phase of NS, especially accompanied by intrarenal inflammation. As already seen, sodium retention alone is not enough to cause edema. So let us review the other proposed mechanisms.

Increased Capillary Permeability

With extracellular fluid (ECF) volume expansion, the fluid tends to be distributed more toward the interstitial compartment in patients with NS. This is due to increased vascular permeability of endothelial capillary barriers, probably due to the release of vascular permeability factors and other cytokines.[16,17] **Flowchart 1** shows the pathophysiology of edema in NS considering all proposed mechanisms.

ACUTE GLOMERULONEPHRITIS

In AGN, an injury to the glomerular capillaries leads to the reduction in GFR due to reduced blood flow through the hypercellular and occluded glomerular capillaries. As a result of the variable reduction in GFR, with a normal tubular function, there is decreased filtered load of sodium and water stimulating tubuloglomerular feedback causing enhanced tubular sodium and water reabsorption via the renin-angiotensin-aldosterone mechanism. This will lead to expanded extracellular volume, particularly if sodium intake is not restricted. Blood volume expansion leads to a rise in the hydrostatic pressure at the venular end, which results in minimal or no reabsorption of fluid leading to edema.[18] Edema is usually periorbital, pedal, and occasionally ascites. Scrotal edema is not characteristically seen in AGN.

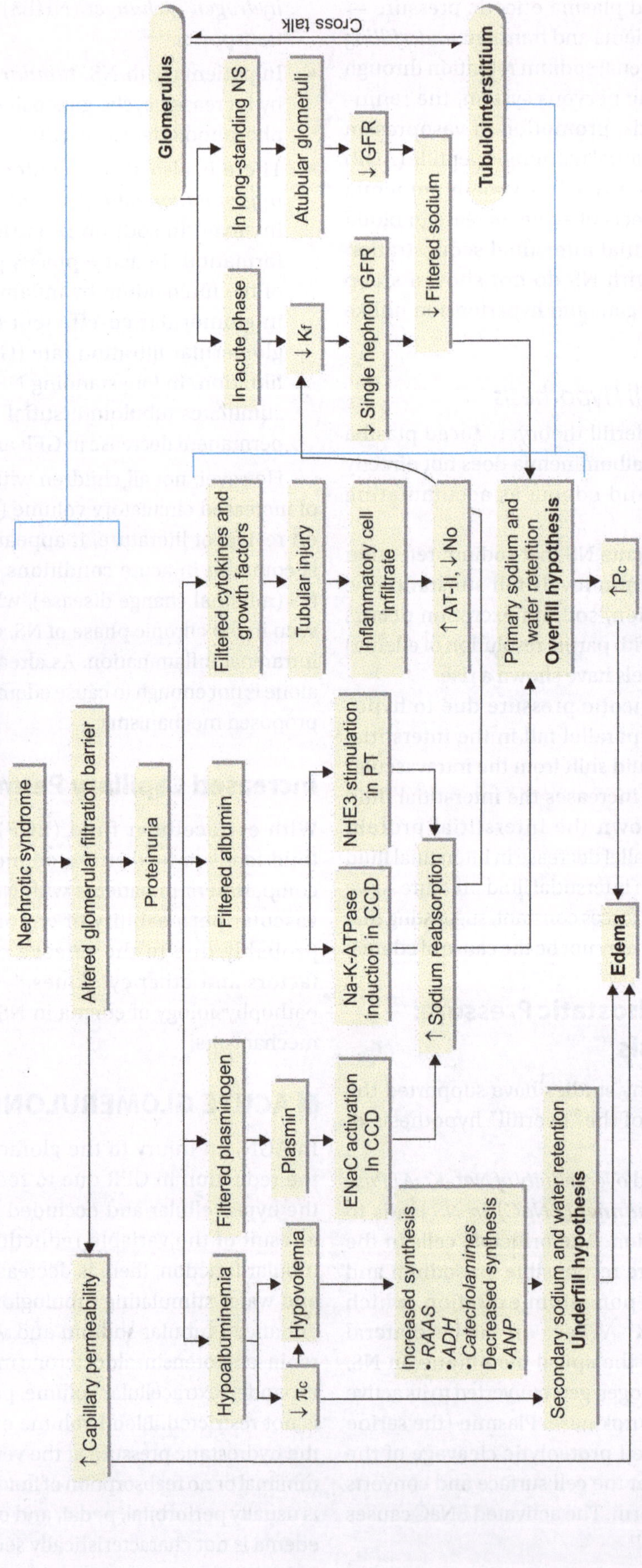

Flowchart 1: Pathophysiology of edema

(ADH: antidiuretic hormone; ANP: atrial natriuretic peptide; AT-II: angiotensin II CCD: cortical collecting duct; ENaC: epithelial sodium channel; GFR: glomerular filtration rate; NS: nephrotic syndrome; PT: proximal tubule; RAAS: renin–angiotensin–aldosterone system)

ACUTE KIDNEY INJURY

In AKI, the edema is due to retention of salt and water secondary to decline of GFR, tubular damage, and iatrogenic fluid resuscitation leading to fluid overload. An abrupt fall in glomerular filtration in AKI causes an accumulation of sodium and water, resulting in an increased blood volume, hypertension, and edema formation. The damaged tubules lose their capacity for selective reabsorption and concentration of the glomerular filtrate resulting in increased reabsorption and oliguria. Oliguria could also be due to tubular backleak of the glomerular filtrate into the interstitium secondary to loss of lining tubular epithelial cells or obstruction due to casts formed by the shredded epithelial cells. It is still debatable whether fluid overload is a cause or effect of AKI. Fluid overload causes endothelial glycocalyx damage and increased capillary permeability which causes AKI. This further increases fluid overload and edema (thus a vicious cycle). Altered capillary permeability due to inflammation and hypoalbuminemia due to critical illness are other contributing factors for edema.[19,20]

END-STAGE KIDNEY DISEASE

In end-stage kidney disease (ESKD) with the progressive loss of nephrons, the fall in the glomerular filtration of water and sodium becomes evident.[21] Blood volume is increased, leading to edema formation and hypertension, especially after an abrupt increase of salt intake. In the early stages of tubulointerstitial cause of CKD, edema formation is uncommon with polyuria and polydipsia being more evident. The ability to dilute the urine is well preserved in the tubulointerstitial disease, and urine output does not diminish. Thus, water depletion and sodium wasting may ensue in the inadvertent restriction of water and sodium intake in such cases.[1]

DIAGNOSIS OF EDEMA

A detailed history regarding the onset, site of first appearance of edema, and associated symptoms should be elicited.[22,23]

Renal

Edema of renal origin appears initially in parts of the body with loose connective tissue and is gravity dependent. Hence, it has a characteristic feature of onset around the eyelids during awakening ("early morning puffiness") and disappearing with erect posture to accumulate in legs by the end of the day. With increasing severity of edema, effusion and anasarca develop. The presence of either hematuria or oliguria with or without hypertension is suggestive of renal edema.

Cardiac

Edema seen more in legs with associated breathlessness and tachycardia is suggestive of cardiac edema. Other features such as cardiomegaly, tender hepatomegaly, S3 gallop, and elevated jugular venous pressure (JVP) may be present.

Hepatic

Disproportionate abdominal distension with features of portal hypertension and jaundice is suggestive of cirrhosis.

Miscellaneous

Hypothyroidism should be considered after ruling out other causes. Unilateral edema is more likely due to lymphedema, which is nonpitting.

Protein-energy malnutrition, especially Kwashiorkor, can present with edema and such children will have other features of poor nutrition.

The extent of edema is semiquantitatively assessed as 1+ for feet and ankles, 2+ for up to the knees, 3+ for all of the legs, and 4+ for the entire body, or anasarca.[4]

Assessing intravascular/effective circulatory volume status: Knowing the effective circulatory volume (ECV) status aids in deciding the treatment modality in NS. Three methods of intravascular volume assessment have been utilized in the NS literature:[5]

- Blood volume measurement with radioactive labeling techniques
- Presence or absence of hypovolemic symptoms and signs clinically
- Neurohumoral hormone assays and their corroborative urinary indices

In practice, radioactive labeling techniques are not readily available and it is difficult to assess volume status based on clinical judgment alone in NS. Hypotension, increased hematocrit, and prerenal AKI may be a clue to low volume status. A high renin and aldosterone state indicates hypovolemia, which corroborates with urine indices; low fractional excretion of sodium (FeNa) of <1% and high excretion of potassium of >60% ($U_K/U_K + U_{Na}$) tend to have a low intravascular volume. Such patients should not receive oral or intravenous diuretics, before correction of their intravascular volume with either crystalloids or colloids. Patients with edema and no clinical or laboratory features of hypovolemia (normal levels of blood urea, FeNa > 1% and $U_K/U_K + U_{Na} < 60\%$) can safely be treated with potent diuretics.[24] It is, however, important to understand that sodium wasting due to prior therapy with diuretics often limits the practical utility of these indices. The features to differentiate overfill versus underfill hypothesis (volume status) are given in **Table 1**.

TREATMENT

The treatment of edema involves the following:

- Symptomatic management
- Treating the specific cause for edema

Bed Rest

Bed rest alleviates orthostatic activation of the renin-angiotensin and sympathetic nervous systems that accompany upright posture and facilitate the transfer of interstitial fluid to

TABLE 1: Difference in clinical and laboratory features of underfill and overfill hypothesis.

Characteristics	*Overfill hypothesis (high ECV)*	*Underfill hypothesis (low ECV)*
Clinical: Blood pressure	Hypertension	Normotensive/ hypotensive/ postural hypotension
Serum albumin	↓ (>2 g/dL)	↓↓ (<2 g/dL)
AKI	Intrinsic renal	Prerenal
GFR	↓↓	↓
Urinary indices	FeNa >1% $U_K/(U_K + U_{Na}) < 60\%$	FeNa <1% $U_K/(U_K + U_{Na}) > 60\%$
Renin and aldosterone	Low	High
Histology	Usually nonminimal change	Usually minimal change disease

(AKI: acute kidney injury; ECV: effective circulatory volume; GFR: glomerular filtration rate)

the vascular compartment expanding circulatory volume. But prolonged bed rest causes venous stasis and is associated with an increased risk of thromboembolic complication, especially in nephrotic children due to an underlying hypercoagulable state. So, a careful balanced decision of bed rest and activity is to be advised.

Salt and Fluid Restriction

As the primary mechanism of renal edema is salt and water retention, combined salt and fluid intake restriction aids in slowing down the rate of edema formation. The therapy is ineffective, if salt and fluids are not restricted concurrently. In children, sodium restriction to the more modest levels is achievable. The practical advice is to say "No added/extra salt" to diet. Use of table salt and processed food with high salt content is to be avoided.[25,26] It is only in refractory edema (edema not responding to diuretics) that strict dietary sodium restriction to 1-2 mEq/kg/day is advised (for a rough idea, 1 tsp of salt = 6 g of salt = 100 mEq of sodium). It should be ensured that diet is practical and not unnecessarily restrictive.[27]

Fluids are restricted either to insensible water loss (400 mL/m²/day) or to insensible water loss added to previous days' urine output depending on the severity of edema.[1] A fluid balance chart should be maintained along with twice-daily weight recording. Fluid restriction after disease remission when the child becomes dry is futile. Hence, cautious advice of liberalizing fluid intake based on urine output once the spontaneous diuresis phase begins is crucial.

Diuretics

Diuretics are the cornerstone in management of moderate-to-severe nephrotic edema (>10% ECF volume). They act by limiting further sodium retention along with excretion of sodium and water retained in the body.

Diuretics → initial fluid and salt loss from intravascular space → reduction in capillary hydrostatic pressure → mobilization of extracapillary edema fluid into intravascular space → refilling plasma volume. Hence, diuretics are useful only when the intravascular volume status is maintained.[4]

The choice, route, and dose of diuretic administration should be decided and titrated based on the severity of edema and response to therapy. Although most sodium reabsorptions occur in the proximal tubule (55–60%) and loop of Henle (25–30%), and only minimal reabsorption occurs in the distal tubule and collecting duct, the efficacy of proximally acting diuretics (e.g., acetazolamide) is offset by compensatory increased distal resorption of sodium and water in the ascending limb of Henle. Hence, loop diuretics (furosemide, torsemide, and bumetanide) are highly potent (FENa 30%) and are the first choice of diuretic in nephrotic edema followed by moderately potent (FENa 5–10%) thiazides and less-potent potassium-sparing diuretics (FENa 2–3%).[28] Among the loop diuretics, equipotent doses of all diuretics (furosemide 40 mg = torsemide 20 mg = bumetanide 1 mg) are equally efficacious. However, loop diuretics can have blunted or absent diuretic action in NS.[29-31] This is due to changes in the pharmacokinetics and pharmacodynamics of loop diuretics in NS as follows **(Table 2)**:

- Delayed absorption of the diuretic (bowel wall edema)
- Reduced secretion of the diuretic into the tubular lumen (its site of action) due to hypoalbuminemia
- Compensatory distal sodium retention after the effective period of the diuretic due to ENaC and Na^+-K^+-ATPase induction and hypertrophy and hyperplasia of the epithelial cells of the distal convoluted tubule.

  The mechanism, dose and duration of action of different diuretics are given in **Table 3**.

Management of Diuretic Resistance

- *Rule out noncompliance*: Noncompliance with either salt restriction or medication intake should first be excluded.
- *Dose adjustment*: Increasing the dose to reach ceiling dose.
- Intravenous bolus injection or continuous infusion after the maximum ceiling dose of oral loop diuretic.
- *Combination diuretic therapy:* Thiazide diuretic combined with a loop diuretic. Thiazide should be given an hour before loop allowing the solute transport in the distal tubule to be blocked fully before it floods with solute from the loop of Henle, ensuring sustained and effective diuresis.[32-34]

Albumin

In refractory edema (edema not responding to effective diuretic dose), plasma volume expansion with salt poor albumin (20 or 25%) infusion might play an adjunctive role. It is given at a dose of 0.5–1 g/kg/day as infusion over 2–4 hours (giving a slower rate causes equilibration of albumin to interstitium decreasing the effect). It is usually given with

TABLE 2: General characteristic of diuretics and its alteration in nephrotic syndrome (NS).

Characteristic	***General principle***	***Issue with use in NS***	***Remedy***
Route: Oral vs IV	• Oral: Sustained diuresis (absorption-limited kinetics—absorption slower than clearance, and hence longer effective blood concentration) • Low postdiuretic sodium retention	Impaired oral absorption and decreased oral bioavailability due to bowel wall edema	Intravenous route is preferred when there is significant edema
Dose			
Loop diuretics have a sigmoid dose–response curve	Sigmoid curve implies that increasing dose beyond a threshold dose shows increased diuretic response (slope) till a plateau or ceiling dose reached at which further increase in dose does not increase diuresis	Sigmoid dose curve shifted down and right in NS	Higher dose is required to produce a similar effect as in normal children
Loop diuretics are highly protein bound	Protein binding helps them stay intravascular, get secreted through the organic anion secretory pathway into proximal tubule to act on the luminal side	Hypoalbuminemia causes the diuretics to get secreted into the interstitial space slowing secretion into tubules. Once secreted, its action decreases because of its binding to tubular fluid albumin	Coadministration with albumin if inadequate diuretic response (especially in significant edema with low intravascular volume) after high dose of oral diuretic and combination diuretic tried
Frequency: Short plasma half-life		• Postdiuretic • Sodium retention after its action ends	• Two or three daily doses with each dose exceeding the threshold dose • IV bolus or infusion—if inadequate diuresis after maximum ceiling dose of oral diuretic • Continuous infusion better over bolus to avoid postdiuretic sodium retention
Efficiency: Natriuretic effect based on distal sodium delivery and compensatory reabsorption	In general setting, produce good natriuresis as distal sodium reabsorption is limited	Distal reabsorption increased in NS due to activation of ENaC, Na^+–K^+-ATPase, and compensatory hypertrophy of distal epithelial cells (*Braking phenomenon*—functional and structural alteration in distal segments leading to decreased natriuresis, especially during chronic administration)	Coadministration with diuretics blocking distal sodium reabsorption (thiazides, amiloride) inhibiting the distal sodium reabsorption and thereby overcomes furosemide resistance

(ENaC: epithelial sodium channel; IV: intravenous)

furosemide at the end of infusion to prevent pulmonary edema. The major drawback with this approach is that the infused albumin is rapidly excreted in the urine. This makes albumin administration an expensive therapy with only short-lasting benefit, and therefore it should be reserved for patients with only the most resistant, severe, symptomatic edema (tense ascites, significant pleural effusion with breathing difficulty, severe scrotal/vulval edema at risk for skin breakage), or for severely intravascular volume-depleted children with significant edema presenting with AKI.[35,36]

Aquaretics

They are a newer group of diuretics producing solute-free diuresis (aquaresis) unlike conventional diuretics. Increased ADH levels and hyponatremia in some NS children suggest water retention in excess of Na^+ retention. This is the rationale for using aquaretics to manage nephrotic edema. Few case reports show efficacy of such aquaretics (V2R antagonist—tolvaptan, somatostatin analog—octreotide) in inducing aquaresis. They act by inhibiting their common intracellular mediator, cyclic adenosine monophosphate (cAMP), thereby decreasing aquaporin channel insertion in the renal collecting duct epithelium and causing diuresis.[28,35]

Urea channels in collecting duct help in accumulating urea in renal medullary interstitium preventing urea-induced osmotic diuresis. Urea channel inhibitors thereby help in managing edema in children with NS with signs of excess water retention.[35]

TABLE 3: Mechanism, dose, and duration of diuretics.

	Mechanism	Bioavailability	Onset (min)	Duration (h)	Dose
Loop					
Furosemide	Inhibits Na+/K+/2Cl− channel in TAL TAL of the loop of Henle	20–80% Oral: IV 2:1	Oral: 40 IV: 5	6–8	• Oral: 1–6 mg/g/day two to three times a day • IV 1–4 mg/kg/day two to three times a day • IV infusion 0.1–1 mg/kg/h
Bumetanide		85%	Oral: 40 IV: 5	4	0.02–0.04 mg/kg/day 12–24 hourly
Torsemide		80% Oral: IV 1:1	Oral: 60 IV: 5	12	5–10 mg/day
Thiazide					
Hydrochlorothiazide	Inhibits NaCl cotransporter in early DCT	70%	120	12–24	2–4 mg/kg/day
Thiazide-like					
Metolazone	Similar to thiazides with additional proximal tubular sodium uptake inhibition	65%	60	24	0.2–0.4 mg/kg/day 12–24 hourly
Potassium sparing					
Spironolactone	Inhibits sodium uptake in collecting duct by blocking mineralocorticoid receptor or ENaC channel	65%	120–180	48–72	2–3 mg/kg/day as single dose
Amiloride		15%	120	24	0.1–0.6 mg/kg/day

(DCT: distal convoluted tubule; ENaC: epithelial sodium channel; IV: intravenous; TAL: thick ascending limb)

Head-out Water Immersion

Head-out water immersion maneuver increases sodium excretion in patients with NS through central blood volume expansion, stimulating ANP release, and suppressing plasma renin activity and plasma aldosterone. It is of only limited practicality similar to the diuretic technique. Sodium excretion decreases to basal values immediately after the patients are removed from the immersion tank, and it is possible that even more avid sodium retention during the time out of the tank offsets the natriuresis that is occurring, as a result of the immersion.[1,7,25]

Support Stockings

Support stockings are also of some use by favoring the distribution of blood to the central blood volume. They alleviate some of the stimuli for sodium retention in a manner analogs to the effects of head-out water immersion.[1,25]

Ultrafiltration

Ultrafiltration (UF) is the movement of water across a membrane due to a hydrostatic pressure gradient (or transmembrane pressure). As the water diffuses, it creates a solute concentration gradient causing solute diffusion (convection). Isolated UF or UF along with dialysis can be used in children with edema resistant to all other treatments.[37] Sustained low efficiency continuous UF/continuous kidney replacement therapy is effective in the removal of excess water without significant hypotension. This technique is offered to hospitalized children in the critical care setting, many of whom have acute renal failure. But NS being a prothrombotic state, having a central vascular catheter and creating a hemoconcentration are risky. Peritoneal dialysis also provides a means of fluid removal (UF) along with dialysis and is a safer alternative to extracorporeal UF in children. It is especially useful in children with refractory ascites.[38,39]

CONCLUSION

Fluid balance is an important function of the kidneys, and edema is a cardinal sign of renal disease. The pendulum of mechanism of edema formation sways between the overfill and the underfill theories. These theories govern the approach to management of edema.

KEY POINTS

- Renal edema could result from a range of disease entities such as NS, AGN, AKI, and chronic kidney disease.
- Understanding the mechanism of edema is critical for the supportive management for individual renal diseases.
- Fluid management, albumin infusion, and diuretics are the mainstay therapies in the care of a patient with nephrotic edema.
- Diuretics and dialysis are essential therapies for those with AKI and chronic kidney disease.

REFERENCES

1. Sudha E, Prahalad N. Approach to edema. In: Nammalwar BR, Vijayakumar M (Eds). Principles and Practice of Pediatric Nephrology, 2nd edition. New Delhi: Jaypee Brothers Medical Publishers; 2013. pp. 195-201.
2. Haemodynamic disorders, thromboembolic disease and shock. In: Kumar V, Abbas AK, Aster JC, Turner JR (Eds). Robbins & Cotran Pathologic Basis of Disease, 10th edition. Philadelphia: Elsevier; 2020. pp. 115-40.
3. Hisano S, Hahn S, Kuemmerle NB, Chan JC, De Santo NG. Edema in childhood. Kidney lnt. 1997;51(S59):S100-4.
4. Krzesinski JM, Cohen EP. Approach to the patient with oedema. In: Turner N, Lamiere N, Goldsmith DJ, Winearls CG, Himmelfarb J, Remuzzi G. (Eds). Oxford Textbook of Clinical Nephrology, 4th edition. United Kingdom: Oxford University Press; 2016. pp. 272-81.
5. Siddall EJ, Radhakrishnan J. The pathophysiology of edema formation in the nephrotic syndrome. Kidney Int. 2012; 82:635-42.
6. Taylor AE. Capillary fluid filtration. Starling forces and lymph flow. Circ Res. 1981;49:557-75.
7. Bobkova I, Chebotareva N, Kozlovskaya L, Shilov E. Edema in renal diseases - current view on pathogenesis. Nephrol Point Care. 2016;2(1):e47-e55.
8. Schrier RW, Fassett RG. A critique of the overfill hypothesis of sodium and water retention in the nephrotic syndrome. Kidney Int. 1998;53(5);1111-7.
9. Koomans HA, Braam B, Geers AB, Roos JC, Dorhout Mees EJ. The importance of plasma proteins for blood volume and blood pressure homeostasis. Kidney Int. 1986;30:730-5.
10. Koomans HA. Pathophysiology of oedema in idiopathic nephrotic syndrome. Nephrol Dial Transplant. 2003;18(6): vi30-2.
11. Ray EC, Rondon-Berrios H, Boyd CR, Kleyman TR. Sodium retention and volume expansion in nephrotic syndrome: implications for hypertension. Adv Chronic Kidney Dis. 2015;22:179-84.
12. Camici M. Molecular pathogenetic mechanisms of nephrotic edema: progress in understanding. Biomed Pharmacother. 2005;59(5):215-23.
13. Besse-Eschmann V, Klisic J, Nief V, Le Hir M, Kaissling B, Ambuhl P. Regulation of the proximal tubular sodium/proton exchanger NHE3 in rats with puromycin aminonucleoside (PAN) induced nephrotic syndrome. J Am Soc Nephrol. 2002;13(9):2199-206.
14. Valentin JP, Ying WZ, Sechi LA, Ling KT, Qiu C, Couser WG, et al. Phosphodiesterase inhibitors correct resistance to natriuretic peptides in rats with Heymann nephritis. J Am Soc Nephrol. 1996;7:582-93.
15. Rodriguez-Iturbe B, Herrera-Acosta J, Johnson RJ. Interstitial inflammation, sodium retention, and the pathogenesis of nephrotic edema: a unifying hypothesis. Kidney Int. 2002;62: 1379-84.
16. Rostoker G, Behar A, Lagrue G. Vascular hyperpermeability in nephrotic edema. Nephron. 2000;85:194-200.
17. Brenchley PE. Vascular permeability factors in steroid-sensitive nephrotic syndrome and focal segmental glomerulosclerosis. Nephrol Dial Transplant. 2003;18(6):21-5.
18. Kurtzman NA. Nephritic edema. Sem Nephrol. 2001;21(3): 257-61.
19. Ostermann M, Straaten HM, Forni LG. Fluid overload and acute kidney injury: cause or consequence? Crit Care. 2015;19:443.
20. Godin M, Bouchard J, Mehta RL. Fluid balance in patients with acute kidney injury: emerging concepts. Nephron Clin Pract. 2013;123:238-45.
21. Khan YH, Sarriff A, Adnan AS, Khan AH, Mallhi TH. Chronic kidney disease, fluid overload and diuretics: a complicated triangle. PLoS One. 2016;11(7):e0159335.
22. Cho S, Atwood JE. Peripheral edema. Am J Med. 2002;113(7): 580-6.
23. Trayes KP, Studdiford JS, Pickle S, Tully AS. Edema: diagnosis and management. Am Fam Physician. 2013;88(2):102-10.
24. Iyengar AA, Kamath N, Vasudevan A, Phadke KD. Urinary indices during relapse of childhood nephrotic syndrome. Indian J Nephrol. 2011;21:172-6.
25. Vasudevan A, Mantan M, Bagga A. Management of edema in nephrotic syndrome. Indian Pediatrics. 2004;41:787-95.
26. Watson AR, Coleman JE. Dietary management in nephrotic syndrome. Arch Dis Child. 1993;69(2):179-80.
27. Humphreys MH. Mechanisms and management of nephrotic edema. Kidney Int. 1994;45:266-81.
28. Gupta S, Pepper RJ, Ashman N, Walsh SB. Nephrotic syndrome: oedema formation and its treatment with diuretics. Front Physiol. 2019;9:1868.
29. Ellison DH. Clinical pharmacology in diuretic use. CJASN. 2019;14(8):1248-57.
30. Brater DC. Resistance to loop diuretics: Why it happens and what to do about it. Drugs. 1985;35:27-43.
31. Cadnapaphornchai MA, Tkachenko O, Shchekochikhin D, Schrier RW. The nephrotic syndrome: pathogenesis and treatment of edema formation and secondary complications. Pediatr Nephrol. 2014;29:1159-67.
32. Hoorn EJ, Ellison DH. Diuretic resistance. Am J Kidney Dis. 2017;69:136-42.
33. Meena J, Bagga A. Current perspectives in management of edema in nephrotic syndrome. Indian J Pediatr. 2020;87:633-40.
34. Oster JR. Epstein M, Smoller S. Combined therapy with thiazide type and loop diuretic agents for resistant sodium retention. Ann Intern Med. 1983;99:405-6.
35. Ellis D. Pathophysiology, evaluation, and management of edema in childhood nephrotic syndrome. Front Pediatr. 2016; 3:111.
36. Fliser D, Zurbrüggen I, Mutschler E, Bischoff I, Nussberger J, Franek E, et al. Co-administration of albumin and furosemide in patients with the nephrotic syndrome. Kidney Int. 1999;55:629.
37. Davenport A. Ultrafiltration in diuretic resistant volume overload in nephrotic syndrome and patients with ascites due to chronic liver disease. Cardiology. 2001;96:190-5.
38. Barman H, Sirie R, Duwarah SG. Effective ultrafiltation with acute peritoneal dialysis in a child with diuretic resistant nephrotic edema. Saudi J Kidney Dis Transpl. 2015;26:743-6.
39. Fauchald P, Noddeland H, Norseth J. An evaluation of ultrafiltration as treatment of diuretic-resistant oedema in nephrotic syndrome. Acta Med Scand. 1985;217:127-31.

CHAPTER

3.4

Hematuria

Amish Udani

INTRODUCTION

Red blood cells (RBCs) >3–5 per high power field (HPF) in a urine sample by microscopy examination are required to diagnose significant hematuria.[1,2] Hematuria often indicates glomerular or nonglomerular abnormality unless proved otherwise. Whether macroscopic or microscopic hematuria, it is brought to the notice of the doctor as it frightens both the patient and the parents. Microscopic hematuria represents one of the most frequently encountered genitourinary abnormalities in children, occurring in 4–6% of school-age children undergoing routine screening, which may on repeat testing decrease to 0.5%.[3] In the absence of concomitant significant proteinuria, hypertension, and renal failure, if the cause of hematuria is not found in initial evaluation, then such children are kept under regular follow-up and re-evaluated if needed.

MACROSCOPIC HEMATURIA

Parents bring the child with a history of blood in urine and need both dipstick and microscopic examination of urine to confirm hematuria. Urine in glomerular hematuria is tea, cola, dirty brown, or rust colored due to oxidation of the heme pigment. Bright red color or blood clots suggest a nonglomerular cause.

MICROSCOPIC HEMATURIA

To avoid RBC lysis in freshly voided uncentrifuged urine with a specific gravity of >1.007, presence of >6 RBC/0.9 mm^3 is abnormal while >3–5 RBC/HPF in a centrifuged specimen (10 mL urine, 2,000 rpm for 5 minutes) will denote significant hematuria.[1,2,4] Microscopic hematuria may be asymptomatic with or without proteinuria or symptomatic according to glomerular or nonglomerular involvement. Glomerular symptoms are usually oliguria, edema, hypertension, rash, or arthralgia. Symptoms of dysuria, frequency, urgency, or pain suggest nonglomerular etiology.

TRANSIENT HEMATURIA

It happens due to an inciting event and resolves once the causative factor disappears. Drugs, infections, trauma, and exercise are common causes and are usually microscopic and benign.[5]

PERSISTENT HEMATURIA

The presence of microscopic hematuria in at least two to three urine analyses obtained during a 2- to 3-week period denotes persistent hematuria.[6] Persistent microscopic hematuria interspersed with episodes of gross bleeding or with proteinuria signifies a serious illness.

ISOLATED HEMATURIA

The presence of RBCs in the urine with no other urinary abnormalities (e.g., proteinuria) or raised serum creatinine or high blood pressure is called isolated hematuria. This definition includes both gross and microscopic hematuria. Severe renal histologic abnormalities in children with persistent isolated hematuria are unusual. These children need long-term follow-up as hematuria can disappear, or the child can develop additional renal or systemic abnormalities, or rarely isolated hematuria can persist.[7,8]

INITIAL HEMATURIA

Hematuria at the start of urination suggests urethral injury distal to the external urinary sphincter because of foreign body or trauma.

TERMINAL HEMATURIA

Presence of blood at the end of micturition is called terminal hematuria. It is seen as few drops of fresh blood at the end with or without dysuria. It indicates either bladder involvement or bulbar or prostatic urethral injury.

TOTAL HEMATURIA

Blood present throughout the act of micturition due to glomerular or nonglomerular cause is defined as total hematuria.[9]

MECHANISM OF HEMATURIA

Hematuria may originate from the glomeruli, renal tubules and interstitium, or urinary tract (including collecting system, ureter, bladder, and urethra).[6] In glomerular hematuria, RBCs cross the glomerular endothelial–epithelial barrier and enter the capillary lumen through structural discontinuities seen at the capillary wall–mesangial cell reflection. In hematuria due to glomerulonephritis (GN) along with RBCs, proteinuria, RBC casts, or dysmorphic RBCs might be seen in the urine examination. The renal papillae are susceptible to necrotic injury from microthrombi and anoxia in patients with a hemoglobinopathy or in those exposed to toxins. RBC sickling and microvascular thrombosis due to medullary hypertonicity, low-oxygen tension, and acidosis followed by rupture of vasa recta into the collecting system lead to microscopic or macroscopic hematuria. Patients with renal parenchymal lesions may have episodes of transient microscopic or macroscopic hematuria during systemic infections or after moderate exercise postulated due to altered renal hemodynamic responses. Rarely, following exercise, RBC casts were documented in few of them and urine analysis was otherwise found to be normal; hence, such children were kept under surveillance. Children with benign familial hematuria (BFH), in contrast to children with Alport syndrome (AS), may have a first-degree relative with hematuria without chronic kidney disease (CKD) or sensorineural deafness. BFH usually runs a nonprogressive course and CKD is very rarely reported. Electron microscopy (EM) of kidney biopsy shows a thin glomerular basement membrane (TBM). Calculi or crystalluria may cause mechanical erosion of mucosal surfaces in the urinary tract and result in nonglomerular hematuria. Diffuse inflammation of bladder mucosa due to infectious or noninfectious etiology results in hematuria.

ETIOLOGY

In our clinical setting, disseminated intravascular coagulation, thrombocytopenia, trauma, and bleeding diathesis are the common causes.[5] Among the glomerular diseases, infection-related GN (IRGN) is most common followed by chronic GN (CGN) with primary glomerular diseases such as IgA nephropathy (IgAN) or with multisystem involvement such as hemolytic uremic syndrome (HUS) or lupus nephritis (LN; **Table 1**). Among nonglomerular disorders, acute cystitis due to adenovirus, crystalluria, or urolithiasis and finally tumors are the frequent causes **(Table 2)**.

TYPES

Hematuria can be divided into the following types:[3]

- Macroscopic (gross) hematuria due to glomerular or nonglomerular cause **(Flowchart 1)**
- Microscopic hematuria with glomerular or nonglomerular symptoms **(Flowchart 2)**
- Asymptomatic microscopic isolated hematuria **(Flowchart 2)**
- Asymptomatic microscopic hematuria with proteinuria **(Flowchart 2)**

EVALUATION

Based on history, clinical features, and urine examination, a clinician should be able to decide if hematuria is due to a glomerular or a nonglomerular cause **(Table 3)**.

History

Nonsteroidal anti-inflammatory drug use for fever or pain may cause hematuria due to interstitial nephritis. Painless hematuria, edema, oliguria, hypertension, and history of preceding or associated infection are commonly seen in glomerular hematuria. History of recurrent or persistent fever, arthralgia, arthritis, recurrent wheeze, recurrent jaundice, and abdominal pain may be present pointing toward secondary GN. Dysuria and increased frequency point toward a nonglomerular cause. Features of renal stone disease such as abdominal pain, vomiting, and passage of gravel may be present. Prolonged or irregular fever can be seen with urinary

TABLE 1: Glomerular causes of hematuria.

Primary glomerulonephritis	*Secondary/multisystem glomerulonephritis*	*Familial*
Postinfective GN	Lupus nephritis	Alport syndrome
IgA nephropathy	Henoch–Schönlein purpura	Benign familial hematuria
C3 glomerulopathy	Hemolytic uremic syndrome	
Focal segmental glomerulosclerosis	Wegener granulomatosis, Goodpasture syndrome	

(GN: glomerulonephritis; IgA: immunoglobulin A)

TABLE 2: Nonglomerular causes of hematuria.

Renal parenchymal	*Vascular/malformation*	*Crystalluria*	*Infectious*	*Extrarenal*
Hydronephrosis	Renal artery or venous thrombosis	Hypercalciuria	Cystitis	Wilms tumor
Ureterovesical junction obstruction	Arteriovenous aneurysms	Hyperuricosuria	Pyelonephritis	Tuberous sclerosis
Polycystic kidney disease	Nutcracker syndrome	Hyperoxaluria	Tuberculosis, HIV nephropathy	Hematological diseases

(HIV: human immunodeficiency virus)

Flowchart 1: Algorithm for evaluation of macroscopic hematuria.

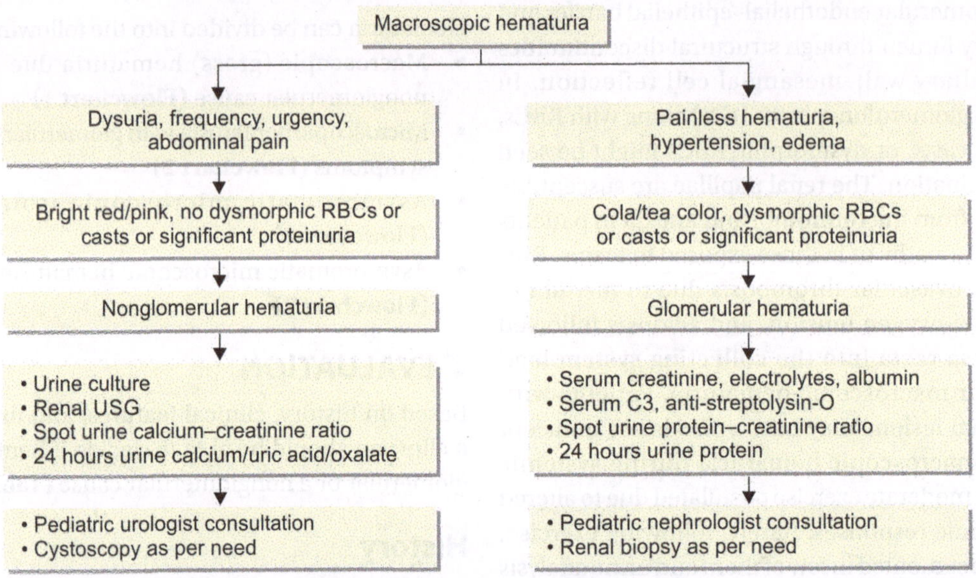

(RBCs: red blood cells; USG: ultrasound)

Flowchart 2: Algorithm for evaluation of microscopic hematuria.

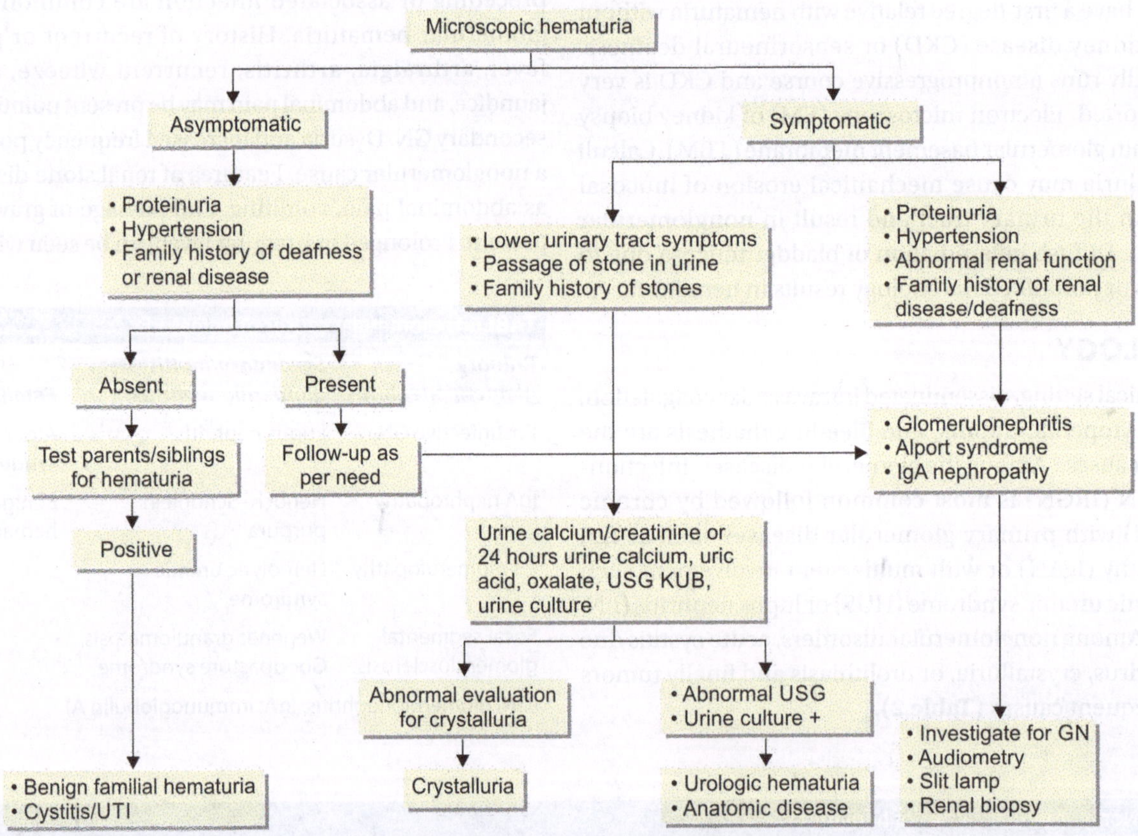

(GN: glomerulonephritis; KUB: kidney, ureter, bladder; USG: ultrasound; UTI: urinary tract infection)

tract infection (UTI).[6] Special stress should be given to a family history of renal disease/deafness, identification of anatomic abnormalities, and presence of macroscopic hematuria. Conditions known to have familial association are AS, BFH, systemic lupus erythematosus (SLE), IgAN, urolithiasis, hemophilia, and sickle cell disease.

Examination

Periorbital edema is the first site of edema with glomerular disease. Raised jugular venous pressure (JVP) or crackles present in lung bases indicating fluid overload denotes GN. Nephrotic edema usually has ascites and may not have features of fluid overload. Renal angle tenderness may indicate upper

TABLE 3: Distinguishing features in glomerular versus nonglomerular hematuria.

Features	***Glomerular causes***	***Nonglomerular causes***
History		
Dysuria, frequency, urgency	Absent	Present in urethritis, cystitis, crystalluria
Pharyngitis, impetigo	Infection-related glomerulonephritis	Absent
Painless, synpharyngitic	IgA nephropathy	Absent
Edema, oliguria	Glomerulonephritis	Absent
Systemic complaints	Fever, rash, arthralgia	Fever with UTI, pain with crystalluria
Dysentery, pallor	Hemolytic uremic syndrome	Absent
Bleeding from other sites	Pulmonary hemorrhage in Wegener granulomatosis, Goodpasture syndrome	Coagulation disorder
Family history	Deafness, eye abnormalities in Alport syndrome	May be positive with calculi and crystalluria
Physical examination		
Hypertension, edema	Usually present	Less common
Abdominal mass	Absent	Present in Wilms tumor, obstructive uropathy, renal vein thrombosis
Rash, arthritis	Systemic lupus erythematosus, Henoch–Schönlein purpura, vasculitis	Absent unless part of drug-induced interstitial nephritis
Urinalysis		
Color	Brown, tea, cola	Bright red
Proteinuria	2+ or more	<2+
Dysmorphic RBCs	>20%	Not common, <15%
RBC casts	Common	Absent
Clots	Absent	May be present

(IgA: immunoglobulin A; RBC: red blood cell; UTI: urinary tract infection)

UTI. Recent trauma can be detected by findings of flank bruises and pain. Examining the abdomen for masses suggests tumors, polycystic kidneys, renal vein thrombosis, or hydronephrosis. The examination of the skin can give evidence of pallor or rash. Pallor indicating anemia may signify either acute loss of blood as in trauma or HUS or CKD. Butterfly rash over the face or photosensitive rash points toward SLE, whereas palpable purpuric rash over buttocks and extensor surface of the limbs suggests Henoch–Schönlein purpura (HSP).

Urine Examination

The presence of RBC casts in urine signifies glomerular hematuria and is associated with persistent or heavy proteinuria >2+ or spot urine protein creatinine ratio >0.5. The RBCs are dysmorphic by phase-contrast microscopy, and >5% acanthocytes have 50% sensitivity and 95% specificity for glomerular hematuria.[10] The absence of RBC casts and <15% dysmorphic RBCs in urine may signify nonglomerular hematuria. Although proteinuria is seen, it is not heavy and is <2+ or spot urine protein creatinine ratio is <0.5.[5,6]

Dipstick is positive for true hematuria, myoglobinuria, or hemoglobinuria and negative in pseudohematuria due to rifampicin, pyridium, nitrofurantoin, metronidazole, colored food dyes, blackberries, rhubarb, fava beans, or beetroot, while microscopic examination shows RBCs or RBC casts or dysmorphic RBC in true hematuria. Dipsticks are readily available for screening purpose which depends on peroxidase like chemical reaction between hemoglobin (and myoglobin) and a chemical tetramethylbenzidine present in the strip producing a blue color. It is capable of detecting 3–10 RBC/μL of uncentrifuged urine with 100% sensitivity and 99% specificity. Absence of RBC on microscopic examination with a positive dipstick test suggests hemoglobinuria or myoglobinuria which can be confirmed by spectrophotometry. A simple bedside test to identify hemoglobinuria is to centrifuge urine and evaluate the color of the supernatant fluid; if it is uniformly pink, it indicates hematuria whereas in true hematuria it is dirty brown. False-positive dipstick reactions occur with oxidizing contaminants such as bacterial peroxidases from UTI, delay in reading the dipstick, and alkaline urine pH > 9.0. False-negative results are seen with the presence of formalin and high amounts of ascorbic acid.[3] Contamination from menstrual blood or Munchausen syndrome in older children should be excluded. In infants, red-diaper syndrome is due to development of red color in soiled diapers after 24–36 hours because of either *Serratia marcescens* or urate crystals.

Baseline investigations other than urine examination such as complete blood count (CBC), serum creatinine, and ultrasound (USG) of abdomen should be done in all children. Further investigations should be done to prove the underlying etiology **(Box 1)**. Pertinent to GN, laboratory investigations include a serum estimation of C3, C4 levels, albumin, and electrolytes. The C3 level is low in acute poststreptococcal GN (PSGN), subset of C3 glomerulopathy (C3G) or HUS and LN. Microscopic hematuria always warrants referral to a pediatric nephrologist. The indications for renal biopsy are persistent microscopic hematuria for >1 year, recurrent gross or microscopic hematuria with decreased renal function, proteinuria or hypertension for >4 weeks, secondary GN, and persistent low C3 beyond 12 weeks.[11] In crystalluria or urolithiasis, screening by a spot urine calcium creatinine ratio or estimation of 24-hour urine calcium, uric acid, oxalate and citrate excretion, serum electrolytes, and calcium levels

BOX 1: Advanced specific evaluation.

Complement studies

Infection-related glomerulonephritis, systemic lupus erythematosus (SLE), C3 glomerulopathy, hemolytic uremic syndrome

Anti-streptolysin-O and anti-DNase B
Acute poststreptococcal glomerulonephritis

Antinuclear antibody (ANA), anti-dsDNA

SLE

Audiogram/ophthalmology evaluation

Alport syndrome

Antiglomerular basement membrane antibodies

Goodpasture syndrome

Antineutrophil cytoplasmic antibodies (ANCA)

Wegener granulomatosis c-ANCA or proteinase 3 (PR3) ANCA

Microscopic polyangiitis p-ANCA or myeloperoxidase (MPO) ANCA

Peripheral smear, reticulocyte count, LDH

Hemolytic uremic syndrome

Spot urine calcium–creatinine ratio

Hypercalciuria

24 hours urine calcium, uric acid, oxalate, citrate

Crystalluria (hypercalciuria, hyperuricosuria, hyperoxaluria, hypocitraturia)

Urine culture, RT-PCR viral studies

Pyelonephritis, viral hemorrhagic cystitis

Kidney biopsy

IgA nephropathy, Alport syndrome

Renal Doppler/CT/MRI abdomen and angiography

Thrombosis, trauma, tumors, vascular malformation, nutcracker syndrome

Spot urine protein creatinine ratio or 24 hours urine protein

Chronic glomerulonephritis

(IgA: immunoglobulin A; LDH: lactate dehydrogenase; RT-PCR: reverse transcription polymerase chain reaction)

should be done. A comprehensive approach to evaluating a child with hematuria is shown in **Flowchart 3**. A recent review on the approach to evaluation including indications for prompt referral to a pediatric nephrologist is a useful resource for pediatricians.[12]

MANAGEMENT

The common causes of hematuria due to glomerular diseases are discussed in the following text.

Infection-related GN is usually PSGN where GN is generally preceded by sore throat or impetigo 7–28 days earlier. Other infections such as staphylococcal, gram-negative bacteria, and viral, fungal and parasitic agents cause postinfectious GN (PIGN) or syn-infection GN. Typical laboratory findings are positive antistreptolysin-O (ASO) and anti-DNase B antibodies, transient hypocomplementemia (C3) for 6–8 weeks, subnephrotic proteinuria, and mild elevation of serum creatinine. Isolated asymptomatic microscopic hematuria may persist for 1 year in PSGN. In atypical cases, renal biopsy should be done.[13] PSGN treatment is usually supportive as it is self-limiting in most of the children. Edema and hypertension are managed with fluid and salt restriction along with diuretics. In severe renal failure or refractory electrolyte disturbance or fluid overload, kidney replacement therapy may be needed. Immunosuppressive agents are used in crescentic PSGN.

The noninfectious GN is classified as slowly progressive GN or CGN. These include IgAN and AS. Gross hematuria is seen in 40–55% of children with IgAN and isolated asymptomatic persistent microscopic hematuria in 30–40%. IgAN may present with microscopic hematuria with glomerular symptoms of hypertension, edema with or without proteinuria, and renal failure. It is diagnosed by granular IgA deposits in mesangium on immunofluorescence studies of kidney biopsy. Codominant deposition of other immunoglobulins may also be seen. Recently, a reliable lectin-based enzyme-linked immunosorbent assay (ELISA) for determining serum galactose-deficient IgA1 has been developed which was elevated in 77% of children with IgAN.[14] There is no specific treatment for IgAN presenting with isolated gross or microscopic hematuria. Fish oil/omega 3 fatty acids are used for anti-inflammatory property without enough evidence in literature to support its use. Antiproteinuric drugs may slow disease progression in presence of hypertension or subnephrotic proteinuria. Immunosuppressive drugs are used in crescentic IgAN, nephrotic range proteinuria, and severe histologic lesions.[15]

Alport syndrome is another condition which may present with either type of hematuria. Collagen IV alpha 5 mutation has X-linked inheritance; mutation in collagen IV alpha 3 or 4 chains results in an autosomal recessive form and aberrant alpha 3 or 4 chains are responsible for a rare autosomal dominant form of AS. Sensorineural deafness and eye abnormalities may be present. Progression to CKD is usually seen in AS. EM of kidney biopsy reveals thickening of the basement membrane or splitting of the lamina densa or basket weave pattern. In BFH, kidney biopsy is rarely done in the absence of recurrent macroscopic hematuria or significant proteinuria. AS and TBM disease are two ends of the clinical spectrum of hereditary nephropathy due to varying severity of type IV collagen gene mutation.[16]

There are other GNs that are moderately progressive in nature such as LN, HSP nephritis, C3G, and HUS. LN may present with macroscopic hematuria, microscopic hematuria with glomerular symptoms, or asymptomatic microscopic hematuria with significant proteinuria. Apart from serology, kidney biopsy is needed to diagnose, guide treatment, and prognosticate the disease.[17]

Flowchart 3: Approach to a child with hematuria.

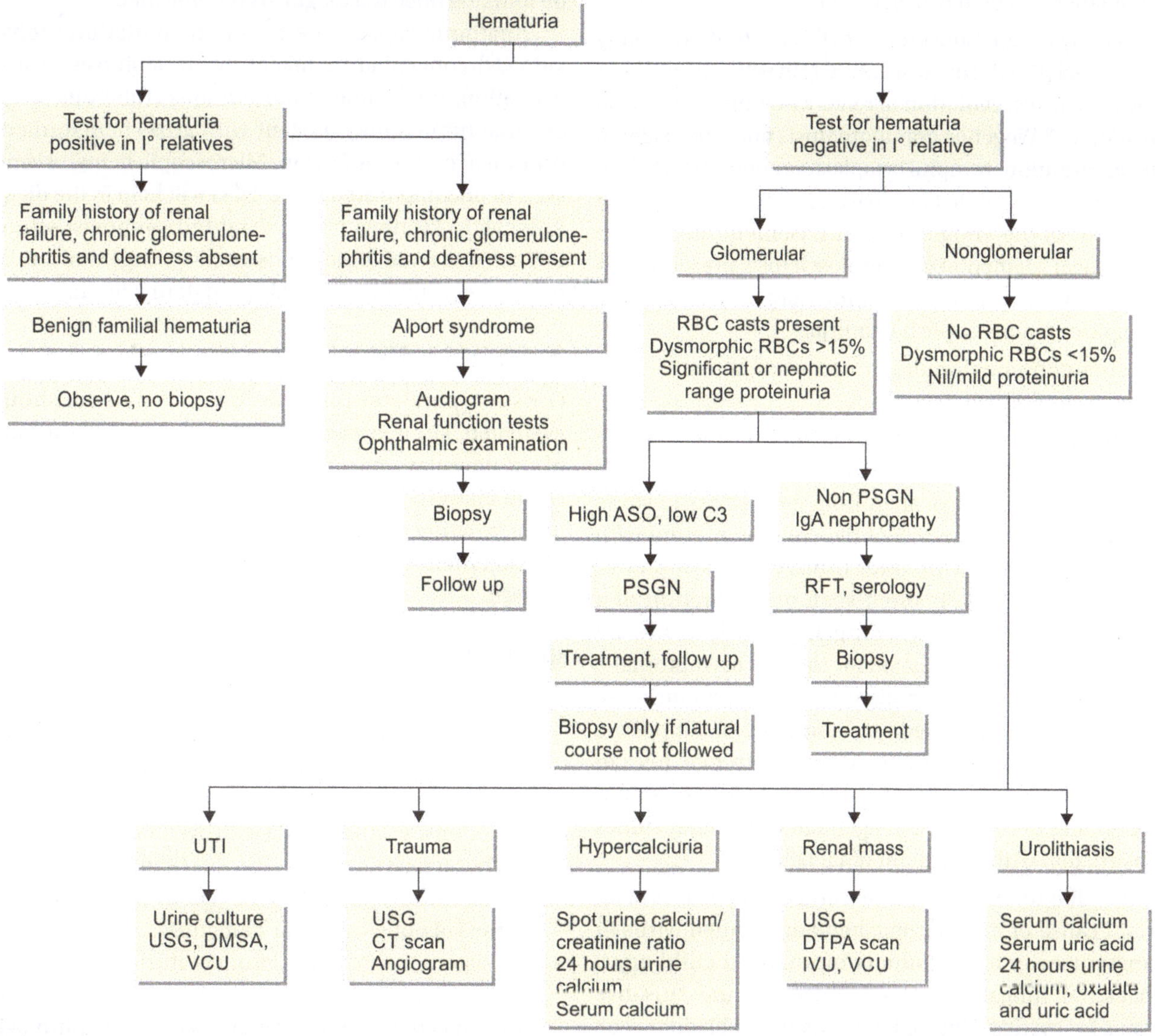

(ASO: antistreptolysin O; DMSA: dimercaptosuccinic acid; DTPA: diethylenetriamine pentaacetate; IVU: intravenous urography; KUB: kidney, ureter, bladder; PSGN: poststreptococcal glomerulonephritis; RBC: red blood cell; RFT: renal function test; USG: ultrasound; VCU: voiding cystourethrograms)

Henoch–Schönlein purpura nephritis is small vessel vasculitis with renal involvement appearing either along with systemic symptoms of nonthrombocytopenic purpuric rash over buttocks and legs, arthralgia, and gastrointestinal manifestations or within 6–8 weeks of the onset of the triad. Hematuria is often microscopic with or without proteinuria and rarely may present with gross hematuria along with hypertension, edema, or renal failure. The pathogenesis, kidney biopsy findings, and treatment are almost similar to IgAN. Apart from mesangium, IgA, C3, or fibrin deposits may be seen along the capillary walls of skin and kidney biopsy as well. In pediatric patients, HSP nephritis is often self-resolving with supportive management of rest, adequate hydration, and paracetamol if pain is present.[13]

C3 glomerulopathy is a group of conditions where persistent low C3 is seen in 80–95% of cases and is diagnosed on immunofluorescence of kidney biopsy with predominant deposition of C3. Half of the patients with C3G present with microscopic hematuria and subnephrotic proteinuria. About 30% present with steroid-resistant nephrotic syndrome with microscopic hematuria and the remaining with gross hematuria along with other glomerular symptoms of oliguria, edema, hypertension, or renal failure. Antiproteinuric drugs along with immunosuppressive agents are used, but long-term prognosis is poor in C3G.[18]

Hemolytic uremic syndrome is a triad of nonimmune hemolytic anemia, thrombocytopenia, and acute kidney injury. It can be triggered with infections, genetic factors, drugs, malignancy, or post-transplant. Thrombotic microangiopathy secondary to microvascular injury and endothelial cell damage is the characteristic pathology of HUS. Most of the children with HUS present with macroscopic hematuria along with signs of acute kidney injury. Treatment should be done under guidance of a pediatric nephrologist.[19]

The rapidly progressing groups of GN are termed rapidly progressing GN (RPGN) or crescentic GN in which in addition to the above causes, evolution of renal vasculitis should also be considered.[20] Wegener granulomatosis and microscopic polyangiitis are antineutrophil cytoplasmic antibody (ANCA)-mediated vasculitis while Goodpasture syndrome is due to development of the antiglomerular basement membrane antibody. Focal segmental glomerulosclerosis presenting as steroid-resistant nephrotic syndrome may have associated microscopic or macroscopic hematuria.

The common nonglomerular causes of hematuria are discussed in the following text.

Urolithiasis is increasing in children due to changes in diet, use of calcium supplements, antibiotics or furosemide, UTI, and decreased water intake apart from genetic risk to stone formation. Approximately 55% of the children present with gross hematuria along with lower urinary tract symptoms. Microscopic hematuria is often seen on evaluation of a child with dysuria, frequency, or urgency. Rarely stones are detected on USG when evaluated for isolated asymptomatic microscopic hematuria. Investigations for crystalluria are done to plan dietary and medical management. Supportive treatment with hydration and control of pain may help in passage of small stones. Surgery is reserved for large stones not responding to medical management or bilateral stones with obstruction with or without renal failure.[21]

Cystitis due to infectious or noninfectious causes is an important cause of macroscopic hematuria. Adenovirus or polyomaviruses in an immunocompromised child apart from bacterial, fungal, or parasitic infections are causative organisms for cystitis. Diffuse inflammation of bladder seen as thickening of the bladder wall is the usual finding on USG. Urine culture or reverse transcription polymerase chain reaction (RT-PCR) studies for virus confirm the diagnosis. It is self-limiting in most of the children with supportive care. Antiviral drugs may be used in immunocompromised children or antibiotics in culture-proven bacterial infection.[22] Acrolein, a metabolite of chemotherapy drugs, after binding to bladder mucosa causes inflammation and hematuria. Supportive treatment with hydration, withdrawal of drug, and Mesna is usually sufficient. Rarely surgical removal of clots or instillation of drugs in bladder is needed to control hematuria.[22]

In the neonatal period, hematuria due to thrombosis of the renal vein or artery can occur, especially after umbilical catheterization. Predisposing factors for renal vein thrombosis include perinatal asphyxia, polycythemia, dehydration, septicemia, shock, nephrotic syndrome, and prothrombotic state secondary to factor V Leiden mutation. Clinically, they present as gross hematuria with unilateral or bilateral renal mass. Renal Doppler studies of renal vessels help in the diagnosis. Anticoagulation therapy or thrombolysis should be initiated once the diagnosis is confirmed.[13]

Anatomic causes due to genetic mutation (polycystic kidneys), congenital anomalies (hydronephrosis, obstructive uropathy), syndromic malformations (tuberous sclerosis), or renal tumors may present with gross hematuria due to rupture of cysts or infection. Microscopic hematuria may be seen in uncomplicated cases. USG will help in the diagnosis. Polycystic kidneys have variable prognosis; surgery is indicated in renal tumors, obstructive congenital anomalies, nutcracker syndrome, and large angiomyolipoma.

CONCLUSION

Gross or persistent microscopic hematuria should be evaluated. The approach to evaluation is to make a diagnosis of a glomerular versus nonglomerular etiology of hematuria. Urine analysis and specific clinical features are useful in differentiating glomerular from nonglomerular hematuria. Management of hematuria is guided by the underlying disease.

KEY POINTS

- Gross or macroscopic hematuria is cola-colored or bright red urine containing RBCs. Microscopic hematuria is noted with >5 RBCs/HPF of urine sediment.
- Painless hematuria that is associated with proteinuria, hypertension, and edema with dysmorphic RBCs in urine is characteristic of GN. Painful hematuria, eumorphic RBCs, features of urinary infection, or stone disease are typical of nonglomerular hematuria.
- Persistent macro- or microhematuria, need for a renal biopsy, and presence of a genetic basis for kidney disease are indications for referral to a pediatric nephrologist.

REFERENCES

1. Dodge WF, West EF, Smith EH, Bunce H. Proteinuria and hematuria in schoolchildren: epidemiology and early natural history. J Pediatr. 1976;88:327-47.
2. Rao PR, Jones JS. How to evaluate dipstick hematuria: what to do before you refer. Cleveland Clin J Med. 2008;75(3):227-33.
3. Diven SC, Travis LB. A practical primary care approach to hematuria in children. Pediatr Nephrol. 2000;14:65-72.
4. Vehaskari VM, Rapola J, Koskimies O, Savilahti E, Vilska J, Hallman N. Microscopic hematuria in school children: epidemiology and clinicopathologic evaluation. J Pediatr. 1979;95:676-84.
5. Phadke KD, Vijayakumar M, Sharma J, Iyengar A. Indian Pediatric Nephrology Group. Consensus statement on evaluation of hematuria. Indian Pediatr. 2006;43(11):965-73.
6. Meyers KE. Evaluation of hematuria in children. Urol Clin N Am. 2004;31(3):559-73.
7. Chow KM, Kwan BC, Li PK, Szeto CC. Asymptomatic isolated microscopic hematuria: long term follow-up. Q J Med. 2004;97:739-45.
8. Vivante A, Afek A, Frenkel-Nir Y, Tzur D, Farfel A, Golan E. Persistent asymptomatic isolated microscopic hematuria in

Israeli adolescents and young adults and risk for end-stage renal disease. JAMA. 2011;306(7):729-36.
9. Kher K, Moxey-Mims M. Hematuria and proteinuria. In: Kher K, Schnaper HW, Greenbaum LA (Eds). Clinical Pediatric Nephrology, 3rd edition. Boca Raton: CRC Press; 2017. pp. 127-52.
10. Hebert LA, Parikh S, Prosek J, Nadasdy T, Rovin BH. Differential diagnosis of glomerular disease: a systematic and inclusive approach. Am J Nephrol. 2013;38:253-66.
11. Vijayakumar M. Acute and crescentic glomerulonephritis. Indian J Pediatr. 2002;69:1071-5.
12. Vedula R, Iyengar AA. Approach to diagnosis and management of hematuria. Indian J Pediatr. 2020;87:618-24.
13. Brown DD, Reidy KJ. Approach to the child with hematuria. Pediatr Clin N Am. 2019;66:15-30.
14. Lau KK, Wyatt RJ, Moldoveanu Z, Tomana M, Julian BA, Hogg RJ, et al. Serum levels of galactose-deficient IgA in children with IgA nephropathy and Henoch-Schonlein purpura. Pediatr Nephrol. 2007;22:2067-72.
15. Nicoara O, Twombley K. Immunoglobulin A nephropathy and immunoglobulin A vasculitis. In: Stanton BF, Chan JC (Eds). Clinical Disorders of the Kidney. Pediatr Clin N Am. 2019;66: 101-10.
16. Kashtan CE. Familial hematuria. Pediatr Nephrol. 2009;24: 1951-8.
17. Wenderfer SE, Eldin KW. Lupus nephritis. Pediatr Clin N Am. 2019;66:87-100.
18. Thomas S, Ranganathan D, Francis L, Madhan K, John GT. Current concepts in C3 glomerulopathy. Indian J Nephrol. 2014;24(6):339-48.
19. Waters AM, Licht C. aHUS caused by complement dysregulation: new therapies on the horizon. Pediatr Nephrol. 2011;26:41-57.
20. Brogan P, Eleftheriou D, Dillon M. Small vessel vasculitis. Pediatr Nephrol. 2010;25:1025-35.
21. Gillespie RS, Stapelton FB. Nephrolithiasis in children. Pediatr Rev. 2004;25(4):131-9.
22. Manikandan R, Kumar S, Dorairajan LN. Hemorrhagic cystitis: a challenge to the urologist. Indian J Urol. 2010;26(2):159-66.

CHAPTER

3.5 Proteinuria

S Prabha, Kalaivani Ganesan

INTRODUCTION

Proteinuria is a marker of kidney disorders of diverse etiologies. Although proteinuria is the result of kidney disease, it also hastens the progression of renal damage.[1] During the time of Hippocrates, uroscopy was the sole diagnostic tool for detecting renal diseases. He described the relation between "bubbles on the surface of the urine" and kidney disease. In the 17th century, Frederick Dekkers found that urine samples became caseous after exposure to heat. 200 years later, Richard Bright described the association of proteinuria with kidney disease.[2] Presently, proteinuria is routinely and easily assessed in clinical practice. The prevalence of isolated asymptomatic proteinuria in children is 0.6–6.3%. Usually, proteinuria is transient and intermittent and when a single urine specimen is tested, prevalence is much higher. On follow-up, <1% will show persistent proteinuria after 6–12 months.[3,4]

NORMAL URINARY PROTEIN EXCRETION IN INFANTS AND CHILDREN

Small amounts of protein in urine are normal and are described as physiological proteinuria. The protein excretion is highest in neonates when corrected for the body surface area. In newborn babies, the normal protein excretion in urine is high, up to 300 mg/m²/day. The reabsorption of filtered proteins is low due to immature renal tubular function at this age.[5,6] Physiological proteinuria varies with the age and size of the child. It is relatively constant after the first year of life and is <4 mg/m²/h or <100 mg/m²/24 h. The physiological proteinuria decreases with age until late adolescence, when an adult level of 150 mg/day is reached.

In children older than 2 years of age, a urine protein to urine creatinine ratio (UPr/UCr or UPCR) < 0.2 on a random urine sample is considered normal. The normal UPCR for infants less than 6 months of age is not clearly defined though a value <0.8 is considered normal. In children between 6 and 24 months of age, UPCR < 0.5 is considered normal.[5] About 15% of the total protein in urine is albumin, while immunoglobulins, amino acids, and low-molecular-weight (LMW) proteins such as beta-2 microglobulin account for approximately 35%. About 50% of the urinary protein is Tamm–Horsfall protein, referred to as uromodulin, secreted by proximal tubules. Renal plasma flow, hydrostatic and oncotic forces, molecular size, charge and configuration of proteins as well as intrinsic properties of capillary wall regulate the movement of proteins across the glomerular capillary wall. Majority of the proteins filtered at the glomerulus is reabsorbed by the proximal tubular cells.

ABNORMAL PROTEIN EXCRETION

Pathological proteinuria is defined as protein excretion in urine of >100–150 mg/m²/day in children.[5] Nephrotic range proteinuria is >40 mg/m²/h in an overnight specimen of urine or >50 mg/kg body weight per 24 hours or a UPr/UCr > 2.0.

MEASUREMENT OF PROTEINURIA

Qualitative Methods

Urine Dipstick

Dipstick method is an inexpensive basic screening test for proteinuria. The standard dipstick detects albumin in urine by a pH-dependent colorimetric reaction between the dye indicator tetrabromophenol blue and albumin. Depending on the albumin concentration in the sample, a sequential color change from pale green to blue occurs. Albumin binds to the dye at a pH between 5 and 7. The dipstick testing is essentially albumin specific as the urinary pH is usually between 5 and 6. The lower limit of sensitivity of albumin for the urine dipstick test is about 250 mg/L, and hence microalbuminuria is not detected by the dipstick test.[7]

The semiquantitative assessment based on the color is as follows. There will not be any change, if protein is nil or negative.

- Trace: 15–30 mg/dL
- 1+: 30–100 mg/dL
- 2+: 100–300 mg/dL
- 3+: 300–1,000 mg/dL
- 4+: Above 1,000 mg/dL

Alkaline urine (pH > 7) or when urine is mixed with mucus, pus, blood, vaginal secretions or semen, false-positive results may be obtained. When urine is dilute, albumin concentration is decreased and dipstick may give false-negative results. Although dipstick is a useful screening test for proteinuria, it should be remembered that it is insensitive to proteins such as gamma globulins and Bence Jones protein in urine.[5]

Precipitation Tests

Precipitation tests assess the turbidity that occurs when proteins in urine are precipitated by reagents such as sulfosalicylic acid (SSA) or trichloroacetic acid or acetic acid and sodium acetate buffer in the presence of heat. The SSA test is performed by mixing one part of urine with three parts of 3% SSA, creating an acidic pH. Precipitation of proteins causes turbidity and is noted by visual inspection. The SSA test detects all types of urinary proteins including LMW proteins, such as immunoglobulin light chains, that is missed by urine dipstick. The sensitivity is high, and as low as 2.5 mg/L of protein is detected. However, a variety of exogenous compounds interfere with this test and hence is sparingly used in clinical practice.[7]

Quantitative Methods

For quantification of proteinuria, spot urine analysis for UPr/UCr and urine albumin-to-creatinine ratio (UA/UCr or UACR) are currently preferred to 24-hour urine collection because of the ease of spot urine sampling. The UA/UCr is used to assess for albumin excretion of 30–300 mg/day in an adult.[8]

Nephelometric, turbidimetric, radioimmunoassay, and enzyme immunoassay techniques are used for measuring albumin in urine. When >300 mg/day of protein in urine is suspected, UPr/UCr can be used. First morning specimens are preferable. When lower grades of proteinuria are suspected, UA/UCr or UACR is preferred as it is a more sensitive screening test. The UPCR is less expensive and can be used to assess the treatment response on follow-up.

The accuracy of estimating the degree of proteinuria in a random urine sample is diminished if creatinine excretion is different from the expected normal levels. The steady-state creatinine excretion in children from 1 to 12 years of age is 20 mg/kg/day and 22–25 mg/kg/day in older children. The lower value corresponds with creatinine excretion in girls. In a muscular individual with a high rate of creatinine excretion, UPr/UCr will underestimate protein excretion while in severe malnutrition, low muscle mass, and cachexia there will be overestimation of urinary protein excretion.[3]

The presence of albumin in urine above the normal range but below the detectable range by the conventional urinary dipstick method is called microalbuminuria. UACR is calculated in the same way as UPCR, and <20–30 mg of urine albumin per gram of creatinine is normal. Microalbuminuria is defined as excretion of 20–200 μg/min/1.73 m^2 or 30–300-mg albumin per gram creatinine a day. Microalbuminuria suggests microvascular disease and is predictive of mortality and morbidity in diabetes mellitus.[9]

The 24-hour urine protein estimation is considered as the "gold standard" for quantitative evaluation of proteinuria, but it is technically difficult and cumbersome in children. Several colorimetric methods are available to quantify protein in a 24-hour urine sample. In children, a way of quantifying urinary protein excretion is to measure protein in a timed urine sample, e.g., for a 12-hour period. Quantitative measurements estimate all the proteins in urine and hence, will be greater than the actual amount of albumin in urine. It is only in special situations that urine protein electrophoresis and direct measurements of LMW proteins, such as beta-2 microglobulin, are performed and are not part of evaluation of a child with proteinuria.[3]

The selectivity index (SI) of protein clearance is estimated by immunonephelometry. This is calculated by the ratio of the clearance of immunoglobulin G (IgG; molecular weight 160,000) to the clearance of transferrin (molecular weight 88,000) by the formula:

SI = (urinary IgG/plasma IgG)/(urinary transferrin/plasma transferrin).

In children with nephrotic syndrome, when the SI is <0.1, proteinuria is highly selective and indicates minimal-change nephrotic syndrome (MCNS). The response is moderate if the ratio is between 0.11 and 0.20, and anything >0.21 is nonselective proteinuria and indicates steroid resistance as seen in focal segmental glomerulosclerosis. Currently, this investigation is not in vogue.[10]

A qualitative protein analysis of urine is done to differentiate glomerular from tubular proteinuria. Tubular proteinuria markers, such as beta-2 microglobulin, alpha-1-microglobulin, retinol-binding protein, and lysozyme, may be measured by immunonephelometry and help to distinguish glomerular from tubular proteinuria. In tubular proteinuria, the level of index proteins in urine will be 10–100 times higher than normal.[7]

MECHANISMS OF PROTEINURIA

Increased protein excretion in urine occurs by three main mechanisms: Glomerular, tubular, and overflow proteinuria.[7]

Glomerular Proteinuria

Increased filtration of proteins, especially albumin, across the glomerular capillary wall secondary to anatomical or functional abnormalities of the filtration barrier causes glomerular proteinuria. Glomerular diseases or conditions such as exercise, fever, and orthostatic (or postural) proteinuria are the common causes. In the normal kidney, the glomerular capillary wall and its adjacent structures form the main barrier to the passage of molecules such as globulin and albumin. The movement of proteins across the filtration barrier is regulated by several factors such as configuration, molecular size and charge of proteins, glomerular plasma flow, and hydrostatic and oncotic forces. Proteinuria indicates perturbation in the permeability and selectivity properties of the glomerular filtration barrier.[11]

Tubular Proteinuria

In healthy children, LMW proteins, such as lysozyme, retinol-binding protein, light chains of immunoglobulin, alpha-1 microglobulin, and beta-2 microglobulin, and hormones such as vasopressin, insulin, growth hormone, and parathyroid hormone are freely filtered at the glomerulus. These proteins are subsequently reabsorbed and catabolized by the proximal tubular cells before returning them to the circulation. Injury to the proximal tubular cells results in inability of the tubule to reabsorb these proteins leading to tubular proteinuria. Tubular proteinuria is often associated with generalized proximal tubular dysfunction as in Fanconi syndrome.[3]

Overflow Proteinuria

When the plasma concentration of certain LMW proteins exceeds the capacity of the tubules to reabsorb the filtered protein, overflow proteinuria results. The presence of immunoglobulin light chains in urine in multiple myeloma, hemoglobinuria in intravascular hemolysis, myoglobinuria in rhabdomyolysis, and amylasuria in acute pancreatitis are some examples of overflow proteinuria.[3] Overflow proteinuria is not common in children.

CLASSIFICATION OF PROTEINURIA

Nonpathological Proteinuria

Transient Proteinuria

It can occur with strenuous exercise, congestive heart failure, or abdominal surgery. It is also seen in febrile illnesses and after seizures. The proteinuria is <2+ and not associated with edema, hematuria, hypertension, or renal failure. It is benign and disappears on subsequent urine examination when the basic condition abates. Hence, no further investigations and treatment are required.

Orthostatic Proteinuria

Isolated proteinuria without hematuria occurring in a random specimen collected during daytime in an asymptomatic child is orthostatic proteinuria (OP). It can be confirmed by repeating the test on a morning urine sample collected immediately after waking up. OP is defined as a 24-hour urine protein of >100 mg/m^2 with a normal protein excretion in a supine sample (<4 mg/m^2/h). The child must completely empty his or her bladder before going to bed so that no residual urine remains in the bladder. In children with OP, the first morning UPCR will be in the normal range, while a random daytime value is high. In OP, 24-hour urine protein is <1 g or UPCR is <1.0.

Orthostatic proteinuria is common, found in 20% of children; it is more common in boys, above 10 years of age and body mass index (BMI) > 85th percentile.[12] OP is a benign condition without clinical significance. However, testing for proteinuria on an annual basis is prudent, until the third decade of life.[3]

Pathological Proteinuria

Pathological proteinuria occurs by three mechanisms—(1) glomerular, (2) tubular disorders, and (3) overflow proteinuria. The causes of proteinuria are given in **Table 1**.

Glomerular Proteinuria

The main function of the glomerulus is to restrict the filtration of proteins across the glomerular capillary wall. Glomerular proteinuria comprises large-molecular-weight proteins, mostly albumin. In glomerular proteinuria, the urinary protein excretion is >100 mg/m^2/day or >4 mg/m^2/h in children. If it persists for >3 months, it is called persistent proteinuria. Urine protein excretion > 40 mg/m^2/h or a UPCR greater than 2.0 indicates nephrotic range proteinuria.

TABLE 1: Causes of proteinuria in children.

Proteinuria	*Causes*
Transient proteinuria	Fever, exercise, seizures, hypovolemia
Orthostatic proteinuria	
Persistent proteinuria—Glomerular proteinuria	*Primary glomerular diseases* • Congenital nephrotic syndrome (Finnish type, DMS) • Minimal-change nephrotic syndrome • Focal segmental glomerulosclerosis • Membranoproliferative GN • Membranous nephropathy • Rapidly progressing GN • IgA nephropathy • Alport syndrome *Secondary glomerular diseases* • Infection-related glomerulonephritis • Lupus nephritis • Henoch–Schönlein purpura • Hepatitis B nephropathy • Hemolytic uremic syndrome • Diabetic nephropathy • HIV nephropathy • Chronic interstitial nephritis • Renal dysplasia or hypoplasia • Drugs—penicillamine, NSAID, heavy metals such as gold, mercury, and lead
Tubular proteinuria	*Primary diseases* • Cystinosis • Lowe syndrome • Tyrosinemia • Galactosemia • Wilson's disease • Polycystic kidney diseases • Mitochondrial disorders *Secondary diseases* • Reflux nephropathy • Ischemic injury—ATN • Drugs and toxins—NSAIDs, aminoglycosides • Heavy metals

(ATN: acute tubular necrosis; DMS: diffuse mesangial sclerosis; GN: glomerulonephritis; HIV: human immunodeficiency virus; IgA: immunoglobulin A; NSAID: nonsteroidal anti-inflammatory drug)

Tubular Proteinuria

Normally, freely filtered LMW proteins are reabsorbed at the proximal convoluted tubule (PCT). Diseases causing injury to the proximal tubular cells result in decreased reabsorptive capacity and subsequent loss of LMW proteins in the urine. Such proteinuria may show trace or 1+ on dipstick, contain little or no albumin, and rarely exceeds 1 g/day or will be <40 mg/m²/h on quantitative analysis. It is not associated with hypoalbuminemia or edema. Glomerular and tubular proteinuria can be distinguished by urine electrophoresis. In glomerular proteinuria, albumin is the major protein in urine, whereas in tubular proteinuria, little or no albumin is detected and LMW proteins migrate in the alpha and beta regions. Tubular proteinuria may be caused by inherited and acquired disorders **(Table 1)**. Tubular proteinuria rarely presents a diagnostic dilemma, because the underlying disease is usually detected before proteinuria. Other defects of proximal tubular function with bicarbonate wasting and phosphaturia manifest early as in Fanconi syndrome.

Overflow Proteinuria

Low-molecular-weight proteins filtered by the glomerulus are almost entirely reabsorbed in the proximal tubule. During states of overproduction of a particular LMW protein and hyperfiltration, the amount of filtered protein exceeds the normal proximal tubular reabsorptive capacity, leading to proteinuria. Overflow proteinuria is not common in children but could occur in myoglobinuria, hemoglobinuria, and repeated albumin transfusions.

Microalbuminuria

Microalbuminuria is a level of albumin excretion in urine that is not detected by dipstick. It is an early marker of systemic vascular endothelial cells dysfunction and kidney disease. In older children, microalbuminuria is defined as a daily excretion of 30–300 mg of albumin per day. The UA/UCr on random urine samples can also be used. With this method, microalbuminuria is defined as a ratio greater than 0.03 mg albumin/mg creatinine.[9]

For the quantitation of albuminuria, a sensitive and specific assay for albumin is used. Microalbuminuria is assessed by using specialized test strips. 24-hour urine collection is considered as the "gold standard" for the measurement of microalbuminuria. The proteinuria, albuminuria, risk assessment, detection, and elimination (PARADE) program initiated by the National Kidney Foundation underscores the importance of asymptomatic microalbuminuria as a risk factor for progressive kidney and cardiovascular diseases.[13]

CLINICAL EVALUATION OF PROTEINURIA

A positive dipstick for protein in a random sample of urine is common in children. Urine dipstick will be positive (defined as ≥1+) in 5–10% of normal school-aged children and adolescents on general screening. However, proteinuria is persistent in only 0.1% of children.[14]

Good history and physical examination help to determine the cause of proteinuria. A urine sample collected at the time of febrile illness or after intensive physical exercise or a seizure episode suggests the possibility of transient proteinuria. Children with proteinuria (particularly if 2+ or less), in the absence of any identifiable source or cause for proteinuria, should have one additional urine analysis performed and a UPr/UCr ratio on the first morning specimen. If the urinalysis and UPr/UCr ratio are normal, then it is likely that the patient has transient proteinuria **(Flowchart 1)**. A large proportion of children show resolution of proteinuria subsequently and need no further evaluation. A negative urine protein in the first morning void and a positive urine protein in the midmorning specimen are indicative of OP.

Flowchart 1: Evaluation of asymptomatic proteinuria in children.

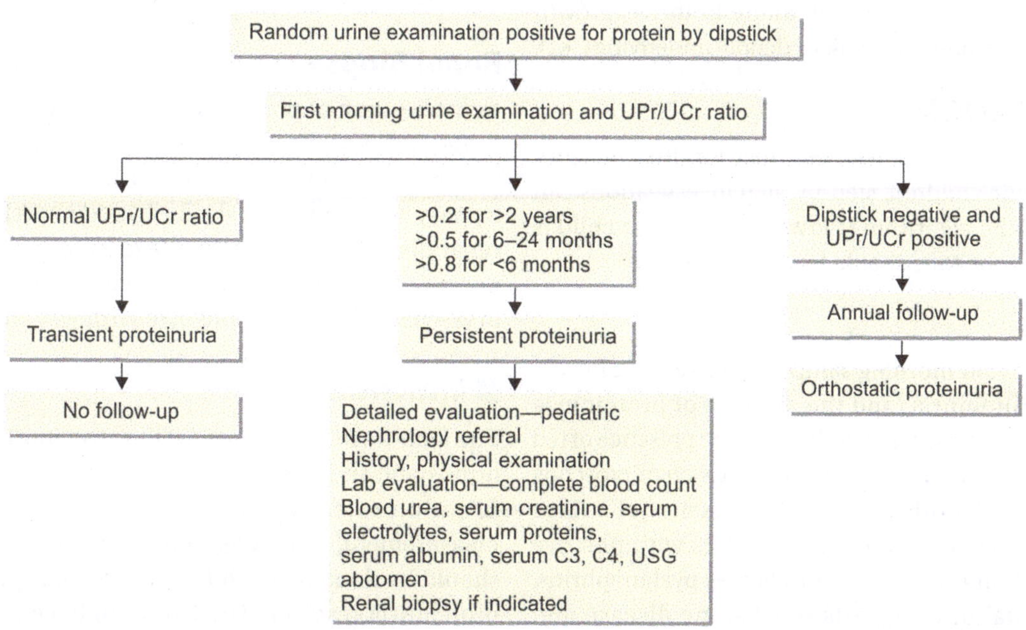

(UPr/UCr: urine protein to urine creatinine ratio)

If both subsequent test results are positive, the child should be considered as persistent proteinuria and subjected to clinical and laboratory evaluation, particularly in the presence of renal symptoms, or systemic clinical features and investigations favoring renal involvement. Once persistent proteinuria is documented, evaluation should begin with history and physical examination focusing on the presence of signs and symptoms of systemic diseases that can affect the kidney. Manifestations of renal disease such as hematuria, both visible and invisible, edema, hypertension, oliguria, or polyuria form a strong basis for further evaluation, even if there is no renal dysfunction. Consanguineous marriage, family history of childhood renal disease, renal anomalies, renal cause of death, deafness, visual defects (Alport syndrome), and polycystic kidney disease are to be enquired. Diabetes, eclampsia, and hypertension during pregnancy can injure the developing fetal kidneys. LBW is associated with significantly higher blood pressure and 24-hour urine albumin excretion compared to healthy controls. Angiotensin-converting enzyme inhibitor (ACEI), angiotensin-receptor blockers (ARBs), and nonsteroidal anti-inflammatory drugs (NSAIDs) during early and late pregnancy cause permanent fetal kidney damage. Perinatal morbidities needing neonatal intensive care unit (NICU) care can be associated with neonatal acute kidney injury, partial recovery, and progression to chronic kidney disease (CKD).

Presence of early morning facial edema, rapid weight gain, reduced urine output, hematuria, history of skin infection, typhoid, mumps, measles and chickenpox, persistent erythematous maculopapular rashes over the face or lower limbs, joint pains (vasculitis), and hypertension indicate the glomerular origin of proteinuria. Recurrent urinary tract infection (UTI), polyuria, nocturia, preceding drug intake such as NSAIDs, aminoglycosides, and cephalosporins indicate a tubular cause for hematuria. Vigorous exercise may cause transient proteinuria. Presence of failure to thrive, growth failure, anemia, and bony deformities denote underlying CKD.

INVESTIGATION

All the investigations need not be performed for all the patients. For asymptomatic children, step-by-step investigations can be done as per the algorithm **(Flowchart 1)**. If the child is symptomatic, all the tests should be performed.

Urinalysis

Urinalysis (first void morning sample) is rewarding for the presence of proteinuria, and the amount of proteinuria reflects the severity of glomerular disease. The presence of red blood cell (RBC) casts and dysmorphic RBCs on microscopy confirms glomerular origin, while the presence of a large number of leukocytes and leukocyte casts with positive bacterial growth in urine cultures indicates pyelonephritis. Persistent crystalluria suggests renal stone disease and tubulointerstitial origin of proteinuria.

Blood Chemistry

Blood urea, nitrogen, serum creatinine, serum electrolytes, serum cholesterol, serum total proteins, and albumin are the basics investigations in glomerular disease.

Immunological Profile

Abnormalities in serum complements C3 and C4, antinuclear antibodies, anti-double-stranded DNA antibody, and antinuclear cytoplasmic antibodies (ANCAs) suggest the diagnosis of systemic vasculitis. An elevated serum globulin on electrophoresis is a reliable screening test for immunologically mediated glomerular injury. Antistreptolysin O (ASO) titer is done in suspected poststreptococcal glomerulonephritis.

Microbiology

Throat, urine, and blood cultures are indicated if infections are a possibility.

Imaging

Sonography of the kidneys and urinary tract is an appropriate, noninvasive screening test for anatomic abnormalities and should be considered in patients with suspected CKD. A voiding cystourethrography (VCUG) should be considered if vesicoureteral reflux is suspected in a child with persistent proteinuria and past history of febrile UTI. A dimercaptosuccinic acid (DMSA) scan is the preferred study to detect renal scars in suspected reflux nephropathy.

Audiometry

In the presence of a family history of nephritis, renal failure, deafness, or visual defects, then the Alport syndrome is considered and audiometry is done to rule out sensorineural hearing loss.

Renal Biopsy

In the workup of proteinuria, renal biopsy is not routinely indicated. Kidney biopsy is considered if proteinuria is accompanied by gross hematuria, hypertension, active urinary sediments, persistent hypocomplementemia, and renal insufficiency (CKD > stage 2) for >3 months with a normal or enlarged kidney or signs and symptoms suggestive of vasculitis. The indications of renal biopsy are given in **Box 1**.

MANAGEMENT

The family can be reassured if the proteinuria is transient or orthostatic and has normal blood pressure and glomerular filtration rate. Regular follow-up with blood pressure measurement, urinalysis, and serum creatinine estimation should be done in a child with persistent proteinuria until proteinuria resolves. The child can have normal diet and physical activity.

BOX 1: Indications of renal biopsy in proteinuria.

- Proteinuria with active urine sediments
- Significant persistent proteinuria >1 g/1.73 m^2/day
- Proteinuria with microscopic hematuria, hypertension, or renal failure
- eGFR < 80 mL/1.73 m^2/min for >3 months with a normal or enlarged kidney
- Presence of systemic features suggesting SLE, HSP, and ANCA vasculitis
- Persistently low C3 for >3 months

(ANCA: antinuclear cytoplasmic antibody; eGFR: estimated glomerular filtration rate; HSP: Henoch–Schönlein purpura; SLE: systemic lupus erythematosus)

Diet

Avoid excessive salt intake as it will contribute to fluid retention and edema. It is prudent to avoid a high-protein diet in children with proteinuric kidney disease as high dietary protein intake may worsen proteinuria and disease progression. Children with proteinuria should receive the recommended daily allowance of protein for age.[3]

Medications

In children with CKD and proteinuria, ACEI and ARB are the preferred antihypertensive drugs as these drugs, in addition to reducing systemic blood pressure, exert other beneficial effects such as reduction in urinary protein excretion and the risk of renal fibrosis. The need for serial monitoring of serum potassium and creatinine needs to be emphasized while on these drugs.[15]

CONCLUSION

The presence of proteinuria can have different significance depending on the underlying cause. At one end are children with false-positive, transient, or intermittent proteinuria in whom the proteinuria is harmless. At the other end are children with persistent proteinuria, hematuria, and renal failure who are at a considerable risk of having a serious renal disease. In between are children with asymptomatic proteinuria without hematuria or renal failure who are at a mild risk of renal disease. The clinician's responsibility remains in recognizing these situations and then planning evaluation, therapy, and follow-up to improve the outcome.

KEY POINTS

- Proteinuria may be a marker of kidney damage and needs attention to differentiate benign forms from significant proteinuria associated with kidney disease.
- In children, urine protein excretion >100 mg/m^2/day >4 mg/m^2/h is abnormal.
- Transient proteinuria and OP are benign and require no detailed evaluation.
- Children with persistent proteinuria need further evaluation including kidney function tests; serum electrolytes, cholesterol, albumin, and total protein; serological tests; imaging; and renal biopsy as indicated to rule out significant renal disease.
- Children with nephrotic proteinuria will most often have idiopathic nephrotic syndrome and must be treated promptly in consultation with a pediatric nephrologist.
- Children with persistent non-nephrotic proteinuria along with hypertension, an abnormal urinalysis, or deranged renal function test (RFT) need prompt pediatric nephrology referral for detailed evaluation including kidney biopsy.

REFERENCES

1. Cravedi P, Remuzzi G. Pathophysiology of proteinuria and its value as an outcome measure in chronic kidney disease. Br J Clin Pharmacol. 2013;76(4):516-23.
2. Cameron JS. 2003 Milk or albumin? The history of proteinuria before Richard Bright. Nephrol Dial Transplant. 2003;18(7):1281-5.
3. Prabha S. Approach to proteinuria. Indian J Pract Pediatr. 2012;14:190-8.
4. Gattineni J. Highlights for the management of a child with proteinuria and hematuria. Int J Pediatr. 2012;2012:768142.
5. Mi Jang K, Cho KH. Clinical approach to children with proteinuria. Child Kidney Dis. 2017;21:53-60.
6. Leung AKC, Wong A, Barg SSN. Proteinuria in children: evaluation and differential diagnosis. Am Fam Physician. 2017;95(4):248-54.
7. Barratt J, Topham P. Urine proteomics: the present and future of measuring urinary protein components in disease. CMAJ. 2007177(4):361-8.
8. Jafar TH, Chaturvedi N, Hatcher J, Levey AS. Use of albumin creatinine ratio and urine albumin concentration as a screening test for albuminuria in an Indo-Asian population. Nephrol Dial Transplant. 2007;22:2194-200.
9. Zabeen B, Nahar J, Islam N, Azad K, Donaghue K. Risk factors associated with microalbuminuria in children and adolescents with diabetes in Bangladesh. Indian J Endocr Metab. 2018;22:85-8.
10. Bazzi C, Petrini C, Rizza V, Arrigo G, D'Amico G. A modern approach to selectivity of proteinuria and tubulointerstitial damage in nephrotic syndrome. Transferrin ratio does not show this type of association. Kidney Int. 2000;58:1732-41.
11. Garg P, Rabelink T. Glomerular proteinuria: a complex interplay between unique players. Adv Chronic Kidney Dis. 2011;18(4):233-42.
12. Brandt JR, Jacobs A, Raissy HH, Kelly FM, Staples AO, Kaufman E, et al. Orthostatic proteinuria and the spectrum of diurnal variability of urinary protein excretion in healthy children. Pediatr Nephrol. 2010;25(6):1131.
13. Hogg RJ, Portman RJ, Milliner D, Lemley KV, Eddy A, Ingelfinger J. Evaluation and management of proteinuria and nephrotic syndrome in children: recommendations from a pediatric nephrology panel established at the National Kidney Foundation conference on proteinuria, albuminuria, risk, assessment, detection, and elimination (PARADE). Pediatrics. 2000;105:1242-9.
14. Vehaskari VM, Rapola J. Isolated proteinuria: analysis of a school-age population. J Pediatr. 1982;101:661-8.
15. Litwin M, Grenda R, Sladowska J, Antoniewicz J. Add-on therapy with angiotensin II receptor I blocker in children with chronic kidney disease already treated with ACE inhibitors. Pediatr Nephrol. 2006;11:1716-22.

CHAPTER

3.6

Failure to Thrive and Growth Retardation due to Renal Disease

Susan Uthup

INTRODUCTION

Failure to thrive (FTT) or growth retardation has long been a major focus of attention and therapeutic challenge. The term "failure to thrive" has been used regularly in clinical medicine for poor weight gain or "faltering growth" in infants and toddlers. FTT is an abnormal pattern of weight gain due to lack of sufficient usable nutrition and documented by inadequate weight gain over time.[1] The term FTT should be used as a clinical finding and not as a diagnosis. FTT may occur in up to 10% of children in primary care and in approximately 5% of hospitalized children.[2] Early identification and management of the issues causing undernutrition are critical as persistent severe malnutrition can cause short stature, secondary immune deficiency, and permanent damage to the brain.[1,3]

Failure to thrive may be sometimes the only manifestation in kidney disease in infants and toddlers. Timely identification of these diseases is important in instituting appropriate treatment. The clinical suspicion and appropriate evaluation are crucial in reaching proper diagnosis.[4] Renal diseases causing FTT and evaluation in suspected renal disease are discussed briefly in this chapter. Detailed discussion and management of these diseases will be discussed in the appropriate sections.

DEFINITION

Failure to thrive is defined as weight less than the 3rd percentile for gestation-corrected age and sex, approximately equivalent to a Z-score of –2 when plotted on an appropriate growth chart and decreased velocity of weight gain that is disproportionate to growth in length. There is decelerated or arrested physical growth. Height and weight measurements fall below the 5th percentile or there is a downward trend in growth falling two major percentile lines due to inadequate caloric intake, inadequate caloric absorption, or excessive caloric expenditure.[5,6] Recognition of FTT depends on reliable accurate and serial measurements of weight and height which are charted on an appropriate reference scale (growth charts).[7] The World Health Organization (WHO) international growth charts for children can be used to record a child's measurement against children of the same age and sex as a reference standard.

The following deviations from the norm are typical of FTT:[8]

- Abnormal weight-to-length ratio with weight-for-length <70–79% or body mass index (BMI) < 3rd percentile
- Weight <3rd percentile
- Lack of increase in length and/or weight with percentile deviations >2 main percentiles (3rd, 10th, 25th, 50th, 75th, 90th, 97th).

ETIOLOGY OF FAILURE TO THRIVE

Failure to thrive and growth retardation occur due to a wide variety of medical and psychosocial stressors. The most common cause of FTT is inadequate caloric intake. Other causes are inadequate nutrient absorption, increased energy requirements (metabolic demands), or a combination of mechanisms.[9] The risk factors for FTT are traditionally classified as psychosocial or nonorganic and organic. Usually, multiple complex factors operate resulting in inadequate caloric intake. The prevalence of various causes of FTT may differ based on the patient's age and the underlying cause.[4] Although the major cause is behavioral or psychosocial, it is prudent to assess for underlying organic causes. The risk factors for poor weight gain include prematurity, developmental delay, congenital anomalies, genetic or chromosomal disorders, intrauterine infections, congenital heart diseases, chronic kidney disease (CKD), anemia, and any medical condition that results in inadequate intake, increased metabolic rate, maldigestion, or malabsorption.[10,11]

FAILURE TO THRIVE AND RENAL DISEASE

Failure to thrive due to renal disease may commence in early infancy or at any time during childhood. It may be due to hereditary or acquired renal diseases, and pathology may be involving the glomerular or tubulointerstitial compartment. CKD associated with renal hypodysplasia, obstructive/refluxing anomalies, cystic diseases, metabolic diseases such as cystinosis and oxalosis, and salt-wasting tubulopathies are the common renal diseases associated with FTT.[5] Except in renal tubulopathy, a common accompaniment in all other renal diseases associated with FTT is reduced glomerular filtration rate (GFR).

Based on the pathophysiology and clinical presentation, the renal causes for FTT and growth retardation may be considered under three broad categories for ease of approach and intervention:

1. Chronic kidney disease with the triad of manifestations—growth failure, anemia, and bony deformities.
2. Congenital anomaly of kidneys and urinary tract (CAKUT)—especially the obstructive anomalies and vesicoureteral reflux. Obstructive voiding symptoms, poor urinary stream, dribbling, recurrent episodes of fever, and pyuria will be the associated symptoms in these babies.
3. Renal tubulopathies—FTT will be associated with polyuria, dehydration, and nephrocalcinosis.

PATHOPHYSIOLOGY OF FAILURE TO THRIVE IN RENAL DISEASES

Chronic Kidney Disease and Growth Failure

Growth failure is a major complication in children with CKD. Poor growth in children with CKD is associated with significant morbidity and mortality. Growth failure, anemia, and bony deformities **(Fig. 1)** comprise the classical triad of manifestation in pediatric CKD. As per the 2008 North American Pediatric Renal Trials and Collaborative Studies (NAPRTCS) registry, >35% of children at the time of enrolment in the CKD registry had impaired growth defined as a height less than the 3rd percentile for age and gender (*Z*-score for height below –1.88). The risk of growth impairment was greatest in infants (58%) and lowest in children older than 12 years. The risk for poor growth increased with decreasing renal function, although even children with mild renal impairment (GFR > 60 mL/min/1.73 m^2) are at a risk for poor growth.[12]

Children who develop renal failure in infancy are more growth impaired than those who acquire renal disease later in childhood. Since 30% of the final adult height is attained during the first 2 years of life, the onset of renal failure during this critical period has been associated with markedly diminished adult height. Height deficit is maximum in the initial postnatal months. Cumulative height deficit will be to the extent of 3 standard deviation (SD) by 3 years. During childhood, the growth rate in CKD mostly correlates with GFR and patients maintain an adequate growth pattern if their GFR is >25 mL/min/1.73 m^2.[13]

Poor nutrition, metabolic acidosis, fluid and electrolyte abnormalities, renal osteodystrophy, anemia, and disturbances of the growth hormone/insulin-like growth factor-1 (GH/IGF-1) axis are important risk factors for growth failure in these children. Disturbances of the somatotropic hormone axis play an important pathogenic role in growth retardation and catabolism in children with CKD.[13,14]

Another important factor influencing growth in CKD is the primary renal disease. Presence of genetic metabolic disorders, such as cystinosis and hyperoxaluria, is associated with worst growth outcomes. Children with cystinosis remain below the 3rd percentile in both height and weight throughout life. Patients with renal dysplasia and congenital obstructive disorders may develop growth retardation due to associated tubular dysfunction even before decline in GFR due to impaired urine concentrating ability, dehydration, acidosis, and salt wasting.[13,14]

Congenital Anomaly of Kidneys and Urinary Tract

Congenital anomaly of kidneys and urinary tract is the leading cause of kidney failure in the young. But babies with obstructing or refluxing anomalies involving the urinary system may present in the neonatal period or infancy with poor weight gain even when the GFR is normal. Detailed history may reveal oligohydramnios or fetal renal anomaly on antenatal sonography which was not evaluated postnatally. Breech delivery and history of respiratory distress soon after birth may be present. Poor urinary stream, straining on micturition, dribbling, foul-smelling cloudy urine, and recurrent episodes of fever without a focus are important clues to the underlying urinary tract obstruction. There may be history of recurrent febrile episodes treated empirically. Sometimes, the presentation may be catastrophic with severe urosepsis, dehydration, acute kidney injury (AKI), severe acidosis, dyselectrolytemia, and hyperkalemia. The obstruction may be due to posterior urethral valve, ureteropelvic junction stenosis, bilateral terminal ureteral stenosis, ectopic ureterocele, or meatal stenosis. Infants and children with vesicoureteral reflux, Prune-Belly syndrome, and pelviureteric junction and megaureter may also present in a similar manner. 20% of the children with CAKUT in CKD stages I–III had FTT with weight or height or both <3 SD.[15]

Renal Tubulopathies

Renal tubular disorders form a significant cause of FTT in children. Salt-losing tubulopathies can affect all tubular segments, from the proximal tubule to the collecting duct. Common renal tubular disorders associated with FTT are distal renal tubular acidosis (d-RTA) and Bartter-like (Bartter and Gitelman) syndromes followed by hereditary Fanconi syndrome (cystinosis and idiopathic Fanconi syndrome) and nephrogenic diabetes insipidus[16,17] **(Table 1)**.

The preservation of electrolyte, volume, and acid-base homeostasis balance is vital for optimum growth. The optimum pH of body fluids is absolutely essential for cellular functions and metabolism. Both metabolic acidosis and alkalosis interfere with normal metabolism. Renal disorders of acid-base balance interfere with cellular metabolism and growth. In all these diseases, apart from acid-base imbalance, there will be polyuria with dehydration, hypokalemia, and hyponatremia. Persistent vomiting and polydipsia interfere with caloric intake and caloric absorption. Caloric utilization

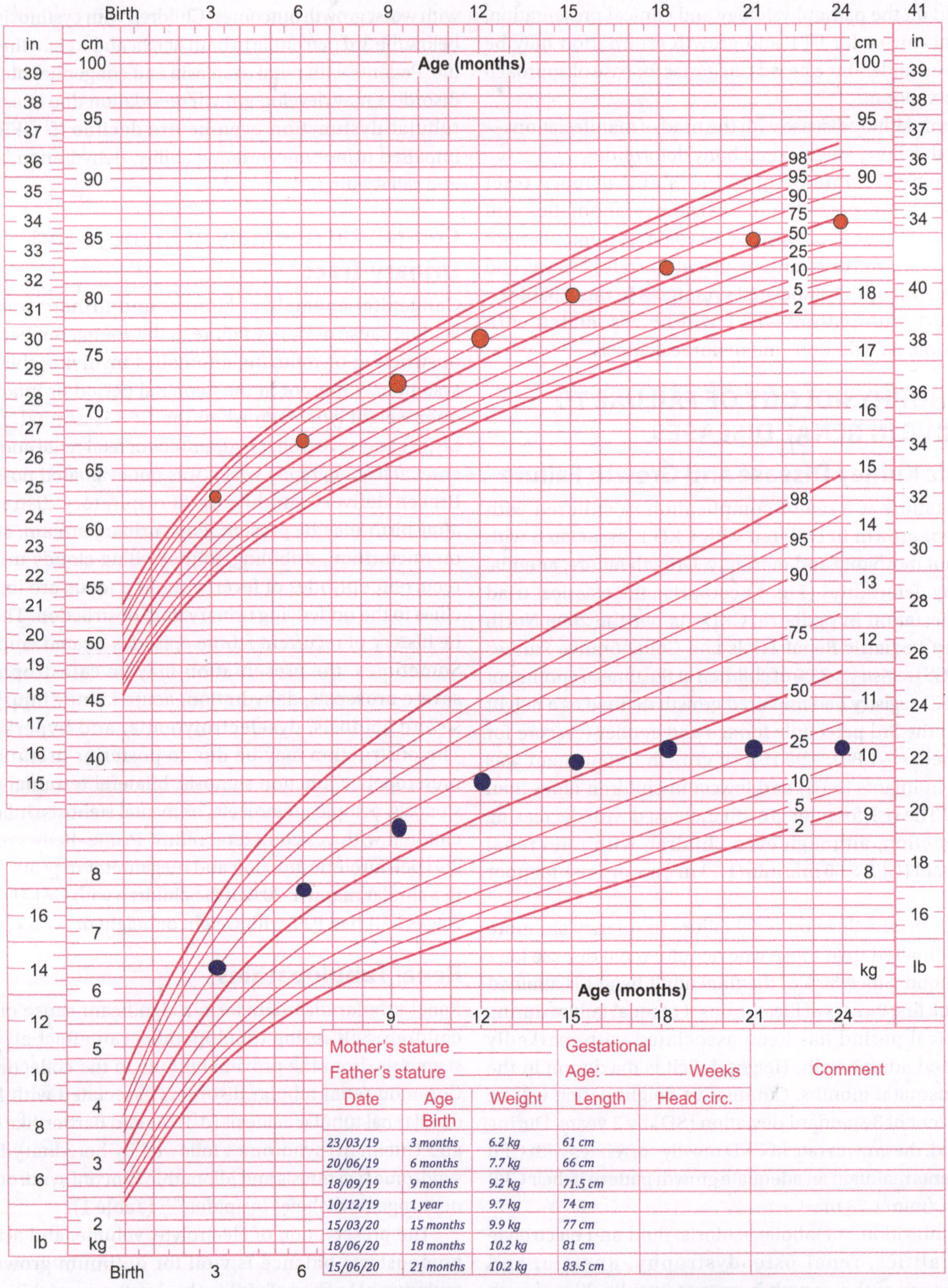

Date	Age	Weight	Length	Head circ.	Comment
	Birth				
23/03/19	3 months	6.2 kg	61 cm		
20/06/19	6 months	7.7 kg	66 cm		
18/09/19	9 months	9.2 kg	71.5 cm		
10/12/19	1 year	9.7 kg	74 cm		
15/03/20	15 months	9.9 kg	77 cm		
18/06/20	18 months	10.2 kg	81 cm		
15/06/20	21 months	10.2 kg	83.5 cm		

Fig. 1: A growth chart depicting serial anthropometry measurements that reveal failure to thrive in an infant with untreated proximal renal tubular acidosis.

will be affected by acidosis or alkalosis as in RTA and Bartter-like syndromes, respectively.[18]

Failure to thrive in infancy is usually the presenting feature in RTA, especially d-RTA and Fanconi syndrome. These children are often polyuric, dehydrated, hypokalemic, constipated, and often anorectic. The cause of growth retardation in RTA could include chronic hypokalemia and metabolic acidosis and rickets. Children with Fanconi

TABLE 1: Renal tubular disorders associated with failure to thrive.

Affected site	*Disorder*	*Transport defect*
Proximal tubule	• Proximal RTA • Fanconi syndrome	• Bicarbonate • Amino acid, bicarbonate, glucose, phosphate • Phosphate
Ascending limb of loop of Henle	Bartter syndrome	Sodium, potassium, chloride
Distal tubule	Distal RTA	Proton (H^+) secretion
Collecting duct	• Pseudohypoaldosteronism • Nephrogenic DI	• Sodium, potassium transport • Water transport

(DI: diabetes insipidus; RTA: renal tubular acidosis)

syndrome and underlying metabolic disorders, such as cystinosis, often will have severe FTT.

Acidosis also interferes with major aspects of the GH-IGF axis. Acidosis-induced anorexia and reduced nutrition contribute to decreased GH secretion. Acidosis also inhibits the GH pulse amplitude, pulse area, and total GH secretion. Serum IGF, hepatic IGF-1 messenger ribonucleic acid (mRNA), hepatic GH receptor mRNA, and gene expression of IGF at the growth plate of the long bone all are suppressed in the presence of metabolic acidosis.[19]

Children with Bartter syndrome generally present in early infancy or early childhood with FTT, persistent polyuria, persistent vomiting, feeding difficulties, constipation, dehydration, and electrolyte imbalance. Nearly all patients with Bartter syndrome have growth failure and are below the 5th percentile for age.[20] Although polyuria, polydipsia, hypokalemia, and salt loss may be responsible for growth retardation, the exact pathogenesis of short stature in the Bartter syndrome is not known. Hypokalemia in the Bartter syndrome may interfere with the action of GH. GH deficiency is also sometimes seen associated with the Bartter syndrome.

The autosomal recessive form of pseudohypoaldosteronism type 1 caused by loss-of-function mutations in any of the subunits of the epithelial sodium channel (ENaC) is yet another rare cause of FTT. Affected infants typically present in the first few days with excessive weight loss and are found to have life-threatening hypovolemia with hyperkalemia and acidosis.[21]

EVALUATION OF FAILURE TO THRIVE

Children with organic FTT often show symptoms and signs of an underlying disease. Antenatal, natal, and postnatal history and comprehensive physical examination often give clues to the underlying disease causing FTT. The first consideration in examining a child with presumed FTT is ensuring accurate measurements. Height (or length), weight, weight for length, and head circumference should be measured correctly and plotted on an appropriate growth chart.[1,7] **Figure 1** depicts serial measurements on a growth chart of an infant who is failing to thrive with RTA.

TABLE 2: Red flag signs indicating organic cause for failure to thrive.

Renal causes	*Nonrenal causes*
• Recurrent UTI • Poor urinary stream • Anemia • Bony deformities • Polyuria • Dehydration • Persistent vomiting	• Cardiac murmur • Dysmorphism • Microcephaly • Developmental delay • Organomegaly • Recurrent infections Lymphadenopathy • Diarrhea • Malabsorption • Persistent vomiting

(UTI: urinary tract infection)

There are certain clinical features which may be considered as red flag signs to identify the underlying disease process. The diagnosis of organic FTT depends on prompt identification of these red flag signs **(Table 2)**. If the history and physical examination rule out these signs, then the problem is nonorganic, and appropriate evaluation and management of caloric intake and correction of psychosocial factors are warranted. If red flag signs are present, then appropriate evaluation of an underlying organic disease is planned based on the clinical presentation. An algorithmic approach to evaluation of renal causes of FTT is shown in **Flowchart 1**.

Anemia, bony deformities, fluid imbalance with polyuria and dehydration, or fluid overload with edema and hypertension in a child with growth failure point to probable CKD as the underlying disease. Any child presenting with urosepsis and FTT should be evaluated for a congenital structural abnormality of kidneys and the urinary system.

Polyuria, excessive thirst, dehydration, and salt craving are the clinical features suggestive of renal tubular disorders in FTT. Renal tubulopathies often present in the neonatal period or infancy with FTT and polyuria. GFR is often normal in these children. Normal anion gap metabolic acidosis and hypokalemia with an alkaline urine points to the diagnosis of RTA. A child with generalized proximal tubular dysfunction will have phosphaturia, glycosuria, and generalized aminoaciduria. Severe FTT is common in cystinosis and other metabolic diseases with generalized proximal tubular dysfunction and Fanconi syndrome. The clinical presentation in distal RTA is polyuria, rickets, and FTT. Nephrocalcinosis is another differentiating feature in d-RTA. Refractory rickets and FTT may be the presentation in RTA, Fanconi syndrome, or familial hypophosphatemia.

Hypochloremic metabolic alkalosis with polyuria, hypokalemia, and nephrocalcinosis in an infant or child with FTT suggest the diagnosis of Bartter syndrome. There may be a history of polyhydramnios and premature delivery.

Flowchart 1: Algorithm on differential diagnosis of failure to thrive due to renal disease.

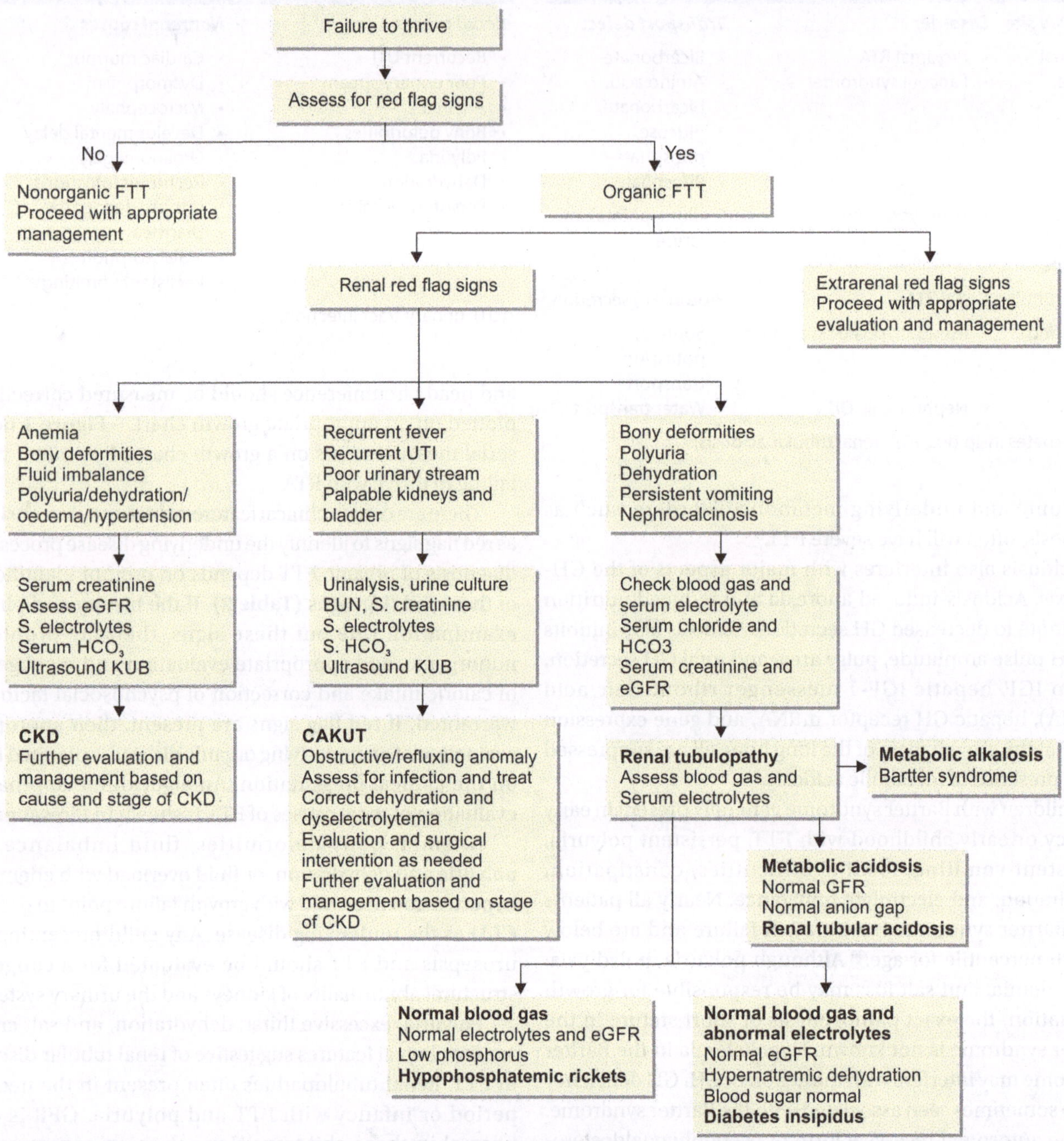

(BUN: blood urea nitrogen; CKD: chronic kidney disease; eGFR: estimated glomerular filtration rate; FTT: failure to thrive; GFR: glomerular filtration rate; KUB: kidney, ureter, bladder; UTI: urinary tract infection)

In an infant or child presenting with polyuria, excessive thirst, dehydration, hypernatremia, irritability, recurrent episodes of fever without an apparent cause, weight loss, constipation, and FTT, the possibility of diabetes insipidus is to be considered. Anorexia due to preference of water over food results in loss of weight and FTT. Irritability and fatigue due to disturbed sleep and affection of linear growth are seen. Seizures due to severe hypernatremia, hyperosmolar dehydration, and potential hypoxia may lead to intracranial bleed and mental retardation.[22] The detailed evaluation and diagnosis of individual conditions are discussed in respective chapters. A comprehensive approach to history-taking, examination, and evaluation for the diagnosis of renal disorders manifesting with FTT is illustrated in **Flowchart 2**.

MANAGEMENT

Management of growth failure in pediatric CKD requires optimization of nutrition, fluid balance, correction of metabolic disorders such as acidosis (bicarbonate therapy), electrolyte imbalance, anemia (iron, recombinant human erythropoietin), renal osteodystrophy (vitamin D and calcium supplementation and phosphate restriction), and GH therapy. Optimization of nutrition is the most important factor in optimizing the growth. Nutritional intake

Flowchart 2: A detailed approach to pointers on history, clues on examination, and evaluation to the diagnosis of various renal disorders presenting as failure to thrive.

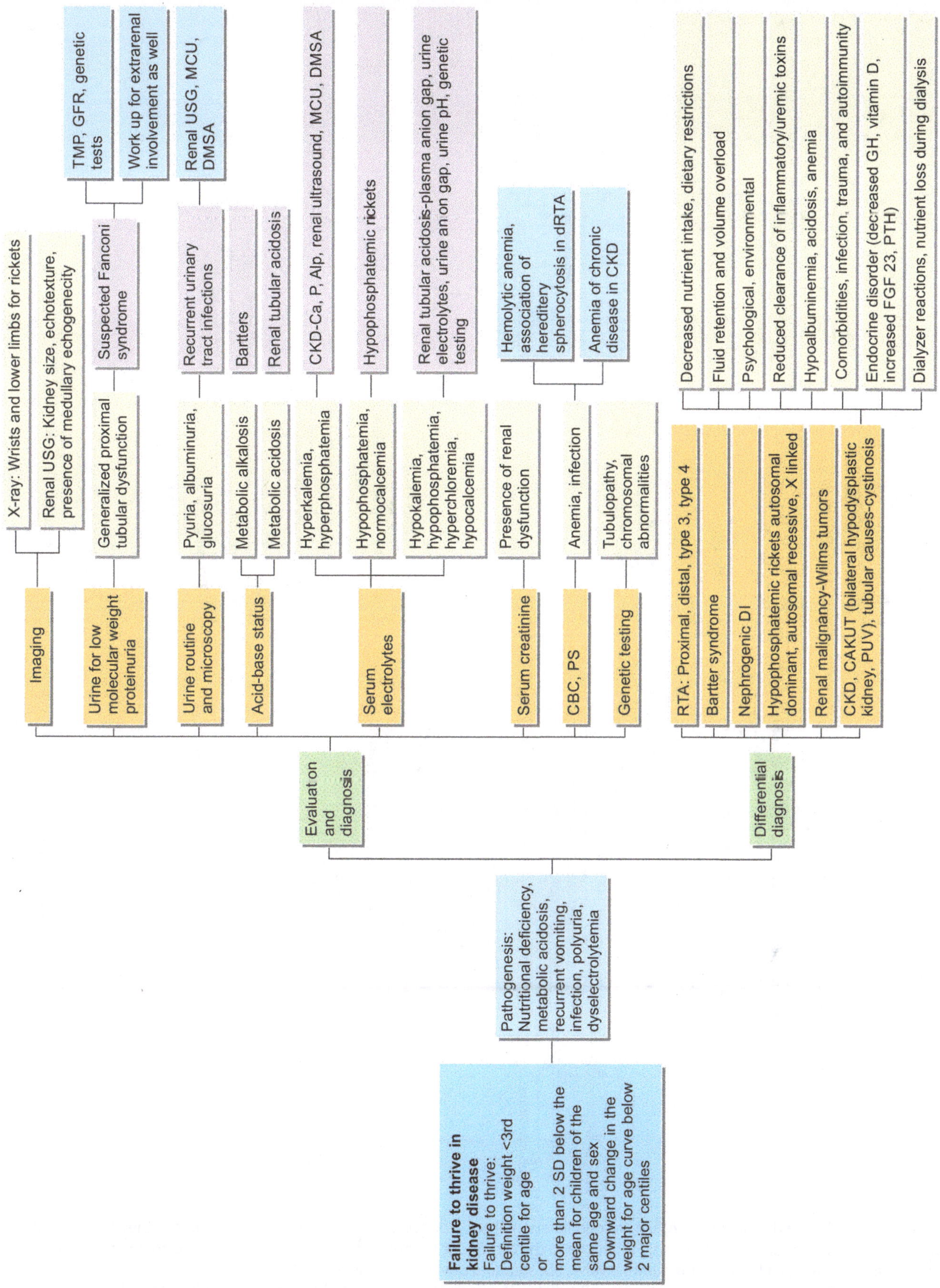

Contd...

Contd...

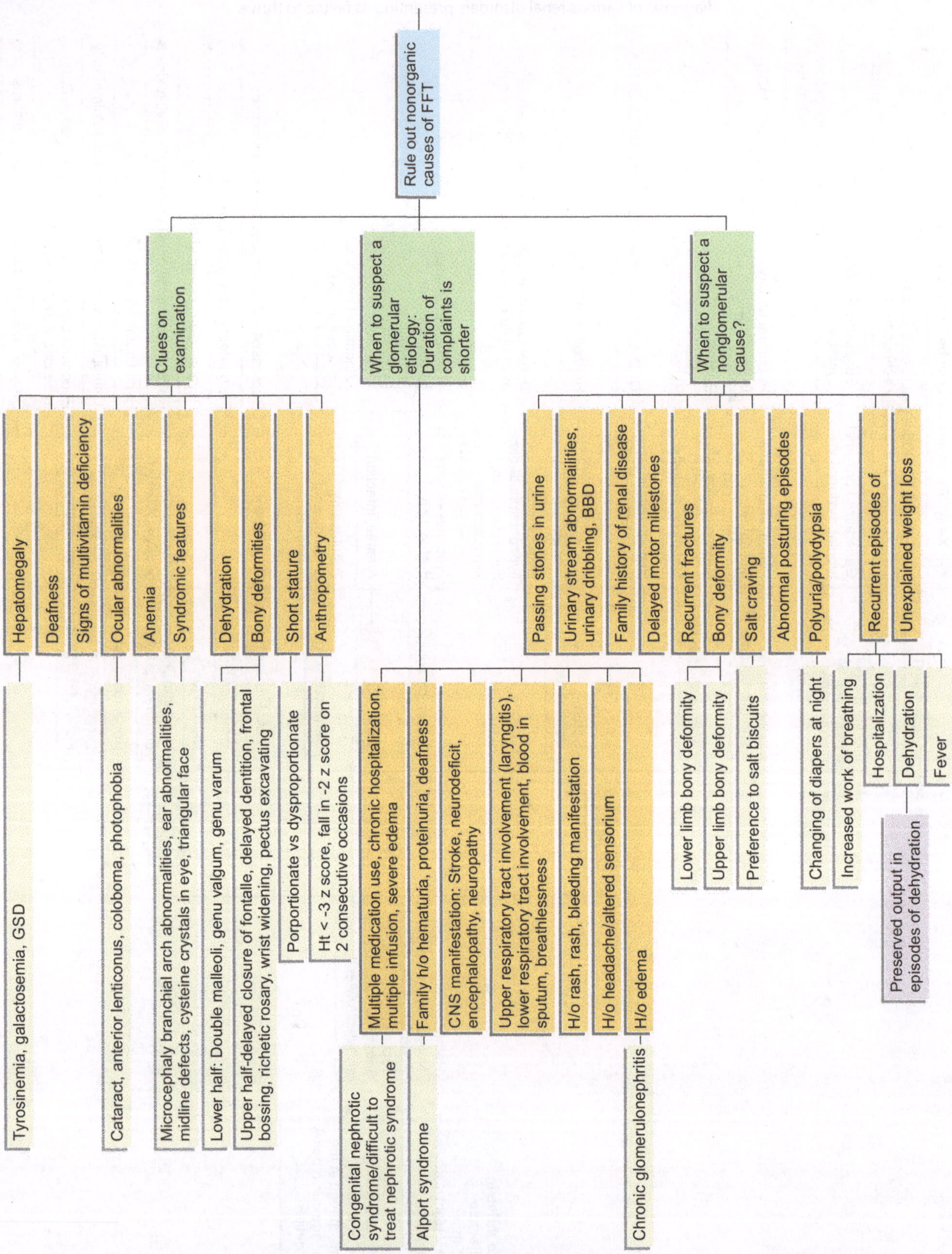

(BBD: bladder and bowel dysfunction; CAKUT: congenital anomaly of kidneys and urinary tract; CKD: chronic kidney disease; DI: diabetes insipidus; d-RTA: distal renal tubular acidosis; FTT: failure to thrive; FGF 23: fibroblast growth factor-23; GH: growth hormone; H/o: history of; PTH: parathyroid hormone; PUV: posterior urethral valve; SD: standard deviation; VD: vitamin D)

Courtesy: Dr Seher Kamal, MD, Fellow, Department of Paediatric Nephrology, St John's Medical College Hospital, Bengaluru.

of 100–120% of Recommended Dietary Allowance (RDA) each of energy and protein should be ensured utilizing oral/nasogastric/G-tube feeding. After the correction of nutritional and metabolic factors, recombinant human GH may be initiated if the height standard deviation score (SDS) is below –2 SD and the epiphysis is open. Recombinant growth hormone (rGH) is given as a subcutaneous injection at a dose of 0.045–0.05 mg/kg or 4 IU/m^2/day. Timely initiation of kidney replacement therapy (KRT) in children with stage 5 CKD optimizes the fluid electrolyte and acid–base balance, but ensuring adequate nutrition is of prime importance in children on dialysis. Renal transplantation is the optimal KRT modality to prevent and correct growth failure.

Neonates and infants with congenital obstructive/refluxing anomalies and FTT need emergency care if they present in urosepsis and AKI. Catheterization of bladder, relief of obstruction, correction of dehydration, electrolyte imbalance, acidosis, prompt initiation of appropriate antibiotics, and surgical intervention as needed will be lifesaving. After initial stabilization, corrective interventions may be planned along with attention to nutrition, fluid, electrolyte, and acid–base balance as in children with CKD.[23]

In RTA, bicarbonate therapy is initiated to correct metabolic acidosis; the aim is to maintain serum total CO_2 above 22 mEq/L in children and above 20 mEq/L in infants. Attention should also be given to correction of dehydration and electrolyte imbalance.

Treatment of the Bartter syndrome is directed at preventing dehydration, maintaining nutritional status, correcting hypokalemia with potassium supplements, and use of potassium-sparing diuretics. Indomethacin, a prostaglandin inhibitor, is effective in ameliorating polyuria and maintaining electrolyte balance. Early diagnosis and proper attention to dehydration, electrolyte balance, and use of drugs such as indomethacin have improved the outcome in Bartter syndrome.[18,21]

A detailed discussion on the management of renal tubulopathies is given in respective sections.

PROGNOSIS

Severe prolonged FTT can negatively affect the long-term outcome. Children with CKD stages 4 and 5 and those with metabolic disorders, such as cystinosis, tend to remain short with little catch-up growth. With adequate treatment, good catch-up growth occurs in CAKUT after correction of obstruction, infection, dehydration, and electrolyte imbalance. Children with d-RTA also do well with significant catch-up growth compared to all other tubular disorders.[16] Regular follow-up with periodic assessment of growth and modification of treatment, as needed, is essential for optimal outcomes.

CONCLUSION

Failure to thrive in infants and children poses a diagnostic dilemma and therapeutic challenge. Only 10% children have an underlying organic disease as the cause for FTT. Diagnosis of organic FTT depends on prompt identification of these red flag signs. FTT may be sometimes the only manifestation in kidney disease in infants and toddlers. CKD associated with renal hypodysplasia, obstructive/refluxing anomalies, and salt-wasting tubulopathies are the common renal diseases associated with FTT. Antenatal, natal, and postnatal history; comprehensive physical examination; and targeted evaluation help to diagnose the underlying disease causing FTT. Timely initiation of definitive treatment and regular follow-up help to improve the outcome.

KEY POINTS

- FTT is an abnormal pattern of weight gain due to lack of sufficient usable nutrition and documented by inadequate weight gain over time.
- FTT is defined as weight less than the 2nd percentile for gestation-corrected age and sex, approximately equivalent to a *Z*-score of –2 when plotted on an appropriate growth chart and decreased velocity of weight gain that is disproportionate to growth in length.
- Presence of red flag signs suggest FTT due to underlying organic causes.
- Common renal diseases associated with FTT include CKD, CAKUT (obstructive/refluxing anomalies), and renal tubular disorders.
- Comprehensive clinical assessment followed by targeted evaluation, management tailored to the underlying disorder, and periodic follow-up help to optimize the outcome.

REFERENCES

1. Cole SZ, Lanham JS. Failure to thrive: an update. Am Fam Physician. 2011;83(7):829-34.
2. Racine AD. Failure to thrive: Pediatric Nutrition. Textbook of Pediatric Care, 7th edition. Elk Grove Village, IL: American Academy of Paediatrics; 2014. pp. 663-700. [online] Available from https://pediatriccare.solutions.aap.org/chapter.aspx?sectionId=108723833&bookId=1626 [Last accessed August, 2021].
3. Yoo SD, Hwang EH, Lee YJ, Park JH. Clinical characteristics of failure to thrive in infant and toddler: organic vs. nonorganic. Pediatr Gastroenterol Hepatol Nutr. 2013;16(4):261-8.
4. Friedman J, Lewy JE. Failure to thrive associated with renal disease. Pediatr Ann. 1978;7(11):73-4, 76-7, 80-2.
5. Olsen EM. Failure to thrive: still a problem of definition. Clin Pediatr (Phila). 2006;45(1):1-6.
6. Casey PH. Failure to thrive. In: Carey WB, Crocker AC, Elias E, Feldman H, Coleman WL (Eds). Developmental-Behavioural Paediatrics, 4th edition. Philadelphia, PA: Saunders Elsevier; 2009. p. 583.
7. Olsen EM, Petersen J, Skovgaard AM, Weile B, Jørgensen T, Wright CM. Failure to thrive: the prevalence and concurrence of anthropometric criteria in a general infant population. Arch Dis Child. 2007;92(2):109-14.
8. Nützenadel W. Failure to thrive in childhood. Dtsch Arztebl Int. 2011;108(38):642-9.

9. Rybak A. Organic and nonorganic feeding disorders. Ann Nutr Metab. 2015;66(Suppl 5):16-22.
10. Schwartz ID. Failure to thrive: an old nemesis in the new millennium. Pediatr Rev. 2000;21:257.
11. Krugman SD, Dubowitz H. Failure to thrive. Am Fam Physician. 2003;68:879.
12. North American Pediatric Renal Trials and Collaborative Studies. 2008 Annual Report: renal transplantation, dialysis, and chronic renal insufficiency. [online] Available from https://web.emmes.com/study/ped/annlrept/Annual%20Report%20-2008.pdf [Last accessed April, 2012].
13. Salas P, Pinto V, Rodriguez J, Zambrano MJ, Mericq V. Growth retardation in children with kidney disease. Int J Endocrinol. 2013;2013:8. Available from http://dx.doi.org/10.1155/2013/970946.
14. Kaspar CDW, Bholah R, Bunchman TE. A review of pediatric chronic kidney disease. Blood Purif. 2016;41:211-7.
15. Biswas A, Bose T, Kalra S. A snapshot of children with congenital anomalies of the kidneys and urinary tract at three tertiary care centers of the armed forces. J Mar Med Soc. 2020;22(2):156-60.
16. Kiran BV, Barman H, Iyengar A. Clinical profile and outcome of renal tubular disorders in children: a single center experience. Indian J Nephrol. 2014;24(6):362-6.
17. Chang CY, Lin CY. Failure to thrive in children with primary distal type renal tubular acidosis. Acta Paediatr Taiwan. 2002;43(6):334-9.
18. Gil-Peña H, Mejia N, Alvarez-Garcia O, Loredo V, Santos F. Longitudinal growth in chronic hypokalemic disorders. Pediatr Nephrol. 2010;25:733-7.
19. Green J, Maor G. Effect of metabolic acidosis on the growth hormone/IGF-I endocrine axis in skeletal growth centers. Kidney Int. 2000;57(6):2258-67.
20. Chadha V, Alon US. Hereditary renal tubular disorders. Semin Nephrol. 2009;29(4):399-411.
21. Kleta R, and Bockenhauer D. Salt-losing tubulopathies in children: what's new, what's controversial? J Am Soc Nephrol. 2018;29(3):727-39.
22. Mishra G, Chandrashekhar SR. Management of diabetes insipidus in children. Indian J Endocrinol Metab. 2011;15(suppl3):S180-7.
23. Gharpure V. Posterior urethral valves in neonate. J Neonatal Surg. 2013;2(3):37.

SECTION

4

Approach to Management of Fluid, Electrolyte and Acid-base Disorders

CHAPTER

4.1

Fluid Therapy: Basics and in Special Situations

Sheeja Sugunan

INTRODUCTION

Intravenous (IV) fluid therapy is the one of the most common interventions in acutely ill children. IV fluids should be considered as any other pharmacological prescription. Administration of appropriate IV fluids is often life-saving in critically ill but it is also the drug associated with most number of adverse events in clinical practice ranging from extravasation, electrolyte imbalances to fluid overload and sepsis.[1] Children, especially newborns and young infants, are particularly more prone for fluid and electrolyte imbalances. The reasons for this include higher total body water, higher metabolic rate, higher insensible loss, and a less mature regulatory mechanism.[2,3] Choice of the right fluid, in the right dose, for the right duration is of paramount importance. Disease processes are dynamic. The need and response to fluid may change over time. Meticulous clinical and laboratory monitoring and frequent revision of fluid prescriptions are often needed in critically ill children.

PHYSIOLOGICAL BASIS OF FLUID MANAGEMENT

About 50–80% of human body is composed of water. Total body water is 80% of body weight in neonates and 60% of body weight in children above 6 months of age. Extracellular fluid (ECF) accounts for one-third of total body water and is larger in children than adults. ECF ranges from 45% in term neonates to 30% by age 1 to 20% in adults.[4] The relative decrease in ECF is due to decrease in interstitial fluid, while the percentage of intravascular fluid is fairly constant.[5]

Sodium is the primary cation and chloride is the primary anion in plasma and is predominantly extracellular. The intracellular compartment primarily consists of potassium, magnesium, proteins, and organic/inorganic phosphate. Interstitial fluid has a composition similar to ECF except for lower protein content. Glomerular filtration increases to adult levels by 2 years of age. The low glomerular filtration rate (GFR) is due to low systemic arterial pressure, high renal vascular resistance, low ultrafiltration pressure, and decreased capillary surface area for filtration. The concentrating ability of renal tubules is low at birth because of hypotonicity of renal medulla. The tubular mechanisms for acids are also poorly developed at birth and increases to adult levels by 12–18 months.

Tonicity is the measure of effective osmolality. Solutes which have restricted permeability like sodium remain in ECF compartment and create an osmotic pressure gradient and drive water movement from intracellular to extracellular compartment. Solutes like dextrose, urea, etc. which are freely permeable across cell membranes, distribute equally between ECF and intracellular fluid (ICF) compartment and do not create osmotic pressure gradient. Tonicity of a fluid primarily depends on the electrolyte content. Hence both sodium and dextrose contribute to osmolality of a fluid, while it is sodium which mainly contributes to tonicity of a fluid. Fluids with a tonicity (Na + K) of less than approximately 145–150 mEq/L are considered as hypotonic.

There is a higher risk of developing hospital-acquired hyponatremia in patients receiving hypotonic fluids. Hyponatremia related to high circulating antidiuretic hormone (ADH) can occur in patients receiving isotonic fluids also. ADH causes absorption of water in the collecting duct and excretion of concentrated urine with urine osmolality >100 mOsm/L. In case of syndrome of inappropriate antidiuretic hormone (SIADH), if ECF is expanded with isotonic fluids, sodium is excreted in the urine and free water retained, leading to hyponatremia. Hence volume of fluid administered needs to be restricted in conditions associated with SIADH.

Endothelial glycocalyx is an integral part of vascular barrier. The glycocalyx interacts with plasma components like albumin to form endothelial surface layer. This layer separates circulating blood and endothelium of blood vessels and regulates endothelial permeability. It also has important role in leukocyte diapedesis and inhibition of intravascular thrombosis. In conditions such as sepsis and trauma this layer is disrupted leading to altered endothelial permeability and favors edema formation.

The important hormonal axes contributing to fluid balance and osmolarity maintenance include ADH, renin-angiotensin-aldosterone system, and atrial natriuretic peptide (ANP).

Drug Therapy and Body Water Distributions

Changes in body water have important implications in drug therapy, especially for water-soluble drugs such as aminoglycosides. Preterm babies need higher dose to achieve the same serum concentration as term neonates due to higher total body water, while interval between doses is longer because of immaturity of the neonatal kidney.[6] Drugs usually distribute into the extracellular space, hence larger the extracellular component of fluid higher the dose required to achieve the desired concentration. This is one of the reasons why in critically ill children with capillary leak and increase in ECF higher doses of drugs are recommended.

Intravenous Fluids: Indications and Choice

Inappropriate fluid prescription and administration can lead to local and systemic side effects such as infection, electrolyte imbalance, fluid overload, etc. Hence, it is of paramount importance that fluids are used judiciously in clinical practice. IV fluids are used in clinical practice mainly for three indications: resuscitation, maintenance, and replacement. Impact of fluid administration as drug diluent or to preserve catheter patency, i.e., fluid creep, should also be taken into account. In critically ill children on multiple infusions, the impact of fluid creep may be considerable on the net fluid balance. Just like for antibiotics, the four Ds (drug, dose, duration, de-escalation) of fluid therapy need to be considered in all situations.[7]

Fluids are categorized into crystalloids and colloids. Crystalloids are the most commonly used IV fluids in clinical practice. The various fluids available and their compositions are shown in **Table 1**. Crystalloids are solutions of ions that are capable of passing through semipermeable membranes.

Balanced and Unbalanced Crystalloids

Crystalloids are considered as the fluids of first choice in clinical practice. Crystalloids that are commonly used for fluid resuscitation are normal saline (NS) and balanced salt solutions. In 0.9% NS, the concentration of sodium and chloride are present in equal concentrations and the strong ion difference is zero. As it contains supraphysiological amount of chloride (154 mEq/L), large volume administration can cause hyperchloremic metabolic acidosis. Studies have shown that high renal tubular chloride concentration leads to afferent vasoconstriction leading to decreased renal blood flow and decreased GFR.[8-10]

Balanced crystalloids like plasmalyte or Ringer's lactate (RL) are buffered by anions other than chloride like lactate, acetate, etc. These metabolizable anions are incorporated to substitute bicarbonate with the aim to achieve a fluid which more closely resembles the constituents of plasma. The chloride content of balanced solutions, more closely approximate plasma.[11] NS was found to cause greater increase in interstitial volume than plasmalyte.[12]

TABLE 1: Composition of commonly used intravenous fluids.

Solutions	*Na^+ (mEq/L)*	*K^+ (mEq/L)*	*Cl^- (mEq/L)*	*Other anions (mEq/L)*	*Osmolarity (mOsm/L)*
Crystalloids					
• *Unbalanced:*					
– NaCl 0.9%	154	0	154	–	308
– NaCl 3%	510	0	510	–	1026
– NaCl 7.5%	1275	0	1275	–	2395
• *Balanced:*					
– Lactate Ringer	130	4	108	Lactate (27.6)	277
– Acetate Ringer	132	4	110	Acetate (29)	
– Acetate Gluconate (Plasmalyle®)	140	5	98	Acetate (27) Gluconate (23)	294
– Acetate Malate (Isofundin®)	145	4	127	Acetate (24) Malate (5)	304
Colloids					
• *Unbalanced:*					
– Hydroxyethylstarch (Voluven®)	154	o	154	–	308
– Albumin	154	0	154	–	308
• *Balanced:*					
– Hydroxyethylstarch (Tetraspan®)	140	4	118	Acetate (24) Malate (5)	297
– Hydroxyethylstarch (Hextend®)	143	3	124	–	307
– Gelatins 4% (Plasmion®)	154	0	120	–	307
– Gelatins 3% (Gelofusin®)	150	0	100	–	284

Lactate-containing fluid should be avoided in patients with severe liver dysfunction and in patients with suspected inborn errors of metabolism. Acetate is metabolized via extrahepatic pathways, and its use in hemodialysis solutions has been associated with myocardial dysfunction.[13]

The evidence against NS remains inconclusive. The possible risk associated with its use is not balanced by much therapeutic advantage. Among crystalloids, balanced fluids may be preferred over NS, especially in situations where large volume resuscitation is needed as they limit acid-base alterations and chloride load.

Normal saline is specifically indicated in few clinical scenarios. In patients with acute central nervous system events, 0.9% saline is preferred due to its higher tonicity and higher osmolality (308 mOsm/L) when compared to traditional balanced solutions like RL. For patients with metabolic alkalosis due to upper gastrointestinal (GI) disease, chronic vomiting or gastric suction NS is an appropriate fluid of choice.

Colloids

Colloids are macromolecules, which are expected to cause a greater degree of volume expansion than crystalloids. It is expected that 3 liters of isotonic crystalloid causes the same volume expansion as 1 liter of colloid. But high-quality blinded randomized controlled trials (RCTs) comparing the safety and efficacy of colloids and crystalloids have shown only modest volume-sparing effect. Recent studies have shown that ratio of colloid to saline needed to achieve hemodynamic stability is 1:1.6 to 1:1.2.[14] Synthetic colloids have its limitations due to its adverse impact on coagulation, increased risk of allergy, and renal injury. Gelatin, hexa starch, and albumin are the commonly used colloids. Colloids are still recommended for use in certain subgroup of patients with severe dengue.

Albumin

Albumin is a natural colloid. It accounts for 50% of plasma protein content. It is the main determinant of oncotic pressure, playing a crucial role in microvascular fluid dynamics. It remains unclear whether albumin confers benefit or risk in terms of mortality and renal function. Given the high cost of albumin and doubtful benefit it should not be generally considered the first choice for fluid replacement unless there is a specific indication. In certain subset of patients like septic shock with severe capillary leak, patients with pre-existing hypoalbuminemia requiring large volume fluid resuscitation or in patients with spontaneous bacterial peritonitis, it may have a role. 20% albumin is essentially a redistribution fluid while 5% albumin is used as resuscitation fluid. In patients with advanced hepatic failure, albumin-containing fluids and albumin dialysis can be beneficial. In patients with traumatic brain injury, use of albumin has been found to be associated with increased mortality.[15]

Hexa Starch

It has been found to be associated with increased incidence of acute kidney injury (AKI) and need for kidney replacement therapy (KRT) in certain patient population. It is currently not a preferred fluid for use in sick children.[16]

Gelatin

Gelatin is a synthetic colloid with relatively short half-life of approximately 2–3 hours. Urea-linked gelatin is associated with higher incidence of allergic reaction than modified fluid gelatin. The evidence on gelatin remains insufficient. Synthetic colloids are not recommended for resuscitation of patients with septic shock.

Dextran

Dextran may interfere with cross matching. There is lack of evidence to support its use in critically ill children.

MAINTENANCE FLUIDS

Whenever possible, enteral route, if available, should be used to provide fluids and nutrition. Routine maintenance fluids do not contain proteins, lipids, vitamins, or minerals. A child on IV fluid will lose 0.5% of body weight daily as routine maintenance fluids provide only 20% of the daily requirement of calories. The goals of maintenance fluids are to prevent dehydration, protein breakdown, ketosis, and electrolyte imbalance.[17] In patients who are prescribed IV fluids the following needs to be documented:

- Indication for fluid administration
- Clinical assessment of fluid status
- Type and volume of fluid
- Daily weight
- Intake output chart (hourly recording with 12 hours subtotal and 24 hours total)
- 24 hours fluid overload % [fluid in – fluid out (liters) × 100/weight (kg)]
- Blood glucose and serum electrolytes at the start of IV fluids and at least once everyday

Type of Fluid

Historically children have been prescribed hypotonic IV fluids based on electrolyte composition of human and animal milk. Administration of hypotonic IV fluids was found to be associated with hospital-acquired hyponatremia often leading to hyponatremic encephalopathy. Children are more prone to develop symptomatic hyponatremia because of their large brain/skull ratio.

Isotonic crystalloids with sodium content between 131 and 154 mEq/L is used for initial maintenance with appropriate KCL and dextrose.[18] Subsequent fluid composition should depend on blood glucose and serum electrolyte concentrations. 5% dextrose and 20 mEq/L of potassium are often added to maintenance fluids, if there is no risk

TABLE 2: Formulas for calculating maintenance fluid requirements.[18]

Holliday-Segar formula		4-2-1 formula	
Weight	**Daily**	**Weight**	**Hourly**
<10 kg	100 mL/kg/day	<10 kg	4 mL/kg/h
10–20 kg	1,000 mL + 50 mL/kg/day for every kg above 10 kg	10–20 kg	40 mL + 2 mL/kg/h for every kg above 10 kg
>20 kg	1,500 mL + 20 mL/kg/day for every kg above 20 kg	>20 kg	60 mL + 1 mL/kg/h for every kg >20 kg
Example for 25 kg child	100 × 10 + 50 × 10 + 20 × 5 = 1,600 mL/24 h	Example for 25 kg child	4 × 10 + 2 × 10 + 1 × 5 = 65 mL/h

for hyperkalemia. Dextrose normal saline (DNS), NS, and plasmalyte are the commonly used maintenance fluids with appropriately added potassium and dextrose. Children with severe acute malnutrition (SAM) are unable to handle extra sodium; hence, isolyte P is the recommended IV fluid in this subgroup of patients.

Dose

Maintenance fluid is the fluid required to replenish the anticipated loss from basal metabolism. Holliday-Segar formula is used to calculate daily fluid requirement and 4-2-1 formula is used to calculate hourly fluid requirement in children **(Table 2)**.[18]

Critically ill children in intensive care unit (ICU) and children with meningitis and pneumonia are usually started on two-thirds maintenance. In normal health, 60% of fluid is passed as urine and 35% is lost through lungs and skin. Children in ICU are in a controlled environment and often on humidified oxygen, which decreases the respiratory and dermal loss of fluid. Two-thirds maintenance in a ventilated child is like full maintenance in otherwise normal child. Critical illnesses such as meningitis, pneumonia, etc. are often associated with nonosmotic secretion of ADH, leading to decrease in urine output. Hence, critically ill children are initially started on two-thirds maintenance and fluid titrated up or down depending on clinical condition and fluid status.

Duration

It depends on the indication of IV fluid. Child should be clinically reassessed and readiness to use enteral route should be assessed periodically. Enteral route should be used as early as possible.

If patients on isotonic fluids develop hyponatremia look for other sources of free water administration like as drug vehicles. Presence of SIADH or adrenal insufficiency can also cause hyponatremia. In case of occurrence of hypernatremia look for renal and extrarenal water loss. Children with SAM can also develop hypernatremia while on isotonic fluids as they are unable to handle extra sodium.

RESUSCITATION FLUIDS

Fluid administration is one of the most important measures in the hemodynamic resuscitation of a sick child. Inadequate fluid resuscitation and fluid overload both are associated with increased incidence of multiorgan dysfunction and adverse outcome. Positive fluid balance is not always iatrogenic. It is often a marker of disease severity. Capillary endotheliopathy in severe diseases causes increased capillary permeability, leading to positive fluid balance. Positive fluid balance is associated with delayed wound healing, increased extravascular lung water, decreased gut motility, ascites, and circulatory overload. It can also cause tense ascites causing intra-abdominal hypertension. This in turn may lead to decreased splanchnic and renal perfusion, decreased venous return, and decreased cardiac output. A restrictive continuous fluid administration alongside cautious bolus administration to achieve hemodynamic targets is considered the preferred mode of resuscitation.

SEPTIC SHOCK

The cause of shock in sepsis is multifactorial. Capillary endotheliopathy, abnormal vasodilatation, cardiac dysfunction, and associated endocrine abnormalities may all contribute to shock. Capillary endothelial glycocalyx contributes to 20% of intravascular volume and is responsible for maintaining vascular barrier, hemostasis, prevention of cell adhesion to endothelium, and transmission of shear stress. Shedding of glycocalyx occurs in the presence of cytokines, endotoxin, hyperglycemia, and reactive oxygen species. All these factors play a role in capillary endotheliopathy seen in critically ill children. Volume loading in normal health and in surgical patients is not found to be associated with glycocalyx shedding. In septic shock patients, amount of glycocalyx shedding was found to be proportional to volume of fluid given. Both hypoperfusion and fluid overload are equally deleterious **(Fig. 1)**. Hence, meticulous monitoring and careful fluid titration to achieve hemodynamic targets with a restrictive fluid administration protocol are preferred.

Type of Fluid

An ideal resuscitation fluid is one which causes predictable and sustained rise in intravascular volume, has composition similar to ECF, is completely metabolized and excreted, and has no systemic or metabolic side effects. Unfortunately, there is no such ideal fluid.

Isotonic crystalloids are the fluid of choice for initial resuscitation. NS, RL, and plasmalyte are the commonly used crystalloids. RL should be avoided in patients with hepatic failure as lactate may not be metabolized and contribute to lactate pool. RL should also be avoided in patients with inborn errors of metabolism associated with lactic acidosis. Large volume resuscitation with NS can cause hyperchloremic metabolic acidosis. Hyperchloremia causes renal vasoconstriction and may increase the need for KRT. Balanced crystalloid use in critically ill adult patients has shown to be associated with decreased incidence of major kidney events on day 30 (MAKE30). Hence balanced crystalloids are the preferred crystalloids for resuscitation.

Dextrose-containing fluids should not be used for resuscitation as it may lead to hyperglycemia. Hyperglycemia leads to glycosuria and delay in correction of shock. Glucose will contribute to lactate pool and worsen the metabolic acidosis in poor perfusion states. Hyperglycemia also favors bacterial growth and causes damage to capillary endothelium.

Albumin is the main determinant of plasma oncotic pressure. It also performs other functions such as stabilization of glycocalyx, antioxidant effects, transport of molecules, immunomodulation, and positive inotropic effects. These functions may be relevant for septic patients. 5% albumin can be used as resuscitation fluid. High cost and absence of robust scientific data showing mortality benefit for albumin are the limiting factors. The subgroup analysis of septic patients (planned a-priori) in SAFE (Saline versus Albumin Fluid Evaluation) trial[19] showed an adjusted odds ratio for death of 0.71 (95% CI: 0.52, 0.97, $p=0.03$) for albumin. The ALBIOS (Albumin Italian Outcome Sepsis) trial[20] which compared administration of albumin to crystalloids showed no difference in outcomes in the study population as a whole. However, patients with septic shock who were randomized to receive albumin had higher 90-day survival rates (6.3% $p=0.04$). Hence 5% albumin may be used as a resuscitation fluid especially in cases where large volume crystalloid resuscitation is needed.

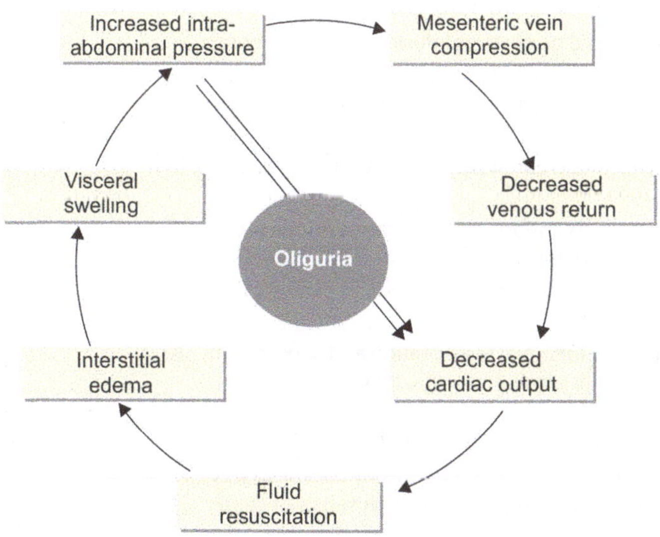

Fig. 1: Vicious cycle of fluid resuscitation and organ injury.

Synthetic colloids such as hexa starch, gelatin, and dextran are usually not used as resuscitation fluids especially in septic shock. These have been found to interfere with coagulation and have increased risk of allergy. Synthetic colloids are also associated with increased need for KRT and increased risk of mortality.

Dose and Duration

Sepsis is a dynamic disease with varying fluid needs during various stages of the disease. The ROSE conceptual model summarizes a dynamic approach to fluid therapy (Resuscitation, Optimization, Stabilization, and Evacuation) as shown in **Table 3.**[21,22]

Resuscitation Phase

This phase focuses on patient rescue and administration of early and appropriate fluid for restoration of circulating blood volume. Aim of this phase is rapid correction of shock with achievement of adequate perfusion pressures. This phase usually lasts for minutes. During this phase, the patient should be resuscitated with 20 mL/kg crystalloid (NS, plasmalyte, or RL) boluses. Surviving sepsis campaign guidelines 2020, now recommends administration of 20 mL/kg boluses (up to 60 mL/kg may be given in the first hour) as fast IV infusion in centers with access to critical care.[23] Fluid boluses may be repeated if child continues to be hypotensive without features of fluid overload. In centers without access to critical care, it is preferable to administer fluids more slowly as 10–20 mL/kg boluses over 20–30 minutes (up to 40 mL/kg in an hour). As rapid fluid administration in this setting may lead to development of fluid overload and adverse outcome especially in children with coexisting comorbidities such as anemia and malnutrition. In hypotensive children in

TABLE 3: ROSE concept of fluid therapy in shock.

	Resuscitation phase	*Optimization phase*	*Stabilization phase*	*Evacuation phase*
Time frame	Minutes	Hours	Days	Days to weeks
Clinical presentation	Hypotensive shock	Unstable shock	Stable	Shock recovery/risk of GIPS
Fluid therapy	Fluid boluses guided by indices of fluid responsiveness	Fluid challenges guided by static, dynamic and hemodynamic parameters	• Maintenance/replacement • Oral therapy preferred	Reversal of fluid balance either spontaneous or active
Fluid balance	Positive	Neutral	Neutral to negative	Negative
Result of treatment	Patient salvage	Organ rescue	Organ support	Organ recovery

low-resource settings, World Health Organization (WHO) recommends 10–20 mL/kg of isotonic crystalloid over 30–60 minutes, followed by an additional 10 mL/kg over 30 minutes if condition has not improved and signs of fluid overload, cardiac failure, or neurologic deterioration have not developed.[24]

Many recent studies (ProCESS, ARISE, ProMISE) have showed no improvement in outcome with early goal-directed therapy,[25-27] while some studies have pointed toward harm of protocolized treatment for all cases of septic shock.[28,29] Hence, it would be prudent to individualize fluid administration in every patient based on fluid needs, physiological status, and patient's premorbid condition.

Many centers now prefer to administer bolus by rapid infusion without a push pull method of administration as it is believed to cause shear pressure on the capillary endothelium increasing capillary leak and is found to be associated with increased need for mechanical ventilation. Monitor and document heart rate, respiratory rate, blood pressure, basal crepitations, and liver size after every bolus to look for signs of improvement and signs of fluid overload. Blood sugar, electrolytes, organ function, and coagulation profile should be checked in all sick children. Sample for blood culture should be taken and the first dose of appropriate antibiotic must be given in the first hour of admission itself if septic shock is suspected. Various fluid resuscitation guidelines with level of evidences are shown in **Table 4**.

Optimization Phase

Once the blood pressure picks up, the patient enters the optimization phase. This phase focuses on *organ rescue* and avoidance of fluid overload. This phase lasts for hours. Appropriate vasoactive agents are started and instead of fluid boluses careful fluid challenges are given. In fluid challenges, smaller volumes of fluid are given over a longer period of time.[22] Aim is to achieve a neutral fluid balance. Echo,

TABLE 4: Fluid resuscitation recommendations with grades of evidence.

Guidelines	*Recommendations*	*Grade of evidence*
ACCM guidelines pediatric and neonatal septic shock. Davis, AL et al. 2017[32]	Fluid resuscitation with 20 mL/kg boluses (up to 40–60 mL/kg may be needed in 1st hour)	1C
	Isotonic crystalloid or 5% albumin may be used for resuscitation	1C
	10% dextrose-containing isotonic intravenous solution can be run at maintenance fluid rate	1C
	Beyond 1st hour Crystalloids are fluid of first choice for those with Hb >10 g/dL. Those with Hb < 10 g/dL PRC transfusion may be given. FFP if used for correction of prolonged INR should be given as infusion and not as bolus	1C
	Following shock resuscitation, diuretics/peritoneal dialysis/high flux CKRT can be used to remove fluid in patients who are 10% fluid overloaded and unable to maintain fluid balance with native urine output/extrarenal losses	1C
Surviving sepsis campaign international guidelines for management of sepsis and septic shock. Rhodes A, et al. 2017[33]	Fluid challenge technique to be applied where fluid administration is continued as long as hemodynamic factors continue to improve	1B
	Crystalloids are the fluid of choice for initial resuscitation and subsequent intravascular volume replacement in patients with sepsis and septic shock	1B
	Either balanced crystalloids or saline can be used for fluid resuscitation of patients with sepsis or septic shock	2C
	Albumin in addition to crystalloids can be used for initial resuscitation and subsequent intravascular volume replacement in patients with sepsis and septic shock when patients require substantial amounts of crystalloids	2C
	Hydroxyethyl starches (HESs) should not be used for intravascular volume replacement in patients with sepsis or septic shock	1A
	Crystalloids to be used over gelatins when resuscitating patients with sepsis or septic shock	2C
Pediatric ARDS: Consensus Recommendations from the Pediatric Acute Lung Injury Consensus Conference.[34]	Pediatric patients with PARDS should receive total fluids to maintain adequate intravascular volume, end-organ perfusion and optimal delivery of oxygen	*Strong agreement*
	After initial fluid resuscitation and stabilization, goal-directed fluid management is recommended. Fluid balance should be monitored and titrated to maintain adequate intravascular volume while aiming to prevent positive fluid balance	*Strong agreement*
European Guideline on Management of Major Bleeding and Coagulopathy following Trauma. Rossaint et al., 2016[35]	Fluid therapy using isotonic crystalloid solutions to be initiated in the hypotensive bleeding trauma patient	1A
	Excessive use of 0.9% NaCl solution be avoided	2C
	Hypotonic solutions such as Ringer's lactate to be avoided in patients with severe head trauma	IC
	Use of colloids to be restricted due to adverse effects on hemostasis	2C

Contd...

Contd...

Guidelines	Recommendations	Grade of evidence
AKI in the perioperative period and in ICU: French expert recommendations. Ichai C et al. 2016[36]	To avoid administering HES in the ICU	1B
	Crystalloid to be preferred over colloid for fluid loading	2A
	Balanced solutions to be preferred in case of large volume loading	2A
	After hemodynamic stabilization, avoid fluid overload in the ICU	2A
Surviving sepsis campaign international guidelines for the management of septic shock and sepsis-associated organ dysfunction in children. Weiss SL, 2020[23]	In healthcare systems with availability of intensive care, administer up to 40–60 mL/kg in bolus fluid (10–20 mL/kg per bolus) over the first hour, titrated to clinical markers of cardiac output and discontinued if signs of fluid overload develop	Weak recommendation, low quality of evidence
	In healthcare systems with no availability of intensive care and in the *absence of hypotension*, bolus fluid administration to be avoided while starting maintenance fluids	Strong recommendation, high quality of evidence
	In healthcare systems with no availability of intensive care, if *hypotension* is present, administering up to 40 mL/kg in bolus fluid (10–20 mL/kg per bolus) over the first hour with titration to clinical markers of cardiac output is suggested and discontinued if signs of fluid overload develop	Weak recommendation, low quality of evidence
	Crystalloids, rather than albumin, are preferred for the initial resuscitation of children with septic shock or other sepsis-associated organ dysfunction	Weak recommendation, moderate quality of evidence
	Starches are not recommended in the acute resuscitation of children with septic shock or other sepsis-associated organ dysfunction	Strong recommendation, moderate quality of evidence

(ACCM: American College of Critical Care Medicine; AKI: acute kidney injury; CKRT: continuous kidney replacement therapy; FFP: fresh frozen plasma; INR: international normalized ratio; PARDS: pediatric acute respiratory distress syndrome; PRC: packed red cell)

USG, and central venous oxygen saturation ($ScvO_2$) help in titrating fluids.

During this phase, the need for further fluid is determined by static hemodynamic parameters such as heart rate, blood pressure, central venous pressure (CVP), and dynamic hemodynamic measures like, inferior vena cava (IVC) variability, passive leg raising (PLR) test, pulse pressure variability (PPV), and peak aortic flow velocity variations. Dynamic hemodynamic parameters are preferred over static hemodynamic parameters in deciding the need for additional fluids. Some of the commonly used methods for predicting fluid responsiveness include:

- *Pulse pressure variability:* PPV has 88% sensitivity and 89% specificity in predicting fluid responsiveness at a median threshold of 12%. It is unreliable in spontaneously breathing patients, arrhythmia, increased intra-abdominal pressure (false positive), and in patients on small tidal volume ventilation and high respiratory rates (false negative).
- *Respiratory variability of IVC and superior vena cava (SVC) diameter:* It has a low sensitivity (76%) and specificity (86%) with a median threshold of 12%. It cannot be used in spontaneously breathing patients and in those on low tidal volume/reduced compliance ventilation. In patients with spontaneous breathing only respiratory variation of high amplitude indicates fluid responsiveness.
- *Passive leg raising test:* It is useful in low tidal volume ventilation and spontaneously breathing patients also. It is in fact a reversible preload challenge without giving any extra fluid. A PLR-induced increase in cardiac output > 10% predicts fluid responsiveness. It has a pooled sensitivity of 85% and specificity of 91%.
- *End-expiratory occlusion test:* A 15-second end-expiratory hold can be done in ventilated patients to predict fluid responsiveness. An increase in cardiac output by 5% predicts fluid responsiveness. It can also be used in patients with acute respiratory distress syndrome (ARDS).

Stabilization Phase

This phase focuses on *organ support*. This is the phase of late conservative fluid management, which lasts for days. Aim is to provide adequate fluid and electrolyte and maintain a zero or negative fluid balance. During this phase, IV fluids if possible are tapered and stopped and oral/RT feeds are started. Blood gas and USG help in optimizing fluid administration.

Evacuation Phase

This is the *organ recovery* phase. It is also known as the de-escalation phase. Most children will achieve diuresis of their own in this phase. Some may require active late goal-directed fluid removal with the help of diuretics or ultrafiltration to attain a negative fluid balance. Use of diuretics in fluid overloaded patients has shown to recruit microcirculation and lead to improved oxygen extraction.

Three-hit Model of Sepsis (Flowchart 1)

Ebb phase: This is the initial phase following an insult-like sepsis or burns. This is the critical life-threatening phase of severe circulatory shock either due to strong vasodilatation leading to fall in mean arterial pressure, sepsis-induced cardiomyopathy, or hypovolemia. This is the first hit of sepsis leading to microcirculatory impairment.[22]

Flowchart 1: Three-hit model of shock and fluid resuscitation.

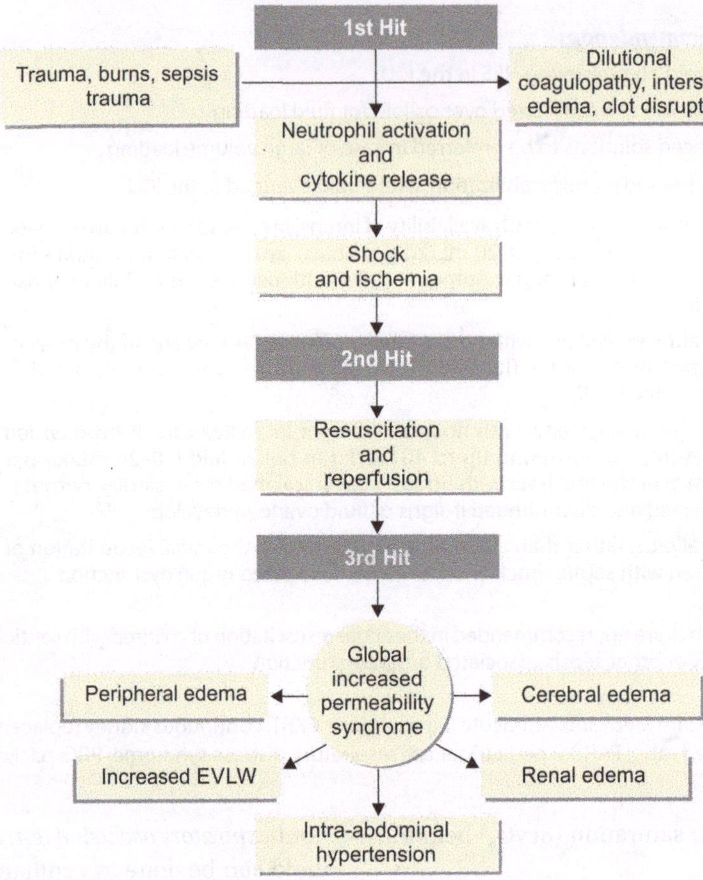

(EVLW: extravascular lung water)

Second hit: This is the phase of ischemia reperfusion which occurs after the initial ischemic phase of shock. In this phase as reperfusion of ischemic region occurs, there is release of cytokines and free radicals which may damage the endothelium cause capillary leak and organ injury. In this phase reperfusion injuries can occur.

Flow phase: Following appropriate fluid, antibiotics, and source control there is usually resolution of shock and reestablishment of organ perfusion. This is known as the flow phase.

Global increased permeability syndrome (GIPS): Some patients do not proceed to the flow phase and instead remain in the increased permeability state with unresolved shock and positive fluid balance. This leads to increased interstitial edema leading to swelling of visceral organs leading to cerebral edema, intestinal edema causing decreased gut motility, decreased wound healing, intra-abdominal hypertension, decreased venous return, and decreased cardiac output. This is known as the *third hit* of sepsis. In this phase, active de-escalation may have an important role by preventing further fluid overload and worsening of organ function. Use of 20% albumin aiming for a target serum albumin of 3 g/dL with diuretics, combined with other measures to decrease intra-abdominal pressure has been suggested as treatment options in this phase. Goal-directed fluid removal with ultrafiltration may have role in some patients.[30,31]

Risk of hypoperfusion/fourth hit: Too much of fluid removal can cause organ hypoperfusion leading to worsening of organ functions. This is considered as the fourth hit of sepsis. Hence, cautious and appropriate fluid administration and removal is of paramount importance in the management of critically ill children.

REPLACEMENT FLUID

Ongoing losses should be replaced to prevent fluid and electrolyte imbalances **(Table 5)**. NS with added potassium can be used to replace fluid losses from the body.[37] The electrolyte composition should be subsequently altered according to serum concentrations. In patients with renal failure serum potassium level should be measured before adding potassium in replacement fluid.

ACUTE DIARRHEAL DISEASE

In patients with acute diarrheal disease need for fluid resuscitation depends on the hydration status. Sensorium, skin turgor, thirst, presence or absence of tears, sunken eyes, and oral mucosa help one to assess the hydration status.[24]

TABLE 5: Electrolyte composition of various body fluids.

Site	*Composition*
Vomiting or nasogastric (NG) tube loss	*Sodium:* 20–60 mEq/L *Potassium:* 14 mEq/L *Chloride:* 140 mmol/L H^+: 50–80 mmol/L
Biliary drainage	*Sodium:* 145 mEq/L *Potassium:* 5 mEq/L *Chloride:* 105 mmol/L HCO_3: 30 mmol/L
Diarrhea	*Sodium:* 30–140 mEq/L *Potassium:* 30–70 mEq/L HCO_3: 20–80 mmol/L
Pancreatic drain or fistula	*Sodium:* 125–138 mEq/L *Potassium:* 8 mEq/L *Chloride:* 56 mmol/L HCO_3: 85 mmol/L
Jejunal stoma or fistula	*Sodium:* 140 mEq/L *Potassium:* 5 mEq/L *Chloride:* 135 mmol/L HCO_3: 8 mmol/L
Polyuria	Sodium and potassium concentrations are very variable

No Dehydration (Plan A)

(Active child without any features of dehydration)

Estimated fluid deficit is <5% of body weight. ORS is given at 10 mL/kg/per purge. Mothers should be encouraged to continue breastfeeding and give home available fluids and food.

Some Dehydration (Plan B)

(Child with any two or more of the following: Restless/irritable, sunken eyes, increased thirst, skin pinch goes back slowly)

Estimated fluid deficit is 5-10% of body weight. ORS is given in sips at 75 mL/kg over 4 hours. Mothers of young infants should be advised to continue breastfeeding during rehydration whenever child demands. If a child is not on breastfeed, then formula feed or plain water 100-200 mL should be given during some dehydration correction. This is mainly required when noncholera diarrhea is treated with ORS in a young infant <6 months of age. These children are at risk of developing hypernatremia, if ORS alone is given for rehydration without breast milk. Assess hydration status at the end of 4 hours, if child is better, he/she can be shifted to plan A. If the child continues to have signs of dehydration, choose plan B again.

Severe Dehydration (Plan C)

(Child with diarrhea with any two or more of the following: lethargic/unconscious, sunken eyes, drinks poorly, or not able to drink, skin pinch goes back very slowly >2 seconds)

In severe dehydration, estimated fluid deficit is >10% body weight. Start IV fluid immediately according to the treatment plan showed in **Table 6**. RL is the preferred fluid for rehydration. If RL is not available 0.9%, then NS may be given. If IV access is not available, ORS may be given through nasogastric (NG) tube at a rate of 20 mL/kg/h. All children should start receiving ORS at 5 mL/kg/h, once they can drink. This provides additional base and potassium, which may not be adequately supplied by the IV fluid. Reassess the child after completion of plan C and further treatment may be continued according the dehydration status (plan A, B, or C).

TABLE 6: Treatment of severe dehydration (plan C).

Age	*First 30 mL/kg in*	*Next 70 mL/kg in*
<12 months of age	1 hour*	5 hour
12 months to 5 years	30 minutes*	2½ hour

*Repeat once if radial pulse weak, not detectable or patient continues to be hypotensive.

CHILDREN WITH SEVERE ACUTE MALNUTRITION

Children with SAM have limited glucose reserve and high total body sodium. The compromised physiological state makes it difficult for these children to handle large volumes of fluid. Hence, this subgroup of patients needs to be monitored meticulously and dehydration states corrected slowly over longer period of time. Whenever feasible use enteral route for rehydration.[24]

Diarrhea in Children with Severe Acute Malnutrition

The assessment of dehydration is extremely difficult in children with SAM. Malnutrition itself can cause delayed skin turgor due to loss of subcutaneous fat, eyes may be dry due to vitamin deficiency or atrophy of lacrimal glands, and oral mucosa may be dry due to mouth breathing or atrophy of salivary glands. The best way to assess the hydration status of these children is periodic monitoring of weight and targeting attainment of pre-diarrheal weight. ORS should be prescribed and not freely available in the unit. The diagnosis of dehydration is often provisional in children with SAM. Response to treatment is the best way to confirm diagnosis.

In case of dehydration, ReSoMaL or half strength ORS should be used for rehydration. Half strength ORS is prepared by diluting 1 liter packet of WHO ORS in 2 liter of water and adding 50 g of sucrose and 45 mL of potassium chloride. ReSoMaL contains approximately 45 mEq/L of sodium, 40 mEq/L of potassium, and 3 mmol/L of magnesium.

Rehydration is started at 5 mL/kg/30 minutes of ReSoMal for first 2 hours. Treatment has to proceed according to changes in weight and clinical status during rehydration.

- If there is weight gain with improvement in vitals, continue rehydration till prediarrheal weight is attained. It may take 8-10 hours to correct dehydration.

- If the weight remains same, with no improvement in vitals after 1 hour of resuscitation, increase the fluid rate by 5 mL/kg/h.
- If there is weight loss, increase the fluid rate by 10 mL/kg/h.

Closely monitor for signs of fluid overload. Increase in weight with no improvement in vitals often indicates shock due to sepsis rather than dehydration. In such children, rehydration should be stopped and appropriates actions taken to treat septic shock. Continue giving 2 hourly feed alternating with ORS during rehydration. In situations where enteral route is not feasible, IV correction may be given using either RL with 5% dextrose or ½ DNS at a rate of 15 mL/kg/h.

Septic Shock in Children with SAM

Severe acute malnutrition children with septic shock find it difficult to tolerate large volume resuscitation. The efficacy of inotropes may also be suboptimal. Resuscitate SAM children with glucose containing fluids, 15 mL/kg/h of ½ DNS or RL with 5% dextrose. Closely monitor respiratory rate, heart rate, and liver size every 15 minutes. If at the end of 1 hour, child shows signs of improvement repeat bolus of 15 mL/kg over 1 hour. Sepsis and dehydration often coexist, in that case rehydration can subsequently be continued with 10 mL/kg/h of ReSoMal through NG tube for up to 10 hours. Continue feeding with starter formula 2 hourly, alternating with ORS.

If at the end of 1 hour of fluid bolus, child does not show signs of improvement, start maintenance fluid at 4 mL/kg/h. Arrange for 10 mL/kg fresh whole blood transfusion and administer it slowly over 3 hours. If patient has features of cardiac failure use packed cells for transfusion. Monitor vitals closely. If respiratory rate increases by 5 breaths/min or heart rate by 25 beats/min stop transfusion. Start feeding with F75 (formula containing 75 calories and 0.9-1 g protein per 100 mL). Administer appropriate antibiotic within first hour of admission.

PERIOPERATIVE FLUID MANAGEMENT

The aim of perioperative fluid administration is to maintain effective circulating blood volume and avoid both fluid overload and under hydration.[37] Fasting, bowel preparation, inflammation associated with underlying infection, and hemorrhage may all contribute to fluid deficit in a surgical patient. Fluid gain depends both on the volume of fluid administered and the capacity of kidneys to excrete excessive fluids.[38]

Perioperative fasting time for children should be as short as possible to improve patient comfort and prevent dehydration and ketoacidosis. Optimized fasting and liberal clear fluid until 2 hours often prevent metabolic and hemodynamic derangements after induction of anesthesia. In children undergoing short procedures (<1 hour) with venous access in place, IV fluid therapy is not needed beyond neonatal period if fasting has been short with normal preoperative hydration status. Fasting guidelines for elective surgery is shown in **Table 7**. If child is fasting for more than 6 hours, appropriate fluid should be administered based on degree of dehydration (1% dehydration = 10 mL/kg fluid loss).

TABLE 7: Fasting guidelines for elective surgery.

Fasting guidelines for elective surgery	*Hours*
Clear liquids	2
Breast milk	4
Infant formula	4 (<3 months), 6 (>3 months)
Light meal	6
Nonhuman milk	6

Intraoperative Fluids

Children require fluids during surgery to meet the fluid requirement arising due to perioperative deficits arising due to fasting, GI, renal or cutaneous loss, intraoperative fluid loss, hemorrhage, and third space losses.

For intraoperative maintenance, usually 1–2% glucose is sufficient to avoid hypoglycemia and hyperglycemia.[39,40] Isotonic IV fluids should be used for maintenance except in special situations. Replacement for intraoperative losses should be done with isotonic solutions or blood based on child's hematocrit. Commonly used isotonic crystalloids in the intraoperative period include NS, RL, or balanced solutions like plasmalyte. Balanced crystalloids are preferred when large volume resuscitation is needed due to its limited acid–base alterations and less chloride load. The role of intraoperative colloid use in children is debatable and sparsely studied. Colloids are an option for a massive and acute replacement (albumin, gelatin or hexa starch). Its role in nonemergent conditions is not yet clear.

Third space loss due to sequestration of fluid from vascular space into tissues around the surgical site is roughly estimated as 2 mL/kg/h for superficial surgery, 4–7 mL/kg/h for thoracotomy and 5–10 mL/kg/h for abdominal surgery. The existence of third space loss is a matter of debate. In case of circulatory instability isotonic crystalloids without glucose can be given as 10–20 mL/kg boluses till normalization of hemodynamic parameters. If large volume resuscitation is needed in order to minimize interstitial fluid overloading and hemodilution colloids or blood transfusion may be given, as it is retained in the intravascular volume more when compared to crystalloids.

Intraoperative Blood Transfusion

The requirement of blood transfusion during intraoperative period depends on various factors such as baseline hemoglobin concentration, quantity of blood loss, etc. neonates and children have higher blood per weight, but are less tolerant to blood loss. In a bleeding child the aim should be to maintain normovolemia and minimize swelling, edema, and hemodilution. Initially crystalloid may be used to replace blood loss in a 2:1 ratio of estimated blood loss. In case of rapid blood loss with hemodynamic instability, administering colloids in a 1:1 ratio may be required. Required transfusion volume of packed red blood cells (RBCs) can be calculated as:

Body weight × desired increment in hemoglobin (g/dL) × 5.

Restrictive hemoglobin threshold may be used for hemodynamically stable infants and children (hemoglobin target of 7 g/dL). Optimum hemoglobin threshold for neonates is still evolving (12 g/dL). Ideally red blood cell transfusion if indicated should be single donor, leukocyte depleted, irradiated, and fresh.

Postoperative Fluids

In minor surgery and surgeries which were not complicated with adequate intraoperative fluid administration, postoperative fluid is not required unless there is an inability to tolerate oral fluids. Isotonic fluid with 5% dextrose is recommended for children <6 years of age, while those above 6 years often 2% glucose is enough. If hypovolemia is suspected postoperatively isotonic crystalloids (10–30 mL/kg) or colloid (10 mL/kg) may be used for resuscitation. In children requiring IV fluids for more than 24 hours daily blood glucose and serum electrolytes should be monitored. Avoid using hypotonic fluids. Hyponatremia should be suspected in child who develops headache, nausea, vomiting, irritability, altered level of consciousness, seizures, neurogenic pulmonary edema, and apnea. Sodium levels should be measured and appropriate action taken.

FLUID THERAPY IN CHILDREN WITH ACUTE KIDNEY INJURY

Approximately 30% of children admitted to pediatric ICUs develop AKI. Kidneys are sensitive both to insufficient arterial flow and venous congestion.[40] As the kidneys are encapsulated, venous congestion engorges the kidney leading to intracapsular pressure build up reducing arterial inflow and venous and lymphatic outflow. Reduced venous return triggers a greater degree of kidney damage than reduced arterial flow. Studies have shown that ischemia by clamping of vein causes several fold higher creatinine increase than clamping of renal arteries for the same duration. Hence fluid overload can induce severe and sustained renal damage. Multiple studies have shown that increasing cumulative fluid accumulation or increasing fluid overload percentage (FO%) at the time of initiation of KRT is independently associated with mortality.

$$\text{Fluid overload \%} = \frac{\text{Total fluid in} - \text{Total fluid out (in liters)}}{\text{Admission weight in kg}}$$

Mortality was found to increase from 40% to 60% in children with >10–20% fluid overload at KRT initiation, independent of severity of illness. Exogenous pressure to the kidneys due to obesity and ascites can also compromise renal blood flow. Hence, fluid administration needs to be carefully titrated to meet the hemodynamic endpoints in critically ill children. Both hypoperfusion and fluid overload are deleterious.

Multimodal monitoring must be used to titrate fluids and vasoactive medications. Aims of shock resuscitation should be to attain a capillary filling time < 3 seconds, normal perfusion pressures for age (MAP-CVP), urine output >1 mL/kg/h, central venous oxygen saturation ($ScVO_2$) > 70%, cardiac index of 3.3 to 6.0 L/min/m^2, and systemic vascular resistance index (SVRI) 800–1,200 dyne sec/m^2. Isolated CVP measurement is of limited value, trends of CVP or change in CVP in response to fluids may provide useful information. High CVP should be avoided. Fluid therapy should be withheld in patients with increasing CVP and no significant increase in blood pressure or cardiac output. Need for fluid is better assessed by dynamic hemodynamic parameters like PPV, stroke volume variability, peak aortic flow velocity variation, passive straight leg raising test, etc.

Choice of Fluids

In children with AKI balanced crystalloids are preferred over 0.9% saline for IV fluid therapy. NS contains supraphysiological content of chloride leading to hyperchloremic metabolic acidosis when infused in large quantities.[41] This can lead complications such as coagulopathy, hyperkalemia, and more pronounced interstitial fluid retention. Hyperchloremic metabolic acidosis causes renal vasoconstriction leading to decreased renal blood flow.[42] Hence, chloride restrictive balanced fluids are preferable.

Often albumin is used with the aim of recruiting interstitial fluid, but as most critically ill conditions are associated with endothelial barrier failure it in fact leads to albumin leakage into interstitial space worsening interstitial edema. Hence albumin should be used with caution. Semisynthetic colloids are associated with increased occurrence of kidney dysfunction and mortality in certain clinical settings. It also causes osmotic nephrosis due to accumulation of low-molecular-weight fraction in proximal renal tubules.

Intravenous fluids should be used with caution to avoid volume overload and interstitial congestion. Rate of IV fluid is also likely to impact kidney function. Rapid IV infusion can transiently raise atrial pressure leading to release of ANP. It has been found the ANP rapidly degrades endothelial surface glycocalyx, compromising the barrier function. Hence, rate of IV fluids should be judiciously titrated. Once blood pressure picks up, smaller volume of fluid challenges, over longer period of time, are preferred over large volume boluses when aiming to achieve hemodynamic targets.

Acute kidney injury predisposes to fluid infusion-associated alterations in electrolytes, acid–base status and tonicity as kidneys concentration and diluting capacities are widely compromised. For patients who have developed AKI and are in need of fluids, isotonic balanced crystalloids are the fluids of choice. Always aim to keep patients euvolemic.

In case of presence oliguria or polyuria, replacement fluid should aim to replenish urine output plus insensible loss. Injured kidneys often find it difficult to handle sodium and AKI is often associated with hyperkalemia. Hence, electrolytes should be monitored periodically and alterations in fluid prescription made accordingly.

Diuretic use in the setting of AKI and volume overload has not been shown to be nephrotoxic. Presence of acidosis leads to increased ammonium generation, in an attempt to unload acid via urinary ammonia excretion. In the setting of AKI with reduced urine output this would lead to increased ammonia accumulation leading to activation of complement, endothelin and aldosterone causing intrarenal inflammation and worsening of kidney function. Hence, in such conditions acidosis needs to be corrected. Isotonic bicarbonate solution may be used to correct acidosis and meet fluid need.

Assess the Extent and Depth of the Burn

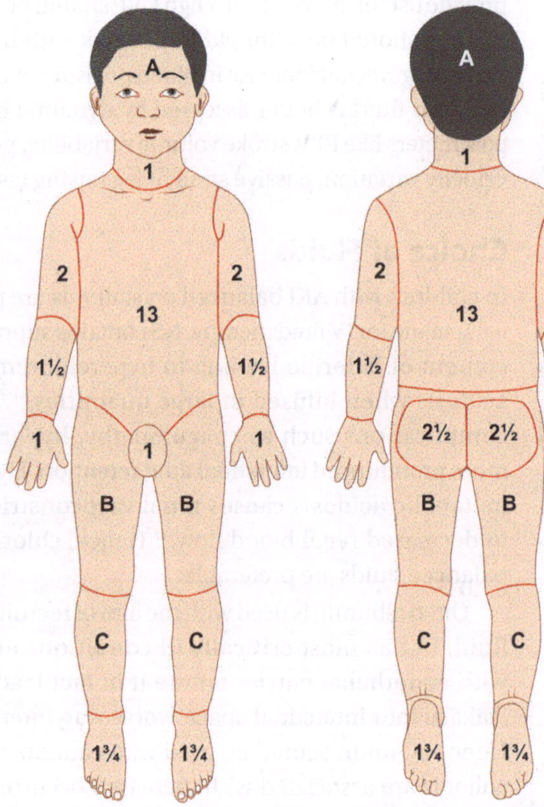

Shade area–indicating depth
Ignore simple erythema

Superficial partial thickness (brisk cap refill, painful, blisters, moist)

Deep partial or full thickness (reduced cap refill, loss sensation, pale mottled, dark, dry)

Region	%
Head	
Neck	
Anterior trunk	
Posterior trunk	
Right arm	
Left arm	
Buttocks	
Genitalia	
Right leg	
Left leg	
Total burn	

Relative Percentage of Body Surface Area Affected by Growth

	Age (years)	0	1	5	10	15	Adult
A	½ of head	9½	8½	6½	5½	4½	3½
B	½ of one thigh	2¾	3¼	4	4½	4½	4¾
C	½ of one leg	2½	2½	2¾	3	3¼	3½

Small Burns: Palm of hand (including fingers together) approximates 1% of body surface area
Palm alone approximates 0.5% BSA

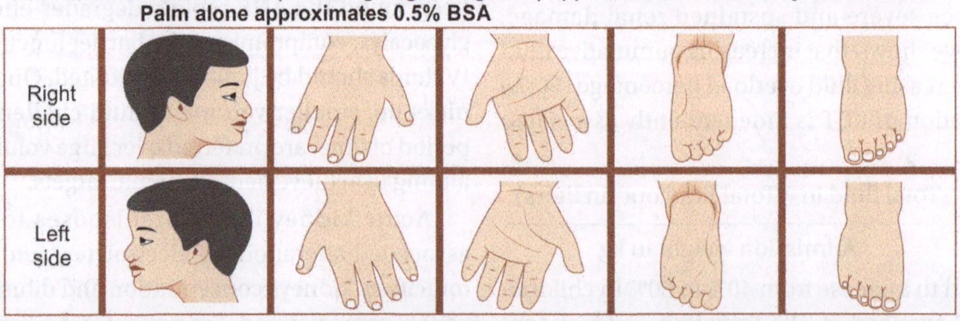

Fig. 2: Lund and Browder chart.

Source: Adapted from Artz CP, JA Moncrief: The Treatment of Burns, 2nd edition. Philadelphia, WB Saunders Company; 1969.

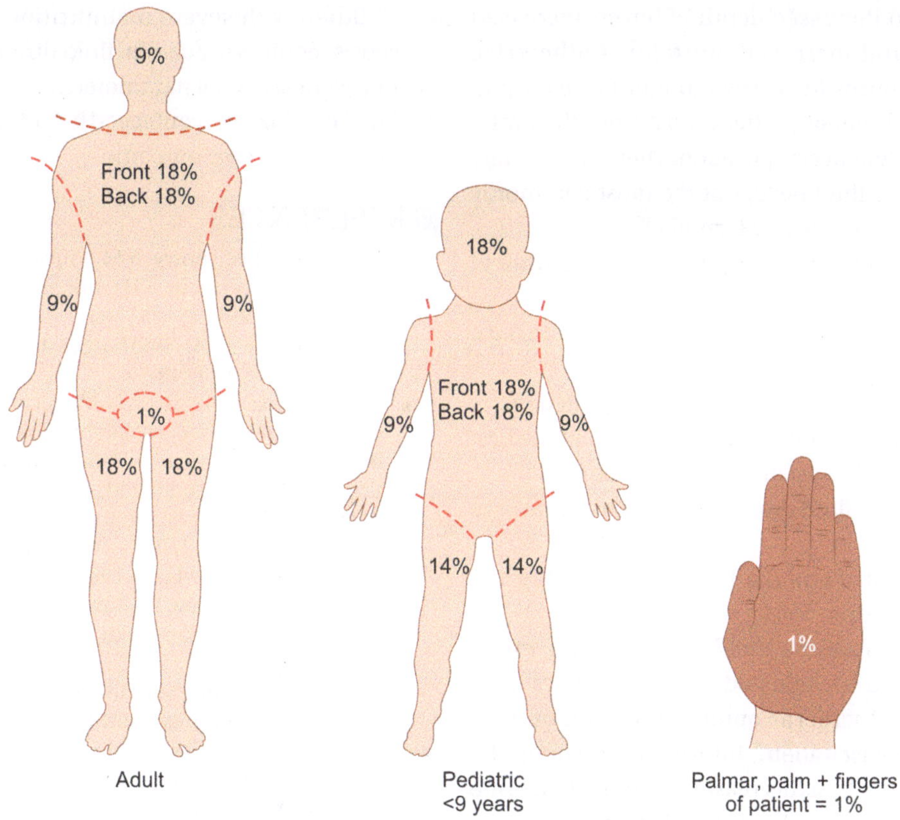

Fig. 3: Rule of nines and palm + fingers method.

Preventing Contrast-induced Nephropathy

In patients with high risk of developing contrast-induced nephropathy use iso-osmolar or low osmolar contrast media NS or isotonic bicarbonate solutions are recommended to be used in adults for prehydration at 1.5 mL/kg/h for 12 hours before and 12 hours after procedure targeting a urine output of more than 150 mL/h. In emergency situations, 3 mL/kg/h may be given for 1 hour before and 6 hours after procedure.

BURNS

Burns not only cause severe local injury, it also causes systemic side effects due to release of inflammatory and vasoactive substances such as cytokines, histamine, prostaglandin, etc. This causes increased capillary permeability, which in turn leads to hypovolemia and hypotension due to fluid shift. These effects usually peak at 6–8 hours. Hence, children with burns should be closely monitored for development of hypoperfusion and shock during the first 24 hours.[43] Aim is to adequately hydrate these children without overhydrating, as "fluid creep" can be as life-threatening as burns injury itself. Too much fluid administration can lead to pulmonary edema and compartment syndrome of abdomen and extremities. Acute renal failure may occur in patients with severe burns due to hypoperfusion and rhabdomyolysis. AKI in burns carry a high mortality risk (about 70%).

Severe burns include:

- 10% total body surface area (TBSA) burns in children <10 years and elderly >50 years.
- 20% TBSA in adults
- 5% full thickness

  Significant burns to eyes, ears, face, genitalia, or joints.

Assessment of a Child with Burns

The time and nature of burns and treatment received prior to admission should be documented. Signs of airway injury due to burns or inhalation injury like hoarseness of voice, stridor, etc. should be specifically looked for. Airway, oropharyngeal, and significant neck injury may need early intubation. Circumferential chest burns may need escharotomy to facilitate chest expansion. If a child develops shock early, consider alternate causes for shock.

Estimate TBSA % of burns, using Lund and Browder chart[44] or rule of nines and hand plus fingers method **(Figs. 2 and 3)**. Do not include areas with epidermal burns (erythema only). Cover the child and wound after assessment. Prevent hypothermia.

Type of Fluid

Ringer lactate is the fluid of choice for resuscitation of children with burns. If unavailable 0.9% NS can be used. Colloid resuscitation have not shown any mortality benefit.

Dose

Children with >10% TBSA burns should undergo fluid resuscitation. Due to their small circulating blood volume, children are at risk of development of shock early. Suboptimal resuscitation leads to increased depth of burns, increased duration of shock, and increased mortality. Catheterize children with severe burns to closely monitor urine output. NG tube insertion and keeping patients nil by mouth may be needed as ileus is a potential complication. There are a variety of formulas to estimate fluid need, but the most commonly used formula is Modified Parkland formula.[45]

- Calculate the estimated fluid requirement from time of injury.
  Total amount of fluid to be given in 24 hours = 3 mL/kg × % TBSA × weight in kg
- Any fluid received previously should be accounted for.
- Half of the calculated amount should be given in the first 8 hours followed by the rest in the next 16 hours.
- Routine maintenance fluid should be added to this in case of children.
- Target a urine output of 1 mL/kg/h for children <30 kg and 0.5 mL/kg/h for children >30 kg weight.

Modified Parkland formula should be taken as a guide only. Fluid rate should be adjusted every 1–2 hours after starting resuscitation, to target an optimal urine output. Take care to avoid "over-resuscitation." Infusion rates should be recalculated on an hourly basis decreasing the rate when urine output target is exceeded. Care should be taken not to increase fluid rates by >20–25% at one time. Close monitoring of vitals and maintenance of intake output chart is mandatory in all patients with severe burns. Ensure children are up-to-date with immunization, as burns is considered a tetanus-prone injury.

CONCLUSION

Fluid therapy in a critically ill child is a double-edged weapon. Both hypoperfusion and fluid overload can be deleterious to the patient. Type of fluid and quantity and duration of fluid therapy are equally important. Principles of fluid stewardship should be followed in all cases. Fluid administration should be individualized based on fluid needs, physiological status, and patient's premorbid condition.

KEY POINTS

- Prescribe IV fluids only when indicated.
- The four Ds (drug, dose, duration, de-escalation) of fluid therapy need to be considered in all situations.
- Avoid using hypotonic fluids for maintenance as critically ill children are at higher risk of hospital-acquired hyponatremia. Fluids with sodium content between 131 and 154 mEq/L is preferred.
- Normal saline can cause hyperchloremic metabolic acidosis. Hence, balanced crystalloids may be preferred in situations where large volume resuscitation is needed.
- Avoid use of albumin in traumatic brain injury.
- A dynamic approach to fluid therapy is preferred in sepsis (ROSE conceptual model).
- Children with severe malnutrition and dehydration or sepsis require very careful fluid titration guided by change in weight and vital parameters.
- Fluid overload percentage >10–20% is an independent risk factor for adverse outcome.

REFERENCES

1. Neale G, Woloshynowych M, Vincent C. Exploring the causes of adverse events in NHS hospital practice. JR Soc Med. 2001;94(7):322-30.
2. O'Brien F, Walker IA. Fluid homeostasis in the neonate. Paediatr Anaesth. 2014;24(1):49-59.
3. Mårild S, Jodal U, Jonasson G, Mangelus L, Odén A, Persson NG. Reference values for renal concentrating capacity in children by the desmopressin test. Pediatr Nephrol. 1992;6(3):254-7.
4. Friis-Hansen BJ, Holiday M, Stapleton T, Wallace WM. Total body water in children. Pediatrics. 1951;7(3):321-7.
5. Bellini C, Boccardo F, Bonioli E, Campisi C. Lymphodynamics in the fetus and newborn. Lymphology. 2006;39(3):110-7.
6. Young TE, Mangum B (Eds). Neofax: A Manual of Drugs Used in Neonatal Care, 20th edition. Montvale, NJ: Thomson Healthcare; 2007.
7. McDermid RC, Raghunathan K, Romanovsky A, Shaw AD, Bagshaw SM. Controversies in fluid therapy: type, dose and toxicity. World J Crit Care Med. 2014;3(1):24-33.
8. Hansen PB, Jensen BL, Skott O. Chloride regulates afferent arteriolar contraction in response to depolarization. Hypertension. 1998;32:1066-70.
9. Wilcox CS. Regulation of renal blood flow by plasma chloride. J Clin Invest. 1983;71:726-35.
10. Chowdhury AH, Cox EF, Francis ST, Lobo DN. A randomized, controlled, double-blind crossover study on the effects of 2-L infusions of 0.9% saline and plasmalyte® 148 on renal blood flow velocity and renal cortical tissue perfusion in healthy volunteers. Ann Surg. 2012;256(1):18-24.
11. Li H, Sun SR, Yap JQ, Chen JH, Qian Q. 0.9% saline is neither normal nor physiological. J Zhejiang Univ Sci B. 2016;17(3):181-7.
12. Reid F, Lobo DN, Williams RN, Rowlands BJ, Allison SP. (Ab) Normal saline and physiological Hartmann's solution: a randomized double-blind crossover study. Clin Sci (Lond). 2003;104(1):17-24.
13. Mercadal L, Franck JE, Metzger M, Yuan W, Kolko A, Monnet E, et al. Improved survival associated with acetate-free haemodialysis in elderly: a registry-based study. Nephrol Dial Transplant. 2015;30(9):1560-8.
14. Guidet B, Martinet O, Boulain T, Philippart F, Poussel JF, Maizel J, et al. Assessment of hemodynamic efficacy and safety of 6% hydroxyethylstarch 130/0.4 vs. 0.9% NaCl fluid replacement in patients with severe sepsis: the CRYSTMAS study. Crit Care. 2012;16(3):R94.
15. Myburgh J, Cooper DJ, Finfer S, Bellomo R, Norton R, Bishop N, et al.; SAFE Study Investigators, Australian and New Zealand Intensive Care Society Clinical Trials Group, Australian Red Cross Blood Service, George Institute for International Health. Saline or albumin for fluid resuscitation in patients with traumatic brain injury. Engl J Med. 2007;357(9):874-84.
16. Serpa Neto A, Veelo DP, Peireira VG, de Assunção MS, Manetta JA, Espósito DC, et al. Fluid resuscitation with hydroxyethyl starches in patients with sepsis is associated with an increased incidence of acute kidney injury and use of renal replacement therapy: a systematic review and meta-analysis of the literature. J Crit Care. 2014;29(1):185.e1-7.

17. Feld LG, Neuspiel DR, Foster BA, Leu MG, Garber MD, Austin K, et al. Clinical Practice guidelines: maintenance intravenous fluids in children. Pediatrics. 2018;142(6):e20183083.
18. Holliday MA, Segar WE. The maintenance need for water in parenteral fluid therapy. Pediatrics. 1957;19:823-32.
19. The SAFE Study Investigators. A comparison of albumin and saline for fluid resuscitation in the intensive care unit. N Engl J Med. 2004;350:2247-56.
20. Caironi P, Tognoni G, Masson S, Fumagalli R, Pesenti A, Romero M, et al. Albumin replacement in patients with severe sepsis or septic shock. N Engl J Med. 2014;370:1412-21.
21. Hoste EA, Maitland K, Brudney CS, Mehta R, Vincent JL, Yates D, et al.; ADQI XII Investigators Group. Four phases of intravenous fluid therapy: a conceptual model. Br J Anaesth. 2014;113(5):740-7.
22. Malbrain MLNG, Van Regenmortel N, Saugel B, De Tavernier B, Van Gaal PJ, Joannes-Boyau O, et al. Principles of fluid management and stewardship in septic shock: it is time to consider the four D's and the four phases of fluid therapy. Ann Intensive Care. 2018;8(1):66.
23. Weiss SL, Peters MJ, Alhazzani W, Agus MSD, Flori HR, Inwald DP, et al. Surviving sepsis campaign international guidelines for the management of septic shock and sepsis-associated organ dysfunction in children. Pediatr Crit Care Med. 2020;21:e52-e106.
24. World Health Organization. (2016). Guideline Updates on paediatric emergency triage, assessment and treatment: care of critically-Ill children. Geneva, Switzerland. [online] Available from https://www.ncbi.nlm.nih.gov/books/NBK350523/ [Last accessed May, 2022].
25. Pro CI, Yealy DM, Kellum JA, Huang DT, Barnato AE, Weissfeld LA, et al. A randomized trial of protocol-based care for early septic shock. N Engl J Med. 2014;370(18):1683-93.
26. Investigators A, Group ACT, Peake SL, Delaney A, Bailey M, Bellomo R, et al. Goal-directed resuscitation for patients with early septic shock. N Engl J Med. 2014;371(16):1496-506.
27. Mouncey PR, Osborn TM, Power GS, Harrison DA, Sadique MZ, Grieve RD, et al. Protocolised Management In Sepsis (ProMISe): a multicentre randomised controlled trial of the clinical effectiveness and cost-effectiveness of early, goal-directed, protocolised resuscitation for emerging septic shock. Health Technol Assess. 2015;19(97):i-xxv, 1-150.
28. Kalil AC, Johnson DW, Lisco SJ, Sun J. Early goal-directed therapy for sepsis: a novel solution for discordant survival outcomes in clinical trials. Crit Care Med. 2017;45(4):607-14.
29. Maitland K, Kiguli S, Opoka RO, Engoru C, Olupot-Olupot P, Akech SO, et al. Mortality after fluid bolus in African children with severe infection. N Engl J Med. 2011;364(26):2483-95.
30. Woodcock TE, Woodcock TM. Revised Starling equation and the glycocalyx model of transvascular fluid exchange: an improved paradigm for prescribing intravenous fluid therapy. Br J Anaesth. 2012;108(3):384-94.
31. Malbrain ML, De Laet I. AIDS is coming to your ICU: be prepared for acute bowel injury and acute intestinal distress syndrome. Intensive Care Med. 2008;34(9):1565-9.
32. Davis AL, Carcillo JA, Aneja RK, Deymann AJ, Lin JC, Nguyen TC, et al. The American college of critical care medicine clinical practice parameters for hemodynamic support of pediatric and neonatal septic shock: executive summary. Pediatr Crit Care Med. 2017;18:884-90.
33. Rhodes A, Evans LE, Alhazzani W, Levy MM, Antonelli M, Ferrer R, et al. Surviving Sepsis campaign: international guidelines for Management of Sepsis and Septic Shock: 2016. Intensive Care Med. 2017;43:304-77.
34. Pediatric Acute Lung Injury Consensus Conference Group. Pediatric acute respiratory distress syndrome: consensus recommendations from the Pediatric Acute Lung Injury Consensus Conference. Pediatr Crit Care Med. 2015;16(5): 428-39.
35. Rossaint R, Bouillon B, Cerny V, Coats TJ, Duranteau J, Fernandez-Mondejar E, et al. The European guideline on management of major bleeding and coagulopathy following trauma: fourth edition. Crit Care. 2016;20:100.
36. Ichai C, Vinsonneau C, Souweine B, Armando F, Canet E, Clec'h C, et al. Acute kidney injury in the perioperative period and in intensive care units (excluding renal replacement therapies). Ann Intensive Care. 2016;6:48.
37. National Clinical Guideline Centre. IV Fluids in Children: Intravenous Fluid Therapy in Children and Young People in Hospital. London: National Institute for Health and Care Excellence (UK). 2015.
38. Malbrain MLNG, Langer T, Annane D, Gattinoni L, Elbers P, Hahn RG, et al. Intravenous fluid therapy in the perioperative and critical care setting: Executive summary of the International Fluid Academy (IFA). Ann Intensive Care. 2020;10(1):64.
39. Sümpelmann R, Mader T, Eich C, Witt L, Osthaus WA. A novel isotonic-balanced electrolyte solution with 1% glucose for intraoperative fluid therapy in children: Results of a prospective multicentre observational post-authorization safety study (PASS). Pediatric Anesthesia. 2010;20(11):977-81.
40. Busto-Aguirreurreta N, Suarez JJJ. Perioperative Fluid Therapy in the Pediatric Patient: Recommendations. J Perioper Crit Intensive Care Nurs. 2016;2:129.
41. Goldstein SL. Fluid management in acute kidney injury. J Intensive Care Med. 2014;29(4):183-9.
42. Yunos NM, Bellomo R, Glassford N, Sutcliffe H, Lam Q, Bailey M. Chloride-liberal vs. chloride-restrictive intravenous fluid administration and acute kidney injury: an extended analysis. Intensive Care Med. 2015;41:257-64.
43. The Royal Children's Hospital, Melbourne. Clinical Practice Guidelines. Burns acute management. [online] Available from https://www.rch.org.au/clinicalguide/guideline_index/Burns/ [Last accessed May, 2022].
44. Lund CC, Browder NC. The Estimation of Areas of Burns. Surgery Gynecology and Obstetrics. 1944;79:352.
45. Zodda D. Calculated decisions: Parkland formula for burns. Pediatr Emerg Med Pract. 2018;15(Suppl 4):1-2.

CHAPTER

4.2

Disorders of Sodium: Hyponatremia and Hypernatremia

Radhika C Radhakrishnan, Mukta Mantan

INTRODUCTION

Sodium is the major cation in extracellular fluid (ECF). Shift in water is mostly a result of changes in plasma sodium concentration; hence, dysnatremias mostly are a reflection of disorders of water balance. A significant portion of our body is constituted by water. The term "total body water" (TBW) denotes the total quantity of fluid in the human body and it varies with age. It is highest (75–80%) in premature infants and decreases with age. Term newborns have TBW of 70% and at the age of 1 year, it is 60%. The correction factors to assess body water according to age is given in **Table 1**.[1]

Total body water is distributed in two major compartments, around two-thirds of TBW is inside the cells, i.e., intracellular fluid (ICF); the rest one-third is outside cells, i.e., ECF. ECF is further distributed in three compartments—interstitial fluid, plasma, and transcellular fluid. In children above 1 year of age, ICF and ECF water are 40% and 20%, respectively, of body weight. Out of the ECF volume, 75% of the volume is present in the interstitial space (i.e., 15% of body weight), and 25% of that water is in the plasma (5% of body weight). The distribution of TBW is depicted in **Figure 1**.[2]

SODIUM AND WATER BALANCE

Normally, the human body maintains plasma osmolality within a relatively narrow range (280–295 mOsm/kg) and serum sodium concentration is between 135 and 145 mEq/L. Complex neurohumoral regulations control sodium homeostasis and water balance. The autonomic nervous system is a key regulator of renin secretion, renal hemodynamics, and tubular fluid reabsorption. Sympathetic stimulation causes renin release and proximal tubular fluid reabsorption. Direct actions of the autonomic nervous system regulate short-term fluid regulation in response to changes in sodium and water balance while aldosterone and antidiuretic hormone (ADH) are responsible for long-term regulation of sodium and water reabsorption.[3]

Antidiuretic hormone is otherwise known as arginine vasopressin (AVP) and is a product of a subset of magnocellular neurons in the paraventricular nuclei (PVN) and supraoptic nuclei (SON) of the hypothalamus. The axons from magnocellular neurons project to posterior pituitary via the pituitary stalk and their terminals contain neurosecretory granules, which store AVP till it is released. AVP has a carrier protein neurophysin II (NPII) and both are coded by a single gene on chromosome 20p13. Both ADH and NPII are produced as a single polypeptide. Then, it is cleaved within the neurosecretory granules and before release, reassembled into AVP-NPII complexes. Posterior pituitary has significant storage capacity of AVP that can last up to 30–50 days under basal circumstances and up to 5–10 days during maximal stimulation. Hence, it takes weeks after a causal insult defect in AVP synthesis to become clinically manifest and partial

TABLE 1: Correction factor to assess total body water (TBW).[1]

Age	*Correction factor*
Newborn	0.8
Infant	0.7
Child	0.6
Adult male	0.6
Adult female	0.5
Elderly male	0.5
Elderly female	0.45

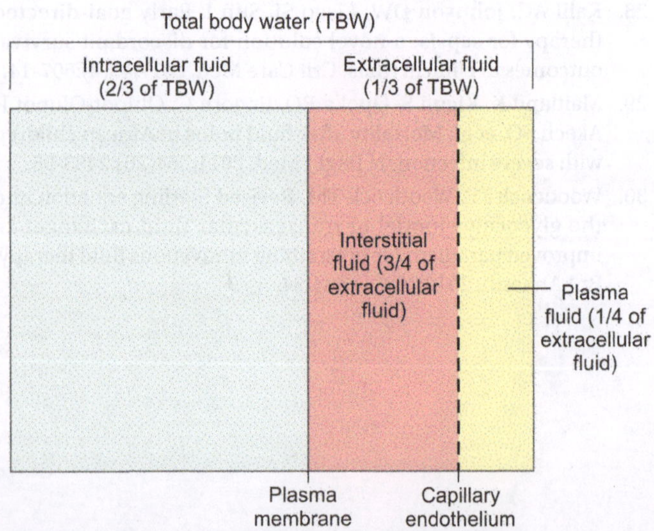

Fig. 1: Distribution of total body water.[2]

defects may be apparent only after prolonged deprivation of water.

Antidiuretic hormone secretion and thirst are both stimulated effectively by a small (1%) increase of osmolality and a high (5–10%) decrease in blood volume.[3] Even 1% increase in plasma osmolality is sensed by osmoreceptors in the hypothalamus (organum vasculosum of the lamina terminalis and anterior hypothalamus) which cause secretion of AVP. Normally, baseline AVP levels are low, 0.5–2 pg/mL, and rises only when plasma osmolality increases to >280 mOsm/kg. Maximal urine concentration (urine osmolality 900–1,200 mOsm/kg) is achieved at plasma AVP levels of 5–6 pg/mL. Even though plasma AVP can increase to >6 pg/mL when plasma hyperosmolality is ongoing, urine osmolality cannot be further increased since renal medullary gradient is limited. AVP secretion is inversely affected by alterations in blood volume that is, it is stimulated by 8–10% reduction in circulating blood volume and inhibited by rises in intravascular volume.

Antidiuretic hormone release is less sensitive to hypovolemia but, whenever there is a significant reduction in intravascular volume, volume takes priority over osmolality. Thus, the body enhances ADH secretion which counteracts the effect of hypo-osmolality. This is mediated via high-pressure baroreceptors located in the carotid sinus and aortic arch and low-pressure baroreceptors located in the atria and pulmonary venous circulation. These receptors are stimulated by stretch due to increase in intravascular volume and send blood volume and pressure signals through glossopharyngeal and vagus nerves, respectively, to the brainstem. From the brainstem, nerve fibers project to hypothalamic PVN and SON causing inhibition of AVP secretion. In addition to osmo- and baroregulation, there are several other factors which affect secretion of AVP. AVP release is stimulated by stress, nausea, pain, and many drugs and is inhibited by various factors.

The antidiuretic effect of AVP is mediated by V2 vasopressin receptor (V2R). This receptor is located on the basolateral side of renal collecting duct epithelial cells and is a G protein-coupled receptor, coded by X chromosome. Activation of V2R causes increase in cyclic adenosine monophosphate (cAMP) inside the cells, causing transport of aquaporin 2 (AQP-2) water channels to the apical membrane of collecting duct epithelial cells, leading to augmented permeability of these cells to water and thus, antidiuresis.

An intact thirst mechanism governs adequate water intake, which in turn is controlled by changes in intravascular volume, plasma osmolality, and blood pressure. An increase in plasma osmolality by 2–3% and decrease in effective blood volume by 4–10% stimulates thirst. Although thresholds that stimulate thirst are more than that for secretion of AVP, adequate thirst is crucial when there is AVP deficiency or insensitivity.

Our body does not have the ability to sense sodium. However, the kidneys have specialized receptors in juxtaglomerular apparatus that can detect flow of tubular fluid and its sodium concentration. This is accomplished by the macula densa cells, which send information to juxtaglomerular cells, situated at the arteriolar walls to reduce glomerular filtration rate (GFR) by a tubuloglomerular feedback mechanism. Similarly, reduced tubular flow leads to a rise in GFR. This mechanism ensures that body fluids are not lost in states with glomerular hyperfusion. In addition, renin-angiotensin-aldosterone system (RAAS) is a critical regulator of blood pressure, intravascular volume, and electrolyte balance.

Atrial natriuretic peptide (ANP) and brain natriuretic peptides result in vasodilation, natriuresis, diuresis, and decrease systemic vascular resistance and arterial blood pressure. They also reduce release of ADH and aldosterone. Sodium excretion is increased both by enhancing GFR and suppressing salt reabsorption. Wall stretch of heart cavities by increased blood volume causes secretion of natriuretic peptides (NPs). Angiotensin II and sympathetic stimulation also boost secretion of NPs, which reach the target organs via blood circulation. NP target receptors have been recognized in several sites including kidneys, adrenal glands, and blood vessels.

Osmolality and Tonicity

Sodium by virtue of being the dominant ECF cation, is the chief determinant of serum tonicity and osmolality. Osmolality is defined as the number of dissolved particles per kilogram of solvent. It is measured by osmometer or calculated as a sum of the solutes present in the solution. Serum osmolality is maintained at a normal range of 285–295 mOsm/kg.

Serum osmolality can be calculated by the formula:

Serum osmolality = (2 × serum Na) + (Glucose/18) + (BUN/2.8)

(Na and K are measured in mmol/L, glucose and BUN are measured in mg/dL).

Tonicity is the effective osmolality, i.e., it indicates the concentration of solutes that can exert osmotic force across the semipermeable membrane. So, only solutes, which cannot freely cross the membrane, will contribute to tonicity. In other words, solutes, which can easily move through the cell membrane like urea, do not contribute to tonicity and are considered as ineffective osmoles. Tonicity can be calculated by the following equation:

Serum tonicity = 2 × [Na] + [glucose]/18 (when glucose is measured in mg/dL)

HYPONATREMIA

Hyponatremia is one of the most common electrolyte abnormalities in children and can lead to significant morbidity and mortality, particularly in subjects in whom change in serum sodium is acute and rapid. Hyponatremia is defined as a serum or plasma sodium <135 mEq/L and severe hyponatremia as a level <125 mEq/L.

Signs and Symptoms

Signs and symptoms of hyponatremia vary based on its duration and severity and can range from mild to severe to life-threatening.

Acute Hyponatremia

Neurologic dysfunction is the most common manifestation of hyponatremia. Rate of change of sodium levels is more important than the absolute degree of hyponatremia. Fast alterations in sodium levels are less well tolerated than slow changes. As the serum sodium decreases, there is development of osmotic gradient between the intravascular and intracellular spaces, leading to movement of water from extracellular space to intracellular space. There acute and chronic cellular regulatory mechanisms attenuate cell volume shifts, which can minimize the volume shifts. This cerebral adaption to hyponatremia is an important factor to consider while we treat hyponatremia. When the change in serum sodium levels are more rapid and of greater degree, regulatory mechanisms do not get enough time to minimize cell volume change but also these changes will be less effective. Since skull is a closed space with limited free space, such rapid fluid shifts causes significant increase in volume of the brain and cause cerebral edema leading to neurologic manifestations.

Serum sodium levels >125 mEq/L may not create any specific clinical manifestations, and patients can have only the symptoms and signs of their underlying acute illness. As the serum sodium decreases acutely to <125 mEq/L, neurologic symptoms begin to appear, beginning with nausea and malaise. Headache, anorexia, restlessness, lethargy, muscle cramps, obtundation, and seizures can appear as serum sodium continues to falls to <120 mEq/L.

Chronic Hyponatremia

Chronic hyponatremia is defined as hyponatremia persisting more than 48 hours. When low plasma sodium levels exist for more than 1 day or develop slowly over several days, cerebral adaptation mechanisms reduce the expansion in cell volume and reduce the occurrence of cerebral edema. These patients may not manifest significant symptoms till the serum sodium gets very much depressed or another acute event leads to a more severe reduction in sodium levels. However, there can be subtle neurologic manifestations such as restlessness, irritability, fatigue, or weakness.

Evaluation and Diagnosis

The first step in evaluation of hyponatremia is to assess the volume status of the patient and measure the plasma osmolality.[1]

True hyponatremia is characterized by reduction in plasma osmolality. Other types of hyponatremia are not associated with low plasma osmolality and are due to fluid shifts as a result of osmotically active substances like urea, glucose, or mannitol, or as a result of high lipid or protein levels. Patients with true hyponatremia may be further classified according to volume status into euvolemic, hypovolemic, or hypervolemic.

The classification of hyponatremia by plasma tonicity is given in **Table 2**.[4]

TABLE 2: Classification of hyponatremia according to plasma tonicity.[4]

	Serum sodium	*Plasma osmolality*	*Typical causes*
Hypotonic	<135 mmol/L	Low (<280 mOsm/kg H_2O)	SIADH; CHF; cirrhosis
Isotonic	<135 mmol/L	Normal (280–295 mOsm/kg H_2O)	Hyperglycemia; pseudohyponatremia (hyperlipidemia, hyperproteinemia)
Hypertonic	<135 mmol/L	High (>295 mOsm/kg H_2O)	Severe hyperglycemia with dehydration; mannitol

(CHF: congestive heart failure; SIADH: syndrome of inappropriate antidiuretic hormone)

Isotonic Hyponatremia (Pseudohyponatremia)

In pseudohyponatremia, hyponatremia is owing to the presence of hypertriglyceridemia, hypercholesterolemia, or hyperproteinemia. In the above conditions, there is reduction in the plasma water fraction and lesser measured sodium concentration. Around 93% of total plasma volume is contributed by plasma water. Assuming that the plasma sodium concentration is 140 mmol/L, the expected plasma water sodium concentration would be 150 mmol/L. The problem of pseudohyponatremia occurs with indirect ion-selective electrode (ISE) method of measuring sodium levels. ISE measures sodium concentration in total serum after diluting the sample. In hyperproteinemia or hypertriglyceridemia, since the nonaqueous fraction of plasma is increased, the serum contains a lesser volume of plasma water and lower sodium. This problem can be avoided by the use of direct ISE methods as it measures sodium activity in plasma of undiluted samples.

Hypertonic Hyponatremia (Translocational Hyponatremia)

In hypertonic hyponatremic conditions, the serum osmolality is raised to more than 295 mmol/L. Increase in osmolality leads to water shifting out of the cells into ECF and ECF dilution. Hypertonic hyponatremias is most commonly caused by hyperglycemia (in the absence of insulin) and can also be associated with intravenous radiocontrast, mannitol, low-molecular weight dextrans, and sucrose. Since urea can easily cross cell membranes, it is considered an ineffective osmole and cannot affect serum tonicity. Hence, uremia does not lead to hypertonic hyponatremia.

Formula for corrected Na calculation in hyperglycemic states:[5]

Corrected Na = measured serum Na + [1.6 × (glucose – 100)/100]

(Na is measured in mmol/L, glucose is measured in mg/dL).

Hypotonic Hyponatremia (True Hyponatremia)

This condition is characterized by decreased serum osmolality (<275 mmol/L). It is further classified depending on the child's extracellular volume status into hypovolemic, euvolemic, and hypervolemic hyponatremia.

Hypovolemic hyponatremia: In hypovolemic hyponatremia, there is a loss of TBW and sodium. Often, the child presents with features of dehydration, like nausea, vomiting, tachycardia, and low blood pressure. Sodium and water loss may be of renal or extrarenal origin. Kidneys can be the source of water loss in conditions like renal failure, overzealous diuretic use, renal tubular acidosis, and mineralocorticoid deficiency.[6] Kidney functions are preserved in extrarenal water losses due to sweating, third-space losses like burns, or pancreatitis, heat exposure, diarrhea, vomiting, pulmonary losses, biliary drains, and high-output gastrointestinal fistulas.[6,7] Urinary sodium can be used to differentiate between these two causes (high in renal water loss and low in extrarenal water loss).

Cerebral salt wasting (CSW) is a cause for hyponatremia arising as a result of intracranial disease and mimics syndrome of inappropriate antidiuretic hormone (SIADH) as both are characterized by elevated urine sodium, concentrated urine, and no edema. But the patient is hypovolemic in CSW while in SIADH the patient is euvolemic. CSW can occur as a result of different conditions like intracerebral hemorrhage, stroke, brain tumors, head injury, tuberculous meningitis, and intracranial surgery. The exact mechanism by which diuresis and natriuresis occur in CSW is not known. Differentiation between CSW and SIADH is described in **Table 3**.

Hypervolemic hyponatremia: Hypervolemic hyponatremia is characterized by an increase in TBW and reduction in sodium levels. Such children have features of fluid overload, including peripheral edema, ascites, anasarca, or pulmonary edema. Causes include nephrotic syndrome, chronic kidney failure, cirrhosis, or congestive heart failure. In renal failure, urinary sodium levels are high, whereas it is low in patients with cirrhosis, congestive heart failure, or nephrotic syndrome.

Euvolemic hyponatremia: In euvolemic hyponatremia, total body sodium levels are normal and intravascular volume is slightly decreased, without clinical features of dehydration.

The various causes and criteria for SIADH diagnosis are given in **Table 4 and Box 1**. SIADH is the most common cause of euvolemic hyponatremia. Other causes are hypothyroidism,

TABLE 3: Difference between SIADH and CSW.

Features	*CSW*	*SIADH*
Dehydration	Present	Absent
Serum sodium	Decreased	Decreased
Urinary sodium excretion	Increased	Variable
Urine osmolality	Increased	Increased
Serum osmolality	Low	Low
Vasopressin	Low	High
Polyuria	Present	Absent
BUN	Increased	Normal
Blood pressure	Low	Normal or increased
ANP	Increased	Normal
Treatment	Saline/3% NaCl	Fluid restriction

(ANP: atrial natriuretic peptide; BUN: blood urea nitrogen; CSW: cerebral salt wasting; SIADH: syndrome of inappropriate antidiuretic hormone)

TABLE 4: Common causes of syndrome of inappropriate antidiuretic hormone (SIADH).[1]

Category	*Cause*
Malignancy	• Bladder carcinoma • Duodenal carcinoma • Ewing sarcoma • Head or neck carcinoma • Leukemia • Lymphoma • Mesothelioma • Pancreatic carcinoma • Pulmonary carcinoma • Prostatic carcinoma • Sarcoma • Thymoma • Ureteral carcinoma
Pulmonary	• Acute respiratory failure • Asthma • Cystic fibrosis • Empyema • Pneumonia • Pneumothorax • Positive pressure ventilation • Tuberculosis
Central nervous system	• Acute intermittent porphyria • Acute psychosis • Agenesis of corpus callosum • Atrophy of cerebrum or cerebellum • Brain abscess • Brain tumors • Cavernous sinus thrombosis • Cerebrovascular accidents • Delirium tremens • Guillain-Barré syndrome • Encephalitis • Head trauma • Hydrocephalus

Contd...

Contd...

Category	Cause
	• Meningitis • Multiple system atrophy • Neonatal hypoxia • Rocky Mountain spotted fever • Subarachnoid hemorrhage
Medications/drugs	• Alcohol abuse and malnutrition • Butyrophenones • Carbamazepine • Cisplatin • Chlorpropamide • Clofibrate • Cyclophosphamide • Cytoxan • Desmopressin • Ecstasy • Interferon α and γ • Methotrexate • Monoamine oxidase inhibitors • Monoclonal antibodies • Morphine • Nicotine • Nonsteroidal anti-inflammatory drugs • Opiates • Oxcarbazepine • Oxytocin • Phenothiazines • Selective serotonin reuptake inhibitors • Sodium valproate • Thiazide diuretics • Tricyclic antidepressants • Vasopressin • Vinca alkaloids
Others	• AIDS • Glucocorticoid insufficiency • Idiopathic • Myxedema • Postoperative period

BOX 1: Diagnostic criteria for syndrome of inappropriate antidiuretic hormone (SIADH).

Bartter and Schwartz criteria for SIADH:
- Hypotonic hyponatremia (effective SOsm < 275 mOsm/kg H_2O)
- Euvolemia
- Less than maximally dilute urine (UOsm > 100 mOsm/kg H_2O)
- Elevated urine sodium excretion (UNa > 30 mEq/L)
- Absence of cirrhosis, chronic kidney failure, heart failure, hypothyroidism, and diuretic usage

Additional data supporting SIADH diagnosis:
- Serum uric acid <4 mg/dL
- Fractional excretion of uric acid >10%
- Worsening of hyponatremia with intravenous normal saline infusion relative to serum osmolality
- Plasma vasopressin level inappropriately elevated relative to serum osmolality
- Abnormal response to water load (excretion <80% of 20 mL/kg load in 4 hours with failure to dilute urine to <100 mOsm/ kg H_2O

nausea, excessive pain, stress, or water intoxication caused by psychogenic polydipsia. Reset osmostat is the second most common form of SIADH and is seen in a subset of patients with SIADH. Such patients are able to adjust urinary water excretion by regulating secretion of ADH, but their threshold for ADH secretion is at a lower serum osmolality set point, leading to premature release of ADH. Patients are still able to suppress ADH and dilute their urine once their set point is reached but only after suffering significant hyponatremia. This preserved ability to secrete ADH is what distinguishes patients with reset osmostat from other types of SIADH.

Clinical Evaluation

History taking and clinical examination should be targeted toward identifying the volume status of the child, history of excessive free water intake, and evidence of ADH effect based on urinary output, and evidence of a concentrated urine.[8]

- History of fluid loss (e.g., vomiting, diarrhea, profound bleeding, diuretic therapy) and signs of extracellular volume depletion (e.g., decreased skin turgor, tachycardia, or orthostatic or persistent hypotension) indicate hypovolemia, which is associated with appropriate ADH secretion and retention of free water. In children, the most common cause of fluid loss associated with hyponatremia is gastroenteritis.
- History or clinical finding of edema and ascites is suggestive of hypervolemic conditions with effective circulatory volume depletion, such as heart failure, cirrhosis, or nephrotic syndrome.
- History suggestive of underlying SIADH like brain injury or infection, and pulmonary disease. In SIADH, there is decrease in urine output and inappropriately concentrated urine due to ADH release in spite of low serum sodium concentration and osmolality.
- History of excess water intake indicate primary or psychogenic polydipsia (e.g., older child with psychiatric disease).
- History of diseases associated with excess renal salt losses like CSW or primary tubular disorders (e.g., renal tubular acidosis, Bartter and Gitelman syndromes), or skin loss like cystic fibrosis.
- History of anuria or oliguria may indicate severe kidney impairment with an inability to excrete free water.

Investigations

Laboratory tests to assess serum and urine osmolality and urine sodium may help in finding the etiology of hyponatremia. Urine osmolality >100 mOsmol/kg in a normovolemic child with hyponatremia should be considered as evidence of impaired water handling as in such situations, normally ADH should be depressed. Such children will most likely have highly concentrated urines with urine osmolality significantly more than plasma osmolality. In contrast, reset osmostat and psychogenic polydipsia are associated with a urine osmolality <100 mOsmol/kg.

An algorithm showing diagnostic approach to hyponatremia is depicted in **Flowchart 1.**[9]

Flowchart 1: Diagnostic approach to hyponatremia.[4]

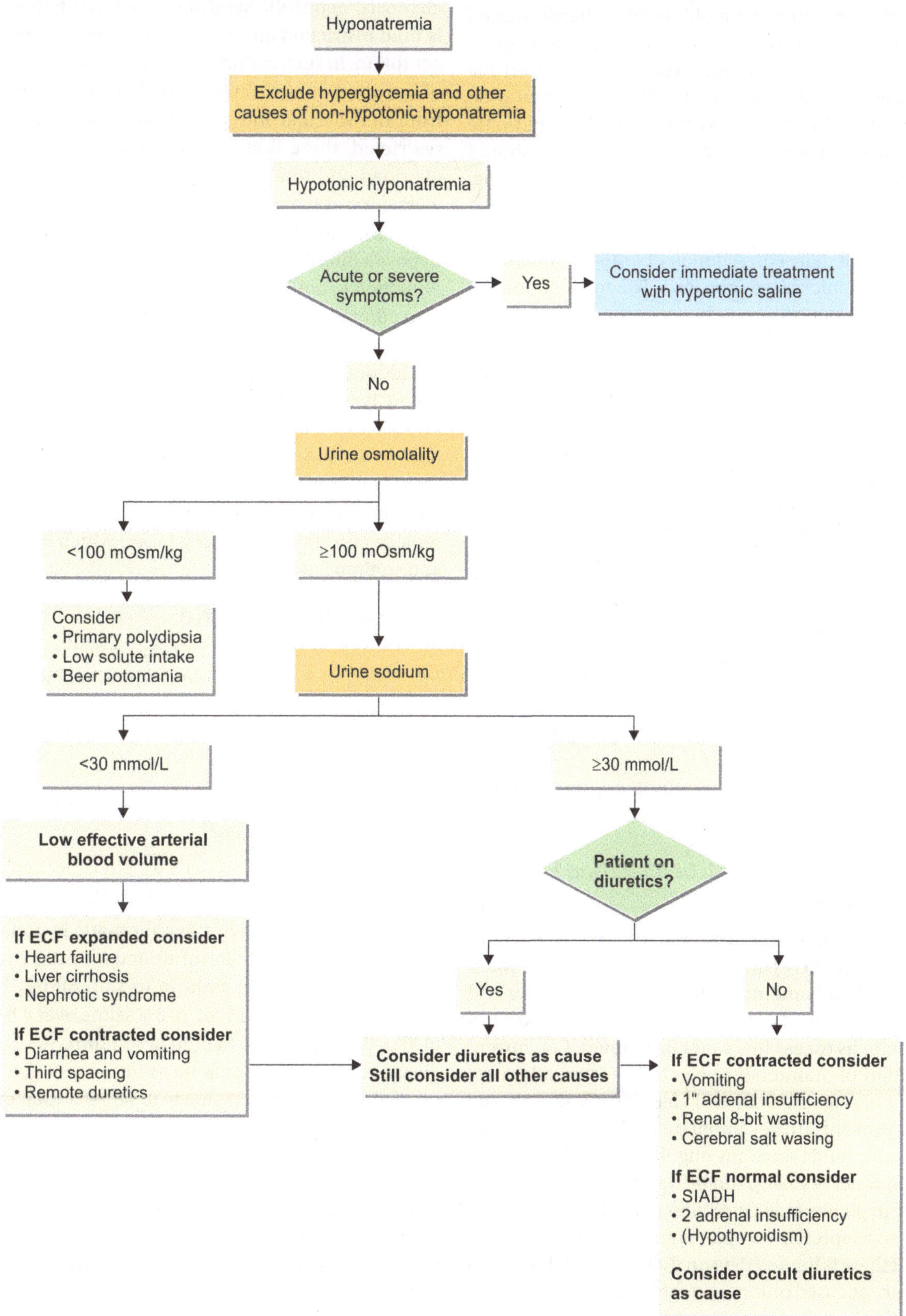

(ECF: extracellular fluid; SIADH: syndrome of inappropriate antidiuretic hormone)

Treatment

The approach to treatment depends on child's:

- Volume status
- Hemodynamic stability
- Presence or absence of symptoms of hyponatremia
- Severity of the symptoms
- Duration of hyponatremia.

Severe Central Nervous System Symptoms

Correction of hyponatremia should be immediately started if the patient has seizures or altered mental status. In such children, 3–5 mL/kg of 3% saline (maximum 100 mL) is recommended as initial treatment.[10] The bolus should be given over 10–60 minutes. After giving the initial hypertonic saline bolus, a repeat measurement of plasma sodium should be done and the bolus is repeated if seizures are ongoing. After acute central nervous system (CNS) symptoms have stopped, further sodium correction is done in a slower manner such that the total daily correction is <12 mEq/L (including the initial hypertonic saline infusion). The most important complication of symptomatic hyponatremia is evolving cerebral edema, and in such cases, the risk of morbidity from delayed therapy is more than that of complication from too fast correction and osmotic demyelination. That is why, aggressive initial correction is indicated for the first 3–4 hours (or until the symptoms resolve) at a rate not to exceed a rise in serum sodium of 2 mEq/L per hour.[11-13] Often, an initial goal is to raise the serum sodium by 5 mEq/L over the first several hours as seizures seem to resolve with this therapeutic approach.[14]

Chronic Hyponatremia

In the child with no symptoms or only mild neurologic symptoms (e.g., nausea and malaise), there is no need for hypertonic saline infusion. The serum sodium deficit is calculated using the equation:

Total body Na deficit = (desired serum Na – actual serum Na) × TBW

The targeted rate of correction in this setting is 6–10 mEq/L over 24 hours.

Hyponatremia with Normal or Increased Effective Circulating Volume

In a hyponatremic patient with normal or increased effective circulating volume (ECV) due to SIADH, restriction of water to 60% of usual daily maintenance fluid requirement will lead to slow correction of fluid overload and normalization of plasma sodium as excess free water is excreted. Concurrent administration of maintenance electrolytes and adequate replacement of ongoing fluid and electrolyte losses should be done to prevent further imbalances. It is important to avoid hypotonic fluids since any ongoing ADH secretion will result in free water reabsorption by the distal tubules which will counter hyponatremia correction of via fluid restriction.

In adults, vasopressin receptor antagonists like tolvaptan are used but there is limited data on their use in children and hence they are not used routinely in the treatment of pediatric hyponatremia.

Hyponatremia with Decreased Effective Circulating Volume

Treatment of hyponatremia in a patient with reduced ECV will depend on the underlying condition.

In a hypervolemic child with decreased ECV due to cirrhosis, nephrotic syndrome, or heart failure, treatment is fluid restriction and treatment of the underlying etiology condition. In such children, edema and ascites are the results of retention of free water by the kidneys and its movement from the vascular into interstitial spaces. When fluids are restricted, there is slow rebalancing of preexisting water overload and total body sodium, thus preventing further worsening of symptoms.

In contrast, children with true depletion of ECV due to hypovolemia, like in gastrointestinal losses, there is usually a reduction in both TBW and salt. In such cases, the treatment is to administer isotonic fluid, which will lead to restoration of circulating volume and improvement in blood flow to the kidneys. The administered isotonic fluid will remain in the ECV, which leads to inhibition of the activated renin-angiotensin-aldosterone axis (RAAS system) and ADH release. This in turn will reduce free water reabsorption which is the mediator for hyponatremia. The patient should then continue to be administered sufficient water and sodium to replace current and ongoing losses which will restore fluid and sodium balance.

Clinical Case Scenario

A 6-year-old girl admitted with suspected intracranial tumor has sudden worsening of sensorium. She is normotensive and normovolemic. Her weight is unchanged at 20 kg. On evaluation, her serum sodium was found to be 115 mEq/L.

Solution:

The total desired correction of sodium level is 10 mEq/L in 24 hours, i.e., to 125 mEq/L.

Sodium deficit = 0.6 × body weight × (desired – observed) sodium = 0.6 × 20 × (125–115) = 120 mEq

Since patient is having symptomatic hyponatremia, we want a fast initial correction of around 4–5 mEq/L over 4 hours. So, to raise his serum sodium to 120 mEq/L, he requires 60 mEq of sodium = 115 mL of 3% saline over 4 hours (1 liter of 3% saline contains 513 mEq of sodium).

Once CNS symptoms have improved, the rest of the correction can be given slowly to target a total of 10 mEq/L correction in 24 hours.

Osmotic Demyelination Syndrome

Osmotic demyelination syndrome (ODS) is an iatrogenic irreversible clinical syndrome consisting of neurologic features which occurs following a very fast correction of serum sodium.[15] It was earlier known as central pontine myelinolysis (CPM), but now CPM is considered as a subset of ODS in which the clinical effects are primarily due to brainstem damage. Other children with ODS can have foci of demyelination anywhere else within the CNS.[15] ODS occurs when the generally agreed safe limits of serum sodium correction are exceeded, that is correction >12 mEq/L in 24 hours, >25 mEq/L in 48 hours, or inadvertent hypernatremia during hyponatremia.[14,15] The neuronal damage is likely due to the result of rapid swelling of brain and nervous system cells during fluid administration, since these cells are not able to adapt quickly to the change in osmolality.[16] Children suffering from chronic hyponatremia are especially vulnerable to ODS, particularly those with underlying hypoxia, malnutrition, alcoholism, toxins, other CNS disease, or other metabolic syndromes. Clinical features of ODS include confusion, fluctuating levels of consciousness, mutism, behavioral changes, dysarthria, dysphagia, and seizures.[15] Patients can progress to a locked-in state, in which they are awake but unable to move or communicate, or quadriparesis.

HYPERNATREMIA

Hypernatremia is defined as serum sodium concentration >145 mEq/L and it is less common in children compared to hyponatremia. Hypernatremia is always associated with intracellular dehydration caused by decrease of TBW.

Etiology

Etiology of hypernatremia can vary depending on the volume status of the patient, i.e., hypovolemic, euvolemic, or hypervolemic.

Hypovolemic Hypernatremia

- Impaired thirst mechanisms—hypodipsia, adipsia
- Inability to acquire adequate free water—elderly, infants, or critically ill patients (e.g., patients on a ventilator, in a coma)
- Gastrointestinal losses—diarrhea, vomiting, nasogastric drainage
- Diuresis—osmotic diuretics, impaired urinary concentration—obstructive uropathy, sickle cell disease, nephronophthisis, cystinosis, and acute or chronic kidney disease.

Euvolemic Hypernatremia

- Diabetes insipidus (DI)
- Hypodipsia.

Hypervolemic Hypernatremia

- Salt poisoning
- Primary hyperaldosteronism
- Formula-fed infants
- Administration of isotonic saline to replete hypotonic losses.

Diabetes Insipidus

Diabetes insipidus is characterized by lack of response to ADH, which can be central or peripheral. Due to deficiency of ADH effect, urine is maximally dilute with low urine osmolality. Even though sodium is excreted in the urine, it is less than the excretion of water and this disproportionate excretion of water compared to sodium leads to hypernatremia.

- *Central DI:* This condition is characterized by insufficient ADH production or release. It may be congenital or acquired. Congenital causes include CNS malformations and genetic syndromes with associated CNS anomalies. Acquired etiologies include infiltrative processes of the hypothalamic-pituitary stalk, CNS tumors, and sequelae from neurological surgeries and trauma.
- *Nephrogenic DI:* This condition is characterized by inadequate renal tubular response to circulating ADH. The causes can be further divided into congenital or acquired.

Clinical Manifestations

Symptoms of hypernatremia are similar to those of hyponatremia, because both affect primarily the CNS. In the presence of hypernatremia, brain cells shrink significantly as water moves from inside the cells into the ECF space. This fluid shift can lead to intracerebral hemorrhage due to tearing of cerebral blood vessels by exertion of shear force. Hypernatremia can also lead to impaired glucose use, reduced left ventricular contractility, hyperventilation, muscle cramps, and rhabdomyolysis. The clinical manifestations include lethargy, weakness, or restlessness; infants can present only with irritability. Clinical findings include nuchal rigidity, hypertonia, brisk reflexes, asterixis, chorea, myoclonus, or seizures. If untreated, the child can progress to seizures, coma, or death. Clinical features are related to increase in serum sodium levels and also rapidity of increase in sodium level, as these determine the degree and rapidity of development of brain cell dehydration.

Evaluation

The first step is to assess the volume status of the patient. Assessment of plasma and urine osmolality may help in identification of underlying etiology of hypernatremia **(Flowchart 2)**.[17] Urine osmolality less than plasma osmolality indicates a concentrating defect, which denotes the possibility of excess urinary water losses. When urine osmolality is more than plasma osmolality, it indicates that such a child has

Flowchart 2: Urine and plasma osmolality in hypernatremia.[17]

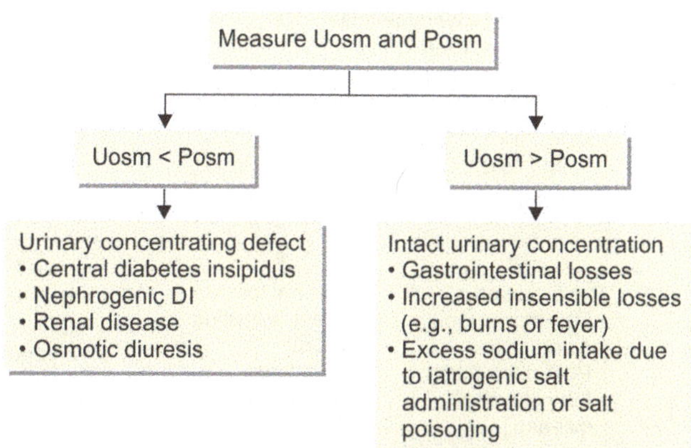

(DI: diabetes insipidus)

intact urinary concentrating mechanisms and points toward extrarenal causes for hypernatremia (gastrointestinal or skin water losses, or excess salt intake).

A detailed algorithm depicting approach to hypernatremia is given in **Flowchart 3.**[18]

Treatment

Treatment depends on the volume status, degree of hypernatremia, and rapidity of its development. Hypovolemia takes precedence over correction of sodium.

Hypovolemia with Hypernatremia

If the patient has significant volume depletion, the first step is to ensure cardiovascular stability. If the child has moderate to severe hypovolemia, initially isotonic fluid is given for fluid resuscitation in order to reinstate blood volume and organ perfusion. At the same time, it is important to avoid overzealous fluid resuscitation so that inadvertent volume overload and its associated cerebral edema can be prevented.

Free Water Correction

When hypernatremia is the sole abnormality, the goal is to correct sodium by replacing the free water deficit, which can be calculated by the formula:

Free water deficit in milliliters = 0.6 × weight × ([current plasma Na/140] – 1)

It can also be calculated by the formula:

Free water deficit in milliliters = (4 mL/kg) × (weight in kg) × (desired change in plasma Na)

This formula is based on the estimate that administration of 4 mL/kg of free water will reduce plasma sodium by roughly 1 mEq/L.

Free water can be delivered as isotonic fluids like half normal saline, 5% dextrose, or as enteral fluids. For children with chronic hypernatremia (plasma sodium ≥ 150 mEq/L for >24 hours) or those with acute severe hypernatremia (plasma sodium >160 mEq/L), the targeted reduction in plasma sodium should not exceed 0.5 mEq/L/h (i.e., 10–12 mEq/L/day). Too rapid treatment of hypernatremia is associated with a risk of cerebral edema.

Ongoing Losses and Maintenance Needs

Hypernatremia correction by the above formulae considers only free water losses that have already occurred up to the time of calculation. In addition, patients have normal maintenance needs and may also have ongoing excess free water losses not so far considered (e.g., continuing diarrhea or persistent fever). Children should receive maintenance fluids as well as replacement of these ongoing losses to prevent further derangements in plasma sodium level.

Clinical Case Scenario

A 3-year-old boy (weight 10 kg) recently diagnosed with DI came to emergency room (ER) with history of stopping medications for the last 5 days. His blood pressure was 100/60 mm Hg and he was apparently euvolemic. His serum sodium was 170 mEq/L.

In this case, free water deficit = 0.6 × weight × ([current plasma Na/140] – 1) = 0.6 × 10 × ([170/140] – 1) = 1,200 mL.

Since the current deficit is 30 mEq/L and the maximal rate of correction should be 10 mEq/L/day, this should be given over 3 days, i.e., 400 mL/day.

Another method of calculation is: Free water to be given over 24 hours = (4 mL/kg) × (weight in kg) × (desired change in plasma Na) = 4 × 10 × 10 = 400 mL/day.

In addition, ongoing losses and maintenance requirements needs to be replaced.

Hypervolemic Hypernatremia

It is important to avoid rapid administration of fluids as it may cause volume overload and pulmonary edema. Extra salt

Flowchart 3: Algorithmic approach to hypernatremia.[18]

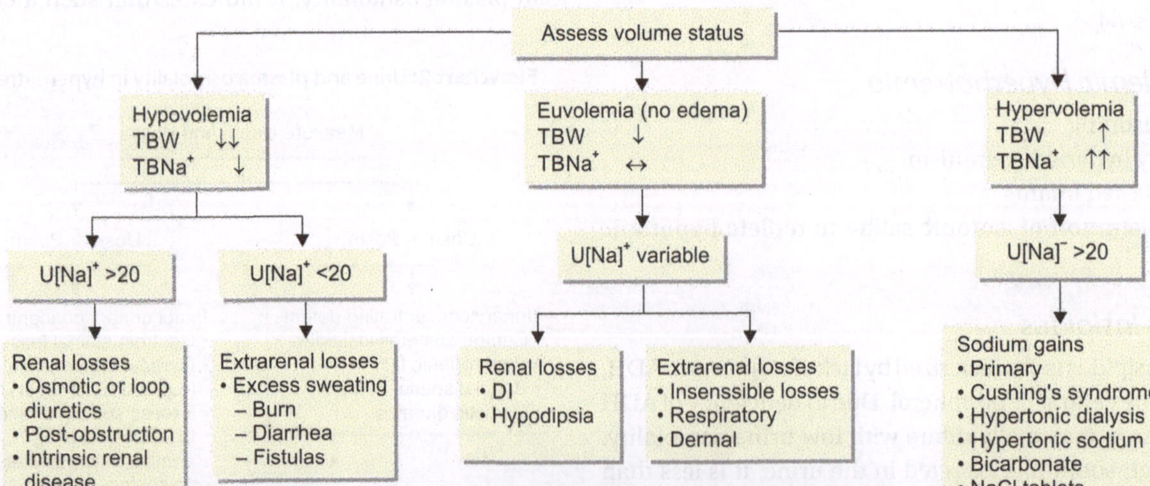

(DI: diabetes insipidus; TBW: total body water)

and water removal can be achieved by use of loop diuretics like furosemide. If there is concomitant renal failure, dialysis will be required.

Treatment of Specific Etiologies

Wherever a definite underlying long-term condition can be identified, such as central or nephrogenic DI, treatment of the etiologic disease should be initiated (e.g., treatment with desmopressin for central DI) in addition to providing free water replacement.

CONCLUSION

Abnormalities in serum sodium level are the most common electrolyte abnormalities in clinical practice and are sometimes multifactorial. Assessment of volume status is the key in managing such patients. Slow and steady correction with frequent laboratory monitoring and avoiding rapid fluctuations in serum sodium levels is paramount for optimal clinical outcomes.

KEY POINTS

- Sodium is the key determinant of serum osmolality and tonicity.
- Dysnatremias reflect disorders of water balance.
- The main manifestations of dysnatremias are related to CNS.
- Classification is based on volume status.
- Treatment depends on volume status, degree, and rapidity of development of dysnatremia.
- Too rapid correction can lead to ODS in hyponatremia and cerebral edema in hypernatremia.

REFERENCES

1. Harring TR, Deal NS, Kuo DC. Disorders of sodium and water balance. Emerg Med Clin N Am. 2014;32:379-401.
2. Dominguez M. (2017). Body Fluid Compartments. [online] Available from: https://step1.medbullets.com/renal/115003/body-fluid-compartments [Last accessed May, 2022].
3. Zieg J. Pathophysiology of hyponatremia in children. Front Pediatr. 2017;5:213.
4. Greenberg A, Rosner MH, Verbalis GJ. Advances in the management of patients with hyponatremia. American Journal of Medicine. Special CME edition.
5. Spasovski G, Vanholder R, Allolio B, Annane D, Ball S, Bichet D, et al. Clinical practice guideline on diagnosis and treatment of hyponatraemia. Eur J Endocrinol. 2014;170(3):G1-47.
6. Kelen G, Hsu E. Fluids and electrolytes. In: Tintinalli J (Ed). Tintinalli's Emergency Medicine: A Comprehensive Study Guide, 7th edition. New York: McGraw Hill Medical; 2011. pp. 117–21.
7. Kaplan LJ, Kellum JA. Fluids, pH, ions and electrolytes. Curr Opin Crit Care. 2010;16:323-31.
8. Saumers MJ, Traum AZ. Hyponatremia in children. Uptodate. 2018.
9. Hoorn EJ, Robert Zietse. Diagnosis and treatment of hyponatremia: compilation of the guidelines. J Am Soc Nephrol. 2017;28:1340-9.
10. Brenkert TE, Estrada CM, McMorrow SP, Abramo TJ. Intravenous hypertonic saline use in the pediatric emergency department. Pediatr Emerg Care. 2013;29:71.
11. Sterns RH, Cappuccio JD, Silver SM, Cohen EP. Neurologic sequelae after treatment of severe hyponatremia: a multicenter perspective. J Am Soc Nephrol. 1994;4:1522.
12. Berl T. Treating hyponatremia: damned if we do and damned if we don't. Kidney Int. 1990;37:1006.
13. Karp BI, Laureno R. Pontine and extrapontine myelinolysis: a neurologic disorder following rapid correction of hyponatremia. Medicine (Baltimore). 1993;72:359.
14. Sterns RH. Severe symptomatic hyponatremia: treatment and outcome. A study of 64 cases. Ann Intern Med. 1987;107:656.
15. Sterns RH, Riggs JE, Schochet SS Jr. Osmotic demyelination syndrome following correction of hyponatremia. N Engl J Med. 1986;314:1535-42.
16. Ayus JC, Krothapalli RK, Arieff AI. Treatment of symptomatic hyponatremia and its relation to brain damage. A prospective study. N Engl J Med. 1987;317:1190-5.
17. Saumers MJ, Traum AZ. Hypernatremia in children. Uptodate 2018.
18. Kim SW. Hypernatremia: successful treatment. Electrolyte Blood Press. 2006;4(2):66-71.

CHAPTER

4.3

Disorders of Potassium

Liji R, Suresh M

INTRODUCTION

Potassium is the major intracellular cation and its levels are crucial to normal homeostasis. Total body K^+ is approximately 40–50 mEq/kg. Of this 98% of exchangeable K^+ is intracellular and only 2% is in the extracellular fluid. The normal plasma concentration of K^+ is 3.5–5.3 mEq/L. The normal distribution between extracellular and intracellular compartments determines the resting membrane potential. Intracellular K^+ participates in various vital processes including cell growth, cell volume maintenance, acid-base balance, and synthetic and enzymatic functions.

POTASSIUM HOMEOSTASIS

Potassium balance is a function of intake and excretion. The homeostasis goal of the adult is to remain in zero K^+ balance. However, a positive K^+ balance is maintained in children to ensure somatic growth. The normal daily potassium requirement varies by age in children and is estimated at approximately 2 mEq/100 kcal of energy requirement throughout most of childhood. Approximately 90% of the daily K^+ intake is excreted in the urine, while 10% is excreted by the gastrointestinal tract.

In the setting of high dietary intake of potassium, normal kidney can maintain potassium homeostasis to a great extent. However, the adjustments in excretion occur over several hours, thus plasma K^+ concentrations may increase transiently that could adversely affect cell voltage. To minimize this body has developed a number of physiological mechanisms to shift K^+ into cells.

Internal Distribution of K^+

Insulin, sympathetic nervous system (via β_2-adrenergic receptors), and acid-base balance are the major determinants of the distribution of K^+ between the intracellular and the extracellular spaces. Factors that regulate potassium homeostasis are given in **Table 1**.

Insulin: Insulin increases the activity of Na-K-ATPase and thereby facilitates potassium uptake primarily in liver and muscles.

TABLE 1: Factors that regulate internal potassium balance.

Increase cell uptake of potassium	*Decrease cell uptake of potassium*
Physiologic factors: • Increase in plasma K^+ concentration • Insulin • β-agonists	*Physiologic factors:* • Decrease in plasma K^+ concentration • α-agonists
Pathologic factor: • Alkalosis	*Pathologic factors:* • Acidosis (normal anion gap >> high anion gap) • Hyperosmolality (enhances cell efflux of K^+) • Cell breakdown (enhances cell efflux of K^+)

Catecholamines: Epinephrine through β_2-receptors stimulates Na-K-ATPase activity and increases K uptake by the cells. However, its effect through the α-receptors is the reverse.[1,2]

Acid-base status: In acidosis, extracellular H^+ is buffered intracellularly and hence positive ions like K^+ from the cells moves into the extracellular fluid to maintain electroneutrality (for each 0.1 change in serum pH, K^+ changes in opposite direction by 0.6 mEq/L. But metabolic acidosis due to organic acids has little effect on serum potassium concentration.

Plasma osmolality: Increase in plasma tonicity by effective osmoles such as glucose in diabetic ketoacidosis (DKA), mannitol or sucrose causes potassium to move from intracellular fluid (ICF) to extracellular fluid (ECF) by solvent drag. However, hyperosmolality caused by solutes that readily cross the plasma membrane like urea does not cause hyperkalemia.

Renal Handling of Potassium

Potassium is freely filtered by the glomerulus and then avidly reabsorbed in the proximal tubule through the paracellular pathway and ascending limb of loop of Henle via $Na^+/K^+/2Cl^-$ cotransporter (NKCC2). Thus, only <10% of the filtered K^+ reaches the distal nephron.

Urinary K^+ excretion results from the secretion of K^+ along the aldosterone-sensitive distal nephron (ASDN). ASDN includes the last portion of the distal convoluted tubule (DCT2), connecting tubule, and collecting duct. This secretory component of K^+ handling is that which varies and is regulated according to physiologic needs.

K^+ secretion occurs via two types of apical K^+ channels: (1) renal outer medullary potassium channel (ROMK) (also called Kir1.1) in principal cells and Maxi-K or BK channels in principal and intercalated cells. The major drive for K^+ secretion is the transepithelial voltage that is oriented in the lumen-negative direction. Aldosterone-sensitive epithelial sodium channel (ENaC) in the principal cells reabsorbs Na which decreases the electropositivity of tubular fluid and facilitates K secretion. The flow-dependent K^+ secretion is mediated by BK channels, which are activated primarily by increase in fluid flow rate.

H-K-ATPase which couples K reabsorption to H^+ secretion in the α-intercalated cells, upregulates under conditions of K depletion to reabsorb K^+. In newborns and infants, there is limited expression of both ROMK and BK channels; however, the activity of H-K-ATPase in intercalated cells is similar to that of adults. This helps in achieving the positive K^+ balance needed for somatic growth and also contributes to the increased incidence of nonoliguric hyperkalemia in preterm infants.

Regulators of Renal K^+ Excretion

Regulators of renal K^+ excretion include:

- Luminal Na^+ delivery and flow rate:
  - Increased distal Na delivery increases sodium reabsorption by the ENaC channels thus creating lumen negativity which aids potassium secretion.
  - Increase in tubular flow rate activates flow-sensitive apical BK channels to secrete potassium and also dilutes luminal fluid K^+ thereby a concentration gradient is maintained for potassium secretion.[3]
- Plasma K^+ concentration
- Circulating aldosterone and arginine vasopressin levels
- Acid-base status

Distal convoluted tubule can alter the rate of K^+ secretion to adjust for the changes in plasma K^+ concentration. Increased plasma K^+ concentration causes depolarization in the proximal DCT through the K^+ channel Kir4.1/5.1. Increased intracellular Cl^- concentration due to the depolarization alters the WNK family of kinases and their regulatory proteins SPAK (Ste20-related proline alanine rich kinase) and OxSR1 (oxidative stress responsive kinase 1), thereby decreasing the activity of Na^+/Cl^- cotransporter (NCC). This resultant increases in Na^+ delivery and flow to the downstream ASDN along with increased aldosterone levels due to increased plasma K^+ drive leads to K^+ secretion. This effect is magnified during long-term high K^+ intake in which K^+ accumulates in the renal interstitium and inhibits Na^+ reabsorption in the thick ascending limb and proximal tubule, resulting in more delivery of Na^+ and flow to the ASDN.

Enteric Sensing of Potassium

K^+ entering the gastrointestinal tract can trigger K^+ secretion without a change in plasma K^+ concentration and aldosterone levels because there is an enteric K^+ sensing mechanism that results in inhibition of NCC activity.[4-6] This rapid natriuretic response to increased dietary K^+ is consistent with the BP lowering effects of K-rich diets. **Figure 1** shows the mechanisms by which kidneys increase potassium excretion following high potassium intake. A reduction in plasma K^+ concentration activates NCC activity. This effect causes salt retention and reduces Na^+ delivery and flow to downstream segments resulting in decreased K^+ secretion.

Aldosterone paradox: The ability of aldosterone to signal the kidney to increase salt retention without K secretion during conditions of volume depletion and stimulate K secretion without Na retention in hyperkalemia is referred to as *aldosterone paradox*. This can be explained by the fact that during volume depletion, there is increased proximal salt and water reabsorption leading to decreased distal Na delivery and decreased flow rate which retards K secretion even though serum aldosterone levels are high.[1] And in conditions where hyperkalemia occurs with normovolemia, direct effects of K^+ lead to inhibition of NCC channels and increased ROMK activity, thus increasing K secretion without Na retention.

HYPOKALEMIA

Hypokalemia is defined as serum potassium concentration, is <3.5 mEq/L. Degrees of hypokalemia are classified as following:[7]

- *Severe:* K^+ level <2.5 mEq/L
- *Moderate:* K^+ level between 2.5 and 3 mEq/L
- *Mild:* K^+ level between 3 and 3.5 mEq/L

Pathogenesis

Hypokalemia occurs due to one or a combination of the following mechanisms:

- Increase in intracellular shift of K^+ (total body K^+ content normal)
- *True potassium depletion (total K^+ body content reduced):*
  - Low potassium intake
  - Increase in loss of K^+:
    - Extrarenal loss via gastrointestinal tract or sweat
    - *Renal loss:* Typically results from increase in aldosterone activity or increased delivery of sodium to distal nephron

Etiology

- *Spurious hypokalemia:* Cells take up potassium when stored at room temperature
- *K^+ redistribution:*
  - Exogenous insulin
  - β-adrenergic agonists
  - Alkalosis

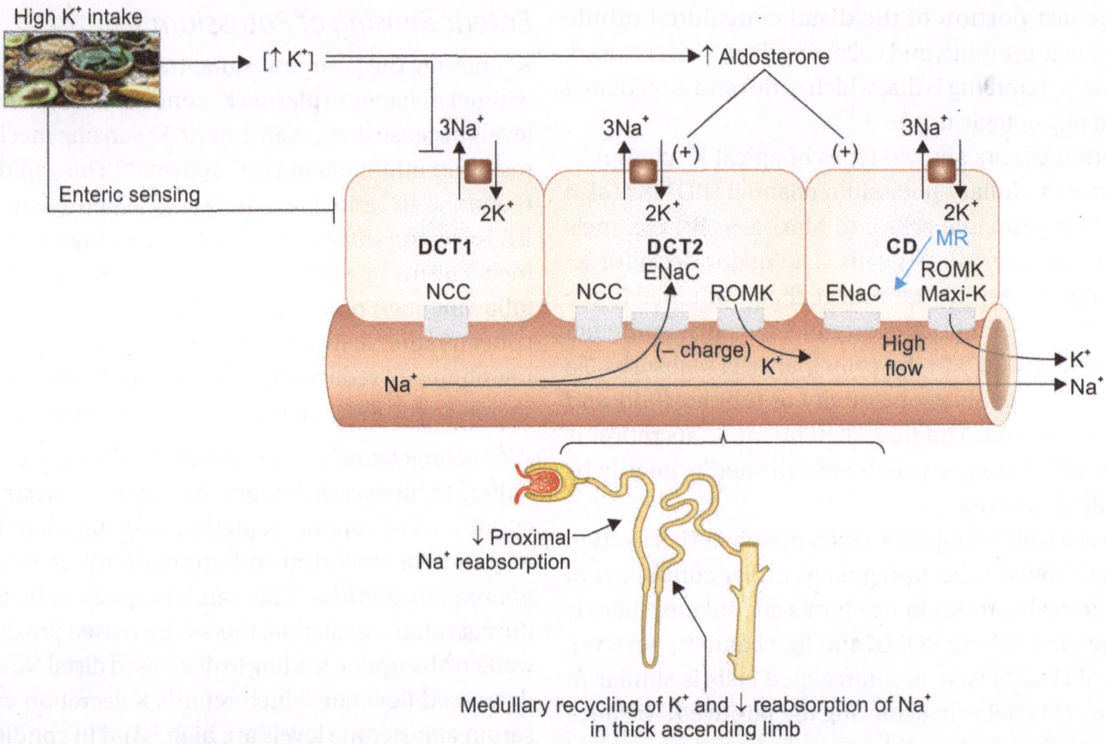

Fig. 1: Bases of the enormous capacity of the normal kidney to excrete K^+. K^+ secretion increases in DCT in response to small changes in plasma K^+ concentration. Long-term high K^+ intake results in K^+ accumulation in the renal interstitium which in turn decreases Na^+ reabsorption in the loop of Henle and proximal tubule. This results in more distal Na^+ delivery thereby further magnifying the K^+ excretion in DCT. The enteric K^+-sensing mechanism inhibits of NCC in DCT when K^+ enters into the gastrointestinal tract, thus augmenting urinary K^+ excretion. (CD: collecting duct; DCT1: proximal portion of distal convoluted tubule; DCT2: distal portion of distal convoluted tubule—aldosterone sensitivity begins here; ENaC: epithelial sodium channel; MR: mineralocorticoid receptor; K^+: potassium; Na^+: sodium; $3Na^+/2K^+$ pump: Na^+/K^+-adenosine triphosphatase; ROMK: renal outer medullary potassium channel)

TABLE 2: Gastrointestinal conditions associated with hypokalemia.

Associated with alkalosis	*Associated with acidosis*	*Acid-base balance unpredictable*
• Vomiting • Nasogastric suction • Congenital chloride diarrhea	• Biliary drainage • Intestinal fistula • Malabsorption • Diarrhea • Radiation enteropathy • Ureterosigmoidoscopy	• Laxatives • Clay ingestion • K^+ binding resin

- Hypokalemic periodic paralysis
- Hyperthyroidism
- Anabolism (treatment of pernicious anemia)
- Barium[8] and chloroquine intoxication, cesium salts

■ *Poor K^+ intake:* It occurs in children with protein energy malnutrition along with hypomagnesemia

■ *Extrarenal K^+ losses:*
- Gastrointestinal conditions **(Table 2)**
- *Skin conditions:* Burns and cystic fibrosis[9]

■ *Renal K^+ loss:*
- Increased aldosterone activity (associated with elevated BP) **(Table 3)**
- Increased sodium delivery to distal nephron **(Table 4)**

TABLE 3: Conditions associated with hypokalemia following renal K loss and hypertension.

Low renin and low aldosterone	*Low renin and high/N aldosterone*	*N/high renin*
• Cushing disease • Congenital adrenal hyperplasia (11-β- or 17-α-hydroxylase deficiency) • Apparent mineralocorticoid excess (defect in 11-β-hydroxysteroid dehydrogenase) • Licorice-ingestion (11-β-hydroxysteroid dehydrogenase blockade) • Liddle syndrome (congenitally increased function of the ENaC channels) • Exogenous mineralocorticoids	• Primary aldosteronism (either hyperplasia or adenoma) • Dexamethasone-responsive aldosteronism (synthesis of aldosterone promoted not only by renin but also by adrenocorticotropin)	• Renal artery stenosis • Malignant hypertension • Renin producing tumor

(ENaC: epithelial sodium channel)

TABLE 4: Conditions associated with hypokalemia following renal K loss due to increased distal sodium delivery.

With acidosis	*With alkalosis*	*Others*
• Renal tubular acidosis (type I or II) • Carbonic anhydrase inhibitors • Amphotericin B • Outdated tetracyclines	• Bartter syndrome • Gitelman syndrome • Loop and thiazide diuretics • Magnesium depletion • Nonreabsorbable anions—high dose of antibiotics such as penicillin, ampicillin, carbenicillin, ticarcillin	• Tubulointerstitial nephritis • Postobstructive diuresis • Recovering AKI • Hypercalcemia

(AKI: acute kidney injury)

- *Others:*
  - Dialysis
  - Plasmapheresis
  - *Drugs:* Risperidone, quetiapine, and chloroquine[10,11]

Pathophysiology

Salient mechanisms associated with the common causes of hypokalemia are mentioned in detail here.

Hypokalemic periodic paralysis is a disorder characterized by muscle weakness or paralysis due to the sudden movement of potassium into the cells. The attacks are precipitated by rest after exercise, high carbohydrate meals, and events accompanied by increased release of insulin or catecholamines. This disorder may be familial or acquired.

Familial periodic paralysis is an autosomal dominant disorder due to the mutation in the gene encoding α-subunit of the dihydropyridine sensitive calcium channel in skeletal muscles. The precise mechanism of K^+ influx is not clear.

The acquired form is associated with thyrotoxicosis. Excess thyroid hormone increases the activity of Na^+-K^+-ATPase activity of the skeletal muscle cells increasing the potassium influx. The acute attacks are treated with intravenous (IV) KCl and propranolol.

Vomiting: Gastric juice contains only 5–10 mEq/L of potassium. Potassium depletion in vomiting is primarily due to increased urinary losses along with the bicarbonaturia associated with metabolic alkalosis due to vomiting. Volume depletion may also increase aldosterone-mediated K secretion in distal tubule.

Diarrhea: Potassium depletion in diarrhea is mainly due to increased gastrointestinal losses. Diarrheal stool contains about 20–50 mEq/L of K^+.[12] However, in case of severe volume depletion the associated α-adrenergic surge will drive K^+ out of cells, thus hypokalemia will not be apparent until after therapy with fluids is initiated.

Diuretics: Thiazides causes more renal K wasting compared to loop diuretics despite its low natriuretic effect. This is because hypercalciuria due to loop diuretics inhibits the ENaC channel and increases lumen positivity thereby restricting K secretion.

Renal tubular acidosis: In distal renal tubular acidosis (RTA), the acidosis inhibits proximal Na^+ handling thereby increasing the distal Na^+ delivery. Hypokalemia normally upregulate activity of the Na^+-K^+-ATPase pump in α-intercalated cells to reabsorb K^+. However, failure to increase pump activity in distal RTA would further increase K^+ wasting.

In proximal RTA, the threshold for bicarbonate reabsorption is decreased resulting in self-limiting bicarbonaturia ($NaHCO_3$). Increased distal delivery of sodium together with increased aldosterone due to volume depletion results in K wasting. When plasma HCO_3 concentration reaches the reduced tubular maximum, bicarbonaturia decreases and K^+ wasting decreases. However, treatment with alkali worsens the hypokalemia because with increase in plasma HCO_3 the distal delivery of $NaHCO_3$ is again increased.

Amphotericin B: Amphotericin B alters the membrane permeability in collecting duct cells causing back diffusion of H^+ from lumen into cells and increased K^+ secretion.[13]

Hypomagnesemia: Mg^{2+} inhibits ROMK-mediated K^+ secretion in the distal nephron, an effect that is overcome by aldosterone-mediated Na^+ entry through ENaC causing cell depolarization. Low Mg^{2+} causes increased renal K^+ excretion causing refractory hypokalemia until the Mg^{2+} deficit is repaired.

Nonreabsorbable anions: In clinical situations where nonreabsorbable anions are excreted in urine, the concomitant increase in distal Na^+ delivery leads to marked increase in potassium excretion. The effect of these anions is likely to be prominent when there is concurrent volume depletion causing high aldosterone levels. The nonreabsorbable anions include bicarbonate in vomiting or proximal RTA, β-hydroxybutyrate in DKA, hippurate following toluene use (glue sniffing), or a penicillin derivative in patients receiving high-dose penicillin therapy.

Symptoms

Hypokalemia causes cell membrane hyperpolarization, rendering the cell less sensitive to excitation which leads to muscle weakness and cardiovascular abnormalities.

Mild hypokalemia may be asymptomatic. Moderate hypokalemia causes muscular weakness, myalgia, and paralytic ileus. Flaccid paralysis, hyporeflexia or respiratory depression may occur with more severe hypokalemia. Rhabdomyolysis may occur with profound hypokalemia with serum potassium <2 mEq/L. Under normal circumstances, exercise is associated with movement of K^+ into the interstitial space which causes rapid vasodilation, allowing increased blood flow to the exercising muscle. Thus, decreased total body K^+ may limit the vasodilation in exercising muscle and causes muscle break down.

Electrocardiographic (ECG) findings of hypokalemia include ST depression, appearance of U wave, decrease in T wave amplitude, ectopic activity, and arrhythmias such as heart block, supraventricular tachycardia (SVT), bigeminy, and ventricular tachycardia.

Hypokalemia may limit the concentrating ability of the kidney resulting in polyuria and polydipsia. Chronic hypokalemia can cause a chronic tubulointerstitial nephritis, referred to as kaliopenic nephropathy, which is characterized by the formation of small renal cysts, polyuria, proteinuria, and renal failure. Histologically there is tubular atrophy, interstitial infiltration with macrophages, and interstitial fibrosis.

Diagnosis

The cause of hypokalemia can be often determined with knowledge of the clinical setting, volume status, acid-base balance, and urine electrolyte levels. The common causes of hypokalemia in children are acute gastroenteritis and intake of medicines causing hypokalemia.

History

- *History of polyuria, failure to thrive, recurrent dehydration:* Tubular disorders
- *Family history of episodic muscle weakness:* Hypokalemic periodic paralysis
- *Symptoms of hyperthyroidism (weight loss, heat intolerance, tremor, palpitations, anxiety, and increased frequency of bowel movements):* Thyrotoxic periodic paralysis

Physical Examination

- *Cardiac rate and rhythm:* To screen for arrhythmias
- Muscle strength, tone, and reflexes
- Effective circulating volume, blood pressure, and respiratory (acid-base) status
  - *Dehydration:* RTA, Bartter syndrome, and Gitelman syndrome
  - *High BP:* Liddle syndrome, apparent mineralocorticoid excess (AME), increased renin and/or aldosterone

Investigations

The following tests may be used in the evaluation of hypokalemia:

24-hour urine K concentration: A 24-hour urinary K^+ of <15 mEq/L suggests an extrarenal cause of hypokalemia.

Transtubular K^+ gradient (TTKG): The main limitation of a spot urine K^+ is its variation with urinary concentration. Two patients with similar renal K^+ excretion would have significantly different urine K^+ concentrations depending on whether the urine was concentrated or dilute. TTKG is designed to overcome this variance and is calculated using the formula:

$$TTKG = (\text{Urine K} \times \text{plasma osmolality})/(\text{plasma K} \times \text{urine osmolality})$$

This calculation requires the urine Na^+ concentration to be at least 25 mEq/L and urine osmolality at least equal to plasma osmolality. TTKG estimates the ratio of potassium in the lumen of the cortical collecting duct to that in the peritubular capillaries at a point where tubular fluid is isotonic relative to plasma. In a patient with hypokalemia, a value of <3 is consistent with an appropriate kidney response to the disorder whereas a value >7 indicates potassium wasting by the kidneys.

Transtubular K^+ gradient has fallen out of favor in recent years, since its calculation assumes negligible absorption of osmoles distal to the cortical collecting duct, thus not accounting for the significant urea and Na^+ reabsorption which occurs in the downstream medulla.

Spot Urine K^+/Creatinine Ratio

Spot urine K^+/creatinine ratio takes advantage of the near constant rate of urinary secretion of creatinine and corrects for the variability in urine concentration. A ratio of <15 mEq/g (<1.5 mEq/mmol) is considered an appropriate response to extrarenal potassium loss or potassium shift into cells. Ratio >15 mg/g suggests renal wasting of potassium.

Urine Chloride Excretion

In patients with hypokalemic metabolic alkalosis and low or normal BP, urinary chloride excretion helps to differentiate between renal and extrarenal causes. In renal causes like Bartter syndrome, urine chloride will be >20 mEq/L whereas in extrarenal causes like vomiting, urine chloride will be <10 mEq/L.

Diagnostic Approach to the Etiology of Hypokalemia

The diagnostic approach to a patient with chronic hypokalemia is given in **Flowchart 1**.

- Obtain a random spot urine potassium to creatinine ratio:
  - *Low urinary potassium excretion:* A spot urine potassium to creatinine ratio of <15 mEq/g (<1.5 mEq/mmol) suggests extrarenal losses of potassium like gastrointestinal loss, inadequate intake or transcellular shifts.
  - *High urinary potassium excretion:* A spot urine potassium to creatinine ratio of >15 mEq/g (>1.5 mEq/mmol) suggests the renal loss of potassium.
- *Children with high urinary potassium excretion:* Assess the effective arteriolar volume status and blood pressure

Flowchart 1: Approach to a child with chronic hypokalemia.

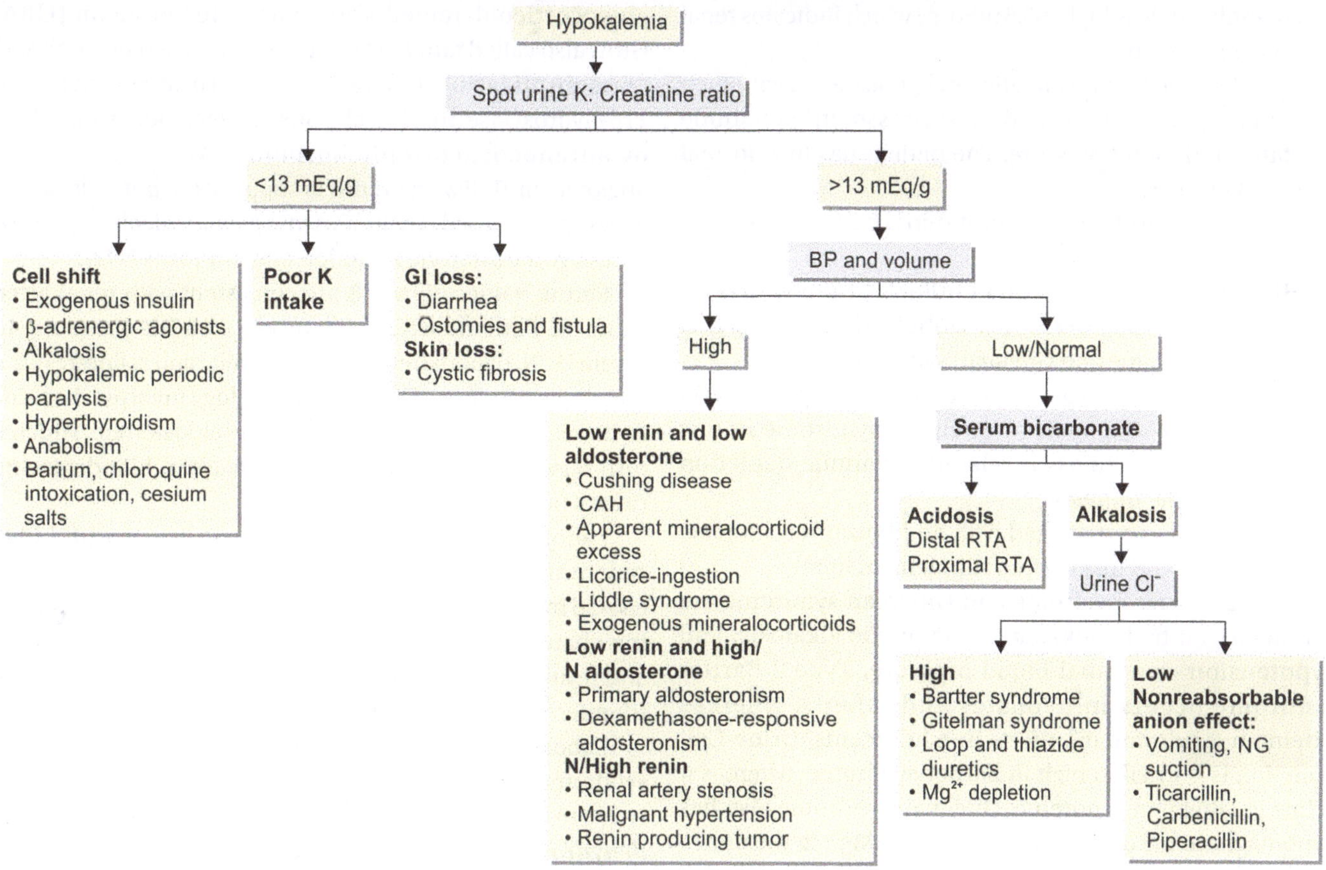

(CAH: congenital adrenal hyperplasia; GI: gastrointestinal; NG: nasogastric; RTA: renal tubular acidosis)

- *Children with high urinary potassium and hypertension (HTN):* Measure the plasma renin activity and aldosterone levels
  - *Low renin and low aldosterone* may suggest Cushing disease, congenital adrenal hyperplasia, AME, Liddle syndrome, exogenous mineralocorticoids
  - *Low renin and high or normal aldosterone* may suggest primary aldosteronism, dexamethasone-responsive aldosteronism
  - *Normal or high renin* may suggest renal artery stenosis, malignant HTN, renin producing tumor
- Children with high urinary potassium and low or normal blood pressure—obtain blood gas analysis
  - *Acidosis* may suggest renal tubular acidosis, DKA
  - *Alkalosis* may suggest:
    - *Urinary chloride >20 mEq/L:* Bartter syndrome and Gitelman syndrome
    - *Urinary chloride <10–15 mEq/L:* Emesis, nasogastric (NG) losses, congenital chloride, diarrhea, cystic fibrosis, and drugs
  - *No acid-base disturbance* may suggest hypomagnesemia, osmotic effect (nonketotic)

Case 1

A 12-year-old male presents with complaints of severe muscle weakness and dizziness. He is not on any medications. His BP is 96/62 mm Hg with orthostatic change. His laboratory results are:

Serum	Urine
Na: 135 mEq/L	Na: 110 mEq/L
K: 2.9 mEq/L	K: 70 mEq/L
Cl: 85 mEq/L	Cl: 35 mEq/L
HCO_3: 30 mEq/L	Ca_2: 20 mg/dL
Ca_2: 8.9 mg/dL	Creatinine: 110 mg/dL
Mg_2: 1.0 mg/dL	
Blood pH: 7.48	

Which one of the following disorders is the most likely diagnosis in this patient?

A. Bartter syndrome with mutation in ROMK channel (type 2)
B. Liddle syndrome
C. Gitelman syndrome
D. Surreptitious vomiting
E. Mineralocorticoid excess syndrome

Approach to Diagnosis

- He has hypokalemic metabolic alkalosis with hypomagnesemia.

- In spite of the hypokalemia, his urinary potassium to creatinine ratio is high (63.6 mEq/g) which indicates renal loss of potassium.
- The next step in the evaluation of hypokalemia with high urinary potassium excretion is assessment of volume status and blood pressure. The patient has low normal blood pressure.
- In the absence of HTN, the next step is blood gas analysis which shows alkalosis.
- High urinary chloride of 35 mEq/L in the setting of hypokalemic alkalosis suggests tubular disorders such as Bartter syndrome and Gitelman syndrome
- The presence of hypomagnesemia and hypocalciuria suggests the diagnosis of Gitelman syndrome in this patient. His dizziness is related to volume depletion caused by Na^+ diuresis.
- The patient was managed with ad libitum NaCl intake, potassium, and magnesium supplementation.

Type 2 Bartter syndrome and Gitelman syndrome are characterized by hypokalemia, metabolic alkalosis, and hypotension or normal blood pressure. Type 2 Bartter syndrome occurs in neonates and infants, whereas Gitelman syndrome manifests in adolescents. Urine Ca^{2+} excretion is normal to high in Bartter syndrome, whereas it is low in Gitelman syndrome. Gitelman syndrome also has hypomagnesemia due to increased loss of Mg^{2+} in the urine.

Case 2

Match the patients all with hypertension and hypokalemic metabolic alkalosis and their clinical diagnoses.

Case	*Na*	*Renin*	*Aldosterone*
1	↑	↓	↑
2	N/↑	↓	↑
3	↓	↑	↑
4	N/↑	↓	↓
5	N/↑	↓	↓

A. Primary aldosteronism
B. Glucocorticoid remediable aldosteronism (GRA)
C. Renal artery stenosis
D. Liddle syndrome
E. Apparent mineralocorticoid excess syndrome

Answers: 1: A; 2: B; 3: C; 4: D; 5: E

Serum values of case 1 are consistent with primary aldosteronism. Primary aldosteronism is associated with low renin and high aldosterone levels. High aldosterone is autonomously produced by adrenal adenoma or adrenal hyperplasia. Aldosterone promotes Na^+ reabsorption causing volume-dependent HTN and K^+ and H^+ secretion in the distal nephron resulting in hypokalemia and metabolic alkalosis. Plasma renin level is low because of volume expansion. Spironolactone or amiloride is the drug of choice for HTN management.

Laboratory values of case 2 are consistent with the glucocorticoid-remediable hyperaldosteronism (GRA). GRA, also called familial GRA type 1, is caused by a chimeric gene duplication between aldosterone synthase and 11β-hydroxylase. In GRA, aldosterone secretion is stimulated by adrenocorticotropic hormone (ACTH) and not by angiotensin II. Plasma renin is suppressed, but aldosterone levels are increased. Treatment with glucocorticoid suppresses excessive aldosterone secretion and improves HTN.

Serum values of case 3 are consistent with renal artery stenosis. Patients with renal artery stenosis present with severe HTN, hyponatremia, hypokalemia, and saline-resistant metabolic alkalosis. The pathophysiology involves that renal ischemia increases renin-angiotensin-aldosterone, which in turn raises blood pressure. This increase in blood pressure causes pressure natriuresis.

Laboratory values of case 4 are consistent with Liddle syndrome, which is an autosomal dominant disorder. It is caused by gain of function mutation of the ENaC. Activation of this channel increases Na^+ reabsorption, K^+ and H^+ excretion and results in low-renin-aldosterone HTN. HTN responds to triamterene or amiloride, but not to spironolactone.

Laboratory values shown in case 5 are consistent with the syndrome of AME, which is an autosomal recessive disorder. It is due to loss-of-function mutation in the *11β-hydroxysteroid dehydrogenase type 2 (11βHSD2)* gene which converts cortisol to the inactive cortisone in renal tubular cells. As a result, cortisol accumulates in renal tubular cells and causes increased Na^+ reabsorption, hypokalemic metabolic alkalosis, and low-renin-aldosterone HTN by its mineralocorticoid activity. Suppression of renin and aldosterone is due to volume excess caused by Na^+ and water retention. HTN responds to salt restriction, amiloride, or triamterene but not to regular doses of spironolactone. Licorice ingestion causes acquired AME.

Case 3

A 14-year-old boy presents with sudden onset generalized weakness and inability to walk. Despite a good appetite, he has lost 4.5 kg in 2 months. His past and family history are unremarkable. In examination, pulse 114 beats/min, BP 138/70 mm Hg, thin built, moist skin, thyroid—palpable and tender, deep tendon reflexes—absent and sensory system—normal.

Laboratory values: Sodium 140 mEq/L, potassium 2.0 mEq/L, chloride 100 mEq/L, bicarbonate 24 mEq/L, blood urea nitrogen (BUN) 10 mg/dL, and creatinine 1.0 mg/dL.

Which one of the following set of urine electrolytes (in mEq/L) would be most consistent with this patient's most likely underlying disorder?

A. Na: 109; K: 10; Cl: 97
B. Na: 60; K: 40, Cl: <10
C. Na: <10; K: 17; Cl: 85

D. Na: 75; K: 52; Cl: 141
E. Na: <10; K: 55; Cl: <10

The correct answer is A.
The patient has thyrotoxic periodic paralysis. Tachycardia, weight loss, and thyromegaly suggest hyperthyroidism. The renal response to the intracellular shift of K is to maximally decrease urinary K excretion. Since the extracellular fluid volume is normal, the urinary Na and Cl are not low and reflect dietary NaCl intake.

The values in choice B (low urine Cl) reflect renal K wasting due to the effect of nonreabsorbable anion, e.g., chronic vomiting.

The urinary K is appropriately low in choice C; however, the low Na and increased urine Cl is suggestive of chronic diarrhea. Increased urine Cl in chronic diarrhea is due to increased urinary excretion of NH_4Cl.

Choice D shows evidence of renal K wasting and concomitant renal Na and Cl wasting is suggestive of ongoing loop or thiazide diuretic use.

The urine K in choice E also suggests renal K wasting. In addition, the low urinary Na and Cl are typical of a patient with volume contraction.

Treatment

The goals of hypokalemia treatment are:
- Treat or prevent life-threatening complications such as cardiac arrhythmias and respiratory muscle weakness
- Correct the potassium deficit
- Treat the underlying cause

Potassium Deficit Correction

The rapidity of potassium supplementation is dependent on the severity of hypokalemia and the presence or absence of symptoms.

Intravenous Potassium

- In the presence of arrhythmias, severe muscle weakness, or respiratory distress, IV KCl should be administered with cardiac monitoring. Oral potassium can be started after stabilizing the serum potassium level.
- The dose of IV KCl is 0.5–1.0 mEq/kg usually given over 1 hour with ECG monitoring, up to a maximum rate of 20 mEq/h. IV potassium should never be administered as bolus since it may cause fatal arrhythmias.
- The peripheral IV concentration should not exceed 40 mEq/L since higher doses may cause phlebitis. Higher concentrations up to 60–80 mEq/L require central veins preferably femoral vein since internal jugular and subclavian routes can cause an acute local rise in K^+ affecting cardiac conduction.
- Avoid dextrose or bicarbonate containing fluids for KCl infusion which may promote intracellular shift of potassium.[14] Also avoid drugs causing hypokalemia such as salbutamol and diuretics.

Oral Potassium

- Symptomatic hypokalemia should be treated with pharmacologic therapy rather than only increasing dietary intake of potassium-rich foods. Oral potassium supplements are available as chloride, phosphate, citrate, gluconate, and bicarbonate salts.
- Use of potassium chloride is preferred in patients with hypokalemia, with associated hypochloremia and metabolic alkalosis. The oral dose of KCl is 0.5–1.5 mEq/kg/dose (maximum 40 mEq/dose), should be given with or just after food to prevent gastric irritation. Potklor syrup contains 20 mEq of K^+ and Cl^-/15 mL solution.
- Potassium bicarbonate and citrate may enhance potassium excretion by increasing bicarbonate excretion; hence, they are not a replacement of choice except in conditions with concomitant metabolic acidosis. Potrate and K-Cit are commercial oral solutions that have 2 mEq of K and HCO_3/mL.
- Potassium phosphate should be considered in patients with both hypokalemia and hypophosphatemia, such as in Fanconi syndrome, DKA, and refeeding syndrome.
- *Refractory hypokalemia*: Serum magnesium should be checked and hypomagnesemia if present, should be treated. The initial dose of IV magnesium sulfate is 50 mg/kg/dose (maximum 2 g) administered over 2 hours and the dose can be repeated if hypomagnesemia persists. Unless magnesium replacement is provided, hypokalemia would not get corrected.
- *Hypokalemia associated with metabolic acidosis:* Avoid correcting acidosis until the serum K reaches approximately 3.0 mEq/L, as correction of acidosis with sodium bicarbonate worsens hypokalemia by driving the K into cells.

HYPERKALEMIA

Hyperkalemia is defined in children and adults as a potassium level >5.5 mEq/L and >6 mEq/L in newborns.

Pathogenesis

Hyperkalemia occurs due to one or a combination of the following mechanisms:
- Increase in extracellular shift of K^+ (total body K^+ content normal)
- *True potassium accretion (total K^+ body content increased):*
  - High potassium intake
  - *Impaired renal K^+ excretion*: Due to reduced filtration or impaired K^+ secretion secondary to reduced distal delivery of Na or impaired activity of Renin-angiotensin-aldosterone system (RAAS).

Etiology

- *Spurious hyperkalemia:*
  - Mechanical trauma during venepuncture
  - Cooling of blood after venepuncture

TABLE 5: Conditions associated with hyperkalemia and impaired renin-aldosterone activity.

Hyperreninemic hypoaldosteronism	*Hyporeninemic hypoaldosteronism*	*Pseudohypoaldosteronism*	
		Primary	***Secondary***
• Adrenal insufficiency (Addison disease) • Salt-losing congenital adrenal hyperplasia (21-hydroxylase deficiency)	• Idiopathic • Complicating acute glomerulonephritis • Mild-to-moderate renal failure (commonly diabetic nephropathy)	• *Type 1 (cortical collecting tubule):* – *Autosomal recessive:* Reduced ENaC activity – *Autosomal dominant:* Mutations in the mineralocorticoid receptor; phenotype—mild and transient • *Type 2 (DCT1):* Familial hyperkalemic hypertension or Gordon syndrome	• Complicating obstructive uropathy (with or without UTI) • SLE • Sickle cell disease • Renal transplantation • Renal amyloidosis

(ENaC: epithelial sodium channel; SLE: systemic lupus erythematosus)

- Hereditary spherocytosis, mutation in red blood cell (RBC) anion exchanger 1 (AE1)
- *Cellular efflux:* Severe leukocytosis and thrombocytosis

▪ *Transcellular shift:*
- Metabolic acidosis (mineral and less so with organic acidosis)
- α-adrenergic stimulation
- Hypertonicity (hyperglycemia, mannitol, and sucrose)
- Tissue injury (rhabdomyolysis, hemolysis, and tumor lysis)
- Hyperkalemic periodic paralysis
- *Drugs*: Digoxin overdose, succinylcholine, and β-blockers
- Hyperkalemia of premature infant

▪ *Increased potassium load*

▪ *Decreased renal excretion:*
- *Decreased filtration (and secretion):* Advanced renal insufficiency—acute or chronic
- *Decreased distal sodium delivery:*
  - Severe volume depletion
  - Congestive cardiac failure
- Impaired activity of renin-angiotensin-aldosterone axis (**Table 5**)
- *Drugs decreasing the activity RAAS axis:* List of drugs causing hyperkalemia is given in **Box 1**.

BOX 1: Drugs causing hyperkalemia.

- *Drugs inhibiting renin release:*
  - Nonsteroidal anti-inflammatory drugs
  - *Calcineurin inhibitors*: Cyclosporine, tacrolimus
- *Inhibition of aldosterone release from the adrenal:*
  - Heparin
  - Ketoconazole
- *Drugs which interfere with RAAS:*
  - Angiotensin-converting enzyme inhibitors like enalapril
  - Angiotensin receptor blockers like losartan
- *Mineralocorticoid receptor blockade:*
  - Spironolactone
  - Eplerenone
- *Blockade of epithelial sodium channel:*
  - Amiloride
  - Triamterene
  - Trimethoprim

(RAAS: renin-angiotensin-aldosterone system)

Pathophysiology

Salient mechanisms associated with the common causes of hyperkalemia are mentioned in detail here.

Pseudohyperkalemia or spurious hyperkalemia refers to a condition in which the increased K^+ concentration is due to K^+ movement out of the cells during or after the blood specimen is drawn.

Insulin deficiency may result in mild hyperkalemia as insulin normally promotes potassium entry into the cells. However, the associated hyperglycemia and hyperosmolality in uncontrolled diabetes mellitus also cause pulling of water out of the cells and parallel movement of potassium into the extracellular fluid.

Tissue catabolism as in trauma, tumor lysis syndrome, rhabdomyolysis, or hemolysis can result in hyperkalemia, especially if there is coexisting renal failure. Hyperkalemia is often associated with hyperphosphatemia, hyperuricemia, and high urea due to release of intracellular phosphate, nucleic acids, and proteins, respectively.

Hyperkalemic periodic paralysis or Gamstrop disease is a rare autosomal dominant disease due to the mutation in the α-subunit of skeletal muscle Na channel gene (*SCN4A*). The condition is associated with flaccid paralysis often associated with increased potassium intake, exposure to cold, and rest after strenuous exercise.

Whole blood transfusion: Potassium is gradually released from RBCs of stored blood, resulting in an extracellular K concentration of up to 30 mEq/L by 21 days in the stored blood. Use of packed red cells (which almost eliminates plasma) or fresh whole blood will minimize this risk.

Renal failure: In acute kidney injury (AKI), acute decrease in glomerular filtration rate (GFR) causes decreased distal delivery of Na^+ and results in decreased K secretion. This is more pronounced in oliguric AKI. Rapid loss of GFR in AKI does not give enough time for normal adaptive mechanisms to come into force.

Hyperkalemia develops slowly in chronic kidney disease (CKD) because the remaining nephrons augment their K^+ secreting capacity and becomes usually evident when the GFR falls below 10 mL/min. Two other defenses against hyperkalemia are the rapid shift of K into the cells after K^+ load and increased colonic excretion of potassium in CKD.

Severe volume depletion can result in hyperkalemia due to decreased delivery of Na^+ to distal nephrons and impaired K entry into the cells. Hyperkalemia is a frequent associated finding of impaired effective circulation in critically ill infants and young children.[15]

Pseudohypoaldosteronism: The autosomal dominant type of pseudohypoaldosteronism (PHA type 1a) is due to loss of function mutation of mineralocorticoid receptor gene (*MRL* gene). The disorder is renal limited and is known to improve with age (2–3 years) due to alternative pathway of K secretion in the distal nephron and with increased oral salt intake. The autosomal recessive type of PHA (type 1b) is due to defect in ENaC that is present in kidneys, colon, lungs, sweat, and salivary glands. This disorder is severe and persists lifelong and is associated with increased sweating and recurrent respiratory infections. Both types of PHA type 1 have markedly elevated plasma renin and aldosterone levels and fail to respond to exogenous mineralocorticoids.

The second type of PHA is PHA type 2 or Gordon's syndrome/familial hyperkalemic hypertension (FHH) which is an autosomal dominant condition, characterized by salt sensitive HTN, hyperkalemia, and nonanion gap metabolic acidosis. This syndrome is due to the mutations in protein kinases WNK1 and WNK4 which result in increased expression of NaCl cotransporter (NCCT) in DCT. Hyperkalemia and HTN in Gordon syndrome are particularly responsive to thiazide diuretics.

Obstructive uropathy: Hyperkalemia occurs due to decreased flow through the renal tubules and collecting duct dysfunction due to chronic obstruction. Patient may sometimes remain hyperkalemic for several weeks following relief of obstruction due to tubular dysfunction.

Sickle cell disease: In children with sickle cell disease and renal tubular injury, there is impaired medullary blood flow and impaired aldosterone sensitivity which leads to reduced urinary potassium excretion.

Pyelonephritis predisposes to hyperkalemia in infants. The interstitial inflammation due to pyelonephritis exacerbates the decrease response to aldosterone that is normally seen in young infants, thus causing decrease in potassium excretion.[16]

Symptoms

Symptoms or signs of hyperkalemia usually tend to occur only with very high potassium levels (>7 mEq/L). Hyperkalemia causes a depolarizing effect on the heart, giving rise to ECG changes **(Fig. 2)**. The usual range of serum/plasma potassium levels in mEq/L and the corresponding ECG changes are:

- *5.5–6.5:* Tall peaked T waves with narrow base and shortening of QT interval
- *6.5–8.0:* Peaked T waves, prolonged PR interval, widening QRS complex, decreased or disappearing P wave, and amplified R wave
- *>8.0:* Absent P wave, bundle branch block, progressive widening of QRS complex that eventually merges with the T wave to form a sinusoidal pattern. This is followed by ventricular fibrillation or asystole.

Hyperkalemia-induced arrhythmias include sinus bradycardia, sinus arrest, ventricular tachycardia, ventricular fibrillation, and asystole.

Hyperkalemia can also lead to neuromuscular manifestations such as paresthesias, fasciculations in the arms and legs, and in some patients may present with muscle weakness and ascending paralysis. Hyperkalemia impairs urinary acidification by lowering the renal ammonium production which serves as a urinary buffer.

Diagnosis

First, exclude spurious hyperkalemia, the most common cause of elevated potassium in asymptomatic and well grown children. This can be differentiated from true hyperkalemia by a normal repeat potassium level that should be obtained from a free flowing venous blood sample to reduce the risk of hemolysis. Then evaluate for the common causes of increased potassium in children such as metabolic acidosis and intake of medicine causing hyperkalemia.

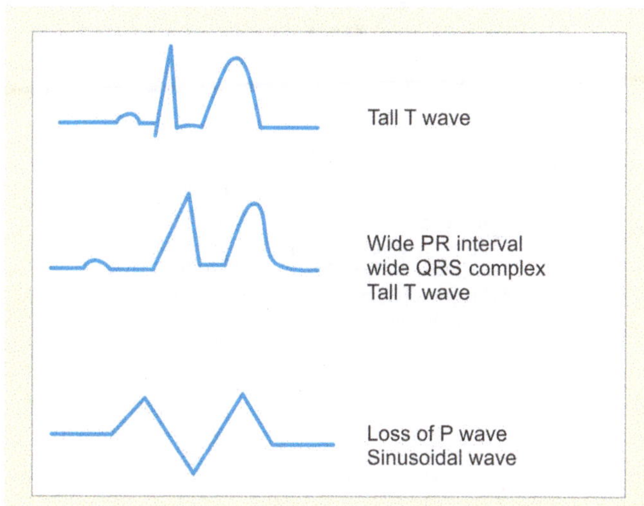

Fig. 2: Electrocardiographic (ECG) changes in hyperkalemia.

The detailed approach to a child with hyperkalemia discussed here.

History

- *Dietary intake:* Potassium rich foods, salt substitutes
- Kidney disease
- Voiding history for obstructive uropathy
- History of polyuria, failure to thrive, recurrent episodes of dehydration—congenital adrenal hyperplasia (CAH).

Physical Examination

- *Volume status:*
  - *Dehydration:* CAH, type IV renal tubular acidosis (IVRTA), pseudohypoaldosteronism
  - *Volume overload/high BP:* Gordon's syndrome
- *Skin hyperpigmentation:* CAH
- *Palpable kidneys/bladder:* Obstructive uropathy
- *Muscle tenderness:* Rhabdomyolysis

Investigations

Investigations include:

- Complete blood count to look for hemolysis, thrombotic microangiopathy, and blood disorders
- Blood glucose to exclude hyperglycemia and DKA
- *Blood urea and creatinine:* To assess GFR
- Serum electrolytes and blood gas
- Urine electrolytes:
  - U_k <20 mEq/L in the setting of hyperkalemia indicates inappropriate K excretion
  - U_{Na} <20 mEq/L is an indicator of reduced distal tubular Na delivery or reduced effective volume
- *TTKG:* In patients with hyperkalemia due to aldosterone deficiency or resistance, TTKG will be <7.
- Ultrasound evaluation of kidneys to look for obstruction
- Electrocardiogram
- If renal function is normal and there is no apparent etiology, patient should be evaluated for mineralocorticoid deficiency such as serum 17-hydroxyprogesterone, serum cortisol, serum testosterone, plasma aldosterone level, and plasma renin activity. The approach to a patient with hyperkalemia is given in **Flowchart 2**.

Approach to Diagnosis

- *Obtain a random spot urine potassium level:*
  - *High urinary potassium excretion:* Urine potassium of >20 mEq/L suggests extrarenal causes of hyperkalemia like increased K^+ intake and transcellular shifts.
  - *Low urinary potassium excretion:* Urine potassium of <20 mEq/L suggests decreased renal excretion of potassium.
- *Children with low urinary potassium excretion:* Assess creatinine and urine output
  - Low urinary potassium excretion and high creatinine and/or low urine output suggest acute kidney injury or chronic kidney.
  - Low urinary potassium excretion and normal creatinine and urine output—check:
    - Serum aldosterone level
    - Low aldosterone:
      - *Hypertension present:* Gordon syndrome
      - *No HTN:* Adrenal insufficiency, salt losing CAH
    - *High aldosterone:* Pseudohypoaldosteronism type 1, obstructive uropathy

Case 1

A 14-year-old boy is referred for evaluation of persistent hyperkalemia (K—6.4 mEq/L) and HTN. His elder sister has

Flowchart 2: Approach to a child with hyperkalemia.

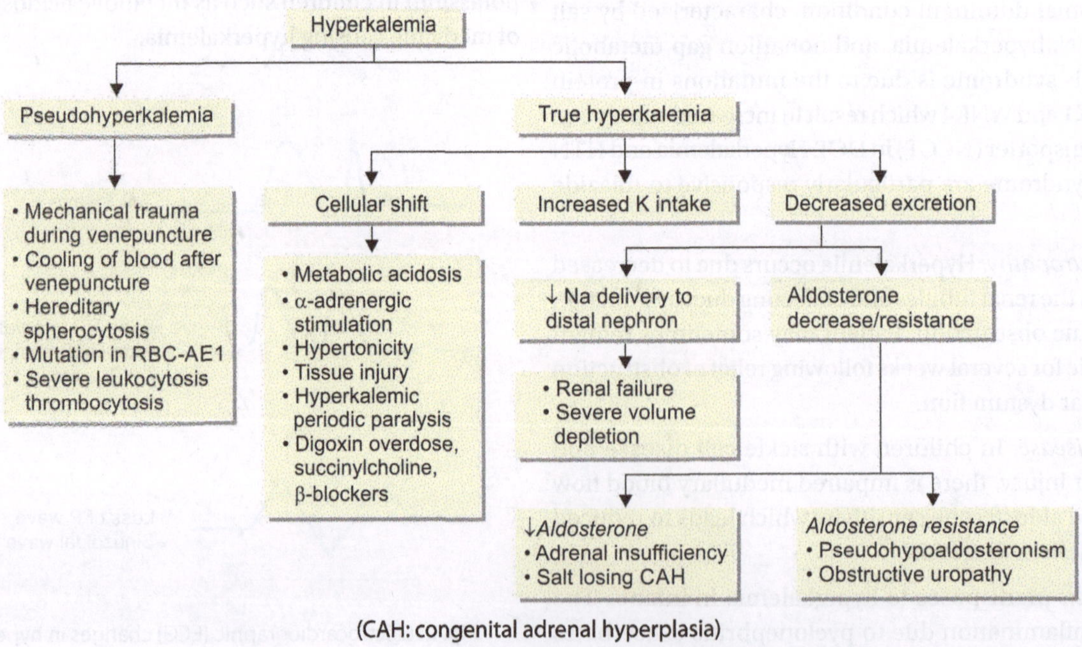

(CAH: congenital adrenal hyperplasia)

similar clinical presentation. Laboratories are as follows: Na—138 mEq/L, Cl—115 mEq/L, HCO_3—20 mEq/L, and creatinine—0.8 mg/dL. His renin and aldosterone levels are low. Urinary: Na—30 mEq/L, K—14 mEq/L. An arterial blood gas (ABG) shows hyperchloremic metabolic acidosis. Which one of the following therapeutic regimen is appropriate for this patient?

A. Furosemide (Lasix)
B. Hydrochlorothiazide (HCTZ)
C. Spironolactone
D. Acetazolamide (Diamox)
E. Salt substitute

Approach to Diagnosis

- *Urine K—14 mEq/L despite hyperkalemia:* Low urinary potassium excretion
- The next step is to check creatinine which is normal.
- In the presence of low urinary potassium excretion and normal creatinine, the next step is to check aldosterone level which is low in this patient.
- He has HTN also, hence his diagnosis is Gordon syndrome.
- The treatment of choice for Gordon syndrome is thiazide diuretic. Hence the answer is B.

Case 2

A 10-year-old female with end-stage kidney disease requiring hemodialysis presents with proximal muscle weakness. The serum potassium is 7.8 mEq/L, and an ECG shows peaked T waves. Which one of the following agents would lower her serum potassium concentration most quickly?

A. Calcium gluconate intravenously
B. Glucose and insulin intravenously
C. Propranolol intravenously
D. Kayexalate in sorbitol orally
E. Sodium bicarbonate intravenously

The correct answer is B. Therapy with glucose and insulin is effective in lowering the serum potassium concentration within minutes.

Propranolol is a β-blocker which may cause hyperkalemia and is therefore contraindicated in this patient.

The site of action of Kayexalate is rectum. Hence oral Kayexalate does not work rapidly.

Sodium bicarbonate may be beneficial, however in end-stage kidney disease (ESKD) potassium falls minimally with bicarbonate therapy.

Treatment

Hyperkalemia is a medical emergency and hence treatment should not be delayed for investigation or to exclude spurious causes.

When serum "K" level is between 5.5 and 6.0 mEq/L, the better approach is treat the cause and discontinue the administration of potassium containing solutions and drugs causing hyperkalemia. And also the dietary intake potassium has to be limited.

Management of severe or symptomatic hyperkalemia has three components:

1. Stabilizing membrane and managing cardiotoxicity
2. Promoting shift of potassium ECF to ICF
3. Elimination of potassium from the body

Stabilizing Membrane and Managing Cardiotoxicity

Intravenous calcium gluconate: Calcium therapy will not alter the serum "K" level, instead it antagonizes the potassium-induced decrease in membrane excitability and restores membrane excitability to normal and its action is immediate.

Intravenous calcium gluconate 0.5–1.0 mL/kg of 10% solution, diluted with equal quantity of 5% dextrose and given as a slow IV for over 10 minutes. Monitoring with ECG or manually checking the heart rate is essential. If the child develops bradycardia, calcium injection should be stopped. This can be repeated in 5–10 minutes if ECG changes persist.

Extreme caution should be taken while using calcium in patients on digitalis since hypercalcemia may precipitate digitalis toxicity. In the clinical setting of a cardiac arrest or impending arrest, calcium chloride is typically used rather than calcium gluconate because it results in a more rapid increase in the serum ionized calcium. The dose of IV calcium chloride is 20 mg/kg (maximum dose 1,000 mg) given over 5–10 minutes. But it should only be given if central venous access is available because administration through a peripheral line is associated with skin necrosis and sloughing.[17]

Promoting Shift of Potassium ECF to ICF

Insulin is administered as 0.1–0.2 units/kg of regular insulin with 0.5–1 g/kg of glucose (10 or 25% dextrose) to prevent hypoglycemia. The effect of insulin is evident within 30–60 minutes and may last for 2–4 hours. An ongoing glucose infusion after the initial insulin-glucose treatment may be necessary to prevent late hypoglycemia.

Nebulized salbutamol is given in the usual dose as for asthma. This can be repeated hourly. The dose of salbutamol is for, neonates—0.4 mg, 1.25 mg for <1 year, 2.5 mg between 1 and 5 years, 5 mg above 5 years. Effect lasts for 20–30 minutes. This intervention has also been shown to be effective and safe in mechanically ventilated preterm neonates.[18] Although widely used for emergency treatment, the fall in potassium concentration is not predictable and is also mild (0.5 mEq/L).

Intravenous sodium bicarbonate can be given if there is concomitant metabolic acidosis. Injection sodium bicarbonate (7.5%) 1–2 mL/kg IV, over 10 minutes diluted with equal volume of 5% dextrose can be given. Sodium bicarbonate may cause CO_2 retention (if there is associated respiratory acidosis), hypernatremia, fluid overload, and fall in ionized calcium levels. Calcium and bicarbonate should never be mixed in syringe or in infusion.

Elimination of Potassium from the Body

Furosemide is given at the dose of 1-2 mg/kg IV if renal function is normal and perfusion is adequate.

Kayexalate (sodium polystyrene sulfonate) or calcium polystyrene sulfonates are cation exchange resins which bind with potassium in the gastrointestinal tract and eliminate it from the body. Each gram of sodium polystyrene sulfonate binds with 1 mEq of potassium and release 2-3 mEq of sodium. It can be given in the dose of 1 g/kg/dose orally or rectally. About 1-2 mmol/kg can be reduced by this intervention. This can be repeated 6-12 hourly. To prevent constipation, polystyrene sufonates are mixed for many years with sorbitol which acts as an osmotic laxative. However reports of colonic necrosis and perforations with this mixture[19] prompted Food and Drug Administration (FDA) to warn that polystyrene sulfonates may be mixed with water and lactulose and not be mixed with sorbitol. In infants with hyperkalemia, resins can be added to milk for 30-60 minutes and filtered milk can be administered to the infant. The resin would bind to potassium in the milk and the complex can be discarded by sieving.

Newer potassium-binding drugs: Patiromer and sodium zirconium cyclosilicate (SZC) are the newer potassium-binding drugs. Patiromer is a nonsystemically absorbed polymer that binds K in exchange for calcium predominantly in the distal colon. SZC is an inorganic crystal that is not systemically adsorbed, and binds K with a strong selectivity in exchange for hydrogen and sodium cations. Although these drugs are approved for use in adults with hyperkalemia, no pediatric data is available.

Dialysis may be used to remove potassium if all these measures fail or potassium is rapidly raising or it is caused by renal failure. Hemodialysis is more efficient than peritoneal dialysis in potassium removal.

Hydrocortisone: If hyperkalemia is part of adrenal insufficiency, hydrocortisone 10 mg/kg/IV should be started.

Treatment of hyperkalemia is summarized in **Flowchart 3**.

Specific Conditions Associated with Hyperkalemia

Congenital adrenal hyperplasia is treated with hydrocortisone and fludrocortisone. In addition, most infants need additional salt supplementation either in the form of 3% saline (3–5 mL/kg/day) or added regular salts in weaning foods. Additional salt intake will allow sufficient delivery of sodium in the distal tubule which in the presence of fludrocortisone permits potassium secretion.

Pseudohypoaldosteronism: Both type 1a and 1b are treated with additional salt intake and potassium binding resins. Gordon's syndrome or type 2 pseudohypoaldosteronism is treated with thiazide diuretics and salt restriction.

Flowchart 3: Treatment of hyperkalemia.

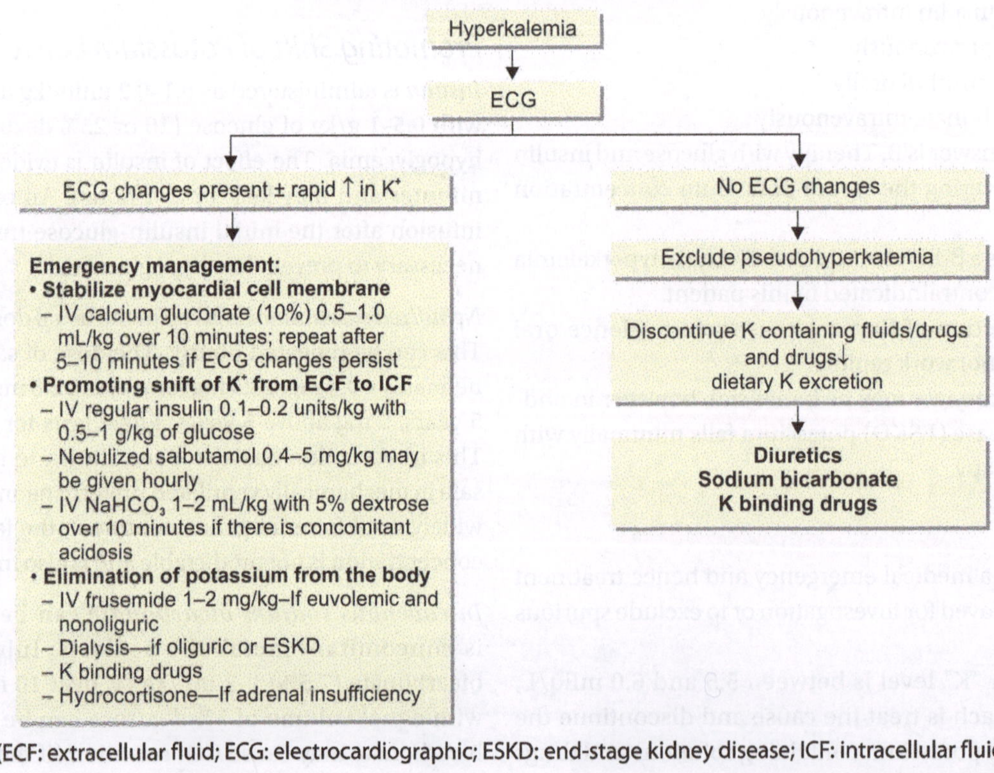

(ECF: extracellular fluid; ECG: electrocardiographic; ESKD: end-stage kidney disease; ICF: intracellular fluid)

Obstructive uropathy is treated with bladder catheterization, normal saline administration, and correction of metabolic acidosis.

CONCLUSION

Potassium is the major intracellular cation and its levels are crucial to normal homeostasis. Disorders of potassium, both hypokalemia and hyperkalemia occurs due to alterations in potassium intake, transcellular shift, and potassium loss—renal or extrarenal. It is of utmost importance to diagnose and treat potassium disorders since the clinical consequences of these disorders are mainly cardiac arrhythmias which may be life threatening.

KEY POINTS

- Urinary K excretion is the result of K secretion in ASDN and distal sodium delivery, tubular flow rate, and aldosterone are the main determinants of urine K excretion.
- Estimation of urine and serum electrolytes, spot urine K to creatinine ratio and acid-base status helps in identifying the cause of potassium disorders.
- Hyperkalemia is a medical emergency and hence treatment should not be delayed for investigation or to exclude spurious causes.

REFERENCES

1. Doucet A, Crambert G. Potassium homeostasis. In: Turner N, Lamieire N, Goldsmith DJ, Winearls CG, Himmelfarb J, Remuzzi G (Eds). Oxford Text Book of Clinical Nephrology, 4th edition. Oxford: Oxford University Press; 2016. pp. 204-17.
2. DeFronzo RA, Bia M, Birkhead G. Epinephrine and potassium homeostasis. Kidney Int. 1981;20(1):83-91.
3. Palmer BF. Regulation of potassium homeostasis. Clin J Am Soc Nephrol. 2015;10(6):1050-60.
4. Palmer BF, DuBose TD. Disorders of potassium metabolism. In: Schrier RW (Ed). Renal and Electrolyte Disorders, 8th edition. Philadelphia: Wolters Kluwer; 2018. pp. 274-324.
5. Thomas L, Kumar R. Control of renal solute excretion by enteric signals and mediators. J Am Soc Nephrol. 2008;19(2):207-12.
6. Oh KS, Oh YT, Kim SW, Kita T, Kang I, Youn JH. Gut sensing of dietary K^+ intake increases renal K^+ excretion. Am J Physiol Regul Integr Comp Physiol. 2011;301(2):R421-9.
7. Cummings BM, Macklin EA, Yager PH, Sharma A, Noviski N. Potassium abnormalities in a pediatric intensive care unit: frequency and severity. J Intensive Care Med. 2014;29(5):269-74.
8. Deepthiraju B, Varma PR. Barium toxicity a rare presentation of fireworks ingestion. Indian Pediatr. 2012;49(9):762.
9. Scurati-Manzoni E, Fossali EF, Agostoni C, Riva E, Simonetti GD, Zanolari-Calderari M, et al. Electrolyte abnormalities in cystic fibrosis: systematic review of the literature. Pediatr Nephrol. 2014;29(6):1015-23.
10. Malik AR, Wolf PK, Ravasia S. Hypokalemia from risperidone and quetiapine overdose. Can J Psychiatry. 2005;50(1):76.
11. Yanturali S, Aksay E, Demir OF, Atilla R. Massive hydroxychloroquine overdose. Acta Anaesthesiol Scand. 2004; 48(3):379-81.
12. Molla AM, Rahman M, Sarker SA, Sack DA, Molla A. Stool electrolyte content and purging rates in diarrhea caused by rotavirus, enterotoxigenic *E. coli*, and *V. cholerae* in children. J Pediatr. 1981;98(5):835-8.
13. Dutta A, Palazzi DL. Risk factors of amphotericin B toxicity in the nonneonatal pediatric population. Pediatr Infect Dis J. 2012;31(9):910-4.
14. Daly K, Farrington E. Hypokalemia and hyperkalemia in infants and children: pathophysiology and treatment. J Pediatr Health Care. 2013;27(6):486-98.
15. Kim M, Somers MJG. Fluid and electrolyte physiology and therapy. In: McMillan JA, DeAngelis CD, Feigin RD (Eds). Oski's Pediatrics, 4th edition. Baltimore: Lippincott Williams and Wilkins; 2006. p.54.
16. Gil-Ruiz MA, Alcaraz AJ, Marañón RJ, Navarro N, Huidobro B, Luque A. Electrolyte disturbances in acute pyelonephritis. Pediatr Nephrol. 2012;27(3):429-33.
17. Broner CW, Stidham GL, Westenkirchner DF, Watson DC. A prospective, randomized, double-blind comparison of calcium chloride and calcium gluconate therapies for hypocalcemia in critically ill children J Pediatr. 1990;117(6):986-9.
18. Singh BS, Sadiq HF, Noguchi A, Keenan WJ. Efficacy of albuterol inhalation in treatment of hyperkalemia in premature neonates. J Pediatr. 2002;141(1):16-20.
19. Bomback AS, Woosley JT, KshirsagarAV. Colonic necrosis due to sodium polystyrene sulfate (Kayexalate). Am J Emerg Med. 2009;27(6):753.e1-2.

CHAPTER

4.4

Metabolic Acidosis and Metabolic Alkalosis

Devi S Sruthi, Susan Uthup

INTRODUCTION

The acid-base status of our body has to be regulated carefully for normal maintenance of the cellular structure, metabolism, and enzymatic function. Maintenance of normal arterial pH between 7.35 and 7.45 and intracellular pH between 7 and 7.3 is essential for normal health, growth, and development.[1] In adults the normal daily nonvolatile acid production is 1–2 mEq of hydrogen ion per kilogram of body weight, while in children, another 1 mEq/kg of H^+ is added to the extracellular fluid due to new bone formation. Thus, the total amount of H^+ to be excreted in a child is 2–3 mEq/kg/day.[2]

The strict maintenance of acid-base balance in the setting of this continuous production of acidic metabolites is accomplished by means of extracellular and intracellular buffers with renal and respiratory regulatory mechanisms. The extracellular buffers include the bicarbonate-carbonic acid buffer system and serum proteins. The intracellular buffers include the bicarbonate-carbonic acid buffer system, hemoglobin, intracellular proteins, and phosphates.[1] Bicarbonate-carbonic acid buffer is the most important and unique buffer system in the body fluid because the acid component of the buffer pair, carbonic acid, is regulated by the lungs and the base component, bicarbonate, is regulated by the kidneys. Bone represents a delayed buffer system. In acidosis, the calcium carbonate binds H^+ in exchange for calcium release.

RESPONSE OF THE BODY TO AN ACID LOAD

Under normal conditions, the H^+ concentration varies little from the normal value of 40 nmol/L (pH 7.4). Immediate extracellular buffering of an acid load is by body buffers, which are able to take up or release H^+.

HCO_3^- combines with H^+ according to the following reaction:

$$H^+ + HCO_3^- \leftrightarrow H_2CO_3 \leftrightarrow H_2O + CO_2$$

Within minutes, respiratory compensation may begin if the acid load is significant, lowering the pCO_2. Intracellular buffering by proteins including hemoglobin, imidazole, and histidine may then occur during the first 1–4 hours period. Finally, renal acid excretion and production of new bicarbonate by the kidney occurs during hours to days to replenish the bicarbonate consumed.

The pH of blood can be calculated using a modified version of the Henderson–Hasselbalch equation which describes the relationship between carbonic acid and bicarbonate. This equation explains how the lungs and kidneys act in concert to modify HCO_3 and pCO_2 to maintain the normal pH.

$$pH = 6.1 + \log \frac{HCO_3^-}{0.03 \times PaCO_2}$$

ACID-BASE DISORDERS

Acid-base disorders causing deviation of pH from the normal range can be classified as either metabolic or respiratory. When an acid-base disorder occurs, physiologic mechanisms attempt to return the extracellular pH back to normal. This involves secondary compensation by the lungs or kidneys. Secondary respiratory compensation for a metabolic disorder begins within minutes and is complete in 12–24 hours. Secondary metabolic compensation for a respiratory disorder begins more slowly, within 1 hour, and requires 2–5 days for completion. Neither, secondary respiratory or metabolic compensation completely returns the pH back to normal, except in cases of respiratory alkalosis.[2]

ROLE OF KIDNEY IN ACID-BASE REGULATION

The renal acid-base handling may be broadly divided into two processes:

1. Reabsorption and reclamation of filtered bicarbonate by the proximal convoluted tubule (PCT).
2. Excretion of fixed acid with a generation of new HCO_3 by the distal nephron.

About 80–90% of filtered HCO_3 is reabsorbed in the proximal tubule. The mechanisms for proximal reabsorption of filtered HCO_3 are shown in **Figure 1**. H_2CO_3 is formed within the proximal tubular cell by the hydration of CO_2. This reversible reaction is catalyzed by cytoplasmic carbonic anhydrase II (CAII). Ionization of H_2CO_3 to H^+ and HCO_3^- follows. H^+ is now

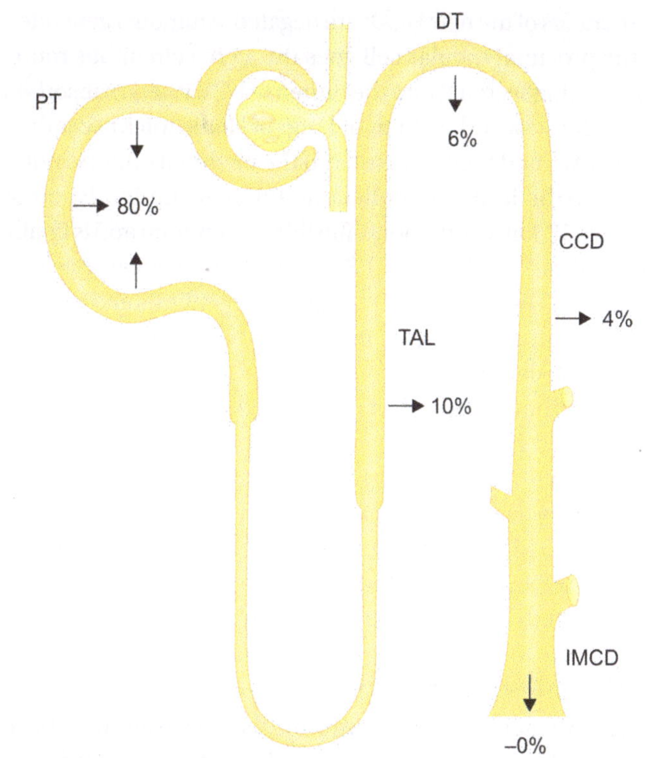

Fig. 1: Segmental reabsorption of HCO_3. (CCD: cortical collecting duct; DT: distal tubule; IMCD: inner medullary collecting duct; PT: proximal tubule; TAL: thick ascending limb)

secreted into the tubular fluid. Almost two-thirds of this apical H^+ secretion occurs through Na^+/H^+ antiporter sodium-hydrogen exchanger 3 (NHE3).[1] This mechanism is electroneutral, driven by a lumen to cell Na^+ gradient and stimulated by intracellular acidosis. A fraction of H^+ is also secreted by vacuolar H^+ ATPase on the luminal membrane. The H^+ secreted into the lumen reacts with filtered HCO_3^- to form luminal H_2CO_3, which quickly dissociates into $CO_2 + H_2O$ in the presence of luminal carbonic anhydrase (CA IV). Luminal CO_2 then freely diffuses into the cell to complete the reabsorption cycle.

Bicarbonate generated within the cell leaves it across the basolateral membrane by electrogenic Na (+)-HCO($_3$) (-) cotransporter NBCe1.[1] In addition, some of the HCO_3 may exit in exchange for chloride via a Cl-HCO_3 antiporter. Also, about 20% of bicarbonate is reabsorbed by passive back-diffusion along the paracellular pathway.[1] The thick ascending limb of the loop of Henle reabsorbs the remaining 10–20% of the filtered HCO_3^-, by a mechanism similar to that in the proximal tubule, through apical Na^+-H^+ exchange and H^+ ATPase **(Fig. 2)**.[3]

DISTAL URINARY ACIDIFICATION

Distal urinary acidification involves secretion (excretion) of acid generated from metabolism as well as new bone formation in children and generation of new bicarbonate to replace the bicarbonate used up in buffering the acids from the above sources. Distal acidification mainly occurs in the collecting tubule. The cellular mechanisms involved in distal acidification are depicted in **Figures 3 and 4**.

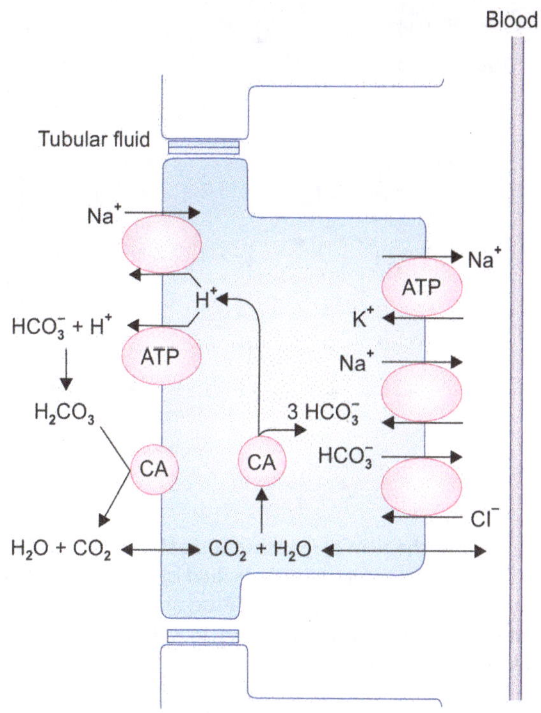

Fig. 2: Cellular mechanism for the reabsorption of filtered HCO_3^- at proximal tubule, ascending loop of Henle, and distal tubule. H^+ secretion occurs by both Na^+- H^+ antiporter and H^+-ATPase. Within the cell, H^+ and HCO_3^- are produced in a reaction catalyzed by CA II. The H^+ is secreted into the tubular fluid and the HCO_3^- enters peritubular capillaries by Na^+-$3HCO_3$ + symporter and Cl^--HCO_3^- antiporter. The CA IV present in the brush border of the PT dehydrates the H_2CO_3 into CO_2 and H_2O. Thus, it causes the entry of CO_2 into the cell and indirectly reabsorption of HCO_3. (ATP: adenosine triphosphate; CA: carbonic anhydrase)

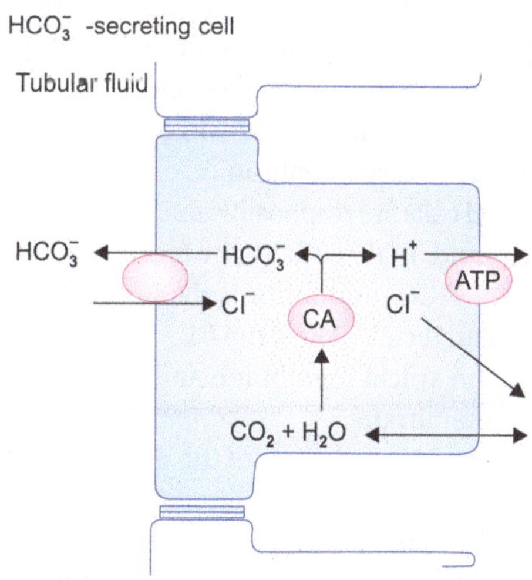

Fig. 3: Cellular mechanism of secretion of HCO_3 by β-intercalated cells of CD. The β-intercalated cells in the collecting duct secrete bicarbonate rather than H^+ into the tubules as the H^+-ATPase is located in the basolateral membrane and Cl^--HCO_3^- antiporter is located in the apical membrane. Their activity is increased in metabolic alkalosis. (ATP: adenosine triphosphate; CA: carbonic anhydrase).

There are three cell types in the collecting tubule:

1. Principal cells are involved in Na^+ reabsorption and K^+ and H^+ secretion.

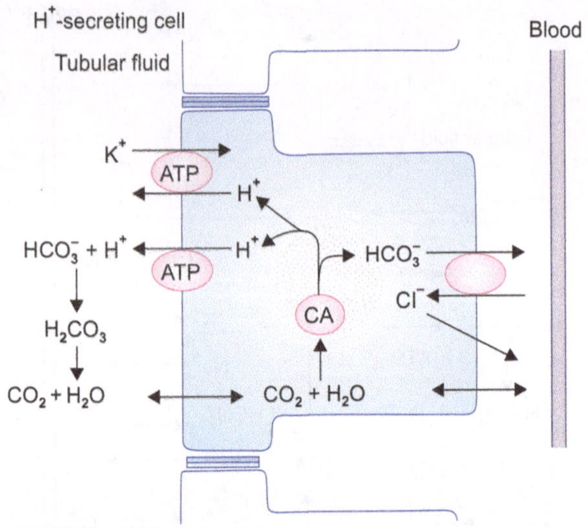

Fig. 4: Cellular mechanism of reabsorption of HCO_3 by α-intercalated cells of CD. H^+ is secreted in the tubule fluid by two mechanisms. The first involves apical membrane H^+-ATPase and the second couples the secretion of H^+ with the reabsorption of K^+ through H^+, K^+-ATPase. (ATP: adenosine triphosphate)

2. α-intercalated cells are mainly responsible for H^+ secretion. In these cells, there are two types of transporters responsible for luminal H^+ secretion cells—H^+ ATPase (main transporter) and H^+-K+-ATPase. H^+ secretion by the H^+ ATPase is an energy-consuming process and occurs against an electrochemical gradient. H^+-K^+-ATPase reabsorbs K^+ and secretes H^+. It plays an important role in patients with hypokalemia. It increases potassium reabsorption and contributes to the maintenance of metabolic alkalosis. Intracellularly formed HCO_3^- leaves the cell by an electroneutral mechanism involving Cl-HCO_3^- an exchange which is the mechanism of new bicarbonate generation in the distal nephron.
3. β-intercalated cells are responsible for HCO_3^- secretion into the tubular fluid. In these cells, the location of H^+ ATPase and the Cl^- – HCO_3 antiporter is diametrically opposite to α-intercalated cells. Thus, the Cl^- - HCO_3 antiporter is located on the apical membrane and H^+ ATPase on the basolateral membrane.[2]

H^+ ions secreted in the lumen of the distal nephron have to be buffered before they can be eliminated. The final urine is electroneutral and not a charged solution. The secreted H^+ ions are buffered by two systems, HPO_4^- and ammonia (NH_3) which facilitate the secretion of more H^+ by combining and decreasing the H^+ concentration in the lumen.

The major form of H^+ ion excretion is as NH_4 combined with anions like Cl^- or SO_4^-. Ammonia (NH3) and HCO_3 are generated in the kidneys through the metabolism of glutamine. Ammonia is excreted, while the new HCO_3 is added to the body. If the ammonia is not excreted in the urine, it is converted into urea by the liver and in the process, new H^+ is generated. This new H^+ needs to be buffered by HCO_3 and thus the benefits of the new HCO_3^- are negated. Ammonia generated in the proximal tubular cell goes through a circuitous route. After getting secreted into the lumen of PCT, it gets reabsorbed in the thick ascending limb of Loop of Henle thick ascending limb (TAL) and then diffuses into the medullary interstitium. It enters the lumen of collecting tubules and binds to the secreted H^+ ion to form nondiffusible ammonium and is finally excreted as NH_4Cl or $(NH_4)_2SO_4$. This forms titratable acidity along with HPO_4^- and $H_2PO_4^-$. Ammonia synthesis and thereby H^+ excretion are increased in situations of metabolic acidosis and hypokalemia.[3]

Phosphate filtered across the glomerulus is mostly reabsorbed in the PCT. Part of the phosphate that is not reabsorbed binds to H^+ in the distal nephron forming monovalent acid form (HPO_4^-). The body has a limited capacity to excrete acid as a titrable acid in the form of HPO_4^-. Phosphate plays an important role in bone formation and hence the body cannot afford to lose phosphate for excreting acid.

METABOLIC ACIDOSIS

Metabolic acidosis is a commonly diagnosed acid-base disorder. It occurs alone, i.e., simple acid-base disorder, or can coexist with other abnormalities such as mixed acid-base disorder. The most common mixed acid-base disorder is a combination of metabolic acidosis with respiratory alkalosis.

Metabolic acidosis is defined as the pathologic process that increases the blood hydrogen ion (H^+) concentration and decreases the serum bicarbonate (HCO_3). Acidemia is defined as a low arterial pH (<7.35) that results from metabolic acidosis, respiratory acidosis, or a combination of both.

Pathophysiology

The primary abnormality in metabolic acidosis is a decrease in bicarbonate concentration, which can occur by means of three mechanisms.

1. An increase in acid concentration is either due to increased acid generation (endogenous production or exogenous intake) or decreased renal acid excretion. This will result in a decrease in serum bicarbonate concentration due to buffering.
2. Loss of bicarbonate via gastrointestinal tract or kidneys.
3. Dilution of bicarbonate in the expanded extracellular fluid (ECF) volume. The normal bicarbonate content gets diluted in larger volumes of ECF.

However, a low plasma bicarbonate concentration is not diagnostic of metabolic acidosis as it also results from the renal compensation in chronic respiratory alkalosis.

Metabolic acidosis stimulates both central and peripheral chemoreceptors controlling respiration, resulting in compensatory hyperventilation and a fall in pCO_2. This will raise the extracellular pH towards normal. An increase in ventilation begins within 1–2 hours and reaches its maximum level at 12–24 hours.[2]

Serum Anion Gap

Anion gap (AGAP) is an important clue to the differential diagnosis of metabolic acidosis. AGAP is the difference between the major measured cations (sodium) and the major measured anions (bicarbonate and chloride) or unmeasured serum anions and "unmeasured serum cations,"[4] as shown in **Figure 5**. At physiological pH, serum albumin is the major contributor to the anion gap since the remaining anions (phosphate, sulfate, and organic anion such as lactate) balance out with "unmeasured" cations (calcium and magnesium). In the body the concentration of total anions equals that of total cations; hence, our body is electroneutral and does not have a "charge."

Measured cations + unmeasured cations = measured anions + unmeasured anions.

$(Na^+) + (K^+, Ca^{2+}, Mg^{2+}) = (Cl^-, HCO_3^-) + (\text{proteins}, PO_4^{2-}, SO_4^{2-}, \text{organic acids})$.

Anion gap = unmeasured anions - unmeasured cations.

The anion gap usually is estimated from the difference in measured cations and anions by the formula: serum $Na^+ - (Cl^- + HCO_3^-)$. The normal range is 8–16 mEq/L.[4]

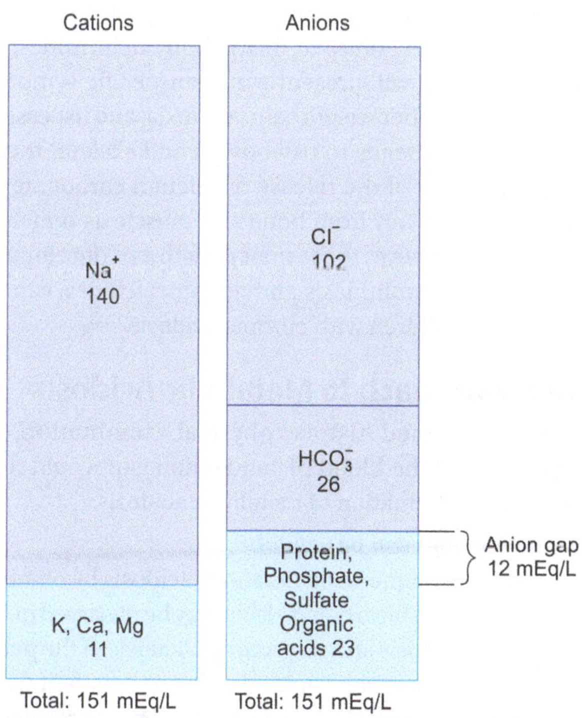

Fig. 5: Anion gap. It is the difference in unmeasured serum anions and cations, which are shown here in the blue shaded portion of the bar for total serum cations and anions. The "unmeasured" serum cations—potassium, calcium, and magnesium are actually readily measurable in the clinical laboratory but are called "unmeasured" for ease of calculation of the anion gap. The anion gap usually is estimated from the difference in measured cations and anions by the formula: serum $Na^+ - (Cl^- + HCO_3^-)$; the normal range is 8–16 mEq/L.[4]
Source: Clinical physiology of acid-base and electrolyte disorders, by Burton Rose

Increased anion gap can be rarely due to an increase in serum protein or sodium concentration or due to a decrease in plasma $K^+/Ca^{2+}/Mg^{2+}$ concentration.

The decreased anion gap is usually seen in patients with hypoalbuminemia or rarely due to an increase in the concentration of K^+, Ca^{2+}, and Mg^{2+} or due to the presence of lithium in blood.[2]

The anion gap can be underestimated in children with hypoalbuminemia. To adjust for hypoalbuminemia the following equation is used:

Corrected anion gap = anion gap + [0.25 × (4 – albumin in g/dL)]

Based on anion gap, metabolic acidosis can be classified into anion gap metabolic acidosis (AGMA) and nonanion gap metabolic acidosis (NAGMA). Anion-gap metabolic acidosis (high anion gap metabolic acidosis) results from the retention of fixed acids, which depletes the HCO_3 stores by releasing protons. Two mechanisms can lead to AGMA, i.e., the addition of strong acids which may be endogenous acids such as ketoacid and lactic acid or exogenous acids or precursors of an acid such as alcohol. The second mechanism is decreased capacity to excrete the normal load of fixed acids as occurs with renal failure. Normal anion-gap metabolic acidosis (hyperchloremic metabolic acidosis) results from a primary loss of HCO_3 or failure to replenish bicarbonate stores depleted by the daily production of fixed acids in subjects with renal tubular acidosis (RTA). In either case, the concentration of the other major measured anion, Cl^- will increase proportionately in the serum resulting in hyperchloremia and the anion gap will be normal.

Causes of Metabolic Acidosis in Children

- *Anion gap metabolic acidosis:*
  - Increase in endogenous production or addition of exogenous acid/acid precursors
    - Diabetic ketoacidosis
    - Lactic acidosis as in shock, mitochondrial dysfunction, crush injury, etc.
    - Methanol poisoning
    - Ethylene glycol poisoning
    - Salicylate toxicity
    - Iron overdose
    - Isoniazid (INH) overdose
    - Inborn errors of metabolism (IEM)
    - Paraldehyde ingestion (rare)
  - Inability to excrete acids as in acute or chronic renal failure.

A frequently used mnemonic to remember the more common causes of anion gap metabolic acidosis in children is MUDPILES, where M = methanol; U = uremia; D = diabetic ketoacidosis; P = paraldehyde; I = iron, INH, and inborn metabolic errors; L = lactic acid; E = ethylene glycol; and S = salicylates.

- *Normal anion gap metabolic acidosis*:
  - Loss of bicarbonate through the gastrointestinal (GI) tract
    - Diarrhea
    - Enterocutaneous fistula
    - Ureteric diversion through colon or augmentation cystoplasty using small bowel (e.g., ileal loop bladder)
    - Use of bile acid sequestrants like cholestyramine
  - Loss of bicarbonate through kidneys
    - Renal loss of HCO_3^- as in proximal RTA (type 2) and use of carbonic anhydrase inhibitor
    - Failure of renal H^+ secretion as in distal RTA (type 1), hyperkalemic RTA (type 4)
  - Other causes
    - Acid infusion—ammonium chloride, hyperalimentation
    - Rapid volume expansion with normal saline.

Causes of non-AG metabolic acidosis can be remembered with the mnemonic ACCRUED [(Ammonium chloride, Carbonic anhydrase inhibitors, Cholestyramine, Renal tubular acidosis (RTA), Ureteroenterostomy, Enterocutaneous fistula, Diarrhea, Dilutional acidosis].

Mixed High Anion and Normal Gap Acidosis

Occasionally, both high and normal anion gap causes coexist as in the following situations:

- *Children recovering from ketoacidosis:* In the recovery phase, keto acids are excreted in urine as sodium or potassium salts before getting metabolized to bicarbonate, normal anion gap metabolic acidosis can occur.
- Children with diarrhea and hypovolemia can have high anion gap metabolic acidosis due to hypoperfusion in addition to normal anion gap metabolic acidosis.

Metabolic Acidosis in Neonates and Infants

Preterm babies younger than 34 weeks gestation have a lower plasma bicarbonate concentration of 16–18 and term babies have a bicarbonate level of 18–20 mEq/L in the first few weeks of life. This is mainly due to a lower renal threshold for bicarbonate reabsorption secondary to the immaturity of $Na+/H^+$ exchange on the luminal membrane and Na^+/HCO_3^- cotransporter on the basolateral membrane of PCT.[5] The daily production of H^+ ions in babies is higher than in adults related to H^+ release by the growing skeleton. Thus, newborns and infants have a limited capacity to compensate for low bicarbonate. Neonates with perinatal asphyxia are at-risk for metabolic acidosis due to high lactic acid concentration.[6,7] Also, neonates on parenteral fluids (normal saline) are at risk for dilutional metabolic acidosis. Serum chloride-sodium ratio (<0.75) is useful in identifying these infants as they have hyperchloremic metabolic acidosis.[8] The tendency towards metabolic acidemia is compensated by the large intake of milk with high alkali content. Infants are therefore more prone to develop metabolic acidosis if the milk intake is low.[2]

Symptoms and Consequences of Metabolic Acidosis

Symptoms of metabolic acidosis are not specific. There will be an increased rate and depth of breathing (Kussmaul breathing) as the respiratory center is stimulated. Hyperventilation develops in an effort to compensate for acidosis. Tachypnea, varying degrees of dyspnea, palpitation, headache, confusion, generalized weakness, nausea, vomiting, and abdominal pain may be the presenting symptom in acute metabolic acidosis. Neurological changes like lethargy, confusion, seizures, and coma occur due to changes in cerebrospinal and brain pH. Peripheral vasodilatation and impaired cardiac function lead to low cardiac output in severe metabolic acidosis. Metabolic acidosis can precipitate hyperkalemia and cardiac conduction abnormalities. For every decrease in the blood pH by 0.1, the serum potassium increases by 0.6 mEq/L. Ionized calcium and magnesium increase with increasing academia. Calcium and magnesium get displaced from the protein binding sites on albumin, as H^+ ions compete with them for these binding sites resulting in an increase in ionized calcium and magnesium ions.[9]

In chronic metabolic acidosis, children may present with decreased appetite, failure to thrive, bony deformities, and bone pain. Infants will present with nonspecific symptoms such as vomiting, poor weight gain, anorexia, and listlessness. Chronic acidemia leads to osteopenia and skeletal muscle wasting as a result of the release of calcium carbonate and glutamate respectively from bone and muscle as buffers for H^+ ion. This contributes to the poor growth and development of rickets.[10,11] Nephrolithiasis and nephrocalcinosis can also occur in some children with chronic acidosis.[12,13]

Clinical Approach to Metabolic Acidosis

A carefully obtained history, physical examination, and determination of the blood pH and anion gap would direct an appropriate evaluation of metabolic acidosis.

The following steps can be helpful:

- Confirm the diagnosis of metabolic acidosis by obtaining blood gas. A low bicarbonate level may be observed in both metabolic acidosis and respiratory alkalosis. If the patient has a simple metabolic acidosis, then the patient will be acidemic with a pH <7.35, and if the patient has respiratory alkalosis with compensated metabolic acidosis, the patient is alkalemic with a pH >7.45.
- Confirm that the respiratory compensation is adequate. Expected pCO_2 in metabolic acidosis can be calculated using the following methods:
  - On average, the pCO_2 will fall 1.2 mm Hg for every 1 mEq/L reduction in the plasma HCO_3^- down to a minimum pCO_2 of 10–15 mm Hg.

- The rule of thumb to assess the adequacy of respiratory compensation is that the pCO_2 in acute metabolic acidosis should be approximately the last 2 digits of pH (e.g., pH = 7.20 here a pCO_2 of 20–22 mm Hg indicates adequate respiratory compensation. Any number above or below 20 ± 3 would suggest additional respiratory acid-base disorder).
- Winters formula: Expected $pCO_2 = [(HCO_3 \times 1.5)] + 8 \pm 2$

- Calculate the anion gap.
  - If the anion gap is high, assess renal function, blood glucose, blood lactate, and urinary ketones. Ask for a history of ingestions and check for evidence of reduced tissue perfusion. A history of severe hypotonia, seizures, developmental delay, or apnea in a newborn infant can be suggestive of an inborn error of metabolism. A serum ammonia level and lactic acid and pyruvic acid ratio help in the differentiation of the IEM.
  - For normal anion gap metabolic acidosis, the most common etiology is diarrhea followed by RTA (approach to NAGMA given later).
- Remember about the possibility of mixed acid-base disorders. The delta gap ratio is calculated in the presence of high anion gap metabolic acidosis to identify a mixed disorder. The delta gap ratio = change in anion gap (from a normal of 12 mmol/L)/change in bicarbonate (from a normal of 24 mmol/L). The calculated delta gap ratio may be used to separate the various forms of metabolic acidosis based on the delta gap ratio:
  - *0.4–0.99:* Mixed high and normal anion gap metabolic acidosis
  - *1.0–1.6:* High anion metabolic acidosis
  - *>1.6:* High anion metabolic acidosis mixed with metabolic alkalosis.

Normal Anion Gap Acidosis

- Diarrhea is the most common cause of normal anion gap acidosis in children. The diarrheal fluid contains a high HCO_3^- and low Cl^- concentration relative to the plasma. Diarrhea results in considerable loss of HCO_3^-, and K^+ leading to metabolic acidosis and hypokalemia. This stimulates renal ammonia genesis to bind to free H^+ ions forming NH_4^+. This combination of hypokalemia and hyperchloremic metabolic acidosis with normal AGAP and high urine pH (>6.0) is also seen in distal RTA. Distal RTA can be excluded based on the history of diarrhea and if required, by measurement of the urinary anion gap. The urinary anion gap is an indirect assessment of urinary ammonium excretion and is calculated as follows:

$$\text{Urinary AGAP} = (Na^+ + K^+) - (Cl^-)$$

The normal urinary AGAP is close to zero. In diarrhea because of increased urinary ammonium excretion, the urinary AGAP is negative (>20), whereas, in distal RTA, urinary AGAP is positive (>10) suggestive of decreased ammonium excretion.[14]

- Renal tubular acidosis in children presents with failure to thrive, polyuria, and polydipsia. A high level of suspicion is required to evaluate for RTA. Simple investigations can identify the type of RTA. In a few cases, additional acidification tests may be required. Therapy of type 1 and type 4 RTA is easier compared to type 2 RTA. Early diagnosis and treatment can improve growth and minimize long-term complications of nephrocalcinosis and metabolic bone disease.
- Ureteral diversion using a colon or small bowel augmentation cystoplasty can result in hyperchloremic metabolic acidosis. Urine contains a relatively higher concentration of chloride compared to bicarbonate. When this urine comes in contact with the colonic or intestinal mucosa, chloride in the lumen is reabsorbed and bicarbonate secreted, leading to loss of bicarbonate in the urine. The use of the stomach, instead of the colon or ileum, may ameliorate the problem. Small bowel or pancreatic drainage can also cause gastrointestinal loss of bicarbonate
- Cholestyramine is an oral chloride-containing anion exchange resin used to treat biliary pruritus and low-density lipoprotein (LDL) hypercholesterolemia. In the bowel, Cl^- is exchanged for HCO_3^-, which is excreted in the stool. If the patient also has renal insufficiency, the net loss of HCO_3^- cannot be compensated by an increase in renal acid excretion and the patient will develop hyperchloremic metabolic acidosis.[2]
- Drugs like acetazolamide inhibit carbonic anhydrase enzyme which decrease the conversion of carbonic acid to water and carbon dioxide at the renal tubule brush border resulting in bicarbonate loss and subsequently metabolic acidosis
- *Dilutional metabolic acidosis*—dilutional acidosis occurs due to expansion of the intravascular fluid volume with large volumes of IV fluids containing neither bicarbonate nor sodium salts of organic anions that can be metabolized to bicarbonate (such as lactate or acetate). This usually occurs in children receiving parenteral fluids following trauma or those undergoing surgery and is often mild.[15-18] There will be clinical signs of fluid overload such as periorbital and pretibial edema, pleural effusions, and ascites. The serum uric acid, blood urea nitrogen (BUN), and serum osmolality are low. Beta-type natriuretic peptide (BNP) is often elevated.

An approach to a child with normal AGAP metabolic acidosis is shown in **Flowchart 1**.

Approach to a Child with Renal Tubular Acidosis

- Obtain blood gas to confirm that the low serum HCO_3^- is due to metabolic acidosis.

Flowchart 1: Approach to a child with NAGMA.

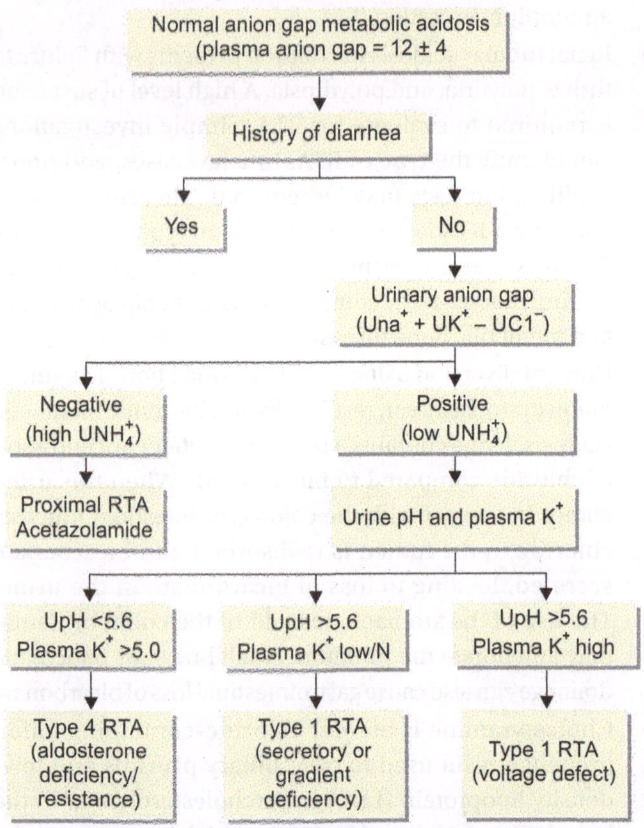

(NAGMA: nonanion gap metabolic acidosis RTA: renal tubular acidosis; UCl^-: urine chloride; Una: urine sodium; UNH: urine ammonia excretion; UpH: urinary pH)

- Calculate plasma anion gap: $[Na^+ - (Cl^- + HCO_3^-)]$ normal 10 ± 2 mEq/L (based on ion specific electrode method of estimating electrolytes).
- If diarrhea is ruled out, the next step in the evaluation of normal AGAP metabolic acidosis is to obtain fresh urine pH and calculate the urine anion gap

  Urine anion gap = $(U\,Na^+ + UK^+ - U\,Cl^-)$
- Urine pH <5.5 with a negative urinary AGAP indicates proximal RTA. Fractional excretion of bicarbonate in urine above 15% is also seen in children with proximal RTA.[14]
- If the urinary AGAP is positive, it denotes low levels of urinary ammonium and favors distal or type 4 RTA. Remember that a positive U AGAP does not always indicate ammonium deficiency.
- Evaluation of urine pH and serum potassium will further differentiate between type 1 and IV RTA. Urinary pH <5.5 with plasma potassium >5.5 favors type 4 RTA, whereas high urine pH (>5.6) with low plasma potassium is suggestive of a type 1 RTA.
- Presence of proteinuria, glycosuria, aminoaciduria, phosphaturia, and hyperuricosuria in addition to proximal RTA suggests Fanconi syndrome.[14]
- Nephrolithiasis and nephrocalcinosis are seen commonly in distal RTA. Skeletal abnormalities can occur in both Fanconi syndrome and distal RTA.
- In patients with subtle changes in pH and HCO_3 tests of urinary acidification are needed (*see* Chapter 8.1 on renal tubular acidosis).

High Anion Gap Metabolic Acidosis

- *Diabetic ketoacidosis (DKA):* In DKA, β-hydroxybutyric acid and acetoacetic acid accumulate due to insulin deficiency. Metabolic acidosis is often associated with significant hypokalemia.
- *Lactic acidosis:* There is an accumulation of lactate in blood, usually >5 mEq/L. The commonest cause is tissue hypoxemia from hypotension, hypovolemia, or sepsis. Rarely, it may be due to an underlying mitochondrial dysfunction or inborn error of carbohydrate metabolism.[19]
- *Uremia:* The metabolic acidosis in uremia is due to the inability of the diseased kidney to excrete the daily dietary acid load. There are two important factors involved in the pathogenesis:
  1. Decrease in total ammonium excretion, especially when the GFR falls below 50 mL/min. This is due to the limited number of functioning nephrons and not due to a decrease in the ammonium production by the individual proximal tubules.
  2. Decreased titratable acidity (primarily as phosphate) contributes to the decline in net acid excretion especially when the GFR falls below 30 mL/min, when the urinary phosphate excretion is decreased. This results in the accumulation of lactic acid, hippuric acid, amino acids, pyroglutamic acid, guanidinosuccinic acid, short-chain fatty acids, and sulfuric acid.[20,21] Usually, the plasma bicarbonate concentration stabilizes around 10–12 mEq/L in most cases. Further reduction in plasma HCO_3^- is prevented by buffering of the excess acid, primarily by the bone buffer calcium carbonate.
- *Salicylate ingestion:* Salicylate overdose initially produces respiratory alkalosis due to stimulation of the respiratory center. Subsequently, metabolic acidosis ensues due to the accumulation of salicylic acid, lactic acid, and keto acids. Salicylates may also induce vomiting and metabolic alkalosis to further complicate the acid-base picture. Because of their more rapid metabolism of salicylate, children under 5 years of age are more likely to present with high AGAP metabolic acidosis rather than respiratory alkalosis. Also, acidosis occurs more commonly with chronic rather than acute ingestion of salicylates.
- *Methanol and ethylene glycol poisoning:* Methanol (wood alcohol, CH_3OH) is present in varnish, de-icing solution, and other commercial preparations. Methanol ingestion increases serum formaldehyde level, which is converted to formate and formic acid by the action of alcohol dehydrogenase in the liver. These metabolites inhibit cytochrome oxidation, leading to progressive acidosis due

to the rise of blood lactic acid and ketoacid concentrations. Accumulation of formic acid, which is the most toxic metabolite, causes optic atrophy and is responsible for the large anion gap (usually >30 mEq/L). Methanol ingestion is more commonly seen in adult alcoholics who seek a cheaper alternative to ethanol and is uncommon in children. Like ethyl alcohol and methanol, ethylene glycol is metabolized by aldehyde dehydrogenase (ADH) forming glycoaldehyde and then to glycolic acid (GA), which accumulates causing profound metabolic acidosis. *High serum osmolal gap* is another important indicator to the presence of methanol or ethylene glycol in AGAP metabolic acidosis. The osmolal gap is the difference between measured and calculated serum osmolality. An osmolal gap of >10 mOsm/L suggests the presence of unmeasured osmotic particles like methanol, ethylene glycol, or ethanol.

- *Starvation ketosis:* Ketosis due to either starvation or a ketogenic diet is another cause of anion gap metabolic acidosis due to increased serum levels of acetoacetate and beta-hydroxybutyrate.

Inborn Errors of Metabolism

Inborn errors of metabolism especially organic acidemias (methylmalonic, propionic, and isovaleric acidemia, glutaric acidemia type 1, 3-methylglutaconic aciduria) maple syrup urine disease and disorders of carbohydrate metabolism (e.g., pyruvate carboxylase, pyruvate dehydrogenase, and phosphoenolpyruvate carboxykinase deficiency) cause metabolic acidosis. Acidosis develops due to the accumulation of lactic acid, keto acids, and methylmalonic acid depending on the underlying etiology.

- *Iron overdose:* Iron overdose can cause lactic acidosis secondary to complications like intestinal ulceration, fulminant liver failure, and decreased cardiac output caused by dissociated ferrous or ferric molecules.
- *INH overdose:* Isoniazid overdose causes accumulation of keto acids resulting in high anion gap metabolic acidosis, seizures, and coma.

A few clinical scenarios are presented below:

Case 1

A 10-year-old child with type 1 diabetes was admitted with fast breathing.

Lab results: ABG—pH 7.24, pCO_2—28 mm Hg, HCO_3—12 mmol/L, SaO_2—98%, pO_2—86 mm Hg, serum Na—133 mmol/L, K—4 mmol/L, Cl—96 mmol/L.

What is a Metabolic Disorder?

The following steps are used for evaluation:

- Here HCO_3 is 12 which is lower than normal, can be due to either metabolic acidosis or compensated respiratory alkalosis
- Interpret the pH. pH here is 7.24, which is lower than normal, hence has metabolic acidosis
- Expected pCO_2 by Winter's formula: $(1.5 \times 12) + 8 \pm 2 =$ range 24–28 mm Hg. Here the measured pCO_2 falls in the expected range, hence diagnosis is simple metabolic acidosis
- Calculate the anion gap, AG =133 – (96 + 12) = 25, AG is increased, hence it is high anion gap metabolic acidosis
- Delta AG is 25 - 12 = 13
- Delta HCO_3 24 - 12 = 12
- Delta gap ratio is 1.1 so simple high anion gap metabolic acidosis.

Case 2

A 7-year-old child is admitted with diarrhea and dyspnea.

Lab results: Urine albumin nil, blood urea—65 mg/dL, serum creatinine—0.7 mg/dL, serum Na—130 mmol/L, serum K—2.5 mmol/L, serum Cl—112 mmol/L,

ABG: pH—7.14, pCO_2—22 mm Hg, pO_2—96 mm Hg, HCO_3—8 mmol/L

What is the ABG Disorder?

The following steps are used for evaluation:

- HCO_3 is 8 which is lower than normal, can be due to either metabolic acidosis or compensated respiratory alkalosis.
- Interpret the pH. The pH is 7.14 which is lower than normal, hence has a metabolic acidosis.
- Expected pCO_2 by Winter's formula: $(1.5 \times 8) + 8 \pm 2 =$ range 18–22 mm Hg. Here the measured pCO_2 falls in the expected range; hence, diagnosis is simple metabolic acidosis.
- Calculate the anion gap, AG = 130 – (112 + 8) = 10, AG is normal; hence, it is normal anion gap metabolic acidosis.

Case 3

A 5-year-old girl presented to the emergency department in shock. There was a history of profuse watery diarrhea for the past 2 days.

Lab values: Hb—12 g/dL, blood urea—40 mg/dL, serum creatinine—0.7 mg/dL, serum Na—139 mmol/L, serum K—3 mmol/L, serum Cl—112 mmol/L, pH—7.2. pCO_2—20 mm Hg, HCO_3—8 mEq/L

What is the ABG Disorder?

The following steps are used for evaluation:

- Here HCO_3 is 8 which is lower than normal, can be due to either metabolic acidosis or compensated respiratory alkalosis
- Interpret pH. The pH is 7.2, is lower than normal, hence has a metabolic acidosis
- Expected pCO_2 by Winter's formula is $(1.5 \times 8) + 8 \pm 2$ which is the expected range is 18–22 mm Hg. Here the measured

pCO_2 falls in the expected range, hence diagnosis is simple metabolic acidosis

- Calculate the anion gap, AG = 139 - (112 + 8) =19, AG is increased, hence metabolic acidosis is calculated as a high anion gap metabolic acidosis
- Delta AG is 19 - 12 = 7
- Delta HCO_3 24 - 8 = 16
- Delta gap ratio is 0.43, so it is a mixed high and normal anion gap metabolic acidosis.

Principles of Therapy in Metabolic Acidosis

Identify and institute corrective measures for the cause, treat dehydration with normal saline infusion, oxygen for patients with hypoxemia, and antibiotics in sepsis-associated lactic acidosis. The use of IV sodium bicarbonate is reserved for cases of extreme acidosis, when the blood pH is <7.0 or for patients with impaired renal acid excretion (with RTA, acute kidney injury, or chronic kidney disease) when their blood pH is <7.2 or when urine alkalization is needed.[22]

The initial goal in severe acidemia is to raise the pH to 7.25, at which the cardiac contractility and responsiveness to catecholamine will be restored. Emergency correction—8.4% $NaHCO_3$ is administered as IV infusion at a dose of 1 mEq/kg. Repeat blood gas, ionized calcium, and serum electrolytes are repeated 5–15 minutes after administration to determine therapy effectiveness and to assess adverse effects like low ionized calcium and hypokalemia. Excessive use of bicarbonate can cause hypernatremia and hypertonicity.

Also, ionized calcium values decrease when sodium bicarbonate is infused. Pretreatment with IV calcium is advised if the corrected calcium is <8 mg/dL. IV calcium gluconate 100 mg/kg can be slowly infused via a central catheter or a large vein prior to infusing sodium bicarbonate. Failure to correct the calcium prior to the sodium bicarbonate infusion can lead to acute hypocalcemia due to the enhanced binding of ionized calcium to serum proteins as the blood pH increases. An acute decrease in ionized calcium causes cardiac dysrhythmias, seizures, and/or even tetany.

Hemodialysis, peritoneal dialysis, or continuous kidney replacement therapy (CKRT) may be needed for treatment of severe, life-threatening metabolic acidosis unresponsive to medical therapy, especially if it is associated with hyperkalemia.

In a nonemergency setting, the bicarbonate deficit is calculated using the following formula:

Estimated bicarbonate deficit = (target bicarbonate – current bicarbonate) × weight (in kg) × 0.4–0.5. Half of the deficit is infused intravenously over 2–4 hours, mixed in 5% dextrose or one-half normal saline (NS) solution. Remaining half is infused over the following 6–24 hours and repeat blood gas, electrolytes, and calcium is done a few hours after correction.[22]

Potassium depletion is common in patients with metabolic acidosis due to GI and/or renal loss of K^+. There are three clinical settings where metabolic acidosis is associated with potassium depletion—(1) acute diarrheal illness, (2) RTA, and (3) diabetic ketoacidosis. Initial potassium concentration may be relatively normal in all these conditions since metabolic acidosis (except organic acidemia) cause K^+ to move out of the cells into the extracellular fluid. When hypokalemia and metabolic acidosis coexists hypokalemia should be corrected first to maintain K^+ above 3.2 before administration of $NaHCO_3$.

Chronic Metabolic Acidosis

Children with chronic acidosis require the administration of alkali supplements orally to correct the acidosis.[23] Alkali therapy include a number of formulations of sodium bicarbonate, sodium citrate/citric acid, potassium citrate/citric acid, and a combination of sodium citric acid and potassium citrate and citric acid. Citrate preparations are not to be used in children with chronic kidney disease (CKD) as they may enhance aluminum absorption. In addition, potassium-based therapy should be avoided in CKD due to the risk of developing hyperkalemia. The details of treatment in CKD and RTA are discussed in detail in respective sections.

Specific Situations

Diabetic Ketoacidosis

About 0.45% NS is started along with KCl and insulin is administered only after raising the plasma K^+ concentration to >3.5 mEq/L. The shift of K^+ into the cells by insulin will cause profound hypokalemia, cardiac arrhythmias, and sudden death. The role of bicarbonate therapy is uncertain in ketoacidosis as the ketoacid anions will be metabolized into bicarbonate with partial correction of the acidemia when insulin is started. Also, administration of bicarbonate is a risk factor for the development of cerebral edema. There are, however, three settings in which bicarbonate therapy is indicated in diabetic ketoacidosis (DKA):

1. PH < 7.16—goal of alkali treatment is to raise the pH to 7.25, HCO_3^- to 12 and not to normalize the pH.
2. Hyperkalemia and metabolic acidosis persist despite insulin therapy.
3. Presence of relatively normal anion gap acidosis, due to loss of keto acids in urine. Here, the quantity of bicarbonate that can be generated from the organic anion acid metabolism is minimal.[2]

Lactic Acidosis

The role of $NaHCO_3$ administration in lactic acidosis is controversial. In severe metabolic acidosis associated with vasodilatation and decreased cardiac contractility, IV $NaHCO_3$ is administered just enough to raise the pH to 7.25.

METABOLIC ALKALOSIS

Metabolic alkalosis is a commonly encountered, but often unrecognized disorder. It can occur as an isolated disorder or as part of other acid-base disorders.

Metabolic alkalosis is a pathological process where the arterial pH is elevated to greater than 7.45 secondary to some metabolic process. Metabolic alkalemia is arterial pH above the normal range (>7.45) due to a primary increase in plasma bicarbonate concentration.

Pathophysiology

An increase in the plasma bicarbonate concentration can occur due to excessive hydrogen ion loss or intake of bicarbonate salts or volume contraction with a relatively constant amount of extracellular bicarbonate (called a contraction alkalosis).[24-27] Excessive drop in hydrogen ions may occur due to loss in urine or from the gastrointestinal tract or movement into the cells.[28]

The respiratory system will try to compensate for metabolic alkalosis by hypoventilation resulting in the retention of CO_2, thus minimizing the elevation of pH which occurs immediately. For every 1 mEq/L increase in plasma bicarbonate concentration, arterial $PaCO_2$ increases by 0.7 mm Hg. Thus, pH is maintained below 7.5. The respiratory adaptation is followed by renal adaptive mechanism. Since kidneys have an inherent ability to efficiently eliminate bicarbonate (unlike acids) any elevation of bicarbonate levels would get corrected with time. So, ingestion of large amounts of bicarbonate in a normal subject does not result in a measurable increase in the plasma bicarbonate level. This is possible due to the following reasons:

- Plasma HCO_3^- is freely and completely filtered and then reclaimed. There is a threshold (approximately 24–26 mEq/L) above which the filtered HCO_3^- will not be reabsorbed in the proximal tubule.
- In alkalosis, there will be volume expansion which reduces reabsorption of sodium and bicarbonate in the proximal tubule.
- Alkalosis inhibits H^+ secretion by proximal tubule and thick ascending limb.
- It also inhibits proximal tubule ammonia synthesis necessary for H^+ secretion.
- Alkalosis causes hypertrophy of HCO_3^- secreting β-intercalated cells and atrophy of α-intercalated cells in the collecting tubule. The kidneys excrete excess bicarbonate through an apical chloride/bicarbonate exchanger and protons are gained to the systemic circulation via the basolateral H^+ ATPase.[2]

Hence in order to maintain the elevated bicarbonate concentration, conditions that reduce bicarbonate filtration, enhance bicarbonate reabsorption, and/or impair bicarbonate secretion should coexist.

Metabolic alkalemia and hypercarbia are almost always associated with hypokalemia. In the event of the addition of HCO_3^- to extracellular fluid, it is necessary to maintain electroneutrality either by the loss of the anion Cl^- or retention of Na^+. Hence, an increase in circulating bicarbonate may be associated with a contracted "effective" circulating volume and low blood pressure due to loss of anion (saline responsive metabolic alkalosis). This usually occurs due to secondary stimulation of collecting duct ion transport. This is also called *chloride responsive metabolic alkalosis.* An expanded "effective" circulating volume and increased blood pressure (BP) due to retention of sodium occur in saline-resistant metabolic alkalosis.[3] This usually occurs due to primary stimulation of collecting duct ion transport. This is also called chloride-resistant metabolic alkalosis.

Etiology

- *Generation of metabolic alkalosis*
  - *Loss of hydrogen ions—H^+ (acid):*
    - Gastrointestinal loses:
      - Vomiting
      - Nasogastric suction
      - Acid diarrhea (congenital chloridiarrhea, villous adenoma).
    - Renal H^+ loses:
      - Diuretics (thiazides, furosemide)
      - Bartter and Gitelman syndrome
      - Magnesium deficiency
      - Hyperaldosteronism
  - *Ingestion of alkali or infusion of bicarbonate:*
    - Iatrogenic, usually in patients with renal failure
    - Massive transfusion of citrated blood
- *Maintenance of metabolic alkalosis*[29]
  - Volume contraction
  - Potassium deficiency
  - Chloride depletion
  - Mineralocorticoid excess (aldosterone, progesterone, and deoxycorticosterone)
  - Increased sodium delivery to the distal nephron, where enhanced sodium reabsorption through epithelial sodium channels generates the secretion of hydrogen ions and potassium.[30]

Some of the important factors involved in the generation and maintenance of metabolic alkalosis will be discussed in some detail. They are as follows:

- *Vomiting:* The stomach normally secretes HCl, generating extracellular HCO_3^- in the process.
  Loss of HCl by vomiting or nasogastric suction results in increased production of the acid by the stomach, which in turn leads to increased generation of HCO_3^-. Volume contraction from fluid loss also occurs, promoting proximal tubule reabsorption of Na^+, and HCO_3^-. There is a secretion of K^+ and H^+ in the distal nephron, which

also contributes to the generation and maintenance of metabolic alkalosis. The hypokalemia seen in patients with vomiting is not because of gastric potassium loss. This is due to renal K^+ loss initially related to increased secretion in the distal nephron in presence of volume contraction. After a few days, when the dehydration is corrected, hypokalemia is due to loss of K^+ in the urine along with bicarbonate, which is not reabsorbed in the proximal tubule.

- *Bartter syndrome and Gitelman syndrome:* There is defective NaCl reabsorption in the thick ascending limb of the loop of Henle in Bartter syndrome and furosemide administration. In Gitelman syndrome and thiazide administration there is decreased NaCl reabsorption in distal convoluted tubule (DCT). This increases the distal delivery of NaCl. The increase in urinary excretion of NaCl leads to ECF volume contraction, which stimulates renin-mediated aldosterone secretion, which in turn stimulates distal nephron reabsorption of Na^+ in exchange for K^+ and H^+. The result is hypokalemic metabolic alkalosis.
- *Excess mineralocorticoid:* Excess mineralocorticoid results in volume expansion due to increased distal nephron Na^+ reabsorption. This volume expansion decreases proximal renal tubular Na^+ reabsorption and increases the delivery of Na^+ to the distal nephron. In presence of a high mineralocorticoid, Na^+ is reabsorbed and K^+ and H^+ are secreted, resulting in metabolic alkalosis, and persistent volume expansion and hypertension.
- *Extracellular fluid volume contraction with chloride deficiency:* This is often associated with a decrease in glomerular filtration rate (GFR) leading to a decreased filtered load of HCO_3^-. There is stimulation of proximal tubular reabsorption of Na^+ and HCO_3^-. Extracellular fluid volume (ECF) volume contraction activates renin angiotensin aldosterone system (RAAS). Angiotensin II stimulates reabsorption of bicarbonate. Increased mineralocorticoid activity results in increased distal reabsorption of Na^+ and secretion of K^+ and H^+. Decreased distal delivery of Cl^- inhibits HCO_3^- secretion by the β-intercalated cells.
- *Potassium deficiency:* In potassium deficiency, there is an increase in proximal convoluted tubule (PCT) ammonium synthesis. A deficit of potassium is associated with intracellular acidosis in the PCT cells as intracellular potassium shifts out of the cells in exchange for H^+ to replenish the ECF potassium. This augments the production of NH_4^+ and HCO_3^- in PCT. NH_4^+ is excreted in the urine with Cl^- while new HCO_3^- is added to the body. Intracellular acidosis augments the reabsorption of other filtered anions (e.g., citrate) which compromises the dietary elimination of HCO_3. Activity of H^+-K^+ ATPase transporter on apical membrane of α-intercalated cells increases, which increases K^+ reabsorption and H^+ secretion.
- *Posthypercapnic alkalosis:* Chronic respiratory acidosis is associated with compensatory hyperbicarbonatemia. When the pCO_2 in patients with chronic respiratory acidosis is lowered rapidly (e.g., mechanical ventilation), the elevated plasma bicarbonate can cause an acute rise in cerebral pH that can produce serious neurologic sequelae or even death. Consequently, pCO_2 should be lowered slowly and carefully in chronic hypercapnia. Also, in patients with a tendency towards volume contraction (e.g., use of diuretics) when pCO_2 falls to the normal level, there will be a stimulus for persistently increased plasma bicarbonate levels and hypokalemia. Hence, attention to volume and potassium status is important, while taking care of patients with chronic hypercapnia.[31,32]
- *Intake of nonreabsorbable anions:* If a patient has a contracted effective circulating volume and takes a Na^+ salt with an anion that cannot be reabsorbed by the kidney (e.g., penicillinate), he or she may develop hypokalemia and metabolic alkalosis. Hypokalemia develops due to the increased action of aldosterone due to volume contraction, which causes sodium reabsorption and potassium secretion. The delivery of chloride to distal nephron is low in the setting of volume contraction as most of the NaCl will be reabsorbed in the PCT.
  The rise in plasma bicarbonate is the result of both NaCl and K^+ deficits. Urinary chloride will be low and provides the clue. Urinary sodium varies depending upon whether a load of nonreabsorbable anion is recent or remote. When the intake of nonreabsorbable anion is discontinued, the urinary sodium comes down.[2]
- *Magnesium depletion:* Patients with hypomagnesemia may have hypokalemia and metabolic alkalosis. The clinical setting for this deficiency includes malabsorption; diarrhea or drugs that act on the loop of Henle (e.g., loop diuretics, cisplatin, or aminoglycosides). These patients should be differentiated from those with primary hyperaldosteronism with hypertension as well as those with Bartter or Gitelman syndrome who may also have hypomagnesemia.

Clinical Effects and Consequences of Metabolic Alkalosis

Patients with metabolic alkalosis may be asymptomatic or may complain of symptoms that are primarily related to the alkalemia, to the underlying etiology of the metabolic alkalosis, or to accompanying electrolyte abnormalities. Symptoms can be due to volume depletion like easy fatigability, muscle cramps, and postural dizziness. Metabolic alkalosis can cause a shift in the oxygen dissociation curve to the left, which impairs oxygen delivery to the tissues leading to tissue hypoxemia. It also suppresses ventilation and also causes vasoconstriction of all vessels especially cerebral and coronaries. Alkalosis causes decreased ionized calcium and shift potassium into the cells causing hypokalemia, both of which can cause cardiac arrhythmias and muscle weakness. Severe metabolic alkalosis can cause agitation, disorientation, seizures,[33] and coma, especially when metabolic alkalosis develops in patients with chronic liver disease.

Approach to a Child with Metabolic Alkalosis

The approach to a child with metabolic alkalosis is shown in **Flowchart 2**.

- Blood gas analysis (for pH, pCO_2, and HCO_3^-) to confirm the diagnosis. In a child with metabolic alkalosis, for every 1 mEq/L rise in bicarbonate level pCO_2 rises by 0.7 mm Hg.
- Assess effective arteriolar volume status and Blood pressure. The key parameters are—weight loss, heart rate, pulse volume, dry mucosa, and orthostatic hypotension.
- Random urine chloride estimation is more helpful than urine sodium estimation in volume-depleted patients (saline responsive metabolic alkalosis). This is because in volume depletion associated with alkalosis, there will be bicarbonate loss to some extent in the urine, which will drag some sodium along with it, and hence the urine sodium may be high despite volume depletion. In a volume-depleted patient due to a nonrenal source of NaCl loss, urine chloride will be <10 mEq/L, whereas, in renal source for NaCl loss (e.g., Bartter and Gitelman syndrome, recent use of diuretics), the urinary chloride will be more than 20 mEq/L.
- To differentiate Bartter from Gitelman's syndrome urinary calcium and plasma magnesium are done.
    - If 24-hour urinary calcium is >4 mg/kg and plasma magnesium is normal, it is most likely Bartter syndrome.[34]
    - If the child has hypomagnesemia with hypocalciuria diagnosis is Gitelman's syndrome.
- Serum electrolytes (Na^+, K^+, Cl^- and HCO_3^-).
- Blood urea, serum creatinine, uric acid, plasma renin, and serum aldosterone assay in a hypertensive patient with metabolic alkalosis (saline resistant metabolic alkalosis).
- In a child with hypertension, mild hypokalemia and mild metabolic alkalosis are clues to the presence of hyperaldosteronism.

A few clinical scenarios are presented here:

Case 1

A 2-month-old baby boy presents with severe vomiting. Clinically he is dehydrated with blood pressure at 90th centile.

Lab values: Blood urea—23 mg/dL, serum creatinine—0.4 mg/dL, Na—120 mmol/L, K—2.9 mmol/L, chloride—92 mmol/L

Flowchart 2: Approach to a child with metabolic alkalosis.

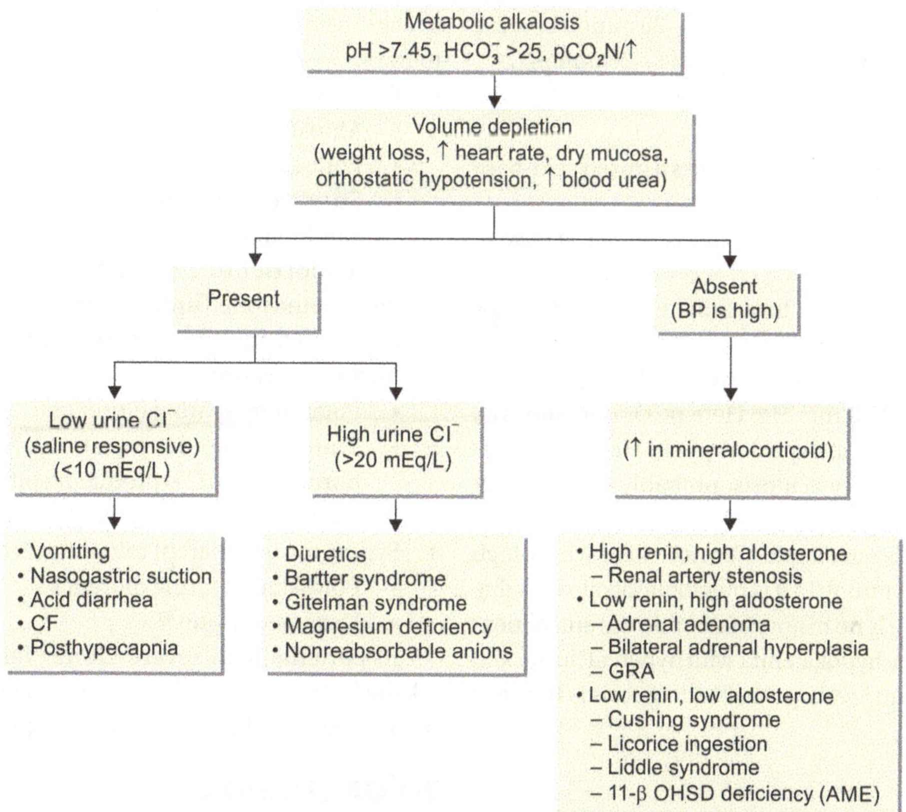

(AME: syndrome of apparent mineralocorticoid excess; CF: cystic fibrosis; GRA: glucocorticoid remediable hyperaldosteronism; OHSD: hydroxysteroid dehydrogenase)

ABG: pH—7.48, pCO_2—47 mm Hg, HCO_3—33 mmol/L, urine chloride—8 mEq/L

Approach to Diagnosis

- pH is 7.48, which indicates alkalemia
- Since bicarbonate level is also high, this is a case of metabolic alkalosis
- For every, 1 mEq/L rise in bicarbonate level pCO_2 rises by 0.7 mm Hg.
  Expected rise in pCO_2 is 6.3 mm Hg [(33 – 24) × 0.7]. Expected pCO_2 is 46.3 mm Hg. Here pCO_2 is 47 mm Hg, which is almost the same as expected pCO_2, hence this is a simple metabolic alkalosis
- Since the patient is clinically hypotensive and hypovolemic, with a low urine chloride (8 mmol/L), it is extrarenal loss, hence most probably hypokalemic hypochloremic metabolic alkalosis with hypokalemia, possibly due to vomiting caused by pyloric stenosis.

Case 2

A 3-year-old child weighing 9 kg is admitted with fever and breathlessness. He has a history of polyuria, polydipsia, growth retardation, and salt craving. He is clinically euvolemic with normal BP for age.

Lab values: Blood urea—22 mg/dL, serum creatinine—0.5 mg/dL, serum Na—120 mmol/L, serum K—3 mmol/L, serum magnesium—1.8 mmol/L

ABG: pH—7.40, PCO_2—46 mm Hg, HCO_3—28 mmol/L, urine calcium—45 mg in 24 hours, urine chloride—28 mmol/L

Approach to Diagnosis

- pH is 7.4 which is normal, and indicates a mixed acid-base disorder.
- Since the bicarbonate level is also high, this is a case of metabolic alkalosis.
- For every, 1 mEq/L rise in bicarbonate level pCO_2 rises by 0.7 mm Hg.
- Expected rise in pCO_2 is 2.8 mm Hg—[(28 – 24) × 0.7] Hg. Expected pCO_2 is 42.8 mm Hg. Here pCO_2 is 47 mm Hg, which is more than the expected pCO_2. Hence, there is a coexistent respiratory acidosis, probably due to lower respiratory infection.
- Since the patient is euvolemic, normotensive with a high urine chloride (20 mmol/L) it is metabolic alkalosis is due to renal loss. There is no history of diuretic use and patient has hyponatremia, hypokalemia with hypercalciuria, and normal magnesium levels, probable diagnosis is Bartter's syndrome.

Treatment

Identify and treat the underlying cause for generation of metabolic alkalosis. Correct the cause of maintenance of metabolic alkalosis. The most common causes of hypokalemic metabolic alkalosis associated with a "contracted effective circulating volume" include gastric fluid loss; diuretic therapy or cutaneous fluid loss. Volume depletion and hypokalemia are the most common factors responsible for the maintenance of alkalosis. These forms of metabolic alkalosis are termed "chloride responsive" because they are reversed by the administration of fluids containing sodium chloride. Correction of volume depletion should be with normal saline and not with Ringer lactate (which has lactate, which gets converted to bicarbonate in the liver), unless if given for the treatment of shock.

In Bartter syndrome salt and potassium chloride supplementation, potassium-sparing diuretics such as spironolactone, amiloride and triamterene, and cyclooxygenase (COX) inhibitors are used. Potassium replacement either oral or parenteral should be provided for the correction of hypokalemia that is invariably associated with metabolic alkalosis of any etiology. Use of carbonic anhydrase inhibitors (such as acetazolamide) or potassium-sparing diuretics in patients who have metabolic alkalosis, but also need diuretics, e.g., cardiac failure. Furosemide and thiazides will further potentiate the problem, whereas acetazolamide will decrease proximal bicarbonate reabsorption by blocking the carbonic anhydrase enzyme.

In alkali ingestion identification and discontinuation of offending alkali is the first approach to treatment. In chloride resistant metabolic alkalosis management is based on the specific cause. The various treatment modalities used are as follows:

- Primary hyperaldosteronism
  - Aldosterone antagonists
  - Potassium-sparing diuretics
  - Surgical removal of tumor in adrenal adenoma/carcinoma
- Glucocorticoid remediable hyperaldosteronism-dexamethasone (unlike cortisol, dexamethasone does not activate mineralocorticoid receptor)
- Cushing's syndrome
  - Potassium-sparing diuretics
  - Trans-sphenoidal resection of adrenocorticotropic hormone (ACTH) producing pituitary adenomas and adrenalectomy for adrenal tumors.
- Syndrome of apparent mineralocorticoid excess
  - Potassium-sparing diuretics
  - Dexamethasone.[34]

In patients with severe kidney failure and metabolic alkalosis, hemodialysis with a low dialysate bicarbonate or hemofiltration with saline infusion has to be done.

CONCLUSION

Maintenance of normal arterial pH between 7.35 and 7.45 and intracellular pH between 7 and 7.3 is essential for normal health, growth, and development. The strict maintenance of acid-base balance in the setting of this continuous production of acidic metabolites is accomplished by means of extracellular and intracellular buffers with renal and respiratory regulatory mechanisms. The total amount of H^+ generated by metabolism is 2–3 mEq/kg/day in a child.[2] the total amount of H^+ to be excreted in a child is 2–3 mEq/kg/day.[2] Metabolic acidosis is the pathologic process that increases the blood hydrogen ion (H^+) concentration and decreases the serum bicarbonate (HCO_3). Metabolic acidosis may be a high anion gap or normal anion gap.

Metabolic alkalosis is a pathological process where the arterial pH is elevated to >7.45 secondary to some metabolic process. The clinical symptomatology is nonspecific and a systematic approach is required for correct diagnosis and treatment in both these disorders.

KEY POINTS

- The primary abnormality in metabolic acidosis is a decrease in bicarbonate concentration.
- Based on anion gap metabolic acidosis can be classified into high and normal anion gap metabolic acidosis.
- The cause of nonanion gap metabolic acidosis can be identified based on urine anion gap, urine pH, and serum potassium values.
- Treatment of underlying conditions forms the basis of therapy. Judicious use of bicarbonate is recommended only in the treatment of specific situations like severe metabolic acidosis.
- The primary abnormality in metabolic alkalosis in an increase in serum bicarbonate level.
- For metabolic alkalosis to develop, both generation of bicarbonate and factors such as volume contraction and hypokalemia which maintains hyperbicarbonatemia are crucial.
- Metabolic alkalosis may be associated with ECF volume contraction, normal ECF or with ECF volume expansion.
- Volume status, blood pressure, and urine chloride levels are important parameters used to identify the etiology of metabolic alkalosis.
- The management of metabolic alkalosis depends upon underlying etiology, volume status, and symptomatology.

REFERENCES

1. Palmer BF, Alpern RJ. Normal acid-base balance. In: Feehally J, Floege J, Johnson RJ (Eds). Comprehensive Clinical Nephrology, 6th edition. Philadelphia: Elsevier; 2010. pp. 142-8.
2. Shah MA. Homeostasis and disorders of sodium, potassium and acid-base balance. In: Vijayakumar M, Nammalwar BR (Eds). Principles and Practice of Pediatric Nephrology, 2nd edition. New Delhi: Jaypee Brothers Medical Publishers (P) Ltd; 2013. pp. 55-78.
3. Hanna JD, Scheinman JI, Chan JC. The kidney in acid-base balance. Pediatr Clin North Am. 1995;42(6):1365-95.
4. Rose BD. Clinical Physiology of Acid-base and Electrolyte Disorders, 4th edition. New York: McGraw-Hill; 1994. pp. 118-85.
5. Manz F, Kalhoff H, Remer T. Renal acid excretion in early infancy. Pediatr Nephrol. 1997;11(2):231-43.
6. Allanson ER, Waqar T, White C, Tunçalp Ö, Dickinson JE. Umbilical lactate as a measure of acidosis and predictor of neonatal risk: a systematic review. BJOG. 2017;124(4):584-94.
7. Allanson ER, Pattinson RC, Nathan EA, Dickinson JE. The introduction of umbilical cord lactate measurement and associated neonatal outcomes in a South African tertiary hospital labor ward. J Matern Fetal Neonatal Med. 2018;31(10):1272-8.
8. Kurt A, Ecevit A, Ozkiraz S, Ince DA, Akcan AB, Tarcan A. The use of chloride-sodium ratio in the evaluation of metabolic acidosis in critically ill neonates. Eur J Pediatr. 2012;171(6):963-9.
9. Wang S, McDonnell EH, Sedor FA, Toffaletti JG. pH effects on measurements of ionized calcium and ionized magnesium in blood. Arch Pathol Lab Med. 2002;126(8):947-50.
10. Lopez-Garcia SC, Emma F, Walsh SB, Fila M, Hooman N, Zaniew M, et al. Treatment and long-term outcome in primary distal renal tubular acidosis. Nephrol Dial Transplant. 2019;34(6):981-91.
11. McSherry E. Acidosis and growth in nonuremic renal disease. Kidney Int. 1978;14(4):349-54.
12. Osther PJ, Bollerslev J, Hansen AB, Engel K, Kildeberg P. Pathophysiology of incomplete renal tubular acidosis in recurrent renal stone formers: evidence of disturbed calcium, bone and citrate metabolism. Urol Res. 1993;21(3):169-73.
13. Norman ME, Feldman NI, Cohn RM, Roth KS, McCurdy DK. Urinary citrate excretion in the diagnosis of distal renal tubular acidosis. J Pediatr. 1978;92(3):394-400.
14. Haque SK, Ariceta G, Batlle D. Proximal renal tubular acidosis: a not so rare disorder of multiple etiologies. Nephrol Dial Transplant. 2012;27(12):4273-87.
15. Sinert R, Zehtabchi S, Bloem C, Lucchesi M. Effect of normal saline infusion on the diagnostic utility of base deficit in identifying major injury in trauma patients. Acad Emerg Med. 2006;13(12):1269-74.
16. Disma N, Mameli L, Pistorio A, Davidson A, Barabino P, Locatelli BG, et al. A novel balanced isotonic sodium solution vs normal saline during major surgery in children up to 36 months: a multicenter RCT. Paediatr Anaesth. 2014;24(9):980-6.
17. Zunini GS, Rando KA, Cox RG. Fluid replacement in craniofacial pediatric surgery: normal saline or ringer's lactate? J Craniofac Surg. 2011;22(4):1370-4.
18. Lima MF, Neville IS, Cavalheiro S, Bourguignon DC, Pelosi P, Malbouisson LMS. Balanced crystalloids versus saline for perioperative intravenous fluid administration in children undergoing neurosurgery: a randomized clinical trial. J Neurosurg Anesthesiol. 2019; 31(1):30-35.
19. Danhauser K, Smeitink JA, Freisinger P, Sperl W, Sabir H, Hadzik B, et al. Treatment options for lactic acidosis and metabolic crisis in children with mitochondrial disease. J Inherit Metab Dis. 2015;38(3):467-75.
20. Sun J, Shannon M, Ando Y, Schnackenberg LK, Khan NA, Portilla D, et al. Serum metabolomic profiles from patients with acute kidney injury: a pilot study. J Chromatogr B Analyt Technol Biomed Life Sci. 2012; 893-894:107-13.
21. Mishima E, Fukuda S, Mukawa C, Yuri A, Kanemitsu Y, Matsumoto Y, et al. Evaluation of the impact of gut microbiota on uremic solute accumulation by a CE-TOFMS-based metabolomics approach. Kidney Int. 2017; 92(3):634-45.

22. Yorgin P, Mak R. (2021). Approach to the child with metabolic acidosis [online]. Available from: https://www.uptodate.com/home [Last accessed May, 2022].
23. Soriano JR. Renal tubular acidosis: the clinical entity, J Am Soc Nephrol. 2002;13(8):2160-70.
24. Rose BD, Post TW. Clinical Physiology of Acid-Base and Electrolyte Disorders, 5th edition. New York: McGraw-Hill; 2001. p. 559.
25. Palmer BF, Alpern RJ. Metabolic alkalosis. J Am Soc Nephrol. 1997; 8(9):1462-9.
26. Galla JH. Metabolic alkalosis. J Am Soc Nephrol. 2000;11(2): 369-75.
27. Khanna A, Kurtzman NA. Metabolic alkalosis. J Nephrol. 2006;19(Suppl 9):S86-96.
28. Halperin ML, Scheich A. Should we continue to recommend that a deficit of KCl be treated with NaCl? A fresh look at chloride-depletion metabolic alkalosis. Nephron. 1994;67(3):263-9.
29. Seldin DW, Rector FC Jr. Symposium on acid-base homeostasis. The generation and maintenance of metabolic alkalosis. Kidney Int. 1972;1(5):306-21.
30. Luke RG, Galla JH. It is chloride depletion alkalosis, not contraction alkalosis. J Am Soc Nephrol. 2012;23(2):204-7.
31. Polak A, Haynie GD, Hays RM, Schwartz WB. Effects of chronic hypercapnia on electrolyte and acid-base equilibrium. I. Adaptation. J Clin Invest. 1961;40(7):1223-37.
32. Schwartz WB, Hays RM, Polak A, Haynie GD. Effects of chronic hypercapnia on electrolyte and acid-base equilibrium. II. Recovery, with special reference to the influence of chloride intake. J Clin Invest. 1961;40(7):1238-49.
33. Brewer ED. Disorders of acid-base balance. Pediatr Clin North Am. 1990;37(2):429-47.
34. Vimala A, Visweswaran RK. Metabolic acidosis and metabolic alkalosis. In: Vimala A (Ed). Fluid, Electrolyte, Metabolic and Respiratory Acid-Base Management, 1st edition. New Delhi: Jaypee Brothers Medical Publishers (P) Ltd; 2014. pp. 275-317.

CHAPTER

4.5 Homeostasis and Disorders of Calcium, Phosphorus, and Magnesium

Deepthi RV, Indira Agarwal

CALCIUM METABOLISM

Role of Calcium in Human Body

Calcium is critical for normal cell function, neural transmission, muscle contraction, membrane stability, bone structure, blood coagulation, intercellular adhesion, and intracellular signaling by acting as second messenger for exocytosis, chemotaxis, hormone secretion, and various enzymatic activities. Recently, its role has been identified in head injury or stroke and cardiopulmonary disorders.

Distribution of Calcium in Human Body

Calcium is the most abundant cation in the body. It constitutes 2% of the body weight (1,300 g). More than 99% is stored as hydroxyapatite in bones, while 0.9% in intracellular (cells and organelles in teeth and soft tissue) and 0.1% is extracellular.

Bone acts as a large reservoir for storing calcium and as a source of calcium when extracellular fluid (ECF) calcium concentration decreases. The distribution of ECF calcium is shown in **Figure 1**. From birth to 20 years of age, calcium content increases by 40-fold. The increase in skeletal weight and density requires the net retention of about 150–200 mg calcium per day. Hence, calcium balance must be positive (formation > resorption) during this age group which ensures healthy skeletal growth.[1]

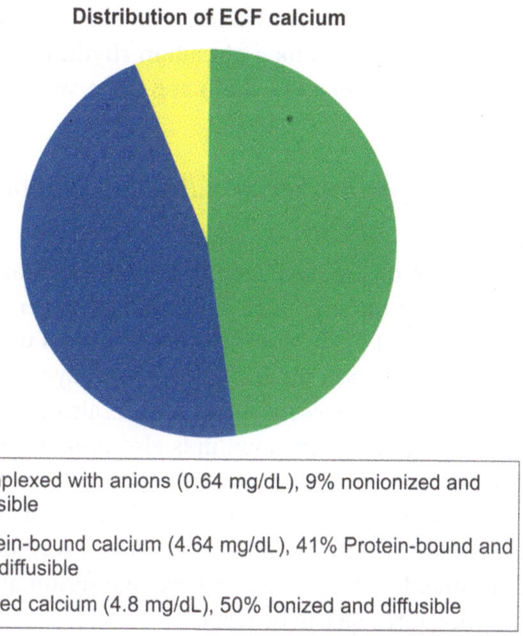

Fig. 1: Distribution of calcium in the extracellular compartment. (ECF: extracellular fluid)

Homeostasis of Calcium in Healthy Adults

Calcium balance is tightly regulated by the interplay between gastrointestinal absorption, renal excretion, and bone resorption. A normal adult ingests 1,000 mg of calcium per day. The net absorption of calcium is only 100–200 mg daily. In the steady state, 100 mg of calcium is excreted in the urine. Net zero calcium balance is the result of net intestinal absorption and urinary excretion which are the same. Entry and exit of calcium between the ECF and intracellular fluid (ICF) spaces are also of identical manner in steady state as shown in the **Figure 2**.

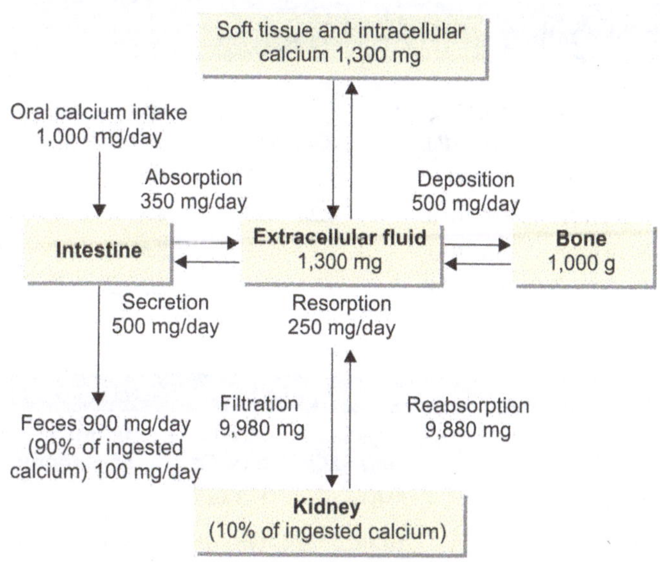

Fig. 2: Calcium flux between body compartments in a healthy adult.

SERUM CALCIUM

Serum calcium is measured as total plasma calcium and the normal range is 9–10.6 mg/dL/4.5–5.1 mEq/L/2.5 mmol/L.

Ionized calcium is the physiologically active form of calcium. Serum ionized calcium is tightly maintained within a physiologic range of 4.4–5.4 mg/dL (1.10–1.35 mEq/L).

Determinants of Serum Calcium

Age

Serum calcium is age-dependent. Normal values of ionized calcium and total calcium concentration in various age groups are shown in **Table 1**. In healthy infants, ionized calcium levels decrease from 5.8 mg/dL at birth to a nadir of 4.9 mg/dL at 24 hours of life and increase slightly during the first week of life. Serum calcium in young children is slightly higher (~0.2 mg/dL) than those in adults.

Circadian Rhythm

There is noted to be diurnal variation in serum calcium levels which is shown in **Table 2**. The blood ionized calcium concentration exhibits a circadian rhythm characterized by a peak at 10 am and a nadir at 6–8 PM, with amplitude of 0.3 mg/dL.[2,3]

Effect of Posture, Serum Albumin, and pH on Serum Calcium

There is no change between fasting and nonfasting serum calcium but there is positional change in serum calcium levels. Upright position causes venous stasis with resultant hemoconcentration and subsequent hemodynamic change in serum albumin.[3] This increases serum calcium by 0.5 mg/dL when upright. Serum calcium is also influenced by serum albumin and blood pH. Serum albumin reduction by 1 g/dL decreases the protein-bound calcium by 0.8 mg/dL. Total measured calcium should be corrected if serum albumin is abnormal. If 4.0 represent the average serum albumin, the following formula can be used:

TABLE 1: Age-dependent normal values of serum ionized (iCa), total calcium (Ca), and phosphorus.

Age	Total Ca (mg/dL)	iCa (mM)	Serum phosphorous (mg/dL)
0–3 months	8.8–11.3	1.22–1.40	4.8–7.4
1–5 years	9.4–10.8	1.22–1.32	4.5–6.5
6–12 years	9.4–10.3	1.15–1.32	3.6–5.8
13–20 years	8.8–10.2	1.12–1.3	2.3–4.5

TABLE 2: Circadian rhythm of serum total and ionized calcium (Ca).

	Serum ionized Ca	Serum total Ca	Serum phosphorus
Nadir	6–8 PM	1–3 AM	11 AM
Peak	10 AM	12–1 PM	2 AM
Amplitude	0.3 mg/dL	0.5 mg/dL	1.2 mg/dL
Fasting concentration	4.67 mg/dL	9.6 mg/dL	3.6 mg/dL
24-hour mean concentration	4.52 mg/dL	9.4 mg/dL	4.0 mg/dL

Corrected calcium (mg/dL) = Measured total Ca (mg/dL) + 0.8 [4.0 – Serum albumin (g/dL)]

Increase or decrease in blood pH by 0.1 respectively increases and decreases the protein-bound calcium by 0.12 mg/dL. The effect of blood pH on ionized calcium is the opposite. Acidosis increases ionized calcium and decreases protein-bound calcium, whereas alkalosis decreases ionized calcium and increases protein-bound calcium.

Clinical Pearl

- In the presence of hypocalcemia and metabolic acidosis, if acidosis is corrected first, it may precipitate tetany.
- When plasma calcium ion concentration is about 50% below normal, the peripheral nerves are excited and discharge spontaneously and initiate the nerve impulses to elicit tetany. Tetany occurs when blood calcium decreases from 9.4 to 6 mg/dL (35% fall) and is lethal at 4 mg/dL.
- Conversely hypercalcemia depresses nervous and musculoskeletal system, decreases QT interval, and causes loss of appetite and constipation. Depressive effect begins at Ca above 12 mg/dL and is marked above 15 mg/dL. Above 17 mg/dL, calcium phosphate crystals precipitate with resultant clinical consequence.

Hormonal Regulation of Serum Calcium Level

Serum levels of ionized calcium are maintained in the normal range by two major calcium-regulating hormones and their receptors namely parathyroid hormone (PTH) and the parathyroid hormone receptor (PTHR), 1,25$(OH)_2$D and the vitamin D receptor (VDR), and the calcium-sensing receptor (CaSR).

Calcium-sensing receptor is a guanosine triphosphate (GTP) or G-protein coupled polypeptide receptor made of 1,084 amino acid residues and encoded by a gene on chromosome 3p13; expressed in the chief cells of parathyroid glands, kidneys, bone marrow, osteoclasts, and osteoblasts.[4] CaSR in the parathyroid glands senses small changes in the serum ionized calcium concentration and then brings about increase in the renal tubular calcium reabsorption through the PTHR and in bone to increase net bone resorption, which is directed at normalizing serum calcium concentration. This receptor is also activated by magnesium. In the kidney, CaSR is located on the basolateral aspect of loop of Henle. Normally filtered sodium chloride enters the cells in the thick ascending limb of the loop of Henle via Na^+K^+2Cl co-transporters in the luminal membrane. Most of the potassium that is reabsorbed by the Na^+K^+2Cl cotransporter leaks back into the lumen through ROMK channel to drive further inward sodium chloride transport. Movement of potassium into the lumen plus the movement of reabsorbed chloride (via a chloride channel) out of the basolateral surface of the cells makes the tubular lumen positive, which drives the passive reabsorption of sodium, calcium, and magnesium via the paracellular pathway between the cells. The apical K channel is inhibited by CaSR resulting in decreased calcium reabsorption. The decrease in serum calcium inactivates the CaSR in kidney to increase calcium reabsorption. With a rise in serum calcium, these actions are reversed and the integrated hormonal response reduces serum calcium. One of the most important regulators of bone uptake and release of calcium is PTH.

Parathyroid hormone maintains serum calcium by directly or indirectly promoting calcium entry into blood at three sites—bone, kidneys, and gut.

- PTH increases bone turnover, resulting in a release of calcium and phosphorus from bone. PTH acts on bone in presence of calcitriol to release calcium in two ways. The immediate effect of PTH is to mobilize calcium from skeletal stores that are readily available. Later, PTH stimulates release of calcium by activation of bone resorption.
- PTH increases renal calcium reabsorption and decreases renal phosphorus reabsorption. It is primarily through these latter distal segments of the kidney that the regulation of urinary calcium excretion occurs.
- PTH increases the conversion of $25(OH)D_3$ (calcidiol) to $1,25(OH)D_3$ (calcitriol) in the kidney, thereby increasing gastrointestinal calcium absorption. The formation of calcitriol is primarily stimulated by PTH and hypophosphatemia. Hypercalcemia impairs and hypocalcemia promotes PTH-induced calcitriol production. The increased PTH also stimulates the kidney to increase secretion of $1,25(OH)D_3$, which activates the VDR in gut to increase calcium absorption.

Parathyroid hormone assay was previously done by caboxyterminal or amino terminal fragment assay and is not in use anymore. Recently, intact PTH is measured by immunoreactive PTH assay using antibodies that detect intact parathyroid hormone (iPTH). The double antibody immune radiometric assay (immune assay) is more sensitive and specific.

Calcitriol is synthesized in the proximal tubule. It is also synthesized by activated macrophages. In the kidney, tubular cells contain two enzymes: 1, alpha-hydroxylase and 24, alpha-hydroxylase that can further hydroxylate $25(OH)D_3$, producing 1,25 dihydroxyvitamin D, the most active form of vitamin D or 24, 25-dihydroxy vitamin D, an inactive metabolite. Normal vitamin D level is >30 ng/mL in adults and >20 ng/mL in children.[5]

Calcitonin participates in calcium and phosphorus metabolism by counteracting PTH. It lowers blood calcium levels by inhibiting the calcium absorption by the intestines, inhibits osteoclast activity in bones, and decreases renal tubular reabsorption of calcium.

Parathyroid hormone-related protein (PTHrP) resembles PTH at N-terminal end. It is longer and more complex than PTH. It is secreted by some tumors as well. During pregnancy, calcium is transferred from maternal circulation to the fetus by a pump regulated by PTHrP. The PTHrP levels increase during lactation and contribute to movement of calcium from maternal skeleton to the mammary glands. PTHrP is implicated in pathogenesis of humoral calcium of malignancy.

Calcium Reabsorption in the Kidneys

Calcium is filtered at the glomerulus. Within the proximal convoluted tubule (PCT) and the proximal straight tubule, 60–70% of the filtered calcium is reabsorbed driven by a gradient generated by sodium and water reabsorption. No reabsorption of calcium occurs within the thin segment of the loop of Henle. The thick ascending limb of the loop of Henle reabsorbs about 20%. Finally, 10% of the filtered calcium is reabsorbed in the distal convoluted tubule, with another 3–10% of reabsorption in the connecting tubule. The reabsorption of calcium by different segments is shown in **Figure 3**.

Tubular Transport of Calcium

Transport of calcium occurs by paracellular and transcellular pathways in proximal tubular cells as shown in **Table 3**.

Paracellular Calcium Reabsorption

In PCT, calcium reabsorption parallels sodium and water reabsorption. Calcium is dissolved in water and carried with the reabsorbed fluids through paracellular pathway.[1,6]

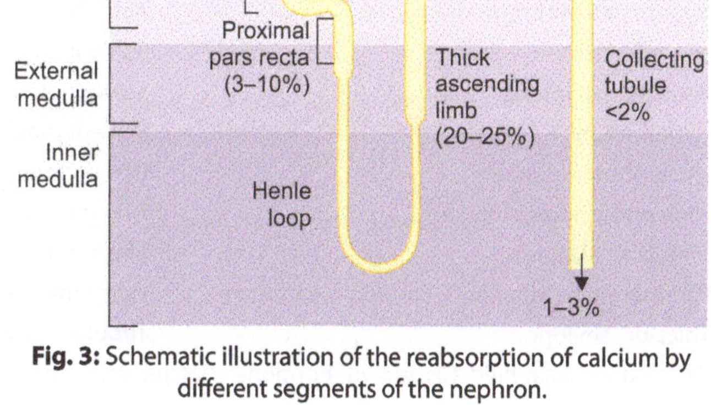

Fig. 3: Schematic illustration of the reabsorption of calcium by different segments of the nephron.

Transcellular Calcium Reabsorption

Transcellular calcium reabsorption involves the following two steps:

1. Calcium diffuses from the tubular lumen into the cell down an electrochemical gradient due to the much higher concentration of calcium in tubular lumen compared with the epithelial cell cytoplasm and because the cell interior has a negative charge relative to tubular lumen.
2. Calcium exits the cell across the basolateral membrane by a calcium adenosine triphosphatase (Ca-ATPase) pump and by Na-Ca counter transport. The distal tubular reabsorption of calcium in kidney depends on the TRPV5 channel and its expression is regulated by PTH.[7]

TABLE 3: Mode of calcium transport in various segments of nephron.

Site of nephron	*Transport mode*	*Fraction*	*Mode of transport*	*Hormonal mediation*
PCT	Passive	80%	Paracellular	PTH independent
	Active	20%	Transcellular	
TALHL	Passive	50%	Paracellular	PTH dependent
	Active	50%	Transcellular	
DCT	Active	100%	Transcellular	PTH dependent

(DCT: distal convoluted tubule; PCT: proximal convoluted tubule: PTH: parathyroid hormone; TALHL: thick ascending limb of Henle's loop)

TABLE 4: Regulators of calcium absorption from gastrointestinal tract (GIT).

Increased GIT calcium absorption	*Decreased GIT calcium absorption*
• Puberty • Pregnancy • Vitamin D excess • Acromegaly • Milk-alkali syndrome	• Advanced age • Chronic kidney disease • Gastrectomy • Intestinal malabsorption • Diabetes mellitus • Corticosteroid • Estrogen deficiency • High fiber or fat content in diet • Low Ca/P ratio in food • Fructose ingestion

The regulators of calcium absorption from GIT and factors affecting the renal calcium excretion are shown in **Tables 4 and 5**, respectively.[8]

Long-term maintenance of calcium homeostasis is dependent on the following factors.[9] This is illustrated in **Flowcharts 1 and 2.**

- Adaptation of intestinal calcium absorption to the needs of the body
- The balance between bone excretion and resorption
- Urine excretion of calcium

PHOSPHORUS METABOLISM

Role of Phosphorus in Human Body

Phosphate is one of the major components of the skeleton. Phosphate is component of DNA and RNA. Phosphate

Flowchart 1: Physiological response to hypercalcemia.

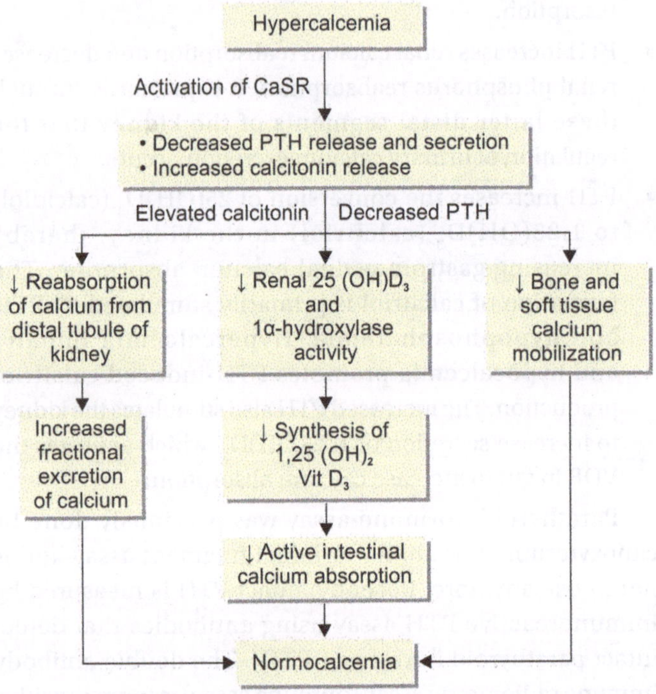

(PTH: parathyroid hormone)

TABLE 5: Factors affecting renal calcium excretion.

Decreased calcium excretion (hypocalciuria)	*Mechanism*	*Increased calcium excretion (hypercalciuria)*
Hyperparathyroidism	Activate Ca channel	Hypoparathyroidism
Low effective ECF volume	Solvent drag	High ECF volume
Reduced salt intake	Solvent drag	High salt intake, NaCl infusion
Hypotension	Solvent drag	Hypertension
Hyperphosphatemia	PTH secretion	Hypophosphatemia
High phosphorous intake	PTH secretion	Low phosphorus intake
Metabolic alkalosis	Effect of pH on calcium	Metabolic acidosis
Parathormone, vitamin D_3 calcitonin, estrogen	Hormonal regulation	Insulin, glucagon, GH thyroid, glucocorticoids
Thiazide, amiloride	Tubular transport	Mannitol, Frusemide

(ECF: extracellular fluid; GH: growth hormone; PTH: parathyroid hormone)

Flowchart 2: Physiological response to hypocalcemia.

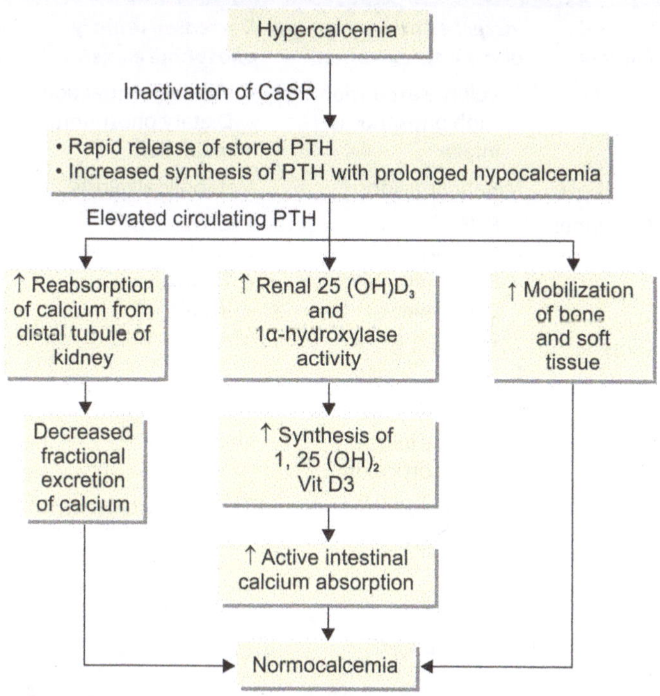

(PTH: parathyroid hormone)

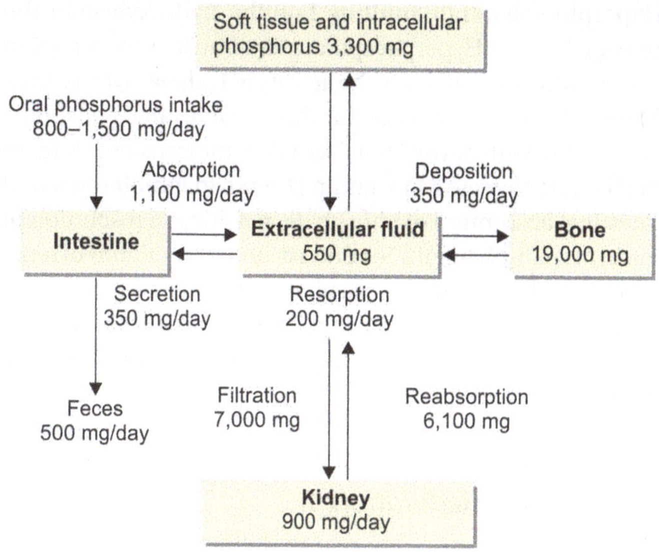

Fig. 4: Phosphate flux between body compartments.

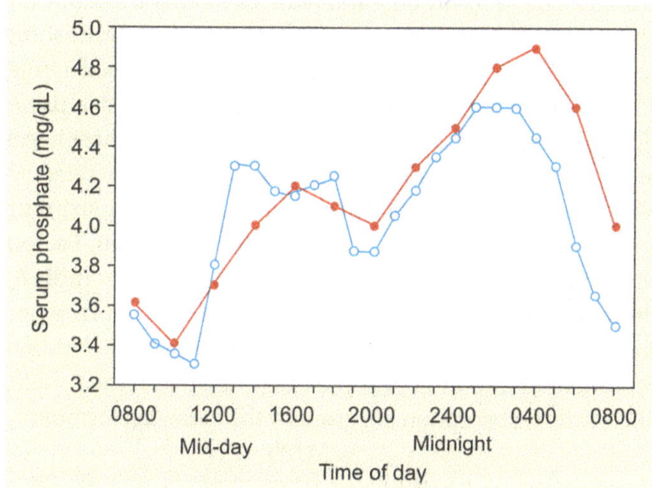

Fig. 5: Circadian variation of serum phosphate levels in normal subjects, as reported by Jubiz et al.[3]

functions as a buffer in bone, serum, and urine. Most intracellular phosphate is either complexed or bound to proteins or lipids. Plasma phosphorus consists of phospholipids, ester phosphates, and inorganic phosphates. The latter are completely ionized, circulating primarily as HPO^{2-} or HPO^{-} in a ratio of 4:1 at a plasma pH of 7.40. 85% of the body phosphate is present in mineralized extracellular matrix in skeleton and teeth, 15% are intracellular (cells and organelles in soft tissue) and <0.1% is extracellular.

Homeostasis of Phosphorus in Healthy Adults

A normal diet provides approximately 1,000 mg of phosphate, two-thirds of which is absorbed, predominantly in the proximal small intestine. Entry and exit of phosphorus between the ECF and ICF spaces occur in a steady state as shown in **Figure 4**.

Determinants of Serum Phosphorus

Age

Serum phosphate concentration is higher in children than adults. As shown in **Table 1**, the reference range is 4–7 mg/dL in children compared with 3–4.5 mg/dL in adults. In the first 3 months of life, P levels are highest (4.8–7.4 mg/dL), and decrease at age 1–2 years to 4.5–5.8 mg/dL (mean 5.0 mg/dL). In mid-childhood, values range from 3.5 to 5.5 mg/dL (mean 4.4 mg/dL) and decrease to adult values by late adolescence.

Circadian Rhythm

Serum phosphate concentration varies with age, time of day, fasting state, and season.[10] The lowest phosphorus was seen at 8–10 AM followed by a small peak and drops during the daytime then a larger nocturnal peak of 45% above the trough level at 12–4 AM as shown in **Figure 5.** The amplitude of nadir to peak phosphorus level is 1.2 mg/dL or 30% of the 24-hour mean level as shown in **Table 2.** Hence to minimize the effect of dietary phosphorus changes on the serum phosphorus concentration, it is advisable to obtain serum samples for analysis in the morning fasting state.

Factors that Regulate the Homeostasis of Phosphorus

Physiologic regulators of renal tubular phosphate reabsorption include the following mentioned here.

Dietary Phosphate and Serum Phosphate Concentration

Mild phosphate depletion and low dietary intake stimulate phosphate reabsorption in the proximal tubule.

Hyperphosphatemia inhibits 1, alpha-hydroxylase in the proximal tubule. Hyperphosphatemia stimulates the secretion of PTH, which will increase the activity of 1, alpha-hydroxylase. The result is generally a neutral effect on intestinal phosphate absorption. With normal renal function, the transient increase in PTH and decrease in vitamin D serve to inhibit renal and intestinal absorption of phosphate, resulting in resolution of the hyperphosphatemia. In contrast, under conditions of renal failure, sustained hyperphosphatemia results in sustained hyperparathyroidism and exacerbates hyperphosphatemia. High vitamin D levels enhance renal proximal tubule phosphate absorption.

Role of Parathyroid Hormone in Phosphate Regulation

Parathyroid hormone increases the activity of 1, alpha-hydroxylase, stimulates fibroblast growth factor (FGF), and promotes bone resorption and reduces tubular maximum of phosphorus by renal tubules and excretion by diminishing activity of Na/P cotransporters in the proximal and distal tubule. So a greater proportion of tubular phosphorus is lost in urine. Hence, whenever plasma PTH is increased, tubular phosphorus reabsorption is decreased and more phosphorus is excreted. As with glucose, renal tubules have a normal tubular maximum for reabsorbing phosphorus of about 0.2 mmol/min. Factors which influence real phosphate excretion are listed in **Table 6.**[1] Under steady state conditions, the urinary phosphate excretion is equivalent to the net phosphate absorption from the intestine. Fractional excretion of phosphorus ($FEPO_4$) and the tubular phosphate reabsorption are given by the following formula:

$$FEPO_4 = \frac{UPh \times Pcr}{Pph \times Ucr}$$

$$\text{Tubular P reabsorption} = 1 - \frac{Uph - Pcr}{Pph \times Ucr}$$

Hormonal Regulation of Phosphorus Homeostasis

- $1,25(OH)_2$ vitamin D stimulates the intestinal phosphorus absorption.
- PTH hormone decreases the renal tubular reabsorption and causes phosphaturia.
- Phosphatonins such as fibroblast growth factor 23 (FGF 23) are phosphaturic factors apart from PTH. The hormonal regulation of serum phosphorus is depicted in **Figure 6**. Renal excretion of phosphorus is controlled by an overflow mechanism. When phosphorus concentration in plasma is below the critical value of about 1 mmol/L, the phosphorus in glomerular filtrate is reabsorbed and no phosphorus is lost in urine. Above the critical concentration, the rate of phosphorus loss is directly proportional to the additional increase. Renal excretion of excess phosphate is responsible for maintenance of serum phosphate.

TABLE 6: Factors affecting renal phosphorus excretion.

Factors	*Increased urinary phosphate excretion*	*Decreased urinary phosphate excretion*
Dietary	• Volume expansion • High phosphorus intake	• Volume contraction • Dietary phosphorus restriction
Metabolic	Metabolic acidosis	Metabolic alkalosis
Hormones	• PTH • $1,25(OH)_2D$ • Phosphatonins • Calcitonin	• GH • GF-1 • Thyroxine • Insulin
Diuretic	• Mannitol • Loop • Thiazide	
Others	• Glucose infusion • Glucocorticoids	Immaturity

(GF: growth factor; GH: growth hormone; PTH: parathyroid hormone)

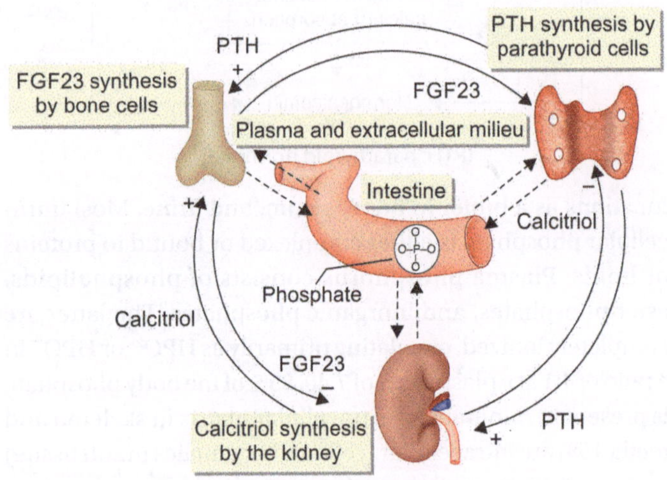

Fig. 6: Three feedback loops showing the regulation of phosphate balance in body. (FGF23: fibroblast growth factor 23; PTH: parathyroid hormone)

Renal phosphate reabsorption is controlled by diet and PTH, both of which affect the number of type 2a Na/P cotransporters in apical membrane of proximal tubules of kidney. High dietary phosphorus decreases the number of Na/P cotransporters in apical membrane and phosphate excretion decreases and vice versa. PTH, in response to high phosphorus concentration or low plasma calcium concentration decrease apical Na/P cotransporters, reduces reabsorption and increases urinary phosphorus excretion.[11] Phosphate absorption in the remainder of the nephron is mediated by type 1 or 3 Na/P cotransporters, which are not regulated. Type 2b Na/P cotransporters are expressed in the small intestine and are upregulated under conditions of dietary phosphate deprivation. Type 2c Na/P cotransporters are expressed exclusively on the S1 segment of the proximal tubule and together with type 2a Na/P cotransporters are essential for normal phosphate homeostasis. Type 2c Na/P cotransporters are also regulated by diet and PTH. The hormonal regulation of phosphate homeostasis is depicted in **Figure 6.**

Parathyroid hormone is upregulated by low plasma calcium and increased plasma phosphate concentrations. It is downregulated by increased plasma calcium and calcitriol levels. PTH acts on the kidney to increase calcium reabsorption and decreases renal phosphate reabsorption. Calcitriol acts on the intestine to increase calcium and phosphate absorption with a net effect to increase plasma calcium and phosphate levels. FGF 23 inhibits renal phosphate reabsorption, suppresses expression of 1,α-hydroxylase activity in the kidney. FGF 23 decreases PTH secretion by acting on the parathyroid glands with primary effect of reducing the plasma phosphate.

Phosphatonins

Phosphatonins are FGF 23, frizzled-related protein4 (sFRP4), and matrix extracellular phosphoglycoprotein (MEPE), which regulate phosphorus metabolism.[12] Phosphate regulating gene with homologies to endopeptidases on the X-chromosome (PHEX), a neutral endopeptidase, regulates phosphorus metabolism. It is responsible for the catabolism of FGF23, which has a phosphaturic role. FGF23 is produced in bone. FGF23 levels rise with decreasing creatinine clearance rates and increasing plasma phosphorus levels. sFRP4 decreases phosphate reabsorption by sodium-phosphate cotransporters. Klotho, a transmembrane protein, is an essential cofactor for the effects of FGF23 on renal proximal tubule cells. FGF23 is cleared by the kidney. Stanniocalcin (STC1) stimulates phosphate reabsorption in the small intestine and renal proximal tubules.[13]

Renal Transport of Phosphate

Phosphorus is freely filtered across the glomerulus and 60–70% of phosphorus is reabsorbed by proximal tubule, 20% by thick ascending limb of loop of Henle, and in the distal tubule, 10–15% of the filtered load being reabsorbed. The renal transport of phosphate is shown in **Figure 7.**

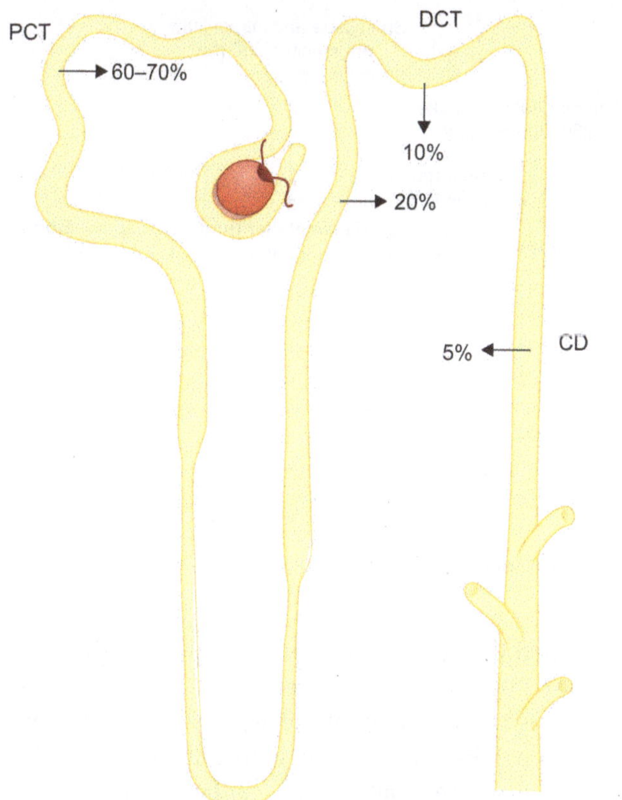

Fig. 7: Schematic illustration of the reabsorption of phosphorus by different segments of the nephron. (CD: collecting duct; DCT: distal convoluted tubule; PCT: proximal convoluted tubule)

MAGNESIUM METABOLISM

Role of Magnesium in Body

Magnesium is the second most abundant cation in intracellular fluid and fourth most abundant cation in the body. Normal magnesium concentration is 0.7–0.95 mmol/L (1.7–2.3 mg/dL) of which 70–80% are filterable.

Distribution of Magnesium in Human Body

Close to half of the body magnesium is stored in bones and remaining half in intracellular compartment. Less than 0.1% is available extracellularly.

The ECF distribution of magnesium is shown in **Figure 8.** Magnesium is involved in regulation of mitochondrial function, inflammatory process, immune defense, allergy, growth, stress response, control of neuronal activity, cardiac excitability, neuromuscular transmission, vasomotor tone, and blood pressure regulation.

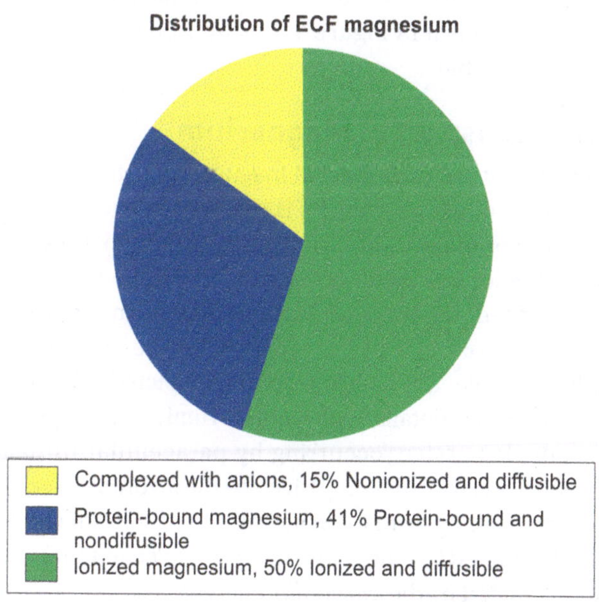

Fig. 8: Magnesium distribution in body fluids. (ECF: extracellular fluid)

Homeostasis of Magnesium in Healthy Adults

The average daily magnesium intake is 250–350 mg; approximately one-third of the ingested magnesium is

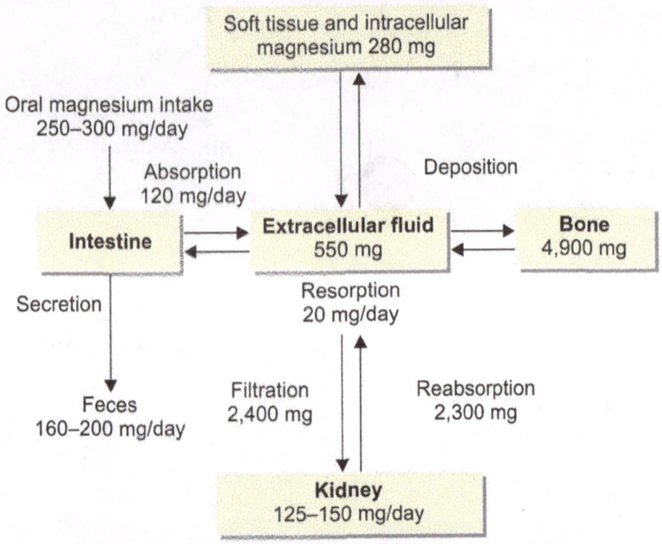

Fig. 9: Magnesium flux between body compartments.

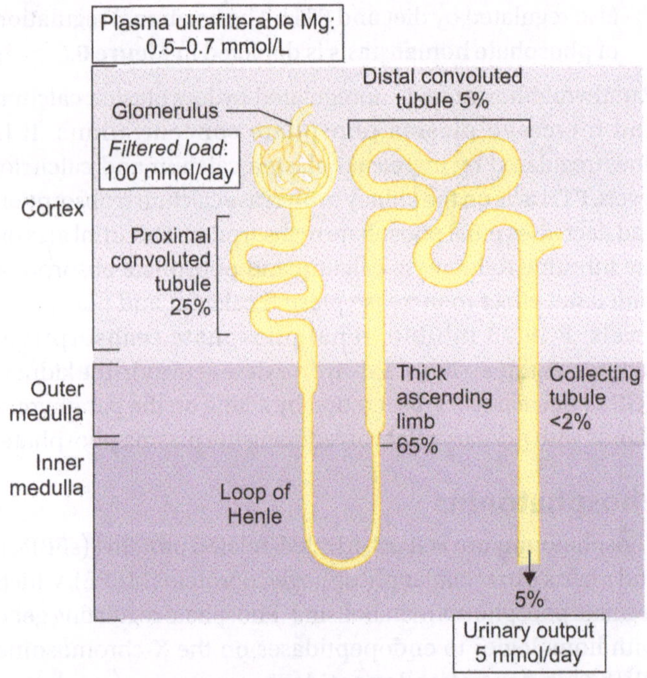

Fig. 10: Schematic illustration of the reabsorption of magnesium by different segments of the nephron.

absorbed in the small bowel through both the channel encoded by the *TRPM6* gene and by passive diffusion.[14] *TRPM6* is specifically localized along the apical membrane of the renal distal convoluted tubule and the brush border membrane of the small intestine epithelium associated with active Mg^{2+} reabsorption.[15] Net zero balance results from net intestinal uptake equaling urinary loss. The daily urinary excretion of the magnesium is 125–150 mg. Entry and exit fluxes between extracellular and intracellular spaces are also identical as shown in **Figure 9**. Precise values of exchanges are still debatable.

Renal Transport of Magnesium

About 80% of the total plasma magnesium is filtered at the glomerulus of which only 3% is excreted in the urine. The major site of magnesium transport is the thick ascending limb of the loop of Henle where 60–70% of the magnesium is reabsorbed, while 15–25% of the filtered magnesium is reabsorbed passively in the proximal tubule and 5–10% in the distal tubule. The renal transport as depicted in **Figure 10** shows the above details. In the loop of Henle, the magnesium transport is passive, occurring by paracellular diffusion between the cells and being driven by the favorable electrical gradient resulting from the reabsorption of sodium chloride and is facilitated by a tight junction protein called Claudin16 that is encoded by the *paracellin 1* gene.[16]

Two conditions are necessary for normal magnesium reabsorption:

1. Generation of an electrical lumen positive gradient induced by sodium and chloride reabsorption
2. Expression of Claudins 16 and 19 which form a cation selective tight junction, facilitating paracellular magnesium transport

The distal reabsorption of magnesium occurs in the cortical collecting tubule. The absorption of filtered magnesium occurs through magnesium channels in the apical (luminal) membrane. This is driven by a favorable transmembrane voltage. Transcellular magnesium reabsorption in the distal convoluted tubule represents the final step before magnesium is excreted. In kidney, CNNM2 is expressed in basolateral membrane with predominant expression in the distal convoluted tubule. Recently, mutations in the *cyclin M2 (CNNM2)* gene were identified to be causative for severe hypomagnesemia. The driving force for this exchanger is the low sodium concentration inside the cell.

Regulation of Plasma Magnesium Concentration

Parathyroid hormone, vasopressin, calcitonin, β-adrenergic agonists, glucagon, and metabolic alkalosis increase magnesium reabsorption in loop of Henle, whereas acetylcholine and atrial natriuretic peptide (ANP) decrease urine magnesium excretion.

The fractional excretion of magnesium, which is between 3 and 5% in subjects with normal renal function ingesting a typical diet, can fall to below 0.5% with magnesium depletion due to extrarenal losses.[17]

Fractional excretion of magnesium is calculated by the following formula:

$$FeMg = \frac{UMg \times SCr}{SMg \times UCr}$$

Factors that increase magnesium excretion are:

- High ECF magnesium concentration
- High ECF calcium concentration
- ECF volume expansion

- Dietary phosphate restriction and phosphate depletion
- Metabolic acidosis
- Hypokalemia

DISORDERS OF CALCIUM PHOSPHORUS AND MAGNESIUM

Hypocalcemia

Neonatal Hypocalcemia

Epidemiology: Hypocalcemia occurs in as many as 30% of infants with very low birth weight (<1,500 g) and in as many as 89% of infants whose gestational age at birth is <32 weeks.[18]

Neonatal hypocalcemia is defined as total serum calcium concentration <8 mg/dL (<2 mmol/L) and ionized calcium <4.4 mg/dL (<1.1 mmol/L) in term infants; <7 mg/dL (<1.75 mmol/L) in preterm infants and ionized calcium <4 mg/dL (<1 mmol/L).

The cessation of placental transfer of calcium at birth is followed by a fall in total blood calcium concentration to 9 mg/dL and ionized calcium to 4.4 mg/dL at 24 hours. Calcium rises postnatally and reaches levels as in older children by 2 weeks of age. Hypocalcemia is usually asymptomatic in newborns.[19] Most common symptom is increased neuromuscular irritability which manifests as jitteriness, muscle jerking, and seizures. Other rare manifestations are stridor, bronchospasm, and pylorospasm. The causes of hypocalcemia in newborns can be classified by the age at presentation as seen in **Table 7**.

Hypocalcemia in Older Children

Definition: Hypocalcemia is defined as a total serum calcium concentration of <8.5 mg/dL in children. In older children, hypocalcemia is usually associated with critical illness, acquired hypoparathyroidism, activating mutations of the calcium-sensing receptor, or defects in vitamin D supply or metabolism and calcium deficiency.

TABLE 7: Contrasting features of early and late neonatal hypocalcemia.

Early neonatal hypocalcemia	*Late neonatal hypocalcemia*
Presents in first 48–72 hours	Presents from 3 to 7 days to 6 weeks postnatal
Etiology: • Prematurity • Infant of diabetic mother • Perinatal asphyxia • Intrauterine growth restriction • Poor oral intake • Hyporesponsiveness to vitamin D • Increased calcitonin • Increased endogenous P load • Alkali therapy • Hypoalbuminemia	*Etiology:* • Transient hypoparathyroidism of newborns • Maternal hyperparathyroidism • Magnesium deficiency • Critically ill newborns • Gentamicin use • Prematurity • High intake of phosphate rich formula or cow's milk

Causes of hypocalcemia: The etiology of hypocalcemia is enlisted in **Table 8** according to the presence of undetectable, normal, or high levels of circulating PTH, an approach that reflects the underlying pathophysiology.[20] Among infants and children, acute hypocalcemia is observed most often in intensive care setting, usually related to an acute illness such as sepsis, cardiac surgery, rhabdomyolysis, pancreatitis, hepatitis, or tumor lysis. Common causes of chronic hypocalcemia are vitamin D deficiency and hypoparathyroidism.

Evaluation of hypocalcemia in children: A detailed history documenting diet, lifestyle, family, and drug history, as well as development and hearing is important. The examination should include an assessment of skin, nails, teeth, and the

TABLE 8: Causes of hypocalcemia in children.

Pathogenesis	*Etiology*
PTH absent	• Hereditary hypoparathyroidism • AR/AD/XL hypoparathyroidism • DiGeorge anomaly (22q11 deletions) • CHARGE association • APECED association • HDR-association • Mitochondrial dysfunction (Kearns–Sayre syndrome) • Acquired hypoparathyroidism • Following neck surgery • Infiltrative disease (Wilson, thalassemia) • Hypomagnesemia • Altered set point (autosomal dominant CaSR-activating mutation)
PTH ineffective	• CKD • Hypovitaminosis D • Decreased intake • Low intestinal absorption (Celiac disease, cystic fibrosis) • Calcium deficiency • Impaired vitamin D metabolism • CLD • Drugs that inactivate vitamin D (anticonvulsants, INH, rifampicin, HAART) • VDDR-I/VDDR-II • Pseudohypoparathyroidism
PTH high	• Tumor lysis syndrome • Rhabdomyolysis • AKI • Hungry bone syndrome • Osteoporosis • Excessive fluoride intake

(AD: autosomal dominant; AKI: acute kidney injury; AR: autosomal recessive; APECED association: Autoimmune Poly-Endocrinopathy-Candidiasis-Ectodermal Dystrophy: CaSR: calcium-sensing receptor; CHARGE association: Coloboma, Heart anomaly, Choanal Atresia, Mental Retardation, Genital hypoplasia, and Ear Anomalies; CLD: chronic liver disease; HDR association: Hypoparathyroidism, Deafness, Renal dysplasia; HAART: highly active antiretroviral therapy; INH: isoniazid; PTH: parathyroid hormone; VDDR: vitamin D-dependent rickets; XL: X-linked dominant)

TABLE 9: Symptoms and signs of hypocalcemia.

System	*Findings*
Neuromuscular	Features of tetany (carpopedal spasm, Chvostek sign, Trousseau sign), myopathy, extrapyramidal symptoms, convulsions, mental retardation, and psychosis
Ocular	Subcapsular cataract, keratoconus, and papilledema
Skin	Dry, scaly skin, and dermatitis
Hair	Coarse, brittle, sparse hair, and alopecia
Nails	Brittle nails with transverse groove
Dental	Enamel hypoplasia, delayed eruption, and abraded carious teeth
Gastrointestinal	Loose stools and gastric achlorhydria
Cardiovascular	Hypotension, myocardial dysfunction, congestive cardiac failure, and prolonged QT interval
Skeletal	• Rachitic features • *Children with hypoparathyroidism:* Increased BMD, osteosclerosis, and thickened calvarium
Endocrine	Impaired insulin release, hypothyroidism, prolactin deficiency, and ovarian failure

(BMD: bone mineral density)

TABLE 10: Investigations in hypocalcemia.[17]

	First line	*Second line*
Blood	• Total and ionized calcium • Phosphorus magnesium • Albumin • Alkaline phosphatase $Na/K/HCO_3$/creatinine • Parathyroid hormone • 25-hydroxy vitamin D	• Autoantibody screen (for polyendocrinopathy) • Biochemical evaluation of family • Family evaluation (FHH) • Maternal vitamin D/Ca/PTH status • 1,25-hydroxyvitamin D (VDDR-II) • Genetic (e.g., 22q del.)
Urine	• Urine (glucose, protein, pH) • Ca/P/magnesium/creatinine	
Imaging	Hand wrist/skull radiograph	• *Renal ultrasound:* – Nephrocalcinosis – Renal dysplasia

(FHH: familial hypocalciuric hypercalciuria; VDDR: vitamin D-dependent rickets)

TABLE 11: Biochemical parameters in various causes of hypocalcemia.

	Total Ca	*iCa*	*Serum P*	*Serum PTH*	*Serum magnesium*	*Urine Ca*	*Vitamin D levels*	
							25(OH) D_3	*1,25 $(OH)_2$ D_3*
Hypoalbuminemia	Low	N	N	N	N	N	N	N
Alkalosis	N	Low	N	N/high	N	low	N	N
Vitamin D deficiency	Low	Low	Low	High	Low/N	low	N	Low
CKD	Low	Low	High	High	N	N	N/low	N/low
Hypoparathyroidism	Low	Low	High	Low	N	Low	N	Low
Pseudohypoparathyroidism	Low	Low	High	High	N	Low	N	Low
Acute pancreatitis	Low	Low	N/low	High	Low/N	N	N	N
Hypomagnesemia	Low	Low	N	Low/N	Low	N	N	N
ADH	Low	Low	N	N	N	High	N	N

(ADH: autosomal dominant hypocalcemia; CKD: chronic kidney disease)

skeleton, as well as the cardiovascular system.[2] The various symptoms and sign of hypocalcemia are shown in **Table 9**. Measuring ionized calcium level is essential to differentiate true hypocalcemia from a mere decrease in total calcium concentration when the albumin is low. Investigations which aid in diagnosis are shown in **Table 10**.

Family history of hypocalcemia is seen in autosomal dominant hypocalcemia (ADH) due to CaSR-activating mutation and hypophosphatemia rickets; hence, biochemistry of first-degree relatives is warranted. **Table 11** shows the biochemical features in various causes of hypocalcemia. Low maternal calcium and vitamin D support the diagnosis of hypocalcemia due to maternal deficiency. PTH is low in hypoparathyroidism and high in chronic kidney disease (CKD), vitamin D deficiency, and pseudohypoparathyroidism. ADH is characterized by normal P, magnesium, PTH, and hypercalciuria (urine calcium/creatinine ratio >0.3). Some patients with ADH who have more marked gain of function mutation have potassium wasting, hypokalemia, and metabolic alkalosis resembling Bartter syndromes.[21] Metabolic acidosis with glycosuria indicates renal tubular acidosis.

Management

- The most important aspect of management is resolution of the primary cause. Intravenous (IV) calcium is indicated in children having seizures and critically ill. Calcium gluconate 10% IV solution contains 9.8 mg/mL elemental calcium. IV calcium chloride is avoided in children. Dose of IV calcium gluconate is 100–200 mg/kg/dose (maximum 1–2 g/dose) IV over 5–10 minutes with cardiac monitoring followed by a continuous infusion of 500–800 mg/kg over 24 hours or intermittently 4–6 hourly.

- In chronic asymptomatic hypocalcemia, oral calcium is prescribed at a dose of 25–50 mg/kg/day of elemental calcium divided 3–4 times/day (maximum 1 g elemental calcium/day). Calcium carbonate is the calcium supplement of choice, because it provides 40% elemental calcium or 400 mg/g of calcium carbonate. In children with concurrent acidosis, hypocalcemia should be corrected first. The various formulations are shown in **Table 12.**
- In hypoparathyroidism, calcitriol is initiated at a starting dose of 0.08 µg/kg/day and increase the daily dose to 0.25–2 µg/day. Adjust the dose as per serum calcium and urinary calcium excretion. Recombinant PTH if available is used for hypoparathyroidism.
- Concomitantly correct hypomagnesemia and vitamin D deficiency if present.
- Administration of phosphate lowering agents may be necessary if hypocalcemia is associated with hyperphosphatemia.
- Infants drinking regular cow's milk must be given humanized infant formula. Children with renal failure should be given a low solute, low phosphate formula.

Hypercalcemia

Definition

Hypercalcemic crisis is defined as marked elevation of serum calcium >14 mg/dL. Majority of adult patients with elevated calcium level will have either primary hyperparathyroidism or malignancy in >90% times. In cases of primary hyperparathyroidism, 80% of cases are due to adenoma or carcinoma and 15% of cases are due to hyperplastic parathyroid gland. In familial hyperparathyroidism, there is possibility of MEN type I/2A.

The use of the mnemonic VITAMINS TRAPS gives the classical causes of hypercalcemia such as vitamin D (or A) intoxication, immobilization, thyrotoxicosis, Addison's disease, Milk-alkali syndrome, inflammatory disorders, neoplasia, sarcoidosis, thiazides or lithium carbonate, rhabdomyolysis, acquired immunodeficiency syndrome (AIDS), and parathyroid diseases.[17]

Children present with hypercalcemia less frequently than adults, but the causes that are common in adults are also common in children as shown in **Table 13.** Some rather rare conditions are seen almost exclusively in younger children and are discussed later in this chapter. Symptoms of hypercalcemia in various organ systems are enumerated in **Table 14.**

Development of symptoms depends on degree of hypercalcemia as shown in **Table 15** and the rate of rise of serum calcium.

Steps in diagnostic workup are:

- *History* is evident in immobilization, thyrotoxicosis, syndromes such as William, Down, Jansen's, metaphyseal chondrodysplasia, and medications. Initial testing is directed at detecting malignancy, hyperparathyroidism, and hyperthyroidism, the most common causes of hypercalcemia.
- *Assess phosphorous*: Hypercalcemia with hypophosphatemia is a feature of:
  - Humoral hypercalcemia of malignancy
  - Primary hyperparathyroidism

Hypercalcemia with normal or high phosphorus indicates:

- Granulomatous disease
- Vitamin D intoxication

TABLE 12: Commonly available oral preparations of calcium.

Calcium preparation	*Tablet strength (mg)*	*Elemental Ca (mg)*
Calcium carbonate	1,250	625
Calcium citrate	950	200
Calcium lactate	650	85
Calcium gluconate	1,000	90
Calcium acetate	667	167
Calcium phosphate	323	125

TABLE 13: Etiology of hypercalcemia in children.

Pathogenesis	*Etiology*
PTH related	• Primary hyperparathyroidism (PHPT)—adenoma, carcinoma, MEN • Familial hypocalciuric hypercalciuria (FHH)—AD-inactivating CaSR mutation
PTHrP related	• Malignancy • Solid tumor with metastasis—breast and myeloma • Humoral hypercalcemic of malignancy—lung, kidney, pheochromocytoma, squamous cell carcinoma, ovary • Hematological malignancy—multiple myeloma, lymphoma, and leukemia • *Others:* – SLE – HIV-associated adenopathy – During late pregnancy and lactation in hypoparathyroidism
Vitamin D related	• Vitamin D intoxication • High 1, $25(OH)_2$ D • Sarcoidosis granulomatosis disease (TB/Wegener's/Crohn's disease/granulomatous pneumonia/lipoid pneumonia/Talc and silicone granulomatosis/cat scratch disease) • Impaired metabolism of vitamin D/$25(OH)_2$ vitamin D

Contd...

Contd...

Pathogenesis	*Etiology*
Associated with high bone turnover	• Hyperthyroidism • Prolonged immobilization • Subcutaneous fat necrosis • Addison's disease • Recovering rhabdomyolysis
Kidney failure	• Secondary hyperparathyroidism • Aluminum intoxication • Milk-alkali syndrome
Drugs	• *Common:* Calcium, vitamin D, vitamin A, lithium, thiazide • *Less common:* Theophylline, recombinant growth hormone, foscarnet, hepatitis B vaccine, omeprazole, manganese toxicity
Unknown mechanism	• *Infections: Nocardia, Brucella*, CMV (in AIDS), berylliosis • Juvenile idiopathic arthritis • Advanced CLD
Rare causes of hypercalcemia in newborn, infancy and young children	• Loss of function mutation of CaSR • Heterozygous—FHH • Homozygous—severe neonatal PTH • Phosphate depletion in severe prematurity • Severe neonatal and congenital hyperparathyroidism • Idiopathic infantile hypercalcemia • Metaphyseal dysplasias—hypophosphatasia, Jansen metaphyseal chondrodysplasia • William syndrome • Down syndrome • Renal tubular acidosis • Infantile hypothyroidism • Adrenal insufficiency • Primary oxalosis • Subcutaneous fat necrosis • Inappropriate dietary formulas • Congenital lactase deficiency • Exchange transfusion and ECMO vitamin A and D supplements

(AIDS: acquired immunodeficiency syndrome; CaSR: calcium-sensing receptor; CMV: cytomegalovirus; CLD: chronic liver disease; ECMO: extracorporeal membrane oxygenation; MEN: multiple endocrine neoplasia; PTH: parathyroid hormone; PTHrP: parathyroid hormone-related protein; TB: tuberculosis; SLE: systemic lupus erythematosus)

TABLE 14: Symptoms and signs of hypercalcemia.

System	*Symptoms*
General	Fatigue, weakness, depression, and anorexia
CNS	Impaired concentration, somnolescence, irritability, confusion, altered sensorium, stupor, coma, headache, and mental retardation
Musculoskeletal	Weakness, joint pain (pseudo gout), bone pain, osteopenia, osteoporosis and osteitis fibrosa cystica, and soft tissue calcifications
Ocular	Band keratopathy, palpebral, and conjunctival calcification
Skin	Pruritus and skin calcification
GIT	Constipation, anorexia, nausea, vomiting, peptic ulcer, pancreatitis, and abdominal cramps
Cardiovascular	Shortened QT interval, cardiac arrhythmia, and hypertension
Renal	Altered urinary concentration ability with polyuria, polydipsia, nephrolithiasis, nephrocalcinosis, renal failure, distal RTA, and dehydration

(CNS: central nervous system; GIT: gastrointestinal tract; RTA: renal tubular acidosis)

TABLE 15: Clinical correlation of serum calcium levels and symptoms of hypercalcemia.

Serum calcium level	*Symptoms*
>11.5 mg/dL (>2.9 mmol/L)	CNS and GIT symptom
>13 mg/dL (>3.2 mmol/L)	Nephrocalcinosis and impaired renal function
>14 mg/dL (>3.5 mmol/L)	Arrhythmias, ST/T changes mimicking MI
>15 mg/dL (>3.7 mmol/L)	Coma/cardiac arrest in severe cases

(CNS: central nervous system; GIT: gastrointestinal tract; MI: myocardial infarction)

- Immobilization
- Metastatic bone disease
- Thyrotoxicosis
- *Assess hypercalciuria:*

Hypercalciuria is seen in	• Hyperparathyroidism • Hypercalcemia of malignancy
Relative hypocalciuria is seen in (FECa <0.01%)	• Thiazide • Familial hypocalciuric hypercalcemia

- *Analyze PTH:* In a child with hypercalcemia, the serum PTH level should be lower than 10 pg/mL. A definitive diagnosis of hyperparathyroidism is confirmed by a PTH level higher than 50 pg/mL.

High PTH indicates	• Primary hyperparathyroidism • Maternal hyperparathyroidism in neonates • Lithium therapy
Low PTH is seen in	• All other non-PTH hormone-related hypercalcemia

- *Analyze vitamin D metabolites*: Vitamin D metabolites are assessed if there is no obvious malignancy and PTH levels are not elevated. An elevated serum concentration of 25,hydroxyvitamin D [25(OH)D] >150 ng/mL indicates intoxication.

High 25(OH) Vit D hints toward	• Vitamin D intoxication • Idiopathic infantile hypercalcemia
High 1,25(OH) Vit D is seen in	• Direct intake of this metabolite • Granulomatous diseases • Lymphoma

- PTHrP is measured in malignancy
- *Thyroid-stimulating hormone (TSH):* To rule out thyrotoxicosis
- Vitamin A level if suspected vitamin A toxicity
- *Electrocardiogram (ECG):* To look for changes
- Increased angiotensin-converting enzyme (ACE) activity is a feature of sarcoidosis.
- *X-ray of the hand:* Long-standing and severe hyperparathyroidism results in bone resorption which involves cortical rather than trabecular bone and is seen in phalangeal bones (osteitis fibrosa cystica).
- Computed tomography (CT) of the head, magnetic resonance imaging (MRI), ultrasonography (USG) or nuclear scan of neck to localize parathyroid adenoma (sestamibi scan)

Difference between Primary Hyperparathyroidism and Familial Hypocalciuric Hypercalcemia

Primary hyperparathyroidism usually presents with severe symptomatic hypercalcemia, hypophosphatemia, and frankly elevated PTH levels, whereas patients with familial hypocalciuric hypercalciuria (FHH) typically have positive family history (autosomal dominant) and asymptomatic or mild hypercalcemia, hypermagnesemia, hypophosphatemia, and normal or mildly elevated PTH. FHH never leads to severe clinical signs of hypercalcemia except in newborn period. The calcium creatinine ratio is the consensus biochemical test to differentiate between primary hyperparathyroidism (PHPT).[21] Hypercalciuria is a feature of PHPT, whereas inappropriately low urine calcium in the setting of hypercalcemia indicated FHH. FECa is usually <0.01%. Demonstration of inactivating mutation in CaSR establishes the diagnosis of FHH.[22]

The importance of identifying FHH is that parathyroidectomy can be avoided.

Rare Causes of Hypercalcemia in Children

Idiopathic Infantile Hypercalcemia (Lightwood Syndrome)

- It is characterized by an increased sensitivity to vitamin D.[23]
- It occurs due to loss of function mutations in the gene that encodes for the inactivation of 25-hydroxyvitamin D.
- Decreased conversion of vitamin D to inactive metabolites

Jansen's Metaphyseal Chondrodysplasia

- Characterized by short limb dwarfism
- Its hereditary form of dwarfism
- There will be associated severe hypercalcemia and hypophosphatemia.
- Metaphyseal chondrodysplasia is characteristic.
- Diagnosed by activating mutation of gene coding for PTHrP receptors.

Management

The mode of therapy and urgency of treatment depend on the degree of hypercalcemia and rate of rise of calcium. Asymptomatic or mildly symptomatic hypercalcemia total calcium <12 mg/dL does not require immediate treatment. Similarly, calcium of 12–14 mg/dL is often well-tolerated chronically, and may not require urgent treatment but acute rise with symptoms will require treatment. Total calcium concentration >14 mg/dL requires immediate treatment, regardless of symptoms.

- The initial step in the care of severely hypercalcemic children is hydration with saline at a rate of 2,800–3,000 mL/m^2 body surface area. Hydration is ineffective in children with kidney failure and dialysis is necessary to correct hypercalcemia. Further medical management is as enumerated in **Table 16**.
- Loop diuretics are used with hydration to increase calcium excretion. The dose of furosemide in children is 0.5–1 mg/kg q6 h. Thiazide diuretics should be avoided. Long term use of loop diuretics increases predisposition to nephrocalcinosis.
- Corticosteroids are useful for treating hypercalcemia caused by vitamin D toxicity, multiple myeloma, lymphoma, sarcoidosis, and other granulomatous diseases. Methylprednisolone is given in children at a dose of 1 mg/kg q6 h and adult dose of 200–400 mg hydrocortisone IV/day for 3–5 days.
- Calcitonin has the most rapid onset of action and most potent among the hypocalcemic agents, but has short duration of action. Hence should be combined with slower-acting agents. Administration of salmon calcitonin

TABLE 16: Various treatment modalities for hypercalcemia.

Treatment of hypercalcemia	*Onset of action*	*Duration of action*
Hydration with NS	Hours	During infusion
Forced diuresis	Hours	During treatment
Pamidronate	1–2 days	2–4 weeks
Zolendronate	12–24 hours	>3 weeks
Denosumab	1–2 days	>3 weeks
Calcitonin	4–6 hours	1–3 days
Oral or IV phosphate	24 hours	During use
Corticosteroids	Days	Days to weeks
Dialysis	Hours	24–48 hours
Gallium nitrate	48 hours	2 weeks
Plicamycin (mithramycin)	24–48 hours	7–10 days

(IV: intravenous; NS: normal saline)

(4 IU/kg) at starting dose and it can be repeated every 6–12 hours (4–8 IU/kg). Patients may develop tachyphylaxis to calcitonin after 24–48 hours, so therapy is usually limited to this time period.

- Bisphosphonates act by binding to hydroxyapatite in bone matrix and inhibiting bone resorption by shortening the lifespan of osteoclasts. Currently, available drugs include etidronate, tiludronate, pamidronate, alendronate, zoledronate, risedronate, ibandronate, and neridronic acid. Pamidronate (0.5–1.0 mg/kg up to a maximum dose 90 mg as infusion over 4–6 hours) is the drug of choice in children. Zoledronic acid (ZA) is preferable because it is superior to pamidronate in reversing hypercalcemia related to malignancy. Bisphosphonates are relatively contraindicated in renal failure.
- For patients with hypercalcemia in whom bisphosphonates are contraindicated (e.g., due to severe renal impairment), denosumab can be administered concurrently with calcitonin.
- A long-acting calcimimetic drug, cinacalcet, is available for the treatment of secondary hyperparathyroidism associated with renal failure, hypercalcemia in parathyroid cancer, neonatal severe primary hyperparathyroidism, FHH, and forms of hyperparathyroidism other than primary hyperparathyroidism. There is no standard dose for cinacalcet in pediatric population. Starting dose is 0.5 mg/kg/day and needs titration of the dose sequentially every 2–4 weeks up to a maximum of 1.5 mg/kg/day.[24] Side effects most commonly reported included nausea, arthralgia, diarrhea, myalgia, paresthesia, and hypocalcemia.
- Dihydrotachysterol 2 (DHT2), doxercalciferol [1,alpha(OH) D_2], paricalcitol, and 22 oxacalcitriol (OCT) inhibit PTH synthesis.
- Inhibition of vitamin D-activation by 1α-hydroxylase is the mechanism by which imidazole derivatives such as ketoconazole act in reducing serum calcium level. Dose of ketoconazole is 3–9 mg/kg/day.
- Children with primary hyperparathyroidism who present with symptoms of severe or moderate elevations of calcium levels are referred for parathyroidectomy.
- Avoidance of calcium-containing foods and supplements and vitamin D

HYPOPHOSPHATEMIA

Definition

A phosphate level below range of phosphate in the blood is called hypophosphatemia. Normal phosphorus in adolescents and adults ranges between 2.9 and 5.4 mg/dL. Moderate hypophosphatemia is 0.96–1.95 mg/dL and severe hypophosphatemia is <0.96 mg/dL.

Etiology

The various causes of hypophosphatemia are shown in **Table 17.** In hospitalized children, (1) malnutrition due to low food intake or anorexia during severe disease, and (2) altered distribution are important causes. It is much more prevalent in diabetic ketoacidosis, sepsis, and alcoholism.

Signs and Symptoms

The manifestations depend upon the severity and chronicity of the phosphate depletion. Two major mechanisms are responsible for these symptoms: (1) Decrease in intracellular adenosine triphosphate and (2) in diphosphoglycerate. The initial response of bone to hypophosphatemia is increased resorption and more prolonged hypophosphatemia leads to rickets and osteomalacia due to decreased bone mineralization.[25] The various symptoms of hypophosphatemia are shown in **Table 18**. Heart failure occurs when serum phosphate falls below 1.0 mg/dL. Clinically significant rhabdomyolysis has been described almost exclusively in children receiving hyper-alimentation without phosphate supplementation and in alcoholics. Rhabdomyolysis with associated release of phosphate from the damaged muscle cells may mask the underlying hypophosphatemia. Hemolysis occurs when the plasma phosphate concentration falls below 0.5 mg/dL.

Evaluation

The diagnosis of hypophosphatemia is usually evident from history. Fractional excretion of filtered phosphate ($FEPO_4$) and tubular reabsorption of phosphorus (TRP) are useful tools for assessing renal phosphorus handling. Daily phosphate excretion should be <100 mg. Normal $FEPO_4$ is <5% (normal value is 5–20%) and TRP ranges from 85 to 95%. In the presence of reduced glomerular function, a more reliable means of measuring phosphate reabsorption is tubular

TABLE 17: Causes of hypophosphatemia in children.

Pathogenesis	*Etiology*
Low dietary intake	Low intake: Severe malnutrition, VLBW babies
Decreased intestinal absorption	• Vitamin D deficiency • Phosphate binders • Malabsorption • Chronic diarrhea
Increased urinary losses	• Fanconi syndrome • Diuretic therapy—acetazolamide • Recovering AKI • Steroid therapy • Tumor-induced osteomalacia • Excess fluid therapy • Vitamin D deficiency • VDDR types I and II • Postrenal transplant • Hyperparathyroidism • XL/AD hypophosphatemic rickets • Bartter syndrome/Gitelman syndrome • Alcoholism
Disturbed redistribution	• Insulin administration for DKA • Hyperalimentation • Refeeding in malnutrition • Acute respiratory alkalosis • Hyperventilation • Hungry bone syndrome • Increased cellular metabolism (androgen, corticosteroid therapy) • Leukemic flare

(AD: autosomal dominant; AKI: acute kidney injury; DKA: diabetic ketoacidosis; VDDR: vitamin D-dependent rickets; VLBW: very low birth weight; XL: X-linked dominant)

TABLE 18: Symptoms of hypophosphatemia.

System	*Symptoms*
Musculoskeletal	Proximal myopathy, rhabdomyolysis, rickets, and osteomalacia
Cardiovascular	Impaired myocardial contractility
GIT	Paralytic ileus
Pulmonary	Respiratory failure
Neurology	Paresthesia, tremors, seizures, Guillain–Barré syndrome, encephalopathy, and coma
Hematology	Hemolysis, impaired chemotaxis, phagocytosis, thrombocytopenia, and platelet dysfunction

(GIT: gastrointestinal tract)

maximum for phosphate corrected for glomerular filtration rate (TmP/GFR).

$$TmP/GFR = Pp - [(Up \times P_{creat})/U_{creat}]$$

Where Pp = plasma phosphate; Up = urine phosphate; P_{creat} = plasma creatinine and U_{creat} = urine creatinine. The normal range for children is 2.8–4.4 mg/dL. Inappropriately high phosphate excretion is defined as above 100 mg/day or a fractional excretion of phosphate above 5%.

Steps in Evaluation of Hypophosphatemia

- *Assess phosphate wasting*: Phosphate wasting is demonstrable in hyperparathyroidism, renal tubular acidosis, and vitamin D deficiency. Conditions with increased cellular uptake (internal redistribution) and reduced net intestinal absorption will have normal phosphate excretion.
- *Others electrolytes*: Concomitant hypomagnesemia is seen in poor dietary intake. Associated hypokalemia is seen in DKA and chronic alcoholism in adults. Primary hyperparathyroidism and intestinal malabsorption have associated hypercalcemia and hypocalcemia respectively. Fanconi syndrome has proteinuria and renal glycosuria.

Management

- Definitive management is treatment of primary cause.
- Hypocalcemia needs to be corrected first.
- Mild hypophosphatemia is treated with oral replacement with milk, oral phosphate, or carbonated beverages. Cow's milk is an excellent source of oral phosphate. 1 L of milk contains 1 g elemental phosphorus. Neutral phosphate solution provides 500 mg of elemental phosphorus/15 mL and is started at 35–45 mg/kg in three to four divided doses. Joulie's solution is a combination of sodium phosphate and phosphoric acid. This preparation provides 30.4 mg of elemental phosphorus/1 mL.
- For severe hypophosphatemia below 1 mg/day, IV phosphate is given at a dose of 0.08–0.16 mmol/kg (elemental phosphate 2.5–5 mg/kg) in 500 mL 1/2 normal saline (NS) IV over 6 hours. Sodium phosphate is preferred for IV therapy (1 mL IV solution contains 3 mmol or 10 mg of phosphorus). Switch to oral replacement when the serum phosphate exceeds 1.5 mg/dL. Side effects of IV phosphorus are hypocalcemia, metastatic calcification, and hyperkalemia (with potassium phosphate, volume excess, hypernatremia, metabolic acidosis, and hyperphosphatemia).
- Dipyridamole can be used to reduce persistent urinary phosphate loss, in addition to increased intake of foods that are rich in phosphates such as dairy items, meat, and beans.
- Children with primary hyperparathyroidism benefit from parathyroidectomy.

HYPERPHOSPHATEMIA

Definition

The normally higher level of serum phosphate in neonates, infants, and children is >6 mg/dL.

Epidemiology

Hyperphosphatemia is rare in the general population. In children with renal failure, the rate of hyperphosphatemia is as high as 70%.

Etiology of Hyperphosphatemia

The causes of hyperphosphatemia are listed in **Table 19.** Among them, the most common cause is renal failure and acute phosphorus loading. Newborns and infants fed on cow's milk is a common cause because phosphate content of cow's milk is six times greater than human milk. When GFR falls below 75% of normal, there will be increasing levels of phosphaturic hormones such as PTH and FGF 23 to maintain phosphate balance. Inadequate nephron mass resulting from drop in GFR below 35 mL/min/1.73 m^2 causes a steady rise in serum phosphorus.

Symptoms and Signs

Most children with hyperphosphatemia are asymptomatic. Some children have hypocalcemic symptoms, bone and joint pain, pruritus, or rash. The long-term complications of chronic hyperphosphatemia result in abnormal bone architecture and increased vascular calcifications, papular rash, uremic pruritus, ischemic ulcers, restricted joint movements, rupture of tendons, and band keratopathy.

Steps in evaluation are:

- *Serum calcium:*

Low calcium with high phosphorus is seen in	• Renal failure • Hypoparathyroidism • Pseudohypoparathyroidism
High calcium with high phosphorus in	• Vitamin D intoxication • Milk-alkali syndrome

TABLE 19: Causes of hyperphosphatemia.

Pathogenesis	*Etiology*
Spurious	• Hemolysis during phlebotomy • Hyperglobulinemia • Hyperlipidemia • Hyperbilirubinemia • Heparinized sample
Decreased urinary phosphate excretion	• Hypoparathyroidism • Pseudohypoparathyroidism • Chronic kidney disease • Familial tumoral calcinosis • Acute kidney injury
Redistribution of phosphate	• Tumor lysis syndrome • Respiratory acidosis • Lactic and ketoacidosis • Increased catabolism • Rhabdomyolysis • Acromegaly
Exogenous phosphate ingestion	• Newborns and infants fed cow's milk • Phosphate laxatives and enemas • Intravenous phosphate • Excessive vitamin D
Malignancy	• Multiple myeloma • Waldenstrom macroglobulinemia
Drugs	• Growth hormone, bisphosphonates, and dipyridamole

- *Serum iPTH:*

High PTH in	Renal failure
Low PTH in	• Vitamin D intoxication (high 25 and 1,25 vitamin D) • Milk-alkali syndrome (associated with low vitamin D)

- *Serum creatinine:*

High creatinine	Renal failure
Normal creatinine	Vitamin D intoxication, laxative abuse, tumor lysis, rhabdomyolysis, and isolated hypoparathyroidism

- *Fractional excretion of phosphate:*

$FEPO_4$ >15%	• Massive ingestion (e.g., laxative abuse) • TLS or rhabdomyolysis
$FEPO_4$ <15%	Renal failure or hypoparathyroidism

Children with pseudohypoparathyroidism have abnormally low levels of 24-hour urine cyclic adenosine monophosphate. Renal ultrasound, bone densitometry, and electron beam CT for vascular calcification can be obtained. The fractional renal excretion of phosphate should be in excess of 15% in hyperphosphatemia. If not, it suggests that renal excretion is impaired either because of renal failure or hypoparathyroidism.

Management

- Specific treatment is provided if cause is determined.
- Dietary phosphate intake needs restriction. Foods rich in phosphorus are dairy products and dark chocolates.
- Oral phosphate binders, calcitriol, calcimimetics, and dialysis are modalities used in secondary hyperparathyroidism. Hyperphosphatemia for children with normal renal function is treated by volume repletion with saline coupled forced diuresis, a loop diuretic such as furosemide. For hypoparathyroidism, calcium and vitamin D are prescribed as mentioned in the treatment of hypocalcemia.
- Severe primary hyperparathyroidism and tertiary hyperparathyroidism need surgical parathyroidectomy. Need close monitoring of calcium and phosphate postoperatively and supplementation for symptomatic hypocalcemia.

HYPOMAGNESEMIA

Definition

Hypomagnesemia is defined as magnesium below the reference range of 1.8–2.1 mEq/L.

Etiology

Hypomagnesemia is common in up to 12% of hospitalized children and 60–65% of children in an intensive care setting. The causes of hypomagnesemia are enumerated in

Tables 20 and 21. *Hypomagnesemia* is commonly associated with chronic disease, gastrointestinal losses, renal losses, and induced by drugs.

Neonatal Hypomagnesemia

Two peculiar causes of neonatal hypomagnesemia are maternal hypomagnesemia and IUGR apart from low intake, renal and intestinal losses. Maternal hypomagnesemia is recognized in maternal diabetes. Circulating magnesium is normally low for first 3–5 days of life in IUGR babies.

Clinical Features

The typical signs and symptoms of hypomagnesemia are tetany, generalized convulsions, muscle weakness, anorexia, and ventricular arrhythmias.

Signs and Symptoms

Clinical features are muscle weakness, tetany, seizures, vasoconstriction causing hypertension (HTN). Magnesium depletion can cause widening of the QRS complex, peaking of T-waves, prolongation of the PR interval, progressive widening of the QRS complex, diminution of the T-wave, Torsades de Pointes, and ventricular arrhythmias. Hypomagnesemia below 1.2 mg/dL causes symptomatic hypocalcemia.

TABLE 20: Etiology of hypomagnesemia.

Pathogenesis	*Etiology*
Gastrointestinal disorders	• Prolonged nasogastric suction vomiting • Acute and chronic diarrhea • Malabsorption syndromes • Bowel resection intestinal/biliary fistulae • Acute hemorrhagic pancreatitis • Primary intestinal hypomagnesemia • PPI therapy • Cisplatin
Renal losses	• Parenteral fluids • Diuresis in DM • Hypercalcemia • *Drugs:* Cyclosporine/tacrolimus, diuretics (loop, thiazides), aminoglycosides, amphotericin, alcohol, pentamidine, and cetuximab • Metabolic acidosis • Hereditary hypomagnesemia with secondary hypocalcemia • *Renal diseases:* – Pyelonephritis – Interstitial nephritis – Glomerulonephritis – Post-obstructive diuresis – Diuretic phase of ATN – Renal tubular acidosis – Post-renal transplantation • *Inherited tubular diseases:* Bartter/Gitelman syndrome • Leptospirosis
Endocrine diseases	Hyperparathyroidism, hyperaldosteronism, and SIADH
Miscellaneous	Foscarnet, citrated blood, hungry bone, vitamin D deficiency, maternal hypomagnesemia, IUGR, refeeding syndrome, following surgery

(ATN: acute tubular necrosis; DM: diabetes mellitus; IUGR: intrauterine growth restriction; PPI: proton pump inhibitor; SIADH: syndrome of inappropriate antidiuretic hormone secretion)

Hypocalcemia in hypomagnesemia is due to the following factors:

- Inappropriately low PTH secretion
- Inappropriately low 1,25(OH) vitamin D
- Renal and skeletal resistance to PTH (magnesium interferes with G protein coupled activation in response to PTH)

In the presence of hypomagnesemia, healthy kidney lowers the magnesium excretion to <0.5 mg/dL. Hence, hypomagnesemia due to intestinal losses or low dietary intake is associated with low urinary magnesium excretion and in renal losses urinary magnesium excretion is inappropriately high or normal. Hypokalemia occurs in 40–60% of hypomagnesemia children due to underlying disorders that cause both magnesium and potassium loss such as diarrhea and diuretic therapy.

Evaluation

History will most often reveal the cause of hypomagnesemia. If no etiology is apparent, the distinction between gastrointestinal and renal losses can be made by measuring the 24-hour urinary magnesium excretion or the fractional excretion of magnesium.

A daily excretion of >10–30 mg or a fractional excretion of magnesium above 2% in a subject with normal renal function indicates renal magnesium wasting. Children with unexplained hypocalcemia and/or hypokalemia should be treated with magnesium.

The possibility of normomagnesemic magnesium depletion (in which there is isolated cellular magnesium depletion) should be considered as a possible cause of refractory hypokalemia or unexplained hypocalcemia in children at high risk for magnesium loss. This syndrome can be detected by demonstrating low urinary magnesium excretion. Another method to detect underlying magnesium depletion is to demonstrate reduced excretion (<80% over 24-hour) of an infused magnesium load (2.4 mg/kg of lean body weight given over the initial 4 hours). Children with malnutrition, cirrhosis, and diarrhea or long-term diuretic use typically have a positive test.

Management

- Primary treatment involves addressing the underlying cause.
- In tetany, seizure and arrhythmia and severe hypomagnesemia below 1.2 mg/dL need IV replacement. 1–2 g magnesium sulfate or 0.15–0.2 mmol/kg magnesium chloride is infused over 5–10 minutes. 1 g magnesium

TABLE 21: Causes of inherited hypomagnesemia.[15]

Conditions	*Mode*	*Chromosome*	*Gene*	*Gene protein*
Gitelman syndrome	AR	16q13	*SLC2A13*	NCCT
Isolated dominant hypomagnesemia (IDH)	AD	11q 23	*FXYD2* *KCNA1*	• Y-subunit of Na-K-ATPase • Apical potassium channel
Isolated recessive hypomagnesemia (IRH)	AR	-	*EGF*	Pro-EGF (epidermal growth factor)
Autosomal dominant hyperparathyroidism	AD	3q21	*CaSR*	CaSR
Familial hypocalciuric hypercalcemia (FHH)	AD	3q21	*CaSR*	CaSR
Neonatal severe hyperparathyroidism (NSHPT)	AR	3q21	*CaSR*	CaSR
*Familial hypomagnesemia with hypercalciuria/nephrocalcinosis (FHHNC)	AR	3q28	*CLDN 16*	Claudin 16 (paracellin 1) tight junction protein
Familial hypomagnesemia with hypercalciuria/ nephrocalcinosis ocular involvement (FHHNC)	AR	1p34	*CLDN 19*	Claudin 19 tight junction protein
Hypomagnesemia with secondary hypocalcemia (HSH)	AR	9q22	*TRPM6*	TRPM6 ion channel
Hypomagnesemia/ metabolic syndrome	Maternal	Mito DNA	*Mito tRNA*	Mitochondrial tRNA
Hypomagnesemia with impaired brain development	AR/AD		*CNNM2*	ACDP2, CNNM2, Cyclin M2
AD hypomagnesemia	AD		*KCNA 1*	Voltage-gated potassium channel (Kv1.1)
HNF1β associated hypomagnesemia	AD		*HNF1β*	Hepatocyte nuclear factor1β

*Stones, young age, hypocalcemia, chronic kidney disease (CKD), nephrogenic diabetes insipidus (NDI), polyuria, hypokalemia, and acidification defect.
(AD: autosomal dominant; AR: autosomal recessive; CaSR: calcium-sensing receptor)

sulfate = 8.12 mEq or 98.6 mg elemental magnesium = 4 mmol of elemental magnesium. Aim is to maintain serum magnesium above 1.0 mg/dL (0.9 mEq/L). This may require repeat doses daily for 3–5 days.

- Oral replacement is given for asymptomatic patient. Oral preparations provide 5–7 mEq (60–84 mg) of magnesium per tablet. Six to eight tablets should be taken daily in divided doses for severe magnesium depletion. Two to four tablets may be sufficient for mild, asymptomatic disease. Oral preparations available are oxide, hydroxide, sulfate, lactate, chloride, and carbonate. Oral magnesium oxide tablet is 400 mg and magnesium hydroxide is 311 mg per tablet.
- Children should be given magnesium-rich diet, e.g., meat, green vegetables, nuts, and seafood.
- In diuretic-induced hypomagnesemia, potassium-sparing diuretic as adjunct may reduce renal magnesium loss. Vitamin D deficiency needs to be treated simultaneously.

HYPERMAGNESEMIA

Etiology

Hypermagnesemia is seen to occur in 15% of inpatients. The causes are listed in **Table 22**. It is common in patients with renal failure after ingestion of magnesium-containing drugs, such as antacids or purgatives.

Signs and Symptoms

Moderate hypermagnesemia inhibits secretion of PTH, leading to a reduction in the plasma calcium. Hypermagnesemia may be associated with nonspecific symptoms such as nausea, vomiting, and flushing. Hyperkalemia is seen due to decreased magnesium-induced blockade of renal potassium channels. Manifestations depend on the severity of hypermagnesemia. **Table 23** shows the clinical correlation of clinical manifestations to serum magnesium level.

Management

- Children in renal failure should not receive magnesium containing medications.
- Stop all magnesium-containing preparation. Clear the intestine of residual offending laxatives or antacids with magnesium-free enema.
- IV calcium gluconate to ameliorate cardiac effects
- Promote urinary magnesium excretion using loop diuretics
- IV hydration as in management of hypercalcemia
- In case of renal dysfunction, peritoneal dialysis, hemodialysis, or exchange transfusion (in neonates) should be done.

CONCLUSION

Calcium is the most abundant cation in the body and bone acts as a large reservoir. Ionized calcium is the physiologically

TABLE 22: Causes of hypermagnesemia in children.

Pathogenesis	*Etiology*
Net increase in magnesium load	• Magnesium-containing laxatives, antacids, enemas, infusions • Treatment of preeclampsia/eclampsia (mother) • Diabetic ketoacidosis • Tumor lysis syndrome • Rhabdomyolysis • AKI • CKD
Increased renal magnesium absorption	• Hyperparathyroidism • Familial hypocalciuric hypercalcemia • Lithium ingestion • Milk-alkali syndrome • Hypothyroidism • Mineralocorticoid deficiency • Adrenal insufficiency • Acromegaly

(AKI: acute kidney injury; CKD: chronic kidney disease)

TABLE 23: Clinical correlation of serum magnesium levels and symptoms of hypermagnesemia.

Serum magnesium level	*Clinical manifestation*
Up to 3.6 mg/dL	Asymptomatic
4.8–7.2 mg/dL	Diminished deep tendon reflexes, bradycardia, and hypotension
>7.2 mg/dL	• Loss of deep tendon reflexes, prolongation of the PR interval • An increase in QRS duration and an increase in QT interval
>12 mg/dL	Respiratory paralysis, hypotension, and loss of consciousness
>15 mg/dL	Asystole, respiratory arrest, and coma

active form that accounts for 50–60% of total calcium concentration.

Phosphorus is a major constituent of the skeleton. Serum calcium and phosphorus is regulated by PTH, calcitriol, calcitonin, and FGF-23 through CaSR. Low effective ECF volume, reduced sodium intake, hyperphosphatemia, and metabolic alkalosis reduce urinary calcium excretion. Calculation of fractional excretion of phosphorus ($FEPO_4$) and the tubular phosphate reabsorption helps in evaluation of urinary phosphate excretion.

In contrast to calcium and phosphorus, the major site of magnesium transport is the thick ascending limb of the loop of Henle where 60–70% of the magnesium is reabsorbed.

Common causes of hypocalcemia are vitamin D deficiency and hypoparathyroidism and a common cause of hypercalcemia is hyperparathyroidism.

Phosphate content of cow's milk is six times greater than human milk making newborns and infants fed on cow's milk vulnerable to hyperphosphatemia.

Hypomagnesemia is a common entity occurring in up to 12% of hospitalized children and in 60–65% in children in an intensive care setting. Clinical features are muscle weakness, tetany, seizures, widening of the QRS complex, and HTN.

KEY POINTS

- Serum calcium and phosphorus are age-dependent and has a circadian rhythm. Serum calcium is also dependent on posture and serum albumin. Serum calcium level is corrected for serum albumin level before confirming the diagnosis of hypercalcemia or hypocalcemia.
- Circadian rhythm of serum calcium is characterized by a peak at 10 AM and a nadir at 6–8 PM, whereas phosphorus with the lowest phosphorus seen at 8–10 AM and a nocturnal peak of 45% above the trough level at 12–4 AM.
- Two-third of the filtered calcium is reabsorbed in PCT and 10–20% in loop of Henle. In hypocalcemia with normal PTH, it is a good practice to rule out familial hypocalcemic hypercalciuria.
- Evaluation of hypercalcemia includes assessment of phosphorus, PTH, vitamin D, urinary calcium, and imaging of bones, parathyroid gland, and kidneys.
- Mild asymptomatic hypocalcemia with normal PTH should raise the suspicion for FHH.
- Hydration with loop diuretics is the initial therapy in hypercalcemia followed by maintenance long-acting therapies such as steroids, bisphosphonates, and cinacalcet.
- Most common cause of hyperphosphatemia is renal failure and acute phosphorus loading. Drop in GFR below 35 mL/min/1.73 m^2 causes a steady rise in serum phosphorus.
- The consequences of chronic hyperphosphatemia are life-threatening, if left untreated.
- Severe hypomagnesemia below 1.2 mg/dL with tetany, seizure, and arrhythmia needs IV replacement.

REFERENCES

1. Kestenbaum B, Houillier P. Disorders of calcium, phosphate and magnesium metabolism. In: Johnson RJ, Feehally J (Eds). Comprehensive Clinical Nephrology, 6th edition. Philadelphia: Mosby; 2019. pp. 124-6.
2. Portale AA, Perwad F. Calcium and phosphorous. In: Avner ED, Harmon WE, Niaudet P, Yoshikawa N (Eds). Pediatric Nephrology, 6th edition. Heidelberg: Springer; 2009. pp. 231-305.
3. Jubiz W, Canterbury JM, Reiss E, Tyler FH. Circadian rhythm in serum parathyroid hormone concentration in human subjects: correlation with serum calcium, phosphate, albumin, and growth hormone levels. J Clin Invest. 1972;51:2040-6.
4. Loupy A, Ramakrishnan SK, Wootla B, Chambrey R, de la Faille R, Bourgeois S, et al. PTH-independent regulation of blood calcium concentration by the calcium-sensing receptor. J Clin Invest. 2012;122(9):3355-67.
5. From Indian Academy of Pediatrics 'Guideline for Vitamin D and Calcium in Children' Committee.; Khadilkar A, Khadilkar V, Chinnappa J, Rathi N, Khadgawat R, et al. Prevention and treatment of vitamin D and calcium deficiency in children and adolescents: Indian Academy of Pediatrics (IAP) Guidelines 2017. Indian Pediatrics. 2017;54(7):567-73.

6. Mensenkamp AR, Hoenderop JG, Bindels RJ. Recent advances in renal tubular calcium reabsorption. Curr Opin Nephrol Hypertens. 2006;15:524-9.
7. Peacock M. Calcium metabolism in health and disease. CJASN. 2010;5(Suppl 1):S23-30.
8. Lambers TT, Bindels RJ, Hoenderop JG. Coordinated control of renal Ca^{2+} handling. Kidney Int. 2006;69(4):650-4.
9. McKay CP. Disorders of Calcium metabolism. In: Feld Lg, Kaskel FJ (Eds). Fluid and Electrolytes in Pediatrics: a Comprehensive Handbook, 1st edition. New York: Springer; 2010. pp. 14971.
10. Markowitz M, Rotkin L, Rosen JF. Circadian rhythms of blood minerals in humans. Science. 1981;213:672-74.
11. Blaine J, Chonchol M and Levi M. Renal control of calcium, phosphate, and magnesium homeostasis. CJASN. 2015;10(7): 1257-72.
12. White KE, Larsson TE, Econs MJ. The roles of specific genes implicated as circulating factors involved in normal and disordered phosphate homeostasis: Frizzled related protein-4, matrix extracellular phosphoglycoprotein, and fibroblast growth factor 23. Endocr Rev. 2006;27(3):221-41.
13. Shaikh A, Berndt T, Kumar R. Regulation of phosphate homeostasis by the phosphatonins and other novel mediators. Pediatr Nephrol. 2008;23(8):1203-10.
14. Kerstan DQG. Physiology and pathophysiology of intestinal absorption of magnesium. In: Massry SG MH, Nishizawa Y, (Eds). Calcium in Internal Medicine. Surry: Springer-Verlag; 2002. p. 171-83.
15. Houillier P. Mechanisms and regulation of renal magnesium transport. Annual Rev Physiol. 2014;76:411-30.
16. Quamme GA, de Rouffignac C. Epithelial magnesium transport and regulation by the kidney. Front Biosci. 2000;5:D694-711.
17. Konrad M, Schlingmann KP. Disorders of Calcium and Magnesium Metabolism. In: Geary (DF), Schaefer F (Eds). Pediatric Kidney Disease, 2nd edition. Berlin Heidelberg; Springer-Verlag; 2016 .pp. 921-52.
18. Loughead JL, Mimouni F, Tsang RC. Serum ionized calcium concentrations in normal neonates. Am J Dis Child. 1988;142(5): 516-8.
19. David L, Anast CS. Calcium metabolism in newborn infants: The interrelationship of parathyroid function and calcium, magnesium, and phosphorus metabolism in normal, "sick," and hypocalcemic newborns. J Clin Invest. 1974;54(2):287-96.
20. Pepe J, Colangelo L, Biamonte F, Sonato C, Danese VC, Cecchetti V, et al. Diagnosis and management of hypocalcemia. Endocrine. 2020;69(3):485-95.
21. Roszko KL, Bi RD, Mannstadt M. Autosomal dominant hypocalcemia (Hypoparathyroidism) types 1 and 2. Front Physiol. 2016;7:458.
22. Thakker RV. Diseases associated with the extracellular calcium-sensing receptor. Cell Calcium. 2004;35(3):275-82.
23. Davies JH, Shaw NJ. Investigation and management of hypercalcaemia in children. Arch Dis Child. 2012;97(6):533-8.
24. Alharthi AA, Kamal NM, Abukhatwah MW, Sherief LM. Cinacalcet in pediatric and adolescent chronic kidney disease: a single-center experience. Medicine (Baltimore). 2015; 94(2):e401.
25. Felsenfeld AJ, Levine BS. Approach to treatment of hypophosphatemia. Am J Kidney Dis. 2012;60(4):655-61.

SECTION

5

Neonatal Nephrology

CHAPTER

5.1

Neonatal Kidney Function, Fluid and Electrolyte Balance

Hamsa V Reddy, Sukanya Govindan

INTRODUCTION

Transition of the fetus from the aqueous environment to extrauterine life is a fascinating and complex process. Renal functions in utero are borne by maternal placenta. The excretory and homeostatic functions of kidneys begin only after birth. Neonates are born with immature glomerular and tubular functions that are dependent on gestational age predisposing them to renal injury and fluid/electrolyte imbalance. Body composition and fluid distribution change dynamically during the intrauterine life, intrapartum phase, and early postnatal period. Hence, a sound understanding of the immature renal function, changes in tubular function, changes in body composition, and fluid compartments is essential.

DEVELOPMENTAL RENAL PHYSIOLOGY

Human kidneys start developing from the 5th week of gestation from three embryological units—pronephros, mesonephros, and metanephros. The first two embryological units involute, whereas the metanephros forms the ureteric bud. Through reciprocal induction between the ureteric bud and the metanephric mesenchyme, the primitive collecting system and the nephrons develop. A series of epithelial-mesenchymal interactions occur in the metanephric mesenchyme giving rise to the glomeruli, which are seen by around 9th week of gestation. Nephrogenesis is complete by 34–36 weeks of gestation, resulting in 0.7–1 million nephrons per kidney. Maturation starts from the juxtamedullary nephrons, with the superficial ones following and maturing after delivery at term.[1]

Fetal urine production begins around 10–12 weeks of gestation, contributing majorly to amniotic fluid volume by approximately 20 weeks of gestation. Mean urine flow rates are high, approximating 5 mL/h at 20 weeks, increasing up to 50 mL/h at 40 weeks' gestation. Hence, fetal oliguria/anuria leads to demonstrable oligohydramnios by 20–24 weeks' gestation with the resultant oligohydramnios sequence.[2]

RENAL BLOOD FLOW

Adult kidneys receive 20–25% of cardiac output, whereas fetal kidneys receive 3–4% of cardiac output, which increases to 8–10% in 1-week-old infants. The maturational increase in the proportion of cardiac output distributed to the kidneys correlates with the redistribution of renal blood flow (RBF) from the medulla to the outer cortex, as fetal kidney growth occurs centrifugally. The RBF is 20 mL/min at 25 weeks and increases to 50–60 mL/min by 40 weeks of gestation. The RBF doubles by 2 weeks of age and reaches mature levels by 2 years of age. The RBF is dependent on renal perfusion pressure (equal to systemic arterial blood pressure) and renal vascular resistance (RVR; dependent on afferent and efferent arteriolar pressure). Renal perfusion pressure is low and RVR is high, resulting in low RBF in neonates. With increasing age, a larger fraction of cardiac output reaches the kidneys leading to higher renal perfusion pressures. The RVR also reduces with the increase in diameter and the total number of renal blood vessels and to the production of vasoactive factors, such as angiotensin II (AII), catecholamines, prostaglandins (PGs), and NO (3).

Glomerular Filtration Rate

The glomerular filtration rate (GFR) is dependent on the glomerular capillary flow rate, the Starling forces across the capillary beds, and the surface area and permeability of the basement membrane. The GFR is represented mathematically by the following formula:

$$\text{GFR} = \text{Kf} \times [P_{GC} - (P_{IT} + \pi_{GC})]$$

where Kf = ultrafiltration coefficient, P_{GC} = hydrostatic pressure at the glomerular capillary, P_{IT} = proximal intratubular hydrostatic pressure, and π_{GC} = oncotic pressure in the glomerular capillary.

The ultrafiltration coefficient is dependent on the glomerular surface area, whereas the Starling forces are partly dependent on the RBF. In the fetal kidneys, the glomerular surface area is increased by the recruitment of glomeruli located in the outer cortex of fetal kidneys. The postnatal increase in systemic arterial blood pressure and reductions in RVR along with an increase in the glomerular surface area leads to an increase in GFR. Until 36 weeks of gestation, GFR is dependent on the increasing number of glomeruli. With the completion of nephron endowment, GFR increases with an increase in the renal mass changes in renal hemodynamics.[3]

The GFR in a fetus is dependent on the gestational age and the birth weight. The GFR increases three- to five-fold around 34 weeks of gestation. Newborns born premature also experience this increase when they reach 34 weeks of gestation. Once born, the GFR correlates directly with the gestational age and the postnatal age. In the term infant, the GFR at birth is approximately 30 mL/min/1.73 m^2, and it typically doubles in the first 2 postnatal weeks, reaching adult levels by 2 years of age. In preterm infants, GFR maturation is markedly diminished, mostly due to incomplete nephrogenesis and it matures more slowly due to the delayed nephrogenesis.

Serum creatinine (SCr) concentration, which is the measure of GFR in the neonates, despite its limitations peaks during the first few postnatal days, although the GFR rapidly increases after birth. This initial increase in SCr is due to multiple factors such as reflection of maternal SCr concentrations, reduced clearance resulting from immature glomerular filtration, and reabsorption of filtered creatinine in the leaky renal tubules of the neonates. The reference values of SCr in newborn babies are provided in **Table 1.**[4,5]

Cystatin C, a nonglycosylated low-molecular-weight protein of 13.3 kD produced in all nucleated cells with relative constancy, can be used to estimate GFR in newborns. It is freely filtered through the glomerulus and completely reabsorbed and catabolized by tubular cells. SCr are less significantly influenced by age, gender, body habitus, or composition compared to creatinine. The reference ranges for serum cystatin C for preterm neonates and neonates are available **(Table 2)**.[6] Because of the cost factors and nonavailability of the test in most places, cystatin C measurement is limited mostly to research purposes.

TABLE 1: Normal serum creatinine values (mg/dL) in term and preterm infants [mean ± standard deviation (SD)].

Age (day)	*<28 weeks*	*28–32 weeks*	*32–37 weeks*	*>37 weeks*
3	1.05 ± 0.27	0.88 ± 0.25	0.78 ± 0.22	0.75 ± 0.2
7	0.95 ± 0.36	0.94 ± 0.37	0.77 ± 0.48	0.56 ± 0.4
14	0.81 ± 0.26	0.78 ± 0.36	0.62 ± 0.4	0.43 ± 0.25
28	0.66 ± 0.28	0.59 ± 0.38	0.40 ± 0.28	0.34 ± 0.2

Sources: Rudd PT, Hughes EA. Reference ranges for plasma creatinine during the first month of life. Arch Dis Child. 1983;58:212-5; van den Anker JN, de Groot R. Assessment of glomerular filtration rate in preterm infants by serum creatinine: comparison with inulin clearance. Pediatrics. 1995;96(6):1156-8.

TABLE 2: Reference values for serum cystatin C in neonates and children.

Age	*Cystatin C (mg/L)*
24–28 weeks' GA	1.48 (0.65–3.37)
29–36 weeks' GA	1.65 (0.62–4.42)
0–3 months	1.37 (0.81–2.32)
4–11 months	0.98 (0.65–1.49)
1–3 years	0.79 (0.50–1.25)

(GA: gestational age)
Source: Finney H, Newman DJ. Reference ranges for plasma cystatin C and creatinine measurements in premature infants, neonates, and older children. Arch Dis Child. 2000;82(1):71-5.

Developmental Changes of the Body Composition and Fluid Compartments

Before birth, fetal fluid and electrolyte balance are largely the function of maternal placenta. Total body water (TBW) is approximately 95% in a 16-week-old fetus, with approximately two thirds in the extracellular compartment and one third in the intracellular compartment. By term, the TBW reduces to 75% of the body weight, of which almost 50% is in the intracellular compartment. During labor and delivery, with an increase in the blood pressure, catecholamine, vasopressin, and cortisol plasma concentrations increase and capillary permeability increases due to intrapartum hypoxia; a shift of fluid from the intravascular to the interstitial compartment occurs, resulting in approximately 25% reduction in circulating plasma volume in the fetus. After birth, with the increase in oxygenation and changes in vasoactive hormone production restore the capillary membrane integrity favoring absorption of interstitial fluid into the intravascular compartment, maintaining the intravascular volume during the first 24–48 hours postnatally, when oral fluid intake may be limited. However, prematurity, pathologic conditions, or both can disrupt this transitional process interfering with the physiologic contraction of the extracellular fluid (ECF) compartment in the immediate postnatal period.[7]

Insensible Water Losses

Insensible water loss (IWL) occurs through the skin, respiratory tract, and stool. IWL is highly variable and is higher in preterm babies than in term infants. IWL is obligate-free water losses, as neonates cannot modulate IWL in response to water balance. IWL is directly proportional to the gestational age; very immature preterm infants (<1,000 g) may lose as much as 2–3 mL/kg/h, partly because of immature skin, lack of subcutaneous tissue, and a large exposed surface area. IWL is more with increased environmental and body temperatures, skin breakdown, radiant warmers, phototherapy, and extreme prematurity. The loss is diminished when an infant is clothed, is covered by an acrylic resin inner heat shield, breathes humidified air, or is of advanced postnatal age. A larger premature infant (2,000–2,500 g) nursed in an incubator may have an IWL of approximately 0.6–0.7 mL/kg/h. Stool water loss is usually small and usually <5 mL/kg/24 h in the first days after birth.[7]

Neonatal Tubular Function

The neonatal period sees changes in the GFR and there is a parallel increase in the delivery of water and solutes to the renal tubules. The GFR of a term newborn is around 20–30 mL/min/1.73 m^2 and it increases to an adult value of 100–120 mL/min/1.73 m^2 by 2 years of age, and this happens due to the postnatal increase in the glomerular filtration surface area. This change should be accompanied by increased water and solute absorption by the tubules, otherwise the neonate will be dehydrated due to solute and water loss even with minor changes in GFR. The tubuloglomerular feedback in the adult kidney helps to maintain a balance between GFR and tubular reabsorption. However, in neonates, especially in preterm babies, this process is immature. There are major changes in the renal tubular transport in the postnatal period including abundance of transporters, developmental changes in hormonal levels, signal transduction, etc.[8]

Proximal tubule: The proximal tubule reabsorbs the majority of water and solutes in the glomerular filtrate including glucose, amino acids, phosphates, bicarbonate, and chloride. The basolateral Na^+/K^+-ATPase pump provides the driving force for tubular transport in this segment. The proximal tubule in the neonatal kidney has a significantly less rate of absorption than the adult kidney, and this is due to the lower activity of the Na^+/K^+-ATPase pump. However, the activity of the Na^+/K^+-ATPase pump progressively increases in the postnatal period due to increased sodium delivery to the tubules and also due to the influence of glucocorticoid and thyroid hormones.[9]

The major channel for bicarbonate and NaCl reabsorption is the Na^+/H^+ exchanger (NHE) and the H^+-ATPase channel. Unlike in adults in whom the NHE3 isoform is the most abundant, in the neonatal kidney most of the NHE activity is attributed to NHE8 isoform and there is no H^+-ATPase activity noted in the neonatal tubules. There is lower activity of sodium-glucose cotransporter 1 (SGLT1) and SGLT2 glucose transporters at birth, and there is a maturational increase in the number and function in the postnatal period.

Neonates have a higher serum phosphate level than adults and are in a state of positive phosphate balance, which is essential for growth. The proximal tubule is the primary site of phosphate reabsorption, and this is mediated by two sodium-phosphate cotransporters NaPi-2a and NaPi-2c. Neonates have a lower GFR than adults, and hence a reduced filtered load of phosphate is not the cause for a positive phosphate balance. It is at least in part due to increased tubular phosphate reabsorption and is hypothesized to be due to higher Vmax of phosphate transporters. There is also a blunted response to the effects of parathormone (PTH) resulting in less phosphate excretion in neonates compared to adults.[9]

Thick ascending limb: The thick ascending limb (TAL) is the diluting segment of the renal tubule, and the tubular fluid can achieve an osmolarity of ~50 mOsm/kg of water. The TAL reabsorbs ~25% of the filtered NaCl and is impermeable to water. The luminal transporter Na^+-K^+-$2Cl^-$ cotransporter (NKCC2) reabsorbs sodium which exits the TAL through the Na^+-/K^+-ATPase pump on the basolateral side. Chloride is transported out of the cell by the ClC-Kb channel, and potassium is recycled into the lumen by the ROMK (renal outer medullary potassium) channel. There are many postnatal changes in the TAL including increased expression of NKCC2, Na^+/K^+-ATPase, and ROMK, resulting in an increase in sodium reabsorption in the TAL. Despite the lower concentration or activity of transporters, the neonate is able to dilute urine probably due to drinking breast milk, a hypotonic fluid. Neonates are able to dilute urine up to an osmolarity of ~50 mOsm/kg of water like adults.

Distal tubule and cortical collecting duct: There is limited data available regarding the postnatal changes in the distal tubule (DT). Despite the reduced sodium reabsorption in all the segments of the nephron, the renal sodium excretion is less in neonates than in adults suggesting increased distal sodium reabsorption. Even though the neonate is able to dilute urine to an osmolarity of ~50 mOsm/kg of water, there is a limited ability to excrete a free water load due to the low GFR. Urinary concentration depends on the vasopressin activity enabling water absorption through aquaporin-2 channels in the collecting duct. The neonatal kidney can concentrate urine only up to an osmolarity of 600 mOsm/kg of water and not beyond that due to the lower intracellular cyclic adenosine monophosphate (cAMP) generated when vasopressin binds to its receptor and also due to the lower expression of aquaporin-2 in the collecting duct.

There is less sodium reabsorption at the cortical collecting duct (CCD) in the neonate compared to adults due to paucity of epithelial Na channels (ENaCs) and the relative resistance to the effect aldosterone has on ENaCs. The neonate needs positive K^+ balance for growth. Potassium secretion primarily occurs through the ROMK channel in the CCD. The driving force for K^+ excretion is the flow-mediated sodium absorption through ENaC, which is limited in the neonate resulting in less K^+ secretion.[9]

The neonatal kidney has fewer intercalated cells in the CCD compared to that of the adult. The type A intercalated cell has a H^+-ATPase as well as a H^+/K^+-ATPase on the apical membrane and basolateral Cl^-/HCO_3^- exchanger and anion exchanger 1 (AE1). The type-B intercalated cells have the H^+-ATPase on the basolateral membrane and a different Cl^-/HCO_3^- exchanger, designated pendrin, on the apical membrane for base secretion. Postnatally, there is a progressive increase in the number of intercalated cells.

Acid–base Balance in the Neonates

Neonates have lower serum bicarbonate compared to adults with values of 20–22 mmol/L in the term infant, 18–20 mmol/L in preterm infants, and as low as 14 mmol/L in extremely preterm infants. Similar to adults, most of the bicarbonate reabsorption occurs in the proximal tubule. However, there is lesser reabsorptive capacity at the proximal convoluted tubule

(PCT) due to lower activity of the basolateral Na^+/K^+-ATPase pump and the apical NHE. Postnatal maturational increase in bicarbonate reabsorption occurs due to an increase in number, activity, and hormonal activation of these transporters.[10]

Neonates have increased acid load from protein intake and formation of new bone and hence need two to three times higher net acid excretion by ammoniagenesis and titratable acid compared to adults. The process of ammoniagenesis undergoes complex developmental changes. At birth, the enzyme for ammoniagenesis glutaminase has lower activity and its substrate glutamine is also available in lower levels in the kidney resulting in less ammonia production and hence less acid excretion. All these factors together limit the ability of neonates to recover from acidosis.[11]

Hormonal Influences of Neonatal Tubular Transport

Glucocorticoid and thyroid hormones are responsible for postnatal maturational changes in the tubular transport. Antenatal dexamethasone administration is shown to increase the Na^+/K^+-ATPase, NKCC, and ROMK and aquaporin-2 channels in the tubules in animal studies. Both glucocorticoid and thyroid hormones appear to increase NHE3 activity postnatally.

In the intrauterine period, fetal water flow occurs from the maternal circulation through the placenta, and this is facilitated through aquaporin channels aided by osmotic gradient set by transport of sodium. In the neonatal period, arginine vasopressin (AVP) secretion occurs triggered by changes in plasma osmolality due to excess or deficient body water. All neonates, including preterm, are able to adequately dilute urine. However, the concentrating ability of preterm neonates is limited and they are only able to concentrate urine to 600–700 mOsm/L in comparison to ~1,300 mOsm/L achieved by adults.[8]

Fluid Prescription for Neonates

The goal of fluid and electrolyte therapy in the immediate postnatal period is not only to maintain fluid and electrolyte balance, but also to allow for appropriate changes to occur without detrimental perturbations in fluid and electrolyte status.[12]

Based on the estimated transepidermal losses and anticipated urine output, the starting fluid volume for newborn babies can be suggested as per the gestational age and birth weight **(Table 3)**. A rational initial intravenous fluid volume would be the sum of an allowance for urinary water of 30–60 mL/kg/day plus estimated IWL.

Intravenous sodium in maintenance fluid should be avoided until the physiological postnatal diuresis/natriuresis is underway, marked clinically by the onset of weight loss. A 10–20% weight loss is common in preterm infants during the first postnatal week. After initiating fluids on the first day, the adjustment for water and electrolytes are done as per **Table 4**. Glucose should be initiated at 7 μg/kg/min. The

TABLE 3: Estimated starting intravenous intake, at an ambient humidity of 50%.*

Gestational age (weeks)	*Birth weight (kg)*	*Approximate trans epidermal water loss (mL/kg/24 h)*	*Allowance for urine output (mL/kg/24 h)*	*Estimated intake range (mL/kg/24 h)*	*Suggested starting volume (mL/kg/24 h)*†
<27	<1	120	30–60	150–180	150
27–31	1–1.5	40	30–60	70–90	90
31–36	1.5–2.5	20	30–60	50–80	80
>36	>2.5	10	30–60	40–70	60

A cautious approach, commencing at the lower end of the estimated requirement, is recommended.
*At higher ambient humidity, transepidermal water losses will be reduced and requirements will be lower.
†Once sustained weight loss of at least 5% is achieved, proceed to the intravenous volume necessary to support nutritional goals without stepwise increments.

TABLE 4: Guidelines for adjusting fluid and electrolyte therapy in newborns.

	Postnatal day 1	*Adjustment during the prediuretic phase (birth to 2 days)*	*Adjustment during the diuretic/natriuretic phase (1–5 days)*
Water	As per gestational age and birth weight **(Table 3)**	*Increase if:* Weight loss is >2%/day or serum sodium increases *Decrease if:* Weight increases or serum sodium decreases	*Increase by 10–30 mL/kg/day if:* Weight loss is >5%/day or serum sodium is >150 mEq/L with no sodium intake *Decrease by 10–30 mL/kg/day if:* Weight loss is <1%/day
Sodium	None	Usually no sodium is required	*Begin 1–2 mmol/kg/day if:* Serum sodium is <135 mEq/L with weight loss or serum sodium is <130 mEq/L with no change or gain in weight
Potassium	None	Usually, no potassium is required	*Begin 1–2 mmol/L/day if* serum potassium is <5 mEq/L and not increasing and urine output is <1 mL/kg/h

Source: Lorenz J. Fluid and electrolyte therapy in the very low-birthweight neonate. NeoReviews. 2008;9(3):e102-8.

glucose in fluids should be adjusted as per the blood sugar measurements by adjusting the glucose infusion rate.

Fluid and electrolyte balance should be monitored carefully, with daily monitoring of the serum sodium, potassium, creatinine, and bodyweight. Urine output has to be monitored continuously with 4–6 hourly assessment. Satisfactory fluid management is marked by a urine flow rate of at least 0.5–1 mL/kg/h on the first day, rising to 2–3 mL/kg/h thereafter and daily weight loss of the order of 1–2%, followed by a weight gain of the order of 14–16 g/kg/day.[13]

CONCLUSION

Development of neonatal GFR is a complex, multifactorial process consisting of fetal and newborn hemodynamics, nephron endowment, gestational age at birth, and birth weight. GFR, RBF, and tubular functions increase with renal growth and nephrogenesis. The first week of life is a very dynamic period for body water and electrolytes during which the risk of perturbations of body water and electrolytes is great. Frequent clinical and laboratory monitoring is essential to ensure correct fluid therapy in neonates.

KEY POINTS

- Nephrogenesis is complete at around 36 weeks of gestation.
- The estimated GFR in the new born ranges from 20 to 40 mL/min/1.73 m^2 depending on the gestational age.
- Serum cystatin C is a useful marker of renal function in the new born.
- Immature neonatal kidneys, though maintain good urine output, are at a risk to develop fluid, electrolyte, and metabolic disturbances.

REFERENCES

1. Guignard JP. Renal morphogenesis and development of renal function. In: Ballard RA, Seri I, Taeusch HW, Gleason CA (Eds). Avery's Diseases of the Newborn, 9th edition. Philadelphia, PA: Elsevier Saunders; 2012. pp. 1165-75.
2. Kelly LK, Seri I. Renal developmental physiology: relevance to clinical care. NeoReviews. 2008;9(4):e150-61.
3. Su SW, Stonestreet BS. Core concepts: neonatal glomerular filtration rate. NeoReviews. 2010;11(12):e714-21.
4. Rudd PT, Hughes EA. Reference ranges for plasma creatinine during the first month of life. Arch Dis Child. 1983;58:212-5.
5. Van den Anker JN, de Groot R. Assessment of glomerular filtration rate in preterm infants by serum creatinine: comparison with inulin clearance. Pediatrics. 1995;96(6):1156-8.
6. Finney H, Newman DJ. Reference ranges for plasma cystatin C and creatinine measurements in premature infants, neonates, and older children. Arch Dis Child. 2000;82(1):71-5.
7. Lorenz J. Fluid and electrolyte therapy in the very low-birth weight neonate. NeoReviews. 2008;9(3):e102-8.
8. Gattineni J, Baum M. Developmental changes in renal tubular transport—an overview. Pediatr Nephrol. 2013;30(12):2085-98.
9. Suarez-Rivera M, Bonilla-Felix M. Fluid and electrolyte disorders in the newborn: sodium and potassium. Curr Pediatr Rev. 2014;10(2):115-22.
10. Iacobelli S, Guignard JP. Renal aspects of metabolic acid-base disorders in neonates. Pediatr Nephrol. 2020;35(2):221-8.
11. Quigley R, Baum M. Neonatal acid base balance and disturbances. Semin Perinatol. 2004;28(2):97-102.
12. Grace E, Keir AK. Fluid therapy: friend or foe? Clin Perinatol. 2020;47(3):515-28.
13. Lindower JB. Water balance in the fetus and neonate. Semin Fetal Neonatal Med. 2017;22(2):71-5.

CHAPTER

5.2

Approach to a Neonate with Renal Disease

Jayati Sengupta

INTRODUCTION

The etiology of renal diseases in neonates ranges from congenital problems and acquired causes that contribute to perinatal morbidity. Both acute presentation and chronic nature of disease are witnessed in the newborn population.

Acute kidney injury and chronic kidney disease have been observed in both developing and developed countries.[1-3] In the developed world, the neonatal chronic kidney disease was noted to have an estimated incidence of 1 in 10,000 live births, and end-stage kidney disease was estimated in about 7.1 per million age-related population.[3]

Congenital anomalies and hereditary nephropathies comprise about two-thirds of cases of renal disease in the developed countries, whereas acquired causes such as sepsis and perinatal hypoxia add to the burden of renal disease in developing countries.[4,5] These newborns can present at birth with difficulty in micturition, oliguria, edema, and rising serum creatinine, as part of symptoms of acute kidney injury or may have problems such as hydronephrosis or hydrops, pulmonary hypoplasia, vesicoureteral reflux detected antenatally, or as in cystic kidney disorders, may run a chronic course and end up with end-stage disease in the next few months.

The common etiological causes of newborn renal disease are due to the following:

- Developmental anomalies during embryogenesis, also known as the spectrum of congenital anomalies of the kidney and the urinary tract (CAKUT)
- Genetic cystic kidney diseases, hereditary tubulopathies, etc.
- Nephrotic syndrome, e.g., congenital nephrotic syndrome (CNS)
- Syndromic and inborn errors of metabolism involving the kidney
- Infections acquired perinatally such as urinary tract infection or renal involvement as part of sepsis
- Neonatal hypertension
- Acquired vascular thrombosis
- Renal damage due to perinatal causes and nephrotoxic medications used by mother in pregnancy or after birth

APPROACH TO A NEWBORN WITH SUSPECTED RENAL DISEASE

Antenatal Diagnosis

Prenatal ultrasound scans have become the mainstay of diagnosis and differentiation of structural renal anomalies in the fetus. The main points to look for are as follows:

- Oligohydramnios, which may be associated with pulmonary hypoplasia with renal dysplasia, renal agenesis, and tubular dysgenesis.
- Hydronephrosis of the fetal kidneys—as early as 15–18 weeks of gestational age (second trimester), fetal hydronephrosis can be picked up and classified and prognosticated based on the anteroposterior diameter (APD) of the fetal renal pelvis. According to most guidelines, antenatal hydronephrosis (ANH) is present if the APD of the fetal kidney is ≥4 mm in the second trimester and ≥7 mm in the third trimester.
- Fetal hydrops may be due to CNS, severe proteinuria, and hypoalbuminemia.[6]
- Polyhydramnios may be the presenting features in some varieties of Bartter syndrome.
- Other features detected in fetal ultrasound are the presence of calyectasis; dilated ureters; echogenicity of kidneys; the variation in size, number, and position of the kidneys; the bladder wall thickness; the urethral flow; and the dilatation of the posterior urethra.[7]

Increased sagittal length of the kidney, presence of cyst-like lesion in the upper pole, and ureterocele in the bladder are clinically diagnostic of a duplex kidney system.

The triad of megacystis, keyhole sign, and hydronephrosis almost certainly point toward a lower urinary tract obstruction (LUTO), and considering other factors such as gestational age, sex, presence of anhydramnios, bladder volume, and urethral size help in improving the accuracy in diagnosis of LUTO.[8]

So, in summary, the various renal abnormalities that can be assessed from the antenatal fetal ultrasound include the following:

- Hydronephrosis—unilateral or bilateral, often due to pelvic-ureteric junction obstruction (PUJO)

- Number and position of kidneys—solitary kidney, horseshoe kidney, renal ectopia, renal agenesis
- Hydroureteronephrosis—as in or vesicoureteric reflux
- Bladder anomalies such as bladder exstrophy, thickened bladder wall in post urethral valves, prune belly syndrome with associated hydronephrosis
- Renal cystic disorders—polycystic kidney disease and multicystic dysplastic kidneys
- Potter syndrome with oligohydramnios, dilated thick-walled bladder due to LUTO
- Duplex kidneys with ureterocele in the bladder

Figures 1 and 2 show antenatal ultrasound images of kidneys with multicystic dysplasia and urinary tract obstruction, respectively.

When antenatal ultrasounds point toward the presence of a renal anomaly, some soft signs are also looked for, which predict the presence of other systemic involvements, especially in the cardiovascular, neurological, musculoskeletal, and gastrointestinal systems. These are also pointers toward some syndromic conditions. These include:

- Increased nuchal translucency
- Absent nasal bone
- Choroid plexus cyst
- Ventriculomegaly
- Shortened bones of extremities—femur and humerus
- Echogenic bowel

So, detection of anomaly in the antenatal scans, presence of soft signs along with increased maternal age, and triple test help determine the risk of chromosomal disorders in the baby.[7]

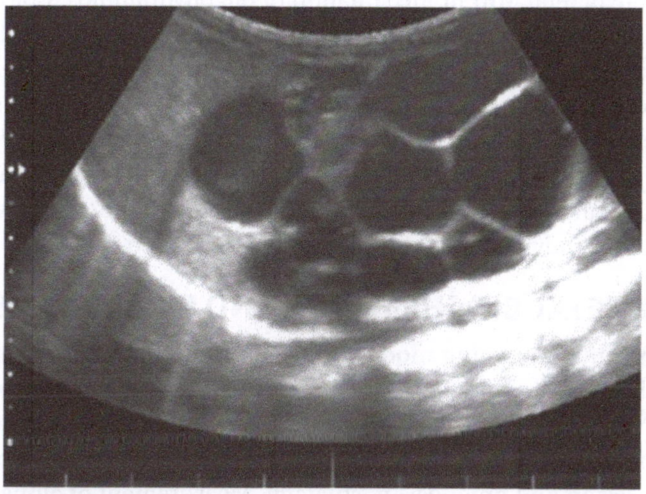

Fig. 1: Multicystic dysplastic kidney. Ultrasonogram scan shows a kidney with multiple cysts of different sizes arranged in no recognizable pattern.

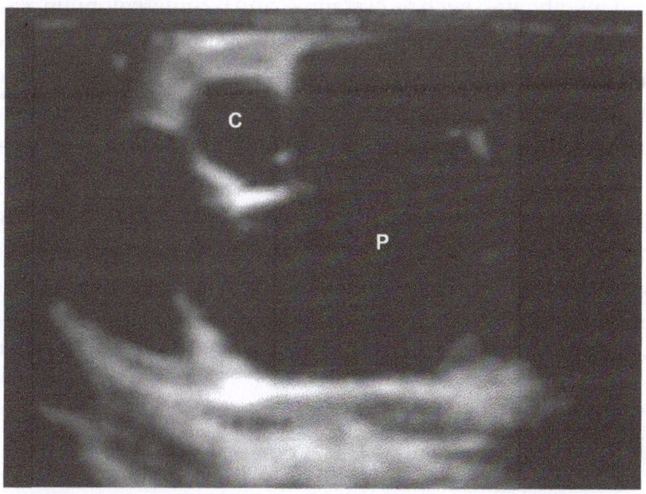

Fig. 2: Ureteropelvic obstruction leading to hydronephrosis showing dilated pelvis (P) and calyces (C).

Maternal Drug History

Maternal use of several drugs has been shown to have deleterious effects on the development of the fetal kidney and subsequent cause of renal failure. History of maternal drug intake in pregnancy and in lactation is therefore of utmost importance.[9] **Table 1** lists the names of some common groups of drugs and their possible effects on the kidney tissue.

GENETICS IN PRENATAL DIAGNOSIS OF RENAL DISORDERS

The most common hereditary kidney diseases are the polycystic kidney diseases. Autosomal dominant polycystic kidney disease (ADPKD) and autosomal recessive polycystic kidney disease (ARPKD) are the most common types of renal dysplasia, although other ciliopathies may mimic these diseases and may be a reason for cyst formation in the kidneys. ADPKD is usually associated with the *PKD1* and *PKD2* genes. If the fetal ultrasonogram (USG) shows enlarged, bilateral bright echogenic kidneys, a family history is to be sought and parental renal USGs may be offered to detect the presence of cystic changes. If, however, the family history is unavailable, an amniocentesis with a chromosomal microarray is advisable. If the microarray is also normal, a targeted gene panel for ADPKD or clinical exome is considered for establishing the diagnosis.

Autosomal recessive polycystic kidney disease is a more severe disease, with autosomal recessive inheritance that also involves the biliary tract. The gene involved is *PHKD1*, which codes for the protein fibrocystin. If ARPKD is suspected based on USG findings in the second or third trimester showing the presence of large echogenic kidneys and possible involvement of other systems, a genetic diagnosis should be offered to parents, and parents should be counseled about continuation or termination of pregnancy based on their choice. **Figure 3** shows USG features of kidneys in the neonate with polycystic kidney disease.

Other cystic disorders due to ciliopathy, such as Bardet-Biedl syndrome, Meckel-Gruber syndrome, and multicystic dysplastic kidney, can be suspected from ultrasound findings and genetic diagnoses offered to parents.

TABLE 1: Drugs and their possible effects on the kidney tissue.

Name of drugs	*Effect on fetal kidney due to maternal use in pregnancy*	*Effect on neonatal kidney due to use during lactation*
ACE inhibitors/ARB	Renal insufficiency	Renal papilla atrophy, low nephron count, tubular changes
Aminoglycosides	Tubular changes, reduced nephron count	Tubular damage, low nephron count
Dexamethasone	Disturbance in tubular transporters	No effect
Antiepileptics	Increased risk of congenital renal anomaly like horseshoe kidney, MCDK	No effect
Cyclophosphamide	Hydronephrosis	No effect
Cyclosporine A	Tubular changes, reduced nephron number	Tubular and glomerular damage
Ergotamine	Renal agenesis, urethral atresia	
Mycophenolate mofetil	Renal ectopia, renal damage	No effect
Furosemide	Renal concentrating defect	None
Adriamycin	Hydronephrosis, bladder agenesis	None

(ACE: angiotensin-converting enzyme; ARB: angiotensin II receptor blocker; MCDK: multicystic dysplastic kidney)

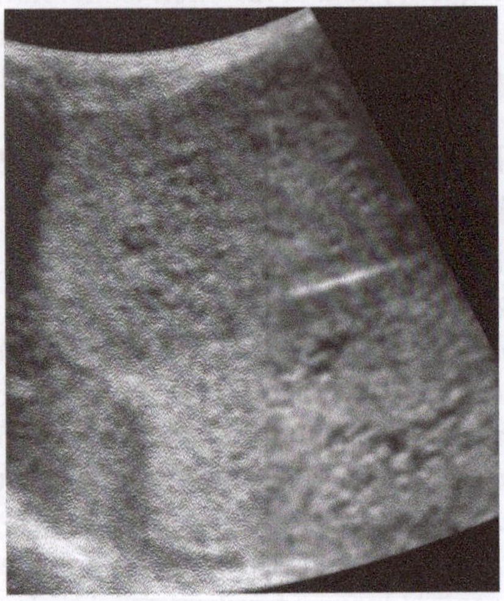

Fig. 3: Autosomal recessive polycystic renal disease in an 11-hour-old term male newborn. Ultrasonogram scan shows bilaterally enlarged and echogenic kidneys.

Renal agenesis, both unilateral and bilateral, detected on USG can point to various syndromic disorders. Bilateral renal agenesis carries an extremely poor prognosis due to anhydramnios leading to fetal pulmonary hypoplasia. Renal agenesis may be associated with genetic syndromes in about 30% cases, and hence genetic diagnosis should be offered to the parents. Common single-gene disorders associated with renal agenesis include Kallmann syndrome, Smith–Lemli–Opitz syndrome, etc.[9]

MRI IN THE FETUS

Prenatal USG images also have their limitations. In cases of renal agenesis and oligohydramnios, ultrasound images can be sometimes inconclusive. To improve the image quality and diagnostic possibilities, MRI has been used in the fetus.[10] The diagnostic capability of fetal MRI to detect congenital anomalies has been underscored in renal agenesis and ectopia.[11] But due to paucity of larger systemic reviews, no statements or guidelines are available as yet regarding the role of fetal MRI in the situation of oligohydramnios. Color Doppler imaging is used to calculate the renal artery length from the division of the internal iliac artery using the femur length as a variable. If the renal arteries are not located as expected, a diagnosis of renal agenesis is considered likely.[12] Tuberous sclerosis complex has been diagnosed through fetal USG and MRI by identifying fetal cardiac rhabdomyoma, subependymal nodules, and renal cysts.[13]

FETAL BIOCHEMISTRY AND BIOMARKERS

Although imaging modalities remain the first choice for diagnosis and prognostication of fetal renal anomalies, several biomarkers from the fetal urine and fetal serum samples have been studied to evaluate their role in assessing the severity of a lesion and prognosis postnatally. Measurement of alpha-fetoprotein in the amniotic fluid and even in maternal serum has been in practice for the diagnosis of CNS for quite some time.[14] Electrolytes, such as sodium, potassium, and chloride, and metabolites, such as cystatin C and β2-microglobulin, can be collected from fetal urine (aspirated from fetal bladder, fetal renal pelvis, or ureter) or from fetal blood through sampling from the umbilical vein. There is always a risk of infection, premature rupture of membranes, preterm delivery, and even fetal demise.

Sodium in the fetal urine of <100 mEq/mL and urinary chloride of <90 mEq/mL in the second trimester have a good prognosis.[15] Several studies conducted since then, and the studies of fetal intervention with decompression in severe obstructive uropathy, have yielded better results, if fetal urine was hypotonic (<100 mEq/mL Na, osmolarity <210 mOsm).[16]

ROLE OF PROTEOMES IN ANTENATAL DIAGNOSIS

Proteomics is the study of the entire set of different proteins produced by or present in the actual functional milieu of a cell or an organ. Courtesy the Human Genome Project, more and more monogenic causes of diseases are being identified and the proteomic study of the defective genes can serve as a marker for the identification of an abnormality. It is more complex and advanced than genomics, because the genetic structure is more or less constant, but proteomes can change from cell to cell or from time to time. Urinary proteome in a pediatric cohort of renal cyst and diabetes was analyzed and found to be different from other similar diseases, such as ADPKD, congenital nephrotic syndrome, and other disorders, that cause chronic kidney disease suggesting different pathophysiology of these conditions.[17]

DNA methylation is a new biomarker shown to identify rare renal disorders. Abnormalities in DNA methylation have been noted in immunoglobulin A (IgA) nephropathy, ADPKD, membranous nephropathy, and renal agenesis.[18]

POSTNATAL ASSESSMENT

Because renal diseases are not an uncommon cause of morbidity and mortality in the newborn population, an understanding of the various presentations of these diseases in the newborn postnatally, or renal problems already diagnosed in the fetus, will help in expediting the management process.

So, a detailed postnatal clinical evaluation of a newborn is very important if renal diseases are suspected. A newborn with a renal disease can present in various ways:

- Antenatally diagnosed congenital renal problems
- Signs and symptoms related to the kidney, such as anuria, hematuria, edema, and proteinuria
- Infections of the urinary tract
- Renovascular problems, such as hypertension
- Fluid and electrolyte abnormalities
- Involvement of the kidney in systemic diseases
- Kidney damage due to perinatal causes

Examination of the newborn can start with looking for features that are known to be associated with renal problems.

- *Dysmorphic features* such as vertebral column anomalies, cardiac problems, single umbilical artery, supernumerary nipples, hypospadias, anorectal malformations, facial asymmetry, cleft palate, coloboma of iris, and distal limb anomalies, such as polydactyly, are often associated with kidney disorders. Prune belly syndrome with laxity of the abdominal wall is almost always associated with anomalies of the urinary tract and hydronephrosis.
- *Potter syndrome:* Severe obstructive uropathy leading to severe oligohydramnios resulting in pulmonary hypoplasia and associated renal agenesis is the prototype of Potter syndrome. The babies have a characteristic look in the form of dry and thick leathery skin, flattened nose, low set ears, retrognathia, and arthrogryposis. The degree of pulmonary hypoplasia, which is dependent on the degree of urinary obstruction and the severity and duration of oligohydramnios, is the key to future prognosis.
- *Palpable masses and bladder:* Flank fullness and palpable masses at birth point toward hydronephrosis, renal vein thrombosis, multicystic kidneys, rarely Wilms tumor, or neuroblastoma. Newborn bladders are hardly ever palpable, and palpable bladders are a clue to obstruction distally like posterior urethral valves and ureterocele.
- *Ascites*: A newborn can seldom present with ascites and generalized edema as a part of hydrops in CNS or urinary ascites due to rupture of bladder by any obstructed distal lesion.
- *Anuria or oliguria:* 90% of newborns usually pass urine within the first 24 hours of birth, but 10% do not. If urine is not passed by 48 hours or a newborn passes urine <1 mL/kg/h, it is a pointer to a renal disease. Poor stream and excessive straining during micturition also point toward a renal pathology.[19]
- *Hydronephrosis:* One of the most common renal problems faced in the newborn is the presence of *hydronephrosis* detected antenatally. If the APD of the renal pelvis was >7 mm in the third trimester, a diagnosis of hydronephrosis can be made and all such babies should have a repeat postnatal scan after 48–72 hours after birth. If normal, they should have a repeat scan at 4 weeks to substantially prove or disprove the presence of hydronephrosis. If, however, the immediate postnatal scan shows the presence of hydronephrosis (APD > 7 mm), then further investigations like a cystogram and mercaptoacetyltriglycine/diethylenetriaminepentacetate (MAG3/DTPA) scan may be required. It is well known that approximately 50% of antenatally detected hydronephrosis can resolve spontaneously after birth.[7] A simplistic approach to postnatal hydronephrosis is depicted in **Flowchart 1**.[20]
- *Infections of the urinary tract* are common in presence of obstructive lesions of the urinary tract and as part of sepsis in the newborn. The typical features of dysuria, frequency is usually lacking. Instead, the baby may have refusal to suck, vomiting, and fever (often afebrile) and generally look sick with poor perfusion, irritability, and failure to thrive. A urinalysis and culture establish the diagnosis.
- *Nephrotic syndrome:* CNS may present in the newborn with ascites and edema and even hydrops. Primary causes such as autosomal recessive Finnish variety or secondary causes due to several congenital infections may be the causative factor. Premature babies with placentomegaly and raised alpha-fetoprotein in the mother gives a clue to the diagnosis. There is proteinuria, anemia, and pitting edema either at birth or within the first 3 months. Newborns with ambiguous genitalia and nephrotic syndrome with mutation in the *WT1* gene may be diagnosed as the Frazier/Denys–Drash syndrome, while those with central nervous system involvement with microcephaly, seizures, and hiatal hernia may be suffering from the Galloway-Mowat syndrome.

Flowchart 1: Approach to hydronephrosis detected antenatally.

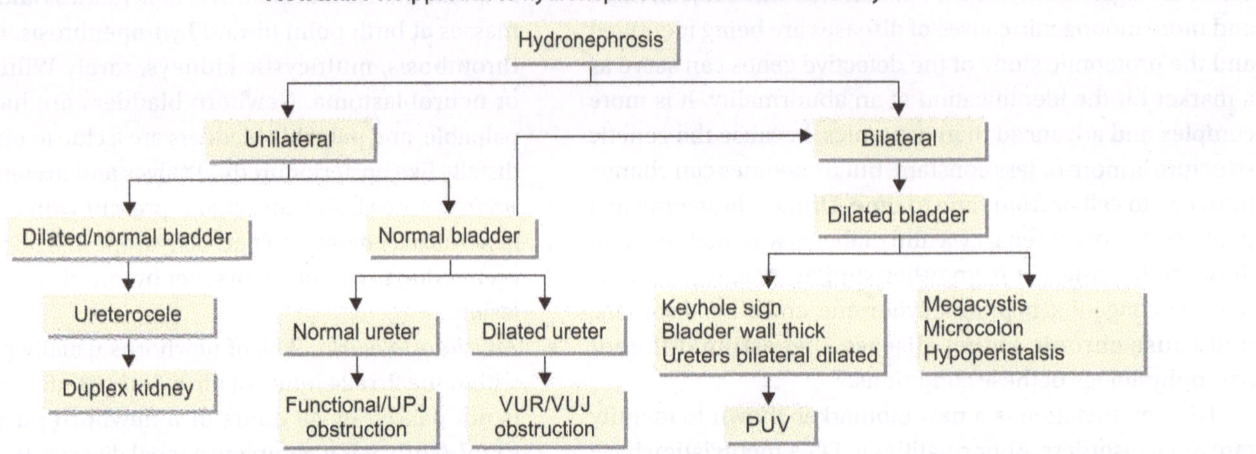

(PUV: posterior urethral valve; UPJ: ureteropelvic junction; VUJ: vesicoureteral junction; VUR: vesicoureteral reflux)

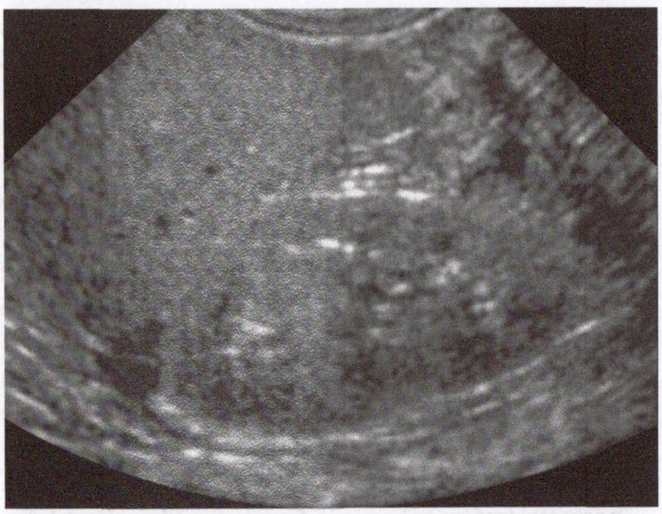

Fig. 4: Severe perinatal asphyxia in a 6-day-old boy. US scan shows increased echogenicity of the renal parenchyma, with loss of corticomedullary differentiation.

- *Metabolic diseases* with renal involvement that can present early include cystinosis (infantile nephropathic variety) and occasionally oxalosis.[21] Neonates can also present with tubular defects associated with storage disorders and mitochondrial cytopathies.
- *Perinatal causes* such as hypoxia, sepsis, hypovolemia, surfactant deficiency, diarrhea, excessive evaporative loss from radiant warmers, severe varieties of congenital heart disease, and patent ductus arteriosus can lead to renal hypoperfusion injury leading to the prerenal or later the intrinsic renal type of acute kidney injury. Obstructive causes, especially posterior urethral valves, can also lead to the postrenal type of acute renal failure in the newborn. Nephrotoxic medications such as nonsteroidal anti-inflammatory agents, aminoglycosides, and vancomycin used on the newborn can also lead to renal ischemia and tubular damage and subsequently renal failure.[22] **Figure 4** shows changes in perinatal hypoxia.
- *Fluid and electrolyte disturbances:* These are also common presentations due to the poor concentrating ability of the kidneys, low glomerular filtration rate (GFR) of the neonatal kidney, and immaturity of the nephrons, especially in low-birth-weight and premature newborns. Hypernatremic dehydration due to excessive evaporative heat loss, especially with use of radiant warmers, is well known. Healthy exclusively breastfed infants can also suffer from hypernatremic dehydration due to inadequate breast milk, which if unnoticed and severe may lead to venous and arterial thrombosis and even renal failure.
- *Neonatal hypertension* is a relatively rare occurrence in normal term newborns. It is more prevalent in neonatal intensive care unit (NICU) graduates who may have renovascular complications of renal arterial thrombosis following umbilical artery catheterization, antenatal steroid administration, acute patent ductus arteriosus, and bronchopulmonary dysplasia. A detailed discussion on this entity is available in the next section of this chapter.

Evaluation of a Newborn with Suspected Renal Disease

A thorough maternal history is of utmost importance. Special points to note include:

- History of the present and past pregnancies—congenital disorders, genetic diseases, maternal sepsis, maternal infections such as cytomegalovirus, and preterm delivery.
- Prenatal screening tests including ultrasound scans, biomarkers, and genetic studies.
- Labor and delivery—gestation, duration of labor, condition of baby at birth, need for resuscitation, need for NICU care, etc.
- Maternal drug history

A detailed physical examination of newborn is of utmost importance in any situation. Special emphasis on screening eyes for coloboma and cataract, ears for malformations and congenital defect, Potter sequence, cardiac and vertebral anomalies, and umbilicus for the presence of two arteries is given as they are often associated with renal problems.

The abdomen is examined thoroughly for any renal lump, palpable bladder, atypical genitalia and male genitalia for hypospadias, tight phimosis, testes number, and position, female for proper urethral and vaginal opening. The anus is examined for correct location and patency. The vertebral column is examined for presence of neural tube defects, sacral dimple, and extremities for poly or syndactyly. Physiological abnormalities, such as fever, anuria, oliguria, proteinuria, leukocyturia, edema, ascites, and respiratory distress, point to a renal disease.

If any of the above signs and symptoms are present, more detailed investigations such as abdominal ultrasound, micturating cystourethrogram (MCU), blood urea, serum creatinine and electrolytes, urine routine, and microscopy are advised. The diagnosis and management of the specific problem would be required for a good prognosis.

CONCLUSION

Newborn kidneys can suffer from a variety of insults, both antenatally and postnatally. Paucity of signs and symptoms can often mask a serious underlying disease. Proper antenatal history, ultrasound scans, and a high index of suspicion are required to diagnose and manage newborn renal disorders promptly and efficiently.

KEY POINTS

- Congenital anomalies of the kidney and urinary tract, CNS, metabolic diseases, genetic tubular diseases, cystic diseases, urinary tract infection, acute kidney injury, and hypertension are the commonly encountered kidney disorders in the newborn.
- Prenatal diagnosis of kidney disease has evolved with time with more precision.
- Specific physical markers of kidney disease should be identified in a neonate at birth to initiate prompt evaluation.

REFERENCES

1. Chan JCM, Williams DM, Roth KS. Kidney failure in infants and children. Pediatr Rev. 2002;23(2):47–60.
2. Airede A, Bello M, Weerasinghe HD. Acute renal failure in the newborn: incidence and outcome. J Paediatr Child Health. 1997;33(3):246-9. [Erratum in: J Paediatr Child Health. 1997; 33(6):550].
3. Misurac J. Chronic kidney disease in the neonate: etiologies, management, and outcomes. Semin Fetal Neonatal Med. 2017;22(2):98-103.
4. Kari JA, Sharief SN, El Desoky SM, Alhasan KA, Albanna AS. Etiology, ethics, and outcomes of chronic kidney disease in neonates. Saudi Med J. 2018;39(4):361-7.
5. Harambat J, van Stralen KJ, Kim JJ, Tizard EJ. Epidemiology of chronic kidney disease in children. Pediatr Nephrol. 2012;27(3):363-73. [Erratum in: Pediatr Nephrol. 2012;27(3): 507].
6. Kleinman LI, Stewart CL, Kaskel FJ. Renal disease in the newborn. In: Edelmann CM Jr (Ed). Pediatric Kidney Disease, 2nd edition. Boston: Little, Brown and Co; 1992. p. 1043.
7. Sinha A, Bagga A, Krishna A, Bajpai M, Srinivas M, Uppal R. Revised guidelines on management of antenatal hydronephrosis. Indian J Nephrol. 2013;23(2):83-97.
8. Fontanella F, Duin LK, Adama van Scheltema PN, Cohen-Overbeek TE, Pajkrt E, Bekker M. Prenatal diagnosis of LUTO: improving diagnostic accuracy. Ultrasound Obstet Gynecol. 2018;52(6):739-43.
9. Talati AN, Webster CM, Vora NL. Prenatal genetic considerations of congenital anomalies of the kidney and urinary tract (CAKUT). Prenat Diagn. 2019;39(9):679-92.
10. Poutamo J, Vanninen R, Partanen K, Kirkinen P. Diagnosing fetal urinary tract abnormalities: benefits of MRI compared to ultrasonography. Acta Obstet Gynecol Scand. 2000;79(1):65-71.
11. Gupta S, Mohi JK, Gambhir P, Mohi MK. Prenatal diagnosis of congenital anomalies of genito-urinary system on fetal magnetic resonance imaging. Egypt J Radiol Nucl Med. 2020; 51:155.
12. DeVore GR. The value of color Doppler sonography in the diagnosis of renal agenesis. J Ultrasound Med. 1995;14(6):443-9.
13. Dragoumi P, O'Callaghan F, Zafeiriou DI. Diagnosis of tuberous sclerosis complex in the fetus. Eur J Paediatr Neurol. 2018;22(6):1027-34.
14. Seppälä M, Rapola J, Huttunen NP, Aula P, Karjalainen O, Ruoslahti E. Congenital nephrotic syndrome: prenatal diagnosis and genetic counseling by estimation of amniotic-fluid and maternal serum alpha-fetoprotein. Lancet. 1976;2(7977):123-5.
15. Glick PL, Harrison MR, Golbus MS, Adzick NS, Filly RA, Callen PW, et al. Management of the fetus with congenital hydronephrosis II: prognostic criteria and selection for treatment. J Pediatr Surg. 1985;20(4):376-87.
16. Crombleholme TM, Harrison MR, Golbus MS, Longaker MT, Langer JC, Callen PW, et al. Fetal intervention in obstructive uropathy: prognostic indicators and efficacy of intervention. Am J Obstet Gynecol. 1990;162(5):1239-44.
17. Ricci P, Magalhães P, Krochmal M, Pejchinovski M, Daina E, Caruso MR, et al. Urinary proteome signature of renal cysts and diabetes syndrome in children. Sci Rep. 2019;9(1):2225.
18. Kerr K, McAneney H, Flanagan C, Maxwell AP, McKnight AJ. Differential methylation as a diagnostic biomarker of rare renal diseases: a systematic review. BMC Nephrol. 20(1):320.
19. Roy RN, Sinclair JC. Hydration of the low birth-weight infant. Clin Perinatol. 1975;2:393.
20. Hindryckx A, De Catte L. Prenatal diagnosis of congenital renal and urinary tract malformations. Facts Views Vis Obgyn. 2011;3(3):165-74.
21. Bäumner S, Weber LT. Nephropathic cystinosis: symptoms, treatment, and perspectives of a systemic disease. Front Pediatr. 2018;6:58.
22. Selewski DT, Charlton JR, Jetton JG, Guillet R, Mhanna MJ, Askenazi DJ, et al. Neonatal acute kidney injury. Pediatrics. 2015;136(2):e463-73.

CHAPTER

5.3

Neonatal Acute Kidney Injury

Hamsa V Reddy, Gurinder Kumar, Arpana A Iyengar

INTRODUCTION

Critically ill neonates are at a risk to develop acute kidney injury (AKI). The challenges of detecting AKI in neonates are related to evolving diagnostic criteria, reflection of maternal creatinine in the first 72 hours of birth, and presence of specific risk factors unique to neonates.[1] Across the spectrum of very low birth weight premature neonates to full-term babies, there exist differences in the physiological range of urine output (UO) as well as in serum creatinine. Single-center studies suggest that neonatal AKI (nAKI) affects 18–70% of critically ill neonates and is associated with poor outcomes.[2-9] The actual incidence of nAKI is likely to be higher than reported, as earlier studies used higher cutoff values of creatinine for diagnosis and frequent nonoliguric presentation. The AWAKEN (Assessment of Worldwide Acute Kidney injury Epidemiology in Neonates) study, a large, multicenter, retrospective study, revealed 30% of AKI in critically ill neonates being an independent risk factor for mortality and increased length of hospital stay.[5] The relevance and importance of nAKI need focus as new-born kidneys are susceptible to hypoperfusion, low glomerular filtration rate (GFR), high renal vascular resistance, high plasma renin activity, decreased intercortical perfusion, and decreased reabsorption of sodium in the proximal tubules. Newborns with congenital diseases (with potential for renal insult during gestation) are bound to have renal maladaptations that differ from those presenting with acute events (after normal fetal development).[6]

DEFINITION AND STAGING OF ACUTE KIDNEY INJURY IN NEONATES

In 2012, the Kidney Disease Improving Global Outcomes (KDIGO) clinical practice guidelines workgroup proposed a criterion for pediatric and adult AKI.[7] In 2012, Jetton and Askenazi proposed a standardized nAKI definition based on the KDIGO definition for adults and children that identifies three levels of severity of AKI based on graded changes in both serum creatinine and UO.[8] A definition only based on UO was proposed by Torres et al., called the neonatal risk injury failure (nRIFLE) criteria, that proposed UO of <1.5 mL/kg/h for 24 hours to be an indicator of AKI. In 2017, Zappitelli et al. proposed the neonatal modified KDIGO definition (mKDIGO) (**Table 1**), wherein UO of <1 mL/kg/h for 24 hours was used to define AKI, instead of <0.5 mL/kg/h. In addition, a lower cutoff value of serum creatinine was used to define stage 3 AKI (2.5 mg/dL instead of 4 mg/dL).[10] There are very few studies that compare the performance of these different available diagnostic criteria. A study comparing nRIFLE with neonatal KDIGO classification found that in sick neonates, the mKDIGO criteria performed better than nRIFLE in detecting AKI with comparable mortality rates. However, nRIFLE diagnosed a higher proportion of neonates with mild AKI compared to KDIGO, suggesting that nRIFLE could probably be useful in detecting mild AKI in situations where repeated sampling for serum creatinine estimation is a constraint.[11]

DIFFICULTIES IN USING THE CURRENT DIAGNOSTIC CRITERIA

The diagnosis of AKI poses challenges as the current diagnosis is based on changes in serum creatinine and UO that vary with gestational age (GA).[8] Both these parameters are late effects of injury and not early markers of the injury itself. Serum creatinine in the first 48 hours of life reflects the maternal serum creatinine in addition to being dependent on the muscle mass. Most neonates have nonoliguric renal failure, making UO an unreliable diagnostic parameter.[12] Unlike children, there are limitations to frequent sampling of neonates leading to under-recognition of AKI.

TABLE 1: Neonatal acute kidney injury KDIGO classification.[10]

Stage	*Serum creatinine (S Cr)*	*Urine output*
0	No change in S Cr or rise <0.3 mg/dL	>1 mL/kg/h
1	S Cr rise ≥0.3 mg/dL within 48 hours or S Cr rise ≥1.5–1.9× reference S Cr* within 7 days	>0.5 mL/kg/h and ≤1 mL/kg/h
2	S Cr rise ≥2–2.9× reference S Cr*	>0.3 mL/kg/h and ≤0.5 mL/kg/h
3	S Cr rise ≥3× reference S Cr* or S Cr ≥2.5 mg/dL or receipt of dialysis	≤0.3 mL/kg/h

*Reference S Cr defined as the lowest previous S Cr value.

RISK FACTORS, ETIOLOGY, AND CLINICAL MANIFESTATIONS

The risk factors for AKI are unique to neonates and constitute both perinatal and postnatal events. nAKI can result from prerenal causes, intrinsic renal disease including vascular insults, and obstructive uropathy.[13] Perinatal risk factors associated with nAKI are outlined in **Table 2.** Neonatal renal dysfunction could result from a preexisting kidney disease as seen with congenital abnormalities of kidney and urinary tract (CAKUT), genetic diseases such as polycystic kidney diseases, and maternal exposure to nephrotoxic agents such as nonsteroidal anti-inflammatory agents and angiotensin-converting enzyme (ACE) inhibitors, depending on the time and duration of exposure. The presence of antenatal hydronephrosis, solitary kidney, renal cysts, and small/large kidneys on prenatal ultrasound gives a clue to underlying CAKUT/cystic renal diseases. Oligohydramnios caused by decreased fetal UO is suggestive of an underlying chronic renal pathology. Neonates with a prenatal onset of renal dysfunction can present with Potter syndrome due to associated oligohydramnios. Potter syndrome may have life-threatening pulmonary insufficiency, flattened nasal bridge, low-set ears, joint contractures, and other orthopedic anomalies.

Similar to older children, acquired causes of AKI in newborns are multifactorial. **Box 1** gives an overview of the causes of nAKI. Neonates with prerenal causes of AKI present with excessive weight loss. They may suffer from poor feeding, lethargy, dehydration, and fever. Newborns with prerenal AKI due to hypoxic/ischemic insults or cortical necrosis are more likely to have oligoanuria. Otherwise, most often, neonates have nonoliguric AKI. Hypernatremic dehydration is an important cause for nAKI as a consequence of inadequate breast-feeding, especially during the summer season.[11]

Neonates with intrinsic AKI present with dyselectrolytemia and acidosis. Hypertension, oliguria, and gross hematuria in a newborn with umbilical vessel catheterization are features of renal vein/arterial thrombosis. Babies with obstructive AKI may present with antenatally detected hydronephrosis, poor urinary stream, thickened palpable bladder, and palpable kidneys with urinoma/urinary ascites.

EVALUATION

Clinical evaluation consists of a directed history and detailed physical examination including evaluation of fluid status. The history is directed toward uncovering risk factors or causes for AKI. The physical examination should include assessment of hydration status (hypovolemia or hypervolemia) and measurement of blood pressure (BP). The neonate should be examined for any weight changes or signs of heart failure. It is important to identify neonates with systemic or pulmonary fluid overload (elevated BP, edema, weight gain, diaphoresis, and tachypnea) as it impacts fluid management.

Laboratory evaluation is not very useful in identifying the etiology of nAKI.[21] Fractional excretion of sodium (FeNa) could be used to differentiate between prerenal AKI and intrinsic disease due to acute tubular necrosis (ATN).

TABLE 2: Risk factors for neonatal acute kidney injury.

Study	*Population*	*Study size*	*Risk factors*
Cataldi et al. (2005)[14]	Premature infants	172	Low Apgar scores, exposure to ampicillin, ceftazidime, ibuprofen
Mathur et al. (2006)[15]	Neonatal sepsis	200	Lower birth weight, meningitis, disseminated intravascular coagulation, and shock
Koralkar et al. (2011)[16]	Very low birth weight infants	229	Lower birth weight, lower gestational age, lower Apgar scores, umbilical artery catheterization, mechanical ventilation, inotrope support
Viswanathan et al. (2012)[17]	Extremely low birth weight infants	472	High mean airway pressures, lower mean arterial pressures, higher exposure to cefotaxime
Selewski et al. (2013)[18]	Asphyxiated neonates undergoing therapeutic hypothermia	96	Asystole at the time of birth, clinical seizures before cooling, persistent pulmonary hypertension, elevated gentamicin or vancomycin levels, pressor support, transfusions
Askenazi et al. (2013)[3]	Birth weight <2,000 g, gestational age <34 weeks, 5-minute Apgar <7	58	Lower birth weight, male, lower Apgar scores at 5 minutes, lower cord pH, mechanical ventilation
AWAKEN Study (2017)[19]	Critically ill neonates	2022	Outborn babies, lower/large gestational age, lower birth weight, lower Apgar scores, prematurity, sepsis, asphyxia, seizures, congenital heart disease, necrotizing enterocolitis, and need for surgical evaluation
Shalaby et al. (2019)[20]	Sick neonates	214	Lower birth weight, lower gestational age, perinatal depression, higher CRIB II score in neonates <32 weeks
Hamsa et al. (2020)[11]	Sick neonates	163	Outborn neonates, very LBW neonates, presence of shock requiring inotropes, neonatal sepsis, need for mechanical ventilation, use of NSAIDs, NEC, hypernatremic dehydration, underlying cardiac or renal anomaly

(CRIB: Clinical Risk Index for Babies; LBW: low birth weight; NEC: necrotizing enterocolitis; NSAID: nonsteroidal anti-inflammatory drug)

BOX 1: Etiology of neonatal acute kidney injury (AKI).

Prerenal causes
- *Decreased true intravascular volume*:
  - Excess insensible losses
  - Poor feeding
  - Dehydration
  - Salt wasting renal or adrenal disease
  - Central or nephrogenic diabetes insipidus
  - Third space losses (sepsis)
- *Decreased effective intravascular volume blood volume*: Congestive heart failure

Intrinsic causes
- *Acute tubular necrosis/acute tubulointerstitial nephritis*:
  - Hypoxic ischemic encephalopathy
  - Nephrotoxic drug exposure
  - Sepsis
  - Pyelonephritis
- *Vascular lesions*:
  - Renal artery thrombosis
  - Renal vein thrombosis
- *Obstructive uropathy*:
  - Posterior urethral valves
  - Prune belly syndrome
- *Renal dysfunction due to preexisting fetal kidney disease*:
  - Congenital abnormalities of kidney and urinary tract—associated with dysplasia/hypoplasia and/or obstruction
  - Cystic renal diseases
  - Maternal factors

Source: Adapted from Andreoli SP. Acute renal failure in the newborn. Semin Perinatol. 2004;28(2):112-23.

TABLE 3: Normal FeNa levels as per gestational age.

Gestational age	*Prerenal AKI (%) FeNa**	*Intrinsic AKI (%) FeNa**
Term infants	<2	>2.5
Preterm >31 weeks GA	<2	>3
Preterm 29–30 weeks GA	<2	>6

$$\text{*FeNa (\%)} = \frac{\text{Urine sodium} \times \text{serum creatinine}}{\text{Serum sodium} \times \text{urine creatinine}} \times 100$$

(AKI: acute kidney injury)

Renal Functions

Serum creatinine is inversely related to body weight and GA. Determination of renal function is also important for fluid management and drug dosing in preterm and term neonates. The GFR is low at birth with a value close to 20 mL/min/1.73 m^2 in term neonates and even lower in premature infants. It improves rapidly after birth, its value doubling within the first 2 weeks of life. This improvement is comparatively at a lower rate in very premature infants.[22] Serum creatinine crosses the placenta resulting in high serum levels at birth, especially for the first 72 hours of life. Thereafter, the values show a steady decline and reach stable levels by 1–2 weeks of age in term neonates. However, preterm infants show higher serum creatinine values at birth compared to term infants coupled with a slower decline over the first 3–4 weeks of life. This observation is most likely due to tubular secretion and creatinine reabsorption by immature tubular cells. In addition, serum creatinine is insensitive to detect mild or moderate reductions in GFR.[23] Most clinical laboratories now align their creatinine measurements against a new standardized isotope dilution mass spectrometry (IDMS) method to measure serum creatinine. The National Kidney Disease Education Program (NKDEP) guidelines recommend that all laboratories convert their systems to use a newer and more accurate method for standardization, called the isotope dilution mass spectrometry.[24] The IDMS does not detect noncreatinine chromogens, resulting in a more accurate but lower serum creatinine value than the conventional assay.

Serum electrolytes (sodium, potassium, chloride), serum bicarbonate, calcium, and phosphorous need to be monitored. In the initial acute phase or in the presence of oliguria, dilutional hyponatremia, hyperkalemia, hyperphosphatemia, hypocalcemia, hypomagnesemia, uremia, and acidosis are fairly common. Hypernatremic dehydration is a well-recognized complication of unrecognized lactational insufficiency in exclusive breastfed babies.

Renal Ultrasound

Prenatal ultrasound is helpful for detecting CAKUT and in other organs. For example, severe bilateral fetal hydronephrosis is indicative of poor kidney function. In males, the most common diagnosis is posterior urethral valves with additional findings of a dilated bladder and posterior urethra. Postrenal AKI may also be associated with severe unilateral hydronephrosis in a solitary kidney.

Postnatal ultrasound: Renal ultrasound is the initial postnatal imaging study undertaken to evaluate all newborns with AKI. It can differentiate AKI from chronic kidney disease by detecting findings (e.g., cysts, hypoplasia) that are consistent with congenital or genetic conditions. Kidney number, size, presence of hydronephrosis, and bladder capacity can be assessed. Doppler studies can allow assessment of renal blood flow and help diagnose occlusion of the major renal vessels (e.g., renal arterial or venous thrombosis).

Urine Analysis

The utility of urine analysis in neonates is limited. The presence of microscopic hematuria, muddy brown granular casts, and epithelial cell casts is highly suggestive of ATN. Leukocyturia could be a clue toward an underlying urinary tract infection. However, the absence of these urinary findings does not preclude the diagnosis. FeNa, though not used commonly in routine practice, can differentiate prerenal from intrinsic AKI. The cutoff values are higher in neonates due to lower renal tubular sodium reabsorption, especially in neonates with GA < 28 weeks. As shown in **Table 3**, FeNa cutoff values increase with decreasing GA, as the threshold for sodium reabsorption decreases with decreasing GA.[25]

Flowchart 1: Algorithm for workup of a neonate with acute kidney injury.

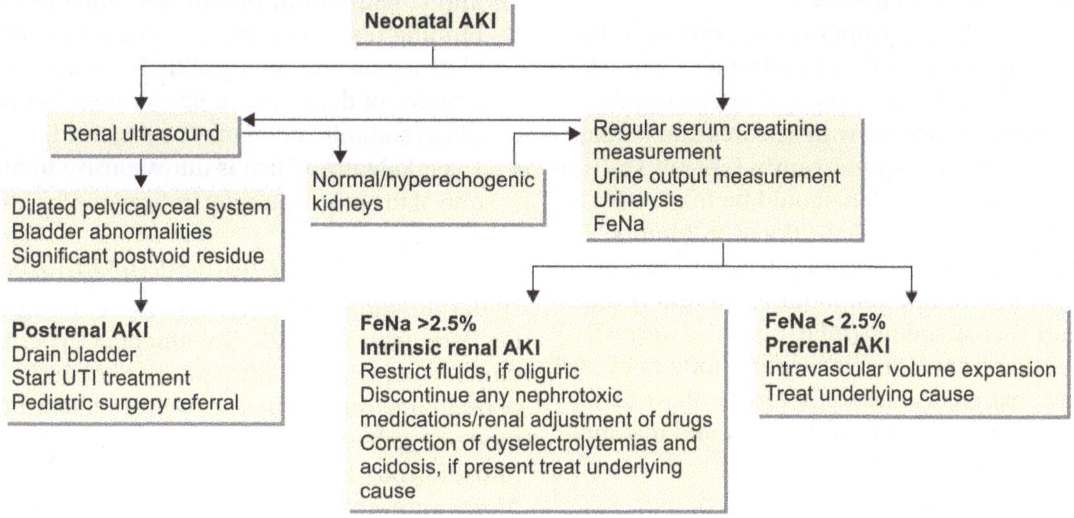

(AKI: acute kidney injury; FeNa: fractional excretion of sodium; UTI: urinary tract infection)

An algorithm for initial workup for a neonate with AKI is summarized in **Flowchart 1**.

MANAGEMENT

The general management of nAKI includes the following:
- Specific treatment of an underlying cause
- Fluid and electrolyte management
- Nutritional support
- Dose adjustment of the drugs as per renal function
- Kidney replacement therapy (KRT)

After the diagnosis of AKI has been established, identifying the cause is extremely important with an aim to detect and revert reversible causes. For example, if an obstruction is identified, it should be promptly relieved by catheterization (urethral or suprapubic), and urological consultation should be sought for further management. Similarly, neonates with volume depletion and AKI should receive prompt fluid resuscitation **(Flowchart 1)**.

Fluid Management

The goal of fluid management is to achieve a euvolemic state. All neonates should be weighed every 12 hours and intake/output should be monitored strictly.[26] In addition, serum sodium may be useful in assessing changes in water balance and readjusting fluid intake. For neonates with prerenal AKI, a fluid challenge may be given which has a diagnostic as well as a therapeutic value. A bolus of isotonic saline 10–20 mL/kg may be given over 1–2 hours and the response assessed. A positive response is any UO in an anuric patient or an increase in UO to ≥1 mL/kg/h in an oliguric baby or improvement in serum creatinine. Continued efforts to achieve and maintain adequate hydration should be made in neonates who respond to fluid challenge by replacing deficits and ongoing losses. However, if there is hypervolemia or clinical signs of fluid overload (heart failure, respiratory distress, or edema), fluids should be restricted to insensible losses plus replacement of UO. The insensible water losses are shown in **Table 4**.

TABLE 4: Insensible water losses in neonates.

Weight of neonate (g)	*Insensible water losses (mL/kg/day)*
<750 g	100–150
750–1,000	60–70
1,000–1,500	20–65
1,500–2,500	20–50
>2,500	20–40

The insensible fluid requirement for infants under radiant warmers rather than incubators may increase by 25–100%.[27,28] During the diuretic phase of intrinsic AKI, fluid requirement increases. In babies with postrenal AKI, relief of obstruction increases UO that warrants close and meticulous monitoring.

Electrolyte Imbalances

Electrolyte abnormalities are commonly encountered in nAKI and are often asymptomatic. Hence, routine monitoring is very important to detect and treat them early.

Hypernatremia

Neonates have increased loss of insensible water, and this is pronounced in low birth weight and premature neonates. Neonates nursed under the radiant heaters and those with faulty breastfeeding during summer months are prone to develop dehydration and hypernatremia. The severity of hypernatremic dehydration, accompanied by high urinary osmolality, may not be evident on physical examination.

Hyponatremia

Hyponatremia is most often due to dilution secondary to water retention; hence, it must be corrected with fluid restriction rather than provision of supplemental sodium. Babies with nonoliguric AKI may have very large urinary sodium losses of up to 10 mmol/kg/day due to immature kidneys or postobstructive diuresis, and these must be replaced either parenterally or through enteral feeds.[29]

In asymptomatic mild hyponatremia (serum sodium 125–135 mEq/L), restriction of fluids will suffice with close monitoring of serum sodium. Serum sodium concentration <125 mEq/L may be associated with seizures and lethargy. In symptomatic severe hyponatremia (serum sodium <120 mEq/L), prompt correction should be made with 3% hypertonic saline in a dose of 5 mL/kg over 2 hours. The amount of sodium needed to correct the hyponatremia can be estimated by the formula: Amount of sodium (mEq) = [desired sodium – actual sodium (mEq/L)] × 0.8 × weight (kg). Care should be taken not to increase serum sodium by >0.5 mEq/L/h.[29] Hyponatremia unresponsive to the above therapy or associated with refractory hyperkalemia and metabolic acidosis are indications for dialysis.[30]

Hyperkalemia

Neonates maintain a net positive potassium balance, which is fundamental to ensure somatic growth but places these infants, especially those born preterm, at risk for life-threatening hyperkalemia.[31] Serum potassium of >6.5 mEq/L is defined as hyperkalemia in neonates. Hyperkalemia (K >7 mEq/L) is one of the most dangerous complications associated with nAKI. An electrocardiogram (ECG) should be immediately taken in the setting of hyperkalemia. Tall, peaked T waves are the first manifestation of cardiotoxicity, followed by prolongation of PR interval, flattening of P waves, and widening of QRS complexes which can subsequently lead to ventricular tachycardia and ventricular fibrillation. Injection calcium gluconate 10% has to be given (0.5–1 mL/kg over 5–10 minutes) under cardiac monitoring to reduce the myocardial excitability. This should immediately be followed by other therapeutic options such as:

- *Glucose and insulin infusion*: 0.5 g/kg of glucose and 0.05–0.1 U/kg of regular insulin over 30 minutes stimulate the cellular uptake of potassium. Close monitoring for hypoglycemia is required while on glucose insulin infusion.
- *Sodium bicarbonate*: This is not routinely indicated for hyperkalemia and should be administered in the presence of metabolic acidosis. 1 mEq/kg IV over 10–30 minutes shifts potassium into cells. [Use 2 mL/kg of 0.5 mEq/mL (4.2%) solution to decrease osmotic load.] Administration of sodium bicarbonate in neonates has been associated with intraventricular hemorrhage (IVH), fluctuations in cerebral blood flow, diminished tissue oxygenation, worsening intracellular acidosis, aggravated myocardial injury, and deterioration of cardiac function.[32]
- *Furosemide*: 1–2 mg/kg IV increases urinary excretion of potassium. Inj. Furosemide should be considered only when the neonate is hemodynamically stable.
- *Cation exchange resin (Na/Ca polystyrene sulfonate)*: 1 g/kg intrarectal q6h. It exchanges sodium for potassium across the colonic mucosa. Each gram of resin can potentially bind up to 0.5–1 mEq of potassium. Sodium polystyrene sulfonate should be used cautiously because of potential complications, including hypernatremia and constipation. In addition, the use of potassium-binding resins in preterm infants has been associated with necrotizing enterocolitis. Because of this reason, the practice of decanting milk with these resins rather than direct administration may be preferred.
- Hyperkalemia, which is unresponsive to medications, is one of the most common indications for instituting KRT.

Calcium and Phosphate Perturbations

Hyperphosphatemia and hypocalcemia may develop in neonates who have AKI. Treatment of hyperphosphatemia consists of dietary phosphate restriction, using low phosphorous milk formulas as well as addition of phosphorous binders, such as calcium carbonate, to the formula to bind phosphorous and decrease gastrointestinal absorption. Aluminum-containing phosphate binders are avoided because of aluminum toxicity. Symptomatic hypocalcemia should be corrected by infusing 10% calcium gluconate at a dose of 0.5–1 mL/kg over 5–10 minutes under cardiac monitoring.[28] Injection is available as 10% calcium gluconate (0.45 mEq Ca^{2+}/mL). The maintenance dose for neonates is 200–800 mg/kg/24 h q6h.

Drug Therapy

The principles of therapy for specific causes of AKI in neonates are described in **Table 5**. Prompt initiation of antibiotics in situations of sepsis or urinary tract infection is mandatory. One should be cautious regarding the use of nephrotoxic drugs (ibuprofen, indomethacin, and diuretics) in the presence of renal failure. All antibiotics, when indicated, need to be adjusted to renal-corrected doses with close monitoring of renal functions. Daily evaluation of medications and participation of the clinical pharmacist are important in a critically ill neonate to monitor the drug levels and hence avoid nephrotoxicity. If the use of nephrotoxic drugs is unavoidable,

TABLE 5: Specific treatment of the underlying cause of acute kidney injury (AKI) in neonates.

Etiology of AKI	*Treatment*
Hypovolemia/prerenal AKI	Fluid resuscitation to restore renal perfusion
Decreased renal perfusion due to critical congenital cardiac defect	Prostaglandin E1 for a ductal-dependent heart lesion followed by corrective surgery
Sepsis	Antibiotics and renal correction if the baby is on nephrotoxic drugs
Perinatal asphyxia	Therapeutic cooling, theophylline, caffeine
Hypoalbuminemia/capillary leak	IV albumin and furosemide for symptomatic neonates
Renal vein thrombosis	Thrombolytic therapy
Obstructive uropathy	Decompression and drainage of urinary tract

a careful inventory of risk factors should be done, which includes GA, prior nephrotoxicity, renal function, severity of illness, volume status, and nephrotoxic medication (NTMx) burden. Care should be taken to optimize the intravascular volume, using minimal effective dose (daily vs. multiple daily aminoglycoside dose), and avoid harmful drug interactions [e.g., simultaneous use of nonsteroidal anti-inflammatory drugs (NSAIDs) and ACE inhibitors]. It is important to monitor kidney function and drug levels regularly for the development and progression of AKI.[33]

Metabolic Acidosis

Acute kidney injury impairs the neonates' ability to regulate acid–base status due to tubular immaturity. The most important intervention for neonatal metabolic acidosis is to treat the underlying cause, and sodium bicarbonate is not used routinely to correct acidosis in preterm neonates as it is associated with IVH, deterioration of cardiac function, myocardial injury, and worsening of intracellular acidosis. Acidosis may be transiently managed by the use of intravenous or oral sodium bicarbonate supplementation. In newborns receiving intravenous fluids or parenteral nutrition, acetate may be favored over chloride to help address metabolic acidosis. Sodium bicarbonate is indicated only if pH is <7.2 or plasma bicarbonate concentration is 12 mEq/L or less. The required bicarbonate dose is calculated as HCO_3 (mEq) = 0.6 × wt (kg) × base deficit (mEq/L). The calculated dose is diluted to a maximum concentration of 0.5 mEq/mL in dextrose or sterile water for injection and infused over 4–6 hours with a maximum rate of 1 mEq/kg/h. Inj. sodium bicarbonate should not be mixed with or be in contact with calcium, norepinephrine, or dobutamine. Babies with persistent metabolic acidosis will require dialysis.[30] It is important to note that treatment of acidosis decreases the amount of ionized calcium. Hence, attention to the serum ionized calcium level is essential to prevent the development of tetany and seizures.

Hypertension

Approximately 10–20% of the neonates with AKI have hypertension secondary to fluid overload, which can be controlled with fluid restriction, furosemide, and/or antihypertensive agents. Neonatal hypertension is defined as systolic BP of at least the 95th percentile for GA, birth weight, and sex on three separate occasions. The development of severe hypertension in the setting of nAKI should raise the suspicion for renal artery or venous thrombosis.

The gold standard for reliable measurement of BP, especially in critically ill neonates, remains invasive arterial BP monitoring through an indwelling radial or umbilical catheter. However, in the absence of other indications for catheter insertion, noninvasive BP monitoring has become the clinical mainstay for diagnosis. Sphygmomanometry is not recommended in neonates because Korotkoff sounds are often barely audible and hence unreliable in neonates. Ultrasonic Doppler can underestimate systolic BP.

Noninvasive BP monitoring is usually performed with automated oscillometric devices, in which pulsatile blood flow sends oscillations to the arterial wall, which are then transmitted to the cuff. The mean arterial pressure measured is then converted through an algorithm to provide projected systolic and diastolic BP values. Although the readings vary slightly from an indwelling catheter, the BP trends are reliable and easily accessed at the bedside. It is important to note that the oscillometric devices are accurate only when used with a proper cuff size; a cuff that is too small gives falsely high BP readings. Of note, BP measurement should be standardized to create uniform results by selection of an appropriate cuff size, minimizing infant activity measurement in the right upper extremity, placement of the infant in the supine position, and timing at least 1.5 hours after feeding or medical intervention.[34]

No definitive normal BP values have been determined for term and preterm neonates because of discrepancies in BP measurement techniques, different definitions of BP used, and variations in neonatal clinical status when measurements were taken. However, for neonates 26–44 weeks' postconception age, useful normative data have been established based on GA, birth weight, and sex.[35]

Nutrition

Neonates with AKI are in a catabolic state, and release of amino acids from increased muscle protein breakdown can further strain on the already limited protein stores of the babies, especially preterm neonates. Instead of utilizing protein for anabolism for growth, the released amino acids are utilized by the liver to synthesize acute-phase proteins. Therefore, nutrition is vital in management of these sick babies to prevent excessive tissue breakdown. If the baby is tolerating oral feeds, breast milk or a special renal formula that has a low renal solute load and phosphorous should be used. Oliguric infants who are on fluid restriction and cannot receive adequate calories should be started on high caloric additives that have low osmolality to provide enough calories. The nutritional intake is targeted to provide a minimum of 100 kcal/kg/day. Term infants with AKI, not receiving KRT, should receive amino acids up to a maximum of 1.5 g/kg/day while a requirement for a preterm is 1.5–2.5 g/kg/day. The protein requirements may need frequent readjustment based on individual need and laboratory data values including electrolytes, acid–base status, and presence of uremia.[36] It should be noted that babies on continuous kidney replacement therapy (CKRT) have higher protein needs due to increased catabolism and amino acid losses across the hemofilters.

Role of Diuretics

Diuretics are commonly used in neonates with AKI to maintain UO. Although studies in critically ill patient populations have not demonstrated a beneficial effect of diuretics on outcomes, a trial of diuretics in oliguric hemodynamically stable newborns with AKI is warranted given the complexity of KRT. Furosemide is a potent loop natriuretic agent commonly used to improve UO in oliguric neonates in the hope of increasing diuresis and improving renal blood flow and GFR by stimulating the production of vasodilator prostaglandins. Use of furosemide should be limited to treating oliguric neonates presenting with edematous states and congestive heart failure. The dose of furosemide in neonates is 0.5 mg/kg/dose given every 8th hour (maximum 2 mg/kg/dose). Prolonged use in premature infants may result in nephrocalcinosis.[37]

Role of Dopamine

Dopamine and dopaminergic agonists (fenoldopam) are not recommended for routine use in AKI with the aim of improving GFR and UO.

Role of Adenosine Antagonists in Preventing Neonatal AKI in Preterm Babies

Methylxanthines (theophylline/aminophylline/caffeine, etc.) are adenosine antagonists that act via A1 and A2A receptors present in the brain, heart, blood vessels, respiratory system, gastrointestinal tract, and kidneys.[38] Recent studies have shown that early administration of caffeine citrate could reduce the risk of AKI in preterm newborns.[39] The researchers analyzed data on a multicenter cohort of 675 preterm neonates enrolled in the AWAKEN study and found that the incidence of AKI was 11.2% in infants treated with caffeine, compared to 31.6% in those not treated with caffeine. Among neonates who developed AKI, caffeine was associated with a lower risk of stage 2 or 3 AKI. Further studies will be needed to identify the optimal timing and dosage of caffeine citrate therapy as well as the effects on long-term renal outcomes.

In neonates with perinatal asphyxia, adenosine receptor antagonists (theophylline) may prevent AKI by inhibiting adenosine-induced vasoconstriction. The KDIGO guidelines recommend a single dose of theophylline for asphyxiated neonates at risk of AKI. Caution is advised as theophylline has potentially harmful neurologic effects. Some of the previous studies and randomized controlled trials (RCTs) have shown a renoprotective role of theophylline and aminophylline in term and preterm neonates with severe birth asphyxia, in children undergoing cardiac surgery, and in preterm neonates with respiratory distress syndrome. A recent systematic review and meta-analysis showed that a single dose of prophylactic theophylline helps in prevention of AKI/severe renal dysfunction in term neonates with severe birth asphyxia.[38]

Role of Therapeutic Hypothermia in Infants with Hypoxic Ischemic Encephalopathy

Neonates with hypoxic-ischemic encephalopathy (HIE) are at a high risk of AKI with several reports of an incidence as high as 40%.[40] Nour et al., studied 34 full-term neonates with HIE and concluded that therapeutic hypothermia was associated with less renal impairment when compared to infants with HIE who were not cooled.[41] Chock et al. further found that aminophylline exposure in neonates cooled for HIE was associated with increased UO and a similar decline in serum creatinine when compared to control infants unexposed to aminophylline.[40]

KIDNEY REPLACEMENT THERAPY

The indications for initiation of KRT in nAKI are given in **Box 2**. The modality used most often to dialyze neonates worldwide is peritoneal dialysis (PD), though hemodialysis (HD) and continuous veno-venous hemodiafiltration (CVVHDF) are other feasible options in the best of centers.

The three different KRT modalities are discussed as follows:

1. *Peritoneal dialysis*: This has traditionally been preferred over hemodialysis in the newborn. The peritoneal catheter (12 Fr) is placed either percutaneously or surgically, after emptying the urinary bladder and creating artificial ascites by instilling the abdomen with 20–30 mL/kg of peritoneal fluid. In resource-limited settings, intercostal drainage tube and suction catheters maybe used. The common sites of insertion are in the midline below umbilicus, above the umbilicus, and the right or left lower quadrant of the abdomen. The PD cycles are initiated after securing the PD catheter by instilling 20–30 mL/kg of dialysis fluid (1.7% dextrose with lactate) over 10 minutes, followed by a dwell period of 20–30 minutes, and the fluid is drained over the next 10–15 minutes. The dwell time/volume may be reduced in case of respiratory compromise. Blood sugar and serum electrolytes must be monitored every 6 hourly and serum creatinine every 24 hourly. If the baby develops hypokalemia, Inj. KCl 1.5–2 mL has to be added to 1 L of dialysate fluid. The contraindications for PD are necrotizing enterocolitis, recent abdominal surgery, abdominal wall defects, local infection, and severe respiratory compromise as it may worsen with abdominal distension. The complications of PD are hyperglycemia, bleeding, perforation of abdominal viscera, peritonitis, adhesion of the catheter tip to the omentum leading to obstruction of the dialysis catheter, leaking dialysate, and inguinal or umbilical hernias.
2. *Hemodialysis*: This is technically challenging in newborns, and hence most of the centers do not have the infrastructure, equipment, and expertise to undertake the procedure. It offers a rapid change in plasma solute composition and rapid removal of excess body water and is not well tolerated in hemodynamically unstable neonates.
3. *Continuous veno-venous hemodiafiltration*: The use of CVVHDF is increasing in newborns. As compared to hemodialysis and PD, CVVHDF has the following benefits:
   - It can be used in states of hemodynamic instability.
   - It allows precise fluid and metabolic control.
   - In babies with sepsis, it enhances the removal of cytokines.

BOX 2: Indications of kidney replacement therapy.

- Severe metabolic acidosis (serum bicarbonate concentration <12 mEq/L), refractory to medical management
- Hyponatremia (serum sodium concentration ≤120 mEq/L)
- Hyperkalemia (refractory to medical management)
- In oligoanuric neonates who require fluid restriction but need nutrition to meet their caloric and metabolic demands
- Volume overload with heart failure, pulmonary edema

The biggest challenge in providing HD and CKRT to newborns is the need for specialized equipment. The equipment should be designed with low circuit volumes running at slow blood flow rates and associated with more precise ultrafiltration scales. A small circuit ultrafiltration machine, Aquadex®, has been adapted to provide continuous veno-venous hemofiltration (CVVH) in neonates. In the past decade, two miniaturized machines—Newcastle Infant Dialysis and Ultrafiltration System (NIDUS®) and Cardio-Renal Pediatric Dialysis Emergency Machine (CARPEDIEM®)—have been developed which can provide KRT to neonates. NIDUS® provides hemodialysis to infants as small as 800 g (range 800 g to 8 kg). CARPEDIEM® (licensed in Italy in 2013) is a pump-driven machine which was designed to provide multiple therapies, including CKRT, to infants 2.5–10 kg in size. It can also provide multiple extracorporeal therapies including CVVH/continuous veno-venous hemodialysis (CVVHD)/CVVHDF, plasma exchange, and blood exchange. Though it requires a double-lumen catheter, it was developed for use with small catheters (4–4.5 Fr). The extracorporeal circuit volume has been reduced to 27 mL excluding the filter which may range in volume from 27.2 to 41.5 mL (three filters available with surface areas of 0.075, 0.15, and 0.25 m^2, respectively). Low blood flow rates ranging from 5 to 50 mL/min can be achieved with excellent accuracy using miniaturized roller pumps, which reportedly cause little microhemolysis. More accurate fluid balance can be achieved by gravimetric control along with improved ultrafiltration (UF) scale sensitivity to 1 g.[42]

SPECIAL CIRCUMSTANCES

Acute Kidney Injury in Neonates Requiring Extracorporeal Membrane Oxygenation

Critically ill neonates who require extracorporeal membrane oxygenation (ECMO) are at a risk for multiple organ failure, including AKI. AKI in these patients is often multifactorial due to an underlying illness as well as from the ECMO itself. The pathophysiology of AKI can be due to altered renal perfusion, systemic inflammation, hypoxic and oxidative injury during ischemia-reperfusion, and NTMx. Further complicating this pathophysiology is the interplay between the kidneys and organs such as the heart and lungs that contribute to multiorgan dysfunction. A significant number of neonates require ECMO after congenital heart surgery and cardiopulmonary bypass (CPB). There is evidence that AKI and fluid overload can be managed effectively on ECMO with KRT, and there is widespread use of KRT on ECMO. KRT can be performed safely and efficiently in neonatal ECMO patients.[43]

AKI Following Cardiac Surgery

Acute kidney injury associated with congenital heart surgery has been well studied. In the majority, AKI occurs in the perioperative period. Intraoperative factors influence the predilection of postoperative AKI as longer bypass times and the use of circulatory arrest are associated with a higher incidence of AKI. Recent studies have demonstrated that earlier use of PD in infants after CPB is associated with a shorter duration of mechanical ventilation and intensive care unit (ICU) stay, less inotropic medication use, and lower mortality.[44,45]

PROGNOSIS

Acute kidney injury increases the risk of mortality and morbidity among neonates. Higher mortality rates and significant morbidity (neurodevelopment impairment and chronic kidney disease) due to AKI are seen in particularly very low birth weight neonates (<1,500 g), perinatal asphyxia, and neonates requiring cardiac surgery and ECMO. In short, the prognosis of AKI in newborn is highly dependent on the etiology of the condition and on GA. Despite appropriate treatment, 25–50% of the newborns with AKI die[46] and long-term problems appear in the survivors.[47] In a multicenter, multinational, observational cohort study on the incidence and outcomes of nAKI (AWAKEN), infants with AKI had higher mortality (9.7%) compared to those without AKI.[19] Long-term follow-up care is required for all neonates with AKI as they are at a risk of chronic kidney disease and hypertension later in life. Though there are a very few studies which have studied the long-term effects of CKD in nAKI survivors, the risk factors associated with progression of AKI are low birth weight, prematurity (by affecting the nephron endowment), and babies with perinatal asphyxia and congenital heart disease (by hypoxia and causing abnormal renal hemodynamics).

Use of Urinary Biomarkers

Efforts to diagnose AKI early will ultimately aid in improving neonatal outcomes. Being cognizant of the limitations of serum creatinine, a search for better AKI biomarkers is ongoing. The most promising biomarkers are cystatin C (Cys C), neutrophil gelatinase-associated lipocalin (NGAL), interleukin-18, and kidney injury molecule-1.

Cys C is a cysteine proteinase inhibitor with a molecular mass of 13 kDa, which is produced in all nucleated cells at a constant rate, with almost complete filtration across the glomerulus, and gets completely reabsorbed and catabolized in the proximal tubule. As Cys C does not cross the placental barrier, it allows for a more accurate reflection of neonatal kidney function. However, available data on the value of Cys C as an AKI biomarker have been inconsistent.[48]

Biomarkers, such as serum Cys C, beta 2-microglobulin (β2-MG), urinary NGAL, and alpha 1-microglobulin (α1-MG), have been found to be useful in detecting AKI in asphyxiated neonates.[49]

Children with congenital heart disease undergoing CPB have been an ideal population for studying AKI because the timing of injury is known, and they do not have an underlying chronic kidney disease. While several urinary biomarkers have been studied, among preterm neonates, urine NGAL is inversely related to both GA and birth weight.[50]

BOX 3: Preventive measures for neonatal acute kidney injury (AKI).

- Serum creatinine should be monitored in high-risk neonates, especially babies with
  - Prematurity with a gestational age (GA) <32 weeks
  - Exposure nephrotoxic medication
  - Critical congenital heart disease
  - Perinatal asphyxia
  - Sepsis
  - Polycythemia
  - Hydrops fetalis
- Efforts should be made to avoid nephrotoxic medications or, if they are absolutely indicated, then levels should be closely monitored
- Adequate management of conditions that result in poor renal perfusion such as systemic hypotension, hypovolemia, PDA, sepsis, and hypoxemia are important in the prevention of established AKI
- Avoid hypovolemia by ensuring balanced fluid and electrolyte intake and output. Appropriate readjustment of fluid intake should be based on the assessment of accurate measurements of intake and output (urinary volume), weight (at least daily), and serum sodium concentration

(PDA: patent ductus arteriosus)

PREVENTION OF ACUTE KIDNEY INJURY

Prevention of AKI in neonates is extremely challenging as they are more vulnerable to AKI than older individuals. This is attributable to the functional and developmental immaturity of the neonatal kidney that affects glomerular filtration and tubular function (e.g., concentrating ability), hemodynamic changes that occur at delivery, and risk of hypovolemia due to large insensible water losses. **Box 3** lists the clinical measures that one could undertake to prevent AKI in neonates.

Nephrotoxic medication exposure is a common cause of AKI in hospitalized children. Successful application of the Nephrotoxic Injury Negated by Just-in-time Action (NINJA) program to multiple pediatric institutions yielded decreased AKI rates. The NINJA program decreased Nephrotoxic medication-associated Acute Kidney Injury (NTMx-AKI) by 62%. NINJA screens all noncritically ill hospitalized patients for high NTMx exposure (over three medications on the same day or an intravenous aminoglycoside over 3 consecutive days) and then recommends obtaining a daily serum creatinine level in exposed patients for the duration of, and 2 days after, exposure ending. Additionally, substitution of equally efficacious but less NTMx for exposed patients starting on the day of exposure is recommended when possible.[51]

CONCLUSION

Neonates are especially vulnerable to the development of AKI which, in turn, is associated with a high mortality. Early identification of babies at risk and prevention of AKI are important strategies to prevent morbidity and mortality among neonates. Close attention to hemodynamic status/fluid and electrolyte balance is critical. Babies requiring KRT should be referred early to centers where expertise are available to manage them.

KEY POINTS

- AKI occurs commonly in neonates and is associated with increased mortality and morbidity.
- Advances in neonatal intensive care have resulted in improved patient survival, but this has not been accompanied by improved outcomes for neonates with AKI.
- Early identification of risk factors for AKI that are unique to the neonate is critical.
- Specific medications and interventions have proved to be effective in the management of AKI in neonates.

REFERENCES

1. Libório AB, Branco KMPC, Torres de Melo Bezerra C. Acute kidney injury in neonates: from urine output to new biomarkers. Biomed Res Int. 2014;2014:1-8.
2. Gadepalli SK, Selewski DT, Drongowski RA, Mychaliska GB. Acute kidney injury in congenital diaphragmatic hernia requiring extracorporeal life support: an insidious problem. J Pediatr Surg. 2011;46:630-5.
3. Askenazi DJ, Koralkar R, Hundley HE, Montesanti A, Patil N, Ambalavanan N. Fluid overload and mortality are associated with acute kidney injury in sick near-term/term neonate. Pediatr Nephrol. 2013;28(4):661-6.
4. Kaur S, Jain S, Saha A, Chawla D, Parmar VR, Basu S, et al. Evaluation of glomerular and tubular renal function in neonates with birth asphyxia. Ann Trop Paediatr. 2011;31(2):129-34.
5. Charlton JR, Boohaker L, Askenazi D, Brophy PD, D'Angio C, Fuloria M, et al. Incidence and risk factors of early onset neonatal AKI. Clin J Am Soc Nephrol. 2019;14(2):184-95.
6. Ricci Z, Ronco C. Neonatal RIFLE. Nephrol Dial Transplant. 2013;28(9):2211-4.
7. KDIGO clinical practice guideline for acute kidney injury. Off J Int Soc Nephrol. 2012;2(1). [online] Available from https://kdigo.org/wp-content/uploads/2017/02/KDIGO_2012_CKD_GL.pdf [Last accessed August, 2021].
8. Jetton JG, Askenazi DJ. Update on acute kidney injury in the neonate. Curr Opin Pediatr. 2012;24(2):191-6.
9. de Melo Bezerra CT, Cunha LCV, Libório AB. Defining reduced urine output in neonatal ICU: importance for mortality and acute kidney injury classification. Nephrol Dial Transplant. 2013;(4):901-9.
10. Zappitelli M, Ambalavanan N, Askenazi DJ, Moxey-Mims MM, Kimmel PL, Star RA, et al. Developing a neonatal acute kidney injury research definition: a report from the NIDDK neonatal AKI workshop. Pediatr Res. 2017;82(4):569-73.
11. Hamsa V, Nesargi SV, Prashantha YN, John MA, Iyengar A, Nesargi SV, et al. Acute kidney injury in sick neonates: a comparative study of diagnostic criteria, assessment of risk factors and outcomes. J Mater Neonatal Med. 2020:1-7.
12. Charlton JR, Guillet R. Neonatal acute kidney injury: diagnosis, exposures, and long-term outcomes. NeoReviews; 2018;19(6):e322-6.
13. Andreoli SP. Acute renal failure in the newborn. Semin Perinatol. 2004;28(2):112-23.
14. Fanni D, Fanos V, Gerosa C, Sanna A, Van Eyken P, Cataldi L. Acute kidney injury in the newborn: the role of the perinatal pathologist. J Pediatr Neonatal Individ Med. 2014;3(2):e030262.
15. Mathur NB, Agarwal HS, Maria A. Acute renal failure in neonatal sepsis. Indian J Pediatr. 2006;73(6):499-502.

16. Koralkar R, Ambalavanan N, Levitan EB, Mcgwin G, Goldstein S, Askenazi D. Acute kidney injury reduces survival in very low birth weight infants. Pediatr Res. 2011;69(4):354-8.
17. Viswanathan S, Manyam B, Azhibekov T, Mhanna MJ. Risk factors associated with acute kidney injury in extremely low birth weight (ELBW) infants. Pediatr Nephrol. 2012;27(2):303-11.
18. Selewski DT, Jordan BK, Askenazi DJ, Dechert RE, Sarkar S. Acute kidney injury in asphyxiated newborns treated with therapeutic hypothermia. J Pediatr. 2013;162(4):725.e1-9.e1.
19. Jetton JG, Boohaker LJ, Sethi SK, Wazir S, Rohatgi S, Soranno DE, et al. Incidence and outcomes of neonatal acute kidney injury (AWAKEN): a multicentre, multinational, observational cohort study. Lancet Child Adolesc Heal. 2017;1(3):184-94.
20. Shalaby MA, Sawan ZA, Nawawi E, Alsaedi S, Al-Wassia H, Kari JA. Incidence, risk factors, and outcome of neonatal acute kidney injury: a prospective cohort study. Pediatr Nephrol. 2018;33(9):1617-24.
21. Nada A, Bonachea EM, Askenazi DJ. Acute kidney injury in the fetus and neonate. Semin Fetal Neonatal Med. 2017;22(2):90-7.
22. Baum M. Neonatal nephrology. Curr Opin Pediatr. 2016;28(2):170-2.
23. Lee JH, Hahn WH, Ahn J, Chang J-Y, Bae C-W. Serum cystatin C during 30 postnatal days is dependent on the postconceptional age in neonates. Pediatr Nephrol. 2013;28:1073-8.
24. National Kidney Disease Education Program. Chronic kidney disease and drug dosing: information for providers. [online] Available from http://www.nkdep.nih.gov/.../CKD_DrugDosing_508.pdf. [Last accessed August, 2021].
25. Gubhaju L, Sutherland MR, Horne RS, Medhurst A, Kent AL, Ramsden A, et al. Assessment of renal functional maturation and injury in preterm neonates during the first month of life. Am J Physiol Renal Physiol. 2014;307(2):F149-58.
26. Pandey V, Kumar D, Vijayaraghavan P, Chaturvedi T, Raina R. Non-dialytic management of acute kidney injury in newborns. J Renal Inj Prev. 2017;6(1):1-11.
27. Bhatia J. Fluid and electrolyte management in the very low birth weight neonate. J Perinatol. 2006;26:S19-21.
28. Oh W. Fluid and electrolyte management of very low birth weight infants. Pediatr Neonatol. 2012;53:329-33.
29. Chua AN, Sarwal MM. Acute renal failure management in the neonate. NeoReviews. 2005;6:e369-e76.
30. Chawla D, Agarwal R, Deorari AK, Paul VK. (2008). Fluid and electrolyte management in term and preterm neonates. AIIMS-NICU Protocols 2008. [online] Available from https://www.ontop-in.org/ontop-pen/Week-8-9/fluid_electrolytes_bablance_150308.pdf [Last accessed August, 2021].
31. Bonilla-Félix M. Potassium regulation in the neonate. Pediatr Nephrol. 2017;32(11):2037-49.
32. Collins A, Sahni R. Uses and misuses of sodium bicarbonate in the neonatal intensive care unit. Semin Fetal Neonatal Med. 2017;22(5):336-41.
33. Hanna MH, Askenazi DJ, Selewski DT. Drug-induced acute kidney injury in neonates. Curr Opin Pediatr. 2016;28(2):180-7.
34. Giri P, Roth P. Neonatal hypertension. Pediatr Rev. 2020;41(6): 307-11.
35. Dionne JM, Abitbol CL, Flynn JT. Hypertension in infancy: diagnosis, management, and outcome. Pediatr Nephrol. 2012;27(1):17-32.
36. Prince A, Viswanathan S, Groh-Wargo S. Nutritional issues surrounding acute kidney injury and chronic kidney disease in newborn infants. J Clin Pediatr Nephrol. 2014;2(1):39.
37. Moghal NE, Shenoy M. Furosemide and acute kidney injury in neonates. Arch Dis Child Fetal Neonatal Ed. 2008;93(4):F313-6.
38. Bhatt GC, Gogia P, Bitzan M, Das RR. Theophylline and aminophylline for prevention of acute kidney injury in neonates and children: a systematic review. Arch Dis Child. 2019;104(7): 670-9.
39. Harer MW, Askenazi DJ, Boohaker LJ, Carmody JB, Griffin RL, Guillet R, et al. Association between early caffeine citrate administration and risk of acute kidney injury in preterm neonates: results from the AWAKEN Study. JAMA Pediatr. 2018;172(6):e180322.
40. Chock VY, Cho SH, Frymoyer A. Aminophylline for renal protection in neonatal hypoxic-ischemic encephalopathy in the era of therapeutic hypothermia. Pediatr Res. 2021;89:974-80.
41. Nour I, Elmaghraby R, Shehata R, El-Refaey A, Aldomiaty H, Mosbah A, et al. Selective head cooling and acute kidney injury in neonates with hypoxic ischemic encephalopathy. J Neonatal Perinatal Med. 2020;13(1):21-30.
42. Ronco C, Garzotto F, Brendolan A, Zanella M, Bellettato M, Vedovato S, et al. Continuous renal replacement therapy in neonates and small infants: development and first-in-human use of a miniaturised machine (CARPEDIEM). Lancet. 2014;383(9931):1807-13.
43. Bridges BC, Selewski DT, Paden ML, Cooper DS, Zappitelli M, Fleming GM, et al. Acute kidney injury in neonates requiring ECMO. NeoReviews 2012;13(7):e428-33.
44. Yuan SM. Acute kidney injury after pediatric cardiac surgery. Pediatr Neonatol. 2019;60(1):3-11.
45. Gist KM, Kwiatkowski DM, Cooper DS. Acute kidney injury in congenital heart disease. Curr Opin Cardiol. 2018;33(1):101-7.
46. Agras PI, Tarcan A, Baskin E, Cengiz N, Gurakan B, Saatci U. Acute renal failure in the neonatal period. Renal Failure. 2004;26:305-9.
47. Abitbol CL, Bauer CR, Montane B, Chandar J, Duara S, Zilleruelo G. Long-term follow-up of extremely low birth weight infants with neonatal renal failure. Pediatr Nephrol. 2003;18:887-93.
48. Gorga SM, Murphy HJ, Selewski DT. An update on neonatal and pediatric acute kidney injury. Curr Pediatr Rep. 2018;6:278-90.
49. Zhang Y, Zhang B, Wang D, Shi W, Zheng A. Evaluation of novel biomarkers for early diagnosis of acute kidney injury in asphyxiated full-term newborns: a case-control study. Med Princ Pract. 2020;29(3):285-91.
50. Marin T, DeRossett B, Bhatia J. Urinary biomarkers to predict neonatal acute kidney injury. J Perinat Neonat Nurs. 2018;32(3):266-74.
51. Goldstein SL, Dahale D, Kirkendall ES, Mottes T, Kaplan H, Muething S, et al. A prospective multi-center quality improvement initiative (NINJA) indicates a reduction in nephrotoxic acute kidney injury in hospitalized children. Kidney Int. 2020;97(3):580-8.

CHAPTER

5.4

Neonatal Hypertension

Gurinder Kumar, Jayati Sengupta

INTRODUCTION

Neonatal hypertension was first described in the late 1970s, and advances in the practice of neonatology have led to an increased awareness of hypertension in modern neonatal intensive care units. Evidence-based guidelines on the management of neonatal hypertension are lacking. It is very important for pediatricians and neonatologists to be aware of normal range of blood pressure (BP) among neonates of different gestational ages, weights, and postnatal ages for a timely correct diagnosis of hypertension.

Hypertension in a neonate is defined as BP of >2 standard deviations above the baseline as per gestational age or systolic BP >95% for infants with similar size and gestational and postnatal age.[1] There is paucity of studies documenting normative BP values in healthy term and preterm neonates in India. Normative neonatal BP values based on gestational age are provided for Indian neonates.[2]

INCIDENCE AND RISK FACTORS

Neonatal hypertension is a relatively rare entity with an incidence ranging from 0.2 to 3%. In full-term newborns the incidence is closer to 0.2%, whereas in critically ill premature neonates, low birth weight, and neonatal intensive care unit (NICU) graduates, the incidence ranges from 1 to 3%.[3] Antenatal steroids, umbilical arterial catheter (UAC) placement, maternal hypertension, postnatal acute renal failure, and chronic lung disease are common conditions in neonates associated with elevated BP.[4]

BLOOD PRESSURE MEASUREMENT IN INFANCY

Measurement of BP in a neonate remains a challenge despite advances in devices for noninvasive measurement. Accurate measurement of BP is essential to correctly diagnose hypertension.

The gold standard for BP measurement is invasive intra-arterial measurement. The commonly used sites for invasive BP monitoring include umbilical artery catheters followed by peripheral radial artery or posterior tibial artery. The major challenge in small preterm neonates to obtain accurate readings is that the artery is prone to spasm after the placement of catheter, and transducer positioning can significantly alter readings if not placed at the heart level.

In clinical practice, noninvasive measurement of BP is more practical by oscillometric devices, which is based on the principle that pulsatile blood flow through a vessel will produce oscillation of the arterial wall which can be transmitted to a BP cuff.

The accuracy of BP measurement can be affected by many factors in neonates such as crying and feeding which can result in elevated BP readings. Hence, standardized protocols for measuring BP are available to ensure accurate recording. The technique for proper BP measurement includes the following:

- Infant should be prone or supine, resting comfortably. It is advisable to take readings when the infant is asleep or in quiet awake state.
- Measure BP >1.5 hours after feeding or a medical procedure.
- Use an appropriate-sized cuff and measure BP in the right arm. The cuff bladder width should be at least 40% of the arm circumference (AC) at a point midway between the olecranon and the acromion, and the bladder length should cover 80–100% of the circumference of the arm at that point. After cuff placement, the infant is left undisturbed for 15 minutes.
- Obtain three BP readings in succession using oscillometric device at a 2-minute interval.[5]

Table 1, which is based on the best available data through 2010 (Dionne et al.), can be used clinically to identify infants with abnormal BP values that may require further evaluation and/or treatment.

ETIOLOGY OF HYPERTENSION IN NEONATES

There are a multitude of potential etiologies of neonatal hypertension **(Box 1)** with the largest percentages of cases caused by catheter-associated thromboembolism, renal parenchymal disease, and chronic lung disease.[6] The common causes of hypertension (HTN) in neonates have been discussed in the following text.

TABLE 1: Neonatal blood pressure centiles.

Postmenstrual age	*50th percentile*	*95th percentile*	*99th percentile*
44 weeks			
SBP	88	105	110
DBP	50	68	73
MAP	63	80	85
42 weeks			
SBP	85	98	102
DBP	50	65	70
MAP	62	76	81
40 weeks			
SBP	80	95	100
DBP	50	65	70
MAP	60	75	80
38 weeks			
SBP	75	90	95
DBP	45	60	65
MAP	55	70	75
36 weeks			
SBP	70	85	90
DBP	40	55	60
MAP	50	65	70
34 weeks			
SBP	68	83	88
DBP	40	55	60
MAP	48	62	69
32 weeks			
SBP	65	80	85
DBP	40	55	60
MAP	48	65	68
30 weeks			
SBP	60	75	80
DBP	38	50	54
MAP	45	58	63
28 weeks			
SBP	55	72	77
DBP	30	50	56
MAP	38	57	63
26 weeks			
SBP	50	70	76
DBP	30	48	53
MAP	38	55	61

(DBP: diastolic blood pressure; MAP: mean arterial pressure; SBP: systolic blood pressure)

Source: Reprinted with permission from Springer Nature: Dionne JM, Abitbol CL, Flynn JT. Hypertension in infancy: diagnosis, management and outcome. Pediatric Nephrol. 2012;27(1):17-32.

BOX 1: Various causes of neonatal hypertension.

Renovascular causes: Thromboembolism, renal artery stenosis, renal venous thrombosis, compression of renal artery, idiopathic arterial calcification, congenital rubella syndrome

Renal parenchymal disease:
- *Congenital:* Polycystic kidney disease, multicystic dysplastic kidney disease, severe renal dysplasia, ureteropelvic junction obstruction, unilateral renal hypoplasia, congenital nephrotic syndrome, renal tubular dysgenesis, ACE inhibitor fetopathy
- *Acquired:* Acute kidney injury, cortical necrosis, interstitial nephritis, hemolytic uremic syndrome, obstruction (stones, tumors)

Endocrine: Congenital adrenal hyperplasia, hyperaldosteronism, hyperthyroidism, pseudohypoaldosteronism type II

Pulmonary: Bronchopulmonary dysplasia, pneumothorax

Cardiovascular system: Coarctation of aorta

Medications
- Dexamethasone, adrenergic agents, vitamin D intoxication, caffeine, theophylline, phenylephrine, pancuronium
- Maternal intake of cocaine, heroin

Tumors: Wilms tumor, mesoblastic nephroma, neuroblastoma, pheochromocytoma

Neurologic: Pain, intracranial hypertension, seizures, subdural hematoma, familial dysautonomia

Miscellaneous: Closure of abdominal wall defect, adrenal hemorrhage, hypercalcemia, extracorporeal membrane oxygenation, birth asphyxia

(ACE: angiotensin-converting enzyme)

Renovascular Causes

One of the unique causes of neonatal hypertension is vascular-associated UAC thrombosis. Several studies have shown that thrombus formation is common in patients with UAC which can embolize into renal parenchyma. Notably, HTN can develop especially in preterm neonates even when actual thrombi are not found in renal arteries, which could be explained by vascular endothelium disruption at the time of catheter placement. Other renovascular causes include renal vein thrombosis (which can present with flank mass, hematuria, and thrombocytopenia), fibromuscular dysplasia, and renal artery stenosis.

Congenital Renal Anomalies

Congenital renal anomalies are the second most common cause of neonatal hypertension and include conditions such as polycystic kidney disease (both autosomal dominant and autosomal recessive). Less frequently, HTN may be seen with unilateral multicystic dysplastic kidneys, possibly due to excess renin production.

Obstructive Uropathy

Hypertension may accompany obstructive uropathy, such as ureteropelvic junction obstruction, which often normalizes after surgical correction but may occasionally persist.

Acquired Renal Parenchymal Diseases

These include conditions such as cortical or acute tubular necrosis which may result in volume overload or high renin levels resulting in hypertension.

Bronchopulmonary Dysplasia

Systemic hypertension is common in infants with bronchopulmonary dysplasia (BPD) indicating the need to closely monitor BP both during NICU stay and after hospital discharge. It is one of the more common associations with neonatal hypertension with an incidence ranging from 5 to >40%. The precise etiology is unknown but likely includes catecholamine excess and decreased pulmonary clearance, upregulation or excess of angiotensin-converting enzyme, exposure to systemic steroids, and altered systemic vascular tone.

Disorders of Endocrine System

Endocrinologic disorders in infancy which can produce hypertension include congenital adrenal hyperplasia with 11-β-hydroxylase or 17-α-hydroxylase deficiency, primary hyperaldosteronism, and hyperthyroidism.

Tumors

Tumors including neuroblastoma, Wilms tumor, and mesoblastic nephroma may produce hypertension due to either production of vasoactive substances such as catecholamines or compression of renal vessels or ureters.

Medications

Maternal cocaine or heroin use can lead to hypertension associated with neonatal abstinence syndrome.

Medications given to infants such as corticosteroids for chronic lung disease, bronchodilators, prolonged uses of pancuronium, and phenylephrine ophthalmic drops can elevate BP.

Neurologic Conditions

Seizures, intracranial hypertension, and pain can all cause hypertension.

It is important to provide adequate analgesia, especially for postoperative patients.

Extracorporeal Membrane Oxygenation-related Hypertension

Extracorporeal membrane oxygenation (ECMO) is one of the primary reasons systemic hypertension is experienced in hospitalized neonates. The pathogenesis is multifactorial and could be due to fluid overload and impaired water and renal sodium handling.

CLINICAL PRESENTATION

The clinical presentation of a neonate with hypertension is most frequently asymptomatic and diagnosed with high BP readings monitored at multiple time points. In rare circumstances, the neonates may present with life-threatening consequences such as heart failure or cardiogenic shock which can result in massive cardiovascular collapse. In a sick neonate, manifestations include feed intolerance, failure to thrive, unexplained tachypnea, lethargy, irritability, apnea, and seizures. These are frequently appreciated in retrospect. It is important to look for unexplained irritability or failure to thrive in babies discharged from nursery as this could be a manifestation of hypertension.

DIAGNOSTIC APPROACH TO HYPERTENSION

In most of newborn babies, the cause of hypertension can be identified by history and physical examination. A focused history includes prenatal history of maternal medications, delivery details for concerns of perinatal asphyxia, neonatal history for any concurrent medical conditions associated with hypertension, medications (current and past), and procedure history (UAC placement).

Physical examination includes a thorough examination to look for any dysmorphic features such as William syndrome and Turner syndrome. One should pay close attention to other vital signs, such as irregular respiratory rate or bradycardia, which could indicate raised intracranial hypertension.

Cardiac examination should focus on features of congestive cardiac failure with four limb BP readings in all four extremities to rule out coarctation of aorta or an aortic thrombus occluding the abdominal or thoracic aorta. Cardiac murmur, four-extremity BP, femoral pulses, and brachiofemoral delay may be important clues to underlying diagnosis of coarctation of aorta. An abdominal examination positive for abdominal distension or mass may be indicative of polycystic kidney disease, obstructive uropathies, or abdominal tumors. The presence of an epigastric bruit or flank mass could be due to renal artery stenosis or ureteropelvic junction obstruction, respectively.

End-organ damage due to hypertension, such as neurologic abnormalities or hypertensive retinopathy, should be looked for.[7]

It is important to assess renal function (blood urea, creatinine, and electrolytes) and quantitative measurement of urine protein, creatinine, and microalbumin as an evidence of renal parenchymal injury. Other diagnostic tests such as cortisol, aldosterone, or thyroxine levels should be done based on the pertinent history. Measurement of plasma renin activity may be deferred unless other electrolyte abnormalities such as persistent hypokalemia are rarely seen (suggesting a monogenic form of hypertension).

This is because of the following reasons:

- Plasma renin concentrations are high in infancy, especially in preterm neonates with direct correlations with gestational age.

- Disease conditions which are typically considered high renin states such as renal artery stenosis and thromboembolism may not show elevated peripheral plasma renin activity in neonates.
- Plasma renin activity may be falsely elevated by medications such as caffeine, methylxanthines, and aminophylline.
- Plasma renin activity may be suppressed in neonates with pulmonary disease.[4]

Most hypertensive babies would require one or more imaging to determine the etiology of hypertension. The initial relatively inexpensive, noninvasive imaging modality of choice is renal ultrasound with Doppler evaluation. This may help to identify anatomic renal abnormalities or congenital renal diseases such as renal masses, renal cystic disease, and obstructive uropathies.

Renal Doppler flow studies are helpful to diagnose renal vessel thrombosis.

Babies with severe hypertension may require an angiogram to accurately diagnose renal artery stenosis, although this is technically challenging in neonates. Many centers unfortunately lack the expertise and equipment to perform this procedure in newborns.

It should be noted that CT or MR angiography should not be ordered as it will not detect branch stenosis in neonates. Due to the above reasons, it may be more appropriate to control hypertension medically till the baby is large enough for an arteriogram for definitive diagnosis and endovascular treatment.

Specific imaging studies such as micturating cystourethrogram (if suspicion for urinary tract malformation), nuclear medicine scans such as diethylenetriamine pentaacetate (DTPA), and mercaptoacetyltriglycine (MAG3; to detect perfusion abnormalities) in arterial infarction can be done if indicated.

Echocardiography may be helpful to evaluate coarctation of aorta and features of end-organ damage (hypertensive cardiomyopathy manifesting as left ventricular hypertrophy, dilation, and/or dysfunction).[8]

The list of investigations which may be required to investigate a hypertensive neonate is summarized in **Box 2**.

BOX 2: Diagnostic testing in neonatal hypertension.

Routine studies
- CBC/platelet count
- Electrolytes, BUN, creatinine
- Calcium
- Urine analysis and urine albumin/creatinine ratio

Imaging
- Chest X-ray
- Renal ultrasound with Doppler
- Echocardiogram
- VCUG
- Arteriogram
- Renal angiography
- Nuclear scan (DTPA/Mag-3)

Additional studies if indicated
- Thyroid studies
- Urine VMA/HVA
- Aldosterone
- Cortisol
- Plasma renin activity

(BUN: blood urea nitrogen; CBC: complete blood count; DTPA: diethylenetriamine pentaacetate; HVA: homovanillic acid; VCUG: voiding cystourethrography; VMA: vanillylmandelic acid)

TREATMENT

Treatment of hypertension in neonates should be individualized depending on severity and etiology.

Reversible and treatable factors which contribute to hypertension should be addressed such as management of fluid overload, hypercalcemia, adjusting inotrope medication, or reducing dosage of steroids.[9] Treatment of pain in postoperative patients, correction of hypoxemia in babies with BPD, and hormonal replacement in babies with endocrine disorder could alleviate hypertension.

The initiation of treatment should be guided by a pediatric nephrologist in conjunction with a neonatologist.

Treatment depends on three main factors including BP percentile for postmenstrual age, clinical status, and evidence of end-organ damage. As per the recent update to the fourth report on BP management in children, treatment of BP to below the 90th centile is recommended.

Before initiating pharmacotherapy, few specific situations require special mention:
- Treat the intracranial hypertension first prior to treating BP.
- Patients with intermittent severely elevated BPs should be investigated for moving clot (with detailed renovascular imaging) and pheochromocytoma [urine vanillylmandelic acid (VMA) and homovanillic acid (HVA)].
- Obtain aldosterone and renin levels prior to initiating therapy if the etiology of hypertension is not confirmed as the levels may get altered after initiating treatment.

Initiation of antihypertensive medications depends on the clinical expertise as data on the treatment of HTN in neonates are limited. The clinical criteria for initiating therapy are not well defined. There is lack of robust normative data on BP thresholds at which treatment needs to be initiated. **Table 2** summarizes the doses of medications including their side effects in the acute and chronic management of neonatal hypertension.[3,4,6,7]

An infant with acute severe hypertension, defined as hypertension with evidence of end-organ dysfunction, needs intravenous infusions of antihypertensives. Oral agents may not be helpful due to their variable duration of effect, onset of action, and an unpredictable response.

On the contrary, continuous IV infusions can be quickly titrated as per the response to achieve BP control. Care should be taken to avoid rapid reduction of BP which may result in

TABLE 2: Recommended doses for selected antihypertensive agents for treatment of a hypertensive infant.

Class	Drug	Route	Dose	Interval	Comment
ACE inhibitor	Captopril	Oral	<3 months 0.01–0.5 mg/kg/dose (max 2 mg/kg/day) >3 months: 0.15–0.3 mg/kg/dose (max 6 mg/kg/day)	Three times daily	• First dose may cause rapid drop in BP (especially if the baby is on diuretics) • Monitor creatinine and K
	Enalapril	Oral	0.08–0.6 mg/kg/day	Once daily to BID	
	Lisinopril	Oral	0.07–0.6 mg/kg/day	Once daily	
Alpha- and beta-antagonist	Labetalol	Oral	0.5–1 mg/kg/dose (max 10 mg/kg/day)		
		IV	0.2–1 mg/kg/dose 0.25–3 mg/kg/h	Q4–6h Infusion	Caution in chronic lung disease; heart block, unstable heart failure, and neurological injury
	Carvedilol	Oral	0.1 mg/kg/dose up to 0.5 mg/kg/dose	Twice daily	Useful in heart failure
Beta-antagonist	Esmolol	IV	100–500 µg/kg/min	Infusion	Ultra-short-acting needs constant infusion. Caution in chronic lung disease; heart block and unstable heart failure
	Propranolol	Oral	0.5–1 mg/kg/dose (max 8–10 mg/kg/day)	TID	• Monitor heart rate; avoid in BPD • Monitor glucose
Calcium channel blockers	Amlodipine	Oral	0.05–0.3 mg/kg/dose (max 0.6 mg/kg/day)	OD-BID	Reflex tachycardia
	Isradipine	Oral	0.05–0.15 mg/kg/dose (max 0.8 mg/kg/day)	QID	Caution with QTc prolongation
	Nicardipine	IV	0.5–4 µg/kg/min	Infusion	Caution in perinatal asphyxia; prefer central line
Central alpha-antagonist	Clonidine	Oral	5–10 µg/kg/day (max 25 µg/kg/day)	TID	May cause mild sedation, rebound hypertension, and xerostomia
Diuretics	Chlorothiazide	Oral	5–15 mg/kg/dose	BID	Monitor electrolytes
	Hydrochlorothiazide	Oral	1–3 mg/kg/dose	OD	Useful in BPD
	Spironolactone	Oral	0.5–1.5 mg/kg/dose	BID	
Vasodilators	Hydralazine	Oral	0.25–1 mg/kg/dose (max 7.5 mg/kg/day)	TID-QID	• Side effects include tachycardia and fluid retention • Rare granulocytosis
		IV	0.15–0.6 mg/kg/dose	Q4h	
	Minoxidil	Oral	0.1–0.2 mg/kg/dose	BID-TID	Tachycardia and fluid retention are common side effects; prolonged use causes hypertrichosis. Pericardial effusion may occur
	Sodium nitroprusside	IV	0.5–10 µg/kg/min	Infusion	• Beware of thiocyanate toxicity with prolonged use (>72 h) or in kidney disease • Caution in hepatic failure

(ACE: angiotensin-converting enzyme; BP: blood pressure; BPD: bronchopulmonary dysplasia)

cerebral ischemia and hemorrhage, especially in preterm babies who are already at risk of due to immaturity of their periventricular circulation. Ideally, the BP should be reduced by one third of planned reduction over the first 6 hours, the next one third over following 24-36 hours, and the final third over the following 48-72 hours.[10] Published reports suggest that calcium channel blocker nicardipine may be particularly useful in babies with severe acute hypertension. Other drugs include nitroprusside, esmolol, and labetalol. Intermittently administered intravenous agents such as hydralazine and labetalol may be used in neonates with mild-to-moderate HTN who cannot tolerate oral therapy due to gastrointestinal (GI) intolerance.

Neonates with less severe hypertension or chronic HTN controlled with IV medications can transition to oral antihypertensives.

Common oral antihypertensives include the following:

- Calcium channel blockers such as is radipine or amlodipine
- Vasodilators including hydralazine and minoxidil
- Diuretics may be used in babies with BPD.
- Beta-blockers should be avoided in babies with chronic lung disease.

Use of angiotensin-converting enzyme (ACE) inhibitors is controversial. Captopril may cause an exaggerated fall in BP in preterm, hyperkalemia, acute kidney injury, and severe hypotension due to renin–angiotensin–aldosterone system (RAAS) activation in neonates.

Infants with urinary tract obstruction, renal artery stenosis, Wilms tumor, neuroblastoma, and coarctation of aorta are most likely to require surgical intervention. Although most cases of renal thrombosis (arterial or venous) are managed medically, they may require surgical intervention. Very rarely, removal of multicystic dysplastic kidney or bilateral nephrectomy in autosomal recessive polycystic kidney (malignant or resistant HTN) may be required to control BP.[11]

OUTCOMES

The outcome of neonatal hypertension depends on the etiology and severity of the condition. For instance, hypertension associated with renal venous thrombosis, umbilical catheterization, or acute renal tubular necrosis is transient and resolve as the underlying disorder ameliorates. However, the presence of end-organ damage is associated with poor prognosis. Most newborns generally require drug therapy for a short period.[12] Long-term therapy is needed in conditions such as HTN secondary to polycystic kidney disease which persists beyond infancy. HTN may persist in children despite vascular repair in children with renal vessel thrombosis as well as aortic coarctation. They are also at a risk of re-stenosis.

Long-term monitoring of the babies with neonatal HTN is essential till HTN resolves. Serial ultrasound may be helpful to follow renal growth parameters or progression of renal parenchymal disease.

It is important to follow-up BP of preterm neonates and growth restriction neonates. Although nephrogenesis is completed at 36 weeks of gestation, it may continue in preterm babies for up to 40 days following birth. These nephrons are abnormal and age at an accelerated rate. Hence, reduced nephron mass is a risk factor for the development of adult HTN.

CONCLUSION

Maintaining normal BP in neonates depends on multiple factors such as gestational age, birth weight, postmenstrual age, and maternal health. HTN is frequently observed in neonates undergoing UAC placement or with underlying diseases such as BPD and renal parenchymal disease. The diagnosis of hypertension poses a big challenge due to difficulties in measuring BP in neonates. Treatment should be guided by the severity of hypertension. Data pertaining to pharmacokinetics and pharmacodynamics of antihypertensive drugs in newborns need further study.

KEY POINTS

- Determination of BP in neonates is challenging. The gold standard of BP measurement is intra-arterial measurement, but the common method used is the oscillometric method.
- Neonatal hypertension is most commonly a consequence of renal or aortic artery thrombosis following umbilical artery catheterization.
- Neonatal hypertension is defined as systolic BP of at least the greater 95th percentile for gestational age, birthweight, and gender on three separate occasions.
- Treatment of hypertension should be tailored to the severity of hypertension and may include oral or intravenous therapy. Care should be taken not to drop BP too quickly in hypertensive neonates as cerebral perfusion pressure will be adversely affected.

REFERENCES

1. Sharma D, Farahbakhsh N, Shari S, Sharma P. Neonatal hypertension. J Matern Fetal Neonatal Med. 2017;30(5):540-50.
2. Samanta M, Mondal R, Ray S, Sabui T, Hazra A, Kundu C, et al. Normative blood pressure data for Indian neonates. Indian Pediatr. 2015;52(8):669-73.
3. Harer MW, Kent AL. Neonatal hypertension: an educational review. Pediatr Nephrol. 2019;34(6):1009-18.
4. Dionne JM, Abitbol CL, Flynn JT. Hypertension in infancy: diagnosis, management and outcome. Pediatr Nephrol. 2012;27(1):17-32.
5. Nwankwo MU, Lorenz JM, Gardiner JC. A standard protocol for blood pressure measurement in the newborn. Pediatrics. 1997;99(6):E10.
6. Starr MC, Flynn JT. Neonatal hypertension: cases, causes, and clinical approach. Pediatr Nephrol. 2019;34(5):787-99.
7. Flynn JT. The hypertensive neonate. Semin Fetal Neonatal Med. 2020;25(5):101138.
8. Sharma D, Farahbakhsh N, Shastri S, Sharma P. Neonatal hypertension. J Matern Fetal Neonatal Med. 2017;30(5):540-50.
9. Mistry K, Gupta C. Neonatal hypertension. NeoReviews 2017;18(6):e357-71.
10. Dionne JM, Flynn JT. Management of severe hypertension in the newborn. Arch Dis Child. 2017;102(12):1176-9.
11. Batisky DL. Neonatal hypertension. Clin Perinatol. 2014;41(3): 529-42.
12. Nickavar A, Assadi F. Managing hypertension in the newborn infants. Int J Prev Med. 2014;5(Suppl 1):S39-43.

SECTION

6

Glomerular Diseases

CHAPTER

6.1

Podocytopathy: Spectrum and Pathogenesis

Anil Vasudevan

INTRODUCTION

Podocyte or the visceral epithelial cell is a key component of the glomerular filtration barrier (GFB). Podocytopathy is a group of kidney diseases in which podocyte injury is the only or a major cause of the disease. They are characterized by massive selective proteinuria and edema manifesting as nephrotic syndrome or as massive proteinuria with or without renal dysfunction. Development of powerful new animal, cellular, molecular, and newer imaging tools has facilitated enormous progress in our understanding of podocyte in health and disease. A variety of genetic and nongenetic causes such as immune-related, infection-related, toxic and hemodynamic factors, and obesity lead to podocytopathy in children and form the basis of newer classification of podocytopathy. The knowledge of podocyte biology and the underlying mechanisms of podocyte disease is helping in discovering targeted therapy, many of which are being tested in clinical trials.

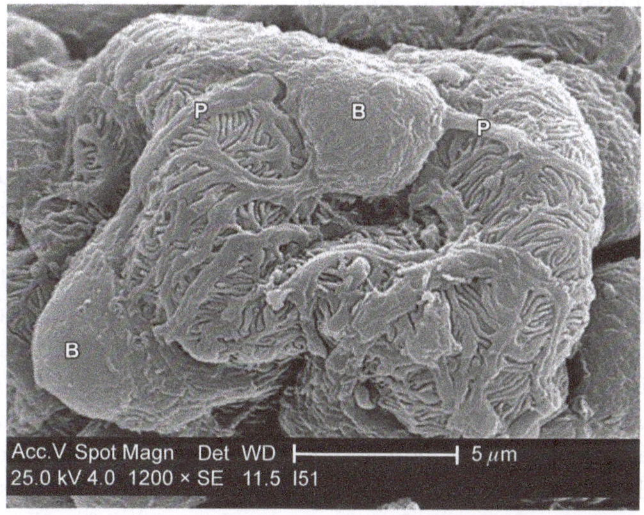

Fig. 1: Podocyte structure. Scanning electron micrograph illustrating the structure of podocytes. It completely covers the external side of the glomerular capillary. From the cell body (B) primary processes (P) grow further arborizing into tiny ramifications that intertwine with processes coming from neighboring cells to form the slit diaphragm. *Source:* Armelloni S, Corbelli A, Giardino L, Li M, Ikehata M, Mattinzoli D, et al. Podocytes: recent biomolecular developments. Biomol Concepts. 2014;5(4):319-30.

STRUCTURE, DEVELOPMENT, AND FUNCTION OF PODOCYTES

Structure of Podocytes

The filtration barrier includes three layers—glomerular epithelium, glomerular basement membrane (GBM), and podocytes which are "octopus-like" terminally differentiated epithelial cells.[1] Podocytes form the visceral layer of Bowman's capsule separating capillary blood from the nephron tubular system. A fully differentiated podocyte has a complex cellular organization consisting of a cell body, major extending processes, and foot processes **(Fig. 1)**. Slit diaphragms, which span the 200-nm gap between adjacent foot processes, serve as an ~60-kDa size-selective filter and is the final barrier in preventing the passage of proteins into the urinary filtrate. Injury to this region has been implicated in the initiation and progression of various podocytopathy.

The podocyte has two domains: (1) apical or luminal domain located above slit diaphragm and (2) a completely embedded part in GBM known as basolateral or abluminal domain. Podocytes exhibit a unique cytoskeletal architecture with the constitution of cytoskeletal elements of cell body, major or primary processes, and foot processes being composed of different proteins. The thick primary processes contain microtubules (MTs) which are tube-like polymers of α- and β-tubulin as well as vimentin intermediate filaments. The foot processes contain actin filaments (AFs) composed of actin monomers (G-actin) exhibiting different actin-based structures—broad membrane protrusions called lamellipodia and long, thin, sharp structures called filopodia.[2,3] Cell bodies and primary processes are devoid of AFs. Actin cytoskeleton and MT dynamics are needed for polarization, podocyte motility, and interaction with adjacent foot processes, all of which help maintain podocyte structure and function. Basal surface of podocyte anchors to underlying basement membrane by several receptors and proteins, including integrins (an essential adhesion molecule; αVβ3 and α3β1), syndecans, tetraspanins, dystroglycan, and focal adhesion complex (FAC). FACs are formed by a complex array of adaptor and linker molecules, interacting with integrin-based adhesion sites.[4] FAC not only anchors podocytes to the underlying GBM or extracellular matrix (ECM) but also serves as signaling hubs by integrating physical and biologic signals termed outside-in/inside-out signaling. Thus, a variety of cellular functions ranging from cell migration to metabolism are influenced and also facilitate the movement of these processes over the GBM.[5]

Embryology of Podocyte Development (Figs. 2A to D)

Podocyte development is a stepwise process with these cells being first visible at the S-shaped body stage as a layer of cuboidal cells beneath the vascular cleft.[6] The differentiation of visceral epithelial cells into podocytes begins in a segmental fashion. In the early stage of development, podocytes are connected by apical junctions with no cytoplasmic branching. The primitive podocytes are flat and are in close contact, without clear boundaries in the S stage of glomerular development. The cells begin to establish their characteristic shape and complex cell architecture once they enter the capillary loop stage wherein there is separation of the cell bodies and development of cytoplasmic processes. The cells become spherical, with gradual separation of cells. The cuboidal cell flattens and acquires cytoplasmic buds on the cell margin of podocyte bases. The buds gradually elongate and grow to form the thick primary processes and then further arborize to form the secondary foot processes, which interdigitate with each other on the surface of capillary loops. The insertion of thick processes under the cell body of podocytes results in separation of cell body from GBM and formation of the subpodocyte space. Foot processes derived from adjacent podocytes form complex interdigitations with adjacent foot processes from neighboring podocytes to develop specialized cell junctions—the slit diaphragms. At this stage, the podocytes permanently stop their mitotic activity and exit the cell proliferation cycle to become terminally differentiated cells which no longer express the proliferation marker.

Molecular Players in Podocyte Development and Function

The molecular signaling and regulation by which glomerular podocyte differentiation occurs remain unclear and is a subject of continued research. Master regulatory genes include *PAX2*, *LMX1B*, and *WT1*.[7] PAX2 is an important regulatory protein that induces cellular proliferation and is also antiapoptotic. The cessation of expression of PAX2 in podocytes results in their definitive loss of ability to divide. WT1, a key transcription factor, begins expression in the undifferentiated blastema followed by increased expression in the condensed blastema, renal vesicles, and S-shaped body stage. Later during podocyte development, it is restricted to mature podocytes and plays a key role in maintaining normal function of podocyte throughout life. WT1 downregulates PAX2 which prevents proliferation leading to WT1-controlled terminal differentiation of podocytes.[8] The formation of MT-based processes and that of AFs-based processes are closely related to Rho family small GTPases (RAC1, RhoA, cdc42, etc.) regulating various events in cells, including process formation.[9] RAC1 activity plays a crucial role in the formation of a branched actin network as present in the lamellipodia, while RhoA is involved in actin polymerization and the formation of actin bundles. Stability of foot processes is represented by a stationary phenotype, whereas their instability corresponds to a motile phenotype. A fine balance between active RAC1 and active RhoA helps to maintain normal foot process morphology and function.[10]

The terminally differentiated podocytes express podocyte-specific proteins that include podocalyxin and glomerular epithelial protein-1 (GLEPP-1) on the luminal membranes; nephrin, podocin, and CD2-AP associated with slit diaphragms and TRPC6, synaptopodin, and actinin-4 in association with cytoplasmic cytoskeleton.[11] Slit diaphragms are specialized intercellular junctions that bridge adjacent foot processes. They are made up of special proteins which play an important

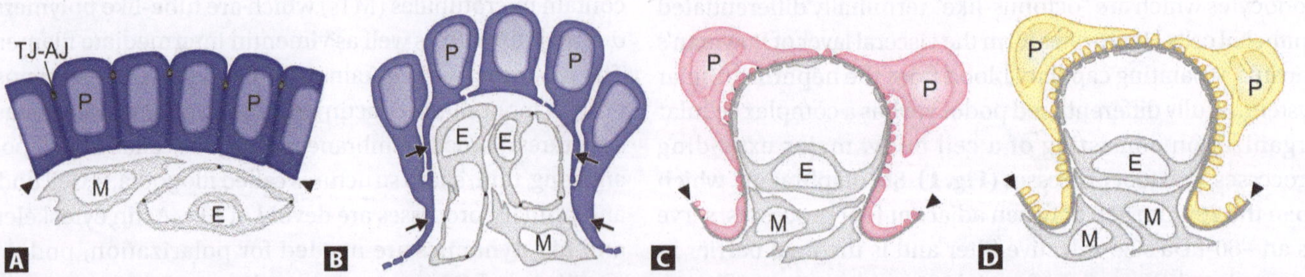

Figs. 2A to D: Schematic development of podocyte. (A) S-shaped body stage. Podocytes form a simple columnar epithelium. Primitive glomerular capillaries and mesangial cells are already detected beneath the glomerular basement membrane (GBM); (B) Capillary loop stage. Primitive glomerular capillaries and mesangium have developed and invaginated into the epithelial layer formed by podocytes and GBM. The lateral surface of capillary walls is covered with the tongue-like portion of the podocyte cell body (arrows); (C) Maturing glomerulus stage. The intercellular space between podocyte cell bodies widen. As a result, the glomerular wall is covered by the immature primary and foot processes; (D) Mature stage. Podocytes cover the urinary surface of the GBM mainly with their numerous mature foot processes. (E: glomerular endothelial cell; M: mesangial cell; P: podocyte). Arrowheads denote GBM.

Source: Hanlon CD, Andrew DJ. Outside-in signaling—a brief review of GPCR signaling with a focus on the *Drosophila* GPCR family. J Cell Sci. 2015;128(19):3533-42.

role in filtration, sensing, and signaling functions of the podocyte. Protein complexes formed by phosphorylation of nephrin and internalization via adaptor proteins such as Nck1/2, Grb2, and Crk1/2 regulate actin polymerization and are an event needed for podocyte foot process development and maintenance.[12]

CD2AP is a scaffold protein functioning as a multifunctional adaptor molecule that interacts with nephrin and podocin. CD2AP modulates cytoskeletal dynamics through actin nucleation-promoting factors as well as links actin assembly to formation of podocyte slit diaphragm.[13] Podocalyxin is a sialoglycoprotein which imparts negative charge to the filtration barrier and plays a critical role in the formation and maintenance of the characteristic cellular architecture of podocytes.[14] The negative charge helps to keep foot processes apart from each other and prevents attachment of podocytes to the parietal epithelium of Bowman's capsule. The Ca^{2+}-permeable channel TRPC6 has a broad role in chemosensation and mechanosensation that helps podocytes sense changes in the external environment, such as alterations in pressure and filtration rate leading to remodeling of cytoskeleton and contraction of foot processes.[15] Podocytes also contribute to the maintenance of filtration barrier by expression of vascular endothelial growth factor-A (VEGF-A), which is necessary for the maintenance of the glomerular endothelium and also by expression of angiopoietins (specifically Ang1).[16]

Functions of Podocytes

Apart from its key role in the maintenance of glomerular permselectivity, podocytes are also involved in regulation of glomerular filtration, GBM-turnover, support of the capillary tuft, endocytosis of filtered proteins, and immunobiological functions. Podocyte function depends on (1) the slit diaphragm complex, (2) the actin-based cytoskeleton, (3) and interactions with other components of GBM to which podocytes adhere. Podocytes help in the synthesis of extracellular matrix proteins which are components of basement membranes such as type IV collagen, heparan sulfate proteoglycan, fibronectin, and laminin. Podocytes also clear materials that may deposit in the GBM. Podocytes play an important role in providing structural support to the glomerular tuft and protect the capillary tuft by counterbalancing the expanding forces exerted on the capillary wall by the transmural pressure gradient tuft. Podocytes also play an active role in immune response as evidenced by localization and isolation of CD80, complement receptor 1 (CR1), and toll-like receptors (TLRs).

ETIOLOGY AND CLASSIFICATION OF PODOCYTOPATHY

Etiology

Depending on the stage of podocyte development and associated genetic or environmental factors (immune mediated, infectious, metabolic, obesity, toxins), podocyte injury or loss can result in a broad spectrum of clinical diseases **(Box 1 and Fig. 3)**.

BOX 1: Etiology of podocytopathy.

Idiopathic

Genetic:
- *Syndromic* (e.g., Denys–Drash syndrome, Galloway-Mowat syndrome)
- *Nonsyndromic* (NPHS1, NPHS2, PLCe1, CD2AP)

Immunological:
- IgA nephropathy
- Systemic lupus erythematosus
- Membranous nephropathy—antibody to PLAR2, thrombospondin

Adaptive:
- Reduced nephron mass—dysplasia, reflux nephropathy, surgical reduction, low birth weight
- Normal nephron mass—obesity, hypertension, sickle cell anemia, CCHD

Infections:
- Hepatitis B, hepatitis C, HIV
- CMV, parvovirus 19, syphilis

Medications:

Pamidronate, IFN-α, β, NSAID, lithium, penicillamine, gold

Metabolic:
- Diabetes mellitus
- Metabolic storage disease (e.g., α-galactosidase deficiency in Fabry disease)

Others:
- Light chain and amyloid A amyloidosis
- Monoclonal gammopathies
- Fibrillary glomerulonephritis

(CCHD: critical congenital heart disease; CMV: cytomegalovirus; HIV: human immunodeficiency virus; IFN: interferon; IgA: immunoglobulin A; NSAID: nonsteroidal anti-inflammatory drug)

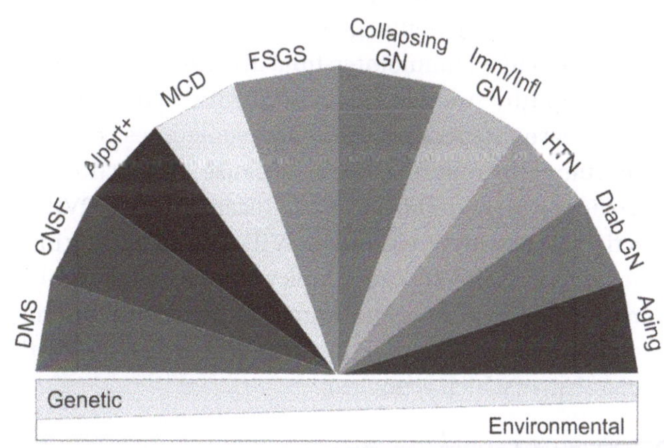

Fig. 3: Spectrum of diseases secondary to podocyte injury. Glomerular diseases can be considered as a consequence of podocyte dysfunction caused by genetic and/or environmental factors. Depending on when during glomerular development and progression they occur and how significantly and rapidly they impact the glomerulus, the clinical phenotype will vary. The clinical syndromes associated with podocyte dysfunction of various types include the following: diffuse mesangial sclerosis (DMS), congenital nephrotic syndrome, Alport's syndrome and variants, minimal change disease (MCD), focal segmental glomerulosclerosis (FSGS), collapsing glomerulonephropathy [collapsing glomerulonephritis (GN)], immune and inflammatory glomerulonephropathies (Imm/Infl GN), hypertensive nephropathy (HTN), diabetic glomerulonephropathy (Diab GN), and glomerulonephropathy (aging). Together these conditions account for 90% of end-stage kidney disease (ESKD).
Source: Wiggins RC. The spectrum of podocytopathies: a unifying view of glomerular diseases. Kidney Int. 2007;71(12):1205-14.

Genetic Disorders

More than 70 genes have now been identified to cause podocytopathy.[17] These include monogenic forms of steroid-resistant nephrotic syndrome, syndromic forms of nephrotic syndrome with extrarenal features, and phenocopies such as Alport syndrome and Dent disease. Also, diseases involving multiple organs as in Fabry disease may manifest as isolated podocytopathy with minimal or no extrarenal features.

Immune or Circulating Factor-associated Diseases

Circulating permeability factors and adaptive immunity (T cells and cytokines) have been implicated in childhood nephrotic syndrome. However, the precise nature of circulating factors and how adaptive immunity plays a role in the pathogenesis of nephrotic syndrome are not completely elucidated. Immune complex deposition or in situ formation as observed in immunoglobulin A nephropathy, systemic lupus erythematosus, and membranoproliferative glomerulonephritis can result in podocyte injury and sclerosis.[18] Membranous nephropathy is associated with podocyte injury secondary to insertion of complement C5b-9 complex into plasma membranes of podocytes.

Infections

Viral infections also cause podocyte injury-related diseases. Human immunodeficiency virus (HIV) infection can cause collapsing focal segmental glomerulosclerosis (FSGS) with or without marked tubulointerstitial disease, a characteristic podocytopathy presenting as nephrotic syndrome and rapid disease progression. FSGS and sometimes collapsing glomerulopathy may also occur because of infection with parvovirus B19, malaria, and more recently with COVID-19 infection. SARS-CoV-2, cause of COVID-19, can directly infect podocytes or indirectly cause injury by promoting cytokine secretion.[19] Apart from several immune-mediated glomerular diseases, hepatitis C infection can also cause FSGS, the mechanism of which is unclear.

Drugs and Toxins

Some drugs can cause podocytopathies by direct toxic effects. Interferon therapy and bisphosphonate therapy can cause collapsing FSGS. Lithium, sirolimus, doxorubicin, and daunomycin can cause podocytopathy with FSGS lesions.[20] VEGF antagonists have been associated with podocytopathy which is usually transient.

Malignancy

Minimal change disease (MCD) has been reported in association with lymphomas and solid tumors such as lung and colorectal cancers. Th2-related cytokines such as interleukin (IL)-13 has been causally implicated in podocytopathy in Hodgkin lymphoma.

Risk Factors

Apart from specific etiology, genetic and nongenetic factors may increase susceptibility for podocytopathy.

Genetics

Of the several susceptibility genes associated with podocytopathies identified using genome-wide studies, *APOL1* (encoding apolipoprotein L1) risk alleles (G1 and G2 alleles) is an important risk factor for FSGS and chronic kidney disease (CKD). These risk alleles are common in African population in America and Africa with frequency ranging from 26 to 50%. FSGS, collapsing glomerulopathy, and nonspecific focal global glomerulosclerosis with arterionephrosclerosis are the common APOL1-associated diseases.[21] Individuals with risk alleles carry a three- to fivefold higher risk for FSGS.

Low Nephron Number

Low nephron number as seen in children with single kidney, hypodysplastic kidney, and low birth weight predispose to podocytopathy with secondary FSGS lesions due to hyperfiltration injury.[22] Animal studies indicate that loss of >75% of nephrons is associated with the greatest risk for developing FSGS, proteinuria, hypertension, and sometimes progressive loss of kidney function.

Obesity, Diabetes Mellitus, and Hypertension

There is an increase in body mass in obesity which causes an increase in single nephron glomerular filtration rate (GFR) and hyperfiltration, predisposing to podocyte hypertrophy and increased shear stress. The earlier stages of this process are potentially reversible as remission of proteinuria has been observed following bariatric surgery.[23] A similar mechanism is also seen in diabetes mellitus. The hyperfiltration is due to increased proximal tubular glucose and sodium reabsorption by sodium/glucose cotransporters [sodium-glucose-linked transporters (SGLTs)] leading to inhibition of tubuloglomerular feedback.[24]

Morphology

The histopathology spectrum associated with podocyte injury [minimal change nephropathy (MCN), FSGS, diffuse mesangial sclerosis (DMS), and collapsing glomerulopathy, membranous nephropathy, lupus podocytopathy] varies with the underlying etiology. Globally and including all age groups, FSGS is the most common lesion, representing 10–40% of all the biopsies, except in Asia, where immunoglobulin A (IgA) nephropathy is prevalent. The histomorphology represents different patterns of podocyte injury rather than defining a unique diagnosis **(Flowchart 1)**. The pathological patterns observed in podocytopathy can be associated with many different pathophysiological processes (e.g., FSGS could be due to genetic or infectious cause) or the same pathobiology can be associated with many different morphological patterns

Flowchart 1: Response to podocytes to injury. Distinct pathways of injury and repair characterize the podocytopathies. In minimal-change nephropathy (MCN), podocyte injury is limited to foot process effacement, and podocyte number remains normal. Second, a more severe form of podocyte injury may occur, leading to podocyte detachment and death. This event initiates an injury cascade that results in the segmental scar characteristic of focal segmental glomerulosclerosis (FSGS). Third, podocyte injury may lead to delayed cellular maturation [diffuse mesangial sclerosis (DMS)], dedifferentiation (CG), and proliferation, with either low rates of podocyte proliferation (manifesting as DMS) or high rates of proliferation [manifesting as collapsing glomerulopathy (CG)].

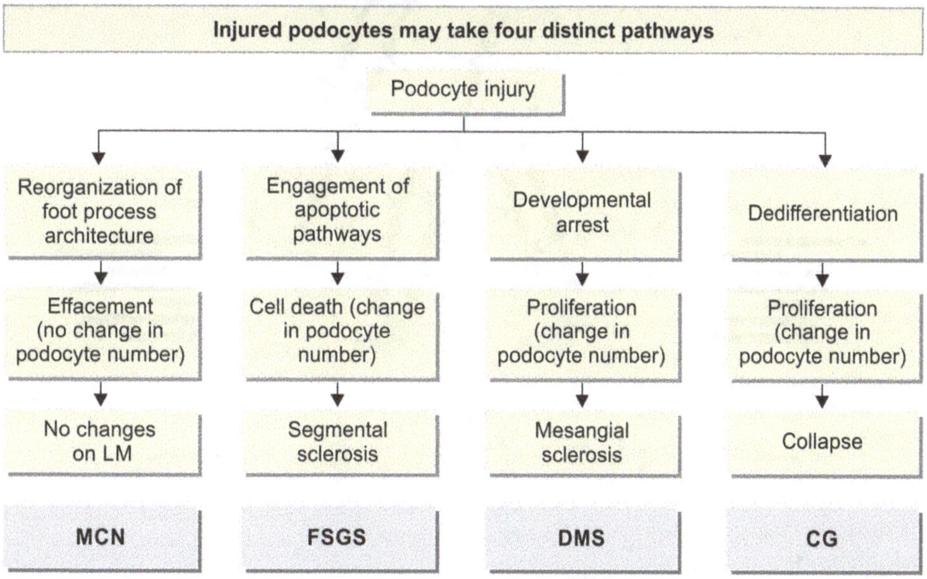

Source: Barisoni L, William Schnaper H, Kopp JB. A proposed taxonomy for the podocytopathies: a reassessment of the primary nephrotic diseases. Clin J Am Soc Nephrol. 2007;2(3):529-42.

or treatment responses. For example, podocin mutation can result in MCD or FSGS and *WT1* mutation can result in DMS or FSGS.

Taxonomy

Taxonomy for podocytopathies that combines histopathology, including podocyte phenotype, glomerular morphology, and etiology (idiopathic, genetic, and reactive forms), is more appropriate **(Table 1)**. The newer classification makes injury to the podocyte central and implies a target for therapy. It helps overcome the misleading notion that MCN, DMS, and FSGS are diseases. Such a classification facilitates a diagnostic workup to identify the etiology or triggers of podocyte injury and to individualize prognosis and treatment.

TABLE 1: Etiology and histomorphology in podocytopathy.

Etiology	*Histomorphology*
Idiopathic	MCD, FSGS, collapsing
Genetic form	MCD, FSGS, DMS, collapsing
Infection associated (hepatitis B, hepatitis C, HIV, parvovirus B19)	Collapsing glomerulopathy Membranous nephropathy FSGS
Adaptive (obesity, sickle cell anemia, reduced nephron mass, reflux nephropathy, surgical reduction)	FSGS
Medications: • Nonsteroidal anti-inflammatory medication, pamidronate, penicillamine, lithium, IFN-α, β • Calcineurin inhibitors, IFN-α, lithium • Pamidronate, IFN-α	 • MCD • FSGS • Collapsing glomerulopathy
Malignancy (Hodgkin's lymphoma)	MCD

(DMS: diffuse mesangial sclerosis; FSGS: focal segmental glomerulosclerosis; HIV: human immunodeficiency virus; IFN: interferon; MCD: minimal change disease)

Pathogenesis of Podocytopathy (Fig. 4)

Podocyte Effacement, Detachment, and Loss

Podocytes react to injurious stimuli in various ways as follows: (1) foot process effacement which can only be visualized by ultrastructural analysis [minimal change nephrotic syndrome (MCNS)], (2) apoptosis and loss of podocytes (FSGS and progression of disease), (3) developmental arrest accompanied by podocyte hypertrophy (DMS), and (4) dedifferentiation and re-entrance into the cell cycle with marked proliferative activity (collapsing glomerulopathy as in HIV).

Common mechanisms drive disease progression when podocytes are injured although injury can result from numerous different causes and risk factors. A common feature of podocyte injury is foot process effacement which is the earliest morphological pattern of podocyte injury and can be reversible. It is associated with massive proteinuria even without podocyte loss as observed in MCD. The foot

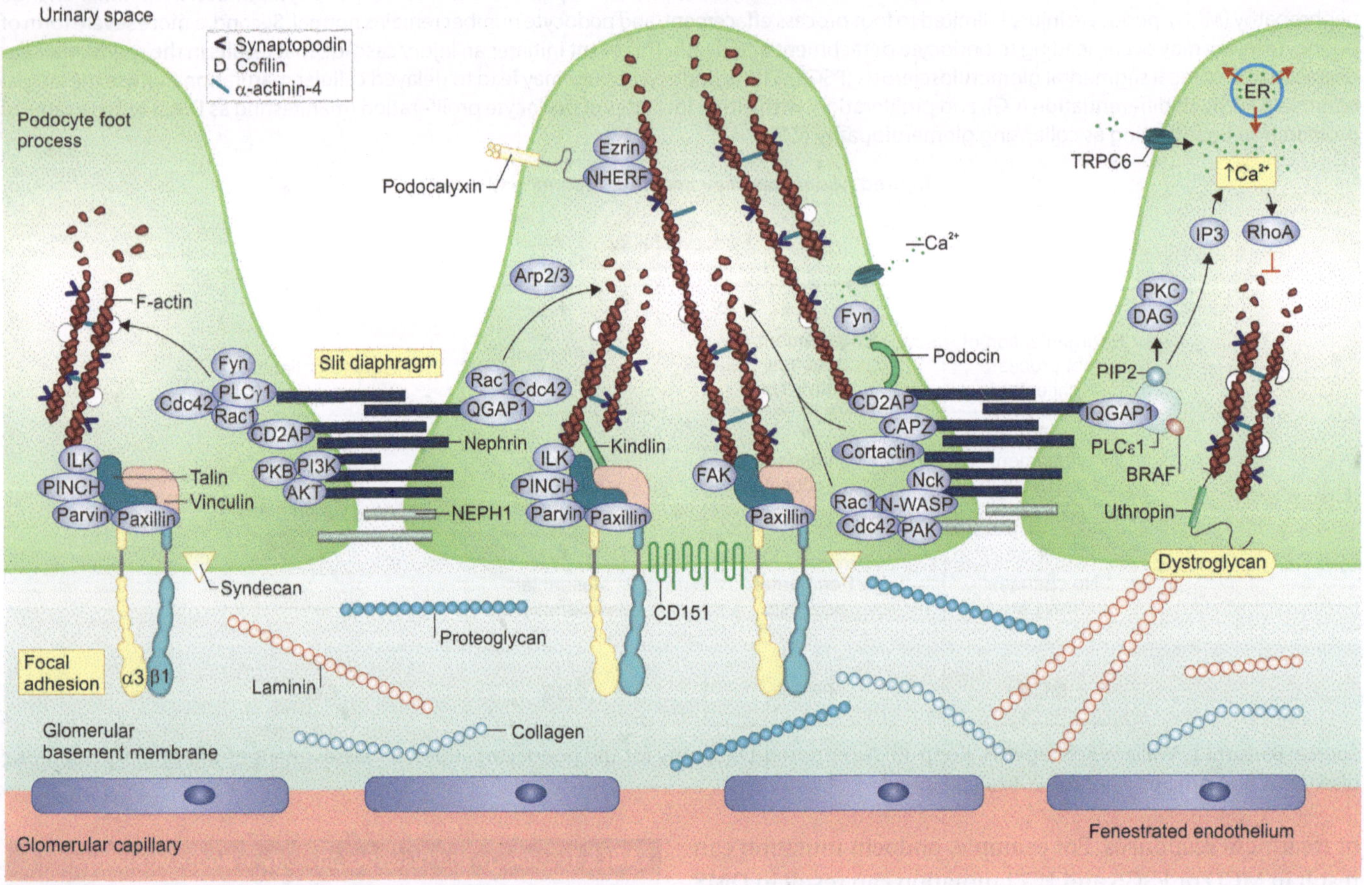

Fig. 4: Podocyte structure and function—integrative signaling molecules enable interactions between podocyte focal adhesions, the slit diaphragm, and actin dynamics.
Source: Perico L, Conti S, Benigni A, Remuzzi G. Podocyte-actin dynamics in health and disease. Nat Rev Nephrol. 2016;12:692-710.

process loses its normal three-dimensional interdigitating architecture structure and spread out, leading to a reduction in filtration barrier function. The effacement is chiefly due to loss of actin polymerization. This leads to reorganization of cytoskeleton from normal circular F-actin arrangement to formation of stress fibers that condense into a narrow band in the cytoplasm adjacent to the abluminal domain.[25] There is redistribution of the slit diaphragm components to the cytoplasm. The effacement can result from the absence of one of the critical architectural components described as in genetic forms of nephrotic syndrome, or it might represent the rearrangement of actin cytoskeleton in response to cytokine stimulation as in MCD. Irrespective of the underlying trigger, the common pathway leading to effacement involves functional imbalance among key regulators of the actin cytoskeleton, such as the Rho family of small GTPases, including RhoA, CDC42, and RAC1.

In podocyte depletion hypothesis, whatever the initial insult to the podocyte (immune, toxic, infectious, ischemic, hyperfiltration, etc.), the outcome depends on the severity of podocyte depletion **(Table 2)**.[26] As injury becomes severe and damage progresses, podocyte detaches from GBM leading to podocyte depletion and proportion of podocyte

TABLE 2: Consequences of podocyte depletion.[26,27]

Podocyte loss (%)	*Consequences*
<20	Mesangial expansion
20–40	• Synechiae formation—adhesion of the glomerular capillary loop to Bowman's capsule in denuded areas of GBM • Segmental sclerosis—scarring limited to part of loop devoid of podocytes
40–60	Progressive sclerosis of glomerulus and impairment of filtering function
>60	Global sclerosis and progressive decline in filtration

loss correlates with the development of glomerular sclerosis and CKD. Data from podocyte depletion study performed in rats by Wharram et al. show that podocyte loss of >20% leads to the development of glomerulosclerosis and CKD.[27] Due to its location in the GBM, there is constant exposure to fluid flow and associated pressures and stress. The loss of some podocytes following injury not only increases local shear stress but also increases mechanical stress on the remaining podocytes triggering a vicious cycle leading to the loss of more podocytes. Increasing filtration of albumin into Bowman's space generates a fluid drag of oncotic pressure which increases shear stress on podocytes and hyperfiltration. With increasing nephron loss as disease progresses, the total glomerular filtration surface is reduced leading to increased filtration and the vertical podocyte shear stress in each of the remaining nephrons.

Podocytes protect themselves from cell death under injury in three ways. One by dedifferentiation into an earlier developmental stage which is regulated by increased expression of NOTCH and WNT/β-catenin.[28] However, this results in concomitant loss of slit diaphragm proteins such as nephrin and podocin, leading to functional defects and impaired filtration. This also contributes to podocyte detachment and loss. The mature podocyte has limited capacity to divide. Potential mechanism for podocyte replacement following podocyte loss demonstrated in in vitro studies is either stem cell immigration from the bone marrow or migration of cells from the parietal epithelial cell layer along Bowman's capsule with a switch to the podocyte phenotype, the second mechanism for repair. Chemokine CXCL12 helps maintain local podocyte progenitors in a quiescent state and prevents generation of new podocytes in normal state.[29] Reduced expression of CXCL2 following podocyte loss activates NOTCH signaling in parietal podocytes driving migration into denuded regions of GBM and proliferation. Retinoic acid formed from retinol leaked into Bowman's space and also synthesized by parietal cells plays a key role in the final process of differentiation into podocytes by downregulating NOTCH pathway. However, the process of migration, proliferation, and differentiation is slow and mostly inefficient. The activated parietal epithelial cells cannot properly differentiate into visceral podocyte as retinoic acid is sequestered by albumin in Bowman's space leading to scarring. The third mechanism to limit the consequence of podocyte depletion and protect GFB is by podocyte hypertrophy to cover the denuded GBM.[19] Although podocytes are postmitotic cells, studies have shown that adjacent foot process migrates along the GBM to close the gaps between the remaining podocytes. However, in presence of persistent injurious stimuli, hypertrophic podocyte could move from an "adaptation" stage to a "decompensation" stage which are characterized by expression of different proteins before becoming detached from the underlying GBM indicating that the extent to which podocytes can undergo hypertrophy is limited. Exceeding this capacity may be one of the causes for glomerulosclerosis observed in experimental models of partial nephrectomy, and high calorie intake and in clinical situations of low nephron mass as in low birth weight and hypodysplastic kidneys.

Autophagy in Podocytopathy

Autophagic activity in podocytes plays an essential role in maintaining podocyte function and survival. Defect in autophagy has shown to be associated with the development of glomerulosclerosis and the pathogenesis of pathological conditions, including MCD and FSGS. Studies in mouse show high basal level of autophagy in podocytes. Podocyte-specific deletion of *Mtor* gene (Mtor pod-KO) resulted in severe foot process effacement and progressive podocyte depletion due to inhibition of autophagic flux, leading to nephrotic range proteinuria by 3 weeks of age and progression to end-stage kidney disease (ESKD) 2 weeks later.[30] Absence or decrease in autophagic activity leads to high oxidative stress and is associated with higher apoptosis, glomerulosclerosis, and worsening of podocytopathy. Decreased autophagic activity is one of the mechanisms of podocytopathy in individuals with *APOL1* risk alleles. Wild-type and risk variant *APOL1* differentially localizes to intracellular lipid droplets and the endoplasmic reticulum (ER), respectively, and results in the reduction of autophagic flux and cytotoxicity.[31]

Mitochondria Biogenesis and Function in Podocytopathy

Podocytes are specialized cells with high energy demands required for maintaining the cytoskeletal and extracellular matrix organization, motility, and remodeling of foot processes. Recent studies demonstrate a critical role for mitochondria that regulate energy homeostasis in podocytes.[32] Mitochondrial dysfunction leads to reduced adenosine triphosphate (ATP) generation and calcium signaling, generation of intracellular reactive oxygen species (ROS), and increased oxidative stress and finally apoptosis.

The generation of ATP is orchestrated by a series of electron and proton transfers by electron transport chain formed by mitochondrial complexes located in the inner mitochondrial membrane. Coenzyme Q10 (CoQ10) is a key player in shuttling electrons between various complexes. Mutations in genes coding mitochondrial respiratory chain proteins such as ADCK, PDSS2, and COQ6 are associated with FSGS.[33] These proteins are required for the biosynthesis of CoQ10. Similarly, mitochondrial dysfunction has also been reported in patients with monogenic forms of nephrotic syndrome not directly related to mitochondria. Mutations in podocyte-specific genes like nephrin lead to defects in the mitochondrial respiratory chain functions resulting in increased ROS generation and accumulation of lipid peroxidation products leading to podocyte injury and dysfunction of GFB.

Studies have shown that activity of podocytes increases when exposed to high glucose and in situations with increased activation of transforming growth factor beta (TGF-β). Since the capacity to increase oxidative phosphorylation or glycolysis by podocytes is limited, it is postulated that the observed changes in mitochondrial function consequent to increased podocyte activity may lead to metabolic conditions that sensitize the podocyte toward apoptosis. Podocyte endothelin-β1 acts on glomerular endothelial mitochondria and causes oxidative damage leading to glomerulosclerosis. Peroxisome proliferator-activated receptor gamma coactivator 1-alpha (PGC-1α) is a major regulator of mitochondrial biogenesis and oxidative metabolism. Overexpression of PGC-1α or peroxisome proliferator-activated receptor-γ (PPARγ) in setting of podocyte stress has shown to protect podocyte against injury by prevention of mitochondrial dysfunction.[34]

Role of TGF-β

Transforming growth factor beta is one of the most important and widely studied regulators of renal fibrosis. It also plays an important role in podocyte injury by suppressing podocyte genes (nephrin, podocin, etc.) and activating fibrotic and mesenchymal genes via Smad-dependent and Smad-independent pathways. TGF-β induces reorganization of actin skeleton as well as podocyte dedifferentiation via Smad2/3 signaling and by activating non-Smad pathways such as mitogen-activated protein kinases (MAPKs) and its downstream molecules such as extracellular regulated kinases (ERKs), p38, and Jun kinase and integrin-linked kinase (ILK).[35]

Podocytopathy in Obesity and Diabetes Mellitus

High plasma free fatty acid (FFA) is one of the characteristics features of obesity and may contribute to obesity-associated podocytopathy. In vitro experiments using human podocyte cell culture has shown that FFA treatment induced human podocyte apoptosis and dysfunction by increased expression of a matricellular protein, thrombospondin-1 (TSP1), and the interaction with its receptor CD36.[36] In diabetes mellitus angiotensin II whose expression is stimulated by high glucose, and mechanical stretch, increases expression of podocyte-derived VEGF and also induces TGF-β signaling leading to podocyte apoptosis.[37]

CONCLUSION

Podocytopathies encompass a broad array of clinicopathologically defined syndromes caused by direct or indirect podocyte injury. Podocyte plays an important role as both a regulator of glomerular development and the determinant of progression to glomerulosclerosis and renal failure. Podocyte biology is impacted by immune, genetic, infectious, and environmental factors. The broad spectrum of clinical syndromes secondary to podocyte injury depends on the stage of glomerular development, underlying cause, and severity of podocyte dysfunction or loss. Typical kidney biopsy features are minimal change lesions and FSGS lesions. The mainstay of treatment for primary podocytopathies includes glucocorticoids and other immunosuppressive drugs and treating the underlying cause such as in diabetes mellitus and HIV. Symptomatic management using diuretics, statins, infection prophylaxis, and anticoagulation along with angiotensin-converting enzyme inhibitor (ACEI) and angiotensin receptor blocker (ARB) forms the mainstay of treatment in inherited forms of podocytopathy. Development of specific podocyte-directed therapies to protect podocytes from injury, detachment, and loss is a research priority.

KEY POINTS

- Podocytopathy is a group of kidney diseases in which podocyte injury is the only or a major cause of the disease.
- A variety of genetic and nongenetic causes such as immune-related, infection-related, toxic, and hemodynamic factors and obesity lead to podocytopathy in children.
- Standard treatment for primary podocytopathies manifesting with FSGS lesions includes glucocorticoids and other immunosuppressive drugs. Nonresponders have poor prognosis with progression to ESKD.
- Renin–angiotensin system antagonists help to control proteinuria and slow the progression of fibrosis.
- Recent research has resulted in a shift in paradigm from stratification based on histology findings toward personalized management guided by clinical, pathophysiological, morphological, and genetic study results.

REFERENCES

1. Scott RP, Quaggin SE. Review series: the cell biology of renal filtration. J Cell Biol. 2015;209:199-210.
2. Schell C, Huber TB. The evolving complexity of the podocyte cytoskeleton. J Am Soc Nephrol. 2017;28:3166-74.
3. Drenckhahn D, Franke RP. Ultrastructural organization of contractile and cytoskeletal proteins in glomerular podocytes of chicken, rat, and man. Lab Invest. 1988;59:673-82.
4. Geiger B, Spatz JP, Bershadsky AD. Environmental sensing through focal adhesions. Nat Rev Mol Cell Biol. 2009;10:21-33.
5. Sachs N, Sonnenberg A. Cell-matrix adhesion of podocytes in physiology and disease. Nat Rev Nephrol. 2013;9:200-10.
6. Ichimura K, Miyazaki N, Sadayama S, Murata K, Koike M, Nakamura K, et al. Three-dimensional architecture of podocytes revealed by block-face scanning electron microscopy. J Cell Sci. 2017;130:132-42.
7. Rascle A, Suleiman H, Neumann T, Witzgall R. Role of transcription factors in podocytes. Nephron Exp Nephrol. 2007; 106(2):e60-6.
8. Chugh SS. Transcriptional regulation of podocyte disease. Transl Res. 2007;149: 237-42.
9. Blattner SM, Hodgin JB, Nishio M, Wylie SA, Saha J, Soofi AA, et al. Divergent functions of the Rho GTPases Rac1 and Cdc42 in podocyte injury. Kidney Int. 2013;84:920-30.
10. Armelloni S, Corbelli A, Giardino L, Li M, Ikehata M, Mattinzoli D, et al. Podocytes: recent biomolecular developments. Biomol Concepts. 2014;5:319-30.
11. Perico L, Conti S, Benigni A, Remuzzi G. Podocyte-actin dynamics in health and disease. Nat Rev Nephrol. 2016;12: 692-710.
12. Garg P, Holzman LB. Podocytes: gaining a foothold. Exp Cell Res. 2012;318:955-63.
13. Lynch DK, Winata SC, Lyons RJ, Hughes WE, Lehrbach GM, Wasinger V, et al. A Cortactin CD2 associated protein (CD2AP) complex provides a novel link between epidermal growth factor

receptor endocytosis and the actin cytoskeleton. J Biol Chem. 2003;278:21805-13.

14. Vitureira N, Andrés R, Pérez-Martínez E, Martínez A, Bribián A, Blasi J, et al. Podocalyxin is a novel polysialylated neural adhesion protein with multiple roles in neural development and synapse formation. PLoS One. 2010;5:e12003.
15. Dryer SE, Reiser J. TRPC6 channels and their binding partners in podocytes: role in glomerular filtration and pathophysiology. Am J Physiol Renal Physiol. 2010;299:F689-701.
16. Schrijvers BF, Flyvbjerg A, De Vriese AS. The role of vascular endothelial growth factor (VEGF) in renal pathophysiology. Kidney Int. 2004;65:2003-17.
17. Pardeshi VC, Narikot A, Vasudevan A. Next-generation sequencing-based genetic diagnosis of steroid-resistant nephrotic syndrome: benefits and challenges. Asian J Pediatr Nephrol. 2019;2:16-24.
18. Singh L, Singh G, Dinda AK. Understanding podocytopathy and its relevance to clinical nephrology. Indian J Nephrol. 2015;25:1-7.
19. Nasr SH, Kopp JB. COVID-19-associated collapsing glomerulopathy: an emerging entity. Kidney Int Rep. 2020;5:759-61.
20. Kopp JB, Anders HJ, Susztak K, Podesta MA, Remuzzi G, Hildebrandt F, et al. Podocytopathies. Nat Rev Dis Primers. 2020;6:68.
21. Siemens TA, Riella MC, Moraes TP, Riella CV. APOL1 risk variants and kidney disease: what we know so far. J Bras Nefrol. 2018;40:388-402.
22. Luyckx VA, Perico N, Somaschini M, Manfellotto D, Valensise H, Cetin I, et al. A developmental approach to the prevention of hypertension and kidney disease: a report from the Low Birth Weight and Nephron Number Working Group. Lancet. 2017;390:424-8.
23. Xu T, Sheng Z, Yao L. Obesity-related glomerulopathy: pathogenesis, pathologic, clinical characteristics and treatment. Front Med. 2017;11:340-8.
24. Vallon V, Thomson SC. The tubular hypothesis of nephron filtration and diabetic kidney disease. Nat Rev Nephrol. 2020;16:317-36.
25. Shirato I, Sakai T, Kimura K, Tomino Y, Kriz W. Cytoskeletal changes in podocytes associated with foot process effacement in Masugi nephritis. Am J Pathol. 1996;148:1283-96.
26. Wiggins RC. The spectrum of podocytopathies: a unifying view of glomerular diseases. Kidney Int. 2007;71:1205-14.
27. Wharram BL, Goyal M, Wiggins JE, Saden SK, Hussain S, Filipiak WE, et al. Podocyte depletion causes glomerulosclerosis: diphtheria toxin-induced podocyte depletion in rats expressing human diphtheria toxin receptor transgene. J Am Soc Nephrol. 2005;16:2941-52.
28. Jing Z, Wei-jie Y, Yi-Feng ZG. Down-regulation of Wt1 activates Wnt/β-catenin signaling through modulating endocytic route of LRP6 in podocyte dysfunction in vitro. Cell Signal. 2015;27:1772-80.
29. Romoli S, Angelotti ML, Antonelli G, Kumar Vr S, Mulay SR, Desai J, et al. CXCL12 blockade preferentially regenerates lost podocytes in cortical nephrons by targeting an intrinsic podocyte-progenitor feedback mechanism. Kidney Int. 2018;94:1111-26.
30. Cina DP, Onay T, Paltoo A, Li C, Maezawa Y, De Arteaga J, et al. Inhibition of MTOR disrupts autophagic flux in podocytes. J Am Soc Nephrol. 2012;23:412-20.
31. Venkatachalam MA. Could autophagic exhaustion be a final common pathway for podocytopathy in FSGS? J Am Soc Nephrol. 2015;26:999-1001.
32. Müller-Deile J, Schiffer M. The podocyte power-plant disaster and its contribution to glomerulopathy. Front Endocrinol (Lausanne). 2014;5:209.
33. Ashraf S, Gee HY, Woerner S, Xie LX, Vega-Warner V, Lovric S, et al. ADCK4 mutations promote steroid-resistant nephrotic syndrome through CoQ10 biosynthesis disruption. J Clin Invest. 2013;123:5179-89.
34. Yuan Y, Huang S, Wang W, Wang Y, Zhang P, Zhu C, et al. Activation of peroxisome proliferator-activated receptor-γ coactivator 1α ameliorates mitochondrial dysfunction and protects podocytes from aldosterone-induced injury. Kidney Int. 2012;82:771-89.
35. Leeuwis JW, Nguyen TQ, Dendooven A, Kok RJ, Goldschmeding R. Targeting podocyte-associated diseases. Adv Drug Deliv Rev. 2010;62:1325-36.
36. Cui W, Maimaitiyiming H, Zhou Q, Norman H, Zhou C, Wang S. Interaction of thrombospondin1 and CD36 contributes to obesity-associated podocytopathy. Biochim Biophys Acta. 2015;1852:1323-33.
37. Badal SS, Danesh FR. New insights into molecular mechanisms of diabetic kidney disease. Am J Kidney Dis. 2014;63:S63-83.

CHAPTER

6.2 Steroid-sensitive Nephrotic Syndrome

Aditi Sinha, Anil Vasudevan, Arvind Bagga

INTRODUCTION

Nephrotic syndrome is one of the most common kidney diseases in children. It is characterized by edema, heavy proteinuria (>1 g/m^2/day; >40 mg/m^2/h), and hypoalbuminemia (serum albumin <3 g/dL, and is a rare disease affecting 1.2–16.9 per 100,000 children annually.[1,2] Most cases in childhood are idiopathic, and an underlying systemic illness (e.g., lupus, Henoch-Schönlein purpura, amyloidosis) is revealed in <10% of patients. More than 80% of children with idiopathic nephrotic syndrome show remission following therapy with oral corticosteroids.[3] While a small proportion of patients may never relapse or relapse infrequently (1–2 relapses a year), 40–60% of patients show frequent relapses or steroid dependence **(Table 1)**. Patients with frequent relapses and steroid dependence are at risk of complications associated with disease relapses, as well as corticosteroid toxicity. The prognosis in steroid sensitive disease is overall favorable. In the majority of cases, the disease is quiescent by adolescence; however, a fair proportion of cases may experience relapse(s) in adulthood.[4]

About 10–15% of patients do not respond to corticosteroids, either at onset (initial steroid resistance) or following a subsequent relapse (late steroid resistance).

TABLE 1: Definitions of disease course.

Remission	Urine protein nil or trace (Up/Uc <0.2 mg/mg) for three consecutive early morning specimens
Relapse	Urine protein >3+ (Up/Uc >2 mg/mg) for three consecutive early morning specimens, having been in remission previously
Frequent relapses	Two or more relapses in the first 6 months after stopping initial therapy; ≥3 relapses in any 6 months; or ≥4 relapses in a year
Steroid dependence	Two consecutive relapses when on alternate day steroids, or within 14 days of its discontinuation
Steroid resistance	Lack of complete remission despite therapy with daily prednisolone at a dose of 2 mg/kg (or 60 mg/m^2) daily for 6 weeks

(Uc: urine creatinine; Up: urine protein)

Management of steroid-resistant nephrotic syndrome is challenging, particularly if the disease does not respond to immunosuppression. Together with the subsequent chapter, this chapter summarizes current understanding of the pathogenesis of nephrotic syndrome and principles of evidence-based management of steroid-sensitive and steroid-resistant disease, as detailed in the revised 2021 guidelines of the Indian Society of Pediatric Nephrology (ISPN).[5,6]

PATHOLOGY

The majority of patients with nephrotic syndrome have insignificant glomerular changes on light microscopy, no deposits on immunofluorescence examination, and effacement of podocytes with disruption and disorganization of actin filaments on electron microscopy, termed minimal change disease.[1,7]

About 40–70% patients with steroid-resistant nephrotic syndrome and 5–10% cases with sensitive nephrotic syndrome have focal segmental glomerulosclerosis (FSGS), characterized by sclerosis involving a segment of the glomerular tuft.[8] A small proportion of patients with steroid resistance, particularly older (>12-year-old) children, show features of membranous nephropathy, membranoproliferative glomerulonephritis, or IgA nephropathy.

PATHOGENESIS

The glomerular filtration barrier consists of capillary endothelial fenestrations, glomerular basement membrane (GBM), and interdigitating podocyte foot processes. Proteinuria in nephrotic syndrome results from dysfunction of podocytes, leading to loss of the selective filtering function. In a significant proportion of cases of initial steroid resistance, this is caused by mutations in genes encoding structural elements of the podocyte slit diaphragm or cytoskeleton (*NPHS1*, *NPHS2*, *CD2AP*, *TRCP6*, and *ACTN4*), GBM proteins (*LAMB2*, *COL4A5*), mitochondrial genes (*COQ2*), or transcription factors (*WT1*, *LMX1B*).[9] While certain loci on major histocompatibility complex (MHC) class II molecules are reported as risk alleles, currently there is no role for genetic testing in patients with SSNS.[10]

The vast majority of cases of nephrotic syndrome, particularly steroid-sensitive disease, is considered to be associated with immune dysfunction. Experimental evidence suggests that alterations in cell-mediated immunity may lead to T helper type 2 (Th2) polarization and the release of an uncharacterized circulating factor that increases glomerular permeability. Studies also suggest an imbalance between Th17 and regulatory T cells[11] that potentially causes persistent activation of Th2 cells; alternatively, deficient action by regulatory T cells might be responsible for inadequate censoring of podocyte CD80 (B7-1) expression, which is known to be upregulated in models of minimal change disease.[12,13] The rapidity with which relapses follow minor infections suggests the involvement of innate immunity, likely involving activation of toll-like receptors and nuclear factor kappa signaling in antigen-presenting cells, which might influence humoral immune responses.[14]

Steroid-resistant nephrotic syndrome is considered to be mediated by a "soluble mediator", a hypothesis that is supported by recurrence of nephrotic range proteinuria immediately post-transplant in 30–50% of patients with idiopathic FSGS who develop kidney failure.[15] It is supported by experimental evidence in which nephrotic plasma induces changes in distribution of podocyte cytoskeletal and slit diaphragm proteins, foot process effacement, and increase in vascular permeability. Proposed circulating factors have included interleukin-13, cardiotrophin-like cytokine-1, tumor necrosis factor-α, hemopexin, c-maf-inducing protein, soluble urokinase-type plasminogen activator receptor, vascular endothelial growth factor, anti-CD40 antibody, and soluble CD40 ligand.[16] However, none of these factors has been shown to be implicated unequivocally.

The precise immune perturbations underlying nephrotic syndrome and the identity of the circulating factor remain elusive. Given lack of understanding of the pathogenesis of proteinuria, the rationale for using immunosuppressive therapies remains empiric and is guided chiefly by clinical studies. These drugs are expected to act by inhibiting or altering humoral or cellular immune responses; however, podocytes are also proposed as the potential targets for antiproteinuric interventions, including steroids, levamisole, calcineurin inhibitors (CNIs), and rituximab.[17]

DEFINITIONS

Nephrotic syndrome is defined by the occurrence of edema in the presence of hypoalbuminemia and nephrotic range proteinuria. **Table 1** provides key definitions of disease course of nephrotic syndrome. "Frequent relapses" include patients with "steroid dependence", a term that identifies a subgroup of patients who fail to sustain remission of steroids. While implied previously, the ISPN definition now explicitly includes the occurrence of three relapses in any 6 months as frequent relapses.[5] Further, the definition of frequent relapses was modified to include patients with fewer relapses (three relapses in a year or two in any 6 months) in the presence of significant corticosteroid toxicity or while on long-term steroids or steroid-sparing therapies. In order to identify patients in definite need of avoiding relapses, two terms were introduced. The term "complicated" refers to any relapse that is associated with a life-threatening complication, such as hypovolemia requiring inpatient care, severe bacterial infection (peritonitis, cellulitis, meningitis), or thrombosis. "Significant steroid toxicity" identifies patients with hyperglycemia (fasting glucose >100 mg/dL, postprandial glucose >140 mg/dL, or HbA1c > 5.7%), obesity (body mass index more than the equivalent of 27 kg/m^2 in adults), short stature [height <–2 standard deviation score (SDS) for age with height velocity <–3 SDS for age], raised intraocular pressure, cataract, myopathy, osteonecrosis, or psychosis.[5]

Given the natural history of disease, relapses may continue to occur even while on immunosuppressive therapy; hence, both sustained remission and infrequent relapses are considered acceptable, and imply "stable remission". The subgroup of patients who continues to manifest frequent relapses (or infrequent relapses in the presence of significant steroid toxicity) despite the use of two or more steroid-sparing agents [such as levamisole, cyclophosphamide, or mycophenolate mofetil (MMF)] is termed "difficult-to-treat" steroid-sensitive disease and merits consideration of more potent but potentially toxic agents.[5]

The diagnosis of steroid resistance is based on demonstration of nonresponse (3–4+ proteinuria, edema, or hypoalbuminemia) despite therapy with prednisone in adequate doses for 6 weeks.[6] Therapy with pulse corticosteroids is not required to confirm steroid resistance. The evaluation and management of steroid-resistant nephrotic syndrome is discussed in Chapter 6.3. Patients with frequent relapses and steroid resistance are at high risk of complications due to the morbidities associated with the illness and toxicity of medications. These patients, and those below the age of 1 year, should be managed by pediatric nephrologists.

EVALUATION

Investigations at the onset of illness must include urinalysis, blood levels of urea, creatinine, albumin, cholesterol, serum electrolytes, and complete blood counts. Quantitative estimation of urine protein, by repeated early morning spot urine protein to creatinine ratios or a timed (12- or 24-hour) collection, is required if nephrotic range proteinuria is uncertain. Urine microscopy is normal, except for occasional hyaline or granular casts and/or microscopic hematuria. A tuberculin test is recommended in view of the risk of activation of latent infection in young children.[5,18] Additional investigations are rarely necessary. Patients with positive tuberculin test or history of contact should undergo chest radiography. Serologies to rule out lupus (antinuclear antibody), antistreptolysin O, and/or complement C3 and C4 are only needed in patients with atypical presentation suggesting glomerulonephritis, such as gross or persistent microscopic hematuria, sustained hypertension, or extrarenal features (rash, arthralgias). An ultrasonography is not necessary unless the child is planned for kidney biopsy or has gross hematuria or acute kidney injury (AKI). Routine screening for chronic viral infections is not recommended.[5]

Most patients with SSNS do not require a kidney biopsy. A biopsy is required at onset if a cause other than minimal change disease is suspected, such as clinical features suggesting a secondary cause, or presence of gross or persistent microscopic hematuria or AKI not attributable to hypovolemia. Age thresholds do not appear to be relevant in mandating the need for kidney biopsy at disease onset. Young infants presenting with nephrotic syndrome and older infants with steroid resistance are considered for next-generation sequencing to determine a genetic cause, the most likely diagnosis in these patients; therefore, a kidney biopsy is avoided. Adolescents presenting with nephrotic syndrome should receive a trial of corticosteroids before considering biopsy, unless there are atypical features (hematuria, hypertension, extrarenal features, or low C3). A kidney biopsy is essential in patients with steroid-resistant nephrotic syndrome, except in patients with syndromic or familial disease, where genetic screening has a higher diagnostic and prognostic role. Kidney biopsy is also suggested before initiating therapy with CNIs and, following prolonged use, to rule out histological nephrotoxicity.

Since relapses might occur throughout childhood and timely intervention prevents morbidities, parents must be taught to maintain a record of proteinuria (by dipstick or boiling), infections, and medications received. During subsequent relapses, blood investigations may be required if complications are suspected. Complete blood counts help rule out systemic infection and hypovolemia. Blood urea, creatinine, albumin, and electrolytes are recommended in children presenting with severe edema, hypovolemia, dehydration, or oligoanuria and following prolonged use of diuretics. Annual reevaluation is recommended even in patients with infrequent relapses in order to monitor growth and detect hypertension. Blood levels of creatinine, albumin, and electrolytes should be assessed every 1–2 years in patients with relapsing illness, and more frequently if on immunosuppressive medications, as discussed later.

MANAGEMENT

Initial Episode

Collaborative efforts by the International Study of Kidney Diseases in Children (ISKDC)[19] and Arbeitsgemeinschaft für Pädiatrische Nephrologie (APN)[20] defined the therapy of nephrotic syndrome in the 1970s to 1990s. Subsequent randomized controlled trials (RCTs) using varying doses and duration of predniso(lo)ne therapy formed the basis for recommendations by the Kidney Disease: Improving Global Outcomes (KDIGO) Glomerulonephritis Work Group[21] and the 2008 recommendations of the ISPN.[22] A 2007 meta-analysis of these studies estimated that, compared to 3 months, therapy for 6 months led to reduced risk of frequent relapses [relative risk (RR) 0.55; 95% confidence interval (CI) 0.39, 0.80] and reduced number of annual relapses (mean difference –0.44; 95% CI –0.82, –0.07).[23] However, the majority of the included RCTs had major methodological flaws, conferring a high risk of bias. The first episode is treated with prednisolone 2 mg/kg (60 mg/m^2) daily for 6 weeks and then 1.5 mg/kg (40 mg/m^2) on alternate days (AD) for 6 weeks.

Four recent well-designed RCTs contest the previously held view.[24-27] Results from these studies that enrolled almost 800 patients emphasize that prolongation of initial therapy to beyond 8–12 weeks is not useful in modifying the course of the disease or reducing subsequent needs for corticosteroids and other agents. All four studies were at low risk of bias and three were placebo controlled. While delaying the time to first relapse, intensive initial therapy did not alter the risk of frequent relapses at 1–2 years' follow-up when analysis was limited to studies at low risk of bias (≥3 months vs. 2 months: RR 0.99; 95% CI 0.82, 1.19; ≥5 months vs. 3 months: RR 0.99; 95% CI 0.74, 1.33).[28] Given these results and the risk of adverse effects associated with therapy with steroids, prolonging initial therapy beyond 8–12 weeks is not recommended. Post hoc analyses in two studies suggest some benefit with prolonged therapy in children below 4–6 years old, this finding requires confirmation.[25,27]

Flowchart 1 shows the approach to managing patients with nephrotic syndrome. Only prednisolone or prednisone is recommended and is administered in single or divided doses[29]; there is no evidence to support the use of deflazacort compared to other corticosteroids. Prednisolone may be dosed by body surface area (BSA) or weight. Weight-based dosing is more convenient since estimating BSA is cumbersome and/or often inaccurate. However, BSA-based dosing is preferred in young children to avoid relative underdosing which was associated with increased risk of frequent relapses in a few studies.[30-32]

Therapy for Relapse

Almost 70–80% of the patients with steroid-sensitive disease exhibit disease relapses, often within a year since onset. Almost half of the relapses are precipitated by minor, usually upper respiratory tract, infections. Proteinuria during infections may be transient; hence, it is advisable to await resolution of infection, thus avoiding the need for corticosteroid therapy. However, 3+/4+ proteinuria that lasts for 3 days or longer is unlikely to resolve spontaneously, and is conventionally, albeit empirically, been treated with prednisolone at 60 mg/m^2/day (2 mg/kg/day; maximum 60 mg) in single or divided doses

Flowchart 1: Immunosuppressive agents in management of nephrotic syndrome, including the initial episode, disease relapses, and management of frequent relapsing or steroid-dependent nephrotic syndrome. The approach to managing patients with steroid resistance is discussed in Chapter 6.3. Decisions on choice of noncorticosteroid immunosuppressive agents should be made following considerations of efficacy, safety, and costs of various therapies (see text).

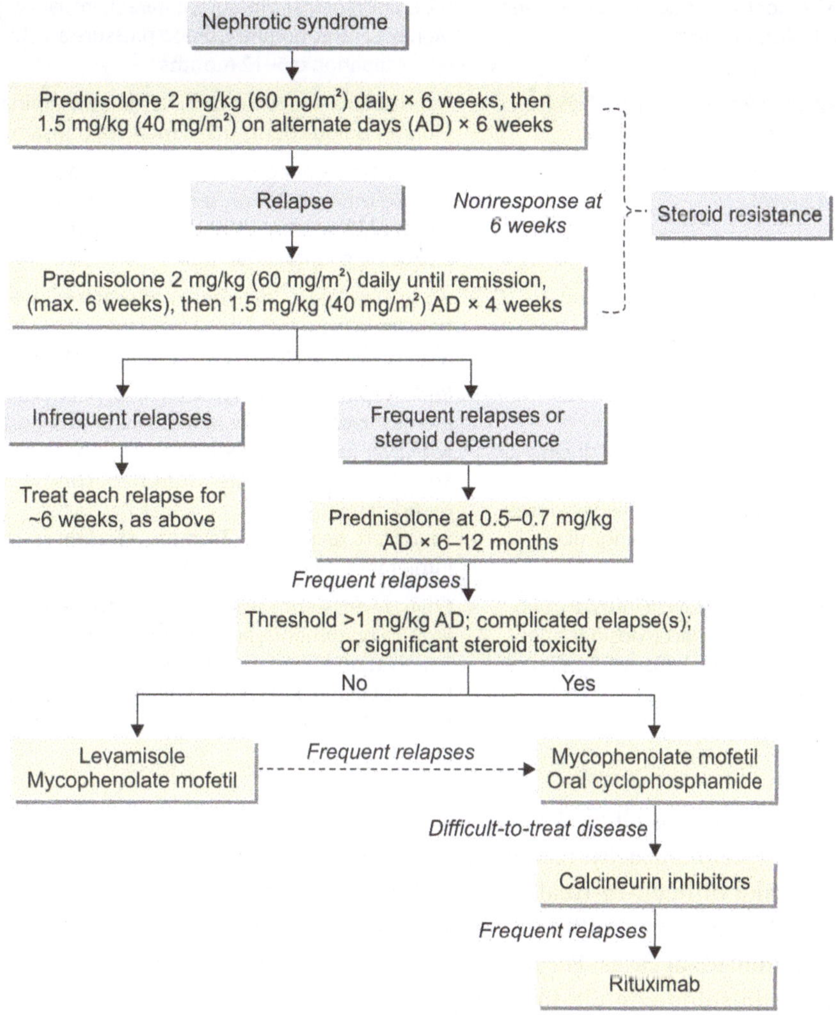

until remission (protein trace/nil for 3 consecutive days), followed by 40 mg/m² (1.5 mg/kg, maximum 40 mg) on AD for 4 weeks **(Flowchart 1)**. Dosing based on BSA and weight is associated with similar outcomes.[33]

Usually, daily therapy is required for <2 weeks. If proteinuria persists, daily therapy with prednisolone is extended to a maximum of 6 weeks; lack of remission despite such treatment indicates late steroid resistance which is managed similar to initial resistance (*see* Chapter 6.3).[6] Recent RCTs suggest that reduced dose or abbreviated duration of therapy with prednisolone is effective in inducing and maintaining remission.[34,35] The optimal dose and duration of prednisolone therapy for relapses require examination in adequately powered RCTs with prolonged follow-up.

Management of Frequent Relapses

Frequent relapses and steroid dependence are more common in patients with age at onset below 3 years, delayed time to initial remission, brief corticosteroid therapy at onset, and short duration of initial remission.[1,3,4] Prolonged therapy with high-dose prednisolone is associated with significant steroid toxicity, as discussed previously, as well as behavior problems, cataract, glaucoma, hypertension, osteoporosis, compression fracture of the spine, avascular hip necrosis, and diabetes. Relapses are associated with significant complications, including infections, thrombosis, and dyslipidemia. Hence, patients with frequent relapses or steroid dependence are treated with long-term AD steroids or alternative steroid-sparing agents to maintain remission while limiting exposure to steroids. While few RCTs have compared the relative efficacy of these medications and most guidelines do not specify the order or choice of therapy, the revised ISPN guidelines on SSNS do advise on the choice of therapies based on steroid threshold for relapses, severity of relapses, presence of adverse effects of corticosteroid therapy, patient age, cost of therapy, and parental preference.[5]

Table 2 summarizes recommendations on dose, duration, adverse effects, and precautions during therapy, while **Flowchart 2** indicates the choice and order of therapies for frequently relapsing or steroid-dependent disease.[5] This

TABLE 2: Immunosuppressive agents for frequently relapsing and steroid-dependent nephrotic syndrome.

Drug	*Dose and duration*	*Adverse effects; precautions*
Prednisolone	0.5–0.7 mg/kg on alternate days for 6–12 months; the same dose is given daily during infections	• Weight gain, Cushingoid features; reduced height velocity; hypertension; raised intraocular pressure; cataract; impaired glycemic tolerance • Monitor anthropometry, blood pressure and blood glucose q 3–6 months; eye evaluation q 6–12 months
Levamisole	2–2.5 mg/kg on alternate days for 2–3 years	• Neutropenia, vasculitic rash; raised transaminases, seizures • Monitor blood counts q 2–3 months; transaminases q 3–6 months
Cyclophosphamide	2–2.5 mg/kg/day orally for 8–12 weeks	• Leukopenia, alopecia, blue nails; risk of gonadal toxicity and malignancies • Initiate therapy during remission; maintain hydration; monitor blood counts q 2 weeks; withhold drug during serious infection or if total leukocyte count <4,000/mm^3
Mycophenolate mofetil	600–1,200 mg/m^2/day in divided doses for 2–3 years	• Abdominal pain, diarrhea, nausea; viral warts; leukopenia; elevated transaminases • Monitor blood counts q 2–3 months; transaminases q 3–6 months
Calcineurin inhibitors • Cyclosporine • Tacrolimus	Given for 2–3 years, in doses as below: 4–5 mg/kg/day in divided doses; target 12-h trough 80–120 ng/mL 0.1–0.2 mg/kg/day in divided doses; target 12-h trough 4–8 ng/mL	• *Both:* Nephrotoxicity, hyperkalemia, hepatotoxicity • Monitor creatinine, potassium at 2 weeks, and then q 3–6 months along with liver function tests, glucose, uric acid, magnesium, and lipids • *Specific to cyclosporine:* Gum hyperplasia, hirsutism; hypertension; dyslipidemia • *Specific to tacrolimus*: Tremors, seizures, headache; diarrhea; glucose intolerance; hypomagnesemia
Rituximab	375 mg/m^2 as slow IV infusion, two doses 1 week apart (consider one to two additional doses if B cells not depleted)	• Chills, fever; serum sickness; bronchospasm; neutropenia; *Pneumocystis jirovecii* pneumonia; acute lung injury; hypogammaglobulinemia; reactivation of hepatitis B or JC virus • Rule out acute and chronic infections before therapy • Monitor CD19 counts; blood counts; IgG levels; consider cotrimoxazole prophylaxis

categorization relies on the definitions alluded to earlier, namely presence of significant steroid toxicity, complicated relapses, stable remission, and difficult-to-treat steroid-sensitive disease. Overall, the approach suffices in most conditions but may vary in individual cases. For example, long-term therapy with prednisolone on alternate days is advocated as the first-line therapy; however, patients diagnosed with steroid dependence soon after initial therapy or with significant steroid toxicity at diagnosis of frequent relapses are considered directly for steroid-sparing therapies. Therapy with cyclophosphamide is avoided in young patients and in pubertal or postpubertal boys, and therapy with CNI is preferred to MMF in very young patients with significant steroid toxicity.

Long-term, Alternate-day Steroids

Prednisolone is tapered to a dose of 0.5–0.7 mg/kg on alternate days to keep the disease in remission without significant adverse effects and maintained for 6–12 months.[5] The dose may be lowered further, to 0.2–0.3 mg/kg on alternate days and given for 6–18 months if it is effective in reducing relapses or maintaining remission without causing steroid toxicity.[5] Patients on long-term therapy with prednisolone require close monitoring for toxicity through frequent assessment of weight, height, blood pressure, ocular toxicity, and hyperglycemia **(Table 2).**

Relapses are precipitated following minor infections and based on recent RCTs that demonstrated that administering the dose of prednisolone daily for 5–7 days during infections effectively prevents infection-related relapses, the ISPN and KDIGO advise that the frequency of administration of prednisolone be increased from alternate day to daily during episodes of fever and/or upper respiratory tract infection.[5,21] While most studies enrolled patients who were already on therapy with prednisolone on alternate days, one published crossover RCT[36] and a placebo-controlled RCT (PREDNOS2; ISRCTN10900733) have examined the role of this intervention in preventing relapses in patients off corticosteroids; while the former study supports the intervention, the latter casts doubts on the utility of giving low dose daily prednisone in preventing relapses after infections.

Based on the hypothesis that suppression of the hypothalamic-pituitary axis is a risk factor for relapses,[37] a retrospective study[38] and one small open-label RCT[39] suggest that compared to therapy on alternate days, prednisolone intake at low doses (0.2–0.3 mg/kg) daily may reduce the frequency of relapses. As of now, the ISPN guidelines do not suggest therapy with low-dose daily prednisone.[5]

Corticosteroid-sparing Agents

The additional use of an alternative agent should be considered in patients with prednisolone threshold for maintaining remission >0.7 mg/kg on alternate days or

Flowchart 2: Management of edema. Hypovolemia needs to be excluded in all children presenting in relapse state with or without edema, particularly in a setting of vomiting, diarrhea, reduced oral intake, or unsupervised diuretic use. Suggestive clinical features include history of abdominal pain, vomiting or postural hypotension; lethargy, prolonged capillary refill time, cold extremities, tachycardia, low volume pulses, or hypotension. Biochemical parameters that indicate hypovolemia include an elevated hematocrit and an increased blood urea to creatinine ratio >100, in mg/dL units, low fractional excretion of sodium (<0.5%), and high urinary potassium index (>0.6). Patients with mild edema usually do not require diuretics and edema resolves with reduction in salt intake and therapy of relapse leading to steady improvement. Doses of commonly used diuretics are provided in Chapter 6.3.

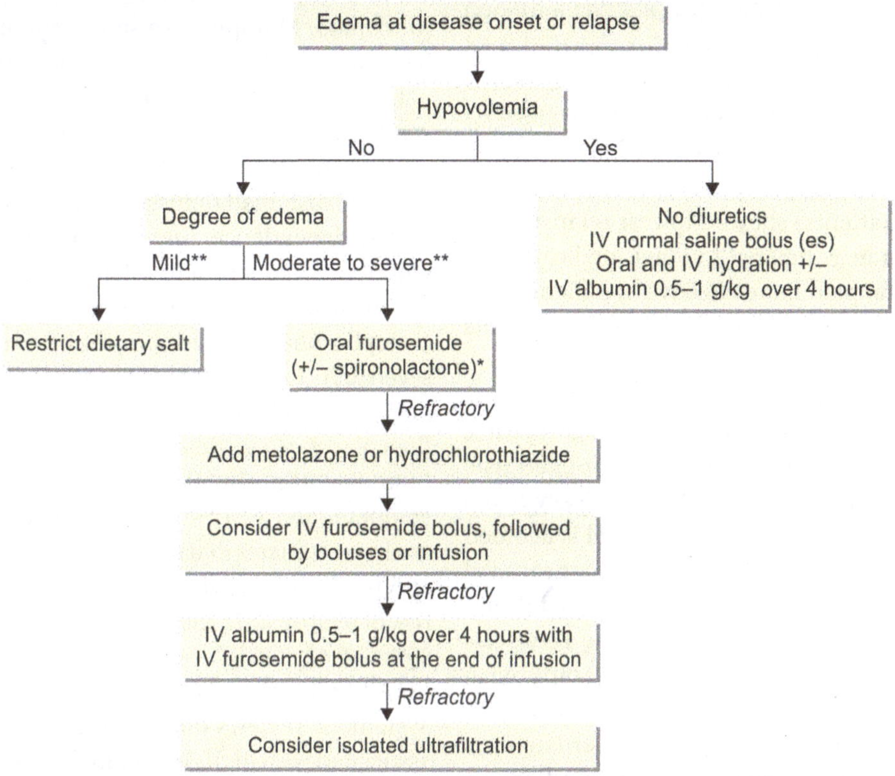

*Spironolactone (1–4 mg/kg/day) should be added to prevent hypokalemia if furosemide use is prolonged (>48 hours).
**Severity of edema graded empirically as: mild if ≤7% increase in body weight, moderate if 7–15% increase in body weight, and severe if 15% increase in body weight.

features of corticosteroid toxicity.[5] The agents used are listed in **Table 2.** Based on the findings of meta-analysis that indicate lack of efficacy of mizoribine and azathioprine and concerns with toxicity of chlorambucil,[40] these agents are no longer recommended for the management of frequent relapses or steroid dependence.[5,21]

Levamisole: This is an effective steroid-sparing agent, especially in patients with frequent relapses or mild steroid dependence.[41] Results of meta-analysis on data from eight RCTs including 462 patients suggest 35% reduction in risk of relapses following 6–12 months of therapy with levamisole (RR 0.65; 95% CI 0.48–0.88).[40] Based on results of three RCTs, the risk of relapses appears to be comparable for levamisole and either MMF or cyclophosphamide.[40] Levamisole is given at a dose of 2–2.5 mg/kg on alternate days **(Table 2).** Since levamisole does not reduce steroid requirement substantially, patients with high threshold or marked steroid toxicity do not do well, and require the use of potent agents. Uncontrolled retrospective studies on the daily use of levamisole appear to indicate its efficacy versus therapy on alternate days; however, the safety of this strategy should be examined in controlled studies with close monitoring for adverse effects **(Table 2).**[5]

Mycophenolate mofetil: MMF inhibits inosine monophosphate dehydrogenase, thus inhibiting lymphocyte proliferation. Several uncontrolled, retrospective, and prospective studies report that MMF (dose 600–1,200 mg/m^2/day or 20–33 mg/kg/day) has steroid-sparing effects and reduces relapse rates without causing significant toxicity in patients with frequent relapses or steroid dependence.[40,42] MMF was comparable to levamisole but inferior to cyclosporine in maintaining satisfactory remission or reducing the frequency of relapses in three open-label RCTs.[40] MMF is perhaps more effective in young children,[43] and may be more effective than levamisole in patients with steroid dependence.[44]

Therapy with MMF is given in two divided doses, 600–1,200 mg/m^2/day (20–30 mg/kg).[5] Side effects include leukopenia, abdominal pain, and diarrhea. There is evidence that therapy with MMF should be monitored by drug levels; targeting area under the curve >45–60 µg.h/mL or trough levels >2–3 µg/mL ensures satisfactory remission.[45-47] In the absence of facilities for therapeutic drug monitoring, therapy may be initiated at the lower end of dose range and escalating as tolerated to 1,000–1,200 mg/m^2, if patients continue to relapse.[5]

Alkylating agents: Oral cyclophosphamide is the most commonly used steroid-sparing agent in SSNS. A systematic review or 38 prospective and retrospective studies including 1,504 patients administered cyclophosphamide or chlorambucil indicated significant reduction in relapses and high proportions in sustained remission at 1–2 years of follow-up.[48] A meta-analysis of six RCTs (n = 202 patients) comparing cyclophosphamide or chlorambucil and prednisone to prednisone alone shows that these agents reduce the risk of relapse at 6–12 months (RR 0.44; 95% CI 0.32–0.60) and 12–24 months (four studies, 59 patients; RR 0.20; 95% CI 0.09–0.46).[40] A Bayesian network analysis (seven reports, 391 patients) showed lowest relapse rates with cyclophosphamide, compared to other medications.[49] Overall, these agents appear more effective in patients with frequent relapses than in steroid dependence and in patients older than 5–7 years.[5]

Adverse effects are common with both alkylating agents, including leukopenia (most common), hemorrhagic cystitis, alopecia, nausea and vomiting, and with prolonged use, gonadal toxicity and malignancies. While the efficacy of the two agents is similar, therapy with chlorambucil is avoided due to high toxicity, including seizures. Given concerns of toxicity, therapy with cyclophosphamide usually follows failure of levamisole or MMF, and limited to one 12-weeks' course (cumulative dose ~168 mg/kg). Therapy with cyclophosphamide is initiated during remission. Prednisolone is coadministered at a dose of ~1 mg/kg on alternate days during therapy with cyclophosphamide; the medication may be stopped after 1–2 months. The efficacy of IV and oral cyclophosphamide is perhaps similar; the former might be a choice if there are concerns about compliance with oral therapy.[5]

Calcineurin inhibitors: Cyclosporine A (CsA) and tacrolimus maintain remission and enable steroid sparing in 60–90% patients with steroid-dependent nephrotic syndrome who fail treatment with alkylating agents.[50-52] The efficacy of these agents relative to placebo or to each other has not been examined for steroid-sensitive disease. One RCT each found that cyclosporine was associated with reduced risk of relapse as compared to prednisolone, alkylating agents, or MMF; patients usually relapsed when therapy was discontinued.[40] Experience on use of tacrolimus is limited to nonrandomized studies but the agent is preferred due to lack of cosmetic adverse effects (hirsutism, gum hyperplasia; **Table 2**).[5]

Chief adverse effects include acute and chronic nephrotoxicity (both agents); hypertension and hyperlipidemia (chiefly CsA); and diarrhea, hypomagnesemia, and hyperglycemia (chiefly tacrolimus). Given their superior efficacy but high risk of toxicity, therapy with CNI, either cyclosporine or tacrolimus, is reserved for patients with difficult-to-treat SSNS.[5] These agents may also be preferred in patients with high threshold relapses or significant corticosteroid toxicity if other agents cannot be used. With either agent, therapy should be given for at least 12 months with monitoring of drug levels (target trough 4–7 ng/mL for tacrolimus; 80–150 ng/mL for CsA).[5] Renal biopsy is indicated before initiating therapy with CNIs and following their prolonged use.

Rituximab: Multiple case series, summarized in a review,[53] have reported benefits of B-cell depletion with rituximab in patients with difficult-to-treat steroid-dependent nephrotic syndrome. Treatment with one or more doses of rituximab results in remission lasting 3–12 months, with 25–83% patients showing sustained remission. In a series of 101 patients with steroid dependence, therapy with rituximab was associated with 81.8% reduction in relapse rates.[54] In nonrandomized comparisons, the efficacy of rituximab was superior to cyclophosphamide and comparable to tacrolimus.[5] Data from seven RCTs in patients with frequent relapses and steroid and/or CNI dependence indicates that rituximab is more effective than placebo (2 studies, 71 patients) or no additional therapy (2 studies, 91 patients) and has similar or superior efficacy as compared to CNI (2 studies, 174 patients).[40] A recent meta-analysis estimates that therapy with rituximab along with CNI and prednisolone, versus the latter two agents, reduced the risk of relapse at 12 months (3 studies, 198 patients; RR 0.63, 95% CI 0.42–0.93).[40]

Adverse effects are common after therapy with rituximab. Systematic reviews indicate that therapy with rituximab is associated with high risk of infusion reactions (4 studies, 252 children; RR 5.8, 95% CI 1.3–25.3),[40] delayed adverse events,[53] serious infections (incidence: 5.3 per 100 patient-years),[55] and risk of reactivation of hepatitis B virus infection (9%; 95% CI 5–15%).[56] Hypogammaglobulinemia is common, particularly in young children and following repeated doses.[57-59]

Based on considerations of safety as well as efficacy, the revised ISPN guidelines recommend that treatment with rituximab be reserved for patients with steroid-dependent nephrotic syndrome who fail to respond to conventional agents (difficult steroid-sensitive disease) and follow therapy with CNI.[5] Therapy is administered while in steroid-induced remission, after ensuring that acute infections, tuberculosis, and chronic viremia have been ruled out. Therapy should be avoided in young children (<5–7 years old). The medication is given as a slow IV infusion in a dose of 375 mg/m² IV once a week for two doses, under the supervision of a pediatric nephrologist. If B-cell depletion (CD19+ cells <1% of CD45+ cells, or <5 cells/μL) is not achieved,[57] a maximum of four infusions may be given. Patients should be monitored for infections, leukopenia, and hypogammaglobulinemia during follow-up. B-cell recovery usually occurs by 6–9 months and is associated with risk of relapses. Options to sustain remission include redosing after recurrence of frequent relapses (redosing when B-cell repopulation is detected) or additional immunosuppression (e.g., with MMF); however, the optimal strategy is not clear. Prophylactic antibiotics (e.g., cotrimoxazole, at 150 mg/m² or 5 mg/kg of trimethoprim on alternate days) should be considered in patients receiving intense immunosuppression.[5]

Supportive Care

Patients with SSNS are at a significant risk of complications associated with disease relapses as well as adverse effects due to medications. The principles of management of supportive care are outlined in **Table 3**. Parents should be explained the natural history of the disease and the need for long-term monitoring, while emphasizing on ensuring normal diet and physical activity as for healthy children. Patients with frequently relapsing illness requiring repeated use of corticosteroids in high doses should be monitored closely for development of hypertension, growth retardation, obesity, and ocular complications. Given the risk of hypothalamic-pituitary suppression, patients who have been treated with oral corticosteroids for more than 2 weeks within the past 1 year should receive prednisolone at 15 g/m² (0.5 mg/kg) during conditions associated with physiological stress (fever ≥38°C, systemic infections, inadequate oral intake, lethargy, dehydration, invasive surgery, dental surgery, trauma, and large burns). "Stress" dosing is not required during uncomplicated viral or bacterial infections.

Disease relapses are associated with risk of hypovolemia, edema, severe infections, and AKI. The revised guidelines on SSNS discuss the management of these conditions and provide guidance on immunization.[5] **Flowchart 2** outlines the management of patients presenting with edema, the most common complication associated with relapses. Hypovolemia needs to be excluded in all children presenting in a relapse state with or without edema, particularly in a setting of vomiting, diarrhea, reduced oral intake, or unsupervised diuretic use.[60,61] Suggestive clinical features include history of abdominal pain, vomiting, postural hypotension, lethargy, prolonged capillary refill time, cold extremities, tachycardia, low-volume pulses, or hypotension. Biochemical parameters that indicate hypovolemia include an elevated hematocrit and an increased blood urea (mg/dL) to creatinine (mg/dL) ratio >100, low fractional excretion of sodium (<0.5%), and high urinary potassium index (>0.6).[36,37] The severity of edema was graded empirically as mild if ≤7% increase in body weight, moderate if 7–15% increase in body weight, and severe if >15% increase in body weight.[37,62] Patients with mild edema usually do not require diuretics; edema resolves with reduction in salt intake and therapy of relapse leading to steady improvement. Oral furosemide is usually sufficient in managing moderate edema associated with steroid-sensitive disease. Spironolactone should be added to prevent hypokalemia if furosemide use is prolonged (>48 hours). More severe cases benefit for the additional use of a thiazide diuretic or switch to IV furosemide; IV albumin is required in a subgroup of patients, particularly those with concomitant hypovolemia and nonresponse to hydration.[37,61]

OUTCOMES

Most patients with SSNS show satisfactory outcomes. The frequency of relapses declines with age; however, a fair proportion continue to have active disease in adulthood, particularly in children with early age at onset and frequently relapsing disease course.[3,4,63,64] Less than 1% children develop kidney failure. Morbidity due to severe infections, associated with disease relapses and immunosuppression, has declined with prompt diagnosis and immunization practices; however, they remain the chief cause of hospitalization and

TABLE 3: Principles of supportive care to reduce symptoms and/or complications.

Diet and lifestyle	• Ensure adequate caloric and protein intake; avoid restricting physical activity • During moderate-to-severe edema: Increase protein intake and restrict salt intake
Growth	Monitor anthropometry q 6–12 months
Hypertension	Monitor blood pressure q 6–12 months; prefer ACEI/ARB to treat hypertension
Infections	• Vaccinate against common pathogens as in national program; avoid live vaccines while on immunosuppression • Ensure vaccination against *Pneumococcus*, varicella, influenza, and hepatitis B infections • Consider IV VZIG or oral acyclovir in susceptible patients exposed to varicella or zoster • Consider cotrimoxazole prophylaxis in patients receiving immunosuppression with more than one nonsteroidal medication
Hypovolemia	• Rule out in all patients with edema, particularly in a setting of vomiting, diarrhea, low intake, or fever **(Flowchart 2)** • Avoid diuretics and ACEI/ARB; administer oral or IV fluids, consider IV albumin (20–25%; 0.5–1 g/kg over 4 hours)
Edema	Rule out hypovolemia; manage as outlined in **Flowchart 2**
Thrombosis	Rule out in the setting of hypovolemia with specific clinical features; administer low-molecular-weight heparin for 3 months
Acute kidney injury	Monitor for during relapse with edema or hypovolemia, particularly if receiving/received ACEI/ARB, diuretics, NSAIDs, radiocontrast, or nephrotoxic drugs recently; manage as per standard guidelines

(ACEI: angiotensin-converting enzyme inhibitor; ARB: angiotensin receptor blocker; IV: intravenous; NSAIDs: nonsteroidal anti-inflammatory drugs; VZIG: varicella-zoster immunoglobulin)

mortality.[3,4,39,40] Steroid toxicity remains a major concern, particularly in patients with frequent relapses or steroid dependence, including short stature, obesity, hypertension, metabolic bone disease, diabetes mellitus, and ocular complications.[39,40] Patients who continue to relapse in adolescence or have features of steroid toxicity should be transitioned into care by nephrologists.

CONCLUSION

Research on pathogenesis emphasizes the importance of immune dysregulation and circulating factors that alter podocyte function and permselectivity of the filtration barrier; however, a unifying pathway to explain disease causation is lacking. The initial episode of nephrotic syndrome is treated with a 12-week course of prednisolone, and tapering of therapy over a prolonged period is not recommended. Relapses are conventionally managed with a short course of prednisolone; future studies are likely to confirm whether a lower dose and shorter duration of therapy may suffice. Management of patients with frequently relapsing and steroid-dependent disease course is challenging. Evidence from clinical studies on safety and efficacy of levamisole, cyclophosphamide, MMF, CNIs, and rituximab has allowed for a stepwise approach to the use of these agents in managing patients with frequent relapses or steroid dependence. Ongoing studies are necessary to consolidate recommendations on the relative effectiveness and safety of therapies as well as inform on long-term outcomes.

KEY POINTS

- Nephrotic syndrome is characterized by edema, heavy proteinuria (>1 g/m²/day; >40 mg/m²/h), and hypoalbuminemia (serum albumin <3 g/dL).
- The first episode of nephrotic syndrome is treated with prednisolone 2 mg/kg (60 mg/m²) daily for 6 weeks and then 1.5 mg/kg (40 mg/m²) on alternate days for 6 weeks.
- More than 80% of children with idiopathic nephrotic syndrome show remission following therapy with oral corticosteroids.
- Almost 70–80% of patients with steroid-sensitive disease exhibit disease relapses, often within a year since onset.
- Frequent relapses and steroid dependence are more common in patients with age at onset below 3 years, delayed time to initial remission, brief corticosteroid therapy at onset, and short duration of initial remission.
- Patients with SSNS are at significant risk of complications associated with disease relapses as well as adverse effects due to medications.
- Levamisole, cyclophosphamide, MMF, CNIs, and rituximab are used in the management of frequent relapses or steroid dependence.

REFERENCES

1. Noone DG, Iijima K, Parekh R. Idiopathic nephrotic syndrome in children. Lancet. 2018;392:61-74.
2. Banh THM, Hussain-Shamsy N, Patel V, Vasilevska-Ristovska J, Borges K, Sibbald C, et al. Ethnic differences in incidence and outcomes of childhood nephrotic syndrome. Clin J Am Soc Nephrol. 2016;11:1760-8.
3. Tarshish P, Tobin JN, Bernstein J, Edelmann CM Jr. Prognostic significance of the early course of minimal change nephrotic syndrome: report of the International Study of Kidney Disease in Children. J Am Soc Nephrol. 1997;8:769-76.
4. Sinha A, Hari P, Sharma PK, Gulati A, Kalaivani M, Mantan M, et al. Disease course in steroid sensitive nephrotic syndrome. Indian Pediatr. 2012;49:881-7.
5. Sinha A, Bagga A, Banerjee S, Mishra K, Mehta A, Agarwal I, et al; Expert Group of Indian Society of Pediatric Nephrology. Steroid sensitive nephrotic syndrome: revised guidelines. Indian Pediatr. 2021;58:461-81.
6. Vasudevan A, Thergaonkar R, Mantan M, Sharma J, Khandelwal P, Hari P, et al; Expert Group of The Indian Society of Pediatric Nephrology. Consensus guidelines on management of steroid-resistant nephrotic syndrome. Indian Pediatr. 2021;58:650-66.
7. Churg J, Habib R, White RH. Pathology of the nephrotic syndrome in children. A report for the International Study of Kidney Disease in Children. Lancet. 1970;760:1299-302.
8. D'Agati V, Fogo A, Bruijn J, Jennette J. Pathologic classification of focal segmental glomerulosclerosis: a working proposal. Am J Kidney Dis. 2004;43:368-82.
9. Watanabe A, Feltran LS, Sampson MG. Genetics of nephrotic syndrome presenting in childhood: core curriculum 2019. Am J Kidney Dis. 2019;74:549-57.
10. Lane BM, Cason R, Esezobor CI, Gbadegesin RA. Genetics of childhood steroid sensitive nephrotic syndrome: an update. Front Pediatr. 2019;7:8.
11. Wang L, Li Q, Wang L, Li C, Yang H, Wang X, et al. The role of Th17/IL-17 in the pathogenesis of primary nephrotic syndrome in children. Kidney Blood Press Res. 2013;37:332-45.
12. Ishimoto T, Cara-Fuentes G, Wang H, Shimada M, Wasserfall CH, Winter WE, et al. Serum from minimal change patients in relapse increases CD80 expression in cultured podocytes. Pediatr Nephrol. 2013;28:1803-12.
13. Ishimoto T, Shimada M, Gabriela G, Kosugi T, Sato W, Lee PY, et al. Toll-like receptor 3 ligand, polyIC, induces proteinuria and glomerular CD80, and increases urinary CD80 in mice. Nephrol Dial Transplant. 2013;28:1439-46.
14. Zhang SY, Audard V, Fan Q, Pawlak A, Lang P, Sahali D. Immunopathogenesis of idiopathic nephrotic syndrome. Contrib Nephrol (Basel, Karger). 2011;169:94-106.
15. Kienzl-Wagner K, Waldegger S, Schneeberger S. Disease recurrence: the sword of Damocles in kidney transplantation for primary focal segmental glomerulosclerosis. Front Immunol. 2019;10:1669.
16. Königshausen E, Sellin L. Circulating permeability factors in primary focal segmental glomerulosclerosis: a review of proposed candidates. Biomed Res Int. 2016;2016:3765608.
17. Savin VJ, Sharma M, Zhou J, Genochi D, Sharma R, Srivastava T, et al. Multiple targets for novel therapy of FSGS associated with circulating permeability factor. Biomed Res Int. 2017; 2017: 6232616.
18. National Strategic Plan for Tuberculosis Elimination 2017–2025. Available from: https://tbcindia.gov.in/WriteReadData/NSP%20Draft%2020.02.2017%201.pdf. [Last accessed November 1, 2020].

19. The primary nephrotic syndrome in children. Identification of patients with minimal change nephrotic syndrome from initial response to prednisolone. A report of the International Study of Kidney Disease in Children. J Pediatr. 1981;98:556-64.
20. Ehrich JH, Brodehl J. Long versus standard prednisone therapy for initial treatment of idiopathic nephrotic syndrome in children. Arbeitsgemeinschaft fur Padiatrische Nephrologie. Eur J Pediatr. 1993;152:357-61.
21. Lombel RM, Gipson DS, Hodson EM; Kidney Disease: Improving Global Outcomes. Treatment of steroid-sensitive nephrotic syndrome: new guidelines from KDIGO. Pediatr Nephrol. 2013;28:415-26.
22. Indian Pediatric Nephrology Group, Indian Academy of Pediatrics, Bagga A, Ali U, Banerjee S, Kanitkar M, Phadke KD, Senguttuvan P, et al. Management of steroid sensitive nephrotic syndrome: revised guidelines. Indian Pediatr. 2008;45:203-14.
23. Hodson EM, Willis NS, Craig JC. Corticosteroid therapy for nephrotic syndrome in children. Cochrane Database Syst Rev. 2007;4:CD001533.
24. Teeninga N, Kist-van Holthe J, van Rijskwijk N, de Mos NI, Hop WC, Wetzels JF, et al. Extending prednisolone therapy does not reduce relapse in childhood nephrotic syndrome. J Am Soc Nephrol. 2012;24:149-59.
25. Sinha A, Saha A, Kumar M, Sharma S, Afzal K, Mehta A, et al. Extending initial prednisolone treatment in a randomized control trial from 3 to 6 months did not significantly influence the course of illness in children with steroid-sensitive nephrotic syndrome. Kidney Int. 2015;87:217-24.
26. Yoshikawa N, Nakanishi K, Sako M, Oba MS, Mori R, Ota E, et al; Japanese Study Group of Kidney Disease in Children. A multicenter randomized trial indicates initial prednisolone treatment for childhood nephrotic syndrome for two months is not inferior to six-month treatment. Kidney Int. 2015;87: 225-32.
27. Webb NJA, Woolley RL, Lambe T, Frew E, Brettell EA, Barsoum EN, et al; PREDNOS Collaborative Group. Long term tapering versus standard prednisolone treatment for first episode of childhood nephrotic syndrome: phase III randomized controlled trial and economic evaluation. BMJ. 2019;365:l1800.
28. Hahn D, Samuel S, Willis NS, Craig JC, Hodson EM. Corticosteroid therapy for nephrotic syndrome in children. Cochrane Database Syst Rev. 2020; CD001533.
29. Ekka BK, Bagga A, Srivastava RN. Single- versus divided-dose prednisolone therapy for relapses of nephrotic syndrome. Pediatr Nephrol. 1997;11:597-9.
30. Emma F, Montini G, Gargiulo A. Equations to estimate prednisone dose using body weight. Pediatr Nephrol. 2019;34: 685-8.
31. Hirano D, Fujinaga S. Two dosing regimens for steroid therapy in nephrotic syndrome. Pediatr Nephrol. 2014;29:325.
32. Saadeh SA, Baracco R, Jain A, Kapur G, Mattoo TK, Valentini RP. Weight or body surface area dosing of steroids in nephrotic syndrome: is there an outcome difference? Pediatr Nephrol. 2011;26:2167-71.
33. Raman V, Krishnamurthy S, Harichandrakumar KT. Body weight-based prednisolone versus body surface area-based prednisolone regimen for induction of remission in children with nephrotic syndrome: a randomized, open-label, equivalence clinical trial. Pediatr Nephrol. 2016;31:595-604.
34. Kainth D, Hari P, Sinha A, Pandey S, Bagga A. Short-duration prednisolone in children with nephrotic syndrome relapse: a noninferiority randomized controlled trial. Clin J Am Soc Nephrol. 2021;16:225-32.
35. Sheikh S, Mishra K, Kumar M. Low-dose versus conventional-dose prednisolone for nephrotic syndrome relapses: a randomized controlled non-inferiority trial. Pediatr Nephrol. 2021;36:3143-50.
36. Abeyagunawardena AS, Thalgahagoda RS, Dissanayake PV, Abeyagunawardena S, Illangasekera YA, Karunadasa UI, et al. Short courses of daily prednisolone during upper respiratory tract infections reduce relapse frequency in childhood nephrotic syndrome. Pediatr Nephrol. 2017;32:1377-82.
37. Leisti S, Hallman N, Koskimies O, Perheentupa J, Rapola J, Vilska J. Association of postmedication hypocortisolism with early first relapse of idiopathic nephrotic syndrome. Lancet. 1977;2:795-6.
38. Srivastava RN, Vasudev AS, Bagga A, Sunderam KR. Long-term, low-dose prednisolone therapy in frequently relapsing nephrotic syndrome. Pediatr Nephrol. 1992;6:247-50.
39. Yadav M, Sinha A, Khandelwal P, Hari P, Bagga A. Efficacy of low-dose daily versus alternate-day prednisolone in frequently relapsing nephrotic syndrome: an open-label randomized controlled trial. Pediatr Nephrol. 2019;34:829-35.
40. Larkins NG, Liu ID, Willis NS, Craig JC, Hodson EM. Non-corticosteroid immunosuppressive medications for steroid-sensitive nephrotic syndrome in children. Cochrane Database Syst Rev. 2020;4:CD002290.
41. Mühlig AK, Lee JY, Kemper MJ, Kronbichler A, Yang JW, Lee JM, et al. Levamisole in children with idiopathic nephrotic syndrome: clinical efficacy and pathophysiological aspects. J Clin Med. 2019;8:860.
42. Querfeld U, Weber LT. Mycophenolate mofetil for sustained remission in nephrotic syndrome. Pediatr Nephrol. 2018;33: 2253-65.
43. Jellouli M, Fitouhi S, Abidi K, Hammi Y, Naija O, Zarrouk C, et al. Mycophenolate mofetil in treatment of childhood steroid-dependent nephrotic syndrome. Tunis Med. 2016;94:221-5.
44. Sinha A, Puraswani M, Kalaivani M, Goyal P, Hari P, Bagga A. Efficacy and safety of mycophenolate mofetil versus levamisole in frequently relapsing nephrotic syndrome: an open-label randomized controlled trial. Kidney Int. 2019;95:210-8.
45. Fujinaga S, Ohtomo Y, Umino D, Takemoto M, Shimizu T, Yamashiro Y, et al. A prospective study on the use of mycophenolate mofetil in children with cyclosporine-dependent nephrotic syndrome. Pediatr Nephrol. 2007;22:71-6.
46. Fujinaga S, Ohtomo Y, Hirano D, Nishizaki N, Someya T, Ohtsuka Y, et al. Mycophenolate mofetil therapy for childhood-onset steroid dependent nephrotic syndrome after long-term cyclosporine: extended experience in a single center. Clin Nephrol. 2009;72:268-73.
47. Gellermann J, Weber L, Pape L, Tönshoff B, Hoyer P, Querfeld U, for the Gesellschaft für Pädiatrische Nephrologie (GPN). Mycophenolate mofetil versus cyclosporin A in children with frequently relapsing nephrotic syndrome. J Am Soc Nephrol. 2013;24:1689-97.
48. Latta K, von Schnakenburg C, Ehrich JH. A meta-analysis of cytotoxic treatment for frequently relapsing nephrotic syndrome in children. Pediatr Nephrol. 2001;16:271-82.
49. Fu HD, Qian GL, Jiang ZY. Comparison of second-line immunosuppressants for childhood refractory nephrotic syndrome: a systematic review and network meta-analysis. J Investig Med. 2017;65:65-71.
50. Arslansoyu Camlar S, Soylu A, Kavukçu S. Cyclosporine in pediatric nephrology. Iran J Kidney Dis. 2018;12:319-30.
51. Hao GX, Song LL, Zhang DF, Su LQ, Jacqz-Aigrain E, Zhao W. Off-label use of tacrolimus in children with glomerular disease: effectiveness, safety and pharmacokinetics. Br J Clin Pharmacol. 2020;86:274-84.

52. Sinha A, Bagga A, Gulati A, Hari P. Short-term efficacy of rituximab versus tacrolimus in steroid-dependent nephrotic syndrome. Pediatr Nephrol. 2012;27:235-41.
53. Sinha A, Bagga A. Rituximab therapy in nephrotic syndrome: implications for patients' management. Nat Rev Nephrol. 2013;9:154-69.
54. Sinha A, Bhatia D, Gulati A, Rawat M, Dinda AK, Hari P, et al. Efficacy and safety of rituximab in children with difficult-to-treat nephrotic syndrome. Nephrol Dial Transplant. 2015;30: 96-106.
55. Tony HP, Burmester G, Schulze-Koops H, Grunke M, Henes J, Kötter I, et al; GRAID investigators. Safety and clinical outcomes of rituximab therapy in patients with different autoimmune diseases: experience from a national registry (GRAID). Arthritis Res Ther. 2011;13:R75.
56. Tang Z, Li X, Wu S, Liu Y, Qiao Y, Xu D, et al. Risk of hepatitis B reactivation in HBsAg-negative/HBcAb-positive patients with undetectable serum HBV DNA after treatment with rituximab for lymphoma: a meta-analysis. Hepatol Int. 2017;11: 429-33.
57. Khojah AM, Miller ML, Klein-Gitelman MS, Curran ML, Hans V, Pachman LM, et al. Rituximab-associated hypogammaglobulinemia in pediatric patients with autoimmune diseases. Pediatr Rheumatol Online J. 2019;17:61.
58. Parmentier C, Delbet JD, Decramer S, Boyer O, Hogan J, Ulinski T. Immunoglobulin serum levels in rituximab-treated patients with steroid-dependent nephrotic syndrome. Pediatr Nephrol. 2020;35:455-62.
59. Colucci M, Carsetti R, Serafinelli J, Rocca S, Massella L, Gargiulo A, et al. Prolonged impairment of immunological memory after anti-CD20 treatment in pediatric idiopathic nephrotic syndrome. Front Immunol. 2019;10:1653.
60. Büyükavci MA, Çivilibal M, Elevli M, Selçuk Duru HN. Hypo- and hypervolemic edema in children with steroid sensitive nephrotic syndrome. Turk J Med Sci. 2015;45:178-83.
61. Meena J, Bagga A. Current perspectives in management of edema in nephrotic syndrome. Indian J Pediatr. 2020;87:633-40.
62. Kaku Y, Ohtsuka Y, Komatsu Y, Ohta T, Nagai T, Kaito H, et al; Japanese Society for Pediatric Nephrology. Clinical practice guideline for pediatric idiopathic nephrotic syndrome 2013: General therapy. Clin Exp Nephrol. 2015;19:34-53.
63. Hjorten R, Anwar Z, Reidy KJ. Long-term outcomes of childhood onset nephrotic syndrome. Front Pediatr. 2016;4:53.
64. Marchel DM, Gipson DS. Adult survivors of idiopathic childhood onset nephrotic syndrome. Pediatr Nephrol. 2021;36: 1731-7.

CHAPTER

6.3 Steroid-resistant Nephrotic Syndrome

Anil Vasudevan, Aditi Sinha, Arvind Bagga

INTRODUCTION

Therapy with oral prednisolone is the treatment of choice in children with nephrotic syndrome (NS). More than 80–85% of children with NS respond to corticosteroids; 15–20% remain unresponsive to steroids and is associated with unfavorable prognosis; 36–50% of the children with steroid-resistant nephrotic syndrome (SRNS) progress to end-stage kidney disease (ESKD) within 10 years of diagnosis.

DEFINITION

Steroid resistance is a clinical diagnosis and is defined as lack of complete remission despite 6 weeks of therapy with prednisolone **(Box 1)**. Those children who do not achieve complete remission in the first episode is referred to as initial SRNS and form majority of SRNS. Children who develop steroid resistance later in the clinical course is referred to as late-onset SRNS. The common histopathological entities observed in SRNS are focal and segmental glomerulosclerosis (FSGS), minimal change disease (MCD), and mesangial proliferative glomerulonephritis. The most common histological variant of NS in children is MCD, accounting for approximately 80% of cases.[1]

BOX 1: Definitions related to steroid-resistant nephrotic syndrome.

- *Steroid-resistant nephrotic syndrome**: Failure to achieve complete remission after 6 weeks of therapy with prednisolone at a dose of 60 mg/m^2/day (2 mg/kg/day; maximum 60 mg/day)
- *Complete remission:* Urine protein nil-trace by dipstick for 3 consecutive days, Up/Uc <0.2, or 24-hour protein <100 mg/m^2/day
- *Partial remission:* Urine protein 1+/2+ (dipstick), Up/Uc between 0.2 and 2, or 24-hour urine protein 100–1,000 mg/m^2/day; serum albumin ≥3.0 g/dL; and absence of edema
- *Nonresponse:* Urine protein 3+/4+ (dipstick), Up/Uc >2, or 24-hour urine protein >1,000 mg/m^2/day; albumin <3.0 g/dL or edema
- *Monogenic disease:* Pathogenic or likely pathogenic variation, defined by American College of Medical Genetics and Genomics, in a gene associated with nephrotic syndrome **(Tables 1 and 2)**
- *CNI-resistant disease:* Nonresponse to cyclosporine or tacrolimus, given in adequate doses and titrated to blood levels, for 6 months
- *Recurrence of nephrotic syndrome postrenal transplantation:* Persistent proteinuria (Up/Uc >1) if previously anuric; or increase of Up/Uc >1 if proteinuria at time of transplant (in the absence of other apparent causes)

*Similar definition for initial and late-onset resistance; patients with steroid toxicity may receive daily prednisolone for 4 weeks, followed by alternate-day therapy for 2 weeks.

(CNI: calcineurin inhibitor; Up/Uc: urine protein to creatinine ratio [mg/mg])

EPIDEMIOLOGY

The proportion of FSGS in India ranges from 15.3 to 39.1%.[2-4] The estimated prevalence of SRNS is 0.5–2/100,000.[5] However, disease burden varies with geographical location and ethnicity. In an analysis of studies published from 1946 to 2014 from different regions of the world, the average incidence of NS was 4.7 (range 1.15–16.9) per 100,000 persons and proportion with steroid resistance varied between 2.1 and 27.3% (average of 12.4%).[6] Asians, particularly south Asians, are reported to have higher proportion of SRNS when compared to those from Europe and Africa with the proportion being 20, 16–27, and 27–54% among Europeans, Africans, and Asians, respectively. Although publication bias and variation in definition of SRNS may account for variability, yet to be discovered environmental and genetic factors may also play a significant role. For example, apolipoprotein L1 (APOL1) G1/G2 risk variants are strongly associated with sporadic FSGS in populations with African ancestry.[7]

ETIOLOGY AND PATHOGENESIS

Research in the last two decades highlighted the podocyte injury as the central event in NS.[8] The diffuse effacement of podocyte foot processes observed by electron microscopy in SRNS suggests a key role for the podocyte in the pathogenesis of idiopathic SRNS. This may be either due to alteration of a structural component of the foot process from mutation in a gene coding the protein or as a target of a circulating immunological factor. The distinction between the two mechanisms has a major impact on immunosuppressive management and outcomes. In literature, FSGS has been used as a corollary to SRNS. While single-gene defects and circulating factor cause idiopathic primary SRNS or FSGS, podocyte may also be the target of injury through several other mechanisms that leads to secondary SRNS or FSGS including infections [e.g., human immunodeficiency virus (HIV) infection, hepatitis B and C], medications (e.g., pamidronate, interferon), metabolic disorders (e.g., mitochondrial disorders, diabetes mellitus), malignancy (e.g., lymphomas), and deposition of an abnormal protein (e.g., amyloid) **(Box 2)**.

Monogenic Causes of Steroid-resistant Nephrotic Syndrome

Steroid-resistant nephrotic syndrome is caused by mutations in genes encoding components of the slit diaphragm, podocyte actin cytoskeleton, mitochondrial proteins, lysosomal proteins, nuclear transcription factors, and glomerular basement membrane (GBM; **Fig. 1**). The advent and rapid advances in next-generation sequencing (NGS) technology have greatly facilitated the identification of numerous novel causative genes. More than 80 genes are associated with the monogenic cause of SRNS **(Tables 1 and 2)**. These genes encode either proteins that are part of the structural component of slit diaphragm or are intracellular proteins involved in regulating establishment and maintenance of podocyte structure and function. The genetic mutations may be acquired in an autosomal recessive (e.g., *NPHS1*, *NPHS2*, and *PLCe1*) or dominant fashion (e.g., *INF2*, *TRPC6*, and *ACTN4*) or both (e.g., *WT1*). SRNS caused by mutations in autosomal-recessive genes tend to present early in childhood while SRNS due to autosomal-dominant genes tend to have varying degrees of penetrance and severity and typically present later in childhood or in young adulthood. Although the prevalence of monogenic SRNS is unknown due to the dearth of population-based studies, cohort studies indicate that 25–30% of the children with SRNS have an underlying genetic cause with a higher proportion in familial SRNS (50–70%).[9] However, there is limited information on the prevalence of monogenic variations in Indian patients with SRNS.[10,11]

BOX 2: Etiology of steroid-resistant nephrotic syndrome.

- Primary/idiopathic
- Hereditary diseases **(Tables 1 and 2)**
- *Infections:* Hepatitis C, hepatitis B, HIV infection, parvovirus B19, malaria
- *Drugs/toxic agents:* Interferon-α, pamidronate, lithium, gold, heroin
- *Hyperfiltration**: Bilateral or unilateral renal dysplasia, obesity, reflux nephropathy
- *Others:* Mitochondrial diseases, amyloidosis

(HIV: human immunodeficiency virus)
*Causes secondary focal and segmental glomerulosclerosis (FSGS).

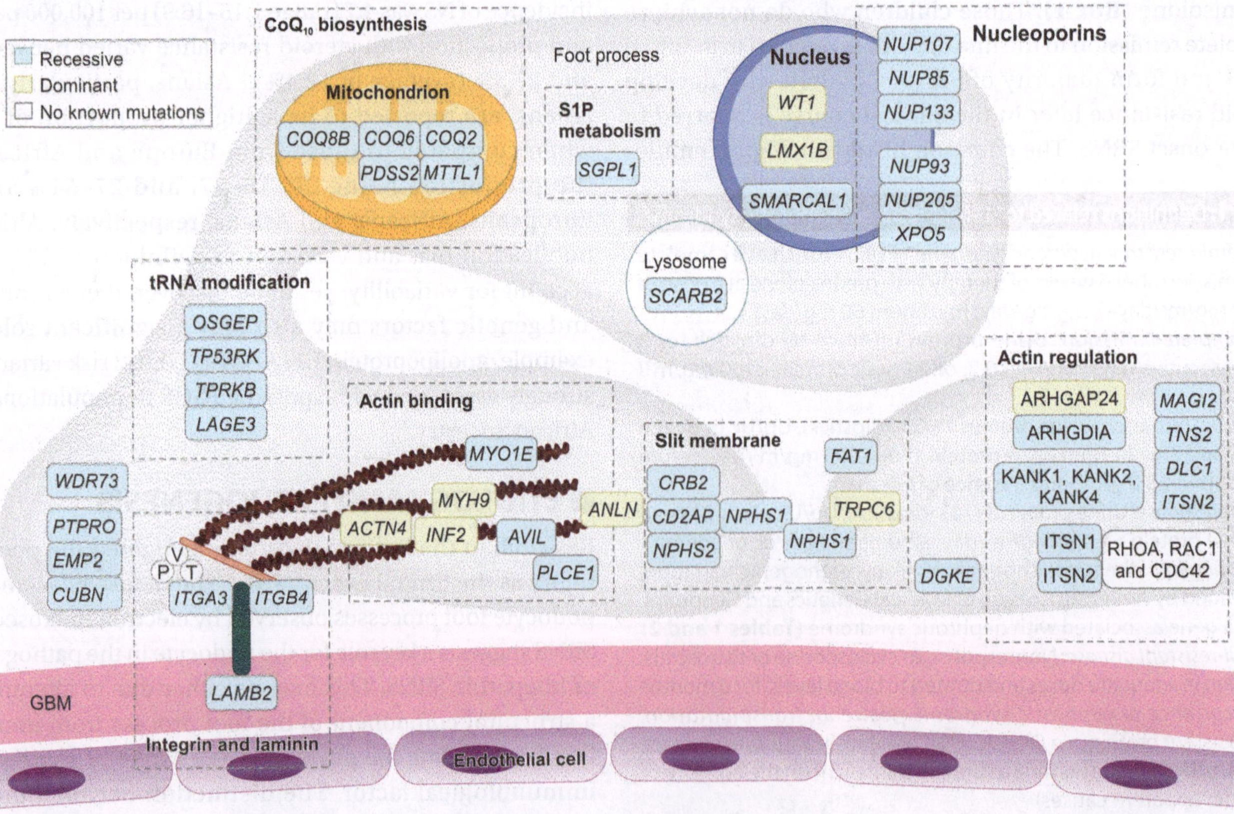

Fig. 1: Monogenetic causes of steroid-resistant nephrotic syndrome (SRNS). Figure represents the foot process of podocyte. Foot processes interdigitate with those from neighboring podocytes, forming the glomerular slit membrane, which is critical for filtering and retention of protein in the bloodstream. Its integrity is lost in nephrotic syndrome. Proteins encoded by genes that, if mutated, cause monogenic SRNS localize to specific subcellular sites of podocytes depicted here.
Source: Kopp JB, Anders HJ, Susztak, K, Podestà MA, Remuzzi G, Hildebrandt F, et al. Podocytopathies. Nat Rev Dis Primers. 2020;6:68.

TABLE 1: Genes associated with steroid-resistant nephrotic syndrome grouped according to the location of corresponding proteins in podocyte.

Location of proteins	*Genes*
Slit diaphragm–associated proteins	*NPHS1, NPHS2, PLCE1, CD2AP, TRPC6, CRB2, FAT1*
Cytoskeletal and membrane proteins	*ACTN4, INF2, MYH9, MYO1E, MAGI2, ANLN, ARHGAP24, ARHGDIA, KANK, 1/2/4, SYNPO, PTPRO, EMP2, APOL1, CUBN, PODXL, TNS2, DLC1, CDK20, ITSN1, ITSN2*
Glomerular basement membrane–associated proteins	*LAMB2, ITGB4, ITGA3, COL4A3/4/5, GPC5, CD151*
Mitochondrial proteins	*COQ2, COQ6, PDSS2, ADCK4, MTTL1*
Lysosomal and endocytic proteins	*SCARB2, OCRL1*
Metabolic and cytosolic proteins	*ZMPSTE24, PMM2, ALG1, TTC21B, CFH, DGKE*
Nuclear pore proteins and transcription factors	*NUP93, NUP205, XPO5, WT1, LMX1B, SMARCL1, E2F3, NX5, PAX2, WDR73*

TABLE 2: Genes associated with syndromic forms of steroid-resistant nephrotic syndrome with key phenotypic features.

Syndrome	*Gene*	*Protein*	*Function*	*Transmission*	*Histology*	*Associated features*
Denys–Drash syndrome	*WT1*	Wilms tumor protein	Podocyte development	AD	DMS	Male pseudohermaphroditism, Wilms tumor
Frasier syndrome					FSGS	Male pseudohermaphroditism, gonadoblastoma
Pierson syndrome	*LAMB2*	Laminin beta-2	Links GBM to podocyte cytoskeleton	AR	DMS	Microcoria, abnormal lens
Schimke syndrome	*SMARCAL1*	SWI/SNF-related, matrix-associated, actin-dependent regulator of chromatin, subfamily A-like protein 1	Chromatin bundling and gene transcription	AR	FSGS	Bone dysplasia, immune deficiency, ischemic cerebral lesions
Nail-patella syndrome	*LMX1B*	LIM homeodomain transcription factor 1, beta	Podocyte and GBM development	AD	FSGS	Hypoplastic nails and patellae, iliac horns
Charcot-Marie-Tooth disease	*INF2*	Inverted formin 2	Actin regulation	AD	FSGS	Neuropathy, deafness
Galloway-Mowat syndrome	*WDR73, WDR7; OSGEP, TP53RK, TPRKB, and LAGE3*	WD40 repeat-containing protein	Unknown	AR	FSGS	Microcephaly, intellectual disability, hiatal hernia, optic atrophy
Mitochondrial respiratory chain disease	*MTTL1*	Mitochondrial tRNA leucine 1	Mitochondrial tRNA	Maternal	FSGS	MELAS (mitochondrial encephalomyopathy, lactic acidosis, and stroke-like symptoms), diabetes mellitus, deafness
	COQ2	Polyprenyltransferase	Coenzyme Q10 biosynthesis	AR	FSGS	Encephalomyopathy, hypotonia, seizures, lactate acidosis
	COQ6	Ubiquinone biosynthesis monooxygenase COQ6	Coenzyme Q10 biosynthesis	AR	FSGS	Sensorineural deafness
	PDSS2	Decaprenyl diphosphate synthase, subunit 2	Coenzyme Q10 biosynthesis	AR	FSGS	Encephalomyopathy, hypotonia, seizures, lactate acidosis

(AD: autosomal dominant; AR: autosomal recessive; DMS: diffuse mesangial sclerosis; FSGS: focal segmental glomerulosclerosis; GBM: glomerular basement membrane)

The most common genes implicated in SRNS are *NPHS1*, *NPHS2*, *WT1*, *PLCe1*, and *LAMB2* and genes coding coenzyme Q10 biosynthesis pathway, *SMARCAL1*, *INF2*, *TRPC6*, and *CD2AP*.[12,13] In certain populations like African Americans, apart from monogenic causes, FSGS is also associated with two independent sequence variants in the *APOL1* gene on chromosome 22 [FSGS, odds ratio (OR) = 10.5; 95% confidence interval (CI) = 6.0–18.4].[14]

The discovery of genetic forms of SRNS has helped in better understanding of the mechanisms that contribute to podocyte dysfunction and the development of SRNS. Mutations in *NPHS1* gene coding for *nephrin* was the first gene to be discovered as a cause for monogenic forms of NS. Nephrin is an important component of slit diaphragm and acts as an intracellular signaling scaffold. Nephrin signaling occurs predominantly via the cytoplasmic tail and is phosphorylated by Src-family kinases. Nephrin along with Nck forms a complex and regulate actin polymerization via PI3K/Akt/Rac1 signaling pathways.[15] Wilms' tumor 1 (WT1) is a key transcription factor which not only plays an important role in glomerular development but also regulates other important slit diaphragm proteins by binding to the proximal promoters, such as NPHS2, synaptopodin, and Nck2. Podocin encoded by NPHS2 is a lipid raft protein which augments nephrin signaling by recruiting nephrin through interaction with Neph1.[16] Other mutations involving proteins of the slit diaphragm associated with SRNS include transient receptor potential cation channel 6 (TRPC6), a nonselective cationic channel which acts as a mechanic sensor in podocyte foot process, CD2-associated protein (CD2AP), a molècule that links slit diaphragm and actin cytoskeleton, and phospholipase C epsilon 1 (PLCe1).[17,18] Mutation in *TRPC6* can cause both gain of function and loss of function resulting in excess or reduced calcium entry into podocytes.

Glomerular epithelial protein-1 (GLEPP1), a tyrosine phosphatase expressed on podocyte foot processes, regulates glomerular pressure and nephrin content at the slit diaphragm. Mutation in *PTPRO* gene encoding GLEPP1 results in SRNS in children.[19] The specialized shape of podocyte and its foot process is due to the highly organized cytoskeleton consisting of a linearly arranged bundle of actin fibers. Dysregulation of actin cytoskeleton affects cell shape and adhesion to GBM, resulting in impaired function of the glomerular filtration barrier. Mutations that involve structural component (ACTN4, Myo1E, MYH9) or regulatory protein [IFN2, ARHGAP24, ARHGDIA, anilin (ANLN)] result in loss of this characteristic structure and are associated with SRNS.[20] Synaptopodin is a protein that interacts with α-actinin-4 and regulates cross-linking between actin filaments. Loss of synaptopodin leads to delayed stress fiber formation and development of aberrant nonpolarized filopodia leading to podocyte injury and apoptosis. Focal adhesions are specialized complexes consisting of an array of adaptor and linker molecules that connects podocytes to the extracellular matrix and underlying GBM.

Mutations in laminin β2, integrin α3, and integrin β4 genes are associated with syndromic forms of SRNS. Mutations in the structural components of GBM like type IV collagen genes (*COL4A3*, *COL4A4*, *COL4A5*) and laminin alpha 5 (*LAMA5*) can also present with SRNS.[21-24]

Mutations in genes encoding proteins involved in the nuclear function of podocytes have been implicated in genetic forms of syndromic or isolated SRNS. SMARCA-like protein (SMARCAL1) and LMX1B homeobox transcription factor 1B is associated with Schimke immuno-osseous dysplasia and nail patella syndrome, respectively.[25,26] Rho/Small GTPases, RhoA, Rac1, and Cdc42, are involved in signal cascades, endocytic pathways, and interactions of podocytes with other structures such as basement membrane. Mutations in genes that interfere with Rho GTPase signaling lead to disruption in cytoskeletal dynamics by affecting actin nucleation promoting factors, including the formin protein and WASP families leading to SRNS with variable response to immunosuppressive therapy.[27] Variants in nuclear genes encoding proteins involved in coenzyme-Q10 biosynthesis in mitochondria, i.e., *COQ2*, *PDSS2*, *COQ6*, and *COQ8B*, have also been identified in isolated or syndromic form of SRNS.

Circulating Factors

In disease not due to single-gene defect, poorly characterized soluble "circulating factor" resulting from immune dysregulation has been shown by clinical and experimental studies to be involved in the development of SRNS. The pathologic role of circulating permeability factors in causing podocyte injury and dysfunction in SRNS is supported by evidences of recurrence of proteinuria, within hours following renal transplantation and disruption of podocyte focal complexes via immunofluorescence by sera from patients with FSGS recurrence.[28,29] In ex vivo studies, sera from patients with FSGS-induced proteinuria or increased permeability of glomeruli to albumin, as compared to normal control plasma supporting the possibility of a systemic factor, involved in the pathogenesis of SRNS. However, identifying the putative factor remains elusive. Numerous factors have been identified including heparanase, hemopexin, angiopoietin-like 4 (ANGPTL4), cardiotrophin-like cytokine-1 (CLCF-1), and soluble urokinase plasminogen activator receptor (suPAR) **(Table 3)**. How these factors might cause podocyte injury and impact glomerular permeability has not been completely elucidated? Hemopexin reduces endothelial glycocalyx resulting in actin cytoskeleton disruption and causing increase in albumin diffusion. CLCF-1 isolated by galactose affinity chromatography from sera of patients with FSGS increased albumin permeability in isolated rat glomeruli through the activation of the JAK/STAT pathway, which was reversed by incubation with JAK/STAT inhibitors. A hyposialylated form of Angptl-4 secreted from podocytes

TABLE 3: Putative circulating factors identified in steroid-resistant nephrotic syndrome.

Circulating factor	*Molecular weight (kDa)*	*Major targets*
VPF	60–160	Anionic charges of endothelium
FSGS factor	30–50	Podocyte
Hemopexin	54–70	Anionic charges of podocyte endothelium
CD80 (B7-1)	55–60	Podocyte
suPAR	20–50	Podocyte integrin
CLCF-1	22	Podocyte
Angptl-4	45–65	Anionic charges
IL-13	10–17	Podocyte adaptors
IL-8	11	Anionic charges
CD40 autoantibody	150	Podocyte integrin
Heparanase	57–60	Anionic charges

(angptl-4: angiopoietin like-4; CD: cluster of differentiation; CLCF-1: cardiotrophin-like cytokine factor-1; FSGS: focal segmental glomerular sclerosis; IL-13: interleukin-13; IL-8: interleukin-8; MCD: minimal change disease; suPAR: soluble urokinase plasminogen activator receptor; VPF: vascular permeability factor)

can induce proteinuria by reducing the anionic charges of the filtration barrier. Experiments using immortalized human podocyte cell lines suggest that circulating plasma proteases in patients with active disease activate a signaling pathway downstream of protease-activated receptor 1 (PAR-1), which involves vasodilator-stimulated phosphoprotein (VASP) phosphorylation as well as phosphorylation of JNK and p38MAP kinases.[30] Apart from circulating factors, dysfunction or dysregulation of T lymphocytes have also shown to be involved in the pathogenesis of SRNS. Increase in podocyte B7-1 expression has been shown to cause podocyte dysfunction due to actin reorganization in a variety of animal models of proteinuria as well as in post-transplant FSGS recurrence.[31]

Phenotype-based on Etiology

Nephrotic syndrome caused by monogenic mutations is distinct from disease mediated by circulating factors that target the podocyte. Children with single-gene defects form a subgroup of SRNS who are initial steroid resistant, do not respond to immunosuppression, and may have a family history of SRNS and low probability of post-transplant recurrence (<5%) while the nongenetic group may initially be late-steroid resistant, demonstrate variable response to immunosuppression, and 30–40% may have recurrence of NS post renal transplantation.[32]

The likelihood of identifying a monogenic cause of SRNS decreases with increasing age with two thirds of those presenting before 1 year of age detected with a genetic cause. After 1 year of age, the chance of identifying a genetic cause for SRNS decreases substantially to 25% between the ages of 1 and 6 years, 18% between 7 and 12 years, and as low as 11% in those aged 13–18 years.[12] The probability of identifying a genetic cause increases to 50% in children with familial SRNS. In addition to isolated SRNS, several single-gene defects (monogenic mutations) also result in a syndromic form of SRNS **(Table 2)**.

CLINICAL FEATURES AND EVALUATION

Steroid-resistant nephrotic syndrome is usually diagnosed following nonresponse to steroids in the initial episode or later in the course of illness. A diligent evaluation to determine the underlying etiology and complications should be performed at the time of diagnosis of SRNS **(Box 3)**.

History and Physical Examination

Evaluation includes a thorough history including family history along with physical examination for possible underlying genetic or secondary causes. Extrarenal manifestations such as skeletal, neurological, eye, ear, and urogenital abnormalities; developmental delay; dystrophic nails; and small or absent patella indicate a syndromic cause, while history of jaundice and systemic manifestations such as rash, joint pains, and palpable purpura indicate a secondary cause. Hypertension, gross hematuria, and some degree of persistent renal insufficiency may be observed with SRNS. In contrast to rapid development of proteinuria, edema, or hypoalbuminemia, which may occur over the course of days to weeks, a more indolent course with varying degrees of proteinuria that is incidentally detected, with or without edema and presenting with features of chronic kidney disease (CKD), may be seen in children with an inherited cause. A family history of SRNS/FSGS or early onset of ESKD may be present in these groups of children.

Laboratory Investigations

Serologic testing for hepatitis B and C, HIV, and tests for lupus nephritis and other glomerular disease with antinuclear antibody (ANA) and serum complement levels also form a part of the evaluation. Quantitation of proteinuria, serum creatinine, and calculating estimated glomerular filtration rate (eGFR) should be performed in all children with SRNS. Assessment of proteinuria by spot urine protein creatinine (Up/Uc) ratio in a morning specimen or 24-hour protein excretion, at diagnosis and 6 monthly follow-up, helps determine response to therapy **(Box 1)**. In addition, parents are counseled regarding urinary dipstick analysis for home monitoring of proteinuria. Serum creatinine and eGFR should be obtained at baseline and follow-up as it helps identify acute kidney injury (AKI) secondary to hypovolemia, fluid loss, infections, and drug toxicity and also in monitoring progression of the disease to CKD.

BOX 3: Initial evaluation in steroid-resistant nephrotic syndrome.

Key tests:
- Urinalysis, including microscopy; spot urine protein to creatinine ratio; or 24-hour urine protein excretion
- Complete blood count
- Serum creatinine (eGFR), albumin, electrolytes, fasting glucose, glycosylated hemoglobin (HbA1c)
- Total, low-density and high-density cholesterol; triglycerides
- Calcium, phosphate, alkaline phosphatase, liver function test
- Ultrasonography of kidneys
- Kidney biopsy (light, immunofluorescence, electron microscopy); avoided in selected patients*

Additional tests:
- Hepatitis B surface antigen, hepatitis C, and human immunodeficiency virus antibodies
- Complement C3, C4; antinuclear antibody

Genetic test: Initial steroid-resistance with: (1) onset during infancy, (2) family history of steroid-resistance, (3) extrarenal features, (4) nonresponse to calcineurin inhibitors, and (5) prior to transplantation

*Biopsy may be avoided in patients with familial steroid-resistance or with extrarenal features, where genetic diagnosis is preferred. (eGFR: estimated glomerular filtration rate)

Renal Biopsy

Renal biopsy, an important diagnostic and prognostic tool, is mandatory for children with SRNS except in familial and/or syndromic cases or those with an identified genetic cause. A biopsy helps in (1) identifying secondary cause such as IgA nephropathy, membranous nephropathy, C3 glomerulopathy, and lupus nephritis; (2) predicting response to therapy; and (3) prognostication. Biopsies are examined by light, immunofluorescence, and electron microscopy to characterize histological features which are shown to be variable in different series depending on the age group and the population studied. Light microscopy shows three morphological patterns: MCD in one-fourth and FSGS in 35–55% of patients and mesangial proliferation in 10–15%.[33] Diffuse mesangial sclerosis is another histopathology observed in young children and is characterized by progression to ESKD in early childhood. More than 80% of children with diffuse mesangial sclerosis have an identifiable causal variant in *NPHS2*, *WT1*, *PLCe1*, or *LAMB2* gene in about 10–20% of patients; the histology shows a secondary cause such as membranous nephropathy, immunoglobulin A nephropathy (IgA-N), or membranoproliferative glomerulonephritis. Early onset FSGS may be missed if the number of glomeruli obtained in renal biopsy is <20.[34] Diffuse foot process effacement on electron microscopy supports an idiopathic cause while focal foot process effacement indicates a secondary cause of SRNS.

Focal and segmental glomerulosclerosis may have several distinctive patterns and based on the Columbia classification system, FSGS is classified into five histological variants: not otherwise specified (NOS), tip, perihilar, collapsing, and cellular (**Table 4 and Fig. 2**).[35] The collapsing glomerulopathy variant of FSGS is a major histomorphology of HIV nephropathy and may also be seen with parvovirus B19 infection, cytomegalovirus (CMV), intravenous drug abuse, and as an idiopathic process.[36] A perihilar pattern is observed

TABLE 4: Columbia classification and clinical correlates.

Columbia classification variant	*Morphology*	*Clinical correlates*
Collapsing	Hyperplasia of parietal podocyte cells with collapse of glomerular tuft	Presents with abrupt onset of severe nephrotic syndrome with poor response to steroids and CNIs; poor prognosis; seen with HIV nephropathy, parvovirus, cocaine abuse
Tip	Segmental sclerosis at the proximal tubular pole	Usually primary and frequently responds to steroids and CNI. Good outcomes
Cellular	Hyperplasia of parietal podocyte sometimes endocapillary proliferation with severe foot process effacement	Least common variant and seen in mostly with primary FSGS and sometimes in other causes of FSGS
Perihilar	Segmental sclerosis at the vascular pole	Usually seen with adaptive FSGS (single kidney, obesity); may not have the classical features of nephrotic syndrome and may only present with subnephrotic or nephrotic range of proteinuria
Not otherwise specified (NOS)	Segmental sclerosis, not meeting the features of other variants	Most common variant and could be found in any form of FSGS

(CNI: calcineurin inhibitor; FSGS: focal and segmental glomerulosclerosis; HIV: human immunodeficiency virus)

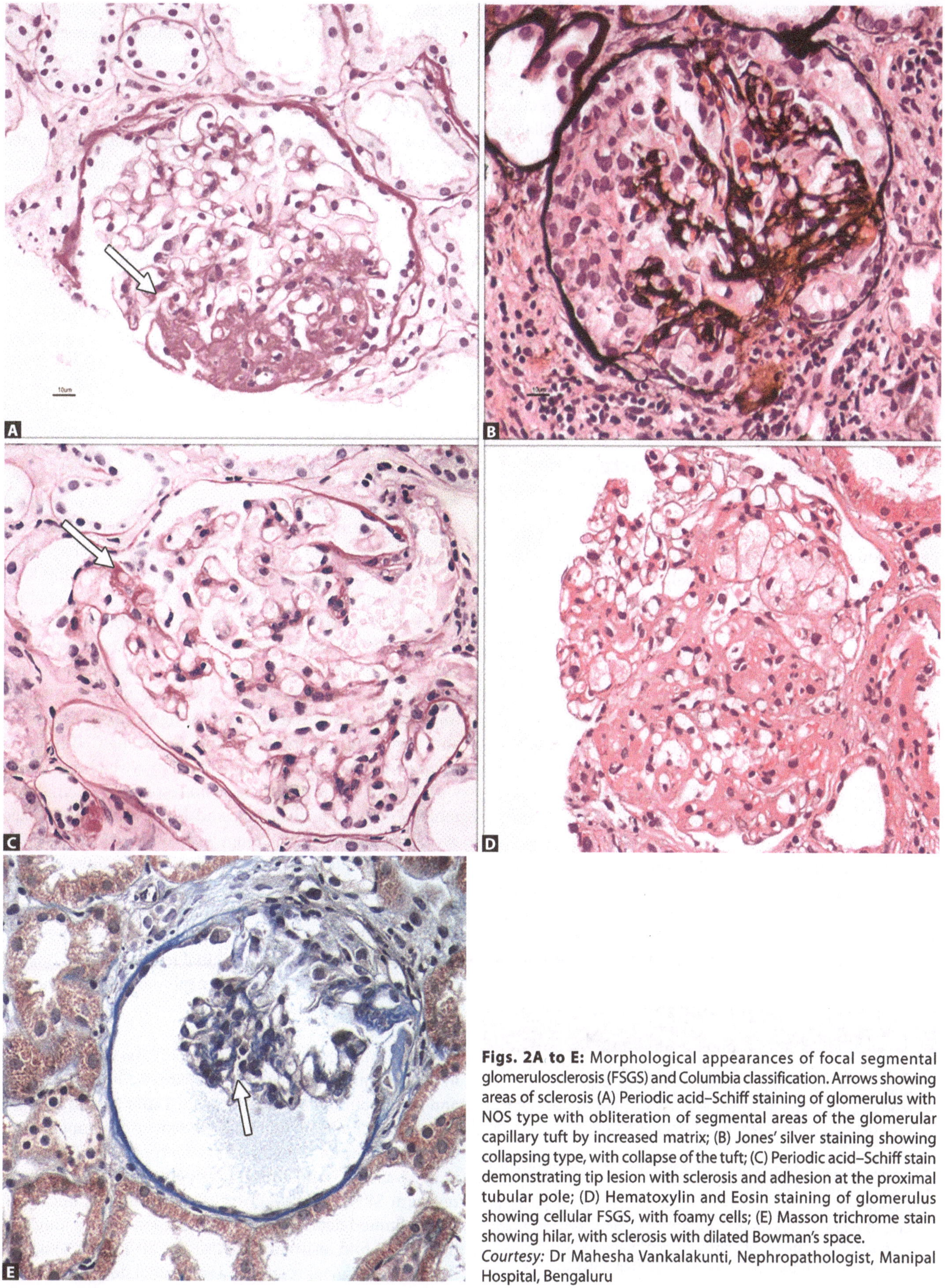

Figs. 2A to E: Morphological appearances of focal segmental glomerulosclerosis (FSGS) and Columbia classification. Arrows showing areas of sclerosis (A) Periodic acid–Schiff staining of glomerulus with NOS type with obliteration of segmental areas of the glomerular capillary tuft by increased matrix; (B) Jones' silver staining showing collapsing type, with collapse of the tuft; (C) Periodic acid–Schiff stain demonstrating tip lesion with sclerosis and adhesion at the proximal tubular pole; (D) Hematoxylin and Eosin staining of glomerulus showing cellular FSGS, with foamy cells; (E) Masson trichrome stain showing hilar, with sclerosis with dilated Bowman's space.
Courtesy: Dr Mahesha Vankalakunti, Nephropathologist, Manipal Hospital, Bengaluru

in FSGS secondary to obesity or reduced number of nephrons and is accompanied by glomerular enlargement. In an FSGS clinical trial cohort, FSGS NOS was the most common variant, observed in 68% of all cases, with collapsing, tip, perihilar, and cellular variants observed in 12, 10, 7, and 3%, respectively. In the same study at the end of 3-year follow-up, collapsing FSGS had the worst prognosis (47% with ESKD), while the NOS and tip variant had better prognosis (20 and 7% with ESKD in NOS and tip variants, respectively).[37] In PODONET cohort, minimal change histology had a better therapeutic response to calcineurin inhibitors (CNIs) as well as better renal survival when compared to FSGS.[38] The information regarding the degree of glomerulosclerosis, interstitial fibrosis, and tubular atrophy obtained from renal biopsy helps in the assessment of prognosis of children with SRNS. Biopsy at diagnosis of SRNS also forms a comparator for repeat biopsy during the course of disease for evaluation of CNI toxicity and progression of the disease.

Genetic Testing in Steroid-resistant Nephrotic Syndrome and its Utility

Genetic testing forms an important component in the evaluation of pediatric SRNS as it has significant impact on clinical management and counseling **(Box 4)**. The Indian Society of Pediatric Nephrology 2021 guidelines recommends genetic testing in congenital NS, initial resistance in children with age of onset less than 1 year, NS with extrarenal features or known syndromes, familial steroid resistance, CNI resistance, and prior to transplantation.[39] Genetic testing is not indicated in children with late SRNS. Since a large number of genes with poor phenotype-genotype correlation are associated with monogenic forms of SRNS, clinical exome sequencing (Mendelian exome panel), which includes all exons of genes listed in Online Mendelian Inheritance of Man (OMIM) database, is the method of choice for genetic testing. Such an approach facilitates not only targeted gene analysis but also in searching variants in the remaining genes of clinical exome if targeted gene analysis fails to identify causal variants. Sanger sequencing is the method of choice for testing if a disease-causing mutation is highly likely in a specific gene as in syndromic forms of SRNS or in positive family history with a known genetic cause. Sanger sequencing is essential to confirm segregation and confirm variants detected on NGS.

BOX 4: Benefits of genetic testing in steroid-resistant nephrotic syndrome.

- Enables specific diagnosis of monogenic disorders, and occasional phenocopies (e.g., Alport syndrome, Dent disease)
- Monitoring for extrarenal complications, e.g., patients with WT1—gonadal dysgenesis, LMX1B—glaucoma, SMARCAL1—skeletal abnormalities
- Predict response to immunosuppressive therapy and recurrence post-renal transplantation
- Provide targeted therapy [e.g., coenzyme Q10 for defect(s) in CoQ10 pathway, eplerenone for *ARHGDIA*, and corticosteroids for mutations in genes of Rho/Rac/Cdc42 network]
- Counseling for future pregnancies and antenatal diagnosis

TREATMENT

Because of the complexity of decision making and the potential for serious adverse effects of immunosuppressive agents, the care of children with SRNS should be supervised by a clinician with expertise in the management of these patients. The initial management goal is to determine if complete remission is achievable by administering additional immunosuppressive therapy. Besides reducing complications of NS, patients with complete remission are unlikely to progress to kidney failure.

Therapy with CNI cyclosporine or tacrolimus is recommended as the initial therapy for children with SRNS along with tapering of prednisolone therapy over 6–9 months.[39] Data from randomized controlled trials (RCT) and cohort studies indicate that therapy with CNI results in complete remission in 30–40% and complete or partial remission in 60–80% patients.[5,40,41] Although tacrolimus and cyclosporine show similar efficacy, tacrolimus might be preferred because of the absence of cosmetic side effects including hypertrichosis and gingival hyperplasia which are common with cyclosporine. Cyclosporine is preferred in children who are unable to swallow tablets (cyclosporine is available as suspension) and in patients with seizures or at risk for diabetes. The dose, adverse effects, and monitoring while on CNI therapy are summarized in **Table 5**. Trough levels are used for monitoring treatment with cyclosporine and tacrolimus; the target 12-hour trough levels are between 80 and 150 ng/mL for cyclosporine and 4 and 8 ng/mL for tacrolimus. Following CNI-induced remission, ~60% patients may have relapses which are treated with steroid therapy. If there is no response to CNI after 6 months, despite adequate dose and drug level they are labeled as CNI resistant and CNI therapy is discontinued. In those who achieve complete or partial remission, CNI is continued for at least 24–36 months with careful monitoring for adverse effects. Nephrotoxicity is observed in 10–25% patients receiving prolonged CNI treatment.[42] Duration of heavy proteinuria, hypertension during therapy, initial resistance, and dose of CNI used are major risk factors for nephrotoxicity. CNI therapy is contraindicated in children with severe impaired kidney function (i.e., GFR <30 mL/min/1.73 m^2).

Other immunosuppressive therapies that have been used in SRNS include intravenous cyclophosphamide, rituximab, and mycophenolate mofetil (MMF; **Table 5**). Intravenous cyclophosphamide is offered to patients who cannot afford CNI or is contraindicated due to adverse effects. Rituximab is used as a second-line therapy in children with CNI-resistant SRNS. However, the efficacy remains uncertain due to limited data. A review of published studies indicates that late steroid resistance (57.7%) and MCD (63.6%) have a higher remission rate compared with initial steroid resistance

TABLE 5: Immunosuppressive therapy in steroid-resistant nephrotic syndrome.

Medication	*Indications*	*Dose*	*Adverse effects*	*Monitoring*
Tacrolimus	First-line therapy	0.1–0.2 mg/kg/day in two divided doses; maximum initial dose 4 mg/day; trough level 4–8 ng/mL	• *Both:* acute kidney injury, nephrotoxicity, hyperkalemia, hepatotoxic • *Tacrolimus*: tremors, seizures, headache; diarrhea; glucose intolerance; hypomagnesemia • *Cyclosporine:* gingival hyperplasia, hypertrichosis; hypertension; dyslipidemia	• Screen for cosmetic side effects, tremors, diarrhea, hypertension • Creatinine, potassium at 2–4 weeks, q 3–6 months • Liver function tests, uric acid, magnesium, lipids q 3–6 months • Blood glucose q 3–6 months (with tacrolimus)
Cyclosporine	First-line therapy in small children who cannot swallow tablet; seizure disorder; diabetes	3–5 mg/kg/day in two divided doses; maximum initial dose 200 mg/day; trough level 80–120 ng/mL		
Prednisolone on alternate days		1.5 mg/kg for 4 weeks; 1 mg/kg for 4 weeks; taper to 0.3–0.5 mg/kg for ~6–9 months	Weight gain, Cushingoid habitus, glucose intolerance, hypertension, raised intraocular pressure, cataract, myopathy, osteoporosis	• Blood pressure, screen for cosmetic effects; eye evaluation q 12 months • Blood glucose every 6–12 months
Cyclophosphamide	Adverse effects of CNI; Not affording long-term CNI	500–750 mg/m² IV; every month for 6 months	Leukopenia, hemorrhagic cystitis, vomiting, alopecia, risk of infections, gonadal toxicity, malignancies	• Blood counts prior to infusion; withhold if total leukocyte count <4,000/mm³ • Ondansetron, MESNA prevent adverse effects
Rituximab	CNI-resistant SRNS, switch over after 24 months of CNI or CNI-related adverse effects	375 mg/m² every week for two to four doses	• Infusion reactions: chills, fever, serum sickness, bronchospasm • *Neutropenia: Pneumocystis jirovecii* pneumonia; reactivation of hepatitis B; JC virus; acute lung injury; hypogammaglobulinemia	• *Predose*: Hemogram, transaminases; hepatitis, and HIV serology; immunoglobulin (IgG) level • Monitor CD19 count, hemogram, IgG level
Mycophenolate mofetil	CNI-resistant SRNS as monotherapy or in combination with CNI; switch over after 24 months of CNI or CNI-related adverse effects	600–1,200 mg/m²/day in two-divided doses	Leukopenia; liver dysfunction; pain abdomen; nausea; diarrhea; headache; warts; weight loss	Hemogram, liver functions q 3–6 months

(CNI: calcineurin inhibitor; JC virus: John Cunningham virus)
Source: Modified from Vasudevan A, Thergaonkar R, Mantan M, Sharma J, Khandelwal P, Hari P, et al; Expert Group of the Indian Society of Pediatric Nephrology. Consensus guidelines on management of steroid-resistant nephrotic syndrome. Indian Pediatr. 2021;58(7):650-66.

(43.9%) and patients with FSGS (41.5%).[43] Mycophenolate with or without CNI has been used in children with CNI-resistant NS and in children with eGFR <60 mL/min/1.73 m² in whom CNI is contraindicated. Complete remission, partial remission, and nonresponse to combined therapy of CNI and MMF were 11.8–47.7, 8.7–38.2, and 43.5–58.8%, respectively.[44,45] Use of adalimumab, abatacept, ofatumumab and adrenocorticotropic hormone, oral galactose, and low-density lipoprotein (LDL) apheresis in patients with CNI-resistant SRNS have not yielded encouraging results and should only be used in the context of clinical trials.[39]

Besides immunosuppression, therapy is directed at decreasing proteinuria using pharmacologic agents and management of related symptoms and complications of NS **(Table 6)**. Blockade of the renin–angiotensin–aldosterone system (RAAS) with either angiotensin-converting enzyme (ACE) inhibitors or angiotensin II receptor blockers (ARBs) to decrease proteinuria and slow the progression of CKD is an important component of supportive care. Genetic testing is advised before planning further immunosuppressive therapy.[46]

In CNI-resistant SRNS, further immunosuppressive therapy is based on genetic testing results. In children with single-gene defects, additional immunosuppressive therapy is not advised because it is not effective and has significant adverse effects. The likelihood of nonresponse to CNI in genetic disease compared to nongenetic disease is higher [relative risk (RR) 4.00; 95% CI 2.52–6.51].[39] In these children, treatment is limited to supportive care and preparing for renal transplantation. However, some patients with a genetic cause for steroid resistance, especially those with *WT1* variants, might show partial remission following treatment with CNI. Targeted therapy is possible for specific mutations, e.g., coenzyme Q10 for defect(s) in CoQ10 pathway, eplerenone

TABLE 6: Supportive care in steroid-resistant nephrotic syndrome.

Complication	*Pathophysiology*	*Comments*
Hypertension	• Target blood pressure 50–75th percentile for age • Lifestyle measures; restrict salt intake • ACE-Is, ARBs are preferred • Enalapril 0.08– 0.6 mg/kg one to two doses • Ramipril 1.6–6 mg/m²/day OD • Losartan 0.7–1.4 mg/kg OD • Other antihypertensives: • Amlodipine 0.1–0.6 mg/kg one to two doses • Nifedipine 0.2–3 mg/kg one to two doses • Metoprolol 1–6 mg/kg one to two doses • Atenolol 0.5–2 mg/kg OD • Prazosin ER 0.05–0.5 mg/kg one to two doses • Clonidine 5–25 µg/kg/day two to three doses	• Monitor serum creatinine and potassium while on ACE-I or ARB • Withhold ACE-I and ARB during vomiting, diarrhea, hypovolemia, and severe illness • Withhold ACE-I and ARB I serum creatinine increases >0.3 mg/dL from baseline • Avoid ACE-I/ARB when eGFR <30 mL/min/ 1.73 m²
Dyslipidemia	Modify lifestyle (dietary change, physical activity, weight control) ≥8-year-old with LDL cholesterol >160 mg/dL, or >130 mg/dL with risk factors*: atorvastatin 10–20 mg daily	In addition to contributing to cardiovascular morbidity, dyslipidemia aggravates glomerulosclerosis and proximal tubular damage and is associated with progression of CKD
Thromboembolism	• *Prevention:* Ensure ambulation, optimal hydration; remove central venous catheters, avoid arterial punctures; use compression stockings • Enoxaparin at a dose of 1.5 mg/kg/dose (<2 months age) or 1 mg/kg/dose (>2 months) subcutaneously, every 12 hours • Maintenance therapy with enoxaparin or warfarin (0.2 mg/kg/ dose started concurrently with enoxaparin) • *Preventive anticoagulation:* If previous thrombosis risk factors present	• For warfarin therapy, the target INR for prothrombin time is between 2.0 and 3.0 • The duration of anticoagulation therapy is for 3 months or until remission
Acute kidney injury	*Supportive care:* Attention to fluid and electrolytes; management of complications of acute kidney injury	Withhold ACE-I and ARB Medications should be dosed based on eGFR IV albumin therapy to be avoided
HPA suppression	Oral prednisolone 0.5–1.0 mg/kg/day OD or IV hydrocortisone 30–50 mg/m²/day;	Stress dose if receiving oral steroids >2 weeks within past 1 year
Bone health	Vitamin D (400–800 IU); calcium (250–750 mg) supplements	Loss of vitamin D protein due to persistent proteinuria; long-term steroids also leads to osteoporosis
Hypothyroidism	Levothyroxine 5–6 µg/kg once a day	Low free T4, TSH >10 mU/L needs to be treated No treatment if remission is expected, follow-up borderline levels

*Risk factors: Chronic kidney disease stage 3–5; blood pressure >90th centile for age; body mass index (BMI) >95th centile; family history of cardiovascular disease.

(ACE-I: angiotensin-converting enzyme inhibitor; ARB: angiotensin receptor blocker; CKD: chronic kidney disease; eGFR: estimate glomerular filtration rate; INR: international normalized ratio; HPA: hypothalamic–pituitary axis; LDL: low-density lipoprotein; TSH: thyroid-stimulating hormone)

for *ARHGDIA*, and corticosteroids for mutations in genes of Rho/Rac/Cdc42 network. The management approach is outlined in **Flowchart 1**.

Newer Therapeutics in Management of Steroid-resistant Nephrotic Syndrome

With better understanding of molecular pathobiology of SRNS, clinical trials evaluating novel molecules targeting the podocyte cytoskeleton, immunological, hemodynamic, and metabolic pathways are in progress **(Table 7)**.[47] In the DUET trial, sparsentan, a dual receptor AT1 and endothelin receptor blockade, reduced proteinuria more effectively compared to irbesartan.[48]

Kidney Transplantation

Kidney transplantation is offered for patients with SRNS and stage 5 CKD. Genetic screening of the recipient is necessary, particularly those with initial resistance or unclear diagnosis since it stratifies the risk for allograft recurrence and helps in donor screening. In children with genetic forms of SRNS that have an autosomal-dominant inheritance pattern, donors demonstrating the same variant as that observed in the recipient are not eligible to donate their kidney. Similarly,

Flowchart 1: Approach to the management of steroid-resistant nephrotic syndrome. Kidney biopsy is necessary, except in patients in whom genetic testing may obviate the need for biopsy (**Box 3**). Patients with monogenic cause for steroid resistance should not receive immunosuppression. Lack of remission despite adequate therapy with CNI for 6 months is an indication for genetic screening, if not performed earlier. Patients with CNI-resistant disease who do not show a monogenic defect may be treated with IV rituximab or combined therapy of CNI and MMF. Immunosuppression is withdrawn in patients with continued nonresponse.

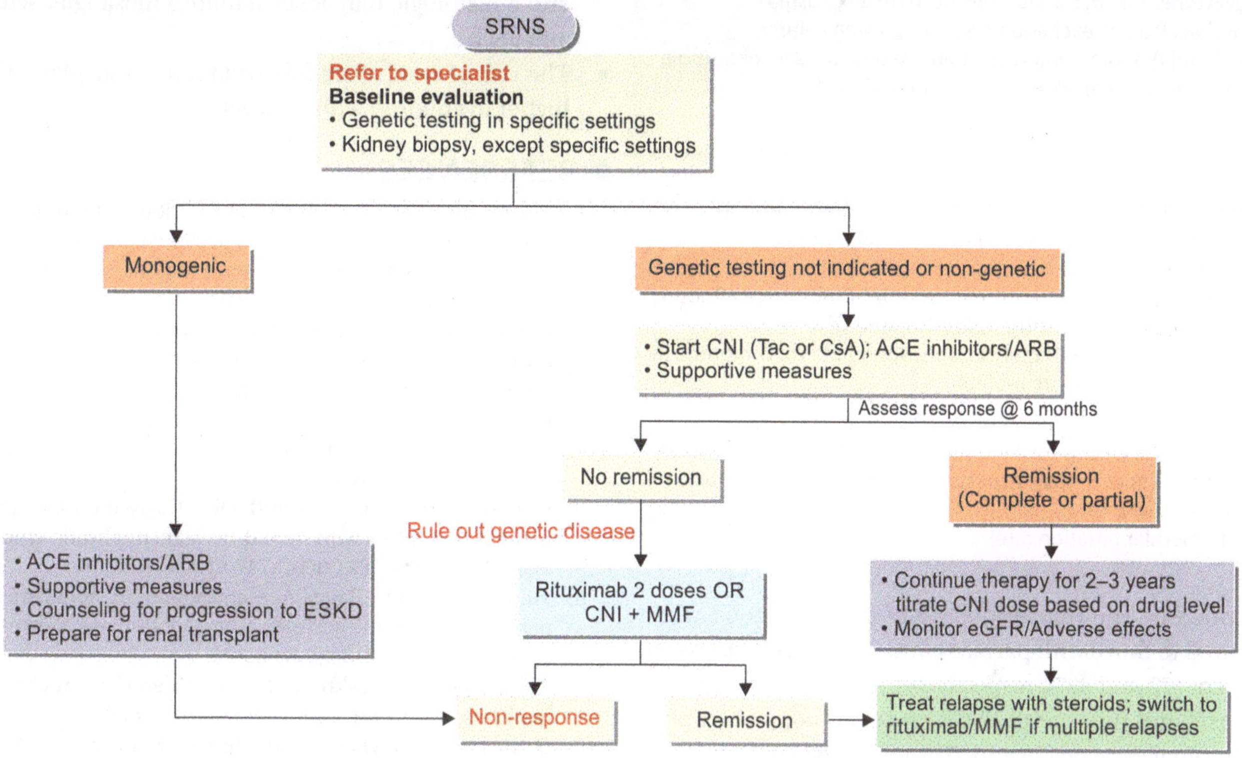

(ACE: angiotensin-converting enzyme; ARB: angiotensin II receptor blocker; CNI: calcineurin inhibitor; CsA: cyclosporine A; eGFR: estimate glomerular filtration rate; ESKD: end-stage kidney disease; MMF: mycophenolate mofetil; SRNS: steroid-resistant nephrotic syndrome)
Source: Vasudevan A, Thergaonkar R, Mantan M, Sharma J, Khandelwal P, Hari P, et al; Expert Group of The Indian Society of Pediatric Nephrology. Consensus guidelines on management of steroid-resistant nephrotic syndrome. Indian Pediatr. 2021;58(7):650-66.

TABLE 7: Therapeutics in phase 2 and 3 trials.

Molecule	*Mechanism of action*	*Route of administration*
Sparsentan	Blockade of AT1 and ETA receptors	Oral
Voclosporin	Calcineurin inhibitor	Oral
GFB-887	TRCP5 inhibitor	Oral
CXA-10	Nrf2 activator	Oral
PF-06730512	Robo2 inhibitor	Intravenous

Source: Trachtman H. Emerging drugs for treatment of focal segmental glomerulosclerosis. Expert Opin Emerg Drugs. 2020;25(3): 367-75.

heterozygous carriers of causal variants in *COL4A3* and *COL4A4* and female hemizygous carriers of variants in *COL4A5* are not accepted as donors since they are at risk of kidney failure.[39]

One of the main challenges of kidney transplantation is the risk of recurrence of proteinuria post renal transplantation, which occurs usually within hours to days after transplant. Recurrence is diagnosed in patients with proteinuria and Up/Uc ≥ 1 mg/mg if anuric prior to transplant or increase of ratio by ≥1 in those with proteinuria at transplantation.[39] The overall risk of recurrence is estimated to be 30–50%.[32] Recurrence is associated with increased risk of delayed graft function and early and late graft losses. Children with late SRNS or recurrent NS in a prior transplant is at the highest risk of recurrence (~80%) while those with confirmed genetic mutation underlying SRNS have the lowest risk (<5%). Children with initial resistance and no identified genetic cause are at a moderate risk of recurrence (~50%).[49,50] Plasma exchange with high-dose CNI and corticosteroids, with or without cyclophosphamide, are the common strategies used for managing patients with allograft recurrence (**Box 5**).

OUTCOME

Children with SRNS are at risk of progression to ESKD. Risk factors for ESKD include a genetic diagnosis, failure to respond to intensified immunosuppressive therapy, and a histologic diagnosis of diffuse mesangial sclerosis and FSGS. In a large multicenter cohort of SRNS, the overall kidney failure-free survival rates were 74% (95% CI 71–77%) at 5 years, 58% (95% CI 53–61%) at 10 years, and 48% (95% CI 43–53%) at 15 years.[38] The 10-year renal survival in children who

BOX 5: Management of recurrence postrenal transplantation.

Plasma exchange:
- Membrane filtration or centrifugation based; heparin or citrate anticoagulation
- Replacement fluid: 5% albumin; fresh frozen plasma
- Schedule: Plasma exchange 1.5 times plasma volume (60–75 mL/kg) per session on alternate days for 2 weeks; single volume (40 mL/kg) once per week for 4–6 weeks

Medications:
- IV methylprednisolone 250 mg/m^2/day for 3 days; taper to previous dose of oral prednisolone
- Increase dose of calcineurin inhibitors: Tacrolimus trough 8–12 ng/mL; cyclosporine trough 150–200 ng/mL
- Rituximab 375 mg/m^2 two doses, 1 week apart
- Add angiotensin-converting enzyme inhibitor once allograft function established with stable estimated GFR
- Consider therapy with oral cyclophosphamide for 3 months in place of mycophenolate mofetil

Monitor proteinuria by urine protein to creatinine (Up/Uc) ratio: daily for 1 week; weekly for 4 weeks; monthly for 1 year; then every 3–6 months; renal biopsy, especially if low-grade proteinuria or graft dysfunction.
(GFR: glomerular filtration rate)

responded to immunosuppression (94%) was good when compared to those with partial remission or nonresponse to treatment (72 and 43%, respectively).[38] Those with a genetic diagnosis and those with FSGS on renal biopsy had poor 10-year renal survival (29 and 52%, respectively).

CONCLUSION

Steroid resistance is a clinical diagnosis and is defined as lack of complete remission despite 6 weeks of therapy with prednisolone. 15–20% of children with NS remain unresponsive to steroids and are associated with unfavorable prognosis; 36–50% of children with SRNS progress to ESKD within 10 years of diagnosis. Podocyte injury plays the central role in the pathogenesis of idiopathic SRNS. This may be either due to alteration of a structural component of the foot process from mutation in a gene coding the protein or as a target of a circulating immunological factor. CNIs are the mainstay of therapy of SRNS. In CNI-resistant SRNS, further immunosuppressive therapy is based on genetic testing results. In children with single-gene defects, additional immunosuppressive therapy is not advised because it is not effective and has significant adverse effects. Renoprotective strategies are initiated in multidrug-resistant NS. They are at risk of progression to ESKD and recurrence of proteinuria after renal transplantation.

KEY POINTS

- SRNS is seen in 15–20% children with NS.
- Monogenic form of SRNS is observed in 25–30% of the children diagnosed with SRNS.
- CNIs are the mainstay of therapy of SRNS. Therapy with ACE inhibitors or ARBs is also an important component of treatment.
- CNI resistance and monogenic SRNS have been associated with unfavorable renal prognosis.
- Risk factors for ESKD include a genetic diagnosis, failure to respond to intensified immunosuppressive therapy, and a histologic diagnosis of diffuse mesangial sclerosis and FSGS.
- The risk of recurrence following renal transplantation is higher in children without a genetic cause.

REFERENCES

1. The primary nephrotic syndrome in children. Identification of patients with minimal change nephrotic syndrome from initial response to prednisone. A report of the International Study of Kidney Disease in Children. J Pediatr. 1981;98(4):561-4.
2. Das U, Dakshinamurty KV, Prayaga A. Pattern of biopsy-proven renal disease in a single center of south India: 19 years experience. Indian J Nephrol. 2011;21(4):250-7.
3. Gulati S, Sharma AP, Sharma RK, Gupta A. Changing trends of histopathology in childhood nephrotic syndrome. Am J Kidney Dis. 1999;34(4):646-50.
4. Lee JM, Kronbichler A, Shin JI, Oh J. Current understandings in treating children with steroid-resistant nephrotic syndrome. Pediatr Nephrol. 2021;36(4):747-61.
5. Tullus K, Webb H, Bagga A. Management of steroid-resistant nephrotic syndrome in children and adolescents. Lancet Child Adolesc Health. 2018;2(12):880-90.
6. Chanchlani R, Parekh RS. Ethnic differences in childhood nephrotic syndrome. Front Pediatr. 2016;4:39.
7. Gribouval O, Boyer O, Knebelmann B, Karras A, Dantal J, Fourrage C, et al. APOL1 risk genotype in European steroid-resistant nephrotic syndrome and/or focal segmental glomerulosclerosis patients of different African ancestries. Nephrol Dial Transplant. 2019;34(11):1885-93.
8. Büscher AK, Weber S. Educational paper: the podocytopathies: the podocytopathies. Eur J Pediatr. 2012; 171(8):1151-60.
9. Watanabe A, Feltran LS, Sampson MG. Genetics of nephrotic syndrome presenting in childhood: core curriculum 2019. Am J Kidney Dis. 2019;74(4):549-57.
10. Siji A, Karthik KN, Pardeshi VC, Hari PS, Vasudevan A. Targeted gene panel for genetic testing of south Indian children with steroid resistant nephrotic syndrome. BMC Med Genet. 2018; 19:200.
11. Ramanathan ASK, Vijayan M, Rajagopal S, Rajendiran P, Senguttuvan P. WT1 and NPHS2 gene mutation analysis and clinical management of steroid-resistant nephrotic syndrome. Mol Cell Biochem. 2017;426(1-2):177-81.
12. Sadowski CE, Lovric S, Ashraf S, Pabst WL, Gee HY, Kohl S, et al. A single-gene cause in 29.5% of cases of steroid-resistant nephrotic syndrome. J Am Soc Nephrol. 2015;26(6):1279-89.
13. Bierzynska A, McCarthy HJ, Soderquest K, Sen ES, Colby E, Ding WY, et al. Genomic and clinical profiling of a national nephrotic syndrome cohort advocates a precision medicine approach to disease management. Kidney Int. 2017;91(4):937-47.
14. Friedman DJ, Pollak MR. APOL1 nephropathy: from genetics to clinical applications. Clin J Am Soc Nephrol. 2021;16(2):294-303.
15. Jones N, Blasutig IM, Eremina V, Ruston JM, Bladt F, Li H, et al. Nck adaptor proteins link nephrin to the actin cytoskeleton of kidney podocytes. Nature. 2006;440(7085):818-23.
16. Huber TB, Simons M, Hartleben B, Sernetz L, Schmidts M, Gundlach E, et al. Molecular basis of the functional podocin-nephrin complex: mutations in the NPHS2 gene disrupt

nephrin targeting to lipid raft microdomains. Hum Mol Genet. 2003;12(24):3397-405.

17. Winn MP, Conlon PJ, Lynn KL, Farrington MK, Creazzo T, Hawkins AF, et al. A mutation in the TRPC6 cation channel causes familial focal segmental glomerulosclerosis. Science. 2005;308(5729):1801-4.
18. Gbadegesin R, Hinkes BG, Hoskins BE, Vlangos CN, Heeringa SF, Liu J, et al. Mutations in PLCE1 are a major cause of isolated diffuse mesangial sclerosis (IDMS). Nephrol Dial Transplant. 2008;23(4):1291-7.
19. Ozaltin F, Ibsirlioglu T, Taskiran EZ, Baydar DE, Kaymaz F, Buyukcelik M, et al. Disruption of PTPRO causes childhood-onset nephrotic syndrome. Am J Hum Genet. 2011;89(1):139-47.
20. Lepori N, Zand L, Sethi S, Fernandez-Juarez G, Fervenza FC. Clinical and pathological phenotype of genetic causes of focal segmental glomerulosclerosis in adults. Clin Kidney J. 2018;11(2):179-90.
21. Has C, Sparta` G, Kiritsi D, Weibel L, Moeller A, Vega-Warner V, et al. Integrin alpha3 mutations with kidney, lung, and skin disease. N Engl J Med. 2012;366:1508-14.
22. Matejas V, Hinkes B, Alkandari F, Al-Gazali L, Annexstad E, Aytac MB, et al. Mutations in the human laminin beta2 (LAMB2) gene and the associated phenotypic spectrum. Hum Mutat. 2010;31:992-1002.
23. Kambham N, Tanji N, Seigle RL, Markowitz GS, Pulkkinen L, Uitto J, et al. Congenital focal segmental glomerulosclerosis associated with beta4 integrin mutation and epidermolysis bullosa. Am J Kidney Dis. 2000;36:190-6.
24. Becherucci F, Landini S, Cirillo L, Mazzinghi B, Romagnani P. Look alike, sound alike: phenocopies in steroid-resistant nephrotic syndrome. Int J Environ Res Public Health. 2020; 17(22):8363.
25. Boerkoel CF, Takashima H, John J, Yan J, Stankiewicz P, Rosenbarker L, et al. Mutant chromatin remodeling protein SMARCAL1 causes Schimke immunoosseous dysplasia. Nat Genet. 2002;30:215-20.
26. Sweeney E, Fryer A, Mountford R, Green A, McIntosh I. Nail patella syndrome: a review of the phenotype aided by developmental biology. J Med Genet. 2003;40:153-62.
27. Ashraf S, Kudo H, Rao J, Kikuchi A, Widmeier E, Lawson JA, et al. Mutations in six nephrosis genes delineate a pathogenic pathway amenable to treatment. Nat Commun [Internet]. 2018; 9(1):1960.
28. Zimmerman SW. Increased urinary protein excretion in the rat produced by serum from a patient with recurrent focal glomerular sclerosis after renal transplantation. Clin Nephrol. 1984;22:32-8.
29. Fine RN. Recurrence of nephrotic syndrome/focal segmental glomerulosclerosis following renal transplantation in children. Pediatr Nephrol. 2007;22:496-502.
30. Saleem MA. Molecular stratification of idiopathic nephrotic syndrome. Nat Rev Nephrol. 2019;15(12):750-65.
31. Alachkar N, Carter-Monroe N, Reiser J. Abatacept in B7-1-positive proteinuric kidney disease. N Engl J Med. 2014;370(13): 1263-4.
32. Bierzynska A, Saleem MA. Deriving and understanding the risk of post-transplant recurrence of nephrotic syndrome in the light of current molecular and genetic advances. Pediatr Nephrol. 2018;33:2027-35.
33. Nammalwar BR, Vijayakumar M, Prahlad N. Experience of renal biopsy in children with nephrotic syndrome. Pediatr Nephrol. 2006;21(2):286-8.
34. Corwin HL, Schwartz MM, Lewis EJ. The importance of sample size in the interpretation of the renal biopsy. Am J Nephrol. 1988;8(2):85-9.
35. D'Agati VD, Fogo AB, Bruijn JA, Jennette JC. Pathologic classification of focal segmental glomerulosclerosis: a working proposal. Am J Kidney Dis. 2004;43(2):368-82.
36. Fogo AB. Causes and pathogenesis of focal segmental glomerulosclerosis. Nat Rev Nephrol. 2015;11(2):76-87.
37. D'Agati VD, Alster JM, Jennette JC, Thomas DB, Pullman J, Savino DA, et al. Association of histologic variants in FSGS clinical trial with presenting features and outcomes. Clin J Am Soc Nephrol. 2013;8(3):399-406.
38. Trautmann A, Schnaidt S, Lipska-Ziętkiewicz BS, Bodria M, Ozaltin F, Emma F, et al. Long-term outcome of steroid-resistant nephrotic syndrome in children. J Am Soc Nephrol. 2017;28(10): 3055-65.
39. Vasudevan A, Thergaonkar R, Mantan M, Sharma J, Khandelwal P, Hari P, et al. Consensus guidelines on management of steroid-resistant nephrotic syndrome. Indian Pediatr. 2021;58(7);650-66.
40. Gipson DS, Trachtman H, Kaskel FJ, Greene TH, Radeva MK, Gassman JJ, et al. Clinical trial of focal segmental glomerulosclerosis in children and young adults. Kidney Int. 2011; 80(8):868-78.
41. Mason AE, Sen ES, Bierzynska A, Colby E, Afzal M, Dorval G, et al. Response to first course of intensified immunosuppression in genetically stratified steroid resistant nephrotic syndrome. Clin J Am Soc Nephrol. 2020;15(7):983-94.
42. Sinha A, Sharma A, Mehta A, Gupta R, Gulati A, Hari P, et al. Calcineurin inhibitor induced nephrotoxicity in steroid resistant nephrotic syndrome. Indian J Nephrol. 2013;23(1): 41-6.
43. Kamei K, Ishikura K, Sako M, Ito S, Nozu K, Iijima K. Rituximab therapy for refractory steroid-resistant nephrotic syndrome in children. Pediatr Nephrol. 2020;35(1):17-24.
44. Wu B, Mao J, Shen H, Fu H, Wang J, Liu A, et al. Triple immunosuppressive therapy in steroid-resistant nephrotic syndrome children with tacrolimus resistance or tacrolimus sensitivity but frequently relapsing. Nephrology (Carlton). 2015;20(1):18-24.
45. Okada M, Sugimoto K, Yagi K, Yanagida H, Tabata N, Takemura T. Mycophenolate mofetil therapy for children with intractable nephrotic syndrome. Pediatr Int. 2007;49(6):933-7.
46. van den Belt SM, Heerspink HJL, Gracchi V, de Zeeuw D, Wühl E, Schaefer F, et al. Early proteinuria lowering by angiotensin-converting enzyme inhibition predicts renal survival in children with CKD. J Am Soc Nephrol. 2018;29(8):2225-33.
47. Trachtman H. Emerging drugs for treatment of focal segmental glomerulosclerosis. Expert Opin Emerg Drugs. 2020;25(3): 367-75.
48. Trachtman H, Nelson P, Adler S, Campbell KN, Chaudhuri A, Derebail VK, et al; DUET Study Group. DUET: a phase 2 study evaluating the efficacy and safety of sparsentan in patients with FSGS. J Am Soc Nephrol. 2018;29(11):2745-54.
49. Koh LJ, Martz K, Blydt-Hansen TD, NAPRTCS Registry Investigators. Risk factors associated with allograft failure in pediatric kidney transplant recipients with focal segmental glomerulosclerosis. Pediatr Transplant. 2019;23:e13469.
50. Ding WY, Koziell A, McCarthy HJ, Bierzynska A, Bhagavatula MK, Dudley JA, et al. Initial steroid sensitivity in children with steroid-resistant nephrotic syndrome predicts post-transplant recurrence. J Am Soc Nephrol. 2014;25:1342-8.

CHAPTER

6.4

Secondary Nephrotic Syndromes in Children

Mukta Mantan

INTRODUCTION

Nephrotic syndrome is the most common glomerular disease in children. Secondary nephrotic syndrome is caused primarily by an infection, systemic disease, or a drug reaction. While diabetes is the most common systemic cause of secondary nephrotic syndrome among adults, in children other causes such as infections and systemic lupus erythematosus (SLE) predominate. The infections associated with nephrotic syndrome are primarily chronic hepatitis B virus (HBV), hepatitis C virus (HCV), and human immunodeficiency virus (HIV) diseases. Various causes of secondary nephrotic syndrome are given in **Box 1**. In this chapter, primarily hepatitis B, C, HIV, and drug-related nephropathy shall be further dealt with.

HEPATITIS B NEPHROPATHY

Hepatitis B virus infection is an important public health problem and an important cause of morbidity and mortality in children. It is estimated that there are more than 240 million HBV carriers worlwide.[1] The prevalence of hepatitis B surface antigen (HBsAg) carriers is 0.3–1% in North America, 1% in Western Europe, 7% in Africa, and up to 10% in South-East Asia where it is endemic.

BOX 1: Causes of secondary nephrotic syndrome.

Conditions

Infections
- Hepatitis B and C
- HIV
- Malaria
- Toxoplasmosis
- Syphilis

Drugs
- NSAIDs
- Penicillamine
- Gold
- Pamidronate
- Lithium
- Interferons

Malignancies
- Lymphomas
- Leukemias

Multisystem diseases
- Diabetes mellitus
- Systemic lupus erythematosus
- Vasculitis
- Amyloidosis
- Sarcoidosis

(NSAIDs: nonsteroidal anti-inflammatory drugs)

Hepatitis B virus is a member of *Hepadnaviridae* family. It is a double-stranded DNA virus that is hepatotrophic. HBV has a double-shelled virion 42–47 nm in diameter and has a 27-nm internal core, an excess of incomplete 22-nm spheres, and a circular DNA genome that encodes four viral proteins. It contains four genes—core, surface, X, and polymerase. HBV is not a cytopathic virus.

The manifestations of hepatitis B primarily occur due to the immunological response of the host. In resolving acute infection, there is robust T-cell response with resultant production of tumor necrosis factor and interferon (IFN), induction of B cells-producing protective antibodies, and hepatic cell death leading to clearance of infection. Failure to mount an adequate immune response leads to persistent infection. Patients who acquire infection in infancy or early childhood are more likely to develop chronic infection.

Extrahepatic manifestations of hepatitis B also occur as a result of immune response and circulating immune complexes are responsible in most instances. Common extrahepatic manifestations are glomerulonephritis, arthritis, and vasculitis. Extrahepatic manifestations can also occur without overt hepatic involvement.[1] Common renal diseases related to hepatitis B are membranous glomerulonephritis (MGN), membranoproliferative glomerulonephritis (MPGN), and vasculitis [polyarteritis nodosa (PAN)]. Others reported are mesangioproliferative GN, immunoglobulin A (IgA) nephropathy, and amyloidosis.[2] Evidence for association of these renal lesions with hepatitis B comes from the fact that the prevalence of these lesions, especially MGN, closely follows that of hepatitis B and widespread immunization with hepatitis B has led to the reduction in the occurrence of MGN.

Definition of Hepatitis B Virus-related Glomerulonephritis

By definition, HBV-associated GN indicates the direct pathogenic relationship between active viral replication and the development of glomerulonephritis. Diagnosis of HBV-related GN is made by the presence of circulating HBsAg, characteristic histology with exclusion of other causes of GN, and the presence of hepatitis B antigen in renal biopsy.

Pathology of Hepatitis B Virus Glomerulonephritis

Hepatitis B virus-associated GN is an immune complex-mediated disease. Three different antigens, HBsAg, hepatitis B core antigen (HBcAg), and hepatitis B e antigen (HBeAg), have been detected by immunofluorescence studies in renal biopsies from patients with HBV-associated GN. Almost all morphological forms of renal diseases including membranous nephropathy (MN), MPGN, mesangial proliferative glomerulonephritis, minimal change disease (MCD), IgA nephropathy, and focal segmental glomerulosclerosis have been described though MN appears to be the most common in published series.[2,3] The association between chronic HBV infection and other renal pathologies such as focal glomerulosclerosis, minimal change nephropathy, and PAN remains unclear.[2]

In HBV-related MN glomerular capillary depositions of HBsAg, HBcAg, and HBeAg have been observed using immunohistochemistry on frozen renal tissue. A typical biopsy picture of HBV-associated MGN shows features of MN with thickened basement membranes and spikes on PAS and silver methenamine stain (**Figs. 1A and B**) and less commonly MPGN and focal segmental glomerulosclerosis (FSGS; cardiotrophin) (**Figs. 1C and D**). The immunofluorescence may show immunoglobulin G (IgG), immunoglobulin M (IgM), and C3 along glomerular capillary walls.

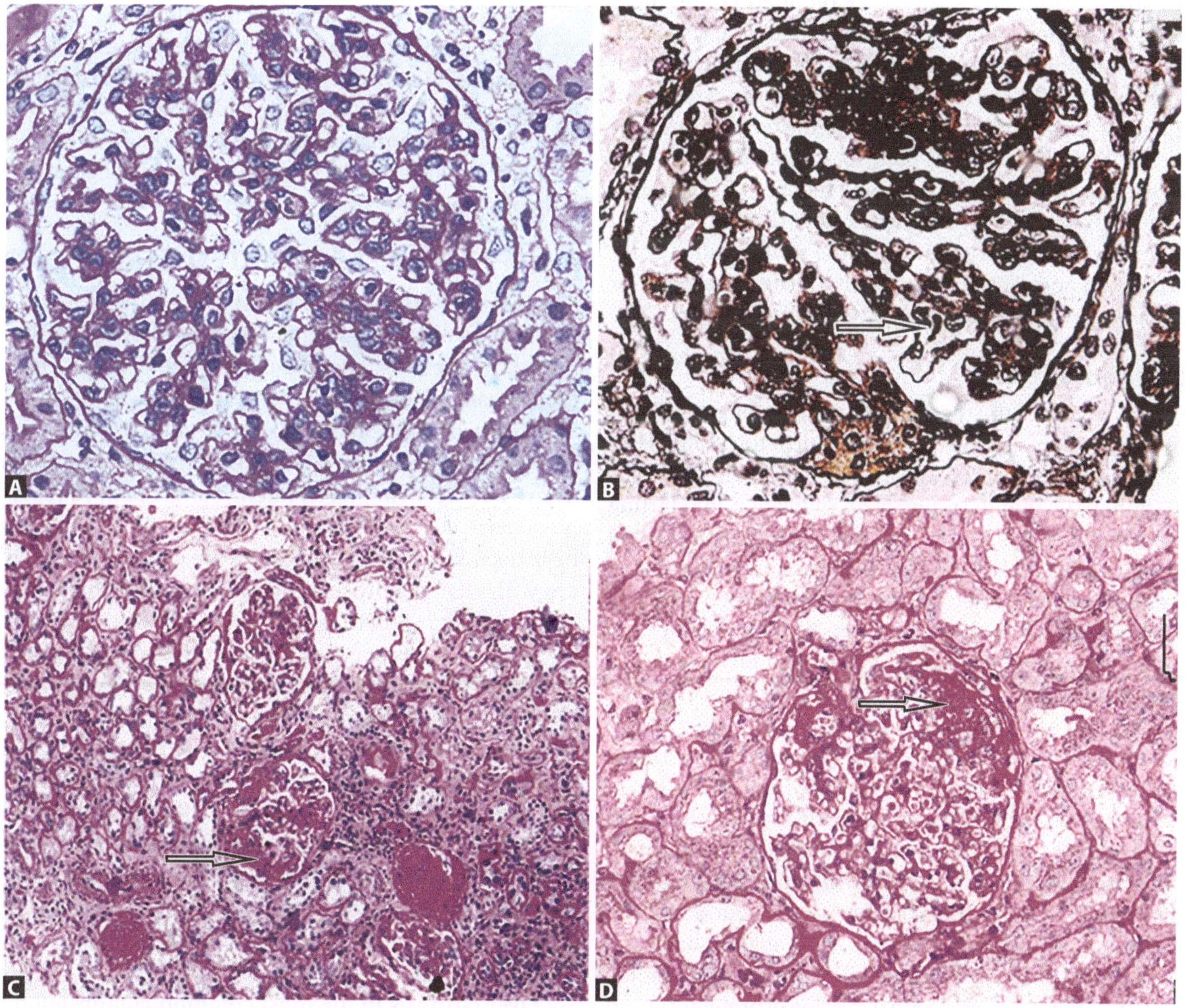

Figs. 1A to D: (A and B) Periodic acid–Schiff (PAS) and Jones silver methenamine (JMS)-stained sections of kidney biopsy showing thickened basement membranes with duplication and focal spikes (arrow) (membranous nephropathy) (40×); (C) PAS-stained slides at low power showing glomeruli with segmental sclerosis and chronic parenchymal damage (FSGS) (10×); (D) PAS-stained slides in high power showing the segmental sclerosed tuft (20×).

Clinical Manifestations

Most patients would present with features of nephrotic or nephritic syndrome. There is strong male preponderance in children and they tend to present commonly as nephrotic syndrome. A history of associated liver disease is uncommon compared to adults. The natural history of HBV-associated MN is not well defined. In children, HBV-associated MN has a favorable prognosis with a high spontaneous remission rate, although some patients may remain proteinuric for 12 months or longer. Adults with hepatitis usually recover and rarely develop chronic hepatitis or the HBsAg carrier state. In contrast, HBV infection in neonates and infants usually leads to the chronic carrier state.

Investigations

The investigations for evaluation include kidney function tests, serum albumin, globulin, cholesterol, and liver function tests. The serology for HBV includes HBsAg, HBeAg, anti-HBe, and anti-HBc antibodies which are required at the initial diagnosis and then for follow-up of the condition; also, HBV DNA levels should be done prior to start of treatment and then at follow-up. Besides urine routine microscopy, an assessment of timed or spot sample is required for the quantification of proteinuria. A renal biopsy is done for all patients with HBV-associated proteinuria or active urine sediment. However, in patients with an underlying chronic liver disease it should be carefully done after monitoring the prothrombin time/international normalized ratio (PT/INR). The indications for liver biopsy are primarily deranged liver function tests.

Management

The primary aim of the therapy is to achieve long-term viral DNA suppression. The decision to treat depends on the HBV DNA levels, liver enzymes, and liver histology. The presence of extra-hepatic manifestation is an indication for starting the antiviral therapy.[1] The Kidney Disease Improving Global Outcomes (KDIGO) guidelines recommend treatment of hepatitis B–related glomerulonephritis with IFN or nucleoside analogs as per the recommendations for the treatment of chronic hepatitis B infection.[1,4] Unlike chronic liver disease due to hepatitis B, for which well-designed placebo-controlled clinical trials are available, studies on the treatment of HBV-related GN are usually case reports or small-sample uncontrolled trials. There are reports of complete remission of hepatitis B–related MN with entecavir in children as well as in adults.[5,6] A meta-analysis concluded that the treatment with antivirals significantly increased the chances of complete remission in HBV-MGN, and no difference was found between IFN and entecavir therapy.[7] Another meta-analysis by Zhang et al. showed that therapy with antivirals but not with steroids was significantly associated with remission of proteinuria and with HBeAg clearance.[8]

Although the data suggest that the antivirals are sufficient for the treatment of HBV-GN, there is a concern regarding uncertain duration of therapy with nucleoside analogs and chances of disease progression. This led to trial of combination therapies with antivirals and immunosuppression. Ochi et al. reported an adult with HBV-MGN presenting as a nephrotic syndrome whose proteinuria worsened on entecavir therapy and the patient achieved remission after therapy with steroids and cyclosporine; no worsening of viral replication was observed after addition of immunosuppressive therapy.[9] Tacrolimus has been shown to reduce HBV replication by inhibiting HBV receptor on hepatocytes. Wang et al. reported 42 adult patients with HBV-MGN who were treated either with tacrolimus and entecavir combination therapy or with entecavir alone. They found that those who received combination therapy had significantly higher proteinuria remission rate and lower time to remission. None of the patients in either cohort had viral reactivation during therapy.[10] A meta-analysis of 12 studies showed that combined therapy with steroids and antivirals significantly reduced the proteinuria in HBV-GN without having an adverse effect on viral replication.[11]

The recommended antivirals in children >2 years of age are lamivudine and entecavir, the doses being 3 mg/kg to a maximum of 100 mg/day for lamivudine and 0.5 mg tablet of entecavir for children <30 kg and 1 mg for >30 kg weight. The duration of antivirals is not clearly defined but should be given for at least 6–12 months after achieving serological seroconversion.

HEPATITIS C–ASSOCIATED NEPHROPATHY

According to the World Health Organization (WHO) globally, an estimated 71 million people have chronic HCV infection. The most affected regions are the WHO Eastern Mediterranean Region and the WHO European Region, with an estimated prevalence in 2015 of 2.3 and 1.5%, respectively. Prevalence of HCV infection in other WHO regions varies from 0.5 to 1.0%. Among children younger than 16 years, the prevalence is <0.5% in Europe. While eight HCV genotypes have been identified, globally, the most common infections are with HCV genotype 1 in 44%, genotype 3 in 25%, and genotype 4 in 15% of the patients.[12]

Hepatitis C virus causes both acute and chronic infection, new HCV infections being usually asymptomatic. Around 30% (15–45%) of the infected persons spontaneously clear the virus within 6 months of infection without any treatment. However, the remaining 70% (55–85%) will develop chronic HCV infection over a variable period of time. The risk of the development of chronicity in children appears to be similar to adults (55–80%); spontaneous resolution of infection after vertical transmission may occasionally occur until the age of 5 years. However, cirrhosis due to HCV infection in the pediatric age group is uncommon.

Liver cirrhosis in thė most common complication of a chronic hepatitis C infection; extrahepatic manifestations include mixed cryoglobulinemia, lymphoproliferative disorders, and renal disease.[12] The proposed mechanism of cryoglobulinemia is persistence of HCV infection leading to chronic overstimulation of B-lymphocytes and production of mixed cryoglobulins mainly composed of a polyclonal Ig, either IgG or IgM. They get deposited in the mesangium and glomerular capillaries and trigger endothelial and complement activation. They can be identified as subendothelial deposits on immunofluorescence of the biopsy specimens.[13]

Glomerulonephritis develops many years after the initial infection with HCV, the most common HCV-related nephropathy being MPGN while rarely MN, FSGS, and proliferative changes too have been described.[14,15] Cryoglobulinemia vasculitis is also observed in about 10% patients affecting skin, nerves, and the kidneys predominantly. Renal involvement in cryoglobulinemia is characterized by proteinuria, hematuria, and deranged function. Hypertension is common in HCV-associated glomerulonephritis, and renal biopsy is consistent mostly with MPGN changes. The lesions in biopsy specimens are characterized by endocapillary proliferation, monocytic infiltration, double contour in basement membranes, large eosinophilic and PAS-positive intraluminal deposits, and vasculitis of small- and medium-sized renal arteries. On electron microscopy, subendothelial deposits are often seen that may have tubular and crystalline patterns similar to those of cryoglobulins in some patients.

Hepatitis C virus positivity has also been linked to lower graft and patient survivals after kidney transplantation. A link between HCV infection and type 2 diabetes mellitus has been proposed. The prevalence of HCV positivity in type 2 diabetic population ranges between 1.7 and 12.1% and a higher prevalence had been observed in those with diabetic nephropathy. Also, post-transplant HCV infection tends to predispose to diabetic nephropathy.

Investigations

Investigations include kidney function test (KFT), serum albumin, globulin, cholesterol, and evaluation of liver functions that include complete liver function test (LFT) including the enzymes, PT/INR. While kidney biopsy will identify the renal abnormality, a liver biopsy is also indicated for patients with deranged enzymes; a quantification of virus by HCV RNA should also be done. Viral genotype and the presence or absence of cirrhosis are the principal factors governing treatment recommendations; hence, efforts should be made to identify these. However, using the new approved pangenotype drugs has precluded the genotype determination to a large extent. A noninvasive way of identification of liver fibrosis is to use a FibroScan score which can also be repeated at regular intervals.

Management

Directly acting antiviral agents are the first-line therapy for HCV-associated renal disease. The recent American Association for the Study of Liver Diseases (AASLD) guidelines approve the use of these agents beyond 3 years of age and recommend early use in the presence of cryoglobulinemia, glomerulonephritis, or presence of vasculitis.

A 12-week course of the combination of ledipasvir/sofosbuvir (weight-based dosing) is recommended in children aged ≥3 years with HCV genotype 1, 4, 5, or 6 infection, without cirrhosis or with compensated cirrhosis. Further, the same guidelines recommend an 8-week course of the daily fixed-dose combination of glecaprevir (300 mg)/pibrentasvir (120 mg) for the treatment of adolescents aged ≥12 years or weighing ≥45 kg with any HCV genotype, without cirrhosis or with compensated cirrhosis.[16] These drugs are pangenotype protease inhibitors and the recommendations for treatment in adolescents are extrapolated from adult data where the drugs have been found to be safe. The primary endpoint of treatment is to achieve undetectable HCV RNA; >95% patients attain sustained viral response (SVR) within 12 weeks of therapy.

HUMAN IMMUNODEFICIENCY VIRUS NEPHROPATHY

Human immunodeficiency virus nephropathy is an important complication of advanced HIV infection and a leading cause of end-stage kidney disease (ESKD) in these patients. However after the use of effective antiviral agents, its incidence has markedly decreased in the western world. HIV-associated nephropathy is characterized by progressive acute renal failure, often accompanied by proteinuria and ultrasound findings of enlarged, echogenic kidneys. Patients with classical HIV nephropathy are likely to have CD4 counts <200 cells/mm^3 and nephrotic range proteinuria. There is a higher susceptibility of African-Americans to this nephropathy indicating a genetic predisposition (*APOL1* gene mutations).[17]

The definitive diagnosis requires renal biopsy, which demonstrates collapsing focal segmental glomerulosclerosis with associated microcystic tubular dilatation and interstitial inflammation. The glomerular collapse is accompanied by prominent hypertrophy and hyperplasia of the overlying podocytes, that have enlarged, open vesicular nuclei with frequent nucleoli; visceral epithelial cells may be so crowded as to obliterate the urinary space, forming pseudocrescents. Podocyte proliferation is a hallmark of HIV-associated nephropathy and is best appreciated on electron microscopy. Its frequency, however, has decreased in the era of potent antiretroviral drugs. The pathogenesis of HIV-associated nephropathy involves direct invasion of renal epithelial cells by the virus and treatment with antiretroviral drugs changes the disease course.

Tubulointerstitial disease is an invariable component of the nephropathy and often out of proportion to the degree of glomerular injury. Besides tubular atrophy, interstitial fibrosis, edema and inflammation, widespread tubular degenerative and regenerative changes are also seen. Tubular "microcysts" are seen which are mostly dilated tubules (at least threefold larger than normal) containing glassy proteinaceous casts and lined by simplified epithelium. In immunofluorescence, there are segmental to global deposits of IgM, C3, and less commonly C1, in the collapsing segments. The noncollapsed glomeruli may display weaker mesangial staining for IgM and C3. In a pediatric series of HIV nephropathy from South Africa, 49 children (1–16 years) underwent renal biopsy and the most common histopathological finding was FSGS in 32 (65.3%) children; 13 (26.5%) had collapsing glomerulopathy and 19 (38.8%) had classic FSGS.[18]

Patients on antiretroviral therapy (ART) show a non-collapsing variant of FSGS on biopsy and the tubulointerstitial damage is also less marked. Children with perinatal HIV infection can present with MCD or diffuse mesangial hypercellularity with numerous endothelial tubuloreticular inclusions and marked foot process effacement. However, tubular microcysts and interstitial inflammation are usually absent in these patients. In presence of effective ART, these lesions are rather rare nowadays.

Along with ART, the adjunctive therapy for HIV-associated nephropathy includes angiotensin-converting enzyme inhibitors (ACEIs) or angiotensin receptor blockers (ARBs) as well as corticosteroids in selected patients with significant interstitial inflammation or rapid progression. A reduction in HIV viral load leads to an improvement in proteinuria and prevents progression of renal disease.

DRUG-INDUCED NEPHROTIC SYNDROME

Most drugs causing nephrotoxicity exert toxic effects by one or more common pathogenic mechanisms, these being altered intraglomerular hemodynamics, tubular cell toxicity, inflammation, crystal nephropathy, rhabdomyolysis, and thrombotic microangiopathy.[19] While acute kidney injury (AKI) is the most common toxicity caused by various drugs, rarely nephrotic syndrome has also reported.

Oral pamidronate used for the treatment of osteoporosis has been associated with collapsing FSGS causing nephrotic syndrome.[20] The exact mechanism by which pamidronate produces these changes is not known, although the pattern of injury favors direct or indirect podocyte effects. Patients with pamidronate-associated FSGS present with florid nephrotic syndrome and renal insufficiency, and withdrawal of the drug often leads to improvement though some impairment of renal function persists. There are rare reports of MCD and FSGS-NOS with pamidronate; better outcomes are seen in patients with MCD after stoppage of the drug. Intravenous bisphosphonates used in the treatment of metastatic bone disease, hypercalcemia of malignancy, and multiple myeloma are more likely to cause nephrotoxicity.

Lithium carbonate is used for the treatment of bipolar disorder. While its prolonged use is mostly associated with chronic tubulointerstitial damage, rarely it has been described as a cause of new-onset MCD that remits on stoppage of the drug.[20-22] FSGS seen with lithium use is often secondary to tubulointerstitial damage.

Varying degrees of glomerular proteinuria have been reported with the use of nonsteroidal anti-inflammatory drugs (NSAIDs)—indomethacin, naproxen, ibuprofen, and piroxicam, and histological changes are similar to those of minimal change nephropathy. Most NSAIDs inhibit prostaglandins, thus increasing the vasoconstriction in the glomerular capillaries, which may be responsible for the glomerular and tubular changes seen with the prolonged use of these agents. One study also showed decreased collagen synthesis of glomerular basement membrane with indomethacin in a rat model.[23] MCD and MN were the most common findings in patients in whom a kidney biopsy was performed. Also, the NSAID-induced nephrotic syndrome is accompanied by variable degrees of AKI. Kidney biopsies typically show the characteristic pattern of drug-induced acute interstitial nephritis (AIN) characterized by a diffuse interstitial infiltrate composed predominantly of T lymphocytes, eosinophils, macrophages, and plasma cells. The glomeruli appear normal on light microscopy while a diffuse effacement of podocyte foot processes is observed in electron microscopy. The AKI induced due to these drugs is reversible and so are some of the glomerular changes. A short course of steroids for 4–6 weeks improves the outcome of both AIN and nephrotic syndrome.[24]

Interferon-α is used in the treatment of hepatitis B and C and various malignancies. IFN-β is extensively used to treat multiple sclerosis. IFN-γ is indicated for chronic granulomatous disease and malignant osteopetrosis. Use of IFNs has been associated with causation of podocytopathy leading to MCD and FSGS like changes in the kidneys.[25] This damage seems to be more in patients with *APLO1* gene mutations and discontinuation of therapy leads to recovery in most with findings of MCD while patients with FSGS tend to have partial recovery.

Penicillamine is used for the treatment of Wilson's disease, rheumatoid arthritis, and systemic sclerosis. Proteinuria has been reported from 6 weeks to 5 years after starting D-penicillamine therapy, with a median time of 7 months. The renal biopsy from such patients has shown a picture of MN in majority followed by MCD.[26] Stopping of penicillamine leads to a resolution of proteinuria in most patients. The exact mechanism of D-penicillamine-induced nephrotic syndrome is not known. In rheumatoid diseases, the drug may potentiate the glomerular damage from the existing rheumatoid immune complexes and it may act as a potent hapten, enhancing the immunological presentation of glomerular basement or renal tubuloepithelial antigens, leading to Goodpasture's syndrome or MGN, respectively.

CONCLUSION

It is important to identify the cause of secondary nephrotic syndrome so that specific therapy may be initiated early for resolution of the proteinuria. The prognosis of the condition is dependent upon the cause and timing of presentation from the onset.

KEY POINTS

- Secondary nephrotic syndrome is caused primarily by an infection, systemic diseases such as SLE, or a drug reaction.
- Infections associated with nephrotic syndrome are primarily chronic hepatitis B, C, and human immunodeficiency viral diseases.

- Renal diseases related to hepatitis B are MGN, MPGN, vasculitis (PAN).
- KDIGO guidelines recommend treatment of HBV-related GN with IFN or nucleoside analogs as per the recommendations for the treatment of chronic HBV infection. The recommended antivirals in children older than 2 years of age are lamivudine and entecavir.
- The most common HCV-related nephropathy is MPGN, while rarely MN, FSGS, and cryoglobulinemia can also occur.
- HCV positivity has also been linked to lower graft and patient survival after kidney transplantation.
- Directly acting antiviral agents are the first-line therapy for HCV-associated renal disease. The primary endpoint of the treatment is to achieve undetectable HCV RNA.
- HIV-associated nephropathy is characterized by progressive acute renal failure, often accompanied by proteinuria and ultrasound findings of enlarged, echogenic kidneys.
- Podocyte proliferation is a hallmark of HIV-associated nephropathy and is best appreciated on electron microscopy.
- Along with ART, ACEIs/ARBs as well as corticosteroids are used for HIV-associated nephropathy.
- Most drugs causing nephrotoxicity exert toxic effects by altered intraglomerular hemodynamics, tubular cell toxicity, inflammation, crystal nephropathy, rhabdomyolysis, and thrombotic microangiopathy.
- Nephrotic syndrome is caused by use of pamidronate, lithium, penicillamine and NSAIDs.
- It is important to identify the cause of secondary nephrotic syndrome so that specific therapy may be initiated early.

REFERENCES

1. European Association for the Study of the Liver. EASL clinical practice guidelines: management of chronic hepatitis B virus infection. J Hepatol. 2012;57:167-85.
2. Shah AS, Amarapurkar DN. Spectrum of hepatitis B and renal involvement. Liver Int. 2018;38:23-32.
3. Lin CY. Clinical features and natural course of HBV-related glomerulopathy in children. Kidney Int. 1991;40(suppl 35): 46-53.
4. Kidney Disease Improving Global Outcomes (KDIGO) Glomerulonephritis Work Group. KDIGO clinical practice guideline for glomerulonephritis. Kidney Int Suppl. 2012;2: 139-274.
5. Mahajan V, D'cruz S, Nada R, Sachdeva A. Successful use of entecavir in hepatitis b-associated membranous nephropathy. J Trop Pediatr. 2018;64:249-52.
6. Yang Y, Xiong Q, Zhao W, Zhong Y. Complete remission of hepatitis B virus-related membranous nephropathy after entecavir monotherapy. Clin Res Hepatol Gastroenterol. 2012;36:e89-e92.
7. Yang Y, Ma YP, Chen DP, Zhuo L, Li WG. A meta-analysis of antiviral therapy for hepatitis b virus-associated membranous nephropathy. PLoS One 2016;11:e0160437.
8. Zhang Y, Zhou JH, Yin XL, Wang FY. Treatment of hepatitis B virus-associated glomerulonephritis: a meta-analysis. World J Gastroenterol. 2010;16:770-7.
9. Ochi A, Ishimura E, Ichii M, Ohno Y, Nakatani S, Kobayashi I, et al. Successful treatment of hepatitis B virus-associated membranous nephropathy with entecavir and immunosuppressive agents. Asian Pacific Soc Nephrol. 2014; 595-6.
10. Wang L, Ye Z, Liang H, Zhang B, Xu L, Feng Z, et al. The combination of tacrolimus and entecavir improves the remission of HBV-associated glomerulonephritis without enhancing viral replication. Am J Transl Res. 2016;8:1593-600.
11. Zheng XY, Wei RB, Tang L, Li P, Zheng XD. Meta-analysis of combined therapy for adult hepatitis B virus-associated glomerulonephritis. World J Gstroenterol. 2012;18:821-32.
12. Spearman CW, Dusheiko GM, Hellard M, Sonderup M. Hepatitis C. Lancet. 2019;394:1451-66.
13. Lhotta K. Beyond hepatorenal syndrome: glomerulonephritis in patients with liver disease. Semin Nephrol. 2002;22:302-8.
14. Rollino C, Roccatello D, Giachino O, Basolo B, Piccoli G. Hepatitis C virus infection and membranous glomerulonephritis. Nephron. 1991;59:319-20.
15. Altraif IH, Abdulla AS, al Sebayel MI, Said RA, al Suhaibani MO, Jones AA. Hepatitis C associated glomerulonephritis. Am J Nephrol. 1995;15:407-10.
16. Ghany MG, Morgan TR; AASLD-IDSA Hepatitis C Guidance Panel. Hepatitis C guidance 2019 update: American Association for the Study of Liver Diseases–Infectious Diseases Society of America recommendations for testing, managing, and treating hepatitis c virus infection. Hepatology. 2020;71: 686-721.
17. Jotwani V, Atta MG, Estrella MM. Kidney disease in HIV: moving beyond HIV-associated nephropathy. J Am Soc Nephrol. 2017;28:3142-54.
18. Ramsuran D, Bhimma R, Ramdial PK, Naicker E, Adhikari M, Deonarain J, et al. The spectrum of HIV-related nephropathy in children. Pediatr Nephrol. 2012;27:821-7.
19. Markowitz GS, Bomback AS, Perazella MA. Drug-induced glomerular disease: direct cellular injury. Clin J Am Soc Nephrol. 2015;10:1291-99.
20. Markowitz GS, Appel GB, Fine PL, Fenves AZ, Loon NR, Jagannath S, et al. Collapsing focal segmental glomerulosclerosis following treatment with high dose pamidronate. J Am Soc Nephrol. 2001;12:1164-72.
21. Wood IK, Parmelee DX, Foreman JW. Lithium-induced nephrotic syndrome. Am J Psychiatry. 1989;146:84-7.
22. Richman AV, Masco HL, Rifkin SI, Acharya MK. Minimal-change disease and the nephrotic syndrome associated with lithium therapy. Ann Intern Med. 1980;92:70-2.
23. Daha MR, Blok APR, de Graeff J, van Es LA. Effect of indomethacin on the synthesis of glomerular basement membrane and on proteinuria in rats with nephrotoxic nephritis. Nephron. 1977;19:113-8.
24. Porile JL, Bakris GL, Garella S. Acute interstitial nephritis with glomerulopathy due to nonsteroidal anti-inflammatory agents: a review of its clinical spectrum and effects of steroid therapy. J Clin Pharmacol. 1990;30:468-75.
25. Markowitz GS, Nasr SH, Stokes MB, D'Agati VD. Treatment with IFN-{alpha}, -{beta}, or -{gamma} is associated with collapsing focal segmental glomerulosclerosis. Clin J Am Soc Nephrol. 2010;5:607-15.
26. Hall C, Jawad S, Harrison P, MacKenzie J, Bacon P, Klouda P, MacIver A. Natural course of penicillamine nephropathy: a long term study of 33 patients. Br Med J (Clin Res Ed). 1988;296:1083-6.

CHAPTER

6.5 Infection-related Glomerulonephritis

Rehna Rahman, Swathi Shiri, Arpana A Iyengar

INTRODUCTION

Infections are common triggering factors for glomerulonephritis (GN) in children. Infection-related GN (IRGN) is a broad term that encompasses multiple entities of immune complex–mediated GN triggered by infections.[1] Based on the latent period following infection, GN is classified into two types:

1. Postinfectious GN (PIGN) develops after a latent period or infection-free interval following the primary trigger. It can be secondary to bacterial, viral, parasitic, or fungal infections. The classical prototype is poststreptococcal GN (PSGN).[2]
2. IRGN occurs simultaneously with an ongoing infection, mostly bacterial.[2,3]

The etiological approach to IRGN of bacterial origin is depicted in **Flowchart 1**.

The causative organisms associated with IRGN are summarized in **Table 1**. This chapter focuses on bacterial infections causing GN. Other infections, especially viral infections, associated with glomerular disease are addressed in the chapter on secondary nephrotic syndrome.

PATHOPHYSIOLOGY OF INFECTION-RELATED GLOMERULONEPHRITIS

The pathophysiology of GN involves the deposition of immune complexes that is formed by nephritogenic factors from bacteria and corresponding antibodies. These immune complexes are deposited in the subepithelial, subendothelial, or mesangial spaces. Formation and deposition of immune complexes involve multiple complex mechanisms, including entrapment of preformed circulating immune complexes, in situ immune complex formation related to lodged bacterial antigens in the glomerular basement membrane (GBM), or antibodies against native antigens of the basement membrane due to molecular mimicry. Formation of immune complexes leads to the activation of complement and downstream pathways, culminating in glomerular inflammation.[3] The pathophysiology of IRGN is represented in **Flowchart 2** and **Figure 1**. The three phases of IRGN include the following:

- Phase 1—formation of immune complex
- Phase II—deposition of immune complex in the glomerulus
- Phase III—inflammation due to immune complex deposition.

POSTSTREPTOCOCCAL GLOMERULONEPHRITIS

Incidence and Etiological Factors

Poststreptococcal GN is the prototype of PIGN. The overall global incidence is 472,000 cases per year, with a burden of 77% in low-income countries.[4] Risk factors for PSGN include overcrowding, poor hygienic conditions, and immunocompromised states. PSGN commonly occurs following pyoderma or pharyngitis infections.[2,4]

Poststreptococcal GN affects children more often than adults, with a peak age of incidence of 5–15 years. It can

Flowchart 1: Approach to infection-related glomerulonephritis. The flowchart represents the bacterial etiology of infection-related glomerulonephritis (IRGN) which can be poststreptococcal glomerulonephritis, *Staphylococcus*-associated glomerulonephritis, and other infections such as subacute bacterial endocarditis, shunt nephritis, etc.

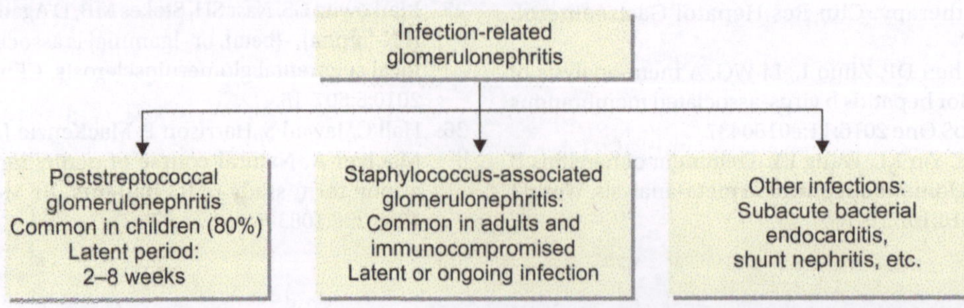

TABLE 1: Causes of infection-related glomerulonephritis.

Group	***Organism***
Bacteria	
Gram positive	Streptococci, staphylococci, pneumococci, *Listeria*
Gram negative	*Haemophilus*, meningococci, *Salmonella*, *Klebsiella*, *Legionella*, *Brucella*
Others	*Mycobacteria*, *Treponema*, *Rickettsia*, *Leptospira*
Viral	Hepatitis A, B, and C Epstein–Barr, CMV, HIV, adenovirus Parvovirus B19, Hantavirus, *Rotavirus*, Coxsackievirus
Parasitic	*Toxoplasma*, *Schistosoma*, Malaria, Filaria
Fungal	Coccidioidomycosis, *Candida*, *Histoplasma*

Note: The table represents the various etiologies of infection-related glomerulonephritis. The organisms are classified as bacterial, viral, parasitic, and fungal.
(CMV: cytomegalovirus; HIV: human immunodeficiency virus)
Source: Adapted from Kambham N. Postinfectious glomerulonephritis. Adv Anat Pathol. 2012;19:338-47.

Flowchart 2: Pathophysiology of infection-related glomerulonephritis (IRGN). The flowchart shows the process of immune complex formation and deposition resulting in GN.

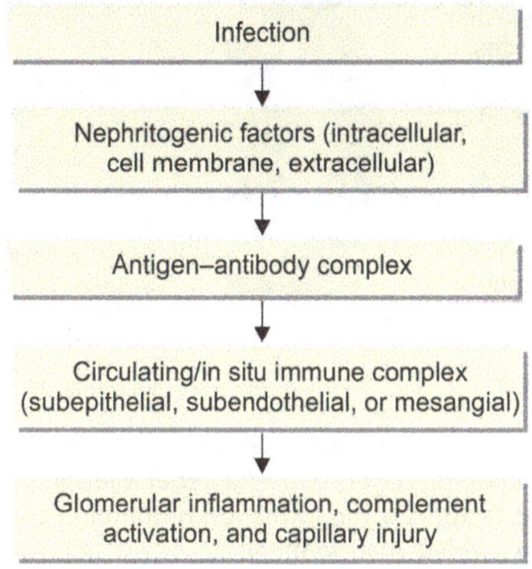

Source: Adapted from Balasubramanian R, Marks SD. Postinfectious glomerulonephritis. Pediatr Int Child Health. 2017;37:240-7.

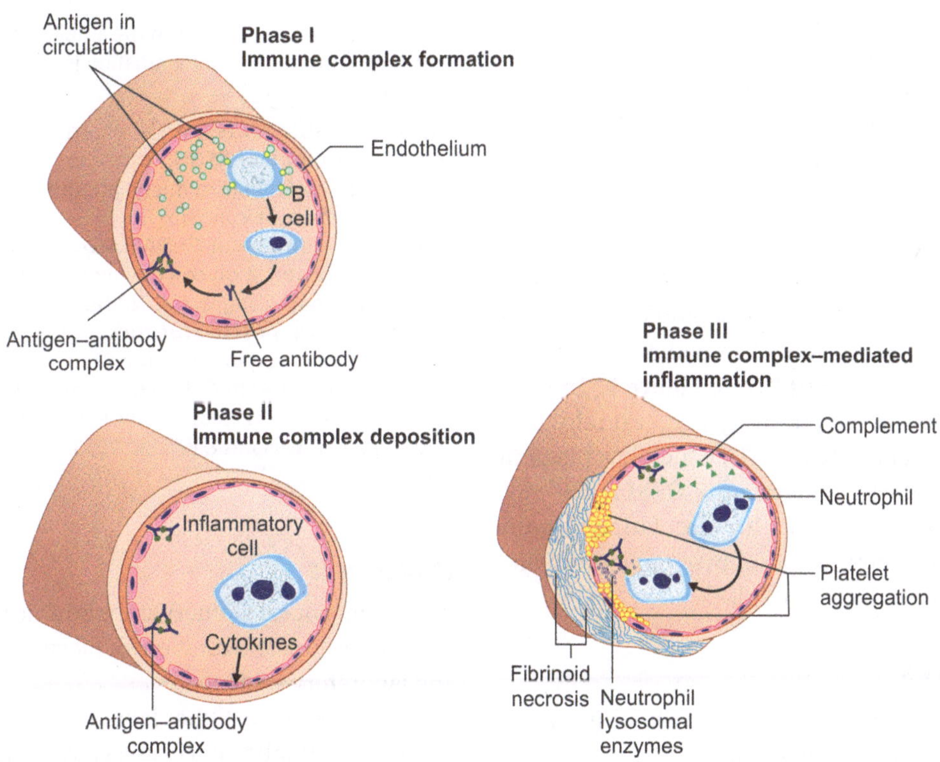

Fig. 1: Structural pathophysiology of infection-related glomerulonephritis (IRGN). The three phases of IRGN: Phase 1 involves formation of immune complex, phase II is the deposition of immune complex in the glomerulus, and phase III is inflammation due to the immune complex deposition.
Source: Adapted from Coffmann T, Falk R, Molitoris B, Neilson E, Schrier R W. Schrier's Diseases of the Kidney, 9th edition. Philadelphia, PA: Lippincott Williams & Wilkins; 2013. pp. 1277-87.

be sporadic or epidemic, sporadic being more common. Children below the age of 2 years account for 5% of cases, especially during epidemics.[4] Adults (over 40 years of age) with risk factors of immunocompromised states such as diabetes mellitus or human immunodeficiency virus (HIV) infection may develop PSGN (5–10%). Subclinical nephritis is more common than overt nephritis in children (4:1 to 10:1, respectively). Overt nephritis is typically seen in males.[5]

Group A beta-hemolytic streptococci M strains are the main causative organisms for PSGN, while group C streptococci are responsible for epidemic outbreaks. The structure of group A beta-hemolytic streptococci is represented in **Figure 2.**

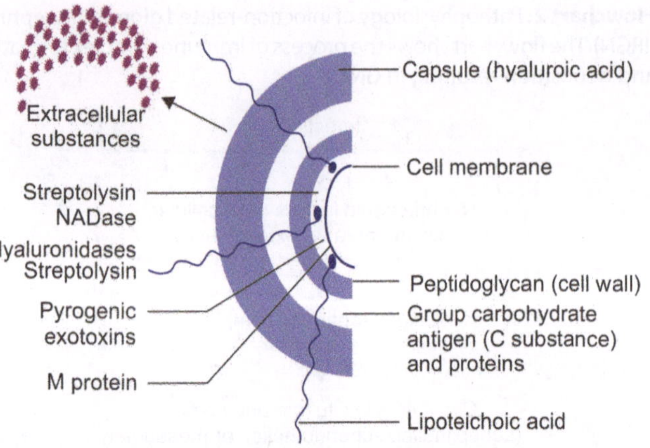

Fig. 2: Structure of group A beta hemolytic *Streptococcus*. The figure represents the various layers of the bacterial wall and proteins which are antigenic factors for the formation of immune complex. (NAD: nicotinamide adenine dinucleotide).
Source: Adapted from Uchida T, Oda T. Glomerular deposition of nephritis-associated plasmin receptor (NAPlr) and related plasmin activity: key diagnostic biomarkers of bacterial infection-related glomerulonephritis. Int J Mol Sci. 2020;21:2595:1-9.

Nephritogenic strains associated with sore throat are M types 1, 2, 4, 12, 18, and 25 and with pyoderma are M types 49, 55, 57, and 60. There is a higher risk of developing nephritis following pyoderma compared to pharyngitis (25 vs. 5%).[5]

Pathophysiology

Certain unique structural properties of group A beta-hemolytic streptococci are responsible for the pathophysiology of PSGN. The various proposed theories for PSGN pathophysiology are described in **Table 2, Flowchart 3, and Figure 3.**[6] Immune complex deposition is mediated by glyceraldehyde-3-phosphate dehydrogenase (GAPDH), which has plasmin-binding capacity and can penetrate the GBM resulting in immune complex formation in situ. Circulating immune complexes, formed by streptococcal pyrogenic exotoxin B (SpeB), are deposited in the glomeruli.[6,7]

Clinical Features

The period of latency depends on the site of infection, 1-3 weeks following pharyngitis and 3-6 weeks after skin infections. Majority (95%) of the children present with features of acute nephritis characterized by the classical triad of oliguria, hematuria (micro/macro), and hypertension.[3] Microscopic hematuria is typically present in all patients and may persist for up to 1 year. Gross hematuria is seen in 25-60% of the patients and usually resolves within 2 weeks. Around 60-80% of patients have hypertension, which may be the only presenting feature. Nephrotic syndrome is a rare presentation (5-10%). In <5%, a rapidly progressive GN (RPGN) requiring kidney replacement therapy (KRT), may be observed.[4,7] The various clinical presentations are summarized in **Table 3.**

TABLE 2: Pathophysiological theories of poststreptococcal glomerulonephritis.

Proposed theory	*Components*
In situ immune complex formation	• Deposition of streptococcal antigens in the glomerulus triggers formation of antistreptococcal antibodies with inflammation
Streptococcal antigens	• NAPlr-GAPDH • SpeB • NPBP • Cationic proteinase • Heparin inhabitable basement membrane protein • Streptococcal-derived kidney-binding protein • Streptokinase
Molecular mimicry	Antistreptococcal antibodies cross-react with glomerular antigens (matrix and cell membrane) due to shared structure
Altered IgG	Streptococcal enzymes alter the immunoglobulin structure. Altered IgG is deposited in the glomerulus and initiates inflammation
Deposition of circulating immune complexes	Role in the amplification of local inflammation in established disease

Note: The table represents the various theories of possible pathophysiology of PSGN. It can be in situ immune complex formation, molecular mimicry, altered IgG, and deposition of circulating immune complex.
(IgG: immunoglobulin G; NAPlr-GAPDH: nephritis-associated plasmin receptor a glycolytic enzyme with glyceraldehyde-3-phosphate dehydrogenase; NPBP: nephritis plasmin-binding protein; PSGN: poststreptococcal glomerulonephritis; SPEB: streptococcal pyrogenic exotoxin B)
Source: Adapted from Coffmann T, Falk R, Molitoris B, Neilson E, Schrier RW. Schrier's Diseases of the Kidney, 9th edition. Philadelphia, PA: Lippincott Williams & Wilkins; 2013. pp. 1277-87.

Diagnosis

Poststreptococcal glomerulonephritis is a clinical diagnosis. The proposed case definition for diagnosis is based on clinical and laboratory evidence.[7,8]

- *Confirmed case:* Either laboratory-definitive evidence or combined laboratory-suggestive evidence and clinical evidence.
- *Probable case:* Only clinical evidence of PSGN.

Laboratory-definitive evidence—kidney biopsy picture of PSGN.

Laboratory-suggestive evidence of PSGN—microscopic hematuria, recent evidence of streptococcal infection [antistreptolysin O (ASO)/anti-deoxyribonuclease B (anti-DNase B)], and low C3.

Clinical evidence—edema, hematuria, and hypertension.

The timeline of manifestations in PSGN is represented in **Figure 4.**

Flowchart 3: Pathophysiology of poststreptococcal glomerulonephritis. The flowchart represents nephritis-associated plasmin receptor and streptococcal pyrogenic exotoxin B–mediated PSGN.

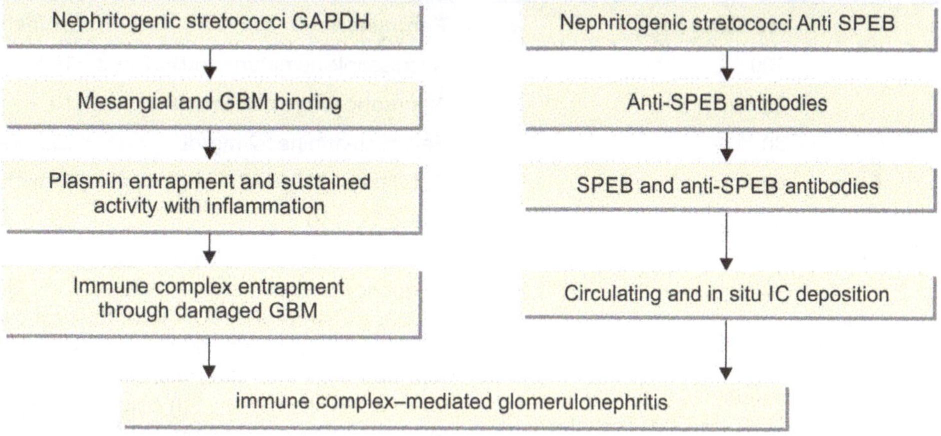

(GAPDH: glyceraldehyde-3-phosphate dehydrogenase; GBM: glomerular basement membrane; PSGN: poststreptococcal glomerulonephritis; SpeB: streptococcal pyrogenic exotoxin B).
Source: Adapted from Balasubramanian R, Marks SD. Postinfectious glomerulonephritis. Pediatr Int Child Health. 2017;37:240-7.

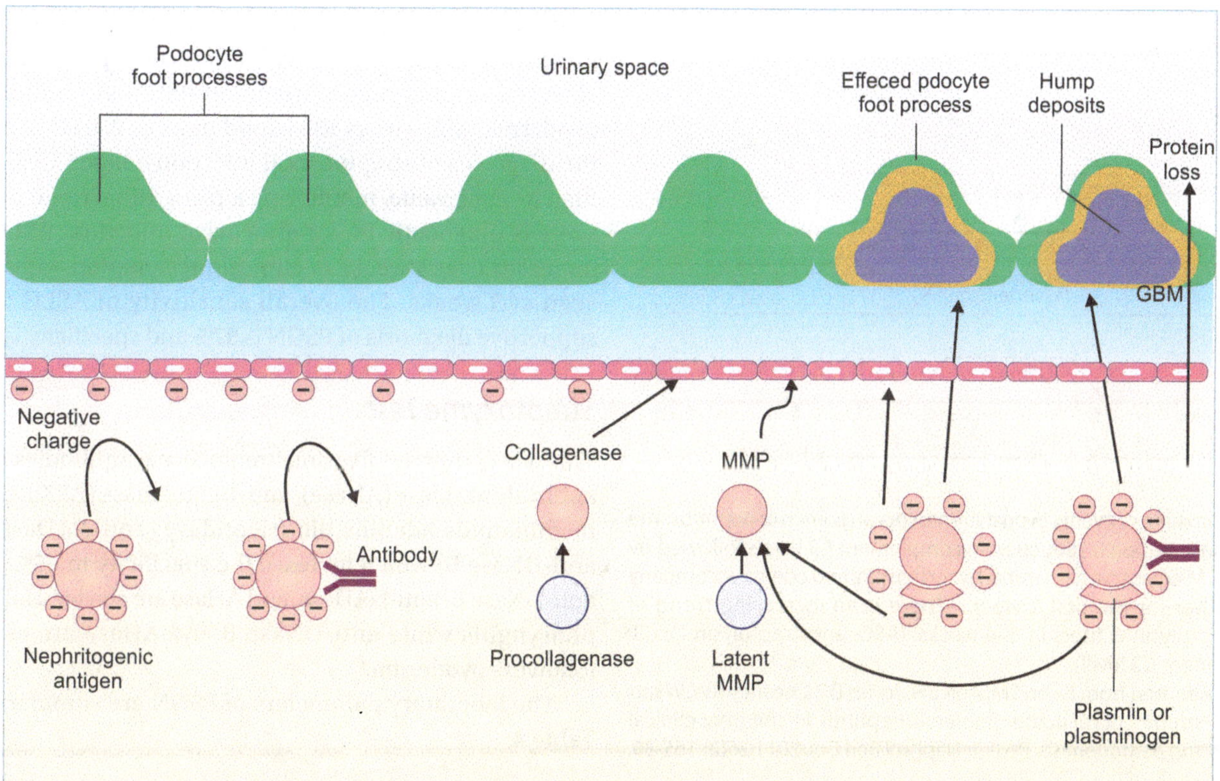

Fig. 3: Structural pathophysiology of poststreptococcal glomerulonephritis (PSGN). The figure represents the stepwise formation and deposition of immune complexes and subepithelial hump deposits and result in structural alteration of the GBM leading to proteinuria and hematuria. (GBM: glomerular basement membrane; MMP: matrix metalloproteinase).
Source: Adapted from Kambham N. Postinfectious glomerulonephritis. Adv Anat Pathol. 2012;19:338-47 and Balasubramanian R, Marks SD. Postinfectious glomerulonephritis. Pediatr Int Child Health. 2017;37:240-7.

Urine

Microscopic hematuria is seen in 100% of cases. On microscopic examination, the presence of red blood cell (RBC) cast is pathognomonic for the diagnosis of PSGN. Presence of dysmorphic RBCs (>20%) and acanthocytes, seen in phase contrast microscopy, is diagnostic of glomerular hematuria. White blood cells (WBCs) and WBC casts may also be seen, attributed to glomerular inflammation. About 70–80% cases have subnephrotic-range proteinuria.[4]

Complement Levels

In the first 2 weeks of active nephritis, C3 and CH50 levels are reduced suggestive of alternate complement pathway activation. C2 and C4 levels are normal or slightly decreased.

TABLE 3: Clinical presentation of poststreptococcal glomerulonephritis.

Clinical parameters	*Incidence (%)*
Microhematuria	100
Edema	85
Gross hematuria	30
Oliguria	60
Hypertension	60
Nephrotic syndrome	5–10
RPGN	<5

Note: The table represents the various clinical presentations of PSGN and their frequency of incidence.
(RPGN: rapidly progressive glomerulonephritis)
Sources: Adapted from Balasubramanian R, Marks SD. Postinfectious glomerulonephritis. Pediatr Int Child Health. 2017;37:240-7; Coffmann T, Falk R, Molitoris B, Neilson E, Schrier RW. Schrier's Diseases of the Kidney, 9th edition. Philadelphia, PA: Lippincott Williams & Wilkins; 2013. pp. 1277-87.

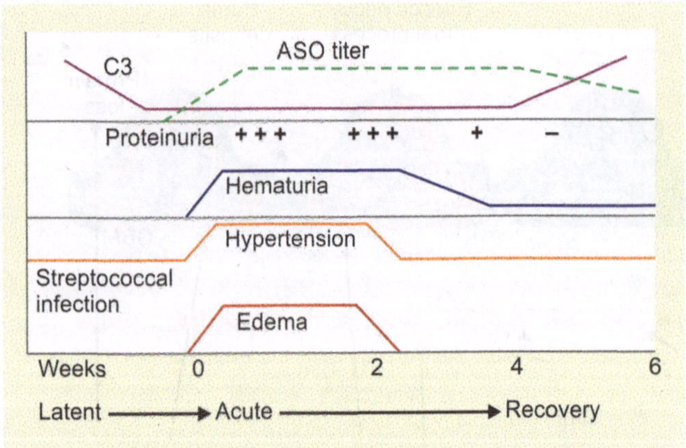

Fig. 4: Timeline of events in poststreptococcal glomerulonephritis. The first manifestation is reduction in complement C3 levels followed by oliguria. Microscopic hematuria, hypertension, and edema accompany each other for the first 2 weeks. There is an increasing trend of antistreptolysin O titers in 2–4 weeks. (ASO: antistreptolysin O; C3: complement C3 level).
Source: Adapted from Eison TM, Ault BH, Jones DP, Chesney RW, Wyatt RJ. Post-streptococcal acute glomerulonephritis in children: clinical features and pathogenesis. Pediatr Nephrol Berl Ger. 2011;26(2):165-80.

By 6–8 weeks, C3 levels normalize. Persistent low levels of C3, beyond 12 weeks, are suggestive of alternative diagnosis such as membranoproliferative GN (MPGN) and complement component 3 GN (C3GN).[5]

Kidney Functions

Although glomerular filtration rate (GFR) is decreased in PSGN, serum creatinine is usually normal and preserved in majority. Around 25% of the children may have acute kidney injury (AKI) with serum creatinine >2 mg/dL and <5% have RPGN course.[5]

TABLE 4: Laboratory evidence of poststreptococcal glomerulonephritis.

Parameters	*Incidence (%)*
Microscopic hematuria and RBC cast	100
Nephrotic-range proteinuria	10
Serum creatinine >2 mg/dL	25 (<5% RPGN)
ASLO titer >250 IU/dL	97 with sore throat
Low C3/CH 50	95

Note: The table represents the laboratory evidence of PSGN and its frequency of incidence.
(ASLO: antistreptolysin O; CH50: classical complement pathway; RPGN: rapidly progressive glomerulonephritis)
Source: Coffmann T, Falk R, Molitoris B, Neilson E, Schrier RW. Schrier's Diseases of the Kidney, 9th edition. Philadelphia, PA: Lippincott Williams & Wilkins; 2013. pp. 1277-87.

Antistreptococcal Antibodies

Antistreptolysin O (ASLO) titer is a supportive evidence for previous or ongoing streptococcal infection. It is significantly elevated in pharyngitis-triggered PSGN as compared to pyoderma. ASLO titers >333 Todd units or 250 IU/L support the diagnosis of streptococcal infection–related GN. Rather than a single value, monitoring a rising serial trend of ASLO titers is diagnostic for streptococcal infection. ASLO titer increases over 4 weeks of clinical presentation with a peak seen at 3 weeks. The overall sensitivity of ASLO titer in supportive diagnosis of PSGN is 97% and specificity is 80%.[5]

Streptozyme Test

This test comprises five antistreptococcal antibodies [ASLO, antihyaluronidase (AHase), antistreptokinase (ASKase), anti-nicotinamide adenine dinucleotidase (anti-NADase), and anti-DNase B] which increase the specificity to 95%. ASLO, anti-DNase B, anti-NADase, and AHase are elevated following pharyngitis while anti-DNase B and AHase are elevated following pyoderma.[6]

The laboratory parameters of PSGN are summarized in **Table 4**.

Histopathology

An alternative diagnosis to PSGN should be considered in children less than 2 years of age, in those with an RPGN presentation, presence of extrarenal features or with normal complement levels. The above features warrant a kidney biopsy. Indications for a kidney biopsy are summarized in **Table 5**. The light microscopy (**Figs. 5A and B**) typically shows diffuse (>50% glomeruli) proliferative and exudative changes. Endocapillary hypercellularity resulting from proliferation of endothelial cells, mesangial cells, and exudative neutrophilic infiltration gives a bloodless appearance to the glomeruli as the glomerular tuft capillary lumen gets obliterated.[4] Crescents

TABLE 5: Indications for kidney biopsy.

At presentation	*Delayed resolution*
• Rapidly progressive GN • Normal C3 levels • Nephrotic syndrome • No evidence of preceding sore throat or pyoderma • Systemic features • Second episode of AGN	• Renal dysfunction persisting >2 weeks • Gross hematuria persisting >4 weeks • Hypertension persisting beyond 3 weeks • Nephrotic-range proteinuria beyond 2 weeks • Low C3 persisting after 12 weeks • Persistent proteinuria beyond 6 months • Persistent microscopic hematuria beyond 12–18 months

Note: The table represents the various indications of kidney biopsy at presentation or delayed resolution.
(AGN: acute glomerulonephritis: GN: glomerulonephritis; C3: complement component C3)
Source: Adapted from Coffmann T, Falk R, Molitoris B, Neilson E, Schrier RW. Schrier's Diseases of the Kidney, 9th edition. Philadelphia, PA: Lippincott Williams & Wilkins; 2013. pp. 1277-87.

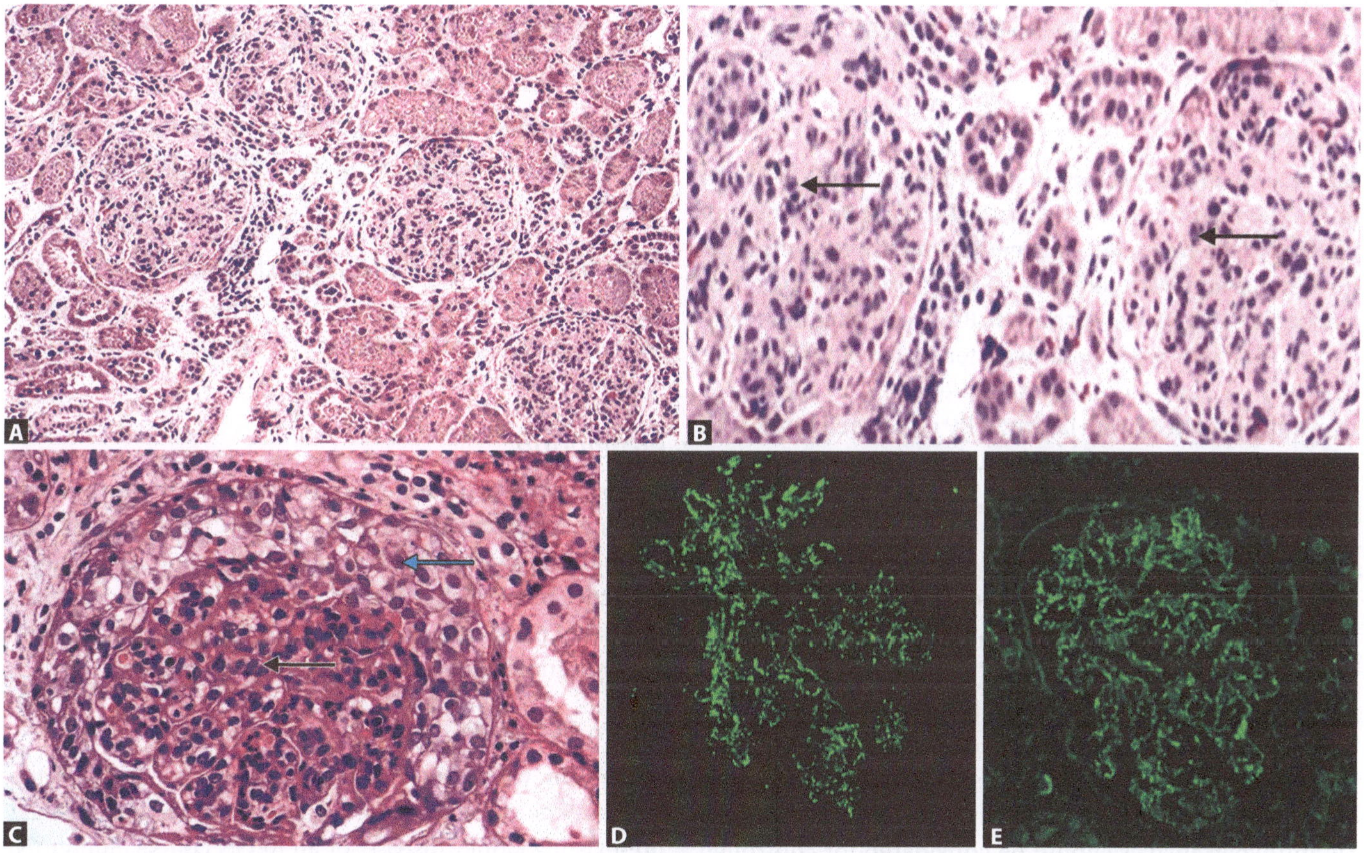

Figs. 5A to E: Light microscopy (LM) and immunofluorescence (IF) images of poststreptococcal glomerulonephritis (PSGN). (A) Light microscopy view in H&E stain showing diffuse exudative proliferation; (B) Light microscopy showing H&E stain with two glomeruli in high power with diffuse endocapillary hypercellularity and arrows showing neutrophils; (C) Light microscopy showing periodic acid–Schiff (PAS) stain of high power view of single glomerulus with crescent. The rest of the glomerulus shows diffuse endocapillary hypercellularity and neutrophilic infiltration giving the glomerulus a bloodless appearance. Blue arrow indicates crescent and black arrow shows neutrophils; (D and E) Immunofluorescence staining shows starry sky appearance of C3 and immunoglobulin G (IgG) deposits.
Courtesy: Dr Anila Abraham, RenopathLabs Pvt Ltd, Chennai.

may be seen occasionally (**Fig. 5C**). Immunofluorescence staining demonstrates discrete, irregular, coarse, and granular deposits of immunoglobulin G (IgG), immunoglobulin M (IgM), and C3 along the glomerular capillary walls and mesangium (**Figs. 5D and E**).[5] Classical patterns described are starry sky appearance, mesangial, and garland patterns. Electron microscopy characteristically shows dense subepithelial deposits or humps. Early in the course of the disease, IgG immune complexes are seen as deposits which resolve in 6 weeks.[6,9] The temporal timeline of kidney biopsy changes is given in **Table 6**.

Management

The goals of managing PSGN are to control hypertension, fluid overload, and treat hyperkalemia. The overall management is supportive. Common emergent manifestations of PSGN include hypertensive cardiac failure, pulmonary edema, hypertensive encephalopathy, and hyperkalemia.

TABLE 6: Timeline of renal biopsy in poststreptococcal glomerulonephritis.

	Early (<2 weeks)	*Typical (2–4 weeks)*	*Late (>4–6 weeks)*
Clinical features	Mild albuminuria, hematuria	Acute nephritic syndrome	Persistent hematuria/proteinuria
Light microscopy	Endocapillary proliferation Focal and segmental	• Diffuse global proliferation • Exudate early, then lymphocytes and monocytes • Endothelial and mesangial proliferation	Mesangial proliferation
Immunofluorescence	C3 and IgG, starry sky pattern	C3 and IgG, starry sky or garland pattern	C3 ± IgG, mesangial pattern
Electron microscopy	Mesangial, subepithelial (humps) deposits	Mesangial/subepithelial/subendothelial deposits	Mesangial, rarely subepithelial

Note: The table represents the timeline of histopathological changes of poststreptococcal GN. The typical changes of PSGN are seen in 2–4 weeks.
(C3: complement C3 level; IgG: immunoglobulin G)

Hypertension

The main pathophysiology of hypertension in PSGN is salt and water retention secondary to reduced GFR. The drug of choice for the treatment of hypertension is a loop diuretic, furosemide administered intravenously (preferred to oral) at a dose of 2–4 mg/kg per dose at 6th–8th hourly time intervals.[8] In case of acute symptomatic hypertension or blood pressure (BP) >95 + 12 mm Hg, sublingual nifedipine at 0.25 mg/kg/dose can be given 6th–8th hourly. If BP remains elevated even after 4–5 days, then long-acting antihypertensives amlodipine can be initiated.

Hypertensive Emergencies

Acute symptomatic hypertension with end-organ involvement can present as congestive cardiac failure [orthopnea, hypoxia, elevated jugular venous pressure (JVP) and on auscultation S3 heart sound with gallop and basal crepitations] or as hypertensive encephalopathy (headache, altered sensorium, persistent vomiting, and seizures). Apart from the above treatment measures of diuretics and oral antihypertensives, IV antihypertensives should be considered for controlled reduction of BP as described in the section on Hypertension.

Fluid and Dietary Restriction

Oral fluid is restricted based on the urine output and response to diuretics. Salt restriction is an important part of management of edema and hypertension (no extra added salt). Potassium restriction in diet is important to prevent life-threatening complication of hyperkalemia.[9]

Hyperkalemia

Besides dietary restriction of potassium, 10% calcium gluconate 2 mL/kg (maximum 10 mL) in 20 mL normal saline is given slowly over 30 minutes under cardiac monitoring. Nebulized salbutamol (3 mg in 2 mL NS) is also started simultaneously. In case of persistent hyperkalemia or serum potassium >6.5 mEq/L injection, regular insulin 0.1–0.5 units/kg in 2 mL/kg of 25% dextrose is given over 30 minutes.[9]

Rapidly Progressive Glomerulonephritis

In case of an RPGN course, KRT with hemodialysis or peritoneal dialysis is initiated. Immunosuppression is usually not indicated for RPGN secondary to PSGN.

Proteinuria

In cases of PSGN, subnephrotic-range proteinuria is self-limiting. Angiotensin-converting enzyme (ACE) inhibitors or angiotensin receptor blocker (ARBs) are contraindicated in the active phase of the illness due to the risk of hyperkalemia. In case of persisting proteinuria beyond 6–8 months, renal biopsy is indicated to exclude alternative diagnosis.

Acute Kidney Injury

Acute kidney injury is seen in 25% of the cases due to factors such as nephrotoxic medications, severe proliferative changes, pre-existing kidney disease, or an RPGN course. Supportive care is given as above. Kidney biopsy is warranted.

Prognosis

Poststreptococcal glomerulonephritis is a self-limiting disease with resolution of symptoms and laboratory findings in >90% of the cases. Resolution of edema is seen within 7–10 days. Gross hematuria clears by 2 weeks and hypertension resolves in 3–4 weeks. C_3 normalizes by 6–8 weeks. Proteinuria and microscopic hematuria resolve by 6 and 18 months, respectively. Recovery of kidney function is seen in 95% of the children. Factors that play a role in the progression of kidney disease are presence of crescents, garland pattern on immunofluorescence, nephrotic syndrome, and AKI. A very rare occurrence of progression to CKD is seen in <5% of affected children.[2,10] Studies have shown that after a follow-up of 5–18 years in those with childhood PSGN, 7–13% have persistent proteinuria, 13–15% have persistent hypertension, 5–12% persistent proteinuria, and abnormal renal function in 0.9–2%.[8,11]

Differential Diagnosis

Poststreptococcal glomerulonephritis should be differentiated from other infectious causes of acute glomerulonephritis (AGN) like *Staphylococcus*-associated GN (SAGN), MPGN, C3GN, and IgA nephropathy (IgAN). The histopathological differences between these entities are presented in **Table 7**.

Prevention

The ideal therapeutic strategy to prevent acute PSGN is to prevent streptococcal infection (pharyngitis or pyoderma). This is relevant to epidemics to curtail the spread of nephritis-associated streptococcal infection. Treatment of active streptococcal infection in the affected patient in sporadic cases prevents spread to other healthy siblings. However, once the streptococcal infection sets in, there is little role of antibiotics in the prevention of PSGN. For an active skin infection with staphylococcal or streptococcal impetigo, the antibiotic of choice is penicillin.[11] In case of sore throat, the diagnosis is difficult as only 10–20% of the infected patients isolate group A *Streptococcus* in throat culture. The McIsaac score aids in the diagnosis of streptococcal pharyngitis. McIsaac score has 1 point each for temperature >38°C, absence of cough, tender cervical lymphadenopathy, tonsillar swelling or exudates, and age 3–14 years. The total score ranges from 0 to 4 with a sensitivity of 85% and specificity of 92%.[12] Antibiotics are recommended in the presence of clinical symptoms when the score is 4. If the score is 2–3, throat cultures are necessary prior to initiation of antibiotics. Prophylactic penicillin is recommended in the following situations: in epidemics within closed communities, for household contacts of index cases in areas where streptococcal infection is highly prevalent. The following medications are recommended as prophylaxis in such situations:[12]

- Benzathine penicillin 0.6 MU dose in small children
- Oral phenoxymethyl penicillin G 125 mg, every 6 hours for 7–10 days
- Erythromycin if allergic to penicillin.

TABLE 7: Comparison of histopathology in poststreptococcal glomerulonephritis, *Staphylococcus*-associated glomerulonephritis, immunoglobulin A nephropathy, and membranoproliferative glomerulonephritis.

Parameter	*PSGN*	*SAGN*	*IgAN*	*MPGN*
LM	• Diffuse endocapillary hypercellularity • Exudative pattern • Crescents rare	• Wide spectrum • Mesangial HC common • Endocapillary HC few cases • Segmental necrotizing lesions • Diabetic changes: nodular hyalinosis • FSGS absent	• Mesangial hypercellularity common • Endocapillary HC common in children • FSGS frequent	• Endocapillary and mesangial hypercellularity • Double contours of GBM
IF	• Coarse granular "lumpy-bumpy" C3 staining along the glomerular capillary • Loops and mesangium with or without IgG • Garland pattern: Dense packed large deposits • Starry sky: Small deposits • Mesangial staining later cases	• Moderate to strong C3 deposits in mesangium • Mild to moderate IgA deposits • 25% no IgA deposits • 13% pauci-immune deposits • 40% co-dominant IgA and IgG deposits	• IgA-dominant deposits in the mesangium than in the capillary wall • C3 uncommon	Variable based on the cause IgG, C3, IgM: Immune complex mediated C3 ≥2 orders: C3GN Full-house pattern with IgG, IgM, IgA, C3, and C1q
EM	Large subepithelial hump deposits	• Mesangial deposits most common • Subepithelial deposits 30% • Few subendothelial deposits	Mesangial deposits most common	Subendothelial and mesangial deposits in immune complex MPGN intramembranous ribbon-like deposit in dense deposit disease

Note: The table shows the histopathological differences between PSGN, SAGN, IgAN, and MPGN.
(C3: complement 3; EM: electron microscopy; FSGS: focal segmental glomerulosclerosis; GBM: glomerular basement membrane; GN: glomerulonephritis; HC: hypercellularity; IF: immunofluorescence; IgA: immunoglobulin A; IgAN: immunoglobulin A nephropathy; IgG: immunoglobulin G; IgM: immunoglobulin M; LM: light microscopy; MPGN: membranoproliferative glomerulonephritis; SAGN: *Staphylococcus*-associated glomerulonephritis)
Source: Adapted from Satoskar AA, Parikh SV, Nadasdy T. Epidemiology, pathogenesis, treatment and outcomes of infection-associated glomerulonephritis. Nat Rev Nephrol. 2020;16(1):32-50.

Vaccination

There is no definitive vaccination strategy to prevent PSGN. The World Health Organization (WHO) has addressed group A beta-hemolytic *Streptococcus* infections as a global health issue and a proposed model for an innovative vaccination strategy is in the pipeline.[13]

Currently, two vaccines are under trial[13]:

1. *MJ8VAX vaccine:* It is under phase 1 of human trial. The antigen is a 29 amino acid peptide of the carboxy terminal of M protein.
2. *StreptAnova:* It is a 30 valent vaccine, with antigen derived from M protein with four recombinant subunits with N terminal fragments with 20–30 mm protein units. It is under phase II of human trial.

The protective efficacy of these vaccines in the prevention of PSGN is yet to be determined.

STAPHYLOCOCCUS-ASSOCIATED GLOMERULONEPHRITIS

Staphylococcus-associated GN is caused by *Staphylococcus aureus* [methicillin-resistant *S. aureus* (MRSA)/methicillin-sensitive *S. aureus* (MSSA)] or *S. epidermidis*. It occurs most commonly in elderly population (after the fifth decade of life), young immunocompromised individuals, and IV drug abusers. The underlying focus of infection is usually a local abscess, cellulitis, or pneumonia.[1]

Clinical Features

Patients with SAGN typically present with hematuria, AKI, and nephrotic-range proteinuria, in the presence of ongoing superficial infection (cellulitis, abscess) or deep infection (osteomyelitis, pneumonia). Patients usually present with worsening of underlying chronic disease or immunocompromised condition. In contrast to other causes of GN, where hypertension and features of fluid overload are common, SAGN can present with features of sepsis like tachycardia, wide pulse pressure, and hypotension.[1,10] The differences between acute PSGN and SAGN are given in **Table 8**.

Diagnosis

The diagnosis of SAGN is not based on a single criterion. Combined clinical, urine, histopathology, and culture results aid in making a diagnosis. Satoskar et al. formulated diagnostic criteria based on clinical and laboratory findings of GN.[1]

Definitive criteria:

- *Staphylococcus* isolated in a recent or ongoing infection site culture
- Acute proliferative GN based on hematuria, proteinuria (nephrotic range), AKI, and kidney biopsy showing proliferative changes with variable crescents, IgA, and C3 deposits.

Additional criteria:

- *Risk factors:* Diabetes mellitus, IV drug users, prosthetic devices, poor oral hygiene, skin cellulitis
- *Low complement levels:* C3 levels may be low in 60% cases
- *Leukocytoclastic vasculitis:* Rare presentation of SAGN (20% cases)
- *Positive antineutrophil cytoplasmic antibody (ANCA) levels:* Mild or atypical ANCA positivity is seen in few cases

TABLE 8: Comparison between poststreptococcal glomerulonephritis and *Staphylococcus*-associated glomerulonephritis.

Parameter	*PSGN*	*SAGN*
Presenting age	Children 5–15 years	Elderly > 60 years Young adults IVDU
Organism	Group A beta-hemolytic streptococci	*S. aureus* and *S. epidermidis*
Focus of infection	Pharyngitis/pyoderma	Endocarditis, skin abscess, cellulitis, osteomyelitis, etc.
Period of latency	1–2 weeks pharyngitis 3–6 weeks pyoderma	No latency Occult skin or bone infection
Clinical presentation	Edema, oliguria, HTN, and gross hematuria (60%) RPGN <5%	AKI (50%), nephrotic-range proteinuria (40%) worsening of diabetes, leukocytoclastic vasculitis rash (20%)
Laboratory	Microscopic hematuria (100%) low C3 (95%) rising ASLO titers	Microscopic hematuria (100%) low C3 in 30–50% pANCA positive in 20%
Treatment and outcome	Symptomatic management Fluid and salt restriction BP control Outcomes: 95% recovery RPGN, crescents, nephrotic syndrome poor outcomes	Treat underlying infection Control diabetes Poor outcomes 50% CKD progression in uncontrolled diabetes, crescents, endocarditis, etc.

Note: The table shows comparison between clinical, laboratory, and treatment differences between PSGN and SAGN.
(AKI: acute kidney injury; ASLO: antistreptolysin O; BP: blood pressure; CKD: chronic kidney disease; IVDU: IV drug user; HTN: hypertension; pANCA: perinuclear antineutrophil cytoplasmic antibody; PSGN: poststreptococcal glomerulonephritis; RPGN: rapidly progressive glomerulonephritis; SAGN: *Staphylococcus*-associated glomerulonephritis)
Source: Adapted from Satoskar AA, Parikh SV, Nadasdy T. Epidemiology, pathogenesis, treatment and outcomes of infection-associated glomerulonephritis. Nat Rev Nephrol. 2020;16(1):32-50.

- Subepithelial humps in electron microscopy
- C3 immunofluorescence in mesangial and capillary wall.

Treatment

The mainstay of treatment of SAGN is to treat the underlying infection with sensitive antibiotics. It is vital to isolate the organism in the culture from blood or any local infection site if accessible. Supportive care consists of fluid management and inotropic support if refractory hypotension. KRT is considered in case of refractory hyperkalemia, metabolic acidosis, anuria, or hyperammonemia.[6,10]

BACTERIAL ENDOCARDITIS-RELATED GLOMERULONEPHRITIS

In the recent era, due to appropriate treatment with antibiotics, there has been a reduction in endocarditis-related GN. The causative organisms are *Streptococcus viridans*, *S. aureus*, and rare organisms such as *Bartonella* and *Brucella*. *S. aureus*-related endocarditis is more common than *Streptococcus*-associated endocarditis. Bacterial endocarditis-related GN is rare in pediatric population and seen only in young adults with IV drug abuse.[6] It is difficult to differentiate between bacterial endocarditis-related GN and SAGN.

Bacterial endocarditis-related GN can be due to:

- *Subacute endocarditis:* It usually affects previously damaged valves secondary to low-virulence organisms like *S. viridans*, *S. mutans*, and HACEK (*Haemophilus*, *Aggregatibacter*, *Cardiobacterium*, *Eikenella*, and *Kingella*). In children, it is seen secondary to rheumatic fever or congenital heart disease. It is less destructive in nature and affects the left-side valves. Histopathology reveals MPGN.[1]
- *Acute endocarditis:* It affects healthy valves, commonly the right-sided valves, and is due to virulent organisms such as MRSA. It has a destructive course. Majority (80%) of cases present with AKI and nephrotic-range proteinuria. Two-thirds have low C3 and one-thirds can have positive ANCA.[1,6]

Histopathology

The histopathological pattern is similar to SAGN. Focal necrotizing crescents and diffuse or focal endocapillary hypercellularity are more common in bacteria endocarditis-related GN. Around 20% cases can have a pauci-immune pattern. Immunofluorescence staining reveals predominant C3 deposits with or without IgG. Electron microscopy shows less mesangial and capillary wall deposits. Few (20% cases) have subepithelial humps.[6,14]

Treatment

The treatment of choice of SAGN is broad-spectrum sensitive antibiotics and supportive care. Pauci-immune RPGN, which requires intensive immunosuppression, is a close differential diagnosis. Prompt management and follow-up of SAGN are crucial as >50% progress to kidney failure or CKD stage V.[15]

SHUNT NEPHRITIS

It is uncommon in children as ventriculoatrial, ventriculojugular, or ventriculovenal shunts for the management of hydrocephalus has become obsolete. When used, around 25–30% of these shunts had risk of infection and up to 5% developed nephritis. The causative organism was *S. epidermidis* in up to 75% of cases.[6]

Clinical Features and Diagnosis

Systemic manifestations include fever, prostration, myalgia, and weight loss weeks to months after shunt creation. Over 50–60% cases have gross hematuria and AKI. Around 30% present with nephrotic syndrome. On evaluation, low C3 and C4 and occasionally cryoglobulins are isolated. Blood cultures are also positive for the causative organisms.[16]

Histopathology

Membranoproliferative glomerulonephritis pattern is seen with granular deposits of C3, IgM, and IgG deposits. Electron microscopy reveals subendothelial and mesangial deposits.[6]

Treatment

Along with initiation of IV antibiotics, it is important to remove the infected shunt along with external drainage of cerebrospinal fluid. Around 70% of the cases recover from GN with normalization of kidney functions. Rare progression to chronic kidney stage V has been reported. There is no role of immunosuppression in shunt nephritis. In the present era, the treatment of hydrocephalus is by ventriculoperitoneal shunt due to which shunt-related nephritis has reduced.[16]

CONCLUSION

Infection-related glomerulonephritis is primarily approached based on clinical presentation along with supportive evidence of complement levels and renal histopathology. PSGN is the most common cause of IRGN in children. It is important to differentiate PSGN from other causes such as SAGN, MPGN, and IgAN. Infective endocarditis and shunt nephritis-related GN are rare causes of GN in children.

KEY POINTS

- PSGN is the prototype of IRGN in children presenting with oliguria, hypertension, gross hematuria and edema.
- Low C3 levels and increasing titers of ASLO support the diagnosis of PSGN.
- A loop diuretic is the treatment of choice for hypertension in PSGN along with strict fluid and dietary restriction of salt and potassium.
- Kidney biopsy is indicated in the presence of atypical features such as normal C3, persistent AKI, nephrotic

syndrome at presentation, persistent gross hematuria or hypertension, and persistent low C3 beyond 12 weeks.

- SAGN although an important cause of IRGN in adults and adolescent IV drug users is rare in children.
- Endocarditis and shunt-related nephritis is extremely rare in children in the present era.

REFERENCES

1. Satoskar AA, Parikh SV, Nadasdy T. Epidemiology, pathogenesis, treatment and outcomes of infection-associated glomerulonephritis. Nat Rev Nephrol. 2020;16(1):32-50.
2. Kambham N. Postinfectious glomerulonephritis. Adv Anat Pathol. 2012;19:338-47.
3. Nast C. Infection-related glomerulonephritis: changing demographics and outcomes advances in chronic kidney disease. Adv Chronic Kidney Dis. 2012;19(2):68-75.
4. Eison TM, Ault BH, Jones DP, Chesney RW, Wyatt RJ. Post-streptococcal acute glomerulonephritis in children: clinical features and pathogenesis. Pediatr Nephrol Berl Ger. 2011;26(2):165-80.
5. Balasubramanian R, Marks SD. Postinfectious glomerulonephritis. Pediatr Int Child Health. 2017;37:240-7.
6. Coffmann T, Falk R, Molitoris B, Neilson E, Schrier R W. Schrier's Diseases of the Kidney, 9th edition. Philadelphia, PA: Lippincott William and Wilkins; 2013. pp. 1277-87.
7. Uchida T, Oda T. Glomerular deposition of nephritis-associated plasmin receptor (NAPlr) and related plasmin activity: key diagnostic biomarkers of bacterial infection-related glomerulonephritis. Int J Mol Sci. 2020;21(7):2595.
8. Chaturvedi S, Boyd R, Krause V. Acute post-streptococcal glomerulonephritis in the northern territory of Australia: a review of data from 2009 to 2016 and comparison with the literature. Am J Trop Med Hyg. 2018;99(6):1643-8.
9. Rodríguez-Iturbe B, Batsford S. Pathogenesis of post-streptococcal glomerulonephritis a century after Clemens von Pirquet. Kidney Int. 2007;71(11):1094-104.
10. Glassock RJ, Alvarado A, Prosek J, Hebert C, Parikh S, Satoskar A, et al. *Staphylococcus*-related glomerulonephritis and poststreptococcal glomerulonephritis: why defining "post" is important in understanding and treating infection-related glomerulonephritis. Am J Kidney Dis Off J Natl Kidney Found. 2015;65(6):826-32.
11. Stratta P, Musetti S, Barecca A, Mazzucco G. New trends of an old disease: the acute post infectious glomerulonephritis at the beginning of the new millennium. J Nephrol. 2014;27:229-39.
12. Rodríguez-Iturbe B, Musser J. The current state of post streptococcal glomerulonephritis. J Am Soc Nephrol. 2008;19: 1855-64.
13. Johan V, Fernando GR, Kim JH, Jean Louis J, Pierre RS, O'Brein KL, et al. The path to group A *Streptococcus* vaccines: World Health Organization research and development technology roadmap and preferred product characteristics. Clin Infect Dis. 2019;69(5):877-83.
14. Boils CL. Endocarditis-associated glomerulonephritis. In: Satoskar AA, Nadasdy T (Eds). Bacterial Infections and the Kidney [Internet]. Cham: Springer International Publishing; 2017 [cited December 2020]. pp. 87-116. Available from: https://doi.org/10.1007/978-3-319-52792-5_4 [Last accessed May, 2022].
15. Boils CL, Nasr SH, Walker PD, Couser WG, Larsen CP. Update on endocarditis-associated glomerulonephritis. Kidney Int. 2015;87(6):1241-9.
16. Haffner D, Schindera F, Aschoff A, Matthias S, Waldherr R, Schärer K. The clinical spectrum of shunt nephritis. Nephrol Dial Transplant Off Publ Eur Dial Transpl Assoc Eur Ren Assoc. 1997;12(6):1143-8.

CHAPTER

6.6

Immunoglobulin A Nephropathy

Manoj G Matnani, Indira Agarwal

INTRODUCTION

Immunoglobulin A nephropathy (IgAN), also called Berger disease, is the most common primary glomerular disease worldwide. It was first described in 1968 by Berger and Hinglais and is now recognized as a distinct clinic-pathologic entity. It is considered to be an immune complex (IC)-mediated or aggregated (polymerized) IgA-mediated glomerulonephritis (GN). It was considered initially as a benign disease with favorable prognosis, but data from long-term follow-up studies indicate that 20–50% of adults would ultimately progress to end-stage kidney disease (ESKD).[1]

INCIDENCE AND PREVALENCE

The prevalence of IgAN varies widely from one country to another. In the Pacific Rim (e.g., Japan, Singapore, Australia, and New Zealand), it accounts for as many as one half of primary GN while around 20-30% in Europe and 2–10% in North America.[2] Racial, genetic, and environmental factors contribute to the geographic differences in the prevalence. The high incidence of IgAN in certain countries may reflect the practice of routine urinalysis. In Japan, all school-going children between the ages of 6 and 18 years are screened annually and those found to have urinary abnormalities are referred for further investigation. IgAN is the most common primary GN in Japanese children detected in approximately 30% of biopsy specimens obtained (*Courtesy:* Kobe University and Wakayama Medical University Hospitals).

ETIOLOGY

Immunoglobulin A nephropathy can be primary or secondary. The exact etiology of primary IgAN is unknown. Infections and genetic factors are implicated in the pathogenesis.

INFECTIONS

Immunoglobulin A is the main immunoglobulin directed against viral and bacterial antigens in the exocrine system. Due to the frequent association noted between upper respiratory and gastrointestinal tract (GIT) infection with the onset of macroscopic hematuria, it has been suggested that certain viral or bacterial infections may lead to IgAN. Many other antigens including herpes simplex virus, cytomegalovirus (CMV), Epstein-Barr virus (EBV) nuclear antigen, adenovirus, and milk antigen have also been identified.

GENETIC FACTORS

Genetic factors may not only determine susceptibility to GN but also influence the pathological severity and natural course of IgAN.

MODE OF INHERITANCE

By multipoint linkage analysis under the assumption of genetic heterogeneity, a close association with the trait under a dominant model of transmission with incomplete penetrance has been observed on chromosome 6q22-23 (locus named *IGAN1*, in 60% of familial IgAN).[3]

DISEASE PATHOGENESIS IN IMMUNOGLOBULIN A NEPHROPATHY

There is substantial evidence that IgAN is an IC disease. The initiating event in the pathogenesis of IgAN is the mesangial deposition of IgA, which is predominantly polymeric IgA of the IgA1 subclass containing J chain. Codominant deposition of immunoglobulin G (IgG) and invariable complement C3 but rarely C1q may also contribute to disease severity.[4]

Genetic and environmental factors increase the susceptibility and risk of disease progression in IgAN. The immunopathogenesis of this disease is a result of a confluence of factors and is described as a multi-"hit" process. There is a genetically determined increase in circulating levels of IgA1, with galactose-deficient O-glycans in the hinge region (Hit 1). Antibodies directed against galactose-deficient IgA1 form ICs that accumulate in the glomerular mesangium (Hits 2 and 3). There is activation of mesangial cells, proliferation and secretion of extracellular matrix, cytokines, and chemokines with resultant renal injury (Hit 4).[4]

The presence of circulating and glomerular ICs comprised of galactose-deficient IgA1, an IgG autoantibody directed against the hinge region O-glycans presence of C3, is the key feature initiating the disease. The predisposition to form aberrantly glycosylated IgA1 may be inherited.[5]

Galactose-deficient IgA1 levels may be detected to be elevated in 25% of blood relatives of IgAN patients. In these individuals, segregation analysis suggested a major dominant gene in the background of additional polygenic abnormalities.[6]

Levels of galactose-deficient IgA1 in a person may be influenced to some extent by environmental factors. It is known that these antibodies are susceptible to bacteria-derived proteases.[7] It has been found that antiglycan autoantibodies are not sequences present in the host germline but are formed by somatic hypermutation and these target IgA *VH* gene segments.[8] ICs thus formed target the kidney and directly cause glomerular inflammation and mesangial proliferation. Glomerulosclerosis and tubulointerstitial fibrosis are caused by the activation of local and systemic renin–angiotensin system (RAS) as well as complement activation resulting in gradual loss of renal function. Presence of coexisting risk factors such as hypertension and smoking contribute to disease progression by causing microvascular injury.[9] Obesity results in maladaptive hyperfiltration injury and glomerulomegaly and may be implicated in nonimmunologically mediated disease progression.[10]

The site of IgA production in IgAN is not established neither are the triggers responsible for production of galactose-deficient IgA1 known. Experimental models suggest that excess production of aberrantly glycosylated IgA in mucosal-associated lymphoid tissue may have environmental triggers. BAFF is a B-cell activation factor of the tumor necrosis factor (TNF) family and is critical but not sufficient for the development of an experimental IgAN phenotype.[11]

Immunotherapy primarily causes reduction in proteinuria, without change in long-term outcome. Based on this, recent studies have questioned the role of antiglycan antibodies in disease immunopathogenesis. These may be explained by the fact that these are short-term treatment interventions, and the formation of antiglycan antibodies are only part of a complex disease process. Brief immunomodulatory intervention may not be sufficient to alter defects in mucosal immune function and microbiota profiles in a sustained fashion as these processes are genetically influenced and environmentally determined.

ROLE OF COMPLEMENT

Activation of complement, including the lectin pathway, is also regarded an important pathogenic contributor in IgAN. This is evidenced by the fact that polymeric IgA1 is capable of activation of this pathway in vitro, and mannose-binding lectin pathway elements are detected in glomerular deposits.[12,13]

The linking of defects in the regulation of the alternative pathway of complement to IgAN immunopathogenesis has been shown by clinical and genetic studies.[14] Evidence of the presence of circulating and ICs containing C3 is shown on immunofluorescence in kidney biopsies. Gharavi et al. proposed the presence of properdin and complement factor H (CFH) in the immune deposits.[15] An allele initially localized to the *CFH* gene that confers protection against the development of IgAN has been identified by genome-wide association studies (GWAS). A deletion of CFH-related (CFHR) genes 1 and 3 in linkage disequilibrium with the identified risk allele is identified. The CFHR1 and CFHR3 proteins titrate CFH activity, and their absence is associated with altered CFH levels and enhanced CFH activity.[15,16]

SECONDARY IMMUNOGLOBULIN A NEPHROPATHY

Secondary deposition of IgA in the glomerular mesangium occurs in a variety of disorders such as thin basement membrane nephropathy, lupus nephritis, minimal change disease, diabetic nephropathy, and IgA-dominant *Staphylococcus*-associated postinfectious GN. Causes of secondary IgAN are given in **Table 1**.

CLINICAL FEATURES

Immunoglobulin A nephropathy may present at any age, but the peak incidence is in the second and third decades of life. It affects boys more than girls. The M:F ratio varies from 2:1 to 6:1. Patients with IgAN typically present in one of the three ways. Approximately 40–50% present with single or recurrent episodes of gross hematuria, usually following bacterial tonsillitis or other viral upper respiratory infections. Less-frequent initiating events include other mucosal system infections (e.g., diarrhea and sinusitis). The interval between the precipitating infection and the appearance of hematuria ranges from 1 to 2 days. This has been called "synpharyngitic hematuria" compared with 1 or 2 weeks in acute postinfectious GN (called postinfectious hematuria). Patients may complain of flank pain during acute episodes, which usually reflects stretching of the renal capsules. Low-grade fever may also be present. These features can mimic urinary tract infection or urolithiasis.

Another 30–40% have incidentally detected microscopic hematuria and mild proteinuria on a routine examination. Gross hematuria may occur later in 20–25% of these patients. Less than 10% present with either nephrotic syndrome

TABLE 1: Causes of secondary immunoglobulin A nephropathy.

Multisystem diseases	HSP, SLE, cystic fibrosis, celiac disease, Crohn disease, dermatitis herpetiformis, ankylosing spondylitis
Neoplasms	Carcinoma of lung, colon, monoclonal IgA gammopathy mycosis fungoides, NHL
Infectious diseases	*Mycoplasma* infections, leprosy, toxoplasmosis
Others	Chronic liver disease, pulmonary hemosiderosis, mixed cryoglobulinemia, polycythemia

(HSP: Henoch–Schönlein purpura; IgA: immunoglobulin A; NHL: non-Hodgkin's lymphoma; SLE: systemic lupus erythematosus)

or rapidly progressive GN. Hypertension is usually mild to moderate. Those with undetected long-standing IgAN may present with malignant hypertension and chronic kidney failure. A subset of patients can have a rapidly progressive course characterized by extensive crescents and tubulointerstitial changes.

Asymptomatic hematuria with minimal proteinuria (i.e., <0.5 g/day) may be incidentally detected during school-screening programs, military draft screens, or insurance programs. The milder symptoms of isolated microscopic hematuria with minimal proteinuria usually have a good outcome, particularly in the white population.[17] Long-term follow-up of these patients is recommended as a small proportion could develop proteinuria, hypertension, and renal failure.[18,19] Amongst those who do develop progressive chronic kidney disease (CKD), renal survival may range according to the time of biopsy and introduction of lead-time bias. The actual 10-year renal survival is reported to be 57–91%.[20] Factors associated with poor prognosis include hypertension, proteinuria, and decreased estimated glomerular filtration rate (eGFR) at diagnosis, the severity of pathologic findings.[21,22] The ethnicity of the patient may also be an important determinant of outcome.[23]

A classical clinical syndrome associated with the first presentation of IgAN is synpharyngitic nephritis with macroscopic hematuria seen in 10–15% of the patients.[24] Presence of gross hematuria at the time of presentation with infection often prompts immediate medical attention. Recurrent macroscopic hematuria is associated with a favorable prognosis in the short-term. Subsequent development of persistent proteinuria is associated with potentially progressive disease.[25]

A rare clinical presentation includes a dual diagnosis of IgAN and minimal change disease. Although nephrotic-range proteinuria >3 g/day is not uncommon in IgAN, coexistence of nephrotic syndrome is rare.[25-27] Renal function in such children is often preserved and overt nephrotic syndrome with edema, dyslipidemia, and hypoalbuminemia is present. The course of disease follows that of minimal change disease and these children respond well to steroids and thus have a favorable outcome.[28] Sometimes, a steroid-sparing agent may also be required to maintain remission. Only 306 out of 11,885 in a cohort of IgAN had renal biopsy findings of diffuse IgA-dominant mesangial deposits with minimal changes in glomeruli on light microscopy. More than 50% podocyte foot-process effacement was seen in all. The prognosis was excellent as none of them reached ESKD at the end of a median of 2.6 years.[28]

A rapidly progressive course which may be demonstrated with biopsy findings of >50% of glomeruli exhibiting crescents and clinically a severe disease is rare. When present the rate of ESKD may be as high as 42.5% at 1 year despite immunosuppressive therapy, as reported in a large case series of 113 subjects.[29]

IMMUNOGLOBULIN A NEPHROPATHY AND HENOCH–SCHÖNLEIN PURPURA NEPHRITIS

A close relationship exists between these two disorders as evidenced by the following observations:

- The morphology and immunopathology features are similar in both the diseases.
- Infective episodes precede Henoch-Schönlein purpura nephritis (HSPN) in 30–50% patients. The presence of *Hemophilus parainfluenzae* antigens have been demonstrated in the glomerular mesangium along with the presence of IgA antibodies in the sera of these patients.
- Both of them are variants of the same process and that IgAN is HSPN without the rash.
- HSPN is an acute disease, with glomerular lesions nonprogressive after the onset. Hence in most patients, the prognosis is associated with the severity of glomerular change at the onset. In contrast, IgAN is a chronic, slowly progressive glomerular lesion that may eventually lead to CKD, whatever is the initial presentation.
- Finally, HSPN occurs mostly in young children and is rare in adulthood, whereas IgAN affects mainly older children and adults.[30]

Diagnosis

Clinical history and laboratory data point to the possible diagnosis of IgAN, but confirmation is by kidney biopsy. The immunofluorescence or immunoperoxidase studies showing IgA deposits within mesangium confirm the diagnosis.

Laboratory Investigations

Urinalysis shows hematuria, proteinuria, and leukocytes. Urine microscopy showing dysmorphic RBCs and RBC casts suggests GN but is not specific for IgAN. Hemogram suggesting anemia, leukocytosis, and thrombocytopenia will suggest other underlying causes for nephritis. *Serial measurement of 24-hour urine protein or urinary protein*: Creatinine ratio and renal function tests including GFR are highly recommended most useful parameters to assess the progression of renal disease. Complement levels C3 and C4 are usually within normal limits, whereas signs of subclinical complement activation can be detected by measuring the C3d breakdown product. High serum levels of IgA are seen in 35–50%. High levels of macromolecular IgA (IgA IC, mixed IgA/IgA-IC, IgA/fibronectin aggregates) are frequently found, particularly during phases of clinical activity.[31] But this is not sufficiently specific to establish the diagnosis. The definitive diagnosis is only made on a histologic basis, which confirms the presence of IgA as a sole or predominant Ig in the glomerular mesangium.

Pathology

Light Microscopy

The characteristic abnormality is mesangial enlargement, caused by various combinations of hypercellularity and increase in mesangial matrix. Biopsies can be graded according to the amount of mesangial cell proliferation on the basis of World Health Organization (WHO) criteria.

Minimal glomerular lesions: The majority of the glomeruli appear normal, whereas a few show slight increase in mesangial matrix, with/without hypercellularity. The number of mesangial cells per peripheral mesangial area does not exceed three (<3).

Focal mesangial proliferation: Up to 80% of the glomeruli show moderate or severe mesangial cell proliferation (>3), with increased matrix. Small cellular or fibrocellular crescents in <20% of glomeruli are frequently found. Tubular atrophy, interstitial fibrosis, and interstitial lymphocyte infiltration are present but not extensive.

Diffuse mesangial proliferation: More than 80% of the glomeruli show moderate or severe mesangial cell proliferation (>3), always accompanied with increased matrix. Cellular and fibrocellular crescents are frequently found affecting <50% of the glomeruli. However, in 10% of patients >50% of the glomeruli are involved. Tubular atrophy, interstitial fibrosis, and interstitial lymphocyte infiltration are frequent and extensive in 10% of the patients. Histologic features associated with an increased risk of progressive disease include markers of more severe inflammatory disease such as crescent formation and immune deposits in the capillary loops in addition to the mesangial deposits and markers of chronic fibrotic disease such as glomerulosclerosis, tubular atrophy, interstitial fibrosis, and vascular disease. The histopathological grading is given in **Box 1**.[32]

Immunofluorescence

The hallmark is the presence of IgA in the glomerular mesangium as the sole or predominant immunoglobulin **(Figs. 1A and B)**. Immunoglobulin M (IgM; 8%), IgG (32%), and C3 (64%) are also present. The early components of the classical complement pathway C4 or C1q are absent. Fibrin- or fibrinogen-related antigens are found in 25–70% patients and are one of the injurious agents in the glomeruli. Peripheral

BOX 1: Histologic subclassification of immunoglobulin A nephropathy.

- Minimal or no mesangial hypercellularity without glomerular sclerosis
- Focal and segmental glomerular sclerosis without active cellular proliferation
- Focal proliferative GN
- Diffuse proliferative GN
- Any biopsy showing ≥40% globally sclerotic glomeruli and/or ≥40% estimated cortical tubular atrophy or loss

(GN: glomerulonephritis).

Source: Haas M. Histologic classification of IgA nephropathy: a clinicopathologic study of 244 cases. Am J Kidney Dis. 1997;29:829-42.

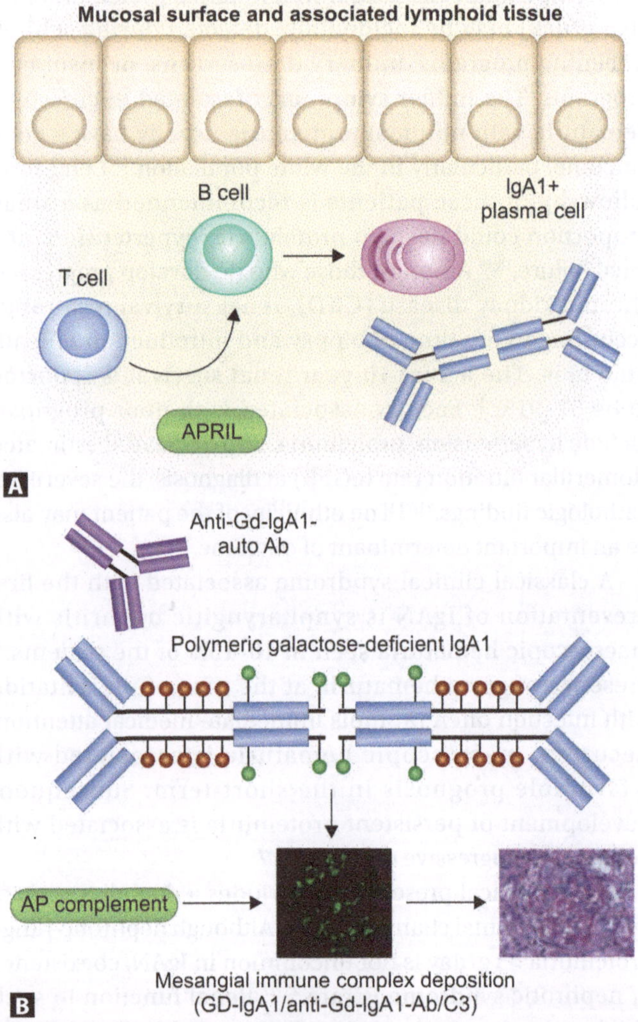

Figs. 1A and B: Understanding the pathogenesis of IgA nephropathy reveals therapeutic targets. (A) Mucosal IgA production by plasma cells occurs by T cell-dependent and-independent process. T cell cytokines such as APRIL promote B cell class switch to IgA1-producing plasma cells. Inhibitors of these cytokines are potential therapeutic targets. B cell and plasma cell inhibitors (e.g., rituximab, bortezomib) may result in decreased IgA production; (B) The IgA1 produced in patients with IgA nephropathy is underglycosylated (Cd-IgA1). Susceptible individuals will also produce anti-Gd-IgA1 autoantibody (auto-Ab).[9] Antiproliferative drugs may affect production of antiglycan autoantibodies. The Gd-IgA1-auto-Ab immune complexes activate the alternative pathway of complement. Complement inhibitors may prevent formation of immune complexes; (C) The immune complexes are nephritogenic, contributing to local inflammation, cellular proliferation, and ultimately fibrosis. Broad-based targeting of process implicated in glomerular and tubulo-interstitial injury (e.g., inflammation, fibrosis) target these final common pathways of kidney damage. Anti-Gd-IgA1-auto-Ab, autoantibody directed at galactose-deficient IgA1. (IgA: immunoglobulin A)

Source: Rodrigues JC, Haas M, Reich HN. IgA nephropathy. Clin J Am Soc Nephrol. 2017;12:677-86.

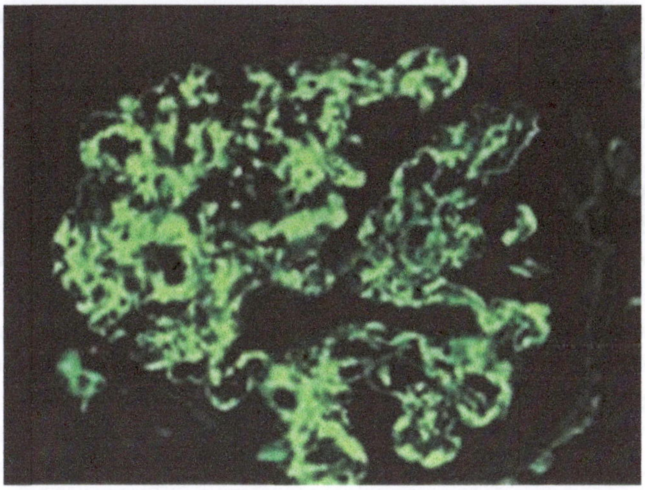

Fig. 2: Immunoglobulin A (IgA) nephropathy. *Granular staining for IgA, predominantly in the mesangium FITC anti-IgA.*
Courtesy: Dr Anila Abraham, Pathologist, Madras Medical Mission, Chennai, Tamil Nadu, India.

capillary wall deposits of IgA seen in 10% of the patients are associated with more severe clinical manifestations and a poor renal outcome **(Fig. 2)**.

Electron Microscopy

Electron dense deposits in the mesangium are the most constant and prominent feature. These are granular masses situated immediately beneath the lamina densa in the perimesangial region and expanded mesangium. Subepithelial deposits and lysis of glomerular basement membrane (GBM) are seen frequently in children.

Clinic–Pathologic Correlation in Immunoglobulin A Nephropathy: Oxford Classification

International IgA Nephropathy Network Group working in collaboration with the Renal Pathology Society developed a consensus on the pathologic classification of IgAN. The design of a structured, standardized, and reproducible pathologic scoring system in IgAN by renal biopsy evaluation has added important prognostic information beyond what is obtained from clinical variables alone. Histologic variables correlating with adverse renal outcomes independent of the clinical features at baseline and the degree of proteinuria and blood pressure control during follow-up include mesangial hypercellularity, segmental glomerulosclerosis, endocapillary hypercellularity, and tubular atrophy/interstitial fibrosis. The Oxford classification has been validated and the predictive value of each histologic variable appears to be similar in adults and children.

The Oxford classification schema was derived studying patients with >0.5 g/day of proteinuria, eGFR > 30 mL/min/1.73 m^2 at renal biopsy, and >1 year of follow-up. The clinical relevance and applicability of the MEST score derived from the renal biopsy has now been validated across multiple populations including, most recently, the European (VALIGA) cohort.[17] Elucidating the relationship between histologic class and treatment response is an important next step. Response to corticosteroids may differ according to histology as evidenced by studies using the MEST score.

The effect of crescents on outcome remains a challenging question in IgAN. The recent data may shed some light on clinical implications of these findings. Although crescents are a common finding in IgAN, the presence of >30% of crescents is considered significant. Patients with crescents involving >50% of the glomeruli are at high risk of progression, with 75% reaching ESKD by 10 years as suggested by some early studies. Crescents portend a poor prognosis with rapid progression of loss of kidney function. The First Oxford Conference on IgAN in 2014 included a working group, which examined the association of crescents with renal outcomes in 3,096 patients combined from four published studies: the original Oxford cohort, the VALIGA study cohort, and two large Asian cohorts, one from China and the other from Japan.[30] On the basis of the findings of this study, crescent scores were added to the Oxford (MEST) classification as follows: C0: no cellular or fibrocellular crescents; C1: cellular/fibrocellular crescents in <25% of glomeruli—identifying patients at increased risk of a poor outcome (compared with C0) among those not given immunosuppressive therapy; and C2: crescents in ≥25% of glomeruli—identifying patients at increased risk of a poor outcome even if given immunosuppression.[33,34]

Treatment

The optimal treatment of IgAN is controversial as the slow progression of the disease hinders the ability to perform adequate studies. There are two important aspects in the management of IgAN. General measures to slow the progression of CKD including blood pressure control, reduction of proteinuria with angiotensin-converting enzyme inhibitors (ACEIs) or angiotensin II receptor blockers (ARBs) and statins to correct dyslipidemia are not specific to IgAN. The specific therapy is focused on two principles. The first is anti-inflammatory drugs including corticosteroids and immunosuppressant drugs for the systemic immune reaction and renal histologic activity. Antisclerogenic drugs to inhibit progressive renal fibrosis is the second. Warfarin and dipyridamole are used to inhibit the mediators of glomerular damage.

Conservative Therapy

The mainstay of treatment in IgAN is supportive measures and conservative therapy to reduce proteinuria and slow the rate of renal function decline. RAS blockade medications, ACEIs, and ARBs reduce proteinuria, but this combination therapy may increase the risks of hyperkalemia and hence should be closely monitored if used.[35] Statins also decrease the severity of the disease as has been demonstrated by some clinical trials.

Mycophenolate

The data on the efficacy of mycophenolate as in the treatment of IgAN is mixed, and hence current clinical guidelines do not recommend its use[36] except in low-risk renal disease where it has better applicability. In a randomized, double-blind, placebo-controlled clinical trial, 44 patients with persistent proteinuria (Urine protein creatine ratio) of >0.6–0.8 and eGFR >50 mL/min/1.73 m² were randomly assigned to mycophenolate mofetil (MMF) or placebo in addition to conservative therapy. Only 7 patients in the treatment group and 10 patients in the placebo group were analyzed as those with a good response to conservative management during the run-in phase (36 of 184) were excluded. The trial did not see completion as there was a lack of observed benefit.[37]

A trial of the use of mycophenolate in patients with more advanced and high-risk disease was conducted—this included a double-blind, controlled trial of 32 patients with 1 g/day of proteinuria and at least two additional risk factors (male sex, hypertension, clearance <80 mL/min/1.73 m², glomerulosclerosis, tubulointerstitial fibrosis, or ≥25% of glomeruli affected by crescents).[38] This study also showed a worse renal outcome in the MMF group compared to placebo with RAS blockade and was thus terminated early.

However, another small, randomized, nonblinded trial of 40 patients with >1 g/day of persistent proteinuria showed a better response. The MMF group demonstrated remission of proteinuria (16 vs. 6) and had overall less proteinuria (1.1460.23 g/24 hours vs. 2.460.40 g/24 hours).[39] In the long term also, improved renal survival was seen in the MMF-treated patients (90 vs. 55%, $P = 50.01$).[40]

Most of the studies were limited by small sample size and the possibility of race-specific variability in response to MMF may be present as seen in lupus nephritis.[41] Systematic reviews and meta-analyses of the randomized trials of MMF also suggest mixed results.[42-44]

Rituximab

The usefulness of rituximab for the treatment of IgAN is not promising, unlike its success in other glomerular disease as it failed to show reduction in proteinuria in a pilot trial. The outcome of 34 patients with proteinuria >1 g/day and eGFR < 90 mL/min/1.73 m² randomized to rituximab versus conservative management was not favorable to its continued use.[45]

Combination Therapy

Patients with progressive disease need stronger immunosuppression of corticosteroids along with an additional agent. Improved renal survival after 2 years was demonstrated by a single-center, prospective, randomized, controlled trial of 38 patients with "high-risk" IgAN (hypertension, >15% rise in creatinine in prior year) in patients receiving prednisone and cyclophosphamide/azathioprine as compared to those with no immunotherapy.[46]

Dual agent immunotherapy does not always afford an advantage. A multicenter, open-label, trial of 207 patients with creatinine <2.0 mg/dL and proteinuria >1.0 g/day for at least 3 months was given dual-agent immunotherapy. Patients were randomized to receive corticosteroids alone (1 g intravenously for 3 consecutive days at months 1, 3, and 5, and then continued at 0.5 mg/kg) or corticosteroids in addition to azathioprine 1.5 mg/kg. The primary outcome of time to 50% decrease in creatinine or secondary outcome of change in proteinuria over time did not show a major difference. In addition, major side effects were noted in the azathioprine group.[47]

Another randomized study by the same investigators on additional 46 patients with advanced disease (creatinine ≥2.0 mg/dL)[48] showed no difference in renal survival at 6 years, although multivariable survival analysis showed azathioprine therapy to have improved renal survival. A drawback was that due to complications of the therapy, a substantial number of patients did not complete the study, highlighting the potential toxicity of immunosuppression in patients with renal insufficiency.

Novel Agents

A novel potential therapy for IgAN is a modified formulation of oral budesonide (Nefecon). This new medication modulates IgA production in the mucosal lymphoid tissue in the distal ileum and proximal large intestine. Systemic effects are minimal due to high first-pass metabolism.[49] A phase 2 double-blind, placebo-controlled trial had a 6-month run-in phase where patients were randomized to receive placebo, 8, or 16 mg/day of budesonide. The selected patients were those with proteinuria > 0.5 or 0.75 g/day and eGFR > 45 mL/min/1.73 m². The drug was proved to be successful in significantly reducing proteinuria in 27% of patients treated with the budesonide while in contrast there was a 3% rise in proteinuria in the placebo group. The change in eGFR was far less in the budesonide group (24.7 mL/min/1.73 m² for placebo vs. 0.32 and 1.95 mL/min/1.73 m² for 8 and 16 mg/day, respectively $P < 0.05$; secondary endpoint). The lower dose in the budesonide group was more effective than the higher dose, which in addition was also noted to have more adverse events, the latter necessitating treatment cessation in 22% of patients (ClinicalTrials.gov NCT01738035).

Acthar gel, a purified form of adrenocorticotropic hormone, is currently under trial (ClinicalTrials.gov NCT02382523) for patients with IgAN and nephrotic syndrome who failed previous immunosuppression. This is an open-label efficacy/safety study in which the recruiting criteria include patients with eGFR >30 mL/min/1.73 m². Another open-label pilot study is being conducted on patients with >1 g/day of proteinuria and no eGFR restriction to analyze the efficacy/safety of bortezomib, a proteasome inhibitor (ClinicalTrials.gov NCT01103778).[50] Both studies examine proteinuria at 12 months as the primary outcome with varying requirements for RAS blockade. Spleen tyrosine kinase is a nonreceptor tyrosine kinase which might regulate the amount of key pathogenic pathways in IgAN. A double-blind randomized study with criteria of >0.5 g/day of proteinuria and eGFR >30 mL/min/1.73 m^2 to study the safety/efficacy of fostamatinib, an oral spleen tyrosine kinase inhibitor versus a placebo with the primary outcome of proteinuria at 24 weeks, is underway (ClinicalTrials.gov NCT02112838).[51]

Follow-up

There are no specific markers to assess the disease activity. So clinical parameters are used to identify continued immunologic activity. Urinalysis with emphasis on hematuria and proteinuria, serum creatinine, and estimated glomerular filtration rate are serially monitored. Persistent hematuria is generally a marker of persistent immunologic activity but not necessarily of progressive disease. Hematuria alone does not require any form of therapy but follow-up is essential as proteinuria may develop over time. Protein excretion above 1 g/day is a marker of more severe disease and is a major risk factor for disease progression unless the degree of proteinuria is reduced.

Prognosis and Outcome

The natural history of IgAN in children represents the early phase of the overall natural history of the disease. Several clinical signs usually develop after 5–15 years, indicating the need for long-term follow-up. 9% of 169 Japanese children with IgAN developed kidney failure by 15 years when followed up for more than 10 years. Persistent hypertension, persistent heavy proteinuria, and reduced GFR at presentation are regarded as poor prognostic indicators. The pathologic features associated with a poor outcome include diffuse mesangial proliferation, a high proportion of glomeruli with sclerosis, crescents or capsular adhesions, the presence of moderate or severe tubulointerstitial changes, the presence of subepithelial electron-dense deposits, and lysis of GBM by electron microscopy.

CONCLUSION

Immunoglobulin A nephropathy, also called Berger disease, is the most common primary glomerular disease worldwide. It is considered to be an IC-mediated or aggregated (polymerized) IgA-mediated GN. Clinical history and laboratory data point to the possible diagnosis of IgAN, but confirmation is by kidney biopsy. The immunofluorescence or immunoperoxidase studies showing IgA deposits within mesangium confirm the diagnosis. International IgA Nephropathy Network Group working in collaboration with the Renal Pathology Society developed a consensus on the pathologic classification of IgAN that gives important prognostic information beyond what is obtained from clinical variables alone. The mainstay of the treatment in IgAN is supportive measures and conservative therapy to reduce proteinuria and slow the rate of renal function decline. RAS blockade medications, ACEIs, and ARBs reduce proteinuria. Immunosuppressive therapy with corticosteroids and drugs such as MMF is considered in those with increase in serum creatinine or persistent nephrotic proteinuria and histologic evidence suggesting active inflammation. IgAN, though considered a benign condition, may lead to significant kidney damage, and progressive disease develops in 20–30% of children 15–20 years after the disease onset.

KEY POINTS

- IgAN, also called Berger disease, is the most common primary glomerular disease worldwide.
- A post-translational glycosylation defect leads to aberrant O-linked glycosylation in the hinge region of IgA1. Abnormal polyclonal IgA production and impaired clearance of IgA from the blood lead to abnormal deposition of IgA in the mesangium.
- Genetic and environmental factors increase the susceptibility and risk of disease progression in IgAN.
- The immunopathogenesis is the result of a confluence of factors and is described as a multi-"hit" process.
- IgAN may present at any age, but the peak incidence is in the second and third decades of life. It affects boys more than girls.
- Recurrent episodes of gross hematuria precipitated by episodes of upper respiratory tract or other infections or asymptomatic microscopic hematuria with or without proteinuria is the most common clinical presentation in children.
- A structured, standardized, and reproducible pathologic classification and scoring system in IgAN by the International IgA Nephropathy Network Group—the Oxford Histologic Classification System—has added important prognostic information beyond what is obtained from clinical variables alone.
- Histologic variables correlating with adverse renal outcomes independent of the clinical presentation and the degree of proteinuria and blood pressure control are mesangial hypercellularity, segmental glomerulosclerosis, endocapillary hypercellularity, and tubular atrophy/interstitial fibrosis.
- Renoprotective interventions to slow progression, though not specific to IgAN, are control of hypertension and proteinuria with ACEI/ARB.
- Immunosuppressive therapy with corticosteroids and drugs such as MMF is considered in those with hematuria plus an increase in serum creatinine or persistent nephrotic proteinuria after maximal antiproteinuric therapy and histologic evidence suggesting active inflammation (e.g., proliferative or necrotizing or crescentic GN).

Hypertension, proteinuria, and impaired renal function at presentation are poor prognostic indicators.

REFERENCES

1. Goodman G, Reid-Adam J. Immunoglobulin A nephropathy. Pediatr Rev. 2019;40(8):439-41.
2. Coppo R. Pediatric IgA nephropathy in Europe. Kidney Dis. 2019;5:182-8.
3. Kiryluk K, Julian BA, Wyatt RJ, Scolari F, Zhang H, Novak J, et al. Genetic studies of IgA nephropathy: past, present, and future. Pediatr Nephrol. 2010;25(11):2257-68.
4. Magistroni R, D'Agati VD, Appel GB, Kiryluk K. New developments in the genetics, pathogenesis, and therapy of IgA nephropathy. Kidney Int. 2015;88:974-89.
5. Kiryluk K, Moldoveanu Z, Sanders JT, Eison TM, Suzuki H, Julian BA, et al. Aberrant glycosylation of IgA1 is inherited in both pediatric IgA nephropathy and Henoch-Schönlein purpura nephritis. Kidney Int. 2011;80:79-87.
6. Gharavi AG, Moldoveanu Z, Wyatt RJ, Barker CV, Woodford SY, Lifton RP, et al. Aberrant IgA1 glycosylation is inherited in familial and sporadic IgA nephropathy. J Am Soc Nephrol. 2008;19:1008-14.
7. Lamm ME, Emancipator SN, Robinson JK, Yamashita M, Fujioka H, Qiu J, et al. Microbial IgA protease removes IgA immune complexes from mouse glomeruli in vivo: potential therapy for IgA nephropathy. Am J Pathol. 2008;172:31-6.
8. Huang ZQ, Raska M, Stewart TJ, Reily C, King RG, Crossman DK, et al. Somatic mutations modulate autoantibodies against galactose-deficient IgA1 in IgA nephropathy. J Am Soc Nephrol. 2016;27:3278-84.
9. Yamamoto R, Nagasawa Y, Shoji T, Iwatani H, Hamano T, Kawada N, et al. Cigarette smoking and progression of IgA nephropathy. Am J Kidney Dis. 2010;56:313-24.
10. Kataoka H, Ohara M, Honda K, Mochizuki T, Nitta K. Maximal glomerular diameter as a 10-year prognostic indicator for IgA nephropathy. Nephrol Dial Transplant. 2011;26:3937-43.
11. Schiemann B, Gommerman JL, Vora K, Cachero TG, Shulga-Morskaya S, Dobles M, et al. An essential role for BAFF in the normal development of B cells through a BCMA-independent pathway. Science. 2001;293:2111-4.
12. Roos A, Rastaldi MP, Calvaresi N, Oortwijn BD, Schlagwein N, van Gijlswijk-Janssen DJ, et al. Glomerular activation of the lectin pathway of complement in IgA nephropathy is associated with more severe renal disease. J Am Soc Nephrol. 2006;17:1724-34.
13. Roos A, Bouwman LH, van Gijlswijk-Janssen DJ, Faber-Krol MC, Stahl GL, Daha MR. Human IgA activates the complement system via the mannan-binding lectin pathway. J Immunol. 2001;167:2861-8.
14. Kiryluk K, Li Y, Sanna-Cherchi S, Rohanizadegan M, Suzuki H, Eitner F, et al. Geographic differences in genetic susceptibility to IgA nephropathy: GWAS replication study and geospatial risk analysis. PLoS Genet. 2012;8:e1002765.
15. Gharavi AG, Kiryluk K, Choi M, Li Y, Hou P, Xie J, et al. Genomewide association study identifies susceptibility loci for IgA nephropathy. Nat Genet. 2011;43:321-7.
16. Zhu L, Zhai YL, Wang FM, Hou P, Lv JC, Xu DM, et al. Variants in complement factor H and complement factor H-related protein genes, CFHR3 and CFHR1, affect complement activation in IgA nephropathy. J Am Soc Nephrol. 2015;26:1195-204.
17. Gutiérrez E, Zamora I, Ballarín JA, Arce Y, Jiménez, S, Quereda C, et al; Grupo de Estudio de Enfermedades Glomerulares de la Sociedad Española de Nefrología (GLOSEN). Long-term outcomes of IgA nephropathy presenting with minimal or no proteinuria. J Am Soc Nephrol. 2012;23:1753-60.
18. Szeto CC, Lai FM, To KF, Wong TY, Chow KM, Choi PC, et al. The natural history of immunoglobulin a nephropathy among patients with hematuria and minimal proteinuria. Am J Med. 2001;110:434-37.
19. Shen P, He L, Huang D. Clinical course and prognostic factors of clinical early IgA nephropathy. Neth J Med. 2008;66:242-7.
20. D'Amigo G. Natural history of idiopathic IgA nephropathy and factors predictive of poor outcome. Semin Nephrol. 2004;24:179-96.
21. Barbour SJ, Reich HN. Risk stratification of patients with IgA nephropathy. Am J Kidney Dis. 2012;59:865-73.
22. D'Amico G. Natural history of idiopathic IgA nephropathy: role of clinical and histological prognostic factors. Am J Kidney Dis. 2000;36:227-37.
23. Barbour SJ, Cattran DC, Kim SJ, Levin A, Wald R, Hladunewich MA, et al. Individuals of Pacific Asian origin with IgA nephropathy have an increased risk of progression to end-stage renal disease. Kidney Int. 2013;84:1017-24.
24. Ibels LS, Győry AZ. IgA nephropathy: analysis of the natural history, important factors in the progression of renal disease, and a review of the literature. Medicine (Baltimore). 1994;73:79-102.
25. Le W, Liang S, Chen H, Wang S, Zhang W, Wang X, et al. Long-term outcome of IgA nephropathy patients with recurrent macroscopic hematuria. Am J Nephrol. 2014;40:43-50.
26. Lai KN, Lai FM, Chan KW, Ho CP, Leung AC, Vallance-Owen J. An overlapping syndrome of IgA nephropathy and lipoid nephrosis. Am J Clin Pathol. 1986;86:716-23.
27. Herlitz LC, Bomback AS, Stokes MB, Radhakrishnan J, D'Agati VD, Markowitz GS. IgA nephropathy with minimal change disease. Clin J Am Soc Nephrol. 2014;9:1033-39.
28. Li XW, Liang SS, Le WB, Cheng SQ, Zeng CH, Wang JQ, et al. Long-term outcome of IgA nephropathy with minimal change disease: a comparison between patients with and without minimal change disease. J Nephrol. 2016;29:567-73.
29. Lv J, Yang Y, Zhang H, Chen W, Pan X, Guo Z, et al. Prediction of outcomes in crescentic IgA nephropathy in a multicenter cohort study. Am J Kidney Dis. 2013;24:2118-25.
30. Pillebout E. IgA vasculitis and IgA nephropathy: same disease? J Clin Med. 2021;10:2310.
31. Glassock RJ. Analyzing antibody activity in IgA nephropathy. J Clin Invest. 2009;119:1450.
32. Haas M. Histologic classification of IgA nephropathy: a clinicopathologic study of 244 cases. Am J Kidney Dis. 1997;29:829-42.
33. Coppo R, Troyanov S, Bellur S, Cattran D, Cook HT, Feehally J, et al; VALIGA Study of the ERA-EDTA Immunonephrology Working Group. Validation of the Oxford classification of IgA nephropathy in cohorts with different presentations and treatments. Kidney Int. 2014;86:828-36.
34. Haas M, Verhave JC, Liu ZH, Alpers CE, Barratt J, Becker JU. A multicenter study of the predictive value of crescents in IgA nephropathy [published online ahead of print September 9, 2016]. J Am Soc Nephrol. 2017;28(2):691-701.
35. European Medicines Agency's Committee for Medicinal Products for Human Use (CHMP). Restriction of combined use of medicines affecting the renin-angiotensin system (RAS). European Medicines Agency, London 2014.
36. Kidney Disease Improving Global Outcomes (KDIGO) Glomerulonephritis Work Group. KDIGO clinical practice guideline for glomerulonephritis. Kidney Int. 2012;2:139-274.

37. Hogg RJ, Bay RC, Jennette JC, Sibley R, Kumar S, Fervenza FC, et al. Randomized controlled trial of mycophenolate mofetil in children, adolescents, and adults with IgA nephropathy. Am J Kidney Dis. 2015;66:783-91.
38. Frisch G, Lin J, Rosenstock J, Markowitz G, D'Agati V, Radhakrishnan J, et al. Mycophenolate mofetil (MMF) vs placebo in patients with moderately advanced IgA nephropathy: a double-blind randomized controlled trial. Nephrol Dial Transplant. 2005;20:2139-45.
39. Tang S, Leung JC, Chan LY, Lui YH, Tang CS, Kan CH, et al. Mycophenolate mofetil alleviates persistent proteinuria in IgA nephropathy. Kidney Int. 2005;68:802-12.
40. Tang SC, Tang AW, Wong SS, Leung JC, Ho YW, Lai KN. Long term study of mycophenolate mofetil treatment in IgA nephropathy. Kidney Int. 2010;77:543-9.
41. Appel GB, Contreras G, Dooley MA, Ginzler EM, Isenberg D, JayneD, et al; Aspreva Lupus Management Study Group. Mycophenolate mofetil versus cyclophosphamide for induction treatment of lupus nephritis. J Am Soc Nephrol. 2009;20:1103-12.
42. Chen Y, Li Y, Yang S, Li Y, Liang M. Efficacy and safety of mycophenolate mofetil treatment in IgA nephropathy: a systematic review. BMC Nephrol. 2014;15:193.
43. Xu G, Tu W, Jiang D, Xu C. Mycophenolate mofetil treatment for IgA nephropathy: a meta-analysis. Am J Nephrol. 2009;29:362-7.
44. Tian L, Shao X, Xie Y, Wang L, Wang Q, Che X, et al. The long-term efficacy and safety of immunosuppressive therapy on the progression of IgA nephropathy: a meta-analysis of controlled clinical trials with more than 5-year follow-up. Expert Opin Pharmacother. 2015;16:1137-47.
45. Lafayette RA, Canetta PA, Rovin BH, Appel GB, Novak J, Nath KA, et al. A randomized, controlled trial of rituximab in IgA nephropathy with proteinuria and renal dysfunction [published online ahead of print November 7, 2016]. J Am Soc Nephrol. 2017;28(4):1306-13.
46. Ballardie FW, Roberts IS. Controlled prospective trial of prednisolone and cytotoxics in progressive IgA nephropathy. J Am Soc Nephrol. 2002;13:142-8.
47. Pozzi C, Andrulli S, Pani A, Scaini P, Del Vecchio L, Fogazzi G, et al. Addition of azathioprine to corticosteroids does not benefit patients with IgA nephropathy. J Am Soc Nephrol. 2010;21:1783-90.
48. Pozzi C, Andrulli S, Pani A, Scaini P, Roccatello D, Fogazzi G, et al. IgA nephropathy with severe chronic renal failure: a randomized controlled trial of corticosteroids and azathioprine. J Nephrol. 2013;26:86-93.
49. Smerud HK, Bárány P, Lindström K, Fernström A, Sandell A, Påhlsson P, et al. New treatment for IgA nephropathy: enteric budesonide targeted to the ileocecal region ameliorates proteinuria. Nephrol Dial Transplant. 2011;26:3237-42.
50. Yeo SC, Liew A, Barratt J. Emerging therapies in immunoglobulin A nephropathy. Nephrology (Carlton). 2015;20:788-800.
51. Ma TK, McAdoo SP, Tam FW. Targeting the tyrosine kinase signalling pathways for treatment of immune-mediated glomerulonephritis: from bench to bedside and beyond. Nephrol Dial Transplant. 2017;32(Suppl 1):i129-38.

CHAPTER

6.7 Henoch–Schönlein Purpura Nephritis

Manoj G Matnani

INTRODUCTION

Henoch–Schönlein purpura (HSP) is a small-vessel, leukocytoclastic vasculitis (LCV) which can cause a large variety of symptoms in different organs.[1] As renal involvement [Henoch-Schönlein purpura nephritis (HSN)] is the main cause of chronic disease, the kidney should be closely observed and significant involvement should be treated in accordance with the best evidence obtainable. Because of its striking similarity with immunoglobulin A (IgA) nephropathy (IgAN) and association with the glomerular deposition of IgA1-containing immune complexes in the mesangium, Henoch-Schönlein vasculitis is also called IgA vasculitis (IgA V).

EPIDEMIOLOGY OF HENOCH–SCHÖNLEIN PURPURA AND HENOCH–SCHÖNLEIN PURPURA NEPHRITIS

Henoch-Schönlein vasculitis is one of most common types of systemic vasculitis in childhood, with a slightly higher incidence in boys than in girls. Between 6 and 24 per 100,000 children below 17 years of age are affected, depending on the ethnic background of the children.[2] The incidence is highest in children aged 4–7 years (up to 70 cases/100,000 children per year) and in children of Asian descent. HSP frequently follows a respiratory tract infection, and a large variety of different viral and bacterial pathogens have been implicated as trigger(s) of the disease. A positive throat culture for group A beta-hemolytic streptococci has been found in 20–30% of patients with HSP and glomerular deposition of a streptococcal antigen may be responsible for some of the cases of HSN.[3] HSP is generally self-limited in children, although relapses occur in one-third of cases. Renal involvement may become chronic and lead to permanent organ damage determining the long-term prognosis of the disease. A high proportion of patients with HSP (30–50%) either have or develop hematuria and/or proteinuria as a symptom(s) of HSN, both of which are mostly of minor extent and self-limited.[1,4] Of all patients with HSP with abnormal urinalysis, a minority develop severe glomerulonephritis, which is associated with an increased risk of long-term chronic kidney disease.[5,6] Children with no urinary pathology during the first 6 months after the onset of HSP do not develop renal impairment during the long-term follow-up.[4]

ETIOPATHOGENESIS

Role of Immunoglobulin A in the Pathogenesis of Henoch–Schönlein Purpura Nephritis

Postulation that HSN is a systemic immune complex-mediated disease is supported by the clinical or histological recurrences of HSN in some patients after transplantation. Although detailed pathogenic mechanisms of HSN have not been fully elucidated, perturbations in the immune system, including elevations in serum levels of IgA1, IgA1-containing circulating immune complexes, and IgA rheumatoid factors have been documented in patients with HSP. Elevated serum levels of IgA and IgA-containing immune complexes were observed in patients with HSN. Furthermore, it was noted that all patients with HSP have IgA1-circulating immune complexes of small molecular mass, but only those with nephritis have additional large-molecular-mass IgA1–immunoglobulin G (IgG)-containing circulating immune complexes.[7]

Abnormal Glycosylation of Immunoglobulin A1 and its Role in the Pathogenesis of Henoch–Schönlein Purpura Nephritis

Henoch–Schönlein purpura nephritis is similar to IgAN in that IgA1 (but not IgA2) is found in the circulating immune complexes and in immune deposits in mesangium. Only humans and higher primates have IgA1. As depicted in **Figure 1**, the human IgA1 molecule has a hinge region containing up to six *O*-linked glycan chains, consisting of *N*-acetyl galactosamine (GalNAc), usually with a β1,3-linked galactose (Gal) attached to it.[8] GalNAc and/or Gal may or may not be sialylated and serum IgA1 from normal healthy subjects predominantly has the Gal-GalNAc disaccharide in its mono- and disialylated forms.

The Biosynthetic Origin of Galactose-deficient Immunoglobulin A1

There are two major sites with IgA1-producing cells: mucosal tissues and bone marrow. Both have been suggested as

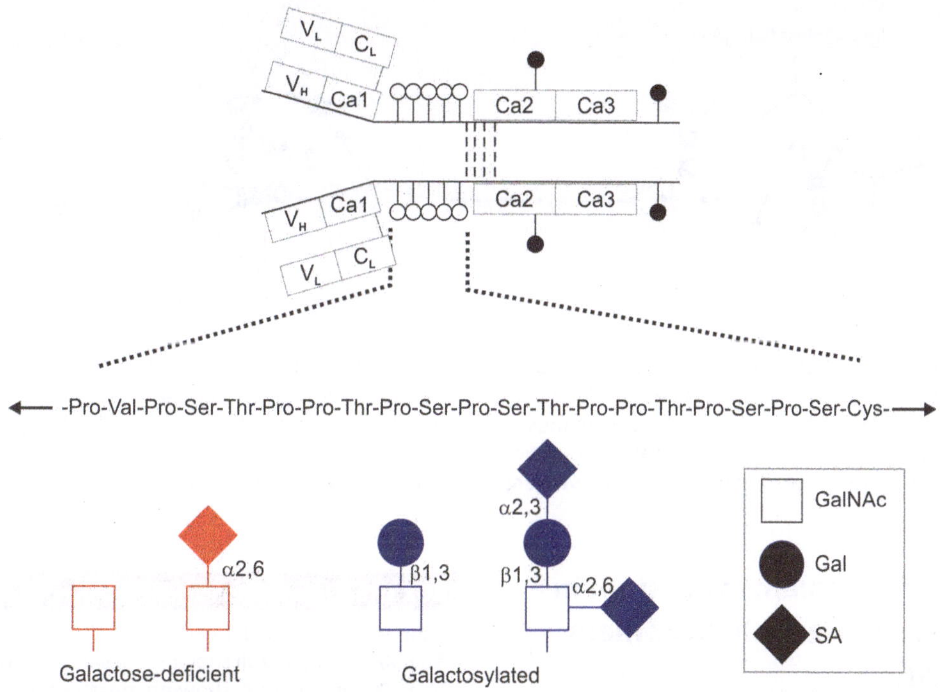

Fig. 1: Immunoglobulin A1 (IgA1) and its hinge region with *O*-linked glycans (white circles) and *N*-linked glycans (black circles). Underlined amino acids denote usual sites of attachment of as many as five *O*-linked glycans. Examples of galactose-deficient (in red color) and galactosylated (in blue color) *O*-linked glycans in the hinge region of human circulatory IgA1 are shown at the bottom. (GalNAc: *N*-acetyl galactosamine; Gal: galactose; SA: sialic acid)

possible sites of production of the aberrantly glycosylated IgA1. The primary defect that leads to the production of such abnormally glycosylated IgA1 is probably heritable. Data also suggest that premature sialylation may contribute to the aberrant IgA1 *O*-glycosylation in IgAN, and these cell lines provide a new model for future studies on the mechanisms leading to aberrant IgA1 *O*-glycosylation in IgAN and HSN.

Sialylation of Immunoglobulin A1 Molecules in Immunoglobulin A Nephropathy and Henoch–Schönlein Purpura Nephritis

As sialic acid carries a high negative charge, the degree of sialylation may alter interactions of IgA1 with other molecules and thus affect clearance of IgA1 and IgA1-containing immune complexes. It is therefore of interest that a portion of IgA1 from patients with IgAN is *Gal-deficient* and *over sialylated.*

Possible Mechanisms Involving Galactose-deficient Immunoglobulin A1 in the Development of Henoch–Schönlein Purpura Nephritis

Flowchart 1 depicts a proposed mechanism how aberrantly glycosylated IgA1 may become nephritogenic.[8] Polymeric galactose-deficient immunoglobulin A1 (Gd-IgA1) molecules are recognized by naturally occurring anti-glycan IgA1 or IgG and circulating immune complexes are formed. Due to their size, Gd-IgA1-containing immune complexes are

Flowchart 1: Possible role of IgA1 and IgA1-containing immune complexes in the pathogenesis of Henoch–Schönlein purpura nephritis (HSN).

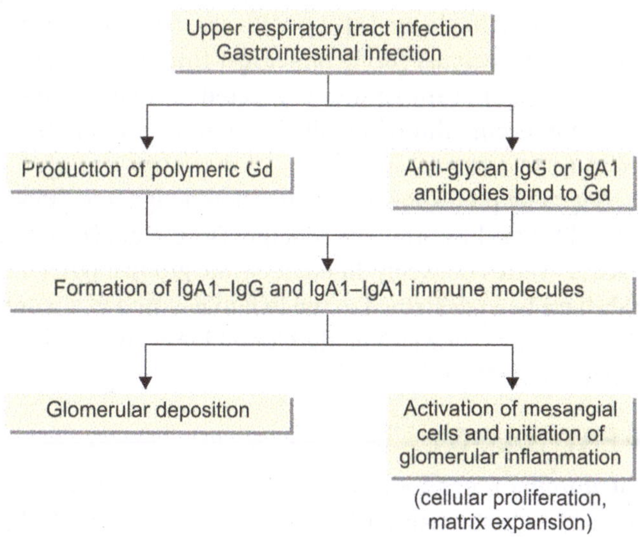

(Gd: galactose-deficient; IgA1: immunoglobulin A1; IgG: immunoglobulin G)

less efficiently taken up by the asialoglycoprotein receptor in the liver and catabolized and their amounts increase in the circulation. These complexes may then deposit in the renal mesangium and incite glomerular injury, likely due to the binding to mesangial cells leading to cellular activation. Consequently, mesangial cells start to proliferate and overproduce extracellular matrix components, cytokines, and chemokines, as shown in **Figure 2.**[9]

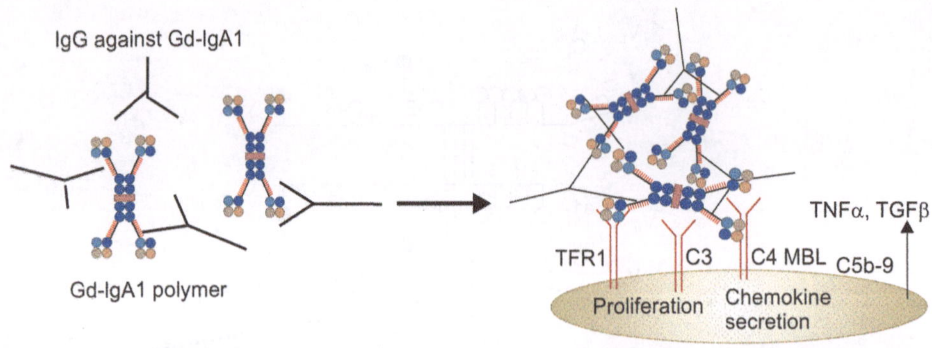

Fig. 2: Possible mechanisms involving Gd-IgA1 in the development of Henoch–Schönlein purpura nephritis (HSN). Gd-IgA1 polymers are recognized by IgG antibodies forming circulating large IgG–IgA1 immune complexes. The immune complexes (>800 kDa) bind to renal mesangial cells, probably at least partially mediated by TFR1, leading to mesangial deposition of complement factors (C3, MBL, C4, C5b-9), mesangial cell proliferation, and chemokine secretion. (Gd-IgA1: galactose-deficient immunoglobulin A1; IgG: immunoglobulin G; MBL: mannose-binding lectin; TFR1: transferrin receptor 1; TGF-β: transforming growth factor-beta; TNFα: tumor necrosis factor alpha)

Potential Role of Complement System in the Pathogenesis of Henoch–Schönlein Purpura Nephritis

Complement activation appears to play an important role in the pathogenesis of IgAN and HSN, as glomerular complement activation may initiate the inflammatory cascade and enhance glomerular injury. Although it has long been known that the alternative complement pathway is activated in patients with IgAN and HSN, attention has shifted to the lectin pathway. This third pathway of complement activation is initiated by mannose-binding lectin (MBL). MBL also forms complexes with MBL-associated serine protease-1 (MASP-1), MASP-2, and MASP-3. Recent studies suggested that complement activation occurs through both the alternate and the lectin pathways in patients with IgAN.

A genetic predisposition for developing IgAN or HSN is highly likely to be part of the etiology. The incidence of both diseases varies between different ethnic groups. IgAN and HSN have been described to run in families, and in a pair of identical twins, one sibling developed IgAN and the other developed HSN.[10,11]

PATHOLOGY

The dominant or predominant finding of glomerular IgA deposition is the hallmark of renal histology in HSN. IgA deposition is mainly present in the mesangium but can also be found in the subepithelial and subendothelial space. In the majority of biopsies, the deposition of IgG, C3, and other complement factors can be found in the glomerulus. In addition, a variable extent of acute inflammation or chronic damage is present. As such, HSN leads to a similar renal pathology to IgAN and can be regarded as a part of the histological spectrum of IgAN. Compared to IgAN, HSN renal biopsy samples are reported to show increased endocapillary proliferation, epithelial crescents, perivascular glomerular IgA, subendothelial/subepithelial IgA deposits and fibrin deposits. The Oxford Classification[12] based on the identification of histopathological features of renal biopsies and assessment of associations between candidate histopathological predictors and renal prognosis, has improved the predictive value of renal biopsies for IgAN; however, patients with HSN were excluded from the analysis. The Oxford Classification **(Box 1)** uses a score of mesangial hypercellularity, endocapillary hypercellularity, segmental glomerulosclerosis, and tubular atrophy/interstitial fibrosis (MEST) score to predict the outcome of the IgAN. The value of this histological classification has shown promise for pediatric IgAN patients, but to date it has not been evaluated in patients with HSN. Since the publication of the International Study of Kidney Disease in Children (ISKDC) classification, in HSN, the percentage of crescents has been used for estimating disease severity and predicting outcome **(Table 1)**.[13] In this clinical context, the extent of the renal pathology appears to correlate with the severity of the clinical presentation and long-term prognosis more so for IgAN **(Table 2)**.

BOX 1: The Oxford classification of immunoglobulin A nephropathy.[13]

Mesangial hypercellularity

M_0 <50% of glomeruli showing mesangial hypercellularity

M_1 >50% of glomeruli showing mesangial hypercellularity

Endocapillary hypercellularity—E_0 absent E_1 present

Segmental glomerulosclerosis/adhesion—S_0 absent, S_1 present (presence or absence of podocyte hypertrophy/tip lesions in biopsies with S_1)

Tubular atrophy/interstitial fibrosis

T_0 ≤25% of the cortical area affected by tubular atrophy or interstitial fibrosis

T_1 26–50% of the cortical area affected by tubular atrophy or interstitial fibrosis

T_2 >50% of the cortical area affected by tubular atrophy or interstitial fibrosis

Cellular/fibrocellular crescents

C_0 absent

C_1 present in at least one glomerulus, C2 present in >25% of glomeruli

TABLE 1: The International Study of Kidney Disease in Children classification of Henoch–Schönlein purpura nephritis.

ISKDC grade	*Description*
Grade I	Minimal alterations
Grade II	Mesangial proliferation
Grade III	Proliferation or sclerosis with <50% crescents [(1) focal or (2) diffuse]
Grade IV	Mesangial proliferation or sclerosis with 50–75%, crescents [(1) focal or (2) diffuse]
Grade V	Mesangial proliferation or sclerosis with >75% crescents [(1) focal or (2) diffuse]
Grade VI	Membranoproliferative like glomerulonephritis

Source: Modified from reference 12.

TABLE 2: Histologic classification of immunoglobulin A nephropathy of Haas.[14]

Haas classification	*Description*
Class I: Minimal histologic lesion	Glomeruli are normocellular, without segmental sclerosis, necrosis, or crescents
Class II: Focal-segmental glomerulosclerosis (FSGS)-like	Glomeruli show focal and segmental sclerosis without mesangial or endocapillary hypercellularity, crescents, or necrosis
Class III: Focal proliferative glomerulonephritis	50% or fewer of the glomeruli (not including globally sclerotic glomeruli) are hypercellular. This hypercellularity may be limited to mesangial areas, or include endocapillary hypercellularity, crescents, or necrosis
Class IV: Diffuse proliferative glomerulonephritis	More than 50% of the glomeruli (not including globally sclerotic glomeruli) are hypercellular. This hypercellularity may be limited to mesangial areas, or include endocapillary hypercellularity, crescents, or necrosis
Class V: Advanced chronic glomerulonephritis	40% or more of the glomeruli are globally sclerotic, and/or there is >40% estimated tubular atrophy or loss in the cortex. If these criteria are met, the biopsy specimen is graded as class V regardless of other histologic feature

SYMPTOMATOLOGY AND DIAGNOSIS

Diagnostic Criteria of Henoch–Schönlein Purpura

Schönlein first described HSP as a triad of purpuric rash, arthritis, and abnormalities of the urinary sediment in 1837.[15] In 1874, Henoch described the association of purpuric rash, abdominal pain with bloody diarrhea, and proteinuria.[16] Up to date, several sets of diagnostic criteria for HSP have been proposed; the detail and comparison of these different classification criteria are further reviewed and discussed as follows:

The European League Against Rheumatism/Paediatric Rheumatology International Trials Organization/Paediatric Rheumatology European Society (EULAR/PRINTO/PRES) 2010 criteria include palpable purpura as a mandatory criterion, together with at least one of the following findings: diffuse abdominal pain, LCV with predominant IgA deposits on skin biopsy, acute arthritis or arthralgias in any joint, and renal involvement as evidenced by proteinuria and/or hematuria **(Table 3)**. The sensitivity and specificity of these classification criteria were 100 and 87%, respectively.[21]

Differential Diagnosis of Henoch–Schönlein Purpura

Henoch-Schönlein purpura must be distinguished from other diseases with similar presentations **(Box 2)**. Thrombocytopenic purpura like immune thrombocytopenic purpura can be easily identified by the detection of low platelet count. If it is difficult to decide the cause of cutaneous purpuric lesions that may be presented in other types of vasculitis such as urticarial vasculitis, cryoglobulinemia, and hypersensitivity vasculitis (HV), a skin biopsy and immunofluorescence study may assist in the diagnosis. Some rheumatic diseases might have presentation of cutaneous vasculitis. Clinical characteristics combined with laboratory abnormalities usually provide assistance to determine the underlying diseases. Furthermore, since abdominal pain is commonly presented in HSP, the more common causes of acute surgical abdomen must be considered.

CLINICAL COURSE OF HENOCH–SCHÖNLEIN PURPURA NEPHRITIS

About 20% of HSP nephritis (7% of all HSP) develop either a nephritic or a nephrotic syndrome. Unfortunately, not all studies use the same definitions. Nephritis has been defined as hematuria plus one or two of the following symptoms: hypertension, renal insufficiency, and/or oliguria. Nephrotic syndrome is diagnosed when proteinuria is >40 mg/m^2/h, but some studies additionally require either edema or a serum albumin of <2.5 g/dL. These differences in study definitions contribute to the differences in reported incidence and variable outcome results.

TABLE 3: Summary of classification criteria for Henoch–Schönlein purpura diagnosis.

Classification	*Diagnostic criteria*
Mills et al. (1990)[17]	≥2 of the following: • Palpable purpura, not thrombocytopenic purpura • Bowel angina • Wall granulocytes on biopsy • Age ≤20 years at disease onset
Michel et al. (1992)[18]	≥3 of the following: HSP; ≤2 of the following: HV • Palpable purpura, not thrombocytopenic • Bowel angina • Gastrointestinal bleeding • Hematuria • Age ≤20 years at disease onset • No history of medication intake at disease onset
CHCC, Jennette et al. (1994)[19]	Vasculitis, with IgA-dominant immune deposits, affecting small vessels (i.e., capillaries, venules, or arterioles); typically involves skin, gut, and glomeruli and is associated with arthralgias or arthritis
Helander et al. (1995)[20]	Palpable purpura, not thrombocytopenic with LCV + ≥3 of the following: • Vascular IgA deposition • Age ≤20 years at disease onset • Gastrointestinal involvement • Upper respiratory tract infection prodrome • Mesangioproliferative glomerulonephritis with or without IgA deposition
EULAR/PRINTO/PRES, Ozen et al. (2010)[21]	Palpable purpura, not thrombocytopenic/petechiae (mandatory) + ≥ one of the following: • Diffuse abdominal pain • *Histopathology:* Typical LCV with predominant IgA deposits or proliferative glomerulonephritis with predominant IgA deposits • Arthritis or arthralgias • *Renal involvement (proteinuria:* >0.3 g/24 h or >30 mmol/mg of urine albumin to creatinine ratio on a spot morning sample; and/or hematuria, red blood cell casts: >5 red cells per high power field or ≥2+ on dipstick or red blood cell casts in the urinary sediment)

(ACR: American College of Rheumatology; HV: hypersensitivity vasculitis; CHCC: Chapel Hill Consensus Criteria; LCV: leukocytoclastic vasculitis; EULAR/PRINTO/PRES: European League Against Rheumatism/Paediatric Rheumatology International Trials Organization/Paediatric Rheumatology European Society)

BOX 2: Differential diagnosis of Henoch–Schönlein purpura.

Thrombocytopenic purpura
- Immune thrombocytopenic purpura
- Thrombotic thrombocytopenic purpura

Other types of vasculitis
- Hypersensitivity vasculitis
- Urticarial vasculitis
- Mixed cryoglobulinemia
- Cutaneous polyarteritis
- ANCA-associated small vessel vasculitis

Rheumatic diseases
- Systemic lupus erythematosus
- Rheumatoid arthritis
- Sjogren's syndrome
- Mixed connective tissue disorder
- Juvenile dermatomyositis
- Antiphospholipid antibody syndrome

Others
- Septicemia
- Disseminated intravascular coagulation
- Papular-purpuric gloves and socks syndrome Mediterranean fever

Causes of acute surgical abdomen

(ANCA: antineutrophil cytoplasmic antibody)

Renal involvement occurs in 85% within 4 weeks of the initial HSP manifestation, in 91% within 6 weeks, and in 97% within 6 months. Therefore, repeated urinary investigations are recommended for 6 months after the onset of HSP, even in patients in whom all other symptoms have subsided. Results from a meta-analysis of 1,133 unselected patients with HSP demonstrated long-term renal impairment, defined as persisting nephritic or nephrotic syndrome, renal insufficiency, or hypertension, in 19.5% with initial nephrotic or nephritic syndrome. Other studies evaluating patients from tertiary care centers with pediatric nephrology services found long-term renal impairment in 33–44% of patients following the development of HSN with nephrotic syndrome or nephritis. The risk of clinically severe HSN with a higher risk of long-term renal sequelae seems to increase with age, but the prognosis of equally severe HSN is not different in children and adults. The time course of renal impairment is unpredictable in patients at the individual level, and active renal disease may develop after an initially mild nephritis or many years after stable minor urinary abnormalities. The severity of renal histological changes also correlates with the renal long-term outcome and, consequently, influences treatment decisions; therefore, a renal biopsy is recommended in the more severe cases of HSN.

INVESTIGATIONS: BIOMARKERS FOR HENOCH–SCHÖNLEIN PURPURA DIAGNOSIS

In HSP, the platelet count is normal or increased. A moderate leukocytosis with a left shift is noted in some patients. Antinuclear antibody is mostly undetectable, and serum levels of C3 and C4 are usually within normal limit. Although some proinflammatory cytokines and chemokines are elevated at acute stage, these laboratory abnormalities are not specific for HSP but can be seen in a variety of inflammatory conditions. The presence of LCV and IgA-immune deposits on skin and/or kidney biopsies significantly increases the diagnostic accuracy for HSP. However, many vasculitis and glomerulonephritis show similar histopathological findings.

A variety of IgA autoantibodies have been found associated with HSP including IgA rheumatoid factor, IgA anticardiolipin antibodies, and IgA antiendothelial cell antibodies. Although aberrant glycosylated IgA1 and some of above IgA autoantibodies are likely to play a pathogenic role in HSP, whether they are diagnostic biomarkers for HSP needs more studies to validate.

TREATMENT

Prevention of Henoch–Schönlein Purpura Nephritis

Although corticosteroids enhance the rate of resolution of the arthritis and abdominal pain, their effectiveness in the prevention of nephritis is debated. Saulsbury in an uncontrolled study of severe HSP cases concluded that the corticosteroid therapy does not prevent nephritis.[22] Conversely, Mollica et al. found that early prednisone treatment reduced the incidence of microscopic hematuria, but this symptom is not associated with a high risk of progression.[23] A randomized controlled trial by Ronkainen et al. concluded that prednisone does not prevent the development of renal symptoms but is effective in treating renal involvement.[24] Dudley et al. in a large randomized, double-blind, placebo-controlled trial found no evidence that early treatment with prednisolone reduces the prevalence of proteinuria 12 months after disease onset.[25] The clinical spectrum of HSN ranges from the relatively common transient isolated microscopic hematuria to nephrotic syndrome, rapidly progressive glomerulonephritis, and renal failure. In mild cases, no treatment is needed if the urine is adequately evaluated, and ambulatory care may suffice. The prolonged bed rest customary in the past occasionally led to complications such as femoral venous thrombosis and psychosocial problems. Although severe abdominal pain and vomiting are self-limiting, resolution can be hastened by means of administration of glucocorticoids. Utani et al.[26] found that factor XIII concentrate replacement resolved severe abdominal symptoms in the care of adults with HSP associated with a decreased level of factor XIII activity.

Evidence

An answer to the question of whether HSN in childhood can be prevented by means of prophylactic treatment prescribed at the time of HSP diagnosis is of fundamental importance. Retrospective and prospective studies have reported on patients with HSP lacking clinical signs of nephropathy at admission who were treated with prednisone at doses ranging from 1.0 to 2.5 mg/kg/day over a period of 7–21 days. Therefore, the existing evidence does not support prednisone in the prevention of nephritis.[22,24]

The currently available data are insufficient to support a recommendation for prophylaxis; 2–4 weeks of prednisone administration failed to prevent renal involvement after 0.5–1 years (grade A recommendation). There is no evidence of benefit of prednisone in preventing serious long-term kidney disease in HSP.

Treatment of Moderately Severe Henoch–Schönlein Purpura Nephritis

There is no therapy of proven value for HSN, although some regimens have been proposed and tested, with controversial results. These include (1) glucocorticoids and immunosuppressive drugs and (2) plasma exchange to remove circulating IgA immune complexes. Retrospective studies suggested that oral glucocorticoids were of no benefit.[27] Similarly, oral glucocorticoids with azathioprine, chlorambucil, or cyclophosphamide do not seem to be beneficial.[27,28] A beneficial effect of methylprednisolone pulse therapy followed by oral prednisone was reported in a prospective case series of severe HSN in comparison with historical controls at the same institution.[29] The beneficial effect of methylprednisolone pulses in combination with immunosuppressive agents such as cyclophosphamide or mizoribine has also been reported. Cyclosporine A therapy has given promising results in case series, although some patients become cyclosporine dependent.

The use of angiotensin-converting enzyme inhibitor or angiotensin receptor blockers may be useful in patients with moderate HSN. Recently, Ninchoji et al.[30] reported the results of retrospective study for the efficacy of treatment for HSN. Renal biopsy was performed in patients with nephrotic syndrome or persistent proteinuria for more than 3 months, and patients were classified by treatment. Patients (n = 31) with moderately severe HSN (histological grades I–III and serum albumin >2.5 g/dL) were treated with angiotensin-converting enzyme inhibitors and/or angiotensin receptor blockers. Patients (n = 19) with HSN exceeding grade III or Alb ≤2.5 g/dL received combination therapy comprising prednisolone, immunosuppressants, warfarin, and dipyridamole.

All patients showed resolution of proteinuria without renal dysfunction during the observation period (3.8 ± 0.4 years).

Treatment strategies for HSN should depend on the histologic and clinical severity. Combination therapy may be effective in clinically and histologically severe HSN. Furthermore, aggressive therapies, particularly combination therapies, are unnecessary for moderate to severe HSN (grade D recommendation). Indeed, a systematic review of 10 randomized controlled trials (RCTs) led to the conclusion that treatment aimed at improving renal outcome in children with HSP is notably sparse, with the sole exception of short-term prednisone, for which proven efficacy has still to be demonstrated.[31]

The majority of reports provide scarce support to the various treatment options identified in cases of severe childhood HSN. One RCT study[32] did not recommend the use of cyclophosphamide in treating severe HSN (grade B). At the present time, however, insufficient data are available to recommend the use of pulse and oral steroids, azathioprine, mycophenolate mofetil (MMF) or cyclosporine A, either alone or in combination (grade D recommendation) in treating severe HSN.

Treatment of Rapidly Progressive or Crescentic Henoch–Schönlein Purpura Nephritis

Plasma exchange combined with glucocorticoids and immunosuppressive drugs may be of value in the care of patients with rapidly progressive crescentic disease.[33] Plasma exchange in patients with HSN, either alone or in combination with immunosuppressant (grade D recommendation), cannot currently be recommended due to the paucity of data available. Further studies should be performed to evaluate the efficacy of azathioprine, cyclosporine A and MMF in this disease.

PROGNOSIS

The results of long-term follow-up studies show that the clinical presentation has no prognostic value for individual patients. However, children with slight proteinuria or hematuria have an excellent prognosis. Those with persistent heavy proteinuria, acute nephritic syndrome, or nephrotic syndrome are at risk of chronic kidney failure. Results of a 23-year follow-up study by Goldstein et al.[5] indicated that approximately 15% of patients with nephritis at onset of HSP or persistent heavy proteinuria, 40% of those with nephrosis, and fewer than 50% of those with a mixed nephritic–nephrotic onset have ongoing urinary abnormalities and that many of these patients ultimately have renal failure The proportion of glomeruli with crescents or segmental lesions (sclerosis, adhesions, thrombosis, or necrosis) seems to be the most important prognostic indicator. The larger the number of glomeruli affected by crescents or segmental lesions, the poorer is the prognosis. The clinic pathological correlation in HSN is discussed in **Table 4**. Long-term follow-up is required in all children with significant renal involvement.

TABLE 4: Clinicopathologic correlation in Henoch–Schönlein purpura nephritis.

Clinical presentation	*Biopsy grade (ISKDC)*	*Approx. risk of renal failure (%)*
Macroscopic or microscopic hematuria, proteinuria—minimal or absent	I–II, rarely III	<5
Hematuria and persistent heavy proteinuria	I–IV	15
Acute nephritic syndrome	II–IV	15
Nephrotic syndrome	II–IV, rarely I or V	40
Nephritic–nephrotic syndrome	II–V, mostly V	>50

CONCLUSION

Henoch–Schönlein vasculitis is one of the most common types of systemic vasculitis in childhood, with a slightly higher incidence in boys than in girls. Renal involvement occurs in up to 75% of the patients with HSP. A minority develop severe glomerulonephritis associated with an increased risk of long-term chronic kidney disease. The Kidney Disease Improving Global Outcome (KDIGO) initiative published guidelines for the treatment of HSN.[34] Due to the lack of evidence-based data for HSN treatment and similarities between HSN and primary IgAN, the KDIGO guidelines proposed the same treatment for both diseases when the clinical conditions are similar.[35,36] Severe renal involvement is associated with an increased risk of long-term chronic kidney disease and kidney failure with the need for kidney transplantation.

KEY POINTS

- Henoch–Schönlein purpura is a relatively common problem in pediatrics with variable clinical presentations but has specific diagnostic criteria as mentioned above.
- Renal involvement occurs in >75% of cases and, in the vast majority, this manifests as hematuria alone or hematuria and low-grade proteinuria. In 10–20% of cases, there may be significant proteinuria, nephrotic syndrome, or acute glomerulonephritis.
- The long-term prognosis for children with HSN is determined by the severity of renal inflammation and the percentage of glomeruli with crescents in a kidney biopsy specimen.
- There is no proven therapy for HSN. Moderate cases may be treated with a prolonged course of oral corticosteroids and mycophenolate mofetil. More severe cases may be treated with intravenous pulse methylprednisolone and other immunosuppressive medications.

- All patients with HSN require extended follow-up. HSN account for <5% of the pediatric population in whom end-stage kidney disease develops. These patients are candidates for kidney transplantation.

REFERENCES

1. Calvino MC, Llorca J, Garcia-Porrua C, Fernandez-Iglesias JL, Rodriguez-Ledo P, Gonzalez-Gay MA. Henoch-Schonlein purpura in children from northwestern Spain: a 20-year epidemiologic and clinical study. Medicine (Baltimore). 2001;80:279-90.
2. Gardner-Medwin JM, Dolezalova P, Cummins C, Southwood TR. Incidence of Henoch-Schonlein purpura, Kawasaki disease, and rare vasculitides in children of different ethnic origins. Lancet. 2002;360:1197-202.
3. Masuda M, Nakanishi K, Yoshizawa N, Iijima K, Yoshikawa N. Group A streptococcal antigen in the glomeruli of children with Henoch-Schonlein nephritis. Am J Kidney Dis. 2003;41:366-70.
4. Narchi H. Risk of long term renal impairment and duration of follow up recommended for Henoch-Schonlein purpura with normal or minimal urinary findings: a systematic review. Arch Dis Child. 2005;90:916-20.
5. Goldstein AR, White RHR, Akuse R, Chantler C. Long-term follow-up of childhood Henoch-Schonlein nephritis. Lancet. 1992;339(8788):280-2.
6. Scharer K, Krmar R, Querfeld U, Ruder H, Waldherr R, Schafer F. Clinical outcome of Schonlein-Henoch purpura nephritis in children. Pediatr Nephrol. 1999;13:816-23.
7. Levinsky RJ, Barratt TM. IgA immune complexes in Henoch-Schönlein purpura. Lancet. 1979;2:1100-3.
8. Lau KK, Suzuki H, Novak J, Wyatt RJ. Pathogenesis of HSP nephritis. Pediatr Nephrol. 2010;25:19-26.
9. Pohl M. Henoch-Schonlein purpura nephritis. Pediatr Nephrol. 2015;30:245-52.
10. Julian BA, Quiggins PA, Thompson JS, Woodford SY, Gleason K, Wyatt RJ. Familial IgA nephropathy. Evidence of an inherited mechanism of disease. N Engl J Med. 1985;312:202-8.
11. Meadow SR, Scott DG. Berger disease: Henoch-Schonlein syndrome without the rash. J Pediatr 1985;106:27-32
12. Trimarchi H, Barratt J, Cattran DC, Cook HT, Coppo R, Haas M, et al. Oxford classification of IgA nephropathy 2016: an update from the IgA nephropathy classification working group. Kidney Int. 2017;91:1014-21.
13. Haas M. IgA nephropathy and Henoch-Schönlein purpura nephritis. In: Jennette JC, Olson JC, Schwartz MM, Silva FG (Eds.). Heptinstall's Pathology of the Kidney. Philadelphia, PA: Lippincott, Williams & Wilkins; 2007. pp. 423-86.
14. Haas M. Histologic sub classification of IgA nephropathy: a clinicopathologic study of 244 cases. Am J Kidney Dis. 1997; 29:829-42.
15. Schönlein JL. Allegemeine und specielle Pathologie und Therapie, Vol. 2. Herisau, Germany: Literatur-Comptoir; 1837.
16. Henoch EH. Uber ein eigenthumliche form von Purpura. Berl Klin Wochenschr. 1874;11:641-3.
17. Mills JA, Michel BA, Bloch DA, Calabrese LH, Hunder GG, Arend WP, et al. The American College of Rheumatology 1990 criteria for the classification of vasculitis. Arthritis Rheum. 1990;33:1114-21.
18. Michel BA, Hunder GG, Bloch DA, Calabrese LH. Hypersensitivity vasculitis and Henoch-Schönlein purpura: a comparison between the 2 disorders. J Rheumatol. 1992; 19:721-8.
19. Jennette JC, Falk RJ, Andrassy K, Bacon PA, Churg J, Gross WL, et al. Nomenclature of systemic vasculitides. Proposal of an international consensus conference. Arthritis Rheum. 1994;37:187-92.
20. Helander SD, De Castro FR, Gibson LE. Henoch-Schönlein purpura: clinicopathologic correlation of cutaneous vascular IgA deposits and the relationship to leukocytoclastic vasculitis. Acta Derm Venereol. 1995;75:125-9.
21. Ozen S, Pistorio A, Iusan SM, Bakkaloglu A, Herlin T, Brik R, et al. EULAR/PRINTO/PRES criteria for Henoch-Schönlein purpura, childhood polyarteritis nodosa, childhood Wegener granulomatosis and childhood Takayasu arteritis: Ankara 2008. Part II: final classification criteria. Ann Rheum Dis. 2010;69:798-806.
22. Saulsbury FT. Corticosteroid therapy does not prevent nephritis in Henoch-Schonlein purpura. Pediatr Nephrol. 1993;7(1):69-71.
23. Mollica F, Li Volti S, Garozzo R, Russo G. Effectiveness of early prednisone treatment in preventing the development of nephropathy in anaphylactoid purpura. Eur J Pediatr. 1992;151(2):140-4.
24. Ronkainen J, Koskimies O, Ala-Houhala M, Antikainen M, Merenmies J, Rajantie J, et al. Early prednisone therapy in Henoch-Schonlein purpura: a randomized, double-blind, placebo-controlled trial. J Pediatr. 2006;149(2):241-7.
25. Dudley J, Smith G, Llewelyn-Edwards A, Bayliss K, Pike K, Tizard J. Randomised, double-blind, placebo controlled trial to determine whether steroids reduce the incidence and severity of nephropathy in Henoch-Schonlein purpura (HSP). Arch Dis Child. 2013;98(10):756-63.
26. Utani A, Ohta M, Shinya A, Ohno S, Takakuwa H, Yamamoto T, et al. Successful treatment of adult Henoch-Schonlein purpura with factor XIII concentrate. J Am Acad Dermatol. 1991;24(3):438-42.
27. White RH, Cameron JS, Trounce JR. Immunosuppressive therapy in steroid-resistant proliferative glomerulonephritis accompanied by the nephrotic syndrome. Br Med J. 1966; 2(5518):853-60.
28. Shin JI, Park JM, Shin YH, Kim JH, Lee JS, Kim PK, et al. Can azathioprine and steroids alter the progression of severe Henoch-Schonlein nephritis in children? Pediatr Nephrol. 2005;20(8):1087-92.
29. Niaudet P, Habib R. Methylprednisolone pulse therapy in the treatment of severe forms of Schonlein-Henoch purpura nephritis. Pediatr Nephrol. 1998;12(3):238-43.
30. Ninchoji T, Kaito H, Nozu K, Hashimura Y, Kanda K, Kamioka I, et al. Treatment strategies for Henoch-Schonlein purpura nephritis by histological and clinical severity. Pediatr Nephrol. 2011;26(4):563-9.
31. Chartapisak W, Opastirakul S, Willis N, Craig JC, Hodson EM. Prevention and treatment of renal disease in Henoch- Purpura: a systematic review. Arch Dis Child. 2009;94(2):132-7.
32. Tarshish P, Bernstein J, Edelmann CM Jr. Henoch-Schönlein purpura nephritis: course of disease and efficacy of cyclophosphamide. Pediatr Nephrol. 2004;19:51-6.
33. Camerone G, Garelli S, Valbonesi M, Mosconi L. Plasma exchange treatment in a patient with severe Schoenlein-Henoch purpura. Minerva Med. 1982;73(18):1185-7.
34. KDIGO guidelines on glomerulonephritis Chapter 11: Henoch-Schönlein purpura nephritis. Kidney Int Suppl. 2012;2:218-20.
35. Davin JC, Coppo R. Pitfalls in recommending evidence-based guidelines for a protean disease like Henoch-Schonlein purpura nephritis. Pediatr Nephrol. 2013;28(10):1897-903.
36. Davin JC, Coppo R. Henoch-Schonlein purpura nephritis in children. Nat Rev Nephrol. 2014;10(10):563-73.

CHAPTER

6.8

Membranoproliferative Glomerulonephritis

Devi S Sruthi, Susan Uthup

INTRODUCTION

Membranoproliferative glomerulonephritis (MPGN), also known as mesangiocapillary glomerulonephritis (GN), is an uncommon cause of chronic progressive GN in children and young adults. MPGN is in fact the name for a general pattern of a histopathological lesion on renal biopsy and not a specific disease entity. It is characterized by a light microscopic pattern of glomerular injury that includes mesangial hypercellularity, endocapillary proliferation, and thickened glomerular capillary wall. The term MPGN itself is derived from the typical histopathological features.[1]

CLASSIFICATION

Traditionally, MPGN has been classified as MPGN types I, II, and III based on the electron microscopic findings. However, the recent advances in the understanding of pathogenetic processes involved in MPGN suggest that this classification can result in considerable overlap among the different types. Hence, more recently MPGN has been reclassified into two diseases—immune complex (IC)-mediated MPGN (IC-MPGN) and complement-mediated MPGN—based on the findings on immunofluorescence microscopy.[2] IC-MPGN is characterized by the deposition of immunoglobulins and complement components, while complement-mediated MPGN is characterized by glomerular deposits of complement components in the absence of significant immunoglobulin deposition.[1]

ETIOPATHOGENESIS

Immune Complex-mediated Glomerulonephritis

This type of MPGN usually occurs in the setting of persistent antigenemia, which results in the deposition of immune complexes or monoclonal immunoglobulins leading to activation of classical complement pathway.[3,4] In adults, the most important antigens identified result from infection, autoimmune disease, or monoclonal gammopathies.[3] An underlying cause can be found in the majority of cases,[5] but despite extensive evaluation, a small minority remains "idiopathic." However, in children, antigenemia in IC-MPGN is mostly idiopathic.[6]

Infections

Viral (hepatitis B and C), chronic bacterial (e.g., endocarditis, shunt nephritis, abscesses), fungal, and, particularly in the developing world, parasitic infections (e.g., malaria, schistosomiasis, echinococcosis) can cause MPGN.[7-9] Hepatitis C virus (HCV)-induced MPGN is typically associated with mixed (type II) cryoglobulinemia.

Autoimmune Disorders

Immune complex-mediated MPGN is observed in patients with systemic lupus erythematosus (particularly in the chronic phase of lupus nephritis) and, less often, Sjögren's syndrome or rheumatoid arthritis.[10]

Neoplasms

Monoclonal gammopathies due to plasma cell dyscrasia and chronic lymphoproliferative disorders is an important cause of MPGN in adults but rare in children. It is associated with either monoclonal immunoglobulin deposition or isolated complement deposition on immunofluorescence microscopy in dense deposit disease (DDD) and C3GN.

Rarer causes of IC-MPGN include chronic liver disease, alpha 1 antitrypsin deficiency, etc.[11] Immunofluorescence microscopy may suggest the underlying etiology of IC/monoclonal immunoglobulin-mediated MPGN. MPGN caused by hepatitis C virus infection usually show granular deposition of immunoglobulin M (IgM), C3, and both kappa and lambda light chains. Immunoglobulin G (IgG) may or may not be present, and C1q is typically negative. These features may also be seen with MPGN induced by other viral infections.[12] MPGN resulting from monoclonal gammopathy is characterized by deposition of monotypic immunoglobulin with kappa or lambda light chain restriction but not both.[13] MPGN resulting from autoimmune diseases, typically SLE is often shows "full house" pattern of immunoglobulin deposition, including IgG, IgM, IgA, C1q, C3, C4, and kappa and lambda light chains.[14]

TABLE 1: Differences between postinfectious glomerulonephritis and C3 glomerulonephritis.

Features	*PIGN*	*C3GN*
Immunofluorescence microscopy	Both bright C3 and IgG deposition	Bright C3 staining alone
Electron microscopy	Well-demarcated subepithelial humps seen especially in poststreptococcal glomerulonephritis	Abundant subendothelial, mesangial, and occasionally subepithelial or intramembranous deposits that have a fuzzy amorphous lobular quality
Antifactor B antibodies	Present in 91%[16]	Present in 14%

(IgG: immunoglobulin G; PIGN: postinfectious glomerulonephritis)

Electron microscopy in immunoglobulin-positive MPGN typically demonstrates subendothelial and mesangial deposits. Subepithelial deposits can also be seen with autoimmune diseases. Tubuloreticular structures in endothelial cells in MPGN are suggestive of lupus nephritis, and a fingerprint pattern associated with cryoprecipitate is seen in mixed cryoglobulinemia or rarely in lupus nephritis associated with cryoglobulinemia.[15]

Hypocomplementemia is common in all types of MPGN.[12] In IC-MPGN, complement activation occurs via the classic pathway and is typically manifested by a normal or mildly decreased serum C3 concentration and a low serum C4 concentration. Low C3 levels common to both infection-related glomerulonephritis (IRGN) and C3GN cannot be used to distinguish these two entities. The salient differences on renal histology of postinfectious GN (PIGN) and C3GN are given in **Table 1**.

Complement-mediated Membranoproliferative Glomerulonephritis

Complement-mediated MPGN results from dysregulation and persistent activation of the alternative complement pathway[5,17] due to impaired regulatory mechanisms which result in the deposition of complement products along the capillary walls and in the mesangium. There are limited data on the epidemiology of these rare disorders with estimates of 1–2 per 10^6 children 5–15 years of age.[18] In children, the most common etiology is the formation of autoantibodies that protect C3 convertase from degradation (C3, C4, or C5 nephritic factors). Genetic mutations resulting in impaired function of complement components/alternative complement pathway regulators are other causes, with the remaining cases considered as idiopathic (which may be due to unidentified genetic mutations).[19-21] Complement-mediated MPGN can be subdivided into C3 glomerulopathy and C4 glomerulopathy based upon the complement product identified within glomerular deposits. In C3 glomerulopathy, immunofluorescence microscopy of kidney sections demonstrates predominantly bright staining for C3, with minimal or no immunoglobulin staining, in the mesangium and along the capillary walls.[2] C4 glomerulopathy is characterized by bright staining for C4d, a degradation product of C4, with minimal or no C3 or immunoglobulin staining.

Complement-mediated MPGN may be further classified based upon ultrastructural features observed on EM as DDD or C3GN [or C4 glomerulonephritis (C4GN)]. Some genetic mutations associated with these disorders are also associated with atypical hemolytic uremic syndrome. C3 glomerulopathy is classified as C3 deposition that is ≥2 orders of magnitude higher than accompanying immunoglobulin if any.[2]

C3 Dense Deposit Disease

C3 DDD is a rare form of MPGN that affects both children and young adults. In most patients, antibody stabilizing C3 convertase, called C3 nephritic factor (C3NeF), is present. On light microscopy, patterns of injury other than MPGN-like mesangial proliferative, diffuse proliferative, crescentic GN, or a sclerosing glomerulopathy can also be seen. EM is needed to confirm the diagnosis and shows the typical sausage-shaped, wavy, densely osmophilic deposits along the glomerular basement membrane (GBM) and mesangium (hence the name of the disease). Other features include acquired partial lipodystrophy (loss of fat in face and upper body) and presence of drusen (macular deposits seen in Bruch's membrane of retina) on fundus.

C3 Glomerulonephritis

C3 glomerulonephritis (also called GN with isolated C3 deposits) is, like C3 DDD, caused by excessive activation of the alternative complement cascade due (in most patients) to mutations in or antibodies to complement regulating protein.[5,22] C3GN has also been reported in association with inherited disease due to mutations in the *CFHR5* gene (CFHR5 nephropathy). Light microscopy often shows an MPGN pattern of injury. Other forms of GN may be seen, such as mesangial proliferative, diffuse proliferative, crescentic GN, and a sclerosing glomerulopathy.[23] Crescentic GN is a rare subtype that more commonly affects children and young adults.[24] EM demonstrates deposits that are similar to those seen with IC/monoclonal immunoglobulin-mediated MPGN but does not show the typical sausage-shaped intramembranous and mesangial deposits observed in DDD. Some patients have C3NeF, as in DDD.[23] The salient differences between DDD and C3 (or C4) GN are shown in **Table 2**.

In complement-mediated MPGN, there are usually low serum C3 and normal C4 levels due to activation of the

TABLE 2: Difference between dense deposit disease and C3 glomerulonephritis.

Features	DDD	C3GN
Mean age (years)	14	24
Sex distribution	Equal	Equal
Associated disorders	Macular degeneration, drusen in Bruch's membrane of retina, type 1 diabetes mellitus, acquired partial lipodystrophy (Barraquer-Simons' or Dunnigan-Koeberling syndrome)	
Electron microscopy	Intramembranous densely osmophilic sausage-shaped or wavy, ribbon-shaped electron-dense deposits along the GBM and mesangium	Mesangial, subepithelial, or subendothelial electron-dense deposits expanding the basement membrane. The material is less electron dense and less well defined than in dense deposit disease
C3 convertase dysregulation	++	+
C5 convertase dysregulation	+	++
C3NeF	+++ (in 80%)	+
Factor H-associated antibody	++	++
Soluble membrane attack complex (sMAC)	+	+++
ESKD	50% in 10 years of diagnosis	10% in 2–3 years. Progression to ESKD appears to be slower in C3GN
Recurrence post-transplant	• Histological DDD nearly universal 50% graft loss in 5 years • Transplant outcome poor	• 60–70% recurrence with graft loss in ~50% • Transplant outcome poor

(C3GN: C3 glomerulonephritis; DDD: dense deposit disease; ESKD: end-stage kidney disease; GBM: glomerular basement membrane)

alternate pathway. However, complement-mediated MPGN is not excluded by a normal serum C3 concentration, and it is not unusual to find a normal C3 concentration with DDD or C3GN.[22]

C4 Glomerulopathy

C4 glomerulopathy, which includes C4 DDD and C4GN, is a rare disorder characterized by the glomerular deposition of C4 in the absence of C3, C1q, and immunoglobulin.[25,26] These patients do not have congenital or acquired defects in the alternative pathway of complement, but they may have an overactive lectin pathway of complement. An observational study by Singh et al. suggests that the presence of glomerular C4d should not exclude a C3 glomerulopathy. In lower intensities, it appears to represent overlying classical/lectin pathway activation with concordant Ig/C1q deposits. A subset of cases, however, displays intense and discordant C4d staining, which raises the possibility of an associated lectin pathway abnormality, a potential future area of study.[27]

Membranoproliferative Glomerulonephritis without Immunoglobulin or Complement Deposition

A histologic pattern that may resemble MPGN on light microscopy can be seen in the healing phase of thrombotic microangiopathies (e.g., thrombotic thrombocytopenia purpura-hemolytic uremic syndrome), antiphospholipid antibody syndrome, nephropathy associated with bone marrow transplantation, chronic kidney allograft nephropathy, radiation nephritis, and malignant hypertension. The common underlying cause of the MPGN pattern in such patients is endothelial injury followed by reparative changes. Immunofluorescence microscopy does not show significant immunoglobulin or complement deposition in the glomeruli, and EM does not show electron-dense deposits along the capillary walls.

Clinical Features

Patients with MPGN with active disease may present as nephrotic syndrome, acute nephritic syndrome, asymptomatic proteinuria, and hematuria detected on routine urinalysis or recurrent episodes of gross hematuria. Patients with chronic disease may have a bland urine sediment with a variable degree of proteinuria and elevation in serum creatinine. A single-center study in children by Khandelwal et al.[28] reported nephrotic syndrome as the chief presentation in 65.2% of children, while 15% of children had acute nephritic syndrome. Majority (86.9%) had hematuria and significant hypertension was found at presentation in 41.3%. Patients with DDD comprised half of the cohort and had rapidly progressive GN (RPGN). An infectious trigger preceded the diagnosis in many of the patients.[28]

The largest pediatric IC-MPGN/C3 glomerulopathy (C3G) cohort in a multicentric, multinational collaborative study, which combines the KidCOM and C3PO registries,[29] found that nearly half of the patients originally diagnosed as MPGN would be reclassified as C3G today as per the recent C3G consensus criteria.[2] Patients in this study had a mean age of 9.3 years at diagnosis and 13.4 years at the last follow-up (the mean follow-up time was 4 years). The cohort was 47.3% male and predominantly white. The majority of patients had hematuria at the time of the initial presentation, and hypertension was present in 57.5% of patients at diagnosis. Only 11.8% of all patients presented with nephrotic syndrome at the initial diagnosis. Patients in the cohort had a moderately depressed mean estimated glomerular filtration rate (eGFR) at presentation. There was a trend toward higher serum creatinine levels at the initial presentation and at the last follow-up in patients with C3GN compared with those with IC-MPGN, although this did not reach statistical significance. The mean serum C3 was low in patients in both groups at diagnosis. Compared with adults, children are more likely to have hematuria at the onset and less likely to have renal insufficiency and hypertension.[30]

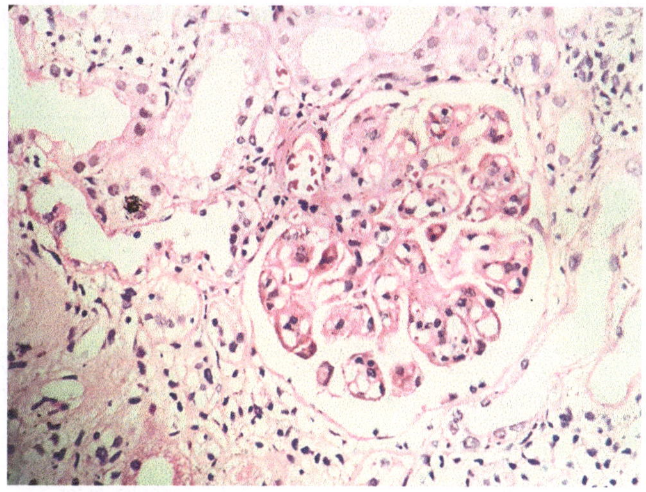

Fig. 1: Light microscopy H & E ×400 showing MPGN pattern: mesangial expansion and basement membrane thickening can be noted.
Courtesy: Dr. Seethalekshmi NV and Jyotsna, Amrita Institute of Medical Sciences, Cochin.

Histopathology

The typical histopathological features of MPGN include the following:

- Thickened GBM leading to a "double contour" or "tram track" appearance of basement membrane in periodic acid–Schiff or silver stains.
- Global and diffuse increase in cellularity of the glomerulus along with mesangial expansion leading to a hyperlobular (or clover leaf-like) appearance of the glomerular tuft on light microscopy **(Figs. 1 and 2)**.

The thickened GBM occurs due to subendothelial deposition of ICs and/or complement factors, cellular entrapment between the GBM and the endothelial cell, and new basement membrane formation.[1] The increased glomerular cellularity is due to increased mesangial and endocapillary cellularity, which results from both proliferation of mesangial cells and influx of circulating monocytes.

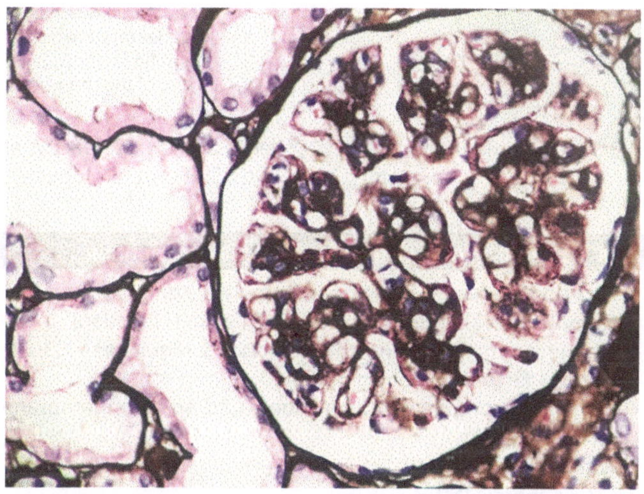

Fig. 2: Light microscopy methenamine silver ×400—membranoproliferative glomerulonephritis (MPGN) basement membrane double contours.
Courtesy: Dr. Seethalekshmi NV and Jyotsna, Amrita Institute of Medical Sciences, Cochin.

Evaluation of MPGN

As such, the discovery of the lesion of MPGN in a kidney biopsy is the start of an exploratory process leading to a diagnosis, not an end in itself. The algorithmic evaluation of MPGN is shown in **Flowchart 1**. Special diagnostic tests for evaluation of C3GN are given in **Box 1**.

Treatment

All patients with a kidney biopsy lesion of MPGN, irrespective of cause, should be treated with general measures including dietary sodium and protein restriction, blood pressure control, minimization of proteinuria with renin–angiotensin system (RAS) inhibition, and treatment of dyslipidemia. Other aspects of therapy include diuretics to control edema and maintenance of adequate nutrition.

Patients with an Underlying Cause

Most patients with IC-mediated MPGN have an identifiable underlying cause, such as a chronic infection, autoimmune disease, etc. Such patients should receive therapy directed against the underlying cause of the MPGN since resolution of the MPGN usually occurs after successful treatment of the primary disease. For example, in patients with infection-associated MPGN, initial therapy should focus on successful treatment of the primary infection, such as antiviral therapy for MPGN due to hepatitis C or B virus. Immunosuppressive therapy may be harmful in patients with hepatitis, except in conditions such as severe HCV-associated mixed cryoglobulinemia or RPGN.[31]

Flowchart 1: Evaluation of membranoproliferative glomerulonephritis.

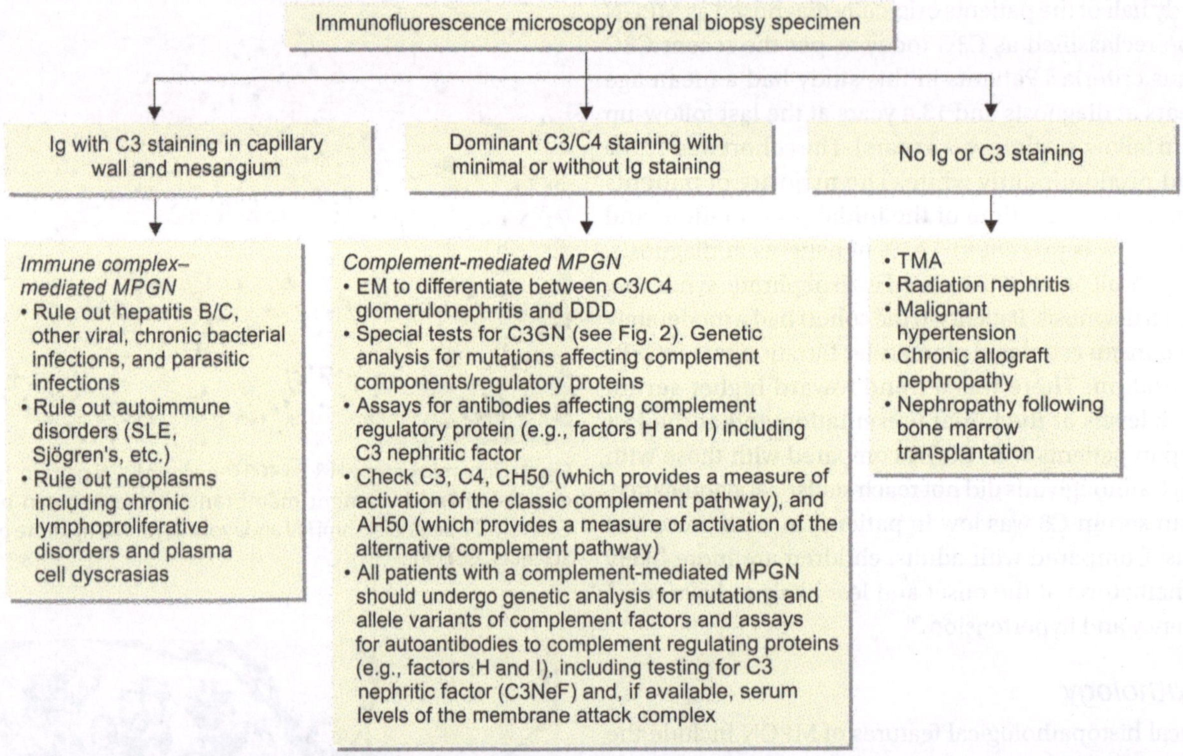

(C3GN: C3 glomerulonephritis; DDD: dense deposit disease; EM: electron microscopy; Ig: immunoglobulin; MPGN: membranoproliferative glomerulonephritis; SLE: systemic lupus erythematosus; TMA: thrombotic microangiopathy)

BOX 1: Special diagnostic tests for C3 glomerulonephritis.

- Functional assays—CH50 (total hemolytic component), AP50 (complement alternate pathway), FHF (factor H function)
- Measurement of complement components, regulators—C3, C4, factor H, factor B, factor I, properdin
- Markers of complement activation—C3d, soluble membrane attack complex
- *Autoantibodies:*
  - C3 nephritic factor
  - C4 nephritic factor
  - C5 nephritic factor
  - Antibodies to factor H&B
- Genetic factors–C3, factor H, I, B, CFHR5
- Test for monoclonal Ig serum and urine electrophoresis, serum-free light chain assay, immunofixation (more important in adults

Patients with no Underlying Cause

The treatment of idiopathic IC-MPGN or C3G is aimed at modifying the underlying immune dysregulation as well as minimizing the complications of hypertension and proteinuria. The present management largely relies on RAS blockade and immunosuppression because much of the evidence for therapy again comes from adult data.[29]

Idiopathic Immune Complex-mediated Membranoproliferative Glomerulonephritis

- In children who present with mild disease, characterized by normal kidney function, non-nephrotic-range proteinuria and no significant hematuria, conservative treatment (including RAS inhibition) alone may be needed. Studies have shown excellent long-term outcomes in such children whether or not they were treated with glucocorticoids.[32] However, if the patient develops worsening proteinuria, hematuria, or kidney function, immunosuppressive therapy may be warranted.
- Children who present with nephrotic syndrome and normal GFR at presentation require corticosteroids for a period of 12–16 weeks in addition to conservative therapy.[33,34] In such cases, calcineurin inhibitors (CNIs) may be used as an alternative if steroid use is contraindicated.
- For patients with idiopathic crescentic glomerulonephritis (ICGN), abnormal kidney function (but without crescentic involvements), and active urine sediment, with or without nephrotic-range proteinuria, add corticosteroids to supportive care. If there is inadequate response to steroids, mycophenolate mofetil (MMF) may be added as a second-line agent after tapering steroids. If there is no improvement in kidney function, hematuria, or proteinuria, discontinue therapy and consider a repeat kidney biopsy. If the kidney biopsy continues to show active GN, consider using cyclophosphamide or rituximab. In patients with persistent disease activity despite at least 6 months of MMF plus low-dose prednisone or after 3–6 months of daily oral cyclophosphamide plus prednisone or rituximab, discontinue corticosteroids and immunosuppression and continue supportive therapy.[35]

- For children presenting with a rapidly progressive crescentic idiopathic ICGN, treatment with high-dose corticosteroids and cyclophosphamide is indicated. Initiate treatment with intravenous (IV) methylprednisolone followed by oral glucocorticoids and oral cyclophosphamide or oral glucocorticoids and rituximab.[35]
- For most patients with idiopathic ICGN presenting with an eGFR <30 mL/min/1.73 m^2, conservative therapy alone is needed, unless kidney biopsy shows an active necrotizing crescentic GN or other reason that could support use of immunosuppression (i.e., minimal interstitial fibrosis or concomitant acute tubulointerstitial nephritis); these patients should be referred for kidney transplant evaluation in due course.[35]

Treatment of C3 Glomerulonephritis

There is no effective disease-specific therapy for C3GN. Supportive measures with plasma therapy and cellular immune suppression, angiotensin-converting enzyme (ACE) inhibitors/angiotensin receptor blockers (ARBs), and lipid-lowering agents are recommended. There is a paucity of data regarding treatment of C3GN in children. In a mixed adult-pediatric cohort study of patients with C3G, Meena et al.[36] showed a significant increase in time to end-stage kidney disease (ESKD) in patients treated with steroids compared with those who did not receive steroid therapy at diagnosis, and the protective effect of steroid therapy remained significant in the multivariate analysis.

- In children with C3GN or DDD who have mild disease, characterized by hematuria, subnephrotic proteinuria, and normal kidney function, treatment with ACE inhibitors (or ARBs) alone is needed.
- In patients with C3GN or DDD who have nephrotic proteinuria (>40 mg/m^2/h) or abnormal kidney function (but not rapidly progressive disease), and who do not have a genetic mutation leading to factor H deficiency, a treatment with MMF plus oral glucocorticoids rather than an ACE inhibitor (or ARB) alone is needed.[37-39] In patients whose proteinuria or kidney function fails to improve after 6 months of MMF therapy, terminal complement blockade with eculizumab[17,39-41] should be tried.
- In patients with C3GN or DDD who have RPGN (i.e., rapidly deteriorating kidney function and crescentic GN on kidney biopsy), immunosuppressive therapy with IV followed by oral glucocorticoids in combination with either cyclophosphamide or MMF should be tried.[39]
- In patients with C3GN or DDD who have identified genetic defects in factor H protein leading to deficient serum levels (regardless of proteinuria or kidney function), periodic infusions of fresh frozen plasma (FFP) to replace the missing or mutant protein should be given rather than treating with immunosuppression.[39]
- Plasma exchange is the first-line therapy for factor H defects and elevated C3NeF. Treatment with FFP/recombinant factor H is recommended for factor H deficiency. C3GN due to autoantibodies to a complement protein may benefit from immunosuppressive therapy with steroids and rituximab. Recombinant humanized monoclonal antibody eculizumab has been found useful in C3GN. It inhibits the cleavage of C5 to C5a and C5b by C5 convertase.[42]

Although indications and guidelines for complement blockade have not yet been firmly established, results by Kirpalani et al. suggest a potential future role for such disease-modifying therapy.[29]

Kidney transplantation is an option for patients with DDD and C3GN, but the disease often recurs, mostly because standard immunosuppression does not correct the underlying abnormality. Thus, whenever possible, patients being prepared for transplantation who have any identifiable abnormalities in complement regulation should be treated to correct these abnormalities prior to transplantation.[39] Family members should be screened for the disease, if being worked up as donors.

PROGNOSIS

Kirpalani et al.[29] reported that in children, advanced chronic kidney disease (CKD) and ESKD were rare findings, with only 7.3% of children with C3GN, 5.7% IC-MPGN, and 12.5% reaching ESKD at mean follow-up at 4 years and no deaths were documented. Bomback et al. also noted a significantly longer time to ESKD or death in pediatric patients compared with adults.[43]

CONCLUSION

Membranoproliferative glomerulonephritis is a histological pattern of glomerular injury on renal biopsy and needs evaluation for any underlying cause. Based on the pathogenesis, MPGN is classified into IC-mediated and complement-mediated MPGN. Immunofluorescence microscopy helps to distinguish between the two entities. In IC-MPGN, both IC and complement staining are seen while in complement-mediated MPGN complement staining is predominant. Though infections and autoimmune disorders are the important causes of IC-MPGN in children, idiopathic MPGN is also seen. Complement-mediated MPGN includes C3 glomerulopathy as well as the very rare C4 glomerulopathy. C3 glomerulopathy is further classified into C3GN and DDD based on electron microscopy and extrarenal findings. Children with MPGN may present with hematuria, proteinuria, nephritic syndrome, nephrotic syndrome, or renal failure and evaluation for alternative complement pathway activation should be performed in complement-mediated MPGN. All patients with MPGN should be treated with general measures including sodium restriction, renin-angiotensin-aldosterone system (RAAS) inhibition, and drugs for dyslipidemia. Therapy should be directed against underlying cause once it is identified. As idiopathic IC-MPGN and C3 glomerulopathy are not very common diseases, there is no consensus guidelines for immunosuppressive therapy in children. Corticosteroids, MMF, cyclophosphamide, and rituximab are the various immunosuppressive agents used. The choice of agents is based on histology, clinical features, degree of proteinuria, renal failure, etc. Terminal complement blockade using eculizumab is an upcoming treatment option in c3 glomerulopathy.

KEY POINTS

- MPGN is a histological diagnosis and not a specific disease entity. It is a pattern of glomerular injury with light microscopic findings including hypercellularity and GBM thickening.
- The traditional electron microscopic classification has been replaced by the classification based on immunofluorescence microscopy, which is based upon the underlying pathogenetic process also. It includes IC-MPGN, complement-mediated MPGN, and MPGN with no complement/IC deposits.
- Identification of an underlying cause is very important as therapy is directed against the underlying cause.
- In complement-mediated MPGN, evaluation of activation of alternative pathway of complement should be performed.
- Immunosuppressive therapy should be considered in patients with idiopathic IC-MPGN and C3 glomerulopathy.
- Plasma exchange is the first-line therapy for factor H defects and elevated C3NeF.
- Recombinant humanized monoclonal antibody eculizumab has been found useful in C3GN.
- The long-term prognosis in children seems better as compared to adults with longer time for progression to ESKD.

REFERENCES

1. Sethi S, Nester CM, Smith RJ. Membranoproliferative glomerulonephritis and C3 glomerulopathy: resolving the confusion. Kidney Int. 2012;81(5):434-41.
2. Pickering MC, D'Agati VD, Nester CM, Smith RJ, Haas M, Appel GB, et al. C3 glomerulopathy: consensus report. Kidney Int. 2013;84(6):1079-89.
3. Noris M, Remuzzi G. Glomerular diseases dependent on complement activation, including atypical hemolytic uremic syndrome, membranoproliferative glomerulonephritis, and C3 glomerulopathy: core curriculum 2015. Am J Kidney Dis. 2015;66(2):359-75.
4. Sethi S, Fervenza FC. Membranoproliferative glomerulonephritis—a new look at an old entity. N Engl J Med. 2012;366(12): 1119-31.
5. Sethi S, Fervenza FC, Zhang Y, Nasr SH, Leung N, Vrana J, et al. Proliferative glomerulonephritis secondary to dysfunction of the alternative pathway of complement. Clin J Am Soc Nephrol. 2011;6:1009.
6. Licht C, Schlötzer-Schrehardt U, Kirschfink M, Zipfel PF, Hoppe B. MPGN II—genetically determined by defective complement regulation? Pediatr Nephrol. 2007;22(1):2-9.
7. Yamabe H, Johnson RJ, Gretch DR, Fukushi K, Osawa H, Miyata M, et al. Hepatitis C virus infection and membranoproliferative glomerulonephritis in Japan. J Am Soc Nephrol. 1995;6(2):220-3.
8. Rodrigues VL, Otoni A, Voieta I, Antunes CSF, Lambertucci JR. Glomerulonephritis in schistosomiasis mansoni: a time to reappraise. Rev Soc Bras Med Trop. 2010;43:638.
9. Rincón B, Bernis C, Garcia A, Traver JA. Mesangiocapillary glomerulonephritis associated with hydatid disease. Nephrol Dial Transplant. 1993;8:783-4.
10. Zand L, Fervenza FC, Nasr SH, Sethi S. Membranoproliferative glomerulonephritis associated with autoimmune diseases. J Nephrol 2014; 27:165.
11. Ichi B, Jayne D. Membranoproliferative glomerulonephritis. Pediatr Nephrol. 2010;25(8):1409-18.
12. Rennke HG. Secondary membranoproliferative glomerulonephritis. Kidney Int. 1995;47:643.
13. Nasr SH, Larsen CP, Sirac C, Theis JD, Domenger C, Chauvet S, et al. Light chain only variant of proliferative glomerulonephritis with monoclonal immunoglobulin deposits is associated with a high detection rate of the pathogenic plasma cell clone. Kidney Int. 2020;97:589.
14. Weening JJ, D'Agati VD, Schwartz MM, Seshan SV, Alpers CE, Appel GB, et al. The classification of glomerulonephritis in systemic lupus erythematosus revisited. J Am Soc Nephrol. 2004;15:241.
15. Su CF, Chen HH, Yeh JC, Chen SC, Liu CC, Tzen CY. Ultrastructural 'fingerprint' in cryoprecipitates and glomerular deposits: a clinicopathologic analysis of fingerprint deposits. Nephron. 2002;90:37.
16. Chauvet S, Berthaud R, Devriese M, Mignotet M, Martins PV, Robe-Rybkine T, et al. Anti-factor B antibodies and acute postinfectious GN in children. J Am Soc Nephrol. 2020;31:829.
17. Sethi S, Fervenza FC. Membranoproliferative glomerulonephritis: pathogenetic heterogeneity and proposal for a new classification. Semin Nephrol. 2011;31:341.
18. Lebreton C, Bacchetta J, Dijoud F, Bessenay L, Fremeaux-Bacchi V, Sellier-Leclerc AL. C3 glomerulopathy and eculizumab: a report on four paediatric cases. Pediatr Nephrol. 2017;32:1023-8.
19. Riedl M, Thorner P, Licht C. C3 glomerulopathy. Pediatr Nephrol. 2017;32:43-57.
20. Zhang Y, Meyer NC, Fervenza FC, Lau W, Keenan A, Cara-Fuentes G, et al. C4 nephritic factors in C3 glomerulopathy: a case series. Am J Kidney Dis. 2017;70: 834-43.
21. Marinozzi M-C, Chauvet S, Le Quintrec M, Mignotet M, Petitprez F, Legendre C, et al. C5 nephritic factors drive the biological phenotype of C3 glomerulopathies. Kidney Int. 2017;92:1232-41.
22. Sethi S, Fervenza FC, Zhang Y, Zand L, Vrana JA, Nasr SH, et al. C3 glomerulonephritis: clinicopathological findings, complement abnormalities, glomerular proteomic profile, treatment, and follow-up. Kidney Int. 2012; 82:465.
23. Servais A, Frémeaux-Bacchi V, Le Quintrec M, Mignotet M, Petitprez F, Legendre C, et al. Primary glomerulonephritis with isolated C3 deposits: a new entity which shares common genetic risk factors with haemolytic uraemic syndrome. J Med Genet. 2007;44:193.
24. Ravindran A, Fervenza FC, Smith RJH, Sethi S. C3 glomerulonephritis with a severe crescentic phenotype. Pediatr Nephrol. 2017;32:1625.
25. Sethi S, Sullivan A, Smith RJ. C4 dense-deposit disease. N Engl J Med. 2014;370:784.

26. Sethi S, Quint PS, O'Seaghdha CM, Fervenza FC, Bijol V, Dorman A, et al. C4 glomerulopathy: a disease entity associated with C4d deposition. Am J Kidney Dis. 2016;67:949.
27. Singh G, Singh SK, Nalwa A, Singh L, Pradeep I, Barwad A, et al. Glomerular C4d staining does not exclude a C3 glomerulopathy. Kidney Int Rep. 2019;4(5):698-709.
28. Khandelwal P, Bhardwaj S, Singh G, Sinha A, Hari P, Bagga A. Therapy and outcomes of C3 glomerulopathy and immune-complex membranoproliferative glomerulonephritis. Pediatr Nephrol. 2021;36(3):591-600.
29. Kirpalani A, Jawa N, Smoyer WE, Licht C; Midwest Pediatric Nephrology Consortium. Long-term outcomes of C3 glomerulopathy and immune-complex membranoproliferative glomerulonephritis in children. Kidney Int Rep. 2020;5(12): 2313-24.
30. Alchi B, Jayne D. Membranoproliferative glomerulonephritis. Pediatr Nephrol. 2010;25(8):1409-18.
31. Elewa U, Sandri AM, Kim WR, Fervenza FC. Treatment of hepatitis B virus-associated nephropathy. Nephron Clin Pract. 2011;119:c41.
32. Somers M, Kertesz S, Rosen S, Herrin J, Clovin R, Palacios de Carreta N, et al. Non-nephrotic children with membranoproliferative glomerulonephritis: are steroids indicated? Pediatr Nephrol. 1995;9:140.
33. Tarshish P, Bernstein J, Tobin JN, Edelmann CM Jr. Treatment of mesangiocapillary glomerulonephritis with alternate-day prednisone—a report of the International Study of Kidney Disease in Children. Pediatr Nephrol. 1992;6:123.
34. Ford DM, Briscoe DM, Shanley PF, Lum GM. Childhood membranoproliferative glomerulonephritis type I: limited steroid therapy. Kidney Int. 1992;41:1606.
35. Fervenza FC, Sethi S, Gassock RJ. (2020). Membranoproliferative glomerulonephritis: treatment and prognosis. Available from https://www.uptodate.com. [Last accessed May, 2022].
36. Meena P, Bhargava V, Gupta P, Rana DS, Bhalla AK, Gupta A, et al. Clinico-pathological features and predictors of end-stage renal disease (ESRD) in C3 glomerulopathy: a retrospective study. Clin Nephrol Res. 2019;3:37-42.
37. Goodship TH, Cook HT, Fakhouri F, Fervenza FC, Frémeaux-Bacchi V, Kavanagh D, et al. Atypical hemolytic uremic syndrome and C3 glomerulopathy: conclusions from a "Kidney Disease: Improving Global Outcomes" (KDIGO) Controversies Conference. Kidney Int. 2017;91:539.
38. Rovin BH, Caster DJ, Cattran DC, Gibson KL, Hogan JJ, Moeller MJ, et al. Management and treatment of glomerular diseases (part 2): conclusions from a Kidney Disease: Improving Global Outcomes (KDIGO) Controversies Conference. Kidney Int. 2019;95:281.
39. Kopel T, Salant DJ, Gassock RJ. (2020). C3 glomerulopathies: dense deposit disease and C3 glomerulonephritis. Available from https://www.uptodate.com [Last accessed May, 2022].
40. Welte T, Arnold F, Kappes J, Seidl M, Häffner K, Bergmann C, et al. Treating C3 glomerulopathy with eculizumab. BMC Nephrol. 2018;19:7.
41. Le Quintrec M, Lapeyraque A-L, Lionet A, Sellier-Leclerc A-L, Delmas Y, Baudouin V, et al. Patterns of clinical response to eculizumab in patients with C3 glomerulopathy. Am J Kidney Dis. 2018;72:84-92.
42. Thomas S, Ranganathan D, Francis L, Madhan K, John GT. Current concepts in C3 glomerulopathy. Indian J Nephrol. 2014; 24:339-48.
43. Bomback AS, Santoriello D, Avasare RS, Regunathan-Shenk R, Canetta PA, Ahn W, et al. C3 glomerulonephritis and dense deposit disease share a similar disease course in a large United States cohort of patients with C3 glomerulopathy. Kidney Int. 2018;93:977-85.

CHAPTER

6.9 Membranous Nephropathy

Radhika C Radhakrishnan, Susan Uthup

INTRODUCTION

Membranous nephropathy (MN) is one of the rare causes of nephrotic syndrome (NS) in children.[1] MN is histologically characterized by uniform thickening of the glomerular capillary wall on light microscopy and subepithelial granular immune complex deposits of immunoglobulin G (IgG) on immunofluorescence (IF).

EPIDEMIOLOGY

Idiopathic MN in children occurs at an incidence rate of 1.2–4.5%.[2,3] An incidence rate of 1.5% was reported by the International Study for Kidney Disease in Children (ISKDC) study in children with NS.[4] Its incidence is more in adolescents compared to children who are younger—1% in children between 1 and 12 years versus 22% in adolescents between 13 and 19 years.[5] The median age of onset ranges from 7 to 12 years.[2,6] There is no definite sex predilection.[6,7] Around 0.5% of childhood chronic kidney disease (CKD) and 0.6% of childhood end-stage kidney disease (ESKD) are attributed to MN. The average age of onset of pediatric ESKD due to MN is reported to be around 16 years.[8,9]

ETIOLOGY

Membranous nephropathy may be primary (idiopathic) or secondary. In adults, primary MN (PMN) is much more common with secondary causes constituting only around 20%. However, in children, secondary MN is more common and varies between 35 and 75%.[2,7] The prevalence of MN is influenced by occurrence of hepatitis B virus (HBV) infection in the community since HBV-related MN is an important cause of secondary MN, especially in children. The important causes of secondary MN are listed in **Table 1**. Primary and secondary MN should be differentiated as they differ in management and outcome. This may be accomplished by the presence of some clinical clues which suggest a possible underlying cause for MN or by histology which can demonstrate features indicative of secondary causes, particularly autoimmune diseases such as lupus nephritis.

TABLE 1: Causes of secondary membranous nephropathy of secondary membranous nephropathy.[10]

General causes	*Specific causes*
Infections	• Hepatitis B • Hepatitis C • Streptococci • Malaria • Schistosomiasis • Syphilis • Leprosy • Tuberculosis • Cytomegalovirus
Drugs	• Captopril • Clopidogrel • Mercury • Penicillamine • Nonsteroidal anti-inflammatory • Gold
Autoimmune causes	• Systemic lupus erythematosus • Rheumatoid arthritis • Autoimmune thyroiditis • Sjögren syndrome • Mixed connective tissue disease
Neoplasms	• Carcinomas of bladder, breast, pancreas, prostate • *Hematological malignancies:* Lymphoma, chronic lymphocytic leukemia
Others	• Diabetes mellitus • Sarcoidosis • Sickle-cell disease • Hematopoietic stem cell transplant • Postrenal transplant

PATHOGENESIS

Recent research has revealed significant insights into etiopathogenesis of MN albeit in adults. The landmark studies done in Heymann models of MN in rats demonstrated that in situ immune complex formation involving megalin, a rat podocyte membrane antigen, led to characteristic subepithelial IgG deposits. Activation of complement pathway through the membrane attack complex C5b-9 was the primary mediator of associated proteinuria.[11] Alloimmune MN in babies of neutral endoproteinase (NEP)-deficient mothers was shown to have an immune mechanism involving maternal anti-NEP antibody. In situ immune complexes with NEP are formed on the infant podocyte membranes.[12]

Beck et al., in 2009, demonstrated IgG4 antibodies to M type phospholipase A2 receptor (PLA2R) on podocytes, in 70% of adults with PMN. These antibodies were present in circulation as well as deposited in glomeruli.[13] Presence of this antibody has been reported by several other groups in 52–78% of MN. An Indian study reported PLA2R-related MN in three fourths of children with PMN.[14] Later, another podocyte antigen thrombospondin type 1 domain containing 7A (THSD7A) was found to be the target of a second IgG4 antibody in a fewer subset of patients with PMN (2–5%).[15] However, both these antibodies can be negative in around 10% of patients with PMN, indicating that further autoantibodies to podocyte membrane antigens will be discovered in future. Double expression of autoantibodies to both PLA2R and THSD7A has also been rarely reported.

Current evidence indicates that antibody response precedes occurrence of proteinuria in PMN by several weeks or months termed preclinical disease. Several etiologic events can precipitate the initiation of antibody response in the presence of compatible immunogenetic risk alleles.[16] This leads to deposition of IgG4 and C5b-9 in the glomerular epithelia, which after reaching a threshold level leads to podocyte activation or injury and increased excretion of urine protein, thus causing NS. Similarly, the antibody disappearance precedes the resolution of proteinuria by several weeks or months, that is, clinical remission lags behind immunologic remission.[16,17] This interval indicate the time taken to form a threshold level of deposits to incite proteinuria at the beginning and that taken to clear subepithelial deposits, repair capillary wall and podocyte damage, and restore permselectivity glomerular filtration barrier.

In Heymann rat models, the primary mediator of antibody-induced podocyte injury and proteinuria is complement activation resulting in sublytic C5b-9 attack on podocytes.[16] This complement activation is mediated by underglycosylated IgG4 acting through the mannose-binding lectin pathway. The sublytic agonistic effect of C5b-9 insertion on the podocyte membrane leads to activation of numerous signaling pathways. This eventually leads to pathogenic processes such as increased synthesis of growth factors, oxidants, proteases, and extracellular matrix components in addition to apoptosis, slit diaphragm disruption, DNA damage with cell cycle arrest autophagy, remodeling of the actin cytoskeleton, and detachment of damaged cells.[17]

Even though PLA2R was initially regarded as specific for PMN, recently secondary MN with PLA2R staining or PLA2R antibody positivity has been reported in systemic lupus erythematosus (SLE), hepatitis C, malignancy, and sarcoidosis.[18-20]

In infants and young children, PLA2R and THSD7A antibodies do not appear to have any major role. Hence, other allo- or autoantigens must be investigated for, after thoroughly excluding other secondary causes, especially malignancy.[18] Antibovine serum albumin (BSA) antibodies are of particular interest in MN as high levels have been found in 7 out of 41 consecutive adults and 4 out of 5 consecutive children of age less than 5 years with MN. They are also commonly prevalent in the general population. Also, high titers of circulating BSA were seen in those children with high titers of anti-BSA antibodies. Several animal models have demonstrated that a cationic form of BSA can induce MN. High levels of circulating cationic BSA and antibodies in children were associated with subepithelial deposits of BSA in the absence of PLA2R.[21]

HISTOPATHOLOGY

Light Microscopy

The histologic hallmark is diffuse global thickening of capillary walls, best seen in methenamine silver-stained sections, which stains glomerular basement membrane (GBM) black and does not stain the subepithelial deposits **(Fig. 1)**. The newly synthesized GBM appears as small black spikes around unstained deposits projecting from the GBM toward the urinary space. All glomeruli are involved. The size of the glomerulus is normal or slightly increased. There is no increase in cellularity or mesangial matrix and capillary loops are patent **(Fig. 2)**.

Immunofluorescence

The hallmark in IF is uniform, granular capillary wall staining for IgG and C3 **(Fig. 3)**. The predominant IgG staining is for IgG4 demonstrated by using monoclonal antibodies. A secondary cause such as SLE should be suspected if mesangial deposits of immunoglobulin A (IgA) or immunoglobulin M (IgM) are seen.

Electron Microscopy

The hallmark is the presence of electron-dense immune complex deposits in the subepithelial space **(Fig. 4)**,

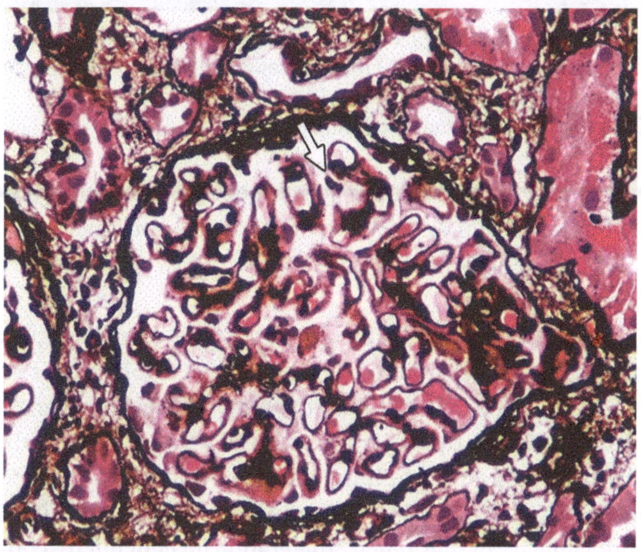

Fig. 1: Photomicrographs (LM) depicting subepithelial argyrophilic spikes along with glomerular basement membrane (arrow) best seen on Jones methenamine silver stain (JMS ×400).
Courtesy: Dr Anila Abraham, Renopath, Chennai.

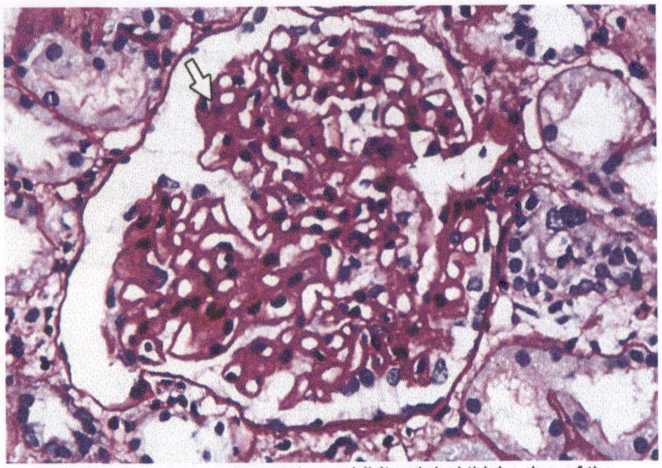

By light microscopy, glomerulus exhibits global thickening of the glomerular basement membrane, in the absence of cellular proliferation (PAS × 400)

Fig. 2: Photomicrographs (LM) depicting thick refractile periodic acid–Schiff (PAS)-positive glomerular basement membrane (arrow).
Courtesy: Dr Anila Abraham, Renopath, Chennai.

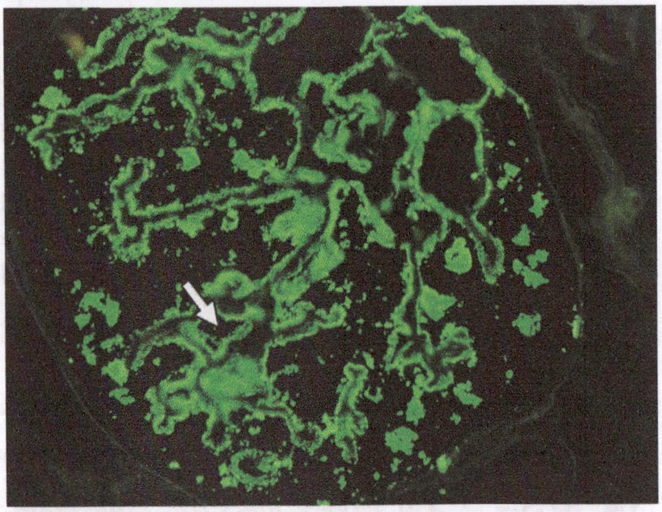

Fig. 3: Photomicrographs depicting immunofluorescence staining for immunoglobulin G (IgG) reveals granular global positivity in the capillary walls (IgG ×400).
Courtesy: Dr Anila Abraham, Renopath, Chennai.

which match the granular IgG deposits demonstrated by IF. Effacement of epithelial foot processes and microvillus transformation is present in all stages of MN where there is heavy proteinuria.

It is pathologically difficult but important to distinguish primary and secondary MN since it has implications for treatment. Presence of extensive subendothelial or mesangial electron dense deposits, absence of PLA2R glomerular staining, and predominance of IgG1-3 are indicative of secondary causes. SLE-associated MN can be associated with endocapillary or mesangial proliferation on light microscopy, a "full-house" pattern of Ig staining, including IgG, IgM, IgA, C1q and non-IgG4 on IF, and tubuloreticular inclusions within the glomerular endothelial cells on EM.

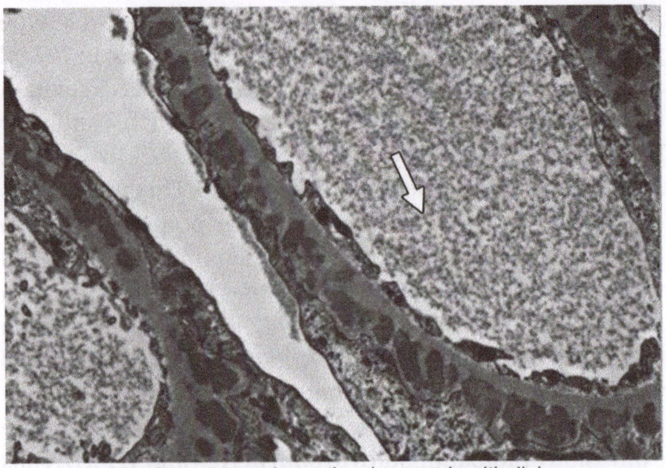

Membranous nephropathy shows subepithelial deposits, which intervening GBM spikes (electron microscopy × 5000)

Fig. 4: Photomicrographs electron microscopy depicting membranous nephropathy showing subepithelial deposits with intervening glomerular basement membrane (GBM) spikes (arrow) ×5,000.
Courtesy: Dr Anila Abraham, Renopath, Chennai.

CLINICAL FEATURES

Children with MN present with either asymptomatic proteinuria or with overt features of frank NS. About 40–75% of the children present with NS and 16–38% of the children have asymptomatic, nephrotic-range proteinuria.[22,23] Microscopic hematuria occurs in 80% and gross hematuria occurs in 40% cases. Acute kidney injury (AKI) is rare and if it occurs, other related conditions or diagnoses such as bilateral renal vein thrombosis (RVT) or the use of nephrotoxic medications or excessive diuretics should be sought for. The most common mode of diagnosis of MN is via biopsy of children with steroid-resistant NS (SRNS) as most children with MN do not respond to standard course of prednisolone therapy. The differences between childhood and adult MN are given in **Table 2.**[24]

INVESTIGATIONS

Investigations include urinalysis (proteinuria, hematuria), urine protein creatinine ratio, serum albumin, creatinine, urea, and cholesterol. Investigations to rule out a secondary cause should always be done and include antinuclear antibody (ANA), anti-double-stranded DNA (anti-dsDNA) to rule out SLE, hepatitis B and C serology, serology for syphilis, complement levels (C3, C4), and cryoglobulins in hepatitis C positive and/or those with low levels of C3.[17-19] Definitive diagnosis requires renal biopsy. If a secondary cause is not found, evaluation should include testing for PLA2R antibody. The sample for PLA2R antibody testing should be collected ideally at the time of kidney biopsy and before starting the treatment. Since some cases of PLA2R-related MN may be missed by antibody detection alone, staining for PLA2R antigen in the kidney should also be done. A preponderance of IgG4 is found in cases with PLA2R-related MN in serum and kidney specimens.

TREATMENT

Guidelines for treatment of MN are expected to change in the near future in light of recent developments in PLA2R antibody testing and new clinical trials. In contrast to adults, all children with SRNS will have to undergo renal biopsy, and PLA2R antibody test should be done in those with kidney biopsy showing MN. Wait and see strategy with supportive treatment alone is usually not adopted in children. A diagnostic strategy based on PLA2R testing, degree of proteinuria, and serum creatinine is depicted in **Flowchart 1**.[24]

Supportive Therapy

General supportive measures include low-salt diet and recommended dietary allowance (RDA) of protein. Fluid restriction and diuretics are used to control edema. Hypertension (HTN) is aggressively treated with angiotensin-converting enzyme (ACE) inhibitors and angiotensin II receptor blockers (ARBs). Both these drugs not only control HTN, but also decrease proteinuria by decreasing the intraglomerular pressure. 3-hydroxy-3-methylglutaryl coenzyme A (HMG-CoA) reductase inhibitors such as atorvastatin help to reduce hypercholesterolemia. Routine anticoagulation is not advisable unless thrombotic complications such as RVT occur.

TABLE 2: Difference between childhood and adult membranous nephropathy.[24]

Features	*Child*	*Adult*
Proportion of NS with MN in biopsy	<5% 5–20% (adolescents)	15–30%
Primary MN	25%	75%
PLA2R	45%	70–80%
Male predominance	Variable	Yes
Microhematuria	75%	50%
Hypertension	<10%	30%
Thromboembolic events	<5%	10–20%
Spontaneous remission	Common	30%
Progression to ESKD	<25%	30–40%

(ESKD: end-stage kidney disease; MN: membranous nephropathy; NS: nephrotic syndrome; PLA2R: phospholipase A2 receptor)

Immunosuppressive Therapy

Children are usually treated with prednisolone for at least 6–8 weeks at standard doses used for idiopathic NS before the diagnosis of MN is made. Kidney Disease Improving Global Outcomes (KDIGO) guidelines suggest that treatment of idiopathic membranous nephropathy (IMN) in children follows the recommendations for the treatment of idiopathic MN in adults.[25] The initial therapy consist of a 6-month course of alternating monthly cycles of oral and IV corticosteroids, and oral alkylating agents (Ponticelli regimen; **Box 1**). Cyclophosphamide is preferred over chlorambucil as an alkylating agent. No more than one course of the cyclical corticosteroid/alkylating-agent regimen should be given in children. Contraindications to this regimen are indicated in **Box 2**. KDIGO guidelines recommend patients be managed conservatively for at least 6 months following the completion of this regimen before being considered a treatment failure if there is no remission, unless kidney function is deteriorating or severe, disabling, or potentially life-threatening symptoms related to the NS are present.

Flowchart 1: Diagnostic approach for membranous nephropathy.[24]

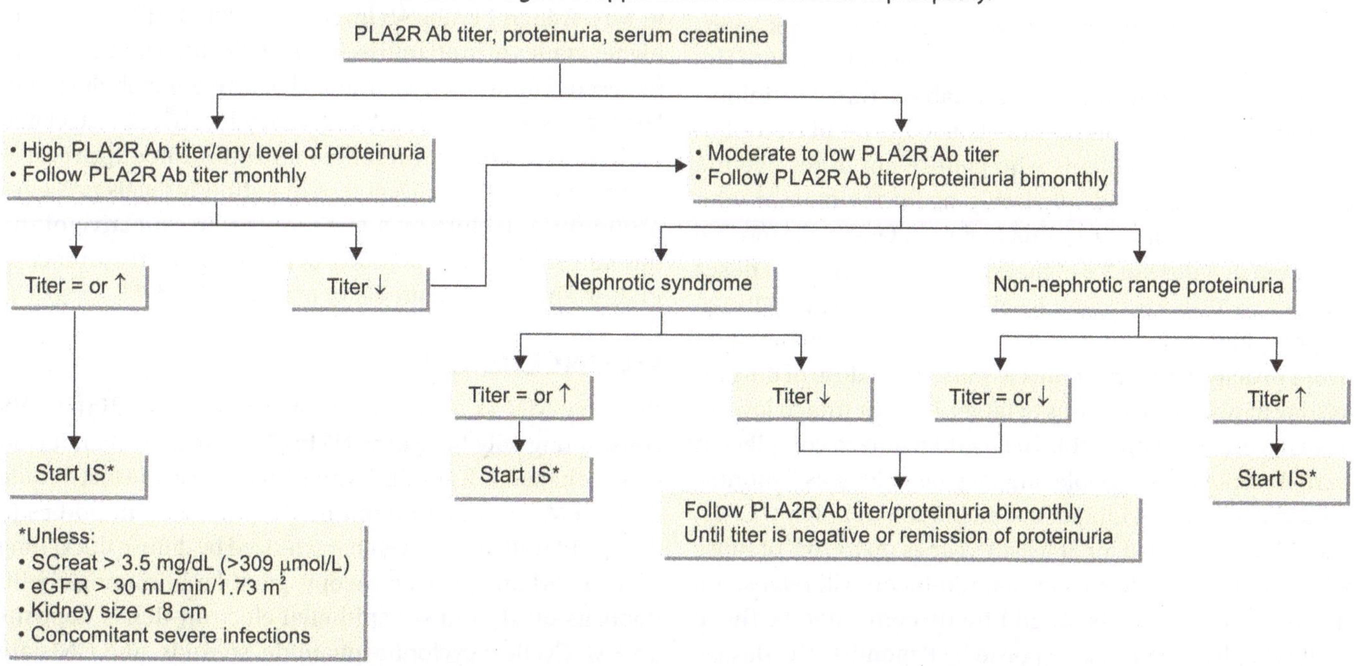

(eGFR: estimated glomerular filtration rate; PLA2R: phospholipase A2 receptor)

BOX 1: Cyclical corticosteroid/alkylating-agent therapy for idiopathic membranous nephropathy (the "Ponticelli Regimen").[26]

- *Month 1*: IV methylprednisolone (1 g) daily for three doses and then oral methylprednisolone (0.5 mg/kg/day) for 27 days
- *Month 2*: Oral chlorambucil (0.15–0.2 mg/kg/day) or oral cyclophosphamide (2.0 mg/kg/day) for 30 days
- *Month 3*: Repeat month 1
- *Month 4*: Repeat month 2
- *Month 5*: Repeat month 1
- *Month 6*: Repeat month 2

Note: Monitor every 2 weeks for 2 months and then every month for 6 months, with serum creatinine, urinary protein excretion, serum albumin, and white blood cell count. If total leukocyte count falls to <3,500/mm³, then hold chlorambucil or cyclophosphamide until recovery to 4000/mm³.

BOX 2: Contraindications to the use of the cyclical corticosteroid/alkylating-agent regimen.[26]

- Untreated infection (HIV, hepatitis B and C, tuberculosis, fungal infection, etc.)
- Neoplasia [lung, skin (except squamous cell)], breast, colon, etc.
- Urinary retention
- Inability to comply with monitoring
- Preexisting leukopenia (<4,000 leukocytes/mm³)
- SCr >3.5 mg/dL (>309 mmol/L)

(HIV: human immunodeficiency virus; MN: membranous nephropathy; SCr: serum creatinine)

Complete remission is defined as urinary protein excretion <0.3 g/day [urine protein/creatinine ratio (uPCR) <300 mg/g or <30 mg/mmol], confirmed by two values at least 1 week apart, accompanied by a normal serum albumin concentration, and a normal serum creatinine. Partial remission is defined as urinary protein excretion <3.5 g/day (uPCR <3,500 mg/g or <350 mg/mmol) and a 50% or greater reduction from peak values, confirmed by two values at least 1 week apart, accompanied by an improvement or normalization of the serum albumin concentration and stable serum creatinine.

Cyclosporine or tacrolimus is used for a period of at least 6 months in patients who choose not to receive the cyclical corticosteroid/alkylating-agent regimen or who have contraindications to this regimen. Oral cyclosporine is started at a dose of 3.5–5 mg/kg/day in two divided doses to target a 12-hour trough level of 60–150 ng/mL (50–125 nmol/L) aiming for lowest levels to maintain remission and avoid toxicity. Oral tacrolimus is started at a dose of 0.1 mg/kg/day in two divided doses to target 12-hour trough level of 5–10 ng/mL (6–12 nmol/L). The median time to complete or partial response is variable and may be as long as 6 months following treatment initiation. Calcineurin inhibitors (CNIs) should be continued for at least 1 year as up to 70% of those who achieve complete or partial remission will relapse on discontinuation. CNIs should be discontinued in those without at least a partial response by 6 months. The dosage of CNI should be reduced at intervals of 4–8 weeks to a level of about 50% of the starting dosage, provided that remission is maintained and no treatment limiting CNI-related nephrotoxicity occurs, and continued for at least 12 months. CNI blood levels should be monitored regularly during the initial treatment period and whenever there is an unexplained rise in serum creatinine (SCr; >20%) during therapy.

Large observational studies have provided encouraging data on use of rituximab for MN. The MENTOR study has confirmed in a randomized, controlled trial that rituximab is efficacious and able to bring about durable remission in the majority of patients with an acceptable safety profile. Because of poor performance of cyclosporin, the MENTOR study suggests that rituximab should be the recommended alternative agent for the treatment of MN when alkylating agents are not suitable.[25,26]

Rituximab is given at a dose of 375 mg/m² as IV infusions on day 1 and 8. Hepatitis B titers may be checked prior to rituximab infusion. Monitoring IgG levels both before and after rituximab infusions can help to identify children at risk of significant infection and decide on immunoglobulin replacement. In adults, patients with very high risk of progression are treated with cyclophosphamide, but data are sparse in children. Adrenocorticotropic hormone (ACTH; synthetic or intact) has been used as a treatment for MN, but larger studies are required before it can be suggested as standard therapy.

PROGNOSIS

Two-thirds of the children and adolescents with PMN respond to conventional immunosuppression.[14] Nephrotic range proteinuria, estimated glomerular filtration rate (eGFR) <60 mL/min/1.72 m², low-molecular-weight proteinuria, and rapid deterioration in GFR are risk factors for poor prognosis in MN. A high PLA2R-Ab level (>250–300 IU/L) is linked to higher grades of proteinuria, lower eGFR/higher SCr, urinary IgG excretion, and serum/urinary beta-2 microglobulin levels. Higher baseline anti-PLA2R antibody levels also correlated with worse kidney outcomes and immunosuppressive treatment resistance. Decrease in antibody levels precedes proteinuria decline by a few months, irrespective of the immunosuppressive measure. In addition, the recurrence of PLA2R-Ab is a strong predictor of relapse in MN.[17]

CONCLUSION

Primary MN is an uncommon cause of pediatric NS constituting only 1–2% of all NS in children. MN secondary to chronic hepatitis B and SLE is more frequent in the first decade of life. PMN is an autoimmune disease with antibodies to M-type PLA2R in 70%. It is characterized by diffuse thickening of the GBM on light microscopy, granular immunoglobulin deposits on IF, and subepithelial electron-dense deposits on EM. Cyclical cyclophosphamide, steroids, and CNIs are the first-line therapies available. More than 60% respond to immunosuppression. Rituximab is useful both as a first-line and as rescue therapy in PMN.

KEY POINTS

- MN is a rare cause of SRNS in children.
- PLA2R antibody may be positive in PMN in >70% and, if positive, helps in diagnosis, monitoring of treatment response, and identification of relapses.
- Higher baseline anti-PLA2R antibody levels are correlated with worse kidney outcomes and immunosuppressive treatment resistance.
- Nephrotic range proteinuria, eGFR < 60 mL/min/1.72 m^2, low-molecular-weight proteinuria, and rapid deterioration in GFR are risk factors for poor prognosis in MN.

REFERENCES

1. Chen A, Frank R, Vento S, Crosby V, Chandra M, Gauthier B, et al. Idiopathic membranous nephropathy in pediatric patients: presentation, response to therapy, and long-term outcome. BMC Nephrol. 2007;8:11.
2. Olbing H, Greifer I, Bennett BP, Bernstein J, Spitzer A. Idiopathic membranous nephropathy in children. Kidney Int. 1973;3:381-90.
3. Kleinknecht C, Levy M, Gagnadoux MF, Habib R. Membranous glomerulonephritis with extra-renal disorders in children. Medicine (Baltimore). 1979;58:219-28.
4. International Study of Kidney Disease in Children. Nephrotic syndrome in children: prediction of histopathology from clinical and laboratory characteristics at time of diagnosis. A report of the International Study of Kidney Disease in Children. Kidney Int. 1978;13:159-65.
5. Moxey-Mims MM, Stapleton FB, Feld LG. Applying decision analysis to management of adolescent idiopathic nephrotic syndrome. Pediatr Nephrol. 1994;8:660-4.
6. Valentini RP, Mattoo TK, Kapur G, Imam A. Membranous glomerulonephritis: treatment response and outcome in children. Pediatr Nephrol. 2009;24:301-8.
7. Lee BH, Cho HY, Kang HG, Ha IS, Cheong HI, Moon KC, et al. Idiopathic membranous nephropathy in children. Pediatr Nephrol. 2006;21:1707-15.
8. North American Pediatric Renal Trials and Collaborative Studies (NAPRTCS). (2007). Annual report. Available from www.naprtcs.org [Last accessed May 2022].
9. U.S. Renal Data System. Atlas of chronic kidney disease and end-stage renal disease in the United States, National Institutes of Health, National Institute of Diabetes and Digestive and Kidney Diseases. In: USRDS 2008 Annual Data Report, Bethesda, MD; 2008.
10. Menon S, Valentini RP. Membranous nephropathy in children: clinical presentation and therapeutic approach. Pediatr Nephrol. 2010;25:1419-28.
11. Kerjaschki D. Pathomechanisms and molecular basis of membranous glomerulopathy. Lancet. 2004;364:1194-6.
12. Debiec H, Guigonis V, Mougenot B, Decobert F, Haymann JP, Bensman A, et al. Antenatal membranous glomerulonephritis due to anti-neutral endopeptidase antibodies. N Engl J Med. 2002;346:2053-60.
13. Beck LH Jr, Bonegio RG, Lambeau G, Beck DM, Powell DW, Cummins TD, et al. M-type phospholipase A2 receptor as target antigen in idiopathic membranous nephropathy. N Engl J Med. 2009;361:11-21.
14. Ramachandran R, Nayak S, Kumar V, Kumar A, Agrawal N, Bansal R, et al. Primary membranous nephropathy in children and adolescents: a single-centre report from South Asia. Pediatr Nephrol. 2021;36:1217-26.
15. Tomas NM, Beck LH Jr, Meyer-Schwesinger C, Seitz-Polski B, Ma H, Zahner G, et al. Thrombospondin type-1 domain-containing 7A in idiopathic membranous nephropathy. N Engl J Med. 2014;371:2277-87.
16. Couser GW. Primary membranous nephropathy. Clin J Am Soc Nephrol. 2017;12:983-97.
17. Francis JM, Beck LH Jr, Salant DJ. Membranous nephropathy: a journey from bench to bedside. Am J Kidney Dis. 2016;68:138-47.
18. Kronbichler A, Oh J, Meijers B, Mayer G, Shin J. Recent progress in deciphering the etiopathogenesis of primary membranous nephropathy. BioMed Res Int. 2017.
19. Larsen CP, Messias NC, Silva FG, Messias E, Walker PD. Determination of primary versus secondary membranous glomerulopathy utilizing phospholipase A2 receptor staining in renal biopsies. Modern Pathol. 2013;26(5):709-15.
20. Xie Q, Li Y, Xue J, Xiong Z, Wang L, Sun Z, et al. Renal phospholipase A2 receptor in hepatitis B virus-associated membranous nephropathy. Am J Nephrol. 2015;41(4-5):345-53.
21. Debiec F, Lefeu MJ, Kemper MJ, Niaudet P, Deschênes G, Remuzzi G, et al. Early-childhood membranous nephropathy due to cationic bovine serum albumin. New Engl J Med. 2011;364(2):2101-10.
22. Kusunoki Y, Itami N, Tochimaru H, Takekoshi Y, Nagasawa S, Yoshiki T. Glomerular deposition of C4 cleavage fragment (C4d) and C4-binding protein in idiopathic membranous glomerulonephritis. Nephron. 1989;51:17-9.
23. Dyer PA, Short CD, Clarke EA, Mallick NP. HLA antigen and gene polymorphisms and haplotypes established by family studies in membranous nephropathy. Nephrol Dial Transplant. 1992;7:42-7.
24. Ayalon R, Beck LH Jr. Membranous nephropathy not just a disease for adults. Pediatr Nephrol. 2015;30(1):31-9.
25. KDIGO clinical practice guideline for glomerulonephritis. 2012;2(2).
26. Trivin-Avillach C, Beck LH Jr. Management of membranous nephropathy after MENTOR. Clin J Am Soc Nephrol. 2020;15(3):415-7.

CHAPTER

6.10 Rapidly Progressive Glomerulonephritis

Anshuman Saha, Susan Uthup

INTRODUCTION

Rapidly progressive glomerulonephritis (RPGN) is a heterogeneous group of clinical syndromes that lead to rapid loss of kidney function over a short period of time (days, weeks, or a few months). It is a renal emergency as irreversible renal damage and progression to end-stage kidney disease (ESKD) is likely if not intervened in time. RPGN is a form of rapidly progressive renal failure (RPRF). The nephritic presentation helps to differentiate RPGN from other causes of RPRF.

DEFINITION

Rapidly Progressive Renal Failure

Rapidly progressive renal failure is a clinical syndrome characterized by a rapid progressive loss of renal function [decrease of estimated glomerular filtration rate (eGFR) by >50%] over days to weeks with a seemingly obvious or unknown etiology.[1] The duration of illness may range from weeks to months. It encompasses a heterogeneous group of clinical syndromes. Renal histology shows lesions involving one or more renal compartments: glomerulus, tubule, interstitium, and vessels.

Rapidly Progressive Glomerulonephritis

Rapidly progressive glomerulonephritis is defined by clinical presentation of RPRF with features of glomerulonephritis such as oliguria or anuria, gross hematuria, hypertension, edema along with dysmorphic erythrocyturia, erythrocyte cylindruria, and glomerular proteinuria.[2,3] RPGN is the most severe manifestation of "nephritic" spectrum of glomerulonephritis which is characterized morphologically by extensive crescent formation (extracapillary proliferation in Bowman's space). For this reason, the clinical term RPGN is often used interchangeably with the pathologic term "crescentic glomerulonephritis."

Crescentic Glomerulonephritis

Crescentic glomerulonephritis (GN) is defined as the presence of crescents in >50% of glomeruli.[2] Glomerular crescents are defined as two or more layers of proliferating parietal epithelial cells in Bowman's space.

Pathogenesis of Crescent Formation

Crescent formation appears to represent a nonspecific response to severe glomerular injury.[2] It denotes the most severe form of glomerulonephritis and there is an initiation, formation, and resolution phase.

Initiation: The initiating event is the development of physical gaps or rents in the glomerular basement membrane and Bowman's capsule. Coagulation factors including fibrinogen enter Bowman's space. Release of proinflammatory cytokines such as interleukin-1 (IL-1) and tumor necrosis factor-alpha (TNF-α) and delayed fibrinolysis due to procoagulant and fibrinolytic inhibitory factors lead to the formation of fibrin polymers. Cellular elements such as monocytes, macrophages, and T lymphocytes (Th1 and Th17 $CD4^+$ T cells) also enter Bowman's space accelerating crescent formation. The contents in Bowman's space can enter the interstitium, via disruption of Bowman's capsule, leading to periglomerular inflammation.[2,3]

Formation: The exudation of coagulation factors and inflammatory mediators such as IL-1, TNF-α, serine proteinases (elastase, PR3), and matrix metalloproteinases released by mononuclear cells leads to proliferation of parietal epithelial cells, macrophages, and fibroblasts resulting in crescent formation. The release of proteases causes further lysis of the GBM proteins and facilitates entry of other inflammatory mediators in Bowman's space. Upregulated expression of adhesion molecules by IL-1 and TNF-α leads to macrophage recruitment and proliferation.[3]

Resolution: The stage of inflammation and cellular proliferation is followed by the development of fibrocellular and fibrous crescents. The transition from cellular to fibrocellular and fibrous crescents is due to production of type 1 collagen and proliferation of fibroblasts mediated by fibroblast growth factors and transforming growth factor β (TGF-β). Development of fibrocellular and fibrous crescent suggests chronicity and poor response to immunosuppression. The plasminogen-plasmin system is responsible for fibrinolysis and resolution of crescents.[3]

Etiology and Classification of Crescentic GN

Diseases **(Table 1)** leading to crescentic GN can be categorized into three broad categories based on histopathology and immunofluorescence (IF) staining in renal biopsy.[2]

1. *Immune complex crescentic GN* with immunoglobulin and C_3 deposits along capillary wall and mesangium
2. *Pauci-immune necrotizing and crescentic GN* with scant or no immunoglobulin or complement deposits
3. *Anti-GBM crescentic GN* with linear deposition of anti-GBM antibodies along the glomerular basement membrane

Sometimes, RPGN may be both antineutrophil cytoplasmic antibody (ANCA) and anti-GBM positive. This is called "double-antibody" positive disease or double-positive vasculitis.[4]

Immune complex crescentic GN: These are a group of diseases in which infections and systemic immune complex diseases lead to proliferative GN with formation of crescents. It is defined by the presence of immune deposits in the glomeruli. The serologic and histologic findings will point to the underlying disease. Immunohistology shows granular deposits of immunoglobulin and complement along the capillary walls and in the mesangium. Infection-related GN (IRGN) includes postinfectious GN (PIGN), *Staphylococcus*-associated GN, shunt nephritis, infective endocarditis, hepatitis, syphilis, etc. Common systemic immune complex diseases causing crescentic GN include lupus nephritis and immunoglobulin A (IgA) vasculitis. Primary glomerular diseases such as IgA nephropathy, immune complex membranoproliferative glomerulonephritis (MPGN), and C_3 glomerulopathy also can present as crescentic GN. About 25% of immune complex crescentic GN are ANCA positive, whereas <5% of noncrescentic immune complex GN have ANCA).[3] This suggests that the presence of ANCA in immune complex GN may predispose to more aggressive disease.

Pauci-immune crescentic GN: It is characterized by paucity of immunoglobulin or complement deposits in IF staining of biopsy. The diseases are mediated by antineutrophilic cytoplasmic antibodies (ANCAs). ANCA-associated small vessel vasculitis includes microscopic polyangiitis (MPA), granulomatous polyangiitis (GPA), and eosinophilic GPA (EGPA). Some cases of ANCA-positive disease are induced by drugs such as penicillamine, propylthiouracil, and hydralazine.[3] <5% of cases of pauci-immune crescentic GN is ANCA negative but behave like ANCA disease and are called idiopathic RPGN.[5]

Anti-GBM crescentic GN: It is characterized by linear immunoglobulin G deposit in IF and positive anti-GBM antibody. It is exceedingly rare in children accounting for <10% of crescentic GN.[2] The anti-GBM autoantibody is directed against a 28-kDa monomer located on the α3 chain of type IV collagen (Goodpasture antigen). Pulmonary involvement (Goodpasture syndrome) is rare. Very rarely (5% of cases) anti-GBM antibody can develop in patients of Alport syndrome after renal transplantation causing anti-GBM nephritis.[6] Pulmonary hemorrhage, however, is rare in these patients.

Immune complex GN is the most common cause of RPGN in children accounting for 45–75% of cases. Pauci-immune crescentic GN though common in adults accounts for 25–42% of cases.[2,7-10] In recent series, pauci-immune crescentic GN was reported as frequently as immune complex GN.[2,11]

TABLE 1: Etiology and classification of rapidly progressive glomerulonephritis.

Immune complex crescentic glomerulonephritis	
Postinfectious	Poststreptococcal nephritis, infective endocarditis, shunt nephritis, other bacterial infections, human immunodeficiency virus, hepatitis B and C
Systemic disease	Systemic lupus erythematosus, IgA vasculitis
Primary GN	IgA nephropathy, C3 glomerulopathy, immune complex membranoproliferative glomerulonephritis, membranous nephropathy
Pauci-immune crescentic glomerulonephritis	
Systemic vasculitis	• Microscopic polyangiitis (MPA) • Granulomatosis with polyangiitis (GPA) • Eosinophilic granulomatosis with polyangiitis (EGPA)
Idiopathic/renal limited vasculitis	ANCA-negative vasculitis
Medications	Penicillamine, hydralazine, propylthiouracil
Anti-GBM crescentic glomerulonephritis	
Goodpasture syndrome	Anti-GBM with pulmonary hemorrhage
Anti-GBM GN	

(ANCA: antineutrophil cytoplasmic antibody; GBM: glomerular basement membrane; GN: glomerulonephritis; IgA: immunoglobulin A)

CLINICAL FEATURES

Rapidly progressive glomerulonephritis usually presents like acute nephritic syndrome with gross hematuria, oliguria or anuria, edema, and hypertension. The onset can be insidious with initial nonspecific symptoms such as fatigue, anorexia, and edema. Renal insufficiency is usually present at the time of presentation. Sometimes, they may have a catastrophic presentation with hypertensive emergency, left ventricular failure, and uremia. Presence of systemic symptoms such as prolonged fever, arthralgia, arthritis, malar rash, oral ulcers, and seizures will indicate an underlying systemic illness like systemic lupus erythematosus (SLE). Presence of respiratory tract involvement such as hemoptysis, epistaxis, and chronic sinusitis will suggest underlying ANCA-associated vasculitis. Pulmonary hemorrhage can also be a manifestation of anti-GBM disease, SLE, and IgA vasculitis.[7-9]

Hemolytic uremic syndrome (HUS) is an important differential in the diagnosis of RPGN as it presents as RPRF with hematuria, oliguria, and hypertension. It may sometimes coexist with many primary GN like C_3 glomerulopathy and lupus nephritis. Presence of microangiopathic hemolytic anemia (MAHA) and thrombocytopenia points to the diagnosis of HUS. Acute tubulointerstitial nephritis can also manifest as RPRF and can be differentiated by nonoliguric renal failure and history of intake of nephrotoxic medications.

INVESTIGATIONS

The investigations required are delineated in **Table 2**. The urinalysis typically reveals hematuria, dysmorphic red blood cells (RBCs), RBC cast, other casts, and a variable degree of proteinuria. Nephrotic range proteinuria is uncommon. Leukocyturia is common. Presence of eosinophil in urine will suggest interstitial nephritis. Anemia and thrombocytopenia should raise the suspicion for HUS or SLE. Presence of schistocytes, reticulocytosis, and elevated lactate dehydrogenase (LDH) will suggest presence of MAHA. Direct Coombs Test (DCT) is negative in HUS but will be positive in SLE. Renal insufficiency is invariably present and is usually severe.[7]

Complement Analysis

A level of C_3 and C_4 in blood gives an important clue to underlying etiology. Complements are normal in anti-GBM disease and pauci-immune GN but could be normal in immune complex diseases such as IgA nephropathy, IgA vasculitis, or membranous nephropathy. Low C_3 along with normal C_4 suggests alternate complement pathway activation in PIGN or C_3 glomerulopathy. Both low C_3 and C_4 suggest classical complement pathway activation in lupus nephritis, immune complex MPGN, cryoglobulinemic vasculitis, and some IRGN. C_3 may be normal in 10% cases of PIGN and C_3 GN.[8,9]

TABLE 2: Diagnostic evaluation of children with rapidly progressive glomerulonephritis.

Hematology	Complete blood count, peripheral smear, reticulocyte count, DCT
Renal function tests	serum creatinine, urea, sodium, potassium, calcium, phosphorous
Infection workup	Hepatitis B antibody, anti-HCV antibody, antistreptolysin O titer, blood cultures
Immunology	*Complement levels:* C3, C4 • ANA, dsDNA • cANCA, pANCA
Imaging	Renal ultrasound
Renal biopsy	LM, IF, EM
Special investigations	• Anti-GBM IgG antibodies • Hepatitis serology • Blood cryoglobulin levels • X-ray chest, CT chest and sinuses

(ANA: antinuclear antibody; c-ANCA: cytoplasmic antineutrophil cytoplasmic antibody; DCT: direct Coombs test; dsDNA: double-stranded DNA; EM: electron microscopy; HCV: hepatitis C virus; IF: immunofluorescence; LM: light microscopy; p-ANCA: perinuclear antineutrophil cytoplasmic antibody)

Serology

Positive antistreptolysin O (ASO) titer and anti-deoxyribonuclease B suggest poststreptococcal glomerulonephritis (PSGN). Patients with SLE show antinuclear antibody (ANA) and anti-double-stranded DNA (dsDNA) autoantibodies. Elevated levels of ANCA suggest an underlying pauci-immune vasculitis. Most ANCA have specificity for myeloperoxidase (MPO) or proteinase 3 (PR3). ANCA should be screened by indirect IF and positive tests confirmed by both PR3-ELISA and MPO-ELISA. GPA is usually associated with PR3 ANCA, which produces a cytoplasmic staining pattern on indirect IF (c-ANCA). Microscopic polyangiitis and drug-induced ANCA have MPO ANCA that shows perinuclear staining on indirect IF (p-ANCA). Approximately 10% of patients with pauci-immune crescentic GN have negative assays for ANCA.[11,12]

High titer of anti-GBM immunoglobulin G (IgG) antibody, demonstrated by IF or ELISA, is seen in anti-GBM nephritis or Goodpasture's syndrome which correlates with disease activity. About 5% of ANCA-positive samples are also anti-GBM positive and approximately 20–30% of anti-GBM-positive samples are ANCA positive. Serology for ANCA is therefore recommended in all patients with either anti-GBM antibodies in blood or linear IgG deposition along the GBM. The initial clinical outcome for these patients is similar to that of anti-GBM disease, although relapses may occur as in systemic vasculitis.[2,5,11]

Renal Histology

The hallmark light microscopic feature of crescentic GN is presence of crescents. Crescents are defined as the presence of two or more layers of proliferating parietal epithelial cells that are filling totally (circumferential) or partially (circumscribed) Bowman's space.[2,3,13] When more than half of glomeruli are affected, it is called crescentic glomerulonephritis. When the crescent is made of proliferating cells, then it is called cellular crescent (**Fig. 1**). Fibrocellular crescent is made of both proliferating cells and fibrosis. A crescent is called fibrous when it has very few cells and mostly has fibrosis. Fibrous crescents suggest chronic injury and is less amenable to treatment.[11,13] Three categories of crescentic GN can be differentiated by proportion of glomeruli involved, aging of crescent, severity of glomerular inflammation, presence of periglomerular inflammation, cellularity in unaffected glomeruli and glomerular tuft, involvement of vessels, IF, and electron microscopic picture (**Table 3**).

Since anti-GBM disease is a single hit disease, all glomeruli show similar aging of crescent, and 85–100% of glomeruli may be involved. Glomerular tuft of affected glomeruli is unremarkable and IF shows linear IgG deposits. Pauci-immune necrotizing glomerulonephritis is characteristic of ANCA disease. Tubulointerstitial nephritis and necrotizing arteritis are common. Periglomerular inflammation with granuloma is more commonly seen in ANCA disease but can be seen in any severe crescentic GN; however, interstitial granuloma is typically found in GPA.[12,13]

In patients enrolled in European Vasculitis Study Group (EUVAS) trials, renal outcomes appeared to depend on the severity of the glomerular lesions and the degree of glomerular sclerosis on renal histology, with the best outcome in those who had predominant focal necrotizing lesions and the worst in those with mainly sclerotic lesions. This formed the basis of a new histological classification system.[13,14]

Immune complex crescentic GN shows varying degrees of glomerular involvement with crescents in different stages of aging. There will be mesangial and endocapillary proliferation involving unaffected glomeruli and glomerular tuft of affected glomeruli. IF shows granular immunoglobulin and complement deposits and electron microscopy shows extensive electron-dense deposits **(Figs. 2A to C)**.[13] The diagnostic algorithm of crescentic GN is depicted in **Flowchart 1**.

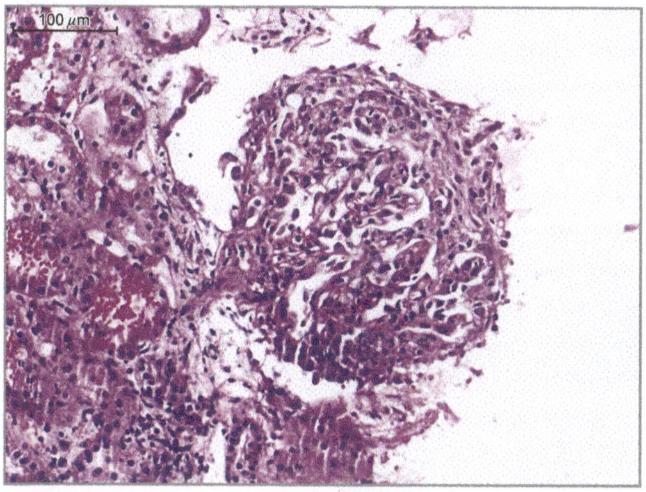

Fig. 1: A 9-year-old boy with rapidly progressive glomerulonephritis (RPGN). *Renal histology*—Light microscopy with periodic acid–Schiff (PAS) stain in high resolution showing single glomerulus with diffuse endocapillary and mesangial hypercellularity and cellular crescent. *Courtesy:* Dr Alok Sharma, Lal PathLabs

TREATMENT

Rapidly progressive glomerulonephritis is a medical emergency which can be life-threatening or can progress rapidly to ESKD if treatment is delayed. A high degree of clinical suspicion followed by serological evaluation and renal histology forms the basis of diagnosis. As the biopsy results may be delayed, the treatment decision is usually taken pending the renal histology. A clinical diagnosis of RPGN should prompt important serological investigations as discussed above for proper etiological diagnosis and management. The treatment aims to achieve remission with induction immunosuppression and maintain remission preventing relapses with the maintenance immunosuppression.

Induction Immunosuppression

Irrespective of the etiology of crescentic GN, the treatment regimen followed for induction immunosuppression almost remains the same. The treatment regimen discussed here will be the one for ANCA-associated vasculitis.

Intravenous pulse methylprednisolone is widely used as an induction agent and is administered as soon as a clinical diagnosis of RPGN is made. However, it has never been tested in a randomized controlled trial (RCT). The dose and duration

TABLE 3: Pathologic features of crescentic glomerulonephritis.

	Immune complex GN	*Pauci-immune GN*	*Anti-GBM*
Glomeruli			
Crescents >50%	25%	50%	85–100%
Aging of crescents	Pleomorphic	Pleomorphic	Monomorphic
Necrotizing lesion	+	+++	++
Rupture of GBM/Bowman's capsule	±	++	++
Periglomerular granuloma	–	++	++
Endocapillary and mesangial proliferation	+++	–	–
Double contour BM	++	–	–
Tubulointerstitium			
Interstitial granuloma	–	++	±
Interstitial inflammation	Lymphocytic + PMN	Lymphoplasmacytic	Lymphoplasmacytic + PMN
Arteritis	±	++	–
IF	Granular IgG ± C3	Scant/-	Linear IgG
EM	Extensive electron dense deposits in subendothelial, mesangial, subepithelial	–	–

(BM: basement membrane; EM: electron microscopy; GBM: glomerular basement membrane; GN: glomerulonephritis; IF: immunofluorescence; IgG: immunoglobulin G; PMN: polymorphonuclear neutrophil)

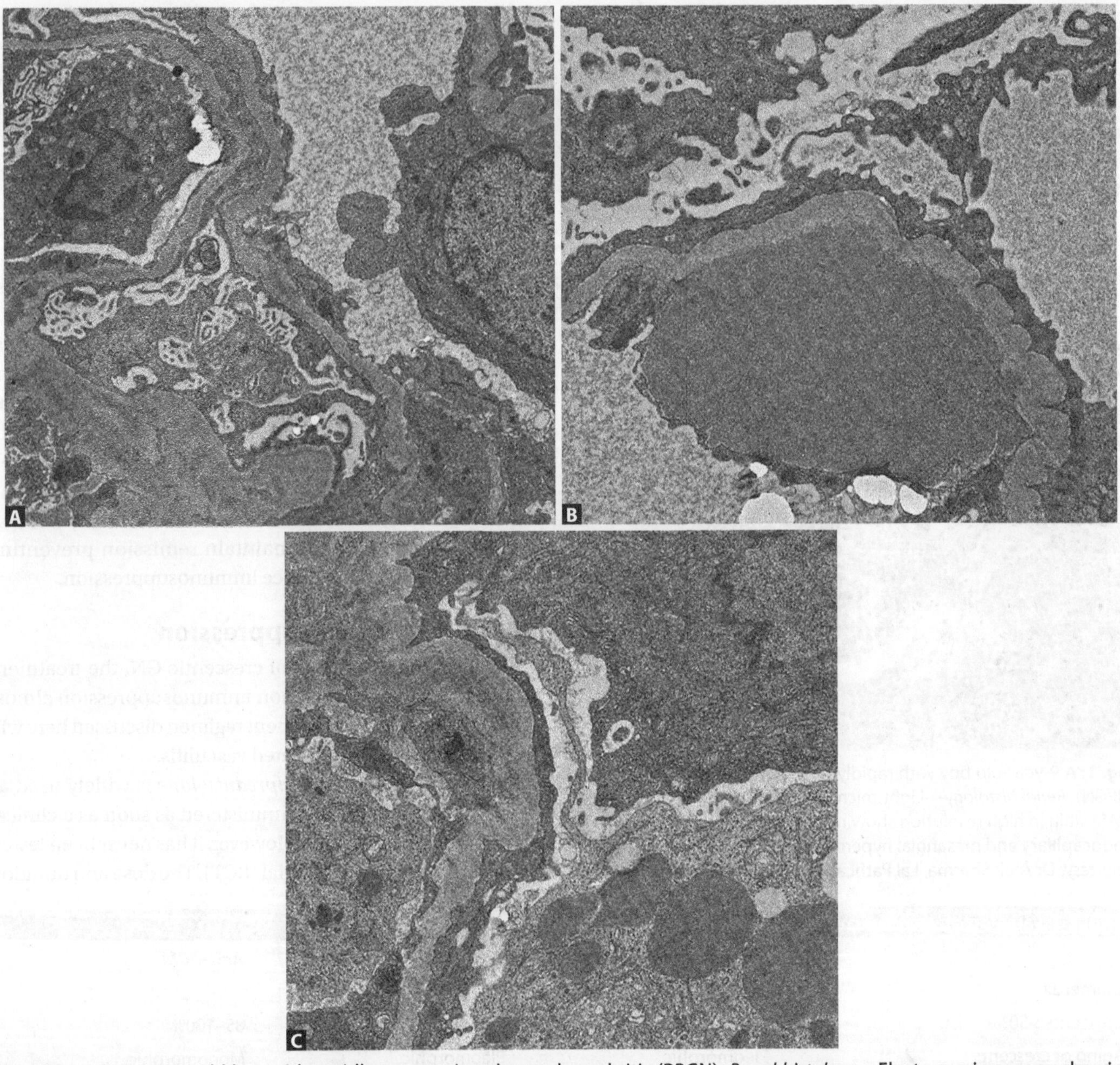

Figs. 2A to C: A 9-year-old boy with rapidly progressive glomerulonephritis (RPGN). *Renal histology*—Electron microscopy showing subendothelial and mesangial electron dense deposits. Subendothelial rarefaction and accumulation of granular deposits in few glomerular capillaries.
Courtesy: Dr Alok Sharma, Lal PathLabs.

also vary and range from 10 to 30 mg/kg (max adult dose of 1–3 g) for 3–5 days. This is followed by oral prednisolone 1 mg/kg which is tapered over months. In the most recent PEXIVAS trial, a more rapid reduction of steroid was found to be as effective but safer as a "standard" corticosteroid tapering regimen.[15] In the RAVE trial, the rituximab group had a lower corticosteroid exposure, and observational studies have supported early corticosteroid removal when rituximab is used.[16] A dose of 5 mg can be reached by 6 months and is continued for 18–24 months when cyclophosphamide is used along with corticosteroid to induce remission. Steroid can be withdrawn by 6 months if rituximab is used for induction immunosuppression.[15,16]

The best evidence for induction in ANCA-associated crescentic GN is for intravenous *cyclophosphamide*. The dose used in the CYCLOPS trial is 15 mg/kg every 2 weeks for three doses initially followed by every 3 weekly for three more doses.[14] Another three doses may be considered if required. Alternately a monthly pulse of 500–750 mg/m^2 for six doses as in the modified National Institute of Health (NIH) regimen can be used as in class 4 lupus nephritis.[17] The dose of cyclophosphamide for IgA nephropathy and C_3 glomerulopathy is similar to ANCA vasculitis.[17,18] Intravenous pulse and oral cyclophosphamide have shown similar outcome.[19] However, the cumulative dosage of cyclophosphamide is lower with intravenous cyclophosphamide with lesser incidence of leukopenia and is hence preferred in crescentic GN.[19]

Flowchart 1: Diagnostic algorithm of crescentic glomerulonephritis (GN).[12]

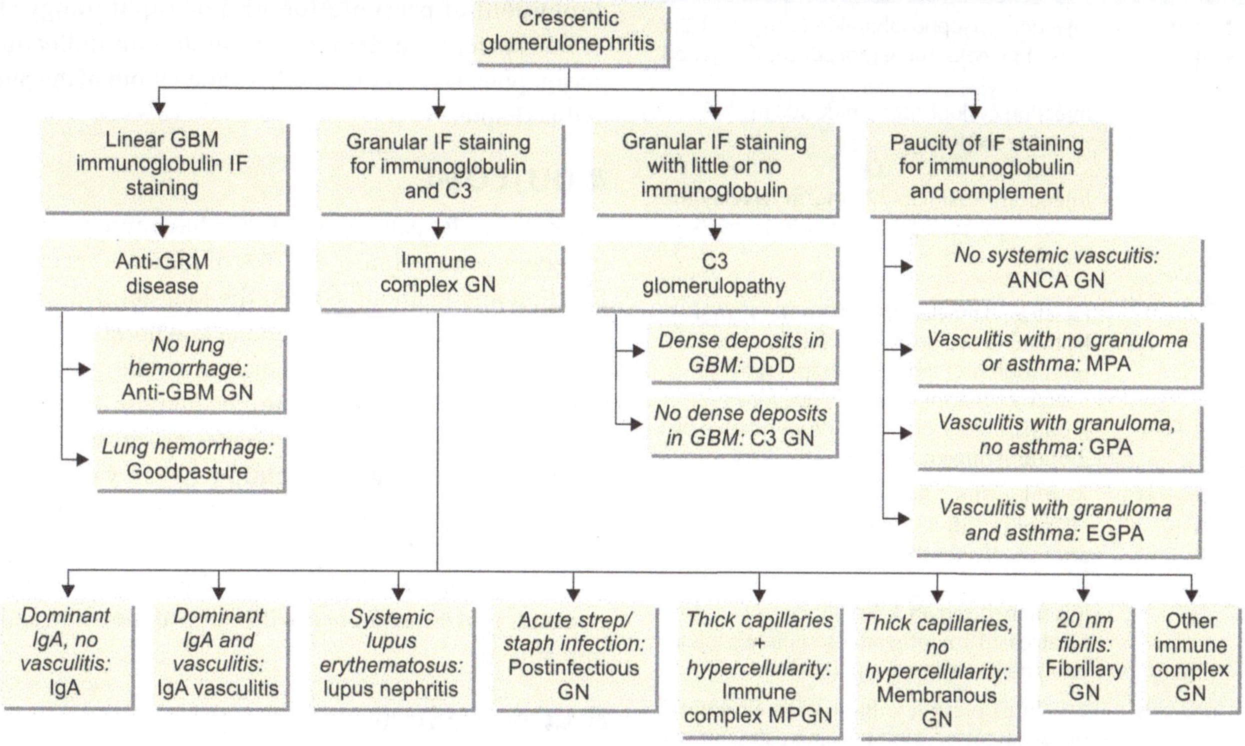

(ANCA: antineutrophil cytoplasmic antibody; DDD: dense deposit disease; EGPA: eosinophilic granulomatous polyangiitis; GBM: glomerular basement membrane; GN: glomerulonephritis; GPA: granulomatous polyangiitis; IF: immunofluorescence; MPA: microscopic polyangiitis; MPGN: membranoproliferative glomerulonephritis)

Source: Modified from Jennette JC, Thomas DB. Crescentic glomerulonephritis. Nephrol Dial Transplant. 2001;16(Suppl 6):80-2.

Rituximab has been shown equally effective when compared to cyclophosphamide in inducing remission in two RCTs. The RITUXVAS study included patients with severe renal failure (serum creatinine > 4 mg/dL). Rituximab combined with two pulses of cyclophosphamide plus glucocorticoids was comparable to steroid and cyclophosphamide for remission induction. The number of adverse events was also comparable.[20] Rituximab was used at a dose of 375 mg/m^2/wk, four doses along with two doses of cyclophosphamide 15 mg/kg at 0 and 2 weeks.[20] It, however, has failed to improve outcome at 1 year when used as an induction agent in lupus nephritis.[21]

Achieving remission should be the target of the induction regimen as it provides the best outcome in patient and renal survival. Remission is defined as absence of activity of vasculitis in ANCA disease and absence of proteinuria and renal dysfunction.[17] Immunosuppression should be stopped after 3 months if the patient remains dialysis dependent.[17]

Maintenance Immunosuppression

The aim of maintenance immunosuppression is to prevent relapses. As per the Kidney Disease Improving Global Outcomes (KDIGO) controversy conference and new unpublished KDIGO guideline for GN, following cyclophosphamide induction, either azathioprine plus low-dose glucocorticoids or rituximab without glucocorticoids should be used to prevent relapse.[22] Following rituximab induction, maintenance immunosuppressive therapy should be given to most patients. The European League Against Rheumatism (EULAR)/European Dialysis and Transplant Association (EDTA) prefers azathioprine and glucocorticoids over rituximab for remission maintenance.[23] Rituximab maintenance after cyclophosphamide induction has been shown to be superior to azathioprine for preventing relapses in one RCT. It probably decreases major relapses; no difference in adverse events was reported (MAINRITSAN).[24]

Azathioprine maintenance up to 18 months after induction of remission with cyclophosphamide has been shown to be equally effective as continuing cyclophosphamide (CYCAZAREM) for 1 year and then switching to azathioprine.[25,26] Mycophenolate mofetil (MMF) has not been shown to be more effective than azathioprine.[27] Rituximab when used as maintenance is used at a fixed interval or guidance based on CD19 level. The duration of maintenance is a minimum of 2 years as per EULAR/EDTA. A fixed duration of maintenance treatment is not advocated by KDIGO but suggest continued immunosuppression for 18 months to 4 years following induction of remission, tailored according to an individual's risk of relapse and the drug used for maintenance.

Mycophenolate mofetil is used for maintenance in class 4 lupus nephritis and c3 glomerulopathy.[17,18] Treatment regimen is similar to ANCA disease in IgA nephropathy.[17] The overall

TABLE 4: Treatment of crescentic glomerulonephritis.[22]	
Induction of remission	• Injection cyclophosphamide 15 mg/kg 0, 2, 4, 7, 10, 13 weeks. Three more doses if required Or Injection cyclophosphamide 500 mg/m² monthly six doses Or • Injection rituximab 375 mg/m² weekly four doses + Inj cyclophosphamide 15 mg/kg 0, 2 weeks And • Injection methylprednisolone 10–30 mg/kg three to five doses followed by oral prednisolone 1 mg/kg and rapid taper to 5 mg by 6 months and continue for 18–24 months. Prednisolone can be withdrawn by 6 months if rituximab is used as induction
Maintenance of remission	• Azathioprine 1.5–2 mg/kg/day for at least 18 months after complete remission. Taper after 24–48 months Or • Injection rituximab 375 mg/m² every 6 months for at least 18 months after complete remission or on demand based on CD19 levels
Plasmapheresis	• 1.5 times plasma volume with albumin as replacement for at least seven treatments over 14 days for ANCA disease • Daily with albumin or fresh frozen plasma as replacement till bleeding stops in pulmonary hemorrhage • Daily for 14 days or till anti-GBM antibody is undetectable in anti-GBM disease
Supportive treatment	SMX-TMP prophylaxis during induction for 6 months

(ANCA: antineutrophilic cytoplasmic antibody; GBM: glomerular basement membrane; SMX-TMP: sulfamethoxazole trimethoprim)

treatment of crescentic glomerulonephritis is presented in **Table 4.**

Plasmapheresis

The recent PEXIVAS trial in adults failed to demonstrate benefit in reducing death or delaying ESKD in ANCA disease over a median follow-up of 2.9 years.[15] However, it excluded children less than 15 years. Earlier, the MEPEX trial showed improved kidney outcome after plasma exchange.[28] Hence, plasma exchange can be considered for severe disease where RPGN coexists with pulmonary hemorrhage and hypoxemia or overlap syndrome of ANCA disease and anti-GBM.[22,23]

TREATMENT OF ANTIGLOMERULAR BASEMENT MEMBRANE DISEASE

Early diagnosis and initiation of treatment are the prime determinants of response to therapy and long-term prognosis in children with anti-GBM disease. Plasmapheresis and induction immunosuppression with pulse methylprednisolone and cyclophosphamide are recommended. Treatment, however, should not be initiated when the patient is dialysis dependent at presentation and histopathology shows 100% crescent.[17] A detailed discussion on indications of plasmapheresis and treatment regimen is out of the purview of this chapter.

OUTCOME

The outcome for patients with RPGN has improved drastically in recent years. Almost 60–70% of patients recover renal function and maintain GFR in the long-term. Severe renal failure at presentation, fibrocellular and fibrous crescents on histology, and dependence on dialysis are the most important predictors of poor outcome. The outcome also depends on the underlying etiology. PIGN has better prognosis and usually recovers without any intervention. ANCA vasculitis, anti-GBM disease, lupus nephritis, and dense deposit disease are associated with less favorable outcome. Fibrous crescents, glomerulosclerosis, and interstitial fibrosis on biopsy are portenders of nonresponse to immunosuppression and poor outcome.

CONCLUSION

Rapidly progressive glomerulonephritis is characterized clinically with features of severe glomerulonephritis and morphologically by crescentic glomerulonephritis. There is progression to end-stage kidney disease in untreated patients within a period of weeks to months. Early diagnosis with kidney biopsy, serologic testing, and early initiation of appropriate therapy are essential to minimize the degree of irreversible kidney injury. Empiric therapy may be started in severe disease and more specific therapy can be given once the diagnosis is established.

KEY POINTS

- RPGN is a heterogeneous group of clinical syndromes that lead to rapid loss of kidney function over a short period of time (days, weeks, or a few months).
- It is the most severe manifestation of "nephritic" spectrum of glomerulonephritis and is characterized morphologically by extensive crescent formation.
- Diseases leading to crescentic GN can be categorized into three broad categories: anti-(1) GBM disease, (2) immune complex crescentic GN, and (3) pauci-immune crescentic glomerulonephritis.
- RPGN presents usually with RPRF. Extrarenal manifestations give a clue to the underlying etiology.
- An accurate early diagnosis with kidney biopsy and serologic testing is crucial in initiating early treatment.
- Early initiation of appropriate therapy is essential to minimize the degree of irreversible kidney injury.
- Empiric initial therapy consists of intravenous pulse methylprednisolone and cyclophosphamide.

- Plasmapheresis is considered in severe renal and extrarenal involvement, especially pulmonary involvement with hemoptysis.
- KDIGO guideline recommends maintenance immunosuppression with either azathioprine plus low-dose glucocorticoids or rituximab without glucocorticoids to prevent relapse.
- With early therapy, almost 60–70% of patients recover renal function and maintain GFR in the long-term.
- Severe renal failure at presentation, fibrocellular and fibrous crescents on histology, and dependence on dialysis are the most important predictors of poor outcome.

ACKNOWLEDGMENT

We acknowledge and sincerely thank Dr Alok Sharma, Consultant Pathology at Lal PathLabs, for the biopsy images.

REFERENCES

1. Bhowmik D, Sinha S, Gupta A, Tiwari SC, Agarwal SK. Clinical approach to rapidly progressive renal failure. J Assoc Physicians India. 2011;59:38-41.
2. Jennette JC. Rapidly progressive crescentic glomerulonephritis. Kidney Int. 2003;63(3):1164-77.
3. Saha MK, Pendergraft WF III, Jennet JC, Falk RJ. Primary glomerular disease. In: Yu Alan SL, Chertow GM, Luyckx VA, Marsden PA, Skorecki K, Taal MW (Eds.). Brenner and Rector's The Kidney, 11th edition. Philadelphia, PA: Elsevier; 2020. pp. 1007-92.
4. McAdoo SP, Tanna A, Hrušková Z, Holm L, Weiner M, Arulkumaran N, et al. Patients double-seropositive for ANCA and anti-GBM antibodies have varied renal survival, frequency of relapse, and outcomes compared to single-seropositive patients. Kidney Int. 2017;92(3):693.
5. Eisenberger U, Fakhouri F, Vanhille P, Beaufils H, Mahr A, Guillevin L, et al. ANCA-negative pauci-immune renal vasculitis: histology and outcome. Nephrol Dial Transplant. 2005;20(7):1392-9.
6. Kashtan CE. Renal transplantation in patients with Alport syndrome. Pediatr Transplant. 2006;10(6):651-7.
7. Southwest Pediatric Nephrology Study Group: A clinicopathologic study of crescentic glomerulonephritis in 50 children. Kidney Int. 1985;27(2):450-58.
8. Srivastava RN, Moudgil A, Bagga A, Vasudev AS, Bhuyan UN, Sundraem KR. Crescentic glomerulonephritis in children: a review of 43 cases. Am J Nephrol. 1992;12(3):155-61.
9. Jardim HM, Leake J, Risdon RA, Barratt TM, Dillon MJ. Crescentic glomerulonephritis in children. Pediatr Nephrol. 1992;6(3):231-5.
10. Niaudet P, Levy M. Glomerulonephritis a croissants diffuse. In: Royer P, Habib R, Mathieu H, Broyer M (Eds.). Nephrologie Pediatrique, 3rd edition. Paris: Flammarion; 1983. pp. 381-94.
11. Sinha A, Puri K, Hari P, Dinda AK, Bagga A. Etiology and outcome of crescentic glomerulonephritis. Indian Pediatr. 2013;50(3):283-8.
12. Jennette JC, Thomas DB. Crescentic glomerulonephritis. Nephrol Dial Transplant. 2001;16(Suppl 6):80-2.
13. Berden AE, Ferrario F, Hagen EC, Jayne DR, Jennette JC, Joh K, et al. Histopathologic classification of ANCA-associated glomerulonephritis. J Am Soc Nephrol. 2010;21(10):1628-36.
14. de Groot K, Harper L, Jayne DR, Flores Suarez LF, Gregorini G, Gross WL, et al; EUVAS (European Vasculitis Study Group). Pulse versus daily oral cyclophosphamide for induction of remission in antineutrophil cytoplasmic antibody-associated vasculitis: a randomized trial. Ann Intern Med. 2009;150(10):670-80.
15. Walsh M, Merkel PA, Peh CA, Szpirt WM, Puéchal X, Fujimoto S, et al.; PEXIVAS Investigators. Plasma exchange and glucocorticoids in severe ANCA-associated vasculitis. N Engl J Med. 2020;382(7):622-31.
16. Stone JH, Merkel PA, Spiera R, Seo P, Langford CA, Hoffman GS, et al; RAVE-ITN Research Group. Rituximab versus cyclophosphamide for ANCA-associated vasculitis. N Engl J Med. 2010;363(3):221-32.
17. KDIGO clinical practice guideline for glomerulonephritis. Kidney Int Supplements. 2012;2:140.
18. Goodship TH, Cook HT, Fakhouri F, Fervenza FC, Frémeaux-Bacchi V, Kavanagh D, et al; Conference Participants. Atypical hemolytic uremic syndrome and C3 glomerulopathy: conclusions from a "Kidney Disease: Improving Global Outcomes" (KDIGO) Controversies Conference. Kidney Int. 2017;91(3):539-51.
19. Walters GD, Willis NS, Cooper TE, Craig JC. Interventions for renal vasculitis in adults. Cochrane Database Syst Rev. 2020;1(1):CD003232.
20. Jones RB, Tervaert JW, Hauser T, Luqmani R, Morgan MD, Peh CA, et al; European Vasculitis Study Group. Rituximab versus cyclophosphamide in ANCA-associated renal vasculitis. N Engl J Med. 2010;363(3):211-20.
21. Rovin BH, Furie R, Latinis K, Looney RJ, Fervenza FC, Sanchez-Guerrero J, et al; LUNAR Investigator Group. Efficacy and safety of rituximab in patients with active proliferative lupus nephritis: the Lupus Nephritis Assessment with Rituximab study. Arthritis Rheum. 2012;64(4):1215-26.
22. Rovin BH, Adler SG, Barratt J, Bridoux F, Burdge KA, et al. Executive summary of the KDIGO 2021 Guideline for the Management of Glomerular Diseases. Kidney Int. 2021;100(4): 753-79.
23. Yates M, Watts RA, Bajema IM, Cid MC, Crestani B, Hauser T, et al. EULAR/ERA-EDTA recommendations for the management of ANCA-associated vasculitis. Ann Rheum Dis. 2016;75(9):1583-94. Erratum in: Ann Rheum Dis. 2017;76(8):1480.
24. Guillevin L, Pagnoux C, Karras A, Khouatra C, Aumaître O, Cohen P, et al; French Vasculitis Study Group. Rituximab versus azathioprine for maintenance in ANCA-associated vasculitis. N Engl J Med. 2014;371(19):1771-80.
25. Walsh M, Faurschou M, Berden A, Flossmann O, Bajema I, Hoglund P, et al. Long-term follow-up of cyclophosphamide compared with azathioprine for initial maintenance therapy in ANCA-associated vasculitis. Clin J Am Soc Nephrol. 2014;9(9):1571-6.
26. Sanders JS, de Joode AA, DeSevaux RG, Broekroelofs J, Voskuyl AE, van Paassen P, et al. Extended versus standard azathioprine maintenance therapy in newly diagnosed proteinase-3 anti-neutrophil cytoplasmic antibody-associated vasculitis patients who remain cytoplasmic anti-neutrophil cytoplasmic antibody-positive after induction of remission: a randomized clinical trial. Nephrol Dial Transplant. 2016;31:1453-9.
27. Hiemstra TF, Walsh M, Mahr A, Savage CO, de Groot K, Harper L, et al; European Vasculitis Study Group (EUVAS). Mycophenolate mofetil vs azathioprine for remission maintenance in antineutrophil cytoplasmic antibody-associated vasculitis: a randomized controlled trial. JAMA. 2010;304(21):2381-8.
28. Jayne DR, Gaskin G, Rasmussen N, Abramowicz D, Ferrario F, Guillevin L, et al; European Vasculitis Study Group. Randomized trial of plasma exchange or high-dosage methylprednisolone as adjunctive therapy for severe renal vasculitis. J Am Soc Nephrol. 2007;18(7):2180-8.

CHAPTER

6.11 Hemolytic Uremic Syndrome

Priyanka Khandelwal, Geetika Singh, Arvind Bagga

INTRODUCTION

Hemolytic uremic syndrome (HUS) is clinically defined by the triad of microangiopathic hemolytic anemia, thrombocytopenia, and acute kidney injury (AKI). HUS is a type of thrombotic microangiopathy (TMA), a histopathological vasculopathy that chiefly affects the kidney in HUS and includes the presence of platelet and fibrin thrombi in capillaries and arterioles, and endothelial swelling and detachment. Although HUS is a rare disorder (incidence 0.7–8 cases per 100,000 population), it is an important cause of severe AKI in children.[1-4]

ETIOLOGY AND CLASSIFICATION

Thrombotic microangiopathy chiefly includes thrombotic thrombocytopenic purpura (TTP) and heterogeneous conditions causing HUS **(Box 1 and Flowchart 1)**. Worldwide, gastroenteritis caused by Shiga toxin-producing organisms, chiefly *Escherichia coli*-HUS (STEC-HUS) and *Shigella dysenteriae*, leads to majority of HUS (85–90%).[2] HUS can also follow invasive infection with *Streptococcus pneumoniae* (Sp-HUS) or influenza A/H1N1 and might mimic or be triggered by tropical infections such as dengue, malaria, and leptospirosis.[5] Recently, HUS has been reported to be triggered by severe acute respiratory syndrome coronavirus 2 infection. Cobalamin C (cblC) deficiency is a rare genetic form of HUS, with distinct clinical features and management.[2] Atypical HUS is less common (5–10%) and associated with uncontrolled activation of the alternate complement pathway due to genetic or acquired defects. Occasionally, HUS is associated with autoimmune disorders, e.g., systemic lupus erythematosus, malignant hypertension, medications, and malignancy or pregnancy.[6] TTP is a related disorder caused by severe congenital or acquired deficiency of von Willebrand protease, a metalloproteinase with thrombospondin motifs 13 (ADAMTS13).[7]

BOX 1: Classification of thrombotic microangiopathy.

Hemolytic uremic syndrome
- Infection-associated HUS
  - *Shiga toxin-associated HUS:* Shiga toxin-producing *Escherichia coli, Shigella dysenteriae* type 1
  - Invasive infection with neuraminidase-producing *Streptococcus pneumoniae*
  - *Other infections:* Influenza A, coronavirus-19, human immunodeficiency virus, leptospira, malaria, dengue and rickettsia, cytomegalovirus, Epstein–Barr virus, *Salmonella typhi, Campylobacter, Citrobacter*
- Secondary HUS
  - Systemic lupus erythematosus; antiphospholipid antibody syndrome
  - Hematopoietic stem cell or solid organ transplant
  - Malignancy
  - Malignant hypertension
  - *Drugs:* Quinine, mitomycin, ticlopidine, clopidogrel, calcineurin inhibitors, sirolimus, oral contraceptives, bevacizumab
- *Defective cobalamin metabolism:* Homozygous or compound heterozygous mutation in *MMACHC*

Atypical HUS
- Homozygous or heterozygous mutations in *CFH, CFI, CFB, C3, CD46, THBD*, or *DGKE*
- Autoantibodies to factor H
- Unexplained

Thrombotic thrombocytopenic purpura
- *Inherited:* Homozygous or compound heterozygous mutations in *ADAMTS13* (Upshaw–Schulman syndrome)
- *Acquired ADAMTS13 deficiency:* Inhibitory antibodies to ADAMTS13

(ADAMTS13: a metalloproteinase with thrombospondin motifs 13; *C3:* complement C3; *CD46:* membrane cofactor protein; *CFB*: factor B; *CFH*: complement factor H; *CFI*: factor I; *DGKE*: diacylglycerol kinase ε; HUS: hemolytic uremic syndrome; *MMACHC*: methylmalonic aciduria and homocystinuria type C; *THBD:* thrombomodulin)

INCIDENCE AND EPIDEMIOLOGY

Shiga Toxin-producing *E. coli* Hemolytic-uremic Syndrome

The most common infectious agent causing HUS, especially in children younger than 3–5 years, is STEC. Rarely, other Shiga toxin-producing bacteria *S. dysenteriae, S. flexneri, S. sonnei*, and *Citrobacter* might be isolated. Diarrhea or dysentery due to Shiga toxin-producing enteropathogens is followed by HUS in 5–15% cases, a proportion that can reach 20–30% during outbreaks.[2,8] The predominant STEC serotype causing HUS is O157:H7, responsible for ~2,000 cases of STEC-HUS worldwide annually.[8] While the non-O157 serogroups are a heterogeneous group with lesser risk of HUS (~1%), they are perhaps more commonly encountered in patients with

Flowchart 1: Thrombotic microangiopathy (TMA) syndromes in children comprise TTP and HUS. STEC-HUS and acquired deficiency of a metalloproteinase with thrombospondin motifs 13 (ADAMTS13) are the most common primary TMA syndromes in children and adults, respectively.

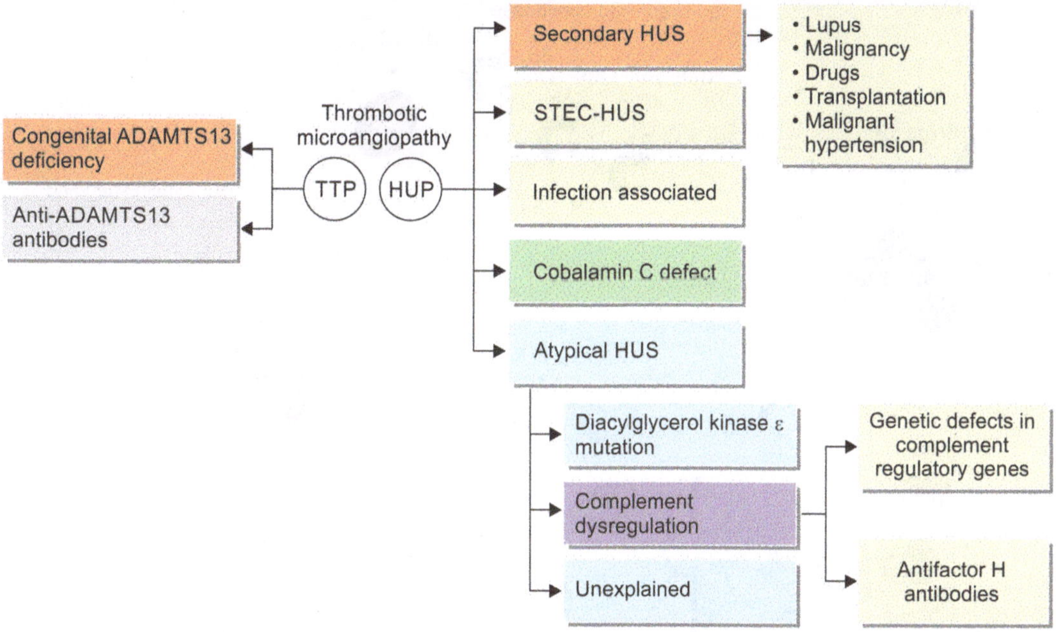

(HUS: hemolytic uremic syndrome; STEC-HUS: Shiga toxin-producing *E. coli* hemolytic-uremic syndrome; TTP: thrombocytopenic purpura)

diarrhea or dysentery.[8] STEC-HUS is mostly sporadic, the incidence being highest in children 3–5 years old, at 2–3 per 100,000 per year.[8] STEC colonize cattle, and transmission is feco-oral by contaminated meat, raw milk products, municipal drinking water, or vegetables. Among the epidemics caused by STEC, the 2011 German epidemic, caused by O104:H4 serotype, was unique due to several reasons: chiefly adults were affected, typical history of dysentery was lacking, HUS occurred in 20–22% with frequent neurological complications and high mortality, and an enteroaggregative *E. coli* (EAEC) that acquired a prophage-encoding *Stx2* was responsible.[9] The O80:H2 serotype is emerging in Europe that causes unusually severe HUS. HUS associated with *S. dysenteriae* has a higher morbidity and mortality rate than STEC-HUS. Epidemiological data of STEC-HUS in India are limited, and the current rates of transmission of *S. dysenteriae* are remarkably low.[10]

Atypical Hemolytic Uremic Syndrome

The estimated annual incidence of atypical hemolytic uremic syndrome (aHUS) is 2.3–4.2 cases per 100,000, of which children comprise 1–1.1 cases per 100,000. About 40–60% patients with aHUS have genetic or acquired dysregulation of the alternative complement pathway.[11] Genetic abnormalities associated with aHUS are rare with ~500 variants reported in more than 3,000 patients.[11,12] Not all patients with genetic defects develop aHUS, and other environmental triggers (viral infection, pregnancy, medications, cancer, etc.) may be required for the disease to manifest; ~30% of aHUS results from unknown mechanisms.[13] Anti-factor H (FH) antibodies-associated aHUS is a distinct disease and is responsible for 5–25% cases of aHUS in Caucasian patients and ~50% of pediatric patients in south Asia, chiefly affecting 5–15-year-old.[14] Data from the global aHUS registry from centers in Europe, North America, and Australia have shown that anti-FH antibodies were identified in 45% of children with aHUS aged 6–17 years.[15]

PATHOGENESIS

Shiga Toxin-producing *E. coli* Hemolytic-uremic Syndrome

The mechanism of cytotoxicity and complement activation by the Shiga toxins (Shiga toxins 1 and 2 encoded by *stx1* and *stx2* genes) is shown in **Figure 1**. Shiga toxins bind to its receptor, globotriaosylceramide (Gb3), on target cells and inhibit protein synthesis by disrupting ribosomal function. Internalization of toxins in the endothelial cells leads to stimulation of proapoptotic pathways, release of inflammatory cytokines, increased expression of adhesion molecules, and activation of the procoagulant pathway triggering endothelial dysfunction, fibrin deposition, thrombosis, and sequestration of red cells and platelets.[16,17] There is growing evidence of activation of the alternate complement system in patients with STEC-HUS. Levels of complement degradation products, soluble membrane attack complex (sMAC), and complement-coated microvesicles have been found to be elevated in patients with STEC-HUS.[18]

Atypical Hemolytic Uremic Syndrome

Complement dysregulation at the surface of endothelial cells is the main mechanism of aHUS that incites inflammation, prothrombotic state, and microvascular thrombosis, especially

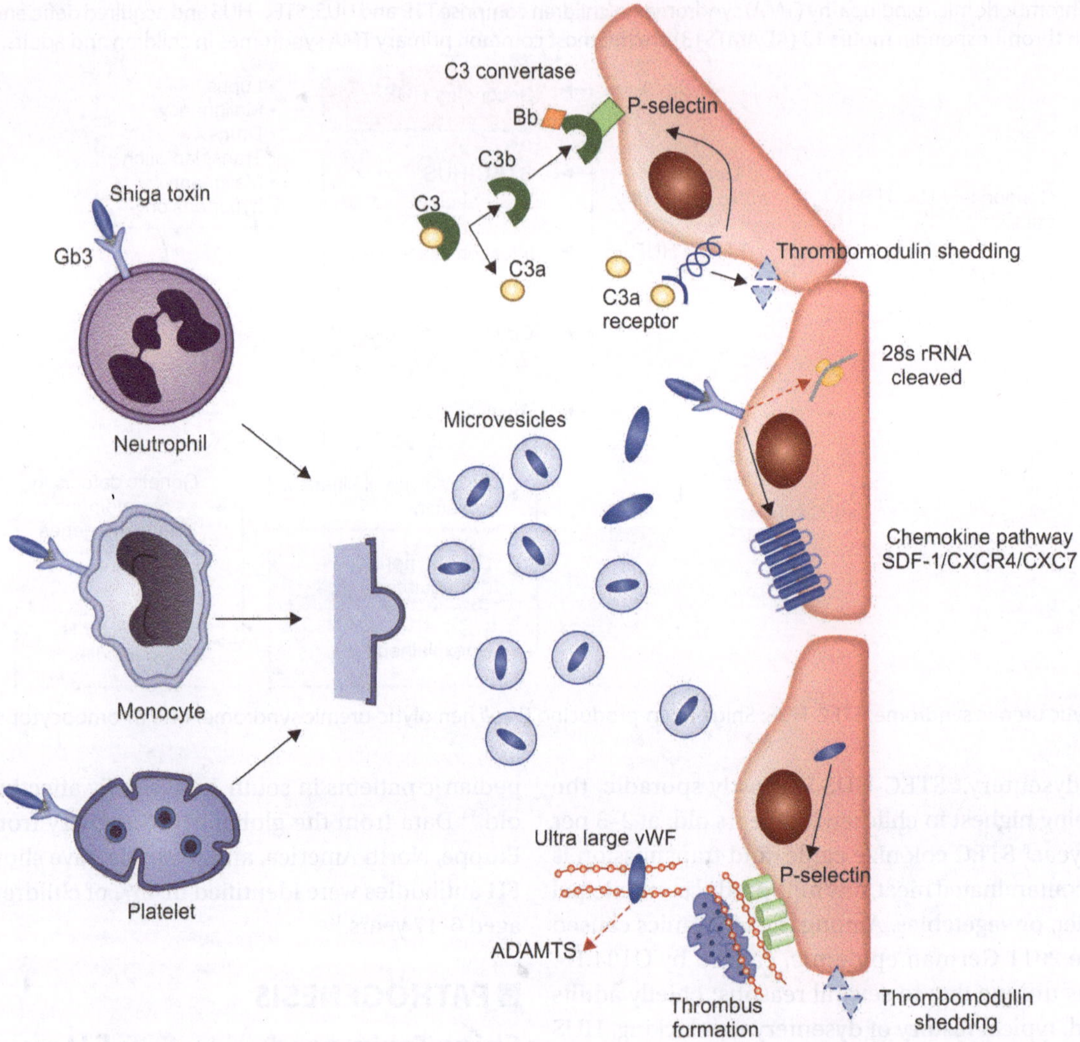

Fig. 1: Shiga toxin produced by bacterial infection of the colon binds the enterocytes and crosses the brush border to enter the circulation. The pentameric B subunit binds to globotriaosylceramide 3 (Gb3) and toll-like receptor 4 expressed on circulating blood cells. This causes activation of neutrophils, monocytes, platelets, and erythrocytes inducing budding of microvesicles containing the toxin within and on its surface. Microvesicles are endowed with activated complement factors C3b, C9, and tissue factor. The key pathogenic mechanism in STEC-HUS is targeting by Shiga toxin and/or Shiga toxin associated with microvesicles to Gb3 expressing endothelial cells, followed by docking and release of toxin by microvesicles. The A1 subunit of the toxin causes depurination of adenosine in a highly conserved region of the 28s ribosomal subunit of 60s ribosomal RNA that alters its binding to tRNA, interrupting the synthesis of proteins and leading to cell death. Other mechanisms of cytotoxicity include increased synthesis of chemokines (SDF-1/CXCR4/CXCR7 pathway) and adhesion molecules. Shiga toxin induces surface mobilization of P-selectin that favors C3 activation and assembly of alternative C3 convertase (C3bBb) on cell surface. The anaphylatoxin C3a interacts with its endothelial receptor (C3aR), potentiating P-selectin expression and thrombomodulin shedding with thrombus formation. Shiga toxin also binds ultralarge multimers of von Willebrand factor (vWF) and reduces their cleavage by ADAMTS13 which leads to further thrombosis.

involving the glomerular capillaries. Complement system is composed of three distinct pathways—classical, lectin, and alternative—which play an important role in innate immunity. The three pathways converge to form the C3 convertase that triggers the assembly of terminal complement complex or MAC (C5b-9) for lysis of target cells. The alternative pathway is continuously active by hydrolysis of C3 to generate C3b and has a self-amplifying loop that is triggered by complement deposition on cell surfaces. The amplification loop is strictly regulated at the surface of the endothelium by fluid phase (factors H and I) and membrane-bound (membrane cofactor protein, CD46) regulators.[19,20] **Figure 2** illustrates the key proteins that regulate activation of the alternate complement pathway.

Complement Genetics

Approximately 20–45% patients with aHUS show an inherited complement defect including loss of function of factor H (*CFH*), factor I (*CFI*), and *CD46* and gain-of-function variants in complement 3 (*C3*) and factor B (*CFB*) or rearrangements in FH-related proteins (*CFHR 1-5*).[11] Mutations in diacylglycerol kinase ε (*DGKE*), an intracellular protein with no direct role in the complement cascade, are described in 2–3%, chiefly those below 2 years of age. The pathogenic role of variants in thrombomodulin (*THBD*), a protein in the coagulation system, is debated.[11] Antibodies to FH prevent its binding to C3b, and decrease protection from complement-dependent cell lysis.[21] Genes encoding FH and FH-related proteins (CFHR1-5) are

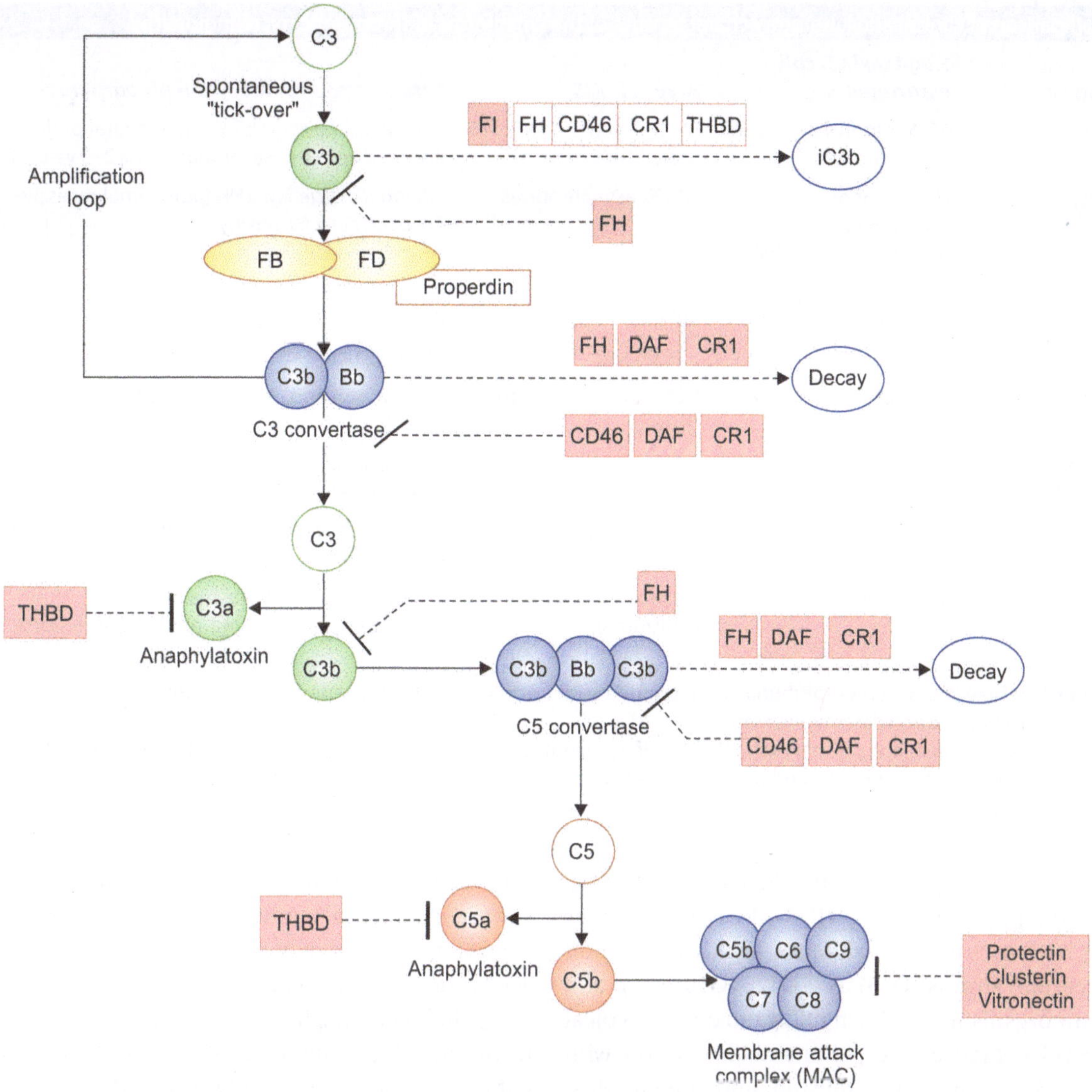

Fig. 2: Regulators of the alternative pathway of complement activation. Complement activation occurs in a sequential manner by initiation of complement activation, formation and amplification of C3 convertase (C3bBb), formation and amplification of C5 convertase (C3bBbC3b), and the assembly of the terminal complement complex or membrane attack complex (MAC; C5b-9). The self-amplifying process of the alternative pathway is inhibited by multiple regulator molecules. Factor H (FH) is a fluid-phase inhibitor of the C3 convertase. FH competes with factor B (FB) for binding to C3b and displaces Bb from the C3bBb convertase (decay-accelerating activity). It acts as a a cofactor for factor I (FI) in the cleavage of C3b to iC3b. Three membrane glycoproteins, C3b receptor (CR1, CD35), membrane cofactor protein (MCP, CD46), and decay accelerating factor (DAF, CD55), act as inhibitors of C3 and C5 convertases, whereas protectin (CD59) inhibits the assembly of MAC. CR1 and DAF have decay-accelerating activity toward C3 and C5 convertase. CR1 and MCP act as cofactors for CFI-mediated cleavage of C3b. Clusterin and vitronectin are plasma proteins that prevent the insertion of terminal complement complexes into cell membranes. The activity of the alternative pathway C3/C5 convertase, C3bBb, can be enhanced by the only known physiological positive complement regulator, properdin.

highly homologous and prone to nonallelic homologous recombination resulting in large deletions and hybrid genes such as *CFH/CFHR1*. Anti-FH-associated aHUS is strongly associated with a polymorphism resulting from such recombination: an 84-kb homozygous deletion of the *CFHR1* gene in 80–90% patients.[21] Variants in other genes encoding plasminogen (*PLG*), inverted formin-2 (*INF2*), vitronectin (*VTN*), and clusterin (*CLU*) have also been recently reported in aHUS.[22-24]

The genetic predisposition of aHUS is complex, and development of the disease is multifactorial requiring an environmental or infectious trigger. Inheritance of aHUS can be monogenic (autosomal recessive or dominant transmission) or rarely polygenic. Since penetrance is variable and most mutations are heterozygous, only 20% patients report a family history.

CLINICAL FEATURES

The distinguishing features of STEC-HUS, aHUS, and TTP are given in **Table 1**.

Shiga Toxin-producing *E. coli* Hemolytic-uremic Syndrome

Profuse, usually bloody, diarrhea (hemorrhagic colitis) occurs in ~90% patients about 3–7 days after ingestion of

TABLE 1: Comparison of clinical and laboratory characteristics of the chief forms of thrombotic microangiopathy.

Characteristic	*Shiga toxin E. coli-associated HUS*	*Atypical HUS*	*Thrombotic thrombocytopenic purpura*
Age at onset	65% 6 months–3 years; 5% <6 months	55% <2 years; 45% 2–15 years	*Inherited deficiency:* ≥75% in neonatal period *Acquired defect:* 62% >9 years; 16% 2–9 years; 22% <2 years
Family history	Uncommon; simultaneous occurrence if familial contamination	~15%; asynchronous	*Inherited deficiency:* 25% (autosomal recessive) *Acquired defect:* Unlikely
Diarrhea at onset	95% (bloody in >80%)	40%	Possible
Platelet count	>30,000/µL	>30,000/µL	<30,000/µL
Acute kidney injury	85%; 60% require dialysis	95%; 50–60% require dialysis	Uncommon and mild*; rarely require dialysis
Neurological symptoms	~20%	~20%	*Inherited deficiency:* ~35% *Acquired defect:* ~70%
Relapses	No	~45%	*Inherited deficiency:* ≥80% (without plasma infusions) *Acquired defect:* ~ 30% if treated
Therapy	Supportive care†	Plasma exchanges‡ Eculizumab§	*Inherited deficiency:* Plasma infusion *Acquired defect:* Plasma exchanges + corticosteroids ± rituximab

*Chiefly as transient hematuria, hemoglobinuria, or proteinuria with normal or slightly elevated serum creatinine
†Eculizumab if neurological or cardiac involvement
‡Complement blockade is first line; plasma exchange only if eculizumab is unavailable or autoantibody-associated disease
§Immunosuppression if anti-factor H (FH) antibody–mediated disease
(HUS: hemolytic uremic syndrome)

contaminated food. After a week, when diarrhea is resolving, ~5–15% infected patients develop HUS. The risk factors for developing HUS include age <5 years, high white blood cell count, certain strains (O157:H7; O126; O104:H4), and infection with organisms producing Shiga toxin 2.[25] Typical features of HUS include fatigue, pallor and oligoanuria, with or without fluid overload, hypertension, and edema. Most patients have mild disease managed with optimizing fluid balance, nutrition support, and control of hypertension. However, severe cases with anuria often require dialysis in 30–60% and show signs of extrarenal involvement. Cerebral involvement, the most important cause of mortality, manifests as irritability, altered consciousness, and seizures and is noted in 3–50% cases.[8,26] Other organs including myocardium, pancreas, and gastrointestinal tract may be involved.[26]

Atypical Hemolytic Uremic Syndrome

Atypical HUS is usually a rapidly progressive illness. The onset is insidious with hypertension, AKI, and without thrombocytopenia in 20%. While distinguished from STEC-HUS by absence of dysenteric prodrome, the disease is often triggered by febrile, respiratory, and even diarrheal infections. The chief renal manifestations are azotemia, proteinuria, hematuria, and stage 2 hypertension; 70–80% patients require dialysis. Nephrotic range proteinuria may occur, especially in patients with *DGKE* mutations. Low serum C3 with normal C4 levels indicates activation of the alternative complement. However, hypocomplementemia found in one-third of the patients does not correlate with disease severity. Extrarenal manifestations occur in 20–50% patients. Neurological involvement is common and includes altered sensorium, seizures, diplopia, cortical blindness, hemiparesis, or hemiplegia. Imaging shows bilateral symmetrical lesions in the basal ganglia, deep white matter, and brainstem. Other complications include myocarditis, cardiomyopathy, pancreatitis, hepatocellular injury, peripheral vascular disease, pulmonary hemorrhage, and ischemic colitis. aHUS has a chronic and relapsing course and risk of progressive kidney disease. Important features of patients with various forms of HUS are summarized in **Table 2**. Patients with pathogenic variants in *FH* and *FI* have worse outcome than those with *CD46* variants and anti-FH-associated aHUS; recurrence of disease in the allograft is found in 80–100% of the former.[15,27,28]

DIAGNOSIS

All the following are required for the diagnosis of HUS: (1) microangiopathic hemolytic anemia: hemoglobin <10 g/dL and fragmented red cells on peripheral smear (schistocytes ≥2%) with either increased lactate dehydrogenase (LDH) >450 IU/L or undetectable haptoglobin, (2) thrombocytopenia (platelets <150,000/µL), and (3) AKI (rise in creatinine by 50% over baseline).[29] Urine sediment may be normal or show red cells and variable degree of proteinuria. Coombs test is positive in *S. pneumonia*-associated HUS. Sepsis and disseminated intravascular coagulation (DIC) should be ruled

TABLE 2: Important causes of atypical hemolytic uremic syndrome.

Abnormal or deficient factor	*Function*	*% of aHUS**	*Minimum age*	*Low C3 (%)*	*ESKD† (%)*	*Relapses (%)*	*Post-transplant recurrence (%)*
Factor H	Binds C3b as cofactor for FI-mediated cleavage to inactive iC3b; prevents assembly of C3 convertase; decays accelerating activity for C3 and C5 convertase	20–30	<1 month	30–50	70–80	50	75–90
Membrane cofactor protein or CD46	Binds C3b and has cofactor activity for FI-mediated cleavage to inactive iC3b	5–15	>12 months	0–27	0–10	70–90	15–20
Factor I	Serine protease; requires a cofactor to cleave C3b	4–10	<1 month	20–30	50–80	10–30	60–80
C3	Central role in the complement cascade; substrate for C3 convertase; active form C3b is required for enzymatic complexes	2–10	>1 year	70–80	60	50	40–70
Factor B	Provides catalytic site for the C3 convertase	1–4	<12 months	100	50		100
Thrombomodulin	Accelerates CFI-mediated inactivation of C3b in presence of cofactors; helps inactivate C3a and C5a	3–5	1 month	50	50	30	NA
Diacylglycerol kinase ε	Not linked directly to the complement cascade; loss of function activates of protein kinase C and causes prothrombotic state	25–30% of <1 year	<12 months	20–30	15–20	60	None of 5
Anti-FH antibody	Binds to factor H to reduce its cell surface complement regulatory activity	6–56	5–15 years	40–60	30–40	20–30	Low

Note: All inheritance is autosomal dominant, except *DGKE* which is autosomal recessive
*No abnormality detected in ~40% cases
†Or death within one year from onset
(ESKD: end-stage kidney disease; FH: factor H; NA: not available)

out in patients with suspected HUS. Elevated D-dimer and neutrophilic leukocytosis are common in patients with severe STEC-HUS and shigellosis.[30] HUS and TTP might be difficult to differentiate clinically. TTP is rare in children but should be suspected in case of persistent severe thrombocytopenia (<30,000/μL) and mild/no AKI **(Table 1)**.[7]

Box 2 lists important investigations for diagnosis and etiological evaluation in patients of HUS. An approach to patients with HUS is shown in **Flowchart 2**. *STEC-HUS* is suspected in patients above 6 months of age if occurring within 2–3 weeks of bloody diarrhea and/or occurring during a known outbreak of STEC-HUS.[29] The diagnosis is confirmed by positive stool or rectal swab culture, combined with either detection of (1) virulence genes (*stx1*, *stx2*) on fecal extracts or cultures by polymerase chain reaction (PCR), (2) free fecal Shiga toxin by enzyme-linked immunoassay (ELISA), or (3) serum immunoglobulin M (IgM) antibodies to serogroup-specific lipopolysaccharide (by ELISA, passive hemagglutination assay). The most sensitive and specific analysis is PCR on stool cultures.[31] However, the ability to isolate the bacteria by culture declines after the first 7–10 days of illness and following antibiotic administration. In case of delayed presentation when culture is noncontributory, detection of serum IgM antibodies against specific *E. coli* lipopolysaccharide suggests recent infection.[32] *CblC deficiency* should be screened in all cases by estimating the total homocysteine level. The condition is suspected by the detection of elevated levels of total homocysteine (>50–100 μM/L by chromatography, immunoassay) with normal blood levels of vitamin B_{12} and folate.[33] Genetic sequencing shows homozygous or compound heterozygous mutation in *MMACHC*.[33] Plasma and urine methylmalonic acid levels are elevated. Screening for *secondary causes*, especially systemic lupus, malignant hypertension, and antiphospholipid antibody syndrome, should be done. *Atypical HUS* is diagnosed in patients in whom coexisting conditions,

BOX 2: Evaluation in patients with hemolytic uremic syndrome.

Diagnosis
- Complete blood count; peripheral smear for schistocytes; reticulocyte count*
- Lactate dehydrogenase, haptoglobin*
- Direct Coombs test†
- *Blood:* Creatinine, electrolytes, transaminases, bilirubin, complement C3*
- Urinalysis
- Rapid test for malaria, dengue; IgM antibodies for dengue, leptospirosis (if suspected)
- Coagulation profile* (suspected systemic sepsis)
- Ultrasound abdomen
- *If clinical features present:* Echocardiogram, neuroimaging, amylase, troponin T

Determining cause of HUS
- Essential
  - Investigate for infection associated or secondary HUS, *if clinically suspected* (see **Box 1**)
  - Anti-factor H antibodies (ELISA)*; antinuclear antibodies
  - CD46 expression on neutrophils (flow cytometry)
  - ADAMTS13 activity assay*,‡
  - Total homocysteine*,‡
- Selected patients
  - *Suspected Shiga toxin-associated HUS:* Stool or rectal swab for culture; PCR for Shiga toxin genes (*stx1*, *stx2*); ELISA for free Shiga toxin in stool; IgM antibodies to specific lipopolysaccharide(s)
  - *Suspected pneumococcal HUS:* Blood, pleural fluid or cerebrospinal fluid culture, PCR or ELISA; peanut lectin agglutination assay (Thomsen–Friedenreich antigen detection)
  - *Sequencing genes: CFH, CFI, CFB, C3, CD46, DGKE, THBD, PLG, VTN, INF2, MMACHC*
  - *Multiplex ligation-dependent probe amplification:* Copy number variations *CFHR1-5*

*Blood samples should be drawn before plasma exchanges or infusion
†Positive with pneumococcal infection, lupus; must be tested prior to administering blood products
‡Plasma to be separated from fresh citrated blood (ADAMTS13) and EDTA blood (homocysteine) within 1-hour of collection and frozen at –20 to –70°C.
(ADAMTS13: A disintegrin and metalloproteinase with a thrombospondin type 1 motif, member 13; *CD46:* membrane cofactor protein; *CFHR:* complement factor H related; ELISA: enzyme-linked immunosorbent assay; HUS: hemolytic uremic syndrome; IgM: immunoglobulin M; PCR: polymerase chain reaction)

specific infections (STEC-HUS, Sp-HUS, tropical infections), cobalamin defects, ADAMTS13 deficiency, and secondary forms have been excluded.[6,34-39]

Based on age, the following etiologies are suspected: (1) below 6 months of age: hereditary ADAMTS13 deficiency, methylmalonic aciduria; (2) infants and young children: STEC-HUS, *S. pneumonia*-associated HUS, factor H deficiency, *DGKE* mutations; (3) school-age children and adolescents: anti-FH antibody-associated HUS, CD46 deficiency, autoantibodies to ADAMTS13. Presence of nonsynchronous family history or recurrent disease suggests aHUS or ADAMTS13 deficiency.

All patients with suspected aHUS, especially those with low complement C3, require detailed analysis of the complement pathway. Samples for complement studies should be taken before plasmapheresis or infusing blood products. It is important to screen patients for a defect in cell surface expression of CD46 by flow cytometry;[40] such patients do not benefit from plasmapheresis. Prompt screening for anti-FH antibodies is recommended given the therapeutic implication; titers in the acute phase are considerably higher than the positive threshold (1,000–20,000 arbitrary units (AU)/mL vs. normal levels of 100–150 AU/mL).[21,41]

Genetic testing guides management, prognosis, risk of relapses, genetic counseling, and risk of recurrence following transplant. Patients with aHUS without anti-FH antibodies require sequencing of implicated genes and multiplex ligation-dependent probe amplification (MLPA) for copy number variations in *CFHR1-5*. Targeted next-generation sequencing (NGS) panels facilitate simultaneous screening for multiple genes.[42] A database of genetic variants is available at http://www.complement-db.org/home.php. Sanger sequencing is essential to confirm variants detected on NGS, screen parents to confirm segregation, and for antenatal counseling. The need for additional genetic screening in patients with anti-FH-associated aHUS is debated; genetic sequencing is suggested in patients with a refractory, relapsing, familial or atypical illness, and prior to transplantation.

HISTOLOGY

Kidney biopsy is not routinely indicated since the diagnosis and classification of HUS are clinical.[29] Histological diagnosis is required in patients with unclear diagnosis of HUS or unsatisfactory clinical response and to distinguish between causes of allograft dysfunction. TMA on histology may be acute, subacute, or chronic and can involve glomerular capillaries, arterioles, or both. In its acute form, marked endothelial swelling, subendothelial widening, and presence of luminal fibrin with entrapped fragmented red blood cells are classical; significant luminal occlusion in glomerular capillaries and arterioles occurs **(Figs. 3A to D)**.[3] As lesions progress toward a subacute or chronic stage in the arterioles, organization of fibrin occurs with intimal fibroblastic proliferation resulting in an "onion skin" appearance. Arteriolar TMA results in glomerular ischemia resulting in loss of mesangial substance (mesangiolysis) with ballooning and congestion of capillaries; patchy acute cortical necrosis is seen in its severest form.[3] Chronic lesions show reduplication of the glomerular basement membrane and mesangial proliferation causing a "membranoproliferative" pattern without immune complexes and complement staining on direct immunofluorescence.[3] Chronic cases may also show tuft shrinkage, wrinkling of the capillary walls, and expansion of Bowman's space. Ultrastructural evaluation shows glomerular endothelial swelling, fenestral fusion, subendothelial expansion with electron-lucent material, and later reduplication of the glomerular basement membrane.[3]

Flowchart 2: Proposed algorithm for approach to patients with HUS.

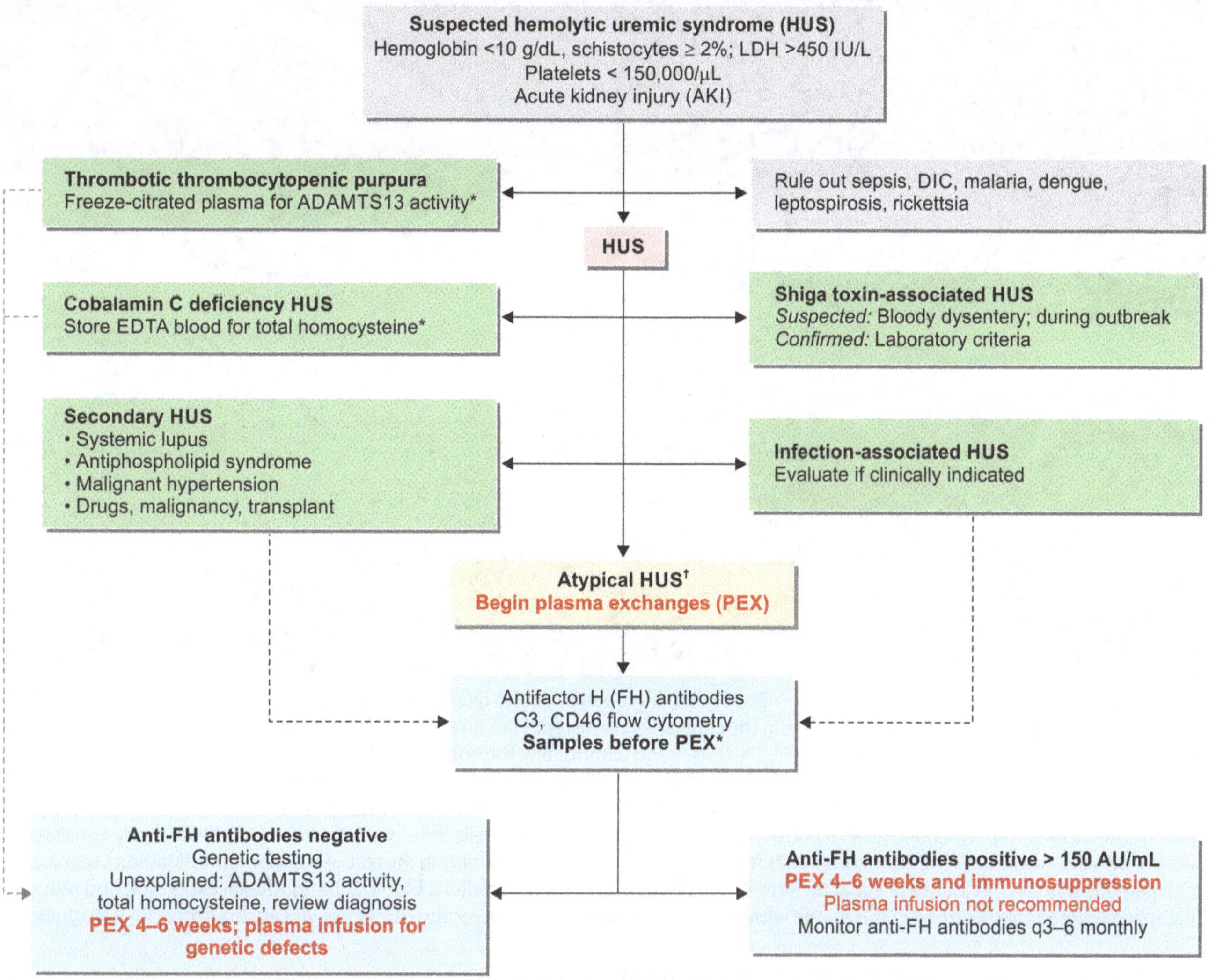

**See* Box 2 for evaluating patients with HUS, including storing and processing of samples.
†Also consider atypical HUS if positive nonsynchronous family history or recurrent disease
(ADAMTS13: a disintegrin and metalloproteinase with a thrombospondin type 1 motif, member 13; CD46: membrane co-factor protein; DIC: disseminated intravascular coagulation; EDTA: ethylenediaminetetraacetic acid; HUS: hemolytic uremic syndrome; LDH: lactate dehydrogenase)
Source: Reprinted by permission from Bagga A, Khandelwal P, Mishra K, Thergaonkar R, Vasudevan A, Sharma J, et al. Hemolytic uremic syndrome in a developing country: Consensus guidelines. Pediatr Nephrol. 2019;34:1465-82.

MANAGEMENT

General management focuses on supportive care. This includes attention to fluid and electrolyte balance, management of hypertension, monitoring for extrarenal involvement, nutritional support, and provision of kidney replacement therapy as required.[43] Most children develop some renal insufficiency and approximately two-thirds require dialytic support. Patients with severe anemia may need packed red cells. Platelet transfusions are limited to children with active bleeding since they might increase the risk of microthrombi.

Shiga Toxin-producing *E. coli* Hemolytic-uremic Syndrome

There is no specific treatment for STEC-HUS; management focuses on best supportive therapy. Epidemiological data have shown an association between dehydration and adverse outcomes in patients with STEC infection. Prompt volume expansion with isotonic fluids, given till the day of onset of HUS, is therefore recommended in patients with dysentery;[44] monitoring for fluid overload is important in patients with AKI. There is conflicting evidence that administration of antibiotics might increase the risk of HUS by inducing expression of the toxin;[45] the role of antibiotics in STEC gastroenteritis is therefore controversial. Conversely, patients with shigellosis require prompt antimicrobial treatment (with oral ciprofloxacin, azithromycin, or cefixime for 5 days) to reduce mortality and complications. While used anecdotally in patients with refractory illness and severe neurological symptoms, current evidence does not support the use of plasma exchanges (PEXs).[46] Analysis of the German STEC-HUS registry did not show benefit of eculizumab,

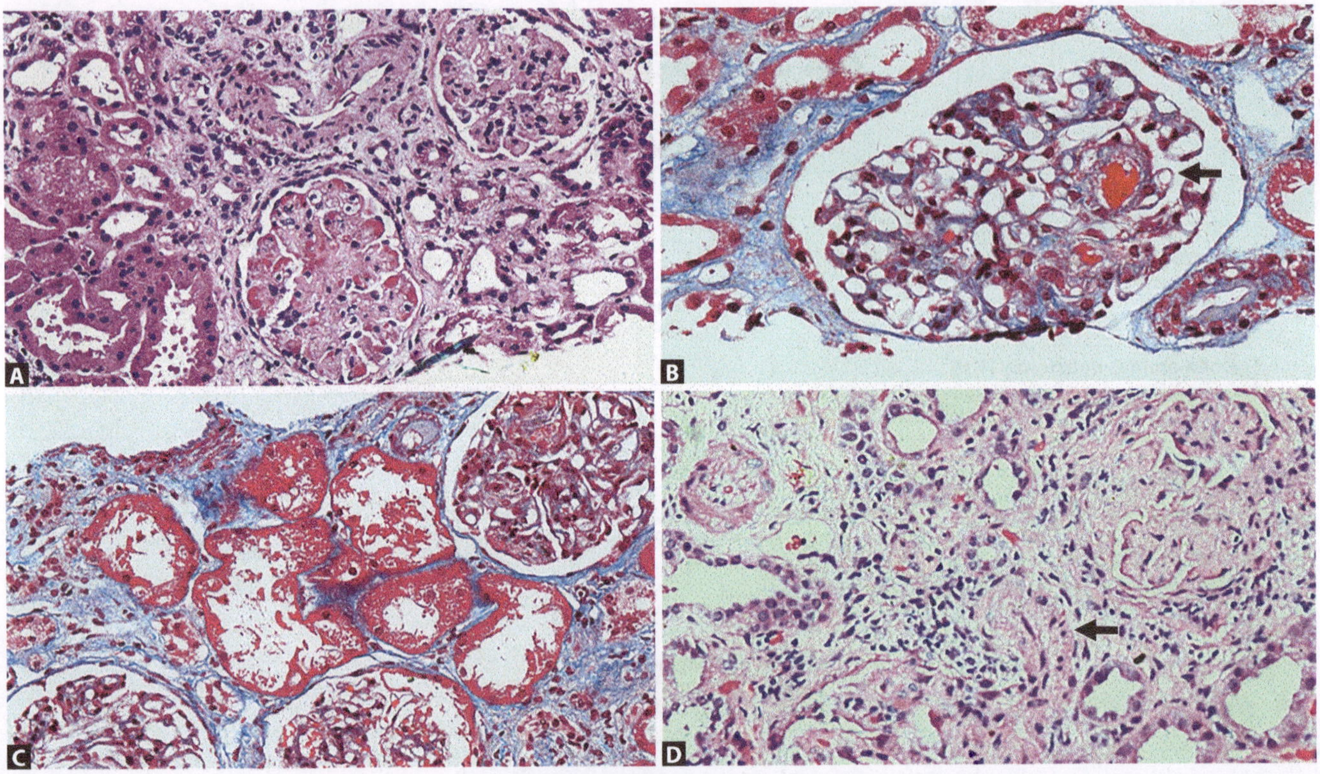

Figs. 3A to D: Spectrum of acute and subacute thrombotic microangiopathy. (A) The glomeruli in this case show evidence of mesangiolysis (loss of mesangial structure) with accumulation of fibrin in the capillaries consistent with an acute glomerular thrombotic microangiopathy (TMA). The small artery included in this field shows mild medial thickening without any thrombosis. [Hematoxylin eosin, 20x original magnification]; (B) Masson's trichrome highlights fibrin as intensely fuchsinophilic in this glomerular thrombus: black arrow, with loss of endothelial cells. Note the acute tubular injury in the background. [Masson's trichrome, 40x original magnification]; (C) The glomerulus on the top right of the image shows endothelial swelling, subendothelial expansion and fragmented red blood cells indicative of acute endothelial injury consistent with glomerular TMA even without frank fibrin thrombi. Note the ischemic mesangial 'pruning' in the rest of the glomeruli. [Masson's trichrome, 20x original magnification]; (D) Evidence of subacute arteriolar TMA with endothelial swelling, lifting, subendothelial expansion and reduction in luminal space is noted (black arrow) in this image with ischemic sclerosis of the glomerulus. [Hematoxylin eosin, 20x original magnification].

an anti-C5 monoclonal antibody that blocks the terminal complement complex, although early treatment was useful in children with neurological involvement.[47] Randomized trials (NCT02205541; EudraCT 2016-000997-39) are examining the therapeutic role of eculizumab in STEC-HUS. Plasma infusions, antimotility agents, heparin, urokinase, dipyridamole, STEC gastroenteritis, and glucocorticoids do not ameliorate the disease course.[48]

Atypical Hemolytic Uremic Syndrome without Anti-FH Antibodies

The standard of care for patients without anti-FH antibodies, especially with inherited defects in complement regulation, is complement blockade with eculizumab. However, eculizumab is an expensive medication that is currently unavailable in India and other developing countries. In the absence of complement blockers, prompt and intensive PEX is the only alternative.

Complement Blockade

Eculizumab is preferred as the first-line therapy as well as in patients with unsatisfactory response to 3–5 days' PEXs or inability to perform PEXs due to difficult vascular access or other complications. Prospective trials show an efficacy of 65% in inducing complete response, with substantial improvements in estimated glomerular filtration rate on medium-term follow-up.[49] Compared to patients administered plasma therapy, fewer patients (6–15%) progressed to end-stage kidney disease (ESKD) or died on medium-term follow-up, when administered eculizumab.[2] Prevention of meningococcal infection is crucial in eculizumab-treated patients and requires timely vaccination and antibiotic prophylaxis. The role of eculizumab for noncomplement disorders, e.g., *DGKE* mutations is unclear.[50] Eculizumab is conventionally administered lifelong; however, there is emerging data on abbreviated therapy. Withdrawal of therapy is associated with relapses in almost half the patients with inherited complement genetic defects, but in ~10% with no identified defect, suggesting that discontinuation of therapy is possible.[51] While the use of a CH50 level <10% is recommended for monitoring of sufficient complement blockade on eculizumab therapy, recent data suggest feasibility of reducing the dose to target incomplete complement blockade (CH50 of <30–70%).[52]

Ravulizumab, a long-acting C5 inhibitor that requires administration once in 8 weeks, has been shown to be effective and safe in pediatric and adult patients with aHUS.[49] Studies utilizing other agents that block the complement cascade (C3 activation, formation of MAC, or block C5 RNA) are in progress.[53] These medications are expensive and not freely available across the world. In countries with limited resources, intensive PEX is the only alternative to complement blockade.

Plasmapheresis (Plasma Exchange)

In many countries, timely institution of PEX, performed with 60–75 mL/kg fresh frozen plasma as exchange fluid, to replace absent or mutated complement regulators, is most appropriate for aHUS.[29] PEX should begin as soon as possible, preferably within 24 hours of the diagnosis of aHUS, without awaiting biopsy diagnosis or results of complement studies. PEX is performed daily till hematological remission, defined as platelets >100,000/µL, schistocytes <2%, LDH less than the upper limit of normal for 2 consecutive days, and then tapered over 4–6 weeks.[29] Subsequently, long-term plasma infusions are advised every 10–14 days for patients with pathogenic variants in complement regulatory genes (*CFH, CFI, CFB*, or *C3*; limited benefit of plasma therapy for *CD46* and *DGKE*). Adverse reactions to plasma or filter, blood-borne infections, and complications related to central venous catheter including infection or thrombosis might occur in ~10% patients.[54] Renal outcome in patients managed with plasma therapy alone is unsatisfactory, with almost 30–50% rate of progression to ESKD in large aHUS cohorts at 1–5 years' follow-up.[2]

Anti-FH Antibody-associated Hemolytic Uremic Syndrome

Intensive PEX enables significant reduction of the anti-FH immunoglobulin G (IgG) antibodies and is associated with clinical and hematological remission.[46,55] Plasma infusions are not a substitute for PEX, since they do not remove autoantibodies. A combination of PEX and immunosuppressive therapy is most useful to improve long-term outcomes.[14,41] Immunosuppression comprises oral prednisolone usually administered for 10–12 months (1 mg/kg/day for 4 weeks and then alternate day followed by tapering) and induction with cyclophosphamide (five to six doses of 500 mg/m^2 IV once in 3–4 weeks). This is followed by maintenance immunosuppression with mycophenolate mofetil or azathioprine for 18–24 months. Relapses occur in about 15–30% of the patients, usually within the first 12–24 months' follow-up.[14,41] High titers of anti-FH antibodies (>1,300 AU/mL), low levels of free factor H, and lack of administration of maintenance immunosuppression increase the risk of relapses.[14] Therefore, antibody titers should be carefully monitored, especially in the first year of illness. Some centers, especially in the developed countries, may initiate empiric therapy with eculizumab in all aHUS patients pending results of anti-FH antibody ELISA. In such patients, there is a debate if therapy with eculizumab should be continued or replaced by PEX and immunosuppression.[21] The generation of antibodies is also not affected by administration of eculizumab and additional immunosuppression might be required.

OUTCOME AND MONITORING

Patients should be monitored for hematological remission and for renal dysfunction, proteinuria, and hypertension at follow-up.

Shiga Toxin-producing *E. coli* Hemolytic-uremic Syndrome

The short-term outcome of STEC-HUS is satisfactory, with resolution of renal impairment over a few weeks. Long-term, 20–30% cases have renal sequelae, including proteinuria, hypertension, and deranged renal function; ESKD occurs in approximately 12%. Oligoanuria persisting for >4 weeks, cerebral involvement, and cortical necrosis are associated with adverse prognosis. Mortality rate is 2–5%, primarily due to severe extrarenal involvement.[8,61]

Atypical Hemolytic Uremic Syndrome

The outcome of aHUS, chiefly dependent on the underlying pathogenic mutation, is guarded. Mortality is estimated at 8–14% in children at 3–5 years of follow-up. Progression to ESKD, in the absence of effective treatment, occurs in one-half of the patients, especially those with inherited genetic defects. Those with anti-FH antibodies respond to plasma exchange and immunosuppression; progression to ESKD occurs in 15–20% patients. Patients, particularly those with abnormalities in CD46, should be monitored for relapses, especially following infections **(Table 2)**.[15,28]

DISEASE RECURRENCE AFTER RENAL TRANSPLANTATION

Renal transplantation is associated with 50–80% risk of recurrence in the allograft in patients with aHUS. The risk is highest (~80%) in patients with mutations in *FH, C3*, and *FB*, 50% for mutations in *FI*, 20% for those without an identifiable defect, and below 10% for isolated mutations in *CD46*.[50,62,63] Prophylactic eculizumab or combined liver kidney transplantation is recommended in patients who are at high risk of recurrence. Patients with autoantibody-associated HUS requiring transplantation may need plasma exchanges and immunosuppressive therapy before and during transplantation.[21,64]

SPECIFIC FORMS OF HEMOLYTIC UREMIC SYNDROME

Streptococcus pneumoniae-associated Hemolytic Uremic Syndrome

Streptococcus pneumoniae-associated HUS (SpHUS) is defined by the triad of HUS occurring in a patient with *S. pneumoniae* infection. While the incidence of SpHUS has declined and different serotypes are now implicated due to the widespread use of pneumococcal vaccines, particularly in the developed nations, SpHUS still accounts for ~5–15% of childhood HUS.[56]

Pathogenesis

S. pneumoniae produces neuraminidase that cleaves sialic acid of glycoproteins on erythrocytes, platelets, and glomerular endothelial cells to expose the cryptic Thomsen–Friedenreich antigen (T-antigen). Interaction of the T-antigen with preformed IgM antibodies leads to polyagglutination, Coombs' positive hemolysis, and direct endothelial injury leading to HUS. Other neuraminidase-producing organisms, such as *Capnocytophaga canimorsus* and influenza A, are also known to cause HUS. Further, desialylation by neuraminidase disrupts binding of FH to C3b, causing activation of the complement on cell surface and cytotoxicity. Certain *S. pneumoniae* serotypes also produce proteins (e.g., Hic protein and pneumococcal surface protein C) that directly inhibit factor H activity or binding.[57]

Presentation

The incidence of SpHUS is highest in children below 2 years of age and most frequently seen in patients with pneumonia with empyema or meningitis. Features of HUS develop 3–13 days following presentation with invasive pneumococcal infection. Compared to patients with STEC-HUS, those with SpHUS are usually younger, sicker, and have prolonged oligoanuria and thrombocytopenia and severe hemolysis. Extrarenal involvement may occur, including transaminitis, pancreatitis, purpura fulminans, limb amputation, cholecystitis, thrombosis, or hearing loss. Overall, 2–12% patients die, with lower rates of mortality in patients with pneumonia than those with meningitis. ESKD is noted in 10–15% cases, while 10–30% patients each show hypertension, proteinuria, or neurological sequelae.

Diagnosis

Pneumococcal HUS is suspected (*probable* diagnosis) in patients, usually younger than 2 years, with pneumonia, meningitis, or sepsis and positive direct Coombs' test without features of DIC. Direct Coombs' test is 60% sensitive for SpHUS. Absence of active bleeding and normal fibrinogen levels help distinguish SpHUS from DIC that may be present in patients with invasive streptococcal disease. The diagnosis is *confirmed* by either (1) isolation of *S. pneumoniae* by culture or detection of pneumococcal antigen by PCR or ELISA in body fluids or (2) positive peanut lectin (*Arachis hypogaea*) agglutination assay. This assay evaluates the T-antigen exposure and is 100% sensitive and ~50% specific for the diagnosis of SpHUS.[58,59]

Management

Treatment is with IV cephalosporins; vancomycin is used if prevalence of multidrug resistance is high. While plasma infusions or PEX is best avoided, firm recommendations are lacking. When conducted, 5% albumin rather than plasma should be used as replacement fluid. If required, dextran-washed red cells and platelets should be used to remove anti-Thomsen–Friedenreich antibodies.[58,59]

Cobalamin Deficiency-associated Hemolytic Uremic Syndrome

Cobalamin deficiency occurs in a small (~6–8%) proportion of patients with HUS, but is important to recognize due to its distinct management and lack of response to PEX. The disorder may present at all ages. **Figure 4** depicts the biochemical pathways involved in cblC deficiency. CblC acts as a coenzyme for cytosolic methionine synthase that catalyzes the conversion of homocysteine to methionine, as well as mitochondrial methylmalonyl-CoA mutase, which converts methylmalonyl-CoA to succinyl-CoA. Patients with mutations in cblC may have a functional deficiency of one or both enzymes, resulting in homocystinuria and/or methylmalonic acidemia. The most common inborn error of cobalamin metabolism is biallelic variations in the *MMACHC* gene (cblC deficiency), in which both abnormalities are noted.

Clinical Presentation

Two forms are recognized: (1) classical, early onset type with infantile presentation, severe multisystem disease, and high mortality and (2) late-onset milder type. Typical presentation in neonates is with nonspecific symptoms, including vomiting and failure to thrive; almost all patients eventually have neurological involvement in the form of hypotonia, seizures, lethargy, and developmental delay. HUS is more common in patients presenting later, occurring in approximately 25%. Renal failure may be insidious, with progressive renal insufficiency in almost 50% cases. One-third of the patients with HUS may not have extrarenal manifestations, although neurological (44%) and cardiopulmonary involvement (39%) including pulmonary hypertension (17%) is common.[60]

Diagnosis

Pancytopenia or leukopenia is observed commonly; megaloblastic picture on peripheral smear may occur in 10–25% cases. Elevated total homocysteine levels (>50–100 μM/L) with normal levels of vitamin B_{12} and folate are the hallmark **(Table 2)**. Samples for total homocysteine should be collected (and stored, if not feasible to process immediately) before empiric plasma therapy is initiated.[29] Testing is recommended in all patients with HUS regardless of age. The diagnosis is confirmed by homozygous or compound heterozygous mutation in the *MMACHC* gene. Amino acid and organic acid chromatography reveals elevated levels of plasma and urine methylmalonic acid. While TMA is the most common renal manifestation, tubulointerstitial nephritis and proximal renal tubular acidosis are reported.[33]

Management

The mainstay of therapy is administration of parenteral hydroxocobalamin (1 mg/day) with an aim of reducing homocysteine levels below 40–60 μM/L; cyanocobalamin and oral hydroxycobalamin are ineffective.[33] Given the

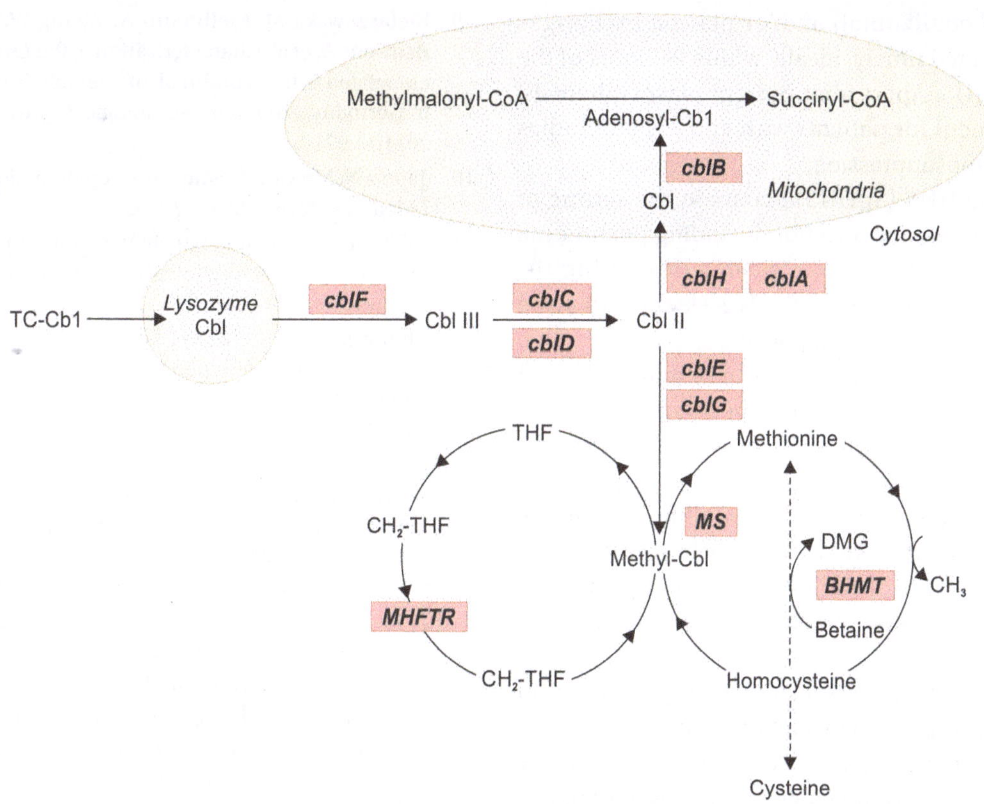

Fig. 4: Vitamin B_{12} (cbl) metabolism. Cobalamin released from its transporter TC in the lysosome is subjected to a series of reduction steps before being adenosylated in the mitochondrion and methylated in the cytosol. These reactions are mediated by enzymes cblA to cblH. Methylcobalamin is a cofactor for MS, the enzyme catalyzing the chief pathway for methylation of homocysteine to methionine. The methyl donor for this reaction is 5-methyl tetrahydrofolate (CH_3-THF). Homocysteine may also be methylated to methionine through a minor pathway using the BHMT or converted to cysteine. Defects in genes encoding individual cobalamin enzymes may result in isolated methylmalonic aciduria, isolated hyperhomocysteinemia or combined defects. (BHMT: betaine homocysteine methyltransferase; cbl: cobalamin; cblA: cobalamin A; cblH: cobalamin H; MS: methionine synthase; TC: transcobalamin)

biochemical bases, adjunctive therapies include betaine (has synergistic effect with hydroxocobalamin, helps methylating homocysteine to methionine) and folate (reduces homocysteine levels). Early initiation of treatment reverses HUS, prevents mortality, and allows renal recovery but may not prevent continued neurological and retinal involvement.[33]

CONCLUSION

Hemolytic uremic syndrome is a rare disease characterized by severe AKI, multiorgan involvement, and high morbidity and mortality that requires urgent therapeutic intervention. A structured approach to evaluation is required to make the correct diagnosis; appropriate collection, storage, and processing of blood specimens are important to prevent diagnostic delays. The management of Shiga toxin-associated HUS, the most common etiology worldwide, is chiefly supportive. While the outcome of atypical HUS has significantly improved with the availability of eculizumab in the developed world, prompt initiation of plasma exchanges is the only alternative where complement blockade is unavailable. Patients with anti-FH-associated illness are satisfactorily managed with a combination of plasma exchanges and immunosuppressive medications. Clinical trials on novel agents that block the complement cascade are ongoing.

KEY POINTS

- HUS is an important cause of severe AKI in children.
- It is characterized by a triad of microangiopathic hemolytic anemia, thrombocytopenia, and AKI.
- Infection with Shiga toxin-producing enteropathogens, including *E. coli* strain O157:H7 and *S. dysenteriae*, is the most important cause of HUS in children.
- Management involves good supportive care, dialysis as required, and avoidance of antimotility drugs and platelet transfusions.
- Most patients show satisfactory renal recovery, although proteinuria and hypertension are common sequelae.
- Atypical HUS though less common (5–10%) is associated with uncontrolled activation of the alternate complement pathway due to genetic or acquired defects.
- The prognosis of atypical HUS is worse than Shiga toxin-associated HUS with high rates of mortality, extrarenal complications, and ESKD.
- Screening for anti-FH antibodies and targeted genetic sequencing is useful in enabling specific diagnosis.

- Therapy with eculizumab and/or plasma exchanges should be initiated timely, ideally within 24 hours of the diagnosis of HUS. Apart from prompt plasmapheresis, specific treatment for patients with anti-FH antibodies involves immunosuppression.
- *S. pneumoniae* HUS (SpHUS) occurs in the setting of invasive *S. pneumoniae* infection including pneumonia with or without effusions/empyema or meningitis. Early identification of these patients is essential to avoid administration of fresh frozen plasma.
- CblC defects such as methylmalonic acidemia and hyperhomocysteinemia should be suspected in all patients presenting with HUS, regardless of age and extrarenal manifestations.
- Diagnosis is suggested by elevated total homocysteine and confirmed by genetic testing for homozygous or compound heterozygous *MMACHC* variants. Therapy involves administration of parenteral hydroxocobalamin, betaine and folate.
- Renal transplantation is associated with 50–80% risk of recurrence in the allograft in patients with aHUS. Prophylactic eculizumab or combined liver kidney transplantation is recommended in patients at high risk of recurrence. Patients with autoantibody-associated HUS requiring transplantation may need plasma exchanges and immunosuppressive therapy before and during transplantation.

REFERENCES

1. Avila Bernabeu AI, Cavero Escribano T, Cao Vilarino M. Atypical hemolytic uremic syndrome: new challenges in the complement blockage era. Nephron. 2020;144:537-49.
2. Fakhouri F, Zuber J, Fremeaux-Bacchi V, Loirat C. Haemolytic uraemic syndrome. Lancet. 2017;390:681-96.
3. Goodship TH, Cook HT, Fakhouri F, Fervenza FC, Frémeaux-Bacchi V, Kavanagh D, et al. Atypical hemolytic uremic syndrome and C3 glomerulopathy: conclusions from a "Kidney Disease: Improving Global Outcomes" (KDIGO) Controversies Conference. Kidney Int. 2017;91:539-51.
4. Sheerin NS, Glover E. Haemolytic uremic syndrome: diagnosis and management. F1000Res. 2019;8:F1000.
5. Sinha A, Singh G, Bhat AS, Mohapatra S, Gulati A, Hari P, et al. Thrombotic microangiopathy and acute kidney injury following vivax malaria. Clin Exp Nephrol. 2013;17:66-72.
6. Loirat C, Fakhouri F, Ariceta G, Besbas N, Bitzan M, Bjerre A, et al. An international consensus approach to the management of atypical hemolytic uremic syndrome in children. Pediatr Nephrol. 2016;31:15-39.
7. Joly BS, Stepanian A, Leblanc T, Hajage D, Chambost H, Harambat J, et al. Child-onset and adolescent-onset acquired thrombotic thrombocytopenic purpura with severe ADAMTS13 deficiency: a cohort study of the French national registry for thrombotic microangiopathy. Lancet Haematol. 2016;3:e537-e546.
8. Joseph A, Cointe A, Mariani Kurkdjian P, Rafat C, Hertig A. Shiga toxin-associated hemolytic uremic syndrome: a narrative review. Toxins (Basel). 2020;12(2):67.
9. Bielaszewska M, Mellmann A, Zhang W, Köck R, Fruth A, Bauwens A, et al. Characterisation of the *Escherichia coli* strain associated with an outbreak of haemolytic uraemic syndrome in Germany, 2011: a microbiological study. Lancet Infect Dis. 2011;11:671-6.
10. Taneja N, Mewara A. Shigellosis: epidemiology in India. Indian J Med Res. 2016;143:565-76.
11. Fakhouri F, Fremeaux-Bacchi V. Thrombotic microangiopathy in aHUS and beyond: clinical clues from complement genetics. Nat Rev Nephrol. 2021;17:543-53.
12. Bhatia D, Khandelwal P, Sinha A, Hari P, Cheong HI and Bagga A. Incomplete penetrance of CD46 mutation causing familial atypical hemolytic uremic syndrome. Pediatr Nephrol. 2015;30:2215-20.
13. Togarsimalemath SK, Si-Mohammed A, Puraswani M, Gupta A, Vabret A, Liguori S, et al. Gastrointestinal pathogens in anti-FH antibody positive and negative hemolytic uremic syndrome. Pediatr Res. 2018;84:118-24.
14. Puraswani M, Khandelwal P, Saini H, Saini S, Gurjar BS, Sinha A, et al. Clinical and immunological profile of anti-factor H antibody associated atypical hemolytic uremic syndrome: a nationwide database. Front Immunol. 2019;10:1282.
15. Schaefer F, Ardissino G, Ariceta G, Fakhouri F, Scully M, Isbel N, et al. Clinical and genetic predictors of atypical hemolytic uremic syndrome phenotype and outcome. Kidney Int. 2018;94:408-18.
16. Lee MS, Yoon JW, Tesh VL. Editorial: recent advances in understanding the pathogenesis of shiga toxin-producing *Shigella* and *Escherichia coli*. Front Cell Infect Microbiol. 2020;10:620703.
17. Menge C. Molecular biology of *Escherichia coli* Shiga toxins' effects on mammalian cells. Toxins (Basel). 2020;12(5):345.
18. Buelli S, Zoja C, Remuzzi G, Morigi M. Complement activation contributes to the pathophysiology of shiga toxin-associated hemolytic uremic syndrome. Microorganisms. 2019;7(1):15.
19. Frazer-Abel A, Kirschfink M, Prohaszka Z. Expanding horizons in complement analysis and quality control. Front Immunol. 2021;12:697313.
20. Merle NS, Church SE, Fremeaux-Bacchi V, Roumenina LT. Complement system part I—molecular mechanisms of activation and regulation. Front Immunol. 2015;6:262.
21. Durey MA, Sinha A, Togarsimalemath SK, Bagga A. Anti-complement-factor H-associated glomerulopathies. Nat Rev Nephrol. 2016;12:563-78.
22. Bu F, Zhang Y, Wang K, Borsa NG, Jones MB, Taylor AO, et al. Genetic analysis of 400 patients refines understanding and implicates a new gene in atypical hemolytic uremic syndrome. J Am Soc Nephrol. 2018;29:2809-19.
23. Challis RC, Ring T, Xu Y, Wong EKS, Flossmann O, Roberts ISD, et al. Thrombotic microangiopathy in inverted formin 2-mediated renal disease. J Am Soc Nephrol. 2017;28:1084-91.
24. Osborne AJ, Breno M, Borsa NG, Bu F, Frémeaux-Bacchi V, Gale DP, et al. Statistical validation of rare complement variants provides insights into the molecular basis of atypical hemolytic uremic syndrome and C3 glomerulopathy. J Immunol. 2018;200:2464-78.
25. Pifer R, Sperandio V. The interplay between the microbiota and enterohemorrhagic *Escherichia coli*. Microbiol Spectr. 2014;2(5).

26. Khalid M, Andreoli S. Extrarenal manifestations of the hemolytic uremic syndrome associated with Shiga toxin-producing *Escherichia coli* (STEC HUS). Pediatr Nephrol. 2019;34:2495-507.
27. Yan K, Desai K, Gullapalli L, Druyts E, Balijepalli C. Epidemiology of atypical hemolytic uremic syndrome: a systematic literature review. Clin Epidemiol. 2020;12:295-305.
28. Raina R, Krishnappa V, Blaha T, Kann T, Hein W, Burke L, et al. Atypical hemolytic-uremic syndrome: an update on pathophysiology, diagnosis, and treatment. Ther Apher Dial. 2019;23:4-21.
29. Bagga A, Khandelwal P, Mishra K, Thergaonkar R, Vasudevan A, Sharma J, et al. Hemolytic uremic syndrome in a developing country: consensus guidelines. Pediatr Nephrol. 2019;34:1465-82.
30. Srivastava RN, Moudgil A, Bagga A, Vasudev AS. Hemolytic uremic syndrome in children in northern India. Pediatr Nephrol. 1991;5:284-88.
31. Gould LH, Bopp C, Strockbine N, Atkinson R, Baselski V, Body B, et al. Recommendations for diagnosis of shiga toxin—producing *Escherichia coli* infections by clinical laboratories. MMWR Recomm Rep. 2009;58:1-14.
32. Wijnsma KL, van Bommel SA, van der Velden T, Volokhina E, Schreuder MF, P van den Heuvel L, et al. Fecal diagnostics in combination with serology: best test to establish STEC-HUS. Pediatr Nephrol. 2016;31:2163-70.
33. Huemer M, Diodato D, Schwahn B, Schiff M, Bandeira A, Benoist J-F, et al. Guidelines for diagnosis and management of the cobalamin-related remethylation disorders cblC, cblD, cblE, cblF, cblG, cblJ and MTHFR deficiency. J Inherit Metab Dis. 2017;40:21-48.
34. Kato H, Nangaku M, Hataya H, Sawai T, Ashida A, Fujimaru R, et al. Clinical guides for atypical hemolytic uremic syndrome in Japan. Clin Exp Nephrol. 2016;20:536-43.
35. Cheong HI, Jo SK, Yoon SS, Cho H, Kim JS, Kim YO, et al. Clinical practice guidelines for the management of atypical hemolytic uremic syndrome in Korea. J Korean Med Sci. 2016;31:1516-28.
36. Campistol JM, Arias M, Ariceta G, Blasco M, Espinosa L, Espinosa M, et al. An update for atypical haemolytic uraemic syndrome: diagnosis and treatment. A consensus document. Nefrologia. 2015;35:421-47.
37. Kavanagh D, Goodship TH. Atypical hemolytic uremic syndrome, genetic basis, and clinical manifestations. Hematology Am Soc Hematol Educ Program. 2011;2011:15-20.
38. Fremeaux-Bacchi V, Fakhouri F, Garnier A, Bienaimé F, Dragon-Durey M-A, Ngo S, et al. Genetics and outcome of atypical hemolytic uremic syndrome: a nationwide French series comparing children and adults. Clin J Am Soc Nephrol. 2013;8:554-62.
39. Bouts AH, Roofthooft MT, Salomons GS, Davin JC. CD46-associated atypical hemolytic uremic syndrome with uncommon course caused by cblC deficiency. Pediatr Nephrol. 2010;25:2547-8.
40. Khandelwal P, Birla S, Bhatia D, Puraswani M, Saini H, Sinha A, et al. Mutations in membrane cofactor protein (CD46) gene in Indian children with hemolytic uremic syndrome. Clin Kidney J. 2018;11:198-203.
41. Sinha A, Gulati A, Saini S, Blanc C, Gupta A, Gurjar BS, et al. Prompt plasma exchanges and immunosuppressive treatment improves the outcomes of anti-factor H autoantibody-associated hemolytic uremic syndrome in children. Kidney Int. 2014;85:1151-60.
42. Thergaonkar RW, Narang A, Gurjar BS, Tiwari P, Puraswani M, Saini H, et al. Targeted exome sequencing in anti-factor H antibody negative HUS reveals multiple variations. Clin Exp Nephrol. 2018;22:653-60.
43. Kidney Disease Improving Global Outcomes (KDIGO) Acute Kidney Injury Work Group. KDIGO clinical practice guideline for acute kidney injury. Kidney Int Suppl. 2012;2:1-138.
44. Grisaru S, Xie J, Samuel S, Hartling L, Tarr PI, Schnadower D, et al. Associations between hydration status, intravenous fluid administration, and outcomes of patients infected with Shiga toxin-producing *Escherichia coli*: a systematic review and meta-analysis. JAMA Pediatr. 2017;171:68-76.
45. Agger M, Scheutz F, Villumsen S, Mølbak K, Petersen AM. Antibiotic treatment of verocytotoxin-producing *Escherichia coli* (VTEC) infection: a systematic review and a proposal. J Antimicrob Chemother. 2015;70:2440-6.
46. Schwartz J, Padmanabhan A, Aqui N, Balogun RA, Connelly-Smith L, Delaney M, et al. Guidelines on the use of therapeutic apheresis in clinical practice-evidence-based approach from the Writing Committee of the American Society for Apheresis: the seventh special issue. J Clin Apher. 2016;31:149-62.
47. Loos S, Ahlenstiel T, Kranz B, Staude H, Pape L, Härtel C, et al. An outbreak of Shiga toxin-producing *Escherichia coli* O104:H4 hemolytic uremic syndrome in Germany: presentation and short-term outcome in children. Clin Infect Dis. 2012;55:753-59.
48. Michael M, Elliott EJ, Ridley GF, Hodson EM, Craig JC. Interventions for haemolytic uraemic syndrome and thrombotic thrombocytopenic purpura. Cochrane Database Syst Rev. 2009;(1):CD003595.
49. Pugh D, O'Sullivan ED, Duthie FA, Masson P, Kavanagh D. Interventions for atypical haemolytic uraemic syndrome. Cochrane Database Syst Rev. 2021;3:CD012862.
50. Azukaitis K, Simkova E, Majid MA, Galiano M, Benz K, Amann K, et al. The phenotypic spectrum of nephropathies associated with mutations in diacylglycerol kinase epsilon. J Am Soc Nephrol. 2017;28:3066-75.
51. Fakhouri F, Loirat C. Anticomplement treatment in atypical and typical hemolytic uremic syndrome. Semin Hematol. 2018;55:150-8.
52. Wijnsma KL, Duineveld C, Wetzels JFM, van de Kar N. Eculizumab in atypical hemolytic uremic syndrome: strategies toward restrictive use. Pediatr Nephrol. 2019;34:2261-77.
53. Zipfel PF, Wiech T, Rudnick R, Afonso S, Person F, Skerka C. Complement inhibitors in clinical trials for glomerular diseases. Front Immunol. 2019;10:2166.
54. Khandelwal P, Thomas CC, Rathi BS, Hari P, Tiwari AN, Sinha A, et al. Membrane-filtration based plasma exchanges for atypical hemolytic uremic syndrome: audit of efficacy and safety. J Clin Apher. 2019;34:555-62.
55. Khandelwal P, Gupta A, Sinha A, Saini S, Hari P, Durey MAD, et al. Effect of plasma exchange and immunosuppressive medications on antibody titers and outcome in anti-complement factor H antibody-associated hemolytic uremic syndrome. Pediatr Nephrol. 2015;30:451-7.
56. Agarwal HS, Latifi SQ. *Streptococcus pneumoniae*-associated hemolytic uremic syndrome in the era of Pneumococcal vaccine. Pathogens. 2021;10(6):727.
57. Scobell RR, Kaplan BS and Copelovitch L. New insights into the pathogenesis of *Streptococcus pneumoniae*-associated hemolytic uremic syndrome. Pediatr Nephrol. 2020;35:1585-91.

58. Loupiac A, Elayan A, Cailliez M, Adra A-L, Decramer S, Thouret M-C, et al. Diagnosis of *Streptococcus pneumoniae*-associated hemolytic uremic syndrome. Pediatr Infect Dis J. 2013;32:1045-9.
59. Spinale JM, Ruebner RL, Kaplan BS, Copelovitch L. Update on *Streptococcus pneumoniae* associated hemolytic uremic syndrome. Curr Opin Pediatr. 2013;25:203-8.
60. Beck BB, van Spronsen F, Diepstra A, Berger RM, Komhoff M. Renal thrombotic microangiopathy in patients with cblC defect: review of an under-recognized entity. Pediatr Nephrol. 2017;32:733-41.
61. Scheiring J, Andreoli SP, Zimmerhackl LB. Treatment and outcome of Shiga-toxin-associated hemolytic uremic syndrome (HUS). Pediatr Nephrol. 2008;23:1749-60.
62. Bresin E, Rurali E, Caprioli J, Sanchez-Corral P, Fremeaux-Bacchi V, de Cordoba SR, et al. Combined complement gene mutations in atypical hemolytic uremic syndrome influence clinical phenotype. J Am Soc Nephrol. 2013;24:475-86.
63. Le Quintrec M, Zuber J, Moulin B, Kamar N, Jablonski M, Lionet A, et al. Complement genes strongly predict recurrence and graft outcome in adult renal transplant recipients with atypical hemolytic and uremic syndrome. Am J Transplant. 2013;13:663-75.
64. Khandelwal P, Sinha A, Hari P, Bansal VK, Dinda AK, Bagga A. Outcomes of renal transplant in patients with anti-complement factor H antibody-associated hemolytic uremic syndrome. Pediatr Transplant. 2014;18:E134-9.

CHAPTER

6.12

Alport Syndrome and Thin Basement Membrane Disease

Sukanya Govindan

INTRODUCTION

Alport syndrome (AS) and thin basement membrane disease (TBMD) are genetic diseases characterized by abnormal type IV collagen. Due to the common molecular basis, the two diseases are grouped together by the term collagen IV nephropathy.[1] These two disorders have a wide clinical presentation ranging from isolated microscopic hematuria to nephropathy leading to end-stage kidney disease (ESKD) along with extrarenal manifestations such as sensorineural hearing loss (SNHL) and ocular anomalies.[2]

MOLECULAR PATHOLOGY

The predominant type of collagen in the body is type I which forms tendons and ligaments and is also responsible for kidney fibrosis. However, type IV collagen is the major collagenous constituent of the mature mammalian glomerular basement membrane (GBM) and is made of three alpha chains (α 3, 4, and 5) in a triple helical structure in a 1:1:1 ratio. There are six distinct types of collagen IV alpha chains identified and are encoded by genes *COL4A1* to *COL4A6* in three different chromosomes: *COL4A1* and *COL4A2* on chromosome 13, *COL4A3* and *COL4A4* on chromosome 2, and *COL4A5* and *COL4A6* on chromosome X.

Alport syndrome and TBMD arise as a result of mutations in genes *COL4A3*, *COL4A4*, and *COL4A5* that affect the synthesis, assembly, deposition, or function (or a combination of these) of the collagen IV α345 molecule. The alpha-3, alpha-4, alpha-5, and alpha-6 (IV) chains are expressed in the basement membrane (BM) of the kidney, cochlea, and eye. Mutations in *COL4A5* cause X-linked AS (XLAS), whereas mutations in *COL4A3* or *COL4A4* gene can cause autosomal dominant AS (ADAS) or autosomal recessive AS (ARAS). Also digenic inheritance can occur when a combination of two mutations in different genes occurs. Mutations in *COL4A3* and *COL4A4* genes are also associated with TBMD.[3]

GENETICS AND MODE OF INHERITANCE

COL4A5 Mutations

Mutation in this gene is transmitted in an X-linked recessive pattern in almost 85% of patients, whereas 10–15% of affected patients can have de novo mutations. Hemizygous males have severe phenotype with almost 100% of patients developing ESKD and do not transmit the mutation to the next generation. Few X-linked families with associated leiomyomatosis have contiguous deletions involving both the *COL4A5* and *COL4A6* genes. The type of mutation influences disease severity in males with deletions, nonsense, and frame shift mutations causing severe disease with complete loss of expression of α345 (IV) in GBM while the effects of splicing and missense mutations are variable. In XLAS, renal disease is often accompanied by SNHL and ocular anomalies such as perimacular flecks and lenticonus. Heterozygous females or carriers have a milder phenotype and offspring have 50% chance of inheriting the mutation. Females have a 25% lifetime risk of progression to ESKD and those with history of gross hematuria, proteinuria, deafness, and GBM lamellation and thickening have higher risk of progressive nephropathy.[1,3]

COL4A3 and *COL4A4* Mutations

Mutations in both alleles of *COL4A3* or *COL4A4* cause ARAS and autosomal inheritance is clinically suspected by similar disease severity in males and females in the family, parental consanguinity, or microscopic hematuria in the father and lack of severe renal disease in both the parents of an affected patient. Like in XLAS, deafness and ocular abnormalities are frequently seen in patients with ARAS and patients have 100% risk of ESKD, but rate of progression and development of extrarenal manifestation are influenced by genotype. However, unlike in XLAS genotype–phenotype correlations are less robust in ARAS.[1,3]

Heterozygous mutations in *COL4A3* or *COL4A4* are inherited in an ADAS fashion and are associated with a spectrum of clinical presentations from complete absence of disease manifestation, asymptomatic microscopic hematuria, progressive kidney disease, deafness, and ocular abnormalities. Within families, the clinical features can vary significantly and are influenced by lifestyle factors such as smoking, high salt intake, and high blood pressure and also due to possible effect of modifier genes that can either exacerbate or dampen the clinical outcome of mutations.[1,3] TBMD is also associated with heterozygous mutations in

COL4A3 or *COL4A4*, and there is emerging evidence that these patients should be considered to have ADAS and the condition is not entirely benign as once thought.[4]

Digenic Inheritance

Recently, AS phenotype has been recognized in patients with coexisting mutation in *COL4A3*, *COL4A4*, or *COL4A5* with digenic inheritance. This is a form of non-Mendelian inheritance simulating either an autosomal dominant or autosomal recessive (AR) pattern depending on the modifying effect of transcription factors. Clinical features and risk of progressive nephropathy need to be assessed individually for a patient and affected families.[1,3]

CLINICAL FEATURES

Clinical manifestations depend upon the mode of inheritance, gender, and the type of genetic mutation. *Microscopic hematuria* is the single most and constant feature of AS. It is an early onset symptom and could be the only symptom detected in infancy. Episodes of *macroscopic hematuria* precipitated by exercise or upper respiratory tract infection are observed in children. Abnormal *proteinuria and hypertension* occur with increasing age and progressive renal damage and are strong indicators of the onset of chronic kidney disease (CKD). One-third of the children have nephrotic proteinuria. Progressive *bilateral SNHL* affecting high and middle frequencies can be detected during the first decade of life. It is never present at birth.[3,4]

Anterior lenticonus is a conical protrusion of the lens into the anterior chamber of the eye that develops progressively during adolescence. Anterior lenticonus is pathognomonic of AS and a marker of severity of AS. Retinal changes are characterized by the progressive appearance of asymptomatic *perimacular yellowish flecks*. Both types of ocular lesion are diagnostic specific to AS and are observed in about one-third of the patients. Nontraumatic corneal erosions have been reported in AS. Recurrent corneal erosion is characterized by attacks of acute ocular pain, photophobia, and tearing. Slit-lamp examination discloses localized abrasion of the corneal epithelium and occasionally a detached flap. Endothelial vesicles compatible with posterior polymorphous dystrophy of the cornea is an uncommon ocular finding.[3,4]

In the XLAS, the disease is consistently severe in hemizygous males and less symptomatic in affected females. In the AR form, the disease is very much similar to XLAS and is equally severe in males and females. Carriers who are heterozygous for AR form have no or mild clinical manifestations. In families with autosomal dominant inheritance, each child of an affected individual has a 50% chance of inheriting the mutation and having a collagen IV disorder (ADAS or TBMD).[5]

A juvenile-type XLAS was associated with diffuse esophageal leiomyomatosis, manifested by dysphagia or retrosternal pain. Leiomyomatosis also can involve the tracheobronchial tree and female genitalia and is associated with congenital bilateral cataracts. Leiomyomatosis is as severe in females as in males, whereas renal involvement is milder in females, just as in X-linked forms without leiomyomatosis. The *COL4A6* mutation is implicated in its development.[3]

Table 1 summarizes the genotype–phenotype correlations and the risk of end-stage kidney disease (ESKD).

EVALUATION

Alport syndrome should be considered in every child with unexplained persistent microscopic or episodic macroscopic

TABLE 1: Genotype–phenotype correlations and the risk of ESKD.[1]

Inheritance	*Genes affected*	*Genetic state*	*Risk of ESKD*	*Comments*
X-linked	COL4A5	Hemizygous males	100%	Rate of progression to ESKD and timing of extrarenal manifestations strongly correlates with type of mutation
		Heterozygous females	Up to 25%	*Risk factors for progression:* Gross hematuria, SNHL, proteinuria, GBM thickening and lamellation
Autosomal	*COL4A3* and *COL4A4*	Recessive (homozygous or compound heterozygous	100%	Rate of progression to ESKD and timing of extrarenal manifestations strongly influenced by genotype
		Dominant	20% or more among those with risk factors for progression, <1% in absence of risk factors	Risk factors for progression: Proteinuria, FSGS, GBM thickening and lamellation, SNHL, or evidence of progression in patient or family, genetic modifiers
Digenic	*COL4A3*, *COL4A4*, and *COL4A5*	*COL4A3* and *COL4A4* mutations in trans/cis Mutations in *COL4A5* and in *COL4A3* or *COL4A4*	Variable, 20–100%	Non-Mendelian inheritance simulating AD or AR transmission based on the influence of transcription signals (cis/trans)

(AD: autosomal dominant; AR: autosomal recessive; ESKD: end-stage kidney disease; FSGS: focal segmental glomerulosclerosis; GBM: glomerular basement membrane; SNHL: sensorineural hearing loss)

hematuria of glomerular origin and in older adolescents with chronic glomerulonephritis along with ear and eye manifestations. The presence of an extrarenal abnormality favors AS, but its absence does not rule it out. A thorough history and physical examination must be obtained along with family history. Laboratory evaluation should include urinalysis with urine microscopy and renal function panel. Urinalysis would reveal blood and protein, and urine microscopy should be performed to evaluate for acanthocytes. Any patient with suspected AS should be referred to otorhinolaryngology for high-frequency hearing loss and ophthalmology for the eye examination.[6,7]

Renal Biopsy

Renal biopsy is done when there is proteinuria, presence of red cell casts or acanthocytes, or deranged renal function.

Light microscopy (LM): There are no specific LM findings for AS. Nonspecific findings such as mesangial proliferation, foam cells, focal segmental glomerulosclerosis (FSGS), tubular atrophy, and interstitial fibrosis can be seen.[8]

Electron microscopy (EM): EM is necessary to confirm the diagnosis of AS and will show irregular thinning and thickening of the GBM, lamellations, and splitting of the lamina densa described as a "basket weave pattern." Thinning of GBM in isolation can be present in TBMD and early stages of AS, and hence careful observation of these patients is necessary.[8]

Immunofluorescence/immunohistochemistry: Immunohistology staining for α3, α4, and α5 chains can be done in kidney biopsy specimens to support or refute the diagnosis of AS. In XLAS, α5 staining is absent in about 80% of affected males while in female carriers patchy loss of α5 staining is observed. In ARAS patients, the GBM is negative for α3, α4, and α5 staining, while Bowman's capsule is α5 positive; this is because the GBM consists of α3–α4–α5, but Bowman's capsule consists of α5–α5–α6 and *COL4A3*/*COL4A4* mutations do not influence α5 expression in Bowman's capsule. In ADAS patients, both the GBM and Bowman's capsule exhibit a normal pattern of α5 expression. α5 staining is a useful auxiliary method for diagnosis but normal α5 staining in GBM in up to 20% of males with XLAS.[8]

Skin BM α5 staining can also be used for supportive diagnosis in XLAS as skin consists of type IV collagen α5–α5–α6 triple helix. Male XLAS cases show negativity for α5 expression, while female XLAS cases show a mosaic expression pattern, as observed in GBM.[9]

Genetic Testing

Genetic testing is being used more in recent times to diagnose or confirm the diagnosis of AS. It is accurate and give important prognostic information as it also identifies the type of mutation in the affected gene. Next-generation sequencing (NGS) of *COL4A3*, *COL4A4*, and *COL4A5* genes is recommended in all patients with no family history.[4] While using gene panels for NGS it is important to include genes that cause diseases similar to AS. Examples include branchiootorenal syndrome (BOR) with nephritis and deafness, Fechtner syndrome with macrothrombocytopenia, presenile cataracts, deafness, nephritis due to *MYH9* mutation, and renal diseases with GBM lamellation such as Pierson syndrome and nail patella syndrome.[1] In patients with a positive family history, testing for the target gene can be performed to confirm the diagnosis. If a pathogenic variant is not detected by NGS, screening for copy number variants (CNVs) can be performed by pair analysis or multiplex ligation-dependent probe amplification (MLPA).[1,4]

DIFFERENTIAL DIAGNOSIS

Conditions causing recurrent or persistent microscopic or gross hematuria should be ruled out before diagnosing a child with AS. Differential diagnosis of AS includes IgA nephropathy, membranoproliferative glomerulonephritis (MPGN), mesangioproliferative glomerulonephritis (MesPGN), and TBMD. A positive family history with extrarenal manifestations of hearing loss and ocular anomalies differentiates AS from the above conditions. A kidney biopsy is useful in ruling out these disorders.[7]

TREATMENT

Unfortunately, there is no specific treatment for AS. Treatment is focused primarily on delaying the progression of CKD with renoprotective drugs including angiotensin-converting enzyme inhibitors (ACEIs) or angiotensin receptor blockers (ARB) to reduce proteinuria. Lifestyle modification such as smoking cessation, restricting salt intake, and avoiding over-the-counter medication intake should be advised in all patients to prevent rapid progression to ESKD.[10,11]

Kidney transplantation is the best therapy available for ESKD due to AS and has a good success rate comparable to other kidney diseases. There is a 2–5% risk of developing anti-GBM disease post-transplant which can result in rapid graft loss. Nevertheless, kidney transplant should be offered to all patients with AS for its significant benefit over dialysis.[10,12] There is currently no cure for SNHL and ocular abnormalities seen in AS. Gene therapy, stem cell treatments, and agents including statins and metalloproteinase inhibitors are being evaluated in early phase trials, and much progress is needed before these therapies are available for clinical use.[10]

THIN BASEMENT MEMBRANE DISEASE

The main feature of TBMD is the presence of recurrent hematuria with or without proteinuria associated with thinning of GBM demonstrated in kidney biopsy. The disease is thought to be benign and there is no progressive decline in renal function. Nephrotic range of proteinuria, hypertension, or renal failure is never seen in children with thin basement membrane nephropathy (TBMN). Presence of severe proteinuria, hypertension, and renal failure should suggest the possibility of AS. Also unlike AS, there are no extrarenal anomalies seen in TBMD. However, there is no clear delineation between AS and TBMD and *COL4A3* and *COL4A4* mutations are known to be associated with almost 40% of patients with TBMD.[5] Recently, there is more and more literature to suggest that TBMD is not benign as once thought, and these patients should be considered as part of AS spectrum (carriers in ARAS or patients with ADAS) and monitored frequently for glomerular filtration rate (GFR) decline.[3,4,8]

Renal Biopsy

Light Microscopy

Light microscopy of renal samples in TBMD shows almost normal glomerular architecture with occasional mesangial cellular proliferation and matrix expansion. Slight attenuation of the GBM sometimes can be observed by Jones methenamine silver or periodic acid-Schiff stains, suggestive of GBM thinning. Erythrocytes may be identified in the urinary space.[8]

Immunofluorescence Microscopy

Immunofluorescence staining is invariably negative for immunoglobulin or complement deposition.

Immunochemical Studies

Evaluation of the type IV collagen α 3-5 chains in renal biopsy is used in differentiating between TBMD and early stages of AS with microscopic hematuria and thin GBM. These chains are usually absent in the GBM in AS. In TBMD, the staining is positive as in normal kidneys.[8]

Electron Microscopy

The characteristic finding is the uniform thinning of the GBM in majority of the glomerular capillaries. The podocytes with their foot process are normal. The GBM thickness should be assessed relative to the age of the patient. According to various authors, the GBM thickness increases progressively in children until the age of 11 years. At age 2 days to 1 year, the thickness is 132–208 nm, at age 1–6 years 208–245 nm, and at age 6–11 years 244–307 nm. Generally, in children, the GBM thickness is 150 nm at birth, 200 nm at the age of 1 year, and approaches thickness in adults at the age of 11 years. The mean thickness in male adults is 370 + 50 nm and in female adults is 320 + 50 nm. They have recommended the criteria for TBMD in children to be <200 nm and in adults <264 nm.[5,8]

Treatment

There is no specific therapy for TBMN. The child needs to be monitored for the appearance of hypertension, proteinuria, or renal insufficiency and patients who develop these complications should be treated accordingly.[10]

CONCLUSION

Alport syndrome and TBMDs are genetic diseases due to abnormal collagen IV and can have lifelong renal and extrarenal consequences. Genetic diagnosis and renal biopsy help in the diagnosis and the risk of ESKD is significant in these patients. Current treatment options include renin-angiotensin-aldosterone system (RAAS) blockade to prevent progression to CKD and renal transplant in end-stage renal failure.

KEY POINTS

- AS and TBMD are genetic diseases characterized by mutations in genes *COL4A3*, *COL4A4*, and *COL4A5*.
- These two disorders have a wide clinical presentation ranging from isolated microscopic hematuria to nephropathy leading to ESKD along with extrarenal manifestations. The risk of ESKD varies with the type of inheritance.
- Renal biopsy and genetic analysis remain the cornerstone for accurate diagnosis in suspected patients.
- Currently, renoprotection with RAAS blockade is offered to retard progression, and kidney transplantation can be successfully done in patients with ESKD.

REFERENCES

1. Kashtan CE, Ding J, Garosi G, Heidet L, Massella L, Nakanishi K, et al. Alport syndrome: a unified classification of genetic disorders of collagen IV α345: a position paper of the Alport Syndrome Classification Working Group. Kidney Int. 2018;93(5):1045-51.
2. Kashtan CE. Alport syndrome. Kidney Int. 1997;58:S69-71.
3. Nozu K, Nakanishi K, Abe Y, Udagawa T, Okada S, Okamoto T, et al. A review of clinical characteristics and genetic backgrounds in Alport syndrome. Clin Exp Nephrol. 2019;23(2):158-68.
4. Savige J, Ariani F, Mari F, Bruttini M, Renieri A, Gross O, et al. Expert consensus guidelines for the genetic diagnosis of Alport syndrome. Pediatr Nephrol. 2019;34(7):1175-89.
5. Savige J, Rana K, Tonna S, Buzza M, Dagher H, Wang YY. Thin basement membrane nephropathy. Kidney Int. 2003;64(4):1169-78.
6. Hanson H, Storey H, Pagan J, Flinter F. The value of clinical criteria in identifying patients with X-linked Alport syndrome. Clin J Am Soc Nephrol. 2011;6:198-203.
7. Brown DD, Reidy KJ. Approach to the child with hematuria. Pediatr Clin North Am. 2019;66(1):15-30.
8. Heidet L, Gubler MC. The renal lesions of Alport syndrome. J Am Soc Nephrol. 2009;20:1210-5.
9. van der Loop FT, Monnens LA, Schröder CH, Lemmink HH, Breuning MH, Timmer ED, et al. Identification of COL4A5 defects in Alport's syndrome by immunohistochemistry of skin. Kidney Int. 1999;55(4):1217-24.
10. Savige J, Gregory M, Gross O, Kashtan C, Ding J, Flinter F. Expert guidelines for the management of Alport syndrome and thin basement membrane nephropathy. J Am Soc Nephrol. 2013;24(3):364-75.
11. Proesmans W, Van Dyck M. Enalapril in children with Alport syndrome. Pediatr Nephrol. 2004;19:271-5.
12. Kashtan CE. Renal transplantation in patients with Alport syndrome. Pediatr Transplantation. 2006;10:651-7.

SECTION

7

Kidney Manifestation of Systemic Diseases

CHAPTER

7.1

Tropical Infections, Toxins, and the Kidney

Nivedita Kamath

INTRODUCTION

The tropical regions are geographically described as regions on either side of the equator between the tropics of Cancer and Capricorn. Ecologically, these regions are unique as they receive heavy rainfall and have a high temperature throughout the year. Most importantly, they are home to almost 40% of the world's population. The tropical region also has the most number of countries in the low and lower middle-income categories. The climatic conditions as well as the ecology of the region contribute to a unique spectrum of diseases, including infections and toxin-mediated diseases among others. Several of these diseases affect the kidney with a wide spectrum of renal manifestations ranging from transient urinary abnormalities, acute kidney injury (AKI), and chronic kidney disease (CKD).[1-3] The mechanism of renal involvement, clinical spectrum, and evaluation and management of common infections and toxin-mediated diseases are discussed in this chapter.

TROPICAL INFECTIONS

Tropical infections affecting the kidneys may be attributable to bacteria, viruses, rickettsiae, or parasites.

Mechanisms of Renal Involvement in Tropical Infections

The mechanism of renal involvement in tropical infections is usually multifactorial. Renal involvement may be secondary to pre-renal factors, direct invasion by the infective organism, activation of the immune system, or injury to the capillary endothelium. Often, renal involvement is seen as a consequence of systemic disease.[2,4]

- *Direct invasion of the renal parenchyma/genitourinary system*: Direct invasion by bacterial organisms may result in pyelonephritis or renal abscesses. It is also typically described in schistosomal infections and genitourinary tuberculosis.
- *Immune mediated*: Activation of the immune system by the infective organism could affect the kidney. Bacterial infections result in activation of the T and B cells, resulting in the formation of immune complexes as seen in infection-related glomerulonephritis. Viral infections, such as dengue, trigger the immune system, resulting in tubulointerstitial damage, causing acute interstitial nephritis and acute tubular injury.
- *Injury to the capillary endothelium*: Injury to the capillary endothelium results in microangiopathic hemolysis and thrombotic microangiopathy. This is seen with bacterial infections, such as shigellosis, and parasitic infections, such as falciparum malaria.
- *Systemic effects*: Often, the kidney may be affected secondary to the systemic disease. This may be seen in severe hypovolemic shock, causing acute tubular injury as seen in bacterial sepsis and severe falciparum malaria.[2]

Spectrum of Renal Manifestations

Tropical infections often present as an acute febrile illness with systemic features.[2,4] Renal manifestations in tropical diseases can vary from subtle to life threatening. Tropical diseases could present with a wide spectrum of renal manifestations ranging from asymptomatic proteinuria and hematuria to AKI and CKD. The spectrum of renal manifestations depends on the mechanism of injury and the part of the kidney affected. Glomerular involvement presents as acute glomerulonephritis or nephrotic syndrome, often associated with proteinuria or abnormal urinary sediment, e.g., malarial nephropathy and leptospirosis. Predominant tubulo-interstitial involvement often presents as abnormal urinary sediments alone without symptoms, AKI following acute tubular necrosis, or acute tubulointerstitial nephritis, e.g., leptospirosis and falciparum malaria. Some diseases such as tuberculosis, schistosomiasis, hepatitis B, and hepatitis C virus infections have been implicated to result in CKD in adult patients from tropical regions. The spectrum of renal manifestations in common tropical infections is described in **Table 1**.

Renal Involvement in Specific Conditions

Bacterial Infections

Leptospirosis

Etiology: Leptospirosis, caused by the spirochete *Leptospira interrogans*, is prevalent as both an epidemic and an endemic zoonosis in the tropics. Leptospira is excreted in the urine of the rat, which is its major reservoir. In the human host, the blood-borne spirochete enters the kidney by invading the

TABLE 1: The spectrum of renal manifestations in common tropical infections.[2,4]

Infection	Proteinuria	Abnormal urine sediment*	Acute kidney injury	Chronic kidney disease	Renal histology
Bacterial					
Leptospira	++++	++++	++++	–	ATN, AIN
Enteric fever	++	++	+	–	MPGN, AIN
Cholera	–	–	++	–	ATN
Scrub typhus	++	+	+	–	ATN, AIN
Tuberculosis	+	++	–	++	AIN
Viral					
Dengue	+	++	++	–	ATN, MPGN
Yellow fever	–	–	++	–	ATN
Hanta	+	+	++	–	ATN
Parasitic					
Malaria	+	+	+++	+	ATN, AIN, MPGN
Filariasis	++	++	+	–	MPGN, FSGS
Schistosomiasis	++	++	++	++	MGN, FSGS
Leishmaniasis	++	+	++	++	MPGN, Amyloidosis
Trypanosomiasis	++	+	+	–	MPGN

*Abnormal urinary sediment refers to the presence of cells such as red blood cells (RBCs), white blood cells (WBCs), and casts.
(AIN: acute interstitial nephritis; ATN: acute tubular necrosis; FSGS: focal segmental glomerulosclerosis; MGN: membranous glomerulonephritis; MPGN: membranoproliferative glomerulonephritis)
Source: Adapted from Rashad B, Francis Magdi SV. Tropical diseases. In: Atlas of Diseases of Kidney. Vol 4. Philadelphia: Current Medicine Inc.; 1999. pp. 6-18.

capillary endothelium, adheres to the tubular epithelium, and invades into the renal interstitium.[5,6]

Pathophysiology: The pathophysiology of kidney involvement in leptospirosis is acute tubular necrosis or acute tubulo-interstitial nephritis, which is mediated by immune mechanisms as well as a direct invasion of the renal tubules. Hypovolemic shock, hyperbilirubinemia, and rhabdomyolysis which are present in severe disease may contribute to AKI. Prerenal AKI could be due to hypovolemic shock. Occasionally, glomerular involvement due to immune-mediated injury resulting in proteinuria and abnormal urinary sediments may be seen.[7]

Clinical manifestations: The clinical manifestations of Leptospirosis may vary from a mild febrile illness to a severe form—Weil's disease, characterized by severe multisystem involvement including jaundice, hemorrhagic manifestations, and AKI. The initial febrile phase is followed by an immune phase with multisystem manifestations.[4]

The renal manifestations of leptospirosis vary from asymptomatic proteinuria, hematuria, and abnormal urinary sediment to AKI. AKI, the most common manifestation, has been reported in both the icteric and anicteric phases in about 10–60% of patients in various reports.[4,5,7] AKI is often seen in severe disease and is an important predictor of mortality. Leptospiral AKI is often nonoliguric.[8] Studies in experimental animals have shown a significant proximal tubular involvement, resulting in low-molecular-weight proteinuria, phosphaturia, and low fractional excretion of sodium. Overactivity of the sodium–potassium chloride channel (NKCC) in the loop of Henle and medullary resistance to vasopressin result in preservation of the urine output, hypomagnesemia, and hypokalemia.[5]

Evaluation: Dark-field illumination of the urine may show spirochetes in the first few weeks of the illness. Leptospira can be isolated from the blood or cerebro-spinal fluid (CSF) in the first 2 weeks of the illness and from the urine between the second and third weeks. However, it requires special media such as Fletcher's media and is a fastidious organism taking about 4 weeks to grow in culture media.[5] The microscopic agglutination test showing a fourfold rise in antibody titers when performed 2 weeks apart is diagnostic.[5,7] ELISA for rapid testing of IgM antibodies against leptospira may be useful in the first week of the illness. Real-time PCR is a sensitive method to detect leptospiral DNA in the blood of infected persons.

Renal biopsy, if done, shows acute tubular injury. Inflammatory infiltration in the interstitium with interstitial edema is not uncommon. Rarely, bile casts and heme casts may be seen. Though glomeruli are most often normal, occasionally there may be mesangial proliferation, focal necrotizing glomerulonephritis, or hemorrhagic vasculitis.[5]

Management: Antibiotics, such as intravenous penicillin or third-generation cephalosporins, are the first line of the specific therapy. Supportive therapy consists of fluid therapy, inotropic support, respiratory support, and maintenance of electrolyte and acid-base balance. Kidney replacement therapy (KRT) is reported to be required in about 60% of adults with severe renal dysfunction. There is no consensus on the optimal modality of KRT in leptospiral AKI. In children, peritoneal dialysis, hemodialysis, and hemofiltration have been used.[7] Timely initiation of dialysis may reduce mortality. Plasmapheresis has also been tried in severe forms of leptospiral AKI.[7]

Rickettsial infection: Rickettsial infections are endemic infections transmitted by fleas, ticks, or mites. Renal involvement is typically seen in scrub typhus, Rocky Mountain spotted fever, tick typhus, and Q fever. The endothelial cells of the capillaries in the kidney are the target cells for rickettsia.[9-11]

Scrub typhus caused by *Orientia tsutsugamushi* is an important cause of rickettsial infection in India. Renal involvement has been reported in about 80% of patients with scrub typhus.[4] AKI is not only the most common renal manifestation but also an important predictor of outcome.

Acute kidney injury is the most common renal manifestation in other rickettsial infections as well. Acute proliferative glomerulonephritis with immune complex deposition, acute tubulo-interstitial nephritis, asymptomatic proteinuria, and hematuria have also been reported.

Though commonly used in clinical practice, serological assays such as the Weil-Felix test have poor sensitivity. Real-time polymerase chain reaction (PCR) has a higher sensitivity for the detection of rickettsial infection. Doxycycline is the drug of choice in the treatment of rickettsial infection. Management of AKI is usually supportive.

Tuberculosis

Epidemiology: Urogenital tuberculosis (UTB) accounts for 15–20% of extrapulmonary tuberculosis. Though rare in children, UTB may be seen in immunosuppressed children and adolescents.[12]

Pathophysiology: UTB occurs by hematogenous/lymphatic spread from a primary focus, most often from a pulmonary focus. The seeding of the bacteria occurs most often in the kidney, resulting in the formation of granulomas. Granulomatous inflammation results in chronic tubulo-interstitial nephritis, papillary necrosis, ulcers, and cavitatory fibrosis. The dissemination of infection to the pelvis can result in tubercular pyelonephritis and pyonephrosis. Extensive necrosis of the renal parenchyma results in caseation and formation of a "putty kidney." Calcification occurs in the areas of necrosis.

Ureteric involvement occurs secondary to renal involvement by the spread of the bacilli downstream. Ureteric inflammation with ulceration, granulomas, and necrosis resulting in fibrosis are common. There may be multiple ureteric strictures giving a corkscrew appearance on imaging. Obstruction along the ureter results in hydronephrosis.

Bladder involvement may be secondary to renal and ureteric tuberculosis or by lymphatic spread from the primary focus. The initial presentation may be as cystitis, resulting in sterile pyuria. Chronic inflammation of the bladder and vesicoureteric junction result in a golf-hole appearance and vesicoureteric reflux. Chronic inflammation and fibrosis of the bladder result in a small-capacity, thickened bladder called "thimble bladder." Rarely, a fistula may be formed between the bladder and other pelvic organs.

Clinical features: Clinical manifestations vary from an asymptomatic presentation to features of chronic cystitis, obstructive uropathy, and CKD.

Evaluation: Diagnosis is confirmed by demonstration of the bacilli in three consecutive early morning specimens of urine. Real-time quantitative PCR is a highly sensitive test for the diagnosis of bacilli in the urine. Histological demonstration of acid-fast bacilli with granulomatous inflammation also confirms the diagnosis of tuberculosis.

Radiological evaluation of the urogenital tract may demonstrate a wide variety of abnormalities. Abdominal X-rays and intravenous urogram are no longer used as common modalities for imaging. Ultrasonographic evaluation and CT scan may show characteristic abnormalities attributable to UTB.

Management: Treatment consists of antitubercular therapy typically given as four drugs (isoniazid, rifampicin, pyrazinamide, and ethambutol) for 2 months as intensive-phase therapy followed by 4 months of continuation phase with two drugs (isoniazid and rifampicin).

Surgical intervention may be required for drainage of obstructive hydronephrosis and reconstruction of bladder and ureters.

Viral Infections

Dengue: Dengue, a flavivirus is transmitted by the bite of the female *Aedes aegypti* mosquito. The severe forms of dengue—dengue hemorrhagic fever and dengue shock syndrome—are often associated with multisystem involvement.[13,14] AKI is the most common renal manifestation in severe dengue infection. The wide spectrum of other renal manifestations includes asymptomatic proteinuria, hematuria, and glomerulonephritis. The prevalence of AKI in dengue has been reported to be about 0.9–10% in children and around 2.2–35.7% in adults. AKI in dengue infection may be pre-renal in the early phase of the disease and may progress to acute tubular necrosis due to ischemia associated with hypotension or inflammatory cytokines. Nephrotoxic medications, hemolysis, and rhabdomyolysis are other important risk factors for AKI. Electrolyte abnormalities, such as hyponatremia, are frequently seen due to fluid overload or inappropriate fluid therapy. Asymptomatic hematuria and proteinuria may be prevalent in one third of patients with dengue infection. Glomerulonephritis is often mild, caused by the cytotoxic effects of the virus itself or due to immune complex deposits. Thrombotic microangiopathy also has been rarely reported.[15]

The diagnosis of dengue infection is made by antigen detection (NS1 antigen) early in the course of the disease from the time of onset of symptoms or by antibody detection (IgM by ELISA) after 4 days from the onset of symptoms. Other supportive evidence to the diagnosis of dengue may be leucopenia with relative lymphocytosis, severe thrombocytopenia, hemoconcentration (rising hematocrit), and abnormal coagulation parameters.[4]

The WHO guidelines discuss the fluid therapy and supportive management of dengue in adults and children. KRT may be required in cases of fluid overload or to facilitate the provision of fluid therapy. Studies from southeast Asian countries show that about 50% of children with dengue and severe AKI require KRT. Though there is no evidence-based consensus on the modality of dialysis, slower therapies such as continuous KRT and slow low-efficiency dialysis may be required in children with dengue shock syndrome. In low-resource countries, peritoneal dialysis may be the feasible modality of dialysis. Mortality is about 12–44% in children and adults. AKI is an important risk factor for mortality.[14]

Hanta virus:[16,17] It belongs to the family Bunyaviridae and is transmitted by bites or exposure to aerosolized droppings of infected rodents. Hanta virus infection results in hemorrhagic fever. Severe manifestations are reported as hemorrhagic fever with renal syndrome (HFRS) from Asia and Europe and hemorrhagic fever cardiopulmonary syndrome in South America. The clinical presentation of the infections typically follows five phases: febrile, hypotensive, oliguric, polyuric, and convalescent. The renal manifestations may vary from mild hematuria and proteinuria to AKI. AKI is often associated with thrombocytopenia, proteinuria, and elevated C reactive protein. Renal biopsy shows acute tubular necrosis with interstitial edema and hemorrhage.

The diagnosis of Hanta virus infection may be made by the demonstration of immunoglobulin M (IgM) by ELISA (enzyme-linked immunoassay), usually in the first 3 weeks of the illness. Later in the course, a fourfold rise in IgG titers may be helpful in the diagnosis.

Treatment is mainly supportive. Ribavirin has been used to reduce the severity of illness and is found to be useful early in the course of the disease. KRT is rarely required.

Yellow fever:[13] It is caused by a flavivirus and transmitted by the bite of the *Aedes aegypti* mosquito. Yellow fever is endemic in certain regions of Africa and South America.

It manifests as a hemorrhagic febrile illness with multi-organ involvement. Hepatic disease, hemorrhagic manifestation, disseminated intravascular coagulation, and shock are seen in severe disease. Severe disease is often associated with AKI, which may be pre-renal or due to acute tubular necrosis. Yellow fever is diagnosed by the demonstration of IgM antibodies on ELISA or isolation of the virus by PCR. Liver biopsy, when done, may show the characteristic Councilman bodies.

Treatment is predominantly supportive. Yellow-fever vaccination is recommended for all travelers going to endemic areas.

Parasitic Infections

Malaria:

Etiology: Malaria, a parasitic infection caused by *Plasmodium vivax*, *P. falciparum*, *P. ovale*, and *P. malariae*, is spread by the bite of the Anopheles mosquito. The sporozoites in the salivary gland of the mosquito enter the bloodstream of the host during a bite and reach the liver of the host. In the liver, they multiply and form merozoites that are released into the bloodstream. They then attack the RBCs and go through the phases of trophozoite, schizont, and merozoites that are released back into circulation by the rupture of RBC. Some merozoites transform into gametocytes that are taken up by the mosquito. The male and female gametocytes fuse to form the zygote, the ookinete, and then the sporozoite, and the life cycle continues.

Pathophysiology: Malarial AKI is a common complication of severe malaria caused by *P. falciparum* or *P. vivax*. Nonendemic population, high parasite load (infected RBC > 5%), children, HIV infection, and travelers visiting endemic areas are important risk factors for severe malaria. AKI is often associated with multisystem involvement, typically cerebral malaria.

The pathophysiology of AKI in malaria is multifactorial. The RBCs affected by *P. falciparum* are less deformable and more prone to hemolysis. The erythrocyte membrane protein of the parasite is expressed on the surface of these RBCs, making them prone to adhesion and aggregation. The adhesion of parasitized RBC to the vascular endothelial cell results in occlusion of the microvasculature, resulting in hypoxia to major organs. There is also a significant release of inflammatory cytokines that play an important role in causing AKI. Also, complicated malaria is often associated with fluid loss, reduced fluid intake, and hypotension, resulting in renal hypoperfusion. Massive hemolysis causes hemoglobinuria (blackwater fever) that may, by itself, cause pigment-induced nephrotoxicity. Rarely, rhabdomyolysis or thrombotic microangiopathy may contribute to AKI in children with severe malaria.[18,19]

Clinical features: Severe malaria is a systemic illness that often presents with severe anemia, jaundice, hypoglycemia, lactic acidosis, and cerebral malaria. AKI is seen in the first 3–7 days of onset of symptoms and is usually oligoanuric. Hyponatremia, hyperkalemia, and metabolic acidosis are often present. The spectrum of renal involvement in malaria is varied and is usually seen in infections secondary to *P. vivax*, *P. falciparum*, and *P. malariae*. Renal involvement is seen in about 62.5% of *P. falciparum*, and 28.6% of *P. vivax* and *P. falciparum* are often associated with severe malaria and AKI.[18] Malarial AKI was seen in 0.6–2% of children with AKI from centers in India; however, in certain African countries, malaria is the third most common cause of AKI in children. Rarely, acute glomerulonephritis and thrombotic microangiopathy may also be seen with these infections. *P. malariae* is associated with chronic malarial nephropathy. Children with severe malaria are often hypercatabolic and require KRT.

Evaluation: The demonstration of the parasite on a peripheral smear examination or a rapid antigen detection by ELISA is required for the diagnosis of malaria. Intravenous artesunate is the initial drug of choice in severe malaria. A single dose of primaquine is given to prevent relapse of *P. falciparum* infection. In situations where artesunate is not available, intravenous quinine may be used with strict monitoring.

Management: Provision of appropriate fluids and inotropic support, correction of electrolytes, acid-base imbalance, and hypoglycemia is the supportive care of children with severe malaria. Dialysis is indicated in progressive or severe renal failure with features of pulmonary edema, refractory hyperkalemia, or refractory metabolic acidosis. The choice of modality depends on hemodynamic stability, feasibility, and availability of dialysis modality. There is some data from developing countries on the use of peritoneal dialysis in children with severe malaria. Mortality in children with malarial AKI ranges from 5 to 25%. Severe AKI requiring dialysis along with younger age, hypotension, and severe anemia are poor prognostic factors.[4]

Acute glomerulonephritis: P. falciparum and *P. vivax* may be associated with acute glomerulonephritis. Although it is often asymptomatic, mild proteinuria and microscopic hematuria may be seen on urinalysis. Usually, the renal function is not deranged and hypertension is rare. The glomerulonephritis is self-limiting. Renal biopsy is often not indicated, but when done, it may show mild mesangial proliferation and basement membrane changes with deposits of C3 and IgM along the capillary wall and mesangium. Electron microscopy shows mesangial and subendothelial electron-dense deposits.[19]

Malarial nephropathy:[20] Chronic malarial nephropathy was described in tropical regions, especially in African countries, as a progressive disorder characterized by persistent proteinuria. About 3–4 decades ago, quartan malaria caused by *P. malariae* was reported to cause 80% of nephrotic syndrome in children who responded poorly to immunosuppression and progressed to renal failure. However, in more recent times, there are no reports of chronic malarial nephropathy and that is perhaps attributable to effective treatment of malaria with antimalarial drugs.

Chronic malarial nephropathy is considered an immune complex disease characterized by thickening of the glomerular capillary wall, frequent splitting, and double contour of the basement membrane with deposits of complement, IgM, and IgG along the capillary membrane. Electron microscopy shows the flaking or fibrillary splitting of the basement membrane.[19]

Schistosomiasis:[21,22] Schistosomiasis caused by the parasite schistosoma is seen in tropical countries of Africa and South America. The common species causing disease in humans are *Schistosoma mansoni, S. japonicum,* and *S. hematobium.*

Involvement of the urinary tract is usually seen in *S. hematobium* infection. The adult forms of the parasite reside in the mesenteric and perivesical venules, and the eggs are released into the bladder. The eggs produce proteolytic enzymes which cause inflammation and ulceration of the bladder. In the initial stages, this manifests as hematuria, dysuria, pollakiuria, and proteinuria. The symptoms may often be treated as urinary tract infection. Cystoscopy would reveal the presence of polyps, nodules, and inflammation of the bladder mucosa. The eggs hatch and release miracidia which penetrate the snail (intermediate host), where they undergo asexual reproduction and cercaria are released. The cercaria enters the bloodstream by penetrating the skin and reaches the mesenteric and perivesical venous plexus.

Chronic infection results in chronic inflammation and fibrosis of the bladder and ureters, causing hydronephrosis. Secondary bacterial infections and calculi are common secondary complications. Chronic inflammation is also a risk factor for bladder carcinoma later in life.

Rarely, chronic schistosomiasis may present as glomerulopathy. This is typically seen in hepatosplenic schistosomiasis. Often, it is asymptomatic, though rarely, it may present as persistent proteinuria, hematuria, or hypocomplementemic acute glomerulonephritis. Renal biopsy may show mesangioproliferative or membranoproliferative glomerulonephritis. Rarely membranous nephropathy, focal segmental glomerulosclerosis, and amyloidosis have been reported.

Diagnosis of schistosomiasis is made by demonstration of the eggs of the parasite in a centrifuged sample of urine. Cystoscopy and contrast urography show the sequelae of chronic inflammation.

Praziquantel is used in the treatment of schistosomiasis. It paralyses the adult form but does not affect the eggs. Steroids may be added to control the inflammatory response.

Toxins

Toxins derived from local flora and fauna are an important cause of renal injury in the tropics. In addition, exposure to certain chemicals and traditional medicines also contribute to renal disease. These conditions are reported commonly from the adult population. The mechanism of renal involvement and evaluation and management of commonly reported toxin-mediated renal disease are discussed below.

Snake envenomation

Etiology: Snake envenomation is an important cause of community-acquired AKI in tropical countries. Renal manifestations are seen following envenomation by snakes belonging to the Elapidae, Colubridae, and Viperidae families.

Pathophysiology: Snake venom contains several enzymes such as proteases, hydrolases, and phospholipases which cause direct cell toxicity and tissue injury. Also, it contains toxins that incite an inflammatory response. The immunological reaction to toxins can cause anaphylaxis, release of inflammatory cytokines, and free-radical generation, which results in hemodynamic changes, activation of complement, increased vascular permeability, and altered coagulation profile. The direct cell toxicity results in the modulation of ion channels, membrane lysis, and disruption of cytoskeleton.[23]

Clinical manifestations: The spectrum of renal manifestations is varied. AKI is the most common manifestation and is often due to acute tubular necrosis. Acute tubular necrosis may be secondary to the hemodynamic effect of the venom and could also be pigment induced, following massive hemolysis or rhabdomyolysis and resulting in hemoglobinuria and myoglobinuria, respectively. AKI may be secondary to toxic acute interstitial nephritis **(Fig. 1)**, thrombotic microangiopathy, and rarely cortical necrosis. Glomerulonephritis and vasculitis are rare manifestations and may be secondary to direct toxicity of the venom. Asymptomatic hematuria and proteinuria have been described, and rarely proteinuria may be in the nephrotic range. Hypersensitivity to antivenom could also result in interstitial nephritis.[24]

Management: Acute kidney injury is seen after hemotoxic or myotoxic bites. The incidence of AKI ranges from 5 to 29% in adults. AKI can be seen within a few hours of the bite to as late as 96 hours. AKI is usually severe, oligoanuric, and often requires dialysis. Early and frequent dialysis is required in AKI secondary to snake envenomation. There is little evidence on the best modality for dialysis in adults or children with snake bite-induced AKI. Monovalent antivenom is the treatment of choice. Early administration of antivenom results in a significant improvement in outcome.[23]

Bites of other animals and insects

Bee and wasp sting:[25] Multiple stings by honeybees and hornets are reported to cause severe rhabdomyolysis, resulting in AKI. AKI may be multifactorial, resulting from renal vasoconstriction, direct cellular toxicity, and hemolysis, and mediated by inflammatory cytokines. The most common histopathological manifestation is acute tubular necrosis.

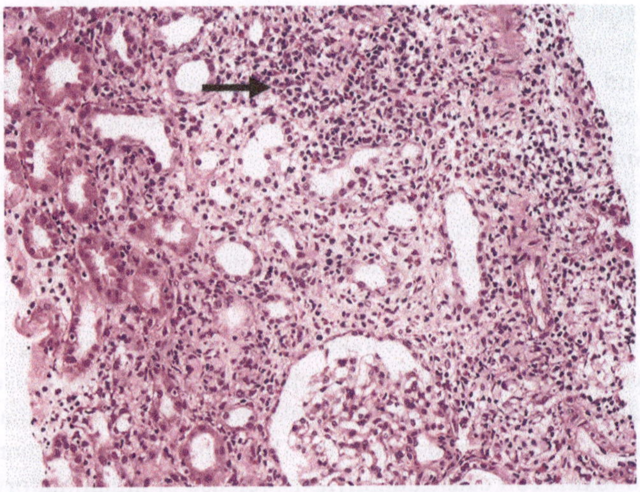

Fig. 1: Renal histopathology (H and E stain) depicting acute interstitial nephritis following a snake bite. The arrow points to an area of lymphocytic infiltrate and edema in the interstitium with widely separated tubules.

Source: With permission from Dr Anila Abraham, Nephropathologist, Renopath, Chennai.

Plasmapheresis and continuous kidney replacement therapy have been used in the treatment of oliguric AKI resulting from bee stings. Wasp stings are also associated with severe rhabdomyolysis and AKI in tropical countries.

Scorpion sting: It is common in tropical rural areas, especially in summer. The venom contains toxins which cause an increased adrenergic and cholinergic activity resulting in cardiac and multiorgan dysfunction. Though renal involvement is rare, severe vasoconstriction, rhabdomyolysis, and direct cellular toxicity have been reported to result in acute tubular necrosis, interstitial inflammation, and thrombotic microangiopathy on renal histology.[25]

Plant toxins: Several plant toxins when consumed alone or as traditional medicines are reported to have nephrotoxic effects.

Djenkol beans can cause loin pain, gross hematuria, oliguria, nausea, and vomiting, and AKI in severe cases. Poisonous mushrooms (*Amanita* species) contain phallotoxins which can cause necrosis of the liver and kidney, resulting in hepatic and renal failure. Liquorice contains glycyrrhizic acid which can result in life-threatening hypokalemia.

Aristolochia is a common herb used in traditional Chinese remedies and can cause chronic interstitial nephritis/aristolochic acid nephropathy (previously known as Chinese herb nephropathy). Balkan endemic nephropathy is also attributable to aristolochic acid. Aristolochic acid, the active ingredient, is a known carcinogen and causes urothelial cancers.[26]

Star fruit (*Averrhoa carambola*) consumption has been documented to result in neurotoxicity (confusion, seizures, status epilepticus) and nephrotoxicity. The fruit contains high levels of oxalate which, in addition to precipitation in the renal tubules resulting in calcium oxalate production and causing acute oxalate nephropathy, also have cytotoxic effects on the renal tubular cells.[27]

Traditional medicines: These are widely used in tropical countries. These medicines contain plant products which may have nephrotoxic properties, e.g., aristolochic acid, and heavy metals such as lead, mercury, and arsenic which can cause both AKI and CKD. In addition, traditional medicines promote polypharmacy with unknown drug interactions, and result in delay in diagnosis and treatment of the underlying disease.[28]

Chronic Kidney Disease of Unknown Origin

CKD of unknown origin (CKDu) in the tropical regions of Asia (Sri Lanka and India) and Latin America (Mesoamerican nephropathy) are now included under the term "chronic interstitial nephritis in agricultural communities (CINAC)." The etiology is multifactorial—exposure to agro-chemicals, contaminated water, heat stress, repeated episodes of dehydration, use of traditional medicines, and genetic susceptibility are all possible risk factors. This condition affects young men and women in agricultural communities and is characterized by the absence other risk factors for kidney disease such as diabetes, hypertension, glomerular disease, or other known causes of CKD. This is a slowly progressive disease with minimal proteinuria. Tubular proteinuria, polyuria, metabolic alkalosis, tubular wasting of sodium, potassium, phosphate, and magnesium may be seen in early stages of CKD. The renal histology shows chronic tubulointerstitial nephritis, glomerulosclerosis, fibrous intimal thickening, and arteriolar hyalinosis.[29]

CONCLUSION

Tropical infections and toxin-mediated diseases, though prevalent in the tropics, are emerging as a global concern with an increase in travel and immigration. The kidney and the urinary tract are frequently involved in these diseases, and the manifestations of renal involvement are protean. A high index of suspicion is often required for early diagnosis and management. These diseases contribute significantly to the incidence of AKI and require timely management, including KRT in children as well as adults. Many of these diseases are preventable by improving hygiene and living conditions in these regions.

KEY POINTS

- Tropical infections, animal- and plant-related toxins are important causes of kidney diseases, especially AKI in the tropical zones.
- Infections are caused by a wide spectrum of organisms ranging from bacteria, viruses, and parasites, the most common being leptospirosis, tuberculosis, dengue, malaria, and schistosomiasis.
- The spectrum of kidney manifestations in tropical infections is varied. These diseases may present as asymptomatic proteinuria or hematuria, AKI, nephrotic syndrome, or CKD.
- Animal- and plant-related toxins present with a wide spectrum of renal manifestations and require a high index of suspicion for diagnosis and appropriate management.

REFERENCES

1. Jha V, Parameswaran S. Community-acquired acute kidney injury in tropical countries. Nat Rev Nephrol. 2013;9(5):278-90.
2. Rashad B, Francis Magdi SV. Tropical diseases. In: Atlas of Diseases of Kidney. Philadelphia: Current Medicine Inc.; 1999. pp. 6-18.
3. Jha V, Chugh KS. Community-acquired acute kidney injury in Asia. Semin Nephrol. 2008;28(4):330-47.
4. Kamath N, Iyengar A. Infections and the kidney: a tale from the tropics. Pediatr Nephrol. 2017;33(8):1317-26.
5. Andrade L, de Francesco Daher E, Seguro AC. Leptospiral nephropathy. Semin Nephrol. 2008;28(4):383-94.
6. Haake DA, Levett PN. Leptospira in humans. Curr Top Microbiol Immunol. 2015;387:65-97.
7. Visith S, Kearkiat P. Nephropathy in leptospirosis. J Postgrad Med. 2005;51(3):184-8.
8. Abdulkader RCRM, Silva MV. The kidney in leptospirosis. Pediatr Nephrol. 2008;23(12):2111-20.
9. Mahajan SK. Rickettsial diseases. J Assoc Physic India. 2012;60: 37-44.
10. Rathi N, Kulkarni AYV. IAP guidelines on rickettsial diseases in children. Indian Pediatr. 2017;54:223-9.
11. Cowan G. Rickettsial diseases: the typhus group of fevers—a review. Postgrad Med J. 2000;76(895):269-72.
12. Muneer A, Macrae B, Krishnamoorthy S, Zumla A. Urogenital tuberculosis—epidemiology, pathogenesis and clinical features. Nat Rev Urol. 2019;16(10):573-98.
13. Lima EQ, Nogueira ML. Viral hemorrhagic fever-induced acute kidney injury. Semin Nephrol. 2008;28(4):409-15.
14. Country Office for India, World Health Organization. (2015). National guidelines for clinical management of dengue fever. WHO Country Office for India. [online] Available from https://apps.who.int/iris/handle/10665/208893 [Last accessed September, 2021].
15. Vachvanichsanong P, Thisyakorn U, Thisyakorn C. Dengue hemorrhagic fever and the kidney. Arch Virol. 2016;161(4):771-8.
16. Ferluga D, Vizjak A. Hantavirus nephropathy. J Am Soc Nephrol. 2008;19:1653-8.
17. Latus J, Schwab M, Tacconelli E, Pieper FM, Daniel W, Rettenmaier B, et al. Acute kidney injury and tools for risk-stratification in 456 patients with hantavirus-induced nephropathia epidemica. Nephrol Dial Transplant. 2015;30(2): 245-51.
18. Mishra SK, Das BS. Malaria and acute kidney injury. Semin Nephrol. 2008;28(4):395-408.
19. Ehrich JHH, Eke FU. Malaria-induced renal damage: facts and myths. Pediatr Nephrol. 2007;22(5):626-37.
20. Olowu WA, Adelusola KA, Adefehinti O, Oyetunji TG. Quartan malaria-associated childhood nephrotic syndrome: Now a rare clinical entity in malaria endemic Nigeria. Nephrol Dial Transplant. 2010;25(3):794-801.
21. da Silva GB, Duarte DB, Barros EJG, De Francesco Daher E. Schistosomiasis-associated kidney disease: a review. Asian Pacific J Trop Dis. 2013;3(1):79-84.
22. Barsoum RS. Schistosomal glomerulopathies. Kidney Int. 1993;44(1):1-12.
23. Sitprija V. Snakebite nephropathy. 2006;11(5):442-8.
24. Sitprija V. Animal toxins and the kidney. 2008;4(11):616-27.
25. de Oliveira NA, Cardoso SC, Barbosa DA, da Fonseca CD. Acute kidney injury caused by venomous animals: inflammatory mechanisms. J Venom Anim Toxins Incl Trop Dis. 2021;27:20200189.
26. Jha V, Chugh KS. Nephropathy associated with animal, plant, and chemical toxins in the tropics. Semin Nephrol. 2003;23(1):49-65.
27. Wijayaratne DR, Bavanthan V, de Silva MVC, Nazar ALM, Wijewickrama ES. Star fruit nephrotoxicity: a case series and literature review. BMC Nephrol. 2018;19(1):288.
28. Luyckx V, Naicker S. Acute kidney injury associated with the use of traditional medicines. Nat Rev Nephrol. 2008;4:664-71.
29. Weaver VM, Fadrowski JJ, Jaar BG. Global dimensions of chronic kidney disease of unknown etiology (CKDu): a modern era environmental and/or occupational nephropathy? BMC Nephrol. 2015;16:145.

CHAPTER

7.2 Lupus Nephritis

Susan Uthup

INTRODUCTION

Systemic lupus erythematosus (SLE) is a chronic, systemic autoimmune disease with pleomorphic manifestations. It is characterized by immune dysregulation and formation of a variety of autoantibodies directed against different cell components, causing chronic inflammation and damage to target organs such as kidneys, joints, skin, pleura, heart, hematopoietic system, liver, lung, and brain. The clinical course is chronic and is characterized by exacerbations or flares and periods of remissions.[1] Pediatric-onset SLE (pSLE) accounts for 10–20% of all SLE. It is usually more severe with a higher disease activity over time and renal and neurological involvement.[2] Lupus nephritis (LN) affects 50–75% of all children with SLE, mostly within the first 2 years of diagnosis, with a higher prevalence in Asians. It remains a major contributor to morbidity and mortality in childhood-onset lupus.[2-4]

EPIDEMIOLOGY

The incidence rates of pSLE have been reported to be 0.3–0.9 per 100,000 children-years, with prevalence rates of 3.3–8.8 per 100,000 children. The median age of onset of pSLE is between 11 and 12 years.[2] The disease is quite rare in children under the age of 5 years. Peak incidence is around puberty. The disease is often more acute and severe in children less than 16 years. The occurrence of nephritis varies from 30 to 80%. Girls are affected more than boys even in prepubertal age. The female/male ratio increases from 2:1 in prepubertal children to 4.5:1 in adolescents and 8:1 in adults.[1,5]

ETIOPATHOGENESIS

The exact pathogenesis of SLE is not clear. SLE occurs in genetically predisposed individuals who are exposed to environmental triggers. A complex interaction between genetic susceptibility factors, environmental triggers, viral and bacterial antigens, antigen–antibody responses, B-cell and T-cell interactions, and immune clearance processes leads to loss of self-tolerance and subsequent autoimmune responses in SLE.[1,6]

The familial prevalence is 1.3–12%.[7] First-degree relatives are more often affected. Concordance rates are higher in monozygotic twins (20–40%) than in dizygotic twins and siblings (2–5%).[8] Monogenic forms of SLE have been identified in children mainly due to defects in the complement system; type I interferon pathway; aberrant nucleic acid repair, degradation, and sensing; or abnormal B-cell development.[9,10]

HLA-B8, HLA-DR2, and HLA-DR3 occur with increased frequency in SLE. Complement C4 and Fc receptor genes are also implicated. Congenital deficiencies in the early components of the classical pathway (C1q, C1r, C1s, C2, or C3) and low copy numbers of C4 predispose to the development of SLE. Inherited or acquired C1q deficiency is particularly important due to functional consequences, including the defective clearance of apoptotic bodies and reduced phagocytosis. The cellular debris may persist longer and contribute to the loss of self-tolerance and to the development of autoimmunity.[1,11]

Environmental factors induce epigenetic alterations, i.e., variations in gene expression that may trigger the onset of SLE. Epigenetic changes may be caused by factors such as viral infection like Epstein–Barr virus (EBV), sun exposure, hormonal alterations, nutrition, drugs like anticonvulsants, and antiarrhythmic physical and mental stress. Sunlight exposure and UV radiation cause inflammation and apoptosis of keratinocytes, thus triggering SLE. The strong predominance of SLE in females underlines the influence of hormonal factors, especially estrogen.[1,12] The initial trigger for SLE is loss of immune tolerance. The T-cell-dependent autoimmune response is mainly driven by nucleosome. Nucleosome is the fundamental unit of chromatin and is composed of DNA wrapped around histones. Abnormal regulation of apoptosis and impaired clearance of apoptotic products have been demonstrated in lupus. Neutrophil apoptosis (NETosis) is normally a host defense mechanism to trap and kill microorganisms. NETosis results in release of neutrophil extracellular traps (NETs) composed of chromatin fibrils, histones, and neutrophil antibacterial and immunostimulatory proteins. The released nuclear self-antigens will be processed by antigen-presenting cells (APCs) normally. This is delayed in SLE, thereby exposing self-antigen to immune system.[13,14]

Genetic defects of complement system also lead to flaws in opsonization, thus impairing the clearance of self-antigens.

Dendritic cells, the key regulators of immune system, are also affected in SLE. Nuclear self-antigen internalization and recognition by toll-like receptors promote the conversion of dendritic cells into APCs and lead to activation of autoreactive T cells. The autoreactive T cells amplify the immune response by increasing the production of T and B cells in the bone marrow and lymphoid organs. Active B cells differentiate into plasma B cells or memory B cells. Human regulatory T cells (Tregs) normally suppress B- and T-cell-mediated autoantibody production. Tregs are reduced in number and functionally defective in SLE. Autoreactive B cells process and present self-antigens to T cells, promoting proinflammatory cytokine activation. Abnormalities in B-cell tolerance thus lead to autoantibody production.[9,10,15]

AUTOANTIBODIES IN SYSTEMIC LUPUS ERYTHEMATOSUS

The hallmark of lupus is antibody production against self-antigens, particularly antinuclear antibodies (ANAs) to DNA and other nuclear antigens such as ribosomes, small nuclear (anti-Sm) and cytoplasmic (anti-Ro, anti-La) ribonuclear proteins, platelets, coagulation factors, immunoglobulin, erythrocytes, and leukocytes.[16] These are associated with circulating and tissue-bound immune complexes, which lead to complement fixation and recruitment of inflammatory cells, culminating in tissue injury. Presence of ANA is not unique to SLE because they can be detected in other rheumatologic disorders such as chronic juvenile arthritis, scleroderma or mixed connective tissue disease, autoimmune hepatitis, thyroiditis, or after taking certain medications. High levels of ANA are highly suggestive of SLE.[17]

Anti-dsDNA antibodies are more specific to SLE. They can be detected in the serum by measuring their capacity to bind radio-labeled native DNA (Farr test), immunoenzymatic technique, or by indirect immunofluorescence (IF) on the microorganism *Crithidia luciliae*. Farr assay is better correlated with the presence and severity of nephritis and helps to monitor disease activity. Anti-Sm antibodies are highly specific for lupus, but they are positive in only 30%. It is often associated with a less severe form of the disease. Antiphospholipid (APL) antibodies, including anticardiolipin and the lupus anticoagulant, may be found in SLE and are responsible for an increased risk of thrombotic complications.[17]

CLINICAL MANIFESTATIONS

Children with SLE present with diverse and often severe manifestations. Usual presenting symptoms include prolonged fever (58%), fatigue, anorexia, weight loss, lymphadenopathy, musculoskeletal problems (64%), such as arthralgia (80%) or arthritis, malar rash, discoid lesions, livedo reticularis, renal (50%), nervous system (37%), pulmonary (75%), and cardiac (16%) and hematologic (72%) abnormalities. Coombs positive hemolytic anemia, anemia of chronic disease, thrombocytopenia, and leukopenia are the hematologic manifestations. Neuropsychiatric manifestation is the most serious extrarenal manifestation of SLE. Seizures, psychosis, stroke, cerebral venous thrombosis, pseudotumor cerebri, aseptic meningitis, chorea, global cognitive deficits, mood disorders, transverse myelitis, and peripheral neuritis (mononeuritis multiplex) are the nervous system manifestations. Antiphospholipid antibodies (APLAs) occur in 30% and chorea may be seen in these children. Serositis occurs in 40% and affects pleura, pericardium, and peritoneum. Hepatosplenomegaly and lymphadenopathy are common. Gastrointestinal manifestations include pain, diarrhea, melena, infarction, inflammatory bowel disease, and hepatitis. Cardiac manifestations are cardiomegaly, myocarditis, conduction abnormalities, heart failure, coronary artery vasculitis, valvular thickening, verrucous endocarditis (Libman–Sacks disease), and thrombosis. Pulmonary manifestations include acute pulmonary hemorrhage, pulmonary infiltrates (sometimes with superimposed infection), and chronic fibrosis.[18]

DIAGNOSIS OF SYSTEMATIC LUPUS ERYTHEMATOSUS

The diagnosis of SLE is often clinically established by the presence of clinical and laboratory features defined by the 1997 modified American College of Rheumatology (ACR) criteria. Eleven diagnostic criteria developed by the ACR were used to establish the diagnosis of SLE. Some children with SLE may not satisfy the criteria at the onset but may develop more manifestations subsequently and satisfy the full criteria for the diagnosis. Development of four of the 11 criteria over a lifetime gives a 96% sensitivity and specificity for the diagnosis of SLE.[19]

Systemic Lupus International Collaborating Clinics (SLICC) SLE classification criteria later developed have better sensitivity and use clinical and immunologic criteria **(Table 1)**. The SLICC criteria for SLE classification require the following: (1) fulfillment of at least four criteria, with at least one clinical criterion and one immunologic criterion, or (2) lupus nephritis as the sole clinical criterion in the presence of ANA or anti-dsDNA antibodies. The criteria are cumulative and need not be present concurrently.[20]

In 2019, European League against Rheumatism (EULAR)/ACR[21] developed classification criteria for SLE (**Flowchart 1**). The EULAR/ACR classification criteria include positive ANA at least once as the obligatory entry criterion followed by additive weighted criteria grouped in seven clinical (constitutional, hematologic, neuropsychiatric, mucocutaneous, serosal, musculoskeletal, and renal) and three immunologic (APLA, complement proteins, SLE-specific antibodies) domains.[21] These criteria are weighted from 2 to 10. Patients accumulating ≥10 points are classified as SLE. The new criteria have a sensitivity of 96.1% and specificity of 93.4%, compared

TABLE 1: Systemic Lupus International Collaborating Clinics (SLICC) SLE classification criteria.

Clinical criteria	*Immunological criteria*
• Acute or subacute cutaneous lupus • Chronic cutaneous lupus • Oral, nasal, or palate ulcers • Nonscarring alopecia • Synovitis involving two or more joints, characterized by swelling or effusion OR tenderness in two or more joints and 30 minutes or more of morning stiffness • Serositis • *Renal:* Urine protein/creatinine (or 24-h urine protein) representing 500 mg of protein/24 h or red blood cell casts • *Neurologic:* Seizures, psychosis, mononeuritis multiplex, acute confusional state in the absence of other causes • Hemolytic anemia • Leukopenia (<4,000/mm^3 at least once) in the absence of other known causes • Thrombocytopenia (<100,000/mm^3) at least once in the absence of other known causes	• ANA above laboratory reference range • Anti-dsDNA above laboratory reference range except ELISA that is twice above reference range • Anti-Sm antibody • *Antiphospholipid antibody:* Any of the following: – Lupus anticoagulant – False-positive rapid plasma reagin – Medium or high titer anticardiolipin (IgA, IgG, or IgM), anti-β-2-glycoprotein I (IgA, IgG, or IgM) • Low complement C3, C4, or CH50 • Direct Coombs test in the absence of hemolytic anemia

Requirement: ≥4 criteria with at least one clinical criterion AND one immunologic criterion OR biopsy-proven lupus nephritis with positive ANA or anti-dsDNA antibodies
(ANA: antinuclear antibody; ELISA: enzyme-linked immunosorbent assay)

with 82.8% sensitivity and 93.4% specificity of the ACR 1997 and 96.7% sensitivity and 83.7% specificity of the SLICC 2012 criteria.[22]

DISEASE ACTIVITY SCORES

As no single measure can assess disease activity in lupus, several standardized indices have been created to evaluate disease activity. The Systemic Lupus Erythematosus Disease Activity Index (SLEDAI)[23] and British Isles Lupus Assessment Group (BILAG) index[24] are most often used. The irreversible organ damage is quantified by SLICC/ACR index.[25]

RENAL INVOLVEMENT IN SYSTEMATIC LUPUS ERYTHEMATOSUS

Kidney disease is one of the most common and serious features of SLE. Although LN can occur at any age, 10–20% patients have onset in childhood with higher rates of renal involvement reported in Asian population.[26] LN is a major risk factor for morbidity and mortality. Renal disease often develops concurrently or shortly after the onset of SLE, generally within the first 6–36 months. LN may be occasionally the only manifestation of SLE in children. The risk factors for the development of LN include younger age, male sex, juvenile onset lupus, and serologically active disease, including positivity for anti-C1q antibodies. It is more severe in children and tends to sustain severe damage secondary to aggressive disease and treatment-associated toxicity.[27]

The clinical manifestations of LN in childhood are often subtle and range from minor abnormalities detected on urinalysis to hypertension with headache, dizziness, visual disturbances, signs of cardiac decompensation, edema, hematuria, proteinuria, nephrotic syndrome, and even severe renal failure or electrolyte abnormalities.[28] Acute kidney injury in SLE is often due to crescentic glomerulonephritis. Besides LN, kidney injury could be due to thrombotic microangiopathy (TMA)/APL nephropathy, nonimmune complex podocytopathy, tubulointerstitial nephritis, acute tubular necrosis, renovascular disease, or nephrotoxicity from medications. Distal renal tubular acidosis may be sometimes the initial manifestation. The course of LN may be protracted with periods of remissions and exacerbations. Clinical renal involvement usually correlates well with the degree of glomerular involvement in SLE. Severe hypertension, heavy proteinuria, and generalized edema are more common in diffuse proliferative or membranous LN. SLE in patients clinically presenting with nephrotic syndrome and glomerular morphology of minimal change disease (MCD), mesangial proliferation (MsP), or focal segmental glomerulosclerosis (FSGS) is now classified as lupus podocytopathy.[29] About 10–50% of children with LN progress to end-stage kidney disease (ESKD). Early detection and treatment can significantly improve the renal outcome.[30]

PATHOGENESIS OF LUPUS NEPHRITIS

Glomerular involvement in SLE is often considered as a human prototype of classic immune complex-induced glomerulonephritis. Nephritogenic autoantibodies mediate renal damage by two mechanisms. Anti-dsDNA antibodies cross-react with the glomerular basement membrane, mesangium, endothelium, and epithelium followed by activation of complement cascade, especially by the classical pathway. Higher affinity autoantibodies form intravascular immune complexes which are deposited in glomeruli. Alternatively, immune complexes form in situ with autoantibodies binding to the glomerular basement membrane antigens.[31]

Flowchart 1: European League against Rheumatism/American College of Rheumatology classification criteria for SLE 2019.

Antinuclear antibody (ANA) at a titer of ≥1:80 on HEP-2 cells or an equivalent positive test (ever)

↓

If absent, do not classify as SLE
If present, apply additive criteria

↓

Additive criteria
- Do not count a criterion if there is a more likely explanation than SLE
- Occurrence of a criterion on at least one occasion is sufficient
- SLE classification requires at least one clinical criterion and ≥10 points
- Criteria need not occur simultaneously
- Within each domain, only the highest weighted criterion is counted toward the total score

Clinical domain and criteria	Weight	Immunological domain and criteria	Weight
Constitutional: Fever	2	*Antiphospholipid antibodies:* • Anticardiolipin antibodies or • Anti-β2GP1 antibodies or • Lupus anticoagulant	2
Hematologic: • Leukopenia • Autoimmune hemolysis • Thrombocytopenia	 3 4 4	*Complement proteins:* • Low C3 or low C4 • Low C3 and low C4	 3 4
Neuropsychiatric: • Delirium • Psychosis • Seizure	 2 3 5	*SLE-specific antibodies:* • Anti-dsDNA antibody* or • Anti-Smith antibody	6
Mucocutaneous: • Nonscarring alopecia • Oral ulcers • Subacute cutaneous or discoid lupus • Acute cutaneous lupus	 2 2 4 6		
Serosal: • Pleural or pericardial effusion • Acute pericarditis	 5 6		
Musculoskeletal: Joint involvement	6		
Renal: • Proteinuria > 0.5 g/24 h • Renal biopsy—class II or V lupus nephritis • Renal biopsy—class III or IV lupus nephritis	 4 8 10		

↓

Classify as SLE with a score of 10 or more if entry criterion fulfilled

(IV: intravenous; SLE: systemic lupus erythematosus)

Neutrophil extracellular traps and NETing neutrophils are found in the kidneys of patients with SLE which facilitate inflammation, cause endothelial damage, and induce plasmacytoid dendritic cells to produce interferon alpha (IFN-α). IFN-α promotes B-cell differentiation into plasma cells and facilitates production of TH1 and TH2 cells. B cells also present autoantigens to T cells, which leads to T-cell activation and release of proinflammatory cytokines, such as interleukin 6 (IL-6). B- and T-cell proliferations are dependent upon costimulation that occurs independently from antigen presentation through interactions between CD28:B7 and CD40L:CD40 located on T and B cells, respectively.[32]

Additionally, B-lymphocyte stimulators (BLyS) and A proliferation-inducing ligand (APRIL) function to activate B cells and prolong survival. Autoreactive plasma cells produce autoantibodies that bind autoantigens and form immune complexes. These immune complexes deposit in the renal parenchyma, activate the alternative complement pathway, and recruit proinflammatory cells to the kidney, leading to tissue damage and inflammation.[33]

Complement system is generally activated in LN and may directly mediate kidney injury through the terminal pathway or indirectly increase renal inflammation by recruiting leukocytes to the kidney. Autoantibodies to C components C1q and to C3b are found in LN. Anti-C1q antibodies may enhance autoantigen exposure and may facilitate immune-complex deposition in kidneys. The clearing ability of the mesangium and local hemodynamic factors may also play a role. Intraglomerular immune complexes activate complement and engage leukocyte Fc receptors and procoagulant factors. They attract inflammatory cells, including lymphocytes and macrophages; activate neutrophils; and release proteolysis enzymes, various cytokines such as tumor necrosis factor α (TNF-α), IL-6, transforming growth factor beta (TGF-β), IFN-γ, and chemokines regulating cellular proliferation and matrix synthesis in glomeruli. In severe forms of LN, proliferation of endothelial, mesangial, and epithelial cells and the production of matrix proteins lead to fibrosis.[34] APLA positivity with intraglomerular thrombosis and rarely peripheral arterial and venous thrombosis occurs in children with SLE and APLA syndrome.[35]

DIAGNOSIS OF LUPUS NEPHRITIS

Lupus nephritis is most commonly discovered by examination of urine as opposed to physical examination. All patients with SLE should be evaluated for kidney involvement at initial diagnosis and at least yearly thereafter even if they do not have symptoms of kidney disease. Evaluation should include a urinalysis and measurement of serum creatinine or estimated glomerular filtration rate (eGFR). Reevaluation for LN is also recommended in lupus flares.

Laboratory tests to evaluate renal function include urinalysis [to check for protein, red blood cells (RBCs), and cellular casts and spot test for creatinine and protein concentration] and 24-hour urine test for creatinine clearance and protein excretion and assessment of blood urea, creatinine, and GFR. Clinically relevant LN is associated with a 30% decrease in eGFR, proteinuria of >1,000 mg/day, and renal biopsy findings indicating active LN.

According to the ACR, renal involvement in SLE is defined by the following: Persistent proteinuria, i.e., 24-hour urinary protein ≥500 mg or urine protein to creatinine ratio (PCR) ≥0.5, or urine dipstick ≥3 and/or active urine sediment. Active urine sediment is defined by >5 RBCs/hpf, >5 white blood cells (WBCs)/hpf in the absence of infection, or cellular casts (consisting of erythrocyte, hemoglobin, granular, tubular, or mixed casts). An ideal additional criterion is renal biopsy showing immune complex nephritis associated with complement deposition.[36]

Immunologic Tests

Positive ANA is seen in almost all children with LN. Anti-dsDNA antibodies are more specific to SLE. Hypocomplementemia is universal in active LN. Complement components C4 and C1q are more depressed than C3, indicating classical complement pathway activation. CH50 is also low in active lupus. Anti-C1q antibodies are associated with proliferative LN and higher titers correlate with active renal disease. They are more specific and in combination with low C3 and C4, predict renal flares. The lupus activity can be evaluated with anti-dsDNA titers, complement levels (C3, C4, and CH50), erythrocyte sedimentation rate (ESR), or C-reactive protein (CRP). CRP is generally not elevated in SLE, even with active disease, unless the patient has significant arthritis or infection.

BIOMARKERS IN LUPUS NEPHRITIS

Serologic and urinary biomarkers such as neutrophil gelatinase–associated lipocalin (NGAL) and TNF superfamily cytokine [TNF-like weak inducer of apoptosis (TWEAK)] help in early diagnosis of LN. Urinary monocyte chemoattractant protein-1 (UMCP-1) is specific for renal activity, sensitive to predict renal flares, and correlates with severity of flares and proliferative types of LN.[37-39]

High urinary NGAL predicts disease activity and renal flares and has higher sensitivity and specificity compared to dsDNA antibodies.[40]

RENAL BIOPSY IN LUPUS

Early recognition of renal involvement and performance of a diagnostic renal biopsy are essential to ensure optimal outcomes in LN. Histology is mandatory in deciding the class, severity, activity, chronicity of renal disease and extent of irreversible chronic alterations. Also it helps in guiding appropriate optimal treatment and assessing prognosis.[41,42] Indications for renal biopsy as per ACR are given in **Box 1**.

The WHO classification system of LN combined light microscopic (LM) findings with the IF and electron microscopic (EM) findings to present an accurate and precise system. In 2003, the International Society of Nephrology/Renal Pathology Society (ISN/RPS) developed a new classification schema **(Table 2)** to address the limitations of the older WHO classification.[43] LN is classified into six classes by the ISN/RPS. Revision of the International Society of Nephrology/Renal Pathology Society classification for LN was made recently. A more effective, reproducible, and valuable classification system is proposed with the modifications as outlined in **Table 2**.[44]

BOX 1: Indications for renal biopsy in systematic lupus erythematosus as per American College of Rheumatology (ACR).

- Confirmed proteinuria of ≥1 g/24 h urine specimen or spot urine protein urine creatinine ratio > 0.5
- Combination of the following, assuming the findings are confirmed in at least two tests:
  1. Proteinuria ≥0.5 g/24 h plus hematuria defined as ≥5 RBCs/hpf
  2. Proteinuria ≥0.5 g/24 h plus cellular cast
- Increasing serum creatinine without compelling alternative cause
- Repeat biopsy if persistent nephrotic proteinuria or active sediment despite adequate therapy, lupus flare with recurrent proteinuria or hematuria to assess for class transformation

(hpf: high-power field; RBCs: red blood cells)

TABLE 2: International Society of Nephrology/Renal Pathology Society (ISN/RPS) classification of lupus nephritis and proposed modifications in revised ISN/RPS classification.

Classification	*Category*	*Description*	*Modification proposed*
ISN/RPS	Class I	• Minimal mesangial lupus nephritis • Normal glomeruli by LM • Mesangial immune deposits on IF or EM	No change recommended
ISN/RPS	Class II	• Mesangial proliferative lupus nephritis • Purely mesangial hypercellularity of any degree or mesangial expansion by LM and mesangial deposits by IF or EM	Definition for mesangial hypercellularity is adjusted as four or more nuclei fully surrounded by matrix in the mesangial area not including hilar region
ISN/RPS	Class III	• Focal lupus nephritis • Active or inactive focal, segmental, or global endo- or extracapillary GN involving <50% of all glomeruli • *Class III(A):* Active lesions: Focal proliferative LN • *Class III(A/C):* Active and chronic lesions: Focal proliferative and sclerosing LN • *Class III(C):* Chronic inactive lesions with glomerular scars: Focal sclerosing LN	In class III and IV: • Term endocapillary proliferation is replaced by endocapillary hypercellularity • Term crescent is used for a lesion consisting of extracapillary hypercellularity, composed of a variable mixture of cells occupying >10% of Bowman's capsular circumference Cellular crescent is defined as >75% cells and fibrin and <25% fibrous matrix Fibrous crescent has > 75% fibrous matrix and <25% cells and fibrin. Fibrocellular crescent **(Fig. 3)** is with 25–75% cells and fibrin and the remainder fibrous matrix. • Adhesion is defined as an area of isolated continuity of extracellular matrix material between the tuft and capsule even when the underlying segment does not have overt sclerosis. • *Fibrinoid necrosis:* Fibrin associated with glomerular basement membrane disruption and/or lysis of the mesangial matrix; this lesion does not require the presence of karyorrhexis. There was no definition for fibrinoid necrosis. • The segmental and global subdivisions of class IV eliminated • Indicate whether tubulointerstitial lesions occur in presence or absence of interstitial fibrosis.
ISN/RPS	Class IV	• Diffuse proliferative LN—active or inactive diffuse, segmental, or global endo- or extracapillary GN involving ≥50% of all glomeruli, typically with diffuse subendothelial immune deposits, with or without mesangial alterations. Diffuse wire loop deposits but with little or no glomerular proliferation. • Diffuse segmental (IV-S) when ≥50% of the involved glomeruli have segmental lesions Diffuse global (IV-G) when ≥50% of the involved glomeruli have global lesions. Segmental is defined as a lesion that involves less than half of the glomerular tuft. • *Class IV-S(A)*: Active lesions: Diffuse segmental proliferative lupus nephritis • *Class IV-G(A)*: Active lesions: Diffuse global proliferative LN • *Class IV-S (A/C)*: Active and chronic lesions: diffuse segmental proliferative and sclerosing LN • *Class IV-G (A/C)*: Active and chronic lesions: Diffuse global proliferative and sclerosing LN • *Class IV-S (C)*: Chronic inactive lesions with scars: Diffuse segmental sclerosing LN • *Class IV-G (C)*: Chronic inactive lesions with scars: Diffuse global sclerosing LN	
ISN/RPS	Class V	• Membranous lupus nephritis • Global or segmental subepithelial immune deposits by LM and by IF or EM May occur in combination with class III or IV in which case both will be diagnosed • Have any degree of mesangial hypercellularity and can show advanced sclerosis	No change recommended

Contd...

Contd...

Classification	***Category***	***Description***	***Modification proposed***
ISN/RPS	Class VI	Advanced sclerosing lupus nephritis >90% sclerosed glomeruli without active lesions	No change recommended
NIH activity scores	• Glomerular endocapillary hypercellularity • Glomerular leukocyte infiltration • Glomerular fibrinoid necrosis, karyorrhexis • Glomerular subendothelial deposits—wire loop lesions • Glomerular cellular crescents • Interstitial inflammation	• *Active lesions scoring:* 0–24 • *Each lesion scored:* 0–3 • *For glomerular lesions:* – 1+:<25% of glomeruli involved – 2+ 25–50% glomeruli involved – 3+ 50% of glomeruli involved • *For interstitial lesions:* – 1+:<25% interstitial leukocytes – 2+: 25–50% interstitial leukocytes – 3+: >50% interstitial leukocytes – Fibrinoid necrosis and crescents are given double the weight (0–3 × 2)	• Modified NIH injury indexes reported with each biopsy and replaces active and chronic designations for proliferative (class III/IV lesions) • *Active lesion proposed changes:* – Separate fibrinoid necrosis from karyorrhexis – Fibrocellular recognized with cellular crescent as active lesion – Leukocyte infiltration is removed
NIH chronicity scores	• Glomerular sclerosis • Glomerular fibrous crescents • Tubular atrophy • Interstitial fibrosis	• *Chronic lesions scoring:* 0–12 • *Each lesion scored:* 0–3: • *For glomerular lesions:* – +: <25% of glomeruli involved – 2+: 25–50% glomeruli involved – 3+: 50% of glomeruli involved • *For interstitial lesions:* – 1+:<25% tubular atrophy and/or interstitial fibrosis – 2+: 25–50% tubular atrophy and/or interstitial fibrosis – 3+:>50% tubular atrophy and/or interstitial fibrosis	Modification of the NIH lupus nephritis activity and chronicity scoring system **(Table 3)** to be used instead of "A," "C," and "A/C" parameters; preference for a semiquantitative approach to describe active and chronic lesions

(EM: electron microscopy; GN: glomerulonephritis; IF: immunofluorescence; LM: light microscopy; LN: lupus nephritis; NIH: National Institutes of Health)

Source: Adapted from Parikh SV, Almaani S, Brodsky S, Rovin BH. Update on lupus nephritis: core curriculum 2020. Am J Kidney Dis. 2020;76(2):265-81.

The disease activity in LN is classified into active and chronic based on various histological renal lesions. Active histological renal lesions can be seen in the glomeruli as well as in the tubulointerstitium. Active glomerular lesions include endocapillary hypercellularity **(Fig. 1)**, fibrinoid necrosis, karyorrhexis, hyaline thrombi, wire loops (subendothelial deposits; **Fig. 2**), hematoxylin bodies, cellular crescents **(Fig. 3)**, and leukocyte infiltrates. Mononuclear cell infiltrates and tubular necrosis are active tubulointerstitial lesions. Chronic glomerular lesions include glomerular sclerosis (segmental or global), fibrous crescents, fibrous adhesions, and extramembranous deposits.

Interstitial fibrosis and tubular atrophy are the essential chronic tubulointerstitial features. Active lesions are each graded 0-3 except necrosis and cellular crescents which are graded 0-6 to give an activity index (AI) graded 0-24 **(Table 3)**. Active lesions are potentially reversible with the treatment.[44]

The chronicity index (CI) is assessed based on irreversible lesions including glomerular sclerosis, fibrous crescents, tubular atrophy, and interstitial fibrosis. These lesions do not respond to treatment. AI and CI quantify mainly glomerular injury, and tubulointerstitial activity index (TIAI) quantifies extraglomerular kidney disease. The risk factors for poor outcome in childhood-onset SLE (cSLE) include AI ≥ 7, CI ≥ 4, and TIAI > 5 as in adults.[45,46]

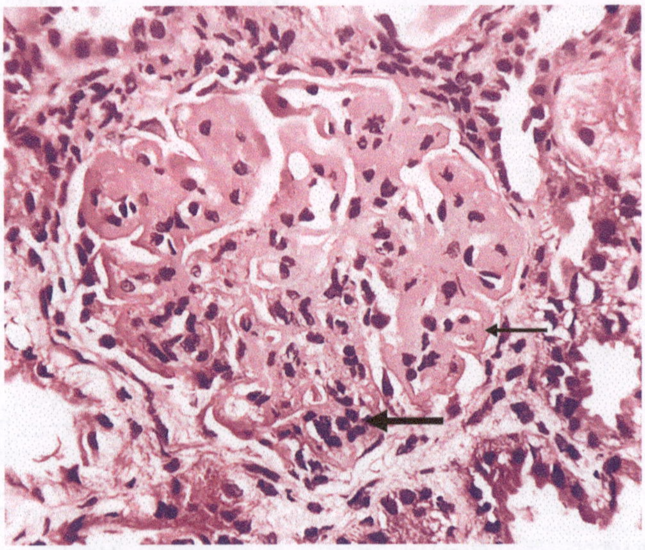

Fig. 1: Class IV lupus nephritis—endocapillary hypercellularity (thick arrow) and wire loop lesions (thin arrow). Light microscopy—H&E stain ×400.

Courtesy: Dr Seethalekshmy NV, Amrita Institute of Medical Sciences, Kochi and Pediatric Nephrology, Government Medical College, Thiruvananthapuram.

In LN, IF microscopy will show immune deposits in the mesangium, subendothelial, or subepithelial space **(Figs. 4A and B)**. Immunoglobulin G (IgG) is the dominant

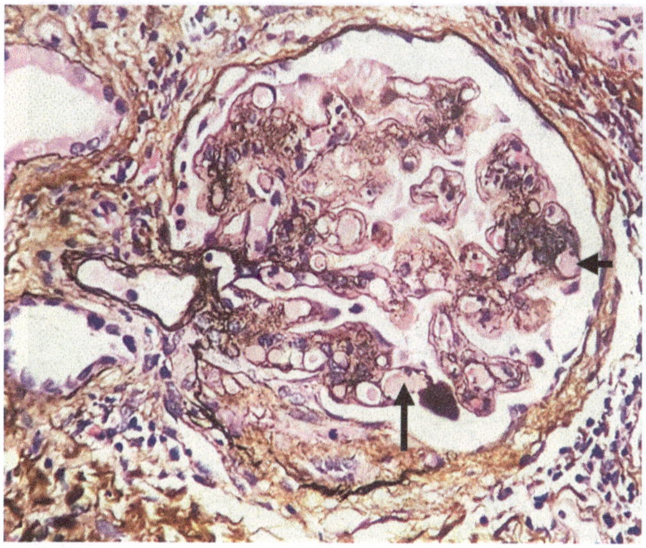

Fig. 2: Hyaline "thrombi," Jones silver stain ×400.
Courtesy: Dr Seethalekshmy NV, Amrita Institute of Medical Sciences, Kochi and Pediatric Nephrology, Government Medical College, Thiruvananthapuram.

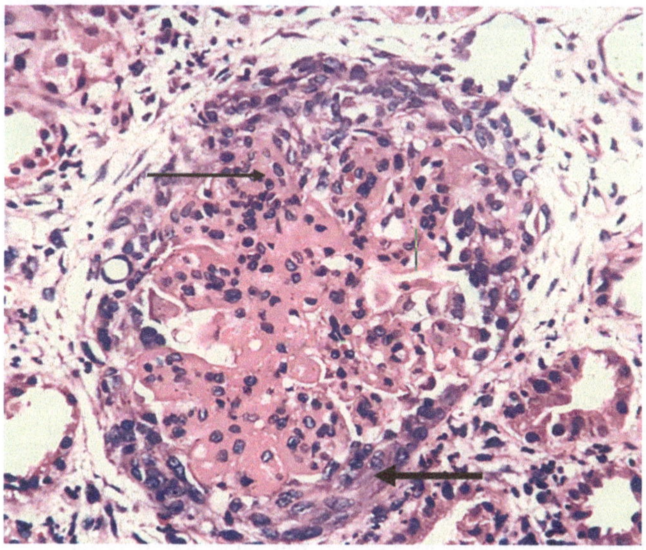

Fig. 3: Endocapillary hypercellularity (thin arrow) and cellular crescent (thick arrow). H&E ×400.
Courtesy: Dr Seethalekshmy NV, Amrita Institute of Medical Sciences, Kochi and Pediatric Nephrology, Government Medical College, Thiruvananthapuram.

immune deposit, especially IgG1 and IgG3. IgA and IgM are also present, as well as early complement components, C4 and C1q, along with C3. Such positivity for all three isotypes of immunoglobulin together with C3, C4, and C1q is called full house IF. This is seen in majority of LN and is considered diagnostic.[43]

Lupus podocytopathy is a unique form of LN seen in approximately 1% of LN biopsies. Glomeruli are normal or show FSGS with or without MsP on light microscopy with negative IF, absence of subepithelial or subendothelial deposits, and diffuse foot process effacement on electron microscopy.[29]

TABLE 3: Proposed modified NIH LN activity and chronicity scoring system.

Modified activity index score (0–24)	
Histology	***Score***
Endocapillary hypercellularity	<25% (1), 25–50% (2), or >50% (3) of glomeruli (score: 0–3)
Neutrophils and/or karyorrhexis	<25% (1), 25–50% (2), or >50% (3) of glomeruli (score: 0–3)
Fibrinoid necrosis	<25% (1), 25–50% (2), or >50% (3) of glomeruli (score: 0–3 × 2)
Wire loop lesions and/or hyaline thrombi	<25% (1), 25–50% (2), or >50% (3) of glomeruli (score: 0–3)
Cellular and/or fibrocellular crescents	<25% (1), 25–50% (2), or >50% (3) of glomeruli (score: 0–3 × 2)
Interstitial leukocytes	<25% (1), 25–50% (2), or >50% (3) in the cortex (score: 0–3)
Modified chronicity index score (0–12)	
Total glomerulosclerosis score, global and/or segmental sclerosis	<25% (1), 25–50% (2), or >50% (3) of glomeruli (score: 0–3)
Fibrous crescents	<25% (1), 25–50% (2), or >50% (3) of glomeruli (score: 0–3)
Tubular atrophy	<25% (1), 25–50% (2), or >50% (3) of the cortical tubules (score: 0–3)
Interstitial fibrosis	<25% (1), 25–50% (2), or >50% (3) in the cortex (score: 0–3)

(LN: lupus nephritis; NIH: National Institutes of Health)
Source: Bajema IM, Wilhelmus S, Alpers CE, Bruijn JA, Colvin RB, Cook HT, et al. Revision of the International Society of Nephrology/Renal Pathology Society Classification for lupus nephritis: clarification of definitions, and Modified National Institutes of Health Activity and Chronicity Indices. Kidney Int. 2018;93:789-96.

TREATMENT

The ultimate goal of treatment in LN is inducing and maintaining complete remissionon (CR) of disease or maximal decrease in disease activity with long-term preservation of renal function. Prevention of disease flares; avoidance or minimization of drug toxicity; allowing normal growth, development, and fertility is important thus ensuring survival with improved quality of life. Renal histology is mandatory and therapy differs depending on the pathology. Optimal treatment includes induction of remission, maintenance treatment for preventing flares and prevention of progressive renal failure. Most effective regimens with least toxicity should be used. Extrarenal manifestations also need prompt attention and management to improve the outcome.[43,44,47–50] The induction and maintenance treatment regimens and a comparison between different protocols for the management of LN are given in **Tables 4 and 5**, respectively. The initial induction phase of the treatment typically lasts 3–6 months.

Kidney Disease Improving Global Outcomes (KDIGO) clinical practice guidelines suggest that treatment for class I/II LN be dictated by extrarenal manifestations, except that

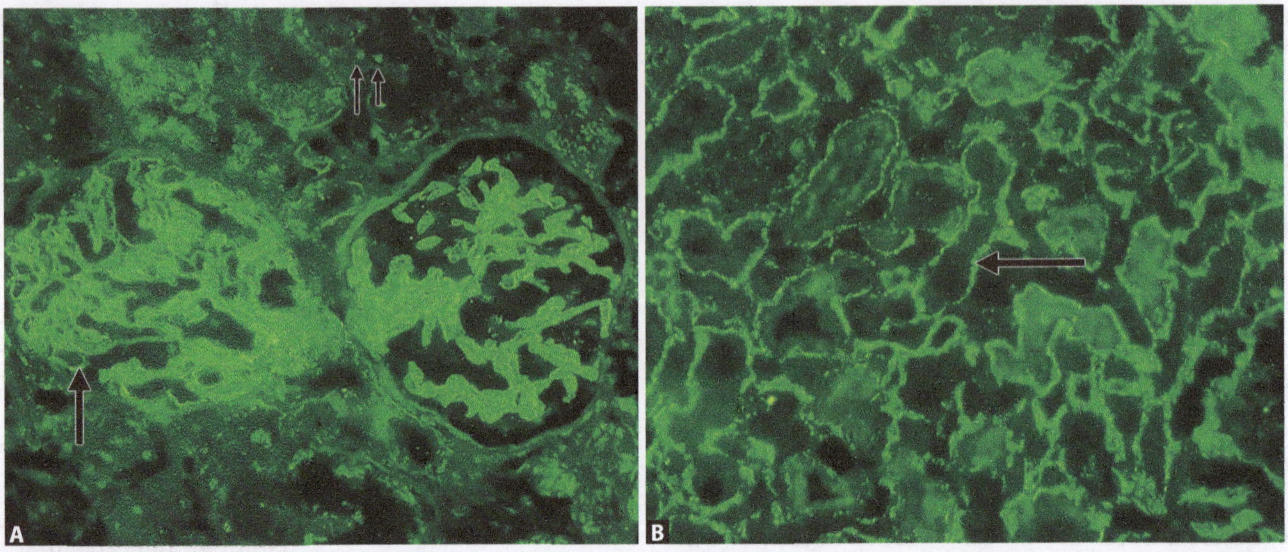

Figs. 4A and B: Immunofluorescence microscopy—lupus nephritis. (A) IgG—granular capillary wall staining and "tissue ANA" staining; (B) IgG—tubular basement membrane staining.
Courtesy: Dr Seethalekshmy NV, Amrita Institute of Medical Sciences, Kochi and Pediatric Nephrology, Government Medical College, Thiruvananthapuram.

TABLE 4: Induction and maintenance treatment regimens for management of lupus nephritis (LN).

Class	***Treatment regimen***
LN class I	Prednisone/prednisolone (<0.5 mg/kg/day—no more than 30 mg/day) hydroxychloroquine (HCQ) based on the clinical manifestation of SLE
LN class II	• Prednisone/prednisolone (0.25–0.5 mg/kg/day—no more than 30 mg/day), with gradual decrease • HCQ in persistent proteinuria, if there is no remission after 3 months of low-dose prednisolone or to manage extrarenal manifestations
LN classes III and IV with or without associated LN class V	*Induction therapy:* Mycophenolate mofetil (MMF) or CYP + corticosteroids *Three protocols:* 1. Euro-Lupus: IV CYP (fixed 500 mg doses, every 15 days for 3 months—total dose of 3,000 mg) followed by maintenance therapy with AZA or MMF43 2. NIH: Intravenous CYP (500 mg/m^2, increased to 750 mg/m^2—1,000 mg/m^2 if tolerated, every 30 days for 6 months—no more than 1 g) followed by 3 monthly doses for another 18 months[43,44] 3. SHARE (Single Hub and Access point for Pediatric Rheumatology in Europe): Oral MMF (1,200 mg/m^2/d to a maximum 1,800 mg/m^2/day for 6 months—no more than 3,000 mg/day)[45] *Corticosteroid therapy—two options:* 1. Intravenous methylprednisolone (30 mg/kg/dose for 3 consecutive days—maximum dose 1 g. This is followed by oral prednisolone; 0.5–1 mg/kg/day (no more than 40 mg/day for 4 weeks), with gradual withdrawal 2. High-dose oral prednisolone (1–2 mg/kg/day—no more than 60 mg/day for 4 weeks), with gradual withdrawal *Maintenance therapy:* • Oral AZA: Doses of 2–3 mg/kg/day, maximum 150 mg/day • Oral MMF: 1,200 mg/m^2/day to a maximum 1,800 mg/m^2/day
LN class V	*Induction therapy:* • SHARE: Oral MMF + prednisone/prednisolone in doses of 0.5 mg/kg/day, with gradual withdrawal • CYP, CNI (cyclosporine/tacrolimus), or rituximab must be considered as options for nonresponders *Maintenance therapy:* SHARE: Oral MMF or oral AZA
Recurrence and refractory cases	LN class III or IV associated or not with LN class V *Recurrence:* • Intravenous methylprednisolone • High-dose oral prednisolone/prednisone (1–2 mg/kg/day—no more than 60 mg/day), with gradual withdrawal after response *Refractory disease:* • Check compliance to treatment • If compliant, replace therapeutic agent (MMF, intravenous CYP, or rituximab) • Multitarget regimen—consider CNI (cyclosporine or tacrolimus) in selected cases

(AZA: azathioprine; CNI: calcineurin inhibitor; CYP: cyclophosphamide; NIH: National Institutes of Health; SHARE: Single Hub and Access point for Pediatric Rheumatology in Europe)

TABLE 5: Comparison of lupus nephritis treatment guidelines.

LN class as per the ISN/ RPS system	*Modified NIH regimen*	*Euro-lupus regimen*	*KDIGO 2020*	*SHARE*	*ACR*
Class 1	Treatment guided by extrarenal manifestations	Treatment guided by extrarenal manifestations	Treatment guided by extrarenal manifestations	Treatment guided by extrarenal manifestations	
Class 2			• *Low-level proteinuria:* Treatment guided by extrarenal manifestations • *If nephrotic proteinuria:* Evaluate for lupus podocytopathy and treat as MCD • If relapse, steroids plus MPA or AZA or CNI to maintain	Prednisone/ prednisolone (0.25–0.5 mg/kg/day—no more than 30 mg/day), with gradual decrease HCQ in persistent proteinuria, if there is no remission after 3 months of low-dose prednisolone or to manage extrarenal manifestations	
Class 3/4	Pulse MP × 3 followed by prednisolone 0.5–1 mg/kg per day, PLUS high-dose CYP 500–1,000 mg/m² BSA IV every month × 6 doses followed by MMF 1–2 g/day or AZA 2 mg/kg/day + low-dose daily GC tapered after a few weeks to lowest effective dose	IV CYP (fixed 500 mg doses, every 15 days for 3 months—total dose of 3,000 mg) followed by maintenance therapy with AZA or MMF	• Induction with IV MP for—one to three doses followed by oral prednisolone 0.6–1 mg/kg/day and MPA or IV or oral cyclophosphamide • Maintenance treatment with MPA for at least 3 years. Prednisolone tapered to 5–7.5 mg/day	• Induction treatment with MMF or IV cyclophosphamide combined with corticosteroids • Maintenance treatment with MMF or azathioprine for at least 3 years	• Induction treatment with MMF or IV CYP (high/low dose) combined with IV MP for 3 days followed by oral prednisolone 0.5–1 mg/kg/day tapered after a few days to the lowest possible dose • Maintenance treatment with MMF/AZA with +/– low-dose oral prednisolone
Class 5	MMF 1,200 mg/m² plus prednisolone in doses of 0.5 mg/kg/day. CYP, CNI (cyclosporine/ tacrolimus) or rituximab must be considered as options for nonresponders	MMF with low-dose prednisone as induction and MMF as maintenance treatment	MMF with low-dose prednisone as induction and MMF as maintenance treatment. In nonresponders, CYP, CNI (cyclosporine/ tacrolimus) or rituximab	Pure class V LN, MMF with low-dose prednisone as induction and MMF as maintenance treatment	• MMF with oral prednisolone 0.5–1 mg/kg/day for 6 months • *If not improved:* IV CYP high dose with oral prednisolone 0.5–1 mg/kg/day • *If improved:* MMF or AZA maintenance

(ACR: American College of Rheumatology; AZA: azathioprine; BSA: body surface area; CNI: calcineurin inhibitor; CYP: cyclophosphamide; GC: glucocorticoid; HCQ: hydroxychloroquine; ISN/RPS: International Society of Nephrology/Renal Pathology Society; KDIGO: Kidney Disease: Improving Global Outcomes; LN: lupus nephritis; MCD: minimal change disease; MMF: mycophenolate mofetil; MP: methylprednisolone; MPA: mycophenolic acid; NIH: National Institutes of Health; SHARE: Single Hub and Access point for Pediatric Rheumatology in Europe)

patients with nephrotic range proteinuria receive steroid or calcineurin inhibitor (CNI) therapy.[47] Focus should also be given to blood pressure control with renin-angiotensin system blockade and immunomodulation with antimalarials [e.g., hydroxychloroquine (HCQ)]. Use of immunosuppressive medications is guided by extrarenal manifestations.

Class III (focal proliferative) and class IV (diffuse proliferative) lesions are the most frequent and severe findings in childhood LN.[48] Patients with proliferative lesions have the highest risk of end-stage kidney disease (ESKD) and are treated with aggressive immunosuppression.[2,30] Combination of class III or class IV with class V (membranous) LN is prevalent, and treatment strategies used for proliferative nephritis should be followed.[30]

Induction of Remission

The concept of vigorous initial treatment—an induction phase, followed by maintenance phase immunosuppressive treatment with at least two drugs—is now widely accepted. Reduction of proteinuria and improvement in renal function can be achieved through prompt institution of appropriate treatment. The aim of the therapy should be complete renal remission, which will require longer treatment duration, often more than 12–24 months. At least partial remission should be achieved by 6–12 months. A complete renal response is defined as urine PCR < 50 mg/mmol and normal or near-normal renal function (within 10% of normal GFR, if previously abnormal). Partial renal response is defined as >50% reduction in proteinuria to subnephrotic levels, and normal or near-normal renal function should be achieved preferably by 6 months but no later than 12 months of initiation of treatment.

Corticosteroids remain the cornerstone of treatment for children with SLE. Initial induction regimen depends on the severity of the disease and the renal biopsy findings. The dose and route of administration depend on the type and severity of organ involvement. The addition of cytotoxic agents to corticosteroid treatment has improved both long- and short-term prognoses.[51] An algorithmic approach to treatment is shown in **Flowchart 2.**

Children with class I and class II biopsies have an excellent renal prognosis and need no specific treatment directed at the kidney. The treatment depends on extrarenal manifestations. However, these children need careful follow-up as transformation to a more severe renal disease is possible. Transformation to another histologic class is usually heralded by increasing proteinuria and urinary sediment activity. A repeat renal biopsy serves as a guide to therapy.

Lupus podocytopathy responds to steroid treatment even though 90% will relapse on maintenance treatment. A combination of steroids with immunosuppressive agents will significantly decrease the relapse rate. Acute kidney injury is common in lupus podocytopathy with FSGS and is less sensitive to corticosteroid therapy. The long-term outcome of lupus podocytopathy is good, but pathological transition may occur during relapses.[29]

Immunosuppressive regimen in proliferative LN consists of high dose daily or alternate-day corticosteroids, intravenous (IV) pulse methylprednisolone, oral or IV cyclophosphamide (CYP), azathioprine (AZA), cyclosporine, mycophenolate mofetil (MMF), and rituximab (RTX). The induction therapy is started with IV methylprednisolone, given as daily pulses for 3 consecutive days at a dose of 0.6–1 g/m²/day infused over at least 30 minutes. Methylprednisolone has potent and rapid anti-inflammatory and immunosuppressive effects. After IV methylprednisolone pulses, extrarenal symptoms disappear rapidly and serum creatinine rapidly returns to normal. Furthermore, these pulses permit initiation of oral prednisone

Flowchart 2: Algorithm for treatment of lupus nephritis.

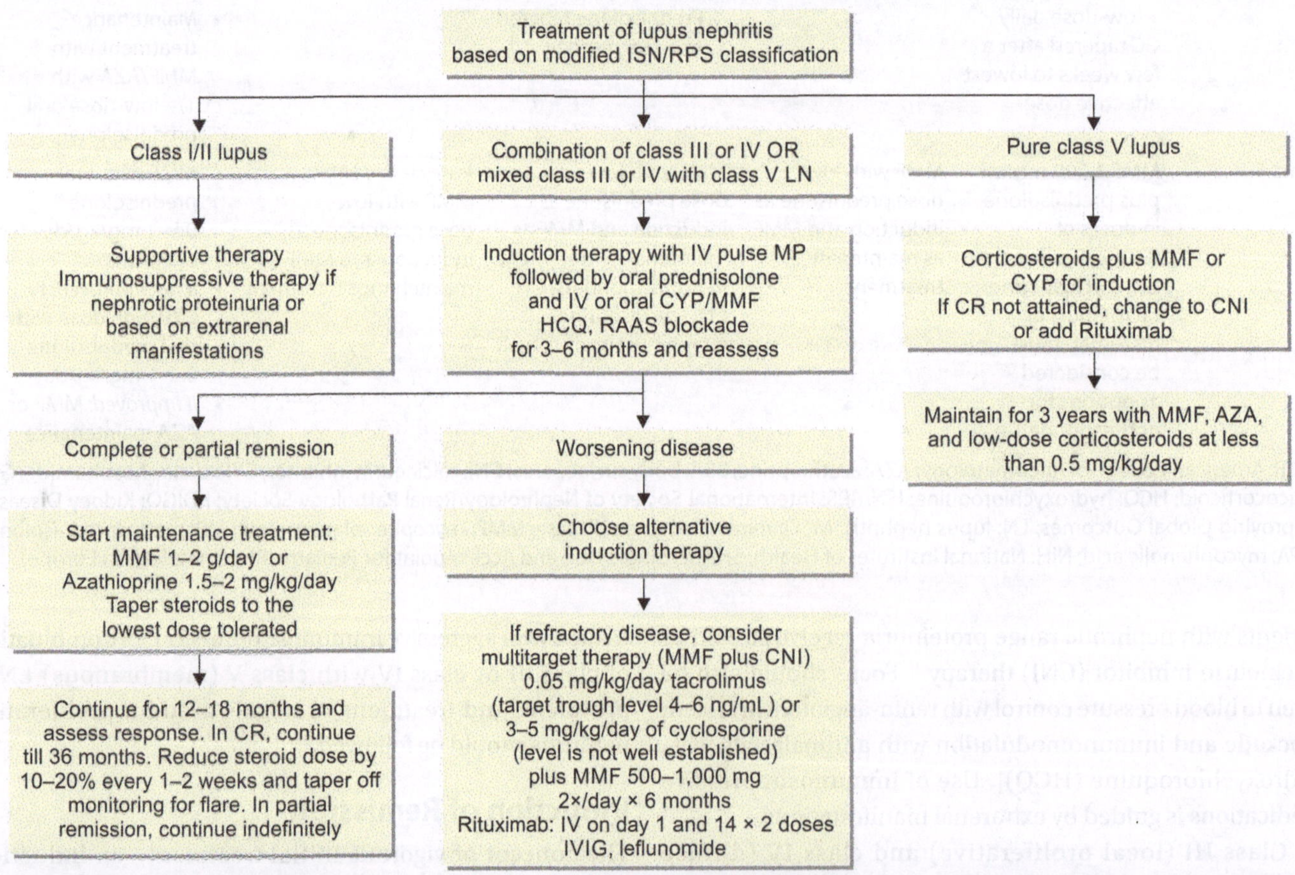

(AZA: azathioprine; CNI: calcineurin inhibitor; CR: complete remission; CYP: cyclophosphamide; HCQ: hydroxychloroquine; ISN/RPS: International Society of Nephrology/Renal Pathology Society; IV: intravenous; IVIG: IV gammaglobulin; LN: lupus nephritis; MMF: mycophenolate mofetil; MP: methylprednisolone; RAAS: renin-angiotensin-aldosterone system)

at a lower dose, thus reducing complications of long-term treatment. In severe cases, these pulses may be repeated. This should be followed by high doses of oral prednisolone at a dose of 1–2 mg/kg/day to a maximum dose of 60–80 mg/day.

As per the Euro-LN group, after 3 days of consecutive IV methylprednisolone pulses of 750 mg, prednisolone is given 0.5–1 mg/kg/day for 1 month and then tapered by 2.5 mg/day every 2 weeks to reach a maintenance dose of 5–7.5 mg/day at 4–6 months.[41,51]

Addition of immunosuppressive drugs improved renal survival significantly. Mycophenolate or low-dose IV CYP is recommended as initial induction agents as they have the best efficacy/toxicity ratio. Aggressive induction therapy is mandatory in severe life-threatening renal disease associated with extrarenal multiorgan involvement. The response is assessed clinically and by laboratory assessment.

In the National Institute of Health (NIH) protocol, IV CYP is the standard initial management of class IV LN along with steroids. It is administered monthly for 6 months, starting at a dose of 500 mg/m^2, and the dose given as boluses may be increased to 1,000 mg/m^2 if the WBC count remains above 3,000/mm^3. After 6 months, the pulses are repeated every 3 months for 18 months, depending on the clinical response. The adverse effects include marrow suppression, gonadal toxicity, and hemorrhagic cystitis.

The Euro-Lupus Group tried to decrease the risk of side effects from CYP therapy without sacrificing efficacy in patients with diffuse or focal proliferative LN or membranous plus proliferative disease by giving either standard 6-monthly pulses of CYP (0.5–1 g/m^2) followed by every third monthly infusions of CYP (0.5–1 g/m^2) as per the NIH protocol or a shorter treatment course consisting of 500 mg of IV CYP every 2 weeks for six doses (total dose, 3 g) followed by AZA maintenance therapy (2 mg/kg/day). Both regimens were equally effective, but the shorter regimen is associated with less toxicity and significantly less severe infections. Low-dose CYP (Euro-Lupus regimen) is preferred as it has comparable efficacy and lower risk of gonadal toxicity.

Mycophenolate mofetil and high-dose CYP are recommended in severe forms of LN associated with adverse prognostic factors and increased risk of progression to ESKD (reduced eGFR, acute deterioration of renal function, presence of fibrous crescents or fibrinoid necrosis, or tubular atrophy/interstitial fibrosis). An early significant drop in proteinuria to ≤1 g/day at 6 months or ≤0.8 g/day at 12 months is a predictor of favorable long-term renal outcome. RTX may be considered in refractory or relapsing disease.

2019 EULAR recommendations have endorsed the need for inducing and maintaining remission or low disease activity and prevention of flares in all organs with the lowest possible dose of glucocorticoids. Class IIIA or IIIA/C (+V) and class IVA or IV A/C(+V) LN are treated with MMF 300–600 mg/m^2/dose twice daily (maximum 3 g/day) for 6 months or equivalent doses of mycophenolic acid (MPA) sodium or low-dose IV CYP 3 g over 3 months in combination with glucocorticoids. In patients with adverse prognostic factors, CYP can be given monthly at higher doses (0.75–1 g/m^2) for 6 months or orally (2.0–2.5 mg/kg/day) for 3 months. To increase the efficacy and to reduce cumulative glucocorticoid doses, treatment regimens should be combined initially with three consecutive pulses of IV methylprednisolone followed by oral prednisolone 0.5 mg/kg/day for 4 weeks, reducing to <10 mg/day by 4–6 months.[51]

In pure class V nephritis with nephrotic proteinuria, MMF in combination with oral prednisolone (0.5 mg/kg/day) is used as initial treatment. In nonresponders, CNIs (tacrolimus/cyclosporine) or RTX are recommended. CNIs may be considered as the second-line agents for induction or maintenance therapy mainly in membranous LN, lupus podocytopathy, or proliferative disease with refractory nephrotic syndrome, despite protocol-based treatment given for 3–6 months. They may be used alone or in combination with MMF. Monitoring blood levels of CNI and periodic assessment of serum creatinine and potassium are essential.[51] Voclosporin, a novel cyclosporine derivative with a more stable pharmacokinetic profile, is under trial.[27]

In LN without adverse prognostic factors or when these drugs are contraindicated or not tolerated, AZA (2 mg/kg/day) may be considered as an alternative, even though there is a higher risk of flare. If there is no response to initial treatment, switch to the alternative induction agent. MMF may be switched to CYP or vice versa. If the kidney function worsens despite induction therapy, consider repeat biopsy to confirm diagnosis and rule out a secondary process such as TMA.

Rituximab is a chimeric monoclonal antibody against the B7 antigen, which acts on B lymphocytes and depletes CD20 B cells. It is a potentially successful therapy for complicated SLE in children. RTX is typically considered following failure of first-line therapies (CYP, MMF) or in relapsing disease. Four weekly infusions of RTX (375 mg/m^2) with oral prednisolone are tried in severe focal or diffuse proliferative LN.[2,28,30,52,53] Other therapies include total lymphoid irradiation, thromboxane inhibitors, and IV gamma-globulin.

Plasmapheresis

Plasmapheresis removes immune complexes involved in the pathogenesis of LN. It is reserved for very severe and refractory cases of SLE with cerebral lupus and/or crescentic glomerulonephritis, severe pulmonary hemorrhage, TMA, and APLA syndrome with clotting episodes, especially catastrophic APLA.[54]

Maintenance Treatment

Once remission has been induced, maintenance therapy is started for managing the chronic, indolent phase of the disease. The goal is to avoid relapses or flares as well as avoid smoldering disease causing chronic irreversible renal scarring. Undue side effects of prolonged immunosuppressive therapy are to be avoided. The choice and length of maintenance therapy in severe SLE are debatable. Maintenance therapy is required for at least 2–3 years in cases of severe SLE and LN or at least 12 months from the time the disease is inactive.[50,51]

Corticosteroids remain a major component of treatment in the maintenance phase of LN. After inducing remission, it is tapered over 6–8 weeks and continued at 10–15 mg/day. To minimize the side effects, long-term steroids are given as a single dose in the morning, switching to alternate days, whenever possible. Glucocorticoids should be minimized and, when possible, withdrawn. Then steroid is gradually reduced by 10–20% every 1 or 2 weeks to attain doses to <7.5 mg/day over 6 months. Osteoporosis prophylaxis should be given concomitantly. Prompt initiation of immune modulatory agents can expedite the tapering/discontinuation of glucocorticoids.[51]

The first-line maintenance therapy in mild SLE is oral AZA at a dose of 2.0–2.5 mg/kg/day as it is well tolerated. The side effects include macrocytosis, leukopenia at high doses, risk of infection, and hepatotoxicity. The total WBC count should be monitored every 4 weeks. Before initiating AZA, thiopurine methyltransferase (TPMT) activity is assessed. Azathioprine use should be avoided in the setting of TPMT deficiency because it can lead to potentially life-threatening bone marrow toxicity at usual doses. Interaction of AZA with allopurinol limits its use in patients with gout. Azathioprine can be safely used in pregnancy as there is very low oncogenic potential.

Along with corticosteroids, children with severe SLE and LN require long-term maintenance therapy with antiproliferative drugs such as MMF or AZA. The former is associated with fewer relapses. MMF is a reversible inhibitor of inosine monophosphate dehydrogenase. It is a more potent, safe, and effective long-term maintenance therapy in focal or diffuse proliferative LN. Maintenance dose is 300–600 mg/m^2 dose twice daily (maximum daily dose 3 g). It may be used along with steroid for induction or sequentially after a 6-month course of IV CYP and is shown to be as effective as IV CYP with less toxicity in patients with stable renal function. The side effects include leukopenia, gastrointestinal discomfort, and diarrhea. Total count is monitored every 4 weeks, and the drug is discontinued if TC is <3,000/mm^3. Lack of renal, hemodynamic, and metabolic toxicity makes MMF an attractive alternative to CYP. Maintenance MMF therapy has been advocated in children with SLE and LN after induction therapy with low-dose IV CYP. Other commonly used immunosuppressive agents include cyclosporine (4–6 mg/kg/day) and tacrolimus (0.15–0.2 μg/kg/day).

After 12–18 months of treatment, if complete response is achieved, consider slow taper of maintenance therapy. If partial response is achieved, continue treatment indefinitely, but consider repeat biopsy to determine whether active lesions are still present. In cases with stable or improved renal function but incomplete renal response as evidenced by persistent proteinuria >0.8–1 g/24 h after at least 1 year of immunosuppressive treatment, repeat biopsy can distinguish chronic from active kidney lesions. Mycophenolate may be combined with low dose of a CNI in severe nephrotic syndrome or incomplete renal response in the absence of uncontrolled hypertension, high CI at kidney biopsy, and/or reduced GFR.

Hydroxychloroquine is recommended for all patients with SLE, unless contraindicated, at a dose not exceeding 5 mg/kg/real body weight. In the absence of risk factors for retinal toxicity, ophthalmological screening (by visual fields examination and/or spectral domain-optical coherence tomography) should be performed at baseline, after 5 years, and yearly thereafter. It helps to improve cardiovascular outcomes and reduces the incidence of atherosclerosis. Also, there is evidence of renoprotective effect of HCQ in LN.

RELAPSE OR FLARE

It is diagnosed by worsening of renal symptoms, serology, or extrarenal flares. Some children may present with an increase in serum creatinine associated with active urinary sediment and often increased proteinuria. Presence of cellular casts is predictive of a renal relapse. Increase in proteinuria is the only renal symptom in relapses in some children. An elevation in anti-dsDNA titer and a decrease in complement levels (C4 and C3) are most often associated with renal flares. These serologic parameters should be checked regularly, at least every 6 months, as their changes often precede clinical relapse. In cases with worsening of renal symptoms, repeat renal biopsy may also be of help before deciding a change in therapy. Flares of SLE can be treated according to the severity of organ involvement by adjusting ongoing therapies to higher doses, switching or adding new therapies.[51,54,55]

Follow-up

During maintenance phase, children are followed up monthly with assessment of weight, height, blood pressure, urinalysis, proteinuria (either 24 hours or UP/UC), and complete blood count and albumin levels. eGFR estimation by modified Schwartz formula, C3 and C4 along with dsDNA is determined every 3 months. Antiphospholipid and lipid profiles should be checked at baseline and thereafter at least 6 monthly. After the initiation of the therapy once the patient's condition stabilizes, monitoring may be done less frequently. Even in children who are stable for many months or years, lupus flares with renal deterioration can occur and hence the clinician should be vigilant with flares of LN.[47,48] Clinical visit is needed every 2–4 weeks for the first 6 months. Children on steroids should be regularly monitored for linear growth. Disease activity is measured with SLEDAI-2K score at presentation and then yearly. All patients with pSLE should have access to an ophthalmologist and should have at least annual eye screening if the patient is on HCQ.

Treatment response is assessed by clinical, biochemical, and serological criteria and is defined clinically and generally stratified into CR, PR, or no response. Proteinuria is the most important clinical variable used to define response. A reduction in protein excretion to <0.5 g/day based on a 24-hour urine collection or urine spot PC ratio (UPCO) with normal serum creatinine or serum creatinine level within 15% of the previous baseline is considered a CR. PR requires >50% reduction in proteinuria and to non-nephrotic levels, with serum creatinine level within 25% of the previous baseline. Patients who do not achieve CR or PR are considered nonresponders.[55] Repeat biopsy may be considered for worsening (particularly nephritic flare or refractory nephrotic flare) parameters or refractory LN with no response beyond 12 months. It is also often done for a rising creatinine level without any obvious cause.

Adjunctive Therapy

ACR and EULAR/ERA-EDTA (European League Against Rheumatism and European Renal Association European Dialysis and Transplant Association) recommend that all SLE patients with nephritis be treated with a background of HCQ to improve outcomes by reducing renal flares and limiting the accrual of renal and cardiovascular damage.[43,49,50]

Additionally, all patients with proteinuria >0.5 g/day (or >0.5 urine PCR) should have blockade of the renin-angiotensin system to reduce intraglomerular pressure unless otherwise contraindicated. This forms an important aspect of managing children with LN. A balanced diet, adequate in protein (1.5–2 g/kg), calories, and fiber, is recommended. Restrict protein intake if renal function is significantly impaired. Salt and fluid restriction is necessary in children with hypertension, edema, or renal failure. No potassium restriction is required in children with normal GFR. Ensure physical activity and avoid excessive weight gain. Only up to 30% calories should be derived from fat. Avoid saturated fats.

Treat hypertension aggressively. Angiotensin-converting enzyme inhibitors (ACEIs) or angiotensin II receptor blockers (ARBs) are used to treat hypertension and to reduce proteinuria in LN. Avoid drugs that affect renal function, including nonsteroidal anti-inflammatory drugs (NSAIDs), especially in patients with elevated serum creatinine.

Monitoring for normal growth and physical and pubertal development is important in children with SLE. Calcium and vitamin D supplements have a beneficial effect along with adequate dietary calcium in preventing osteoporosis. The serum levels of 25-OH-vitamin D should be maintained above 30 ng/mL. Periodic assessment of bone density is also important. The main preventive strategy is aggressive treatment to minimize disease activity and at the same time trying to minimize corticosteroid doses.

Thromboembolic risks are significant for patients with SLE. Antiplatelet doses of "aspirin" are given in children with APLA. Premature cardiovascular disease (CVD) is the most common cause of death in adult SLE. Apart from the classical risk factors such as hypertension and hyperlipidemia, these children also have proteinuria, vasculitis, low-grade systemic inflammation, antiphospholipid syndrome, hypertension, elevated levels of homocysteine, and the impact of prolonged corticosteroid therapy.

Systematic lupus erythematosus is an independent risk factor for CVD in young adults. Atherosclerosis may start in children with lupus due to inflammatory vascular disease, persistent disease activity, LN, presence of APL antibodies, dyslipidemia, renal failure, and use of steroids.[1]

Infections are the most important cause of death in SLE. Both disease-related and treatment-related factors including high-dose steroids, CYP, MMF, and RTX increase the risk. High disease activity, severe leukopenia, and presence of renal involvement also contribute independently. Sometimes, it is difficult to differentiate infections from lupus flares. CRP is useful as these children have normal levels except during infections. A regular immunization protocol for killed vaccine is followed, but live vaccines should be avoided during immunosuppressive therapy. Influenza and pneumococcal vaccines (both PCV13 and PPSV23) should be given during the stable phase. Development of malignancy can be of concern, including skin cancers and lymphoma with long-term immunosuppression. Bladder cancer is reported to be associated with the use of CYP.

Novel Therapeutic Approaches

A number of new immunomodulatory agents are currently being studied to improve outcomes in LN **(Table 6)**. These agents are being studied as additive therapy on top of the standard induction regimen combining corticosteroids with either MMF or IV CYP. Several novel approaches with more specific effects on the immune system have been studied in LN with disappointing results. Total marrow ablation with stem cell rescue therapy may offer clear short-term benefits, but it is unclear whether they prevent chronic kidney failure for long term. Several B-cell-directed therapies have been recently found to be of promise in the treatment of LN. Costimulatory blockers like humanized anti-CD40L monoclonal antibodies

TABLE 6: Emerging novel agents in lupus nephritis treatment.

Biological agent	*Target of action*
Obinutuzumab	B-cell depletion
Belimumab	B-cell growth and survival inhibitor
Atacicept	B-cell growth and survival inhibitor
Anifrolumab	Type 1 interferon
Tocilizumab	Interleukin 6
Eculizumab	Complement
Abatacept	T-cell costimulatory pathway
Dapirolizumab	T-cell anti-CD40L
Bortezomib, ixazomib	Proteasome inhibitors

and B-cell-depleting agents such as anti-CD20 monoclonal antibodies [ocrelizumab (humanized) and ofatumumab (human)], epratuzumab (anti-CD22 monoclonal antibody), belimumab (anti-BLyS monoclonal antibody), atacicept (TACI-Ig fusion protein that inhibits BLyS and APRIL), abetimus, infliximab, tocilizumab, abatacept, and rigerimod are being tried. But belimumab is the only targeted therapy approved so far for the treatment of SLE. Proteasome inhibitors (bortezomib, ixazomib) that particularly affect plasma cells and B-cell activating factor (BAFF, also known as BLyS), antagonists (belimumab, tabalumab), tolerance-inducing molecules (abetimus sodium), blockers of lymphocyte CD28/CD80 costimulation (abatacept), monoclonal antibody against IFN-α receptor 1 (anifrolumab), anti-C5 monoclonal antibody eculizumab, and a small molecule C5a receptor blocker (CCX168) have also been tried.[52,55] Current EULAR recommendation reserves biological therapy for those with persistent disease activity despite standard treatment.

Renal Transplantation in Lupus Nephritis

End-stage kidney disease occurs in 10–50% patients with severe renal disease. Kidney transplantation is possible after achieving clinical and serologic remission or at a low level for at least 3–6 months. Anticoagulation is indicated in lupus with APLA syndrome perioperatively to prevent thrombotic complications. After renal transplantation, the activity of the disease declines and recurrence in the graft is unusual.[56]

Prognosis and Outcome

Renal survival in children with LN is 93% at 5 years, 85% at 10 years, and 80% at 15 years. Renal survival for class IV LN is approximately 10% lower at each of these time points.[52] Poor prognostic indicators are given in **Box 2**.

For children with LN, intense immunosuppressive treatment combining steroids with CYP/MMF/AZA has greatly improved the outcome. With current treatment regimens, the incidence of ESKD in patients with proliferative LN has improved and the 5-year renal survival of children ranges from 77 to 93%. Recent advances in treatment using targeted biological therapies may further improve the outcomes.[55,57,58] Meticulous attention is necessary to optimize patient outcome in childhood LN. New strategies using genomics and proteomics give hope for identification of biomarkers that can be used for early disease detection and treatment.[39] However, LE and its treatment have a major detrimental impact on growth, psychological development, and quality of life. Current guidelines recommend maintenance treatment for at least 3 years with 1 year of CR before stopping immunosuppression.[59] Noncompliance to therapy, particularly during adolescence, is a major cause of treatment resistance and poor outcome.[57] It is important to promote a multidisciplinary approach to SLE to assure better individual treatment of patients.

BOX 2: Poor prognostic factors in lupus nephritis.

- Young age at onset of nephritis
- Male sex
- Black race
- Hypertension
- Nephrotic syndrome
- Initial serum creatinine >3 mg/dL
- Renal biopsy
  - Diffuse proliferative lupus nephritis
  - High chronicity index
- Delay between onset of renal disease and treatment
- Nephritis exacerbations
- Poor response to therapy by the end of the first year
- Persistently elevated anti-dsDNA
- Persistently low C3 and C4 levels

CONCLUSION

Systemic lupus erythematosus is a chronic systemic autoimmune disease characterized by immune dysregulation. Children with SLE present with diverse and often severe manifestations. Histology is mandatory in deciding the class, severity, activity, and chronicity of renal disease and the extent of irreversible chronic alterations. The goals of treatment in LN are complete remission of disease or maximal decreases in disease activity with long-term preservation of renal function. Prevention of disease flares; avoidance or minimization of drug toxicity; allowing normal growth, development, fertility; and ensuring survival with improved quality of life is the final goal in children and adolescents with SLE. Optimal treatment includes induction of remission, maintenance treatment for preventing flares, and prevention of progressive renal failure. For children with LN, intense immunosuppressive treatment combining steroids with CYP/MMF/AZA has greatly improved the outcome. A multidisciplinary team approach to SLE is needed to ensure standard protocol-based treatment and follow-up in pediatric lupus.

KEY POINTS

- SLE is a systemic autoimmune disorder associated with formation of a variety of autoantibodies directed against different cell components, causing chronic inflammation and damage to various organ systems, including kidney.
- The clinical manifestations of LN in childhood are often subtle and range from minor abnormalities detected on urinalysis to hypertension, edema, hematuria, proteinuria, nephrotic syndrome, and even severe renal failure.
- Renal histology is mandatory and will guide appropriate optimal treatment and assess prognosis.
- Corticosteroids remain the cornerstone of treatment for children with SLE.
- Initial induction regimen depends on the severity of the disease and the renal biopsy findings.
- Immunosuppressive regimen in proliferative LN consists of high-dose daily or alternate-day corticosteroids; IV pulse methylprednisolone; or oral or IV CYP, AZA, cyclosporine, MMF, and RTX.
- Along with corticosteroids, children with severe SLE and LN require long-term maintenance therapy with antiproliferative drugs.

- Adjunctive therapy with HCQ has improved the outcome by reducing renal flares and limiting the accrual of renal and cardiovascular damage.
- Treatment response is assessed by clinical, biochemical, and serological criteria and is defined clinically.
- A number of new immunomodulatory agents are currently being studied to improve outcomes in LN.
- With current treatment regimens, the incidence of ESKD in patients with proliferative LN has improved.
- New strategies using genomics and proteomics give hope for identification of biomarkers that can be used for early disease detection and treatment.

REFERENCES

1. Niaudet P, Meunier BB, Salomon R. Renal involvement in children with systemic lupus erythematosus. In: Avner ED, Harmon WE, Niaudet P, Yoshikawa N, Emma F, Goldstein SL (Eds). Pediatric Nephrology, 7th edition. Berlin, Heidelberg: Springer-Verlag; 2016. pp. 1449-88.
2. Kamphuis S, Silverman ED. Prevalence and burden of pediatric-onset systemic lupus erythematosus. Nat Rev Rheumatol. 2010;6:538-46.
3. Levy DM, Kamphuis S. Systemic lupus erythematosus in children and adolescents. Pediatr Clin North Am. 2012;59:345-64.
4. Hiraki LT, Benseler SM, Tyrrell PN, Hebert D, Harvey E, Silverman ED. Clinical and laboratory characteristics and long-term outcome of pediatric systemic lupus erythematosus: a longitudinal study. J Pediatr. 2008;152:550-6.
5. Cameron JS. Lupus nephritis. J Am Soc Nephrol. 1999;10(2): 413-24.
6. Tsokos GC. Systemic lupus erythematosus. N Engl J Med. 2011; 365(22):2110-21.
7. Alarcon-Segovia D, Alarcón-Riquelme ME, Cardiel MH, Caelro F, Massardo L, Villa AR, et al. Familial aggregation of systemic lupus erythematosus, rheumatoid arthritis, and other autoimmune diseases in 1,177 lupus patients from the GLADEL cohort. Arthritis Rheum. 2005;52:1138-47.
8. Crow YJ. Lupus: how much "complexity" is really (just) genetic heterogeneity? Arthritis Rheum. 2011;63(12):3661-4.
9. Iwamoto T, Niewold T. Genetics of human lupus nephritis. Clin Immunol. 2017;185:32-9.
10. Monroe M, James J. Genetics of lupus nephritis: clinical implications. Semin Nephrol. 2015;35(5):396-409.
11. Chen M, Daha MR, Kallenberg CG. The complement system in systemic autoimmune disease. J Autoimmun. 2010; 34(3):J276-86.
12. Lahita RG. Sex hormones and systemic lupus erythematosus. Rheum Dis Clin North Am. 2000;26(4):951-68.
13. Bosch X. Systemic lupus erythematosus and the neutrophil. N Engl J Med. 2011;365(8):758-60.
14. Villanueva E, Yalavarthi S, Berthier CC, Hodgin JB, Khandpur R, Lin AM, et al. Netting neutrophils induce endothelial damage, infiltrate tissues, and expose immunostimulatory molecules in systemic lupus erythematosus. J Immunol. 2011;187:538-52.
15. Lou H, Wojciak-Stothard B, Ruseva MM, Cook HT, Kelleher P, Pickering MC, et al. Autoantibody-dependent amplification of inflammation in SLE. Cell Death Dis. 2020;11:729-44.
16. Dema B, Charles N. Autoantibodies in SLE: specificities, isotypes and receptors. Antibodies (Basel). 2016;5(1):2.
17. American College of Rheumatology Ad Hoc Committee on Immunologic Testing Guidelines; Kavanaugh AF, Solomon DH. Guidelines for immunologic laboratory testing in the rheumatic diseases: anti-DNA antibody tests. Arthritis Rheum. 2002;47(5):546.
18. Bader-Meunier B, Armengaud JB, Haddad E, Salomon R, Deschênes G, Koné-Paut I, et al. Initial presentation of childhood-onset systemic lupus erythematosus: a French multicenter study. J Pediatr. 2005;146(5):648-53.
19. Hochberg MC. Updating the American College of Rheumatology revised criteria for the classification of systemic lupus erythematosus. Arthritis Rheum. 1997;40(9):1725.
20. Petri M, Orbai AM, Alarcon GS, Gordon C, Merrill JT, Fortin PR, et al. Derivation and validation of the Systemic Lupus International Collaborating Clinics classification criteria for systemic lupus erythematosus. Arthritis Rheum. 2012;64(8):2677-86.
21. Aringer M, Costenbader K, Daikh D, Brinks R, Mosca M, Ramsey-Goldman R, et al. 2019 European League Against Rheumatism/American College of Rheumatology classification criteria for systemic lupus erythematosus. Ann Rheum Dis. 2019;78 (9):1151-9.
22. Sag E, Tartaglione A, Batu ED, Ravelli A, Khalil SMA, Marks SD, et al. Performance of the new SLICC classification criteria in childhood systemic lupus erythematosus: a multicentre study. Clin Exp Rheumatol. 2014;32(3):440-4.
23. Bombardier C, Gladman DD, Urowitz MB, Caron D, Chang CH. Derivation of the SLEDAI. A disease activity index for lupus patients. The Committee on Prognosis Studies in SLE. Arthritis Rheum 1992;35:630-40.
24. Hay EM, Bacon PA, Gordon C, Isenberg DA, Maddison P, Snaith ML, et al. The BILAG index: a reliable and valid instrument for measuring clinical disease activity in SLE. Q J Med 1993;86:447-58.
25. Gladman D, Ginzler E, Goldsmith C, Isenberg DA, Maddison P, Snaith ML, et al. The development and initial validation of the Systemic Lupus International Collaborating Clinics/American College of Rheumatology damage index for systemic lupus erythematosus. Arthritis Rheum. 1996;39:363-9.
26. Jakes RW, Bae S-C, Louthrenoo W, Mok C-C, Navarra SV, Kwon N. Systematic review of the epidemiology of systemic lupus erythematosus in the Asia-Pacific region: prevalence, incidence, clinical features, and mortality. Arthritis Care Res. 2012;64:159-68.
27. Parikh SV, Almaani S, Brodsky S, Rovin BH. Update on lupus nephritis: core curriculum 2020. Am J Kidney Dis. 2020;76(2):265-81.
28. Almaani S, Meara A, Rovin BH. Update on lupus nephritis. Clin J Am Soc Nephrol. 2017;12:825-35.
29. Chen D, Hu W. Lupus podocytopathy: a distinct entity of lupus nephritis. J Nephrol. 2018;31(5):629-34.
30. Scobell R, Pradhan M. Management of lupus nephritis in children. Indian Pediatr. 2020;57(15):401-6.
31. Cortes-Hernandez J, Ordi-Ros J, Labrador M, Buján S, Balada E, Segarra A, et al. Antihistone and anti-double-stranded deoxyribonucleic acid antibodies are associated with renal disease in systemic lupus erythematosus. Am J Med. 2004;16:165-73.
32. Hakkim A, Fürnrohr BG, Amann K, Laube B, Abed UA, Brinkmann V, et al. Impairment of neutrophil extracellular trap degradation is associated with lupus nephritis. Proc Natl Acad Sci USA. 2010;107:9813-18.
33. Cancro MP, D'Cruz DP, Khamashta MA. The role of B lymphocyte stimulator (BLyS) in systemic lupus erythematosus. J Clin Invest. 2009;119(5):1066-73.

34. Birmingham DJ, Bitter JE, Ndukwe EG, Dials S, Gullo TR, Conroy S, et al. Relationship of circulating anti-C3b and anti-C1q IgG to lupus nephritis and its flare. Clin J Am Soc Nephrol. 2015;11: 47-53.
35. Lee T, von Scheven E, Sandborg C. Systemic lupus erythematosus and antiphospholipid syndrome in children and adolescents. Curr Opin Rheumatol. 2001;13(5):415-21.
36. Dooley MA, Aranow C, Ginzler EM. Review of ACR renal criteria in systemic lupus erythematosus. Lupus. 2004;13:857-60.
37. Torres-Salido MT, Cortés-Hernández J, Vidal X, Pedrosa A, Vilardell-Tarrés M, Ordi-Ros J. Neutrophil gelatinase-associated lipocalin as a biomarker for lupus nephritis. Nephrol Dial Transplant. 2014;29(9):1740-9.
38. Liu ZC, Zhou QL. Tumor necrosis factor-like weak inducer of apoptosis and its potential roles in lupus nephritis. Inflamm Res. 2012;61(4):277-84.
39. Bennett M, Brunner HI. Biomarkers and updates on pediatrics lupus nephritis. Rheum Dis Clin North Am. 2013;39:833-53.
40. Wenderfer S, Ruth N, Brunner H. Advances in the care of children with lupus nephritis. Pediatr Res. 2017;81:406-14.
41. Bertsias GK, Tektonidou M, Amoura Z, Aringer M, Bajema I, Berden JHM, et al. Joint European League Against Rheumatism and European Renal Association European Dialysis and Transplant Association (EULAR/ERA-EDTA) recommendations for the management of adult and paediatric lupus nephritis. Ann Rheum Dis. 2012;71:1771-82.
42. Hahn BH, McMahon MA, Wilkinson A, Wallace WD, Daikh DI, Fitzgerald JD, et al. American College of Rheumatology Guidelines for screening, treatment, and management of lupus nephritis. Arthritis Care Res. 2012;64:797-808.
43. Weening JJ, D'Agati VD, Schwartz MM, Seshan SV, Alpers CE, Appel GB, et al. The classification of glomerulonephritis in systemic lupus erythematosus revisited. Kidney Int. 2004; 65:521-30.
44. Bajema IM, Wilhelmus S, Alpers CE, Bruijn JA, Colvin RB, Cook HT, et al. Revision of the International Society of Nephrology/ Renal Pathology Society Classification for lupus nephritis: clarification of definitions, and Modified National Institutes of Health Activity and Chronicity Indices. Kidney Int. 2018; 93:789-96.
45. Brunner HI, Bennett MR, Abulaban K, Klein-Gitelman MS, O'Neil KM, Tucker L, et al. Development of a novel renal activity index of lupus nephritis in children and young adults. Arthritis Care Res. (Hoboken). 2016;68:1003-11.
46. Zappitelli M, Duffy CM, Bernard C, Gupta IR. Evaluation of activity, chronicity and tubulointerstitial indices for childhood lupus nephritis. Pediatr Nephrol. 2008;23:83-91.
47. Cattran DC, Feehally J, Cook HT, Liu ZH, Fervenza FC, Mezzano SA, et al. Kidney disease: Improving Global Outcomes (KDIGO) Glomerulonephritis Work Group. KDIGO clinical practice guideline for glomerulonephritis. Kidney Int Suppl. 2012;2:139-274.
48. Houssiau FA, Vasconcelos C, D'Cruz D, Sebastiani GD, de Ramon Garrido Ed E, Danieli MG, et al. Immunosuppressive therapy in lupus nephritis: the Euro-Lupus Nephritis Trial, a randomized trial of low-dose versus high-dose intravenous cyclophosphamide. Arthritis Rheum. 2002;46:2121-31.
49. Castro-Santana LE, Colón M, Molina MJ, Rodríguez VE, Mayor AM, Vilá LM. Efficacy of two cyclophosphamide regimens for the treatment of lupus nephritis in Puerto Ricans: low vs. standard dose. Ethn Dis. 2010;20(1 Suppl 1):S1-116-21.
50. Groot N, de Graeff N, Marks SD, Brogan P, Avcin T, Bader-Meunier B, et al. European evidence-based recommendations for the diagnosis and treatment of childhood-onset lupus nephritis: the SHARE Initiative. Ann Rheum Dis. 2017;76:1965-73.
51. Fanouriakis A, Kostopoulou M, Alunno A, Aringer M, Bajema I, Boletis JN, et al. 2019 update of the EULAR recommendations for the management of systemic lupus erythematosus. Ann Rheum Dis. 2019;78:736-45.
52. Parikh SV, Rovin BH. Current and emerging therapies for lupus nephritis. J Am Soc Nephrol. 2016;27(10):2929-39.
53. Rovin BH, Furie R, Latinis K, Looney RJ, Fervenza FC, Sanchez-Guerrero J, et al. LUNAR Investigator Group. Efficacy and safety of rituximab in patients with active proliferative lupus nephritis: the lupus nephritis assessment with rituximab study. Arthritis Rheum. 2012;64:1215-26.
54. Pagnoux C. Plasma exchange for systemic lupus erythematosus. Transfus Apher Sci. 2007;36:187-93.
55. Samotij D, Reich A. Biologics in the treatment of lupus erythematosus: a critical literature review. Biomed Res Int. 2019;2019:8142368.
56. Gipson DS, Ferris ME, Dooley MA, Huang K, Hogan SL. Renal transplantation in children with lupus nephritis. Am J Kidney Dis. 2003;41(2):455-63.
57. Wu JY, Yeh KW, Huang JL. Early predictors of outcomes in pediatric lupus nephritis: focus on proliferative lesions. Semin Arthritis Rheum. 2014;43:513-20.
58. Oni L, Wright RD, Marks S, Beresford MW, Tullus K. Kidney outcomes for children with lupus nephritis. Pediatr Nephrol. 2021;36(6):1377-85.
59. Morales E, Galindo M, Trujillo H, Praga M. Update on lupus nephritis: looking for a new vision. Nephron. 2021;145:1-13.

CHAPTER

7.3

Systemic Vasculitis

Susan Uthup

INTRODUCTION

Vasculitis is a group of heterogeneous disorders with multiorgan involvement resulting from inflammation of blood vessels. Large vessels such as the aorta and its branches; medium-sized vessels such as visceral arteries; and small vessels such as arterioles, venules, and capillaries may be affected causing necrosis, vascular occlusion, stenosis, aneurysm, rupture, and ischemic damage to the supplied organ or tissues. Vasculitis may be primary or secondary. Primary vasculitis is autoimmune in etiology, while secondary vasculitis may be due to infection, drugs, malignancy, and connective tissue diseases such as systemic lupus erythematosus (SLE) or rheumatoid arthritis.[1] The most common vasculitis in children are Henoch–Schönlein purpura (HSP)/immunoglobulin A (IgA) vasculitis and Kawasaki disease (KD).[2] In this chapter, the epidemiology, classification criteria, renal manifestations, evaluation, and management of various vasculitis in children will be discussed.

EPIDEMIOLOGY

Primary systemic vasculitis, though rare in children, carries significant morbidity and mortality despite advances in diagnostic modalities and treatment. The annual incidence of primary vasculitis in children and adolescents is approximately 23 per 100,000.[3] Primary systemic vasculitis is not uncommon in India. But there is paucity of data from the Indian subcontinent. HSP and KD are the common childhood vasculitis in India.[4]

CLASSIFICATION

Primary vasculitis may be classified according to the pathogenesis or clinical, serological, or pathological features. In 1994, the International Chapel Hill Consensus Conference (CHCC) developed a nomenclature system for vasculitis based on the size of the predominantly affected vessels. In 2012, this nomenclature was updated by replacing most of the eponyms with terms describing main groups of vasculitis based on the pathogenesis **(Box 1)**.[5]

BOX 1: International Chapel Hill Consensus Conference on the Nomenclature of Vasculitides (2012).[5]

- Large vessel vasculitis (LVV)
  - Takayasu arteritis (TAK)
  - Giant cell arteritis (GCA)
- Medium-vessel vasculitis (MVV)
  - Polyarteritis nodosa (PAN)
  - Kawasaki disease (KD)
- Small-vessel vasculitis (SVV)
  - Antineutrophil cytoplasmic antibody (ANCA)-associated vasculitis (AAV)
    - Microscopic polyangiitis (MPA)
    - Granulomatosis with polyangiitis (Wegener's) (GPA)
    - Eosinophilic granulomatosis with polyangiitis (Churg–Strauss) (EGPA)
  - Immune complex small vessel vasculitis
    - Anti-GBM disease (anti-GBM)
    - Cryoglobulinemic vasculitis
    - IgA vasculitis (Henoch–Schönlein vasculitis) (IgA V)
    - Hypocomplementemic urticarial vasculitis (Anti-C1q vasculitis)
  - Variable vessel vasculitis (VVV)
    - Behçet's disease (BD)
    - Cogan's syndrome (CS)
  - Single organ vasculitis
    - Cutaneous leukocytoclastic angiitis
    - Cutaneous arteritis
    - Primary central nervous system vasculitis
    - Isolated aortitis
  - Vasculitis associated with systemic disease
    - Lupus vasculitis
    - Rheumatoid arthritis
    - Sarcoid vasculitis
    - Others
  - Vasculitis associated with probable etiology
    - Hepatitis B virus-associated vasculitis
    - Hepatitis C-associated cryoglobulinemic vasculitis
    - Syphilis-associated aortitis
    - Drug-associated immune complex vasculitis
    - Drug-associated ANCA-associated vasculitis
    - Cancer-associated vasculitis
    - Others

The American College of Rheumatology (ACR) criteria proposed for vasculitis in adults in 1990 have never been validated in children. The European League Against Rheumatism (EULAR) and the Pediatric Rheumatology European Society (PRES) developed the first pediatric-specific classification of vasculitis in 2005 based upon the size of

BOX 2: EULAR/PRES endorsed consensus classification of childhood vasculitis 2006.[6]

- Predominantly large-vessel vasculitis
  - Takayasu arteritis
- Predominantly medium-sized vessel vasculitis
  - Childhood polyarteritis nodosa
  - Kawasaki disease
  - Cutaneous polyarteritis
- Predominantly small vessel vasculitis
  - Granulomatous
    - Wegener's granulomatosis
    - Churg–Strauss syndrome
  - Nongranulomatous
    - Microscopic polyangiitis
    - Henoch–Schönlein purpura
    - Isolated cutaneous leukocytoclastic vasculitis
    - Hypocomplementemic urticarial vasculitis
- Other vasculitides
  - Behçet's disease
  - Vasculitis secondary to infection (including hepatitis B-associated PAN), malignancy, and drugs including hypersensitivity vasculitis
  - Isolated vasculitis of the CNS
  - Cogan syndrome
  - Unclassified

(CNS: central nervous system; EULAR/PRES: European League Against Rheumatism/Pediatric Rheumatology European Society; PAN: polyarteritis nodosa)

affected vessels and the presence or absence of granuloma **(Box 2)**.[3,6] The 2008 Ankara Consensus Conference endorsed by EULAR, Pediatric Rheumatology International Trials Organization (PRINTO), and PRES developed and validated the classification criteria for most common vasculitides in childhood such as IgA vasculitis/HSP, KD, polyarteritis nodosa (PAN), granulomatous polyangiitis/Wegener granulomatosis (GPA/WG), and Takayasu arteritis (TA).[7]

CLINICAL MANIFESTATIONS

The clinical manifestation in vasculitis is determined by the size of the affected vessels, organs involved, the extent of vascular injury, and underlying pathologic characteristics. Depending on the organ systems involved, there will be renal, sinopulmonary, dermatologic, gastrointestinal, and musculoskeletal manifestations. As the kidney is a highly vascular organ, renal involvement is common in systemic vasculitis. Though renal manifestation usually forms part of generalized symptomatology, it is likely to be delayed or remain subclinical. Vasculitis affecting the kidney may be systemic or renal limited. Most often, it presents as acute glomerulonephritis with kidney failure, severe hypertension or persistent proteinuria, and hematuria. Small-vessel vasculitis (SVV) involves glomerular capillaries and results in crescentic glomerulonephritis with rapidly progressive renal failure. Involvement of larger vessels such as in TA and medium vessels as in classic polyarteritis nodosa (cPAN) will cause renal ischemia and hypertension. Focal lesions cause aneurysm, and segmental ones result in stenosis or occlusion.[8,9] Common vasculitis syndromes and their renal manifestations are briefly discussed in this chapter.

LARGE-VESSEL VASCULITIS

Takayasu Arteritis

In 1908, Mikito Takayasu, a Japanese ophthalmologist, reported the association of retinal arteriovenous anastomoses and absent upper extremity pulses. TA, also called pulseless disease, is a large-vessel vasculitis of unknown origin. It is a chronic inflammatory granulomatous arteritis that affects the aorta, its main branches on either side of the diaphragm, and also coronary and/or pulmonary arteries. Vessel wall dissection, aneurysm, or stenosis with thrombosis and occlusion may occur in areas weakened by inflammation. The development of collateral circulation will minimize the impact of vascular occlusion.[8-10]

Epidemiology

It is the third most common childhood vasculitis and is the most common large-vessel vasculitis of adolescence. It is the most common cause of renovascular hypertension in the Indian adolescents and young adults. The mean age of onset is 11 years, but it has been reported in children as young as 6 months. It is more common in the Asian population and has a strong female preponderance most often affecting young women in the second and third decades of life.[10,11]

Pathology

Segmental and patchy granulomatous inflammation involves all three layers of the aorta (pan arteritis) and its major branches. Inflammatory infiltrate is often composed of T cells and shows predominantly mononuclear cell inflammation with a variable admixture of multinucleated giant cells and formation of granuloma. Mononuclear infiltration of the adventitia with perivascular cuffing of the vasa vasorum occurs early. Granulomatous changes may be observed in the tunica media with Langerhans cells and central necrosis of elastic fibers and smooth muscle cells. Concentric thickening of all layers of the artery wall (intima, media, and adventitia) occurs. The inflammation leads to arterial stenosis, thrombosis, and aneurysms. Focal destruction of the wall leads to aneurysms or fibrosis of the wall with narrowing of the major arteries. The corresponding organ shows ischemic changes.[1,10,11]

Clinical Features

The clinical features can be divided into an early pre-pulseless systemic phase and a late occlusive phase. The difficult-to-diagnose early phase is characterized by nonspecific features such as low-grade fever, malaise, night sweats, weight loss, arthralgia, and fatigue and is seen in 50%. This active phase may remit or progress insidiously into the chronic or late occlusive phase. Hypertension is the most common manifestation in this phase and may lead to cardiac failure, visual disturbances, headache, or seizures. Most patients have asymmetric pulses, usually along with a blood pressure differential in the arms. Renal artery stenosis with vascular insufficiency is the cause of hypertension.[12,13] Neurologic symptoms occur secondary to hypertension or ischemia. Lower extremity claudication, bruit, or missing pulse may be seen in an asymptomatic child. Raynaud's phenomenon may also be seen. Systemic symptoms are seen in a high proportion of children.[14,15]

Diagnostic Criteria

EULAR and the PRES consensus criteria for the diagnosis of TA are given in **Table 1**.[7]

Investigations

There are no specific markers for the confirmation of the diagnosis or for the assessment of activity of the disease. Elevated acute-phase reactants, including C-reactive protein (CRP) and erythrocyte sedimentation rate (ESR), are seen in almost all children and they correlate poorly with disease activity. There is normochromic normocytic anemia (50%), leukocytosis, and thrombocytosis. Antinuclear antibody (ANA) and antineutrophil cytoplasmic antibody (ANCA) are negative. Rheumatoid factor is positive in 15%. Antiendothelial cell antibodies are often positive. Conventional, digital subtraction angiography, CT, or MR angiography is necessary for the diagnosis. Angiography shows luminal irregularity, vessel stenosis, occlusion, dilatation, or aneurysms in the aorta or its primary branches **(Figs. 1A to C)**. Digital subtraction angiography has allowed the diagnosis to be made with less dye. Arteriography often demonstrates long, smooth, tapered narrowing or occlusion **(Fig. 2)**.[9,15] Positron emission tomography (PET) scan is useful to differentiate renovascular disease in TA from fibromuscular dysplasia.[1]

Treatment

The goals of medical therapy are to control active inflammation and to normalize clinical and laboratory parameters while preventing further vascular damage. The mainstay of the initial therapy is prednisolone 1 mg/kg daily for 3 months and then taper to an alternate-day schedule [National Institutes of Health (NIH) Protocol], which is continued for 1 year following clinical remission. Patients who do not respond to 3 months of corticosteroids or who relapse during tapering of

TABLE 1: EULAR/PRES classification criteria for Takayasu arteritis.[7]

Criterion	*Description*
Mandatory criterion	Angiographic abnormalities (conventional, CT, or MRI) of the aorta or its major branches and pulmonary arteries–aneurysm/dilatation, narrowing, occlusion, or thickened arterial wall
Plus one of these five criteria	• Pulse deficit or claudication (activity related) of the extremities • Blood pressure discrepancy in four limbs (>10 mm Hg) • Bruit over the aorta and/or its major branches • Systolic/diastolic hypertension >95th centile for height • Elevated acute phase reactants (ESR >20 mm/h or CRP)

(CRP: C-reactive protein; ESR: erythrocyte sedimentation rate; EULAR/PRES: European League Against Rheumatism/Pediatric Rheumatology European Society)

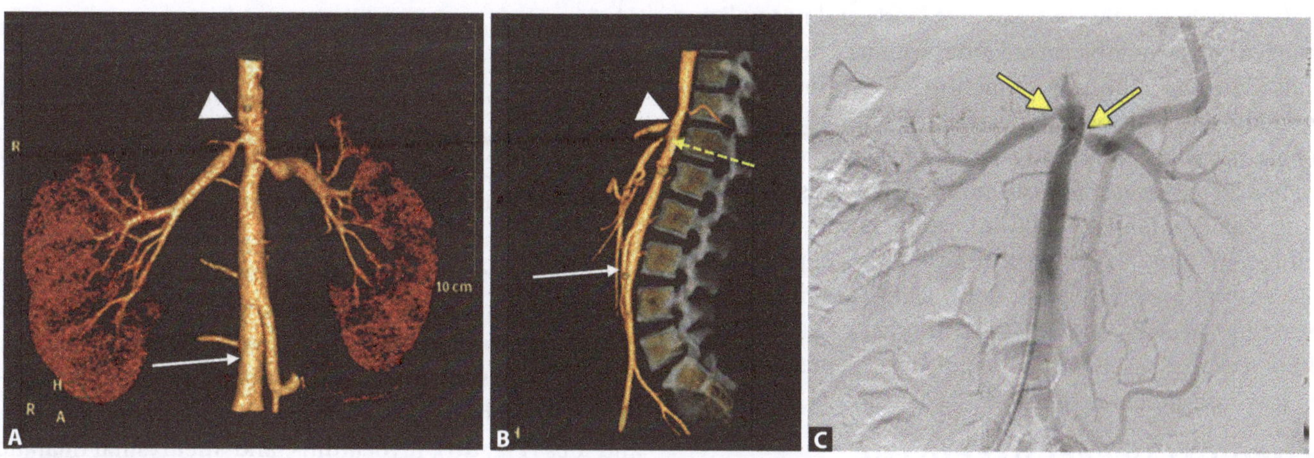

Figs. 1 A to C: Abdominal CT angiogram of a 15-year-old girl with hypertension. (A and B) Anterior and lateral projections showing a narrowed viscerorenal segment (arrow heads) of abdominal aorta with relatively normal-sized aortic bifurcation (white arrow). Narrowing of the origins of both renal arteries in (A) and celiac artery and superior mesenteric artery in (B) (yellow dotted arrows) suggesting middle aortic syndrome; (C) Digital subtraction angiogram—anterior projection showing bilateral ostioproximal narrowing with normal distal renal arteries (solid arrows). *Courtesy:* Dr Anoop A. Sree Chitra Tirunal Institute for Medical Sciences & Technology, Thiruvananthapuram, Kerala, India.

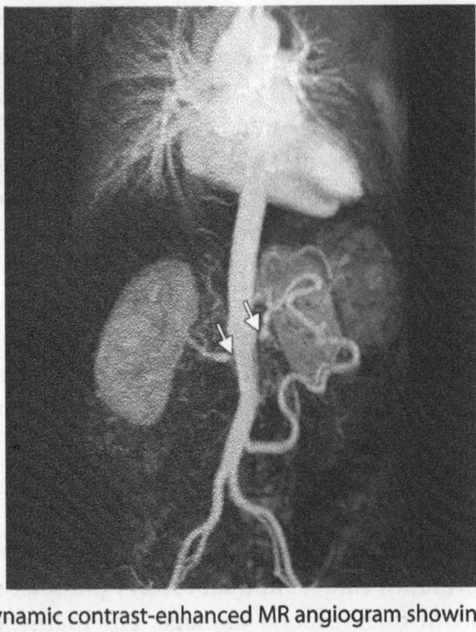

Fig. 2: Dynamic contrast-enhanced MR angiogram showing bilateral renal artery stenosis (white arrows) in aortoarteritis.
Courtesy: Dr Bejoy Thomas, SCTIMST, Thiruvananthapuram, Kerala, India.

corticosteroids require second-line cytotoxic drugs.[15] Weekly methotrexate, daily cyclophosphamide (maximum total dose 150 mg/kg), cyclosporine, or mycophenolate mofetil may be beneficial in glucocorticoid-resistant disease. Leflunomide has been used in glucocorticoid and methotrexate-resistant disease. Tumor necrosis factor (TNF) inhibition with etanercept or infliximab,[16] TNF-α receptor blocker or adalimumab, interleukin-6 (IL-6) inhibitor tocilizumab, or B-cell-depleting agent rituximab has been used in children with TA. Cyclophosphamide is reserved for refractory or life-threatening diseases. Hemodynamically significant vascular stenosis requires surgical or endovascular interventions.[8,9,12,15]

Hypertension is controlled by drugs. Renovascular hypertension is usually resistant and needs intervention. Percutaneous transluminal angioplasty of the aorta and renal artery is effective in treating stenosis and normalizing systolic and diastolic blood pressures within 24 hours. Bypass grafts are used for the improvement of long-segment stenosis or aneurysm. Multiple endovascular stenting is now used in children with renovascular hypertension to relieve long-segment renal artery stenosis. Immunosuppressant-eluting stents could potentially deliver local treatment at the sites of inflammation. The 10-year survival rate is approximately 85% with appropriate treatment. Children have a more severe course of disease with a high mortality rate of 10–30%. Although the disease may be rapidly fatal, it may also burn out leaving a good outcome.[12,14,15]

MEDIUM-VESSEL VASCULITIS

Kawasaki Disease

Kawasaki disease is a type of medium- and small-vessel necrotizing vasculitis affecting skin and mucosa. Also known as mucocutaneous lymph node syndrome, it shows predilection for the involvement of coronary arteries. It is an acute multisystem disease affecting infants and children younger than 5 years of age with a peak at 1 year. The disease is more common in boys.[1,7]

Epidemiology

Kawasaki disease is one of the common vasculitis in children with an estimated annual incidence of 5.5 per 100,000 in children younger than 5 years and was highest in the Indian subcontinent (14.6 per 100,000).[2]

Etiopathogenesis

The etiology is not known. Abnormal immune response to environmental or infectious triggers and superantigens in genetically predisposed is implicated. There is suggestion of a microbial respiratory infection as the inciting factor. Immunological factors are also implicated and include proinflammatory mediators and circulating IgG and IgM antiendothelial cell antibodies that cause endothelial inflammation. IgM ANCAs are also found in KD. Skewed T-cell receptor Vβ repertoire has been reported.[1]

Pathology

Arteritis of medium-sized vessels leads to aneurysmal dilatation, especially of coronary arteries. Coronary arteritis is seen 6–8 days after the onset of KD. All layers of the artery are involved, and the inflammatory infiltrate is composed of neutrophils, monocytes, and macrophages. Progressive destruction of adventitia results in arterial dilatation, formation of saccular aneurysms with thrombosis, or rupture of the vessel sometimes. Parenchymal inflammation involving kidneys presents as mild glomerulonephritis and tubulointerstitial dysfunction.[17,18]

Clinical Manifestations

Kawasaki disease is a triphasic disease consisting of an acute febrile period that lasts up to 14 days, a subacute phase of 2–4 weeks, and a convalescent phase that can last months to years. The acute period is characterized by a persistent and high (>38.5°C) fever. The fever is typically minimally responsive to antipyretics. The fever is likely related to elevated concentrations of proinflammatory cytokines, particularly IL-6 and TNF-α.[3] Other clinical features include nonpurulent conjunctivitis (**Fig. 3A**), morbilliform rashes, cervical lymphadenopathy, tender hepatomegaly, mucocutaneous lesions, redness of lips, strawberry tongue (**Fig. 3B**), redness of oral and pharyngeal mucosa, desquamation of fingers and toes (**Fig. 3C**), myocarditis, and aneurysmal dilatation of the coronary arteries.[16,17] Renal involvement is observed as proteinuria and hematuria. Acute kidney injury with tubulointerstitial involvement and spontaneously remitting nephrotic syndrome have been reported.[1] Focal aneurysm

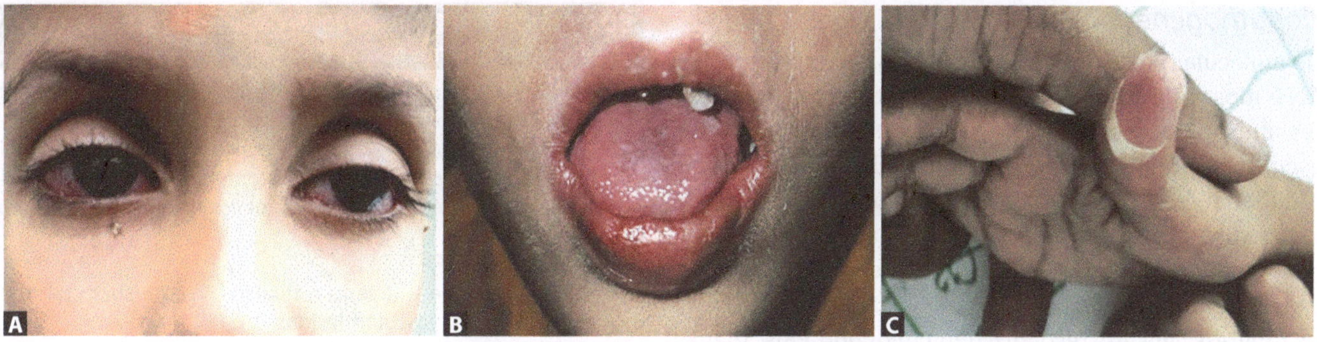

Figs. 3A to C: Kawasaki disease—clinical features. (A) Bilateral nonpurulent conjunctivitis; (B) Injected fissured lips, strawberry tongue; (C) Desquamation— fingertips.

may involve large arteries and common iliac and internal iliac arteries **(Fig. 4)**. The clinical diagnostic criteria by the American Heart Association (AHA) for the diagnosis of KD[19] are given in **Box 3**.

Investigation

Marked polymorphonuclear leukocytosis and normocytic anemia are usual. Thrombocytosis occurs by the second week. Acute-phase reactants, CRP (≥30 mg/dL) and ESR (≥40 mm/h), are elevated. Elevated liver enzymes (≥50 U/L) and hypoproteinemia are other features. An echocardiography will identify coronary artery abnormalities.[17]

Treatment and Outcome

Early and aggressive treatment is decisive in preventing coronary involvement which dictates prognosis and long-term outcome. Coronary aneurysms develop in 15-25% if treatment is delayed. IV gamma globulin (2 g/kg) within the first 7–10 days of illness reduces the occurrence of coronary artery aneurysm. Aspirin is the principal therapeutic agent because of its anti-inflammatory and antithrombotic effects. Aspirin is started at a dose of 30–50 mg/kg/day till the child is afebrile for 48–72 hours and is then reduced to 3–5 mg/kg/day and continued for 6–8 weeks. Prednisolone is indicated in treatment-resistant KD. Recovery is good if there is no cardiac involvement.

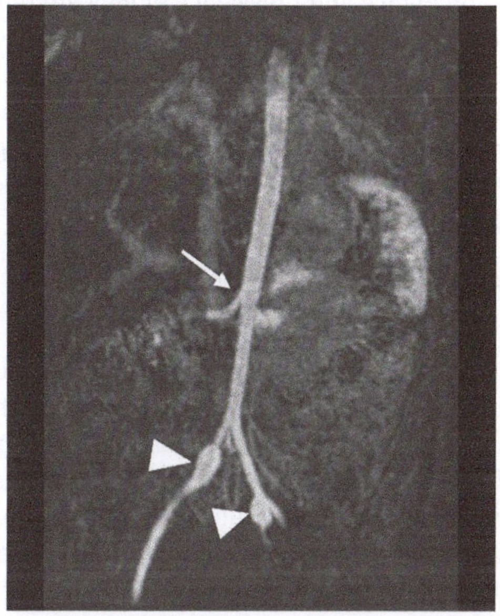

Fig. 4: A 5-year-old boy with diagnosis of Kawasaki disease underwent MR aortic angiogram for evaluation of hypertension showing normal origin of right renal artery (arrow) and focal aneurysms in right common iliac artery and left internal iliac artery (arrowheads). The patient had coronary artery aneurysms in echocardiogram.
Courtesy: Dr Anoop A, Sree Chitra Tirunal Institute for Medical Sciences & Technology, Thiruvananthapuram, Kerala, India.

BOX 3: American Heart Association (AHA) classification criteria for Kawasaki disease.[8]

Fever persisting for at least 5 days (mandatory criterion) plus four of the following five features:

1. Changes in peripheral extremities or perineal area (erythema and/or edema of the hands and feet and subsequent periungual desquamation and perineal area desquamation)
2. Polymorphous exanthema involving the trunk
3. Bilateral nonpurulent conjunctival injection
4. Changes of lips and mucosa of oral cavity (red cracked lips, "strawberry" tongue, or diffuse erythema of oropharynx)
5. Cervical lymphadenopathy (often >1.5 cm)

In the presence of coronary artery involvement (detected on echocardiography) and fever, fewer than four of the remaining five criteria are sufficient

Polyarteritis Nodosa

Polyarteritis nodosa is defined as the necrotizing vasculitis of medium-/small-sized arteries without glomerulonephritis or vasculitis in arterioles, venules, and capillaries, and it is not associated with ANCA.[1,7,8] Although any organ system may be involved, the most common manifestations include peripheral neuropathy, mononeuritis multiplex, intestinal ischemia, renal ischemia, testicular pain, and livedo reticularis. Renal involvement is due to the vasculitis of lobar and arcuate arteries.[7]

Epidemiology

Childhood PAN is a rare and severe multisystemic vasculitic disease predominantly affecting medium-sized vasculitis and accounts for 3% of all childhood vasculitides.[3,20] PAN is found in children between 3 and 16 years of age with a median age of 9–10 years. The disease is more common in men.[7,20]

Etiopathogenesis

The molecular pathophysiology of PAN is currently unclear. PAN is most often idiopathic. An immune complex-mediated mechanism has been suggested as an instigating factor for vasculitis. An autoantibody is produced against vascular endothelial cells triggered by an infection in a genetically predisposed child. Well-recognized associations are cryoglobulinemia, hairy cell leukemia, rheumatoid arthritis, Sjogren's syndrome, and hepatitis B. Association with hepatitis B is progressively less recognized in childhood PAN, thanks to the improvement in hepatitis B vaccination. Streptococcal infections are frequently implicated in childhood diseases. Increased incidence and prevalence of PAN are reported in individuals with familial Mediterranean fever (FMF), one of the most common autoinflammatory disorders in childhood. Autosomal recessive loss-of-function mutations in the adenosine deaminase 2 (*ADA2* or formerly *CECR1*) gene are reported in a subset of particularly early onset cases of PAN (deficiency of *ADA2*: *DADA2*).[9]

Pathology

"Classic" PAN affects the medium-sized muscular arteries. There is focal, often circumferential fibrinoid necrosis, pan mural infiltration, and destruction of segments of the vessel wall by inflammatory exudates composed of neutrophils and eosinophils within the vessel walls. There is extravasation of erythrocytes, macrophages, neutrophils, and less commonly mononuclear cells. Thrombosis and aneurysms preferentially occur at sites of the vessel bifurcation. Mononuclear cells are seen in the subacute stage, and fibroblast proliferation with eventual fibrosis occurs in the chronic stage. In the kidneys, aneurysms, thrombosis and disruption of the segmental renal arteries lead to ischemic injury and scar formation. Interstitial inflammation, which is also necrotizing in character, causes considerable tubular atrophy. The glomerular changes can be focal and segmental though occasionally diffuse proliferation may occur.[1,21]

Clinical Manifestations

The onset is often insidious with fever, weight loss, weakness, arthralgia, myalgia, and abdominal pain. Skin manifestations include tender erythematous nodules, purpura, livedo reticularis, ulcers, and bullous or vesicular eruption. The nodules in PAN are reminiscent of erythema nodosum or nodular panniculitis. Hypertension is the common presenting symptom in classical PAN. Renal involvement frequently leads to variable degrees of renal insufficiency and hypertension. Renal infarctions may occur in severe vasculitis. Mononeuritis multiplex with motor and sensory deficits, digital gangrene, orchitis, pancreatitis, mesenteric arteritis with ischemia, and bloody or nonbloody diarrhea are other manifestations.[22] The 2005 EULAR/PRES consensus classification criteria for childhood PAN are given in **Box 4**.

BOX 4: EULAR/PRES (Ankara, 2008) classification criteria for childhood polyarteritis nodosa.[6]

A systemic illness characterized by the presence of one major plus one out of five minor criteria

- *Major criteria/mandatory criteria:* Evidence of necrotizing vasculitis of small and mid-sized artery on histopathology or angiographic abnormality—aneurysm, stenosis, or occlusion of a medium or small artery
- *Minor criteria:*
  - Skin involvement (livedo reticularis, tender subcutaneous nodules, other vasculitic lesions)
  - Myalgia or muscle tenderness
  - Systemic hypertension (systolic/diastolic blood pressure >95th centile for height)
  - Peripheral neuropathy (sensory neuropathy or motor mononeuritis multiplex)
  - Renal involvement (proteinuria, hematuria, or impaired renal function) (GFR <50% normal for age)
  - Testicular pain or tenderness
  - Signs or symptoms suggesting vasculitis of any other major organ system (gastrointestinal, cardiac, pulmonary, or central nervous system)

(GFR: glomerular filtration rate)

Investigations

Anemia, leukocytosis, thrombocytosis, and elevated acute-phase reactants are seen in active disease. Proteinuria, hematuria, and abnormal glomerular filtration rate (GFR) indicate renal involvement. Evidence of vascular involvement is established by biopsy of skin, sural nerve, testis, or skeletal muscle. Arteriography offers an alternative to biopsy for diagnosis. Conventional mesenteric or renal arteriography will demonstrate multiple aneurysms and irregular constrictions in the larger vessels with occlusion of smaller penetrating arteries. CT or MR angiography is a less invasive angiography technique. Angiography demonstrates arterial aneurysms or narrowing **(Fig. 5)** and pruning of peripheral vascular trees in the kidney and/or liver. The most reliable nonaneurysmal signs in angiography are perfusion defects, presence of collateral arteries, lack of crossing of small peripheral arteries, and delayed emptying of small renal arteries.[23]

Treatment and Outcome

According to the latest EULAR recommendation for the management of SVV and medium-vessel vasculitis (MVV), high doses of corticosteroids and cyclophosphamide (CYP) are used for remission induction for PAN.[24] Induction of remission of systemic PAN is with high doses of corticosteroids (1–2 mg/kg/day with or without initial corticosteroid pulses of 30 mg/kg) and cyclophosphamide in combination with antiplatelet doses of aspirin. Cyclophosphamide is given usually as IV monthly pulses of 750 mg/m^2 for 6 months. In life-threatening or organ-threatening situations, plasmapheresis is indicated. Following successful induction of remission, maintenance therapy with azathioprine, methotrexate, or mycophenolate mofetil is instituted along with low dose

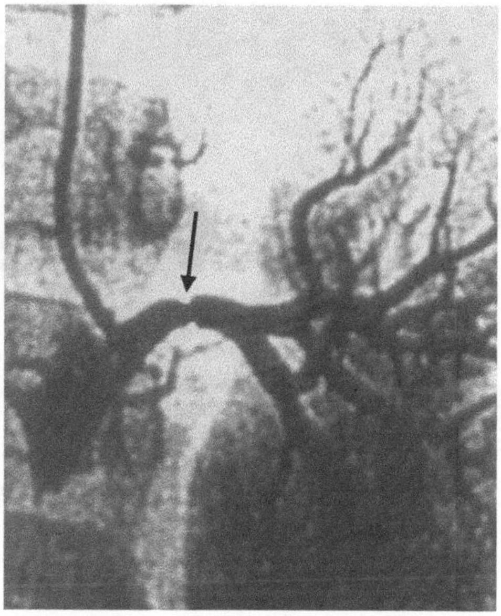

Fig. 5: Angiography showing stenosis of left renal artery in polyarteritis nodosa.
Courtesy: Adhisivam B, et al. Department of Nephrology and Pediatrics, Kanchi Kamakoti CHILDS Trust Hospital, Chennai, Tamil Nadu, India.

daily or alternate-day prednisolone. The total treatment duration is for 2–3 years.[3] Although relapse can occur during the maintenance phase, it is less common as compared to other vasculitis. Recently, biologicals such as infliximab or rituximab, have been tried successfully in the treatment of systemic PAN.[25]

Small-vessel vasculitis may be classified into two groups based on the pathogenesis, i.e., immune complex vasculitis and pauci-immune SVV.[1]

Immune Complex Vasculitis

The two most common immune complex-mediated SVV in childhood with renal involvement are HSP and SLE. Renal manifestations in SLE are discussed in Chapter 8.3 and HSP is discussed in Chapter 7.5.

Pauci-immune Small-vessel Vasculitis

Pauci-immune SVV is a group of potentially life-threatening vasculitis associated with circulating ANCAs and are collectively called ANCA-associated SVV (AASV). They include granulomatosis with polyangiitis (GPA, formerly known as WG), microscopic polyangiitis (MPA), Churg-Strauss syndrome (CSS), and renal-limited vasculitis (RLV). They involve capillaries, venules, arterioles, and small arteries and share pathogenic, pathological, and clinical features. Renal manifestation in AASV is pauci-immune necrotizing crescentic glomerulonephritis which presents as rapidly progressive glomerulonephritis (RPGN) with acute kidney injury. Although rare in children, it carries significant morbidity with potential long-term disability or early mortality.[3,6]

The characteristic feature of AASV is the presence of circulating ANCAs. Serum tested on ethanol-fixed neutrophils by indirect immunofluorescence (IIF) shows two staining patterns—perinuclear or cytoplasmic. The antibody directed against proteinase 3 in neutrophils causes staining limited to the perinuclear region of the neutrophil and is called perinuclear ANCA (P-ANCA). P-ANCA is often associated with MPA. The antibody directed against myeloperoxidase (MPO) in neutrophils causes a fluorescence pattern distributed throughout the cytoplasm of the neutrophil and is called cytoplasmic ANCA (C-ANCA). C-ANCA is seen in approximately 90% of pediatric patients with GPA .[1,6]

Antineutrophil cytoplasmic antibody-associated SVV develops in genetically predisposed children who have been exposed to causative environmental factors. The mechanism by which ANCAs cause vasculitis involves ANCA-mediated excessive activation of neutrophils that subsequently release inflammatory cytokines, reactive oxygen species, and lytic enzymes. The excessive activation of neutrophils by ANCAs induces the formation of neutrophil extracellular traps (NETs). NETs are involved not only in ANCA-mediated vascular injury but also in the production of ANCAs themselves. Therefore, a vicious cycle of NET formation and ANCA production is considered to be involved in the pathogenesis of ANCA-associated vasculitis (AAV). ANCA alone is not sufficient to induce vasculitis. Microenvironmental factors may induce the proinflammatory cytokines, such as TNF-α. Neutrophil priming by TNFα causes the mobilization of PR3 and MPO from granules to the cell surface, which allows ANCAs to bind and activate neutrophils. The primed neutrophils have increased expression of activation markers and superoxides. Once a vasculitic lesion begins, other inflammatory cells including mononuclear cells, such as monocytes and lymphocytes, are quickly recruited and contribute to endothelial cell damage.[26]

Clinical manifestations of ANCA-SVV are protean. A high index of suspicion and targeted investigation are required for prompt diagnosis. The manifestations may be limited to the kidney alone or may involve the upper respiratory tract, the lungs, the skin, or a number of other organs in various combinations. When glomerular capillaries are affected, the clinical manifestation is necrotizing crescentic glomerulonephritis and frequently presents as RPGN. The renal histologic findings include "pauci-immune" (i.e., little immune deposition on immunofluorescence) necrotizing glomerulonephritis with large circumferential crescents **(Figs. 6A and B)**, segmental loss of basement membrane, and tubulointerstitial inflammation. AASV follows a severe course with pulmonary hemorrhage, respiratory failure, rapidly progressive glomerular nephritis, and acute renal failure. Mortality is near 100%, if untreated with a mean survival of 5 months. Renal failure at presentation confers a high risk of end-stage kidney disease despite potent immunosuppressive

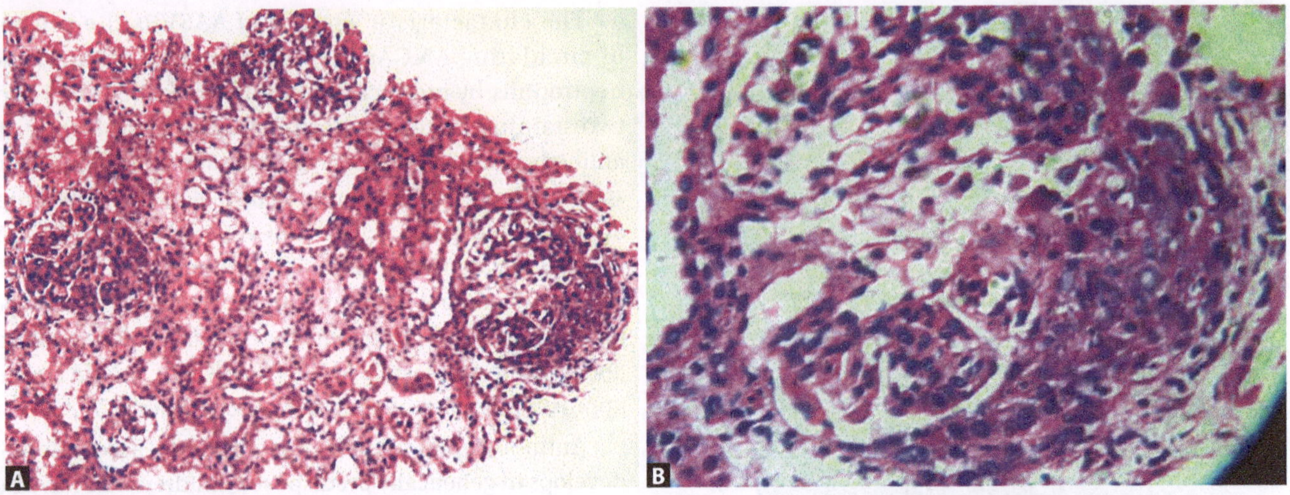

Figs. 6A and B: Necrotizing crescentic glomerulonephritis in microscopic polyangiitis (light microscopy H&E stain × 400).
Courtesy: Dr Hiran KR, Amrita Institute of Medical Sciences, Cochin and Pediatric Nephrology, Government Medical College, Thiruvananthapuram, Kerala, India.

therapy. Relapses are very common and occur in up to 60% of patients. Children are more likely to have multiple organ involvement, renal involvement, and subglottic stenosis.[3,27] Various SVVs are discussed briefly below.

Granulomatosis with Polyangiitis/ Wegener Granulomatosis

Wegener granulomatosis is an idiopathic systemic SVV with predilection for the upper and lower respiratory tracts and kidneys. It is the most common granulomatous vasculitis in children and is recently named as granulomatosis with polyangiitis. It is defined according to the Chapel–Hill criteria as granulomatosis inflammation involving the respiratory tract, with necrotizing vasculitis affecting small- to medium-sized vessels (e.g., capillaries, venules, arterioles, and arteries). Necrotizing glomerulonephritis is common.[1,27-29]

Epidemiology: Wegener granulomatosis is rare in the pediatric age group. The incidence of pediatric-onset GPA was 1.8 cases/million person-years.[28]

Etiopathogenesis: The etiology of WG is an exaggerated immunologic response to an inhaled environmental antigen. No specific antigen, exogenous or endogenous, has been identified. The immune complexes formed in situ or cell-mediated immune mechanism may be the cause of granulomatous vasculitis.[1]

Pathology: The typical renal lesion is a focal segmental necrotizing glomerulonephritis, with pauci-immune crescentic glomerular changes. There is acute proliferation and necrosis in the glomeruli, focal in distribution, with thrombosis of glomerular capillary loops (focal necrotizing glomerulonephritis). In the severe type, there is diffuse proliferation and necrosis of the majority of glomeruli with the formation of epithelial crescents. Clinical manifestations relating to this lesion include hypertension, significant proteinuria, and nephritic and nephrotic syndrome and, ultimately, the protean clinical manifestations of renal failure in the lungs and granulomatous inflammation with mononuclear infiltrates (T cells, macrophages, histiocytes, and giant cells) occur.[1,29] In the lungs, granulomatous pulmonary nodules with or without central cavitation occur.

Clinical manifestations: Wegener granulomatosis typically affects the upper and lower respiratory tracts and is associated with glomerulonephritis. The disease can affect any organ system in the body. The clinical presentation may be a predominantly granulomatous form with localized chronic disease or a florid, acute small vessel vasculitic form characterized by severe pulmonary hemorrhage and/or RPGN.[29] The classic triad of manifestations involves the upper and lower respiratory tract and kidneys. The disease classically progresses from ear, nose, throat, and eyes (E) through lungs (L) to kidney (K) and is briefly remembered as ELK syndrome. Constitutional symptoms include headache, malaise, weight loss, anorexia, weakness, and fever. In addition, symmetrical, polyarticular arthralgia involving small and large joints is frequent.

The upper respiratory tract involvement includes epistaxis, recurrent sinusitis, otalgia, and hearing loss (conductive and sensorineural). Sinusitis involves the maxillary, sphenoid, and ethmoid sinuses. There is mucosal thickening and rarely total obliteration may be seen. Destruction of the cartilaginous nasal septum causes the characteristic "saddle nose" deformity. Granulomatous inflammation occurs anywhere in the mouth, pharynx, larynx, or trachea causing pseudotumors, glottis, and subglottic polyps. Large- or medium-sized airway stenosis may result from granulomatous inflammation and ulceration. Pulmonary involvement dominates with cough, dyspnea, chest pain, and hemoptysis. Single or multiple, unilateral or bilateral, nodular cavitating infiltrates, pneumothorax, pleuritis, and pleural effusions are seen on X-ray.[5]

BOX 5: EULAR/PRINTO/PRES criteria for Wegener's granulomatosis.[6]

Three of the following six features should be present:

1. Renal involvement (proteinuria or hematuria or red blood cell casts)
2. Granulomatous inflammation within the wall of an artery or in the perivascular or extravascular area
3. Upper airway involvement (nasal discharge or septum perforation, sinus inflammation)
4. Laryngotracheobronchial involvement (subglottic, tracheal, or endobronchial stenosis)
5. Pulmonary involvement [abnormal chest X-ray or computed tomography (CT)]
6. Proteinase 3 (PR3)-ANCA or MPO-ANCA positivity [by immunofluorescence, or by enzyme-linked immunosorbent assay (ELISA)]

(ANCA: antineutrophil cytoplasmic antibody; MPO: myeloperoxidase)

The renal manifestation is an acute nephritic syndrome or RPGN. Other renal manifestations include hypertension, significant proteinuria, nephritic-nephrotic syndrome, and renal failure. Renal involvement occasionally precedes the typical signs of respiratory tract disease.[29]

Skin manifestations include painful subcutaneous modules, papules, ulcers, vesicles, petechiae, and palpable purpura. Complete heart block results from granulomatous inflammation of the conducting system with nodal arteritis. Eye involvement may take the form of episcleritis, uveitis, proptosis related to orbital granulomas, and retinal vasculitis.[29]

The 2008 consensus classification definition for WG is given in **Box 5**. Three of the newly defined set of six criteria are required for the classification of WG in a child. The sensitivity and specificity of the new EULAR/PRINTO/PRES criteria are 93 and 99%, respectively.[1,6,27]

Increased ESR, leukocytosis, thrombocytosis, and anemia are common hematological abnormalities. Hematuria, sterile pyuria, and red blood cell (RBC) casts along with proteinuria are present. Serum IgG and IgA and occasionally IgM and IgE are elevated. Circulating immune complexes have been demonstrated by positive rheumatoid factor, cryoprecipitates, positive C1q binding assay, and positive Raji cell assay. The serum is negative for antinuclear antibodies, anti-dsDNA, LE cells, antistreptolysin O, and hepatitis B surface antigen. CRPs have been found to parallel disease activity.

Microscopic Polyangiitis

Microscopic polyangiitis is a necrotizing pauci-immune vasculitis affecting predominantly small vessels and is often associated with a high titer of MPO-ANCA or P-ANCA. The vascular beds of one or more organs may be involved simultaneously or at different times including the kidneys, lungs, skin, spleen, liver, heart, and muscle. MPA commonly presents as pulmonary hemorrhage and glomerulonephritis. Renal manifestations include acute nephritic syndrome, nephritic nephrotic syndrome, or RPGN with renal histology showing focal necrotizing glomerulonephritis with crescents **(Figs. 6A and B)**. Urinary sediment reveals proteinuria and microscopic hematuria. Some have gross hematuria. Renal insufficiency may be present initially or may develop later in the course of the disease. The disease may be limited to the kidneys alone causing a necrotizing and crescentic glomerulonephritis (RLV). Pulmonary symptoms are due to nongranulomatous arteriolar vasculitis and capillaritis. Other manifestations include cutaneous (palpable purpura, petechiae, ulcers, nodules, ecchymosis), neurological (peripheral neuropathies typically mononeuritis multiplex), or gastrointestinal vasculitis.[5,6,29]

Eosinophilic Polyangiitis/Churg-Strauss Syndrome

Eosinophilic granulomatosis with polyangiitis (EGPA) is a necrotizing vasculitis characterized by eosinophilic infiltrates in small- and medium-sized vessels. It is characterized by asthma, blood eosinophilia, and pulmonary infiltrates along with rhinitis, sinusitis, and nasal polyposis.[1,5,6] Eosinophil-rich and granulomatous inflammation involve the respiratory tract, and necrotizing vasculitis affects small- to medium-sized vessels. Peripheral neuropathy, coronary arteritis, and gastrointestinal involvement are common. Glomerulonephritis is uncommon, and cavitary lung nodules do not occur. Renal involvement may occur as acute renal failure due to renal vasculitis and respond well to steroids. Obstructive uropathy can occur because of eosinophilic granulomatous inflammation of the urinary tract. RPA/CSS is very rare in childhood.[5] Reliable demographic information and/or classification criteria for the pediatric age group do not exist, and diagnosis is confirmed by ACR criteria for adults. As compared with adults, cardiac and pulmonary manifestations are more severe in children and the mortality is high.[30]

For classification as EGPA, four of six criteria must be fulfilled: (1) asthma, (2) eosinophilia (peripheral blood) >10%, (3) mono- or polyneuropathy, (4) pulmonary infiltrates, (5) paranasal sinus anomalies, and (6) biopsy with extravascular eosinophilic infiltrates.[28] Laboratory findings include eosinophilia, elevated ESR, CRP, high serum IgE levels, and white blood cell (WBC) counts. Anemia is common. Proteinuria and hematuria are seen. Histology shows prominent eosinophils and granulomas. Antineutrophil cytoplasmic antibodies were found in only 25% of children with CSS.[1,28]

Renal Limited AAV

Renal limited AAV describes those patients with RPGN, often with ANCA positivity (usually MPO-ANCA) but without other organ involvement.[3]

ANCA-negative Glomerulonephritis

ANCA-negative WG, MPA, and RLV are well described in children as in adults. The disease is usually localized and may later seroconvert.[6,27]

DIAGNOSIS OF SMALL-VESSEL VASCULITIS

The pauci-immune SVV may be indistinguishable clinically from other causes of acute-onset renal failure with similar urinary findings such as acute interstitial nephritis, lupus nephritis, antiglomerular basement membrane (anti-GBM) disease, thrombotic microangiopathy, HSP, and diffuse proliferative glomerulonephritis. Exposure to drugs such as penicillamine, hydralazine, and propylthiouracil may provoke vasculitis. The absence of immune deposits on histology and ANCA helps in the diagnosis. Sometimes, simultaneous infection of kidneys and lungs may occur in systemic SVV causing crescentic glomerulonephritis with severe renal failure and pulmonary hemorrhage. This is the pulmonary-renal syndrome. The differential diagnosis includes WG, MPA, CSS, anti-GBM disease, SLE, HSP, and renal vein thrombosis with pulmonary embolus.

As the clinical manifestations of ANCA-SVV are protean, diagnosis can be challenging. A high index of suspicion and targeted investigation are required for prompt diagnosis. The basic diagnostic workup in all cases of suspected AASV should include a full blood count and tests for inflammatory markers such as ESR and CRP. Urinalysis, renal function tests, and the appropriate organ-specific investigations should be planned depending on the clinical manifestations. Chest X-ray or computed tomography helps to assess the respiratory tract involvement.[1,5,6]

Antineutrophil cytoplasmic antibodies are very useful for making the diagnosis of AASV. Both IIF and enzyme-linked immunosorbent assays (ELISAs) are highly sensitive (>95%) and specific (>99%) in active systemic diseases. Typically, WG is associated with a cytoplasmic staining pattern of ANCA by IIF with cANCA, and ELISA reveals specificity against PR3 (PR3-ANCA). MPA and renal-limited AAV are typically associated with pANCA by IIF and with MPO-ANCA by the ELISA. As ANCAs are not diagnostic, organ-specific involvement should be assessed by biopsy. Tissue diagnosis, in particular renal biopsy and also a biopsy of skin, nasal septum, or other tissue, helps not only in the diagnosis but also in assessing the stage of the disease for therapeutic decision-making.[1,27,29]

MANAGEMENT OF VASCULITIS

The priorities in the management of a child with vasculitis are prompt recognition and timely treatment, as many of the vasculitis can be severe and life-threatening. The long-term prognosis primarily depends on the rapid diagnosis, and prompt institution of therapy. Specific treatment is determined by the type of vasculitis, the severity of inflammation, and the particular organ systems affected. There is improvement in treatment regimens with introduction of newer agents including biologicals.[31] The principles in management include differentiating vasculitis from other conditions that mimic vasculitis or secondary vasculitis, defining disease activity and severity and weighing the benefits and risks of therapy.[32]

The treatment can be divided into specific treatment against the inflammatory renal injury and the management of pathophysiological consequences of glomerular disease, such as fluid retention, hypertension, hyperkalemia, and uremia.

Specific Treatment

Specific treatment involves three phases—induction, maintenance, and treatment of relapses.[27,32,33]

Induction Phase

Combination therapy with high-dose corticosteroids and cyclophosphamide is the current standard induction treatment. Methylprednisolone is given intravenously 7–15 mg/kg/day to a maximum of 1 g/day as an infusion for 3 days followed by oral prednisolone 1 mg/kg daily for the first month. Then the dose is tapered to an alternate-day regimen during the second month and the steroid is discontinued by the next 6–12 months.[27,32]

Cyclophosphamide regimen usually consists of six pulses of intravenous doses of 500–1,000 mg/m^2 per dose every 3–4 weeks. Alternatively, oral doses at 2 mg/kg/day can be given for 2–3 months. The dose should be adjusted to maintain a nadir of leukocyte count above 4,000 cells/mm^3 2 weeks post-treatment. Intravenous cyclophosphamide has equal efficacy in inducing remission with a lesser risk of side effects. The total dose of intravenous cyclophosphamide is two to three times smaller than the oral regimen. This regimen induces improvement in over 90% and complete remission in 75%. Intravenous methylprednisolone combined with plasma exchange is given in life-threatening pulmonary hemorrhage, dialysis-dependent renal failure, and severe disease not responding to conventional therapy.[24,27,32]

Alternative agents: Recently biologic therapy is used to treat children with both AAV and ANCA-negative vasculitides. Such agents include rituximab, antitumor necrotizing factor-α (etanercept, infliximab, and adalimumab), and anakinra (recombinant interleukin 1 receptor antagonist). These agents are reserved for those with severe disease not responding to standard treatment or when cumulative cyclophosphamide and/or corticosteroid toxicity is of particular concern.[25,27,34]

Maintenance Phase

The induction phase is followed by azathioprine (1.5–3 mg/kg/day) and low-dose corticosteroids to maintain remission. Mycophenolate mofetil (MMF) can be given as maintenance therapy instead of azathioprine. The maintenance therapy should be continued for several years, and the child should be monitored for relapse with clinical follow-up, renal function tests, and ANCA. Treatment of relapses is similar to the induction regimen.[25,34]

Supportive Management

Salt and water restriction and diuretic therapy are instituted for the control of hypertension and edema. A variety of vasodilators are also effective in reducing blood pressure. Angiotensin-converting enzyme inhibitors may be less effective because of renin-angiotensin system suppression. If there is severe oliguria, dialysis and ultrafiltration are required. Early dialysis may also be indicated for hyperkalemia not responding to conservative therapy, metabolic acidosis, and uremic syndrome. All children on immunosuppressive therapy receive *Pneumocystis jiroveci* prophylaxis with trimethoprim-sulfamethoxazole or pentamidine. Calcium supplements of 1 g daily along with 800 IU vitamin D should be used to prevent negative calcium balance.[6,32-34]

DISEASE ACTIVITY MEASUREMENT

Standardized tools, such as Birmingham Vasculitis Activity Score (BVAS), are used to measure disease activity and damage in clinical practice and trials. Pediatric Vasculitis Activity Score (PVAS) is modified from BVAS. These scores help to guide treatment decisions and assess prognosis.[34]

PROGNOSIS

The AAV still carries considerable disease-related morbidity and mortality, particularly due to progressive renal failure or aggressive respiratory involvement and therapy-related complications, such as sepsis. The mortality for pediatric WG and MPA is 10–15%. 40% develop chronic renal failure despite therapy. Necrotizing pauci-immune glomerulonephritis with positive ANCA suggests an overall poor renal prognosis in children.[33,34]

CONCLUSION

Vasculitis is a group of heterogeneous disorders with multi-organ involvement resulting from inflammation of blood vessels. Vasculitis may be primary or secondary. Primary systemic vasculitis, though rare in children, carries significant morbidity and mortality despite advances in diagnostic modalities and treatment. Primary vasculitis may be classified according to the pathogenesis or clinical, serological, or pathological features.

As the kidney is a highly vascular organ, renal involvement is common in systemic vasculitis. Renal manifestations depend on the size of the vessel involved and may vary from glomerular disease as in SVV to renovascular involvement in large and medium vessel vasculitis. The priorities in the management of a child with vasculitis are prompt recognition and timely treatment, as many of the vasculitis can be severe and life-threatening. The long-term prognosis primarily depends on the rapid diagnosis and prompt institution of therapy with steroids and cytotoxics.

KEY POINTS

- Vasculitis is a heterogeneous group of disorders resulting from inflammation of blood vessels.
- Primary vasculitis is autoimmune in etiology while secondary vasculitis may be due to infection, drugs, malignancy, and connective tissue diseases such as SLE or rheumatoid arthritis.
- Large vessels such as the aorta and its branches, medium-sized vessels such as visceral arteries, and small vessels such as arterioles, venules, and capillaries may be affected causing necrosis, vascular occlusion, stenosis, aneurysm, rupture, and ischemic damage to the supplied organ or tissues.
- Renal manifestations depend on the size of the vessel involved and may vary from glomerular disease as in SVV to renovascular involvement in large- and medium-vessel vasculitis.
- The goals of medical therapy are to control active inflammation and to normalize clinical and laboratory parameters while preventing further vascular damage.
- Prognosis depends on early aggressive treatment with steroids, cytotoxics, and plasmapheresis when indicated as in rapidly progressive renal failure.

REFERENCES

1. Sez O, Declehan O. Renal involvement in children with vasculitis. In: Avner ED, Harmon WE, Niaudet P, Yoshikawa N, Emma F, Goldstein SL (Eds). Pediatric Nephrology, 7th edition. Berlin Heidelberg: Springer-Verlag; 2009, 2016. pp. 1431-88.
2. Gardner-Medwin JM, Dolezalova P, Cummins C, Southwood TR. Incidence of Henoch-Schönlein purpura, Kawasaki disease, and rare vasculitides in children of different ethnic origins. Lancet. 2002;360(9341):1197-202.
3. Weiss PF. Pediatric vasculitis. Pediatr Clin North Am. 2012; 59(2):407-23.
4. Saha A, Sarkar S, Mondal T. Profile of pediatric vasculitides – prospective hospital-based data from eastern India. Indian J Rheumatol. 2021;16(2):127-32.
5. Jennette JC. Overview of the 2012 revised International Chapel Hill Consensus Conference nomenclature of vasculitides. Clin Exp Nephrol. 2013;17:603-6.
6. Ozen S, Ruperto N, Dillon MJ, Bagga A, Barron K, Davin JC, et al. EULAR/PReS endorsed consensus criteria for the classification of childhood vasculitides. Ann Rheum Dis. 2006;65:936-41.
7. Ozen S, Pistorio A, Iusan SM, Bakkaloglu A, Herlin T, Brik R, et al. EULAR/PRINTO/PRES criteria for Henoch-Schönlein purpura, childhood polyarteritis nodosa, childhood Wegener granulomatosis and childhood Takayasu arteritis: Ankara 2008. Part II: final classification criteria. Ann Rheum Dis. 2010;69:798-806.
8. Sag E, Batu ED, Ozen S. Childhood systemic vasculitis. Best Pract Res Clin Rheumatol. 2017;31:558-75.
9. Schnabel A, Hedrich CM. Childhood vasculitis. Front Pediatr. 2019;6:421.
10. Gedalia A, Cuchacovich R. Systemic vasculitis in childhood. Curr Rheumatol Rep. 2009;11(6):402-9.

11. Serra R, Butrico L, Fugetto F, Chibireva MD, Malva A, De Caridi G, et al. Updates in pathophysiology, diagnosis and management of Takayasu arteritis. Ann Vasc Surg. 2016;35:210-25.
12. Chugh KS, Sakhuja V. Takayasu's arteritis as a cause of renovascular hypertension in Asian countries. Am J Nephrol. 1992;12(1e2):1e8.
13. De Pablo P, Garcia-Torres R, Uribe N, Ramón G, Nava A, Silveira LH, et al. Kidney involvement in Takayasu arteritis. Clin Exp Rheumatol. 2007;25(1 Suppl 44):S10-4.
14. Goel R, Kumar TS, Danda D, Joseph G, Jeyaseelan V, Surin AK, et al. Childhood-onset Takayasu arteritis experience from a tertiary care center in South India. J Rheumatol. 2014;41(6):1183e9.
15. Gulati A, Bagga A. Large vessel vasculitis. Pediatr Nephrol. 2010;25:1037-48.
16. Buonuomo PS, Bracaglia C, Campana A, Insalaco A, Pardeo M, Cortis E, et al. Infliximab therapy in pediatric Takayasu's arteritis: report of two cases. Rheumatol Int. 2009;31(1):93-5.
17. Hedrich CM, Schnabel A, Hospach T. Kawasaki disease. Front Pediatr. 2018;6:198.
18. Takahashi K, Oharaseki T, Yokouchi Y, Naoe S, Saji T. Kawasaki disease: basic and pathological findings. Clin Exp Nephrol. 2013;17(5):690-3.
19. Newburger JW, Takahashi M, Gerber MA, Gewitz MH, Tani LY, Burns JC, et al. Diagnosis, treatment, and long-term management of Kawasaki disease: a statement for health professionals from the committee on rheumatic fever, endocarditis and Kawasaki disease, Council on Cardiovascular Disease in the Young, American Heart Association. Pediatrics. 2004;114(6):1708-33.
20. Dillon MJ, Eleftheriou D, Brogan PA. Medium-size-vessel vasculitis. Pediatr Nephrol. 2010;25:1641-52.
21. Eleftheriou D, Dillon MJ, Tullus K, Marks SD, Pilkington CA, Roebuck DJ, et al. Systemic polyarteritis nodosa in the young: A single-center experience over thirty-two years. Arthritis Rheum. 2013;65(9):2476-85.
22. Mondal R, Sarkar S, Pal P, Nandi M, Hazra A, Sabui TK. Childhood polyarteritis nodosa: A prospective multicentre study from eastern India. Indian J Pediatr. 2014;81(4):371-4.
23. Brogan PA, Davies R, Gordon I, Dillon MJ. Renal angiography in children with polyarteritis nodosa. Pediatr Nephrol. 2002;17(4):277-83.
24. Mukhtyar C, Guillevin L, Cid MC, Dasgupta B, de Groot K, Gross W, et al. European Vasculitis Study Group. EULAR recommendations for the management of primary small and medium vessel vasculitis. Ann Rheum Dis. 2009;68(3):310-7.
25. Eleftheriou D, Melo M, Marks SD, Tullus K, Sills J, Cleary G, et al. Biologic therapy in primary systemic vasculitis of the young. Rheumatology. 2009;48:978-86.
26. Nakazawa D, Masuda S, Tomaru U, Ishizu A. Pathogenesis and therapeutic interventions for ANCA-associated vasculitis. Nat Rev Rheumatol. 2019;15:91-101.
27. Brogan P, Eleftheriou D, Dillon MJ. Small vessel vasculitis. Pediatr Nephrol. 2010;25:1025-35.
28. Panupattanapong S, Stwalley DL, White AJ, Olsen MA, French AR, Hartman ME. Epidemiology and outcomes of granulomatosis with polyangiitis in pediatric and working-age adult populations in the United States: analysis of a large national claims database. Arthritis Rheumatol. 2018;70(12):2067-76.
29. Akikusa JD, Schneider R, Harvey EA, Hebert D, Thorner PS, Laxer RM, et al. Clinical features and outcome of pediatric Wegener's granulomatosis. Arthritis Rheum. 2007;57:837-44.
30. Zwerina J, Eger G, Englbrecht M, Manger B, Schett G. Churg-Strauss syndrome in childhood: a systematic literature review and clinical comparison with adult patients. Semin Arthritis Rheum. 2009;39:108-15.
31. Eleftheriou D, Dillon MJ, Brogan PA. Advances in childhood vasculitis. Curr Opin Rheumatol. 2009;21(4):411-8.
32. Yates M, Watts RA, Bajema IM, Cid MC, Crestani B, Hauser T, et al. EULAR/ERA-EDTA recommendations for the management of ANCA-associated vasculitis. Ann Rheum Dis. 2016;75(9):1583-94.
33. Lee JJY, Alsaleem A, Chiang GPK, Limenis E, Sontichai W, Yeung RSM, et al. Hallmark trials in ANCA-associated vasculitis (AAV) for the pediatric rheumatologist. Pediatr Rheumatol. 2019;17:31.
34. Jayne D. Progress of treatment in ANCA associated vasculitis. Nephrology. 2009;14:42-8.

CHAPTER

7.4 Juvenile Diabetes and Kidney Injury

Vijay Viswanathan, Reshma Mirshad, Leema George

INTRODUCTION

Type 1 diabetes, hitherto known as juvenile diabetes, is a multifactorial disease with genetic predisposition and autoimmune pathogenesis, and it predominantly affects children and young adults.[1] The peak age of onset is approximately 10 years, but this disorder may occur shortly after birth through midlife.[2] Diabetic nephropathy (DN) is one of the microvascular complications of diabetes, which is characterized by elevated urinary albumin excretion rate (UAER) and blood pressure (BP) with a decline in renal function. The prevalence of the onset of DN is 25–40% after a disease duration of at least 10 years in type 1 diabetes mellitus (T1DM) or type 2 diabetes mellitus (T2DM).[3,4]

Kidney failure caused by diabetes is infrequent during childhood. However, many years of hyperglycemia contribute to long-term complications, both microvascular and macrovascular. Hence, all children with diabetes warrant assessment of glomerular filtration rate (GFR), BP, and urine albumin excretion. Screening of the aforementioned factors should begin after 5 years of the onset of T1DM or at puberty. The advanced stages of nephropathy, such as overt proteinuria or end-stage kidney disease (ESKD), take decades to develop and are rare in children and adolescents with T1DM. The kidney biopsies showed structural changes characteristic of diabetic kidney disease (DKD) as early as 1.5–5 years after diabetes onset in adults and children, which often progresses during puberty.[5-7] It is known that a significant increase in mortality is observed in diabetes with nephropathy and is primarily due to cardiovascular disease (CVD) and not only the result of ESKD.[8]

EPIDEMIOLOGY

The incidence of T1DM varies in different ethnicities; it is much lower in Caucasians than in Asians. In India, T1DM is equal to 10.2 per 100,000 population from 1991 to 2015, with a higher prevalence in urban than in rural areas.[9] According to the International Diabetes Federation (IDF), the overall annual increase is estimated to be around 3%, with strong indications of geographic differences. The epidemiological data stated that 25–30% of people with T1D would progress to ESKD. However, not everyone develops progressive nephropathy that ultimately requires dialysis or transplantation; <1–1.5% of children with diabetes show overt proteinuria.[10] From 2001 to 2009, the prevalence of type 1 diabetes in youth increased by 21.1% with comparable increases for both sexes and in most racial/ethnic and age groups.[11] The lifetime risk of kidney disease in T1DM has, by tradition, been estimated at 50%, but it may exceed 70%.[12]

In North America, DKD remains the leading cause of ESKD.[13,14] It is projected that among 100 million European children aged 0–14 years, around 10,000 will develop insulin-dependent diabetes mellitus (IDDM) each year. A subset of 10–30% of patients with IDDM develop DN depending on the metabolic control.[15] There is a constant increase in the annual incidence of T1DM and T2DM among persons aged <20 years. But the increase in the rates of incidence is lesser for T1DM (1.9%) compared to T2DM (4.8% per year).[16]

Maturity-onset diabetes of the young (MODY) is a form of monogenic diabetes, often misdiagnosed as T1DM. Hepatocyte nuclear factor 1-alpha (HNF1A) (responsible for MODY3) and HNF1B (MODY5 or RCAD) molecular defects have been associated with a specific renal phenotype independent of DN.[17] Hence, children with monogenic diabetes (diabetes caused by single-gene mutation) can have renal involvement as a part of the disorder. More frequent use of genetic studies would increase the diagnosis of MODY.

PATHOGENESIS

Kidney injury and overt DN caused by either type of diabetes are very infrequent during childhood or adolescence. In predisposed T1DM patients, DKD almost certainly begins soon after T1DM diagnosis and may accelerate during adolescence. The various pathomechanisms involved in chronic kidney disease (CKD) progression render it increasingly difficult to disentangle their specific roles in the development of kidney injury. DN is a multifactorial disease with the involvement of multiple pathways. Several complex molecular interactions are implicated in the process that is also genetically regulated.[18,19] However, the precise pathomechanism of DN is not represented. There are several factors which lead to the development of DN.

Hyperglycemia has a crucial effect on glomerular and mesangial cells and is associated with increased mesangial cell proliferation and hypertrophy with increased matrix production. This, in turn, results in basement thickening. Hyperglycemia may also increase the expression of vascular endothelial growth factor (VEGF) in podocytes resulting in increased vascular permeability.

Chronic hyperglycemia is known to activate several deleterious pathways, such as diacylglycerol (DAG)-protein kinase C (PKC) pathway and polyol pathway. The mechanism by which hyperglycemia leads to PKC activation involves de novo formation of DAG and oxidative stress.[20] PKC activation induces the activity of mitogen-activated protein kinases (MAPK) in response to extracellular stimuli through dual phosphorylation at conserved threonine and tyrosine residues.

Hyperglycemia is also associated with the glycosylation of tissue proteins that are nonenzymatic, which results in the initial production of reversible glycosylation end products followed by irreversible advanced glycosylation end products (AGEs). Excess intracellular glucose results in increased glucose flux through alternative polyol and hexosamine pathways and increased oxidative stress, stimulating secondary intracellular signaling pathways, leading to the production of growth factors, cytokines, and inflammatory factors.[21]

Hyperglycemia stimulates VEGF expression and, therefore, acts as a mediator of endothelial injury in human diabetes.[22-24] It also increases the expression of transforming growth factor β 1 (TGF-β1) in the glomeruli and of matrix proteins specifically stimulated by this cytokine.[25] Inflammatory cytokines, such as interleukin-1 (IL-1), IL-6, and IL-18 and tumor necrosis factor, have also been implicated in the progression of DN. IL-6 has a strong association with the development of glomerular basement membrane thickening as well as possible relationships with increased endothelial permeability and mesangial cell proliferation. IL-18 induces the production of other inflammatory cytokines, such as IL-1, interferon γ, and tumor necrosis factor, and might be associated with endothelial cell apoptosis. Tumor necrosis factor causes direct renal injury and affects apoptosis, epithelial permeability, and cell-cell adhesion.

In addition to the metabolic pathways and cytokines, Rho-kinase has been linked to numerous steps in the ultrastructural damage of DN. This is an effector of small GTPase-binding protein Rho and induces endothelial dysfunction, mesangial excessive extracellular matrix (ECM) production, podocyte abnormality, and tubulointerstitial fibrosis. Endothelial dysfunction, characterized by impaired vasorelaxation, results from reduced bioavailability of endothelial nitric oxide. This is a common finding among people with T1DM and could represent a significant link to the cardiovascular complications.[26] Significant association has been reported between the different microvascular complications of diabetes, and hence patients with one complication often develop a second one, suggesting common risk factors and/or pathogenetic mechanisms.[27] Other factors such as noncoding RNAs, epigenetic mechanisms such as DNA methylation, and histone modifications can also play a crucial role in the pathogenesis of DN (**Fig. 1**).

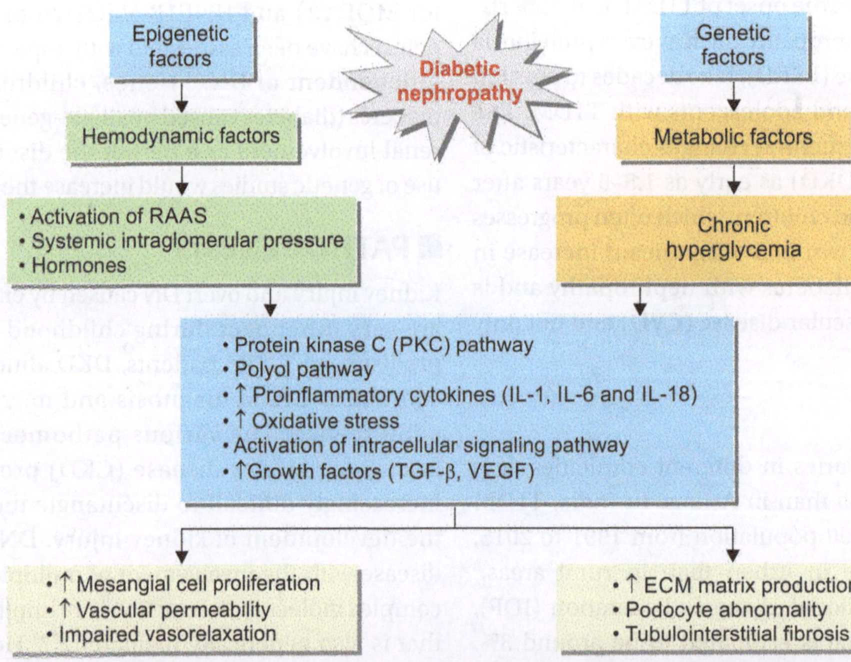

Fig. 1: Pathogenesis of diabetic nephropathy. (ECM: extracellular matrix; RAAS: renin-angiotensin-aldosterone system; TGF-β: transforming growth factor β; VEGF: vascular endothelial growth factor)

CLINICAL PRESENTATION

Diabetic nephropathy is divided into preclinical and clinical phases.

Stage I: Hypertrophic hyperfiltration. In this stage, the kidney is enlarged by 20% and the renal flow is increased by 10–15%. GFR is either normal or increased on an average by 20–40% above the age-matched normal controls. Albuminuria and BP continue to be within the normal range. This stage lasts approximately 5 years from the onset of the disease.

Stage II: The quiet stage. This stage starts approximately 2 years after the onset of the disease and is characterized by kidney damage with basement membrane thickening and mesangial proliferation. This is usually a clinically silent stage with a normal albumin excretion rate despite the structural changes. Many patients remain in this stage until the end of their life. However, 30–40% progress to subsequent stages. The explanation for this variable progression remains obscure and may relate to factors such as the degree of metabolic control, development of hypertension, and genetic factors.

Stage III: The microalbuminuria stage (albumin 30–300 mg/24 h) or initial nephropathy. This is the first clinically visible sign of glomerular damage. It usually occurs 5–10 years after the onset of the disease. Accelerated progression of renal disease is seen in patients with elevated BP. Around 40% of the patients reach this stage.

Stage IV: Chronic kidney failure (CKF) is the irreversible stage (albumin > 300 mg/day). GFR decreases to <60 mL/min/1.73 m^2 with increased BP above normal values. Proteinuria develops once persistent proteinuria is present; the average time until the development of ESKD or death is from 3.3 to 4.8 years.

Stage V: Terminal kidney failure (TKF) or advanced renal failure (GFR < 15 mL/min/1.73 m^2). Nearly 50% of the patients with TKF require kidney replacement therapy (peritoneal dialysis, hemodialysis, kidney transplantation). In contrast with the nondiabetic patients, diabetics with ESKD usually have other systemic degenerative manifestations in addition to their renal disease.[28-31]

Most children with T1DM are clinically silent when histological changes are developing without evidence of kidney dysfunction. Several groups have examined changes in kidney structure in youth with T1DM. Although biopsy studies show that diabetic lesions develop in the kidney before puberty, the onset of sustained microalbuminuria rarely occurs before sexual maturation. Hence, it is essential to clearly understand diabetic kidney injury's clinical presentation in children.

Renal Histology in Diabetic Nephropathy

The utility of renal biopsy in patients with diabetes is currently an object of debate. The most common indications include rapidly worsening renal function and/or unusual clinical features (e.g., sudden appearance of heavy proteinuria in patients with a short duration of DM, hematuria, active urine sediment, no signs of other microvascular complications such as retinopathy) in a patient with diabetes. The biopsy would be crucial for identifying the presence of non-DKD.[32]

Histopathological findings show thickening of the glomerular basement membrane, detected as early as 1.5–2.5 years after the onset of T1DM. It is followed by thickening of the tubular basement membrane, implying that glomerular hemodynamic perturbations are not required for these changes to occur. Afferent and efferent arteriolar hyalinosis may be present within a few years after diabetes onset and correlate significantly with the percentage of sclerosed glomeruli. Abnormalities of the glomerular–tubular junction are late manifestations of the disease, predominantly in patients with proteinuria.[33]

Biomarkers

Novel biomarkers are essential to achieve effective renoprotection and early detection of kidney disease in children. Despite the reliability of the traditional biomarkers of glomerular injury such as albumin/creatinine ratio (ACR) and eGFR which predict DKD, their limitation as diagnostic tools has underscored the need for paradigm shift to biomarkers.

Many abnormalities might reflect early kidney disease in diabetic children. A combination of high levels of serum neutrophil gelatinase-associated lipocalin (sNGAL) and high but normal albumin excretion rate (AER) have a strong prognostic impact on the development and progression of kidney disease in diabetic children with normoalbuminuria. Therefore, sNGAL may allow early identification of those at risk of renal complications. In children with T1DM, NGAL and IL-18 are the most promising tubular biomarkers for the diagnosis of acute and chronic renal diseases without any overt signs of DN.[34] Some of the biomarkers of kidney injury in type 1 diabetes mellitus subject are depicted in **Table 1**.

Early Screening and Prevention of Risk Factors

Diabetic nephropathy is the most frequently observed microvascular complication in T1DM. In T1DM, annual

TABLE 1: Summary of some of the biomarkers of kidney injury in type 1 diabetes mellitus subjects.

Biomarker	*Biospecimen*	*Stage of kidney disease*
N-acetyl-β-D-glucosaminidase	Urine	Predicts the early and late stages of CKD in type 1 diabetics
Liver fatty acid-binding protein	Urine	Predicts early CKD and progression to ESKD in type 1 diabetics
Kidney injury molecule-1	Urine/blood	Predicts CKD progression to ESKD

(CKD: chronic kidney disease; ESKD: end-stage kidney disease)

screening for microalbuminuria should be performed from 11 years of age in children with 2 years' diabetes duration and from the age of 9 years in children with 5 years' diabetes duration. In children with T2DM, screening for microalbuminuria should begin as early as the time of diagnosis as per the International Society for Pediatric and Adolescent Diabetes and the IDF (ISPAD/IDF) consensus for microalbuminuria.[35,36]

Diabetic nephropathy screening and diagnosis are made by measuring albumin in a spot urine sample, collected either in the morning or at random. Extra care should be taken to eliminate the associated conditions that increase urinary albumin excretion (UAE) such as acute febrile illness, urinary tract infection, and hematuria. First-voided urine in the morning is preferable because of the known diurnal variation in albumin excretion and postural effects. A random sample can be used but may be associated with an increased risk of false-positive results. In case of an abnormal result, screening should be repeated with first morning urine collections. Albuminuria is confirmed by finding two or all three abnormal samples over a 3- to 6-month period. In young people with childhood-onset T1DM, increased AERs can predict the future risk of albuminuria and proteinuria within a year of diagnosis.[37]

Even though the UAE measurement is the cornerstone for diagnosis, some patients with T1DM have a decreased GFR in the presence of normal UAE. These findings were more common among female patients with long-standing diabetes, hypertension, and retinopathy.[38] Therefore, GFR is routinely estimated along with the UAE for proper screening. The reference range of GFR values in young individuals ranges from 80 to 130 mL/min.

Persistent albuminuria has been shown to predict end-stage renal failure progression and is associated with an increased risk of macrovascular disease. Regular follow-up is vital to identify rapid or slow progression to albuminuria and cases of regression to normoalbuminuria. Glycated hemoglobin (HbA1c) of >7.5% significantly increases the probability of microalbuminuria after 10 years and macroalbuminuria after 20 years of diabetes onset. Therefore, efforts to normalize metabolic control should be started right from diabetes onset.[30] Children with diabetes and CKD should be assessed at least annually as the renal consequences are noted in the later years of life. The exact frequency of GFR and ACR monitoring will depend on the severity of CKD. GFR and albuminuria categories in CKD are given in **Figure 2.**

Along with attention to good metabolic control to prevent and to delay microvascular complications, early diagnosis and treatment of hypertension, dyslipidemia, and avoidance of smoking are also important in preventing progression of CKD in diabetic children and adolescents. As puberty is an independent risk factor for microalbuminuria, annual screening must be performed after puberty.

				Persistent Albuminuria Categories Description and Range		
				A1	A2	A3
				Normal to mildly increased	Moderately increased	Severely increased
				ACR < 30 mg/g	ACR of 30–300 mg/g	ACR > 300 mg/g
GFR categories (mL/min per 1.73 m^2) Description and range	G1	Normal or high	≥90	1 if CKD	1	2
	G2	Mildly decreased	60–89	1 if CKD	1	2
	G3a	Mildly to moderately decreased	45–59	1	2	3
	G3b	Moderately to severely decreased	30–44	2	3	3
	G4	Severely decreased	15–29	3	3	4+
	G5	Kidney failure	<15	4+	4+	4+

Fig. 2: Glomerular filtration rate and albuminuria categories in chronic kidney disease. (ACR: albumin/creatinine ratio; CKD: chronic kidney disease)
Source: Adapted from Stevens PE, Levin A. Kidney Disease: Improving Global Outcomes Chronic Kidney Disease Guideline Development Work Group Members. Evaluation and management of chronic kidney disease: synopsis of the kidney disease: improving global outcomes 2012 clinical practice guideline. Ann Intern Med. 2013;158(11):825-30.

Kidney failure from either form of diabetes is uncommon during childhood. Still, children with diabetes are at an increased risk of progressive kidney disease and warrant an ongoing assessment of kidney function periodically as advised. Involvement of a pediatric nephrologist should include interpretation of screening as well as evaluation and treatment of those with renal dysfunction or atypical features.[39]

MANAGEMENT

The best approach to deal with this catastrophic condition is timely diagnosis and appropriate intervention. Absence of routine screening is the major hurdle in early diagnosis. There is no effective pharmacological intervention to prevent or reverse kidney injury. Early diagnosis can have lifetime benefits by controlling the disease progression, increasing life expectancy, and decreasing the humanistic and economic burden. Effective management strategies should guide the approach as listed below.

Patient Perspectives and Self-management

The kidney disease: Improving Global Outcomes guidelines implemented a new concept by explicit inclusion of patient perspectives. The importance of including the patient in the decision-making process prioritizes patients' care by improving self-management, self-motivation, diabetes-related knowledge, beliefs, and skills **(Flowchart 1)**. Self-management education should be done on how to improve emotional and mental well-being, treatment satisfaction, and quality of life.

Glucose Monitoring

The aim of the treatment is achieving the best glycemic control possible. HbA1C target of <7.5% (58 mmol/mol) as per the American Diabetes Association (ADA) recommendation should be considered in children and adolescents with T1DM.[40] Daily glucose monitoring helps prevent hypoglycemia and improve glycemic control.[41] Newer insulin analogs, continuous subcutaneous insulin infusion (insulin pump) therapy, and continuous glucose monitoring have dramatically improved care and decreased complications for youths with T1DM.

Lifestyle Interventions

Recent KDIGO guideline recommends that patients with diabetes and CKD consume a diet high in vegetables, fruits, whole grains, and fiber but lower in processed meats, refined carbohydrates, and sweetened beverages. The sodium intake is limited to <2 g/day (or <5 g sodium chloride), consistent with the BP control and CVD prevention.

The general recommendation on physical activity for children and adolescents with T1DM or T2DM includes 60 min/day or more of moderate- or vigorous-intensity aerobic activity, with vigorous muscle-strengthening and bone-strengthening activities at least 3 days/week.[42]

Prospective Pharmacological Treatment

Various strategies are advocated to slow the progression of CKD in children and adolescents with DN including strict BP control, optimizing anemia, reducing proteinuria, and achieving normal 25-hydroxyvitamin D levels.

Management of Hypertension

Lowering BP is another important component of the treatment of DN.

The first-line agent for the treatment of hypertension in adolescents and children with microalbuminuria or

Flowchart 1: Integrated care approach to improve outcomes, self-management, and patient–provider communication in patients with diabetes and chronic kidney disease (CKD).[40]

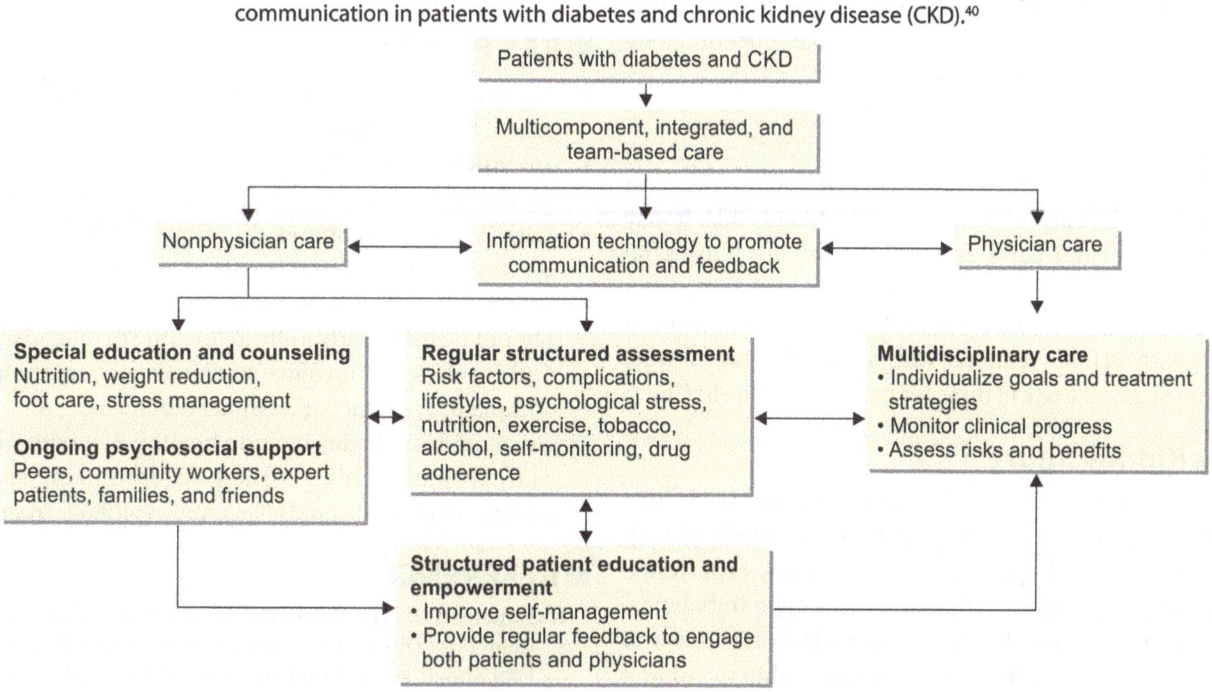

hypertension should be either ACE inhibitors (ACEIs) or angiotensin II receptor blockers (ARBs). ACEI/ARBs help to normalize or reduce microalbuminuria and slow or prevent progression. If ACEI/ARB fails to achieve BP goals below the 90th percentile combination therapy can be considered. To date, no agent is a superior second-line drug, though beta-blockers, calcium channel blockers, and central alpha-blockers have all been used with success. Antihypertensive therapy with either enalapril or metoprolol has been shown to retard glomerulopathy progression and interstitial expansion in normotensive, macroalbuminuric adolescents with DN.[43]

Proteinuria

Proteinuria is defined as urinary protein excretion higher than 100–150 mg/m^2/day in children.[44] It has been described as a risk factor for renal disease progression in CKD. A higher degree of proteinuria lowering during the initial months of treatment with ACEI was independently associated with a lower risk of CKD progression in a large interventional trial analysis in children.[45] However, the long-term effect of proteinuria-lowering drugs on renal survival has not been well established in children. Dietary protein restriction is not usually recommended to avoid harmful effects on the growth and development, and children must receive the appropriate daily protein intake depending on their age.

Vitamin D

Recent studies have suggested that vitamin D may retard the progression by suppressing renin transcription through cross-talk between renin-angiotensin-aldosterone system (RAAS) and vitamin D-fibroblast growth factor-23 (FGF-23)-Klotho pathways.[46] In the post hoc analysis of the ESCAPE (European Study of Cohorts for Air Pollution Effects) cohort, in children with CKD, 25-hydroxyvitamin D ≥ 50 nmol/L was associated with greater preservation of renal function along with concomitant ACEI therapy.

Dyslipidemia

Dyslipidemia is considered as an independent risk factor not only for CVD but also for the progression of CKD. It may damage glomerular capillary endothelial and mesangial cells as well as podocytes. An association between serum cholesterol levels and GFR decline was observed in adult patients with T1DM.[47] Patients with a total cholesterol level > 126 mg/dL are at a risk of three times faster decline in GFR.[48]

Acute Kidney Injury

Acute kidney injury (AKI) is an independent factor associated with higher mortality rate in diabetic ketoacidosis (DKA). Due to osmotic diuresis, children with DKA experience varying degrees of dehydration and electrolyte imbalance. The compensatory mechanism for dehydration is not well established; thus, children are more vulnerable to volume depletion than adults. Prerenal AKI may occur which may progress to acute tubular necrosis in severe volume depletion. When the GFR decreases, renal acid excretion is compromised with resultant metabolic acidosis. The main goal of DKA treatment is to normalize metabolic acidosis, but the presence of AKI may delay a patient's recovery from metabolic acidosis. The intervention of AKI is composed of diagnostic assessment to uncover the underlying etiology, optimize hemodynamics, minimalize exposure to nephrotoxic medications, conservative fluid management after initial resuscitation, and maximize nutrition.[49]

Kidney Transplantation

The preferred treatment for ESKD in children is kidney transplantation which improves the quality of life, growth, and improved rehabilitation than continued dialysis.[50] Live donor kidney transplant (LDKT) and simultaneous pancreas-kidney transplant (SPKT) offer distinct benefits over receiving a deceased-donor kidney transplant (DDKT) alone. A functional pancreas graft may improve the quality of life over kidney transplant alone, eliminate the need for exogenous insulin therapy, and enhance glycemic control.

CONCLUSION

Diabetes is a chronic disease that requires lifelong treatment and management. The goals of the therapy in children and adolescents with IDDM are to maintain optimum metabolic control insulin along with diet modification or lifestyle changes. Aggressive control of BP with ACEI/ARB and monitoring for microalbuminuria enables early institution of therapeutic measures to reduce or even revert microalbuminuria. Future directions may include methods to identify and treat patients at risk of DKD before microalbuminuria by developing new diagnostic tools and therapies.

KEY POINTS

- Children and adolescents with diabetes are at an increased risk of kidney disease later in life.
- In children with T1DM, annual screening for microalbuminuria should be performed from 11 years of age with 2 years of diabetes duration and from the age of 9 years in children with 5 years of diabetes duration.
- In children with T2DM, screening for microalbuminuria should begin as early as from the time of diagnosis.
- UAER assessed in an office setting on early morning urine sample provides accurate information.
- Preventive strategies include healthy diet with physical activity, maintaining normal BP, optimizing glycemic control, controlling lipid levels, and avoidance of smoking.

REFERENCES

1. Daneman D. Type 1 diabetes. Lancet. 2006;367(9513):847-58.
2. Centers for Disease Control and Prevention. National Diabetes Fact Sheet: general information and national estimates on

diabetes in the United States, 2003. Atlanta, GA: Centers for Disease Control and Prevention; 2004.
3. Andersen AR, Christiansen JS, Andersen JK, Kreiner S, Deckert T. Diabetic nephropathy in type 1 (insulin-dependent) diabetes: an epidemiological study. Diabetologia. 1983;25:496-501.
4. Ballard DJ, Humphrey LL, Melton LJ 3rd, Frohnert PP, Chu PC, O'Fallon WM, et al. Epidemiology of persistent proteinuria in type II diabetes mellitus. Population-based study in Rochester, Minnesota. Diabetes. 1988;37:405-12.
5. Osterby R. Morphometric studies of the peripheral glomerular basement membrane in early juvenile diabetes. I. Development of initial basement membrane thickening. Diabetologia. 1972;8:84-92.
6. Mauer SM, Steffes MW, Ellis EN, Sutherland DE, Brown DM, Goetz FC. Structural-functional relationships in diabetic nephropathy. J Clin Invest. 1984;74:1143-55.
7. Rito PL, Fioretto P, Drummond K, Kim Y, Steffes MW, Basgen JM, et al. Proximal tubular basement membrane width in insulin-dependent diabetes mellitus. Kidney Int. 1998;53:754-61.
8. Andrésdóttir G, Jensen ML, Carstensen B, Parving HH, Hovind P, Hansen TW, et al. Improved prognosis of diabetic nephropathy in type 1 diabetes. Kidney Int. 2015;87(2):417-26.
9. Kalra S, Kalra B, Sharma A. Prevalence of type 1 diabetes mellitus in Karnal district, Haryana state, India. Diabetol Metab Syndr. 2010;2:14.
10. Schultz CJ, Konopelska-Bahu T, Dalton RN, Carroll TA, Stratton I, Gale EA, et al. Microalbuminuria prevalence varies with age, sex, and puberty in children with type 1 diabetes followed from diagnosis in a longitudinal study. Oxford Regional Study Group. Diabetes Care. 1999;22:495-502.
11. Chiang J. Hypertension and diabetic kidney disease in children and adolescents. Diabetes Spectr. 2015;28(3):220-4.
12. Costacou T, Orchard TJ. Cumulative kidney complication risk by 50 years of type 1 diabetes: the effects of sex, age, and calendar year at onset. Diabetes Care. 2018;41:426-33.
13. Saran R, Li Y, Robinson B, Abbott KC, Agodoa LYC, Ayanian J, et al. U.S. renal data system 2015 annual data report: epidemiology of kidney disease in the United States. Am J Kidney Dis. 2016; 67(Suppl. 1):S1-S305.
14. Marshall SM. Diabetic nephropathy in type 1 diabetes: has the outlook improved since the 1980s? Diabetologia. 2012;55: 2301-6.
15. Sochett E, Daneman D. Early diabetes-related complications in children and adolescents with type 1 diabetes. Endocrinol Metabol Clin N Am. 1999;28:865-82.
16. Divers J, Mayer-Davis EJ, Lawrence JM, Isom S, Dabelea D, Dolan L, et al. Trends in incidence of type 1 and type 2 diabetes among youths - selected counties and Indian reservations, United States, 2002–2015. MMWR Morb Mortal Wkly Rep. 2020;69(6):161-5.
17. Naylor R, Johnson AK, del Gaudio D. Maturity-onset diabetes of the young overview. In: Adam MP, Ardinger HH, Pagon RA, Wallace SE, Bean LJH, Stephens K, Amemiya A (Eds). GeneReviews® [Internet]. Seattle, WA: University of Washington; 1993-2020.
18. Perrin NE, Torbjornsdotter TB, Jaremko GA, Berg UB. Follow up of kidney biopsies in normoalbuinuric patients with type 1 diabetes. Pediatr Nephrol. 2004;19:1004-13.
19. Rich SS. Genetics of diabetes and its complications. J Am Soc Nephrol. 2006;17:353-60.
20. Kunisaki M, Bursell SE, Umeda F, Nawata H, King GL. Normalization of diacylglycerol-protein kinase C activation by vitamin E in aorta of diabetic rats and cultured rat smooth muscle cells exposed to elevated glucose levels. Diabetes. 1994;43:1372–7.
21. Marshall SM. Recent advances in diabetic nephropathy. Clin Med (London, England). 2004;4:277-82.
22. Hohenstein B, Hausknecht B, Boehmer K, Riess R, Brekken RA, Hugo CPM. Local VEGF activity but not VEGF expression is tightly regulated during diabetic nephropathy in man. Kidney Int. 2006;69:1654-66.
23. De Vriese AS, Tilton RG, Elger M, Stephan CC, Kriz W, Lameire NH. Antibodies against vascular endothelial growth factor improve early renal dysfunction in experimental diabetes. J Am Soc Nephrol. 2001;12:993-1000.
24. Sharma K, Ziyadeh FN. Hyperglycemia and diabetic kidney disease. The case for transforming growth factor-beta as a key mediator. Diabetes. 1995;44:1139-46.
25. Schalkwijk CG, Stehouwer CD. Vascular complications in diabetes mellitus: the role of endothelial dysfunction. Clin Sci (Lond). 2005;109:143-59.
26. Girach A, Vignati L. Diabetic microvascular complications—can the presence of one predict the development of another? J Diabetes Complications. 2006;20:228-37.
27. Bogdanović R. Diabetic nephropathy in children and adolescents. Pediatr Nephrol. 2008;23(4):507-25.
28. Vujičić B, Turk T, Crnčevicć-Orlić Z, Đorđević G, Rački S. Diabetic nephropathy, pathophysiology and complications of diabetes mellitus. In: Oguntibeju OO (Ed). IntechOpen; 2012.
29. Fiorentino M, Bolignano D, Tesar V, Pisano A, Biesen WV, Tripepi G, et al. ERA-EDTA Immunonephrology Working Group. Renal biopsy in patients with diabetes: a pooled meta-analysis of 48 studies. Nephrol Dial Transplant. 2017;32(1):97-110.
30. Stevens PE, Levin A. Kidney Disease: Improving Global Outcomes Chronic Kidney Disease Guideline Development Work Group Members. Evaluation and management of chronic kidney disease: synopsis of the kidney disease: improving global outcomes 2012 clinical practice guideline. Ann Intern Med. 2013;158(11):825-30.
31. American Diabetes Association. 13. Children and adolescents: standards of medical care in diabetes—2019. Diabetes Care. 2019;42(Suppl 1):S148-64.
32. Giannini C, Mohn A, Chiarelli F. Early signs of diabetic nephropathy in childhood. Diabetes Manage. 2012;2(4):337-53.
33. Drummond K, Mauer M; International Diabetic Nephropathy Study Group . The early natural history of nephropathy in type 1 diabetes. II. Early renal structural changes in type 1 diabetes. Diabetes. 2002;51:1580-7.
34. Ellis EN, Warady BA, Wood EG, Hassanein R, Richardson WP, Lane PH, et al. Renal structural-functional relationships in early diabetes mellitus. Pediatr Nephrol. 1997;11:584-91.
35. Donaghue KC, Marcovecchio ML, Wadwa RP, Chew EY, Wong TY, Calliari LE, et al. ISPAD clinical practice consensus guidelines 2018: microvascular and macrovascular complications in children and adolescents. Pediatr Diabetes. 2018;(suppl)27:262-74.
36. Caramori ML, Fioretto P, Mauer M. Low glomerular filtration rate in normoalbuminuric type 1 diabetic patients is associated with more advanced diabetic lesions. Diabetes. 2003;52:1036-40.
37. Hussein M. Early diabetic nephropathy in a pediatric patient. J Royal Med Serv. 2006;13(1):51-3.
38. Lane P, Steffes M, Mauer M. The role of the pediatric nephrologist in the care of children with diabetes mellitus. Pediatr Nephrol. 1991;5:359-63.
39. Raile K, Galler A, Hofer S, Herbst A, Dunstheimer D, Busch P, et al. Diabetic nephropathy in 27,805 children, adolescents, and adults with type 1 diabetes: effect of diabetes duration, A1C,

hypertension, dyslipidemia, diabetes onset, and sex. Diabetes Care. 2007;30(10):2523-8.
40. Kidney Disease: Improving Global Outcomes (KDIGO). (2020). Clinical practice guideline on the diabetes management in chronic kidney disease. [online] Available from https://kdigo.org/wp-content/uploads/2020/10/KDIGO-2020-Diabetes-in-CKD-GL.pdf [Last accessed September, 2021].
41. Colberg SR, Sigal RJ, Yardley JE, Riddell MC, Dunstan DW, Dempsey PC, et al. Physical activity/exercise and diabetes: a position statement of the American Diabetes Association. Diabetes Care. 2016;39(11):2065-79.
42. Samuels J, Samuel J. New guidelines for hypertension in children and adolescents. J Clin Hypertens (Greenwich). 2018;20(5):837-9.
43. Priya Pais ED, Nelson CC. Textbook of Pediatrics, 21st edition. Philadelphia: Elsevier, Inc; 2016.
44. van den Belt SM, Heerspink HJL, Gracchi V, de Zeeuw D, Wühl E, Schaefer F; ESCAPE Trial Group. Early proteinuria lowering by angiotensin-converting enzyme inhibition predicts renal survival in children with CKD. J Am Soc Nephrol. 2018;29(8):2225-33.
45. Shroff R, Aitkenhead H, Costa N, Trivelli A, Litwin M, Picca S, et al. ESCAPE Trial Group. Normal 25-hydroxyvitamin D levels are associated with less proteinuria and attenuate renal failure progression in children with CKD. J Am Soc Nephrol. 2016;27(1):314-22.
46. Mulec H, Johnson SA, Bjorck S. Relation between serum cholesterol and diabetic nephropathy. Lancet. 1990;335:1537-8.
47. Wühl E, Schaefer F. Therapeutic strategies to slow chronic kidney disease progression. Pediatr Nephrol. 2008;23(5):705-16.
48. Huang SK, Huang CY, Lin CH, Cheng BW, Chiang YT, Lee YC, et al. Acute kidney injury is a common complication in children and adolescents hospitalized for diabetic ketoacidosis. PLoS One. 2020;15(10):e0239160.
49. Hart A, Smith JM, Skeans MA, Gustafson SK, Stewart DE, Cherikh WS, et al. OPTN/SRTR 2015 Annual Data Report: Kidney. Am J Transplant. 2017;17(Suppl 1):21-116.
50. Young BY, Gill J, Huang E, Takemoto SK, Anastasi B, Shah T, et al. Living donor kidney versus simultaneous pancreas-kidney transplant in type I diabetics: an analysis of the OPTN/UNOS database. Clin J Am Soc Nephrol. 2009;4(4):845-52.

CHAPTER

7.5

Sickle Cell Nephropathy

Manish Kumar, Kirtisudha Mishra

INTRODUCTION

Sickle cell disease (SCD) is a common hereditary hemoglobinopathy resulting from a point mutation in the β-globin chain, promoting polymerization of deoxygenated hemoglobin, and leading to red cell distortion, hemolytic anemia, microvascular obstruction, and ischemic tissue damage. Based on the type of inheritance of mutated gene and abnormal hemoglobin variant, SCD can be further classified into the following types:

- Homozygous sickle gene inheritance (HbSS disease), where one sickle cell gene ("S") is inherited from both the parents. This is the most severe form of SCD and is also called sickle cell anemia (SCA).
- Heterozygous sickle gene inheritance associated with other abnormal variants of hemoglobin (HbSC disease, HbSD disease, HbSE disease), where one sickle cell gene "S" is inherited from one parent and another abnormal gene "C," "D," or "E" from the other parent. This is a milder variant of SCD.
- Heterozygous sickle gene inheritance with thalassemia (HbS-beta thalassemia disease), where, in addition to one sickle gene "S" from one parent, a beta thalassemia gene is also inherited from the other parent. There are two types of beta thalassemia: "0" and "+." Those with HbS beta^0-thalassemia usually have a severe form of SCD. People with HbS beta$^+$-thalassemia tend to have a milder form of SCD.
- Sickle cell trait (Hb AS), where one sickle cell gene "S" is inherited from one parent and one normal gene "A" from the other parent. This type often remains asymptomatic.[1]

Sickle cell hemoglobin (HbS), which is formed due to a point mutation at the sixth amino acid position of beta globin chain, replacing glutamic acid with valine, has a tendency to undergo polymerization at hypoxic, acidotic, or hyperosmolar conditions. Red blood cells (RBCs) containing polymerized HbS become sickle shaped, losing their flexibility as they pass through the narrow capillaries, thereby resulting in widespread vaso-occlusive episodes. This causes various acute and chronic complications, such as painful sickle crises, dactylitis, acute chest syndrome, leg ulcers, avascular necrosis of bone, and renal involvement.

Sickle cell nephropathy (SCN), one of the most common complications of SCD, is characterized by a wide range of functional and structural renal abnormalities. Renal involvement starts early and manifests as impaired urinary concentrating ability and glomerular hyperfiltration, and it progresses to urine acidification defect, proteinuria, hematuria, acute kidney injury (AKI), and chronic kidney disease (CKD) as age advances. It is usually more severe in homozygous disease (HbSS) than in compound heterozygous (HbSC and HbSβ$^+$-thalassemia) and is typically mild in heterozygous state (sickle cell trait, HbAS).[2] Most of the clinical manifestations in SCN are related to the repeated vaso-occlusive episodes and hemolysis-related vasculopathy.[3]

EPIDEMIOLOGY

Approximately 300,000 babies are born annually with SCA across the world, and the number is likely to get increased to approximately 400,000 by 2050.[4] The frequency of HbS allele distribution is very high in sub-Saharan African countries, Mediterranean basin, Middle East, and India, with Nigeria, India, and Democratic Republic of Congo contributing to half of all the neonates born with AS and SS allele worldwide.[5] The epidemiology of SCD in India is complex, with the disease being more prevalent in tribal population. According to a national survey-based evidence map, the highest distribution of HbS allele frequency (up to >10%) has been predicted across the central belt of India, extending from south-eastern Gujarat to south-western Odisha, with large parts of Madhya Pradesh and Chhattisgarh being predicated to have an HbS allele frequency of ≥4%.[6]

With the diagnostic and therapeutic advancement, the life expectancy in children with SCD has increased considerably, but at the same time chronic problems such as kidney diseases have become more prevalent. In one of the largest and longest longitudinal follow-up studies of 1,056 adults with SCD, the incidence of chronic renal failure was 12%, with the median age for the development of chronic renal failure being 37 years. The mean survival time following the decline in glomerular filtration rate (GFR) to <60 mL/min/1.73 m^2 was 4 years.[7]

The US Renal Data System (USRDS) revealed that only 0.1% of population on chronic dialysis treatment had SCD as a cause of end-stage kidney disease (ESKD) between 1992 and 1997. It also showed that patients with SCN had higher mortality and were less likely to receive renal transplant.[8] North American Pediatric Renal Trials and Collaborative Studies (NAPRTCS) database showed that only 0.5% of ESKD patients and 0.2% of renal transplant population had SCN.[9]

PATHOPHYSIOLOGY

The pathophysiology of renal dysfunction in SCD is driven by two main mechanisms (1) vaso-occlusive phenomenon and (2) hemolysis-related vasculopathy. A relatively hypoxic, acidic, and hyperosmolar environment in the renal medulla leads to sickling of RBCs in the vasa recta as HbS within the RBCs undergoes polymerization. RBCs containing polymerized HbS show both structural (become sickle shaped and rigid) and functional changes (increased endothelial adherence), resulting in vaso-occlusion, ischemia-reperfusion injury, and papillary necrosis. Also, sickled RBCs, being more fragile in comparison to normal RBCs, undergo premature destruction, resulting in widespread intravascular hemolysis (**Flowchart 1**).

Chronic intravascular hemolysis releases free heme into the plasma, which is a potent scavenger of nitric oxide (NO). Hemolysis also releases erythrocyte arginase-1 into the plasma, which consumes plasma arginine, a substrate for NO synthesis, and exacerbates the low bioavailability of NO. Normally, as NO regulates the basal vasodilator tone, its deficiency impairs the appropriate vascular response to oxidative and inflammatory stress due to hemolysis. Chronic hemolysis also results in renal iron deposition, but it does not appear to be related to liver iron overload, a marker of total body iron load. In contrast to thalassemia, iron overload is not associated with significant organ damage in SCD patients. However, children with glomerular hyperfiltration had significantly higher renal iron load as assessed by R2-MRI in comparison to those with normal GFR.[10]

Inhibition of NO signaling by released heme from RBCs leads to platelet and hemostatic activation and transcriptional expression of nuclear factor κB (NF κB)-dependent adhesion molecules, such as vascular cell-adhesion molecule-1, intercellular cell-adhesion molecule-1, and the selectins.[11] In addition, increase in oxygen-free radicals and overexpression of endothelin-1 result in constriction of blood vessels and tissue hypoxia, further exacerbating HbS polymerization. Heme also causes renal injury through its proinflammatory effect by inducing monocyte chemoattractant protein-1

Flowchart 1: Pathophysiology of sickle cell nephropathy.

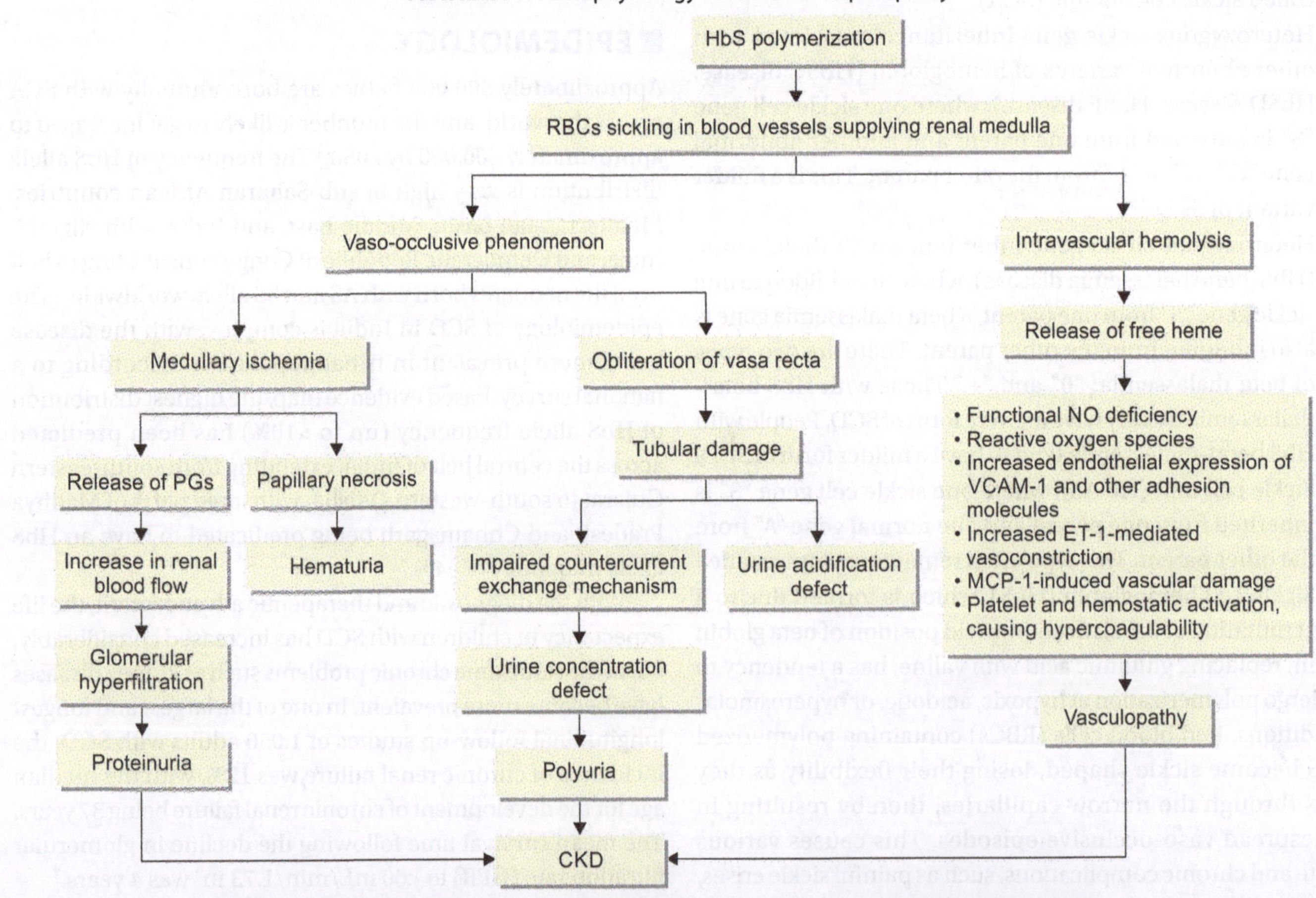

(CKD: chronic kidney disease; ET-1: endothelin-1; MCP-1: monocyte chemoattractant protein-1; NO: nitric oxide; PGs: prostaglandins; VCAM-1: vascular cell adhesion molecule-1)

(MCP-1).[12] Hb released from hemolyzed sickle cells get filtered, enters into the proximal tubule, and interferes with the protein uptake resulting in tubular proteinuria.[13]

Glomerular hyperfiltration, one of the earliest features of SCN, is presumed to occur because of increased production of vasodilating substances, such as prostaglandins (PGs) in the medullary region secondary to ischemia. Indirect measurement of renal PG activity has been assessed by observing the effects of PG inhibitor indomethacin. Studies in adults showing significant decrease in GFR with indomethacin in patients with SCD in comparison to controls suggest that PGs are necessary to maintain GFR in these patients.[14,15] However, such studies are lacking in children. Another possible basis of glomerular hyperfiltration is activation of heme oxygenase (HO) system in the kidney, induced by heme, oxidative stress, and inflammation. Catabolism of heme by HO-1 results in the formation of carbon monoxide (CO), which is a vasorelaxant, leading to renal hyperperfusion. A further mechanism postulated for glomerular hyperfiltration is increased cardiac output secondary to anemia, resulting in increased renal blood flow and thus glomerular hyperfiltration.

CLINICAL PRESENTATION

Various clinical manifestations of SCN depend on the age of the patient and part of the kidney involved. SCN is one of the most severe chronic complications of SCD, with the spectrum of disease ranging from asymptomatic microalbuminuria to ESKD. Renal involvement in SCA starts early in childhood, manifesting as urine concentration defect and glomerular hyperfiltration. Polyuria or nocturnal enuresis, proteinuria, hematuria, hemoglobinuria, AKI, and CKD are common clinical presentations in patients with SCN. Overt renal failure occurs in adulthood. Rarely, renal medullary cell carcinoma may develop in SCD, especially in those with sickle cell trait.

Renal Tubular Dysfunction

Hyposthenuria or impaired urine concentrating ability is one of the earliest features of renal tubular involvement in SCD, manifesting as polyuria or nocturnal enuresis, predisposing these children to dehydration. This condition results from washout of the medullary osmotic gradient due to destruction of vasa recta, the blood vessels supplying the renal medulla, secondary to repeated vaso-occlusive episodes. This is reversible with packed cell transfusion in infancy, partially corrected in an older child, but irreversible in adolescents and beyond.[16]

Both distal and proximal renal tubular abnormalities are seen in children with SCD. Distal renal tubular dysfunction presents as an impaired ability to excrete potassium and subsequent risk of hyperkalemia in conditions associated with increased potassium load, declining renal function and exposure to drugs such as angiotensin-converting enzyme (ACE) inhibitor, beta blockers, and potassium-sparing diuretics. Another manifestation of distal tubular dysfunction is the urinary acidification defect, manifesting as an incomplete form of distal renal tubular acidosis, and this correlates with the severity of hyposthenuria.[17]

Proximal tubular dysfunction manifests as increased maximal tubular reabsorption of phosphorous, though elevation of serum phosphorous is usually mild. Because of the increased tubular excretion of creatinine, low serum creatinine levels are often seen, resulting in overestimation of creatinine clearance. Other features of proximal tubular dysfunction are increased urinary excretion of β2 microglobulin and retinol-binding protein.

Glomerular Dysfunction

Glomerular hyperfiltration is an early marker of renal damage in children with SCN, and the process starts as early as infancy.[18] Prevalence of glomerular hyperfiltration in children with SCD ranges from 40 to 76%.[19,20] Cystatin C-based formula for estimating GFR correlates better with actual GFR, especially with declining renal function. As the child grows older, GFR plateaus during late childhood and then starts declining during adolescence. In majority of children with SCA, glomerular hyperfiltration is the harbinger of the more serious condition, proteinuria, which further potentiates progression to CKD.

Microalbuminuria (spot urine albumin/creatinine ratio of 30–300 mg/g) is an early manifestation of SCN, seen in 9.6–30% of children with SCA.[21-24] Increasing age, high GFR, and low hematocrit are associated with increased risk of development of microalbuminuria.[23] Majority of the children with microalbuminuria progress to overt proteinuria and decrease in kidney function with advancing age. Albuminuria of >100 mg/g is more likely to be persistent, with a higher risk of rapid decline in GFR and development of CKD.[24] Nephrotic syndrome in association with SCA has been rarely reported, with renal histology findings of collapsing FSGS and eventually progressing to renal failure.[25]

Hematuria

Hematuria, microscopic or macroscopic, is a common clinical presentation of SCN, with a prevalence ranging from 4 to 13%.[26,27] Higher prevalence of hematuria is seen in sickle cell crisis. Repeated sickling and vascular obstruction in the renal medulla, with consequent extravasation of red blood cells in crisis, may result in hematuria. Hematuria can also result from renal papillary necrosis secondary to medullary ischemia caused by vaso-occlusion in the vasa recta. Occasionally, sloughed papillae may result in urinary outflow obstruction leading to AKI and urinary tract infection.

Most hematuria episodes are painless, but some patients may complain of abdominal or back pain. Nutcracker phenomenon resulting from increased pressure in left renal vein due to its compression between aorta and superior mesenteric artery causes unilateral bleeding. Repeated episodes of gross hematuria are associated with an increased risk of CKD. Rarely, gross hematuria can be associated with the development of renal medullary carcinoma, especially in sickle cell trait, and is associated with higher mortality.[28]

Acute Kidney Injury

Acute kidney injury has been rarely reported in children with SCA during acute sickle cell painful crisis. Use of nonsteroidal anti-inflammatory drugs (NSAIDs) during acute painful crises may further increase the risk of AKI. In a retrospective review, out of 197 vaso-occlusive pain episodes in 97 patients, 33 (17%) AKI events were identified, as per the Kidney Disease Improving Global Outcomes (KDIGO) classification criteria of AKI. Patients with AKI had a significantly larger acute drop in Hb level (1.21 vs. 0.50 g/dL, $p = 0.008$) in comparison to those without AKI.[29]

Chronic Kidney Disease

Chronic kidney disease is a frequent and a potentially severe complication in children with SCA. It is more common in people with HbSS and HbSβ° than in people with HbSC or HbSβ⁺. The prevalence of CKD increases with age, affecting more than 50% of the people with SCD who are over 40 years of age.[30] Older age, higher baseline severity index for SCD (4+ acute vaso-occlusive pain episodes during the first year), βS-gene haplotype, acute chest syndrome, higher number of prescriptions for NSAIDs, hematuria, hemoglobinuria, nephrotic range proteinuria, low hemoglobin level, vaso-occlusive crises, nocturnal hypertension, pulmonary hypertension, stroke, parvovirus B19 infection, and hyperuricemia are associated with an increased risk of CKD.[31-33] Presence of *MYH9* and *APOL1* genetic variants are strongly associated with progression to CKD.[34,35] In contrast, coinheritance of α-thalassemia and elevated HbF levels are associated with decreased risk of CKD.

HISTOPATHOLOGY

Renal biopsy is not performed routinely in children with SCD, and information on renal histopathology findings is limited. There is no pathognomonic lesion for SCN, but glomerular hypertrophy is a universal finding and may be seen as early as 1–3 years of age. A multicentric retrospective study on renal biopsy in children with SCD performed for isolated proteinuria and acute or chronic renal impairment revealed mesangial hypercellularity (75%) as the most common histopathology finding, followed by focal segmental glomerulosclerosis (30%), membranoproliferative glomerulonephritis (16%), and thrombotic microangiopathy (2%).[36]

MANAGEMENT

Children with SCA should undergo a detailed history, thorough clinical examination, and investigations to assess the degree of renal involvement. Urinalysis for quantification of proteinuria (microalbuminuria in early stage) and microscopic examination for RBCs are required in all cases with SCA. Those presenting with gross hematuria should undergo a renal ultrasound or CT urography (intravenous urography in the absence of CT) for the possible diagnosis of renal papillary necrosis or renal medullary carcinoma. Blood test for antinuclear antibody (ANA)/double-stranded DNA and complement levels should be done to rule out lupus nephritis. Renal biopsy should be offered to those with nephrotic range proteinuria and hematuria with or without proteinuria, if the above investigations are negative. In addition, serology for hepatitis B and C virus and HIV should be done, as these children are at an increased risk of acquiring these infections because of repeated blood transfusions.

Surveillance and early diagnosis, prevention of SCN, avoidance of nephrotoxic agents, and anemia interventions form the basis of management. Unfortunately, there is no specific measure to prevent or retard the progression to CKD in children with SCD. Given that patients with SCD already have some degree of renal involvement, exposure to NSAIDs should be minimized as a measure to retard the progression to CKD. The National Heart, Lung, and Blood Institute (NHLBI) 2014 expert panel report suggests screening for albuminuria annually beginning at 10 years of age in patients with SCD.[37] However, more recent evidence suggests a potential benefit of earlier screening.[38] Treatment options for SCN are limited, namely, repeated blood transfusions, ACE inhibitors/angiotensin receptor blockers (ARBs), and hydroxyurea, either alone or in combination with each other.[39]

Packed Cell Transfusion

Early blood transfusion has been found to protect against microalbuminuria in children with SCD.[40] Red blood cell transfusion, by decreasing the HbS concentration and subsequent RBCs sickling, prevents the vaso-occlusive phenomenon in the renal medulla and thereby glomerular and tubular hypoxic damages to the kidney. However, benefits of chronic blood transfusion must be balanced against the potential adverse effects, such as infections, iron overload, transfusion reactions, and alloimmunization. EPO benefit in SCD and CKD is suboptimal. It may be associated with an increased vaso-occlusive risk. Also, inherent bone-marrow suppressive effect of hydroxyurea may lead to higher ESA dosing.

Polyuria and Enuresis

Because of the urinary concentration defect in these children, adequate hydration status should be maintained to avoid vaso-occlusive events, especially during diarrheal episodes, strenuous physical activity, and high environmental temperature. Management of enuresis is similar to other children, like restriction of oral fluid before bedtime, use of alarm therapy, and DDAVP. However, data on the use of DDAVP for the treatment of nocturnal enuresis in children with SCD are limited.

Glomerular Hyperfiltration

Hydroxyurea is used in children with SCA to reduce the frequency of acute painful episodes and other acute complications such as acute chest syndrome and stroke, and also to decrease the frequency of blood transfusion. It acts by increasing the blood level of HbF and thus decreases the percentage of HbS concentration, resulting in reduced frequency of polymerization and sickling episodes in the kidneys.[41] In a multicentric placebo-controlled trial (BABY-HUG trial), to study the efficacy of hydroxyurea on renal dysfunction in infants (mean age, 13.8 months) with SCA, children who received hydroxyurea (20 mg/kg/day) for 24 months did not show any significant decrease in GFR in comparison to the placebo group. However, children who received hydroxyurea showed a significant improvement in urine concentrating ability and lesser renal enlargement, suggesting some clinical benefit.[42] In another study [HUSTLE (hydroxyurea study of long-term effects) study] to assess the long-term effects of hydroxyurea in children with SCA (age range, 2.5–14 years), there was a significant decrease in GFR after 3 years of treatment, as measured by ^{99m}Tc DTPA clearance (167 ± 46 mL/min/1.73 m^2 to 145 ± 27 mL/min/1.73 m^2, $p = 0.016$), though there was no effect on albuminuria.[43]

Proteinuria

Angiotensin-converting enzyme inhibitor/ARB, as a renoprotective agent, has been used over the years in a variety of clinical conditions, but its effect in patients with SCD is not clear. Existing evidence is not enough to show reduction of proteinuria with the use of ACE inhibitor in SCD, though there is a tendency toward decrease in urinary albumin excretion.[44] In a retrospective study, treatment with ACE inhibitors/ARBs for a minimum of 6 months did not result in significant decline in proteinuria. However, the rate of decline in eGFR was significantly slower in patients on ACE inhibitors/ARBs in comparison to those who did not receive ACE inhibitors/ARBs (2.78 vs. 4.70 mL/min per 1.73 m^2/year), suggesting some benefit in retarding the progression of renal dysfunction.[45] In a phase II multicenter trial, 6 months of Losartan treatment were found effective in decreasing albuminuria in majority of patients with SCA, especially those with macroalbuminuria.[46] The American Society of Hematology guideline suggests ACE inhibitor/ARB in children with SCD and albuminuria, unless contraindicated, along with adequate follow-up and monitoring for possible side effects such as hypotension and hyperkalemia.[47]

Hematuria and Papillary Necrosis

Being a self-limited condition, episodes of hematuria are managed conservatively, such as maintenance of adequate hydration, bed rest, pain relief, and antibiotics, if necessary. Epsilon-aminocaproic acid (EACA) or tranexamic acid, an antifibrinolytic agent, has been previously used to treat hematuria with some efficacy.

Chronic Kidney Disease/End-stage Kidney Disease

Management of CKD/ESKD secondary to SCD is similar to the treatment of CKD due to other causes. Because of a suboptimal increase in the erythropoietin level, these children require higher doses of erythropoietin-stimulating agents to achieve acceptable Hb levels. Dialysis and renal transplantation are viable options in patients with ESKD due to SCD, with graft survival at 1 year being similar to those with ESKD because of other causes. However, there is a several-fold increased risk of mortality in patients on dialysis due to SCD in comparison to those with ESKD due to other causes, with 26% dying within the first year of initiation of dialysis.[48,49] The mean survival time after the development of kidney failure in patients with SCA is approximately 4 years, even in those receiving adequate dialysis.[50] Overall patient survival after renal transplantation is significantly lower in patients with SCD in comparison to control groups.[51] Post-transplantation recurrence of SCN, manifesting as acute intrarenal sickling, is an important cause of graft loss in the perioperative period. A top-up transfusion, if the patient is severely anemic, has been suggested prior to transplantation. Regular exchange transfusion with an aim to decrease HbS < 30% has also been suggested in those with evidence of acute sickle kidney or those who have lost a graft because of recurrent SCN.[52]

CONCLUSION

Sickle cell nephropathy is an uncommon but one of the most severe complications in children with SCD. Repeated vaso-occlusive episodes and hemolysis result in a spectrum of renal complications, ranging from glomerular hyperfiltration and urinary concentration defect to hematuria, microalbuminuria, proteinuria, and progression to CKD/ESKD. In the absence of a definitive treatment, early screening for microalbuminuria and treatment with ACE inhibitor are warranted. Hydroxyurea has shown some benefit in terms of improvement in urine concentrating ability and decrease in GFR, though there was no effect on decrease in albuminuria. Once CKD is developed, treatment is similar to CKD due to other causes. Renal transplantation is a viable option for those with ESKD, with 1-year graft survival being similar to ESKD due to other causes.

KEY POINTS

- Sickle cell nephropathy is a common complication in children with sickle cell anemia.
- Vaso-occlusive episodes and chronic hemolysis-related vasculopathy are two important pathophysiologic mechanisms.

- Renal dysfunction starts early in childhood, with glomerular hyperfiltration being the earliest manifestation, progressing to proteinuria and CKD in the majority by the fourth decade of life.
- Screening for microalbuminuria should start early during childhood.
- Treatment options are ACE inhibitor/ARB, hydroxyurea, and packed cell transfusion.
- Dialysis and transplantation are options for patients with ESKD, with 1-year graft survival similar to those with ESKD due to other causes.

REFERENCES

1. Olaniran KO, Eneanya ND, Nigwekar SU, Vela-Parada XF, Achebe MM, Sharma A, et al. Sickle cell nephropathy in the pediatric population. Blood Purif. 2019;47(1-3):205-13.
2. Derebail VK, Ciccone EJ, Zhou Q, Kilgore RR, Cai J, Ataga KI. Progressive decline in estimated GFR in patients with sickle cell disease: an observational cohort study. Am J Kidney Dis. 2019;74(1):47-55.
3. Nath KA, Hebbel RP. Sickle cell disease: renal manifestations and mechanisms. Nat Rev Nephrol. 2015;11(3):161-71.
4. Piel FB, Hay SI, Gupta S, Weatherall DJ, Williams TN. Global burden of sickle cell anaemia in children under five, 2010–2050: modelling based on demographics, excess mortality, and interventions. PLoS Med. 2013;10(7):e1001484.
5. Piel FB, Patil AP, Howes RE, Nyangiri OA, Gething PW, Dewi M, et al. Global epidemiology of sickle haemoglobin in neonates: a contemporary geostatistical model-based map and population estimates. Lancet. 2013;381(9861):142-51.
6. Hockham C, Bhatt S, Colah R, Mukherjee MB, Penman BS, Gupta S, et al. The spatial epidemiology of sickle-cell anaemia in India. Sci Rep. 2018;8(1):17685.
7. Powars DR, Chan LS, Hiti A, Ramicone E, Johnson C. Outcome of sickle cell anemia: a 4-decade observational study of 1056 patients. Medicine (Baltimore). 2005;84(6):363-76.
8. Abbott KC, Hypolite IO, Agodoa LY. Sickle cell nephropathy at end-stage renal disease in the United States: patient characteristics and survival. Clin Nephrol. 2002;58:9-15.
9. Warady BA, Sullivan EK. Renal transplantation in children with sickle cell disease: a report of the North American Pediatric Renal Transplant Cooperative Study (NAPRTCS). Pediatr Transplant. 1998;2:130-3.
10. Vasavda N, Gutiérrez L, House MJ, Drašar E, St Pierre TG, Thein SL. Renal iron load in sickle cell disease is influenced by severity of haemolysis. Br J Haematol. 2012;157(5):599-605.
11. Potoka KP, Gladwin MT. Vasculopathy and pulmonary hypertension in sickle cell disease. Am J Physiol Lung Cell Mol Physiol. 2015;308(4):L314-24.
12. Tracz MJ, Alam J, Nath KA. Physiology and pathophysiology of heme: implications for kidney disease. J Am Soc Nephrol. 2007;18(2):414-20.
13. Eshbach ML, Kaur A, Rbaibi Y, Tejero J, Weisz OA. Hemoglobin inhibits albumin uptake by proximal tubule cells: implications for sickle cell disease. Am J Physiol Cell Physiol. 2017;312(6): C733-40.
14. De Jong PE, de Jong-Van Den Berg TW, Sewrajsingh GS, Schouten H, Donker AJ, Statius van Eps LW. The influence of indomethacin on renal haemodynamics in sickle cell anaemia. Clin Sci Lond. 1980;59:245-50.
15. Allon M, Lawson L, Eckman JR. Delaney V, Bourke E. Effects of nonsteroidal antiinflammatory drugs on renal function in sickle cell anemia. Kidney Int. 1988;34:500-6.
16. Itano HA, Keitel HG, Thompson D. Hyposthenuria in sickle cell anemia: a reversible renal defect. J Clin Invest. 1956;35: 998-1007.
17. Cazenave M, Audard V, Bertocchio JP, Habibi A, Baron S, Prot-Bertoye C. Tubular acidification defect in adults with sickle cell disease. Clin J Am Soc Nephrol. 2020;15(1):16-24.
18. Ware RE, Rees RC, Sarnaik SA, Iyer RV, Alvarez OA, Casella JF, et al; BABY HUG Investigators. Renal function in infants with sickle cell anemia: baseline data from the BABY HUG trial. J Pediatr. 2010;156(1):66-70.
19. Aloni MN, Ngiyulu RM, Ekulu PM, Mbutiwi FI, Makulo JR, Gini-Ehungu JL, et al. Glomerular hyperfiltration is strongly correlated with age in Congolese children with sickle cell anaemia. Acta Paediatr. 2017;106(5):819-24.
20. Aygun B, Mortier NA, Smeltzer MP, Hankins JS, Ware RE. Glomerular hyperfiltration and albuminuria in children with sickle cell anemia. Pediatr Nephrol. 2011;26(8):1285-90.
21. Alzahrani YA, Algarni MA, Alnashri MM, AlSayyad HM, Aljahdali KM, Alead JE, et al. Prevalence and risk factors for microalbuminuria in children with sickle cell disease at King Abdulaziz University Hospital: a retrospective cross-sectional study. Cureus. 2020;12(1):e6638.
22. Aloni MN, Mabidi JL, Ngiyulu RM, Ekulu PM, Mbutiwi FI, Makulo JR, et al. Prevalence and determinants of microalbuminuria in children suffering from sickle cell anemia in steady state. Clin Kidney J. 2017;10(4):479-86.
23. King L, MooSang M, Miller M, Reid M. Prevalence and predictors of microalbuminuria in Jamaican children with sickle cell disease. Arch Dis Child. 2011;96(12):1135-9.
24. Al-Musawa FE, Al-Saqladi AM. Prevalence and correlates of microalbuminuria in Yemeni children with sickle cell disease. Saudi J Kidney Dis Transpl. 2019;30(4):832-42.
25. Nasr SH, Markowitz GS, Sentman RL, D'Agati VD. Sickle cell disease, nephrotic syndrome, and renal failure. Kidney Int. 2006;69(7):1276-80.
26. Akubuilo UC, Ayuk A, Ezenwosu OU, Okafor UH, Emodi IJ. Persistent hematuria among children with sickle cell anemia in steady state. Hematol Transfus Cell Ther. 2020;42(3):255-60.
27. Anigilaje EA, Adedoyin OT. Correlation between dipstick urinalysis and urine sediment microscopy in detecting haematuria among children with sickle cell anaemia in steady state in Ilorin, Nigeria. Pan Afr Med J. 2013;15:135.
28. Alvarez O, Rodriguez MM, Jordan L, Sarnaik S. Renal medullary carcinoma and sickle cell trait: a systematic review. Pediatr Blood Cancer. 2015;62(10):1694-9.
29. Baddam S, Aban I, Hilliard L, Howard T, Askenazi D, Lebensburger JD. Acute kidney injury during a pediatric sickle cell vaso-occlusive pain crisis. Pediatr Nephrol. 2017;32(8): 1451-6.
30. Gosmanova EO, Zaidi S, Wan JY, Adams-Graves PE. Prevalence and progression of chronic kidney disease in adult patients with sickle cell disease. J Investig Med. 2014;62(5):804-7.
31. Saraf SL, Zhang X, Kanias T, Lash JP, Molokie RE, Oza B, et al. Haemoglobinuria is associated with chronic kidney disease and its progression in patients with sickle cell anaemia. Br J Haematol. 2014;164(5):729-39.
32. Lebensburger JD, Cutter GR, Howard TH, Muntner P, Feig DI. Evaluating risk factors for chronic kidney disease in pediatric patients with sickle cell anemia. Pediatr Nephrol. 2017;32(9): 1565-73.

33. Stallworth JR, Tripathi A, Jerrell JM. Prevalence, treatment, and outcomes of renal conditions in pediatric sickle cell disease. South Med J. 2011;104(11):752-6.
34. Ashley-Koch AE, Okocha EC, Garrett ME, Soldano K, De Castro LM, Jonassaint JC, et al. MYH9 and APOL1 are both associated with sickle cell disease nephropathy. Br J Haematol. 2011;155(3):386-94.
35. Kormann R, Jannot AS, Narjoz C, Ribeil J-A, Manceau S, Delville M, et al. Roles of APOL1 G1 and G2 variants in sickle cell disease patients: kidney is the main target. Br J Haematol. 2017;179(2):323-35.
36. Zahr RS, Yee ME, Weaver J, Twombley K, Matar RB, Aviles D, et al. Kidney biopsy findings in children with sickle cell disease: a Midwest Pediatric Nephrology Consortium study. Pediatr Nephrol. 2019;34(8):1435-45.
37. Yawn BP, Buchanan GR, Afenyi-Annan AN, Ballas SK, Hassell KL, James AH, et al. Management of sickle cell disease: summary of the 2014 evidence-based report by expert panel members. JAMA. 2014;312(10):1033-48.
38. Lebensburger JD, Aban I, Pernell B, Kasztan M, Feig DI, Hilliard LM, et al. Hyperfiltration during early childhood precedes albuminuria in pediatric sickle cell nephropathy. Am J Hematol. 2019;94(4):417-23.
39. Roy NB, Fortin PM, Bull KR, Doree C, Trivella M, Hopewell S, et al. Interventions for chronic kidney disease in people with sickle cell disease. Cochrane Database Syst Rev. 2017;7(7):CD012380.
40. Alvarez O, Montane B, Lopez G, Wilkinson J, Miller T. Early blood transfusions protect against microalbuminuria in children with sickle cell disease. Pediatr Blood Cancer. 2006;47(1):71-6.
41. Nevitt SJ, Jones AP, Howard J. Hydroxyurea (hydroxycarbamide) for sickle cell disease. Cochrane Database Syst Rev. 2017;4(4): CD002202.
42. Alvarez O, Miller ST, Wang WC, Luo Z, McCarville MB, Schwartz GJ, et al; BABY HUG Investigators. Effect of hydroxyurea treatment on renal function parameters: results from the multi-center placebo-controlled BABY HUG clinical trial for infants with sickle cell anemia. Pediatr Blood Cancer. 2012;59(4): 668-74.
43. Aygun B, Mortier NA, Smeltzer MP, Shulkin BL, Hankins JS, Ware RE. Hydroxyurea treatment decreases glomerular hyperfiltration in children with sickle cell anemia. Am J Hematol. 2013;88(2):116-9.
44. Sasongko TH, Nagalla S, Ballas SK. Angiotensin-converting enzyme (ACE) inhibitors for proteinuria and microalbuminuria in people with sickle cell disease. Cochrane Database Syst Rev. 2015;2015(6):CD009191.
45. Thrower A, Ciccone EJ, Maitra P, Derebail VK, Cai J, Ataga KI. Effect of renin-angiotensin-aldosterone system blocking agents on progression of glomerulopathy in sickle cell disease. Br J Haematol. 2019;184(2):246-52.
46. Quinn CT, Saraf SL, Gordeuk VR, Fitzhugh CD, Creary SE, Bodas P, et al. Losartan for the nephropathy of sickle cell anemia: a phase-2, multicenter trial. Am J Hematol. 2017;92(9):E520-8.
47. Liem RI, Lanzkron S, D Coates T, DeCastro L, Desai AA, Ataga KI, et al. American Society of Hematology 2019 guidelines for sickle cell disease: cardiopulmonary and kidney disease. Blood Adv. 2019;3(23):3867-97.
48. McClellan AC, Luthi JC, Lynch JR, Soucie JM, Kulkarni R, Guasch A, et al. High one year mortality in adults with sickle cell disease and end-stage renal disease. Br J Haematol. 2012; 159(3):360-7.
49. Nielsen L, Canouï-Poitrine F, Jais JP, Dahmane D, Bartolucci P, Bentaarit B, et al. Morbidity and mortality of sickle cell disease patients starting intermittent haemodialysis: a comparative cohort study with non- Sickle dialysis patients. Br J Haematol. 2016;174(1):148-52.
50. Powars DR, Elliott-Mills DD, Chan L, Niland J, Hiti AL, Opas LM, et al. Chronic renal failure in sickle cell disease: risk factors, clinical course, and mortality. Ann Intern Med. 1991;115(8): 614-20.
51. Gérardin C, Moktefi A, Couchoud C, Duquesne A, Ouali N, Gataut P, et al. Survival and specific outcome of sickle cell disease patients after renal transplantation. Br J Haematol. 2019;187(5):676-80.
52. Sharpe CC, Thein SL. Sickle cell nephropathy—a practical approach. Br J Haematol. 2011;155(3):287-97.

CHAPTER

7.6 Obesity and Glomerulosclerosis

Karalanglin Tiewsoh, Mukta Mantan

INTRODUCTION

Obesity is known to be a risk factor for various chronic diseases. In this chapter, we will try to outline the definition and incidence of obesity in children, discuss its effects on health and the kidneys, in particular, the pathogenesis behind obesity-related glomerulopathy (ORG), clinical manifestations, and management of such children.

DEFINITION OF OBESITY IN CHILDREN

The World Health Organization (WHO) defines obesity as an excess in fat mass significant to increased risk of morbidity; altered physical, psychological, or social well-being; and/or mortality.[1] Body mass index (BMI), calculated as weight in kg/height in meters^2 is the most practical way to measure obesity. Other body-fat measurements, such as dual-energy X-ray absorptiometry or bioelectrical impedance analysis, are used for research purposes. While adults have BMI cutoffs for defining overweight (25 kg/m^2) and obesity (30 kg/m^2), children are considered overweight or obese, if they cross certain points on the reference BMI curves defined as a function of age and sex. While the West uses the Centers for Disease Control and Prevention (CDC) growth chart, in India, for children under 5 years of age, the WHO Multicentre Growth Reference Study (WHO MGRS) and for those above 5 years, the revised Indian Academy of Pediatrics (IAP 2015) BMI curves have been recommended **(Table 1)**.[2-6]

TABLE 1: Definition of obesity.[2-5]

BMI reference curve	*Methods and cutoffs used*
CDC[2]	Children 2–20 years (US data) • Overweight >85th centile • Obesity >95th centile
WHO[3,5]	Children 0–5 years (WHO Multicentric Growth Reference Study) • *Overweight:* BMI or weight for length/height > +2 SD • *Obesity:* BMI or weight for length/height > +3 SD Children 5–19 years (WHO 2007 Reference Charts) • *Overweight:* BMI > +1 SD • *Obesity:* BMI > +2 SD
IAP-2015[4]	Data from nine Indian studies • Overweight >23 kg/m^2 • Obesity >27 kg/m^2

(BMI: body mass index; CDC: Centers for Disease Control and Prevention; IAP: Indian Academy of Pediatrics; SD: standard deviation; WHO: World Health Organization)

INCIDENCE OF OBESITY

The global incidence of obesity is increasing tremendously, with prevalence of pediatric obesity rising from 4% in 1975 to 18% in 2016 as per the Non-Communicable Disease Risk Factor Collaboration (NCD-RisC) study.[7] Further, contrary to general belief, the low- and middle-income counties are as affected by the obesity epidemic as the high-income countries.[8] Besides, a study revealed that the prevalence of obesity is almost 23.9% in affluent Indian children aged 2–17 years.[9]

HEALTH EFFECTS OF OBESITY

Obesity or increased BMI has been considered to be a risk factor for an array of chronic diseases, mainly cardiovascular disease, endocrine disorders, chronic kidney disease (CKD), certain malignancies, and musculoskeletal disorders.[10]

Effect on the Kidneys

Obesity can have an impact on the kidneys, more so when the child has an underlying renal disease. However, with time, its effect can be seen in normal and healthy kidneys too. As the obesity epidemic increases, nephrologists need to be aware of its effect on the kidneys. While obesity can exacerbate hypertension, insulin resistance, and intrarenal inflammation, ORG has emerged as a direct effect that needs attention. The prevalence of ORG is expected to rise parallel to the obesity epidemic.[11-18]

PATHOPHYSIOLOGY OF OBESITY-RELATED GLOMERULOPATHY

The pathogenesis of ORG is complex and results from an interplay of hemodynamic, hormonal alterations, and abnormal lipid metabolism **(Fig. 1)**.

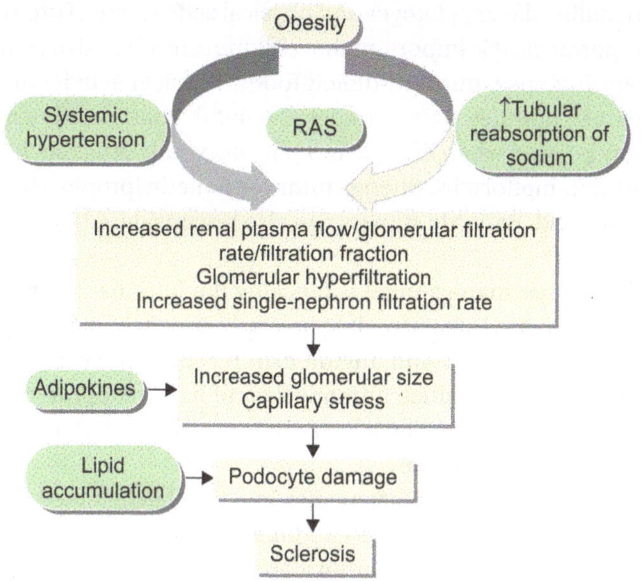

Fig. 1: Pathogenesis of obesity-related glomerulopathy. (RAS: renin-angiotensin system)

Altered Renal Hemodynamics

The most important pathologic change in ORG is glomerular hyperfiltration.[12] The renal plasma flow (RPF), glomerular filtration rate (GFR), and filtration fraction (FF) increase in obesity. In fact, studies have shown that the GFR is 16–61% higher in obese individuals than lean controls, RPF by 9–33%, and FF (GFR/RPF) by 9–29%.[12] This altered renal hemodynamics has been proposed to be due to the systemic hypertension causing relative vasodilatation of the afferent arteriole as compared to the efferent and therefore increased pressure at the glomerular tuft. Further, another theory relates this hemodynamic change to increased proximal tubular sodium reabsorption, deactivation of tubuloglomerular feedback, afferent arteriole dilatation, and increased single-nephron plasma flow.

It has been found that fat cells synthesize components of the renin-angiotensin system (RAS) and obesity itself activates the RAS. This leads to increase in angiotensin II and aldosterone levels. These add up to the glomerular pressure effect by causing efferent arteriole constriction and increased tubular reabsorption. Besides RAS activation, the activated renal sympathetic nervous system and insulin resistance also cause increased tubular reabsorption of sodium leading to hyperfiltration.

Increased glomerular pressure with an increase in filtrate flow (single-nephron filtration rate) stretches the glomerular capillary wall. Further, it causes the glomeruli to enlarge. Subsequently, the capillary stress damages the podocyte, leading to further sclerosis.

Abnormal Cell and Hormone Responses

Adipose tissue secretes chemokines, known as adipokines.[12] These adipokines have angiogenic and inflammatory effects. Such paracrine effects in the kidneys can be seen in response especially to the mechanical forces caused by hyperfiltration. These effects may have either adaptive or maladaptive changes in the glomeruli tuft. There are certain adipokines (leptin, adiponectin, and resistin) that affect cellular hypertrophy and interstitial fibrosis. Other factors, such as angiopoietins and vascular endothelial growth factor (VEGF), affect endothelial-pericyte integrity. The final outcome depends on their interplay.

Interestingly, while BMI is used to diagnose obesity, there is some evidence that those with higher visceral abdominal fat produce more adipokines than those with subcutaneous abdominal fat, thus indicating that waist circumference is a better indicator of renal injury. Further, with increasing BMI, ectopic deposition of lipid in the kidneys occurs, including mesangial and proximal tubular cells. Ectopic lipid leads to insulin resistance that is associated with renal hyperfiltration and CKD.

Abnormal Lipid Metabolism

The abnormal lipid metabolism in obese individuals leads to the accumulation of triglycerides and cholesterol in the renal tissue.[12] Triglyceride accumulates because of a triad of increased synthesis, increased uptake, and decreased fatty acid oxidation. Similarly, cholesterol accumulates due to increased synthesis and uptake with decreased efflux. Accumulation of these substances leads to a proinflammatory state and, therefore, fibrosis and proteinuria.

PATHOLOGY

Obesity-related glomerulopathy is diagnosed when renal histopathology reveals changes ranging from glomerular hypertrophy to focal segmental glomerulosclerosis (FSGS) in obese individuals.[14] The association between obesity and glomerulomegaly was first observed in few autopsy reports of morbidly obese patients.[19] Subsequently, in adults, there has been an increase in ORG diagnosis from 0.2% in 1986–1990 to almost 2.7% in 2001–2015.[18]

The glomerular diameter or the estimated glomerular volume increases due to increased systolic blood pressure, intraglomerular hypertension, and secretion of angiogenesis-promoting factors. Of the five subtypes of FSGS (cellular, tip, perihilar, collapsing, and not otherwise specified), the perihilar type at the vascular pole is the most common in ORG. Usually, the FSGS occurs in the hypertrophied glomeruli. The development of sclerosis has been found to be related to decrease in both nephron mass and glomerular density. Some lesions may have focal or diffuse increase in the mesangial matrix and thickening of the glomerular basement membrane. Tubular atrophy and interstitial fibrosis may exist depending on the degree of sclerosis. Arteriosclerosis is also common. Immunofluorescence is nonspecific with occasional trapping of immunoglobulin M (IgM) and/or C3. The electron microscopy changes show very mild foot process effusion in the presence of podocyte hypertrophy. Lipid vacuoles may also be visible in mesangial cells, podocytes, or proximal tubular cells.[12,18]

CLINICAL MANIFESTATIONS

Obesity-related glomerulopathy presentation ranges from subnephrotic proteinuria to end-stage kidney disease (ESKD). The majority of obese patients will have isolated proteinuria on urinalysis; around 10–48% may have nephrotic range proteinuria and rarely (0–6%) may present as nephrotic syndrome. In those presenting with nephrotic syndrome, differentiating between primary FSGS and ORG becomes important **(Table 2)**. The rarity of nephrotic syndrome presentation with proteinuria, edema, and hyperlipidemia has been proposed to be due to adaptation of the body to the slow podocyte injury and the difference in tubular handling of proteinuria in this hyperfiltrating nephropathy. It is common for obese individuals to have hypertension and dyslipidemia. The incidence of ESKD ranges from 10 to 33%, occurring especially in those obese individuals whose proteinuria had gone undetected or where there was a reduction in the number of nephrons either because of low birth weight or a renal abnormality.[11-18]

MANAGEMENT

There is no consensus on the optimal management of ORG. However, it is suggested that screening for proteinuria in high-risk individuals with a urine albumin-to-creatinine ratio and following up with renal function test and good clinical examination, including blood pressure, among others, would be helpful. While most of the studies on ORG are in adults, weight loss and RAS blockade seems to be the only two measures whereby progression of disease can be altered, though large prospective trials are lacking.[11,12,17,18]

Weight loss is, of course, the most important advice for such patients. The recommendations of pediatric endocrinologists for treating obesity should be followed. Lifestyle modifications, including dietary changes and physical activity, are of utmost importance. It is important that children are advised to avoid calorie-dense, nutrient-deficit foods. Physical activity of at least 60 minutes, 5 days a week is helpful. Pharmacotherapy may be used when lifestyle modifications fail. Drugs such as orlistat, metformin, phentermine, and diethylpropion have been used. Bariatric surgery can also be considered when all else fail.[20]

Another management is blocking the RAS that seems to play a major role in the pathogenesis. Angiotensin-converting enzyme inhibitors and angiotensin receptor blockers have been shown to reduce proteinuria and have renoprotective effects in ORG. Addition of spironolactone in adults has been found to be beneficial.

In adults, various other medications have been studied such as insulin-sensitizing agents, sodium–glucose cotransporter-2 (SLGT2) inhibitors, and antioxidants. However, most of them have yet to be approved for clinical use.

As it is common for such patients to have hypertension, monitoring and control of blood pressure by various medications would be warranted.

TABLE 2: Differentiating between obesity-related focal segmental glomerulosclerosis and primary focal segmental glomerulosclerosis.[11,18]

	Obesity-related FSGS	*Primary FSGS*
Onset	Slow	Rapid
Proteinuria	Sub nephrotic range	Nephrotic range
Edema	Not present	Present
Serum albumin	Normal	Low
Progression	Slow	Rapid
Variant	Perihilar FSGS	Any
Glomerular volume	Increased	Normal
Effacement of foot process	Mild	Severe

(FSGS: focal segmental glomerulosclerosis)

CONCLUSION

As the global incidence of obesity is increasing, pediatric nephrologists should be aware of its effects on the kidneys. The clinical manifestations of ORG ranges from subnephrotic proteinuria to nephrotic syndrome. When undetected, these children may end up in ESKD. While the pathogenesis is mainly due to altered renal hemodynamics leading to glomerular hyperfiltration, certain adipokines and accumulation of lipids add to the damage. Perihilar FSGS is the most common histopathology associated with ORG. Except for the clinical data of obesity and lipid vacuoles in the renal tissue, differentiating ORG from other FSGS variants would be difficult. A consensus on managing such patients is lacking, but screening the same for proteinuria and hypertension in addition to early detection of deranged renal function would be helpful. Weight reduction and RAS blockade are the mainstay of treatment.

KEY POINTS

- Pediatric obesity has risen from 4% in 1975 to 18% in 2016.
- Obesity can lead to the following renal manifestations: isolated proteinuria, nephrotic syndrome, and ESKD.
- ORG is diagnosed when renal histopathology reveals changes ranging from glomerular hypertrophy to FSGS in obese individuals.
- Treatment is mainly supportive.

REFERENCES

1. WHO Technical Consultation. Obesity: preventing and managing the global epidemic. Report of a WHO consultation 2000. Report No.: 0512-3054 (Print) 0512-3054. Geneva: World Health Organization; 2000.

2. Kuczmarski RJ, Ogden CL, Grummer-Strawn LM, Flegal KM, Guo SS, Wei R, et al. CDC growth charts: United States. Adv Data. 2000;314:1-27.
3. Multicentre Growth Reference Study WHO Group. WHO Child Growth Standards based on length/height, weight and age. Acta Paediatr. 2006;450:76-85.
4. Khadilkar V, Yadav S, Agrawal KK, Tamboli S, Banerjee M, Cherian A, et al. Revised IAP growth charts for height, weight and body mass index for 5 to 18 year old Indian children. Indian Pediatr. 2015;52:4755.
5. de Onis M, Onyango AW, Borghi E, Siyan A, Nishida C, Siekmann J. Development of WHO growth reference for school-aged children and adolescents. Bull World Health Organ. 2007;85:660-7.
6. Aggarwal B, Jain V. Obesity in children: definition, etiology and approach. Indian J Pediatr. 2018;85(6):463-71.
7. NCD Risk Factor Collaboration (NCD-RisC). Worldwide trends in body-mass index, underweight, overweight, and obesity from 1975 to 2016: a pooled analysis of 2416 population-based measurement studies in 128.9 million children, adolescents, and adults. Lancet. 2017;390(10113):2627-42.
8. Caprio S, Santoro N, Weiss R. Childhood obesity and the associated rise in cardiometabolic complications. Nat Metab. 2020;2(3):223-32.
9. Khadilkar VV, Khadilkar AV, Cole TJ, Chiplonkar SA, Pandit D. Overweight and obesity prevalence and body mass index trends in Indian children. Int J Pediatr Obes. 2011;6:e216-24.
10. GBD 2015 Obesity Collaborators, Afshin A, Forouzanfar MH, Reitsma MB, Sur P, Estep K, Lee A, et al. Health effects of overweight and obesity in 195 countries over 25 years. N Engl J Med. 2017;377(1):13-27.
11. Praga M, Morales E. The fatty kidney: obesity and renal disease. Nephron. 2017;136(4):273-6.
12. D'Agati VD, Chagnac A, de Vries AP, Levi M, Porrini E, Herman-Edelstein M, et al. Obesity-related glomerulopathy: clinical and pathologic characteristics and pathogenesis. Nat Rev Nephrol. 2016;12(8):453-71.
13. Snyder S, Turner GA, Turner A. Obesity-related kidney disease. Prim Care. 2014;41(4):875-93.
14. Tsuboi N, Utsunomiya Y, Hosoya T. Obesity-related glomerulopathy and the nephron complement. Nephrol Dial Transplant. 2013;28(suppl 4):iv108-13.
15. Kanasaki K, Kitada M, Kanasaki M, Koya D. The biological consequence of obesity on the kidney. Nephrol Dial Transplant. 2013;28(4):iv1-7.
16. Rüster C, Wolf G. The role of the renin-angiotensin-aldosterone system in obesity-related renal diseases. Semin Nephrol. 2013;33(1):44-53.
17. Yang S, Cao C, Deng T, Zhou Z. Obesity-related glomerulopathy: a latent change in obesity requiring more attention. Kidney Blood Press Res. 2020;45(4):510-22.
18. Xu T, Sheng Z, Yao L. Obesity-related glomerulopathy: pathogenesis, pathologic, clinical characteristics and treatment. Front Med. 2017;11(3):340-8.
19. Cohen AH. Massive obesity and the kidney. A morphologic and statistical study. Am J Pathol. 1975;81:117-30.
20. Styne DM, Arslanian SA, Connor EL, Farooqi IS, Murad MH, Silverstein JH, et al. Pediatric obesity-assessment, treatment, and prevention: an endocrine society clinical practice guideline. J Clin Endocrinol Metab. 2017;102(3):709-57.

CHAPTER

7.7

Renal Manifestations of Metabolic Diseases

Banigallapati Vijay Kiran

INTRODUCTION

Kidney diseases in children can be due to anatomical defects [congenital abnormality of kidney and urinary tract (CAKUT), immunologic (autoimmune), infective (pyelonephritis and urinary tract infection—UTI)] or due to metabolic causes. In this chapter, we discuss the metabolic causes and specifically their renal manifestations and available solutions. This can be divided into single-gene defects leading to abnormal cellular function and polygenic diseases affecting the body as a whole and renal involvement being a part of it.

To understand renal involvement in any disorder, we need to be aware of the three components of the kidney, i.e., the glomerular, tubulointerstitial, and vascular components. If the disorder affects the glomerulus, it may lead to proteinuria and eventually to glomerulosclerosis. If the tubulointerstitial component is involved, there will be electrolyte abnormalities and urine concentrating-diluting mechanism imbalance. Furthermore, interstitial fibrosis and tubular atrophy (IFTA) will ensue. Vascular component involvement may lead to microthrombi followed by ischemia. Whatever may be the component involved, the result over time is a rise in creatinine and progression to end-stage kidney disease (ESKD).

The monogenetic defects of inborn errors of metabolism (IEM) can lead to cellular abnormalities in energy metabolism, interfering with adenosine triphosphate (ATP) generation (as in mitochondrial disorders) or lead to tubulopathy either due to abnormal component accumulation as in Fabry disease and cystinosis or solute transport as in Fanconi–Bickel syndrome (FBS). Sometimes, these genetic mutations lead to abnormal excretion/reduced absorption of a specific solute leading to nephrocalcinosis and renal damage (cystinuria and primary hyperoxaluria). Some of these mutations lead to component-induced damage to the tubular epithelium and interstitium of the kidney [methylmalonic acidemia (MMA), uromodulin-associated familial juvenile hyperuricemic nephropathy (FJHN)]. Furthermore, these metabolic disorders may lead to glomerular lesions as in Fabry disease, or defects in the structure of the glomerular basement membrane [congenital disorder of glycosylation type 1 (CDG1)], or toxic damage to glomerular cells as in focal segmental glomerulosclerosis (FSGS) related to mitochondrial disorders, or hemolytic uremic syndrome (HUS) as in cobalamin deficiency. The other polygenic causes of metabolic abnormality are secondary to systemic polygenic diseases such as diabetes, obesity, and metabolic syndrome, which are discussed separately.

Since these genetic diseases are heterogenous, the Society for the Study of the Inborn Errors of Metabolism (SSIEM) developed a systemic classification of these diseases.[1] This taxonomy categorizes diseases based on the principle that defects belonging to the same biological pathway are likely to have similar clinical features and are often treated using similar approaches. The complete list of these diseases is too exhaustive, and we focus only on those crucial diseases that have predominantly renal manifestations during the disease. These are listed in **Table 1**.

DISORDERS OF AMINO ACID METABOLISM

The most common IEMs of amino acid metabolism are as follows:

- Methylmalonic acidemia (MMA)
- Tyrosinemia type 1
- Alkaptonuria (AKU)
- Cystinuria
- Lysinuric protein intolerance
- Cystinosis

Cystinosis is discussed in a separate chapter of this book. The rest of them are discussed here.

Methylmalonic Acidemia

This is the most common inborn error of organic acid metabolism and is caused by the defect of the enzyme methylmalonyl-coenzyme A mutase (MCM).

Pathophysiology

Isolated MMA is an autosomal recessive (AR) organic acidemia due to impaired metabolism of methylmalonyl-coenzyme A (CoA) due to an enzyme defect (MCM-MUT). Cofactor deficiencies due to cobalamin A (Cb1A) and

TABLE 1: Inborn errors of metabolism and clinical manifestations.[1]

Disease	***Gene***	***Main features***	***Renal features***
		Disorders of amino acid metabolism	
Cystinosis	*CTNS*	FTT, rickets, blond hair, corneal cystine crystals, multisystem involvement	Fanconi syndrome, CKD
Tyrosinemia type 1	*FAH*	Liver failure, hepatocellular carcinoma, CLD, rickets, neurologic crisis	Fanconi syndrome, CKD
Lysinuric protein intolerance	*SLC7A7*	FTT, organomegaly, refusal of protein-rich foods, lung involvement, immune dysfunction	Tubulopathy, CKD, immune-mediated glomerulonephritis
Cystinuria	*SLC3A1*	—	Kidney stones
Methylmalonic acidemia	*MUT*	FTT, vomiting, hyperammonemic coma, encephalopathy, cardiomyopathy	Tubulointerstitial changes, CKD
Alkaptonuria	*HGD*	Ochronotic pigmentation of cartilage and collagen	Urine color turns black on standing, calculi
		Disorders of carbohydrate metabolism	
Galactosemia	*GALT*	FTT, jaundice liver failure, hypotonia, cataracts	Fanconi syndrome
Glycogen storage disease type 1a	*G6PC*	FTT, hepatomegaly, lactic acidosis	Fanconi syndrome, nephrocalcinosis, hypercalciuria, FSGS, CKD
Fanconi–Bickel syndrome	*SLC2A2*	FTT, hepatomegaly, rickets, hypoglycemia	Fanconi syndrome, diabetic-like nephropathy
Primary hyperoxaluria	*AGXT/GRHPR*	Optic atrophy, retinopathy	Calculi, CKD
		Disorders of fat metabolism	
Carnitine palmitoyl transferase deficiency[1,2]	*CPT1A, CPT2*	FTT, fasting leading to encephalopathy, seizures, organomegaly, microcephaly	RTA, enlarged polycystic kidney, hydronephrosis, lipid accumulation in PCT
Fatty acid oxidation disorders	Many	Liver disease, multisystem involvement	Renal tubulopathy, myoglobinuria, AKI
		Mitochondrial/energy disorders	
MELAS	mRNA	Stroke-like episodes, encephalopathy, deafness, myopathy, DM	FSGS
Kearns–Sayre syndrome	mtRNA	Ophthalmoplegia, retinal degeneration, heart block, ataxia, hyperparathyroidism	FSGS
Coenzyme Q deficiency		Encephalomyopathy, liver failure, deafness	SRNS
		Disorders of trace elements and metals	
Wilson disease	*ATP7B*	Liver, neurologic disease, KF ring, hemolytic anemia	Fanconi syndrome, tubular proteinuria, dRTA, hypercalciuria, calculi
		Peroxisomal disorders	
Peroxisome biogenesis disorders—Zellweger syndrome	*PEX*	Facial dysmorphism, developmental delay, brain dysplasia, organomegaly	Microcysts/large cortical cysts
		Lysosomal storage disorders	
Fabry disease	*GLA*	X linked, acroparesthesias, anhidrosis, angiokeratomas, corneal/lens opacities, cardiomyopathy	Fanconi syndrome, hyposthenuria, CKD
MPS type 1	*IDUA*	Coarse facies, corneal clouding, visceromegaly, dysostosis multiplex, developmental delay	Nephrotic syndrome, hypertension

(AKI: acute kidney injury; CKD: chronic kidney disease; CLD: chronic liver disease; DM: diabetes mellitus; dRTA: distal renal tubular acidosis; FSGS: focal segmental glomerulosclerosis; FTT: failure to thrive; KF: Kayser–Fleischer; MELAS: mitochondrial encephalopathy, lactic acidosis, and stroke-like episodes; MPS: mucopolysaccharidosis type 1; PCT: proximal convoluted tubule; RTA: renal tubular acidosis)

Flowchart 1: Metabolism of organic acids and pathophysiology of methylmalonic acidemia and cobalamin defects. Increased MMA and propionyl-CoA get deposited in multiple tissues and lead to organ dysfunction. Carbohydrate metabolic defect leads to hypoglycemia and suboptimal growth (failure to thrive).

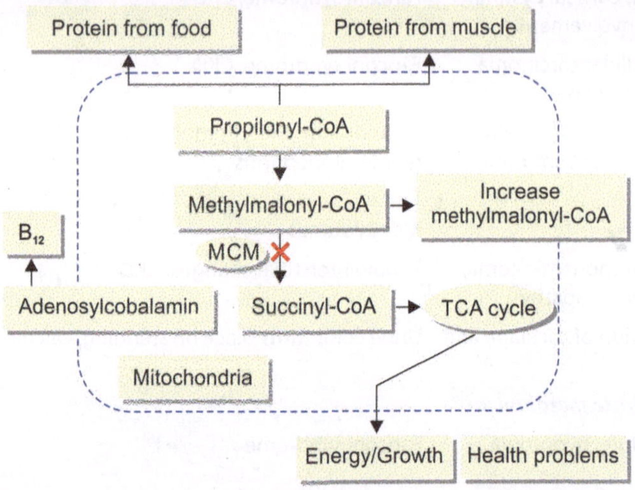

(CoA: coenzyme A; MCM: methylmalonyl-coenzyme A mutase; TCA: tricarboxylic acid cycle)

cobalamin B (Cb1B and Cb1D) can also lead to MMA variants, which respond to vitamin B_{12} therapy and are associated with better prognosis **(Flowchart 1)**. Deficiency of MCM leads to accumulation of MMA, and propionyl-CoA leads to multiple downstream effects on the cellular and mitochondrial function, leading to tubular cell dysfunction and death.[2] Since the TCA cycle is disturbed, growth of these children becomes suboptimal.

Clinical Features and Renal Manifestations

Infants with MMA may present in the neonatal period or early infancy with lethargy, vomiting, and poor feeding (sepsis-like picture). Developmental delay, failure to thrive, and recurrent episodes of metabolic acidosis due to lactate and/or ketones are associated with MMA. Ketonuria, hyperammonemia, and hypoglycemia are also seen. Diagnosis can also be picked up by a positive newborn screen. Cobalamin-unresponsive patients with the classic disease have poor prognosis, with a mortality rate of 50% within the first decade.[3]

Renal manifestations start as tubulopathy, which usually present as severe salt and bicarbonate losses, triggered by episodes of infection, leading to normal anion gap metabolic acidosis. Chronic kidney disease (CKD) intervenes in 50% of the children by 7 years of age.[4] Proteinuria and hematuria are typically absent.

Acute management is required when decompensation is triggered by states that induce catabolism such as fever, prolonged fasting, exercise, and corticosteroids. Additional stressors include general anesthesia, acute trauma, hemorrhage, or excessive protein intake. Management is aimed at treating the underlying cause, stopping catabolism, and stabilizing the patient with dextrose, decreased protein, and increased water intake. Additionally, sodium bicarbonate, ammonia scavengers, and dialysis (if ammonia levels are >400 μM/L) are indicated.

The long-term specific management is by diet limited in protein (low-protein diet is beneficial because amino acids are the precursors of propionyl-CoA) and by supplementing levocarnitine and vitamin B_{12}. Since the enzyme defect is in the liver, some have suggested combined liver and kidney transplant for ESKD patients due to MMA.[5]

Cobalamin Defects

Cobalamin is an essential cofactor for the metabolism of methylmalonyl-CoA to succinyl-CoA. Cobalamin gets converted in the cell's mitochondria to adenosylcobalamin, which is the active form required to convert methylmalonyl-CoA to succinyl-CoA. In the cytosol, it is required for the metabolism of homocysteine.

The genetic defects of cobalamin are usually inherited as an AR inheritance and result in MMA and homocystinuria. This combined with methylmalonic aciduria and homocystinuria (cb1C type) is the most common IEM concerning cobalamin metabolism.

In addition to the classic manifestations of IEM (failure to thrive, hypotonia, retinitis, respiratory distress, cardiomyopathy, etc.), these children may present with HUS.[6,7] Pulmonary hypertension is also observed in infants with cobalamin deficiencies. Therefore, defects in the cobalamin pathway should be suspected when a child with pulmonary hypertension develops thrombotic microangiopathy.[8-10]

Treatment of HUS is hydroxycobalamin administration and not the traditional plasma exchanges. Hence, it is imperative to assess children with atypical HUS having extrarenal manifestations of a systemic metabolic disease to identify the etiology and provide definitive treatment.

Hereditary Tyrosinemia Type 1

Hereditary tyrosinemia type 1 (HT1) occurs due to the deficiency of fumarylacetoacetate (FAA) hydrolase in the liver and the kidney. The lack of this enzyme leads to the accumulation of FAA and succinylacetoacetate (SA; **Flowchart 2**), which damage the cells by rendering them susceptible to free radicals or promoting mutagenesis. As a result, cells in the liver and kidney undergo apoptosis, and liver cells undergo mutation to develop cancers. FAA is the main chemical that causes glomerulosclerosis and interstitial fibrosis,[11] and SA is responsible for tubular dysfunction.[12]

Hereditary tyrosinemia type 1 is characterized by severe, progressive liver disease and renal tubular dysfunction. Patients not diagnosed by newborn screening typically present in early infancy with failure to thrive and hepatomegaly. Some patients develop conjugated hyperbilirubinemia. Liver disease begins prenatally, as evidenced by the common finding of nodularity or cirrhosis in affected neonates. Progression of the

Flowchart 2: Pathway of tyrosine metabolism and pathophysiology of tyrosinemia type 1. Accumulation of fumarylacetoacetate and succinylacetoacetate will lead to cell dysfunction and death.

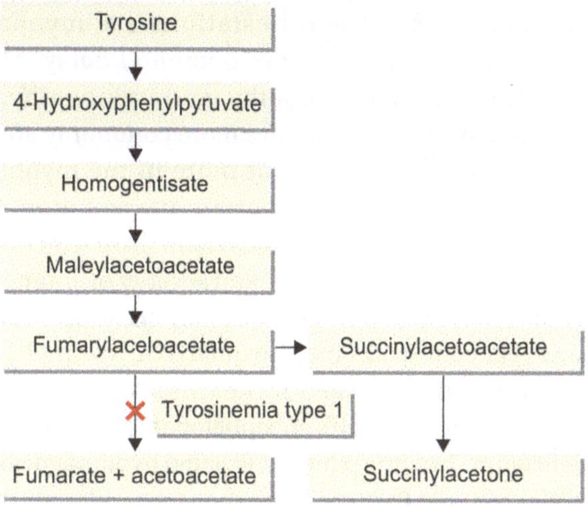

liver disease can be chronic or acute, with rapid deterioration and early death.[13] Liver dysfunction commonly results in hypoglycemia and coagulation abnormalities.

Typical renal presentation is Fanconi syndrome with hypophosphatemic rickets. Later, nephrocalcinosis and IFTA develop, leading to progressive renal failure. Hepatic involvement is more severe compared with the kidney and is the cause of death in these patients.

Treatment with nitisinone, an inhibitor of SA production, has changed the outcome of this disease. With this novel medication, liver failure resolves, and the risk of developing hepatocellular carcinoma reduces. This is also useful in resolving renal damages to some extent.[14,15]

Alkaptonuria

Alkaptonuria is a rare AR amino acid disorder that results from the deficient activity of homogentisic acid dioxygenase (HGD), the third enzyme in tyrosine degradation (*see* **Flowchart 2**). The gene encoding HGD is located on chromosome 3q21-q23, and the description of AKU by Garrod in 1902 led to the recognition of the concept of a single enzyme deficiency resulting in lifelong disease.[16]

Homogentisic acid dioxygenase deficiency results in elevated levels of homogentisic acid (HGA), which polymerizes, forming a pigment that is deposited in connective tissue throughout the body (ochronosis). The only significant finding is that the urine color turns black on standing. At a later stage of life, these patients (27%) develop kidney stones.[17]

Cystinuria

Cystinuria is a genetic condition where bibasic amino acids are not reabsorbed after filtration at the glomerulus. These amino acids are cystine, ornithine, arginine, and lysine. Of these four amino acids, cystine is insoluble in the urine leading to cystine stones. Genetic mutations at *SLC3A1* and *SLC7A9* have been identified, which are the cause of cystinuria in most of the cases.

Cystinuria should be suspected in those who have had their first kidney stone in childhood or adolescence. These are hard stones that may take a staghorn shape. Multiple episodes of stone formations and urological procedures may eventually lead to the development of CKD.

The general approach to treatment includes high fluid intake, restricting sodium and protein intake, and urinary alkalization. These measures are complementary to each other and will help in the prevention of crystallization. The specific management includes use of thiol drugs (tiopronin and D penicillamine) with sulfhydryl groups that convert dimer cystine to monomer cysteine and more water-soluble end products. Captopril may also act in a similar manner.[18,19]

Lysinuric Protein Intolerance

Lysinuric protein intolerance is a rare genetic condition where the body cannot digest cationic amino acids such as lysine, arginine, and ornithine.[20] Also, the transport of these is defective in the renal tubular cells. *SLC7A7* gene is defective, and it is inherited in an AR manner.

After weaning, the symptoms develop and mimic protein intolerance as these amino acids are not digested. Along with it, short stature, muscle weakness, impaired immune function, and osteoporosis develop. Lung and kidney involvement is ominous. Pulmonary alveolar proteinosis, hemophagocytic lymphohistiocytosis, and immune-mediated glomerulonephritis can occur, which can resemble lupus nephritis. Treatment is supportive with extremely low-protein diet.

DISORDERS OF CARBOHYDRATE METABOLISM

- Glycogen storage disease type 1 (GSD1)/Von Gierke disease
- FBS
- Primary hyperoxaluria

Glycogen Storage Disease Type 1

This is an AR disease due to defects in a key enzyme that converts glucose-6-phosphate to glucose and phosphate (glucose-6-phosphatase). Children with this disorder accumulate glycogen in the liver, kidney, and intestinal mucosa and present with poor tolerance to fasting, hypoglycemia, lactic acidosis, hyperuricemia, and hyperlipidemia. Growth retardation with organomegaly is universal. Over time, this may lead to hepatic and renal failure.

Kidney involvement is similar to diabetes. Initially, there is hyperfiltration (leading to renomegaly, proteinuria, and hematuria), which is followed by glomerulosclerosis and a reduction in the glomerular filtration rate (GFR) leading to renal failure by the third decade.[21] The better the metabolic control, the better the renal outcome. Histologically, there is deposition of glycogen in the proximal tubular cells, glomerular enlargement, thickening, and lamellation of the basement membrane.[22,23] FSGS and interstitial fibrosis ensue.

Tubular involvement is usually seen in childhood but is subclinical. Fanconi syndrome may develop, suggesting generalized dysfunction of the proximal tubular cells. Proximal renal tubular acidosis (RTA), Gitelman-like syndrome, and distal RTA (dRTA) are also seen.[24,25] Kidney stones result from both hypercalciuria and hyperuricosuria.

There is no specific treatment, but treatment with angiotensin-converting enzyme inhibitors (ACEi)/angiotensin receptor blockers (ARBs) has shown to reduce the progression. Eating uncooked cornstarch and frequent meals may also help in delaying nephropathy.[26] Liver transplantation is done to prevent the development of malignant hepatic adenoma, and this might also reduce renal deterioration.[27]

Fanconi–Bickel Syndrome

Fanconi–Bickel syndrome is inherited as an AR disease of monosaccharide transport (D-glucose). Glucose transporter 2 (GLUT2) channel is a bidirectional transporter that transports glucose and galactose across the cells from intracellular to extracellular space. This disease occurs due to mutation of the *SLC2A2* gene, located at 3q26, which codes for GLUT2.[28]

Children present with hepatomegaly (due to accumulation of glycogen), recurrent hypoglycemia episodes leading to failure to thrive, and severe proximal tubulopathy leading to rickets. This is associated with glycosuria and galactosuria, and its consequence is osmotic diuresis and polyuria.[29] The difference between GSD1 and FBS is the absence of hypoglycemia and lactic acidosis in the latter.

Treatment is carried out with oral frequent uncooked cornstarch, which maintains blood glucose levels.[30] The rest is supportive with water, electrolytes, and vitamin D supplementation.

Primary Hyperoxaluria

Primary hyperoxaluria is discussed in detail in another chapter.

MITOCHONDRIAL DISORDERS (ENERGY DISORDERS)

Mitochondrial function is dependent upon its own separate DNA. This complex structure helps in the proper transfer of electrons to oxygen, resulting in a proton gradient, which releases energy. These respiratory chain enzyme complexes are coded by mitochondrial DNA, which is inherited from the mother.

Occasionally, specific mutations in these respiratory chain enzymes occur resulting in disorders called mitochondrial disorders. If mutated, the proportion between mutant and nonmutant mtDNA can, therefore, vary from tissue to tissue and can alter over time. Hence, these disorders are quite heterogenous in clinical presentations.

The main clinical manifestations are myopathy, encephalopathy, seizures, developmental delay, retinal degeneration, cardiac myopathy, endocrinopathy, and liver disease. Skeletal muscles are more commonly affected because these mutations occur more in the myoblasts. Exercise intolerance is an important presentation. Over time, these children develop multisystem involvement, with symptoms increasing in number and severity over time.

Renal manifestations result from proximal tubular damage leading to Fanconi syndrome, proximal RTA, low-molecular-weight proteinuria as seen in Kearns–Sayre syndrome, Pearson's syndrome, Leigh's encephalopathy, and coenzyme Q10 deficiency. In some patients, isolated hypomagnesemia, hypercalciuria, and Bartter-like phenotype are also observed. Glomerular involvement may be seen as steroid-resistant nephrotic syndrome with renal histology being FSGS. It has been reported due to mutation in the tRNA *LEU* gene and coenzyme Q10.

MELAS (mitochondrial encephalopathy, lactic acidosis, and stroke-like episodes) syndrome is the most frequent mitochondrial disorder in humans. Renal manifestations are asymptomatic proteinuria and associated maternal family history of diabetes or deafness.[31-33] The age of diagnosis is 15–50 years. Nephrotic syndrome develops in one third with renal histology being FSGS. Renal failure eventually develops due to tubulointerstitial nephritis. Differential diagnoses of renal diseases associated with deafness are Alport syndrome, dRTA, Bartter syndrome with sensorineural deafness, and iatrogenic causes secondary to drug usage like in aminoglycoside/furosemide usage.

Coenzyme Q10 (CoQ10) defects are unique as they are the only treatable mitochondrial defects. These children present with steroid-resistant nephrotic syndrome and progressive renal failure. Extrarenal manifestation, which gives a clue to the diagnosis, includes seizures and neurological deterioration. Histology will be FSGS on renal biopsy. Suggested CoQ10 dosing is 5–30 mg/kg daily (in three divided doses) for infants and children, 300–1,500 mg daily for adolescents, and up to 2,400 mg daily for adults.[34]

CONGENITAL DISORDERS OF GLYCOSYLATION

Congenital disorders of glycosylation result from abnormal N-glycosylation and O-glycosylation of proteins. N-glycosylation of proteins is required in multiple metabolic pathways. The clinical presentation is heterogenous, ranging from fatal multisystem disorders in infancy to multiple exostoses, progeria, or developmental delay in older children. On screening, abnormal isoelectric focusing of serum transferrin can be found. The most common form of CDG is phosphomannomutase 2 (PMM2)-CDG, which presents with facial dysmorphism, failure to thrive, diarrhea, abnormal fat pads, inverted nipples, and abnormal eye movements. Renal manifestation includes incidentally detected renal microcysts and increased echogenicity of the kidney on ultrasound.[35]

Disorders of Uric Acid and Purine Metabolism and Transport

The metabolic end product of purines is uric acid and its immediate precursor xanthine, both of which are insoluble in urine. So, hyperuricemia and hyperuricosuria can predispose to stone formation. This could be due to excessive purine intake, defect in purine metabolism, and/or decreased excretion of these end products.

Examples of inherited enzyme defects leading to purine overproduction are:

- HGPRTase (hypoxanthine-guanine phosphoribosyl-transferase) deficiency
- Glucose-6-phosphatase deficiency (glycogen storage disease type I)

Examples of clinical conditions associated with purine and urate overproduction are

- Myeloproliferative diseases
- Malignancies
- Hemolytic disorders
- Down syndrome
- Glycogen storage diseases (types III, V, and VII)

Uric acid urolithiasis is the most common renal manifestation of abnormal purine metabolism. Defects in the xanthine oxidase result in xanthinuria and xanthine stones. Differential diagnosis of uric acid stones includes 2,8-dihydroxyadenine (DHA) stones—these crystals form as a result of adenine phosphoribosyltransferase deficiency, an AR disorder. DHA crystals may be incorrectly reported as uric acid by some laboratories.

Autosomal Dominant Tubulointerstitial Kidney Disease

ADTKD-UMOD (autosomal dominant tubulointerstitial kidney disease-uromodulin-associated kidney disease), also known as uromodulin kidney disease (UKD), is a group of autosomal dominantly inherited disorders with hyperuricemia and progressive decline in kidney function. The key to identification is the presence of CKD in a parent and a child, both with a bland urinary sediment.

Classification and clinical features:

- ADTKD due to *UMOD* mutations, previously called FJHN. ADTKD is an AD disorder due to a mutation in the *UMOD* gene that encodes for uromodulin (Tamm–Horsfall protein) leading to hyperuricemia, gout, progressive tubulointerstitial damage, and renal failure. Mutation in the same gene causes another disease called medullary cystic kidney disease type 2 (MCKD2), and these two are collectively referred to as uromodulin-associated kidney disease (UAKD). Children present with urinary concentrating defect resulting in polyuria and polydipsia. CKD ensues later by the second and fourth decades of life. There is no specific treatment, but allopurinol can prevent progression in the early stages.[36,37]
- *ADTKD due to REN mutations:* ADTKD-*REN*, which is due to mutations in the *REN* gene encoding renin, produces progressive CKD, low or low-normal blood pressures, anemia that occurs in childhood before the onset of CKD, mild hyperkalemia, and hyperuricemia.[38] In the past, it has been called FJHN type 2. Fludrocortisone may be an effective therapy for this condition.[39]
- *ADTKD due to MUC1 mutations:* ADTKD-*MUC1*, also known as mucin-1 kidney disease (MKD), is caused by mutations in the *MUC1* gene encoding mucin-1 and is associated with progressive CKD but no other distinguishing characteristics (i.e., no precocious gout, childhood anemia, hypotension, or hyperkalemia). It accounts for approximately 30% of ADTKD.[40] In the past, this condition was called MCKD1.

Pathogenesis: Uromodulin is a kidney-specific protein that is exclusively expressed by epithelial cells lining the thick ascending limb (TAL) of Henle's loop. It has many important functions in the kidney, including maintaining water and electrolyte balance in the TAL, protecting against UTIs, preventing kidney stone formation, and activating the innate immunity mechanism in the kidney. Once there is a missense mutation, these abnormal uromodulin proteins cannot assemble properly nor exit the endoplasmic reticulum, resulting in the accumulation and destruction of the cells in the TAL of loop of Henle.

ADTKD due to UMOD should be suspected in a child presenting with a strong family history of kidney disease suggestive of AD inheritance, a family history of gout, and a bland urinary sediment with little proteinuria. ADTKD-*REN* should be strongly considered in a child who presents with one of the following in combination with a family history of CKD plus unexplained anemia that is out of proportion to the reduction in estimated GFR (eGFR) plus CKD in conjunction with hyperkalemia, low or low-normal blood pressure, and hyperuricemia. Confirmation is with genetic testing of the *UMOD/REN* gene by clinical exome sequencing. Treatment is supportive for ADTKD-UMOD. In ADTKD-REN, supportive management plus fludrocortisone helps to retard the progression.

Lecithin Cholesterol Acyltransferase Deficiency

Lecithin cholesterol acyltransferase deficiency (LCAT) is a rare AR disease due to mutation in the *LCAT* gene. LCAT deficiency results in the deposition of the unesterified cholesterol and phosphatidylcholine in plasma and tissues **(Flowchart 3)**.

Cholesterol deposition causes corneal opacities (fish-eye disease), tendon xanthomas, atherosclerosis, hemolytic anemia, proteinuria secondary to mesangial hypercellularity, and deposition of lipids in the glomerular cells.[41,42] These children have low high-density lipoprotein (HDL) cholesterol and proteinuria and develop CKD. The serum lipid profile can be improved by infusions of normal plasma rich in LCAT.

Lysosomal Storage Disorders: Fabry Disease

Fabry disease is the most common lysosomal disease in children. It is inherited as an X-linked error of the glycosphingolipid metabolic pathway that results in the accumulation of globotriaosylceramide (Gb3) in the lysosomes of cells, leading to cellular dysfunction and cell death. The defect in Fabry disease is the deficiency of the lysosomal hydrolase alpha-galactosidase A (alpha-Gal A), which catalyzes the cleavage of the terminal galactose from D galactosyl moieties of the glycolipids such as Gb3 **(Flowchart 4)**. In such enzyme-linked disorders, there is a threshold level below which the clinical features will manifest. In Fabry disease, this threshold level is below 30–35% of the normal values.[43] Since it is an X-linked disease, males are more commonly affected.

Flowchart 3: Cholesterol metabolism and pathophysiology of LCAT deficiency.

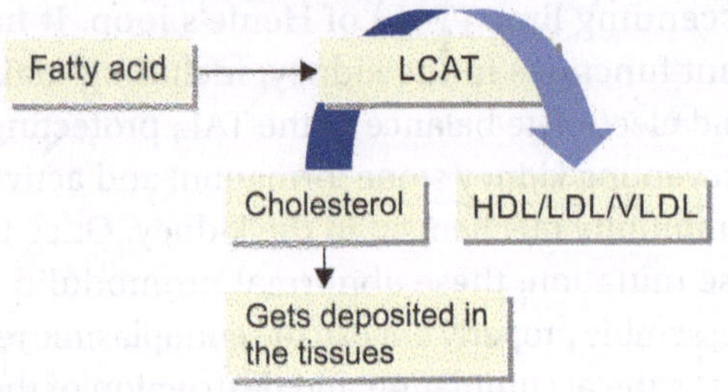

(HDL: high-density lipoprotein; LCAT: lecithin cholesterol acyltransferase deficiency; LDL: low-density lipoprotein; VLDL: very low-density lipoprotein)

Flowchart 4: Metabolism of glycolipids and pathophysiology of Fabry disease—Gb3 cannot get converted to lactosylceramide and gets deposited in the lysosomes.

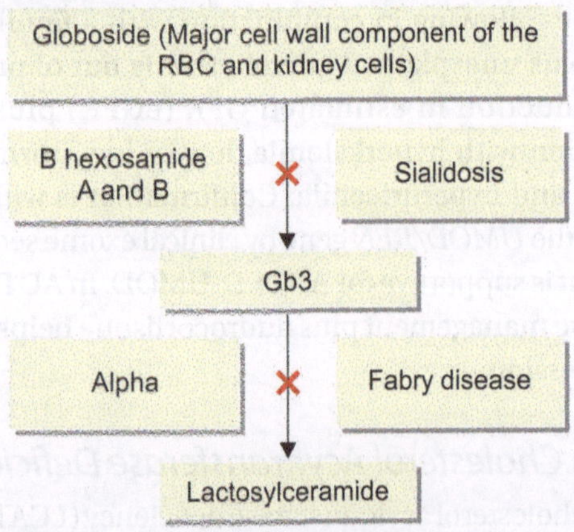

(Gb3: globotriaosylceramide; RBC: red blood cell)

Furthermore, since females carry one mutant gene, clinical manifestations are varied depending upon the lyonization of the mutant gene containing chromosome. Males with the classic form of the disease are "null mutants" with alpha-Gal A activity of <1%. They have a severe form of the disease. Females have a higher alpha-Gal A activity and hence have a varied presentation.

Pathophysiology: The accumulation of Gb3 occurs throughout the body, particularly in the vascular endothelium, vascular smooth muscle cells, and the pericytes.[44] This abnormal deposition of the Gb3 in cells may lead to the death of the smooth muscle cells, vascular occlusion, ischemia, and infarction. Also, the accumulation is seen in autonomic ganglia; renal glomerular, tubular, and interstitial cells; cardiac muscle cells; vascular smooth muscle cells; vascular and lymphatic endothelial cells in the cornea; valvular fibrocytes; and cardiac conduction fibers leading to various manifestations of the disease. Since the sphingolipid metabolism is different in different tissues, and the enzyme activity differs from organ to organ, the clinical manifestations are different, and no two patients have the same presentation.[45] As mentioned earlier, it is not only the deposition that is pathogenic. Occlusion of blood supply leading to ischemia is an important factor contributing to pathology.

Mutation of the alpha-Gal A, galactosidase alpha (*GLA*) gene causes Fabry disease. It is mapped to the long arm of the X chromosome (Xq22.1). Males are hemizygous for the gene, and they pass on the gene to their daughters but not their sons. Furthermore, they have the severe disease compared with females. As females are heterozygous for the gene, they have a 50% chance of passing it on to their progeny. Also, they have a highly variable disease course that ranges from asymptomatic disease to severe variant, as seen in males. This is due to the random inactivation of the X chromosome called lyonization.[46-48] More than 1,000 mutations in the *GLA* gene have been identified till date.[49]

Pathology: The findings on histology are also in proportion to the clinical condition of the patient. Females, children, and individuals with late-onset variants have a lesser histology finding compared with males. Ideally, a kidney biopsy is *not* required for the diagnosis of Fabry, but sometimes the diagnosis is established by electron microscopy (EM) findings seen in the renal biopsy. These characteristic findings are vacuolization of the podocytes and distal tubule epithelial cells **(Fig. 1)**.[45]

Electron microscopy: The classical finding seen on the EM is deposits of Gb3 in the podocytes as lamellated structures called "myeloid or zebra" bodies **(Fig. 2)**. Zebra bodies are considered a hallmark of glycolipid storage disorders—lamellated structures with a 3.5-5-mm-sized onion skin appearance. These are predominant in the podocytes but are also found in endothelial, mesangial, parietal epithelial

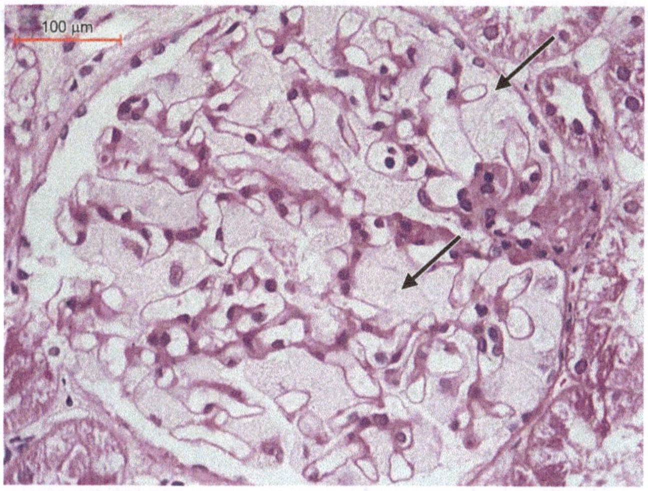

Fig. 1: Fabry disease, kidney biopsy, light microscopy (periodic acid–Schiff). Arrows showing vacuolization of the podocytes and mesangial cells.
Courtesy: Dr Alok Sharma, Dr Lal Path Labs, New Delhi, India.

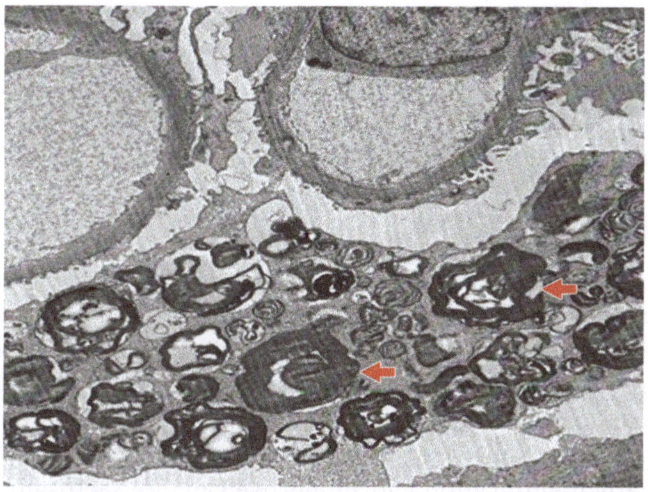

Fig. 2: Electron microscopy of a renal biopsy showing the classic zebra bodies in the parietal epithelium. This accumulation is also seen in the vascular endothelium, leading to progressive ischemia and infarction (arrow heads).
Courtesy: Dr Alok Sharma, Dr Lal Path Labs, New Delhi, India.

cells, distal tubular cells, and vascular smooth muscle cells. Later, degenerative changes are seen in the smooth muscle cells indicating cell death. These EM findings are extremely specific for Fabry disease but can also be seen in silicosis, chloroquine, and hydroxychloroquine usage, and some other drugs such as chlorcyclizine, imipramine, gentamycin, and chlorphentermine.[50-52]

Symptomatology and Clinical Diagnosis

Among the typical manifestations are severe neuropathic pain (accumulation of Gb3 in the nerves), called acroparesthesias, angiokeratomas (deposition of Gb3 in the capillaries), and gastrointestinal presentation with abdominal pain and motility symptoms (Gb3 deposition in the smooth muscles). Corneal verticillate may be seen (due to deposition of Gb3 in the cornea). These manifestations start earlier in life. As the age progresses, other organ involvement is more common.

Renal Manifestation of Fabry Disease

A prominent renal manifestation is proteinuria, and it increases as the patients age. Females have a later onset and slightly less proteinuria compared with males.[48] So, the only renal manifestation seen in homozygous male children is proteinuria. Podocyte Gb3 accumulation increases with age in Fabry disease. Podocyte loss is important in the progression of Fabry nephropathy, and the degree of podocyte loss in the urine (podocyturia) correlates with the clinical severity of renal disease. Even though they present with proteinuria, nephrotic syndrome is rare. In addition to this, they may have oval fat bodies and Maltese crosses in the urine seen under polarized microscopy. Since the distal tubules are also involved in the deposition of Gb3, there is decreased urinary concentrating ability and polyuria may be seen. These may be the earliest symptoms in children with Fabry disease. Some other manifestations are renal sinus cysts and hypertension. CKD develops over time and is not a characteristic feature in children. ESKD occurs by the fifth decade.[44]

The short-term and long-term results of kidney transplantation for Fabry disease are comparable with transplantation for other causes of ESKD. As with other causes of ESKD, survival with transplantation is superior to that observed with dialysis. Thus, transplantation should be the treatment of choice for ESKD due to Fabry disease.[53] In general, clinically significant Fabry kidney disease does not recur in the transplanted kidney, although some recipients may develop Gb3 deposition that typically does not compromise graft function.

Differential diagnosis and evaluation: Fabry disease should be suspected when the patient presents with:

- Intermittent episodes of burning pain in the extremities (acroparesthesias)
- Cutaneous vascular lesion (angiokeratomas)
- Diminished perspiration
- Characteristic corneal and lenticular opacities
- Abdominal pain, nausea, and/or diarrhea of unknown etiology in young adulthood
- Left ventricular hypertrophy or hypertrophic cardiomyopathy of unknown etiology
- Arrhythmias of unknown etiology in young adults
- Stroke of unknown etiology at any age
- CKD and/or proteinuria of unknown etiology
- Multiple renal sinus cysts discovered incidentally

Confirmation of diagnosis is by the following:

- Leukocyte alpha-Gal A levels. Method: Enzyme assay. Units: nmol/h/mg (>60: normal activity, 30–60: possibility of a carrier, <30: deficient activity)[54]

- *Genetic testing*: Gold standard. Next-generation sequencing (NGS) for the coding region and exon–intron boundaries of the *GLA* gene.[55]
- *Tissue biopsy*: Characteristic findings on kidney biopsy or endomyocardial biopsy in the cardiac variant.

Screening of family members[56]: If a child is diagnosed with Fabry disease, his/her male siblings should undergo screening with enzymatic assay, even if asymptomatic. If the blood test reveals low activity of the enzyme, it should be followed up with genetic analysis. His/her female siblings directly need genetic testing to identify the mutation. Enzyme activity should not be used to diagnose females. Prenatal tests for the next child can be offered in the form of chorionic villus sampling analysis for genetic mutation.

Approach to diagnosis: If the clinical findings are suggestive of Fabry disease, the further approach depends on the sex of the patient. If the patient is a female, a genetic mutation analysis of the *GLA* gene is suggested. If the analysis is positive, this establishes the diagnosis. If it is negative, other genetic variants may be looked for. If the clinical diagnosis is still negative, then perform the biopsy of the affected organ. Presence of intracellular Gb3 inclusions will establish the diagnosis.

If the patient is male, measure the leukocyte alpha-Gal A activity. If it is <3%, the diagnosis is established. If it is between 3 and 35%, the diagnosis is likely, and if >35%, then it is not Fabry. Genetic testing for mutation analysis is indicated in cohorts of males having Gal A activity between 3 and 35% only.[57]

Treatment and prognosis: There is no cure for Fabry disease. Recombinant alpha-Gal A, the enzyme that is deficient in patients with Fabry disease and migalastat hydrochloride, an oral pharmacologic chaperone that facilitates trafficking of alpha-Gal A to lysosomes, are the only therapeutic options.[58-60] Enzyme replacement therapy (ERT) has assured good quality of life in these children.

The following recommendations will guide the treatment of these children: ERT or the newer pharmacologic chaperone (migalastat) can be used in the early stages of the disease. This newer molecule can be used in a specific type of Fabry disease with an amenable *GLA* variant. Furthermore, because this is an oral medicine, it should be preferred in this variety. Once the eGFR is <30 mL/min/1.73 m^2, migalastat should not be used.[61] In female carriers and typically affected males who are symptomatic, ERT or migalastat can be used. For those with end-stage kidney disease due to Fabry, extrarenal manifestations will direct ERT usage. The dose of the drugs is as follows:

- *Agalsidase alfa (Replagal):* 0.2 mg/kg as IV infusion every 2 weeks
- *Agalsidase beta (Fabrazyme):* 1 mg/kg IV infusion every 2 weeks
- *Migalastat:* 123 mg orally once on alternate days on an empty stomach[62]

Supportive care with renin-angiotensin system (RAS) inhibitors, such as ACEi or ARB plus standard renal care, is sacrosanct.

Prognosis: There is improved survival with ERT and supportive care. Long-term complications such as CKD, cardiomyopathy, severe neuropathic pain-induced depression, and suicide are the most important factors affecting the quality of life.

Fabry disease is the most common lysosomal disease in humans. It is inherited as an X-linked pattern. Genotype-phenotype variations are seen due to variation of enzyme activity in males and due to skewed X-chromosome inactivation in females. Also, organ accumulation of Gb3 varies. Hence, the clinical manifestations are variable. Renal manifestations are proteinuria, gradual rise in creatinine, and urine concentrating defects. Diagnosis is with leukocyte enzyme levels and genetic analysis for *GLA* gene mutation. Renal biopsy has pathognomonic myeloma/zebra bodies. Treatment is with ERT. Fabry disease is the second lysosomal disease after Gaucher disease to have definitive ERT. Treatment should be lifelong, and once organ failure sets in, transplantation is the only solution.

CONCLUSION

Inborn errors of metabolism, although rare, have significant consequences on children. They are often missed on initial evaluation, challenging to diagnose, and more challenging to treat. Organ damage is ubiquitous, and this affects the growth and longevity of these children. The inheritance pattern is usually AR, but other patterns of inheritance are also noted. Early identification and supportive care are sacrosanct. Some of these diseases have therapeutic interventions available to prevent further organ damage. Kidneys, being the metabolically active organs, are usually affected in these disorders. Although all parts of the kidney are involved, tubular epithelial cells are the first ones to be damaged, hampering these cells' normal function. Over time, without appropriate therapy, glomerulosclerosis and IFTA ensue.

In the inborn error of amino acid metabolism, MMA, tyrosinemia type 1, AKU, cystinuria, and lysinuric protein intolerance are the most common diseases. With regard to carbohydrate metabolism errors, glycogen storage disease type I and FBS are remarkable. Mitochondrial disorders included MELAS, Kearns–Sayre syndrome, and coenzyme Q deficiency leading to multiorgan failure syndromes. Disorders of uric acid metabolism including the AD tubulointerstitial kidney diseases lead to renal failure. Lysosomal storage disorder, such as Fabry disease, was discussed in detail since it is the most common storage disorder leading to organ dysfunction.

TABLE 2: A list of lysosomal storage disorders with FDA-approved ERT.

	Deficient enzyme	*Inheritance*	*ERT*
MPS I (Hurler syndrome)	Alpha-L-iduronidase	Autosomal	Laronidase
MPS II (Hunter syndrome)	Iduronidase sulfatase	X linked	Idursulfase
MPS IV A (Morquio)	NAG 6 sulfatase	Autosomal	Elosulfase
MPS VI (Maroteaux–Lamy)	NAG 4 sulfatase	Autosomal	Galsulfase
Fabry disease	Alpha-galactosidase	X linked	Agalsidase alfa Agalsidase beta
Pompe disease	Alpha-glucosidase	Autosomal	Aglucosidase
Gaucher disease	Beta-glucocerebrosidase	Autosomal	Alglucerase Imiglucerase Velaglucerase Taliglucerase
Lysosomal acid lipase deficiency	Lysosomal acid lipase	Autosomal	Sebelipase

(ERT: enzyme replacement therapy; FDA: Food and Drug Administration; MPS: mucopolysaccharidosis)

KEY POINTS

- IEM are rare inherited diseases affecting the metabolism, leading to multisystem involvement in children.
- These should be suspected in children with failure to thrive and other subtle manifestations such as organomegaly, poor feeding, and polyuria.
- ERT has changed the prognosis of some of these diseases.
- Mucopolysaccharidosis (I, II, IVA, and VI), Fabry disease, Pompe disease, Gaucher disease, and lysosomal acid lipase deficiency disease are the IEM with an Food and Drug Administration (FDA)-approved enzyme replacement therapy available. **Table 2** lists the lysosomal storage disorders with mode of inheritance and ERT, which is FDA-approved.
- Treatment is usually lifelong, and holistic supportive management is sacrosanct for improving the quality of life of these children.

REFERENCES

1. Society for the Study of Inborn Errors of Metabolism. (2011). Inborn errors classification [online]. Available from http://www.ssiem.org/images/centralstore/resources/SSIEMClassificationIEM2011.pdf [Last accessed September, 2021].
2. Morath MA, Okun JG, Müller IB, Sauer SW, Hörster F, Hoffmann GF, et al. Neurodegeneration and chronic renal failure in methylmalonic aciduria—a pathophysiological approach. J Inherit Metab Dis. 2008;31(1):35-43.
3. Fenton WA, Gravel RA, Rosenblatt DS. Disorders of propionate and methylmalonate metabolism. In: The Metabolic and Molecular Bases of Inherited Disease, 8th edition. New York: McGraw Hill; 2001. pp. 2165-93.
4. Cosson MA, Benoist JF, Touati G, Déchaux M, Royer N, Grandin L, et al. Long-term outcome in methylmalonic aciduria: a series of 30 French patients. Mol Genet Metab. 2009;97(3):172-8.
5. Kasahara M, Horikawa R, Tagawa M, Uemoto S, Yokoyama S, Shibata Y, et al. Current role of liver transplantation for methylmalonic acidemia: a review of the literature. Pediatr Transplant. 2006;10(8):943-7.
6. Barlas UK, Kıhtır HS, Goknar N, Ersoy M, Akcay N, Sevketoglu E. Hemolytic uremic syndrome with dual caution in an infant: cobalamin C defect and complement dysregulation successfully treated with eculizumab. Pediatr Nephrol. 2018;33(6):1093-6.
7. Kind T, Levy J, Lee M, Kaicker S, Nicholson JF, Kane SA. Cobalamin C disease presenting as hemolytic-uremic syndrome in the neonatal period. J Pediatr Hematol Oncol. 2002;24(4):327-9.
8. Iodice FG, Di Chiara L, Boenzi S, Aiello C, Monti L, Cogo P, et al. Cobalamin C defect presenting with isolated pulmonary hypertension. Pediatrics. 2013;132(1):e248-51.
9. Kömhoff M, Roofthooft MT, Westra D, Teertstra TK, Losito A, van de Kar NC, et al. Combined pulmonary hypertension and renal thrombotic microangiopathy in cobalamin C deficiency. Pediatrics. 2013;132(2):e540-4.
10. Labrune P, Zittoun J, Duvaltier I, Trioche P, Marquet J, Niaudet P, et al. Haemolytic uraemic syndrome and pulmonary hypertension in a patient with methionine synthase deficiency. Eur J Pediatr. 1999;158(9):734-9.
11. Sun MS, Hattori S, Kubo S, Awata H, Matsuda I, Endo F. A mouse model of renal tubular injury of tyrosinemia type 1: development of de Toni Fanconi syndrome and apoptosis of renal tubular cells in Fah/Hpd double mutant mice. J Am Soc Nephrol. 2000;11(2):291-300.
12. Spencer PD, Roth KS. Effects of succinylacetone on amino acid uptake in the rat kidney. Biochem Med Metab Biol. 1987;37(1):101-9.
13. Weiner DL. Metabolic emergencies. In: Fleisher GR, Ludwig S, Henretig FM (Eds). Textbook of Pediatric Emergency Medicine, 5th edition. Philadelphia, PA: Lippincott, Williams & Wilkins; 2006. p. 1193.
14. De Laet C, Dionisi-Vici C, Leonard JV, McKiernan P, Mitchell G, Monti L, et al. Recommendations for the management of tyrosinaemia type 1. Orphanet J Rare Dis. 2013;8:8.
15. Santra S, Preece MA, Hulton SA, McKiernan PJ. Renal tubular function in children with tyrosinaemia type I treated with nitisinone. J Inherit Metab Dis. 2008;31(3):399-402.
16. Garrod AE. The incidence of alkaptonuria: a study in chemical individuality. Lancet. 1902;2:1616.
17. Phornphutkul C, Introne WJ, Perry MB, Bernardini I, Murphey MD, Fitzpatrick DL, et al. Natural history of alkaptonuria. N Engl J Med. 2002;347(26):2111-21.

18. Chillarón J, Font-Llitjós M, Fort J, Zorzano A, Goldfarb DS, Nunes V, et al. Pathophysiology and treatment of cystinuria. Nat Rev Nephrol. 2010;6:424-34.
19. Stapleton FB. Childhood stones. Endocrinol Metab Clin North Am. 2002;31:1001-15.
20. Mauhin W, Habarou F, Gobin S, Servais A, Brassier A, Grisel C, et al. Update on lysinuric protein intolerance, a multi-faceted disease retrospective cohort analysis from birth to adulthood. Orphanet J Rare Dis. 2017;12(1):3.
21. Martens DH, Rake JP, Navis G, Fidler V, van Dael CM, Smit GP. Renal function in glycogen storage disease type I, natural course, and renopreservative effects of ACE inhibition. Clin J Am Soc Nephrol. 2009;4(11):1741-6.
22. Verani R, Bernstein J. Renal glomerular and tubular abnormalities in glycogen storage disease type I. Arch Pathol Lab Med. 1988;112(3):271-4.
23. Yokoyama K, Hayashi H, Hinoshita F, Yamada A, Suzuki Y, Ogura Y, et al. Renal lesion of type Ia glycogen storage disease: the glomerular size and renal localization of apolipoprotein. Nephron. 1995;70(3):348-52.
24. Rake JP, Visser G, Labrune P, Leonard JV, Ullrich K, Smit GP; European Study on Glycogen Storage Disease Type I (ESGSD I). Guidelines for management of glycogen storage disease type I—European Study on Glycogen Storage Disease Type I (ESGSD I). Eur J Pediatr. 2002;161(Suppl 1):S112-9.
25. Restaino I, Kaplan BS, Stanley C, Baker L. Nephrolithiasis, hypocitraturia, and a distal renal tubular acidification defect in type 1 glycogen storage disease. J Pediatr. 1993;122(3):392-6.
26. Weinstein DA, Wolfsdorf JI. Effect of continuous glucose therapy with uncooked cornstarch on the long-term clinical course of type 1a glycogen storage disease. Eur J Pediatr. 2002;161(Suppl 1):S35-9.
27. Martin AP, Bartels M, Schreiber S, Buehrdel P, Hauss J, Fangmann J. Successful staged kidney and liver transplantation for glycogen storage disease type Ib: a case report. Transplant Proc. 2006;38(10):3615-9.
28. Santer R, Schneppenheim R, Dombrowski A, Götze H, Steinmann B, Schaub J. Mutations in GLUT2, the gene for the liver-type glucose transporter, in patients with Fanconi-Bickel syndrome. Nat Genet. 1997;17(3):324-6. [Erratum in Nat Genet. 1998;18(3):298].
29. Santer R, Steinmann B, Schaub J. Fanconi-Bickel syndrome—a congenital defect of facilitative glucose transport. Curr Mol Med. 2002;2(2):213-27.
30. Lee PJ, Van't Hoff WG, Leonard JV. Catch-up growth in Fanconi-Bickel syndrome with uncooked cornstarch. J Inherit Metab Dis. 1995;18(2):153-6.
31. Guéry B, Choukroun G, Noël LH, Clavel P, Rötig A, Lebon S, et al. The spectrum of systemic involvement in adults presenting with renal lesion and mitochondrial tRNA(Leu) gene mutation. J Am Soc Nephrol. 2003;14(8):2099-108.
32. Jansen JJ, Maassen JA, van der Woude FJ, Lemmink HA, van den Ouweland JM, t' Hart LM, et al. Mutation in mitochondrial tRNA(Leu(UUR)) gene associated with progressive kidney disease. J Am Soc Nephrol. 1997;8(7):1118-24.
33. Seidowsky A, Hoffmann M, Glowacki F, Dhaenens CM, Devaux JP, de Sainte Foy CL, et al. Renal involvement in MELAS syndrome—a series of 5 cases and review of the literature. Clin Nephrol. 2013;80(6):456-63.
34. Rötig A, Appelkvist EL, Geromel V, Chretien D, Kadhom N, Edery P, et al. Quinone-responsive multiple respiratory-chain dysfunction due to widespread coenzyme Q10 deficiency. Lancet. 2000;356(9227):391-5.
35. Scott K, Gadomski T, Kozicz T, Morava E. Congenital disorders of glycosylation: new defects and still counting. J Inherit Metab Dis. 2014;37(4):609-17.
36. Rampoldi L, Scolari F, Amoroso A, Ghiggeri G, Devuyst O. The rediscovery of uromodulin (Tamm-Horsfall protein): from tubulointerstitial nephropathy to chronic kidney disease. Kidney Int. 2011;80(4):338-47.
37. Moro F, Ogg CS, Simmonds HA, Cameron JS, Chantler C, McBride MB, et al. Familial juvenile gouty nephropathy with renal urate hypoexcretion preceding renal disease. Clin Nephrol. 1991;35(6):263-9.
38. Zivná M, Hůlková H, Matignon M, Hodanová K, Vylet'al P, Kalbácová M, et al. Dominant renin gene mutations associated with early-onset hyperuricemia, anemia, and chronic kidney failure. Am J Hum Genet. 2009;85:204-13.
39. Bleyer AJ, Zivná M, Hulková H, Hodanová K, Vyletal P, Sikora J, et al. Clinical and molecular characterization of a family with a dominant renin gene mutation and response to treatment with fludrocortisone. Clin Nephrol. 2010;74:411-22.
40. Kirby A, Gnirke A, Jaffe DB, Barešová V, Pochet N, Blumenstiel B, et al. Mutations causing medullary cystic kidney disease type 1 lie in a large VNTR in MUC1 missed by massively parallel sequencing. Nat Genet. 2013;45:299-303.
41. Gjone E. Familial lecithin: cholesterol acyltransferase (LCAT) deficiency. An updated review Spring 1988. Ophthalmic Paediatr Genet. 1988;9(3):167-9.
42. Imbasciati E, Paties C, Scarpioni L, Mihatsch MJ. Renal lesions in familial lecithin-cholesterol acyltransferase deficiency. Ultrastructural heterogeneity of glomerular changes. Am J Nephrol. 1986;6(1):66-70.
43. Schiffmann R, Fuller M, Clarke LA, Aerts JM. Is it Fabry disease? Genet Med. 2016;18(12):1181-5.
44. Branton MH, Schiffmann R, Sabnis SG, Murray GJ, Quirk JM, Altarescu G, et al. Natural history of Fabry renal disease: influence of alpha-galactosidase A activity and genetic mutations on clinical course. Medicine (Baltimore). 2002;81(2):122-38.
45. Alroy J, Sabnis S, Kopp JB. Renal pathology in Fabry disease. J Am Soc Nephrol. 2002;13(Suppl 2):S134-8.
46. Echevarria L, Benistan K, Toussaint A, Dubourg O, Hagege AA, Eladari D, et al. X-chromosome inactivation in female patients with Fabry disease. Clin Genet. 2016;89(1):44-54.
47. Mauer M, Glynn E, Svarstad E, Tøndel C, Gubler MC, West M, et al. Mosaicism of podocyte involvement is related to podocyte injury in females with Fabry disease. PLoS One. 2014;9(11):e112188.
48. Deegan PB, Baehner AF, Barba Romero MA, Hughes DA, Kampmann C, Beck M; European FOS Investigators. The natural history of Fabry disease in females in the Fabry Outcome Survey. J Med Genet. 2006;43(4):347-52.
49. Saito S, Ohno K, Sakuraba H. Fabry-database.org: database of the clinical phenotypes, genotypes, and mutant α-galactosidase A structures in Fabry disease. J Hum Genet. 2011;56(6):467-8.
50. Reasor MJ, Hastings KL, Ulrich RG. Drug-induced phospholipidosis: issues and future directions. Expert Opin Drug Saf. 2006;5(4):567-83.
51. Houghton DC, Campbell-Boswell MV, Bennett WM, Porter GA, Brooks RE. Myeloid bodies in the renal tubules of humans: relationship to gentamicin therapy. Clin Nephrol. 1978;10(4):140-5.
52. Banks DE, Milutinovic J, Desnick RJ, Grabowski GA, Lapp NL, Boehlecke BA. Silicon nephropathy mimicking Fabry's disease. Am J Nephrol. 1983;3(5):279-84.

53. Mignani R, Feriozzi S, Pisani A, Cioni A, Comotti C, Cossu M, et al. Agalsidase therapy in patients with Fabry disease on renal replacement therapy: a nationwide study in Italy. Nephrol Dial Transplant. 2008;23(5):1628-35.
54. Andrade J, Waters PJ, Singh RS, Levin A, Toh BC, Vallance HD, et al. Screening for Fabry disease in patients with chronic kidney disease: limitations of plasma alpha-galactosidase assay as a screening test. Clin J Am Soc Nephrol. 2008;3(1):139-45.
55. Bennett RL, Hart KA, O'Rourke E, Barranger JA, Johnson J, MacDermot KD, et al. Fabry disease in genetic counseling practice: recommendations of the National Society of Genetic Counselors. J Genet Couns. 2002;11(2):121-46.
56. Schiffmann R, Hughes DA, Linthorst GE, Ortiz A, Svarstad E, Warnock DG, et al.; Conference Participants. Screening, diagnosis, and management of patients with Fabry disease: conclusions from a "Kidney Disease: Improving Global Outcomes" (KDIGO) Controversies Conference. Kidney Int. 2017;91(2):284-93.
57. Desnick RJ, Brady R, Barranger J, Collins AJ, Germain DP, Goldman M, et al. Fabry disease, an under-recognized multisystemic disorder: expert recommendations for diagnosis, management, and enzyme replacement therapy. Ann Intern Med. 2003;138(4):338-46.
58. Schiffmann R, Murray GJ, Treco D, Daniel P, Sellos-Moura M, Myers M, et al. Infusion of alpha-galactosidase A reduces tissue globotriaosylceramide storage in patients with Fabry disease. Proc Natl Acad Sci USA. 2000;97(1):365-70.
59. Schiffmann R, Kopp JB, Austin HA 3rd, Sabnis S, Moore DF, Weibel T, et al. Enzyme replacement therapy in Fabry disease: a randomized controlled trial. JAMA. 2001;285(21):2743-9.
60. Eng CM, Guffon N, Wilcox WR, Germain DP, Lee P, Waldek S, et al.; International Collaborative Fabry Disease Study Group. Safety and efficacy of recombinant human alpha-galactosidase A replacement therapy in Fabry's disease. N Engl J Med. 2001;345(1):9-16.
61. Germain DP, Fan JQ. Pharmacological chaperone therapy by active-site-specific chaperones in Fabry disease: in vitro and preclinical studies. Int J Clin Pharmacol Ther. 2009;47(Suppl 1):S111-7.
62. Germain DP, Hughes DA, Nicholls K, Bichet DG, Giugliani R, Wilcox WR, et al. Treatment of Fabry's disease with the pharmacologic chaperone migalastat. N Engl J Med. 2016; 375(6):545-55.

SECTION

8

Tubular Disorders

CHAPTER

8.1

Renal Tubular Acidosis

Uma S Ali, Gurdeep Dhooria

INTRODUCTION

Renal tubular acidosis (RTA) is a heterogenous group of tubular disorders characterized by hyperchloremic normal anion gap metabolic acidosis, in the absence of any significant decline in the glomerular filtration rate (GFR). Children with RTA often present with one or more of the following symptoms such as short stature, failure to thrive, bony deformities in association with polyuria, and polydipsia.[1,2]

PHYSIOLOGY OF ACID–BASE HOMEOSTASIS

Acid Burden in the Body

Acids are end products of metabolism. The amount of H^+ ions produced daily from the metabolism of foods is approximately 1 mEq/kg/day in adults and 3 mEq/kg per day in children. The additional load of H^+ ions in children comes from the growing bones. The process of forming hydroxyapatite crystals during bone growth in children liberates protons that enter the bloodstream. The H^+ ion concentration in biological fluids is extremely small—about 0.00004 mmol/L. Accumulation of even minute amounts of H^+ ions can have serious adverse effects on various cellular enzymes and functions. Hence, the body has several tightly regulated mechanisms involving different organs and systems to prevent free H^+ ions from increasing. The three main mechanisms are (1) chemical buffering, (2) compensation by lungs, and (3) correction by the kidneys.[3-6]

Chemical Buffering

The most abundant buffer found in both the extracellular and the intracellular compartments is bicarbonate, which combines with H^+ ions to form carbonic acid ($H_2CO_3^-$) that dehydrates into H_2O and CO_2. Phosphates and proteins are the main buffers within cells and hemoglobin in red blood cells. The buffer reaction is immediate, takes only a few seconds, and is aimed at restoring pH to normal.[7]

Compensation

The lung provides compensation within minutes. The complete oxidation of acids produces the volatile acid CO_2, which is excreted by the lungs. In adults, 20,000 mmol of CO_2 are excreted daily.

Correction

Correction is a slower process that takes place in the kidneys over several hours or days. Incomplete oxidation of acids produces nonvolatile acids that need to be excreted by the kidneys. The kidney restores the acid-base balance of the body by four main mechanisms:

1. It reabsorbs the filtered bicarbonate to restore bicarbonate levels to normal.
2. It regenerates new bicarbonate to replace the bicarbonate lost in buffering.
3. It secretes H^+ ions that are produced daily in the body from the metabolism of foods.
4. It generates, recycles, and traps ammonia, which is the most important urinary buffer.

Since the burden of work is large, almost every segment of the renal tubule participates in the process to achieve the fine balance that the body needs.

Bicarbonate reabsorption ***(Fig. 1)****:* The glomerulus, with adjusted glomerular filtration rate (aGFR) of 120 mL/min, filters 4,140 mmol of bicarbonate daily of which 99% is reabsorbed by the renal tubules and only 1% is excreted in the urine. 80% of the HCO_3^- reabsorption occurs in the proximal convoluted tubule (PCT), 10–15% in the thick ascending limb of loop of Henle (TAL), and the remaining in the distal tubules (DT).[8]

The enormous energy needed for this process is provided by the Na^+–K^+-ATPase pumps present abundantly on the basolateral membrane of the PCT. The Na^+–K^+-ATPase pumps three Na^+ ions out of the cell into the peritubular capillaries and imports two K^+ ions into the cells creating a net intracellular negative charge that provides a favorable gradient for entry of sodium from the tubular lumen into the cell. Using this favorable gradient, the sodium-hydrogen exchanger or antiporter (NHE3) present on the apical membrane of the PCT secretes one H^+ ion into the tubule in exchange for one Na^+ ion that enters the cell.

In the lumen, the filtered bicarbonate combines with the secreted H^+ ion to form carbonic acid ($H_2CO_3^-$), which

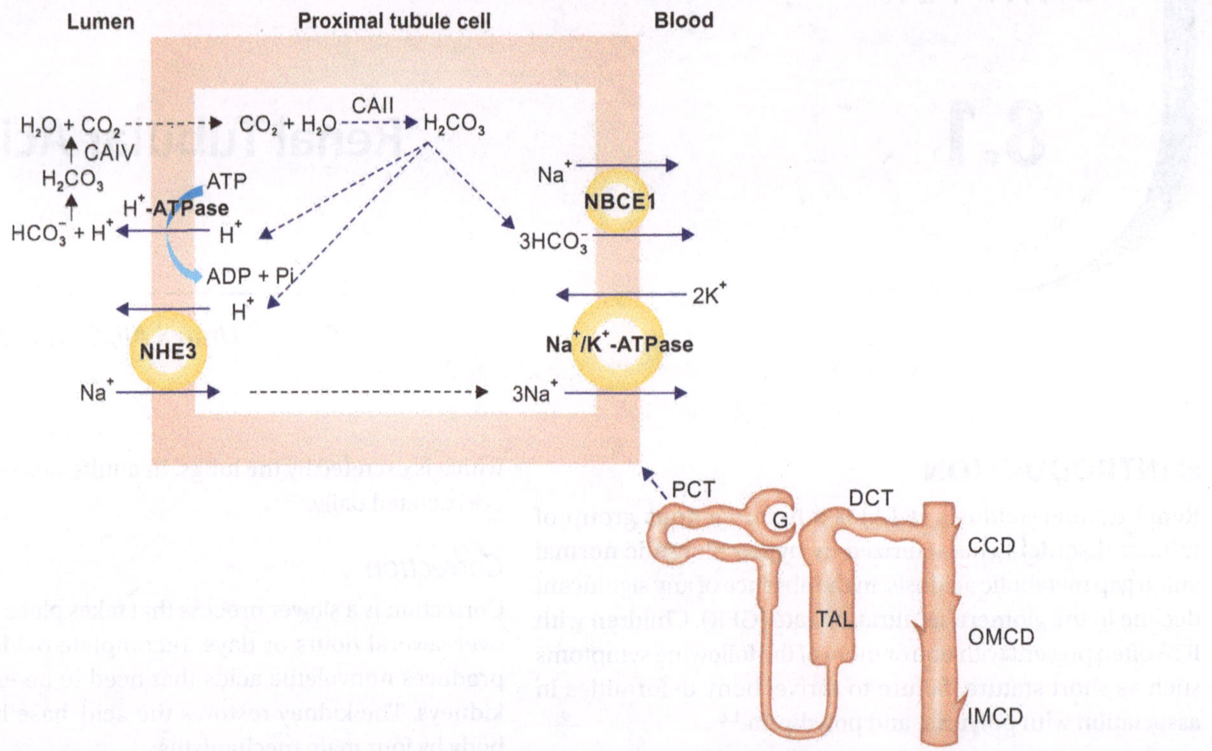

Fig. 1: Bicarbonate reabsorption. (CAIV: catalyzed by carbonic anhydrase IV; CCD: cortical collecting duct; DCT: distal convoluted tubule; IMCD: inner medullary collecting duct; NBCE1: Na+ through the electrogenic sodium bicarbonate symporter ; NHE3: sodium-hydrogen exchanger or antiporter; PCT: proximal convoluted tubule; OMCD: outer medullary collecting duct; TAL: thick ascending limb of loop of Henle)

dehydrates into H_2O and CO_2. This reaction is catalyzed by carbonic anhydrase IV (CAIV) present on the brush border of the apical membrane of the PCT. The presence of CAIV greatly enhances the rate of this reaction, which is needed to reabsorb such large quantities of HCO_3^-. The H_2O enters the PCT through the aquaporin channels *AQP1* present on the apical membrane. The CO_2 was formerly believed to diffuse freely across the apical membrane. It is now known that CO_2 enters the cell through the *AQP1* channels.

Within the cell, the CO_2 is rehydrated to form $H_2CO_3^-$, which dissociates into H^+ and HCO_3^-. This reaction is catalyzed by CAII present within the PCT. Three molecules of HCO_3^- exit the cell along with one of Na^+ through the electrogenic sodium bicarbonate symporter (NBCe1) present on the basolateral membrane. Bicarbonate is never directly reabsorbed by the renal tubule. It is reabsorbed as H_2O and CO_2 through aquaporin channels secondary to H^+ ion secretion. In the PCT, no net secretion of H^+ ions occurs as the H^+ ion secreted is utilized fully to reabsorb bicarbonate.[9]

Regeneration of bicarbonate (Fig. 2): Regeneration of bicarbonate occurs through two processes:

1. Ammoniagenesis
2. Excretion of titratable acid (TA)

New bicarbonate needs to be produced to replace the bicarbonate lost in buffering H^+ ions. The proximal tubule achieves this by ammoniagenesis. Ammonia is formed from the amino acid glutamine within the PCT. Glutamine is largely produced in muscles and is extracted from the blood in the peritubular capillaries by the PCT. Filtered glutamine also enters the PCT through the Na^+-linked amino acid symporter on the apical membrane. Glutamine is converted to α-ketoglutarate in the PCT by the enzyme glutaminase in the mitochondria. The metabolism of one molecule of α-ketoglutarate produces two molecules of NH_4^+ and two of HCO_3^-. Bicarbonate leaves the cell through the NBCe1 transporter on the basolateral membrane and enters the bloodstream while NH_4^+ is secreted into the lumen using the H^+ ion transporter NHE-3 on the apical membrane. Thus, the PCT kills two birds with one stone. It generates ammonia, the most important urinary buffer, and while doing so generates new bicarbonate for the body.[10]

The second mechanism of bicarbonate regeneration is the excretion of titratable acid.

The amount of secreted H^+ ions that is buffered by filtered weak acids is called titratable acidity. The main weak acid in the glomerular filtrate is the mono-protonated phosphate (HPO_4^{2-}). As the pH of the filtrate gets lowered by secretion of H^+ ions in the PCT, 50% of phosphates become diprotonated ($H_2PO_4^-$). For each H^+ ion consumed in this process, one Na^+ enters the cell through the apical membrane and is reabsorbed into the blood along with one mmol of HCO_3^- formed in the cell, thus generating one new molecule of HCO_3^-. The proximal tubule (PT) contributes 60% and the collecting duct (CD) 40% to this process.

The net acid excreted (NAE) equals the new bicarbonate regenerated.

$$NAE = Urinary\ NH_4^+\ (titratable\ acid - HCO_3)$$

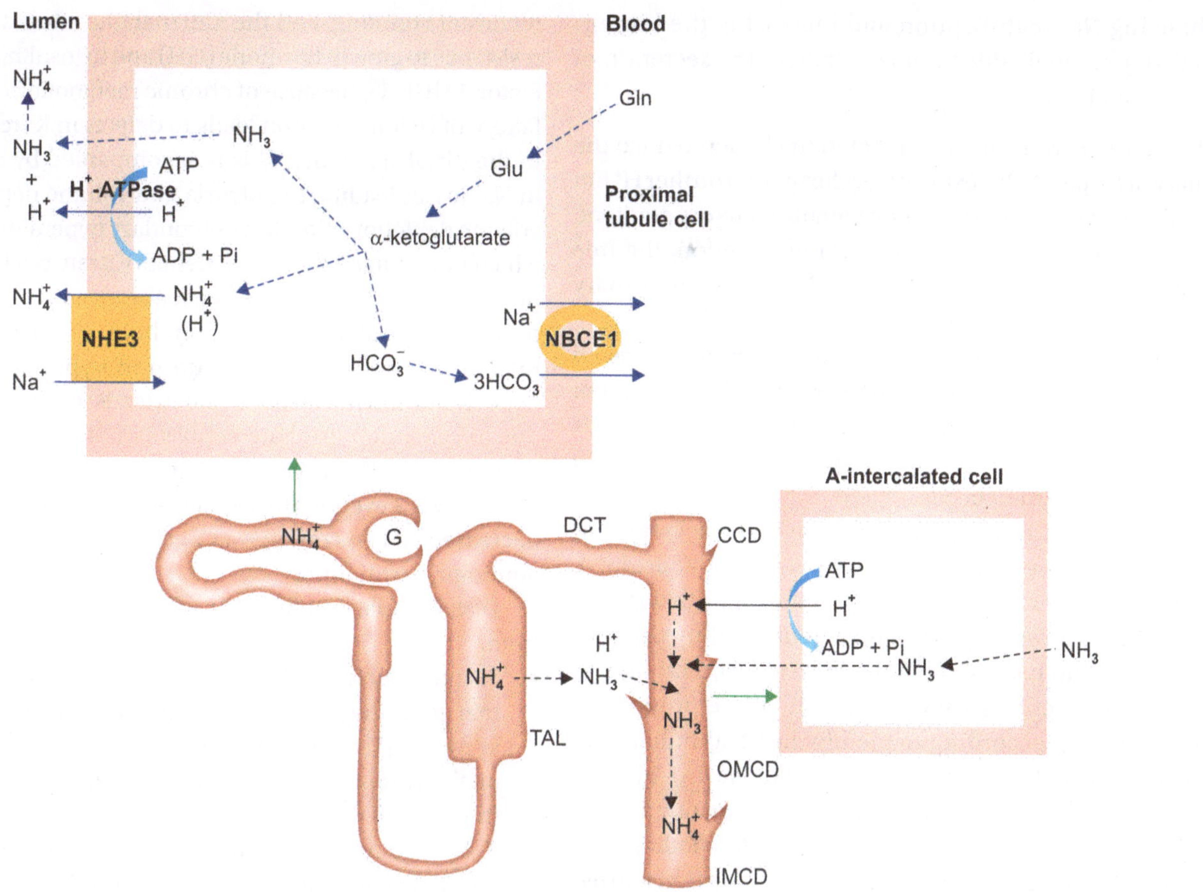

Fig. 2: Regeneration of bicarbonate. (CCD: cortical collecting duct; DCT: distal convoluted tubule; IMCD: inner medullary collecting duct; NBCE1: Na^+ through the electrogenic sodium bicarbonate symporter; NHE3: sodium-hydrogen exchanger or antiporter; OMCD: outer medullary collecting duct; TAL: thick ascending limb of loop of Henle)

H^+ ion secretion ***(Fig. 3)****:* The α intercalated cells (AICs) are the primary cells involved in H^+ ion secretion via the transporter known as the vacuolar H^+-ATPase on the luminal membrane. These cells are present in the distal segments of the nephron—in the late distal tubule, the connecting segment, the cortical collecting duct (CCD), the outer medullary collecting duct (OMCD), and the inner medullary collecting duct (IMCD). In the collecting duct, there are also a K^+–H^+-ATPase antiporter on the luminal surface and a Cl^-–HCO_3^- anion exchanger-1 (AE1) on the basolateral membrane.[11]

The luminal process of dehydrating the formed $H_2CO_3^-$ to H_2O and CO_2 and the intracellular process of rehydrating them back to $H_2CO_3^-$ to liberate H^+ ions and HCO_3^- ions are like the processes in the PCT. However, the CD does not have abundant luminal CAIV; hence, this process is slower in keeping with the lower rates of HCO_3^- reabsorption needed in this segment.

The principal cells (PCs) found in this region adjacent to the AIC are the major facilitators for the H^+ ion secretion. The PCs have an epithelial sodium channel (ENaC) on their luminal surface that reabsorbs Na^+ without any accompanying anion, creating an electronegative gradient in the lumen that favors secretion of positively charged ions such as the H^+ ions and K^+ ions. Aldosterone greatly enhances sodium reabsorption by increasing the number and activity of the ENaC channels on the luminal surface of the PC as well as the Na^+–K^+-ATPase pumps on the basolateral surface. By

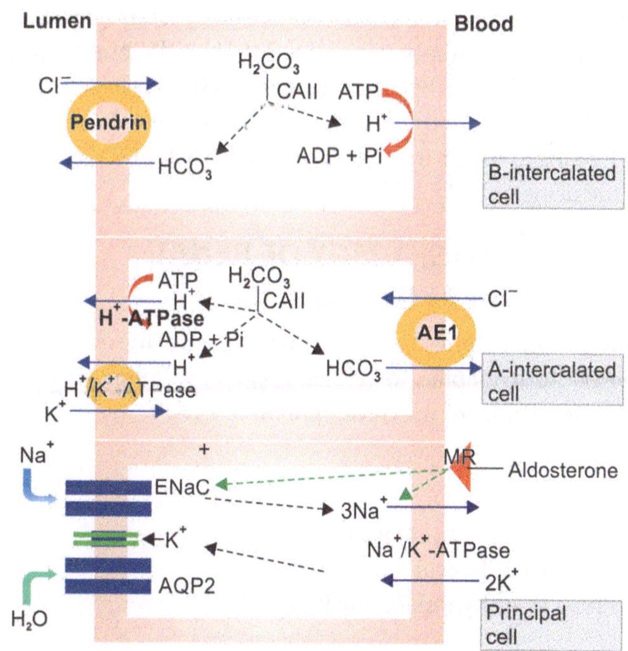

Fig. 3: H^+ ion secretion. (ENaC: epithelial sodium channel; NBCE1: Na^+ through the electrogenic sodium bicarbonate symporter; NHE3: sodium-hydrogen exchanger or antiporter)

enhancing Na^+ reabsorption and increasing the lumen-negative potential, aldosterone enhances the secretion of both H^+ and K^+ ions.[3]

Role of ammonia: H^+ ions secreted in the lumen reduce the urinary pH rapidly. Once the pH reaches 4.5, no further H^+ ion secretion can occur due to an unfavorable secretory gradient. Hence, to maintain the ongoing H^+ ion secretion, the free urinary H^+ ions need to be buffered. The two main urinary buffers are phosphates and ammonia.

One molecule of monohydrogen diphosphate is protonated to one molecule of dihydrogen phosphate with the addition of one H^+ ion. The conversion to dihydrogen phosphate is complete by the time urine pH reaches 5.8. Further buffering by phosphates cannot occur.

The main urinary buffer is ammonia, the secretion of which can increase 10-fold in response to metabolic acidosis. The kidney plays an important role in ammonia generation, recycling, and trapping. Ammonia generated by the PCT from glutamine passes down the lumen of the tubules as NH_3/NH_4, collectively called ammonium, the proportion of each varying according to the biochemical milieu and urine pH. Most of NH_4 is reabsorbed out of the TAL into the medullary interstitium where it exists predominantly as NH_3. Ammonia is recycled as it diffuses into the descending loop of Henle down a concentration gradient and is transported back to TAL from where it is reabsorbed into the medullary interstitium. Ammonia diffuses into the collecting duct due to a favorable gradient as IMCD has low free NH_3. This transport is facilitated by ammonia transporters present on the basolateral membrane of the IMCD. In the lumen of the inner medulla, NH_3 binds to the secreted H^+ ions to form NH_4^+. The IMCD membrane is impermeable to NH_4^+. The trapped NH_4^+ binds to the Cl^- in the lumen of the IMCD and is excreted in the urine as NH_4Cl.[12-14]

PATHOPHYSIOLOGY OF RENAL TUBULAR ACIDOSIS

Inherited or acquired defects in one or more of these pathways give rise to an inability to maintain acid–base homeostasis and are responsible for the development of RTA.

The four varieties of RTA are:

1. Type I or distal RTA
2. Type II or proximal RTA
3. Type III or hybrid RTA
4. Type IV or hyperkalemic RTA

Distal Renal Tubular Acidosis

Distal RTA is called type I as it was the first RTA to be described. Failure of H^+ ion secretion in the distal segments of the nephron leads to metabolic acidosis. The increase in H^+ ions in the body leaches bone buffers resulting in osteopenia and hypercalciuria. Growth failure results from poor appetite, recurrent vomiting, and the antianabolic effect arising from resistance to growth hormone (GH) and to insulin-like growth factor-1 (IGF-1), because of chronic metabolic acidosis. The failure of H^+ ion secretion leads to defects in K^+ reabsorption in the distal segments. This is accompanied by an increase in Na^+ losses leading to polyuria and volume depletion. The volume depletion stimulates secondary hyperaldosteronism, which may worsen the hypokalemia. Citrate is a bicarbonate precursor, and increased citrate reabsorption in the proximal tubule is stimulated by the metabolic acidosis leading to hypocitraturia. The combination of hypercalciuria with hypocitraturia in an alkaline milieu leads to nephrocalcinosis due to calcium phosphate deposits in the IMCD and in the Bellini ducts. The tubules are unable to lower the urinary pH below 5.3 even in the face of systemic acidosis and have decreased NH_4^+ secretion due to abnormal urine/renal vein ammonia partitioning.

Distal tubular acidification defects could therefore arise from:

- Secretory defects of H^+ ions because of genetic mutations that affect the functioning of the vacuolar H^+-ATPase that secretes H^+ ions or due to defects of the AE-1 exchanger on the basolateral membrane that transports HCO_3^- out of the cell into the blood.
- A voltage defect due to failure of generating lumen-negative potential due to defects in sodium reabsorption at the level of the ENaC in the principal cells. Voltage defects could secondarily impair K^+ secretion and led to hyperkalemic RTA.[15]
- A gradient defect due to backleak of H^+ ions as occurs with amphotericin toxicity[16-18]

Proximal Renal Tubular Acidosis

This is also called type II RTA. It manifests most commonly as Fanconi syndrome due to generalized defects affecting the transport of multiple solutes including H^+ ions and HCO_3^- ions along with glucose, phosphate, amino acids, and several other solutes. This generalized defect often occurs secondary to inherited metabolic disorders such as cystinosis, hereditary fructose intolerance, galactosemia, and tyrosinemia. It could also be due to a primary defect in some of the transporters of the PT resulting in failure of cellular energy needed for these transport processes **(Table 1)**.

Isolated proximal RTA is relatively rare. The tubular maximum for HCO_3^- reabsorption is low, leading to bicarbonate wasting that is accompanied by sodium. The increased amount of bicarbonate reaching the distal segments due to the proximal defect is beyond the reabsorptive capacity of these segments leading to bicarbonaturia and high urine pH. Sodium and potassium accompany these losses. However, when serum bicarbonate falls below the threshold, all filtered bicarbonate is reabsorbed and the distal nephrons can acidify the urine in the presence of an acid load, leading to a urine $pH < 5.3$.[19-22]

TABLE 1: Genetic causes of renal tubular acidosis (RTA).

Type of RTA	*Genetic defect*	*Affected transporter*	*Renal features*	*Extrarenal involvement*
Type I: Distal				
AR	*ATP6V1B1*	H-ATPase b1 subunit	Early onset NC	Sensorineural deafness
AR	*ATP6VOA41*	H-ATPase a4 subunit		Late onset deafness
AR	*SLC4A1*	AE-1 HCO_3/Cl exchanger		
AD	*SLC4A1*		Late onset	Spherocytosis and ovalocytosis
Type II: Proximal				
Isolated AR	*SLC4A4*	NBCe-1 Cl–HCO_3 exchanger		• Glaucoma and band keratopathy • Cataracts and mental retardation • Growth retardation • Basal ganglia calcifications, tooth enamel defects, and migraine
Fanconi syndrome				
Primary	*NaP1-II co-transporter*			
	EHHADH	Peroxisomal oxidation of fatty acids		
	HNF4A (R76W)	Nuclear receptor superfamily of ligand-dependent transcription factors	Nephrocalcinosis Renal impairment	• Hyperinsulinism • Macrosomia
Type III: Mixed	*CAII*	Carbonic anhydrase II		• Cerebral calcification • Osteopetrosis • Mental retardation • Deafness • Rod/cone dystrophy and optic N compression
Type IV: Hyperkalemic				
Pseudohypoaldosteronism				
Type I AD	*MLR*	Mineralocorticoid receptor	• Renal type • Neonatal presentation • Salt wasting, hyperkalemia • Metabolic acidosis	
Type I AR	*SNCC1B* *SCNN1G* *SNCC1A*	B ENaC Y ENaC Alpha ENaC	• Neonatal onset • Salt wasting	• Lung, colon, and skin • Increased incidence of respiratory tract infections • Increased sweat chloride
Type II AR	*WNK1* *WNK4*	WNK1 kinase WNK4 kinase	• Hyperkalemia • High BP	

(AD: autosomal dominant; AR: autosomal recessive; ENaC: epithelial sodium channel)

Type IV Renal Tubular Acidosis

This is associated with either aldosterone deficiency or resistance. The lack of aldosterone effect leads to a weak Na^+ reabsorption activity by the ENaC on the luminal surface of the principal cells. This results in a positive lumen voltage and hampers the secretion of both H^+ and K^+ ions that are dependent on the presence of a negative lumen potential. Hyperkalemia causes K^+ to move into the cells with reciprocal shift out of H^+ ions from the cells resulting intracellular alkalosis. This depresses ammoniagenesis, which limits the ability to excrete an acid load. However, in the presence of an acid load, the urine pH can be lowered to below 5.3.

This contrasts with hyperkalemic distal RTA that arises from a voltage defect wherein both the ability to lower pH below 5.3 in the face of an acid load and the secretion of ammonia are impaired.[23-27]

Incomplete Distal Renal Tubular Acidosis

The term incomplete distal RTA refers to an entity characterized by normal serum bicarbonate but with an inability to acidify the urine in response to an acid load. Patients have associated hypercalciuria, hypocitraturia, and may have nephrolithiasis. It should be considered in children who have calcium stones with urine pH > 5.5, in the absence of urinary tract infection.

ETIOLOGY OF RENAL TUBULAR ACIDOSIS

The different types of RTA can result from either genetic or acquired causes. Increasing number of genetic defects leading to RTA have been identified with a genotype–phenotype correlation in many **(Table 1)**. Some of these defects can have extrarenal involvement. Infections, autoimmune disorders, systemic diseases, drugs, toxins, and urological problems, notably obstructive uropathy, are some of the causes that can result in acquired RTA **(Table 2)**. The clinical features of the primary disease are often the presenting manifestations in acquired RTA.

CLINICAL FEATURES

Clinical features that suggest distal RTA include short stature, failure to thrive, polyuria, polydipsia, preference for salty foods, gastrointestinal upsets, and refractory rickets. Clinical features also include muscular weakness that may present as developmental delay. A proportion of cases with autosomal recessive distal RTA have sensorineural deafness, which may be present from birth or manifest in later childhood. Symptoms of stone disease can sometimes be seen. In children, distal RTA is usually observed as a primary entity.

In contrast, proximal RTA often occurs as part of Fanconi syndrome that is often secondary to metabolic diseases such as cystinosis, galactosemia, fructose intolerance, tyrosinemia, Wilson disease, or Lowe's syndrome. The symptoms and signs of the primary metabolic disease usually predominate. Children with Fanconi syndrome have severe failure to thrive, refractory rickets, and polyuria.

Nephropathic cystinosis, the chief cause of Fanconi syndrome, presents at 6–9 months of age with severe illness characterized by growth failure, rickets, and polyuria. Features secondary to multisystem organ dysfunction include photophobia and corneal erosions with cystine crystals on slit-lamp examination. Features of hypothyroidism, diabetes, myopathy, and hypogonadism may evolve with age. End-stage renal disease occurs by 10 years of age. Dent disease is X-linked and has a variable phenotype including rickets, nephrocalcinosis, lithiasis, night blindness, proteinuria, and slow progression to end-stage kidney disease. Lowe's syndrome is also X-linked and has cataract, glaucoma, and intellectual disability. Fanconi–Bickel syndrome has osteoporosis, rickets, nephrolithiasis, neonatal diabetes, and hepatomegaly, while tyrosinemia has severe rickets and often progresses to end-stage liver disease. Galactosemia has jaundice, liver disease, and cataracts and Wilson disease is characterized by neuropsychiatric features, liver failure, and cataracts.

Isolated proximal RTA is rare and presents with stunted growth. Nephrocalcinosis and urolithiasis are usually not seen. Genetic causes may be associated with ocular abnormalities and mental retardation **(Table 1)**.

Type IV RTA is associated with hypoaldosteronism or resistance to the action of aldosterone, either isolated or in the context of chronic kidney disease such as obstructive uropathy. Nephrocalcinosis and urolithiasis are absent and bone lesions are rare. Older children may develop type IV RTA due to advanced tubulointerstitial renal diseases or drugs leading to mineralocorticoid resistance.

LABORATORY DIAGNOSIS OF RENAL TUBULAR ACIDOSIS

Confirm the Presence of Metabolic Acidosis

The presence of metabolic acidosis is confirmed by the analysis of arterial blood gases with the finding of low serum bicarbonate and decreased pH. Venous blood gases are adequate provided the extremity from which the blood is collected is warm and no tourniquet is applied. The bicarbonate is generally <15 mmol/L in distal RTA and >15 in type II and type IV RTA.

TABLE 2: Common acquired causes of renal tubular acidosis (RTA) in children.

Disease category	*Distal RTA type I*	*Proximal RTA type II*	*RTA type IV*
Systemic diseases	• Systemic lupus erythematosus • Hereditary ovalocytosis • Ehlers–Danlos syndrome • Primary hyperoxaluria type 1	• Cystinosis • Wilson disease • Lowe syndrome • Tyrosinemia • Galactosemia	• Congenital adrenal hyperplasia • Addison's disease • Isolated hypoaldosteronism
Renal diseases	• Reflux nephropathy • Medullary sponge kidney • Renal transplant rejection	• Steroid-resistant nephrotic syndrome • Alport syndrome	• Obstructive uropathy • Chronic interstitial nephritis
Drugs and toxins	• Amphotericin B • Trimethoprim • Lithium • Analgesic abuse	• Gentamicin • Valproate • Tetracycline • Acetazolamide • Lead	• Angiotensin-converting enzyme inhibitors • Trimethoprim • K-sparing diuretics

Establish the Presence of Hyperchloremic Nonanion Gap Metabolic Acidosis

Plasma Anion Gap

The anion gap is a laboratory gap found between the most abundant cation and the most abundant anions measured. *Anion gap* = $(Na^+) - [(Cl^-) + (HCO_3^-)]$. The normal plasma anion gap is 8–16 mEq/L. This normal anion gap represents the anions not measured in the usual electrolyte panel and consists of the negatively charged proteins and phosphates in normal health. The accumulation of organic acids due to either defective excretion or abnormal metabolism leads to a wide anion gap acidosis.[28]

Normal anion gap acidosis has no abnormal acid accumulation. It results from failure of H^+ ion excretion and/or increased bicarbonate loss. Important causes of normal anion gap acidosis include RTA and diarrhea. While advanced renal failure shows acidosis with elevated anion gap, normal anion gap acidosis is common at a GFR of 30–50 mL/min, especially in patients with tubulointerstitial diseases.

Check Serum K

Hypokalemia is usually present in proximal RTA, whereas distal RTA may have either normokalemia or hypokalemia. Hyperkalemia indicates the presence of type IV RTA and rarely a distal RTA arising from voltage defect.

Assess the Renal Response to Metabolic Acidosis

The normal response of kidneys to metabolic acidosis involves the excretion of free H^+ ions that lower urine pH and increased production and urinary elimination of NH_4^+, which is the main urinary buffer and enables the excretion of buffered acids.

Urinary pH

Urine pH is measured at the bedside in a freshly passed sample of urine using a pH meter. In the presence of metabolic acidosis, urine pH should drop to <5.3 when no RTA exists. In children with distal RTA, the urine pH remains >5.3 despite metabolic acidosis. In proximal RTA, the urine pH is >5.3 when serum bicarbonate is above the critical threshold. However, when serum bicarbonate falls below the threshold, bicarbonaturia ceases and the urine pH can go <5.3. Urine pH should be estimated after the child is well hydrated and after ensuring that there is no urinary tract infection (UTI).

Urine pH may be elevated, if there is UTI due to urea-splitting organisms. In children with dehydration, there is avid reabsorption of sodium from the proximal tubules. The decreased amount of sodium reaching the distal tubules impairs H^+ ion secretion leading to a higher urinary pH. Urine sodium should be >25 mEq/L for a proper interpretation of urine pH.

It is worth noting that chronic metabolic acidosis gives rise to a marked increase of urinary NH_4^+ excretion. This buffers all the free H^+ ions preventing a fall in urine pH that reflects free H^+ concentrations.[29-31]

Ammonium Excretion in Urine

Since ammonium is not easily measured in routine laboratories, NH_4^+ excretion is estimated by surrogate markers such as urine anion gap or urine osmolar gap.

Urine Anion Gap

The urine anion gap (UAG) is a surrogate marker for ammonium production.

$$UAG = (Urine\ Na^+) + (Urine\ K^+) - (Urine\ Cl^-)$$

Under acidic conditions, patients without renal problems will excrete large amounts of ammonium chloride in urine. Since NH_4^+ is excreted as a chloride salt, urine Cl^- will be greater than the sum of urinary Na and K and the UAG will be negative. Positive values ($Na^+ + K^+ > Cl^-$) in the face of metabolic acidosis indicate inappropriately low NH_4^+ excretion. Patients with distal RTA will have positive UAG because of decreased ammonium chloride excretion.

Urinary Osmolar Gap

Urinary AG does not correlate with NH_4^+ when it is excreted with anions other than Cl^- as in ketoacidosis. In these cases, urinary NH_4^+ is estimated by calculating the urine osmolar gap.

This is calculated as measured urine osmolality – calculated osmolality. Calculated osmolality = ($2Na^+ + 2K^+$ + urea + glucose), with urea and glucose concentrations expressed in mmol/L (to convert from mg/dL to mmol/L, divide by 2.8 and 18, respectively). A value >100 mOsm/kg H_2O suggests high urinary NH_4^+.

Tests to Differentiate Proximal from Distal RTA

Fractional Excretion of Bicarbonate by Bicarbonate Loading Test

In proximal RTA, large amounts of HCO_3^- are excreted when plasma HCO_3^- is above the renal threshold with fractional excretion (FE) of 10–15%, whereas in patients with distal RTA, the FE is <5%. In type IV RTA, FE of HCO_3^- in the setting of normal plasma HCO_3^- is usually between 5 and 10%.

Fractional excretion of HCO_3^- is determined by using the following formula:

$$(Urine\ HCO_3 \times Plasma\ creatinine \times 100)/(Plasma\ HCO_3 \times Urine\ creatinine)$$

Serum bicarbonate levels are normalized to reach 20–22 mmol/L by the administration of sodium bicarbonate orally at 4 mEq/kg/day for 2–3 days or by intravenous infusion of 0.5 M sodium bicarbonate at 1 mEq/kg/h for a few hours to elevate serum bicarbonate to the desired level. Serum and urinary creatinine and bicarbonate are measured before administration of bicarbonate and again when the serum bicarbonate has reached 20 mmol/L or more. Urine should be collected directly in a clean container under mineral oil. Alternatively, freshly passed urine can be collected immediately into a syringe, capped, placed in ice, and transported immediately to the laboratory for analysis as is done for blood gases.[32-36]

Urine pCO_2–Blood pCO_2

This is a sensitive test of distal nephron H^+ secretion. A high urinary pH provides a favorable chemical gradient for H^+ secretion by the collecting duct. In the tubular lumen of the CD, H^+ ions combine with HCO_3^- to form H_2CO_3, which dehydrates slowly into CO_2 and water. The CO_2 diffusion out of the IMCD lumen is limited resulting in high pCO_2 in the renal medulla and final urine. The U-B pCO_2 (partial pressure of carbon dioxide) gradient should be greater than 20 mm Hg in normal individuals. In patients with primary type I distal RTA, the U-B pCO_2 value is around zero or may even be negative, whereas it is expected to be normal in type II RTA and type IV RTA.

This test can be conducted during the bicarbonate loading test by simultaneously monitoring urinary pH and estimating the blood and urine pCO_2 when the urine pH is equal to or more than 7.6.

Ammonium Chloride Loading Test

This test is done to assess the distal tubular acidification in response to acid loading. It is used to differentiate between distal RTA and proximal RTA when the urine pH is >5.3 and the serum bicarbonate is only slightly low. The test is also done in suspected cases of incomplete RTA.

Ammonium chloride is administered to induce acidosis and to assess the renal response to a greater degree of acidosis. Ammonium chloride 100 mg/kg is administered orally with a meal. Urine pH and UAG are measured at the beginning of the test and after 6 hours. At 6 hours following NH_4Cl ingestion, normal patients or those with proximal RTA will develop a negative UAG and urine pH <5.5. If the urine pH remains >5.5 and UAG remains positive at 6 hours, this result is diagnostic of distal RTA. Ammonium chloride has an unpleasant taste and can lead to nausea and vomiting.[36-39]

Furosemide–Fludrocortisone Test

The simultaneous administration of furosemide and fludrocortisone has been used as an alternative to ammonium chloride loading test for assessing distal tubular acidification. Furosemide blocks the Na^+-K^+-Cl^- transporter in the TAL, thus increasing the delivery of sodium chloride to the distal segments of the nephron. This stimulates sodium ion reabsorption by the cortical collecting duct and generates a favorable lumen-negative transtubular voltage that in turn stimulates secretion of H^+ and potassium to urine. The advantage of adding fludrocortisone to furosemide is that the mineralocorticoid action stimulates reabsorption of sodium by the principal cells of the collecting duct a few minutes after its administration, thus facilitating the secretion of H^+ and the decrease of urinary pH.

Fludrocortisone is given orally and furosemide (1 mg/kg) by the intravenous route. Urine samples are collected for a period of 4 hours. Patients with distal RTA fail to acidify their urine to pH <5.3 and do not significantly increase NH_4^+ excretion over the basal values.[40-42]

Additional Workup in RTA

- *Tests for hypercalciuria:* Hypercalciuria is suspected when the value of urinary calcium to creatinine ratio is above the age-related norm and diagnosed in the presence of 24-hour calcium excretion exceeding 4 mg/kg/day. Hypocitraturia is said to be present when the 24-hour urinary citrate is below 2 mg/kg/day. Both hypercalciuria and hypocitraturia are seen in distal RTA.
- Urinary glucose, amino acids, and phosphate excretion should be estimated in all cases of proximal RTA to differentiate isolated proximal RTA from Fanconi syndrome. Patients with inborn errors of metabolism being investigated for RTA should have all these solutes evaluated.
- Ultrasonography (USG) of the kidneys should be done to look for nephrocalcinosis, seen commonly in distal RTA but not in type II or type IV RTA. Evidence of obstructive uropathy may be seen in type IV RTA.
- *Hearing assessment:* All patients with idiopathic distal RTA should undergo a formal hearing evaluation, in view of the association of sensorineural deafness with recessively inherited disease; deafness may not be always be present in infancy and can develop later.
- Peripheral smear for ovalocytes and spherocytes and osmotic fragility in children with distal RTA.
- Genetic testing in RTA patients without an acquired cause to identify the underlying defect. Clinical exome testing with targeted analysis for mutations in genes is likely to enable diagnosis in majority of patients. It helps in prognostication and in antenatal counseling.

TREATMENT

The main goals in the treatment of all RTAs are to control the underlying disease leading to the RTA, if feasible, restore biochemical homeostasis, achieve healing of the bone disease, improve growth, prevent the progression of nephrocalcinosis, and prevent the development of chronic renal failure.

Management of Distal Renal Tubular Acidosis

The primary intervention is to provide adequate alkali to neutralize the daily H^+ ion production. The amount of alkali required ranges from 2–3 mEq/kg/day in older children to 5–8 mEq/kg/day in young infants. The alkali may be given as sodium bicarbonate or as sodium plus potassium citrate. Potassium citrate alone can also be used when the alkali requirement is not >4 mEq/kg/day, as its administration is limited by the amount of K^+ that can be given. Correction of acidosis stops the leaching of bones and gradually allows bone healing to occur over several months. Vitamin D supplementation is not needed unless there is documented deficiency. Deficiency should be corrected only after the correction of the acidosis.

Prevention of progression of nephrocalcinosis requires resolution of hypercalciuria and hypocitraturia with a close attention to urinary pH. A dose of 4 mEq/g/day of K^+ citrate may be sufficient to resolve the hypercalciuria and hypocitraturia and prevent calcium oxalate saturation. However, it does not prevent calcium phosphate saturation due to the alkaline milieu. If the urinary pH is >6.5, thiazides may be added to reduce the hypercalciuria.

Management of Proximal Renal Tubular Acidosis

The goal of treatment in Fanconi syndrome is to stop the causative agent when possible and to replenish the solutes that are wasted in the urine due to the lack of proximal tubular reabsorption.

A primary diagnosis is mandatory for the successful implementation of the treatment in Fanconi syndrome. Specific treatment of the underlying disease helps in achieving resolution or amelioration of the Fanconi syndrome. Therapy may involve medications such as cysteamine in cystinosis, penicillamine in Wilson's disease, or strict omission of the dietary substrates that fuel the metabolic defect as in galactosemia and hereditary fructose intolerance.

Correction of acidosis requires large amounts of bicarbonate to be administered due to the continuous bicarbonate leak that leads to wastage of the administered bicarbonate. High doses of alkali ranging from 5 to 15 mEq/kg/day may be needed. Thiazide diuretics enhance HCO_3^- reabsorption in the PCT and the loop of Henle by reducing extracellular volume and are used to minimize the requirements of HCO_3^-. Potassium supplementation is usually needed and may need to be continued during ongoing alkali therapy, as the ongoing bicarbonaturia causes mandatory sodium and potassium losses. Whereas the secondary hyperaldosteronism helps to maintain sodium balance, the K^+ losses get compounded.

Unlike distal RTA, the bone disease will not be corrected by alkali supplements alone. The correction of bone disease requires supplementation with phosphates and administration of calcitriol. Loss of glucose, uric acid, and amino acids is usually asymptomatic and does not need replacement.

Type IV Hyperkalemic Renal Tubular Acidosis

Treatment depends on the underlying cause. Potassium-retaining drugs should always be withdrawn. Hypoaldosteronism due to adrenal failure may respond adequately to replacement doses of fludrocortisone. Fludrocortisone therapy may also be useful in hyporeninemic hypoaldosteronism, preferably in combination with a loop diuretic such as furosemide to reduce the risk of extracellular fluid volume expansion. In some cases, alkali supplements at 1.5–2 mmol/kg/day are also required.

PROGNOSIS

Patients with RTA are at a risk for life-threatening electrolyte and acid-base abnormalities that could be triggered by minor illnesses. Bone disease, failure to thrive, and short stature are important complications of late diagnosis and inadequate treatment.

Early diagnosis of distal RTA in infancy along with adequate, continuous normalization of the acid-base and electrolyte disturbance helps to heal bones and restore growth. Children who are diagnosed after infancy may have an unsatisfactory final height despite adequate correction. About one third of patients with distal RTA followed beyond puberty show declining kidney function.[42-45]

Progression of nephrocalcinosis and the resultant interstitial inflammation and fibrosis are the main factors for the renal dysfunction.

The outcome of Fanconi syndrome is primarily dependent on the underlying cause. Where the underlying disorder is treatable and can be well controlled, the Fanconi syndrome could resolve or ameliorate with time. In many cases, achieving and maintaining optimal metabolic control in Fanconi syndrome is a challenge, as both the bicarbonate leak and the K^+ losses worsen with therapy necessitating large quantities of alkali and potassium supplements often leading to noncompliance. Adequate growth and stature are often not achieved. Decline in renal function may be seen in some.

Patients with cystinosis and Dent disease show progressive decline in kidney function by the first and third decades, respectively.[46,47]

Long-term outcomes may be also limited by extrarenal comorbidities such as hepatic dysfunction as in tyrosinemia, Wilson disease, galactosemia, hereditary fructose intolerance, or central nervous system disease as in Lowe syndrome and Wilson disease. Untreated patients with Fanconi-Bickel syndrome are at a risk of hepatocellular carcinoma.[48]

As type IV RTA is seen usually with underlying renal or endocrine disorders, the outcome is dependent on the nature of the underlying disease and its response to treatment.

TABLE 3: Differentiating features of the various types of renal tubular acidosis (RTA).

	Proximal RTA (type 2)	Distal RTA (type 1)		Hyperkalemic RTA (type 4)
		Classic	Hyperkalemic	
Serum bicarbonate	>15 mmol/L	<15 mmol/L	<15 mmol/L	>15 mmol/L
Serum K^+	Normal/reduced	Normal/reduced	Raised	Raised
Urine pH	<5.5	>5.5	>5.5	<5.5
Urine anion gap	Negative	Positive	Positive	Positive
NH_4^+ excretion	Normal	Reduced	Reduced	Reduced
Hypercalciuria (>4 mg/kg/day)	Normal	Raised	Raised	Normal or reduced
$FeHCO_3$	>10–15%	<5%	<5%	>5–10%
U-B pCO_2	>20 mm Hg	<20 mm Hg	<20 mm Hg	>20 mm Hg
Nephrocalcinosis	Absent	Often present	Often present	Absent

($FeHCO_3$: fractional excretion of bicarbonate; U-B pCO_2: urine pCO_2–blood pCO_2)

CONCLUSION

Renal tubular acidosis is essentially characterized by normal anion gap and hyperchloremic metabolic acidosis. Primarily, history of polyuria, polydipsia, and liking for salty food are important in all patients. Children with delay in diagnosis also have failure to thrive, short stature, refractory rickets, and bony deformities due to persistent acidosis. RTA can be a primary or secondary defect and results due to either abnormality in bicarbonate ion absorption or hydrogen ion secretion. Primary defects are common in children due to gene mutation or idiopathic nature while secondary forms are more common in adults.

According to their pathophysiological basis, four types of RTA are distinguished. Distal type I RTA, proximal type II RTA, mixed type III RTA, and type IV RTA can be differentiated based on the family history, the presenting manifestations, the biochemical profile, and the radiological findings (**Table 3**). Functional tests to explore the proximal wasting of bicarbonate and the urinary acidification capacity are also useful diagnostic tools. Correction of acidosis with alkaline therapy is indicated in either form of tubular acidosis. Proximal type may require correction of bicarbonate up to 4–6 mEq/kg, while distal type needs less correction doses.

The aims of treatment for RTA are not only to correct as much as possible the biochemical abnormalities but also to fundamentally improve growth in children and to prevent the progression of nephrocalcinosis and the development of chronic renal failure at all ages.

KEY POINTS

- RTA is characterized by normal anion gap hyperchloremic metabolic acidosis.
- RTA arises from the failure of the kidney to reabsorb filtered HCO_3 (proximal RTA), from the inability to excrete sufficient H^+ to balance net endogenous acid production (distal RTA), or from disruption of the renin–angiotensin–aldosterone axis (hyperkalemic RTA).
- The four primary types of RTA can be distinguished on the basis of their clinical manifestations, the presenting biochemical profile, and, if needed, the response to functional tests. Adjunct tests such as the fractional excretion of HCO_3 and UAG clarify the etiology.
- Genetic studies should be performed to identify the involved pathogenic gene but are not strictly necessary for the diagnosis of RTA.

REFERENCES

1. Pereira PC, Miranda DM, Oliveira EA, Silva AC. Molecular pathophysiology of renal tubular acidosis. Curr Genomics. 2009;10(1):51-9.
2. Herrin JT. Renal tubular acidosis. In: Avner ED, Harmon WE, Niaudet P (Eds). Pediatric Nephrology. Philadelphia: Williams & Wilkins; 2003. pp. 757-76.
3. Hamm LL, Nakhoul N, Hering-Smith KS. Acid-base homeostasis. Clin J Am Soc Nephrol: CJASN. 2015;10(12):2232-42.
4. Gregory MJ, Schwartz GJ. Diagnosis and treatment of renal tubular disorders. Semin. Nephrol. 1998;18(3):317-29.
5. Ahn Jin K; Comprehensive Pediatric Hospital Medicine. (2007). Acidosis. [online] Available from https://www.sciencedirect.com/topics/pharmacology-toxicology-and-pharmaceutical-science/acidosis. [Last accessed September, 2021].
6. Soriano J. Renal tubular acidosis: the clinical entity. J Am Soc Nephrol. 2002;13(8):2160-70.
7. Biga LM, Dawson S, Harwell A, Hopkins R, Kaufmann J, LeMaster M, et al. 26.4 Acid-Base Balance. Anatomy & physiology. Oregon State University. [online] Available from https://open.oregonstate.education/aandp/chapter/26-4-acid-base-balance/. [Last accessed September, 2021].
8. Rodriguez Soriano J. New insights into the pathogenesis of renal tubular acidosis—from functional to molecular studies. Pediatr Nephrol. 2000;14(12):1121-36.
9. Soleimani M, Rastegar A. (2016). Core curriculum in nephrology pathophysiology of renal tubular acidosis: Core curriculum 2016. [online] Available from http://dx.doi.org/10.1053/j.ajkd.2016.03.422. [Last accessed September, 2021].
10. DuBose TD, Good DW, Hamm LL, Wall SM. Ammonium transport in the kidney: New physiological concepts and their clinical implications. J Am Soc Nephrol. 1991;1(11):1193-203.

11. Batlle DC, Sehy JT, Roseman MK, Arruda JA, Kurtzman NA. Clinical and pathophysiological spectrum of acquired distal renal tubular acidosis. Kidney Int. 1981;20(3):389-96.
12. Hamm LL, Simon EE. Roles and mechanisms of urinary buffer excretion. Am J Physiol. 1987;253(4 Pt 2):F595-F605.
13. Weiner ID, Verlander JW. Role of NH3 and NH4+ transporters in renal acid-base transport. Am J Physiol Renal Physiol. 2011;300(1):F11-F23.
14. Weiner ID, Hamm LL. Molecular mechanisms of renal ammonia transport. Annu Rev Physiol. 2007;69:317-40.
15. Batlle DC. Segmental characterization of defects in collecting tubule acidification. Kidney Int. 1986;30(4):546-54.
16. Caruana RJ, Barish CF, Buckalew VM Jr. Complete distal renal tubular acidosis in systemic lupus: Clinical and laboratory findings. Am J Kidney Dis. 1985;6(1):59-63.
17. Bonilla-Felix M. Primary distal renal tubular acidosis as a result of a gradient defect. Am J Kidney Dis. 1996;27(3):428-30.
18. DeFranco PE, Haragsim L, Schmitz PG, Bastani B. Absence of vacuolar H-ATPase pump in the collecting duct of a patient with hypokalemic distal renal tubular acidosis and Sjogren syndrome. J Am Soc Nephrol. 1995;6(2):295-301.
19. Brenes LG, Brenes JM, Hernandez MM. Familial proximal renal tubular acidosis. A distinct disease entity. Am J Med. 1997;63(2):244-52.
20. Rodrıguez Soriano J, Boichis H, Stark H, Edelmann CM Jr. Proximal renal tubular acidosis. A defect in bicarbonate reabsorption with normal urinary acidification. Pediatr Res. 1967;1:81-98.
21. Nash MA, Torrado AD, Greifer I, Spitzer A, Edelmann CM Jr. Renal tubular acidosis in infants and children. J Pediatr. 1972;80:738-48.
22. Igarashi T, Ishii T, Watanabe K, Hayakawa H, Horio K, Sone Y, et al. Persistent isolated proximal renal tubular acidosis—a systemic disease with a distinct clinical entity. Pediatr Nephrol. 1994;8(1):70-1.
23. DuBose TD Jr. Hyperkalemic hyperchloremic metabolic acidosis: Pathophysiologic insights. Kidney Int. 1997;51(2):591-60.
24. Geller DS, Rodrıguez-Soriano J, Vallo A, Schiffer S, Bayer M, Chang SS, et al. Mutations in the mineralocorticoid receptor gene cause autosomal dominant pseudohypoaldosteronism type I. Nature Genet. 1998;19(3):279-81.
25. Chang SS, Grunder S, Hanukoglu A, Rosler A, Mathew PM, Hanukoglu I, et al. Mutations of the epithelial sodium channel cause salt wasting with hyperkalaemic acidosis, pseudo-hypoaldosteronism type 1. Nat Genet. 1996;12(3):248-53.
26. Appiani AC, Marra G, Tirelli SA, Goj V, Romeo L, Cavanna G, et al. Early childhood hyperkalemia: Variety of pseudohypoaldo-steronism. Acta Paediatr Scand. 1986;75(6):970-4.
27. Wilson FH, Disse-Nicomede S, Choate KA, Ishikawa K, Nelson Williams C, Desitter I. Human hypertension caused by mutations in WNK kinases. Science. 2001;293(5532):1107-12.
28. Rodríguez-Soriano J, Vallo A. Renal tubular acidosis. Pediatr Nephrol. 1990;4(3):268-75.
29. Elkinton JR, Huth EJ, Webster GD Jr, McCance RA. The renal excretion of hydrogen ion in renal tubular acidosis. I. Quantitative assessment of the response to ammonium chloride as an acid load. Am J Med. 1960;29:554-75.
30. Batlle DC, Hizon M, Cohen E, Gutterman C, Grupta R. The use of the urinary anion gap in the diagnosis of hyperchloremic metabolic acidosis. N Engl J Med. 1988;318(10):594-9.
31. Oh MS, Carroll HJ. Value and determinants of urine anion gap. Nephron. 2002;90(3):252-5.
32. McSherry E, Sebastian A, Morris RC Jr. Renal tubular acidosis in infants: the several kinds, including bicarbonate-wasting classic renal tubular acidosis. J Clin Invest. 1972;51(3):499-514.
33. Rodriguez-Soriano J, Vallo A, Garcia-Fuentes M. Distal renal tubular acidosis in infancy: a bicarbonate wasting state. J Pediatr. 1975;86(4):524-32.
34. Ohlsson A, Cumming WA, Paul A, Sly WS. Carbonic anhydrase II deficiency syndrome: recessive osteopetrosis with renal tubular acidosis and cerebral calcification. Pediatrics. 1986;77(3):371-81.
35. Ismail EAR, Saad SA, Sabry MA. Nephrocalcinosis and urolithiasis in carbonic anhydrase II deficiency syndrome. Eur J Pediatr. 1997;156(12):957-62.
36. Edelmann CM Jr, Boichis H, Rodriguez-Soriano J, Stark H. The renal response of children to acute ammonium chloride acidosis. Pediatr Res. 1967;1:452-60.
37. Walsh SB, Shirley DG, Wrong OM, Unwin RJ. Urinary acidification assessed by simultaneous furosemide and fludrocortisone treatment: an alternative to ammonium chloride. Kidney Int. 2007;71(12):1310-6.
38. Edelmann CM Jr, Rodriguez-Soriano J, Boichis H, Gruskin AB, Acosta MI. Renal bicarbonate reabsorption and hydrogen ion excretion in normal infants. J Clin Invest. 1967;46(8):1309-17.
39. Brenes LG, Sanchez MI. Impaired urinary ammonium excretion in patients with isolated proximal renal tubular acidosis. J Am Soc Nephrol. 1993;4(4):1073-8.
40. Dhayat NA, Gradwell MW, Pathare G, Anderegg M, Schneider L, Luethi D, et al. Furosemide/Fludrocortisone Test and Clinical Parameters to Diagnose Incomplete Distal Renal Tubular Acidosis in Kidney Stone Formers. Clin J Am Soc Nephrol. 2017;12(9):1507-17.
41. Shavit L, Chen L, Ahmed F, Ferraro PM, Moochhala S, Walsh SB, et al. Selective screening for distal renal tubular acidosis in recurrent kidney stone formers: initial experience and comparison of the simultaneous furosemide and fludrocortisone test with the short ammonium chloride test. Nephrol Dial Transplant. 2016;31(11):1870-6.
42. Bagga A, Sinha A. Renal Tubular Acidosis. Indian J Pediatr. 2020;87:733-44.
43. Besouw MTP, Bienias M, Walsh P, Kleta R, Van't Hoff WG, Ashton E, et al. Clinical and molecular aspects of distal renal tubular acidosis in children. Pediatr Nephrol. 2017;32(6):987-96.
44. Watanabe T. Improving outcomes for patients with distal renal tubular acidosis: recent advances and challenges ahead. Pediatric Health Med Ther. 2018;9:181-90.
45. Palazzo V, Provenzano A, Becherucci F, Sansavini G, Mazzinghi B, Orlandini V, et al. The genetic and clinical spectrum of a large cohort of patients with distal renal tubular acidosis. Kidney Int. 2017;91(5):1243-55.
46. Cherqui S, Courtoy PJ. The renal Fanconi syndrome in cystinosis: pathogenic insights and therapeutic perspectives. Nat Rev Nephrol. 2017;13(2):115-31.
47. Ehlayel AM, Copelovitch L. Update on dent disease. Pediatr Clin N Am. 2019;66(1):169-78.
48. Foreman JW. Fanconi Syndrome. Pediatr Clin North Am. 2019;66(1):159-67.

CHAPTER

8.2 Fanconi Syndrome and Cystinosis

Menka Yadav, Abhijeet Saha

FANCONI SYNDROME (FANCONI RENOTUBULAR SYNDROME, LIGNAC–DE TONI–DEBRÉ–FANCONI SYNDROME)

Introduction

Fanconi syndrome (FS) refers to the set of clinical features resulting from a generalized loss or disturbance of the normal transport processes in the renal proximal tubule (PT) of the nephron.[1,2] FS was initially described in the 1930s by the Swiss pediatrician Guido Fanconi. The characteristic features of FS include glycosuria, aminoaciduria, and phosphaturia (hypophosphatemia).

Proximal tubule reabsorbs most of the physiologically filtered load of proteins, including albumin, low-molecular-weight (LMW) proteins, amino acids, glucose, bicarbonate, sodium, chloride, phosphate, and uric acid.[2-4] The PT cells reabsorb, reclaim, and/or degrade the filtered proteins through the extensive luminal receptors and endocytic receptors, such as megalin and cubilin.[5,6] These are also critical for recycling functionally important proteins to the plasma membrane. Alteration in endosomal acidification (e.g., Dent disease) and/or loss of electrochemical gradient for reabsorption (e.g., mitochondrial cytopathies) impair the process of reclaiming the filtered proteins.[7,8] This leads to the urinary wasting of albumin, LMW proteins, electrolytes, and solutes. The generalized proximal tubular dysfunction constitutes the hallmark of FS.

The exact prevalence of the FS remains unknown.[1,9] Cystinosis is the most common cause of FS in children.[10] This chapter will discuss the etiology, clinical presentation, and management of FS. A more detailed description of cystinosis, a treatable yet common cause of end-stage kidney disease (ESKD), is presented.

Etiology and Pathology

The etiology of generalized PT dysfunction and resultant FS can be broadly classified as congenital and acquired causes (**Table 1**).

Albumin and LMW proteins in the glomerular filtrate are endocytosed by PT cells via the megalin–cubilin receptor pathway (**Fig. 1**). Following endocytosis, the endosomes undergo progressive, adenosine triphosphate (ATP)-dependent acidification, which results in the dissociation of the receptor–ligand complexes. The megalin and cubilin are then recycled in the luminal membrane, whereas the ligand is directed to lysosomes for degradation. The defect in this pathway, e.g., endocytosis or acidification of endosomes, clinically manifests as FS.[2,5,6]

The reabsorption of filtered solutes (e.g., glucose, phosphate, amino acids, and bicarbonate) by PT is directly or indirectly coupled to Na^+ movement. Mitochondria provide the energy required by Na^+–K^+-ATPase and thus maintain the electrochemical gradient that allows Na-coupled solutes to enter the cell.[1,2] Therefore, proximal tubule energy production

TABLE 1: Causes of Fanconi syndrome.

Hereditary	*Acquired*
Isolated: • Autosomal dominant (EHHADH) • Autosomal recessive (NaPi2a) *Syndromic/systemic causes:* • Cystinosis • Tyrosinemia • Hereditary fructose intolerance • Galactosemia • Glycogen storage disorder (type 1) • Lowe syndrome • Dent disease • Mitochondriopathies • Fanconi–Bickel syndrome • Wilson disease	*Drug induced:* • Tenofovir, adefovir, lamivudine, stavudine, and didanosine (antiretrovirals) • Ifosfamide, oxaliplatin, cisplatin, and imatinib mesylate (chemotherapeutic agents) • Valproic acid (anticonvulsants) • Aminoglycosides, expired tetracyclines, and cidofovir (antimicrobials) *Others:* • Lead, cadmium, mercury, and copper (heavy metals) • Vitamin D deficiency • Nephrotic syndrome • Amyloidosis • Untreated distal renal tubular acidosis • Renal transplantation • Tubulointerstitial nephritis • Multiple myeloma and dysproteinemia

(EHHADH: enoyl-CoA hydratase and 3-hydroxyacyl CoA dehydrogenase; NaPi2a: sodium-dependent phosphate transport protein 2A)

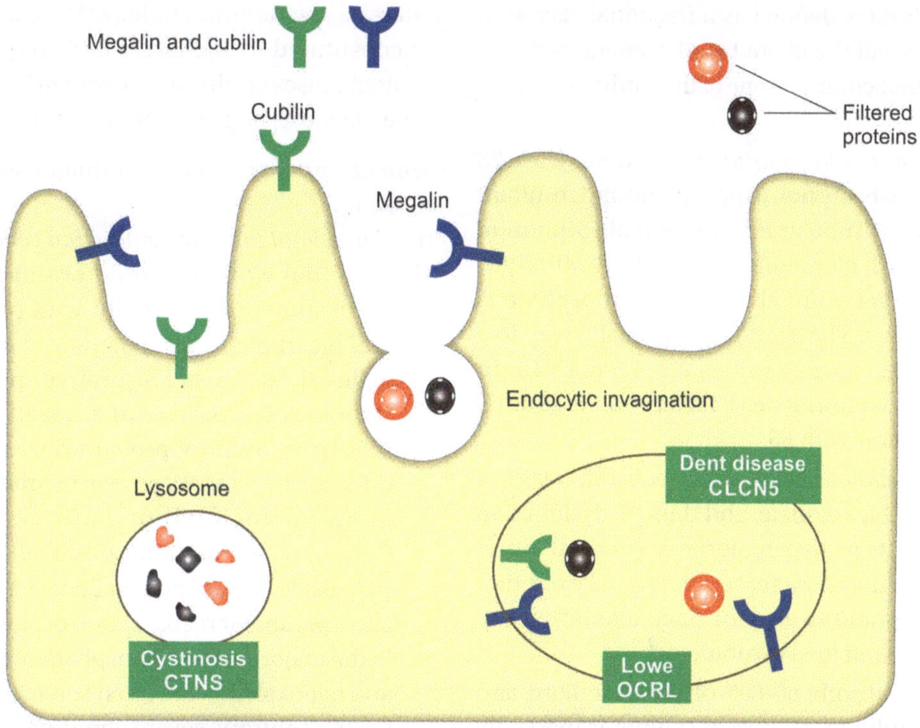

Fig. 1: Reabsorption of filtered solutes by proximal renal tubules is mediated via megalin-cubilin receptor pathway. Following endocytosis, endosomes undergo progressive acidification, resulting in dissociation of receptor-ligand complex. The ligand is directed to lysosome for degradation. The interference in acidification (Dent disease), impaired endocytic transport (Lowe disease) or transport to cytosol (Cystinosis) can manifest as generalized proximal tubular dysfunction, i.e., Fanconi syndrome. (CLCN5: gene encodes chloride-voltage gated channel-5; CTNS: codes for cystinosin; OCRL: gene codes for phosphatidylinositol 4,5-bisphosphate-5-phosphatase)

defects cause nonselective impairment of most transport mechanisms, resulting in FS. In addition, interference with the ATP generation pathway or intracellular ATP content may hamper the reabsorption of the filtered solutes by PT. Thus, FS is one of the common renal manifestations of mitochondrial cytopathies.

Symptomatology and Clinical Diagnosis

Clinical Features

- *Polyuria (urine output >2 L/m²/day), polydipsia, dehydration, and constipation:* Polyuria is primarily secondary to the osmotic diuresis, as excessive solutes are lost in the urine. Urinary concentration defect due to chronic hypokalemia and interstitial calcium deposits also contributes. Recurrent acute episodes of fever and constipation are frequently seen.
- *Rickets and osteomalacia:* Hypophosphatemia secondary to renal wasting and relative 1,25-dihydroxyvitamin D_3 deficiency cause osteomalacia, severe bony changes, and rickets in patients with FS. Metabolic acidosis also impairs the conversion of 25-vitamin D_3 to 1,25-dihydroxyvitamin D_3.[11] Low uptake of vitamin D and vitamin D-binding protein secondary to defective endocytosis also contributes to bone disease.
- *Growth retardation:* Failure to thrive is a common finding in children with FS and may persist in adulthood. The presence of hypokalemia, hypophosphatemia, and metabolic acidosis contributes to growth failure. Hypokalemia and metabolic acidosis reduce circulating growth hormone and insulin-like growth factor-1.[12,13] Besides, hypokalemia can also decrease appetite, leading to undernutrition. Severe rachitic changes, impaired conversion of 25-vitamin D_3 to 1,25-dihydroxyvitamin D_3, and hypophosphatemia worsen the growth retardation. Disease-specific (e.g., cystinosis) bone disease may also contribute to growth failure.[14] Early diagnosis and symptomatic therapy promote growth and may improve final height in patients with FS.

Metabolic Abnormalities

- *Glucosuria:* The filtered load of glucose (molecular weight ≅ 180 Daltons) is almost entirely absorbed by a sodium-coupled active transport located in PT. Glucosuria, in the presence of normal blood sugar levels, is one of the first diagnostic clues to proximal tubular dysfunction.
- *Generalized aminoaciduria:* Amino acids (molecular weight ≤ 204 Daltons) are freely filtered by the glomerulus, but <1% of the filtered load is excreted in urine due to avid reabsorption by apical and basolateral transporters in PT

cells. Aminoaciduria is defined as a fractional excretion of amino acids >5% of the filtered load. Generalized, i.e., nonselective aminoaciduria, is one of the cardinal features of FS.

- *Hypophosphatemia (phosphaturia):* Patients with FS have low tubular reabsorption of phosphate and resultant hypophosphatemia. Tubular maximum reabsorption of phosphate ratio with glomerular filteration (TMP/GFR) reflects the lower set-point above which phosphate is excreted in the urine. The TmP/GFR is usually very low in patients with FS (normal values 2.3–4.3 mg/dL). In addition, parathyroid hormone (PTH) levels are normal or elevated in patients with FS.
- *Hyperchloremic metabolic acidosis:* PT reabsorbs >85% of the filtered load of bicarbonate, and thus PT dysfunction invariably manifests as hyperchloremic (normal anion gap) metabolic acidosis. Increased fractional excretion (>15%) of bicarbonate is evident once alkali therapy replenishes the filtered load to tubules.
- *Hypokalemia:* PT reabsorbs 60–80% of filtered sodium, and thus in FS, distal tubular delivery of sodium is markedly increased. Hypokalemia is secondary to increased distal tubular sodium delivery with resultant renin-angiotensin-aldosterone axis activation. Hyponatremia is seen in few patients. Hypernatremia may also be observed due to increased free water loss and secondary diabetes insipidus in few patients.
- *Hypercalciuria:* Increased production of 1,25-dihydroxy-vitamin D_3, raised urinary vitamin D_3-binding protein, and increased intestinal calcium absorption may underlie hypercalciuria, frequently observed in children with FS. Nephrolithiasis is rarely observed in patients with FS, possibly because of polyuria and alkalized urine. Patients with Dent disease, however, can present with hypercalciuria and nephrolithiasis.[7]
- *Hypouricemia (hyperuricosuria):* Uric acid (molecular weight = 126 Daltons) is freely filtered from the glomerulus, but 90–95% of the filtered load is eventually reabsorbed in the proximal tubules. Hyperuricosuria is commonly seen in FS and leads to lower serum uric acid levels.
- *Low molecular proteinuria:* The glomerular molecular weight cutoff for plasma proteins is approximately 65 kD (kilodaltons), similar to the molecular weight of serum albumin. The PT cells reabsorb almost all of the filtered plasma proteins. In FS, LMW proteinuria is secondary to impaired endocytosis of protein receptor.

Differential Diagnosis and Evaluation for Diagnosis

The proximal renal tubular dysfunction may be isolated or generalized.[3,15] The latter is referred to as FS, which may be an isolated finding or a part of the renal manifestation of more systemic or syndromic etiology. The chief causes in children are constituted by the latter, i.e., syndromic causes, while acquired causes are the more frequent in adults. The approach to the diagnosis begins with a clinical suspicion of FS.[3,4,15]

Clinical approach: Steps to diagnosis of FS include the following:

Q1. *Is proximal tubular dysfunction generalized?*
An initial workup should evaluate other features of PT dysfunction in a child with polyuria, polydipsia, and bicarbonaturia. Generalized aminoaciduria is the hallmark feature of FS. A raised spot protein:creatinine ratio in the presence of a negative urine dipstick is suggestive of LMW proteinuria, as the dipstick testing does not detect LMW protein in urine. Urinary estimation of β2-microglobulin confirms LMW proteinuria. Glucosuria is commonly observed and can be detected by bedside dipstick and/or Benedict's test. Hypercalciuria and low tubular reabsorption of phosphate are observed in the majority. Hypophosphatemia, metabolic acidosis, and hypokalemia are often less marked in Dent disease. On the contrary, severe abnormalities are more evident in other causes of FS.

Q2. *Is an inherited cause likely?*
A history of similar illness in the family and/or sibling deaths may point to an autosomal recessive disorder. Selective involvement of boys and marginal or minimal features in girls (e.g., cataract in mothers in case of Lowe syndrome) may be seen in X-linked disorders. Most of the hereditary causes are syndromic or associated with systemic manifestations. Diagnosis may be confirmed by targeted or clinical exome sequencing in inherited diseases.

Q3. *Is the PT dysfunction accompanied by other systemic manifestations?*
The presence of systemic manifestations is more likely in the case of syndromic causes of FS. Dysmorphism may be evident in certain disorders, e.g., Lowe syndrome. A targeted ocular examination and hearing assessment are crucial. Corneal crystals in cystinosis are diagnostic. Nephrocalcinosis may be evident in Dent disease, cystinosis, and Lowe syndrome while it may result from overzealous therapy in others. Significant hepatic involvement occurs in hereditary tyrosinemia, and untreated patients are at risk of life-threatening hepatocellular carcinoma. The presence of neurological and hepatic manifestations in an older child may point to Wilson's disease. Multisystem and severe neurological manifestations suggest mitochondrial cytopathies where FS is the most common renal manifestations.

Q4. *What could be other causes in the index patient?*
In a child where inherited causes are less likely, and targeted screening fails to point toward any multisystem pathology, uncommon causes should be sought. The drug

history should be carefully reviewed, and environmental or heavy metal exposure needs to be enquired. In an older child or an adolescent with isolated FS and no suggestive family history, acquired causes of FS are more likely.[16,17]

Therapy

Identifying the etiology is crucial as it may allow timely and specific therapy for the patient. Avoidance of certain exposure may have therapeutic significance in few disorders, e.g., galactosemia and hereditary fructose intolerance. Acquired causes may respond after discontinuation of the offending agents.[1,18,19]

General principles of therapy include the following:

- *Counseling:* Parents must be counseled to avoid dehydration, and water availability must be ensured at all times. These patients are at a higher risk of dehydration, and thus early intravenous hydration may be warranted in a child with vomiting or diarrhea.
- Dietary modifications may be required in certain disorders, e.g., low phenylalanine and tyrosine in hepatorenal tyrosinemia, avoidance of foods containing fructose and sucrose in hereditary fructose intolerance, and use of uncooked cornstarch for Fanconi–Bickel syndrome.
- Physical activity and an appropriate diet with calcium, phosphate, and vitamin D alleviate bone disease and bone pains.
- Replacement of the losses of urinary electrolytes and careful vitamin D therapy are the cornerstone of nonspecific treatment in all children. The usual dosages required are:
  - *Bicarbonate:* 2–10 mEq/kg/day, titrate to trough levels (preferably as potassium citrate, sodium bicarbonate as an alternative)
  - *Potassium:* 1–5 mEq/kg/day, titrate to trough levels
  - *Phosphate:* 500–3,000 mg of elemental phosphorus/day, titrate to trough levels
  - *Calcitriol:* 0.1–0.25 μg/day, averts hypophosphatemia and rise in parathyroid hormone. Therapy should be carefully balanced to avoid hypercalciuria.
- Aminoaciduria, glucosuria, proteinuria, LMW proteinuria, and uricosuria usually do not induce clinical symptoms and do not require specific treatments.
- *Growth failure:* While some may benefit from early symptomatic therapy, final adult height is often suboptimal. Supplemental growth hormone may be helpful in selected patients.
- Despite therapy, and more commonly due to lack of timely therapy, children may progress to chronic kidney disease (CKD). Management of these patients is similar to other children with CKD, but special care for fluid and electrolyte imbalance must be followed.

Specific therapy is also available in certain diseases, and timely treatment may prevent disease progression and sequelae. Galactosemia and hereditary fructose intolerance may respond to specific dietary avoidance alone. Cysteamine is a specific therapy that enables the mitigation of systemic effects and CKD in cystinosis. FS is usually unaltered.[20] Nitisinone is available as a specific therapy for hepatorenal tyrosinemia.[21]

Outcome and Prognosis

Identification of a specific cause may enable specific therapy and improve long-term outcomes in these patients. Timely therapy may be crucial in life-limiting disorders. The outcome in inherited causes of FS is variable. Cystinosis invariably progresses to ESKD in early childhood, but many survive to adulthood now as cystine-depleting therapies are available.[22] In hepatorenal tyrosinemia, early therapy with nitisinone, i.e., 2-[2-nitro-4-(trifluoromethyl) benzoyl] cyclohexane-1,3-dione or NTBC, prevents liver failure, renal problems, and neurological attacks and also decreases the risk for hepatocellular carcinoma.

In the case of exogenous causes of FS, the inciting drug or exposure should be stopped or reduced in dose. Recovery from FS can occur after withdrawal of exogenous substances, but it can take months, and chronic damage to the proximal tubular function may persist.

In subsequent sections, we will briefly discuss a few of the causes of FS in more detail. Also, see **Table 2**.

Dent Disease (Dent–Wrong Disease)

Dent disease, an X-linked recessive disorder of PT, is characterized by hypercalciuria, nephrocalcinosis/nephrolithiasis, and LMW proteinuria. It commonly progresses to ESKD, usually by third to fifth decade of life in 30–80% of affected males.[7]

Genetics

Approximately 50–60% of patients have a mutation in the *CLCN5* gene that encodes a voltage-gated chloride transporter, a 746 amino-acid electrogenic $2Cl^-/H^+$ exchanger. This transporter is colocalized with proton-ATPase in subapical endosomes of the PT. These subapical endosomes are involved in the absorption endocytosis of filtered proteins.[6] Progression along the endocytic apparatus is dependent on the endosomal acidification, driven by proton-ATPase with parallel Cl^- conductance to ensure electroneutrality. *CLCN5* may mediate a set point for endosomal acidification. The lack of this channel interferes with protein reabsorption via the megalin–cubilin pathway in PT. Thus, reabsorption of LMW proteins is hampered, leading to loss of LMW proteins in urine. Phosphaturia is also observed, while glycosuria and aminoaciduria are less common. These abnormalities may result from disturbed cycling of cell surface receptors. The reported mutations are scattered throughout the coding region, with no evidence for major mutational hot spots.[7,23,24] Though most mutations result in a truncated or absent protein, no genotype–phenotype correlation has been reported.[25]

TABLE 2: Other causes of Fanconi syndrome.

Disease	*Gene*	*Defect*	*Key features*	*Management*
Hereditary fructose intolerance	*ALDOB*	Deficiency of aldolase B	Hypoglycemia, severe abdominal symptoms	Avoid foods or drugs containing fructose, sucrose, and sorbitol
Galactosemia	*GALT*	Galactose-1-phosphate uridylyltransferase	Lethargy, jaundice, bleeding disorders, cataract, and intellectual disability	Elimination of galactose from the diet
Glycogen storage disease type 1	*G6PC1, SLC37A4*	• 1a: Deficiency in glucose-6-phosphatase-alpha (G6Pase-alpha) • 1b: Deficiency of microsomal glucose-6-phosphatase transporter	Growth retardation, seizures, hepatomegaly, nephromegaly, hypoglycemia, hypercholesterolemia, hypertriglyceridemia, hyperuricemia, lactic acidemia, and neutrophilia	Maintain normoglycemia, uncooked cornstarch is useful
Fanconi–Bickel syndrome	*SLC2A2*	Defect in facilitative glucose transporter	Failure to thrive, "doll-like" face, hepatomegaly, nephromegaly, severe rickets, fasting hypoglycemia, and galactose intolerance	Symptomatic therapy, uncooked starch, and frequent feeding
Tyrosinemia type 1	*FAH*	Fumarylacetoacetate–tyrosine catabolism	Hepatomegaly, cirrhosis, intellectual disability, and high incidence of hepatocellular carcinoma	Low-phenylalanine and low-tyrosine diet; 2-(2-nitro-4-trifluoromethylbenzoyl)-1,3-cyclohexanedione (NTBC)
Wilson disease	*ATP7B*	Copper (Cu) transporting P-type ATPase: failure to excrete Cu into the biliary canaliculi	Liver disease, neuropsychiatric manifestations	The aim is to remove the toxic deposit of Cu from the body to produce a negative Cu balance
Mitochondrial disorders	Multiple	Oxidative phosphorylation	*Heterogeneous phenotype:* Fanconi syndrome, neurological and neuromuscular manifestations, eye, hearing, liver, and heart are commonly affected	Symptomatic, carnitine may be used in some children. Drugs that interfere with mitochondrial function, e.g., valproate should be avoided
Autosomal-recessive Fanconi syndrome	*SLC34A1*	Sodium phosphate co-transport (NaPi2a)	Fanconi syndrome, hypophosphatemic rickets, hypercalciuria, and elevated serum 1,25-dihydroxyvitamin D3	Oral phosphate supplements
Autosomal-dominant Fanconi syndrome	*EHHADH*	Defect in peroxisomal enzyme, EHHADH, that is involved in oxidation of fatty acids	Rickets, impaired growth, and features of Fanconi syndrome	Symptomatic therapy

(ATPase: adenosine triphosphatase; EHHADH: enoyl-CoA hydratase and 3-hydroxyacyl CoA dehydrogenase)

Mutation in the *OCRL1* gene is seen in 15% of Dent disease, referred to as type 2 Dent disease. This X-chromosome inherited gene encodes phosphatase enzyme on the trans-Golgi network. The same gene is mutated in Lowe syndrome, a severe and systemic phenotype of FS. A minority of patients with Dent disease have been observed to have mild intellectual deficit, hypotonia, and subclinical cataract.[23,26,27] However, Lowe syndrome and Dent disease have not been reported in different family members of the same illness. Also, *OCRL1* mutations associated with Dent disease (exon 4–15, first seven exons), in general, do not overlap with those causing Lowe syndrome (exons 9–22). Nevertheless, few overlapping mutations have been reported to occur.

A fraction (25–35%) of patients with Dent disease may not show any mutation on genetic analysis. The genes encoding proteins that interact with *ClC-5* have been suggested, but no putative cause has been confirmed.[23]

Clinical Features

Rickets, difficulty in walking, bony pains, abdominal pain, dysuria, or hematuria secondary to nephrolithiasis is the usual presenting feature. Polyuria or polydipsia with overt FS may be observed. Episodic and vitamin A-responsive night blindness occurs secondary to loss of retinol-binding protein in urine and is one of the pointers to diagnostic suspicion in clinical practice.

Differential Diagnosis

Males with predominantly lower limb deformities with low phosphate may confuse the picture with hypophosphatemic rickets. Besides acidosis, nephrocalcinosis and hypercalciuria may point to distal renal tubular acidosis. However, the degree of hypokalemia and acidosis is relatively less marked with Dent disease. Also, severe hypophosphatemia is uncommon. LMW proteinuria is a key feature in almost all boys. It is the most consistent finding, while there is considerable inter- and intrafamilial variability in the other manifestations of the disease.

Diagnosis: The clinical diagnosis requires the following:

- *LMW proteinuria:* β2-microglobulin is commonly measured. A level, *at least* fivefold above the upper limit of normal, is suggestive. Other LMW proteins include α1-microglobulin, retinol-binding protein, Clara cell protein, and vitamin D-binding protein.
- *Hypercalciuria (>4 mg/kg/day):* Seen in 95% of affected males
- At least one of—nephrocalcinosis, kidney stones, hematuria, hypophosphatemia, or CKD.

Nephrolithiasis and medullary nephrocalcinosis are seen in ~50% and 75% of male patients.[7] The usual stone composition is a mixture of calcium phosphate and calcium oxalate.

Milder features of LMW proteinuria (70%) and hypercalciuria (50%) may be observed in female carriers, while ESKD is rarely reported.

The diagnosis is confirmed with the identification of the mutation in either *CLCN5* or *OCRL1*. However, a minority of patients may not have a mutation in either of the genes. In such cases, clinical presentation and exclusion of other related diseases help to confirm the diagnosis.

The disorder is inherited in an X-linked manner. Though technically feasible, antenatal diagnosis or preimplantation genetic testing is not advised, as the vital prognosis in the majority is good and genotype-phenotype correlation is lacking.[7,25]

Kidney biopsy, if performed, may show progressive, nonspecific lesions, e.g., glomerular hyalinosis, tubular cell degeneration or atrophy, and mild interstitial fibrosis.[7]

Treatment

Unfortunately, Dent disease does not have any specific therapy till date. Management is chiefly supportive, aimed to alleviate symptoms and prevent complications, including nephrolithiasis and disease progression. Increased fluid intake, adequate dietary intake of calcium (avoid restriction), and vitamin D supplementation are advised.[7,26] However, worsening of hypercalciuria and nephrocalcinosis may occur and needs careful monitoring. Oral citrate supplementation is beneficial.

In patients who develop ESKD, kidney transplant cures the disease. Females are obligate carriers of the mutated gene, and some may have a mild Dent's disease phenotype. There may be a reason for concern when considering a female obligate carrier (i.e., the mother) for kidney donation.[28] The decision of mother as a live related donor must be considered after careful assessment of the female obligate carriers.

Lowe Disease

Lowe syndrome (oculocerebrorenal syndrome) is another X-linked disorder like Dent disease but characterized by involvement of the eyes, central nervous system, and kidneys.[26,29] It is caused by pathogenic variation in the *OCRL* gene that encodes inositol polyphosphate 5-phosphatase OCRL. The absence of enzyme leads to high intracellular levels of its substrate. It leads to defects in intracellular protein trafficking and impaired endocytic transport.[27] This manifests in the form of LMW proteinuria and other tubular defects.[29,30]

Though the penetrance of the disease is complete, the severity of phenotype may vary within the same family. Pathogenic variants in early regions of the *OCRL* gene are found in 15% of Dent disease (renal limited phenotype).

- *Eyes:* All boys have vision impairment. Dense congenital cataracts are seen in all boys, while 50% have infantile glaucoma. Microphthalmos, enophthalmos, strabismus, retinal dystrophy, band keratopathy, and corneal scarring are other uncommon findings.
- *Neurological:* Infantile hypotonia (central), seizures (50%), delayed motor milestones, behavioral problems, and intellectual impairment.
- *Kidneys:* FS—LMW proteinuria (earliest marker), albuminuria, nephrocalcinosis, nephrolithiasis, and progressive CKD that leads to ESKD in the second to fourth decade of life.
- *Others:* Rickets, bone fractures, scoliosis, dental malformations, superficial cysts, gastroesophageal reflux, constipation, poor growth, undescended testes, and delayed puberty.

Diagnosis

The diagnosis is suspected on clinical features. Confirmation requires genetic testing. It may include a combination of gene-targeted testing and comprehensive genomic testing. When phenotype suggests Lowe syndrome, sequence analysis of OCRL may constitute the first step, followed by gene-targeted duplication/deletion analysis if no pathogenic variant is found. A multigene panel or clinical exome sequencing may be a preferred approach when the characteristic phenotype is missing. The clinical exome is also increasingly employed with a significant decline in costs involved and the ability to rule out other related differential diagnoses.

Heterozygous postpubertal females have characteristic irregular, punctuate, smooth, off-white opacities in the lens cortex.[26,31] A few may have a dense and visually significant cataract, requiring surgery. Other nonocular manifestations, due to skewed X inactivation, are rarely observed. Given the high rates (4.5%) of germline mosaicism, every mother of a male with Lowe syndrome, even with a negative family history, should be offered prenatal DNA testing, if pathogenic variation in her son is known, irrespective of her eye examination findings.

Management

Therapy is chiefly supportive.[30] Early removal of the cataract may promote proper visual stimulation. However, surgical implantation of artificial lenses is avoided. Infantile glaucoma is often challenging to treat and requires surgical measures. Intraocular pressure needs monitoring on a semiannual basis. Corneal contact lenses are avoided. Oral supplements of potassium citrate, alkali, phosphate, and careful calcitriol therapy are given. Kidney function assessment and urine tests are done on a 3–6-monthly basis. Feeding gastrostomy and/or growth hormone may be needed. Anthropometry should be followed up at 3–6-month intervals in older children and more frequently in infants or growth hormone therapy. Behavior modification programs and/or medications are used for behavioral problems. A dental examination is advised at 6–12 monthly intervals.

Prognosis

ESKD develops by the second to fourth decade of life. Most do not live beyond the fourth decade. Affected males are not known to reproduce. ESKD, dehydration, pneumonia, and other infections contribute to early mortality.

CYSTINOSIS

Introduction

Cystinosis, first described in 1903, was the first treatable lysosomal disorder in the history of clinical medicine.[32] It is an unusual category among the group of lysosomal disorders as evident dysmorphism is lacking.

A leading cause of inherited FS in children (up to 20% of cases of hereditary tubular disorders), cystinosis is a rare autosomal recessive, monogenic lysosomal disorder with an incidence of 1:100,000–1:200,000 live births. A higher incidence has been reported in certain groups (French Brittany, Quebec) due to founder mutations in *CTNS*.[33-35] A 57-kB deletion is the most common cause of cystinosis in more than half of those with northern European ancestry. A higher incidence is also found in the population where consanguinity is widely practiced.[20]

Etiology and Pathology

Cysteine is a sulfur-containing amino acid. In proteins, it usually exists as a cystine by forming a disulfide bond between two cysteine residues, carefully protected inside of the protein in order to function as a stabilizer for high-order structure of the protein. Cystinosin transports cystine from the lysosomal lumen to the cytosol.[36] Cysteine disulfide formation is one of the most important post-translational modifications involved in protein structure. Disulfides play a crucial role in maintaining the structure of many proteins.

Genetics

CTNS gene—which encodes the lysosomal cystine-proton cotransporter, cystinosin—was identified as the causative gene of cystinosis in 1998.[37] The gene is expressed in all tissues, and thus its mutation leads to multisystemic manifestations. It is located on the short arm of chromosome 17. The first two exons are noncoding.

Cystinosin is a cystine-proton symporter that uses the proton gradient to transport cystine from the lysosomal lumen to the cytosol. The abundance of cystinosin is the rate-limiting step for cystine transport, as saturation of cystinosin occurs much below the cystine saturation of lysosomes. This finding explains the reduced transport efficiency in heterozygotes with one defective *CTNS* allele. Genotype-phenotype correlation shows complete disruption of cystine transport in infantile cystinosis compared to the partial preservation of function with juvenile form.[34,38] Data points to possible modifier genes that may influence the renal phenotype and thus account for the variability of the disease severity with identical mutations. The presence of cystinosin, despite impaired transport capability, is associated with a milder phenotype. Thus, cystinosin may have an important role in cell function beyond the cystine transport in lysosomes.[10,34]

The proposed theory for the pathogenesis of cystinosis includes the following **(Fig. 2)**:

- *Cystine accumulation:* Cystine accumulation in lysosomes occurs due to the degradation of filtered disulfide-bearing proteins with impaired cystine transport. Cystine crystal formation is pathognomonic of cystinosis, but the evidence does not suggest the crystals as a pathogenic factor for FS. However, these might be crucial in the subsequent progression of kidney disease through activation of the inflammasome and thus leading to subsequent inflammation and fibrosis.
- Altered cellular energy homeostasis and reduced ATP levels are proposed as the contributory mechanism of FS.[10,39]
- *Increased oxidative stress:* Cystine efflux from lysosomes serves as a source of cysteine, which is used to synthesize

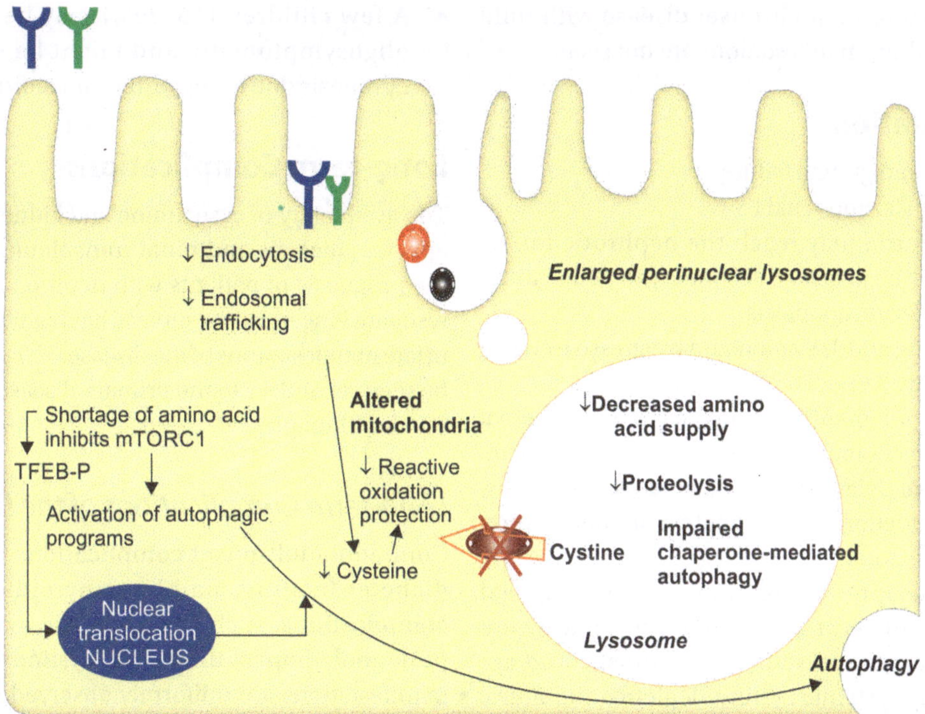

Fig. 2: Pathogenesis of cystinosis is multifactorial. Cystine accumulation, depletion of glutathione with increased oxidative stress, impaired chaperone-mediated autophagy, and altered proteolysis and trafficking are the postulated mechanisms. (mTORC1: mammalian target of rapamycin complex 1; TFEB: transcription factor EB; P: phosphorylated).

glutathione. Altered glutathione metabolism and increased oxidative stress have been proposed to cause the FS in cystinosis.

- *Trafficking and proteolysis defects:* Expression of megalin and cubilin in proximal tubular cells is severely depressed. Besides, impaired lysosomal motility and enlarged lysosomes have been observed in cystinotic cells. The proteolysis in endolysosomes is impaired. The lysosomal membrane is a regulated docking surface for mTORC1 machinery, which integrates cell information to regulate autophagy and cell differentiation. Impairment of mTOR activation has been reported in human cystinotic cells.[40] The impaired mTOR activation may lead to decreased megalin expression in the cystinotic kidney. Chaperone-mediated autophagy (CMA) is impaired in cystinosis, and this may also increase cell sensitivity to oxidative stress.[41] All these features and the fact that cysteamine therapy does not correct alterations in mTOR signaling, transcription factor EB (TFEB) expression, and CMA, despite improvements in cystine clearance, underscore the indirect effects of cystinosin deletion.[10,39]
- Apical dedifferentiation of proximal tubular cells extends longitudinally from the glomerulotubular junction to more distal PT segments. The area earliest involved reflects the area closed to the glomerulus as the filtered disulfide-rich protein is the chief source of lysosomal cystine for proximal tubular cells. Later stages demonstrate PT atrophy (*Swan-Neck deformity*) with interstitial and glomerular fibrosis, which eventually results in atubular glomeruli in ESKD.

Thus, mechanistic studies suggest multifactorial pathogenesis for FS secondary to oxidative stress and impaired vesicular trafficking, autophagy, and mTORC1 and TFEB signaling.

Symptomatology and Clinical Diagnosis

Three forms of the disease are seen:[33-35,42]

1. *Infantile cystinosis:* It is most frequent and severe form of cystinosis. Patients develop marked failure to thrive by 6–9 months, tubular dysfunction, and rickets by 6–18 months with eventual renal insufficiency by median age of 10 years (untreated) or 20 years (treated). Ocular features (photophobia, corneal erosions secondary to crystals) are observed early in the course. Corneal cystine crystals are the first extrarenal finding affecting all patients. It manifests as photophobia and blepharospasm by mid-childhood. In 10–15% of patients, retinopathy leads to retinal blindness. Systemic manifestations, e.g., hypothyroidism, hypogonadism, diabetes mellitus, myopathy, scoliosis, and neurological deterioration, are seen in the second to 3rd decade of life.
2. *Juvenile cystinosis* is a milder and rarer form. It manifests around 12 years of age with variable onset of photophobia and kidney dysfunction.

3. *Ocular cystinosis* is an adult-onset disease with mild photophobia. Kidney manifestations are not seen.

Clinical Presentation

- Failure to thrive and growth failure
- Polyuria, polydipsia, and renal FS
- Tubular proteinuria may reach the nephrotic range. Albuminuria may be observed secondary to podocyturia or increased podocyte apoptosis.
- Impaired sweating and salivation and progressive coarse facial features may be seen.
- Extrarenal systemic manifestations (e.g., photophobia, cognitive and psychological problems, hypothyroidism, diabetes, pubertal delay, male hypogonadism, scoliosis, swallowing dysfunction, and myopathy) are uncommon as a presenting feature.
    - *Ocular:* Photophobia, blepharospasm, corneal erosions, band keratopathy, and retinopathy are reported. Corneal crystals are diagnostic and are unaffected by systemic cystine-depleting therapies. Retinopathy can progress to blindness.
    - *Hypothyroidism:* Progressive cystine accumulation and crystal formation in thyroid follicular cells cause fibrosis and atrophy, leading to primary hypothyroidism in 50–70% from the 2nd decade of life.
    - *Endocrine:* 50% of infantile cystinosis develops slow progressive loss of insulin secretion and C-peptide production. Hypogonadism is frequent in males (70%), and in contrast to males, cystinotic females are usually fertile. Affected males are unable to induce pregnancy. One case of successful conception using percutaneous epididymal sperm aspiration followed by intracytoplasmatic sperm injection has been reported.
    - *Myopathy:* Muscle weakness usually affects patients from the second decade of life, but electromyography (EMG) changes may be found in asymptomatic patients. Swallowing dysfunction (>50% patients) correlates with the number of years without cysteamine therapy.
- Some patients present with characteristic blond hair and white skin. Interestingly, cystinosin has been implicated in the regulation of melanin synthesis. Congenital hypopigmentation and premature skin aging have also been reported.
- Chronic kidney disease may be the first presentation in some children. Cystinosis accounts for ~5% of CKD in children. Nearly 50–90% of children in the reported Indian series present with poor kidney function. ESKD occurs by the end of the first decade of life. Hypertension and vascular damage (juxtaglomerular cell hyperplasia, CKD, and cystine accumulation in blood vessels) are also reported.
- A few children (15–20%) may be asymptomatic or oligosymptomatic and might be suspected to have cystinosis due to suggestive or confirmed family history.

Long-term Complications

The availability of cysteamine and kidney replacement therapy, i.e., dialysis and renal transplantation, has improved the prognosis of patients with nephropathic cystinosis. The resultant longer patient survival has highlighted the emergence of late manifestations of the disease.[22,43] Long-term effects may be seen secondary to the primary disease and/or cysteamine or other therapies.[20,32]

Long-term Complications of the Disease

Common adult-onset complications include myopathy, diabetes mellitus, and hypothyroidism. Less common complications, such as neurologic dysfunction, can still profoundly impact those with cystinosis. Gastrointestinal manifestations are uniformly observed and may be related to the primary disease or cysteamine therapy. Patients with cystinosis may develop pulmonary complications, including respiratory failure caused by muscle weakness, sleep apnea, and aspiration due to swallowing dysfunction.

Some studies have shown that cardiovascular complications can occur on follow-up. The rates of vascular calcification (20–60%) correlate directly with the duration of life without cysteamine and correlate inversely with the duration of life with cysteamine. The amount of time spent on dialysis did not differ between the groups. Neurologic complications of cystinosis are uncommon but heterogeneous and sometimes debilitating. "Cystinosis-associated encephalopathy" can manifest as an encephalopathic form and a stroke-like form. Central nervous system effects of cystinosis may arise from deposition of cystine in the brain, but mixed responses of these symptoms to cysteamine point to other unknown factors. Despite normal IQ scores, patients have significantly poor performance in visuospatial and visual memory skills. Besides, cystinosis has a significant impact on the quality of life, especially in adulthood. Psychosocial support is crucial. It also helps in ensuring therapy compliance, leading to better long-term outcomes.

Long-term Effects of Cysteamine Therapy

Long-term optimal cysteamine treatment is associated with improvements in renal and extrarenal complications. Observation of preserved renal function and reduced incidence of CKD with early initiation are consistent across all studies. The US database study showed that compliance was linearly correlated with age at ESKD onset, and optimal treatment for 1 year preserved 0.9 years of kidney glomerular function. However, the severity of renal FS was unaltered.

In long-term studies, patients who received early and adequate cysteamine therapy had increased life expectancy and fewer complications than inadequately treated patients and those who started treatment later or were untreated. Early initiation reduces the rates of hypothyroidism, diabetes mellitus, pubertal delay, neuromuscular or pulmonary disorders, and swallowing dysfunction. Improved linear growth has been observed when therapy is initiated <3 years of age. Long-term studies indicate that neurocognitive disorders may be preventable, if treatment is cysteamine initiated early. Early initiation (<2 years of age) is associated with significantly higher performance, verbal, and full-scale IQ scores. Visual-spatial skills show improvement, but visual-motor skills were not significantly affected. Intracellular cystine crystal deposition in posterior-segment ocular structures damages retina, choroid, and optic nerve. Long-term cysteamine therapy orally may reduce posterior-segment complications. Treatment for >20 versus ≤10 years decreased the rate of retinopathy (0% vs. 28%). However, corneal deposits are unaffected by oral therapy.

Differential Diagnosis and Evaluation for Diagnosis

Cystinosis is the most common cause of inherited FS in children. Metabolic disorders (tyrosinemia, galactosemia, and glycogen storage diseases), Wilson disease, Dent disease, and Lowe syndrome should be considered among the differential diagnoses.

Atypical presentations, e.g., nephrogenic diabetes insipidus and pseudo-Bartter phenotype, are known to occur. Other causes of CKD should be considered when a child presents as ESKD of an unknown cause.

Early diagnosis is crucial given the availability of specific therapy that may halt or slow down systemic manifestations of the disease.[20,33,34,42,44]

Three chief modalities to confirm the diagnosis include the following:

1. *Elevated leukocyte cystine levels:* First developed as a radioactive assessment of bound cystine, high-performance liquid chromatography (HPLC) or liquid chromatography-tandem mass spectrometry (LC-MS/MS) are the widely used methods. Cystine values are reported as half-molecules because it was originally measured in reducing conditions (as cysteine, i.e., half a molecule of cystine). Now, it is directly measured using mass spectrometry but continues to be reported as half-cystine per milligram of protein. There may be various causes of assay variability, including the technique of leukocyte separation (needs standardization) and sample sensitivity to storage and transportation conditions. Newly diagnosed cystinotic patients have leukocyte cystine levels in the range of 3–20 nmol half cystine/mg protein. In comparison, heterozygous carriers and control individuals have levels <1.0 and <0.2 nmol half cystine/mg protein, respectively.
2. *Visualization of characteristic corneal cystine crystals by slit-lamp examination:* It is the commonly used method in developing nations as a reliable and cheaper diagnostic method. However, an experienced ophthalmologist is required to identify and grade cystine crystals. Cystine crystals do not appear in slit lamp until the second year of life and thus have a limited role in allowing diagnosis and timely therapy in younger children. Reflectance confocal microscopy (RCM) is another possible alternative to evaluate cystine crystal load, e.g., dermal cystine deposits, as a rapid (5 minutes) and painless assessment.[45]
3. *Detection of CTNS mutation:* The gene for cystinosis was first mapped to a 4 cM region of chromosome 17p13 in 1995, followed by the isolation of the cystinosin gene, *CTNS,* by Town et al. in 1998. Molecular testing of the *CTNS* gene, a relatively small gene (12 exons, 10 coding), reveals 95% of disease-causing mutations. It is more time consuming than the above two methods but enables prenatal diagnosis when the mutation is known. Clinical exome sequencing may detect most mutations, but other methods, e.g., direct sequencing of allele or MLPA, may be required in certain mutation/deletions.

A large 57-kB deletion involving the first nine exons and part of exon 10 of the *CTNS* gene, along with two upstream genes (*CARKL* and *TRPV1*), is the most common mutation that causes cystinosis in Northern Europe and North America. Germany is considered to be the country of origin for this 57-kB deletion.[20,33,38] Reduced sensitivity of TRPV1 receptor in patients with Hom 57-kB deletion is associated with reduced sensitivity to capsaicin.[46] The patients tend to have reduced pain sensitivity and attenuated rise in dermal blood flow following capsaicin exposure. The 57-kB deletion has not been reported from the case series from India. Limited data suggest the previously reported p.Thr7PhefsTer7 variant as a putative mutation hotspot in Indian families.[47]

A newborn screening method is not available. Conventional blood spot-based screening methods are challenging given the technical difficulties, low amount of blood in a blood spot, difficulty to prevent spontaneous oxidation of cysteine into cystine in stored spots, and interference from serum cystine levels.[35] Sedoheptulose in dried blood spots of patients with homozygous for 57-kB deletion (simultaneous deletion of *CARKL/SHPK*) is elevated. Still, those without this mutation have a completely normal tandem mass spectrometry, limiting the clinical utility of the test.

Histopathology

A kidney biopsy, if performed, shows tubular flattening and thicker basement membrane with typical changes at the glomerulotubular junction and distal extension. These changes then evolve to tubular atrophy with the development of characteristic *swan-neck deformities*. Multinucleated podocytes, segmental sclerosis, and global collapse are the chief glomerular lesions. The interstitium may demonstrate inflammatory cell infiltration.

Therapy Including Prevention (Table 3)

Symptomatic Therapy

The aims of supportive therapy are as follows:

- Fluid and electrolyte substitution
- Safeguard the acid-base balance
- Nutritional support
- Prevent the development of rickets
- Treatment of hormone deficiency

Cystinosis patients should have access to water and toilets at all times and avoid excessive heat exposure. Oral sodium/potassium citrate, phosphate, and 1,25-dihydroxyvitamin D should begin in early childhood to prevent rickets. The required doses may need frequent reassessment, and serial sodium, potassium, bicarbonate, and phosphate must be monitored.[35] Nephrocalcinosis may result from overzealous therapy. A high-calorie diet (100–130% of the recommended daily intake) is advised, and an early nasogastric tube should be considered. Gastrostomy feeding allows adequate nutrition in children with anorexia and also facilitates drug administration. Thyroid and pancreatic function must be carefully monitored. Growth hormone replacement prevents growth retardation in some patients. Testosterone supplementation may help in primary testicular failure and low plasma testosterone levels. Angiotensin-converting enzyme (ACE) inhibitors may slow the deterioration of renal function but must be used with

TABLE 3: Therapy for cystinosis.

	Medication	*Dose and frequency*	*Remarks*
Fanconi syndrome			
Polyuria		Free water access at all times	Watch for dehydration, especially with illness and diarrhea
Difficult polyuria	Indomethacin	1–3 mg/kg ÷ twice a day	Avoid concomitant ACE inhibitor, stop in case of dehydration
Undernutrition		130% of recommended calorie intake	May necessitate gastrostomy/tube feeding
Salt wasting	Sodium citrate/bicarbonate	2–10 mEq/kg ÷ 3–4 times a day	
Potassium loss	Potassium citrate (prefer) or chloride	2–10 mEq/kg ÷ 3–4 times a day	Target K > 3 mEq/L
Alkali loss	Citrate/bicarbonate (sodium or potassium)	5–15 mEq/kg ÷ 3–4 times a day	Target bicarbonate 21–24 mEq/L
Phosphate loss	Sodium/potassium phosphate	30–60 mg/kg elemental phosphorus ÷ 3–4 times a day	Avoid high doses
Rickets	Calcitriol	0.04–0.08 µg/kg/day	Avoid hypercalcemia
Carnitine	L-carnitine	20–50 mg/kg ÷ three times a day	No clinically relevant effect on muscle health
Proteinuria	ACE inhibitors	0.10–0.25 mg/kg/day	Avoid with indomethacin
Hypothyroidism	Levothyroxine	5 µg/kg/day (2–3 µg/kg/day for >12 years)	Start at 25% and increase to full dose in 4 weeks
Growth retardation	rhGH	0.05 mg/kg/day subcutaneous	Initiate early if growth failure persists despite optimal nutritional intake and control of electrolytes and rickets
Glucose intolerance	Insulin	Subcutaneous	Titrate according to control of blood sugar levels and HbA1c
Cysteamine (systemic)	Immediate release	1.3–1.95 g/m² ÷ four times a day (strict 6 hourly doses)	• Initiate at low dose (1/6th) and increase gradually over 6–8 weeks • Watch for compliance
Cysteamine (systemic)	Delayed release	Start at 80% of immediate release form, dosing at 12-hour interval	As above
Cysteamine (topical)	0.5% eye drops	8–10 times a day	Annual reassessment
Cysteamine (topical)	Eye gel	Four times a day	As above
Gastrointestinal complaints	Proton-pump inhibitor	1 mg/kg, once to twice a day	—

(ACE: angiotensin-converting enzyme; HbA1C: glycated hemoglobin; rhGH: recombinant human growth hormone)

caution in those with salt and volume depletion. Combination with indomethacin must be avoided. Psychosocial support is important.

In case of ESKD, kidney transplantation is the treatment of choice.[44,47,48]

Specific Therapy

Cysteamine (beta-mercaptoethylamine) is the only specific therapy and was first approved for cystinosis patients by the Food and Drug Administration (FDA) in 1994. Early administration has shown to delay the progression of CKD but established FS is not reversible. Cysteamine penetrates the lysosomal membrane by an importer. It reacts with cystine to exchange its disulfide bridge into a mixed (cysteamine-cysteine) disulfide, which exits via the cationic amino-acid exporter (PQLC2). The free cysteine generated exits lysosome through an unknown transporter **(Fig. 3)**.

Oral: It is available as an immediate-release cysteamine bitartrate. Leukocyte cystine content returns to initial levels after 6 hours of dose, and thus immediate-release cysteamine bitartrate must be administered at 6-hour interval.[49]

Dose: Dose is calculated based on the body surface area (1.30 g/m^2/day; maximum of 1.95 g/m^2/day) as weight-based dosing (50 mg/kg/day) may lead to overdosing.

Adverse effects: Gastrointestinal intolerance, bad sweat odor, skin lesions, hyperthermia, lethargy, neutropenia, seizures, and allergic rash are among the reported adverse effects. Reversible cutaneous manifestations (striae, proliferative endothelial lesions) may develop, if high cysteamine doses are administered. Bone pain and myalgia may persist despite a reduction in dosage.

It is advised to discontinue therapy, if a woman plans pregnancy due to teratogenic effects observed in rats. The risks of discontinuation need to be balanced against the potential harm to the developing fetus.[35] There is no evidence that cysteamine dose adjustment is required in patients on dialysis, but metabolism of the drug might be impaired in ESKD.

Therapeutic monitoring: The leukocyte cystine assay is the current gold standard in therapeutic monitoring as leukocytes serve as the best alternative to tissue cystine load (invasive). Granulocyte separation is preferred as it accumulates preferentially in polymorphonuclear leukocytes. However, it is not ideal for long-term follow-up because of the extremely short lifespan of leukocytes.

Pill burden and compliance: Adherence to conventional cysteamine is cumbersome as the pill must be taken 6-hourly including getting up from sleep at night. Also, it causes body odor, halitosis (dimethyl sulfide and methanethiol as metabolized products), and gastrointestinal adverse effects (potent gastric acid-secretagogue), which hamper compliance. Initiating therapy with small doses and proton-pump inhibitors may help. Oral riboflavin and chlorophyll tablets help to reduce body odor. Cysteamine toxicity may be associated with copper deficiency in patients with FS, and copper supplementation may prevent cysteamine-related adverse effects in some patients. The combination of

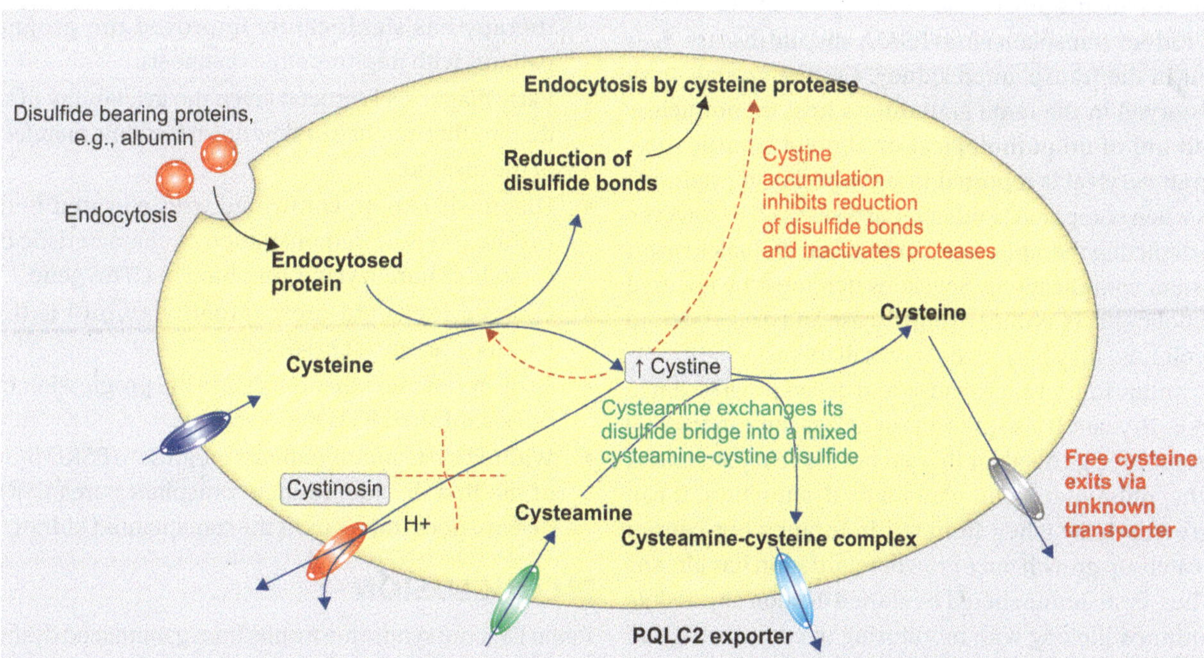

Fig. 3: Mechanism of action of cysteamine. Cysteamine enters the lysosome and reacts with cystine to exchange it's disulfide bridge into a mixed (Cysteamine-cysteine) disulfide. The resulting complex exits via the cationic amino-acid exporter (PQLC2). The free cysteine generated exits lysosome through an unknown transporter.

cysteamine therapy and other supportive therapy requires patients to take 50–60 pills per day. It poses a risk of poor compliance (one third only adhere) and often requires a gastric tube to tolerate medicines while ensuring calorie intake.[50] Twice-daily delayed-release cysteamine bitartrate (DR-CYS) was approved by the FDA in 2013. This enteric-coated tablet enables less frequent dosing and can improve compliance with convenient dosing.

Topical Therapy for Corneal Crystals

Topical cysteamine is used to dissolve corneal crystals as oral therapy is ineffective. The eye drops need to be used frequently (>10 times a day) and may be associated with a burning sensation due to the acidic nature of the formulation. Gel preparation may allow less frequent administration.

Potential Novel Therapies

Hematopoietic stem cell (HSC) transplantation ameliorates renal FS in cystinotic mice. HSCs differentiate into macrophages that transfer cystinosin-bearing lysosomes into proximal tubule cells.[51,52] This transfer occurs via tunneling nanotubes that cross the tubular basement membrane. This approach has also been demonstrated in the eyes and thyroid of *Ctns*-knockout mice with near-complete clearance of corneal cystine crystals and preservation of thyroid follicles.

Outcome and Prognosis

With the availability of cystine-depleting therapies, more patients are increasingly growing into adulthood. Without cysteamine, patients progress to ESKD by the end of the first decade. Kidney transplant cures ESKD, and the disease does not recur in the transplanted kidney. Cystine crystals have been observed in the renal graft due to host mononuclear cells and are of no pathological or clinical significance. Renal graft survival is reported to be superior in cystinotic patients when compared to other renal diseases.[44,48] However, cystine-depleting therapies need to be taken lifelong to avert multisystem complications. Special watch must be ensured for metabolic effects as underlying disease and drugs (steroid and tacrolimus) may hasten the risk of diabetes.

Cysteamine improves prognosis and delays progression to ESKD by 6–10 years. It also prevents or delays some extrarenal manifestations, e.g., need for thyroid hormone replacement, myopathy, pulmonary, and pancreatic dysfunction. It can avoid growth delay when initiated in infancy but cannot induce catch-up growth once growth retardation has already set in. Thus, cysteamine should be started as soon as possible and continued lifelong with monitoring of compliance and leukocyte cysteine levels (<1 nmol ½ cystine/mg protein, i.e., 90th percentile of cystine levels seen in heterozygotes). Nevertheless, it has no effect on renal FS, male infertility, or corneal cystine accumulation.

KEY POINTS

- FS refers to the set of clinical features resulting from a generalized loss or disturbance of the normal transport processes in the proximal renal tubule.
- The characteristic features of FS include glycosuria, aminoaciduria, and phosphaturia (hypophosphatemia).
- Identifying the etiology of FS is crucial, as it may allow timely and specific therapy for the patient.
- Dent disease is an X-linked recessive disorder of PT. It is characterized by hypercalciuria, nephrocalcinosis/nephrolithiasis, and LMW proteinuria.
- Diagnosis of Dent disease is confirmed with the identification of the mutation in either *CLCN5* (50–60%) or *OCRL1* (15%). However, a minority (25–35%) of patients may not have a mutation in either of the genes.
- Lowe syndrome (oculocerebrorenal syndrome) is another X-linked disorder, due to *OCRL1* mutation like Dent 2 disease but with a more systemic phenotype.
- Cystinosis is the most common cause of FS in children.
- *CTNS* gene encodes the lysosomal cystine-proton cotransporter, cystinosin. A 57-kB deletion is the most common cause of cystinosis in more than half of those with northern European ancestry.
- Cystinosin may have an important role in cell function beyond the cystine transport in lysosomes.
- Infantile cystinosis is the most frequent and severe form of cystinosis. Patients develop marked failure to thrive by 6–9 months, tubular dysfunction, and rickets by 6–18 months with eventual renal insufficiency.
- The availability of cysteamine and kidney replacement therapy has significantly improved the prognosis of patients with nephropathic cystinosis.
- Early diagnosis is crucial given the availability of specific therapy that may halt or slow down systemic manifestations of the disease.
- Diagnosis can be confirmed with elevated leukocyte cystine levels or demonstration of characteristic corneal crystals or homozygous mutation in *CTNS* gene.
- Cysteamine (beta-mercaptoethylamine) is the only specific therapy for cystinosis.
- Early cysteamine therapy delays the progression of CKD, but established FS is not reversible.
- Without cysteamine, patients progress to ESKD by the end of the first decade. Kidney transplant cures ESKD, and disease does not recur in the transplanted kidney.

CONCLUSION

Renal Fanconi syndrome results from generalized dysfunction of proximal tubules. It is usually inherited in children, commonly as a part of systemic disorder. Treatment is chiefly supportive. Early diagnosis is crucial as specific therapy is available in some disorders. Cystinosis is the most common cause of Fanconi syndrome in children. Early and specific therapy with cysteamine delays end-stage kidney disease.

REFERENCES

1. Foreman JW. Fanconi syndrome. Pediatr Clin North Am. 2019;66(1):159-67.
2. Klootwijk ED, Reichold M, Unwin RJ, Kleta R, Warth R, Bockenhauer D. Renal Fanconi syndrome: taking a proximal look at the nephron. Nephrol Dial Transplant. 2015;30(9): 1456-60.
3. Quigley R. Proximal renal tubular acidosis. J Nephrol. 2006;19(Suppl 9):S41-5.
4. Chadha V, Alon US. Hereditary renal tubular disorders. Semin Nephrol. 2009;29(4):399-411.
5. Nielsen R, Christensen EI, Birn H. Megalin and cubilin in proximal tubule protein reabsorption: from experimental models to human disease. Kidney Int. 2016;89(1):58-67.
6. Eshbach ML, Weisz OA. Receptor-mediated endocytosis in the proximal tubule. Annu Rev Physiol. 2017;79:425-48.
7. Devuyst O, Thakker RV. Dent's disease. Orphanet J Rare Dis. 2010;5:28.
8. Finsterer J, Scorza FA. Renal manifestations of primary mitochondrial disorders. Biomed Rep. 2017;6(5):487-94.
9. Keefe P, Bokhari SRA. Fanconi syndrome. In: StatPearls [Internet]. Treasure Island (FL): StatPearls Publishing; 2021. [online] Available from http://www.ncbi.nlm.nih.gov/books/NBK534872/. [Last accessed September, 2021].
10. Cherqui S, Courtoy PJ. The renal Fanconi syndrome in cystinosis: pathogenic insights and therapeutic perspectives. Nat Rev Nephrol. 2017;13(2):115-31.
11. Kawashima H, Kraut JA, Kurokawa K. Metabolic acidosis suppresses 25-hydroxyvitamin in D3-1alpha-hydroxylase in the rat kidney. Distinct site and mechanism of action. J Clin Invest. 1982;70(1):135-40.
12. Flyvbjerg A, Dørup I, Everts ME, Orskov H. Evidence that potassium deficiency induces growth retardation through reduced circulating levels of growth hormone and insulin-like growth factor I. Metabolism. 1991;40(8):769-75.
13. Brüngger M, Hulter HN, Krapf R. Effect of chronic metabolic acidosis on the growth hormone/IGF-1 endocrine axis: new cause of growth hormone insensitivity in humans. Kidney Int. 1997;51(1):216-21.
14. Hohenfellner K, Rauch F, Ariceta G, Awan A, Bacchetta J, Bergmann C, et al. Management of bone disease in cystinosis: Statement from an international conference. J Inherit Metab Dis. 2019;42(5):1019-29.
15. Bagga A, Sinha A. Renal tubular acidosis. Indian J Pediatr. 2020;87(9):733-44.
16. Hall AM, Trepiccione F, Unwin RJ. Drug toxicity in the proximal tubule: new models, methods and mechanisms. Pediatr Nephrol. 2021. Online ahead of print.
17. Kitterer D, Schwab M, Alscher MD, Braun N, Latus J. Drug-induced acid-base disorders. Pediatr Nephrol. 2015;30(9): 1407-23.
18. Foreman JW, Roth KS. Human renal Fanconi syndrome—then and now. Nephron. 1989;51(3):301-6.
19. Kashoor I, Batlle D. Proximal renal tubular acidosis with and without Fanconi syndrome. Kidney Res Clin Pract. 2019;38(3): 267-81.
20. Ariceta G, Giordano V, Santos F. Effects of long-term cysteamine treatment in patients with cystinosis. Pediatr Nephrol. 2019; 34(4):571-8.
21. van Ginkel WG, Rodenburg IL, Harding CO, Hollak CEM, Heiner-Fokkema MR, van Spronsen FJ. Long-term outcomes and practical considerations in the pharmacological management of tyrosinemia type 1. Paediatr Drugs. 2019;21(6):413-26.
22. Kasimer RN, Langman CB. Adult complications of nephropathic cystinosis: a systematic review. Pediatr Nephrol. 2021;36:223-36.
23. Ehlayel AM, Copelovitch L. Update on Dent disease. Pediatr Clin North Am. 2019;66:169-78.
24. Gianesello L, Del Prete D, Ceol M, Priante G, Calò LA, Anglani F. From protein uptake to Dent disease: An overview of the CLCN5 gene. Gene. 2020;747:144662.
25. Gianesello L, Del Prete D, Anglani F, Calò LA. Genetics and phenotypic heterogeneity of Dent disease: the dark side of the moon. Hum Genet. 2021;140(3):401-21.
26. Cho HY, Lee BH, Choi HJ, Ha IS, Choi Y, Cheong HI. Renal manifestations of Dent disease and Lowe syndrome. Pediatr Nephrol. 2008;23(2):243-9.
27. De Matteis MA, Staiano L, Emma F, Devuyst O. The 5-phosphatase OCRL in Lowe syndrome and Dent disease 2. Nat Rev Nephrol. 2017;13(8):455-70.
28. Gambaro G, Naticchia A, Ferraro PM, Spagnoletti G, Romagnoli J, Salerno MP, et al. Living kidney donation in a type 1 Dent's disease patient from his mother. Kidney Blood Press Res. 2019; 44:1306-12.
29. Bökenkamp A, Ludwig M. The oculocerebrorenal syndrome of Lowe: an update. Pediatr Nephrol. 2016;31:2201-12.
30. Loi M. Lowe syndrome. Orphanet J Rare Dis. 2006;1:16.
31. Röschinger W, Muntau AC, Rudolph G, Roscher AA, Kammerer S. Carrier assessment in families with Lowe oculocerebrorenal syndrome: novel mutations in the OCRL1 gene and correlation of direct DNA diagnosis with ocular examination. Mol Genet Metab. 2000;69:213-22.
32. Goodyer P. The history of cystinosis: Lessons for clinical management. Int J Nephrol. 2011;2011:e929456.
33. Emma F, Nesterova G, Langman C, Labbé A, Cherqui S, Goodyer P, et al. Nephropathic cystinosis: an international consensus document. Nephrol Dial Transplant. 2014;29(Suppl 4):iv87-94.
34. Veys KR, Elmonem MA, Arcolino FO, van den Heuvel L, Levtchenko E. Nephropathic cystinosis: an update. Curr Opin Pediatr. 2017;29(2):168-78.
35. Elmonem MA, Veys KR, Soliman NA, van Dyck M, van den Heuvel LP, Levtchenko E. Cystinosis: a review. Orphanet J Rare Dis. 2016;11:47.
36. Langman CB. Oh cystinosin: let me count the ways! Kidney Int. 2019;96:275-7.
37. Town M, Jean G, Cherqui S, Attard M, Forestier L, Whitmore SA, et al. A novel gene encoding an integral membrane protein is mutated in nephropathic cystinosis. Nat Genet. 1998;18:319-24.
38. Anikster Y, Shotelersuk V, Gahl WA. CTNS mutations in patients with cystinosis. Hum Mutat. 1999;14:454-8.
39. Wilmer MJ, Emma F, Levtchenko EN. The pathogenesis of cystinosis: mechanisms beyond cystine accumulation. Am J Physiol Renal Physiol. 2010;299:F905-16.
40. Ivanova EA, van den Heuvel LP, Elmonem MA, De Smedt H, Missiaen L, Pastore A, et al. Altered mTOR signalling in nephropathic cystinosis. J Inherit Metab Dis. 2016;39:457-64.
41. Napolitano G, Johnson JL, He J, Rocca CJ, Monfregola J, Pestonjamasp K, et al. Impairment of chaperone-mediated autophagy leads to selective lysosomal degradation defects in the lysosomal storage disease cystinosis. EMBO Mol Med. 2015;7:158-74.
42. Wilmer MJ, Schoeber JP, van den Heuvel LP, Levtchenko EN. Cystinosis: practical tools for diagnosis and treatment. Pediatr Nephrol. 2011;26:205-15.

43. Gahl WA, Balog JZ, Kleta R. Nephropathic cystinosis in adults: natural history and effects of oral cysteamine therapy. Ann Intern Med. 2007;147:242-50.
44. Atmis B, K Bayazit A, Cevizli D, Kor D, Fidan HB, Bisgin A, et al. More than tubular dysfunction: cystinosis and kidney outcomes. J Nephrol. 2021. Online ahead of print.
45. Bengali M, Goodman S, Sun X, Dohil MA, Dohil R, Newbury R, et al. Non-invasive intradermal imaging of cystine crystals in cystinosis. PLoS One. 2021;16:e0247846.
46. Buntinx L, Voets T, Morlion B, Vangeel L, Janssen M, Cornelissen E, et al. TRPV1 dysfunction in cystinosis patients harboring the homozygous 57 kb deletion. Scientific Rep. 2016;6:35395.
47. Raut S, Khandelwal P, Sinha A, Thakur R, Puraswani M, Velpandian T, et al. Infantile nephropathic cystinosis: Clinical features and outcome. Asian J Pediatr Nephrol. 2020;3(1):15.
48. Cohen C, Charbit M, Chadefaux-Vekemans B, Giral M, Garrigue V, Kessler M, et al. Excellent long-term outcome of renal transplantation in cystinosis patients. Orphanet J Rare Dis. 2015;10:90.
49. Levtchenko EN, van Dael CM, de Graaf-Hess AC, Wilmer MJG, van den Heuvel LP, Monnens LA, et al. Strict cysteamine dose regimen is required to prevent nocturnal cystine accumulation in cystinosis. Pediatr Nephrol. 2006;21(1):110-3.
50. Linden S, Klank S, Harms E, Grüneberg M, Park JH, Marquardt T. Cystinosis: Therapy adherence and metabolic monitoring in patients treated with immediate-release cysteamine. Mol Genet Metab Rep. 2020;24:100620.
51. Elmonem MA, Veys K, Oliveira Arcolino F, Van Dyck M, Benedetti MC, Diomedi-Camassei F, et al. Allogeneic HSCT transfers wild-type cystinosin to nonhematological epithelial cells in cystinosis: First human report. Am J Transplant. 2018; 18(11):2823-8.
52. Harrison F, Yeagy BA, Rocca CJ, Kohn DB, Salomon DR, Cherqui S. Hematopoietic stem cell gene therapy for the multisystemic lysosomal storage disorder cystinosis. Mol Ther. 2013;21(2):433-44.

CHAPTER

8.3

Bartter Syndrome and Gitelman Syndrome

Mahantesh V Patil, Jyoti Sharma

INTRODUCTION

Bartter and Gitelman syndromes (BS and GS, respectively) are hereditary salt-losing tubulopathies (SLT) characterized by variable extents of volume depletion, hypokalemic, and hypochloremic metabolic alkalosis. Since the first description of BS by Frederic Bartter in 1962, there have been great advancements in understanding of the pathophysiology and in molecular diagnosis. The initial classification of different subtypes of BS was mainly focused on the age at presentation, distinguishing *antenatal variants of BS* (including BS1, BS2, BS4, and BS5), all typically associated with severe polyhydramnios causing premature birth from *classical BS* (BS3) that has a later milder presentation.[1] At present, mutations in at least seven genes involved in the reabsorption of sodium and chloride in the thick ascending limb of the loop of Henle (TAL) and/or the distal convoluted tubule (DCT) have been implicated in these disorders.[2] Bartter syndrome 1–4, GS, and EAST (epilepsy, ataxia, sensorineural deafness, and tubulopathy) are inherited as autosomal-recessive disorders, while BS type 5 is inherited as an X-linked recessive disorder.

A pathophysiological classification proposes separating the various types into disorders of the TAL, of DCT, or of both segments. *Disorders of the TAL*, present in the antenatal period, are characterized by hypercalciuria and nephrocalcinosis and are equivalent to the use of loop diuretics. They occur due to mutations in *SLC12A1* (NKCC2) or *ROMK* (KCNJ1). In contrast, *disorders of the DCT* are characterized by hypo- or normocalciuria and hypomagnesemia and typically manifest later in childhood or adolescence. They mimic the use of thiazide diuretics and may occur due to mutations in *CLCNKB* or *SLC12A3* (NCCT). The *compound disorders* affecting both segments are usually caused by BSND (Barttin) mutations or combined CLCNK-B/A mutations and typically have a severe antenatal presentation.[3,4] However, there is significant clinical heterogeneity in presentation and a precise genotype-phenotype correlation is not possible.[2] Hence, when a precise diagnosis is required, genetic analysis should be done **(Table 1)**.

PATHOPHYSIOLOGY OF SALT-LOSING TUBULOPATHIES

Physiology of Sodium Chloride and Magnesium Reabsorption

Healthy kidneys reabsorb almost 99% of the filtered load of water and electrolytes, with about 60% of the reabsorption of *sodium* occurring in the proximal tubule, 30% in the TAL, 5–10% in the early DCT, and the remainder in the aldosterone-sensitive distal tubule (ASDT). Approximately 2,500 mg of *magnesium* is filtered per day, of which 96% is reabsorbed along the nephron. Only a small portion (5–15%) is reabsorbed in the proximal tubule and 50–72% is reabsorbed passively through the paracellular pathway in the TAL. Active reabsorption of Mg^{2+} takes place at the apical Mg^{2+} channel, TRPM6, at the DCT and accounts for 10% of the total filtered load and determines the final urinary secretion of Mg^{2+}.[3]

Sodium transport in the TAL and early DCT is accomplished by the active reabsorption of Na^+ with Cl^- from the tubular fluid[5] **(Fig. 1)**. In the TAL, luminal sodium (Na^+) is reabsorbed electroneutrally—half by the sodium-potassium-chloride co-transporter (NKCC2) and half by taking a paracellular route by cation-selective intercellular pathways. The NKCC2 also transports one K^+ and two Cl^- ions for each sodium ion. Potassium that enters the TAL cell via NKCC2 is recycled back to the tubular urine through the luminal renal outer medulla potassium channels (ROMK). This replenishes the urinary K^+ that would otherwise decrease along the TAL and ensures NKCC2 activity along this tubular segment. In addition, it establishes a lumen-positive transepithelial voltage gradient that drives paracellular transport of cations such as Na^+ (50% of the total absorbed in this portion of the tubule), Ca^{2+}, and Mg^{2+} via claudins. Sodium is actively pumped out of the TAL cell by the basolateral sodium-potassium-ATPase pump (Na-K-ATPase) in exchange for K^+. Chloride leaves the cell basolaterally through specific chloride channels (ClC-Ka *and* ClC-Kb). The operation of both chloride channels requires the B-subunit Barttin.[5-7]

TABLE 1: Salient features of salt-losing tubulopathies.

	BS type 1	*BS type 2*	*BS type 4*	*BS type 3*	*BS type 5*	*Gitelman*	*EAST*
Gene	*SLC12A1*	*KCNJ1*	*4a BSND or 4b CLCNKA and CLCNKB*	*CLCNKB*	*MAGED2*	*SLC12A3*	*KCNJ10*
Mode of inheritance	AR	AR	AR	AR	XLR	AR	AR
Segment of tubule	TAL	TAL + CD	TAL + DCT	DCT + (TAL)	TAL	DCT	DCT
Channel	NKCC2	ROMK	4a Barttin ClC-Ka and ClC-Kb	ClC-Kb	MAGED2	NCCT	KCNJ10
Age of presentation	Perinatal	Perinatal	Perinatal	0–5 years	Perinatal	Childhood	Infancy
Polyhydramnios Prematurity	+	+	+	–	+	–	–
Other features at presentation		Hyperkalemia in initial stages	Sensorineural hearing loss Magnesium wasting Deterioration of renal function in infancy	Presentation with polyuria polydipsia dehydration, salt craving	Transient neonatal BS Magnesium wasting	Tetany magnesium wasting, hypocalciuria	Epilepsy, ataxia, sensorineural deafness Hypocalciuria Magnesium wasting
Hypercalciuria and nephrocalcinosis	+	+	–	±	+	–	–

(AR: autosomal recessive; BS: Bartter syndrome; DCT: distal convoluted tubule; EAST: epilepsy, ataxia, sensorineural deafness, and tubulopathy; NKCC: sodium–potassium–chloride co-transporter; ROMK: renal outer medulla potassium; MAGED2: melanoma-associated antigen D2; TAL: thick ascending limb of loop of Henle; XLR: X-linked recessive; SLC12A1: solute carrier family 12 member1; SLC12A3: solute carrier family 12 member 3; CD: collecting duct; NCCT: sodium chloride co-transporter; KCNJ10: potassium inwardly rectifying channel subfamily J member 10; ClC-Ka: chloride channel Ka; ClC-Kb: chloride channel Kb)

One of the major functions of the TAL is to generate and maintain a high tonicity in the interstitium as a prerequisite for countercurrent exchange and the urinary concentration and dilution mechanism. The high osmolality generated here results from the fact that the TAL that is the site for 25–30% NaCl absorption is impermeable to water.

The juxtaglomerular apparatus consists of the macula densa (modified epithelial cells of the tubule in the transition zone between the TAL and DCT), granular cells of the afferent arteriole of the same nephron, and adjacent extraglomerular mesangial cells **(Fig. 2)**. It couples the sodium chloride concentration of the tubular fluid to renal hemodynamics, i.e., the tubuloglomerular feedback (TGF). Sodium chloride concentration in the tubular lumen is sensed via apical sodium chloride uptake by NKCC2 assisted by ROMK and basolateral chloride release (ClC-K and Barttin). This triggers a series of intracellular signaling events and release of paracrine signaling molecules such as prostaglandin E2 (PGE2), ATP, adenosine, and nitric oxide. In case of an increased sodium chloride concentration at the macula densa, the TGF induces afferent arteriole vasoconstriction and a drop in glomerular filtration rate (GFR) and decreases renin release, whereas a decreased macula-dense sodium chloride concentration dilates the afferent arteriole and increases renin release.[8]

In the DCT, fine-tuning of Na concentration occurs with a reabsorptive capacity of 10% of sodium chloride, almost exclusively by the transcellular route mediated by the luminal sodium chloride co-transporter (NCCT) **(Fig. 3)**. The NCCT transports one Na^+ ion with one Cl^-. Active extrusion of Na^+ occurs at the basolateral membrane by the Na-K-ATPase, and the inwardly rectifying potassium channels KCNJ 10 (Kir4.1) complement its activity. These channels allow recirculation of potassium into the tubular cell, thus supplying the Na-K-ATPase pump necessary K^+ for continuous transport of Na^+ and thereby also generating an electrochemical gradient that favors transcellular Cl^- transport. In the DCT, basolateral exit of Cl^- occurs through ClC-Kb. Reabsorption of Ca^{++} and Mg^{++} in the DCT is active and transcellular in nature, consisting of uptake through selective ion channels *TRPV5* and *TRPM6*, respectively. Reabsorption of magnesium is driven by the activity of the basolateral Na-K-ATPase and is directly proportional to the transcellular transport of Na^+. That is why DCT disorders of Na^+ reabsorption are associated with urinary magnesium wasting and hypomagnesemia.[5-7]

In the ASDT, most of the reabsorption of Na^+ occurs via the amiloride-sensitive epithelial sodium channel (ENaC). Chloride is transported separately between the epithelial cells by a passive process. The ubiquitous basolateral Na-K-ATPase that is responsible for electrogenic extrusion of Na^+ at the basolateral membrane creates a lumen-negative transepithelial voltage that drives the paracellular Cl^- transport. In the interest of intracellular electroneutrality, for

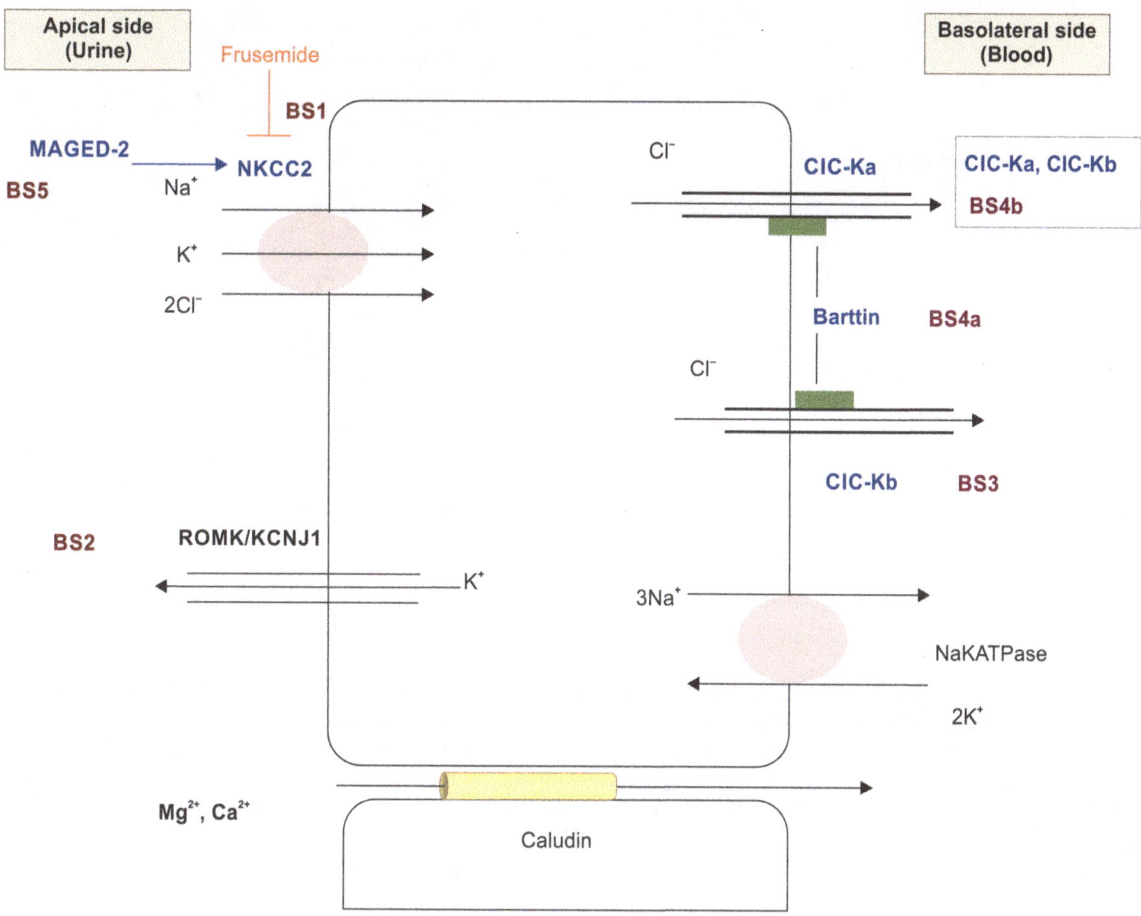

Fig. 1: Electrolyte transport in the thick ascending limb of loop of Henle (TAL). The sodium–potassium–chloride cotransporter (NKCC2) transport imports one sodium, one potassium, and two chloride ions from the lumen into the cell. This transporter can be blocked by loop diuretics. Inherited dysfunction causes Bartter syndrome type 1 (BS1). Potassium leaves the cell via the luminal *KCNJ1* channel, mutations in which cause Bartter syndrome type 2 (BS2). Chloride leaves the cell via the basolateral chloride transporters CLCN-kb and CLCN-ka, both of which need the Barttin subunit in order to function. Mutations in CLCNKB cause Bartter syndrome type 3 (BS3) and in Barttin, these cause Bartter syndrome type 4a (BS4a); combined dysfunction of the CLCN-ka and CLCN-kb channels causes Bartter syndrome type 4b (BS4b). Sodium leaves the cell via the basolateral Na–K-ATPase that exports three sodium ions and imports two potassium ions. Mutations in the gene encoding *MAGED-2* result in a transient decreased expression of NKCC2 in the antenatal period, causing Bartter syndrome type 5 (BS5). Recycling of potassium into the lumen and the resultant lumen-positive transepithelial potential drives paracellular uptake of calcium and magnesium. Therefore, hypercalciuria with nephrocalcinosis and hypermagnesuria is typically seen in Bartter syndromes type 1 (NKCC2), type 2 (KCNJ1), and type 5 (MAGE-D2), while it can be variable in Bartter syndromes type 3 (CLCNKB), type 4a (Barttin), and type 4b (combined CLCNKA and CLCNKB).

each Na^+ ion, which enters the tubular cell via ENaC, secretion of one K^+ ion occurs via luminal ROMK potassium channels. In situations of increased urine flow, K^+ secretion is reinforced by large flow-dependent high-conductance potassium channels (BK), which are expressed at the apical cell membrane.[6,9]

Pathophysiology

In isolated loop disorders, there is upregulation of DCT functions as well as that of the ASDT, whereas in DCT disorders, the ASDT is complemented by upregulation of TAL functions.[10] This upregulation as well as compensatory mechanisms, i.e., secondary hyperaldosteronism, has a major impact on the clinical presentation of patients with salt-losing tubulopathies.

In patients with defects of sodium chloride reabsorption in the TAL or the DCT, there is salt and water wasting resulting in *polyuria* and *polydipsia*. A reduction in extracellular fluid volume activates compensatory mechanisms for sodium conservation, i.e., stimulation of renin secretion, angiotensin II, and aldosterone synthesis. Secondary hyperaldosteronism, in an attempt to increase Na^+ retention at the expense of an increased K^+ excretion, eventually results in *hypokalemia*.

As mentioned above, Na^+ wasting along the TAL and early DCT is accompanied by decreased reabsorption of Cl^-. Though Na^+ is recovered partially by increased reabsorption along the ASDT (by ENaC), Cl^- gets lost in the urine resulting in *hypochloremia*. To maintain electroneutrality, distal Na^+ reabsorption occurs at the cost of excretion of other cations such as NH_4^+ and K^+. Ammonium is the main carrier of protons in the urine, and its secretion results in *metabolic alkalosis*. Potassium loss aggravates *hypokalemia* caused by secondary hyperaldosteronism.

Impaired activity of one of the transport proteins NKCC2, ROMK, ClC-K, and Barttin not only results in salt-wasting due

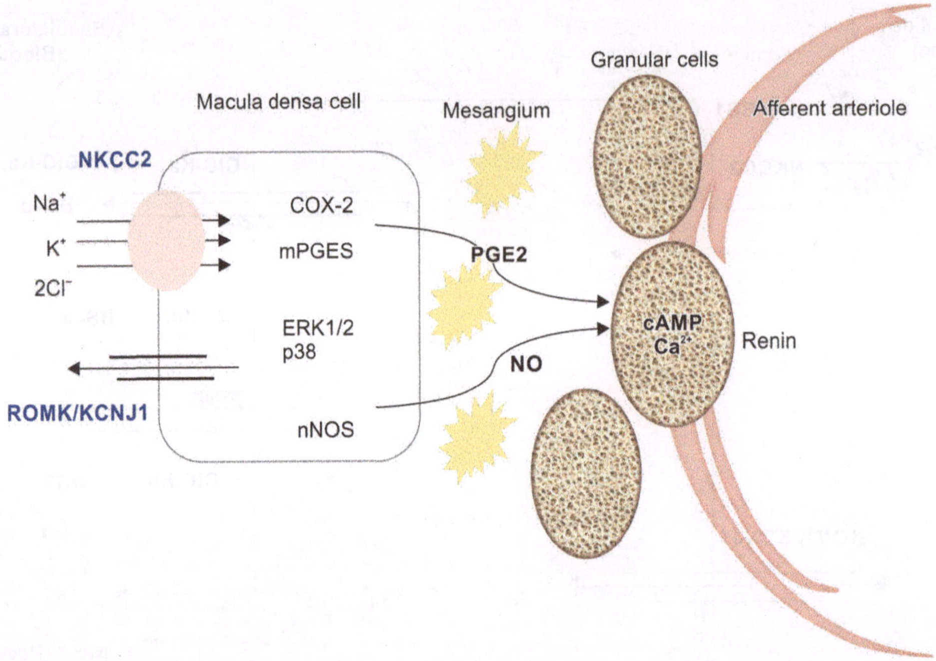

Fig. 2: Schematic diagram of the juxtaglomerular apparatus showing control mechanisms of renin release and elements of the macula densa sensing and signaling apparatus. Macula densa cells can sense variations in tubular fluid sodium chloride. Salt is sensed via the sodium–potassium–chloride cotransporter (NKCC2). Signal transduction includes activation of mitogen-activated protein (MAP) kinases p38 and pERK1/2, prostaglandin E2 (PGE2) synthesis through cyclooxygenase-2 (COX-2), and microsomal prostaglandin E synthase (mPGES). PGE2 via paracrine signaling causes increased renin synthesis and release from adjacent juxtaglomerular cells and activation of the renin–angiotensin system (RAS). (nNOS: neural nitric oxide synthase; NO: nitric oxide; ROMK: renal outer medulla potassium channel)
Source: Adapted from Peti-Peterdi J, Harris RC. Macula Densa Sensing and Signaling Mechanisms of Renin Release: Figure 1. J Am Soc Nephrol. 2010;21(7):1093-6.

to reduced TAL salt-reabsorbing capacity, but also because there is impaired "salt sensing" at the macula densa. This incorrect signal of a low tubular salt concentration leads to increased PGE2 synthesis, a phenomenon that gave the name of *hyperprostaglandin E syndrome* during the initial descriptions of this disease. PGE2 inhibits the TGF and causes afferent arteriole dilatation and promotes renin formation, which aggravates salt wasting by increasing the GFR by angiotensin II-mediated constriction of the efferent arteriole. PGE2 also has diuretic effects, which further aggravate salt wasting. Thus, impaired salt reabsorption in TAL leads to a blinding of the macula densa resulting in increased renin production, which is irrespective of volume status.[2] Increased systemic PGE2 activity causes fever, vomiting, diarrhea, failure to thrive, and osteopenia.[10] These features are not seen in children with GS where the defect is in the TAL.

In patients with TAL defects of the *NKCC*, *ROMK*, or *ClCKB*, the loss of the lumen-positive transepithelial voltage gradient leads to impaired paracellular calcium reabsorption and increased luminal calcium loss. In these patients, there is upregulated DCT Na^+ transport via NCCT, high intracellular Na^+ concentration, which in turn inhibits Ca^{++} extrusion across the basolateral membrane via the Na^+/Ca^{++} exchanger NCX1, resulting in a high intracellular Ca^{++} concentration. This leads to reduced apical Ca^{++} entry through the Ca-selective channel TRPV5 allowing *hypercalciuria* and manifesting as *nephrocalcinosis and osteopenia* even during infancy. On the other hand, expression and activity of the Mg-specific channel TRPM6 are increased, counteracting at least in part urinary magnesium wasting in the upstream tubular segment.[10]

Children with defects in the TAL usually have *hyposthenuria* since dilution of tubular fluid and generation of the interstitial concentration gradient due to the sodium reabsorption are integral to the countercurrent concentrating mechanism. Impaired DCT salt reabsorption and resultant salt loss indirectly increase renal water excretion but do not interfere with urinary concentrating capability so the urinary osmolality may remain normal in patients with isolated mutations in *CLCNKB* or *SLC12A3 (NCCT)*. Compensatory increased reabsorption activity in the proximal tubule and the upregulated TAL segment are responsible for enhanced sodium and chloride reabsorption. These two compensating effects result in *much less salt and water wasting in DCT disorders than in loop disorders*. Moreover, increased Ca^{++} uptake through the activated TRPV5 channel selectively prevents hypercalciuria.[9,10]

Distal convoluted tubule disorders are characterized by *hypocalciuria* though the exact mechanism is not clear. One explanation for this is that reduced intracellular Na^+ concentration due to decreased luminal absorption results in increased Na uptake and increased Ca^{++} extrusion via an Na^+/Ca^{++} exchanger across the basolateral membrane.

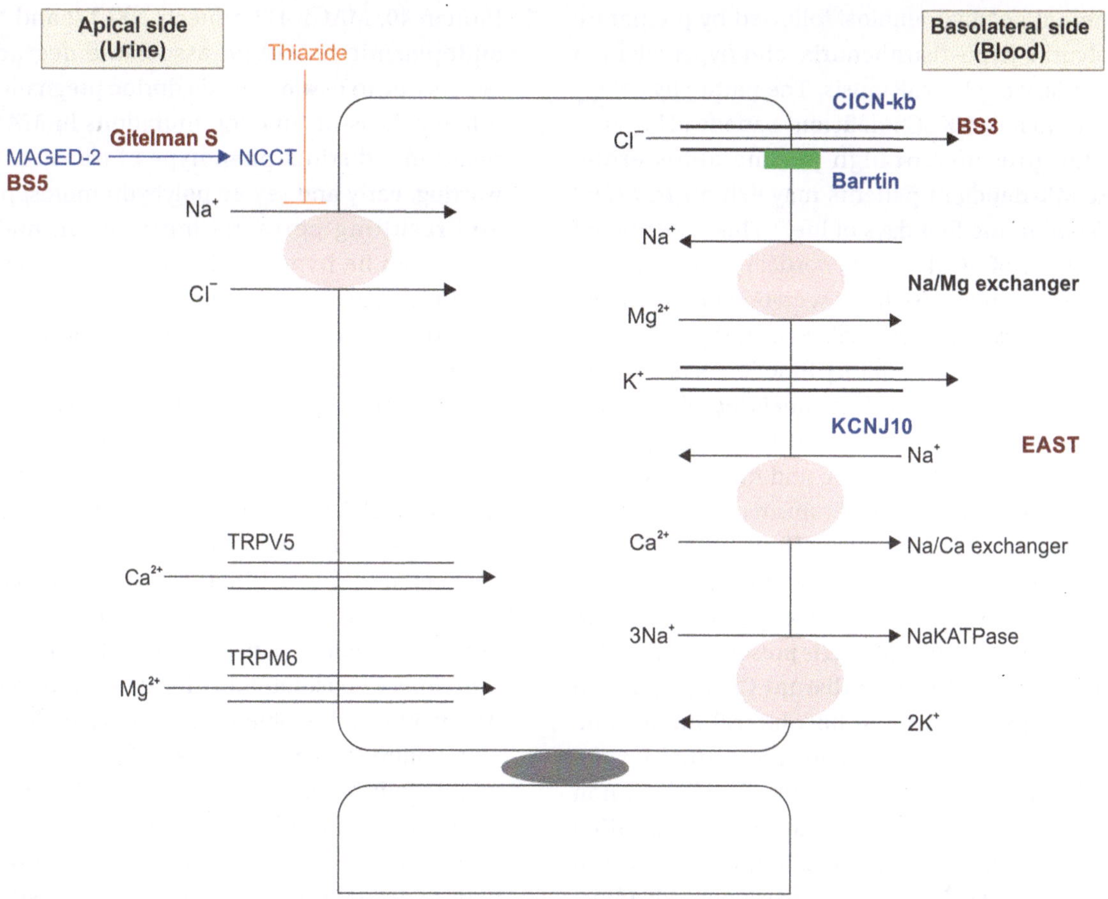

Fig. 3: Electrolyte transport in the distal convoluted tubule (DCT). The NCCT imports one sodium, one potassium and two chloride ion from the lumen into the cell. This transporter can be blocked by thiazide diuretics. Mutations in the gene encoding NCCT cause Gitelman syndrome. Chloride leaves the cell via the basolateral CLCN-kb channel, which needs the Barttin subunit in order to function. Both proteins are expressed in both the thick ascending limb of loop of Henle (TAL) and DCT, and their decreased function can cause Bartter syndrome (types 3 and 4a, respectively). Sodium can exit the cell via the basolateral Na–K-ATPase that actively exports three sodium ions while importing two potassium ions. Potassium is immediately recycled and pumped out of the cell by the basolateral potassium channel KCNJ10, mutations in which cause EAST syndrome. Calcium and magnesium are imported by TRPV5 and TRPM6, respectively. A Na/Mg exchanger is present in the basolateral responsible for extrusion of Mg^{2+}.

The resultant intracellular decrease of Ca^{++} concentration facilitates apical cell membrane Ca^{++} entry through the Ca-selective channel TRPV5. Another explanation is that there is increased calcium reabsorption in the proximal tubule secondary to extracellular volume contraction. Irrespective of the pathophysiology, hypocalciuria is a distinct feature of DCT disorders, whereas hypercalciuria is typical for TAL disorders.

Pathogenesis of hypomagnesemia is explained by downregulation of TRPM6; decreased absorptive surface area for Mg^{2+} has also been seen in experimental studies.[9]

CLINICAL PRESENTATION (TABLE 1)

- *Bartter syndrome 1, antenatal Bartter syndrome: Defect in the furosemide-sensitive Na-K-2Cl⁻ cotransporter:* Antenatal Bartter syndrome (aBS) is a severe phenotype caused by disruption of sodium chloride reabsorption in the TAL. One of the causes is inactivating mutations of *SLC12A1* (solute carrier *12A1* gene), which encodes NKCC2. Onset is within the second trimester with fetal polyuria leading to maternal polyhydramnios and premature delivery around 32 weeks of gestation. These newborns suffer from profound polyuria of about 20 mL/kg/h, and the urine is usually hyposthenuric. They may have life-threatening episodes of dehydration, failure to thrive, and growth retardation. Due to the high urinary calcium excretion, medullary nephrocalcinosis develops within the first months of life. Some children may have typical facies, characterized by a triangular-shaped face, prominent forehead, large eyes, prominent ears, drooping mouth, and strabismus.[9] They may also have fever without a focus, diarrhea, vomiting, generalized seizures, and recurrent urinary tract infections. Osteopenia is also common. Renal function is usually well preserved in aBS with rare children with progressive renal failure leading to end-stage kidney disease (ESKD).
- *Bartter syndrome 2: Defect in the renal outer medullary potassium channel:* Mutations in the *KCNJ1* gene cause deficiency of ROMK channel and antenatal presentation

with maternal polyhydramnios, followed by premature birth, polyuria, hypo-/isosthenuria, and hypercalciuria with secondary nephrocalcinosis. The pathophysiology is similar to that of NKCC2-deficient patients. However, despite the presence of high plasma aldosterone levels, ROMK-deficient patients may exhibit *transient hyperkalemia* in the first days of life.[11] This is attributed to the presence of ROMK in the cortical collecting duct (CCD) where it is responsible for secretion of potassium, and its absence results in hyperkalemia. The hyperkalemia is transient because the secretory function is taken over by the upregulation of the big K channels that also secrete potassium in the CCD. In the immediate neonatal period, the hyperkalemia, hyponatremia, and high aldosterone levels mimic pseudohypoaldosteronism type I.

- *Bartter syndrome 4a: Barttin defect:* The β-subunit Barttin is essential for the function of the chloride channels ClC-Ka and ClC-Kb. While the TAL is populated with both isoforms, in the DCT, only ClC-Kb is present. Inactivating mutations in the *BSND* gene disrupt CLC-K function and chloride exit across the basolateral membrane in both the *TAL and DCT,* a feature essential for the function of NKCC1. Patients with the *BSND* mutation have a severe form of Bartter syndrome resembling that of NKCC2 and ROMK defects. In addition, Barttin defects are also associated with sensorineural deafness because a properly functioning NKCC1 and CLC-K Barttin complex are required for endolymph formation in the inner ear. Hypermagnesuric hypomagnesemia is usually significant due to disruption of both magnesium reabsorption pathways—the paracellular one in the TAL and the transcellular one in the DCT. They usually do not have hypercalciuria and nephrocalcinosis. This could be due to defective NaCl transport in both the TAL and DCT, with divergent effects on urinary calcium excretion. These children have poor response to nonsteroidal anti-inflammatory drugs (NSAIDs) and develop renal dysfunction in infancy and progress to ESKD. Renal biopsy in these children shows focal segmental glomerular sclerosis possibly due to intraglomerular hyperfiltration and elevated angiotensin II levels.
- *Bartter syndrome 4b, digenic disorder: The ClC-Ka/b phenotype*: Inactivating mutations in both the ClC-Ka and ClC-Kb chloride channels result in a clinical picture similar to that of patients who are Barttin deficient (BS4a).[12]
- *Bartter syndrome 5, transient antenatal Bartter syndrome: MAGED2 mutation*: This is a recently described entity, also known as "acute recurrent polyhydramnios." The gene *MAGED2* encodes melanoma-associated antigen D2 (MAGE-D2) and maps to the X chromosome. MAGE-D2 affects the expression and function of the sodium chloride co-transporters NKCC2 and NCCT during fetal development. Through its interaction with Heat Shock Protein 40, MAGE-D2 protects NKCC2 and NCCT from endoplasmic reticulum-associated degradation that occurs due to tissue hypoxia during pregnancy and early infancy. Loss-of-function mutations in *MAGED2* gene result in a distinct phenotype of transient renal salt-wasting, early and severe polyhydramnios, prematurity, and resulting perinatal mortality in male fetuses. There can be hypercalciuria, hypermagnesuria, and nephrocalcinosis. It is postulated that the effect of the mutation is transient because developmental changes permit expression of NKCC2 and NCCT independent of MAGE-D2 beyond a certain stage of renal development.[13]
- *Bartter syndrome type 3, classic Bartter syndrome: Defect in the basolateral chloride channel ClC-Kb*: An isolated defect of ClC-Kb, which is encoded by the *CLCNKB* gene, leads to a more variable and milder phenotype of BS, similar to that originally described by Bartter, hence known as classic BS. ClC-Kb defect results in dysfunction of the DCT mainly, since ClC-Ka takes over some of the functions of basolateral chloride excretion in the TAL. About 50% of the patients present in the first year of life with failure to thrive, episodes of hypokalemic alkalosis and dehydration, muscle cramps and tetany, muscular hypotonia, and lethargy. They may also have growth retardation and osteopenia. An antenatal presentation, with maternal polyhydramnios that is usually mild, is seen in a small percentage of patients. Of note, hearing in children with BS3 is normal because the function of ClC-Kb/Barttin channels in the inner ear can be replaced by ClC-Ka/Barttin.

  Most patients have high urinary magnesium losses, hypomagnesemia, and normal or low urinary calcium excretion. ClC-Kb deficiency thus mimics GS.[14,15]

TREATMENT

Treatment is aimed at maintaining adequate fluid and electrolyte balance and allowing growth to occur.[7]

In children with aBS, in the immediate postnatal period, it is essential to maintain euvolemia and replenish electrolytes with intravenous fluid. Losses are very high, i.e., urine output may be ~50 mL/kg/day, with very large losses of Na^+ (up to 45 mEq/kg/day) and Cl^- in the urine. Potassium replacement is usually required after 2–3 weeks of life. Both sodium and potassium chloride can be then replaced with oral solutions divided in three to four doses and titrated for each neonate's requirement.[16]

Prostaglandin inhibitors inhibit renal and systemic prostaglandin synthesis and decrease polyuria, convert hyposthenuria to isosthenuria, reduce hypercalciuria, and stimulate catch-up growth.[7] NSAIDs are, however, started cautiously to avoid precipitating acute kidney injury and in view of the risks of gastrointestinal ulcers, perforation, and necrotizing enterocolitis in the premature neonate. The drug that may be used is indomethacin, which is started at a dose of 0.05 mg/kg/day and gradually increased to 2.5 mg/kg/day according to its effects on urinary output. Thiazides should not be used to reduce hypercalciuria, since they interfere with compensatory mechanisms in the DCT and further aggravate salt and fluid losses.

Treatment of Classic Bartter Syndrome

The primary aim is to correct hypokalemia and alkalosis by maintaining adequate hydration and by oral potassium chloride supplements in a dose of 1–3 mEq/kg/day. In addition, these children require indomethacin (2–5 mg/kg/day); alternatively ibuprofen in a dose of up to 30 mg/kg/day may be used.[16] Children with hypomagnesaemia may require the addition of magnesium salts.

LONG-TERM FOLLOW-UP OF PATIENTS

Though BS was earlier considered to be a benign disorder that could be managed with salt supplements and NSAIDs, it has now emerged that these children have long-term morbidity seen as growth failure, osteopenia, impaired renal function, and proteinuria on follow-up. Growth hormone deficiency has been demonstrated in some patients, and a positive response observed following therapy with recombinant human growth hormone.

Impaired renal function in BS has been attributed to a combination of long-standing hypokalemia, hypovolemic episodes, nephrocalcinosis, intraglomerular hyperfiltration, chronic activation of the renin–angiotensin–aldosterone system (RAAS), and toxicity of NSAID.[9] Hypokalemic nephropathy manifesting as renal cysts has been seen in patients with classic BS.

Renal biopsy findings in some children with *BSND* have shown focal segmental glomerular sclerosis, mesangial hypercellularity, tubulointerstitial fibrosis, and tubular atrophy.[17]

DIFFERENTIAL DIAGNOSIS OF BARTTER SYNDROME

The differential diagnosis of hypokalemic, metabolic alkalosis includes vomiting in young infants, especially that related to *pyloric stenosis*. Older children with BS present with failure to thrive and the characteristic metabolic abnormalities (hypokalemic and hypochloremic metabolic alkalosis), and this may be closely mimicked by cystic fibrosis. Demonstration of increased urinary chloride excretion in children with BS can help to distinguish between renal and nonrenal causes of chloride loss. The differential diagnosis of metabolic abnormalities of BS includes the surreptitious use of loop diuretics and excessive use of laxatives, but both are rare in children. A Bartter-like syndrome has been described in patients treated with aminoglycosides and resolves 2–6 weeks after stopping the drug.[18,19]

GITELMAN SYNDROME: DEFECT IN *SLC12A3* GENE ENCODING THE Na^+–Cl^- COTRANSPORTER

Gitelman syndrome is very heterogeneous with respect to age at presentation, biochemical abnormalities, and clinical manifestations. Patients usually present toward the end of the first decade or later, variously with short stature, delayed puberty, carpopedal spasms due to hypomagnesemia, muscle weakness, fatigue, poor exercise endurance, salt craving, polydipsia, nocturia or enuresis, and constipation. Hypomagnesemia decreases the solubility of calcium pyrophosphate crystals and promotes their formation in joints and sclera, leading to chondrocalcinosis and sclerochoroidal calcifications.[20,21] Potassium and Mg^{2+} depletion typically causes low blood pressure and prolonged QT interval in ~50% of the patients, which predisposes to an increased risk for ventricular arrhythmias.[22]

Treatment of BS includes liberal salt intake and lifelong oral magnesium and potassium supplementations. Magnesium repletion facilitates K^+ repletion and reduces the symptoms. Though any magnesium salt may be used, $MgCl_2$ is recommended since it will also correct the urinary loss of Cl. Available in India are 25% magnesium sulfate as an injectable formulation and tablet magnesium oxide 400 mg (60% Mg^{2+}) and magnesium citrate 330 mg (16% Mg^{2+}). The dose is 5 mg/kg/day of elemental magnesium, adjusted to requirement and given in three to four daily doses. Diarrhea is the limiting factor. In addition to magnesium, high doses of oral KCl supplements are required. The suggested target for potassium is 3.0 mEq/L and for magnesium 1.46 mg/dL (0.6 mmol/L).[23] Spironolactone, amiloride, or eplerenone can be used to increase serum K^+ levels in patients resistant to KCl supplements. These drugs should be used cautiously to avoid hypotension.

Differential Diagnosis

Differential diagnosis of GS includes, as for BS, diuretic or laxative abuse and chronic vomiting. Similar biochemical abnormalities, i.e., hypokalemic metabolic alkalosis with hypomagnesemia and hypocalciuria, may occur due to use of cisplatin. Classic BS (ClC-Kb defect) is a close mimic of BS. However, the former is more common in children <3 years of age with failure to thrive, polyuria, and normal plasma magnesium levels. Typical features such as GS may also be seen in patients with Sjögren's syndrome. Biochemical features similar to those of BS are seen in children with mutations in the *KCNJ10* gene coding for the inwardly rectifying potassium channel KCNJ10/Kir4.1 that causes a disorder characterized by epilepsy, ataxia, sensorineural deafness, and tubulopathy (or EAST syndrome). The extrarenal features of EAST syndrome distinguish it from GS.

Long-term Follow-up

Though the life expectancy of patients with GS is not affected, not enough is known about the morbidity associated with chronic hypokalemia and hypomagnesemia in terms of metabolic syndrome, cardiac arrhythmias, chronic kidney disease, and propensity to develop chondrocalcinosis.[23]

CONCLUSION

Bartter syndrome and Gitelman syndrome are inherited salt-losing tubulopathies that have in common hypokalemic, hypochloremic metabolic alkalosis. They are inherited as autosomal-recessive disorders except for *MAGED2*-associated aBS that is X linked. Though there exists a great deal of phenotypic variability, BS1 (NKCC2 defect), BS2 (ROMK defect), BS4 (Barttin defect), and BS4b (digenic CLCka, ClCkb defect), considered as antenatal BS, present with maternal polyhydramnios, prematurity, polyuria, hypercalciuria, and nephrocalcinosis.

KEY POINTS

- Classic BS (ClCkb defect) presents in infancy with polyuria, episodes of dehydration, muscle hypotonia, and failure to thrive and may mimic GS.
- Management of BS involves replenishment of fluids and electrolytes and administration of prostaglandin inhibitors (NSAID).
- In the long term, these children have growth retardation, osteopenia, and may develop worsening of renal function and proteinuria.
- Patients with GS mimic the biochemical defects of a patient on long-term thiazides. They present after the first decade with muscle weakness, tetany, poor growth and have hypocalciuria and hypomagnesemia. They require ad libitum salt intake and lifelong supplementation with oral magnesium and potassium.

REFERENCES

1. Seyberth HW. An improved terminology and classification of Bartter-like syndromes. Nat Clin Pract Nephrol. 2008;4(10): 560-7.
2. Besouw MTP, Kleta R, Bockenhauer D. Bartter and Gitelman syndromes: Questions of class. Pediatr Nephrol. 2020;35(10): 1815-24.
3. Seyberth HW, Weber S, Kömhoff M. Bartter's and Gitelman's syndrome. Curr Opin Pediatr. 2017;29(2):179-86.
4. Walsh PR, Tse Y, Ashton E, Iancu D, Jenkins L, Bienias M, et al. Clinical and diagnostic features of Bartter and Gitelman syndromes. Clin Kidney J. 2018;11(3):302-9.
5. Madden N, Trachtman H. Physiology of the developing kidney: sodium and water homeostasis and its disorders. In: Avner ED, Harmon WE, Niaudet P, Yoshikawa N, Yoshikawa N, Emma F (Eds). Pediatric Nephrology. Berlin: Springer-Verlag; 2016. pp. 181-217.
6. Satlin LM, Bockenhauer D. Physiology of the developing kidney: potassium homeostasis and its disorder. In: Avner ED, Harmon WE, Niaudet P, Yoshikawa N, Emma F, Goldstein FL (Eds). Pediatric Nephrology. Berlin: Springer-Verlag; 2016. pp. 219-46.
7. Konrad M, Schlingmann KP. Disorders of calcium and magnesium metabolism. In: Geary DF, Schaefer F (Eds). Pediatric Kidney Disease, 2nd edition. Berlin Heidelberg: Springer-Verlag; 2016. pp. 921-52.
8. Peti-Peterdi J, Harris RC. Macula densa sensing and signaling mechanisms of renin release: Figure 1. J Am Soc Nephrol. 2010;21(7):1093-6.
9. Devuyst O, Belge H, Konrad M, Jeunemaitre X, Zennaro MC. Renal Tubular disorders of electrolyte regulation in children. In: Avner ED, Harmon WE, Niaudet P, Yoshikawa N, Emma F, Goldstein FL (Eds). Pediatric Nephrology. Berlin: Springer-Verlag; 2016. pp. 1202-52.
10. Seyberth HW. Pathophysiology and clinical presentations of salt-losing tubulopathies. Pediatr Nephrol. 2016;31(3):407-18.
11. Finer G, Shalev H, Birk OS, Galron D, Jeck N, Sinai-Treiman L, et al. Transient neonatal hyperkalemia in the antenatal (ROMK defective) Bartter syndrome. J Pediatr. 2003;142(3):318-23.
12. Nozu K, Inagaki T, Fu XJ, Nozu Y, Kaito H, Kanda K, et al. Molecular analysis of digenic inheritance in Bartter syndrome with sensorineural deafness. J Med Genet. 2008;45(3):182-6.
13. Laghmani K, Beck BB, Yang SS, Seaayfan E, Wenzel A, Reusch B, et al. Polyhydramnios, transient antenatal Bartter's syndrome, and MAGED2 mutations. N Engl J Med. 2016;374(19):1853-63.
14. Konrad M, Vollmer M, Lemmink HH, van den Heuvel LP, Jeck N, Vargas-Poussou R, et al. Mutations in the chloride channel gene CLCNKB as a cause of classic Bartter syndrome. J Am Soc Nephrol JASN. 2000;11(8):1449-59.
15. Simon DB, Bindra RS, Mansfield TA, Nelson-Williams C, Mendonca E, Stone R, et al. Mutations in the chloride channel gene, CLCNKB, cause Bartter's syndrome type III. Nat Genet. 1997;17(2):171-8.
16. Amirlak I. Bartter syndrome: an overview. QJM. 2000;93(4): 207-15.
17. Kömhoff M, Laghmani K. Pathophysiology of antenatal Bartter's syndrome. Curr Opin Nephrol Hypertens. 2017;26(5):419-25.
18. Chou CL, Chen YH, Chau T, Lin SH. Acquired Bartter-like syndrome associated with gentamicin administration. Am J Med Sci. 2005;329(3):144-9.
19. Chrispal A, Boorugu H, Prabhakar AT, Moses V. Amikacin-induced type 5 Bartter-like syndrome with severe hypocalcemia. J Postgrad Med. 2009;55(3):208-10.
20. Punzi L, Calò L, Schiavon F, Pianon M, Rosada M, Todesco S. Chondrocalcinosis is a feature of Gitelman's variant of Bartter's syndrome. A new look at the hypomagnesemia associated with calcium pyrophosphate dihydrate crystal deposition disease. Rev Rhum Engl Ed. 1998;65(10):571-4.
21. Bourcier T, Blain P, Massin P, Grünfeld JP, Gaudric A. Sclerochoroidal calcification associated with Gitelman syndrome. Am J Ophthalmol. 1999;128(6):767-8.
22. Bettinelli A, Tosetto C, Colussi G, Tommasini G, Edefonti A, Bianchetti MG. Electrocardiogram with prolonged QT interval in Gitelman disease. Kidney Int. 2002;62(2):580-4.
23. Anne B, Detlef B, Davide B, Lorenzo CA, Etienne C, Olivier D, et al. Gitelman syndrome: consensus and guidance from a Kidney Disease: Improving Global Outcomes (KDIGO) Controversies Conference-Zurich Open Repository and Archive. [online] Available from https://www.zora.uzh.ch/id/eprint/148519/. [Last accessed September, 2021].

CHAPTER

8.4 Nephrogenic Diabetes Insipidus

Kanika Kapoor, Abhijeet Saha

INTRODUCTION

Diabetes insipidus (DI) is a disease in which large volumes of hypotonic urine are excreted due to vasopressin [arginine vasopressin (AVP)] deficiency [central diabetes insipidus (CDI)] or renal resistance to vasopressin [nephrogenic diabetes insipidus (NDI)]. Though DI is a disease which was identified 200 years ago,[1] NDI was recognized only 70 years back by Forssmann[2] and Waring et al.[3] The term "nephrogenic diabetes insipidus" was coined by William and Henry in 1947.[4] There has been immense advancement in basic and molecular research leading to synthesis of vasopressin and cloning of water channels in the last two decades. NDI is a tubular disorder resulting from failure of kidneys to respond to vasopressin, thus causing physiologic inability to concentrate urine and increased excretion of dilute urine. NDI can be congenital or acquired. It is characterized by a clinical triad of polyuria, polydipsia, and hypernatremia. The exact prevalence of hereditary NDI is not known, but it is assumed to be rare. The prevalence of hereditary NDI in Quebec, Canada, is estimated to be 8.8:1,000,000 males.[5]

PATHOGENESIS

Regulation of Water Balance by Kidneys

The kidneys play a central role in maintaining salt and water balance in our body. The urine osmolality is modified between 30 and 1,200 mOsm/kg to maintain serum osmolality between 280 and 300 mOsm/kg by regulating the excretion of water and salt by kidneys. The urinary excretion of water is tightly regulated to allow rapid adaptation to changes in plasma osmolality and intravascular volume. Under physiological conditions, the production of urine is obligatory. The glomerulus filters 180 L/day of plasma but only 1.5 L is excreted as urine. The renal tubule is responsible for the reabsorption of >99% of the water and sodium in the glomerular filtrate. Approximately 90% of the water composing the filtered load is obligatorily reabsorbed in proximal tubules and loop of Henle through the water channel aquaporin 1 (AQP1).[6] The remaining 18–20 L of the forming urine reaching the distal tubules and the collecting ducts is subjected to regulated water reabsorption depending upon plasma osmolality and blood volume, thus defining the final urine volume to be excreted (1.5–2 L/day). Increase in plasma osmolality and decrease in blood volume stimulate secretion of vasopressin from the pituitary gland.

Arginine vasopressin is synthesized by magnocellular neurons of supraoptic and paraventricular nuclei of hypothalamus in a biologically inactive form and cleaved to an active form in storage granules. The active form is transported to the posterior pituitary and released in response to appropriate stimuli. The osmotic stimulus is stronger than that of volume. Even minor changes in plasma osmolality, i.e., less than 1% above the threshold stimulates osmoreceptors in the hypothalamus, leading to secretion of vasopressin from the pituitary gland. A similar response is elicited via baroreceptors due to a decrease in blood volume but at a change of 5–10% of effective circulatory volume.[7] AVP is the key regulator of the water permeability of the collecting ducts. In states of dehydration, AVP is released and exerts its antidiuretic action via binding to type-2 vasopressin receptor (AVPR2), a G protein-coupled receptor located at the basolateral side of the plasma membrane of principal cells of collecting duct. Binding of vasopressin to AVPR2 receptors results in the release of α subunit of heterotrimeric G protein (Gsα), which in turn activates adenylate cyclase (AC), resulting in increased cyclic adenosine monophosphate (cAMP) production and activation of cAMP-dependent protein kinase A (PKA) **(Fig. 1)**. Activated PKA leads to phosphorylation of several residues in the carboxy-terminus of aquaporin 2 (AQP2) and enables trafficking of AQP2 to the apical membrane of the principal cell of collecting duct, thereby markedly increasing water permeability at this site. The water effluxes the cells via AQP3 and -4 on the basolateral side of cell to the extracellular fluid and ultimately to the blood.[8]

Aquaporins (AQPs) are membrane proteins that transport mostly water and, in some cases, glycerol, urea, and small solutes.[9] Each AQP has six membrane-spanning helical domains inserted in the cell membrane and functions as a tetrameric structure. Of 13 AQPs found till date, nine AQPs with distinct roles in regulation of water balance are differentially expressed along renal tubules and collecting ducts in the human kidney. AQP1 is mainly expressed in both apical

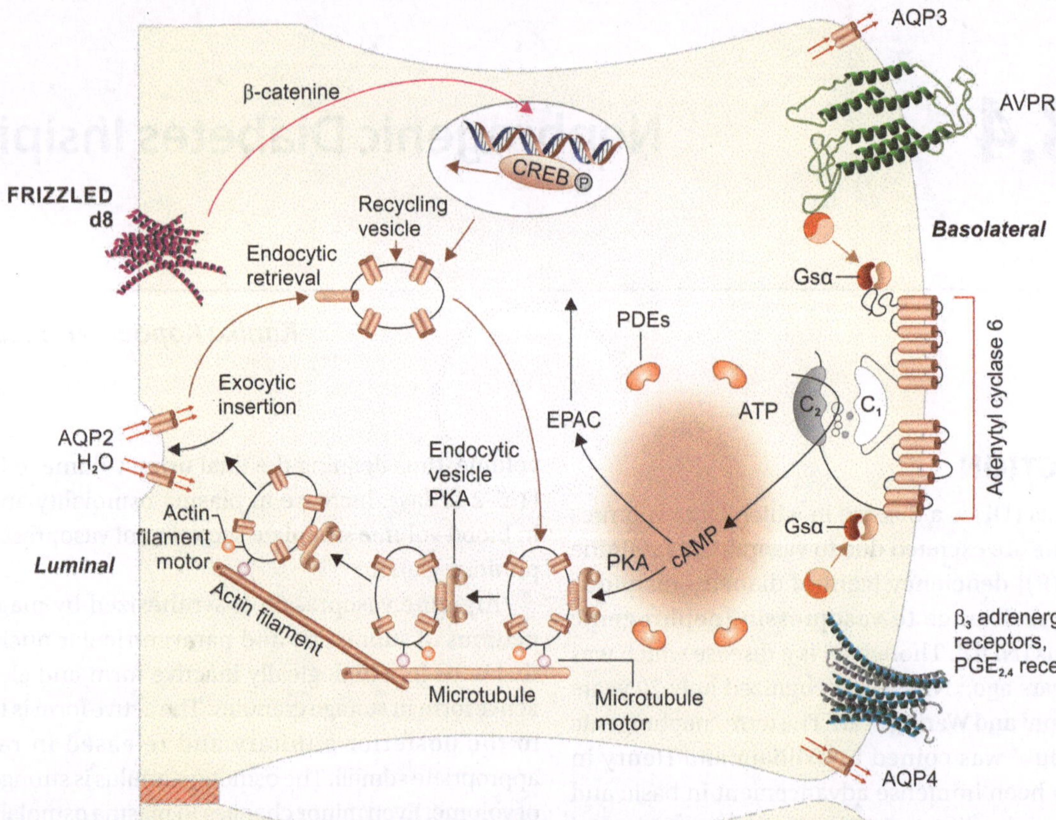

Fig. 1: Schematic representation of the effect of AVP to increase water permeability in the principal cells of the collecting duct. Binding of AVP to AVPR2 receptor (a G-protein-linked receptor) present on the basolateral membrane results in the release of α-subunit of heterotrimeric G protein (Gsα), which in turn activates AC, resulting in increased cAMP production and activation of cAMP-dependent PKA. PKA and possibly the exchange factor directly activated by cAMP (EPAC) are the targets of the generated cAMP. On the long-term, vasopressin also increases AQP2 expression via phosphorylation of the CREB, which stimulates transcription from the AQP2 promoter. Cytoplasmic vesicles carrying the water channel proteins (represented as homo tetrameric complexes) are fused to the luminal membrane in response to AVP, thereby increasing the water permeability of this membrane. Microtubules and actin filaments are necessary for vesicle movement toward the membrane. The β-3 adrenergic receptor and other G protein coupled PGE22 and PGE24 receptors are also expressed in principal cells. The AQP2 expression stimulation through the frizzled d8-β-catenin pathway by AC are potential therapeutic targets to stimulate membrane insertion of AQP2 in the absence of functional AVPR2. (AQP, aquaporin; AVP, arginine vasopressin; AVPR2, vasopressin V2 receptor; CREB, cAMP responsive element binding protein; PGE22, prostaglandin E2 receptor EP2 subtype; PGE24, prostaglandin E2 receptor EP4 subtype; EPAC, exchange protein directly activated by cAMP; PKA, protein kinase A).

and basolateral membranes of the proximal tubule where it constitutively reabsorbs >70% of water in the glomerular filtrate. AQP2 is found in the intracellular vesicles of the cells of the collecting duct and is a "vasopressin-regulated water channel." In the absence of AVP signaling, aquaporin channels are located in apical and subapical vesicles and no apical water permeability exists.

AQP3 and AQP4 are constitutively expressed in the basolateral membrane of cells of the cortical collecting duct (CCD) and the outer medullary collecting duct (OMCD) and facilitate water entry into the interstitium.[10] AQP2 is constantly retrieved from the membrane by endocytosis so that ongoing water permeability depends on the delivery of AQP2 to the membrane, either by recycling or by generation of new channels. Water diffuses via these channels along the concentration gradient from the tubular lumen into the principal cell and exits into the interstitium via the constitutively expressed AQP3 and AQP4 water channels.

Primary Nephrogenic Diabetes Insipidus

Nephrogenic diabetes insipidus is characterized by inability of the kidneys to concentrate urine despite elevated concentration of vasopressin. Renal tubular insensitivity to AVP can be either congenital or acquired. Congenital NDI in the majority of patients results from mutations in *AVPR2* (X-linked) and in some patients is related to mutations in the aquaporin-2 gene (autosomal).[11] Clinically, it is characterized by marked polyuria, polydipsia, and electrolyte imbalance with a constant risk of severe dehydration in infants.

Secondary Nephrogenic Diabetes Insipidus

In addition to primary forms of NDI, there are also secondary forms of NDI (sNDI). In adults, sNDI is much more commonly seen than primary NDI, mostly due to lithium treatment. Secondary NDI is commonly seen in children with obstructive uropathies **(Table 1)**. The increased pressure impairs normal collecting duct function by decreasing AQP2 expression.[11]

TABLE 1: Etiology of nephrogenic diabetes insipidus (NDI).

Causes of nephrogenic diabetes insipidus	
Primary: • X-linked NDI-Xq28 encoding AVPR2 (arginine vasopressin receptor 2) • Autosomal recessive NDI-Ch12q13 encoding AQP2	*Secondary:* • *Inherited:* Nephronophthisis, Bartter syndrome types 1 and 2, distal renal tubular acidosis, apparent mineralocorticoid excess (AME), familial hypomagnesemia with hypercalciuria, nephrocalcinosis, renal Fanconi syndrome • *Acquired:* – *Dyselectrolemia:* Hypokalemia, hypercalcemia, and hypercalciuria – *Renal parenchymal disorders:* Obstructive uropathy – *Drugs:* Foscarnet, amphotericin, aminoglycoside, methicillin, lithium, furosemide, cisplatin, isophosphamide, and vinblastine – *Systemic disorders:* Amyloidosis, sarcoidosis, sickle cell disease and trait, and Sjogren syndrome

Decreased AQP2 expression has been demonstrated in the setting of bilateral ureteric obstruction in animals, and marked decrease in AQP2 expression is seen only in the obstructed kidneys in case of unilateral obstruction. It was observed that this downregulation of AQP2 persists up to 30 days after release of obstruction, which might explain the diuresis often observed after release of severe obstruction in patients.[10] Acquired NDI most commonly is secondary to drugs or metabolic disturbances. Electrolyte abnormalities such as hypokalemia and hypercalciuria can cause secondary NDI by decreasing AQP2 expression. The exact mechanism is, however, not completely understood. Besides altered AQP2 trafficking, it has been postulated that hypercalciuria may be associated with activation of the calcium-sensing receptor (CaSR) in the thick ascending limb of the loop of Henle (LOH), which decreases sodium reabsorption and calcium reabsorption in LOH impairing the medullary concentration gradient, thus hampering the production of concentrated urine.[12-14]

Rarely, sNDI is observed with inherited tubulopathies[15] such as Bartter syndrome-types 1[16] and 2, apparent mineralocorticoid excess, renal Fanconi syndrome, cystic kidney disorders, and distal renal tubular acidosis[17] In many such patients, there was initial misdiagnosis, as NDI symptoms dominated the clinical presentation with presence of low urine osmolality and hypernatremia with identification of the underlying cause being difficult. *The presence of concomitant hypokalemia and hypercalciuria is a clue to the secondary NDI as the underlying disorder.* The most common though not universal biochemical abnormalities in these disorders are presence of hypokalemia and hypercalciuria.[15] As elaborated previously, secondary NDI in these disorders is due to altered AQP2 expression due to these electrolyte disturbances. The reversibility of sNDI in these disorders after correction of dyselectrolemia also suggests their causative role.

GENETICS

Congenital NDI in the majority of patients results from mutations in the arginine vasopressin receptor 2 gene (*AVPR2*) (X-linked) and in some patients is related to mutations in the *AQP2* gene (autosomal).[18] At present, >250 mutations in the *AVPR2* gene and 65 mutations in the *AQP2* gene have been reported in patients with NDI.[20]

Mutations in *AVPR2* Gene

Ninety percent of cases of primary inherited NDI are due to loss-of-function mutations in the *AVPR2* gene resulting in inactive V2 receptor. Loss of function of *AVPR2* results in disruption of water reabsorption in the collecting duct due to a loss of AVP signaling-dependent AQP2 expression and transport to the apical membrane. The gene is located on the long arm of chromosome X (region Xq28).[20] The mode of inheritance is X-linked recessive (MIM304800). Hence, majority of the patients with inherited NDI are males. However, heterozygous females can have variable degrees of polyuria and polydipsia because of skewed X chromosome inactivation. Till date, a total of 287 potential disease-causing mutations in the *AVPR2* gene have been described, with 177 (62%) being missense mutations.[21] Most of the mutations in the *AVPR2* gene encode functional but misfolded proteins, which are retained and degraded in the endoplasmic reticulum.[22,23] Some patients with *AVPR2* pathogenic variants can exhibit partial insensitivity to AVP or 1-deamino-8D-arginine vasopressin (DDAVP). At present, 18 *AVPR2* pathogenic variants resulting in partial NDI have been reported. The disease onset may be later in childhood.[19]

Mutations in *AQP2* Gene

Approximately 10% of cases of congenital NDI are due to loss-of-function mutations in the *AQP2* gene located on long arm chromosome 12 (12q13).[20] The mode of inheritance is often autosomal recessive; few have been known to be inherited as autosomal dominant disease. At least 70 putative disease-causing AQP2 mutations have been reported in 74 families.[24] The majority of *AQP2* gene mutation is missense mutation resulting in misfolded proteins that are retained in the ER.[22] Similar to the *AVPR2* inactivating mutations, those on *AQP2* can affect the proper synthesis, processing, or plasma membrane localization of the gene product, thus preventing the antidiuretic action of AVP in the principal cells of the collecting duct. Those mutations resulting in autosomal dominant inheritance affect amino acids at the carboxyl terminal of *AQP2*. The onset of disease is in later childhood and is less severe in those with autosomal dominant disease (partial NDI).[20]

CLINICAL MANIFESTATIONS

Children with primary or congenital NDI are mostly boys who usually present in the first year of life, with failure to thrive and vomiting. Patients with NDI have normal weight at birth, and antenatal history is unremarkable with no polyhydramnios as AVP-dependent mechanisms are immature at birth and placenta clears the osmolar load.[25] *This helps to distinguish NDI from other tubulopathies such as Bartter syndrome who present with fetal polyuria and antenatal polyhydramnios.* Infants who are exclusively breastfed usually thrive well and do not develop signs of dehydration due to low salt and protein content of human milk, thus reducing osmolar load on kidneys. Parents often report a suspected case of NDI as an infant with vigorous sucking, persistent vomiting, poor weight gain, constipation, and frequent wet and heavy diapers. The vomiting is due to intake of large volumes of milk causing gastroesophageal reflux. Intake of low caloric large volume feeds with feeding intolerance in early months causes failure to thrive in infants. Even in infancy, these patients show preference for cold liquids and refuse solid food. These infants display marked thirst and altered psychosocial development and thus hyperactivity, distractibility, short attention span, and restlessness in ~50% cases.[26,27] History of repeated hospitalizations for possible septicemia may be present as young infants with dehydration often develop moderate-to-high-grade fever. *Preserved urine output or polyuria in a dehydrated child should raise a suspicion of NDI.*

Infants affected by congenital NDI may also present rarely with seizures and episodes of severe hypernatremic dehydration with risk of neurological sequelae. Growth retardation may lead to short stature but bone age is normal.[28] There can be secondary dilatation of the ureters and bladder due to flow uropathy.[29-31] Older children may present with nocturia and nocturnal enuresis.

In contrast, acquired NDI is much more common in adults than primary NDI. The disease being rare is often missed due to false reassurance of normal urine output.[22]

GENOTYPE–PHENOTYPE CORRELATION

Most of the mutations in the *AVPR2* gene result in a uniform clinical phenotype of a male infant in the first week of life with dehydration episodes, excessive irritability, incessant cry, hypernatremia, hyperthermia, preserved urine output, failure to thrive, and inappropriately low urine osmolality.[32] Those who are diagnosed late and remain untreated often present with recurrent fever without focus, seizures, mental retardation, and failure to thrive. However, there are few mutations in the *AVPR2* gene which cause partial NDI and are associated with milder phenotype and present later in childhood. Some of these patients have been successfully treated with high-dose desmopressin.[33,34] Heterozygous female patients may exhibit variable degrees of polyuria and polydipsia because of skewed X chromosome inactivation.

The time of onset of the disease and the clinical symptoms are similar regardless of the molecular defect in *AVPR2* gene (X linked) or *AQP2* gene with autosomal recessive inheritance in majority of patients. However, pathogenic variants in *AQP2* gene causing autosomal dominant NDI are associated with a milder phenotype and later onset. The vasopressive effects of AVP are mediated through AVP1 receptors expressed in vasculature, while the renal effects, especially the increase in water permeability of the collecting duct (CD), are mediated by *AVPR2*. Administration of *AVPR2*-specific agonist desmopressin, however, has extrarenal effects too. Male children with X-linked NDI can be distinguished from autosomal recessive NDI by extrarenal response to intravenous DDAVP administration. DDAVP decreases blood pressure, increases heart rate (vasodilatory), and increases von Willebrand factor, factor VIII, and tissue-type plasminogen activator level (coagulation) responses in autosomal recessive NDI due to *AQP2* mutations, whereas patients with *AVPR2* mutations lack extrarenal responses.[35]

DIAGNOSIS

The first step to diagnose DI is quantification of 24-hour urine output to confirm the presence of polyuria. This can be done by direct collection in older children and weighing the diapers in infants. Polyuria is defined as urine output >2 L/m²/day or >4 mL/kg/h in children and >6 mL/kg/h in neonates. Polydipsia is defined as water intake of more than 2 L/m²/day (or >5 L/day).[36] A thorough history and careful examination should be done to rule out other causes of polyuria-polydipsia syndrome **(Table 2)**. A history about the pattern of drinking, voiding frequency, nocturia, intake of drugs, family history of

TABLE 2: Differential diagnosis of polyuria.

Diagnosis	*Clinical features*
Diabetes mellitus	Weight loss, polyphagia, malaise, fasting hyperglycemia, and glycosuria
Central diabetes insipidus	Growth retardation, skin rash (Langerhans cell histiocytosis), headache, and visual field defects
Nephrogenic diabetes insipidus	Seizures, mental retardation, constipation, and drug intake
Primary polydipsia	Compulsive water drinking

Investigations in child with polyuria-polydipsia syndrome:
- Fasting glucose
- Serum creatinine, sodium, potassium, and calcium
- Early morning serum and urine osmolality
- Urine glucose and ketones

similar complaints, consanguinity, and neurological or renal disease should be sought.

The preliminary investigations include fasting blood glucose, urine glucose, serum potassium, calcium, and creatinine levels to exclude causes of polyuria-polydipsia syndrome due to solute diuresis. Paired early morning serum sodium and osmolality and urine osmolality may be useful to assess renal concentrating ability. First morning urine sample can be used as a screening test in some polyuric patients, because a concentrated first morning urine (urine specific gravity 1.030) excludes NDI in absence of glycosuria and proteinuria.[37] Serum cortisol and thyroid function tests may be done to assess anterior pituitary function in suspected CDI patients.

Normal urinary osmolality values by age are as follows:

- <1 year: >600 mOsm/kg H_2O
- 1–2 years: 600–800 mOsm/kg H_2O
- >2 years: >800 mOsm/kg H_2O

Infants with DI may have normal urine output during episodes of dehydration. Dehydration in a child with normal urine output indicates loss of urine concentrating ability. *A blood biochemistry showing hypernatremia with inappropriately dilute urine is the clue to DI. An early morning paired serum osmolality of >300 mOsm/kg and urine osmolality <300 mOsm/kg confirms DI.* On the contrary, a paired serum osmolality of <270 mOsm/kg and urine osmolality of >800 mOsm/kg rule out DI.[37] Serum sodium levels are elevated in DI while low or normal sodium levels suggest primary polydipsia (PP). Serum osmolality is increased in children with DI while it is decreased in those with PP. In case of congenital NDI due to *AVPR2* mutations, the serum sodium is often >145 mEq/L with corresponding urine osmolality below 200 mOsm/kg; hence, a water deprivation test (WDT) is not indicated and can be hazardous.[32] In newborns and young infants, WDT is not done. If the diagnosis is unclear, DDAVP test should be done. The maximally concentrating ability of an infant a few weeks old is closer to 500 mOsm/kg water.

In older infants and children, if the cause of hypotonic polyuria is indeterminate by these baseline investigations, WDT is performed after admitting patients under close medical supervision **(Box 1 and Table 3)**.

BOX 1: Protocol for water deprivation test and DDAVP test.

Indication: If the initial serum osmolality is <300 mOsm/kg, plasma Na^+ <145 mEq/L and Uosm <Posm

Preparation/prerequisites:

- Admit patient. Place a large-bore IV cannula for obtaining samples
- Patient should be well hydrated and should have normal electrolytes before starting the test
- It is started after morning breakfast and first void volume is recorded and is discarded. Record baseline weight
- Keep the patient semirecumbent except when the patient has to void
- Baseline serum sodium is measured
- Plasma osmolality and urine osmolality are measured
- Baseline vital parameters, HR and BP, are recorded
- Baseline AVP and plasma copeptin levels are obtained where available
- No further fluids are given until the test is terminated

Monitoring:

- Weight and vital signs are measured hourly
- Plasma sodium and osmolality (Posm) at 4 hours and then every 2 hours until test is terminated
- Each void urine volume and Uosm is measured
- Uosm and Posm hourly

Termination of test:

The test is immediately terminated, if any one of following is present:

- Weight loss is >5% or physical signs of dehydration, or
- Serum sodium >145 mEq/L or serum osmolality >295 mOsm/kg, or
- Urine osmolality >750 mOsm/kg
- Duration of test is 6 hours in infants or 8 hours in <2-year-old and 12 hours in >2-year-olds

Record weight, vital signs, and measure plasma sodium, Posm, and Uosm at the end of the test

DDAVP test:

At the end of the dehydration phase, desmopressin is administered either through intranasal or intravenous/subcutaneous route (preferable)

- Intravenous—1 µg in infants and 2 µg in children
- Intranasal spray—10 µg in infants and 20 µg in older children

Urine output, urine osmolality, serum sodium, and plasma osmolality are measured hourly for 1–2 hours after desmopressin administration

(AVP: arginine vasopressin; Uosm: urine osmolality, Posm: plasma osmolality; DDAVP: 1-deamino-8D-arginine vasopressin)

DDAVP Test

The loss of urine-concentrating ability may be due to absolute or partial AVP deficiency (CDI) or renal resistance to AVP-dependent mechanisms of water reabsorption (NDI). Administration of synthetic analog of vasopressin, i.e., desmopressin (deamino-8-D-arginine vasopressin) in patients with NDI, will show little or no increase in urine osmolality. Desmopressin is administered at a dose of 1 µg subcutaneously or intravenously infused over 20 minutes (maximum dose is 0.4 µg/kg).[32] The intranasal dose is 10 µg in infants and 20 µg in children. The urine osmolality and volume are measured at baseline and at 30-minute intervals over the next 2 hours. If the urine osmolality does not increase by >100 mOsmol/kg over baseline, the diagnosis of NDI is made[38,39] **(Box 1 and Table 3)**.

Copeptin Assay

For long, WDT has been considered as a gold standard test to differentiate causes of polyuric polydipsia syndrome. However, it has a low diagnostic accuracy of around 70%, is cumbersome, can be hazardous in young infants, and needs expertise. Standardized assays of AVP are not commercially available and have technical limitations. Copeptin is the C-terminal segment of the AVP precursor peptide pre-pro-vasopressin. Copeptin is a surrogate marker of AVP.[40]

TABLE 3: Interpretation of water deprivation and DDAVP test.

Baseline urine osmolality (mOsm/kg)	*Post-water deprivation Uosm (mOsm/kg)*	*Post-DDAVP administration Uosm (mOsm/kg)*	*Post-DDAVP administration change in Uosm (%)*	*Interpretation*
<300	<300	>800*	>50% rise	Complete central DI
<300	<300	300–800	9–50	Partial CDI
<300	<300	<300	<9	NDI
<300	<300	300–600	9–10	Partial NDI

(CDI: central diabetes insipidus; DDAVP: 1-deamino-8D-arginine vasopressin; DI: diabetes insipidus; NDI: nephrogenic diabetes insipidus; Uosm: urine osmolality)
*>300–500 mOsm/kg in infants

Flowchart 1: Copeptin-based algorithm for approach to diagnosis polyuria-polydipsia syndrome.

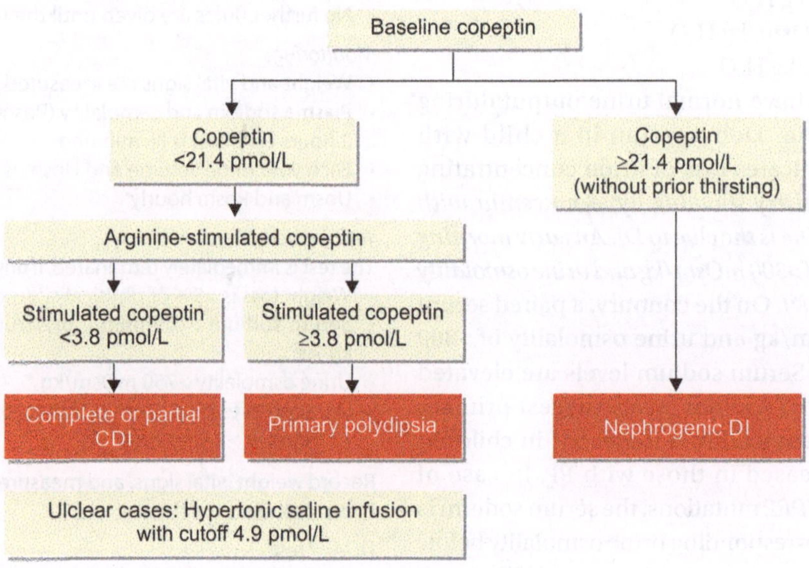

(CDI: central diabetes insipidus)

Plasma copeptin measurements are high in familial NDI, i.e., higher than 21.4 pg/mL,[41,42] reflecting a normal vasopressin response to dehydration. A newer copeptin-based algorithm[42] to differentiate CDI and NDI has been proposed but is not validated in children **(Flowchart 1)**.

MUTATIONAL ANALYSIS

The small sizes of the genomic and coding regions of the involved genes (*AVPR2* and *AQP2*) allow for relatively easy mutational analysis, thereby allowing for carrier, prenatal and perinatal testing. All families with hereditary DI should have their molecular defect identified. Molecular genetic testing approaches include sequential single-gene testing or a multigene panel.

Following establishment of diagnosis of NDI, additional evaluation with renal ultrasound is needed to evaluate for hydronephrosis, dilatation of urinary tract, and megacystis. Genetic counseling should be done by a clinical geneticist. Developmental evaluation and appropriate intervention in case of neurological sequelae are needed.

TREATMENT OF NEPHROGENIC DIABETES INSIPIDUS

The treatment strategies in hereditary NDI are beneficial in ameliorating the symptoms rather than providing a cure for the disease. Symptomatic treatment aims to restore normal intravascular volume by replacing urinary losses and decreasing the urinary volume. Patients with NDI have significant polyuria, and any episode of additional water loss (fever, diarrhea, and vomiting) can lead to life-threatening hypernatremic dehydration. Repeated episodes of hypernatremic dehydration have been associated with mental retardation, intracerebral calcifications, and permanent neurological sequelae. Drugs such as thiazide diuretics, potassium-sparing diuretics, and nonsteroidal anti-inflammatory drugs (NSAIDs)/cyclooxygenase-2 (COX-2) inhibitors have been used for long to decrease urine output, but their efficacy is suboptimal **(Table 4)**. Early diagnosis, liberal fluid intake, and low osmolar diet remain the mainstay of management of primary NDI.

TABLE 4: Drugs used in treatment of nephrogenic diabetes insipidus.

Drug	*Mechanism of action*	*Dose*	*Side effects/caution*	*Monitoring*
Thiazides	Blocks NCCT inducing natriuresis Increases proximal tubular water reabsorption	2–4 mg/kg/day in two divided doses	Hypokalemia, chronic thiazide therapy can result in hyperuricemia, glucose intolerance, and dyslipidemia	Serum sodium, potassium, uric acid, lipid profile, and blood glucose
Amiloride	Blocking of ENaC, increase natriuresis	0.1–0.3 mg/kg/day	Nausea and hyperkalemia	Serum sodium and potassium
Indomethacin	Decrease GFR and decrease urine volume	1–3 mg/kg/day in three to four divided doses	Impairment of renal function, gastrointestinal bleeding, and elevated creatinine neutropenia, thrombocytopenia and, rarely, aplastic anemia	Serum creatinine, blood counts, and serum sodium (concomitant use of thiazide may result in hyponatremia)

(ENaC: epithelial sodium channel: GFR: glomerular filtration rate; NCCT: sodium chloride cotransporter)

Emergent Management

Patients presenting with dehydration should be hospitalized and receive intravenous or enteral hydration. Though most protocols of hypernatremic dehydration use 0.9% saline as the initial fluid for resuscitation to prevent rapid fall of sodium levels, *patients with NDI should receive 5% dextrose in water or 0.22% saline for intravenous and water or milk for enteral hydration.* Isotonic fluids should be administered only in cases of shock which is uncommon in these patients since it may worsen hypernatremia. The principle behind administration of hypotonic fluids is that it is essentially pure water loss in hereditary NDI (urine sodium is ~10 mmol/L). Hence, fluids hyperosmolar as compared to urine will exacerbate the existing hypernatremia. The rate of administration of IV fluids should be slightly more than urine output to gradually decrease sodium levels at 0.5 mEq/h.[22,43]

Fluids

Treatment is challenging in infants who are dependent on caregivers for maintaining hydration. Fluids should be offered every 2 hours in infants. Hence, the calories might suffer. Sometimes, feeding per nasogastric or gastrostomy tube is needed to provide caloric requirement.

Diet

An important component of therapy is decreasing the urinary volume by intake of low solute diet, thus leading to reduction in renal osmolar load.[44] A diet low in sodium (1 mmol/kg/day) and protein (2 g/kg/day) is advised, but stringent protein restriction may hamper growth and cause serious nutritional deficiencies in children.[22] Since urine osmolality is low and fixed in patients with NDI, hence solute load determines urine output. 1 g of salt provides an osmotic load of 34 mOsm (17 mOsm of sodium and 17 mOsm of chloride). The recommended osmotic load is 15 mOsm/kg/day and fluid intake is 150 mL/kg/day.[37] Fats and carbohydrates are metabolized to byproducts which do not need renal excretion; hence, diet rich in these will provide calories without increasing renal osmolar load.

Diuretics

The use of diuretics to decrease urine volume seems contradictory. However, *the first-line regimen in children with NDI is a combination of hydrochlorothiazide and amiloride.*

Thiazides

The proposed mechanism by which thiazides work is blocking of the sodium chloride cotransporter (NCCT) in the distal tubule, thus causing natriuresis and increasing obligatory water losses. This causes volume depletion, thus stimulating the renin–angiotensin II aldosterone system. There is increased proximal tubular water and sodium reabsorption via AQP1. Thereby, less urine reaches the distal tubule and decreases CD-dependent water reabsorption. In animal models, hydrochlorothiazide is found to increase AQP2 upregulation independent of AVP-dependent stimulation.[45-47] Thiazides effectively reduce urine output when associated with a very low sodium diet.

Amiloride

Similar to hydrochlorothiazide, amiloride acts by blocking epithelial sodium channels (ENaC) resulting in lowered sodium reabsorption and increased hypovolemia.[46,47] Amiloride might have an additive effect and also prevent hypokalemia with chronic thiazide use. It is less tolerated in toddlers due to persistent nausea.

Prostaglandin Synthesis Inhibitors

Prostaglandin synthesis inhibitors decrease GFR minimizing urinary losses. Indomethacin is used at a dose of 1-3 mg/kg/day in three to four divided doses.[48,49] Prolonged use of this drug can lead to deterioration of renal function.

Caution is advised for use in NDI in whom it can cause acute kidney injury in dehydrated patients. It is often associated with gastrointestinal side effects such as anorexia, nausea, vomiting, abdominal pain, and ulceration including life-threatening hemorrhage. Hematological complications include neutropenia, thrombocytopenia, and rarely aplastic anemia.

Antireflux medications such as histamine H2-antagonists, (e.g., ranitidine 2–4 mg/kg/dose twice daily) and a prokinetic (e.g., domperidone 0.2–0.5 mg/kg three to four times daily) decrease vomiting in infants with NDI and also prevent Indomethacin-associated GI side effects.

Due to poor tolerance of amiloride in early years, the combination of hydrochlorothiazide with indomethacin is useful with a subsequent switch to thiazide with or without amiloride.

The preferred initial therapy in patients with secondary inherited NDI due to renal tubular disorders as in Bartter-like syndromes is NSAIDs. Patients should be closely monitored for side effects of the drugs and for changes in urinary volume. Growth monitoring is essential in these patients.

Despite all the treatment, there is 50–70% reduction in urine volume and patients fail to achieve urine volume as healthy children.[22] There is flow uropathy reported in 30% of children with NDI. So frequent and "double voiding" should be encouraged to prevent dilatation of bladder and urinary tract.

Due to the insufficient control of the polyuria by conventional treatments, recent focus has been on new and alternative methods to induce antidiuresis in NDI patients. Some of these strategies are currently under clinical evaluation.

Children with NDI undergoing minor procedures or major surgery requiring NPO status, IV fluids 5% dextrose in water approximately the rate of urine flow should be given. In those patients in whom flow uropathy has developed, continuous or intermittent bladder catheterization should be advised in case significant post-void residue is present.

Follow-up

Follow-up every 3 months in infants and 6 monthly in older children is suggested. At each follow-up visit, adherence to low-sodium diet, liberal fluids, and compliance to medications should be emphasized. Growth and development should be monitored and recorded. Renal ultrasound examination to monitor for dilatation of the urinary tract should be done annually.[19]

Genetic Counseling

Families with an affected child should be counseled regarding the nature of disease, risk in future pregnancies, risk to offspring of a proband, and availability of prenatal testing. Hereditary NDI may be transmitted as an X-linked recessive disease in 90%, autosomal recessive in ~9%, or as autosomal dominant in ~1% of families. In X-linked disease, males are affected and females are carriers who may be asymptomatic or have variable degrees of polyuria and polydipsia.[19] There is a 50% chance of transmission in each pregnancy. Affected males transmit the *AVPR2* pathogenic variant to all of their daughters who will be heterozygotes and to none of their sons. In autosomal recessive disease, parents of the affected child are obligate heterozygotes of the *AQP2* pathogenic variant; each conception has a 25% chance of having an affected child, 50% carriers, 25% unaffected, and carriers are asymptomatic.[19]

Novel Therapies

Several treatment approaches for hereditary NDI are under investigation. However, the clinical data available is scarce. These target restoration of AVP signaling upstream of *AQP2* trafficking so are not applicable to patients with mutations in *AQP2* gene. Since most mutations result in misfolded proteins, a molecular chaperone or a nonpeptide *AVPR2* agonist and antagonist which can induce proper folding of the mutant receptor may bypass the ER.[50] Several agents have been tested which can increase cAMP levels and increase *AQP2* trafficking. Agonists for the prostaglandin receptors EP2 and EP4, such as butaprost, could provide an alternative pathway to increase cAMP and AQP2 phosphorylation and target AQP2 to the apical membrane without involvement of V2R. Phosphodiesterase 5 inhibitors have been shown to activate the guanosine monophosphate (cGMP) pathway and promote insertion of AQP2 in vivo and in vitro in the apical membrane of the OMCD but do not change insertion in the CCD which is the major site of water reabsorption.[51]

LONG-TERM PROGNOSIS

Early reports on patients with NDI suggested severe intellectual impairment as an almost invariable feature of the disease, but subsequently it was observed that this complication can be prevented with early diagnosis and by adequate treatment. Most children with NDI are short and underweight during early years of life partly due to limited caloric intake; however, majority of them attain normal adult height.[53] Despite the overall favorable prognosis, patients do have complications due to polyuria. Comorbidities caused by NDI include primary nocturnal enuresis in 40%, short stature in 35%, urologic complications in 35%, persistent failure to thrive in 30%, and chronic kidney disease (CKD) stage 2 or greater in 30% children.[52,53]

CONCLUSION

Neonates and young infants with polyuria-polydipsia syndrome should be immediately referred to specialized centers for rapid diagnosis and treatment of hypernatremic dehydration. Massive free water losses cause significant morbidity, even in treated patients. High fluid intake is necessary to avoid hypernatremic dehydration, which can result in permanent neurologic complications. A variety of medications, including thiazide diuretics, potassium-sparing diuretics, and NSAIDs/COX-2 inhibitors, have been utilized to decrease urine output, although their efficacy is suboptimal. The quality of life is compromised due to mental health issues, polyuria, and constant thirst. Understanding of the pathogenesis of the disease led to the development of in vivo mouse models for testing possible therapies. Future research may show which of these strategies can improve or replace the current standard therapies for patients suffering from different NDI types.

KEY POINTS

- NDI is caused by the inability of the kidney to concentrate urine due to hereditary or acquired renal resistance to the action of vasopressin on the collecting duct.
- NDI can be inherited (X-linked or autosomal) or acquired.
- Hereditary NDI is an X-linked recessive disease due to loss-of-function mutations in the *AVPR2* gene, in 90% cases.
- NDI is suspected in an infant presenting with failure to thrive, repeated episodes of dehydration, hypernatremia, low urine osmolality (<200 mOsm/kg), and confirmed with DDAVP test and mutational analysis.
- Water deprivation test should be done in a patient with urine osmolality between 300 and 600 mOsm/kg and normal serum biochemistries.
- Newer approaches to differentiate CDI and NDI by copeptin-based assays need validation in children.
- Current strategies of management of NDI focus on symptomatic improvement by liberal fluid intake, dietary sodium restriction to decrease osmotic load, and pharmacological treatment with thiazide diuretics with or without amiloride and indomethacin.
- With early diagnosis and appropriate management, complications such as mental retardation and growth failure can be prevented.

REFERENCES

1. Valenti G, Tamma G. History of diabetes insipidus. G Ital Nefrol. 2016;33(Suppl 66):33.S66.1.
2. Forssman H. On hereditary diabetes insipidus with special regard to a sex-linked form. Acta Med Scand. 1945;153:355-196.
3. Waring AJ, Kajdi L, Tappan V. A congenital defect of water metabolism. Am J Dis Child. 1945;69:323-4.
4. Williams RH, Henry C. Nephrogenic diabetes insipidus: transmitted by females and appearing during infancy in males. Ann Intern Med. 1947;27:84-95.
5. Arthus MF, Lonergan M, Crumley MJ, Naumova AK, Morin D, DE Marco LA, et al. Report of 33 novel AVPR2 mutations and analysis of 117 families with X-linked nephrogenic diabetes insipidus. J Am Soc Nephrol. 2000;11(6):1044-54.
6. Kortenoeven ML, Fenton RA. Renal aquaporins and water balance disorders. Biochim Biophys Acta. 2014;1840(5):1533-49.
7. Atherton JC. Regulation of fluid and electrolyte balance by the kidney. Anaesth Intens Care Med. 2006;7(7):227-33.
8. Milano S, Carmosino M, Gerbino A, Svelto M, Procino G. Hereditary nephrogenic diabetes insipidus: Pathophysiology and possible treatment. An update. Int J Mol Sci. 2017;18(11): 2385.
9. Su W, Cao R, Zhang XY, Guan Y. Aquaporins in the kidney: physiology and pathophysiology. Am J Physiol Renal Physiol. 2020;318(1):F193-203.
10. Nielsen S, Frøkiaer J, Marples D, Kwon TH, Agre P, Knepper MA. Aquaporins in the kidney: from molecules to medicine. Physiol Rev. 2002;82(1):205-44.
11. Frokiaer J, Marples D, Knepper MA, Nielsen S. Bilateral ureteral obstruction downregulates expression of vasopressin-sensitive AQP2 water channel in rat kidney. Am J Physiol. 1996;270:F657-68.
12. Khanna A. Acquired nephrogenic diabetes insipidus. Semin Nephrol. 2006;26(3):244-8.
13. Sands JM, Naruse M, Baum M, Jo I, Hebert SC, Brown EM, et al. Apical extracellular calcium/polyvalent cation-sensing receptor regulates vasopressin-elicited water permeability in rat kidney inner medullary collecting duct. J Clin Invest. 1997;99(6):1399-405.
14. Earm JH, Christensen BM, Frokiaer J, Marples D, Han JS, Knepper MA, et al. Decreased aquaporin-2 expression and apical plasma membrane delivery in kidney collecting ducts of polyuric hypercalcemic rats. J Am Soc Nephrol. 1998;9(12): 2181-93.
15. Bockenhauer D, Bichet DG. Inherited secondary nephrogenic diabetes insipidus: concentrating on humans. Am J Physiol Renal Physiol. 2013;304(8):F1037-42.
16. Bettinelli A, Ciarmatori S, Cesareo L, Tedeschi S, Ruffa G, Appiani AC, et al. Phenotypic variability in Bartter syndrome type I. Pediatr Nephrol. 2000;14:940-5.
17. Das D, Sinha R, Dey S. Renal tubular acidosis presenting as nephrogenic diabetes insipidus. Indian Pediatr. 2019;56(4): 325-7.
18. Bichet DG, Bockenhauer D. Genetic forms of nephrogenic diabetes insipidus (NDI): Vasopressin receptor defect (X-linked) and aquaporin defect (autosomal recessive and dominant). Best Pract Res Clin Endocrinol Metab. 2016;30(2): 263-76.
19. Knoers N, Lemmink H. Hereditary nephrogenic diabetes insipidus. In: Adam MP, Ardinger HH, Pagon RA, Wallace SE, Bean LJH, Stephens K, Amemiya A (Eds). Gene Reviews® [Internet]. Seattle (WA): University of Washington, Seattle; 2000. pp. 1993-2020.
20. Babey M, Kopp P, Robertson GL. Familial forms of diabetes insipidus: clinical and molecular characteristics. Nat Rev Endocrinol. 2011;7(12):701-14.
21. Cooper DN, Ball EV, Stenson PD, Phillips AD, Evans K, Heywood S, et al. The Human Gene Mutation Database at the Institute of Medical Genetics in Cardiff. [online] Available from http://www.hgmd.cf.ac.uk. [Last accessed September, 2021].
22. Bockenhauer D, Bichet DG. Pathophysiology, diagnosis and management of nephrogenic diabetes insipidus. Nat Rev Nephrol. 2015;11:576-88.
23. Wesche D, Deen PM, Knoers NV. Congenital nephrogenic diabetes insipidus: the current state of affairs. Pediatr Nephrol. 2012;27(12):2183-204.
24. Gao C, Higgins PJ, Zhang W. AQP2: Mutations associated with congenital nephrogenic diabetes insipidus and regulation by post-translational modifications and protein-protein interactions. Cells. 2020;9(10):2172.

25. Bonilla-Felix M. Development of water transport in the collecting duct. Am J Physiol Renal Physiol. 2004;287(6):F1093-101.
26. Hoekstra JA, van Lieburg AF, Monnens LA, Hulstijn-Dirkmaat GM, Knoers VV. Cognitive and psychosocial functioning of patients with congenital nephrogenic diabetes insipidus. Am J Med Genet. 1996;61:81-8.
27. van Lieburg AF, Knoers NV, Monnens LA. Clinical presentation and follow-up of 30 patients with congenital nephrogenic diabetes insipidus. J Am Soc Nephrol. 1999;10(9):1958-64.
28. Lejarraga H, Caletti MG, Caino S, Jiménez A. Long-term growth of children with nephrogenic diabetes insipidus. Pediatr Nephrol. 2008;23:2007-12.
29. Vest M, Talbot NB, Crawford JD. Hypocaloric dwarfism and hydronephrosis in diabetes insipidus. Am J Dis Child. 1963;105:175-81.
30. Yoo TH, Ryu DR, Song YS, Lee SC, Kim HJ, Kim JS, et al. Congenital nephrogenic diabetes insipidus presented with bilateral hydronephrosis: genetic analysis of V2R gene mutations. Yonsei Med J. 2006;47(1):126-30.
31. Stevens S, Brown BD, McGahan JP. Nephrogenic diabetes insipidus: a cause of severe nonobstructive urinary tract dilatation. J Ultrasound Med. 1995;14(7):543-5.
32. Bichet DG. Genetics in endocrinology: Pathophysiology, diagnosis and treatment of familial nephrogenic diabetes insipidus. Eur J Endocrinol. 2020;183(2):R29-R40.
33. Bockenhauer D, Carpentier E, Rochdi D, Van't Hoff W, Breton B, Bernier V, et al. Vasopressin type 2 receptor V88M mutation: molecular basis of partial and complete nephrogenic diabetes insipidus. Nephron Physiol. 2010;114:1-10.
34. Makita N, Sato T, Yajima-Shoji Y, Sato J, Manaka K, Eda-Hashimoto M, et al. Analysis of the V2 vasopressin receptor (V2R) mutations causing partial nephrogenic diabetes insipidus highlights a sustainable signaling by a non-peptide V2R agonist. J Biol Chem. 2016;291:22460-71.
35. van Lieburg AF, Knoers NVAM, Mallman R, Proesmans W, van den Heuvel LP, Monnens LA. Normal fibrinolytic responses to 1-desamino-8-D-arginine vasopressin in patients with nephrogenic diabetes insipidus caused by mutations in the aquaporin-2 gene. Nephron. 1996;72:544-6.
36. Leung AK, Robson WL, Halperin ML. Polyuria in childhood. Clin Pediatr (Phila). 1991;30(11):634-40.
37. Kavanagh C, Uy NS. Nephrogenic diabetes insipidus. Pediatr Clin North Am. 2019;66(1):227-34.
38. Mishra G, Chandrashekhar SR. Management of diabetes insipidus in children. Indian J Endocrinol Metab. 2011; 15(Suppl3):S180-S187. doi:10.4103/2230-8210.84858.
39. Linshaw MA. Back to basics: congenital nephrogenic diabetes insipidus. Pediatr Rev. 2007;28(10):372-80.
40. Fenske W, Quinkler M, Lorenz D, Zopf K, Haagen U, Papassotiriou J, et al. Copeptin in the differential diagnosis of the polydipsia-polyuria syndrome--revisiting the direct and indirect water deprivation tests. J Clin Endocrinol Metab. 2011;96(5):1506-15.
41. Timper K, Fenske W, Kuhn F, Frech N, Arici B, Rutishauser J, et al. Diagnostic accuracy of copeptin in the differential diagnosis of the polyuria-polydipsia syndrome: A prospective multicenter study. J Clin Endocrinol Metab. 2015;100(6):2268-74.
42. Christ-Crain M, Bichet DG, Fenske WK. Diabetes insipidus. Nat Rev Dis Primers. 2019;5:54.
43. Bockenhauer D, Bichet DG. Nephrogenic diabetes insipidus. Curr Opin Pediatr. 2017;29(2):199-205.
44. Berl T. Impact of solute intake on urine flow and water excretion. J Am Soc Nephrol. 2008;19:1076-8.
45. Kim GH, Lee JW, Oh YK, Chang HR, Joo KW, Na KY, et al. Antidiuretic effect of hydrochlorothiazide in lithium-induced nephrogenic diabetes insipidus is associated with upregulation of aquaporin-2, Na-Cl co-transporter, and epithelial sodium channel. J Am Soc Nephrol. 2004;15:2836-43.
46. Alon U, Chan JCM. Hydrochlorothiazide-amiloride in the treatment of congenital nephrogenic diabetes insipidus. Am J Nephrol. 1985;5:9-13.
47. Knoers N, Monnens LAH. Amiloride-hydrochlorothiazide in the treatment of congenital nephrogenic diabetes insipidus. J Pediatr. 1990;117:499-502.
48. Rasher W, Rosendahl W, Henricho IA, Maier R, Seyberth HW. Congenital nephrogenic diabetes insipidus: vasopressin and prostaglandins in response to treatment with hydrochlorothiazide and indomethacin. Pediatr Nephrol. 1987;1:485-90.
49. Jakobsson B, Berg U. Effect of hydrochlorothiazide and indomethacin on renal function in nephrogenic diabetes insipidus. Acta Paediatr. 1994;83:522-52.
50. Bernier V, Morello JP, Zarruk A, Debrand N, Salahpour A, Lonergan M, et al. Pharmacologic chaperones as a potential treatment for X-linked nephrogenic diabetes insipidus. J Am Soc Nephrol. 2006;17(1):232-43.
51. Assadi F, Ghane Sharbaf F. Sildenafil for the Treatment of Congenital Nephrogenic Diabetes Insipidus. Am J Nephrol. 2015;42(1):65-9.
52. D'Alessandri-Silva C, Carpenter M, Ayoob R, Barcia J, Chishti A, Constantinescu A, et al. Diagnosis, treatment, and outcomes in children with congenital nephrogenic diabetes insipidus: A Pediatric Nephrology Research Consortium Study. Front Pediatr. 2020;7:550.
53. Sharma S, Ashton E, Iancu D, Arthus MF, Hayes W, Van't Hoff W, et al. Long-term outcome in inherited nephrogenic diabetes insipidus. Clin Kidney J. 2018;12(2):180-7.

CHAPTER

8.5 Glycosuria

Brinda Panchal Jain, Karalanglin Tiewsoh

INTRODUCTION

The kidney is a vital organ for glucose homeostasis contributing to both gluconeogenesis and the glucose utilization process. It does so by regulation of glucose reabsorption from the renal tubules after it is filtered in the glomerulus.

GLUCOSE HANDLING BY THE KIDNEY

Gluconeogenesis in the Kidney

Renal gluconeogenesis mainly occurs in the proximal renal tubule, and >90% of it is made from substrates such as glutamine, alanine, glycerol, and lactate. This process is more sensitive to hormones such as insulin and catecholamines; however, glucagon has little effect on it. It adapts to stimuli such as hypoglycemia by increasing the renal uptake of gluconeogenic substrates in the proximal tubule and to diabetes by increasing the renal glucose excretion.[1]

Glucose Reabsorption in the Kidney

Glucose being a small uncharged molecule with a molecular weight of 180 kD is freely filtered in the glomerulus. Therefore, in individuals with a normal glomerular filtration rate (GFR) and blood glucose levels, 160–180 mg of glucose is filtered everyday.[2] This would lead to losses of a large amount of glucose in the ultrafiltrate. Hence, most of this is reabsorbed back in the proximal tubule by an insulin-independent process. This filtration of glucose increases with either an increase in the blood glucose levels or/and increase in the GFR. However, the proximal tubule has a maximum capacity of reabsorption called transport maximum (Tmax) for glucose (Tm glucose). Beyond this point, glucose appears in the urine causing glycosuria.[1]

Glucose Transport Along the Proximal Tubule of Nephron

Glucose transporters (GLUTs) in the proximal tubules are of different types in order to ensure complete reabsorption of glucose. The S1 segment has high flux and low affinity transporters absorbing most of the glucose, while the S3 segment has low flux and high affinity GLUTs, thus ensuring that all the filtered glucose is reabsorbed back.[3]

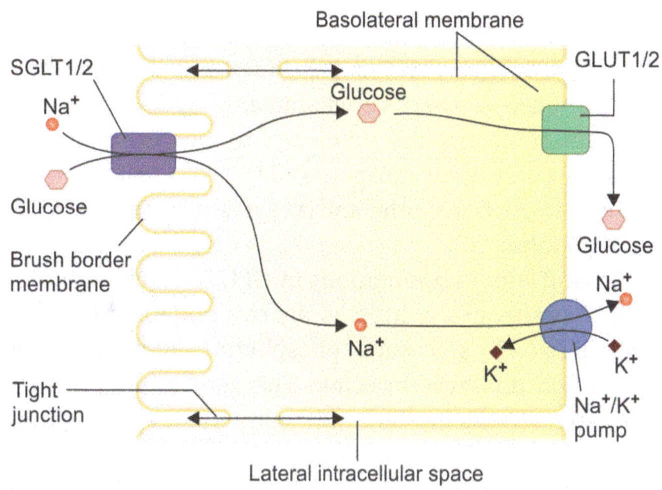

Fig. 1: Glucose absorption from the glomerular filtrate through tubule epithelial cells into blood. (GLUT: glucose transporter; SGLT: sodium-dependent glucose transporter)
Source: Adapted from Int Union Physiol Sci/Am Physiol Soc; 2004.

Glucose absorption across the brush border cells of proximal tubule requires a sodium gradient, which is created by the Na/K-ATPase pump at the basolateral surface. This pump drives sodium outside the cell from the basolateral surface, thus decreasing intracellular concentration of sodium and maintaining the gradient. Glucose is then cotransported with sodium into the cells through special sodium-dependent glucose transporters (SGLTs).[4] Glucose then diffuses into the interstitium once its concentration inside the cell increases through specific facilitative GLUTs located at the basolateral membrane[5] **(Fig. 1)**.

Sodium-dependent Glucose Transporters

There are six types of SGLTs, which belong to a broader SLC5 family.[6] SGLT2 has low affinity and high capacity with a sodium glucose transport ratio of 1:1, reabsorbing 90% of the filtered glucose. It has no affinity for galactose and is abundantly present in the S1 and S2 segments of the proximal tubule. SGLT1 has high affinity and low capacity for glucose with a ratio of sodium to glucose of 2:1 and is abundantly present in the S3 segment of the proximal tubule. It can additionally transport galactose and absorbs the remaining

10% of the filtered glucose.[7-10] Proposed function and location of SGLT3 are yet to be ascertained. Other members such as SGLT4-6 have been named but their structure and function are yet to be determined.[1]

Mutations in SGLT2 result in "familial renal glucosuria," ranging from renal glycosuria of 1 to >100 g/day. However, no other complications (such as impaired kidney function or urinary tract infections) have been consistently observed in individuals with this mutation.[11] Conversely, mutations in SGLT1 cause "intestinal glucose and galactose malabsorption" leading to life-threatening diarrhea on exposure to glucose or galactose with little or no glycosuria.[12]

Facilitative Glucose Transporters

Glucose transporter 2 (GLUT2) (SLC2A2) is a low-affinity glucose transporter and is predominantly expressed in S1/S2 segments of the proximal tubule and to a lesser extent in S3 segment, whereas the transporter GLUT1 (SLC2A1) is a high-affinity glucose transporter and is expressed along the entire proximal tubule.[13,14]

Loss-of-function mutations in GLUT2 cause Fanconi-Bickel syndrome, which is a proximal tubulopathy characterized by glycosuria, phosphaturia, aminoaciduria, proteinuria, and hyperuricemia. This generalized proximal tubulopathy may be due to the glucotoxicity caused by accumulation of glucose in the cell, as its exit from the basolateral membrane is impaired. In contrast, individuals with mutations in GLUT1 primarily present with neurologic problems, in the absence of a renal phenotype.[15]

EVALUATION

While evaluating a case of glycosuria, one should keep in mind that ruling out diabetes mellitus, proximal tubular dysfunction, and acute kidney injury is important. Familial renal glycosuria is a rare genetic disorder and by itself may not need active management.[16]

A careful history of activity of the child, eating habits, sleeping pattern, urinary frequency, any trauma, poisoning, and family history should be taken. Examination of the child should include anthropometry for wasting and stunting, a good general physical examination, and blood pressure besides the systemic examination.

Quantification of the urine output would be important to rule out polyuria. Urine analysis may include a urine dipstick for glucose or more specifically a 24-hour urine glucose. It is important to remember, however, that basal glycosuria is also normally present and would depend on the diet of the child at that particular time. Though basal glycosuria levels have been discussed in adults, there have not been any consensus in children, though a level of 20.1 mg in 24-hour urine with a range of 5.5–43.2 has been considered normal.[17] Thus, anything beyond this level may be considered abnormal.

While in children, a normal fasting glucose level would be sufficient, one can also perform the glucose tolerance test to rule out diabetes mellitus. For ruling out other secondary causes of glycosuria, renal function test, a venous blood gas, serum electrolytes, urine osmolality, 24-hour urine calcium, and PO_4 reabsorption rate may be performed.

Finally, a genetic analysis to rule out mutations in SLC5A2, the SGLT2-coding gene, causing familial renal glucosuria, can be performed.[18] Besides, other inherited causes of renal glycosuria can be confirmed only after a genetic study. Next-generation sequencing of the clinical exome or, if possible, of the whole genome would be appropriate.

MANAGEMENT

While secondary causes of glycosuria would need further management, which would depend on the etiology, familial renal glucosuria needs no active intervention. However, it is preferable that these children be followed up at least annually to assess their glycosuria and have a thorough examination.

CONCLUSION

Glycosuria can be primary due to a defect in channels of the proximal tubule or secondary to another disease. It usually occurs when filtered glucose exceeds the Tmax for its reabsorption in the proximal tubule. Evaluation needs a detailed history and examination, and specific investigations targeted to confirm the etiology. Treatment can vary from being watchful with benign familial glycosuria to specific therapy depending on the etiology.

KEY POINTS

- Glucose handling by the kidney is mainly done by the proximal tubule. The process of gluconeogenesis and glucose reabsorption takes place here.
- There are special channels called SGLT and GLUT on the luminal and basolateral surfaces of these cells, which carry out the process of reabsorption till the Tmax for glucose is reached, beyond which glycosuria occurs.
- Evaluation primarily aims at deciding whether this is due to a primary renal cause or secondary to other diseases such as diabetes mellitus, and treatment is directed accordingly.

REFERENCES

1. Mather A, Pollock C. Glucose handling by the kidney. Kidney Int Suppl. 2011;(120):S1-6.
2. Vallon V. Glucose transporters in the kidney in health and disease. Pflugers Arch. 2020;472(9):1345-70.
3. Barfuss DW, Schafer JA. Differences in active and passive glucose transport along the proximal nephron. Am J Physiol. 1981;10(3):322-32.
4. Sacktor B. Sodium-coupled hexose transport. Kidney Int. 1989;36:342-50.

5. Dominguez JH, Song B, Maianu L, Garvey WT, Qulali M. Gene expression of epithelial glucose transporters: the role of diabetes mellitus. J Am Soc Nephrol. 1994;5(5 Suppl 1):S29-36.
6. Wright EM, Turk E. The sodium/glucose cotransport family SLC5. Pflugers Arch. 2004;447:510-8.
7. Ikeda TS, Hwang ES, Coady MJ, Hirayama BA, Hediger MA, Wright EM. Characterization of a Na+/glucose cotransporter cloned from rabbit small intestine. J Membr Biol. 1989;110(1): 87-95.
8. Turner RJ, Moran A. Heterogeneity of sodium-dependent D-glucose transport sites along the proximal tubule: Evidence from vesicle studies. Am J Physiol. 1982;11(4):F406-14.
9. Lee YJ, Lee YJ, Han HJ. Regulatory mechanisms of Na+/glucose cotransporters in renal proximal tubule cells. Kidney Int Suppl. 2007;(106):S27-35.
10. Quamme GA, Freeman HJ. Evidence of a high-affinity sodium-dependent D-glucose transport system in the kidney. Am J Physiol. 1987;253(1):F151-7.
11. Santer R, Calado J. Familial renal glucosuria and SGLT2: From a Mendelian trait to a therapeutic target. Clin J Am Soc Nephrol. 2010;5(1):133-41.
12. Gorboulev V, Schürmann A, Vallon V, Kipp H, Jaschke A, Klessen D, et al. Na +-D-glucose cotransporter SGLT1 is pivotal for intestinal glucose absorption and glucose-dependent incretin secretion. Diabetes. 2012;61(1):187-96.
13. Chin E, Zhou J, Bondy C. Anatomical and developmental patterns of facilitative glucose transporter gene expression in the rat kidney. J Clin Invest. 1993;91(4):1810-5.
14. Dominguez JH, Camp K, Maianu L, Garvey WT. Glucose transporters of rat proximal tubule: Differential expression and subcellular distribution. Am J Physiol. 1992;262(5 Pt 2):F807-12.
15. Pascual JM, Wang D, Lecumberri B, Yang H, Mao X, Yang R, et al. GLUT1 deficiency and other glucose transporter diseases. Eur J Endocrinol. 2004;50(5):627-33.
16. Serrano Ríos M. Renal diabetes (primary renal glycosuria): a short overview. Verh Dtsch Ges Inn Med. 1987;93:512-7.
17. Brodehl J, Oemar BS, Hoyer PF. Renal glucosuria. Pediatr Nephrol. 1987;1(3):502-8.
18. Calado J, Santer R, Rueff J. Effect of kidney disease on glucose handling (including genetic defects). Kidney Int Suppl. 2011; 120:S7-13.

CHAPTER

8.6 Renal Rickets

Arpana A Iyengar, S Thangavelu

INTRODUCTION

Rickets is a bone disease associated with demineralization of the growing bone and cartilage secondary to defects in calcium and phosphorus homeostasis. Rickets in children is most often seen with nutritional deficiencies of vitamin D and calcium (nutritional rickets). Rickets can result from genetic mutations encoding proteins involved in vitamin D and phosphate metabolism. Acquired defects in vitamin D metabolism due to liver disease or drug toxicity can also lead to rickets.

Kidneys play an important role in maintaining vitamin D, calcium, and phosphorus homeostasis. *Renal rickets* is a terminology used to describe rickets that results commonly from chronic kidney disease (CKD). However, this chapter adopts a broader approach to the clinical entity of renal rickets, describing rickets related to hypophosphatemic rickets (HPR), renal tubular acidosis (RTA), CKD, and vitamin D-dependent rickets (VDDR).

In renal rickets, an expected response to 3 months of vitamin D therapy is not achieved.[1] The spectrum of rickets includes:

- Nutritional rickets
- *Gastrointestinal causes:* Malabsorption, neonatal cholestasis, and Wilson's disease
- *Renal rickets:* CKD, RTA, hereditary HPR (X-linked, autosomal dominant, autosomal recessive, and hypercalciuric HPR)
- *Diseases of vitamin D metabolism:* Medication related, VDDR I and II
- *Miscellaneous*: Oncogenic rickets, rickets of prematurity

Rickets can be broadly classified as *calcipenic rickets* and *phosphopenic rickets.* Disorders due to direct inhibition of mineralization (fluorosis, hypophosphatasia, and aluminum toxicity) are not discussed in this chapter. Calcipenic rickets is a result of hypocalcemia due to decreased intake of calcium and vitamin D or abnormalities in vitamin D metabolism. Phosphopenic rickets occurs when hypophosphatemia is due to impaired renal or gastrointestinal phosphate reabsorption. The common causes for these types of rickets with their manifestations are described in **Table 1**.[2] Renal rickets can manifest as calcipenic or phosphopenic rickets. Besides CKD, the most common causes for renal rickets observed in India are distal renal tubular acidosis (D-RTA), HPR, proximal renal tubular acidosis (P-RTA), VDDR, and Dent's disease.[3,4] It is imperative to suspect rickets that occurs due to non-nutritional causes, and **Box 1** lists the key pointers favoring non-nutritional rickets.

TABLE 1: Types of rickets, associated conditions, and their characteristic clinical features.

Features	*Calcipenic rickets*	*Phosphopenic rickets*
Associated conditions	Nutritional rickets, VDDR, hepatic/drug-induced rickets, and rickets of CKD	Renal phosphate loss (HPR and P-RTA)
Age at onset	Early	Both early and late
Bony deformities	All limbs involved	Predominantly lower limbs
Bone pain	Common	Uncommon
Muscle weakness	Present	Absent
Tetany	Common	Absent
Dental abscess	Absent	Common
Serum calcium	Low/normal	Normal
Serum phosphorus	Low	Low
Alkaline phosphatase	Elevated	Mildly elevated
Parathormone	Elevated	Normal/mildly elevated

(CKD: chronic kidney disease; HPR: hypophosphatemic rickets; P-RTA: proximal renal tubular acidosis; VDDR: vitamin D-dependent rickets)

PATHOPHYSIOLOGY

Osteoblasts mineralize the osteoid and osteoclasts break down bone matrix during remodeling. Bone maturation occurs when the osteoid is mineralized by calcium salts. This process is defective in rickets resulting in demineralized osteoid beneath the growth plate causing softened bones. Serum calcium, phosphorus, vitamin D, parathyroid hormone

BOX 1: Pointers to suspect non-nutritional rickets.

- Age at the time of diagnosis is <6 months or beyond 2 years
- More than one child in the family affected
- When associated with failure to thrive with or without polyuria
- When associated with developmental delay other than selective motor delay
- Presence of clinical clues such as rickets with jaundice, recurrent diarrhea, hypertension, and alopecia
- Presence of biochemical abnormalities such as raised urea, creatinine, acidosis, hypokalemia, urine glycosuria or proteinuria, abnormal liver function, or hypoalbuminemia
- Normal vitamin D level
- Inadequate response to vitamin D therapy

(PTH), and fibroblast growth factor-23 (FGF23) are key players for bone metabolism.[5] The pathogenesis of rickets due to defects in vitamin D metabolism is illustrated in **Figure 1**. Key aspects in the pathophysiology of rickets due to RTA, VDDR, CKD, and HPR are provided here. The genetic forms of renal rickets alongside their mutations are listed in **Table 2**.

Pathogenesis of Calcipenic Rickets

Vitamin D_2 and vitamin D_3 get hydroxylated in the liver by 25-hydroxylase, encoded by *CYP2R1*. Primarily in the kidney, 25(OH)D undergoes 1α-hydroxylation to its active form, 1,25-dihydroxyvitamin D (1,25$(OH)_2$D), by 1α-hydroxylase encoded by *CYP27B1*. Activity of 1α-hydroxylase in the kidney is tightly regulated by PTH, calcium, phosphate, FGF23, and 1,25$(OH)_2$D **(Fig. 1)**. Calcium and phosphate absorption from the intestine is mediated by 1,25$(OH)_2$D binding to VDR. Metabolic inactivation of 1,25$(OH)_2$D and 25(OH)D occurs, primarily in the kidney and intestine by 24-hydroxylase, encoded by *CYP24A1*.[6]

Pathogenesis of Phosphopenic Rickets

Fibroblast growth factor-23 (FGF23) is a phosphaturic hormone produced by osteocytes, plays an important role in bone metabolism, and is regulated by phosphate-regulating neutral endopeptidase homolog (PHEX) and dentin matrix acidic phosphoprotein 1 (DMP1) in the osteocytes. FGF23 binds to FGF receptors with the help of Klotho and decreases the threshold for renal tubular reabsorption of phosphate. It primarily decreases the abundance of renal phosphate transporters NPT2A and NPT2C on the apical surface of the proximal renal cells. FGF23 also inhibits synthesis of 1,25$(OH)_2$D by increasing the expression of *CYP24A1* and downregulating the expression of *CYP27B1 levels.* In addition, 1,25$(OH)_2$D inhibits PO_4 reabsorption from the intestine, and finally the interplay of pathways leads to hypophosphatemia that causes defective chondrocyte differentiation, decreased hydroxyapatite formation, and rickets[5,7] **(Fig. 2)**. Two reviews provide a detailed discussion on the bone metabolism in both calcipenic and phosphopenic rickets.[2,7]

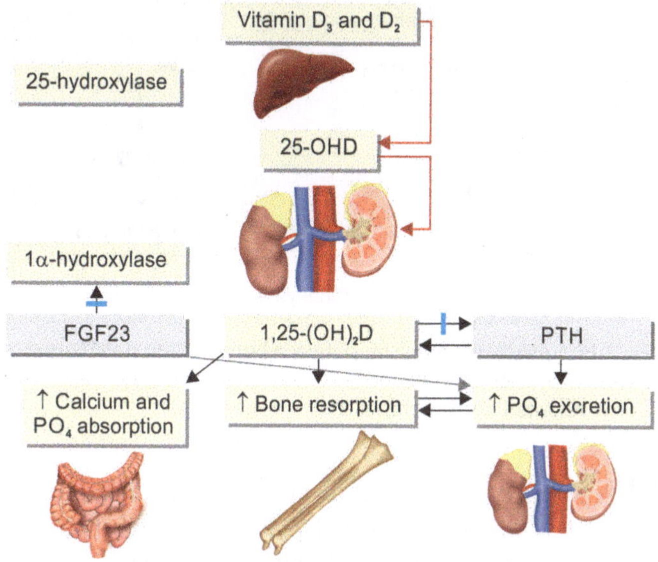

Fig. 1: Regulation of calcium and phosphate homeostasis. (FGF: fibroblast growth factor; PTH: parathyroid hormone)

TABLE 2: Genetic forms of renal rickets.

Renal rickets	***Gene mutation***
RTA:	
• Distal	*SLC4A1* *ATP6V1B1* *ATP6V0A4*
• Fanconi syndrome	*SLC34A3*
• Cystinosis	*CTNS*
• Fanconi–Bickel syndrome	*SLC2A2*
Dent's disease	CLCN5
VDDR:	
• Type IA	*CYP27B1*
• Type IB	*CYP2R1*
• Type II	*VDR*
HPR:	
• XLH	*PHEX*
• ADHR	*FGF23*
• ARHR	*DMP1/ENPP1*
• HHRH	*SLC34A3*

[ADHR: autosomal-dominant hypophosphatemic rickets; ARHR: autosomal-recessive hypophosphatemic rickets; HHRH: hereditary hypophosphatemic rickets with hypercalciuria; HPR: hypophosphatemic rickets (X-linked, autosomal dominant, autosomal recessive, and hypercalciuric hypophosphatemic rickets); RTA: renal tubular acidosis; VDDR: vitamin D-dependent rickets]

Vitamin D-dependent Rickets

1α-hydroxylase deficiency and 25-hydroxylase deficiency: A defect in conversion of 25(OH)D to 1,25$(OH)_2$D owing to *CYP27B1* gene mutation on chromosome 12q13.3 that encodes 25-hydroxyvitamin D_3-1α-hydroxylase results in VDDR type 1A.[8] It is a rare disease with autosomal recessive inheritance that leads to 1α- hydroxylase deficiency and decreased synthesis of calcitriol. Mutations in *CYP2R1* that decrease expression or function of 25-hydroxylase result in VDDR type 1B. It is associated with hypocalcemia, secondary

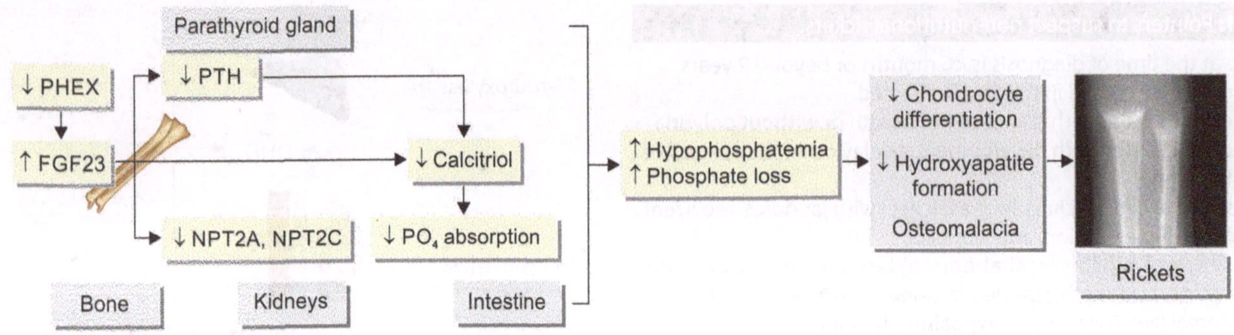

Fig. 2: Interplay of mechanisms between bone, kidney, parathyroid gland, and intestine in phosphopenic rickets. (FGF: fibroblast growth factor; PTH: parathyroid hormone)
Source: Adapted from reference 7.

hyperparathyroidism, and low plasma concentrations of 25(OH)D. Children are affected in the first 2 years of life with severe growth retardation and features of rickets.

1,25(OH)$_2$D resistance: Tissue resistance to vitamin D due to mutations in genes encoding vitamin D receptors (VDR) results in VDDR type IIA, characterized by hypocalcemia, hyperparathyroidism, normal serum concentrations of 25(OH)D, and increased serum 1,25(OH)D levels.[9] VDR is a member of the group of nuclear transcription factors that bind to vitamin D response elements (VDREs). Mutations of VDR interrupt binding of 1,25(OH)$_2$D to VDR (alopecia absent) or interfere with binding of the 1,25(OH)$_2$D-VDR complex to the VDREs in the DNA (alopecia present). Alopecia, rickets with low serum levels of calcium and phosphorus, and elevated serum concentrations of 1,25(OH)$_2$D are typical features. Children with alopecia usually have early onset of rickets and greater resistance to therapy compared to those without alopecia.

The presence of a nuclear ribonucleoprotein that interferes with the vitamin D receptor–DNA interaction results in VDDR IIB. VDDR type III is due to increased inactivation of vitamin D metabolites caused by a recurrent gain-of-function missense mutation in the gene encoding *CYP3A4*.[10]

Renal Tubular Acidosis

In RTA, rickets manifests due to bone resorption secondary to metabolic acidosis.[11,12] In an attempt to buffer the acidosis, leaching of minerals including hydroxyapatite from the bones occurs. Rickets is severe with proximal RTA and milder with distal RTA. Loss of phosphate and vitamin D deficiency predispose to occurrence of rickets in proximal RTA. Proximal tubular dysfunction is also seen with Dent's disease, an X-linked recessive syndrome associated with proximal tubular solute-wasting, hypercalciuria, nephrocalcinosis, kidney stones, renal failure, and occasionally rickets.[13]

CKD-related Rickets

Rickets in CKD occurs due to a combination of defects in calcium, phosphorus, PTH, vitamin D metabolism, abnormalities in bone turnover, mineralization, volume, linear growth, and vascular or soft-tissue calcification. Children with a nonglomerular native kidney disease such as cystinosis, congenital anomalies of the kidney/urinary tract, and Dent's disease present with severe rickets. Recent insights into FGF23 have revolutionized the understanding of the mechanisms of secondary hyperparathyroidism. Plasma FGF23 levels rise with worsening kidney function even before changes in the levels of phosphate and PTH are noted. In the early stages of CKD, high levels of FGF23 reduce hyperphosphatemia at the expense of 1,25(OH)$_2$ vitamin D suppression, initiating secondary hyperparathyroidism.[14] The decrease in serum 1,25(OH)$_2$D3 leads to decreased intestinal calcium absorption. The triad of low levels of calcium, calcitriol, and hyperphosphatemia further increases PTH secretion that leads to mobilization of calcium from the bone and osteitis fibrosa. Other consequences of progressive CKD include metabolic acidosis, hyporesponsiveness of VDR, and reduced expression of the calcium-sensing receptor on the parathyroid gland leading to parathyroid gland hyperplasia.

Hypophosphatemic Rickets

X-linked hypophosphatemic rickets (XLHR) is the most common genetic form of hypophosphatemia due to mutations in the *PHEX* gene impairing inactivation of FGF-23 that results in proximal tubular phosphate wasting and hypophosphatemia. Clinical features include rickets, disproportionate short stature, poor growth, craniosynostosis, lower limb involvement, and dental abnormalities. Low tubular reabsorption (TRP) in the presence of low serum phosphate is the hallmark of XLHR. Autosomal-dominant HPR results from missense mutations in the *FGF23* gene on chromosome 12p13, which renders it resistant to proteases, thus causing phosphaturia. Clinical features are similar to XLHR. Autosomal-recessive hypophosphatemic rickets (ARHR) type 1 occurs due to loss-of-function mutations in dentin matrix protein-1 (DMP1), a bone matrix protein that downregulates FGF23. ARHR type 2 results due to loss-of-function mutations of the ecto-nucleotide *pyrophosphatase/*

pyrophosphodiesterase 1 gene (*ENPP1*). The mutated *ENPP1* gene causes HPR resulting from elevated FGF23 levels and reduced inorganic pyrophosphate levels, a physiologic inhibitor of calcification **(Fig. 2)**. Clinical manifestations and biochemical findings are similar to those with XLHR. Hereditary hypophosphatemic rickets with hypercalciuria (HHRH) is caused by loss-of-function mutation in the *SLC34A3* gene encoding a sodium-dependent phosphate transporter, namely sodium-phosphate co-transporter (NPT2C). This differs from other forms of HPR in that plasma 1,25$(OH)_2$ vitamin D concentration is normal or appropriately elevated for the degree of hypophosphatemia with the presence of hypercalciuria and nephrolithiasis.[7,15-17] Further details on pathogenesis of other extrarenal manifestations (auditory, dental, and neurological manifestations) associated with HPR are described elsewhere.[7]

CLINICAL FEATURES

First, renal rickets should be differentiated from nutritional rickets. Clinical features can guide us to distinguish the two entities **(Table 3)**. Specific manifestations of rickets due to renal disorders are described below:[18,19]

- *Age:* Rickets is evident in infancy with VDDR and P-RTA. Beyond the first year of life, rickets is a manifestation of HPR, RTA, and CKD. It is important to remember that only with maturation of the glomerular filtration rate (GFR) does the urinary phosphate leak become evident, and therefore rickets is usually not seen in infancy with HPR. Rickets in infancy or early childhood can manifest with delayed motor milestones.
- *Polyuria/polydipsia:* In young children, polyuria manifests as recurrent episodes of dehydration, preference to plain water rather than milk, failure to thrive, constipation, and occasionally salt craving. Rickets with polyuria is a typical sign observed with RTA and occasionally with CKD. Children with HPR and VDDR do not present with polyuria.
- *Skeletal deformities:* Involvement of the upper torso (craniotabes, frontal bossing, delayed closure of anterior fontanelle, rachitic rosary, Harrison sulcus, and widening of writs) is common in renal rickets, while disproportionate short stature, abnormal gait, and lower limb deformities are more pronounced in HPR. Bone fractures secondary to trivial impact are seen with VDDR, P-RTA, and rickets due to CKD but not with HPR. In older children, double malleoli, knock-knee deformity (genu valgum), and genu varum are commonly seen with or without bone pain. Muscle weakness and hypotonia are commonly associated with renal rickets, while poor mineralization of teeth, dental defects (enamel hypoplasia, dental abscess, and pulp necrosis), and craniosynostosis are commonly observed with HPR.
- *Systemic features:* Secondary causes of D-RTA and disorders of P-RTA such as cystinosis, Lowe's syndrome, and tyrosinemia manifest with systemic signs of visual and auditory disturbances, hepatosplenomegaly, developmental delay, and neurological and hepatic involvement. HPR can rarely present with raised intracranial tension and craniosynostosis. Children with VDDR characteristically present with recurrent lower respiratory infections and hypocalcemic seizures. Alopecia is a characteristic feature of VDDR II. Anemia and hypertension may be associated with rickets due to CKD.
- *Family history:* Genetic forms of rickets can present with a positive family history. Mild bowing of legs may be evident in the mother of the index child in X-lined HPR.

TABLE 3: Clinical parameters that differentiate renal rickets from nutritional rickets.

Characteristics	*Nutritional rickets*	*Renal rickets*
Typical age at onset	6 months to 2 years	>2 years of age (except for VDDR that presents in infancy)
Polyuria and polydipsia	Absent	Present with RTA
Short stature	Absent	Present
Lower limb deformities	Less common	Predominant in HPR
Bone fractures	Absent	Common with CKD and RTA
Dental abscess	Absent	Present in FHPR
Muscle weakness	Present	Present
Family history	Not common	Common
Tetany	Less common	Common in CKD, RTA, and VDDR
Response to vitamin D therapy	Good	Poor

[CKD: chronic kidney disease; RTA renal tubular acidosis; HPR: hypophosphatemic rickets (X-linked, autosomal dominant, autosomal recessive and hypercalciuric hypophosphatemic rickets); VDDR: vitamin D-dependent rickets]

Response to native vitamin D supplementation is good with nutritional rickets and not necessarily so with renal rickets. **Figures 3A to C** show typical healing response to vitamin D supplementation in nutritional rickets.

EVALUATION

Based on the clinical features and biochemical parameters, a step-wise approach to detecting types of rickets is provided in **Box 2 and Figures 4A to H**.

The biochemical approach to diagnosing the cause for renal rickets is depicted in **Flowchart 1**. Details on evaluating RTA and CKD-related MBD are dealt with in the respective chapters. Evaluation and management of HPR are recently published as clinical practice guidelines.[20] In this section, evaluation for HPR and VDDR is discussed in detail. Reference

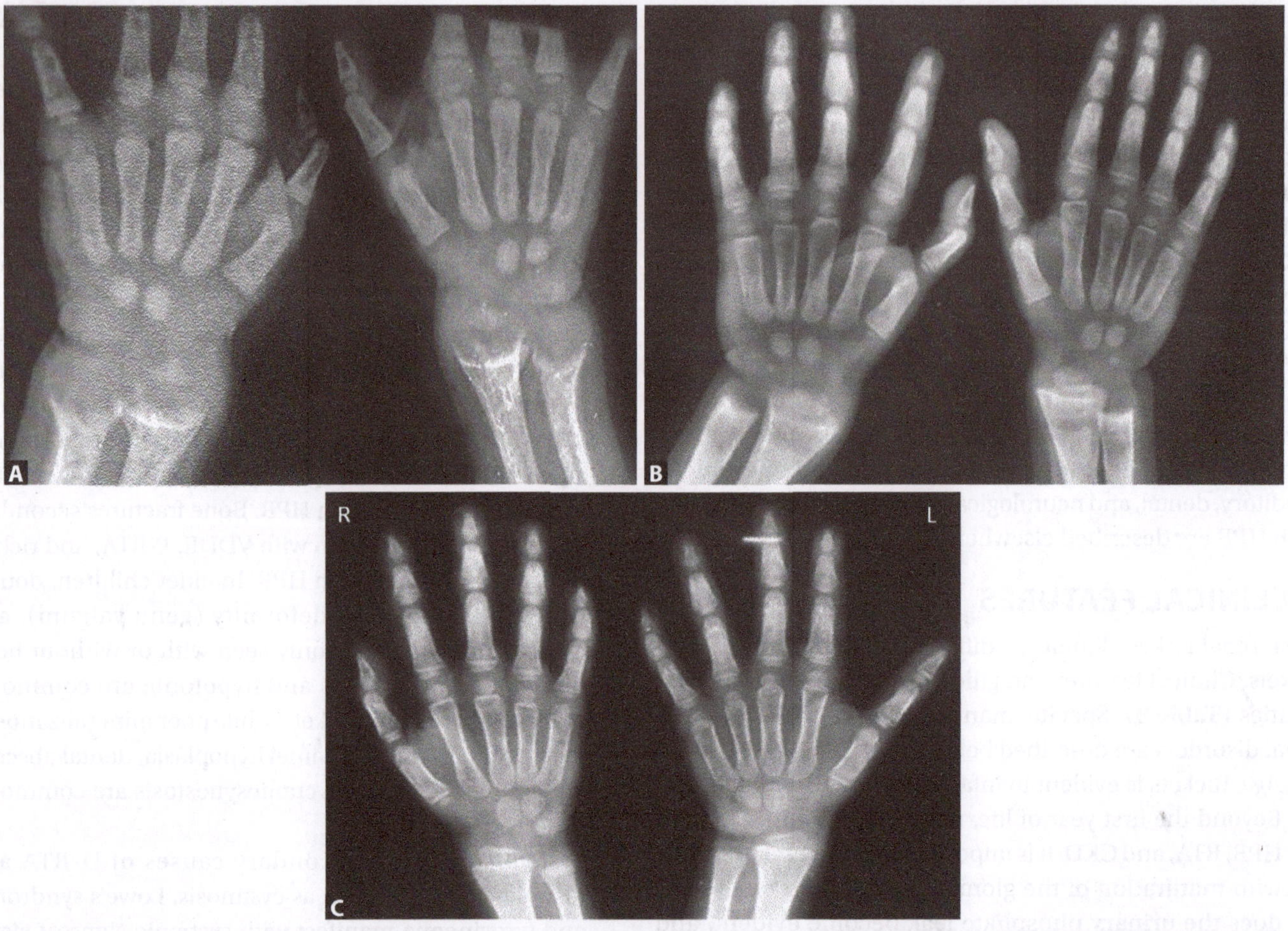

Figs. 3A to C: Serial X-rays showing healing response to vitamin D supplementation. (A) Oct 2017. X-ray: Classical cupping, fraying, and widening of physis; (B) Jan 2018. X-ray: Provisional zone of calcification. Partially healed rickets; (C) Apr 2018. Healed rickets.

BOX 2: Stepwise approach to a child with rickets based on clinical, radiological, and biochemical laboratory results.

Step 1: Child has typical clinical features—Is it rickets or rickets-like state?
- Clinical features present, radiological features similar but serum alkaline phosphatase is low—hypophosphatasia
- Clinical features present, but radiological features are not typical—metaphyseal dysplasia, Morquio's disease. Serum calcium, phosphate, and alkaline phosphatase levels are normal

Step 2: Is it nutritional or non-nutritional rickets?
Refer to **Box 1 and Table 3.**

Step 3: If non-nutritional, whether it is renal or nonrenal?
In this situation, the presence of laboratory data is more helpful to recognize renal etiology.
- Raised urea, creatinine, high serum phosphate (clinical—short stature, hypertension, and anemia)—chronic kidney disease
- Normal anion gap metabolic acidosis, hypokalemia, high chloride with or without USG findings showing nephrocalcinosis (clinical—episodes of dehydration or acidosis)—RTA
- In addition to the above, if the child has severe failure to thrive, albuminuria and glycosuria—Fanconi syndrome
- Low serum phosphate, normal serum calcium, normal parathyroid hormone (clinical—predominant lower limb deformities)—HPR

Step 4: If nonrenal, it could be gastrointestinal (GI), vitamin D metabolism disorders, or miscellaneous causes:
- Usual gastrointestinal causes are malabsorption syndrome, neonatal cholestasis, and Wilson's disease. They are usually obvious, because of their distinct clinical and laboratory features.
- Disorders of vitamin D metabolism. Anticonvulsant drugs such as phenytoin and phenobarbitone interfering with metabolism of vitamin D, They are identified by the history of anticonvulsant therapy and by checking serum levels of 25-hydroxyvitamin D and 1,25-hydroxyvitamin D levels

values for serum phosphate levels vary with age and are important for interpretation. Serum bicarbonate and serum electrolytes are important for diagnosis, while 1,25(OH)D and FGF23 estimation is rarely indicated. Urinary tubular proteinuria, generalized aminoaciduria, and glycosuria are evident with proximal RTA. Urine calcium estimation

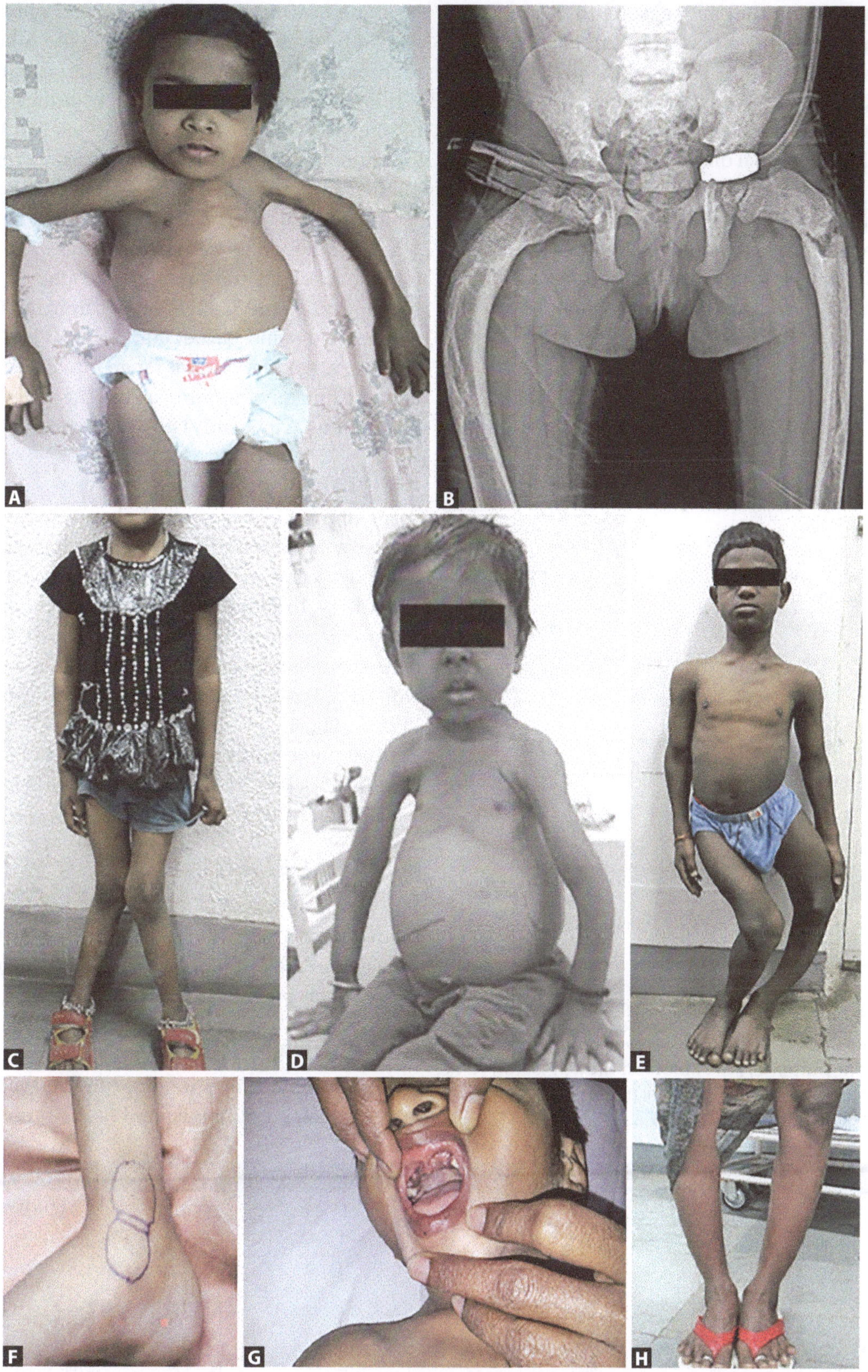

Figs. 4A to H: (A) Child with rickets due to chronic kidney disease; (B) Severe osteopenia and fracture femur in a child on chronic peritoneal dialysis; (C) Knock knees in a child with cystinosis (P-RTA); (D) Rickets with hepatosplenomegaly in a child with tyrosinemia (P-RTA); (E) Windswept deformity in a child with HPR; (F) Double malleoli; (G) Deformed dentition in HPR; (H) Bow legs in the mother of a child with HPR. (P-RTA: proximal renal tubular acidosis; HPR: hypophosphatemic rickets)

is important for RTA, Dent's disease, and HHPR. The biochemical parameters in various types of renal rickets are listed in **Table 4.**

Other disorders mimicking renal rickets, such as fluorosis, metaphyseal dysplasia, and hypophosphatasia, need to be considered in the differential diagnosis.

Urine Phosphate Estimation

To document renal phosphate wasting, a 2-hour urine sample is collected following a 4-hour fast and serum phosphate is obtained after 1 hour. Creatinine and phosphorus are estimated in serum and urine. Renal phosphate wasting should be evaluated by calculating the tubular maximum reabsorption of phosphate per glomerular filtration rate (TmP/GFR). The first step is to calculate the fraction excretion of phosphorus ($FePO_4$), which is—$FePO_4\%$ = (Urine PO_4 × Serum creatinine/Serum PO_4 × Urine creatinine) × 100; Tubular reabsorption of phosphorus (TRP) = 100 – $FePO_4$.

The normal range of TRP in children is between 0.85 and 1.0, depending on the serum phosphorus concentration. The tubular threshold maximum for phosphorus per glomerular filtration rate (TmP/GFR) is derived from the TRP and plotted on the Walton and Bijvoet nomogram **(Fig. 5)**.[21] For a quick interpretation, the normal range for TmP/GFR in children is approximately the same as the normal range for serum phosphorus. A low TmP/GFR is observed in HPR.

Flowchart 1: A simplistic biochemical approach to diagnosis of renal rickets.

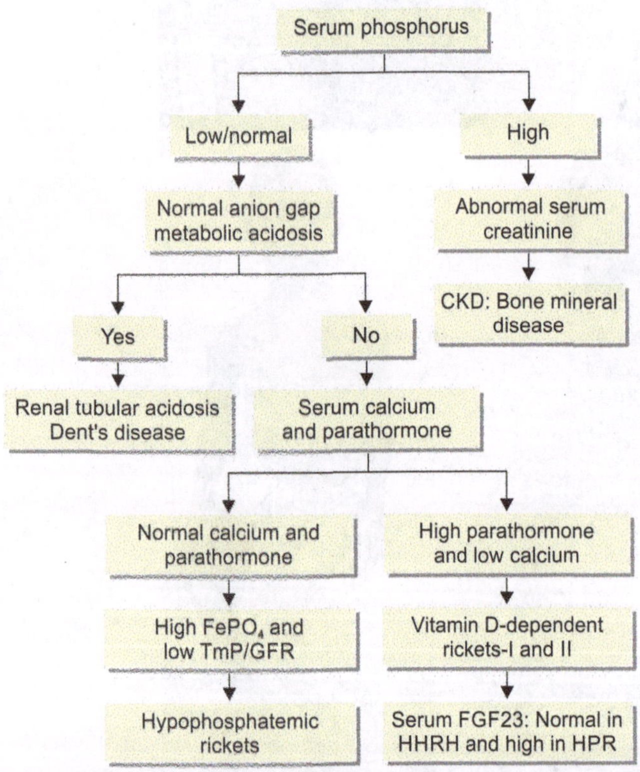

(CKD: chronic kidney disease; FGF: fibroblast growth factor; HPR: hypophosphatemic rickets; TmP/GFR: tubular maximum reabsorption of phosphate per glomerular filtration rate)

Radiography

X-ray of long bones reveals changes with expansion in the growth plate and cupping, fraying, and widening of metaphysis. Osteopenia and fractures are common in children with CKD with additional features of osteitis fibrosa cystica in those with severe hyperparathyroidism. Sclerotic bones and dense vertebrae may be seen in children and young adults with HPR. Typically, features of bone resorption are not seen in HPR **(Fig. 6)**.

A 10-point scoring system for radiographic assessment of severity of rickets (rickets severity score) has been found to be useful in HRP.[22]

MANAGEMENT

The key components of medical therapy for RTA and CKD-related rickets are presented here while further details are provided in the respective chapters. The treatment for HPR and VDDR is provided in detail below.[5,7,20,23]

Renal Tubular Acidosis

Alkali therapy to maintain serum bicarbonate levels of 20–22 mmol/L is administered in the form of oral sodium

TABLE 4: Biochemical parameters in types of renal rickets.

Renal rickets	*S. Ca*	*S. PO_4*	*PTH*	*ALP*	*U. Ca*	*25OHD*	*1,25OHD*	*FGF23*
RTA	↓/N	↓/N	↑	↑	↑	–	–	–
CKD–MBD	↓/N	↑	↑	↑	–	↓	–	↑
VDDR I	↓	↓/N	↑	↑	–	N	↓	–
VDDR II	↓	↓/N	↑	↑		N	↑	–
XLH	N	↓	N/↑	↑	–	N	↓/N	↑
ADHR	N	↓	N	↑	–	N	↓	↑
ARHR	N	↓	N	↑	–	N	↓	↑
HHRH	N	↓	N/↓	↑	↑	N	↑	N/↓

[ALP: alkaline phosphatase; CKD–MBD: chronic kidney disease–mineral and bone disorder; HPR: hypophosphatemic rickets (X-linked, autosomal dominant, autosomal recessive, and hypercalciuric hypophosphatemic rickets); PTH: parathormone; RTA: renal tubular acidosis; S. Ca: serum calcium; S. PO_4: serum phosphorus; U. Ca: urinary calcium; VDDR: vitamin D-dependent rickets]

Source: Adapted from references 5 and 8.

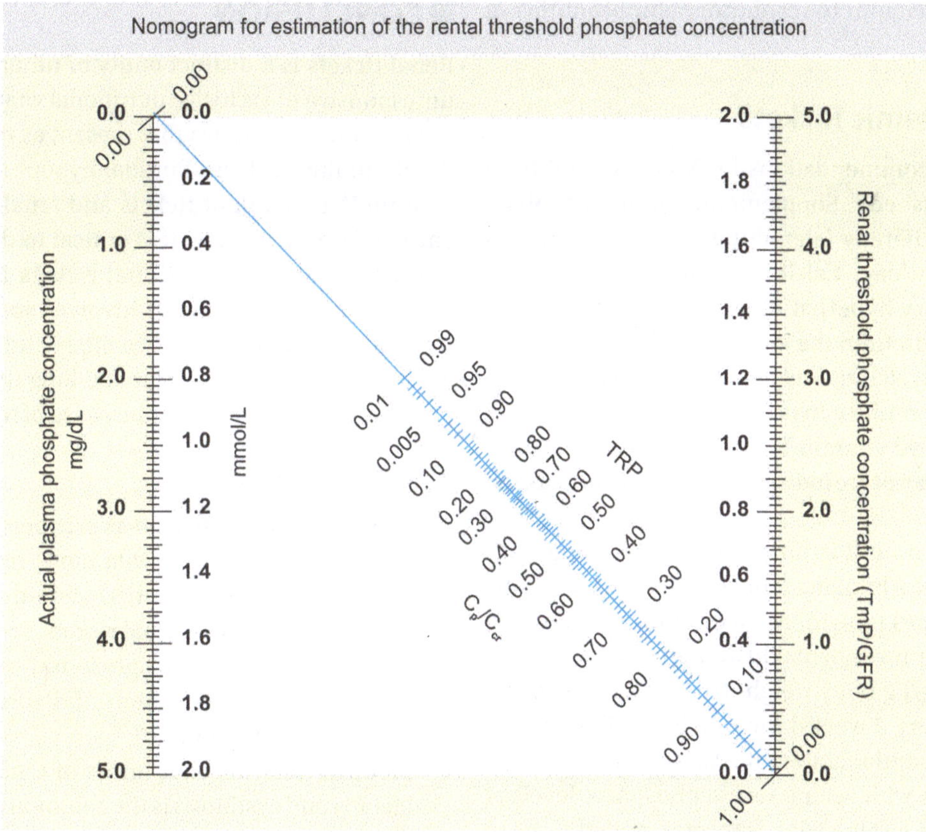

Fig. 5: The nomogram for plotting tubular maximum reabsorption of phosphate per glomerular filtration rate (TmP/GFR).
Source: Adapted from reference 22.

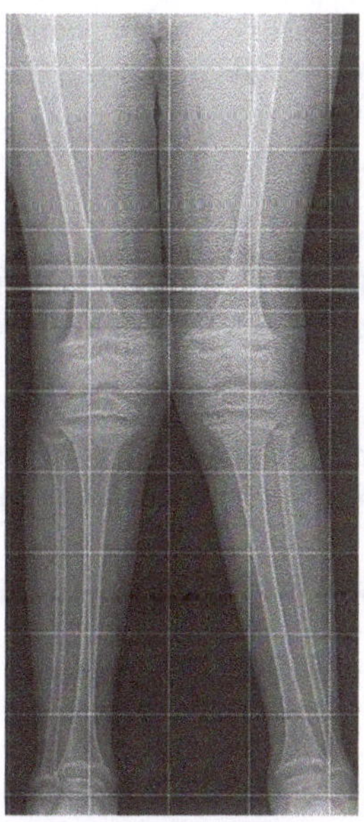

Fig. 6: X-ray of lower limbs that shows no classical features of resorption in hypophosphatemic rickets (HPR).

bicarbonate (4 mEq/tablet) or Shohl's solution (1 mEq/mL) at 2–4 mEq/kg/day in three to four divided doses for distal RTA and 10–15 mEq/kg/day in proximal RTA.

Potassium supplementation in the dose of 1–2 mEq/kg/day as potassium citrate is recommended to correct associated hypokalemia. While there is no indication for active vitamin D therapy in distal RTA, those with proximal RTA need active vitamin D and phosphate supplementation. Bony deformities due to rickets can get corrected with medical therapy in distal RTA. In certain cases of proximal RTA, surgical correction may be indicated when medical therapy has failed.

Chronic Kidney Disease—Mineral and Bone Disorder

Control of hyperphosphatemia, calcium supplementation, restoring stores of native vitamin D, and supplementation of active vitamin D form the cornerstone therapies. Metabolic acidosis also contributes to bone mineral disease and needs to be corrected with oral sodium bicarbonate.

Vitamin D-dependent Rickets

In those with VDDR I, children will respond to calcitriol or 1α-hydroxyvitamin D (1–2 µg daily) with dietary calcium (30–75 mg/kg/day of elemental calcium) supplementation. Monitoring for hypercalcemia, hypercalciuria, and nephrocalcinosis secondary to calcitriol therapy is needed. In children with VDDR II, due to resistant to 1,25-OHD, mega doses of calcitriol and calcium are needed with no assurance of adequate response. High doses of calcitriol that range between 0.05 and 0.2 mcg/kg/day along with calcium and phosphate supplementation are recommended. These children usually succumb to respiratory comorbidities in early childhood.

Hypophosphatemic Rickets

Clinical practice recommendations for X-linked HPR have been recently published.[20] Supplementation of phosphate is the mainstay of therapy (elemental phosphorus in 3–5 doses at 20–60 mg/kg/day). Calcitriol or alfacalcidol is added to prevent secondary hyperparathyroidism and increases phosphate absorption from the gut. With calcitriol therapy, monitoring for hypercalciuria and nephrocalcinosis is crucial. With persistent secondary hyperparathyroidism despite phosphate and active vitamin D treatment, calcimimetic agents such as cinacalcet are indicated with close monitoring for side effects.

A recent development is the effective treatment with burosumab (KRN23), a human monoclonal antibody against FGF-23 that promotes growth, reduces bone pain and leg deformities, and improves dental health. Indications to use burosumab [0.4 mg/kg body weight (maximum 2 mg/kg), subcutaneously every 2 weeks] include bone disease that is refractory to conventional therapy. Close monitoring for hyperphosphatemia with fasting serum phosphate levels at least a week after the last injection is recommended.

With regard to growth and interventions for musculoskeletal abnormalities, children with short stature can be offered growth hormone once the alkaline phosphatase and PTH are well controlled. Orthopedic care includes avoidance of casts or insoles for the limb deformities with elective surgical corrective treatment recommended only in those who have received optimal medical therapy for at least 1-year duration, in those with persisting deformity and with symptoms interfering with limb function or gait. Surgical interventions should consider the remaining growth potential of the child and may prove more effective after skeletal maturity has been achieved. Following surgical correction, regular monitoring is advised for clinical and functional evaluation.

Multidisciplinary follow-up care with dental interventions, orthopedic management, neurosurgical therapies, auditory monitoring, bone pain management, and lifestyle modifications are critical in the long-term care of HPR. In addition, the quality of life of a child with persistent rickets and deformities has gained focus through ongoing studies.

To conclude, renal rickets includes specific disorders that result in demineralization of bone due to disturbances in calcium, phosphorus, vitamin D, PTH, and FGF23. Renal rickets is treatable, if diagnosed early, and long-term therapy is warranted in the majority. With better understanding of the role of FGF23 in HPR, novel therapies have emerged that target FGF23 bioactivity, signaling, and degradation pathways for better clinical outcomes. A multidisciplinary approach will go a long way in managing children with renal rickets and their associated comorbidities.

CONCLUSION

Renal rickets is a distinct entity of tubular disorders that is unresponsive to exclusive nutritional vitamin D supplementation. Common entities that present as renal rickets include renal tubular acidosis, familial hypophosphatemic rickets, vitamin D-dependent rickets and renal osteodystrophy of chronic kidney disease. It is critical to differentiate clinical manifestations of nutritional rickets from renal rickets. Approach to the diagnosis involves specific tests of renal functions, acid–base abnormalities and dyselectrolytemia. Most of the disorders require life-long therapy with specific medications depending on the cause of renal rickets.

KEY POINTS

- Renal rickets can present as calcipenic or phosphopenic rickets and manifests as vitamin D-resistant rickets.
- RTA, HPR, and vitamin D-dependent and CKD are important causes for renal rickets.
- Differences in clinical presentation, evaluation, and approach to management of disorders causing renal rickets need attention.
- Medical treatment for forms of renal rickets is usually lifelong and cystinosis is the common form of renal rickets that can progress to end-stage kidney disease.

REFERENCES

1. Munns CF, Shaw N, Kiely M, Specker BL, Thacher TD, Ozono K, et al. Global Consensus Recommendations on prevention and management of nutritional Rickets. J Clin Endocrinol Metab. 2016;101(2):394-415.
2. Chanchlani R, Nemer P, Sinha R, Nemer L, Krishnappa V, Sochett E, et al. An overview of rickets in children. Kidney Int Rep. 2020;5(7):980-90.
3. Joshi RR, Patil S, Rao S. Clinical and etiological profile of refractory rickets from western India. Indian J Pediatr. 2013; 80(7):565-9.
4. Bharati J, Bhatia D, Khandelwal P, Gupta N, Sinha A, Khadgawat R, et al. C-Terminal fibroblast growth factor-23 levels in non-nutritional hypophosphatemic rickets. Indian J Pediatr. 2019; 86(6):555-7.
5. Carpenter TO, Shaw NJ, Portale AA, Ward LM, Abrams SA, Pettifor JM. Rickets. Nat Rev Dis Primers. 2017;3:17101.
6. Christakos S, Ajibade DV, Dhawan P, Fechner AJ, Mady LJ. Vitamin D: metabolism. Endocrinol Metab Clin North Am. 2010;39(2):243-53.
7. Beck-Nielsen SS, Mughal Z, Haffner D, Nilsson O, Levtchenko E, Ariceta G, et al. FGF23 and its role in X-linked hypophosphatemia-related morbidity. Orphanet J Rare Dis. 2019; 14(1):58.
8. Levine MA. Diagnosis and management of Vitamin D dependent rickets. Front Pediatr. 2020;8:315.
9. Giraldo A, Pino W, Garcia-Ramirez LF, Pineda M, Iglesias A. Vitamin D dependent rickets type II and normal vitamin D receptor cDNA sequence. A cluster in a rural area of Cauca, Colombia, with more than 200 affected children. Clin Genet. 1995;48(2):57-65.

10. Roizen JD, Li D, O'Lear L, Javaid MK, Shaw NJ, Ebeling PR, et al. CYP3A4 mutation causes vitamin D-dependent rickets type 3. J Clin Invest. 2018;128(5):1913-8.
11. Quigley R. Proximal renal tubular acidosis. J Nephrol. 2006;19(Suppl 9):S41-5.
12. Lee JH, Park JH, Ha TS, Han HS. Refractory rickets caused by mild distal renal tubular acidosis. Ann Pediatr Endocrinol Metab. 2013;18(3):152-5.
13. Devuyst O, Thakker RV. Dent's disease. Orphanet J Rare Dis. 2010;5:28.
14. Waziri B, Duarte R, Naicker S. Chronic kidney disease-mineral and bone disorder (CKD-MBD): Current perspectives: Int J Nephrol Renovasc Dis. 2019;12:263-76.
15. Shimada T, Muto T, Urakawa I, Yoneya T, Yamazaki Y, Okawa K, et al. Mutant FGF-23 responsible for autosomal dominant hypophosphatemic rickets is resistant to proteolytic cleavage and causes hypophosphatemia in vivo. Endocrinology. 2002;143(8):3179-82.
16. Feng JQ, Ward LM, Liu S, Lu Y, Xie Y, Yuan B, et al. Loss of DMP1 causes rickets and osteomalacia and identifies a role for osteocytes in mineral metabolism. Nat Genet. 2006;38(11): 1310-5.
17. Bergwitz C, Roslin NM, Tieder M, Loredo-Osti JC, Bastepe M, Abu-Zahra H, et al. SLC34A3 mutations in patients with hereditary hypophosphatemic rickets with hypercalciuria predict a key role for the sodium-phosphate co-transporter NaPi-IIc in maintaining phosphate homeostasis. Am J Hum Genet. 2006;78(2):179-92.
18. Bagga A, Sinha A. Renal tubular acidosis. Indian J Pediatr. 2020;87(9):733-44.
19. Carpenter TO, Imel EA, Holm IA, Jan de Beur SM, Insogna KL. A clinician's guide to X-linked hypophosphatemia. J Bone Miner Res. 2011;26(7):1381-8.
20. Haffner D, Emma F, Eastwood DM, Duplan MB, Bacchetta J, Schnabel D, et al. Clinical practice recommendations for the diagnosis and management of X-linked hypophosphataemia. Nat Rev Nephrol. 2019;15(7):435-55.
21. Goodyer P, Phadke K. Evaluation of renal disease. Manual of Pediatric Nephrology. Berlin, Heidelberg: Springer-Verlag; 2014. pp. 1-65.
22. Thacher TD, Pettifor JM, Tebben PJ, Creo AL, Skrinar A, Mao M, et al. Rickets severity predicts clinical outcomes in children with X-linked hypophosphatemia: Utility of the radiographic Rickets Severity Score. Bone. 2019;122:76-81.
23. Kidney Disease: Improving Global Outcomes (KDIGO) CKD–MBD Update Work Group. KDIGO 2017 Clinical Practice Guideline update for the diagnosis, evaluation, prevention, and treatment of Chronic Kidney Disease–Mineral and Bone Disorder (CKD–MBD). Kidney Int Suppl. 2017;7:1-59.

CHAPTER

8.7 Hypercalciuria and Nephrocalcinosis

Pankaj Pandurang Bhansali

INTRODUCTION

Hypercalciuria, or excessive urinary calcium excretion, is a typical metabolic abnormality, observed in 3–6% of children. It is found in almost 50% of children with renal stones. In 1953, Albright proposed the term, idiopathic hypercalciuria (IH), for defining elevated excretion of urinary calcium despite normal serum calcium and absence of any obvious condition capable of causing it. Various studies have confirmed an important role of kidneys in calcium handling, but the pathophysiology of IH has still eluded us.

Hypercalciuria can be an incidental finding or can have varied presentations such as lower urinary tract symptoms, nephrolithiasis, and decreased bone mineral density. Along with kidney stone disease, bone demineralization is an important morbidity associated with long-term hypercalciuria in adults. So, it is important to recognize the diversity of the disease, associated risks, and the need of instituting timely intervention.

Secondary hypercalciuria is a situation where a recognized condition induces excessive calcium excretion in urine.

DEFINITION

In adults, hypercalciuria is considered if excretion of calcium in urine is in excess of 250 mg/day in women and in excess of 300 mg/day in men, when patients are on their usual diet. In children, it is defined as urinary calcium excretion of >4 mg/kg/day in a timed urine sample. In the 24-hour urine collection, it is important that the patient is free of infection, medicines, and is on an unrestricted diet. Spot urinary calcium creatinine ratio can be used as a screening test or in smaller children when it is difficult to collect the timed urine sample. Empty stomach, first or second morning urine sample shall be collected.

The calcium-creatinine ratio varies with age:

- *0–6 months:* <0.8
- *7–12 months:* <0.6
- *>24 months:* <0.21

PATHOPHYSIOLOGY

The development of hypercalciuria involves a maladaptation of the three main organs involved in calcium homeostasis, namely, gastrointestinal tract, bone and kidney, and the hormonal interplay between parathyroid hormone (PTH), calcitonin, and 1,25-dihydroxyvitamin D.[1,2] Although many aspects of the pathophysiology are still elusive, better understanding has been gained in the last few decades about hypercalciuria.

Idiopathic hypercalciuria has been classified into three subtypes depending on urinary calcium response to fasting or diet with low calcium and to a calcium load.

1. *Absorptive hypercalciuria:* Primarily, an increase in intestinal calcium absorption is responsible for increased urinary calcium excretion along with normal or low PTH. There is a significant fall in calcium excretion following fasting. The probable explanation is increased expression of vitamin D receptor in the intestine or altered metabolism of 1,25-dihydroxyvitamin D. It has been further subdivided into type I (direct absorption of calcium in the gut), type II (excessive 1,25-dihydroxyvitamin D mediated), and type III (secondary to phosphaturia).

   Type III absorptive hypercalciuria is also called renal phosphate leak hypercalciuria. It is suspected if the serum phosphate level is <2.9 mg/dL in case of IH. Active form, 1,25-dihydroxyvitamin D, is stimulated in kidneys secondary to hypophosphatemia and it is liable for increased intestinal calcium absorption alongside phosphate resulting in hypercalciuria.
2. *Resorptive hypercalciuria:* Excess calcium present in the urine is primarily from bone, owing to increased bone turnover or demineralization. It manifests with a normal or high calcium level with aptly suppressed PTH, and fasting hypercalciuria. In fasting hypercalciuria, urine calcium excretion does not lower appropriately after restriction of dietary calcium. Bone loss may be responsible for a compensatory increase in intestinal calcium absorption. Pacifici et al. documented an increased amount of interleukin-1 in the monocytes of the patients. It may be an important mediator of excessive bone resorption.

   Excessive intake of animal protein can be a risk factor as it can lead to acid load and calcium excretion secondary to demineralization.
3. *Renal leak hypercalciuria:* The primary defect in renal tubular calcium transport is responsible for hypercalciuria.

Compensatory mechanisms lead to a rise in PTH and an increase in calcium secondary to mobilization from bone or absorption from the gut, and fasting hypercalciuria. But it is not considered as the main cause of IH.

However, in most cases, the clinical value of the classification appears modest. IH has a generalized effect on calcium metabolism with acceleration of all three processes including gut absorption, mobilization from bone, and renal leak.

GENETICS

Studies among first-degree relatives of stone formers have revealed a higher incidence of nephrolithiasis and hypercalciuria. Several genes differing from individual to individual contributed to IH, therefore, making it a complex polygenic trait.[2,3] Genes encoding vitamin D receptor, calcium-sensing receptor, transient receptor potential vanilloid 5 (TRPV5), and renal epithelial calcium channel, and many more genes have shown a potential association with IH. The gene or genes responsible for IH are still not specifically acknowledged. Besides, the diet of the patient has an enormous influence on the expression of hypercalciuria. At present, there is insufficient data affirming the play of these interrelated mediators in IH.

CLINICAL FEATURES

Hypercalciuria is purely a laboratory diagnosis. It can have varied presentations from accidental diagnosis in asymptomatic children to different clinical manifestations such as hematuria, renal calculi, and symptoms mimicking lower urinary tract infection (UTI). Many children (>50%) have some form of hematuria. It may be microscopic, diagnosed during urine examination or gross, as a presenting symptom. Microcrystallization of calcium with urinary anions has been thought to injure the uroepithelium and produce hematuria. Repeated UTI is another manifestation of hypercalciuria. Frequently, it can present with abdominal pain, urinary frequency, urgency, and dysuria without urinary infection. It is a key reason of renal calculus, colicky abdominal pain, and obstructive uropathy.

In a retrospective review of 288 hypercalciuric children, presenting symptoms were voiding symptoms and gross hematuria (28%), voiding symptoms and microscopic hematuria (30%), urinary frequency (21%), dysuria (22%), and combined urgency-frequency and dysuria (28%).[4]

DIAGNOSIS

Once hypercalciuria is diagnosed, it is important to rule out hypercalcemia and other causes of hypercalciuria predominantly in presence of similar family history, dysmorphic features, failure to thrive, rickets, renal dysfunction, electrolyte and acid-base imbalance, and poor response to therapy. Other common causes of normocalcemic hypercalciuria of renal origin are Bartter syndrome, renal tubular acidosis (RTA), familial hypomagnesemia with hypercalciuria and nephrocalcinosis, Dent's disease, and hereditary hypophosphatemic rickets. Secondary resorptive hypercalciuria is observed in osteogenesis imperfecta and McCune-Albright syndrome. An approach to hypercalciuria is depicted in **Flowchart 1**.

Flowchart 1: Approach to hypercalciuria.

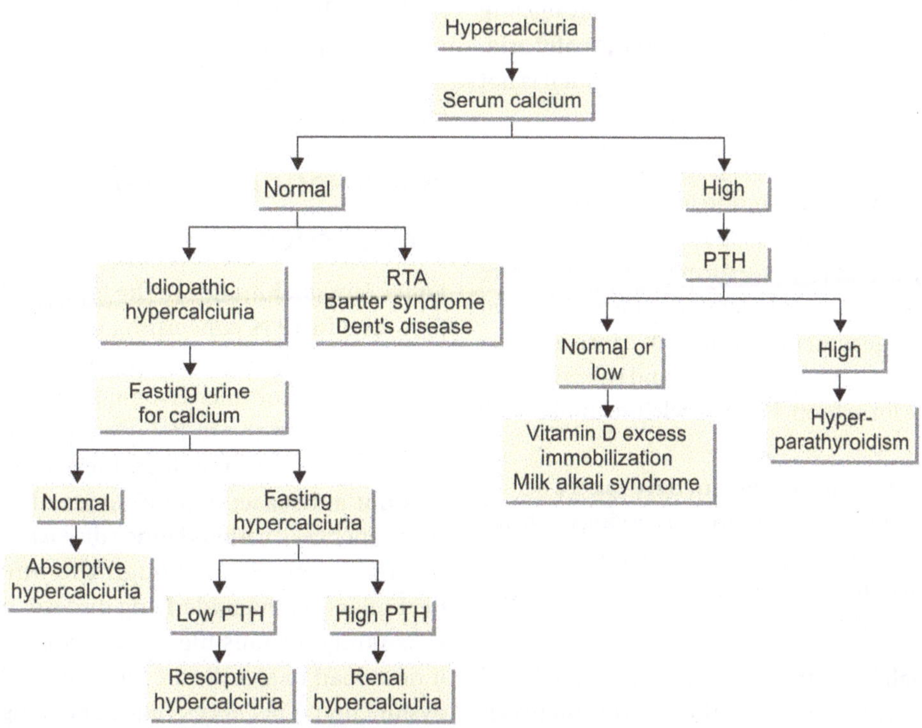

(PTH: parathyroid hormone; RTA: renal tubular acidosis)

For confirming absorptive hypercalciuria, a fasting morning urine sample is collected with normal sodium and protein intake but with low calcium intake. Normalization of the urinary calcium–creatinine ratio confirms absorptive hypercalciuria. Fasting hypercalciuria is diagnosed if hypercalciuria persists despite fasting. Further differentiation between resorptive hypercalciuria and renal hypercalciuria is based on serum calcium and PTH value.

The traditional classification system assumes existence of distinct types of IH and can be differentiated from one another. But practically there is a significant overlap between different types. Furthermore, it is difficult to differentiate them despite extensive, time-consuming, and challenging test, which is usually unnecessary. It hardly affects the treatment plan.[5] The calcium-loading test is generally used for selected cases, mainly for research purposes.

Presences of calcium crystals in urine are not confirmatory of hypercalciuria.

TREATMENT

Diet

Decrease sodium and animal protein in diet:[6] Diet has a vast influence over calcium excretion in urine, not only in children with IH but also in normal subjects. Calcium excretion demonstrates a proportional rise with an increase in salt and protein intake. In healthy subjects, the urine calcium increases by about 1 mmol per 100 mmol increment in urinary sodium excretion and by 0.4 mmol per gram intake of dietary protein. These effects are exaggerated in children with IH. Potassium has been shown to have a negative correlation with calcium excretion. Lowering salt-containing food and increasing potassium-rich food help in decreasing hypercalciuria. Protein restriction can also reduce hypercalciuria, but it is not suggested in children as it can upset growth.

Allow normal calcium intake: Dietary calcium restriction can lead to bone demineralization due to negative calcium balance. It also increases the risk of stone formation. Curhan et al. reported that the risk of stone formation is 34% more in people with calcium-restricted diet than those with good calcium intake. Low ingestion of calcium can cause a rise in oxalate absorption and its urinary excretion and subsequently calcium oxalate stone formation. Normal calcium intake shall be ensured.

The diet of children with IH shall not have excess salt or animal protein. They shall have four to five servings of fruits and vegetables along with normal calcium intake. A urinary Na/K ratio of <2.5 can help us in confirming compliance with dietary recommendations.

Dietary oxalate: It shall be restricted especially with reduced calcium intake. Excessive oxalate excretion in urine increases the risk of calcium oxalate stone.

Medicines: These shall be used when hypercalciuria or symptoms related to hypercalciuria persist beyond 1 month of dietary modifications.[7,8]

Potassium citrate: It increases citrate excretion in urine that helps in inhibiting the crystallization of calcium salt. Citrate therapy has been effective in preventing the growth of residual stone fragments after surgical intervention and also decreases new stone formation. Potassium supplement at 2–3 mEq/kg/day has been shown to reduce hypercalciuria. It remains first-line medicine in the management of IH. But a higher dose can be counterproductive promoting the risk of calcium phosphate stones in alkaline pH.

Thiazide diuretics: These have anticalciuric action. They can be considered, if diet and potassium citrate does not succeed in reducing symptoms or calcium excretion. Hydrochlorothiazide 1.5–2.5 mg/kg/day or chlorothiazide 15–25 mg/kg/day can be used. It is suggested that thiazide-induced mild volume contraction induces paracellular calcium absorption in the proximal tubule. Thiazide also increases the expression of TRPV5 channel in renal epithelial cells that has a significant place in calcium absorption. Prolonged thiazide use warrants monitoring for dyselectrolytemia, hyperglycemia, and hyperlipidemia. Adding potassium citrate along prevents the risk of hypokalemia and hypocitraturia. Addition of amiloride, along with thiazide, has the advantage of increasing calcium reabsorption besides potassium-sparing effect.

Bisphosphonate (alendronate): It has been considered useful in resorptive hypercalciuria. In genetic hypercalciuric rats, it has proved to be effective by reducing urinary calcium excretion and improving bone mineralization despite being on low-calcium diet. Human studies have also shown to reduce urinary calcium excretion along with improved bone mineral content. But further studies need to confirm its long-term benefit.

NEPHROCALCINOSIS

Introduction

Fuller Albright introduced the term nephrocalcinosis for the first time in 1934 concerning calcium deposition into the kidney associated with primary hyperparathyroidism. Initially, it was coined for microscopic finding, while presently it is mostly used for the radiological picture. Nephrocalcinosis is characterized by the deposition of calcium in the kidney. It is not a disease; it is rather a radiological finding as a consequence of various kidney diseases, metabolic disorders, or medicines. Even though the outcome is primarily dependent on the underlying disease, nephrocalcinosis per se is rarely responsible for end-stage kidney disease, but it does lead to significant renal morbidity and progressive dysfunction. This necessitates detecting underlying disease and initiating targeted therapy.

Classification (Table 1)

The term nephrocalcinosis describes the deposition of calcium (both calcium phosphate and calcium oxalate) in renal parenchyma and tubules. Few experts separate the deposition of calcium oxalate as a separate entity, but it is not accepted unanimously. In the clinical setting, where nephrocalcinosis is a radiological diagnosis, it does not seem practical to separate these entities.

In >97% of cases, the medulla is the predominant site for nephrocalcinosis. Cortical nephrocalcinosis is very uncommon, responsible for <3% of cases. It has been linked with severe underlying cortical diseases such as cortical necrosis, pyelonephritis, and chronic glomerulonephritis.[9] It is also found in oxalosis, kidney allograft rejection, and autosomal-recessive polycystic kidney disease. Both medullary and cortical nephrocalcinosis have been described with oxalosis.

Pathogenesis

Increased calcium excretion in urine with or without hypercalcemia is the most important explanation for nephrocalcinosis. It can also have increased phosphate and oxalate excretion or decreased citrate excretion in urine. Both nephrocalcinosis and nephrolithiasis can be observed in cases with these urinary abnormalities. But more frequently, both conditions are observed in the absence of other, for reasons that are not clear.

Numerous monogenic disorders have been identified with metabolic abnormalities responsible for nephrocalcinosis. These have definitely helped in understanding calcium and phosphorus handling by kidneys and renal tubule. But a complete and uniform explanation responsible for nephrocalcinosis still continues to evade experts. The finding of hypocalciuria, instead of hypercalciuria, in the patient with enamel renal syndrome further opens a new window to rethink the underlying mechanism of nephrocalcinosis.

Calcium oxalate and calcium phosphate crystals form when the concentration of the reactants exceeds the saturation limit. Calcium phosphate deposits (Randall's plaques) are primarily noted in the inner medullary (papillary) interstitium in the basement membranes of the thin limbs of the loop of Henle. These calcium phosphate plaques can enlarge into the surrounding interstitial tissue or rupture into the tubule lumen serving as a nidus for luminal calcium oxalate stone formation. Calcium phosphate can promote calcium oxalate crystallization.[10]

TABLE 1: Oliver Wrong's classification.

Molecular or chemical	A significant increase in renal intracellular calcium but is not detectable in microscopy or radioimaging. It is often reversible with improvement in hypercalciuria
Microscopic	Microscopically (with biopsy) detectable calcium deposition but not visible with radiography. It is a precursor of macroscopic nephrocalcinosis
Macroscopic	Calcification is visible by radiographic imaging of either X-ray, ultrasound, or CT scan. This is the usual type, which is observed in clinical practice

Etiology

Various acquired and inherited diseases have the potential to produce nephrocalcinosis. Most of them have hypercalciuria as the underlying factor. IH, various renal tubular defects such as RTA and Bartter syndrome, primary hyperoxaluria, and excess intake of vitamin D are the most common causes. Few causes such as Dent's disease and familial hypomagnesemia with hypercalciuria and nephrocalcinosis are relatively uncommon but have a high potential for progressive renal dysfunction **(Table 2)**.

- Primary hyperoxaluria was not included in study.
  The conditions responsible for nephrocalcinosis can be broadly divided into following categories **(Table 3)**:
- *Hypercalcemia with hypercalciuria*:
  - Primary hyperparathyroidism
  - Vitamin D therapy
  - William's syndrome
  - Congenital hypothyroidism
  - Sarcoidosis
- *Hypercalciuria without hypercalcemia*:
  - Distal RTA
  - Bartter syndrome
  - Medullary sponge kidney
  - Familial hypomagnesemic hypercalciuric nephrocalcinosis
  - Dent's disease
  - Lowe's syndrome
  - Autosomal-dominant hypocalcemia
  - Neonatal nephrocalcinosis and loop diuretics
  - Chronic hypokalemia
- *Hyperphosphaturia*:
  - Hypophosphatemic rickets (XLX, ADHR, and ARHR)
  - Dent's disease and Lowe's syndrome
  - Tumor lysis syndrome

TABLE 2: Incidence of conditions responsible for nephrocalcinosis.[11-13]

Causes	Ronnefarth et al.	Mukta et al.	Kagnur et al.
Idiopathic hypercalciuria	34%	7.5%	9.3%
Distal RTA	17%	20%	33%
Bartter syndrome	6%	5%	13%
Primary hyperoxaluria		7.5%	16.7%
Vitamin D excess	8%	5%	

(RTA: renal tubular acidosis)

TABLE 3: Inheritance, genetic basis, and clinical manifestations.

Disorder	*Inheritance*	*Gene protein/channel defect*	*Clinical manifestations (along with nephrocalcinosis)*
Distal renal tubular acidosis	AR/AD	H^+ pump/AE1	Hyperchloremic acidosis, hypokalemia
Bartter syndrome	AR	NKCC2/ROMK	Alkalosis, hypokalemia, hyponatremia, secondary aldosteronism
FHHNC	AD	Claudin	Urinary losses of Ca and Mg, progressive renal failure
Dent's disease	XR	Chloride channel 5	LMW proteinuria, proximal tubular defect, and progressive kidney failure
Lowe's syndrome	XR	Phosphatidylinositol phosphatase enzyme	Multiple proximal tubular defects, hydrophthalmia, cataract, mental retardation, and progressive kidney failure
Primary hyperoxaluria	AR	AGT/GRHPR enzyme defect	Progressive renal failure, diminished vision, bone pain and fractures, cardiac conduction defects
ADHH	AD	CASR-activating mutation	Hypocalcemia, hypercalciuria, normal PTH, and seizures Nephrolithiasis mainly during calcium and vitamin D therapy
Medullary sponge kidney	AD	*GDNF/RET* gene defect	Incomplete renal tubular acidosis, recurrent UTI, and metabolic bone disease
Enamel renal syndrome	AR	FAM20A	Amelogenesis imperfecta, gingival hyperplasia, and impaired tooth eruption
X-linked hypophosphatemia AD hypophosphatemic rickets AR hypophosphatemic rickets	X-linked AD AR	PHEX FGF23 DMP1	Rickets, growth retardation, decreased tubular reabsorption of phosphate, normal serum and urinary excretion of calcium, PTH, normal. Treatment with vitamin D leads to nephrocalcinosis

(AD: autosomal dominant; ADHH: autosomal dominant hypocalcemia with hypercalciuria; AE1: anion exchanger 1; AR: autosomal recessive; FHHNC: familial hypomagnesemia with hypercalciuria and nephrocalcinosis; LMW: low molecular weight; PTH: parathyroid hormone; UTI: urinary tract infection; XR: X-linked recessive)

- *Hyperoxaluria*:
  - Primary hyperoxaluria
  - Excess vitamin C or oxalate containing food
  - Fat malabsorption

Clinical Presentation

Nephrocalcinosis is mostly an asymptomatic radiographic finding discovered during evaluation for some other problem. It can have coexistent nephrolithiasis. The common symptoms associated with nephrocalcinosis are failure to thrive, polyuria, nocturia, polydipsia, renal colic, repeated UTIs, hematuria, bony deformities, vomiting, and anorexia. Ronnefarth et al. found psychomotor and/or mental retardation in 28% of cases. But most clinical features are related to the primary disease responsible for nephrocalcinosis.

Few symptoms have been attributed directly to nephrocalcinosis. Polyuria and polydipsia can be due to compromised urinary concentrating ability observed in nephrocalcinosis. They can manifest as nephrogenic diabetes insipidus. Nephrolithiasis and, less commonly, nephrocalcinosis are associated with renal colic. Microscopic or gross hematuria can sometimes bring attention to nephrocalcinosis.

Family history of nephrocalcinosis or nephrolithiasis has been observed in 29% by Ronnefarth et al., while consanguinity in almost 50% of cases by Kangur et al.

Investigations

Diagnosis of nephrocalcinosis is frequently an incidental finding during radiographic imaging performed for evaluation of nephrolithiasis, renal tubular dysfunction, or for a cause unrelated to renal disease. It can be diagnosed on abdominal plain film, ultrasonography, or computed tomography (CT) **(Table 4)**. Ultrasound and CT scan are more sensitive than abdominal plain film. Ultrasound is preferred imaging to screen for it, and a typical appearance of nephrocalcinosis is depicted in **Figure 1**.

TABLE 4: Grading by ultrasonography.[14]

Grade	*Sonography findings*
I	Echogenicity of medullary pyramids slightly higher than that of cortex
IIa	White garland at border of pyramids
IIb	Markedly increased echogenicity of whole pyramids without acoustic shadowing
III	Homogenous increase in echogenicity of medullary pyramids with acoustic shadowing

After diagnosing nephrocalcinosis, subsequent evaluation to determining the underlying condition is important. The underlying condition will decide kidney prognosis and it may have systemic implications beyond just renal involvement. Diseases such as primary hyperparathyroidism and primary hyperoxaluria can have significant effects on other organs as well, and diseases such as medullary sponge kidney can have limited effect on kidney function.

If the child has clinical manifestations pointing toward a certain disease, the child shall be investigated accordingly. Investigations include blood samples for pH, bicarbonate,

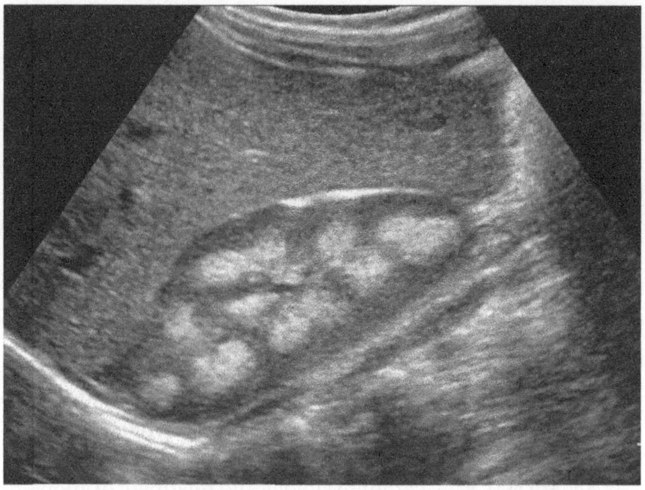

Fig. 1: Nephrocalcinosis on renal ultrasonography.

urea, creatinine, electrolytes, calcium, phosphorous, and magnesium. Urine samples shall be processed for microscopy, infection, and pH. A timed sample of urine shall be collected for the estimation of calcium, oxalate, phosphate, citric acid, and creatinine. If a 24-hour sample is not feasible, a spot sample shall be analyzed. 25-hydroxycholecalciferol and parathyroid hormone assay are necessary for a patient with hypercalciuria. In suspected Dent's disease, urinary β2-microglobulin needs to be assessed.

If the appropriate diagnosis is not apparent despite thorough evaluation, genetic testing for monogenic causes of nephrocalcinosis can be considered, particularly for a child with progressive nephrocalcinosis or worsening renal function.

Treatment

Treatment is focused on the management of an underlying disease wherever possible such as alkali supplements in RTA, parathyroidectomy for primary hyperparathyroidism, glucocorticoid therapy for sarcoidosis, stopping calcium and vitamin D supplement in hypercalcemia secondary to calcium, and vitamin D intake.

Interventions can be undertaken to reduce the concentration of calcium, phosphate, and oxalate in the urine and to increase solubility. Fluid intake can be increased to 2 L/m^2 to produce adequate urine output so that solutes do not saturate in tubules. It is beneficial for all children with nephrocalcinosis and nephrolithiasis. Hypercalciuria is the most common pathology behind nephrocalcinosis. As excess sodium in diet promotes increased calcium excretion, salt intake has to be controlled. Calcium restriction can lower the bone mineral density and increase intestinal oxalate absorption and its excretion in urine. Therefore, calcium shall be continued according to the recommended daily allowance. Protein restriction is not recommended due to risk of growth retardation. But diet high in animal protein can induce increased acid load and subsequently cause hypocitraturia and hypercalciuria.[15] Diet shall have good quantity of fruits and vegetables as they provides potassium and citrate that have inhibitory effect on calcium precipitation.[16] If dietary modifications fail to induce a desired change in hypercalciuria, a thiazide diuretic can be added. Citrate can be administered in patients with hypocitraturia.

Prognosis

Nephrocalcinosis diagnosed on imaging is not likely to be improved, and if primary pathology is not diagnosed and managed appropriately, it can progress and lead to deterioration of kidney function. However, improvement can be observed in few situations such as calcium, vitamin D, or furosemide-related nephrocalcinosis and also in IH, if necessary, measures are initiated in time.

The long-term outcome of the kidney is dependent on underlying etiology. Progression to end-stage kidney disease (ESKD) is not common in nephrocalcinosis, if managed effectively. A higher probability of progression to ESKD has been observed in primary hyperoxaluria, Dent's disease, and familial hypomagnesemia with hypercalciuria and nephrocalcinosis.

Neonatal Nephrocalcinosis

Neonates, especially preterm babies, are very susceptible to nephrocalcinosis. Numerous factors such as immature renal tubules, nutritional supplements, and various medications increase the risk of calcium deposition in the renal tubule and interstitium. In preterm infants, the risk of nephrocalcinosis has been documented up to 7–41%.

Risk Factors

- *Renal tubular immaturity*: Nephrogenesis continues until 36 weeks leading to a markedly low glomerular filtration rate in preterm neonates. The process of tubular proliferation and maturation continues even beyond, making immature tubules susceptible to crystal formation. Both of these factors collectively enhance the risk of nephrocalcinosis in preterm neonates.[17] Tubular bicarbonate reabsorption is affected in preterm neonates <1,500 g causing alkaline urinary pH and risk of calcium phosphate precipitation.
- *Hypercalciuria*:
  - *Hypercalcemia hypercalciuria*:
    - Subcutaneous fat
    - Nutritional supplements with calcium and vitamin D
    - *Genetic disorders*: William's syndrome, idiopathic infantile hypercalcemia, congenital lactase deficiency, and neonatal primary hyperparathyroidism
  - *Normocalcemic hypercalciuria*:
    - Furosemide and dexamethasone
    - *Genetic disorders*: Bartter syndrome, distal RTA, and hypophosphatasia
  - *Hyperoxaluria*

Management

Once nephrocalcinosis is diagnosed, probably responsible factors shall be stopped and treatment of the underlying disease shall be initiated. If the clinical condition permits, furosemide shall be discontinued and a thiazide diuretic can be considered. Calcium or phosphorous intake shall be monitored, particularly when the neonate is on parenteral nutrition or calcium and vitamin D supplement. Adequate fluid intake and urine output shall be ensured.

Follow-up

After discharge from neonatal intensive care unit (NICU), nephrocalcinosis shall be monitored by serial sonography, renal function, and urinary calcium excretion. In preterm neonates without underlying genetic defects, most cases show spontaneous resolution in early childhood.[18] We can expect a good outcome in an infant with nephrocalcinosis secondary to medicines or nutritional supplements. Further studies are required to assess long-term result as follow-up has shown mixed results about creatinine clearance and tubular dysfunction.

CONCLUSION

Hypercalciuria is an important tubular disorder that can manifest with recurrent UTI and lower urinary tract symptoms along with hematuria or abdominal pain. Nephrocalcinosis is the result of calcium deposition within the parenchyma of the kidney and is secondary to a diverse group of disorders. The phenotype presentation of nephrocalcinosis varies based on the genetic makeup of specific disease entities.

KEY POINTS

- Hypercalciuria can be found in 3–6% of children.
- 24-hour urinary calcium estimation shall be preferred over the spot urine calcium-creatinine ratio, whenever possible.
- First or second morning urine shall be collected for the spot calcium-creatinine ratio.
- Most of the children can be managed with dietary modifications.
- Calcium restriction is not recommended, as it can worsen the chances of stone formation.
- Nephrocalcinosis is diagnosed by imaging studies and can be an important manifestation of tubular diseases such as hyperoxaluria, Bartter syndrome, and renal tubular acidosis.
- Vitamin D toxicity is an important preventable cause for nephrocalcinosis.
- Nephrocalcinosis is not reversible and if allowed to progress, can lead to kidney injury.

REFERENCES

1. Tarak S, Alon US. Pathophysiology of hypercalciuria in children. Pediatr Nephrol. 2007;22(10):1659-73.
2. Elaine M, Fredric L. New insights in pathogenesis of idiopathic hypercalciuria. Semin Nephrol. 2008;28(2):120-32.
3. Stechman MJ, Loh NY, Thakker RV. Genetic causes of hypercalciuric nephrolithiasis. Pediatr Nephrol. 2009;24(12):2321-32.
4. Parekh DJ, Pope JI, Adams MC, Brock JW 3rd. The role of hypercalciuria in a subgroup of dysfunctional voiding syndromes of childhood. J Urol. 2000;164(3):1008-10.
5. Bataille P, Fardellone P, Ghazali A, Cayrolle G, Hottelart C, Achard HM, et al. Pathophysiology and treatment of idiopathic hypercalciuria. Curr Opin Rheumatol. 1998;10(4):373-88.
6. Srivastava T, Schwaderer A. Diagnosis and management of hypercalciuria in children. Curr Opin Pediatr. 2009;21(2):214-9.
7. Milliner DS. Urolithiasis. In: Avner ED, Harmon WE, Niaduet P, Yoshikawa N (Eds). Pediatric Nephrology, 6th edition. Berlin Heidelberg: Springer; 2009. pp. 1405-24.
8. Tamilarasi V. Hypercalciuria and renal stone disease. In: Nammalwar BR, Vijayakumar M (Eds). Principles and Practice of Pediatric Nephrology, 2nd edition. New Delhi: Jaypee Brothers Medical Publishers; 2013. pp. 277-88.
9. Wrong O. Nephrocalcinosis. In: Davison AM, Cameron JS, Grünfeld J, Winearls CG, Himmelfarb J, Remuzzi G (Eds). Oxford Textbook of Clinical Nephrology. Oxford: Oxford University Press; 2005. p. 1375.
10. Linda S, Philippe J, Rodert J. What is nephrocalcinosis. Kidney Int. 2015;88(1):35-43.
11. Ronnefarth G, Misselwitz J. Nephrocalcinosis in children: A retrospective survey. Pediatr Nephrol. 2000;14(10-11):1016-21.
12. Mantan M, Bagga A, Virdi VS, Menon S, Hari P. Etiology of nephrocalcinosis in northern Indian children. Pediatr Nephrol. 2007;22(6):829-33.
13. Kagnur R, Sriram K, Palanisamy S. Etiological profile of nephrocalcinosis in children from southern India. Indian Pediatr. 2020;57:415-9.
14. Hoyer PF. Nephrocalcinose. In: Hofmann V, Deeg KH, Hoyer PF (Eds). Ultraschalldiagnostik in Pädiatrie und Kinderchirurgie. Stuttgart: Thieme; 1996. pp. 372-4.
15. Curhan GC, Willett WC, Rimm EB, Stampfer MJ. A prospective study of dietary calcium and other nutrients and the risk of symptomatic kidney stones. N Engl J Med. 1993;328(12):833-8.
16. Carvalho-Salemi J, Moreno L, Michael M. Medical nutrition therapy for pediatric kidney stone prevention, part one. J Ren Nutr. 2017;27(1):e5-8.
17. Schell-Feith EA, Kist-van Holthe JE, van der Heijden AJ. Nephrocalcinosis in preterm neonates. Pediatr Nephrol. 2010;25(2):221-30.
18. Kist-van Holthe JE, van Zwieten PH, Schell-Feith EA, Zonderland HM, Holscher HC, Wolterbeek R, et al. Is nephrocalcinosis in preterm neonates harmful for long-term blood pressure and renal function? Pediatrics. 2007;119(3):468-75.

CHAPTER

8.8 Primary Hyperoxaluria

Aditi Das, Abhijeet Saha

INTRODUCTION

Primary hyperoxalurias (PHs) are a rare autosomal recessive disorder of inborn error of metabolism due to enzymatic defects in glyoxylate metabolism, which leads to overproduction of oxalate.[1,2] Humans cannot degrade oxalate and primarily eliminate it by the renal system and, to some extent, through the gastrointestinal tract. Oxalate is excreted by both passive osmotic and active processes through renal tubules and through active transport from plasma to gut. In physiological conditions, oxalate is primarily excreted by kidneys. When renal functions get deranged, oxalate excretion increases through the gut.[2] Endogenous overproduction of oxalate results in increased urinary oxalate excretion, usually 1 mmol (0.88 mg)/1.73 m^2/day [normal 0.5 mmol (0.45 mg)/1.73 m^2/day conversion factor 1 mmol = 88 mg], which leads to calcium oxalate (CaOx) supersaturation in urine, resulting in nephrocalcinosis and urolithiasis. Crystal deposition in renal parenchyma causes inflammation, fibrosis, and gradual deterioration in renal function.[1,3] When end-stage kidney disease (ESKD) develops, oxalate deposition accelerates, which leads to systemic oxalosis, involving multiple organs, especially in skeleton, heart, and eyes.[4]

CLASSIFICATION

Primary hyperoxaluria is related to three distinct hereditary enzyme deficiencies, which are—type 1 [(PH1, number 259900 in the Online Mendelian Inheritance of Man (OMIM) database], type 2 (PH2; OMIM 260000), and type 3 (PH3; OMIM 613616). Studies revealed that there can be other causes that present as PH, though the causes are yet to be detected, and this group is known as unclassified PH.[1,3] PH1 is the most severe form accounting for 80% of cases. The presentation is varied from infantile oxalosis to recurrent urolithiasis and nephrocalcinosis leading to ESKD by the second decade of life.[1] In PH2, the age of presentation is almost similar and about 20% of patients develop ESKD.[1,5] The PH3 is the least severe form (formerly DHDPS, dihydrodipicolinate synthase) associated with a phenotypically milder form, and the renal function is usually well preserved.[6]

EPIDEMIOLOGY

Primary hyperoxaluria type 1 is reported in around 1–2% of cases from the chronic kidney disease (CKD) registries of USA, UK, and Japan. Higher rates are reported from inbred populations. Among Kuwaiti and Tunisian pediatric populations, around 10% and 13% of kids with ESKD have PH1 (prevalence approximately 1 to 3:1,000,000).[7,8] PH1 has a prevalence of 1–3/million population and is reported more frequently in populations where consanguineous marriage is frequent. The highest prevalence has been reported from North Africa and the Middle East, with around 10% of pediatric ESKD cases.[8]

SOURCES

Dietary oxalate attributes to 24–53% of urinary oxalate. High oxalate-containing foods including cocoa, chocolate, peanut butter, nuts, leafy greens (mainly spinach and rhubarb), black tea, or star fruit result in high urinary oxalate concentration. Therefore, restricted intake of dietary oxalate and use of calcium carbonate or calcium citrate during meals, which binds dietary oxalate, are considered beneficial. Vitamin C mega dose (4 g/day) and ethylene glycol ingestion can also result in hyperoxaluria.[9-11]

PRIMARY HYPEROXALURIA TYPE 1

Biology and Molecular Basis

The first PH1 case was reported by the French clinician Lepoutre in 1925 in an infant, and AGT (alanine:glyoxylate-aminotransferase) deficiency was first described by Danpure and Watts in 1986.[12] The most severe form of PHs is PH1, which accounts for around 80% of genetically determined patients.[7] In PH1, the failure of glyoxylate detoxification leads to overproduction of oxalate by cytosolic lactate dehydrogenase (LDH), resulting in increased urinary oxalate excretion. The enzymatic pathway is depicted in **Figure 1**. Due to poor solubility, this product forms CaOx crystals and when the urine becomes supersaturated, urolithiasis and/or nephrocalcinosis develops. Eventually, patients reach ESKD due to progressive renal parenchyma inflammation and interstitial fibrosis caused by nephrocalcinosis and recurrent urolithiasis.[7]

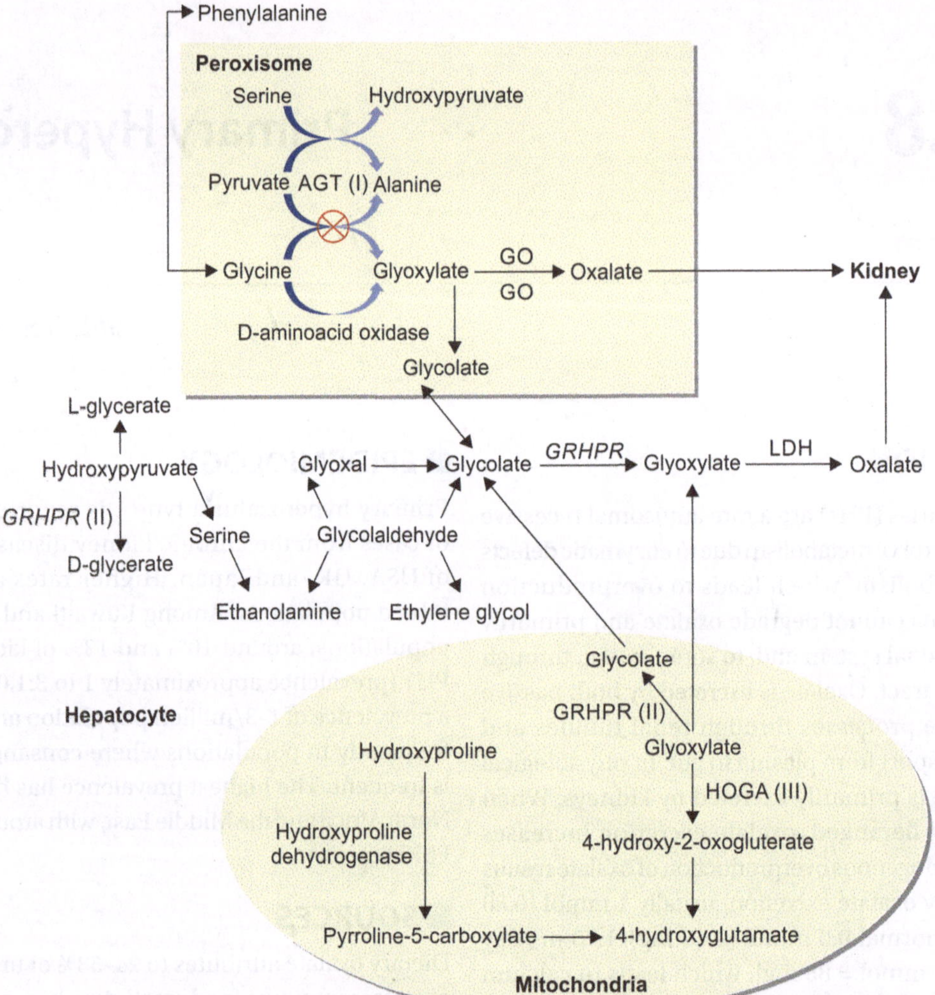

Fig. 1: Enzyme pathway associated with glyoxylate metabolism. (GRHPR: glyoxylate reductase/hydroxypyruvate reductase; HOGA: 4-hydroxy-2-oxoglutarate aldolase; LDH: lactate dehydrogenase)

Absent (nonsense/frameshift mutations/deletions), missense (50%)/splice site mutations of liver-specific AGT enzyme have been described. AGT is a pyridoxine-dependent enzyme and in the peroxisomal compartment, it catalyzes the transamination of glyoxylate to glycine. During the absence of AGT, cytoplasmic LDH converts glyoxylate to oxalate and glycolate. Missense point mutation leads to impaired AGT functions by a direct decrease in catalytic activity, insoluble AGT formation, aggregation or impaired homodimer formation, impaired importation to peroxisome, or combinations of all.[12]

More than 180 mutations have been identified on *AGXT*, the gene encoding AGT; some are frequent. Genetic heterogeneity is responsible for marked heterogeneity in phenotype, and genotype/phenotype correlations have yet to be clearly demonstrated. Pyridoxine is the AGT cofactor, and vitamin B_6 sensitivity has been shown in 10–30% of PH1 population, especially in *G170R* mutation.[4] The dimeric unstable structure can be stabilized by vitamin B_6 component pyridoxal phosphate, and vitamin B_6 also has a role in protein activity and peroxisomal transport. Therefore, some missense mutations show responsiveness to pyridoxine supplement and have a good long-term prognosis.[12] The PH1 mutations "c. 508G>A, c. 33dupC, and c. 731T > C" are more prevalent in European and African countries, whereas in North India "c. 302T > C" is more common.[4] A list of identified mutations is provided in **Table 1**.

Calcium oxalate crystals accumulate in the urinary space, forming urolithiasis. They also form nephrocalcinosis by aggregating in the renal interstitium and interacting with renal tubular epithelium, where they induce an inflammatory response and leads to progressive interstitial fibrosis, which leads to deterioration in kidney function. Ongoing crystallization, injury, and fibrosis in the corticomedullary junction could potentially affect the urinary-concentrating capacity.[1,8] Urinary citrate is generally considered as an inhibitor of CaOx stone formation and is associated with retardation of CaOx crystals maturation. Some studies have reported better glomerular filtration rate (GFR) in those with high urinary citrate excretion. In advanced CKD stages, the urinary citrate level may decrease in nonhyperoxaluric patients. Therefore, lower urine citrate at the baseline may be a consequence of renal injury. Higher urinary calcium is another risk factor for CaOx deposition and supersaturation.[1]

TABLE 1: Mutations associated with primary hyperoxaluria type 1 (PH1) according to pathogenic mechanism.[13]

Mitochondrial mistargeting	***Gly170Arg***
Catalytic	*Arg360Gln, Arg360Trp, Gly41Val, Glu95Lys, Asp183Asn, Tyr260Cys, His261Gln*
Protein aggregation	*Pro319Leu, Leu298Pro, Arg233Cys, Leu284Pro, Leu359Pro, Leu284Pro, Ser158Leu, Gly82Arg, Met195Arg, Ala368Thr, Ala112Asp, Cys253Arg, Pro11Arg, Cys173Tyr, Gly109Val, Gly116Arg, Gly82Glu, His83Arg, Asp201Glu, Arg36His, Arg111Gln, Asp243His, Leu166Pro, Arg233His*
Mistargeting–aggregation	*Phel152Ile, Ile244Thr*
Catalytic–aggregation	*Gly161Cys, Ser205Pro, Ser187Phe, Gly156Arg, Gly161Arg, Gly41Glu, Gly161Ser, Ser275Arg, Trp108Arg, Arg36Cys, Glu274Asp, Leu269Pro, Ser218Leu*
Mistargeting–catalytic–aggregation	*Gly47Arg, Gly41Arg*

Renal tubular epithelial and parenchymal cells get damaged by high concentrations of oxalate in the glomerular filtrate and by CaOx crystals. As the renal function progressively deteriorates, renal oxalate excretion also significantly reduces, but hepatic oxalate production remains high, resulting in a critical saturation point for plasma oxalate (plasma oxalate >30–50 μmol/L). This leads to systemic oxalosis where systemic oxalate deposition occurs in the bones, retina, heart, skin, joints, soft tissues, and nerves. The bone acts as a major compartment of the insoluble oxalate load, and oxalate osteopathy causes severe bone pain, erythropoietin-resistant anemia, spontaneous fractures, and specific oxalate osteopathy on X-ray.[7]

Clinical Spectrum

The presentation of PH1 ranges from early neonatal to the sixth decade of life, typically presenting at 4–7 years of age.[14,15] ESKD within the first years of life is seen in 10–20% of cases (infantile oxalosis).[7,16] There are marked phenotypic, enzymatic, and genotypic heterogeneities in the clinical spectrum, including age at onset, type of presentation, severity of the spectrum, and progression to oxalosis and ESKD.[1,7,12] Some genotypic association, particularly *pGly170Arg* mutation, has better renal survival. Even marked phenotypic variation can be observed within families (discordant family), which can lead to confusion in diagnosis.[17] Though studies suggest that the magnitude of hyperoxaluria primarily determines the course of the disease, other factors for renal outcome are still undetermined and a similar genotype can be manifested in a wide range of clinical courses.[1,18] Higher urinary oxalate excretion indicates poor prognosis at diagnosis and follow-up. The broad spectrum of clinical presentation includes familial or sporadic recurrent urolithiasis and/or nephrocalcinosis (white kidney), dysuria, renal colic, hematuria, frequent urinary tract infection (UTI), failure to thrive, and CKD.[1,12,19] Sometimes, patients experience recurrent urolithiasis with good renal function during adulthood, though asymptomatic individuals may present with ESKD as their first presentation.[1,20] Polyuria at diagnosis usually predicts poor urinary concentrating ability and severity of tubulointerstitial injury.[21] Studies revealed that progression to ESKD is more common and rapid in nephrocalcinosis involving cortex rather than medulla.[7]

When ESKD develops, and the liver continues to produce excess oxalate, plasma oxalate (Pox) levels rise to 80–200 μmol/L predialysis and exceeds the supersaturation threshold for calcium oxalate (ßCaOx >1 relative unit at Pox >30–50 μmol/L).[12] This results in systemic oxalosis involving retina, myocardium, vessel walls, skin, soft tissues, endocrine gland, bone, bone marrow, and the central nervous system. Bone contains the major oxalate burden.[8,22] Consequences include retinopathy, cardiomyopathy, cardiac conduction disturbances/arrhythmia, heart block, vasculopathy, erythropoietin-resistant anemia, oxalate osteopathy involving bone and joint deformation and pain, bone fracture after trivial trauma, and skin infection.[5,7,23-25] Hypothyroidism and hypogonadism can also be seen as secondary to systemic oxalosis.[26,27]

Diagnosis

Positive family history, radiological findings of nephrocalcinosis or nephrolithiasis, and suggestive laboratory features point toward the diagnosis.[15] On fundoscopy, the retina may show white dots. Electroretinography (ERG) findings may be suggestive of subnormal retinal function.[7] The cardiological evaluation includes ECG, echocardiography, and cardiac MRI for confirmation of myocardial deposition of abnormal echogenic dots. Intracardiac calcifications may act as a source of emboli. Due to crystal deposition in tunica media, deposition in the coronary artery may lead to myocardial ischemia ("atherosclerotic oxalosis") or stroke.[8] Oxalate deposition can be demonstrated by bone marrow aspirate. Multiple soft-tissue swellings all over the body are indicative of severe systemic oxalosis.[7,28] Endocrine abnormalities include hypothyroidism. Intestinal and dermal calcification, necrosis, and gangrene have also been described.[8] A diagnostic algorithm is depicted in **Flowchart 1**. Diagnosis of PH1 can be missed due to improper 24-hour urine sample collection. Hyperoxaluria may be missed if oxalate precipitates in the container. Cortical nephrocalcinosis in USG may be misinterpreted as nonspecific parenchymal hyperechogenicity. For systemic oxalosis detection, fundoscopy is required, where retinal abnormalities are often not recognized. Bony changes are often misinterpreted as renal osteodystrophy.[7] When the Pox concentrations are >50 μmol/L irrespective of GFR, they are indicative of PH1.[29,30] A 24-hour urine oxalate level, corrected

Flowchart 1: Diagnostic algorithm to evaluate primary hyperoxaluria.

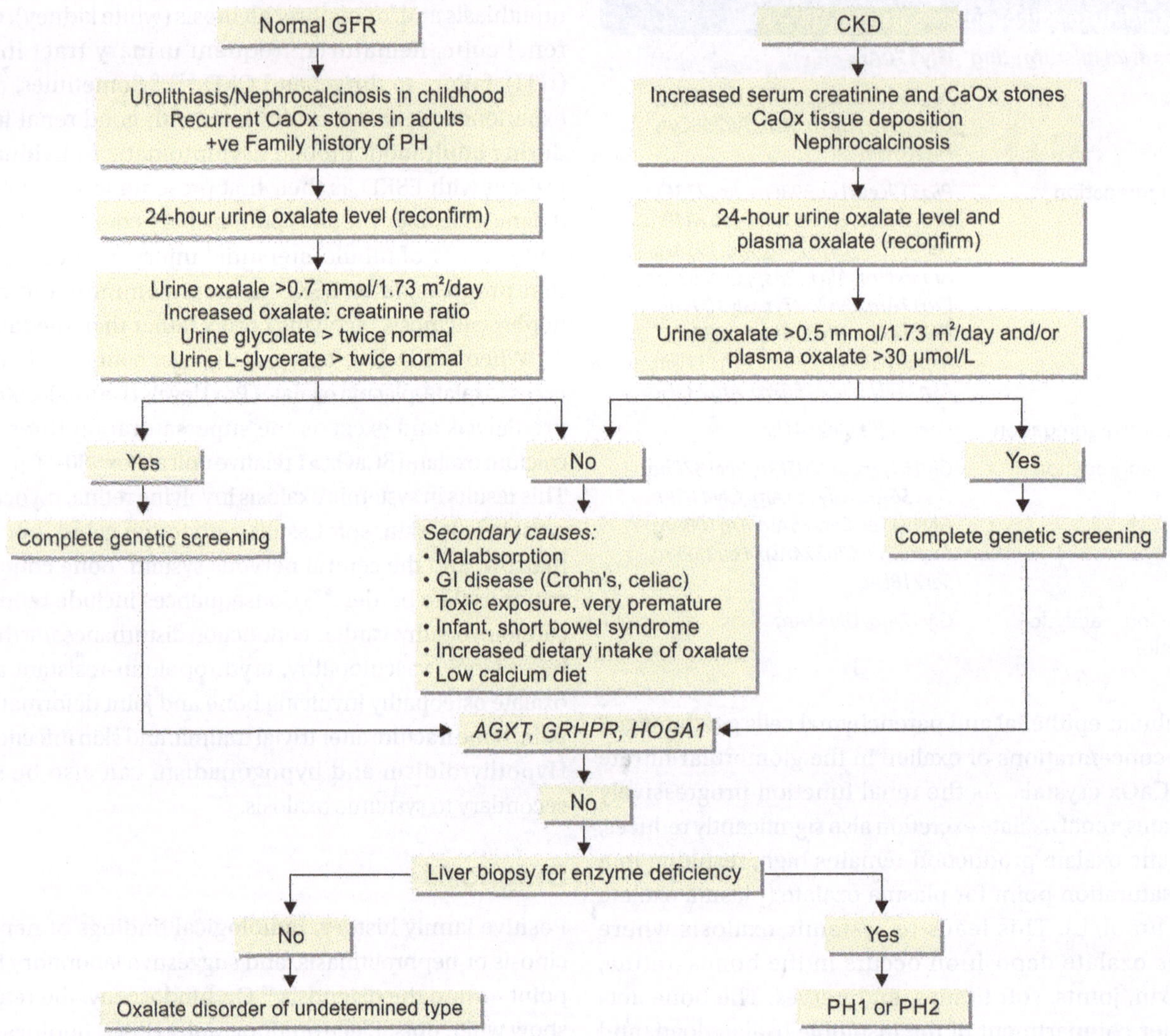

(CaOx: calcium oxalate; CKD: chronic kidney disease; GI: gastrointestinal; GFR: glomerular filtration rate; PH: primary hyperoxaluria)

for the body surface area, is preferred for the diagnosis of PH1. The spot urine oxalate/creatinine ratio is helpful to calculate oxalate excretion, especially where timed sample collection is not feasible, particularly in infants.[31-33] Normal levels are tabulated in **Table 2**. Bone is a major component of insoluble oxalate pool, causing oxalate osteopathy, pain, fractures, and anemia resistance to erythropoietin.[34]

Biochemical Findings

Urine analysis for CaOx monohydrate crystalluria and stone analysis by infrared spectroscopy are required to detect and quantify the composition. With normal and significant residual GFR, hyperoxaluria (urine oxalate >1 mmol/1.73 m²/day, reference value <0.5) and hyperglycoluria (urine glycolate >0.5 mmol/1.73 m², reference value <0.5) are suggestive of PH1. Different biologic fluid and tissue assays may reveal oxalate crystals.[35-38]

Genetic and Mutational Testing

Genetic analysis of *AGXT* gene mutation is preferred over liver biopsy to detect AGT enzyme deficiency. PH1 is confirmed by

TABLE 2: Age-related reference values for urinary oxalate, glycolate, L-glycerate, and hydroxy-oxoglutarate excretion.

	Normal values		
Units	***Oxalate***	***Glycolate***	***L-glycerate***
mmol/1.73 m²/day (all ages)	<0.5 (<45 mg)	<0.5 (<45)	
µmol/L (all ages)			<5
mmol/molcreatinine			
0–6 months	<325–360	<363–425	14–205
7–24 months	<132–174	<245–293	14–205
2–5 years	<98–101	<191–229	14–205
5–14 years	<70–82	<166–186	23–138
>16 years	<40	<99–125	<138

HOG: µmol/1.73 m²/day (all ages): <40

AGXT gene mutations. Genotypes with lower hyperoxaluria and homozygous or heterozygous *AGXT-G170R* mutation have a better long-term prognosis and show complete or partial pyridoxine responsiveness.[39-41]

Liver Biopsy

Liver biopsy to confirm deficiency of AGT enzyme activity may be done.[38] Studies showed that the catalytic activity may reduce to 0.5 mmol pyruvate/s/kg protein (normal values: 490–750).[42]

Radiographs

Oxalate osteopathy changes are usually symmetrical, progressive, and mainly involve long bone metaphysis. At the metaphysis, a sclerotic juxtaphyseal band develops, which is more homogenous and denser than that of secondary hyperparathyroidism. The bandwidth correlates with the duration of ESKD and the distance from physes correlates with the duration the patient is on dialysis. Oxalate crystal deposition induces a granulomatous reaction, which results in bone resorption, cystic changes, and pathological fractures. Thin lucent metaphyseal bands are found at the metaphyseal region of short bone (carpal, tarsal, and patella), between physes, and the metaphyseal sclerotic band, due to slower growth, results in bone within bone appearance. Pathological fractures can persist even after kidney–liver transplant and mainly involve the femoral neck. During advanced bone maturation, diffuse coarsening of trabeculae can be found, known as woolly trabeculation. Renal osteodystrophy leads to short stature, rugger jersey spine, and diffuse vertebral sclerosis. Secondary hyperparathyroidism along with renal osteodystrophy leads to subperiosteal bone resorption, distal phalangeal osteolysis, and soft-tissue calcification. After the liver–kidney transplant, CaOx crystals released from skeletal stores and solid organ and skeletal findings improve. Bone density may normalize, new bone lays down resulting in migration of sclerotic metaphyseal line toward diaphysis.[43,44]

Sonography

Primary hyperoxaluria type 1 typically presents as medullary nephrocalcinosis. An arc-like echogenic area with posterior acoustic shadowing is characteristic. Renal calculi may result in hydronephrosis **(Fig. 2)**. In advanced stages, renal atrophy develops; medullary nephrocalcinosis progressively involves the cortical area and renal parenchyma gradually obscures.[45]

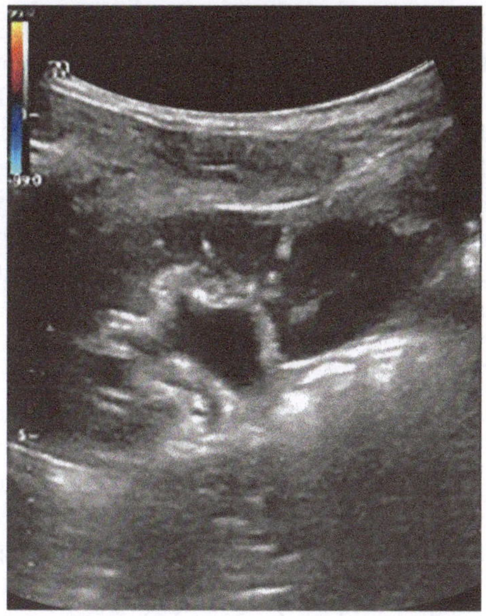

Fig. 2: Renal USG showing multiple calculi in a 9-years-old male with PH1 with hydronephrosis.

Scintigraphy

Calcium oxalate crystal deposition causes diffusely increased radiotracer uptake in bone scan in axial, peripheral skeleton, metaphysis of long bones, calcified bones, and osteoid. It also indicates crystal-induced inflammatory osteoclastic and osteoblastic activity, bone destruction, and secondary hyperparathyroidism-induced osteoclastic activity. Rib, calvaria, and mandibular involvement are usually spared in PH1, unlike renal osteodystrophy. Cardiac, soft-tissue radiotracer uptake reflects advanced systemic oxalosis. These findings reverse after combined liver-kidney transplant.[46,47]

Other Imaging

On echocardiogram, "sparkling" echogenic myocardium reflects myocardial crystal deposition. Associated findings may include concentric myocardial wall thickening, ventricular dilation, and pericardial effusion. Computed tomography findings include renal stones and medullary and/or cortical calcification, increased bone density, and bony erosions and cysts. MRI findings include T2 low-signal intensity in affected organs such as bone, spleen, and liver due to CaOx deposition. After a successful liver kidney transplant, these findings are gradually reverted.[48]

Follow-up

In 30 years' follow-up, among the PH, PH2, and PH3 populations, the renal survival rates are 27%, 92%, and 95%, respectively.[1] A higher degree of oxalate excretion during follow-up is associated with a poor outcome. Therefore, conservative measures to reduce urinary oxalate excretion are necessary for favorable renal outcomes, even if oxalate levels are not entirely normalized. Urine volume is not a significant predictor for ESKD in the long term.[42]

Treatment

Delay in diagnostic and therapeutic measures leads to prolonged exposure to progressively increasing oxalate load, resulting in ESKD, systemic oxalosis-related mortality and morbidity, and need for dialysis and transplant.[7] Timely intervention in the form of optimizing fluid intake, adequate nutrition, urine alkalinization, and oral crystal inhibitors (citrate, magnesium, or phosphate) and pyridoxine treatment for some patients with PH1 can retard progression.[1,8,42] For the patients with GFR > 30 mL/min/1.73 m^2, measures should be taken aiming to delay progression to ESKD. An individual usually progresses to ESKD over time at a median age of 24–35 years. Symptomatic children presenting during infancy typically have a more severe course and develop ESKD before the age of 3 years.[49]

Fluid Intake

High fluid intake (>3 L/1.73 m^2/day) plays a key role in conservative management and is applicable for all types of PH. In infants and toddlers, optimum fluid administration is often problematic, so early consideration for gastrostomy tube placement is preferable. Situations of significant fluid losses (fever, diarrhea and vomiting, UTIs, etc.) or less oral hydration (postsurgery) need to be anticipated, and early initiation of intravenous fluid supplementation is necessary.[12,50]

Pyridoxine

The only specific orally available treatment option is vitamin B_6. With residual AGT activity of 30–50%, pyridoxine is useful. Retrospective studies showed, of 30–50% PH1 cases, that urinary oxalate excretion was reduced; even it could not be normalized always. It includes six active components (vitamers): pyridoxine, pyridoxal, pyridoxol, pyridoxamine and pyridoxal-phosphate (activated phosphate esters), and pyridoxamine 5 phosphate. Pyridoxal phosphate acts as a co-factor of all transaminases, including AGT. When pyridoxine is administered in a pyridoxine hydrochloride form, it interacts with AGT and is activated.[51] In a supraphysiological dose, PLP (pyridoxal phosphate) acts in multiple ways. It is postulated that PLP may increase AGT expression, stabilize mutant AGT protein and subsequently increase AGT enzyme activity, and help in proper AGT targeting into peroxisomes.[8,50,52] The recommended dose of pyridoxine is 5 mg/kg/day, increased by 5 mg/kg to a maximum of 20 mg/kg/day for a period of 6 months. Responsiveness should be determined by the reduction of urinary oxalate by a 30% level at least after 3 months of optimum treatment.[41,53] Sometimes, the optimum response can be noted after 6 months of maximum dose administration. Treatment should be continued even when the patient is on dialysis to decrease the oxalate production and thus to decrease the oxalate load, until liver transplant. Some case series reported adverse effects such as sensory neurotoxicity, though very rare even on maximum dosage.[39]

Variable responsiveness to pyridoxine treatment has been demonstrated even among the same genotypes.[53] Studies revealed that early initiation of treatment with pyridoxine, even since infancy, may reverse the course of the renal disease and help to preserve renal function, especially in missense mutations involving misfolding and peroxisomal import and susceptible genotype (e.g., p.Gly170Arg homo).[7,17,54] Mutations such as Trp108Arg, Ser158Leu, and Asp183Asn need a supraphysiological dose for optimum response. Truncating mutations are less likely to be responsive to pyridoxine treatment. Even without known pyridoxine-responsive mutation, the maximum daily pyridoxine therapy can reduce >30% of urinary oxalate.[7] Other than mutation, various other factors involving uptake and metabolism of vitamin B6 are there to modify the responsiveness, which are yet to be detected.[53]

Urinary Calcium–oxalate Precipitation Inhibitors

Citrate and magnesium impede CaOx nucleation and formation of stones. Citrate is metabolized in liver to bicarbonate and increases urinary pH and reduces citrate reabsorption in the tubule. Thus, urinary citrate excretion increases and urinary pH becomes 6.2–6.8. In higher urinary pH, CaOx solubility is increased by binding of citrate with calcium and decrease crystal precipitation. CaOx dihydrate stone is stable at a pH of 5–7.4. Citrate interacts with crystallizing matter as an inhibitor and increases the solubility of CaOx.[50] The recommended dose of alkali citrate is 0.1–0.2 g/kg/day (0.3–0.6 mmol/kg/day) as sodium or potassium salt. Thiazide administration along with citrate reduces calcium excretion and urinary CaOx saturation. Dietary magnesium reduces oxalate absorption, and it directly interacts with crystallizing matter and reduces crystallization in urine.[55] Orthophosphate also increases urine pH (6.2–6.8) and reduces crystallization.[12,50]

Diet

Oxalate absorption through gut is less in PH1 and PH2 patients and excretion of dietary oxalate is also very less.[12] A recent study showed that PH patients may benefit from low oxalate diet, restricting oxalate-rich items (spinach, chocolate, rhubarb, sweet potatoes, cocoa, nuts, tea).[56] However, vitamin C acts as an oxalate precursor and is metabolized nonenzymatically to oxalate. Vitamin D also increases intestinal oxalate absorption.[57,58] Restriction of oral calcium intake may lead to freer and more absorbable oxalate.[59] Therefore, calcium restriction should not be advised.

Dialysis

Dialysis is usually not sufficient to handle the continuous production of oxalate by liver when the patient develops ESKD.[49] It acts as a temporary measure before transplantation.[12] Frequent, short-duration hemodialysis (HD) sessions with high flux filters, i.e., almost daily 3-hour session, are preferred than long-duration, less-frequent sessions. Rebound rise of the plasma oxalate level is noted after HD.[60] Therefore, an intensified hemodialysis protocol including daily HD or in combination with peritoneal dialysis is sometimes required for oxalate removal.[15,50] Intensive dialysis can reduce the plasma oxalate level by 43% after 1 year and speckle echocardiography showed improved cardiac function.[50] Pre- and post-HD serum oxalate levels should be measured. The post-HD serum oxalate level should be less than the plasma CaOx supersaturation level (<30 μmol/L).[18]

Transplant

In PH1, the ultimate management is transplantation. In the absence of transplantation, 5-year and 9-year survival after the onset of ESKD are 40% and 20%, respectively.[8] Isolated renal transplant can reduce the serum oxalate level, but as oxalate production remains high by liver, the chance of disease recurrence and graft failure is high.[7,49] Therefore, pre-emptive liver transplant or combined liver-kidney transplantation is preferred for a better outcome. Isolated liver transplant can be considered in a pre-end-stage CKD patient (GFR 30–40 mL/min/1.73 m^2), but oxalate excretion leads to progressive deterioration in kidney function.[61] Simultaneous renal transplant becomes necessary when GFR falls <15–30 mL/min/1.73 m^2.[8] Isolated renal transplant can be considered in elderly population and PLP-sensitive genotype.[8,62] Sequential liver–kidney transplant is preferred in infantile oxalosis. 5-year patient and liver allograft survival rate after combined liver–kidney transplant are 80% and 72%, respectively.[49] Early reports from the European Dialysis and Transplant Association (EDTA) Registry suggested a patient survival of 79% at 3 years after the start of kidney replacement therapy (KRT) and a 3-year kidney graft survival ranging from 25 to 50% in recipients aged 15 years. Reports from the United States suggested equally or even better outcomes with kidney transplantation alone.[49] Immediately after transplantation, hemodialysis and hemofiltration should be continued, as the release of CaOx from the bones and other organs results in a sharp rise in serum oxalate that may overwhelm the glomeruli and lead to graft failure.[8] The urine oxalate level may be markedly elevated for several years after combined liver–kidney transplant. High fluid intake and crystallization inhibitors should be continued postoperatively. Most renal graft failure is recorded within the first 3 months of transplant included mortality due to liver transplant-related complications.[49]

Oxalobacter Formigenes

Oxalobacter formigenes is a strictly anaerobic commensal organism that colonizes in the vertebrate intestine.[12] It depends on oxalate for its only source of carbon, and there is a symbiotic relationship in the regulation of absorption in gut.[63] It regulates enteric elimination of oxalate by activating oxalate transport from plasma into intestine. Animal models showed that due to a concentration gradient, oxalate passively flows across the gut epithelium and there is also specific transporter-mediated active flux of oxalate and oxalate is finally excreted through feces. It also facilitates mobilization of systemic deposition of CaOx.[50] Uncontrolled studies have shown that oral *O. formigenes* preparation, when used in subjects with normal or reduced GFR, induces reduction in urine or plasma oxalate levels by 4 weeks.[64] Some case reports on infantile oxalosis also demonstrated the same result. However, some randomized controlled trials (RCTs) did not show similar results.[12] There might be inefficient delivery of drugs to colon, or the human intestine may not be responsive to *O. formigenes* effects on oxalate excretion. The bacteria strain used in the study might have low viability and recovery time, which might have a negative impact on outcome.[50]

Experimental Approaches

- *Enzyme replacement therapy (ERT):* Therapeutic hydrophilic macromolecules AGTs are required to be delivered to hepatocytes through endocytosis and need to be stable in acidic pH and subsequently to be entered into peroxisome by interacting with PEX5P import protein. AGT requires "cell-penetrating peptides," "transactivator of transcription," "polyarginine," "galactose residues," and "asialoglycoprotein receptor" to enter into hepatocytes. "Hemagglutinin inclusions" can facilitate escape from endosomal digestion and polymer-conjugated AGT maximizes peroxisomal delivery. The drawback of this approach is that untargeted hepatocytes will continue to produce an unregulated amount of oxalate.[65] ERT includes "PEG-PGA-AGT" which is in the developmental phase. Substrate substitute therapy includes Nephur [Food and Drug Administration (FDA) approved], OxDC CLEC, Oxazyme, and ALLN-77 which are in phase 1, 2, and 3 trial stages, respectively.[66]
- *Substrate-reduction treatment:* RNA-interference mechanisms (Lumisaran, DCR-PHXC) can be utilized to manipulate glyoxylate metabolism, and thus hepatic oxalate production can be decreased.[50,67]
- *Chaperon-proteostasis regulator therapy:* Misfolded AGT interacts with molecular chaperons resulting in modulations. Studies suggested that administration of PLP enhances AGT activity, folding, expression, and targeting to peroxisome. Pyridoxamine and pyridoxal are also effective.[65]
- *CRID 3, R-7050:* Inhibition of calcium oxalate induces interstitial inflammation and subsequently renal fibrosis, thus prolonging renal survival and improving the quality of the lives of patients with PH.[68]
- *Gene therapy:* Defective gene is replaced by AAV, SVac-vectors ("Adeno associated viral vectors"). It is possibly the first non-transplantation curative approach for PH1 patients.[69] In a mouse model with PH1, helper-dependent AAV is also reported as helpful.[65]
- *Cell therapy:* Genome editing involving *CRISPR/Cas9* is being tested on mouse models to overcome the need for immunosuppression. Studies are ongoing regarding high-quality hepatocyte transplantation, which is a less invasive method, where mutant AGT-deficient host hepatocytes are replaced by competent cells. Some authors described at least 75% mutant host cells to be replaced for the effective outcomes.
- PH1 human-induced pluripotent stem cells (PH1-iPSCS) when differentiated in hepatocyte-like cells (HLC) after transduced with liver-specific lentivirus vector, AGT expression could be restored and disease modification could be possible. However, this transduction is challenging and a possibility of mutagenesis is there.[70]

PRIMARY HYPEROXALURIA TYPE 2

Introduction

Primary hyperoxaluria type 2 (PH2) is inherited in an autosomal-recessive manner and is the least frequent form of PH.[11,71] PH2 is the result of glyoxylate reductase/hydroxypyruvate reductase (GRHPR) deficiency and is caused by mutations in the single copy *GRHPR* gene (OMIM 604296) located on chromosome 9p13.2.[1] The first cloning of *GRHPR* gene was reported in 1999 from the human liver library by Cramer et al. and Rumsby et al.[12] PH2 has a less severe course than PH1, though CKD and ESKD have also been reported. Initially, PH2 was described as L-glyceric aciduria, due to excessive production of urinary L-glycerate.[11] Sometimes, PH2 is associated with elevated L-glycerate levels, which is considered to be pathognomonic.[71] Non-physiologic action of D-glycerate dehydrogenase is causing impairment in dehydrogenation of D-glycerate. Glyoxylate reductase is now the preferred term; due to the glyoxylate reduction reaction, it appears to be more significant.[11]

The genomic location mapping for the *GRHPR* gene is necessary for molecular diagnostics, and till date, 39 mutations have been reported.[11] The most frequent mutations are c.103delG and c.403_404+2delAAGT and predominate in Caucasians and Asians, respectively.[8,72] There are nine exons spanning ca.14 kb, 1.2 kb cDNA, and open reading frame of 984 base pairs, producing 328 amino acid proteins with a molecular weight of 35.4 kDa. All mutations resulting in functionally null alleles lead to loss-of-protein expression and/or no catalytic activity.[73]

Biology and Molecular Basis

Glyoxylate reductase/hydroxypyruvate reductase enzyme activity is mostly demonstrated in liver but also found in leukocytes and the kidney. Primarily, the enzyme activity is located in the cytosol and to some extent in the mitochondria. The enzyme utilizes pyridine nucleotides [phosphorylated nicotinamide adenine dinucleotide phosphate (NADP) and NADPH/unphosphorylated NAD+ and NADH)] as co-factors and acts in the gluconeogenic pathway from serine and in the detoxification of cytosolic glyoxylate.[11,73] *GRHPR* has higher affinity toward NADPH, favoring formation of hydroxypyruvate to D-glycerate in the cytosol. In a normal physiological condition, glyoxylate is mainly distributed in mitochondria and peroxisomes. Mitochondrial GRHPR catalyzes reaction to produce glycolate from glyoxylate and peroxisomal glycolate oxidase catalyzes the reverse oxidation. These reactions are largely preferred over oxidation by cytosolic LDH in physiologic states and thus prevent rapid conversion of reactive glyoxalate to oxalate.[74] Hepatic glyoxylate metabolism is primarily affected causing accumulation of glyoxylate and hydroxypyruvate. LDH metabolizes these accumulated substances to oxalate and L-glycerate, leading to high urine L-glycerate excretion.[11]

Clinical Spectrum

The age of onset of symptoms of PH2 is typically in childhood and clinical presentation can overlap with PH1, mainly those associated with the presence of renal stones including hematuria, renal colic, or obstruction of the urinary tract. Some individuals may remain asymptomatic till adulthood. Though less common, affected individuals may present with nephrocalcinosis or ESKD (20% cases). The clinical course is less severe than PH1. Infantile and systemic oxalosis have been seldom reported.[75,76] In the majority of the cases, calcium oxalate stones were found. Once ESKD (20%) sets in, systemic oxalosis can develop involving bone, bone marrow, joints, retina, and myocardium; it can even manifest as calcified nodules on the fingers. Radiological evidences of the bone involvement are transverse translucent symmetric bands with fixed sclerotic margins at the end of long bones, subsequently developing cystic rarefaction. In the advanced phase, osteodystrophy results in bone pain and pathological fractures. Bone marrow involvement causes erythropoietin-stimulating agent refractory anemia. Oxalate deposition in retina causing retinopathy and/or maculopathy leads to visual disturbance. Myocardium involvement results in cardiac conduction disturbances such as heart block and cardiomyopathy. Joint involvement can be suggested by synovitis secondary to oxalate deposition. Nonhealing cutaneous ulcers can be the manifestation of ischemia due to vascular involvement. Periodontal disease and hypothyroidism are also reported.[11,76-78]

Diagnosis

The molecular approach using genetic testing for biallelic pathogenic variants in *GRHPR* is helpful to detect PH2. When there are no pathogenic variants or only one pathogenic variant is found, to confirm PH2, liver biopsy is necessary to demonstrate deficiency of GRHPR enzyme, or hyperoxaluria along with hyperglyceric aciduria to be documented without an identifiable secondary cause.[1]

Kidney stone analysis predominantly reveals calcium oxalate. The urinary oxalate level is typically > 0.7 mmol/1.73 m²/24 h (normal <0.46 mmol/1.73 m²/24 h). A 24-hour collection in acid is preferable to a random sample. Urinary organic acid screen is helpful to detect high urinary L-glycerate, though a specific method for glycerate detection is preferable. After the onset of ESKD (often with glomerular filtration rate < 20 mL/min/1.73 m²), elevated plasma oxalate concentrations (>50 μmol/L) can be detected.[11] Single-gene testing includes sequence analysis of GRHPR. Gene-targeted deletion/duplication analysis may be required, if one or no pathogenic variant is found. A multigene panel that includes GRHPR and other genes of interest may be considered. The points to be considered are as follows:

- The included genes, diagnostic tests, and their sensitivity can vary in different laboratories and can be changed from time to time.
- Some multigene panels may include genes not associated with the indexed condition; thus, clinicians should be vigilant about the panel to detect the likely genetic cause considering cost-effectiveness and to limit the detection of pathogenic variants of uncertain significance.
- Some laboratories provide customed panel options and exome analysis based on phenotype.
- Methods used in a panel may include deletion/duplication analysis, sequence analysis, and nonsequencing-based analysis.

In 1998, Giafi and Rumsby first described glyoxylate reductase enzyme activity assay in liver tissue. A needle biopsy (~20 mg of tissue) is required, and the sample must be frozen immediately before processing.[79]

Evaluation includes the assessment of renal function, imaging studies including bone X-ray to detect radio-dense metaphyseal bands followed by cystic rarefaction of bones, cardiac evaluation with echocardiography and ECG, and ophthalmic evaluation to look for deposition of oxalate crystals. Genetic evaluation is necessary to evaluate at-risk family members before symptoms occur and to delay disease onset in asymptomatic relatives. Measurement of urinary oxalate excretion is also helpful if pathogenic variants in the family are not known.

Treatment and Prognosis

Management includes general rules for that of nephrolithiasis, to relieve obstruction, and to manage CKD according to the staging. General measures should include adequate fluid intake (>2.5 L/m^2/day). Treatment with orthophosphate (20–30 mg/kg/day) or potassium citrate (0.1–0.15 g/kg/day) can be considered as inhibitors of urinary calcium oxalate crystal formation. There is no supportive evidence for the use of pyridoxine in PH2.

As the plasma oxalate concentration begins to rise when the renal clearance is less than 40 mL/min/1.73 m^2, early initiation of dialysis or preemptive kidney-only transplantation is preferred. Oxalate clearance on hemodialysis is greater than on peritoneal dialysis (120 mL/min on hemodialysis vs. 7 mL/min on peritoneal dialysis): thrice-weekly hemodialysis eliminates 6–9 mmol/1.73 m^2/week oxalate, equivalent to 2–3 days of endogenous production of oxalate. Different combinations of hemodialysis modalities, such as intermittent daily hemodialysis along with overnight peritoneal dialysis, or intense home hemodialysis along with the use of high flux filters and the long duration of dialysis, are helpful for oxalate clearance and prevent rebound rise of oxalate. As ESKD sets in, the more intense the regular dialysis and the longer an individual is on dialysis, the more chance of systemic oxalate deposition is there.[35]

Studies revealed that isolated kidney transplantation is required to manage PH2, as it is less severe and liver transplant cannot completely reduce oxalate load.[80,81] In the postoperative period, judicious diuresis and use of urinary calcium oxalate inhibitors are helpful to prevent oxalate deposition in graft kidney and thus prevent graft loss. Postoperatively, urine glycerate and oxalate and plasma oxalate all are found to be normalized within 1 month and 13-month follow-up.[82]

At least biannual follow-up is necessary to assess renal function, which includes blood pressure, blood count, hematocrit, urinalysis to measure 24-hour urine oxalate excretion or spot urine oxalate-to-creatinine ratio, calcium oxalate saturation, urine protein, and urine routine to rule out hematuria which indicates renal calculi. Renal imaging for stone assessment may be required annually or biannually. When an individual develops CKD stage 3, testings for hemogram, renal function, and electrolytes are needed to be performed quarterly. For systemic oxalosis, evaluation has to be done at least yearly.[11] X-ray examination should be considered to evaluate radiological changes in long bones along with cystic changes and to detect pathological fractures. Every 5 yearly DEXA scanning suffices. MRI or CT scanning of bones is occasionally required. Hematological evaluation should include full blood count, hematocrit, and workup for anemia. Erythropoietin-resistant anemia can be manifested as oxalate crystal deposition in bone marrow, which can be demonstrated in bone marrow aspirate, though this evaluation is seldom required. Fundoscopy is necessary to evaluate for retinopathy and maculopathy. For cardiac conduction defects and contractility evaluation, ECG and echocardiogram are required as appropriate. Dermatological evaluation is necessary to detect subungual oxalate deposition and cutaneous ulcers, which is suggestive of vasculopathy. Clinical examination of joints may be required to rule out synovitis and if suggestive then arthroscopy may be considered. Dental examination for periodontal disease may be required. Thyroid function tests should be considered to rule out hypothyroidism.

Quarterly to biannually plasma oxalate level evaluation is necessary until ESKD sets in, as when GFR falls <15 mL/min/1.73 m^2, the relation between plasma oxalate levels rises with a fall in GFR and it becomes more difficult to interpret. Monthly plasma oxalate measurement is required to change dialysis prescription when the patient is on maintenance hemodialysis.

Prenatal Testing and Preimplantation Genetic Diagnosis

When the *GRPHR* pathogenic variants are found in an affected family member, prenatal testing for a pregnancy at increased risk and preimplantation genetic diagnosis should be considered. Families should be counseled regarding early diagnosis and option for termination to be discussed. Most centers prefer parental choice regarding prenatal testing, especially when termination of pregnancy is being considered. Other issues to be concerned about are complications related to renal and/or liver transplantation and the scarcity of suitable organs for transplantation.[11]

PRIMARY HYPEROXALURIA TYPE 3

Introduction

Primary hyperoxaluria type 3 (PH3) (OMIM 613616)[3] is caused by mutations in the *HOGA1* gene, which encodes the mitochondrial 4-hydroxy-2-oxoglutarate aldolase (HOGA) enzyme.[1] PH3 accounts for 10–15% of all PH cases. Belostotsky et al. in 2010 first described *HOGA1* gene mutations in PH3 patients.[6]

Biology and Molecular Basis

Mitochondrial enzyme *HOGA1* cleaves 4-hydroxy-2-oxoglutarate into pyruvate and glyoxylate, which corresponds to the final step of the hydroxyproline degradation pathway.

Several nonsense mutations and a splice-site variant were detected in *HOGA1* which leads to loss of function of mitochondrial enzyme 4-hydroxy-2-oxoglutarate aldolase,[83] resulting in accumulation of the precursor 4-hydroxy-2-oxoglutarate (HOG) in mitochondria. This event leads to high levels of the HOG metabolite in mitochondria, leaking into the cytosol whereby a nonspecific pyruvate aldolase and LDH could be converted into glyoxylate. Glyoxylate is rapidly oxidized into oxalate, resulting in hyperoxaluria.[3,83] An alternatively proposed mechanism for the production of oxalate is the inhibition of glyoxylate reductase by accumulating HOG. Mutations such as c.769T > G, c.834G > A, c.715G > A, c.208C > T, and c.834_834 + 1GG > TT, c.290G > A, c.554C > T, c.110G > A, c.812G > A, c.841C > T, c.811C > T, c.70delG, and c.406G > C and c.418C > T, c.3G > A, and c.834 + 1G > T substitutions in the *HOGA1* gene have been reported till date.[83]

Clinical Spectrum

In comparison to PH1 and PH2, PH3 patients usually present with a milder phenotype and association with ESKD has not been noted. The pathogenic heterozygous mutations lead to milder forms of PH3.[3] Patients typically present in the first few years of life with nephrolithiasis along with UTI, hematuria, and colic/pain during childhood, but the frequency of nephrocalcinosis is less. Significant impairment of GFR is rarely described. Some individuals may remain asymptomatic.[84,85] Studies revealed that PH3 patients may not have a positive family history for urolithiasis.[83]

Diagnosis

Primary hyperoxaluria type 3 was diagnosed by mutations of *HOGA1*.[1] Studies revealed that 4-hydroxyglutamate (4OHGlu), the immediate precursor of HOG, is useful as a diagnostic biomarker and can be used as a screening method. 4-hydroxy-2-oxogluterate and its reduced forms 2,4-dihydroxyglutaric and 4-hydroxyglutamate, accumulate in urine. For the biochemical diagnosis of PH3, measurement of urine HOG by ion chromatography-mass spectrometry and the simultaneous measurement of HOG and 2,4-dihydroxyglutaric acid by gas chromatography-mass spectrometry are useful.[85]

Treatment

In persistent hypercalciuria, hydrochlorothiazide alone or in combination with amiloride can be used to reduce calcium excretion and urine CaOx saturation. The recommended thiazide dose is 0.5–1 mg/kg/day.[12] Urinary stones can be removed in most cases by less traumatic surgical methods [such as extracorporeal shock wave lithotripsy (ESWL), ureteroscopy, and retrograde intrarenal surgery (RIRS)], thus avoiding percutaneous nephrolithotomy and open surgery, which can lead to further renal damage.[83] Unlike PH1 and PH2, combined liver and kidney transplant is not recommended for PH3 due to uncertainty in the metabolic pathway in this disease.[8]

CONCLUSION

Primary hyperoxaluria is a rare genetic systemic disorder that affects kidneys in the form of urolithiasis, nephrocalcinosis and progressive kidney dysfunction. The three types of primary hyperoxaluria involve loss of function of key enzymes of the hepatic glyoxylate metabolism. Primary hyperoxaluria type 1 is the most common and severe entity that leads to end-stage kidney disease. Genetic testing therefore has clinical implications. For primary hyperoxaluria type 1, the management includes conservative measures followed by combined liver-kidney transplantation.

KEY POINTS

- Primary hyperoxaluria is an autosomal recessive disorder due to enzymatic defects in glyoxylate metabolism leading to overproduction of oxalate.
- There are three distinct types of primary hyperoxaluria and type 1 is the common and severe entity leading to systemic oxalosis, CKD and end-stage kidney disease.
- Nephrocalcinosis, nephrolithiasis, positive family history are evident with confirmatory tests of hyperoxaluria (urine oxalate >1 mmol/1.73 m^2 per day, reference value <0.5) and hyperglycoluria (urine glycolate >0.5 mmol/1.73 m^2, reference value <0.5) in early stages.
- Genetic testing is critical and include *AGXT* gene mutations.
- For type I hyperoxaluria, hydration, stone inhibitors and pyridoxine supplementation form conservative measures followed by the need for combined liver-kidney transplantation.

REFERENCES

1. Zhao F, Bergstralh EJ, Mehta RA, Vaughan LE, Olson JB, Seide BM, et al. Predictors of incident ESRD among patients with primary hyperoxaluria presenting prior to kidney failure. Clin J Am Soc Nephrol. 2016;11:119-26.
2. Milliner D, Hoppe B, Groothoff J. A randomised Phase II/III study to evaluate the efficacy and safety of orally administered *Oxalobacter formigenes* to treat primary hyperoxaluria. Urolithiasis. 2018;46:313-23.
3. Allard L, Cochat P, Leclerc AL, Cachat F, Fichtner C, De Souza VC, et al. Renal function can be impaired in children with primary hyperoxaluria type 3. Pediatr Nephrol. 2015;30:1807-13.
4. Garrelfs SF, Rumsby G, Peters-Sengers H, Erger F, Groothoff JW, Beck BB, et al. Patients with primary hyperoxaluria type 2 have significant morbidity and require careful follow-up. Kidney Int. 2019;96:1389-99.
5. Hoppe B. An update on primary hyperoxaluria. Nat Rev Nephrol. 2012;8:467.
6. Belostotsky R, Seboun E, Idelson GH, Milliner DS, Becker-Cohen R, Rinat C, et al. Mutations in DHDPSL are responsible for primary hyperoxaluria type III. Am J Hum Genet. 2010;87:392-9.
7. Soliman NA, Nabhan MM, Abdelrahman SM, Abdelaziz H, Helmy R, Ghanim K, et al. Clinical spectrum of primary hyperoxaluria type 1: Experience of a tertiary center. Nephrol Ther. 2017;13:176-82.
8. Strauss SB, Waltuch T, Bivin W, Kaskel F, Levin TL. Primary hyperoxaluria: spectrum of clinical and imaging findings. Pediatr Radiol. 2017;47:96-103.

9. Holmes RP, Assimos DG. The impact of dietary oxalate on kidney stone formation. Urol Res. 2004;32:311-6.
10. Nasr SH, Kashtanova Y, Levchuk V, Markowitz GS. Secondary oxalosis due to excess vitamin C intake. Kidney Int. 2006;70:1672.
11. Rumsby G, Hulton SA. (2017). Primary hyperoxaluria type 2: Glyoxylate Reductase/Hydroxypyruvate Reductase Deficiency: US NatLib Med. [online] Available from https://www.ncbi.nlm.nih.gov/books/NBK2692/. [Last accessed September, 2021].
12. Geary D, and Schaefer F. Pediatric Kidney Disease, 2nd edition. Berlin Heidelber: Springer; 2016. pp.1037-59.
13. Fernández-Higuero JÁ, Betancor-Fernández I, Mesa-Torres N, Muga A, Salido E, Pey AL. Structural and functional insights on the roles of molecular chaperones in the mistargeting and aggregation phenotypes associated with primary hyperoxaluria type I. Adv Protein Chem Struct Biol. 2019;114:119-52.
14. Harambat J, Fargue S, Bacchetta J, Acquaviva C, Cochat P. Primary hyperoxaluria. Int J Nephrol. 2011;2011:864580.
15. Al Riyami MS, Al Ghaithi B, Al Hashmi N, Al Kalbani N. Primary hyperoxaluria type 1 in 18 children: genotyping and outcome. Int J Nephrol. 2015;2015:634175.
16. Cochat P, Rumsby G. Primary hyperoxaluria. N Engl J Med. 2013;369:649-58.
17. Harambat J, Fargue S, Acquaviva C, Gagnadoux MF, Janssen F, Liutkus A, et al. Genotype-phenotype correlation in primary hyperoxaluria type 1: the p. Gly170Arg AGXT mutation is associated with a better outcome. Kidney Int. 2010;77:443-9.
18. Hoppe B, Kemper MJ, Bökenkamp A, Portale AA, Cohn RA, Langman CB. Plasma calcium oxalate supersaturation in children with primary hyperoxaluria and end-stage renal failure. Kidney Int. 1999;56:268-74.
19. Frishberg Y, Rinat C, Shalata A, Khatib I, Feinstein S, Becker-Cohen R, et al. Intra-familial clinical heterogeneity: absence of genotype-phenotype correlation in primary hyperoxaluria type 1 in Israel. Am J Nephrol. 2005;25:269-75.
20. Danpure CJ, Valle DL, Beaudet AL, Vogelstein B, Mitchell GA, Antonarakis S. The online metabolic and molecular bases of inherited disease (OMM-BID). New York, NY: McGraw-Hill; 2014. p. 133.
21. Perucca J, Bouby N, Valeix P, Bankir L. Sex difference in urine concentration across differing ages, sodium intake, and level of kidney disease. Am J Physiol Regul Integr Comp Physiol. 2007;292(2):R700-5.
22. Hoppe B, Beck BB, Milliner DS. The primary hyperoxalurias. Kidney Int. 2009;75:1264-71.
23. Di Pasquale G, Ribani M, Andreoli A, Zampa GA, Pinelli G. Cardioembolic stroke in primary oxalosis with cardiac involvement. Stroke. 1989;20:1403-6.
24. Fishbein GA, Micheletti RG, Currier JS, Singer E, Fishbein MC. Atherosclerotic oxalosis in coronary arteries. Cardio Path. 2008;17:117-23.
25. Rao NM, Yallapragada A, Winden KD, Saver J, Liebeskind DS. Stroke in primary hyperoxaluria type I. J Neuroimag. 2014;24:411-3.
26. Karadag S, Gursu M, Aydin Z, Uzun S, Dogan O, Ozturk S, et al. Primary hyperoxaluria in an adult presenting with end-stage renal failure together with hypercalcemia and hypothyroidism. Hemodial Int. 2011;15:573-6.
27. Shatha M, Yuval E. Endocrine manifestations of primary hyperoxaluria. Endocr Pract. 2017;23:1414-24.
28. Leumann EP, Dietl A, Matasovic A. Urinary oxalate and glycolate excretion in healthy infants and children. Pediatr Nephrol. 1990;4:493-7.
29. Cochat P, Nogueira PC, Mahmoud MA, Jamieson NV, Scheinman JI, Rolland MO. Primary hyperoxaluria in infants: medical, ethical, and economic issues. J Pediatr. 1999;135:746-50.
30. Millan MT, Berquist WE, So SK, Sarwal MM, Wayman KI, Cox KL, et al. One hundred percent patient and kidney allograft survival with simultaneous liver and kidney transplantation in infants with primary hyperoxaluria: a single-center experience. Transplant. 2003;76:1458-63.
31. Broyer M, Brunner FP, Brynger H, Dykes SR, Ehrich JH, Fassbinder W, et al. Kidney transplantation in primary oxalosis: data from the EDTA Registry. Nephrol Dial Transplant. 1990;5:332-6.
32. Jamieson NV. A 20-year experience of combined liver/kidney transplantation for primary hyperoxaluria (PH1): the European PH1 transplant registry experience 1984–2004. Am J Nephrol. 2005;25:282-9.
33. Van der Hoeven SM, Van Woerden CS, Groothoff JW. Primary hyperoxaluria type 1, a too often missed diagnosis and potentially treatable cause of end-stage renal disease in adults: results of the Dutch cohort. Nephrol Dial Transplant. 2012;27:3855-62.
34. Bacchetta J, Boivin G, Cochat P. Bone impairment in primary hyperoxaluria: a review. Pediatr Nephrol. 2016;31(1):1-6.
35. Cochat P, Hulton SA, Acquaviva C, Danpure CJ, Daudon M, De Marchi M, et al. Primary hyperoxaluria Type 1: indications for screening and guidance for diagnosis and treatment. Nephrol Dial Transplant. 2012;27:1729-36.
36. Daudon M, Jungers P, Bazin D. Peculiar morphology of stones in primary hyperoxaluria. N Engl J Med. 2008;359(1):100-2.
37. Daudon M, Jungers P. Clinical value of crystalluria and quantitative morphoconstitutional analysis of urinary calculi. Nephr Physiol. 2004;98:31-6.
38. Rumsby G, Williams E, Coulter-Mackie M. Evaluation of mutation screening as a first line test for the diagnosis of the primary hyperoxalurias. Kidney Int. 2004;66:959-63.
39. Monico CG, Olson JB, Milliner DS. Implications of genotype and enzyme phenotype in pyridoxine response of patients with type I primary hyperoxaluria. Am J Nephrol. 2005;25:183-8.
40. Monico CG, Rossetti S, Olson JB, Milliner DS. Pyridoxine effect in type I primary hyperoxaluria is associated with the most common mutant allele. Kidney Int. 2005;67:1704-9.
41. Fargue S, Rumsby G, Danpure CJ. Multiple mechanisms of action of pyridoxine in primary hyperoxaluria type 1. Biochim Biophys Acta. 2013;1832:1776-83.
42. Fargue S, Harambat J, Gagnadoux MF, Tsimaratos M, Janssen F, Llanas B, et al. Effect of conservative treatment on the renal outcome of children with primary hyperoxaluria type 1. Kidney Int. 2009;76:767-73.
43. El Hage S, Ghanem I, Baradhi A, Mourani C, Mallat S, Dagher F, et al. Skeletal features of primary hyperoxaluria type 1, revisited. J Child Orthop. 2008;2:205-10.
44. Brancaccio D, Poggi A, Ciccarelli C, Bellini F, Galmozzi C, Poletti I, et al. Bone changes in end-stage oxalosis. Am J Roentgenol. 1981;136:935-9.
45. Diallo O, Janssens F, Hall M, Avni EF. Type 1 primary hyperoxaluria in pediatric patients: renal sonographic patterns. Am J Roentgenol. 2004;183:1767-70.
46. Schneider P, Rendl J, Börner W, Heidbreder E. Primary hyperoxaluria type 1. Bone scintigraphy, X-ray radiography, and gamma-ray quantitative CT. Clin Nucl Med. 1991;16:681-3.
47. Solmos GR, Ali A, Rodby RA, Fordham EW. Rapid reversal of bone scan abnormalities in a patient with type 1 primary hyperoxaluria and oxalosis. Clin Nucl Med. 1994;19:769-72.
48. Yoshioka J, Park YD, Tanaka Y, Kobayashi Y, Miyajima M, Tani A, et al. Echocardiographic features in a patient with primary oxalosis. Echocardiography. 2001;18:599-602.

49. Harambat J, van Stralen KJ, Espinosa L, Groothoff JW, Hulton SA, Cerkauskiene R, et al. Characteristics and outcomes of children with primary oxalosis requiring renal replacement therapy. Clin J Am Soc Nephrol. 2012;7:458-65.
50. Weigert A, Martin-Higueras C, Hoppe B. Novel therapeutic approaches in primary hyperoxaluria. Expert Opin Emerg Drugs. 2018;23:349-57.
51. Musayev FN, Di Salvo ML, Saavedra MA, Contestabile R, Ghatge MS, Haynes A, et al. Molecular basis of reduced pyridoxine 5′-phosphate oxidase catalytic activity in neonatal epileptic encephalopathy disorder. J Biol Chem. 2009;284:30949-56.
52. Jacob DE, Grohe B, Geßner M, Beck BB, Hoppe B. Kidney stones in primary hyperoxaluria: new lessons learnt. PLoS One. 2013;8:e70617.
53. Hoyer-Kuhn H, Kohbrok S, Volland R, Franklin J, Hero B, Beck BB, et al. Vitamin B6 in primary hyperoxaluria I: first prospective trial after 40 years of practice. Clin J Am Soc Nephrol. 2014;9:468-77.
54. Oppici E, Montioli R, Lorenzetto A, Bianconi S, Voltattorni CB, Cellini B. Biochemical analyses are instrumental in identifying the impact of mutations on holo and/or apo-forms and on the region(s) of alanine:glyoxylate aminotransferase variants associated with primary hyperoxaluria type I. Mol Genet Metab. 2012;105:132-40.
55. Leumann E, Hoppe B, Neuhaus T. Management of primary hyperoxaluria: efficacy of oral citrate administration. Pediatr Nephrol. 1993;7:207-11.
56. Siener R, Hoppe B, Löhr P, Müller SC, Latz S. Metabolic profile and impact of diet in patients with primary hyperoxaluria. Int Urol Nephrol. 2018;50:1583-9.
57. Wong K, Thomson C, Bailey RR, McDiarmid S, Gardner J. Acute oxalate nephropathy after a massive intravenous dose of vitamin C. Aust N Z J Med. 1994;24(4):410-1.
58. Marangella M, Vitale C, Cosseddu D, Petrarulo M, Linari F. Effects of oral and intravenous calcitriol on serum calcium oxalate saturation in dialysis patients. Clin Sci. 1993;85:309-14.
59. Sikora P, Von Unruh GE, Beck B, Feldkötter M, Zajaczkowska M, Hesse A, et al. [13C2] oxalate absorption in children with idiopathic calcium oxalate urolithiasis or primary hyperoxaluria. Kidney Int. 2008;73:1181-6.
60. Illies F, Bonzel KE, Wingen AM, Latta K, Hoyer PF. Clearance and removal of oxalate in children on intensified dialysis for primary hyperoxaluria type 1. Kidney Int. 2006;70:1642-8.
61. Brinkert F, Ganschow R, Helmke K, Harps E, Fischer L, Nashan B, et al. Transplantation procedures in children with primary hyperoxaluria type 1: outcome and longitudinal growth. Transplantation. 2009;87:1415-21.
62. Monico CG, Milliner DS. Combined liver-kidney and kidney-alone transplantation in primary hyperoxaluria. Liver Transpl. 2001;7:954-63.
63. Hatch M, Freel RW, Vaziri ND. Regulatory aspects of oxalate secretion in enteric oxalate elimination. J Am Soc Nephrol. 1999;10:S324-8.
64. Grujic D, Salido EC, Shenoy BC, Langman CB, McGrath ME, Patel RJ, et al. Hyperoxaluria is reduced and nephrocalcinosis prevented with an oxalate-degrading enzyme in mice with hyperoxaluria. Am J Nephrol. 2009;29:86-93.
65. Martin-Higueras C, Torres A, Salido E. Molecular therapy of primary hyperoxaluria. J Inherit Metab Dis. 2017;40:481-9.
66. Dindo M, Conter C, Oppici E, Ceccarelli V, Marinucci L, Cellini B. Molecular basis of primary hyperoxaluria: clues to innovative treatments. Urolithiasis. 2019;47:67-78.
67. Liebow A, Li X, Racie T, Hettinger J, Bettencourt BR, Najafian N, et al. An investigational RNAi therapeutic targeting glycolate oxidase reduces oxalate production in models of primary hyperoxaluria. J Am Soc Nephrol. 2017;28:494-503.
68. Ludwig-Portugall I, Bartok E, Dhana E, Evers BDG, Primiano MJ, Hall JP, et al. An NLRP3-specific inflammasome inhibitor attenuates crystal-induced kidney fibrosis in mice. Kidney Int. 2016;90(3):525-39.
69. Toscano MG, van der Velden J, van der Werf S, Odijk M, Roque A, Camacho-Garcia RJ, et al. Generation of a vero-based packaging cell line to produce SV40 gene delivery vectors for use in clinical gene therapy studies. Mol Ther Methods Clin Dev. 2017;6:124-34.
70. Estève J, Blouin JM, Lalanne M, Azzi-Martin L, Dubus P, Bidet A, et al. Generation of induced pluripotent stem cells-derived hepatocyte-like cells for ex vivo gene therapy of primary hyperoxaluria type 1. Stem Cell Res. 2019;38:101467.
71. Barratt TM, Kasidas GP, Murdoch I, Rose GA. Urinary oxalate and glycolate excretion and plasma oxalate concentration. Arch Dis Child. 1991;66:501-3.
72. Pinapala A, Garg M, Kamath N, Iyengar A. Clinical and genetic profile of Indian children with primary hyperoxaluria. Indian J Nephrol. 2017;27:222.
73. Van Schaftingen E, Draye JP, Van Hoof F. Coenzyme specificity of mammalian liver d-glycerate dehydrogenase. Eur J Biochem. 1989;186:355-9.
74. Belostotsky R, Pitt JJ, Frishberg Y. Primary hyperoxaluria type III—a model for studying perturbations in glyoxylate metabolism. J Mol Med (Berl). 2012;90:1497-504.
75. Johnson SA, Rumsby G, Cregeen D, Hulton SA. Primary hyperoxaluria type 2 in children. Pediatr Nephrol. 2002;17:597-601.
76. Milliner DS, Wilson DM, Smith LH. Phenotypic expression of primary hyperoxaluria: comparative features of types I and II. Kidney Int. 2001;59:31-6.
77. Wichmann G, Passauer J, Fischer R, Weise M, Gross P. A young patient with end-stage renal disease, dyspnoea, weakness, peripheral neuropathy and an unsuspected underlying disease. Nephrol Dial Transplant. 2003;18:1670-2.
78. Yamanouchi M, Ubara Y, Takayama T, Kuhara T, Takaichi K. Calcified nodules on fingers in primary hyperoxaluria type 2. Lancet Diabetes Endocrinol. 2016;4:468.
79. Giafi CF, Rumsby G. Kinetic analysis and tissue distribution of human D-glycerate dehydrogenase/glyoxylate reductase and its relevance to the diagnosis of primary hyperoxaluria type 2. Ann Clin Biochem. 1998;35:104-9.
80. Cregeen DP, Williams EL, Hulton S, Rumsby G. Molecular analysis of the glyoxylate reductase (GRHPR) gene and description of mutations underlying primary hyperoxaluria type 2. Hum Mutat. 2003;22:497.
81. Filler G, Hoppe B. Combined liver-kidney transplantation for hyperoxaluria type II? Pediatr Transplant. 2014;18:237-9.
82. Dhondup T, Lorenz EC, Milliner DS, Lieske JC. Combined liver-kidney transplantation for primary hyperoxaluria type 2: a case Report. Am J Transplant. 2018;18:253-7.
83. Fang X, He L, Xu G, Lin H, Xu M, Geng H. Nine novel HOGA1 gene mutations identified in primary hyperoxaluria type 3 and distinct clinical and biochemical characteristics in Chinese children. Pediatr Nephrol. 2019;34:1785-90.
84. Beck BB, Baasner A, Buescher A, Habbig S, Reintjes N, Kemper MJ, et al. Novel findings in patients with primary hyperoxaluria type III and implications for advanced molecular testing strategies. Eur J Hum Genet. 2013;21:162-72.
85. Greed L, Willis F, Johnstone L, Teo S, Belostotsky R, Frishberg Y, et al. Metabolite diagnosis of primary hyperoxaluria type 3. Pediatr Nephrol. 2018;33:1443-6.

SECTION

9

Ciliopathies and Hereditary Tubulointerstitial Diseases

CHAPTER

9.1

Genetic and Molecular Bases of Renal Ciliopathies

Anil Vasudevan

INTRODUCTION

Motile and nonmotile cilia are hair-like cellular organelles that are ubiquitous in nature and play a major role in various signal transductions and organ development in humans. The first report of cilia is by Antoni van Leeuwenhoek, a Dutch scientist, who observed hair-like structure in microorganisms used for movement.[1] Many of the functions of cilia are context dependent such as polarity, proliferation of cells, determining left–right asymmetry, and differentiation. *Ciliopathy refers to a class of genetic disorders affecting multiple systems in humans, which are caused by many largely unrelated genes regulating ciliary structure/function.*[2] Ciliopathy can be classified according to the structure and function of the affected cilia. The two types of cilia are (1) motile cilia present in organs such as lungs and fallopian tubes which move extracellular fluids (clear mucus secretions from lung) or propel cells (such as ova) or (2) nonmotile cilia (primary cilia) present in organs such as kidney, brain, and skeletal system that function as an "antenna" by helping in relaying signals from the surrounding environment or cells to the interior of cells. Primary cilia are also referred to as sensory cilia. Ciliopathy due to dysfunction of cilia is first-order ciliopathy whereas disruption of nonciliary proteins essential for ciliary function is second-order ciliopathy. While 450 cilia-related genes have been identified, approximately 35 "ciliopathies" are linked to 180 ciliary proteins.[3] There is difference in physiological consequences of disruption of motile and nonmotile cilia with dysfunction of nonmotile cilia affecting multiple organs including kidneys. Defects of motile cilia causing primary ciliary dyskinesia (e.g., Kartagener's syndrome) will not be considered further in this chapter.

STRUCTURE AND FUNCTION OF CILIA

Structure of Cilia

Cilia are found on almost all vertebrate cells and are microtubule-based structures which are highly conserved throughout evolution. The four key important structures of cilia are (1) basal body representing one of the two centrioles of the centrosome, (2) transition zone, (3) microtubule-based axoneme, and (4) membrane which covers the ciliary process **(Fig. 1)**.

Basal Body

Basal body located at the base of the cilia functions as an anchor and docking site. It consists of nine triplet microtubules, subdistal appendages, and nine outward facing structures at the base of cilium, known as distal appendages (or transition fibers), connecting to the cell membrane. Basal body which is surrounded by pericentriolar matrix also contains other specialized accessory structures such as basal feet and ciliary rootlets.

Transition Zone

The region between the proximal-most region of the axoneme and the end of the basal body, which helps to demarcate ciliary and other cell compartments, is called transition zone. Transition zone regulates proteins entering and leaving the cilium through a diffusion barrier formed by Y-shaped structures that connect the ciliary membrane to the underlying axoneme. Septins, a protein that creates barriers between different membrane compartments, also form a part of the diffusion barrier.[4] This zone also houses a variety of large protein complexes that play an important role in cilia formation, trafficking, and gating. The protein complexes are named after ciliopathies associated with their specific gene such as Meckel–Gruber syndrome and nephronophthisis (NPHP) complexes. A distinct molecular subsection located distal to the transition zone is the inversin compartment, housing inversin protein (INV) encoded by *NPHP2* gene.

Axoneme

The axoneme that protrudes from the basal body consists of nine peripheral doublets with or without two central singletons, having radial spokes, dynein arms, and nexin links. The triplets have three kinds of fibers: A, B, and C fibers. A and B fibers forming part of axonemes are made up of 13 and 10 tubulins, respectively, while C fiber is short fiber and limited at the transition zone. Based on whether the axoneme includes an extra central pair of microtubules, cilia are classified as 9 + 2 or 9 + 0.[5] The structural difference between nonmotile and motile cilia is that motile cilia include a central pair of microtubules (9 + 2) along with axonemal inner and outer dynein arms that produce ciliary movement **(Fig. 1)**.

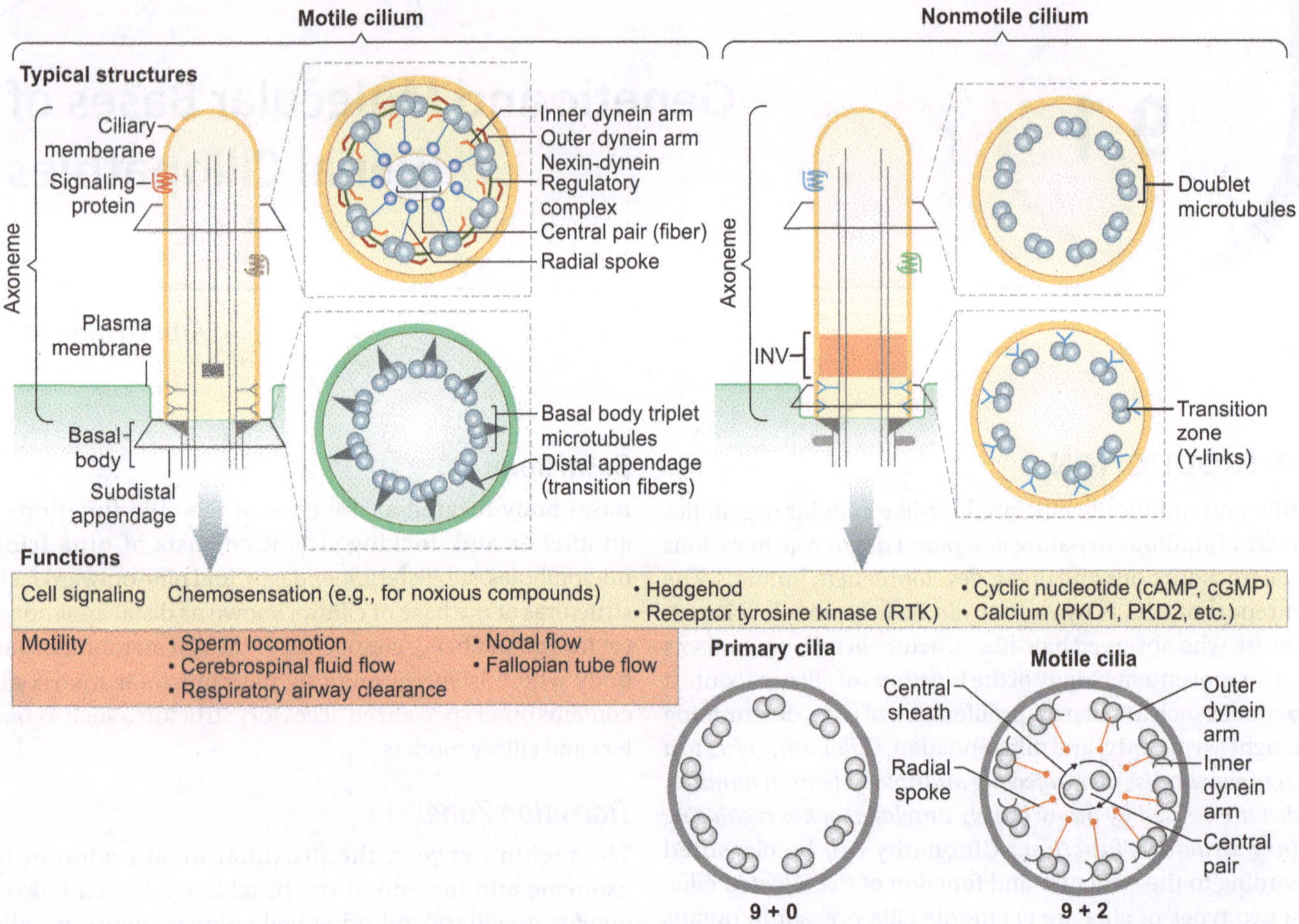

Fig. 1: Cilia extending from basal body typically consist of triplet microtubules and subdistal and distal appendages. Distal appendages (also known as transition fibers) anchor the basal body to the base of the ciliary membrane. Next to the basal body is the transition zone, which contains doublet microtubules that are connected to the ciliary membrane via Y-shaped structures. Axonemes (the ciliary backbone) are composed of doublet microtubules. Motile cilia have in addition a central microtubule (9 + 2) and inner and outer dynein arms. (INV: housing inversin protein)

Ciliary Membrane

The ciliary membrane is in continuity with the plasma membrane with a distinct lipid and protein making up the lipid bilayer. Receptors and signaling molecules are located within primary cilia and separated from the plasma membrane, enabling cilia to move and/or function as a signaling device.

Development of Cilia

Ciliogenesis begins during the interphase with modification of mother centriole to become a basal body. Basal body migrates and attaches to the plasma membrane via distal appendages with basal body-associated membrane becoming the ciliary membrane. This is followed by development of transition zone and extension of rest of the axoneme from the cell body. The axoneme is maintained by the intraflagellar transport (IFT) machinery which mostly contains motor proteins. IFT helps in transporting cargo proteins along the ciliary axoneme.[6] Ciliary proteins are trafficked from the Golgi or cytosol to the base of the cilium and thereon into the ciliary compartment as cilia cannot synthesize their own proteins. The transport process in axoneme is from base to tip (anterograde) and tip to base (retrograde). Components in IFT module that mediate trafficking include IFT subcomplexes A (6 protein subunits) and B (13 protein subunits), kinesin II (anterograde transport), dynein-2 (retrograde) motor proteins, and an accessory module containing Bardet–Biedl syndrome (BBS) proteins (the BBSome) **(Fig. 2)**. BBSome consists of eight BBS proteins (BBS 1, 2, 4, 5, 7, 8, 9, and BBIP10), modulated by Arf and Rab family of proteins.[7] The main functions of BBSome are to stabilize and assemble IFT proteins and support import and export of protein from primary cilium. Sorting and packaging into carrier vesicles followed by docking and fusion of vesicles with base of the cilium and then bidirectional transport to and back from the ciliary base to the tip form the cargo transport process.

Functions of Cilia

Cilia sense a wide variety of extracellular signals and convert them into decisions that regulate polarity, proliferation, differentiation, or tissue maintenance. Signaling receptors located on the ciliary membrane of primary cilia play a key role in transduction of key developmental signaling

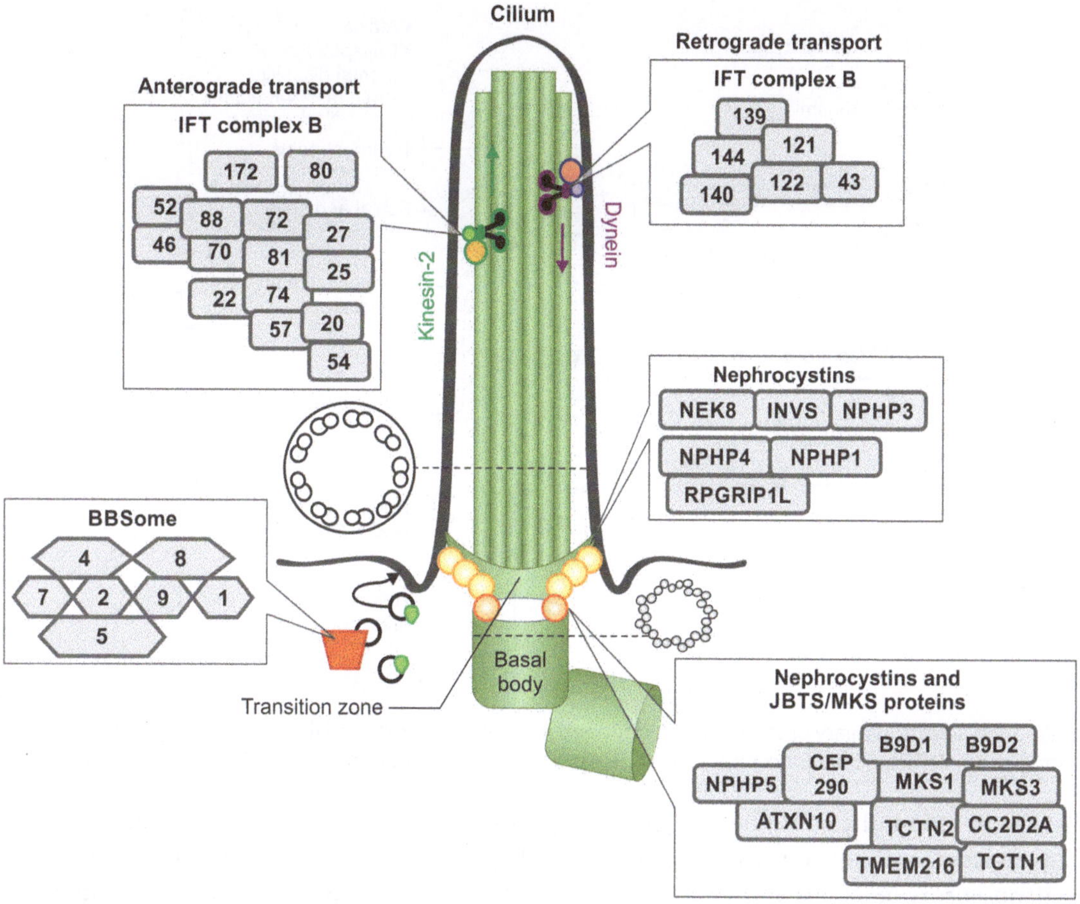

Fig. 2: Kinesin II motors along with axonemal precursors and dynein motor mediate anterograde and retrograde IFT transport, respectively. IFT type A complexes and IFT type B complexes are linked to retrograde and anterograde transport, respectively. (IFT: intraflagellar transport).

pathways such as Notch, Sonic hedgehog (SHH) and Hippo pathways Wnt, platelet-derived growth factor receptor α, and fibroblast growth factor.[8] The subsequent downstream signaling regulates tissue proliferation and differentiation, cellular homeostasis, and growth required for normal organ development and function. Cilia also play a crucial role in the regulation of planar cell polarity (PCP) which is crucial for normal renal tubular development, perturbations of which are observed in cystic kidney diseases. The cilia also perform specialized function as mechanosensors, photosensors, osmosensors, thermosensors, and olfactory sensors.

MOLECULAR AND GENETIC BASES OF CILIARY DYSFUNCTION AND ITS PHENOTYPIC CONSEQUENCES

The physical compartmentalization along with localization of proteins to its complex IFT machinery is fundamental which enables cilia to function as a sensory organelle. Being ubiquitous in nature, disturbance in structure and function of primary cilia results in morphologic features that are broad and overlapping, most commonly involving eye, brain, kidney, skeletal, and liver **(Fig. 3)**. At a molecular level, there is impaired ciliogenesis and compartmentalization (or gating) as well as disruption of different processes such as signaling and dynamic trafficking. The disturbances lead to impairment in cell-cycle regulation, proliferation, apoptosis, and altered developmental patterning and PCP, resulting in distinct phenotypes **(Figs. 4A to C)**. In the kidneys, it leads to various phenotypes such as polycystic kidneys, NPHP, and renal cystic dysplasia (further described in the clinical perspective section).

As stated earlier, cilia perform specialized functions as photosensors, olfactory sensors, and mechanosensors which are cell specific with different signaling mechanisms. In ciliopathy, there is impaired perception of environmental cues which results in specific tissue dysfunction based on the protein or structure involved. In the photoreceptor cells of human retina, cilia are the site for receiving signals and also for initial transduction regulating intracellular levels of cyclic guanosine monophosphate (cGMP).[9] Hence, abnormal development of cilia or disturbance in this pathway leads to retinitis pigmentosa. On the other hand, G protein-coupled receptor (GPCR) on the ciliary membrane of olfactory sensor and cyclic adenosine monophosphate (cAMP) play a role in smell.[10] Hence, mistrafficking of ciliary proteins impairs their function leading to loss of smell as observed in children with Bardet–Biedl syndrome.

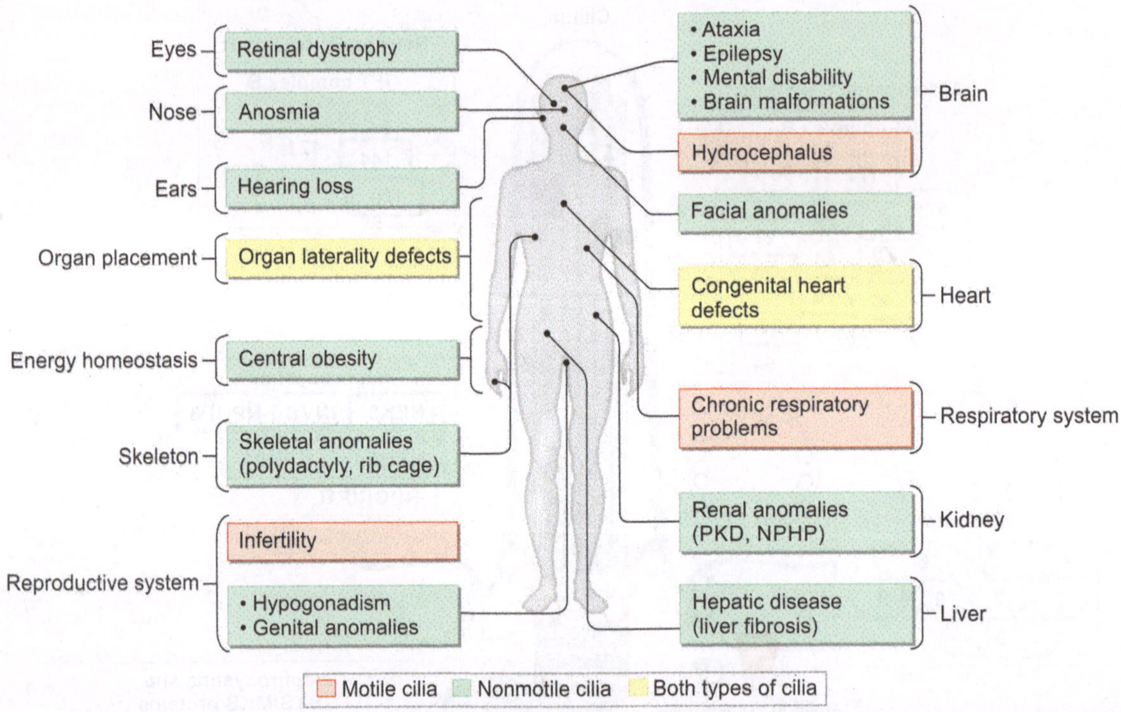

Fig. 3: Single-gene defects in ciliary proteins affect kidney and multiple other extrarenal systems. Primary and secondary clinical phenotypes are depicted here for common renal ciliopathy. (NPHP: nephronophthisis; PKD: polycystic kidney disease)

Kidney disease in ciliopathy could be due to loss of mechanosensory function or its function as a chemosensor. Cilia have mechanosensory functions and a defective fluid flow sensing triggers result in polycystic kidney disease (PKD). Renal ciliopathy as in NPHP may be due to perturbation in function of cilia as a chemosensor in which cilia act as little antennae and sense the external environment through various receptors located on the ciliary membrane such as platelet-derived growth factor AA (PDGF-AA) and somatostatin. Two key processes, PCP and oriented cell division (OCD), help to maintain tubular diameter during tubular development as well as during repair. Primary cilia have an important role in transducing intracellular signaling pathways such as Wnt and sonic hedgehog signaling (SHH) which regulate cell-cycle progression and polarity. Wnt signaling is a key pathway in establishing PCP, which is disturbed in ciliopathy. In animal studies, renal cystogenesis has been observed when PCP signaling is perturbed.[11] Cilia play a key role in mediating the switch between canonical and noncanonical Wnt signaling. PCP signaling also regulates OCD of tubular cells. Whether abnormal OCD precedes cystogenesis or happens during cystogenesis is unclear. Overexpression of β-catenin in transgenic mice leads to renal cysts supporting a role for canonical Wnt activation in cystogenesis.[12]

Polycystic kidney disease is due to abnormal function of proteins polycystin 1 and 2 (PC1 and PC2) and fibrocystin located in cilia. Autosomal dominant polycystic kidney disease (ADPKD) is associated with mutations in *PKD1* and *PKD2* genes that encode PC1 and PC2 while mutations in *PKHD1* gene that encodes for fibrocystin (also known as polyductin) result in autosomal recessive polycystic kidney disease (ARPKD). The molecular mechanisms that contribute to the development of ADPKD are yet to be completely understood. Protein complex formed by interaction of intracellular C-terminal PC1 domain with PC2 and localized to the primary apical cilia membrane acts as a receptor–ion channel. One of the mechanisms is the reduction in channel permeability to ions as a result of disruption of complex formation caused by mutations of *PKD1* or *PKD2* gene. In normal state, Ca^{2+} influx is induced by binding of Wnt ligands to the extracellular PC1 domain in the presence of PC2.[13] Besides disturbance in ion channel activity, the mTOR (mammalian target of rapamycin) pathway has been shown to be inappropriately activated in epithelial kidney cells of ADPKD patients and recapitulated in mouse models.[14] This may be due to disturbance in binding of tuberin, a protein regulating mTOR to the receptor channel complex. Disturbance in these signaling pathways linked to PC1 or PC2 leads to dysregulation of various downstream intersecting pathways resulting in impaired cellular growth, fluid secretion, and tubular morphology. Fibrocystin, implicated in ARPKD, has a long extracellular highly glycosylated N-terminal tail consisting of several IPT and IPT-like domains and multiple parallel beta-helix repeats (PbH1), a short cytoplasmic C-terminus with kinase A phosphorylation sites, and a single transmembrane region.[15] Fibrocystin is involved in trafficking of regulatory proteins to the cilium and acts as a cell surface receptor and is also involved in regulation of cellular proliferation and in cell-cell adhesion. More details on cellular processes leading to cyst formation in ADPKD and ARPKD are provided in Chapter 9.2.

A. Motile cilium structure

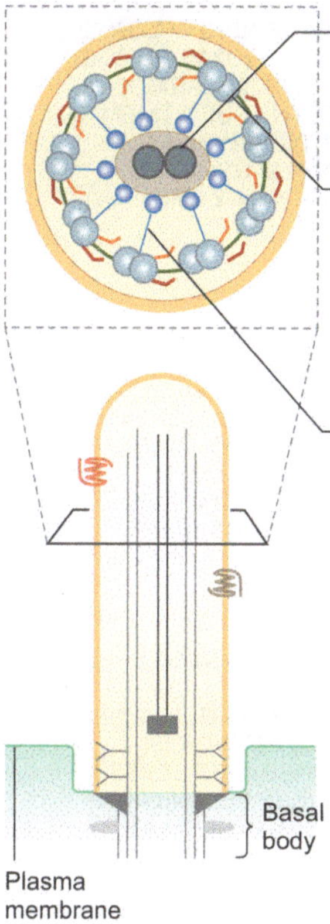

B. Ciliopathy proteins

Motility apparatus ① ⑩

Central pair
- DNAH6
- HYDIN
- RSPH4A

Nexin-dynein regulatory complex
- CCDC39
- CCDC65
- CCDC40
- DRC1
- GAS8

Radial spoke
- DNAJB13
- RSPH1
- RSPH3
- RSPH9

Outer dynein arm, inner dynein arm
- ARMC4
- CCDC103
- CCDC114
- CCDC151
- C21ORF59
- DNAAF1
- DNAAF2
- DNAAF3
- DNAAF5
- DNAH1
- DNAH5
- DNAH11
- DNAI1
- DNAI2
- DNAL1
- DYX1C1
- HEATR2
- LRRC6
- NME8
- SPAG1
- TTC25
- ZMYND10

Cytoplasm

PIH1D3

Regulation of centrioles and transcription in multi ciliated cells
- CCNO
- MCIDAS

Nonmotile cilium structure

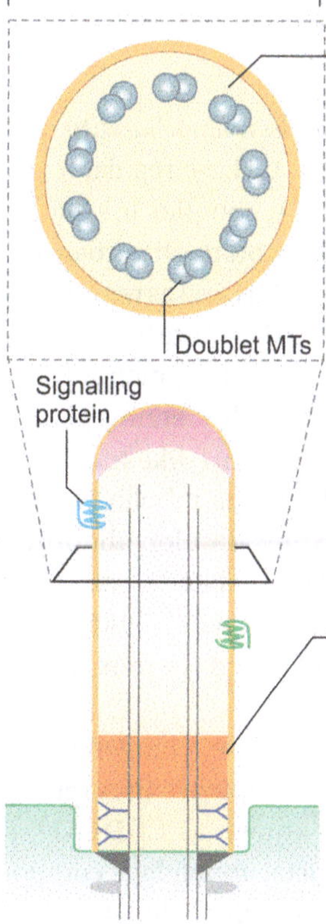

Axoneme and signaling ② ③ ④ ⑤ ⑥ ⑦ ⑧ ⑨ ⑩
- ADCY6
- ANKS3
- ANKS6
- CEP41*
- CNGA1
- CNGA41
- CNGB1
- C2ORF71
- C21ORF2
- DCDC2
- EFHC1
- FLCN*
- GPR161
- ICK*
- INPP5E
- IQCB1*
- LCA5*
- NEK1
- OCRL*
- PIK3R4*
- PKD1
- PKD2
- PKD1L1
- PKHD1
- RAB23
- SDCCAG8*
- SMO
- USP9X

Cilium tip ② ③ ⑧
- CEP104*
- GLI2
- GLI3
- KIF7
- SUFU

INV compartment ② ⑤
- EVC
- EVC2
- INVS
- NPHP3
- NEK8

Transcription factor ③ ④
- CRX
- ZIC2

Other: cytosol, Golgi, nucleus, etc. ① ② ③ ④ ⑤ ⑦ ⑧
- AK7
- DDX59
- GALNT11
- GLIS2
- PIK3R4*
- POMGNT1
- TBC1D32
- XPNPEP3
- ZNF423

C. Associated ciliopathies

① Cilia motility, respiratory, brain, heart, organ placement, sperm

Primary ciliary dyskinesia (PCD)

② Multisystemic (primary cilia), brain, kidney, skeleton, eyes
- Bardet–Biedl syndrome (BBS)
- Carpenter syndrome (CRPT)
- Hydrolethalus ysndrome (HLS)
- Joubert syndrome (JBTS)
- Oculocerebrorenal sysndrome of Lowe (OCRL)
- Meckel syndrome (MKS)
- MORM syndrome
- Pallister–Hall syndrome (PHS)
- Senior–Loken syndrome (SLSN)

③ Brain
- Holoprosencephaly (HPE)
- Juvenile myoclonic epilepsy (JME)
- Medulloblastoma

④ Eyes
- Leber congenital amaurosis (LCA)
- Cone–rod dystrophy (CRD)
- Retinitis pigmentosa (RP)

⑤ Kidney
- Nephronophthisis (NPHP)
- Polycystic kidney disease (PKD)

⑥ Nose

Anosmia, isolated congenital

⑦ Organ placement, heart
- Congenital heart disease (CHD)
- Situs inversus, heterotaxy

⑧ Skeleton
- Ellis-van Creveld syndrome (EVC)
- Greig cephalopolysyndactyly syndrome
- Jeune asphyxiating thoracic dystrophy (JATD)
- Orofaciodigital syndrome (OFD)
- Short-rib thoracic dysplasia (SRTD)

⑨ Ears

Hearing loss

⑩ Various
- Birt–Hogg–Dube syndrome
- Lethal congenital contracture syndrome (LCCS)
- Male infertility
- Pituitary stalk interruption syndrome (PSIS)
- Polycystic kidney disease and hepatic disease

Figs. 4A to C

Contd...

Contd...

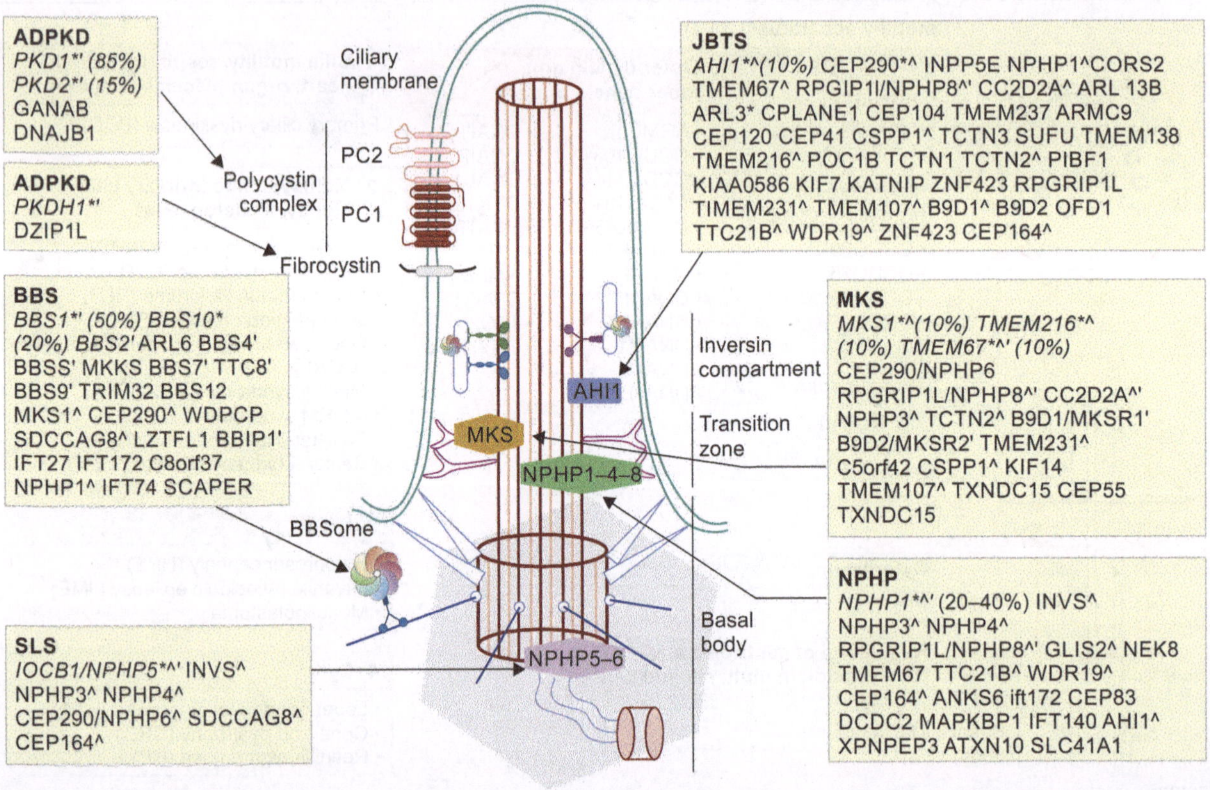

Figs. 4A to C: (A) Components of primary cilia; (B) Ciliopathy proteins associated with basal body, centriolar satellites, or the ciliary apparatus during and/or after development of cilia. Circled numbers indicate ciliopathies (listed in part C) due to defects in these corresponding subcompartments, as well as the affected tissues, organs, or physiological functions. * indicates proteins localized also to other ciliary regions during ciliary development or trafficking; (C) Grouping of ciliopathy into major categories that are associated with the proteins and ciliary compartments shown in part B.

Nephrocystins, encoded by *NPHP* genes, have all been localized to primary cilia, basal bodies, and transition zones and their dysfunction result in NPHP and dysplastic kidneys. These proteins interact with each other forming nephrocystin modules: NPHP1-4-8 (the NPHP complex), NPHP5-6, NPHP2-3-9-ANKS6, NPHP5-6, and MKS.[16] Nephrocystins also interact with other ciliary proteins such as BBSomes and Ofd1 proteins. Some NPHP proteins such as nephrocystin 1, 2, 4, and 10 also localize to adherens junctions and focal adhesion complexes of tubular cells where they regulate junction integrity and polarity. Nephrocystin 1 encoded by NPHP1 localizes to the base of transition zone and is involved in regulation of IFT transport and also binds polycystin-1. Knockdown of NPHP-1 in Madin–Darby canine kidney (MDCK) cells results in abnormal cilia supporting the crucial role of NPHP-1 in maintaining normal ciliary function.[17] Inversin, localized to primary cilium, mediates switch from canonical to noncanonical Wnt signaling which is encoded by *NPHP2* gene.[18] In developing nephrons, the protein helps in maintaining orientation of the cell and its tubular architecture through its interaction with disheveled (Dsh or Dvl1), a PCP signaling protein. The canonical Wnt pathway is also inhibited by nephrocystin 3 encoded by NPHP3. NPHP1 and NPHP4, along with other proteins of MKS/BD9/NPHP modules, are also involved in the early stages of ciliogenesis as observed in studies in *Caenorhabditis elegans*.[19] Calmodulin, retinitis pigmentosa GTPase regulator (RPGR), and nephrocystin 5 form a protein complex in cilia of renal tubular cells as well as in photoreceptors. Disturbance of this complex causes retinitis pigmentosa as well as renal ciliopathy. In a subset of patients with NPHP, mutations in NPHP7 (GLIS2), an intracellular effector of SHH signaling, have been described.[20] *NPHP8/RPGRIP1L* encodes retinitis pigmentosa GTPase regulator interacting protein 1-like located in the centrosome which interacts with gamma-tubulin, NPHP4, and NPHP6.[21] NPHP8 mouse knockouts develop abnormal cilia without axoneme. Never in mitosis A-related kinase 8 encoded by NPHP9/NEK8 forms a complex with ANKS6, NPHP3, and inversin. Knockdown of NEK8 leads to pronephric cysts formation in zebrafish.[22]

As described in a previous section, ciliogenesis begins with docking of basal body to the incipient ciliary membrane. *CEP164*, *CEP89*, *CEP83* (also known as CCDC41), *FBF1*, and *SCLT1* which are the five distal appendage components play important roles in this early step of ciliogenesis. While disruption of CEP164 or CEP83 causes NPHP, mutations in *SCLT1* may also result in orofaciodigital syndrome (OFD), a syndrome characterized by craniofacial abnormalities and polydactyly.[23]

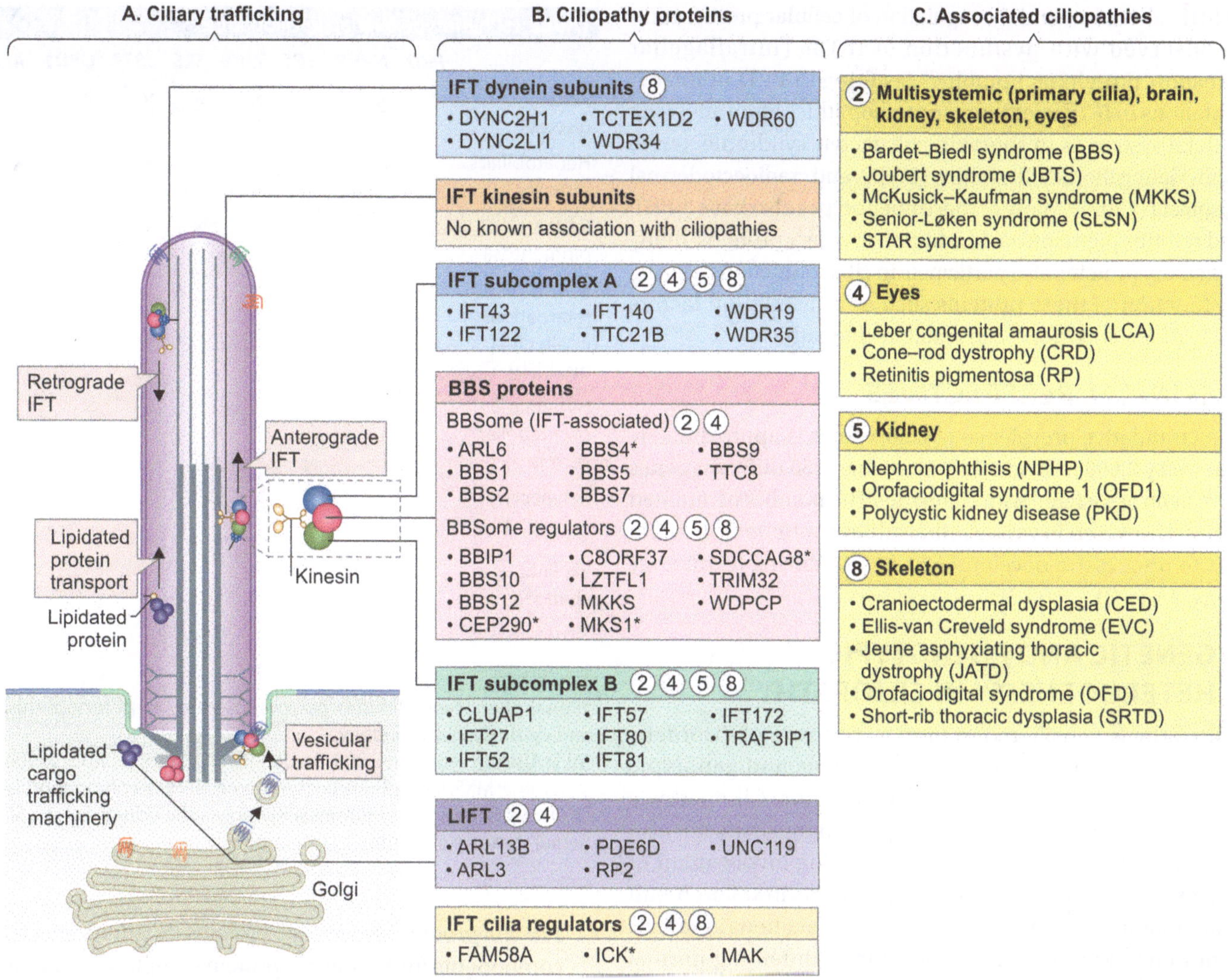

Figs. 5A to C: (A) The functional components of intraflagellar transport (IFT) and lipidated protein intraflagellar targeting (LIFT). IFT modules involved in protein trafficking include anterograde (kinesin-2) and retrograde (dynein-2) motors, IFT subcomplexes A and B, with an accessory module containing Bardet–Biedl syndrome (BBS) proteins (BBSome); (B) Ciliopathy proteins forming or regulating IFT and LIFT trafficking systems. Circled numbers indicate ciliopathies (listed in part C) that result from defects in these ciliary trafficking components. *indicates proteins localized also to other ciliary regions during ciliary development or trafficking; (C) Grouping of ciliopathies into major categories according to tissues affected that are associated with defects in ciliary trafficking.

Bardet–Biedl syndrome (BBS) arises from the disruption of BBSome components (BBS1, BBS2, BBS3, BBS4, BBS5, BBS7, BBS6, BBS8, BBS10, and BBS12). BBSomes are involved in trafficking of ciliary signaling proteins and related functions. Dopamine receptor 1 (DR1), melanin-concentrating hormone receptor 1 (MCHR1), and somatostatin receptor 3 (SSTR3) are three BBS-dependent cargoes.[24] Mutations in genes encoding these proteins result in aberrant ciliary protein localization affecting downstream signaling pathways and is the probable etiology of BBS-associated phenotypes. BBSome also interacts with other major ciliary cystoproteins, such as PC1 and PC2, and NPHP-associated proteins.

Transition zone is a hotspot for ciliopathy and has effects that are generally restricted to single organs such as effects in NPHP but may also has pleiotropic effects as in Meckel syndrome (MKS). While mutations in genes encoding components of MKS complex are associated with MKS, JBTS, and COACH [cerebellar vermis hypoplasia, oligophrenia (mental retardation), ataxia, ocular coloboma, and hepatic fibrosis] syndromes, mutations that affect the NPHP complex cause Senior–Løken syndrome (SLSN) characterized by NPHP with RP. Both IFT (trafficking) and the transition zone (gating) modulate localization of SHH and other signaling components to the cilia.[24] Therefore, disturbance of ciliary Hedgehog signaling may be the cause of many developmental abnormalities such as polydactyly and neural tube defects observed in BBS and MKS, respectively.

Intraflagellar transport plays an important role in maintaining the normal function of cilia. Disruption of this transport machinery also results in pleiotropic ciliopathy **(Figs. 5A to C)**. As mentioned earlier, the SHH pathway helps regulate cellular proliferation. The transport of SHH proteins along cilium is facilitated by IFT and motor proteins. Therefore, mutations in genes coding for IFT proteins lead to SHH alteration and dysregulation of cellular proliferation as observed with dysfunction of IFT88 (intraflagellar transport protein 88 homolog) resulting in PKD in mice.[25] Mutations in *IFT* genes that cause ciliopathies often affect the skeletal system as in short-rib polydactyly syndrome, Jeune asphyxiating thoracic dystrophy (JATD), and cranioectodermal dysplasia (CED).[3] Many of these phenotypes also have NPHP and retinitis pigmentosa. In addition to ciliary proteins, many nonciliary proteins also participate in ciliary functions. Hence, dysfunction of these proteins such as transcription factors (*FX2*, *RFX3*, and *RFX4*) can result in ciliopathies.

CLINICAL PERSPECTIVES

The cumulative prevalence of ciliopathies is approximately 1 in every 2,000 individuals.[26] More than 150 different genes have been associated with ciliopathy. The number of mutated genes discovered in various ciliopathies continue to increase due to progressive developments in sequencing technology (**Figs. 4A to C**).

GENETIC AND PHENOTYPIC HETEROGENEITY IN CILIOPATHY

Ciliopathy is considered to form a spectrum of disorders, with considerable overlap of phenotypic and genotypic characteristics between various conditions. Ciliopathy is characterized not only by phenotypic heterogeneity but also by genetic heterogeneity. There is varying involvement of organs as well as severity of organ dysfunction in children with mutations in the same gene. In addition, mutations in several genes encoding proteins involved in maintaining normal structure and function of cilia cause similar phenotype. **Tables 1 and 2** provide phenotypic and genetic overlap in ciliopathy.

The reasons for phenotypic and genotypic heterogeneity in children with ciliopathy are as follows:

- *Type of mutations:* Truncating mutations are associated with more severe phenotypes than missense mutations. For example, homozygous missense mutations in *NPHP3* result in less-severe phenotype of isolated NPHP while homozygous truncating mutations result in Meckel-Gruber phenotype. Similarly, mutations of different subtypes in *CEP290* gene can lead to phenotypes of varying severity from isolated NPHP to more severe Joubert syndrome to lethal Meckel-Gruber syndrome, which is most severe among the spectrum.
- *"Modifiers" or "oligogenetic inheritance":* Mutations in more than one gene encoding ciliary or nonciliary protein could also cause variability in clinical presentation. Homozygous mutations in 22 pathogenic genes have been identified to cause BBS, an example for genetic heterogeneity in ciliopathy.
- *Mutation load:* Incompletely penetrant or hypomorphic PKD1 allele can affect the severity of PKD and age of presentation in ADPKD.

TABLE 1: Phenotype overlap in ciliopathies.

	PKD	*NPHP*	*BBS*	*MKS*	*SLS*	*JBTS*	*OFD1*	*ALS*
Renal disease*	×	×	×	×	×	×	×	×
Hepatobiliary disease	×	×	×	×		×	×	×
Retinitis pigmentosa		×	×	×	×	×	×	×
Mental retardation/ intellectual disability		×	×	×		×	×	
Hypoplasia of cerebellar vermis						×	×	
Polydactyly			×	×		×	×	
Obesity			×	×		×		×
Skeletal changes		×		×				
Situs inversus		×	×	×	×			
Encephalocele				×		×		

*Renal phenotype includes polycystic kidney, nephronophthisis, and cystic dysplastic kidney.
(ALS: Alström syndrome; BBS: Bardet–Biedl syndrome; JBTS: Joubert syndrome; MKS: Meckel–Gruber syndrome; NPHP: nephronophthisis; OFD1: orofaciodigital syndrome; PKD: polycystic kidney disease; SLS: Senior–Løken syndrome)

- *Protein-protein interactions:* Proteins constituting various components form multiple protein complexes, and these complexes also interact with each other. The complex genetic interactions combined with the interaction of various ciliary proteins with each other provide an explanation for ciliopathies to display extreme phenotypic variation downstream of mutation in a single gene.

Hence, ciliopathy should be considered as a spectrum of disorders with varying severity rather than as distinct syndromes since the amount and type of causal variants in functionally related genes are crucial for the clinical phenotype.

KIDNEY PHENOTYPES IN CILIOPATHY

Ciliopathies, in which the mutations lead to renal disease, are known as a renal ciliopathy. The range of renal phenotypes includes polycystic kidneys, NPHP,, and renal cystic dysplasia (**Table 3**). The underlying mechanisms for various renal phenotypes are incompletely understood as described in previous section.

Polycystic Kidney Disease

Polycystic kidney disease (PKD) is a group of single-gene defect disorders characterized by the presence of multiple cysts, mainly in kidney and liver, presenting from the neonatal

TABLE 2: Genotype overlap in ciliopathies.

Gene/syndrome	*NPHP*	*BBS*	*MKS*	*SLS*	*JBTS*	*OFD*
NPHP1	×			×	×	
NPHP2 (inversin)	×			×		
NPHP3	×		×	×		
NPHP4	×			×		
NPHP5	×			×		
NPHP7/GLIS2	×					
NPHP8/RPGRIPL1	×		×		×	
NPHP11\TMEM67	×	×	×		×	
NPHP12\TTC21B	×					
NPHP13/WDR19	×			×		
NPHP14\ZNF423	×				×	
CEP290	×	×	×	×	×	
NEK8						
AHI1					×	
ARL13B						
BBS1		×				
BBS2		×	×			
BBS3		×		×		
BBS4		×	×			
BBS5		×				
BBS6		×	×			
BBS7		×				
BBS8		×				
BBS9		×				
BBS10		×				
BBS11		×				
BBS12		×				
BBS13		×	×		×	
BBS15		×				
SLSN7\BBS16		×		×		
CCDC28B\ MGC1203				×	×	
MKS1			×	×		
CC2D2A			×	×		
TMEM107			×		×	
TMEM216			×		×	
TMEM231			×		×	
INPP5E						
XNPEP3	×					
OFD1					×	×
OFD6				×	×	×

(BBS: Bardet–Biedl syndrome; JBTS: Joubert syndrome; MKS: Meckel–Gruber syndrome; NPHP: nephronophthisis; OFD: orofaciodigital syndrome; SLS: Senior–Løken syndrome;)

period to adulthood. It is inherited in an autosomal dominant (ADPKD) or a recessive (ARPKD) fashion. ADPKD is typically diagnosed in the second and third decades of life, while ARPKD is usually diagnosed in utero or in the neonatal period with bilateral enlarged kidneys and variable intrahepatic biliary abnormalities such as biliary dysgenesis and hepatic fibrosis with or without bile duct dilatation (Caroli syndrome). ADPKD is caused by a mutation in either of two genes: *PKD1* (75%) or *PKD2* (15%), encoding polycystin-1 (PC-1) and polycystin-2 (PC-2), respectively.[27] PC-1 and PC-2 form a complex and are in cilium and/or its basal body apart from its presence in endoplasmic reticulum. The molecular events leading to cyst formation have been described in a previous section. In addition, mutation in genes not involved in maintaining structure and function of cilia has been described in ADPKD, such as neutral α-glucosidase *AB* (*GANAB*), *SEC63*, *DNAJB11*, and *PRKCSH*.[27] *PKHD1* (polycystic kidney and hepatic disease 1) gene mutated in *ARPKD* encodes fibrocystin, which localizes to primary cilia and basal bodies, and is associated with the polycystin complex.[28] Fibrocystin is a key regulator of cell proliferation, polarization, and apoptosis. Mutation in *DZIP1L* gene that encodes DAZ interacting protein 1-like has been recently known to cause ARPKD.[15] The protein localizes to the mature centriole and is a subdistal and distal appendage marker.

Nephronophthisis ("Wasting of the Nephrons")

Nephronophthisis, an autosomal recessive disease, is one of the most common genetic causes of end-stage kidney disease (ESKD) in children and young adults. Based on the age of onset of kidney failure, three clinical subtypes are recognized: infantile (progress to ESKD by 3 years of age), juvenile (median age of onset of ESKD is 13 years), and adolescent/adult (onset of ESKD by 19 years and later). Renal ultrasonography in children with NPHP usually demonstrates normal-sized kidneys with increased echogenicity and loss of corticomedullary differentiation. In infantile onset, the kidneys may be enlarged cystic kidneys with increased cortical echotexture. Renal biopsy shows corticomedullary cysts, disruption of tubular basement membrane, and tubulointerstitial fibrosis. Unlike PKD, NPHP demonstrates significant genetic heterogeneity with more than 25 genes implicated in NPHP **(Table 4)**. Approximately two thirds of NPHPs are still genetically unclear, while mutations in the *NPHP1* gene are seen in 20–25% of all cases.[26] The function of protein complexes to support ciliogenesis and function overlap with one another, thereby contributing toward the wide phenotypic spectrum observed within NPHP. Apart from mutations in genes coding for various nephrocystins, NPHP can be also caused by mutations in genes encoding other proteins such as CEP164, CEP83, TTC21B, ANKS6,

TABLE 3: Characteristics of renal phenotype in ciliopathy.

	Polycystic kidneys			
	Autosomal dominant	***Autosomal recessive***	***Nephronophthisis***	***Dysplastic kidneys***
Histopathology	Cortex and medulla present numerous spherical cysts—these are saccular expansions of all portions of renal tubule and glomerular capsule which later become disconnected from tubule and are filled with serous, hemorrhagic, or gelatinous fluid; cysts lined by cuboidal or flattened epithelium Functional nephrons exist between cysts with areas of global sclerosis, tubular atrophy, interstitial fibrosis, and chronic inflammation	Radially arranged, elongated cysts from collecting tubules lined by cuboidal or flattened cells that form as dilations of all collecting tubules with fluid accumulation	Interstitial fibrosis and tubular membrane disruptions (thickened, irregular basement membranes) and sporadic corticomedullary cysts	Marked interstitial fibrosis and with or without cysts of different sizes
Imaging characteristics	Bilateral large kidneys with large multiple cysts of varying sizes which appear as dark hypoechoic lesions throughout the kidney	Bilateral enlarged echogenic kidneys with loss of CMD; small cysts arranged radially on high-resolution ultrasonography and variable intrahepatic biliary abnormalities ranging from biliary dysgenesis and fibrosis [congenital hepatic fibrosis (CHF)]	Normal-sized kidneys with loss of corticomedullary differentiation and increased echogenicity in ultrasonography of kidneys. In infantile onset, the kidneys may be enlarged cystic kidneys with cortical hyperechogenicity	Dysplastic kidneys may be small (less than the 50th centile for age), unilateral or bilateral, lack corticomedullary differentiation, and demonstrate increased echogenicity with a variable number of small, subcapsular cysts

(CMD: corticomedullary differentiation)

and DCD2. Approximately 10–20% have been reported to have extrarenal involvement primarily involving retina, liver (fibrocystic disease), brain (cerebellar vermis hypoplasia), and skeletal dysplasia **(Table 5)**. Mutations in NPHP proteins have been associated with retinitis pigmentosa [e.g., Senior-Loken syndrome (SLS)], malformations of central nervous system [e.g., Joubert syndrome and related disorders (JSRD)] and Meckel-Gruber syndrome (MKS), skeletal malformations (Jeune syndrome and related skeletal disorders), and other syndromes such as COACH syndrome and oculomotor apraxia, Cogan type **(Table 6)**.

Renal Dysplasia with or without Cysts

Renal dysplasia with or without cysts is an under-recognized feature of renal ciliopathy and more likely to reflect a severe genotype. In imaging, dysplastic kidneys may be small (less than the 50th centile for age) unilaterally or bilaterally, demonstrate increased echogenicity with a variable number of small, subcapsular cysts, and lack corticomedullary differentiation. Renal dysplasia has been observed in several ciliopathic disorders such as in MKS, JBTS, and BBS as well as in many of the NPHP-related ciliopathy.

Differential Diagnosis

The diagnosis of isolated renal ciliopathy may be challenging, especially if the child presents in advanced stages of CKD. All children presenting with suspected isolated renal ciliopathy should be screened for extrarenal abnormality which may provide clue to underlying etiology. Often, only genetic testing will help in the right diagnosis. Autosomal dominant tubulointerstitial kidney disease (ADTKD), inherited forms of focal segmental glomerulosclerosis (FSGS), Alport's syndrome, medullary cystic kidney disease, and congenital anomaly of the kidney and urinary tract (CAKUT) are the common diagnoses identified by genetic testing in children with clinical diagnosis of NPHP suspected on clinical profile and renal ultrasonography.[29] Occasionally, differentiating ARPKD from ADPKD may be difficult due to overlap in age of presentation and imaging findings. ADPKD can occur in neonatal and early infancy manifesting as enlarged and echogenic kidneys like ARPKD and similarly ARPKD can present in older children, with macrocysts mimicking the renal cysts of ADPKD. Family history, additional imaging such as high-resolution ultrasonography, MRI of kidneys, and genetic testing help in definitive diagnosis.

Genetic Testing in Renal Ciliopathy

Clinical and molecular heterogeneity overlap of clinical features and causative genes make the diagnosis of renal ciliopathy challenging. Causal variants in more than 80 genes are associated with renal ciliopathy. Hence, being

TABLE 4: List of monogenic genes associated with renal ciliopathies.

Gene/ locus	OMIM number phenotype(#)	Protein	Mode of inheritance	Location in primary cilia	Phenotype	Renal phenotype
JBTS3	608629	Abelson helper integration site 1	AR	TZ	Joubert syndrome 3	NPHP
ALMS1	203800	ALMS1, centrosome, and basal body-associated protein	AR	BB	Alstrom syndrome	NPHP and CAKUT
NPHP16	615382	Ankyrin repeat and sterile alpha motif domain containing 6	AR	Axoneme	Nephronophthisis 16	NPHP
BBS3	600151	ADP ribosylation factor such as GTPase 6	AR	BBS–IFT-associated	Bardet–Biedl syndrome 3	Renal cysts, dysplastic kidneys
B9D1	614209; 617120	B9 domain containing 1	AR	TZ	Meckel syndrome 9; Joubert syndrome 27	Renal cysts, dysplastic kidneys
B9D2	614715	B9 protein domain 2	AR	TZ	Meckel syndrome 10; Joubert syndrome 34	Renal cysts
BBS18	615995	BBSome interacting protein 1	AR	BBS–IFT-associated?	Bardet–Biedl syndrome 18	Renal cysts and dysplastic kidneys
*BBS1**	209900	Bardet–Biedl syndrome 1	AR	BBS–IFT-associated	Bardet–Biedl syndrome 1	Renal cysts, dysplastic kidneys
BBS10	615987	Bardet–Biedl syndrome 10	AR	BBS–BB assembly/ folding factor	Bardet–Biedl syndrome 10	Renal cysts, dysplastic kidneys
BBS12	615989	Bardet–Biedl syndrome 12	AR	BBS–BB assembly/ folding factor	Bardet–Biedl syndrome 12	Renal cysts, dysplastic kidneys
BBS2	615981	Bardet–Biedl syndrome 2	AR	BBS–IFT-associated	Bardet–Biedl syndrome 2	Renal cysts, dysplastic kidneys
BBS4	615982	Bardet–Biedl syndrome 4	AR	BBS–IFT-associated; centriolar satellite	Bardet–Biedl syndrome 4	Renal cysts, dysplastic kidneys
BBS5	615983	Bardet–Biedl syndrome 5	AR	BBS–IFT-associated	Bardet–Biedl syndrome 5	Renal cysts, dysplastic kidneys
BBS7	615894	Bardet–Biedl syndrome 7	AR	BBS–IFT-associated	Bardet–Biedl syndrome 7	Renal cysts, dysplastic kidneys
BBS9	615986	Bardet–Biedl syndrome 9	AR	BBS–IFT-associated	Bardet–Biedl syndrome 9	Renal cysts, dysplastic kidneys
C2CD3	615948	C2 calcium-dependent domain containing 3	AR	BB distal centriole	Orofaciodigital syndrome 14	Hydronephrosis
JBTS17	614615	Chromosome 5 open reading frame 42	AR	TZ	Joubert syndrome 17	Renal cysts
JBTS9	#612285; 612284; 216360	Coiled-coil and C2 domain containing 2A	AR	TZ; BB subdistal appendages	Joubert syndrome 9 Meckel syndrome 6 COACH syndrome	Renal cysts
CCDC28B	209900	Coiled-coil domain containing 28B	AR	BBS-associated; centriolar satellite?	Bardet–Biedl syndrome 1 modifier	
JBTS25	616781	Centrosomal protein 104		BB; axoneme (tip)		NPHP

Contd...

Contd...

Gene/ locus	OMIM number phenotype(#)	Protein	Mode of inheritance	Location in primary cilia	Phenotype	Renal phenotype
CEP120	616300; 617761	Centrosomal protein 120	AR	BB (centrosome)	Short-rib thoracic dysplasia; Joubert syndrome 31	NPHP
NPHP15	614845	Centrosomal protein 164	AR	BB distal appendage	Nephronophthisis 15	NPHP
NPHP6	610188; 615991; 610189	Centrosomal protein 290	AR	TZ; centriolar satellite	Joubert syndrome 5, Bardet–Biedl syndrome 14, Meckel syndrome 4	NPHP
NPHP18	615862	Centrosomal protein 83	AR	BB distal appendage	Nephronophthisis 18	NPHP
JBTS21	615636	Centrosome and spindle pole-associated protein 1	AR	BB	Joubert syndrome 21	NPHP
NPHP19	616217	Doublecortin domain containing 2	AR	Axoneme	Nephronophthisis 19	NPHP
DDX59	174300	DEAD-box helicase 59	AR	Nucleus; cytoplasm	Orofaciodigital syndrome 5	Dysplastic kidney
DYNC2H1	613091	Dynein cytoplasmic 2 heavy chain 1	AR	IFT retrograde transport	Short-rib thoracic dysplasia 3	Dysplastic kidney
NPHP7	611498	GLIS family zinc finger 2	AR	Nucleus	Nephronophthisis 7	NPHP
IFT122	218330	Intraflagellar transport 122	AR	IFT-A	Cranioectodermal dysplasia 1	NPHP
NPHP17	615630	Intraflagellar transport 172	AR	IFT-B	Short-rib thoracic dysplasia 10	NPHP
BBS19	615996	Intraflagellar transport 27	AR	IFT-B	Bardet–Biedl syndrome 19	Renal hypoplasia
IFT43	614099	Intraflagellar transport 43	AR	IFT-A	Cranioectodermal dysplasia 3	NPHP
IFT52	617102	Intraflagellar transport 52	AR	IFT-B	Short-rib thoracic dysplasia 16	Tortuous ureters
IFT57	617927	Intraflagellar transport 57	AR	IFT-B	Orofaciodigital syndrome 18	Short urethra
IFT80	611263	Intraflagellar transport 80	AR	IFT-B	Short-rib thoracic dysplasia 2	Multicystic dysplastic kidneys
IFT140	266920	Intraflagellar transport 140	AR	IFT-A	Short-rib thoracic dysplasia 9	NPHP
JBTS1	213300	Inositol polyphosphate-5-phosphatase E	AR	Axoneme-signaling	Joubert syndrome 1	NPHP
NPHP2	602088	Inversin	AR	Inversin compartment	Infantile nephronophthisis 2	NPHP
NPHP5	609254	IQ motif-containing B1	AR	BB; TZ	Senior–Loken syndrome 5	NPHP
KIAA0753	617127	MNR; OFIP	AR	Centriolar satellite	Orofaciodigital syndrome 15	Bilateral hydronephrosis
KIF14	616258	Kinesin-like protein	AR	IFT associated	Meckel syndrome 12	Dysplastic kidneys, renal agenesis

Contd...

Contd...

Gene/ locus	*OMIM number phenotype(#)*	*Protein*	*Mode of inheritance*	*Location in primary cilia*	*Phenotype*	*Renal phenotype*
BBS17	615994	Leucine zipper transcription factor like 1	AR	BBS–IFT-associated	Bardet–Biedl syndrome 17	Renal cysts, dysplastic kidneys
BBS6	605231	McKusick–Kaufman syndrome	AR	BBS–BB; assembly/folding factor	Bardet–Biedl syndrome 6	Renal cysts, CAKUT
MKS1	249000; 617121; 615990	Meckel syndrome, type 1	AR	TZ	Meckel syndrome 1; Joubert syndrome 28; Bardet–Biedl syndrome 13	Renal cysts, dysplastic kidneys, renal agenesis
NEK1	263520	NIMA-related kinase 1	AR	Axoneme; nucleus	Short-rib thoracic dysplasia 6	Renal cysts
NPHP9	615415; 613824	NIMA-related kinase 8	AR	Inversin compartment	Renal-hepatic-pancreatic dysplasia 2, Nephronophthisis 9	NPHP
NPHP1	256100; 609583; 266900	Nephrocystin 1	AR	TZ	Juvenile nephronophthisis 1, Joubert syndrome 4, and Senior–Loken syndrome 1	NPHP
NPHP3	604387; 267010; 208540	Nephrocystin 3	AR	Inversin compartment	Nephronophthisis 3, Meckel syndrome, Renal-hepatic-pancreatic dysplasia	NPHP
NPHP4	606966	Nephronophthisis 4	AR	TZ	Nephronophthisis 4, Senior–Loken syndrome 4	NPHP
OFD1	311200	OFD1, centriole, and centriolar satellite protein	XLD	BB distal end; centriolar satellite	Orofaciodigital syndrome 1	Renal cysts
JBTS22	615665	Phosphodiesterase 6D	AR	Lipidated protein transport	Joubert syndrome 22	Dysplastic kidneys
PKD1		Polycystin 1, transient receptor potential channel interacting	AD	Axoneme-signaling	ADPKD	Cystic kidneys
PKD2		Polycystin 2, transient receptor potential cation channel	AD	Axoneme-signaling	ADPKD	Cystic kidneys
PKHD1	263200	Fibrocystin/ polyductin	AR	Axoneme	ARPKD	Cystic kidneys
NPHP8	611561; 611560; 216360	RPGRIP1 like	AR	TZ	Meckel syndrome 5, Joubert syndrome 7, COACH syndrome	NPHP
NPHP10	615993; 613615	Serologically defined colon cancer antigen 8	AR	BB; TZ	Bardet–Biedl syndrome 16, Senior–Loken syndrome 7	NPHP
JBTS24	616654	Tectonic family member 2	AR	TZ	Joubert syndrome 24	Dysplastic kidneys
JBTS18	614815	Tectonic family member 3	AR	TZ	Joubert syndrome 18	Renal cysts

Contd...

Contd...

Gene/ locus	OMIM number phenotype(#)	Protein	Mode of inheritance	Location in primary cilia	Phenotype	Renal phenotype
TMEM107	617562	Transmembrane protein 107	AR	TZ	Meckel syndrome 13, Joubert syndrome 29	Dysplastic kidneys
JBTS16	614465	Transmembrane protein 138	AR	TZ	Joubert syndrome16	NPHP
JBTS2	603194; 608091	Transmembrane protein 216	AR	TZ	Meckel syndrome 2; Joubert syndrome 2	NPHP
JBTS20	614970; 615397	Transmembrane protein 231	AR	TZ	Meckel syndrome 11; Joubert syndrome 20	Renal cysts
JBTS14	614424	Transmembrane protein 237	AR	TZ	Joubert syndrome 14	NPHP
NPHP11	216360; 613550	Transmembrane protein 67	AR	TZ	COACH syndrome, Nephronophthisis 11	NPHP
TRAF3IP1	616629	TRAF3 interacting protein 1	AR	IFT-B	Senior–Loken syndrome 9	NPHP
BBS11	615988	Tripartite motif-containing 32	AR	BBS; nuclear?	Bardet–Biedl syndrome 11	Renal cysts, dysplastic kidneys
NPHP12	613820	Tetratricopeptide repeat domain 21B	AR	IFT-A	Nephronophthisis 12	NPHP
BBS8	615985	Tetratricopeptide repeat domain 8	AR	BBS-IFT-associated	Bardet–Biedl syndrome 8	Renal cysts, dysplastic kidneys
BBS15	615992	WD repeat containing planar cell polarity effector	AR	BBS; BB; axoneme	Bardet–Biedl syndrome 15	Renal cysts, dysplastic kidneys
NPHP13	614377; 616307	WD repeat domain 19	AR	IFT-A	Nephronophthisis 13, Senior–Loken syndrome 8	NPHP
WDR34	615633	WD repeat domain 34	AR	IFT-dynein	Short-rib thoracic dysplasia 11	Unknown renal phenotype with ESKD
WDR35	613610	WD repeat domain 35	AR	IFT-A	Cranioectodermal dysplasia 2	NPHP
WDR60	615503	WD repeat domain 60	AR	IFT-dynein	Short-rib thoracic dysplasia 8	Cystic kidneys
NPHPL1	613159	X-prolyl aminopeptidase 3	AR	Mitochondria	Nephronophthisis-like nephropathy 1	NPHP
NPHP14	614844	Zinc finger protein 423	AR	Nucleus	Nephronophthisis 14, Joubert syndrome 19	NPHP
NPHP20	617271	JNK-binding protein 1	AR		Nephronophthisis 20	NPHP

(BBS: Bardet–Biedl syndrome; ESKD: end-stage kidney disease; IFT: intraflagellar transport; JNK: c-Jun N-terminal kinase; MKS: Meckel–Gruber syndrome; NPHP: nephronophthisis; OFD: orofaciodigital syndrome)

a multisystem disorder characterized by poor genotype-phenotype correlation, Sanger sequencing of group of genes determined by clinical phenotype, mutation frequency, and ethnicity may be time consuming and less effective. Massively parallel sequencing (MPS), formerly known as next-generation sequencing (NGS) using multigene panel or clinical exome sequencing is expected to be much more effective for genetic testing as a large number of genes can be screened cost effectively and has a higher diagnostic yield. These panels also include genes associated with other renal diseases that may have phenotype similar to ciliopathy (also known as phenocopy). Although using a multigene panel is

TABLE 5: Extrarenal manifestations associated with nephronophthisis (NPHP).

Organ affected	Clinical feature	Associated syndrome
Eye	Retinitis pigmentosa	Senior–Loken syndrome Alstrom syndrome Joubert syndrome Bardet–Biedl syndrome
	Oculomotor apraxia	Cogan syndrome Joubert syndrome
	Nystagmus	Joubert syndrome
	Coloboma	Joubert syndrome COACH syndrome
Central nervous system	Encephalocele	Meckel–Gruber syndrome
	Cerebellar vermis hypoplasia	Joubert syndrome COACH syndrome
Hepatic	Liver fibrosis	Meckel–Gruber syndrome Joubert syndrome COACH syndrome
Bone	Cone-shaped epiphysis	Mainzer–Saldino syndrome
	Polydactyly	Bardet–Biedl syndrome Meckel–Gruber syndrome Joubert syndrome Jeune syndrome

cheaper and minimizes incidental findings, clinical exome sequencing (CES), or Medenliome gene panel, which includes all coding exons of known genes, is preferred. CES facilitates targeted gene analysis and also screen for copy number variations (CNVs). In case a causative variant is not identified in the gene panel **(Table 4)**, search for variants could be extended to the remaining genes in the clinical exome, which is not possible with a targeted multigene panel. In case of negative findings, whole exome sequencing might be considered for novel disease-causing genes. Instead of single nucleotide substitutions or small insertions–deletions, CNVs and large deletions in some of the genes such as *NPHP1* and *CEP290* have been identified as causal variants. These types of variants although could be identified using NGS-based testing, multiplex ligation-dependent probe amplification (MLPA), and a gene-targeted microarray are required to confirm the variant. Genetic diagnostic rates of primary ciliopathies remain around 62% using targeted gene panel sequencing and 44% using whole exome sequencing[30,31] (***see* Table 4** for complete gene list). However, there is significant variability in the detection rate of mutations between various renal phenotypes. The overall detection rate of genetic variant is 77% in ARPKD while positive detection rates of up to 89% have been reported in ADPKD. Combining results from recent studies, genetic testing (single-gene testing and/or multigene panel) identified biallelic causal variants in one of the known

TABLE 6: Genes associated with syndromic nephronophthisis

Disorder	Genes
Bardet–Biedl syndrome	*CEP290, TMEM67, and SDCCAG8*
Joubert syndrome	*NPHP1 (1–2%), CEP290 (10%), RPGRIP1L (2–4%), and TMEM67 (10%)*
Meckel–Gruber syndrome	*NPHP3, CEP290, RPGRIP1L, and TMEM67*
Senior–Loken syndrome	*NPHP1, NPHP3, NPHP4, CEP2990, INVS, SDCCAG8 (3–4%), and IQCB1 (17–18%)*
Jeune syndrome	*TTC21B and WDR19*
COACH syndrome	*RPGRIP1L (4–5%) and TMEM67 (74%)*
Oculomotor apraxia, Cogan type	*NPHP1* and *NPHP4*

NPHP-related genes in only 30–40% of affected individuals leaving 60% of children with NPHP genetically unexplained.[32] Although NGS has emerged as an effective tool in improving diagnosis of renal ciliopathy and better genetic counseling for parents and patients in a clinical setting, there are also challenges with this technology. Since a large number of genes need to be screened in each patient, a major challenge is to analyze and identify disease-causing variants from large volumes of genetic variants that are obtained. This requires expertise as well improving on the existing bioinformatics tool. NGS may identify variants in genes unrelated to phenotype, which leads to ethical issues.

RECENT ADVANCES IN TOOLS TO UNDERSTAND CILIOPATHY AND DEVELOP NOVEL TREATMENT

Identifying the primary ciliary defect using NGS and proteomic-based approaches has contributed to improved understanding of defective cellular processes and identifying potential therapeutic targets. Traditional approaches to modeling primary ciliopathies involve cell line cultures or whole animal studies, typically in *C. elegans*, zebrafish, and mice. 3D organoids derived from human embryonic stem (ES) cells or induced pluripotent stem cell (iPSCs) are also emerging as a valuable alternative to animal models in ciliopathy research.[33] Techniques for genetically editing these cell models are also advancing. It is now possible to replicate a potentially causal variant of unknown clinical significance in an iPSC or human ES cell and differentiate these cells toward cell type relevant to the primary disease tissue to study the effect of variant and evaluate methods of genetic correction. Clustered Regularly Interspaced Short Palindromic Repeats (CRISPR)/*Cas9* genome editing is a popular newer tool to develop specific knockout models relevant to disease phenotype. Targeted therapies for ciliopathies are being explored. Accelerated identification of genes associated with renal ciliopathy has led to more insights into disease mechanisms. This has provided an opportunity for developing targeted therapies using gene therapy and high throughput targeted drug screening assays such as small-molecule screening in zebrafish. Ongoing clinical trials investigating the efficacy and safety of gene therapy for treatment of retinal ciliopathy and syndromic ciliopathies provide hope for newer treatment of ciliopathy.[34] However, extensive genetic heterogeneity in ciliopathy is a hindrance to the development of specific therapies. Repurposing of cyclin-dependent kinase inhibitors could be an appropriate treatment option for ciliopathies, which have a common basis in replication stress. For example, treatment with roscovitine, a cyclin-dependent kinase inhibitor, has been shown to be effective in rescuing ciliary defects in cells derived from patients with Joubert syndrome.[35] Modifying SHH signaling in renal ciliopathy models as a therapeutic strategy has been performed in in vitro models. Treatment with purmorphamine ameliorates the disorganized ciliary phenotype by increasing sonic HH signaling.[36]

CONCLUSION

The nonmotile primary cilia are specialized evolutionary conserved hair-like cellular organelle that plays an important role in kidney health and disease. The functions of cilia are diverse—functioning as a communication hub by transduction of signals from the external environment, promoting cellular proliferation and differentiation, and determining cell polarity. Mutations in ciliary-associated proteins are associated with a spectrum of diseases, collectively known as ciliopathies. Understanding the structural components and developmental process of the cilia has helped in better understanding of the phenotypic spectrum and pathophysiology of renal ciliopathy.

KEY POINTS

- Primary cilia are hair-like cellular organelles that are ubiquitous in nature and play a major role in various signal transductions and organ development in humans.
- The four key important structures of cilia are the basal body, transition zone, microtubule-based axoneme, and membrane.
- Cilia functions as a signaling hub and also regulate polarity, proliferation, tissue differentiation, and maintenance.
- Mutations in ciliary-associated proteins resulting in spectrum of diseases are collectively known as ciliopathies.
- The range of renal phenotypes includes polycystic kidneys, NPHP, and renal cystic dysplasia.

REFERENCES

1. Bloodgood RA. From central to rudimentary to primary: the history of an underappreciated organelle whose time has come. The primary cilium. Methods Cell Biol. 2009;94:3-52.
2. Lee JE, Gleeson JG. A systems-biology approach to understanding the ciliopathy disorders. Genome Med. 2011;3:59.
3. Reiter JF, Leroux MR. Genes and molecular pathways underpinning ciliopathies. Nat Rev Mol Cell Biol. 2017;18: 533-47.
4. Mostowy S, Cossart P. Septins: the fourth component of the cytoskeleton. Nat Rev Mol Cell Biol. 2012;13:183-94.
5. Arts HH, Knoers NV. Current insights into renal ciliopathies: what can genetics teach us? Pediatr Nephrol. 2013;28:863-74.
6. Mourão A, Christensen ST, Lorentzen E. The intraflagellar transport machinery in ciliary signaling. Curr Opin Struct Biol. 2016;41:98-108.
7. Nachury MV, Loktev AV, Zhang Q, Westlake CJ, Peranen J, Merdes A, et al. A core complex of BBS proteins cooperates with the GTPase Rab8 to promote ciliary membrane biogenesis. Cell. 2007;129:1201-13.
8. Santoni M, Piva F, Cimadamore A, Giulietti M, Battelli N, Montironi R, et al. Exploring the spectrum of kidney ciliopathies. Diagnostics. 2020;10:1099.
9. Khanna H. Photoreceptor sensory cilium: traversing the ciliary gate. Cells. 2015;4:674-86.
10. Wachten D, Mick DU. Signal transduction in primary cilia—analyzing and manipulating GPCR and second messenger signaling. Pharmacol Ther. 2021;224:107836.
11. Happé H, Peters D. Translational research in ADPKD: lessons from animal models. Nat Rev Nephrol. 2014:10;587-601.
12. Waters AM, Beales PL. Ciliopathies: an expanding disease spectrum. Pediatr Nephrol. 2011;26:1039-56.
13. Lemos FO, Ehrlich BE. Polycystin and calcium signaling in cell death and survival. Cell Calcium. 2018;69:37-45.
14. Shillingford JM, Murcia NS, Larson CH, Low SH, Hedgepeth R, Brown N, et al. The mTOR pathway is regulated by polycystin-1, and its inhibition reverses renal cystogenesis in polycystic kidney disease. Proc Natl Acad Sci U S A. 2006;103:5466-71.
15. Bergmann C. Genetics of autosomal recessive polycystic kidney disease and its differential diagnoses. Front Pediatr. 2018;5:221.
16. Omran H. NPHP proteins: gatekeepers of the ciliary compartment. J Cell Biol. 2010;190:715-7.
17. Delous M, Hellman NE, Gaude HM, Silbermann F, Le Bivic A, Salomon R, et al. Nephrocystin-1 and nephrocystin-4 are required for epithelial morphogenesis and associate with PALS1/PATJ and Par6. Hum Mol Genet. 2009;18:4711-23.
18. Simons M, Gloy J, Ganner A, Bullerkotte A, Bashkurov M, Kronig C, et al. Inversin, the gene product mutated in nephronophthisis type II, functions as a molecular switch between Wnt signaling pathways. Nat Genet. 2005;37:537-43.
19. Winkelbauer ME, Schafer JC, Haycraft CJ, Swoboda P, Yoder BK. The C. elegans homologs of nephrocystin-1 and nephrocystin-4 are cilia transition zone proteins involved in chemosensory perception. J Cell Sci. 2005;118:5575-87.
20. Attanasio M, Uhlenhaut NH, Sousa VH, O'Toole JF, Otto E, Anlag K, et al. Loss of GLIS2 causes nephronophthisis in humans and mice by increased apoptosis and fibrosis. Nat Genet. 2007;39:1018-24.
21. Arts HH, Doherty D, van Beersum SE, Parisi MA, Letteboer SJ, Gorden NT, et al. Mutations in the gene encoding the basal body protein RPGRIP1L, a nephrocystin-4 interactor, cause Joubert syndrome. Nat Genet. 2007;39:882-8.
22. Hoff S, Halbritter J, Epting D, Frank V, Nguyen TM, van Reeuwijk J, et al. ANKS6 is a central component of a nephronophthisis module linking NEK8 to INVS and NPHP3. Nat Genet. 2013;45: 951-6.
23. Graser S, Stierhof YD, Lavoie SB, Gassner OS, Lamla S, Le Clech M, et al. Cep164, a novel centriole appendage protein required for primary cilium formation. J Cell Biol. 2007;179:321-30.

24. Adamiok-Ostrowska A, Piekiełko-Witkowska A. Ciliary genes in renal cystic diseases. Cells. 2020;9:907.
25. Pazour GJ, Dickert BL, Vucica Y, Seeley ES, Rosenbaum JL, Witman GB, et al. Chlamydomonas IFT88 and its mouse homologue, polycystic kidney disease gene tg737, are required for assembly of cilia and flagella. J Cell Biol. 2000;151:709-18.
26. Braun DA, Hildebrandt F. Ciliopathies. Cold Spring Harb Perspect Biol. 2017;9:a028191.
27. Lanktree MB, Haghighi A, di Bari I, Song X, Pei Y. Insights into autosomal dominant polycystic kidney disease from genetic studies. Clin J Am Soc Nephrol. 2021;16:790-9.
28. Zhang J, Wu M, Wang S, Shah JV, Wilson PD, Zhou J. Polycystic kidney disease protein fibrocystin localizes to the mitotic spindle and regulates spindle bipolarity. Hum Mol Genet. 2010;19:3306-19.
29. Vivante A, Hildebrandt F. Exploring the genetic basis of early-onset chronic kidney disease. Nat Rev Nephrol. 2016;12:133-46.
30. Knopp C, Rudnik-Schoneborn S, Eggermann T, Bergmann C, Begemann M, Schoner K, et al. Syndromic ciliopathies: from single gene to multi gene analysis by SNP arrays and next generation sequencing. Mol Cell Probes. 2015;29:299-307.
31. Sawyer SL, Hartley T, Dyment DA, Beaulieu CL, Schwartzentruber J, Smith A, et al. Utility of whole-exome sequencing for those near the end of the diagnostic odyssey: time to address gaps in care. Clin Genet. 2016;89:275-84.
32. Braun DA, Schueler M, Halbritter J, Gee HY, Porath JD, Lawson JA, et al. Whole exome sequencing identifies causative mutations in the majority of consanguineous or familial cases with childhood-onset increased renal echogenicity. Kidney Int. 2016;89:468-75.
33. Wheway G, Genomics England Research Consortium, Mitchison HM. Opportunities and challenges for molecular understanding of ciliopathies-The 100,000 genomes project. Front Genet. 2019;10:127.
34. Wu Z, Hiriyanna S, Qian H, Mookherjee S, Campos MM, Gao C, et al. A long-term efficacy study of gene replacement therapy for RPGR-associated retinal degeneration. Hum Mol Genet. 2015;24:3956-70.
35. Srivastava S, Ramsbottom SA, Molinari E, Alkanderi S, Filby A, White K, et al. A human patient-derived cellular model of Joubert syndrome reveals ciliary defects which can be rescued with targeted therapies. Hum Mol Genet. 2017:26:4657-67.
36. Devlin A, Sayer JA. Renal ciliopathies. Curr Opin Genet Dev. 2019;56:49-60.

CHAPTER

9.2

Polycystic Kidney Disease

Alpana Ohri, Pankaj Hari

INTRODUCTION

Many kidney disorders are characterized by the presence of multiple cysts in both kidneys that may be genetic, developmental, or acquired in origin. The term polycystic kidney disease (PKD) is, however, restricted to two genetically distinct conditions—autosomal-dominant polycystic kidney disease (ADPKD) and autosomal-recessive polycystic kidney disease (ARPKD), which have in common bilateral multiple cysts, progressive renal disease, and extrarenal involvement. Recent literature implicates primary cilia as a major culprit in cystogenesis. This has led to establishment of multiple clinical trials evaluating emerging therapeutic strategies.[1]

AUTOSOMAL-RECESSIVE POLYCYSTIC KIDNEY DISEASE

Autosomal-recessive polycystic kidney disease is the most common heritable renal cystic disease that manifests in childhood. The hallmark of the disease is diffuse cystic dilatation of the collecting tubules, which is usually associated with hepatic fibrosis.

Epidemiology and Genetics

The incidence of ARPKD in various populations ranges from 1 in 10,000 to 1 in 40,000 births. ARPKD as the name suggests is inherited in an autosomal-recessive fashion with a 25% risk of having another affected offspring. Two main genes—*PKHD1* (polycystic kidney and hepatic disease 1) gene located on 6p21.1-p12 or *DZIP1L* gene located at *3q22.3*—have been implicated. *PKHD1* is one of the largest genes in human genome, which is highly expressed in kidney and at a lower level in the liver. Although a large number of mutations have been described, 80% patients show homozygous or compound heterozygous mutations. While majority of ARPKD sibships display comparable clinical courses, 20% exhibit gross interfamilial phenotype variability possibly due to modifying genes, epigenetic factors, or environmental influences. Recently, mutations in *DZIP1L* have also been reported in some cases manifesting ARPKD-like phenotype.[2]

Pathogenesis

Fibrocystin, the protein product of the *PKHD1* gene, is expressed in the cilia of the renal and bile duct epithelial cells and is important in maintaining the architecture of the renal tubules and the biliary tree. Mutations in the *PKHD1* gene lead to reduced or loss of function of fibrocystin that results in alterations in either the structure with or without dysfunction of the primary cilium. This results in activation of cell proliferation and fluid secretion that leads to cyst formation. In ARPKD, the cyst formation occurs along the collecting duct leading to their fusiform dilatation. The abnormal proliferative epithelium becomes secretory in nature as compared to the normal epithelium that is resorptive. The fluid secreted is rich in epithelial growth factors, which further encourage epithelial proliferation. Animal studies have demonstrated that blocking the epithelial growth factors or their receptors retards cyst formation.[3]

Pathology

Kidneys are symmetrically enlarged up to 10 times the normal size in affected neonates and retain their reniform contour. On gross examination, the cut surface of the kidney shows fusiform spaces or microcysts usually <2 mm in diameter that are arranged radially throughout the parenchyma. These represent the collecting ducts and distal tubules, which are usually connected with urinary space. With the advancing course, macrocysts may form, but they are usually <1.5 cm in diameter and the kidneys do not progress to grow unlimited as opposed to autosomal-dominant PKD. Ectasia of the hepatic bile ducts and bile duct proliferation are invariably present leading to hepatic fibrosis and hepatomegaly.[4]

Clinical Features

There is a wide phenotypic variability in the clinical manifestations of ARPKD. The most severely involved cases present in utero with severe oligohydramnios along with lung hypoplasia and Potter sequence characterized by flat facies and limb deformities. The immediate perinatal problems may be largely respiratory in nature due to pulmonary hypoplasia or due to mechanical compression of the lungs as a result of elevated diaphragms caused by hugely enlarged kidneys. Spontaneous pneumothorax is seen in some neonates. The clinical picture is dominated by respiratory failure that may result in death. Renal insufficiency may be coexistent but is often overshadowed by the lung problems. Hyponatremia related to urine diluting defect is present in newborn period in up to 25% patients but usually resolves with age.

Many children presenting in late infancy or early childhood may be detected because of incidental hematuria, pyuria, or the clinical finding of enlarged palpable kidneys. Hypertension develops in the first few months and is seen in up to 80% of children with ARPKD.

Children detected in later childhood often have a hepatic presentation with firm hepatosplenomegaly or symptoms related to portal hypertension. Liver involvement in the form of congenital hepatic fibrosis or Caroli disease is histologically seen in all patients at birth. However, clinically evident liver disease may be absent in 45% of the affected children. A proportion of children with ARPKD may have liver and splenic enlargement. The hepatic complications include cholangitis, hepatic dysfunction, and portal hypertension. However, cirrhosis and hepatic failure are rare. The renal disease is often mild and may be discovered incidentally during imaging studies of the abdomen. The enlarged kidneys are usually detected during investigations and renal function is often normal at this stage. There seems to be a reciprocal relationship between the severity of the renal and hepatic disease. Children having a severe hepatic involvement manifest with less-severe renal involvement and children with severe renal involvement have a milder liver disease.

There is progression to renal failure and end-stage kidney disease (ESKD) over a variable period of time in most children. More than 50% of affected individuals progress to ESKD by the end of the first decade and the majority by 20 years of age.[5] However, occasional adults with ARPKD may have only mild renal insufficiency. The wide phenotypic variability is the result of the large number of different mutations in the *PKHD1* gene.

Diagnosis

The diagnosis of ARPKD is based on clinical and radiological findings.

Ultrasonography

Ultrasonography (USG) forms the initial and often the only imaging modality needed for the diagnosis of ARPKD (**Fig. 1**). Fetus and small infants have characteristically very large echogenic kidneys without any macrocysts. The cortical echogenicity is greatly increased, when compared with the hepatic parenchyma, and is associated with loss of corticomedullary differentiation. The increased echogenicity

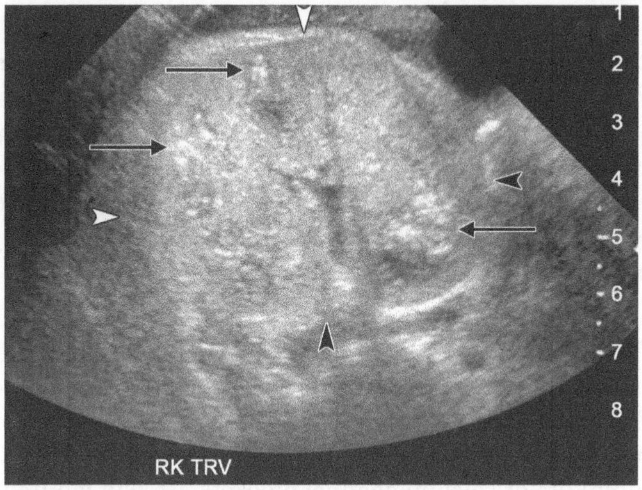

Fig. 1: Renal ultrasonography showing increased echogenicity with loss of corticomedullary differentiation. White arrowheads indicate the normal, thin peripheral cortical rim devoid of collecting ducts. Black arrows and arrowheads indicate the hyper echoic" salt and pepper appearance" in both cortex and medulla (RK: right kidney; TRV: transverse)

is due to the interfaces produced by the walls of ectatic tubules that are too small to be resolved by sonography. There may be a thin, normal, peripheral cortical rim as this portion of the cortex has no collecting tubules. When cysts are not detected, the hyperechoic "salt and pepper appearance" may be mistaken for nephrocalcinosis. The large size of the kidneys and the finding of hyperechoic areas in both the cortex and the medulla and the absence of posterior acoustic shadowing help to arrive at the correct diagnosis. High-resolution USG may be particularly useful in demonstrating the ductal ectasia, which is the hallmark of ARPKD.[6]

Magnetic Resonance Imaging

Magnetic resonance imaging (MRI) shows enlarged kidneys with hyperintense T2-weighted signals. It may be a useful additional diagnostic study in the third trimester of pregnancy in fetuses within conclusive USG, but its accuracy in confirming the diagnosis earlier in pregnancy has not been assessed.

Genetic Testing

Although molecular diagnostic testing by linkage analysis and direct sequencing can establish the diagnosis with 85% certainty, it is an expensive approach. It is difficult as the gene is large with a wide range of different mutations. A previously confirmed ARPKD in the family due to pathogenic and likely pathogenic variants allows preimplantation genetic diagnosis as well as carrier testing of at-risk family members.

Treatment

The treatment of ARPKD is supportive in nature. Prevention and treatment of problems arising out of the lung, kidney, and liver involvement require a coordinated multidisciplinary approach.

Lung

Severely affected newborns may require mechanical ventilation. Pneumothorax may require intercostal drainage. Rarely, unilateral or bilateral nephrectomy may be lifesaving, if massive kidney enlargement impairs diaphragmatic excursion. This can be considered only if the facilities and expertise for continuous dialysis in neonates are readily available.

Renal

Infants with severe renal dysfunction or anuria may require dialytic support. Hypertension is commonly associated and may be treated with angiotensin-converting enzyme (ACE) inhibitors or calcium channel blockers. Growth failure is common in infancy and requires supplemental feeding. Those progressing to end-stage kidney disease (ESKD) require dialysis and renal transplant. Ascending cholangitis resulting in liver failure can be a lethal complication, especially after kidney transplantation.

Liver

Children with esophageal varices require sclerotherapy or banding. A portacaval shunt may be necessary to treat progressive portal hypertension. Liver transplantation can be considered for those with severe portal hypertension.

Kidney transplantation alone may suffice in those with mild hepatic involvement. Combined liver kidney transplantation should be considered for those with severe liver disease and end-stage kidney failure. In an international cohort, the overall survival rate 2 years after kidney transplant was 80% and this might vary in region with limited resources.[7]

Prevention of Secondary Complications

Children with splenic dysfunction should be immunized against encapsulated bacteria. Those who have had ascending cholangitis should be given trimethoprim and sulfamethoxazole for prophylaxis.

Monitoring

Kidney and liver function require regular monitoring. Growth, nutritional status, blood pressure, renal function tests, and glomerular filtration rate (GFR) should be evaluated regularly. Hepatosplenomegaly, development of portal hypertension, varices, and liver function tests also need to be regularly monitored.

Future Perspectives

Therapy against the epidermal growth factor receptor (EGFR)-related growth factor axis has been shown to be efficacious in preclinical studies. Erlotinib, a nonreversible inhibitor of EGFR autophosphorylation, is undergoing phase II clinical studies.

AUTOSOMAL-DOMINANT POLYCYSTIC KIDNEY DISEASE

Autosomal-dominant polycystic kidney disease is the most common inherited disorder leading to renal failure in adults. It is characterized by the progressive development of macrocysts in both the kidneys and is often associated with cystic as well as noncystic malformations in other organs.

Epidemiology

Autosomal-dominant polycystic kidney disease is a fairly common disease with an incidence of 1 in 1,000 in the general population. It is seen in all ethnic and racial groups and affects both sexes equally. The most common age of presentation is in the 3rd or 4th decade of life. Occasionally, cysts may be detected in infants and children but symptomatic presentation is extremely rare in this age group.[8]

Pathogenesis

Cyst formation occurs through three mechanisms: tubular epithelial cell proliferation, fluid secretion, and extracellular matrix abnormalities in structure and/or function.[9] Once formed, cysts continue to grow and detach themselves from the tubule. Even after detachment, cysts continue to increase in size.

Polcystin-1 and polycystin-2 are transmembrane glycoproteins present on the epithelial cells of the renal tubules. The large extracellular domain of polycystin-1 located on the primary cilium of the renal tubular cell functions as a mechanoreceptor. Polycystin-2 contains a cation channel highly permeable to calcium and is linked to polycystin-1. These two proteins regulate calcium entry into the cell.

The flow of urine in the renal tubule stimulates the mechanoreceptor of polycystin-1, resulting in opening of the calcium channel of polycystin-2 and influx of calcium in the cell. The interaction of calcium influx, growth factors, and cyclic adenosine monophosphate (cAMP) through extracellular signal-regulated kinase (ERK) pathway inhibits the cell proliferation.

Polycystin-1 in addition interacts with tuberin and regulates the mammalian target of rapamycin (mTOR) pathway, which is also involved in cell proliferation. In ADPKD, due to dysfunctional polycystins, there is impaired calcium entry into the cell resulting in unopposed proliferative pathways leading to cyst formation.

Unlike ARPKD where cyst formation is restricted to the collecting tubule, in ADPKD, cyst formation can occur in any segment of the nephron because of the ubiquitous presence of polycystins on all renal tubular epithelial cells except the intercalated cells. However, only 5% of the nephron segments undergo cyst formation unlike ARPKD, where 10–90% of the collecting ducts undergo cystic changes. This is because in addition to the inherited germline mutation, for cyst formation to occur, a second hit somatic mutation is needed in the paired normal chromosome. The somatic mutation inhibits polycystin production by the normal allele leading to absent or severely reduced polycystin in the affected cells.

Pathology

The kidneys are enlarged and contain variable-sized cysts scattered in the cortex and medulla with intervening normal parenchyma. These cysts may arise from any part of the nephron or collecting duct. Glomerular cysts may also occur especially in early stages. The cysts are lined with a flattened epithelium and increase in size with age, and therefore the renal enlargement is progressive. Focal hepatic involvement consisting of clusters of dilated tubules is seen in about one-third of patients, but hepatic fibrosis is rare.

Genetics of ADPKD

Autosomal-dominant polycystic kidney disease is a genetically heterogeneous disorder with mutations being reported in *PKD1*, *PKD2*, *GANAB*, *DNAJB11*, and *HNF1B* genes.[10] *PKD1* and *PKD2* gene mutations together attribute for approximately 93% of cases with ADPKD, while in 7% cases, no underlying genetic etiology is discerned even after multigene panel testing.

PKD1 is a large gene of 46 exons that encodes polycystin-1 and responsible for 78% cases of ADPKD. The regions extending between exons 1 and 33 are duplicated, leading to pseudogene formation, thus hindering molecular analysis as they share up to a 98% homology with the wild type *PKD1* gene. This necessitates the need to confirm that identified variants arise from genuine *PKD1* gene and not from the pseudogenes. There is lower sensitivity of whole exome sequencing for these duplicated regions as opposed to long-range polymerase chain reaction (PCR) followed by Sanger sequencing, which allows selective amplification of genuine *PKD1* exons.

The challenges in *PKD1* genetic diagnosis are manifold and include—absence of hot-spot regions (necessitating the need for full gene sequencing) and presence of "private" mutations, hypomorphic alleles, and digenic inheritance (making variant interpretation difficult, especially for nontruncating variants). Truncating *PKD1* mutations lead to more severe phenotype when compared to those with nontruncating or hypomorphic alleles.

Mutations in *PKD2* gene localized on chromosome 4q22.1 account for approximately 15% of cases. It has 15 exons encoding a 968 amino acids protein called polycystin-2 which is involved in calcium transport and calcium signaling in renal epithelial cells. Till date, 318 unique variants belong to this are reported, of which majority lead to protein truncation. Truncating mutations have been associated with increased disease severity.

The penetrance of ADPKD is both age and genotype dependent, although intrafamilial variability is known. Early onset disease due to biallelic hypomorphic variants in *PKD1*/*PKD2* gene as well as due to digenic inheritance in *PKD1* and *HNF1B* has been reported.

Clinical Features

Autosomal-dominant polycystic kidney disease is essentially an adult disease presenting in the 3rd or 4th decade of life, usually with hypertension. In about 2–5% of cases, it can present in childhood and has even been detected in utero. While ADPKD can present in neonatal period and may be difficult to differentiate from ARPKD, it is usually asymptomatic in children with renal cysts detected on ultrasound in adolescents. The presentation in very young children may be atypical with only a few cysts or even with unilateral involvement. As ADPKD progresses, involvement may become bilateral.

Renal Manifestations

Autosomal-dominant polycystic kidney disease in children may have a variable presentation. Most cases are detected in asymptomatic patients by the incidental finding of cysts on USG. Gross hematuria after seemingly minor trauma may be a presenting feature in some children. Hypertension is a common manifestation of ADPKD, occurring in over one-third children and correlates with the severity of structural renal disease. Polyuria and polydipsia secondary to a renal concentrating defect are a common occurrence in children with ADPKD and correlate with the presence of hypertension and the number of renal cysts. Children with ADPKD may have a low-grade proteinuria, which is suggestive of a more severe cystic disease. Pyelonephritis or infection of cyst is seen rarely. Occasionally, older adolescents with relatively large kidneys may have loin pain. Renal insufficiency is rare in childhood but may still occur in 2–5%. Early manifestation of ADPKD is defined as symptomatic disease such as systemic hypertension, proteinuria, and impaired renal function occurring before the age of 15 years. Children diagnosed in utero or within their first 18 months of life are called very early onset (VEO) ADPKD. They are more likely to have hypertension and rapid progression of renal disease compared to a non-VEO ADPKD.

Extrarenal Involvement

Autosomal-dominant polycystic kidney disease is a multisystem disease and both cystic and noncystic involvement of organs is common and may sometimes dominate the clinical picture.

Cystic malformations: These are the most common extrarenal manifestations of ADPKD. Cysts can develop in many organs. Liver is the most common organ involved by cysts. Liver cysts develop in about 80% of adults and are more common in women. These are seen in 55% of cases below 25 years of age; however, hepatic dysfunction is uncommon. Rarely, there may be congenital hepatic fibrosis with ADPKD, which may present as portal hypertension and hypersplenism. Pancreatic cysts may be seen in 10% of patients. Splenic cysts, cysts in arachnoid membranes, and seminal vesicles have been reported in adults, but these are very rare in children.

Noncystic malformations: Intracranial aneurysm is the most important noncystic potentially lethal malformation associated with ADPKD and is seen in 5–8% of adults. Severe headache in a patient with ADPKD can signal a leaking aneurysm causing irritation and warrants emergency care. Cerebral aneurysms are rare in children. Screening for intracranial aneurysms is recommended in high-risk adults by magnetic resonance angiography (MRA).

The most common cardiac abnormality is mitral valve prolapse, which is usually mild, seen in 26% of adults and about 12% of children.

Other associations with ADPKD include umbilical, hiatal, and inguinal hernias. Inguinal hernias can occur in about 10% of children with ADPKD.[11]

ADPKD in children differs greatly from ADPKD in adults in presentation, prognosis, and therapy as detailed in **Table 1**.[12]

Diagnosis of ADPKD

Ultrasound

The imaging modality of choice for the diagnosis of ADPKD is renal ultrasound **(Fig. 2)**.[13] Sonography-based diagnostic criteria are age dependent, based on the fact that simple renal cysts occur increasingly as age advances and are not seen in childhood. The USG criteria for diagnosis of ADPKD are summarized in **Table 2**.[14]

Kidneys are invariably enlarged in adult ADPKD. Cysts on renal ultrasound of the parents and/or grandparents, if the parents are <30 years of age, are suggestive of ADPKD. In the absence of family history, the diagnosis of ADPKD in a child becomes difficult as the cysts are few and may even be unilateral without significant kidney enlargement. In addition to family history, the presence of extrarenal cysts and other characteristic noncystic malformations such as mitral valve prolapse or cerebral aneurysm may support the diagnosis of ADPKD.

Autosomal-dominant polycystic kidney disease may rarely present in utero, when it becomes difficult to differentiate it from ARPKD. Both have enlarged hyperechoic kidneys. Kidneys are echogenic in ARPKD and tend to be larger than in ADPKD. After infancy, nephromegaly is more characteristic of ADPKD as renal size decreases in ADPKD. Liver cysts are suggestive of ADPKD; presence of Caroli disease or hepatic fibrosis goes in favor of ARPKD. These findings may not be seen in utero making the diagnosis more difficult at this age.[6]

Renal cysts with enlarged kidneys are also seen in other inherited disorders such as tuberous sclerosis,

TABLE 1: Clinical manifestations, prognostic indicators, and therapy for autosomal-dominant polycystic kidney disease (ADPKD) in adults and children.[12]

Manifestations	***ADPKD in adults***	***ADPKD in children***
Hematuria	42%	10%
Concentrating defects	100%	58%
Proteinuria	18%	23%
Microalbuminuria	19–40%	30%
Hepatic cysts	85–94%	58% in 15–24 years old
Intracranial aneurysm	5–10%	Rare
Mitral valve prolapse	26%	12%
Hypertension before renal function decline	60–75%	5–44%
Validated prognostic indicators	PKD genotype TKV	No reports [suggested are very early onset (VEO) ADPKD, hypertension, glomerular hyperfiltration, PKD genotype, proteinuria]
Patient stratification scoring systems predicting disease progression	• PRO-PKD score, based on sex, PKD genotype, presence of hypertension and/or urologic events <35 years • Mayo imaging classification, based on htTKV range for age • ADPKD outcomes model, based on disease-progression equations for htTKV and eGFR	No reports
Evidence-based interventions to slow down disease progression	• Rigorous blood pressure control with ACE inhibitors • Tolvaptan	ACE inhibitors if blood pressure > 95th percentile for age, sex, and height

(ACE: angiotensin-converting enzyme; eGFR: estimated glomerular filtration rate; htTKV: height-adjusted total kidney volume; PKD: polycystic kidney disease)

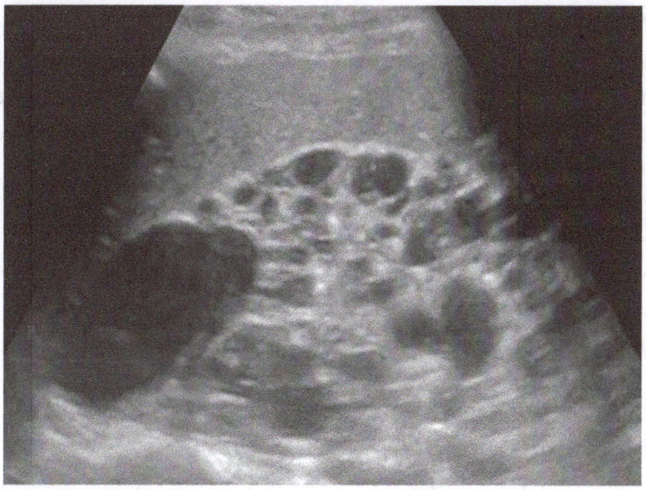

Fig. 2: Renal ultrasonography shows raised echogenicity with multiple scattered cysts of various sizes (seen in ADPKD). (ADPKD: autosomal-dominant polycystic kidney disease)

Bardet–Biedl syndrome, and Meckel–Gruber syndrome. Presence of characteristic extrarenal manifestations facilitates the diagnosis of these disorders as given in **Table 3.**[15]

Other Imaging Modalities

Computed tomography (CT) scan has a better resolution (0.5 cm vs. 1 cm by ultrasound) and is used for complicated cases such as suspected tumor, infection of cysts, etc. MRI is very useful in monitoring renal size and volume and is a recommended modality to determine the rate of progression, monitor the efficacy of disease-specific therapies, and assess asymptomatic potential donors. High-resolution USG can detect even small cyst in neonates and children. No studies have defined a gold standard of imaging in these children. As MRI requires sedation in children, it is not the diagnostic modality.[16]

TABLE 2: Diagnostic criteria for autosomal-dominant polycystic kidney disease (ADPKD) on ultrasonography in those with a positive family history of ADPKD.[14]

	Predicts ADPKD (PPV 100%; sensitivity lower in nontruncating PKD1, PKD2, or GANAB mutations)	***Excludes ADPKD (Negative predictive value 100%)***
Medullary or cortical cysts	<15 years: ≥1 cyst is highly suggestive 15–39* years: ≥3 uni-/bilateral cysts 40–59 years: ≥2 cysts in each kidney >60 years ≥4 cysts in each kidney	Absence of cyst if >15 years (truncating PKD1) Cannot exclude if <40 years with PKD2 or unknown genotype or <30 years (milder genotypes)

*29 years for PKD1.
(PKD: polycystic kidney disease; PPV: positive predictive value)

TABLE 3: Important differential diagnosis of autosomal-dominant polycystic kidney disease (ADPKD).

Disease, gene	***Phenotype***
Classical ADPKD	
PKD1 truncating mutation	B/L cysts ESKD 55 years
PKD1 nontruncating	B/L cysts ESKD 67 years
PKD2	ESKD 79 years
GANAB	B/L cysts preserved renal function
DNAJB1	Small kidneys, multiple cysts, ESKD 60 years
Autosomal-dominant tubulointerstitial kidney disease (ADTKD), HNF1B, MUC1, SEC1A1, UMOD	Normal/small size kidney Few small cysts Variable ESKD
ARPKD *PKHD1, DZIP1L, PMM2*	Enlarged kidneys, mm-sized cysts, ESKD 10–30 years Congenital hepatic fibrosis, Caroli syndrome
Polycystic liver disease (ADPLD)	Few renal cysts, polycystic liver disease
Tuberous sclerosis TSC1, TSC2	Multiple angiomyolipomas, cysts, ESKD CNS (tubers), skin, cardiac rhabdomyoma
Von Hippel–Lindau disease (VHL)	B/L cysts, hemangioblastoma, pheochromocytoma, neuroendocrine tumor
HANAC syndrome COL4A1	B/L cysts, ESKD 50–60 years, hematuria, aneurysms, cramps
Orofaciodigital syndrome (OFD1)	Facial dysmorphism, cleft palate, mental retardation, liver cysts

(ARPKD: autosomal-recessive polycystic kidney disease; B/L: bilateral; ESKD: end-stage kidney disease)

Other Nonrenal Investigations

Other useful investigations include USG of abdomen to detect extrarenal cysts, 2D echocardiography for mitral valve prolapse, and MRA for intracranial aneurysms.

Genetic Testing

Genetic screening of at-risk individuals is possible by exome sequencing. Genetic testing is indicated in patients with suspected PKD and absent family history, patients with inconclusive results on imaging, prenatal diagnosis in families with early onset ADPKD, and evaluation of a potential live related donor for transplant.

Treatment

Treatment of ADPKD can be categorized into disease-specific therapies, management of complications, and other important measures.

Disease-specific Therapies

Significant advances have happened in the treatment of ADPKD, which are aimed at reducing renal cyst size and prevention of decline in kidney function. Several clinical trials have tested novel therapies and genera measures in adults and children, which are summarized in **Table 4**. Of the disease-modifying agents, tolvaptan has been found to be safe and effective in the treatment of adult ADPKD. As a result, the drug is being tested in adolescents with ADPKD for safety and efficacy.[16,17]

Management of Complications

Chronic Kidney Disease

Management of chronic kidney disease (CKD) includes strict control of blood pressure, treatment of metabolic acidosis, and prevention of hyperphosphatemia and associated secondary hyperparathyroidism.

Renal Cysts

Most often, renal cysts are small in size and do not require active management. Therapy for flank pain, cyst decompression, and cyst hemorrhage and infection is needed in adults. Associated nephrolithiasis is uncommon in children.

Liver Disease

Most individuals with polycystic liver disease (PLD) have no symptoms and require no treatment, but rare severe cases may require surgical resection or even liver transplantation.

Other Important Measures in Management of ADPKD

General: Adequate hydration, maintenance of normal BMI and blood pressure, sodium restriction, and regular exercise are suggested as general measures in the management of ADPKD.

Surveillance: Blood pressure monitoring to diagnose hypertension and regular monitoring for proteinuria are indicated in childhood; imaging for intracranial aneurysms may be indicated in high-risk and those with symptoms; echocardiography is indicated, if a heart murmur is detected and those with high risk for thoracic aortic dissection.[18]

Recent Recommendations for Diagnosis, Monitoring, and Genetic Testing for Children with ADPKD

Recently, recommendations have been developed by an international group of experts in ADPKD. An outline of these recommendations is listed here:[16]

- In at-risk children, diagnostic screening should be done by ultrasonography. Detection of one or more cysts in a child with positive family history is suggestive of ADPKD;

TABLE 4: Important therapeutic interventions in autosomal-dominant polycystic kidney disease (ADPKD).

Drug/intervention	*Class*	*Mechanism of action*	*Evidence in trials*
Tolvaptan	Vasopressin receptor agonist	Inhibits fluid secretion and cyst proliferation	Safe and efficacious in slowing TKV increase and decline in GFR in early and late CKD in adults (TEMPO trial)
Lisinopril, telmisartan	Angiotensin-converting enzyme inhibitor, angiotensin receptor blocker	Inhibits renin–angiotensin system	Rigorous BP control better than standard control (HALT-PKD study) in slowing TKV increase
Pravastatin	HMG-CoA reductase inhibitor	Inhibits G protein; cell proliferation	Beneficial in children and young adults
Octreotide, lanreotide	Somatostatin analog	Inhibit fluid secretion and cell proliferation	Slows increase in TKV; effect not sustained (ALADIN study)
Sirolimus, everolimus	Mammalian target of rapamycin (mTOR) inhibitor	Inhibit mTOR signaling pathways; inhibit cell proliferation	Not beneficial
Metformin	AMP-activated protein kinase activator	Antagonizes mTOR activation; cell proliferation	Ongoing

(AMP: adenosine monophosphate; GFR: glomerular filtration rate; HMG-CoA: 3-hydroxy-3-methylglutaryl coenzyme A; TKV: total kidney volume) however, it cannot be ruled out in the absence of cysts in childhood. It is not necessary to screen at intervals <3 years.

- At-risk children, who opt out of diagnostic testing, should undergo yearly screening hypertension and proteinuria.
- Genetic testing is recommended for infants with VEO-ADPKD, those with symptoms, and for children with a negative family history and rapidly progressive disease. Multigene panel rather than testing for single *ADPKD* genes is recommended with adequate coverage for *PKD1* gene.
- If not already known, diagnostic testing for mutations should be done in the affected family member before testing the child.
- Monitoring for hypertension (preferably by ambulatory blood pressure monitor) and proteinuria should be done regularly in children with positive family history.
- Tolvaptan is not recommended routinely in children but off-label use can be considered in adolescents with rapidly progressive disease.
- mTOR inhibitors and somatostatin analogs should not be used for treatment.
- Low dietary salt intake and high water intake are recommended.

Prognosis

Serum creatinine is a late indicator of disease severity as increase in the kidney volume due to cysts and their enlargement with consequent, parenchymal damage precedes the decline in renal function. Recent studies indicate that total kidney volume (TKV) as determined by MRI and its rate of change are reliable predictors of decline in GFR and long-term outcomes.

Proteinuria, polyuria, and impaired urinary concentration have been identified as markers of severe cystic disease in children and associated with larger kidneys. Children with higher blood pressure exhibit greater renal growth rate. Once renal insufficiency sets in, GFR typically decreases at a rate of approximately 2–3 mL/min/1.73 m^2 per year. Although it is a well-known fact that patients with *PKD1* mutations typically progress to ESKD faster than *PKD2* mutations by 10–20 years, in an individual patient, it is difficult to predict the age of onset of renal insufficiency because of significant inter- and intrafamilial phenotypic heterogeneity in the disease.

CONCLUSION

Autosomal-recessive polycystic kidney disease is one of the most common inheritable cystic renal diseases which manifests in childhood. Two main genes implicated in ARPKD are *PKHD1* and *DZIP1L*. In ARPKD, the cyst formation occurs along the collecting duct leading to their fusiform dilatation. Ectasia of the hepatic bile ducts and bile duct proliferation are invariably present leading to hepatic fibrosis and hepatomegaly. There seems to be a reciprocal relationship between the severity of the renal and hepatic disease. Children having a severe hepatic involvement manifest with less-severe renal involvement and children with severe renal involvement have a milder liver disease. There is progression to ESKD over a variable period of time in most children. Combined liver kidney transplantation should be considered for those with severe liver disease and end-stage kidney failure.

The main burden of ADPKD occurs in adulthood. But still a substantial proportion of pediatric patients have treatable disease manifestations. *PKD1* and *PKD2* gene mutations together attribute for approximately 93% of cases with ADPKD. In ADPKD, cyst formation can occur in any segment of the nephron. Monitoring for hypertension and proteinuria should be done regularly in children with positive family history. Tolvaptan has been found to be safe and effective in the treatment of adult ADPKD and is being tested in adolescents with ADPKD for safety and efficacy.

KEY POINTS

- *Autosomal-recessive polycystic kidney disease presents antenatally with enlarged and hyperechoic kidneys.*
- A previously confirmed ARPKD in the family due to pathogenic and likely pathogenic variant allows preimplantation genetic diagnosis as well as carrier testing of at-risk family members.
- *Kidney replacement therapy is required in 50% of patients in the first decade of life.*
- Detection of one or more cysts in a child with positive family history is suggestive of ADPKD.
- Genetic testing is recommended for infants with VEO-ADPKD, for those with symptoms, and for children with a negative family history and rapidly progressive disease.
- Tolvaptan is not recommended routinely in children, but off-label use can be considered in adolescents with rapidly progressive disease.

REFERENCES

1. Beskrovnaya O, Bukanov N. Polycystic kidney diseases: from molecular discoveries to targeted therapeutic strategies. Cell Mole Life Sci. 2008;65(4):605-19.
2. Bergmann C. Early and severe polycystic kidney disease and related ciliopathies: an emerging field of interest. Nephron. 2019;141:50-60.
3. Bergmann C. Genetics of autosomal recessive polycystic kidney disease and its differential diagnoses. Front Pediatr. 2018;5:221.
4. Sweeney WE, Avner ED. Molecular and cellular pathophysiology of autosomal recessive polycystic kidney disease (ARPKD). Cell and Tissue Res. 2006;326(3):671-85.
5. Chandar J, Garcia J, Jorge L, Tekin A. Transplantation in autosomal recessive polycystic kidney disease: liver and/or kidney? Pediatr Nephrol. 2015;30:1233-42.
6. Avni FE, Garel L, Cassart M, Massez A, Eurin D, Didier F, et al. Perinatal assessment of hereditary cystic renal diseases: the contribution of sonography. Pediatr Radiol. 2006;36(5):405-14.
7. Liebau MC. Early clinical management of autosomal recessive polycystic kidney disease. Pediatr Nephrol. 2021;36(11):3561-70.

8. Shamshirsaz AA, Bekheirnia RM, Kamgar M, Johnson AM, McFann K, Cadnapaphornchai M, et al. Autosomal-dominant polycystic kidney disease in infancy and childhood: progression and outcome. Kidney Int. 2005;68(5):2218-24.
9. Braun WE. Autosomal dominant polycystic kidney disease: emerging concepts of pathogenesis and new treatments. Cleve Clin J Med. 2009;76(2):97-104.
10. Rizk D, Chapman A. Treatment of autosomal dominant polycystic kidney disease (ADPKD): the new horizon for children with ADPKD. Pediatr Nephrol. 2008;23(7):1029-36.
11. Sweeney WE Jr, Avner ED. Diagnosis and management of childhood polycystic kidney disease. Pediatr Nephrol. 2011;26(5):675-92.
12. De Rechter S, Bockenhauer D, Guay-Woodford LM, Liu I, Mallett AJ, Soliman NA, et al. ADPedKD: a global online platform on the management of children with ADPKD. Kidney Int Rep. 2019;4:1271-84.
13. Gimpel C, Avni EF, Breysem L, Burgmaier K, Caroli A, Cetiner M, et al. Imaging of kidney cysts and cystic kidney diseases in children: an International Working Group Consensus Statement. Radiology. 2019;290(3):769-82.
14. Cornec-Le Gall E, Alam A, Perrone RD. Autosomal dominant polycystic kidney disease. Lancet. 2019;393(10174):919-35.
15. Chapman AB, Devuyst O, Eckardt KU, Gansevoort RT, Harris T, Horie S, et al. Autosomal dominant polycystic kidney disease (ADPKD): Executive Summary from a Kidney Disease: Improving Global Outcomes (KDIGO) Controversies Conference. Kidney Int. 2015;88(1):17-27.
16. Gimpel C, Bergmann C, Bockenhauer D, Breysem L, Cadnapaphornchai MA, Cetiner M, et al. International consensus statement on the diagnosis and management of autosomal dominant polycystic kidney disease in children and young people. Nat Rev Nephrol. 2019;15:713-26.
17. Cadnapaphornchai MA. Clinical trials in ADPKD. Front Pediatr. 2017;5(53):1-6.
18. Rechter SD, Breysem L, Djalila MI. ADPKD becoming a pediatric disorder. Front Pediatr. 2017;5(272):1-8.

CHAPTER

9.3

Nephronophthisis and Autosomal Dominant Tubulointerstitial Kidney Disease

Deepthi RV, G Sangeetha

NEPHRONOPHTHISIS

Introduction

Nephronophthisis (NPHP) is a heterogeneous group of tubulointerstitial cystic kidney disease, transmitted by an autosomal-recessive inheritance pattern. It is considered to be the most common genetic cause for chronic kidney disease (CKD) in children and young adults, especially in the first three decades of life. The extended clinical and genetic overlap with various syndromes and extrarenal manifestations led to the introduction of the term nephronophthisis complex. Based on the age of onset of CKD grade 5 (CKD-G5), NPHP is described as infantile, juvenile, and adolescent types, which manifest at a median age of 1, 13, and 19 years, respectively. Around 20% of patients with NPHP have associated extrarenal involvement. NPHP is characterized by a reduced urinary concentrating ability with bland urinary sediment. Chronic tubulointerstitial nephritis may progress to CKD-G5, generally before the age of 20 years.[1]

Kidney sizes may be normal or slightly reduced (except in infantile NPHP type 2 where moderate renal enlargement may be there) with the cysts situated at the corticomedullary junction. The renal histology triad of NPHP includes tubular basement membrane (TBM) disruption, tubulointerstitial nephropathy, and cysts.

Epidemiology

Nephronophthisis accounts for 10–25% of CKD-G5 in children. There is no gender predominance noted in NPHP. It has been reported worldwide with an incidence ranging around 1:50000 in Europe and the USA.[2] Smith and Graham first described NPHP in 1945 and Fanconi et al. named it as "familial juvenile NPHP", with the meaning "vanishing of the nephrons".[3,4] The juvenile form, in which patients develop CKD-G5 during childhood or adolescence, is the most common variant. The estimated prevalence for this variant varies from 0.1 to 0.2 per 10,000 live births in reports from Finland and Canada.

Genetics

Nephronophthisis is genetically heterogeneous with several known causative gene mutations that encode components of the ciliary apparatus, which are expressed in primary cilia, basal bodies, or centrosomes. The most common mutation is homozygous deletions of the *NPHP1* gene, reported in approximately 20% of cases. Other gene mutations contribute to <3%. Genetic mutation remains unknown in 70% of patients with NPHP. The gene products have roles in signaling of cell-cell and cell-matrix, and this involves sensing luminal flow rates via ciliary mechanosensory receptors within the renal tubules. As a consequence of the abnormal cell's attempt to compensate for a perceived lack of fluid flow, there is dysregulation of tissue growth and cyst formation in NPHP.[5]

Genetic Mutations

Among the several gene mutations implicated in NPHP, the most notable ones are *NPHP1* to 18.[6]

Clinical correlation of various gene mutations in NPHP:

- All except *NPHP2* gene mutation: Juvenile NPHP
- *NPHP2* gene mutation: Infantile NPHP
- *NPHP3* gene mutation: Adolescent NPHP
- *NPHP5* mutation: Retinitis pigmentosa and Senior–Loken syndrome (SLSN)
- *NPHP6* and *NPHP8* mutations: Joubert syndrome and Meckel–Gruber syndrome (MKS)
- *NPHP7* and *NPHP9* mutations are rare.

Below is a brief summary of the physiological functions of the proteins encoded by NPHP genes:[7,8]

- *NPHP1 gene:* It encodes nephrocystin-1, a 733 amino acid protein, and it is the first gene identified by positional cloning in NPHP.[9] It is expressed primarily in the collecting duct and is located at the cell–cell junction and the cell-matrix interface. It participates in multiple intracellular signaling pathways that involve ciliary function. Large homozygous deletions account for 94% of NPHP mutations while few carry point mutations.[10]
- *NPHP2 gene:* It encodes for the protein inversin (nephrocystin-2). Inversin is important for the normal development of left–right patterning and the signaling mechanisms of planar cell polarity.
- *NPHP3 gene: NPHP3* encodes a protein with a tubulin-tyrosine ligase domain, which interacts with nephrocystin-1.
- *NPHP4 gene: NPHP4* encodes nephrocystin-4 (nephro-retinin) which is situated in the connecting cilium of

photoreceptor cells and interacts with a cone and rod receptor protein, RPGRIP1L (retinitis pigmentosa GTPase regulator interacting protein 1). It is also involved in the intracellular signaling pathway.

- *NPHP5 gene: NPHP5* gene (*IQCB1* gene) encodes nephrocystin-5 and it interacts with calmodulin and the retinitis pigmentosa GTPase regulator (RPGR). Both nephrocystin-5 and RPGR are expressed in the primary cilia of renal epithelial cells and the connecting cilia of photoreceptors. In *NPHP5*, all were truncating mutations.
- *NPHP6 gene:* It encodes a centrosomal protein that interacts with a transcription factor ATF4 that is involved in the control of the cell cycle. Recessive truncating mutations were identified as pathogenic. *ATF4* gene mutations are associated with cyclic adenosine monophosphate (cAMP)-dependent renal cyst formation. *NPHP6* gene mutations were one of the most common causes of Leber's congenital amaurosis (LCA) accounting for 20% of LCA cases.
- *NPHP7 gene:* Gene product of the *GLIS2* gene is Krüppel-like zinc finger protein that appears to be a transcriptional repressor without involvement in ciliary function.
- *NPHP8 gene:* Mutations in the *NPHP8* gene (*RPGRIP1L* gene) and the gene product colocalize to the basal body and centrosomes with nephrocystin-4 and -6. It has an important role in the development of neural tube and limb defects. Mutations identified were missense and truncating types.
- *NPHP9 gene:* Mutations in the *NPHP9* gene (*NEK8* gene) are rare causes of NPHP. It is needed for the regulation of cilia and cell cycle progression.
- *NPHP10 gene:* It encodes *SDCCAG8* (serologically defined colon cancer antigen 8) and is situated at the centrioles of both renal epithelial and retinal photoreceptor cells.
- *NPHP11 gene: NPHP11* gene encodes for *MKS3* and *TMEM67* genes. It also encodes for meckelin, which is located at the base of primary cilia.
- *NPHP12 gene: NPHP12* gene, on chromosome 2, encodes IFT139, a subunit of the intraflagellar transport-A complex, which regulates the retrograde trafficking in the primary cilium.
- *NPHP13 gene:* The *NPHP13* gene encodes for IFT144, another subunit of the intraflagellar transport-A complex. Patients with defects in several other genes that affect components important for ciliary function may also present with NPHP.

Oligogenic inheritance: Mutations in a small number of genes may interact genetically to manifest the disease of the same phenotype, and it is called oligogenic inheritance. It is reported in some patients with Joubert syndrome who had mutations in both the *NPHP1* and *NPHP6* genes.

Pathogenesis

NPHP1-18 gene products are called nephrocystins. The proposed mechanism of the various *NPHP* genes leading to renal disease is ciliary dysfunction. As the nephrocystin proteins are localized in primary cilia or at their base, ciliary function is essential to maintain the renal architecture and integrity.[11,12] Primary cilia present as microtubular projections on virtually all types of cell in the human body. It transmits the information from the extracellular milieu into the cell. Mutations in the *NPHP* genes alter cilia function resulting in the inability of the ciliary mechanosensors to correctly sense luminal flow rates.[13] This results in dysregulated tissue growth and subsequent development of renal cysts due to the inability of renal tubular cells to perceive luminal flow due to dysfunctional ciliary function. As the gene products of some of the *NPHP* genes are also found in the cilia of other organs, they may present with extrarenal manifestations of NPHP.[14] The primary cilia of renal epithelial cells are structurally similar to the connecting cilium of photoreceptor cells in the retina. This explains the renal and eye involvement in Senior–Loken syndrome.[15]

Pathology

The kidneys are grossly normal or shrunken in appearance with around 5–50 cysts of 1–15 mm in diameter, preferentially at the corticomedullary junction. Bilateral renal involvement is universal. The cysts usually arise from the distal convoluted and medullary collecting tubules. Approximately 70% of autopsy cases have cysts and they seem to develop only postnatally and later in the course of the illness. Hence, the presence of cysts is not a prerequisite for making the diagnosis. Infantile NPHP may have enlarged kidney sizes and widespread cysts like in polycystic kidney disease (PKD).

Renal histology of NPHP will show the triad of TBM disruption, tubular cell atrophy with cysts, and tubulointerstitial fibrosis.

Sequence of events in light microscopy includes: TBM disruption, lymphocytic and histiocytic peritubular infiltration. The atrophic tubules predominantly develop at the corticomedullary junction with pronounced thickening and multilayering of the TBM.[16] Diffuse sclerosing tubulointerstitial nephropathy is seen in advanced stages of the disease. The TBM changes and cyst formation are most prominent in the distal tubule of the nephron as the cysts are lined with a single layer of cuboidal or flattened epithelium in that segment. The glomeruli are often normal, but secondary segmental sclerosis and collapsed glomeruli with periglomerular fibrosis and splitting and thickening of Bowman's capsule are seen in advanced disease. On electron microscopy, homogeneous or multilayered thickening of TBMs is prominent along with duplication.[17] Ultrasound reveals normal or small-sized echogenic kidneys with a loss of corticomedullary differentiation.[18]

Clinical Features

Nephronophthisis is characterized by:

- Autosomal-recessive inheritance
- Impaired urinary concentrating ability and sodium reabsorption present as polyuria and polydipsia

- Bland urine sediment with an absence of cells and cellular casts
- Proteinuria is often absent, although some patients may show mild tubular proteinuria in the initial stages and glomerular proteinuria in the late stages of CKD
- Insidious onset of renal insufficiency and progression to chronic tubulointerstitial nephropathy and CKD-G5.

Table 1 enlists some of the important gene loci, their protein products, disease variants, their associations, and extrarenal manifestations of NPHP.[19]

TABLE 1: Nephronophthisis (NPHP) variants, important gene loci, their protein products, their associations, and extrarenal manifestations.

Disease variants/types	*Median and range of onset of ESKD (years)*	*Gene mutation frequency*	*Chromosome*	*Severe retinal degeneration*	*Extrarenal association (10–15%)*
NPHP1/JBTS4/SLSN1	13 (7–29) (juvenile)	Nephrocystin-1 25%	2q12.3	10–15%	OMA, JBTS
NPHP2	3 (0–5) (infantile)	Inversin 1 2%	9q22-q31	10%	VSD, LF situs inversus, HTN
NPHP3/SLSN3/renal hepatic pancreatic syndrome	19 (11–47) (adolescent)	NPHP3 nephrocystin-3 <1%	3q22.1	10%	JBTS, LF, MKS situs inversus CHD (AS, ASD, PDA, RVH)
NPHP4/SLSN4	21 (6–35)	Nephroretinin 2–3%	1p36.31	10–15%	JBTS, OMA, LF, LCA
NPHP5/SLSN5	15 (6–32)	*IQCB1* 3–4%	3q13.33	100%	LCA
NPHP6/JBTS5 SLSN6/MKS4	12 (5–17)	*CEP290* 1%	12q21.32	100%	JBTS, OMA, MKS, BBS, LF, COACH, CHD, MO, bone ABN
NPHP7	8	*GLIS2* 0.1%	16p13.3	–	
NPHP8/JBTS7/MKS5	10 (juvenile)	*RPGRIP1L*0.5%	16q12.2	10%	JBTS, OMA, MKS, LCA, LF, COACH, RHYNS
NPHP9	3 (infantile, juvenile)	*NEK 8* <0.5%	17q11.2	30%	MKS-like
NPHP10//SLSN7	4–24	*SDCCAG8* <0.5%		Rare	BBS-like
NPHP11/JBTS6/MKS3	Infantile	MKS3 TMEM67 (Meckelin) <0.5 %	8q22	–	JBTS, MKS, LF, JATD, COACH
NPHP12/JBTS11	–	*TTC21B* <1%	2	–	JBTS, JATD, MKS, BBS
NPHP13/ Cranioectodermal dysplasia 4	12 (5–17)	*WDR19*		+	JATD, SS
NPHP14/JBTS19	Infantile	*ZNF423*		+	JBTS, situs inversus, LCA, CVH
NPHP15	–	*CEP164*		+	JBTS, LF, obesity, bone ABN, CVH, LCA, NYS, seizures
NPHP16	Infantile, juvenile	*ANKS6*		–	LF, CHD (AS, PS, PDA) Cardiomyopathy
JBTS1	–	*INPP5E*		+	JBTS, OMA
JBTS2	Juvenile	*TMEM216*		+	JBTS, OMA
JBTS3	Juvenile, adult	*AHI1*		+	JBTS, OMA
JBTS8	–	*ARL13B*		–	JBTS, OMA, and MKS

[AS: aortic stenosis; BBS: Bardet–Biedl syndrome; CHD: congenital heart defect; COACH: cerebellar vermis hypoplasia, oligophrenia, cognitive dysfunction, ataxia, coloboma, hypotonia syndrome; COGAN: congenital oculomotor apraxia (impairment of horizontal voluntary eye movements, ocular attraction movements, optokinetic nystagmus); CVH: cerebellar vermis hypoplasia; ELE: elevated liver enzymes; ESKD: end-stage kidney disease; HT: arterial hypertension; JATD: Jeune asphyxiating thoracic dystrophy; JBTS: Joubert syndrome; LCA: Leber congenital amaurosis; LF: liver fibrosis; MKS: Meckel–Gruber syndrome (occipital encephalocele, polydactyly, microphthalmia, and liver fibrosis); MO: microphthalmos; NYS: nystagmus; OH: oligohydramnios; OMA: oculomotor apraxia type Cogan II; PDA: persistent ductus arteriosus; PS: pulmonary stenosis; RVH: right ventricular hypertrophy; SLSN: Senior–Loken syndrome; SS: Sensenbrenner syndrome; VSD: ventricular septal defect]

Extrarenal manifestations consistent with ciliary pathology are seen in 20% of patients and are enlisted in **Table 2.** Other features such as poor growth, primary or secondary enuresis, hyponatremia, and hypovolemia due to loss of sodium conservation might be a hint for the diagnosis. Before the onset of renal failure, blood pressure may be normal. Normocytic normochromic anemia is common prior to renal insufficiency.

Infantile NPHP is a distinct disease entity and CKD-G5 occurs within the first 5 years of life. Kidney size is typically enlarged in infantile NPHP whereas it will be normal or small in "classical NPHP variants". Cardiac manifestations, situs inversus, and ventricular septal defects are commonly seen in NPHP type 2. Patients often have arterial hypertension and AKI. The infantile variant does not have medullary cysts. Enlarged kidneys and cortical microcysts are characteristic of NPHP type 2. Histologically, there is no disruption of TBM. Early onset NPHP is seen with mutations in *NPHP2, NPHP9, NPHP11, NPHP14*, and *NPHP16* while other mutation types present in later life.[20]

TABLE 2: Extrarenal manifestations associated with NPHP.

Extrarenal features	*Associated syndrome*
Ophthalmologic disorders	
Retinitis pigmentosa (RP)	SLSN, Arima syndrome (cerebro-oculo-hepatorenal syndrome), Alstrom syndrome (RP, obesity, DM type 2, hearing impairment), RHYNS (RP, hypopituitarism, NPHP, skeletal dysplasia)
Oculomotor apraxia	COGAN syndrome/congenital oculomotor apraxia (impairment of horizontal voluntary eye movements, ocular attraction movements, optokinetic nystagmus)
Nystagmus, coloboma, ptosis	Joubert syndrome
Skeletal disorders	
Short ribs	Jeune asphyxiating thoracic dystrophy
Cone-shaped epiphysis	Mainzer–Saldino syndrome
Postaxial polydactyly	Joubert syndrome, Ellis-van Creveld syndrome, Bardet–Biedl syndrome (RP, obesity, deafness)
Skeletal dysplasia	Sensenbrenner syndrome (cranioectodermal dysplasia) RHYNS, Ellis-van Creveld syndrome
Neurological disorders	
Occipital encephalocele	Meckel–Gruber syndrome (occipital encephalocele, polydactyly, microphthalmia, and liver fibrosis)
Vermis hypoplasia	Joubert syndrome COACH
Hypopituitarism	RHYNS
Hepatic disorders	
Liver fibrosis	Boichis syndrome (liver fibrosis, bile duct proliferation)
Elevation of hepatic enzymes	Meckel–Gruber syndrome Arima syndrome Joubert syndrome
Others: Situs inversus, cardiac malformation, bronchiectasis, ulcerative colitis	

(COACH: cerebellar vermis hypoplasia, oligophrenia, cognitive dysfunction, ataxia, coloboma, hypotonia; SLSN: Senior–Loken syndrome)

Juvenile NPHP is the most common type of NPHP. In juvenile NPHP, symptoms develop around 4–6 years of age. Progression to CKD-G5 develops at a mean age of around 13 years. Mutations in all except the *NPHP2* gene have been associated with juvenile NPHP. Oculomotor apraxia types Cogan and retinitis pigmentosa are reported as association in a subset of juvenile NPHP with large deletions. Tapetoretinal degeneration is the most common extrarenal disease manifestation in juvenile NPHP.

Adolescent NPHP is due to mutation of *NPHP3*. These children develop CKD-G5 in late adolescence and young adulthood with a median age of 19 years. In patients carrying *NPHP3* mutations, the expression of the gene in the retina and liver causes tapetoretinal degeneration or hepatic fibrosis. *NPHP2, NPHP3*, and *MKS3* gene mutations are known to be associated with congenital hepatic fibrosis.[21]

Syndromic Associations of Nephronophthisis

Senior–Loken Syndrome

Senior–Loken syndrome represents the association of NPHP with retinal degeneration. The most severe variants are *Leber congenital amaurosis* (*LCA*) and milder retinopathy *tapetoretinal degeneration*. LCA is a retinal hereditary disorder. It is characterized by profound visual loss in infancy or from birth. There is associated nystagmus, poor pupillary reflexes, retinal atrophy with varying severity, and pigmentary changes. Children demonstrate pressing, poking, and rubbing the eyes with hands to mechanically stimulate the retina (Franceschetti's oculodigital sign). LCA is a disorder of photoreceptors due to loss of outer segments of the receptor and failed transport of rhodopsin. The genes that can be associated with NPHP and retinitis pigmentosa (RP) are *NPHP5 and NPHP6/CEP290*. All patients with SLSN with *NPHP5* mutations were manifested with early severe LCA.[22] Thus, screening for *NPHP5 mutations* is needed if NPHP patients have an early retinal disease. A milder form of retinopathy termed *tapetoretinal degeneration* presents with severe tunnel vision and night blindness. Fundoscopy reveals varying degrees of pigmentary and atrophic retinopathy.

Joubert Syndrome

Originally described in 1968, Joubert syndrome is characterized by muscular hypotonia in the neonatal period evolving into cerebellar ataxia and psychomotor retardation often associated with intellectual disability, abnormal eye movements such as oculomotor apraxia, rotating nystagmus, head thrusting, and hyperpnea or apnea in infancy. The incidence is around

1:100,000 and has an autosomal recessive inheritance. The most frequent genes that have been identified are *AHI1*, *RPGRIP1L*, and *CC2DA2*, each explaining about 10% of cases.[23,24] Several phenotypes of Joubert syndrome present as neurological signs with multiorgan involvement of the kidneys, retina, liver, and skeleton system. Affected individuals have dysmorphic facies with hypertelorism, a broad forehead, and ptosis. The malformation of the midbrain and hindbrain visible as "molar tooth sign" in MRI brain is pathognomonic of this condition. Regular screening for chronic renal failure is mandatory since approximately 25% of patients with Joubert syndrome-related disease (JSRD) have associated renal disease. The patients develop CKD-5G by the end of the second decade.

Due to clinical and genetic overlap, it may be hard to differentiate Joubert syndrome from other ciliopathies such as MKS. Respiratory and feeding problems need special attention during the neonatal period and infancy. Long-term management is based on the associated organ involvement. The severity of breathing dysregulation in the neonatal period and the extent and severity of renal and hepatic involvement in later life predict the prognosis. Hepatic disease is the major cause of death in Joubert syndrome. Prenatal diagnosis is feasible in families with an identified mutation in the proband.

COACH Syndrome

The acronym COACH stands for cerebellar vermis hypoplasia, oligophrenia, cognitive dysfunction, congenital ataxia, coloboma, and congenital hepatic fibrosis. It is a rare autosomal-recessive disorder that shows substantial overlap with Joubert syndrome. Obligatory liver involvement is the pathognomonic feature, and it may lead to hepatic fibrosis due to malformation of the embryonic ductal plate. Mutations in *MKS3/TMEM67* were identified in 83% of patients with COACH syndrome.[25]

Meckel–Gruber Syndrome

Meckel–Gruber syndrome is a lethal neonatal disorder and affects multiple organ systems. It has autosomal-recessive inheritance with incidence ranging from 1/13,500 to 1/140,000 live births. Typical clinical manifestations are bilateral cystic kidney dysplasia, occipital encephalocele, hepatobiliary ductal plate malformation, and postaxial polydactyly.[26] Associated malformations comprise severe malformations of the central nervous system, cleft palate, microphthalmia, hydrocephalus, developmental disorders of genitalia and skeletal deformities, severe cardiac anomalies, pulmonary hypoplasia, situs inversus, and facial dysmorphism. Prenatal diagnosis is done by documenting the combination of occipital encephalocele and polydactyly by antenatal ultrasonography and increased levels of α-fetoprotein in amniotic fluid by amniocentesis. Enlisted in **Table 1** are several gene mutations responsible for MKS and similar phenotypes. Recent evidence from genetic studies has suggested that severe truncating mutations cause MKS and milder, nontruncating mutations manifest as Joubert syndrome. The defects in various organ systems in MKS are developmental defects whereas defects are of degenerative nature in NPHP and SLSN.

Congenital Oculomotor Apraxia Cogan Type 2

Clinical manifestations include impairment of horizontal voluntary eye movements, ocular attraction movements, and optokinetic nystagmus, which is usually compensated by jerky head movements. It is a nonprogressive disease and can improve with age.[27] Since there is an increased risk of progression to chronic renal failure, it is mandatory to monitor renal function at regular intervals.

Bardet–Biedl Syndrome

This disorder was initially described by Bardet in 1920 and Biedl in 1922. It is a rare multisystem developmental disorder with obesity, polydactyly, hypogonadism, renal dysfunction, retinal defects, and learning disabilities. Supplementary features include developmental delay, behavioral problems, hearing loss, anosmia, diabetes, hypertension, hypogonadism, and cardiovascular defect. The diagnostic criterion which was modified by Beales et al. in 1999 is given in **Table 3.**[28] Renal involvement with polydactyly suggests the diagnosis at birth or in utero. Enlarged hyperechogenic kidneys and loss of corticomedullary differentiation, with or without macrocysts as in PKD, are the renal anomalies seen in Bardet–Biedl syndrome (BBS). Polyuria is the earliest symptom in childhood. CKD develops in 25% of patients by the fifth decade, while 10% developed CKD-G5 in childhood or adolescence.

Electroretinogram, visually evoked responses, renal ultrasound, renal radionuclide scans, electrocardiogram, and

TABLE 3: Diagnostic criteria for Bardet–Biedl syndrome (BBS).

Four primary or three primary plus two secondary features are required for diagnosis of BBS:

Primary features	*Secondary features*
• Rod-cone dystrophy • Postaxial polydactyly • Truncal obesity • Learning disabilities • Hypogenitalism and undescended testis in males • Irregular menstrual cycles in females • Renal anomalies	Speech disorders, developmental delay, and behavior problems, ataxia/poor coordination/imbalance, other ocular anomalies (strabismus, cataracts, astigmatism, optic atrophy, color blindness, macular edema, and degeneration), facial features, anosmia, dental anomalies such as high-arched palate, hearing loss, brachydactyly, syndactyly, congenital heart disease (aortic fibrosis, patent ductus arteriosus, and cardiomyopathy), left ventricular hypertrophy, situs inversus, hepatic fibrosis, polyuria/polydipsia, diabetes mellitus, and Hirschsprung syndrome

Source: Beales PL, Elcioglu N, Woolf AS, Parker D, Flinter FA. New criteria for improved diagnosis of Bardet-Biedl syndrome: results of a population survey. J Med Genet. 1999;36(6):437-46.

echocardiogram need to be done in suspected cases. When the diagnosis is confirmed clinically, molecular diagnosis is done followed by appropriate genetic counseling of the family.

Alström Syndrome

Alström syndrome is an autosomal-recessive disorder that is phenotypically similar to BBS. It was first described in 1959. The characteristic features are obesity, hypogonadism, retinal dystrophy, sensorineural hearing loss, diabetes mellitus, hypothyroidism, hyperlipidemia, and slowly progressive tubule interstitial nephropathy. Dilated cardiomyopathy, progressive pulmonary, and hepatic failure are the other associations. In contrast to patients with BBS who are often mentally retarded, majority with Alström syndrome have normal intelligence. The causative mutation is *ALMS1* located on chromosome 2p13 which encodes for ALMS1 protein that localizes to centrosomes and base of cilia. Confirmation of the genetic diagnosis is possible with sequence analysis of the *ALMS1* gene.

Jeune Asphyxiating Thoracic Dystrophy

Jeune et al. first described Jeune asphyxiating thoracic dystrophy (JATD) in 1954. It has autosomal recessive disease inheritance, characterized by a narrow thoracic cage and short-limbed dwarfism. Types of JATD include lethal, major, minor, and latent forms. Short rib polydactyly syndromes are characterized by perinatal lethality due to respiratory insufficiency secondary to short ribs and narrow chest, which in turn restrict the growth and expansion of the lungs. Further associations are short long bones, polydactyly, trident acetabular roof, and RP.[29]

Diagnosis

It is mandatory to consider the diagnosis of NPHP in any child presenting with polyuria, low specific gravity and osmolality of urine with bland urine sediment, mild or absent proteinuria, progressive renal failure with normal blood pressure, and an ultrasound picture of normal to small kidneys with hyperechogenicity, loss of corticomedullary differentiation, with or without corticomedullary cysts. Routine retinal assessment and additional electroretinography and electro-oculography are done to evaluate the presence and severity of RP. Neurological symptoms warrant MRI to assess the cerebellum. Liver function tests and sonography are useful in ruling out hepatic fibrosis. MRI or computed tomography can also demonstrate medullary cysts in the kidneys. Genetic testing, if possible, negates the need for renal biopsy. Age at presentation and the extrarenal manifestations will be a useful guide for the screening of specific gene mutations.

Differential Diagnosis

Disorders other than NPHP that present with CKD and bland urine sediment are renal dysplasia, PKD, obstructive uropathy, and medullary sponge kidney. Renal imaging can differentiate among these diagnoses.

Treatment

Nephronophthisis-associated ciliopathies have no specific therapy to date. Correction of water and electrolyte imbalances by replacing the ongoing salt and water loss to prevent hypovolemia is the main goal of treatment in children who have no renal impairment. Special attention is needed, especially during periods of intercurrent illnesses. Supportive therapy includes treatment of anemia and nutritional support to promote normal growth. The prognosis depends upon the age of presentation and associated extrarenal manifestations.

Recently, there have been some developments to decrease the progression of cysts in mouse models of NPHP and PKD, which include vasopressin V2 receptor antagonist (tolvaptan), mammalian target of rapamycin (mTOR) inhibitor (rapamycin), and roscovitine.

In advanced CKD, treatment includes erythropoietin, iron supplementation, and management of the metabolic bone disease. Kidney replacement therapy is planned with advanced stages of CKD. Renal transplantation is the definitive therapy of choice in patients with NPHP as recurrence of the primary disease is negligible and prognosis is excellent.

Genetic Counseling

Once the NPHP-related pathogenic variants have been identified in an affected family member, preimplantation genetic testing and prenatal testing for NPHP are possible. Genetic testing is also advised for living-related donor screening. Siblings have a 25% chance of being affected and hence should be kept under follow-up to monitor urinary concentrating ability and renal echogenicity. This prevents the complications such as electrolyte imbalance, dehydration, anemia, and growth retardation, which may be attributed to nonrenal conditions.

AUTOSOMAL-DOMINANT TUBULOINTERSTITIAL KIDNEY DISEASE

Introduction

Autosomal-dominant tubulointerstitial kidney disease (ADTKD) is an uncommon genetic disorder of autosomal-dominant inheritance characterized by a progressive decline in kidney function. ADTKD was previously termed "medullary cystic kidney disease (MCKD)". The term MCKD is a misnomer since medullary cysts are not an obligatory feature of ADTKD.

Currently, the categorization of ADTKD rests upon the underlying genetic mutation, leading to subtypes according to Kidney Disease: Improving Global Outcomes (KDIGO) consensus report that provides standard terminology for these conditions:[30]

- *ADTKD-UMOD:* Mutation in the *UMOD* gene encoding uromodulin (Tamm-Horsfall protein) is the most common subtype of ADTKD. It had been previously referred to as MCKD2 (medullary cystic kidney disease type 2), FJHN (familial juvenile hyperuricemic nephropathy), hereditary nephropathy associated with hyperuricemia and gout, UKD (uromodulin kidney disease), and glomerulocystic kidney disease.[31]

- *ADTKD-MUC1:* Mutations in the *MUC1* gene encoding mucin. This category was referred to as MCKD1 (medullary cystic kidney disease type 1) or mucin-1 kidney disease (MKD) in the past literature.[32]
- *ADTKD-REN:* Mutations in the *REN* gene encoding renin is the least common cause of ADTKD, but they are also the most distinctive. It is the only ADTKD subtype for which a specific treatment is available, and the clinical manifestations resemble other low-renin states. It has also been referred to in the past as FJHN2 (familial juvenile hyperuricemic nephropathy type 2).[33]
- *ADTKD-HNF1B:* Mutations in the *HNF1B* (hepatocyte nuclear factor-1-β) gene were referred to in the past as Maturity Onset Diabetes of the Young type 5 (MODY5) and renal cyst and diabetes syndrome (RCAD).[34]
- *ADKT-NOS:* ADTKD patients with no mutations.

ADTKD should be suspected when a parent and a child both have CKD with bland urinary sediment and absent or minimal proteinuria.

Epidemiology

It is a rare disease. Probably under-reporting contributes to the low estimated prevalence. ADTKD has no gender predilection. There are approximately 500 families in the United States classified as ADTKD and the prevalence is unknown in low- and middle-income countries.

Genetics

There are three known major genetic causes of ADTKD, each of which has distinguishing features as enumerated in **Table 4:**[35]

1. *ADTKD-UMOD (ADTKD due to UMOD mutations): UMOD* gene is located on chromosome 16p12 and encodes for uromodulin. It is autosomal dominant and the majority of patients have a mutation in exon 3, 4, or 5 and few have mutations in other exons. In addition, there are certain polymorphisms in the *UMOD* gene associated with an increased risk of CKD in the general population. Missense mutations due to deletion or addition of a cysteine residue are identified in more than 50% of the *UMOD* gene mutations. In addition to progressive CKD, it is characterized by gout occurring by the teenage years.[36]
2. *ADTKD-MUC1 (ADTKD due to MUC1 mutations):* Also known as MKD, it occurs due to mutations in the *MUC1* gene situated on chromosome 1q21 and encodes for mucin-1. It accounts for approximately 30% of ADTKD. A single cytosine insertion into a variable-number tandem repeat sequence resulting in an abnormal mucin-1 protein is the most common mutation within the *MUC1* coding region. Mucin-1 protein localizes intracellularly in the loop of Henle, distal convoluted tubule, and cortical collecting duct.[37] It is associated with progressive CKD but no other distinguishing characteristics such as precocious gout, childhood anemia, hypotension, or hyperkalemia.
3. *ADTKD-REN (ADTKD due to REN mutations): REN* gene located on chromosome 1 encodes for renin, produces progressive CKD, low- or low-normal blood pressures, anemia that occurs in childhood before the onset of CKD, mild hyperkalemia, and hyperuricemia. This is a less common subtype, accounting for approximately 5% of families with ADTKD.[38]
4. *ADTKD-HNF1B (ADTKD due to HNF1B mutation):* HNF1b is a large group of transcription factors that control many genes expressed in the pancreas, liver, intestines, kidney, genitourinary tract, and lungs. It seems to have a role in their development. *HNF1b* is considered to regulate the *UMOD* gene.

Pathogenesis

ADTKD-UMOD: Uromodulin is produced exclusively in the ascending thick limb of Henle's loop and is the most abundant protein in human urine. It is an insoluble protein and has a role in maintaining the thick ascending limb impermeable to water. Uromodulin also appears to facilitate the intracellular trafficking of both the sodium potassium chloride cotransporter 2 and the renal outer medullary potassium channel to the apical surface of the tubular cells in the thick segment of the ascending limb. Tubular cell atrophy and death occur due to the accumulation of abnormal uromodulin proteins within the cells of the ascending thick limb of Henle's loop. This leads to a decreased number of mitochondria as well as dysregulation in thick ascending limb cells. There is a marked reduction in urinary uromodulin excretion.[39]

The two major pathophysiologic effects of *UMOD* mutations are (1) hyperuricemia and (2) progressive CKD:

1. Hyperuricemia results from reduced fractional excretion of uric acid (FEUA). Uromodulin facilitates the intracellular trafficking of the furosemide-sensitive Na–K–2Cl cotransporter to the apical membrane of the thick ascending limb. Hence, the decreased production of uromodulin leads to a decreased apical expression of the Na–K–2Cl cotransporter, resulting in mild natriuresis. The resultant sodium wasting and volume contraction cause compensatory proximal tubular sodium reabsorption restoring volume status to normal but results in a secondary increase in proximal urate reabsorption.
2. Intracellular accumulation of abnormal uromodulin results in tubular cell death in the thick part of the ascending limb and progressive CKD.[40]

ADTKD-MUC1: The pathophysiology of the renal findings in patients with ADTKD-MUC1 is poorly understood. Though mucin-1 is produced in the skin, breast, gastrointestinal tract,

TABLE 4: Types of autosomal dominant tubulointerstitial kidney disease (ADTKD) (medullary cystic kidney disease) and their distinguishing features.[35]

Characteristic	ADTKD due to UMOD mutations (ADTKD-UMOD)	ADTKD due to MUC1 mutations (ADTKD-MUC1)	ADTKD due to REN mutations (ADTKD-REN)
Inheritance	Autosomal dominant	Autosomal dominant	Autosomal dominant
Chromosome	Chromosome 16p12	Chromosome 1q21	Chromosome 1
Urinalysis results	Bland without protein	Bland without protein	Bland without protein
Renal ultrasound	Normal (50%) or small kidneys, corticomedullary cysts (40%), increased echogenicity (10%)	Normal (50%) or small kidneys, corticomedullary cysts (40%)	Normal or small kidneys, occasional or no cysts
Age of ESKD (years)	20–70 years Median 52 years	5–76 years Median 32 years	40–80 years Median 57 years
Kidney biopsy	Interstitial fibrosis, tubular atrophy	Interstitial fibrosis, tubular atrophy	Interstitial fibrosis, tubular atrophy
Definitive diagnosis	Genetic analysis	Genetic analysis	Genetic analysis
Associated findings	Reduced uromodulin excretion FEUA < 6%	Anemia Salt wasting	Low- or low–normal blood pressure, hyperuricemia, anemia in childhood, mild hyperkalemia Reduced uromodulin excretion
Hypertension	50%	50%	Late, secondary to CKD
Gout	Hyperuricemia: 75% Gout: 65% Juvenile-onset gout at 6–20 years	Hyperuricemia: 40% Gout: 65% Adult-onset gout at 34–66 years	Variable
Treatment	No specific treatment Allopurinol for gout	No specific treatment	High-sodium diet or fludrocortisone
Frequency	Rare	Rare	Very rare
Other names	UKD (uromodulin kidney disease) MCKD2 (medullary cystic kidney disease type 2) FJHN (familial Juvenile hyperuricemic nephropathy)	MKD (mucin-1 kidney disease) MCKD1 (medullary cystic kidney disease type 1)	FJHN2 (familial juvenile hyperuricemic nephropathy type 2) MCKD1 (medullary cystic kidney disease type 1)

(CKD: chronic kidney disease; ESKD: end-stage kidney disease; FEUA: fractional excretion of uric acid)

and respiratory system, it is unclear why the phenotype is manifested only in the kidney.

ADTKD-REN: Renin is expressed in multiple segments of the renal tubule, including the juxtaglomerular complex. Intracellularly, preprorenin is translocated into the endoplasmic reticulum (ER) and converted to prorenin. After secreting some prorenin, the remainder is targeted to lysozymes, where it is further cleaved to active renin. Mutations may affect the segment of the gene encoding the promoter, prosegment, or mature renin peptide.[41]

- Mutations in promoter gene—prevent translocation across the ER.
- Mutations in *REN* prosegment—prevent proper folding of prorenin.
- Mutations in the mature renin peptide—result in deposition of the mutated renin in the ER.

Plasma renin levels in affected patients are low due to decreased production of renin. The low renin, low aldosterone state produces characteristic clinical findings. Intracellular accumulation of preprorenin in renal tubular cells results in ultrastructural damage and apoptosis of renal tubular cells progressing to CKD.

Pathology

The histopathologic features are similar to NPHP. The characteristic tubulointerstitial disease consists of the triad of TBM disintegration with thickening, and attenuation, interstitial infiltration with round cells, and marked interstitial fibrosis with atrophy and ectasia of tubules.[15]

Clinical Features

Autosomal dominant tubulointerstitial kidney disease is characterized by the following features:

- Autosomal-dominant pattern of inheritance
- Slowly progressive renal failure (onset of renal dysfunction in adolescence, but highly variable CKD-G5 onset, between the ages of 20 and 70 years)
- Absence of significant hypertension during early stages of the disease
- Due to loss of renal concentration ability, there is nocturia or enuresis

TABLE 5: Distinguishing features of nephronophthisis (NPHP) and autosomal dominant tubulointerstitial kidney disease (ADTKD).

Distinguishing features	***Nephronophthisis***	***Autosomal-dominant tubulointerstitial kidney disease***
Inheritance	Autosomal recessive	Autosomal dominant
Inherited genes	*NPHP* genes	*UMOD, MUC1, REN, and SEC61A1 genes*
Median onset of CKD-G5	Juvenile *NPHP1:* 13 years Infantile *NPHP2:* 1–3 years Adolescent *NPHP3:* 19 years	ADTKD-*UMOD*: 20–70 years ADTKD-*MUC1*: 20–70 years ADTKD-*REN:* 40–80 years
Extrarenal associations	20% Ophthalmological, neurological, hepatic, skeletal, cardiovascular	Hyperuricemia, gout
Radiological features	Small or normal-sized hyperechogenic kidneys and corticomedullary cyst *Infantile NPHP:* Enlarged kidneys	Small or normal-sized hyperechogenic kidneys and corticomedullary cyst

- A bland urine sediment with nil or minimal proteinuria
- Kidney ultrasound reveals normal kidney size with increased echogenicity in early stage and bilateral shrunken echogenic kidneys as CKD progresses.

UMOD Mutations

Patients have juvenile onset of hyperuricemia, gout, and progressive kidney failure. In a series of 205 patients, 75% of patients had hyperuricemia and 65% had gout. 70% progressed to CKD. 80% of the subjects progressed to CKD-G5 between the ages of 20 and 70 years.[42] The homozygous individuals survived up to adulthood and presented with an earlier onset of hyperuricemia and faster progression to CKD-G5 when compared to heterozygous individuals. Urinary concentrating defects are common and present as persistent enuresis.

MUC1 Mutations

MUC1 mutations present with the predominant symptom of slowly progressive renal failure when compared to *UMOD* or *REN* gene mutations. Hyperuricemia and gout develop late in the course of the disease. The mean age of progression to CKD-G5 is 54 years with the age range between 36 and 80 years. 51% were hypertensive during the course of illness.

REN Mutations

Presentation of patients with *REN* gene mutations is similar to patients with *UMOD* mutations with the development of CKD and early onset gout. Patients with *REN* mutations have late-onset gout for around 20–30 years.[37] Their progression to CKD-G5 is slower and develops after the age of 40 years. *REN* mutations result in additional symptoms such as hypotension and mild hyperkalemia, caused by hyporeninism and an increased risk of acute kidney injury in the setting of volume depletion unlike patients with *UMOD* mutation. Anemia is a feature in early childhood.

Diagnosis

Autosomal dominant tubulointerstitial kidney disease is suspected in a child with CKD having a strong family history of renal disease or gout, bland urine sediment, and no proteinuria.[29] A low FEUA supports the diagnosis. Though cysts are seen at times on ultrasound, they are not an essential requirement for the diagnosis. Medullary cysts are evident on CT, intravenous pyelogram (IVP), or MRI. Renal biopsy findings are nonspecific. The diagnosis is confirmed with a mutational analysis of the *UMOD* gene and a definitive diagnosis is ascertained by linkage analysis.

Although the clinical and histological presentation may show a significant overlap of ADTKD with NPHP, the some contrasting features of the two disorders are given in **Table 5**.

Treatment

As in NPHP, no specific therapy is available for ADTKD. Symptomatic treatment includes the management of hyperuricemia and progressive renal failure. Hyperuricemia is treated with a xanthine oxidase inhibitor. CKD-G5 necessitates kidney replacement therapy. Kidney transplantation is the therapy of choice since it does not recur in recipients after transplantation. Relatives of patients with *UMOD*, *REN*, or *MUC1* mutations should ideally undertake genetic workup as part of screening before living-related donation.

CONCLUSION

Nephronophthisis is a group of tubulointerstitial cystic kidney disease with AR inheritance whereas ADTKD is a rare genetic disorder characterized by AD pattern of inheritance. Both are characterized by nocturia due to impairment of urinary concentrating ability, bland urine sediment with nil or minimal proteinuria, and insidious onset of renal insufficiency.

Although the clinical and histological presentation may show a significant overlap of ADTKD with NPHP, there are some contrasting features of the two disorders which have been summarized in the chapter.

KEY POINTS

- Based on the age of onset of CKD-G5, NPHP is described as infantile, juvenile, and adolescent types.

- The most common mutation is homozygous deletions of the *NPHP1* gene encoding for nephrocystin-1.
- Juvenile variant is the most common type of NPHP.
- Around 20% of patients with NPHP have associated extrarenal involvement.
- NPHP-associated ciliopathies have no specific therapy to date apart from volume and electrolyte replacement and supportive care in CKD.
- ADTKD is suspected in any child with CKD having a strong family history of renal disease or gout, bland urine sediment, and no proteinuria.
- Patients with *UMOD* mutations have juvenile onset of hyperuricemia, gout, and progressive kidney failure.
- Specific treatment is available for ADTKD-REN subtype.
- Diagnosis is confirmed with a mutational analysis and a definitive diagnosis is ascertained by linkage analysis.
- Kidney transplantation is the treatment of choice in CKD-G5.

REFERENCES

1. Bleyer AJ, Hart PS, Kmoch S. Hereditary interstitial kidney disease. Semin Nephrol. 2010;30:366.
2. Levy M, Feingold J. Estimating prevalence in single-gene kidney diseases progressing to renal failure. Kidney Int. 2000;58:925.
3. Smith C, Graham J. Congenital medullary cysts of kidneys with severe refractory anemia. Am J Dis Child. 1945;69:369-77.
4. Fanconi G, Hanhart E, von Albertini A, Uhlinger E, Dolivo G, Prader A. Die familiäre juvenile nephronophthisis. Helv Paediatr Acta. 1951;6:1-49.
5. Srivastava S, Molinari E, Raman S, Sayer JA. Many Genes-One Disease? Genetics of Nephronophthisis (NPHP) and NPHP-Associated Disorders. Front Pediatrics. 2017;5:287.
6. Chaki M, Hoefele J, Allen SJ, Ramaswami G, Janssen S, Bergmann C, et al. Genotype-phenotype correlation in 440 patients with NPHP-related ciliopathies. Kidney Int. 2011;80:1239.
7. Halbritter J, Porath JD, Diaz KA, Braun DA, Kohl S, Chaki M, et al. Identification of 99 novel mutations in a worldwide cohort of 1,056 patients with a nephronophthisis-related ciliopathy. Hum Genet. 2013;132:865.
8. Hildebrandt F, Rensing C, Betz R, Sommer U, Birnbaum S, Imm A, et al. Establishing an algorithm for molecular genetic diagnostics in 127 families with juvenile nephronophthisis. Kidney Int. 2001;59:434-45.
9. Snoek R, van Setten J, Keating BJ, Israni AK, Jacobson PA, Oetting WS, et al. NPHP1 (Nephrocystin-1) Gene Deletions Cause Adult-Onset ESRD. J Am Soc Nephrol. 2018;29:1772-9.
10. Konrad M, Saunier S, Heidet L, Silbermann F, Benessy F, Calado J, et al. Large homozygous deletions of the 2q13 region is a major cause of juvenile nephronophthisis. Hum Mol Genet. 1996;5:367-71.
11. Badano JL, Teslovich TM, Katsanis N. The centrosome in human genetic disease. Nat Rev Genet. 2005;6:194-205.
12. Hildebrandt F, Otto E. Cilia and centrosomes: a unifying pathogenic concept for cystic kidney disease? Nat Rev Genet. 2005;6:928-4.
13. Watnick T, Germino G. From cilia to cyst. Nat Genet. 2003;34:355.
14. Bergmann C. Educational paper: ciliopathies. Eur J Pediatr. 2012;171(9):1285-300.
15. Hildebrandt F, Attanasio M, Otto E. Nephronophthisis: disease mechanisms of a ciliopathy. J Am Soc Nephrol. 2009;20:23.
16. Braun DA, Hildebrandt F. Ciliopathies. Cold Spring Harb Perspect Biol. 2017;9(3):a028191.
17. Zollinger HU, Mihatsch MJ, Edefonti A, Gaboardi F, Imbasciati E, Lennert T. Nephronophthisis (medullary cystic disease of the kidney). A study using electron microscopy, immunofluorescence, and a review of the morphological findings. Helv Paediatr Acta. 1980;35:509.
18. Blowey DL, Querfeld U, Geary D, Warady BA, Alon A. Ultrasound findings in juvenile nephronophthisis. Pediatr Nephrol. 1996;10:22-4.
19. Luo F, Tao YH. Nephronophthisis: A review of genotype-phenotype correlation. Nephrology (Carlton). 2018;23(10): 904-11.
20. Tory K, Rousset- Rouvière C, Gubler MC, Morinière V, Pawtowski A, Becker C, et al. Mutations of NPHP2 and NPHP3 in infantile nephronophthisis. Kidney Int. 2009;75:839.
21. König J, Omran BE, Omran H. Nephronophthisis and autosomal dominant interstitial kidney disease (ADIKD). In: Geary DF, Schaefer F (Eds). Pediatric Kidney Disease, 2nd edition. Heidelberg: Springer-Verlag; 2016. pp. 369-88.
22. Omran H, Sasmaz G, Häffner K, Volz A, Olbrich H, Melkaoui R, et al. Identification of a gene locus for Senior-Løken syndrome in the region of the nephronophthisis type 3 gene. J Am Soc Nephrol. 2002;13:75.
23. Parisi MA, Bennett CL, Eckert ML, Dobyns WB, Gleeson JG, Shaw DWW, et al. The NPHP1 gene deletion associated with juvenile nephronophthisis is present in a subset of individuals with Joubert syndrome. Am J Hum Genet. 2004;75:82.
24. Tory K, Lacoste T, Burglen L, Morinière V, Boddaert N, Macher MA, et al. High NPHP1 and NPHP6 mutation rate in patients with Joubert's syndrome and nephronophthisis: potential epistatic effects of NPHP6 and AHI1 mutations in patients with NPHP1 mutations. J Am Soc Nephrol. 2007;18:1566-75.
25. Doherty D, Parisi MA, Finn LS, Gunay-Aygun M, Al-Mateen M, Bates D, et al. Mutations in 3 genes (MKS3, CC2D2A, and RPGRIP1L) cause COACH syndrome (Joubert syndrome with congenital hepatic fibrosis). J Med Genet. 2010;47(1):8-21.
26. Alexiev BA, Lin X, Sun CC, Brenner DS. Meckel-Gruber syndrome: pathologic manifestations, minimal diagnostic criteria, and differential diagnosis. Arch Pathol Lab Med. 2006;130(8):1236-8.
27. Betz R, Rensing C, Otto E, Mincheva A, Zehnder D, Lichter P, et al. Children with ocular motor apraxia type Cogan carry deletions in the gene NPHP1 for juvenile nephronophthisis. J Pediatr. 2000;136:828-31.
28. Beales PL, Elcioglu N, Woolf AS, Parker D, Flinter FA. New criteria for improved diagnosis of Bardet-Biedl syndrome: results of a population survey. J Med Genet. 1999;36(6):437-46.
29. Halbritter J, Bizet AA, Schmidts M, Porath JD, Braun DA, Gee HY, et al. Defects in the IFT-B component IFT 172 cause Jeune and Mainzer-Saldino syndromes in humans. Am J Hum Genet. 2013;93:915-25.
30. Eckardt KU, Alper SL, Antignac C, Bleyer AJ, Chauveau D, Dahan K, et al. Autosomal dominant tubulointerstitial kidney disease: diagnosis, classification and management-A KDIGO consensus report. Kidney Int. 2015;88:676-83.
31. Hart TC, Gorry MC, Hart PS, Woodard AS, Shihabi Z, Sandhu J, et al. Mutations of the UMOD gene are responsible for medullary cystic kidney disease 2 and familial juvenile hyperuricaemic nephropathy. J Med Genet. 2002;39(12):882-92.

32. Kirby A, Gnirke A, Jaffe DB, Barešová V, Pochet N, Blumenstiel B, et al. Mutations causing medullary cystic kidney disease type1 lie in a large VNTR in MUC1 missed massive parallel sequencing. Nat Genet. 2013;45:299-303.
33. Bleyer AJ, Zivná M, Hulková H, Hodanová K, Vyletal P, Sikora J, et al. Clinical and molecular characterization of a family with a dominant renin gene mutation and response to treatment with fludrocortisone. Clin Nephrol. 2010;74:411-22.
34. Verhave JC, Bech AP, Wetzels JF, Nijenhuis T. Hepatocyte nuclear factor 1 β-associated kidney disease: more than renal cysts and diabetes. J Am Soc Nephrol. 2016;27:345-53.
35. Bleyer A, UpToDate, Curhan GC, Perrone RD. (2020). Autosomal dominant tubulointerstitial kidney disease (medullary cystic kidney disease). [online] Available from: https://www.uptodate.com/contents/autosomal-dominant-tubulointerstitial-kidney-disease-medullary-cystic-kidney-disease. [Last accessed October, 2021].
36. Bollée G, Dahan K, Flamant M, Morinière V, Pawtowski A, Heidet L, et al. Phenotype and outcome in hereditary tubulointerstitial nephritis secondary to UMOD mutations. Clin J Am Soc Nephrol. 2011;6:2429-38.
37. Knaup KX, Hackenbeck T, Popp B, Stoeckert J, Wenzel A, Büttner-Herold M, et al. Biallelic expression of mucin-1 in autosomal dominant tubulointerstitial kidney disease: implications for Nongenetic disease recognition. J Am Soc Nephrol. 2018;29(9):2298-309.
38. Živná M, Kidd K, Zaidan M, Vyleťal P, Barešová V, Hodaňová K, et al. An international cohort study of autosomal dominant tubulointerstitial kidney disease due to REN mutations identifies distinct clinical subtypes. Kidney Int. 2020;98:1589-604.
39. Wei X, Xu R, Yang Z, Li Z, Liao Y, Johnson RJ, et al. Novel uromodulin mutation in familial juvenile hyperuricemic nephropathy. Am J Nephrol. 2012;36:114-20.
40. Köttgen A, Hwang SJ, Larson MG, Van Eyk JE, Fu Q, Benjamin EJ, et al. Uromodulin levels associate with a common UMOD variant and risk for incident CKD. J Am Soc Nephrol. 2010;21:337-44.
41. Dzau VJ, Pratt RE, Paul M, Nakamura N. Molecular studies of human renin synthesis and gene expression. Cardiovasc Drugs Ther. 1988;2:459-62.
42. Scolari F, Caridi G, Rampoldi L, Tardanico R, Izzi C, Pirulli D, et al. Uromodulin storage disease: clinical aspects and mechanisms. Am J Kidney Dis. 2004;44:987-99.

CHAPTER

9.4 Glomerulocystic Kidney Disease

Nisha Krishnamurthy, Uma S Ali

INTRODUCTION

Glomerulocystic kidney disease (GCKD) is a rare type of renal cystic disease. Bernstein defined the glomerular cyst as two to three times dilatation of Bowman's space. It was noted to have a frequent association with glomerular tufts, about 5% in random sections on biopsy, identifying the cysts as glomerulocystic. However, the frequency of these capillary tufts decreased as the size of the cysts increased. Rarely, the cysts were associated with tubular dilatation. He had classified them into three groups: (1) nonsyndromic heritable and sporadic type of cystic kidneys in children and adults, (2) GCKD with heritable malformation syndromes, and (3) glomerular cysts in dysplastic kidneys.[1]

ETIOLOGY AND PATHOGENESIS

Renal development is an interaction between metanephric mesenchyme and ureteric bud. The ureteric bud secretes factors that promote epithelial conversion of the mesenchyme, which in turn promotes the branching of the ureteric bud. Together, this leads to the formation of the nephron and the collecting duct system. The genetic cascade involves transcription factors, signaling factors, and factors that promote ureteric branching. Any defects in these genetically determined pathways lead to abnormal nephrogenesis.

Glomerulocystic kidney disease is an anatomically descriptive term that comes under the broader group of renal cystic diseases, which includes polycystic kidney disease, maturity onset diabetes in the young, nephronophthisis, tuberous sclerosis, and such others. The unifying theory in all these cystic diseases of the kidney is that they have a mutation in the genes, whose proteins are expressed in the primary cilia or basal body of the renal tubules. Ciliary proteins include ion channels, signaling proteins, and intraflagellar transport proteins; the disruption of any of these can lead to renal cyst formation.[2] Polycystin-1 (PC1) is a part of signaling pathway, involved in mechanotransduction. PC1 regulates mammalian target of rapamycin (mTOR) and the activators of transcription (STAT6) pathways. The disruption of its function leads to proliferation or renal epithelial cells. Polycystin-2 (PC2), also called transient receptor potential (TRP), with PC1, is involved in ciliary mechanotransduction.

Tuberin, a product of *TSC2* gene, which is mutated in tuberous sclerosis complex (TSC), along with Hamartin, is an important inhibitor of mTOR activity. It has been found that mTOR and STAT6 play a role in repair of renal injury and renal cystic diseases indicating the presence of a repair response mechanism in the renal epithelial cells. The formation of cysts can be due to an abnormal activation of this mechanism, either due to a genetic mutation or as a response to renal injury secondary to renal ischemia or urinary outflow obstruction.[2]

Mouse models show that an abnormality in ciliary proteins such as Glis3, which is a part of cilium-associated signaling pathway, leads to development of renal cystic disease.[3] Similarly, in mice models, the absence of Wwtr1, a binding protein that regulates transcription factor activity, leads to development of renal cysts and eventually end-stage kidney disease (ESKD). These cysts, like the ones in GCKD, are mainly due to dilatation of Bowman's space with atrophy of the glomerular tufts; a few cysts were seen in collecting ducts also.

Hepatocyte nuclear factor (HNF1β) is a transcription factor that regulates gene expression in liver, pancreas, kidneys, and other epithelial organs. Heterozygous autosomal-dominant mutations of this factor present as maturity-onset diabetes of the young type 5 (MODY5) and cystic abnormalities in the kidneys which were initially called the renal cysts and diabetes (RCAD) syndrome. *HNF1β* inhibits the expression of *Pkhd1*, which is in turn associated with autosomal recessive polycystic kidney disease (ARPKD). This contributes to renal cyst formation in those with *HNF1β* defects. In individuals with MODY5, the spectrum of nondiabetic nephropathic renal involvement includes simple cysts, polycystic kidneys, cystic dysplasia, hypoplastic glomerulocystic kidneys, single kidney, oligomeganephronia, and familial juvenile hyperuricemic nephropathy. These individuals progress to ESKD eventually.[4] The features of the *HNF1β* mutation are not only renal cysts and diabetes, but these are multisystemic to include hyperparathyroidism, elevated liver enzymes, pancreatic atrophy, genital malformations, hyperuricemia, hypocalciuria, renal magnesium wasting, and autism due to the presence of this transcription factor in various organs.[5]

Genes such as *UMOD*, *PKHD1*, and *PKD2* are associated with renal cystic diseases such as multicystic dysplastic kidneys, ARPKD, and autosomal dominant polycystic kidney disease (ADPKD), respectively. It has been shown that HNF1β directly controls the expression of these genes in the tubular epithelial cells.[6]

Glomerulocystic kidney disease is known to be associated with renal dysplasia, which in turn is associated with urinary tract malformations. Cysts in dysplastic kidneys may arise from glomeruli or collecting ducts. These cysts express *PAX2* with persistence of fetal gene patterns. In an ovine model, unilateral obstruction of ureter at a certain developmental stage showed subsequent GCKD, pelvic, and ureteral dilatation on that side.[7] Unilateral ureteral obstruction causes cilium lengthening in the parietal epithelial layer of Bowman's capsule, a marker of renal injury, which in turn affects the epithelial differentiation, thus providing a link between cilia structure and GCKD.[8]

CLASSIFICATION

Glomerulocystic kidney disease is categorized into five major groups **(Table 1)**: (1) Familial GCKD, (2) GCKD associated with heritable diseases and genetic malformation syndromes such as ADPKD/ARPKD and tuberous sclerosis, (3) syndromic, nonhereditary GCKD, (4) sporadic GCKD, and (5) acquired GCKD.[9,10]

The familial type of GCKD is usually inherited in an autosomal dominant fashion. It may or may not be associated with a family history of ADPKD.[11] A large number of these cases are seen in the newborns and young children and fewer cases in adolescents and adults. In an unpublished paper by Bernstein, it has been noted that glomerular tufts were seen in the glomerular cysts in some cases of adult polycystic kidneys and autosomal dominant GCKD might have an asymmetrical onset similar to polycystic kidneys, thus relating the two conditions.

TABLE 1: Classification of glomerulocystic diseases.[9,10]

Familial nonsyndromic GCKD	*Autosomal dominant GCKD*
Associated with heritable disease and genetic malformation syndromes	• Cystic renal dysplasia • ADPKD • Maturity-onset diabetes of the young • Cornelia de Lange syndrome • Medullary cystic kidney disease • Meckel–Gruber syndrome • Down's syndrome • Zellweger's cerebral–renal–hepatic syndrome • Tuberous sclerosis • Juvenile nephronophthisis • Orofacial digital syndrome type 1 • Majewski short rib polydactyly syndrome • Jeune's osteodystrophy • Goldstone syndrome
Syndromic non-Mendelian	Trisomy 9, 13, or 18
Sporadic	New mutations
Acquired	Associated with hemolytic uremic syndrome, maternal ingestion of drugs such as Phenacetin

(ADPKD: autosomal dominant polycystic kidney disease; GCKD: glomerulocystic kidney disease)

Glomerulocystic kidney disease is associated with a fair number of inheritable malformation syndromes such as TSC, MODY, Meckel–Gruber syndrome, nephronophthisis, and Down syndrome. In TSC, the kidneys show severe cystic disease with both glomerular and tubular cysts and angiomyolipomas. The *TSC2* and *PKD1* genes are adjacent on chromosome 16p13; hence, a contiguous deletion or mutation can present as a polycystic kidney phenotype.[11] Nephronophthisis with mutation in *NPHP3* gene is associated with GCKD along with situs inversus, polydactyly, preauricular sinus, and malformation in the cardiac and central nervous systems. Mutations in the HNF-1β are associated with MODY and renal cystic disease.

CLINICAL PRESENTATION, INVESTIGATIONS, AND MANAGEMENT

The presentation of GCKD can be as neonatal hypertension, abdominal mass, and rarely as chronic kidney disease. The clinical features of the associated genetic malformation syndromes should prompt a search for renal cystic presentation. On ultrasound imaging, the kidneys may appear enlarged, with increased echogenicity and poor corticomedullary differentiation. In the familial variety of GCKD, the kidneys may be hypoplastic, small, or normal sized. The presence of punctate cortical cysts and sparing of the medullary region help to differentiate from ARPKD. On computed tomography and magnetic resonance imaging, GCKD is identified as multiple cortical cysts. Renal biopsy is the best diagnostic modality for GCKD. Renal biopsy finding in GCKD is dilatation of Bowman's space, with few showing glomerular tufts, glomerular cysts, minor tubular cysts, and presence of rudimentary medullary pyramids suggestive of an abnormal development of renal medulla. Further depending on the association with other conditions, there may be a few added features. In TSC, the glomerular spaces show large, abnormal parietal epithelial cells piled against Bowman's capsule with atypical podocytes in the tufts. The epithelial cells are hyperplastic and hypertrophic. In medullary cystic kidney disease, the biopsy shows Bowman's space enlargement with fibrosis. There may be other features such as outflow obstruction in the urinary tract, findings suggestive of the malformation syndromes such as angiomyolipomas, and other organ involvement that can be identified by the imaging modalities. The management of GCKD includes antihypertensives, care of chronic kidney disease status, and eventual renal transplant.

CONCLUSION

Glomerulocystic kidney disease has varying phenotypic presentations, associated with a wide array of malformation syndromes, inherited syndromes, congenital or acquired renal diseases, all with a common link to a primary ciliary dysfunction. Further insights into the role of genes and proteins in the renal development and cystogenesis will improve the understanding of this relatively rare and intriguing renal cystic disease.

KEY POINTS

- GCKD is a 2–3-fold dilatation of the Bowman's space with presence of glomerular capillary tufts and rarely tubular obstruction and dilatation.
- GCKD is seen in abnormal kidneys, usually hypodysplastic kidneys.
- The affected kidneys are usually enlarged or may be normal sized.
- GCKD may be sporadic in occurrence or may be a part of genetic malformation syndromes or congenital or acquired renal diseases. It may be a part of other cystic diseases as well.
- The feature that helps to differentiate GCKD from autosomal recessive kidney disease is the presence of abnormal medullary pyramids in the latter.
- Regular monitoring of the patients with GCKD is done to identify and manage hypertension as well as chronic kidney disease.

REFERENCES

1. Bernstein J. Glomerulocystic kidney disease—nosological considerations. Pediatr Nephrol. 1993;7(4):464-70.
2. Weimbs T. Polycystic kidney disease and renal injury repair: common pathways, fluid flow, and the function of polycystin-1. Am J Physiol Renal Physiol. 2007;293(5):F1423-32.
3. Kang H, Beak J, Kim Y, Herbert R, Jetten A. Glis3 is associated with primary cilia and Wwtr1/TAZ and implicated in polycystic kidney disease. Mol Cell Biol. 2009;29(10):2556-69.
4. Hiesberger T, Bai Y, Shao X, McNally B, Sinclair A, Tian X, et al. Mutation of hepatocyte nuclear factor-1β inhibits Pkhd1 gene expression and produces renal cysts in mice. J Clin Invest. 2004;113(6):814-25.
5. Verhave J, Bech A, Wetzels J, Nijenhuis T. Hepatocyte nuclear factor 1β-associated kidney disease: more than renal cysts and diabetes. J Am Soc Nephrol. 2015;27(2):345-53.
6. Gresh L, Fischer E, Reimann A, Tanguy M, Garbay S, Shao X, et al. A transcriptional network in polycystic kidney disease. EMBO J. 2004;23(7):1657-68.
7. Attar R, Quinn F, Winyard PJ, Mouriquand PD, Foxall P, Hanson MA, et al. Short-term urinary flow impairment deregulates PAX2 and PCNA expression and cell survival in fetal sheep kidneys. Am J Pathol. 1998;152(5):1225-35.
8. Wang L, Weidenfeld R, Verghese E, Ricardo S, Deane J. Alterations in renal cilium length during transient complete ureteral obstruction in the mouse. J Anat. 2008;213(2):79-85.
9. Sahay M, Gowrishankar S. Glomerulocystic disease. NDT Plus. 2010;3(4):349-50.
10. Gupta K, Vankalakunti M, Sachdeva M. Glomerulocystic kidney disease and its rare associations: an autopsy report of two unrelated cases. Diagn Pathol. 2007;2(1):12.
11. Bissler J, Siroky B, Yin H. Glomerulocystic kidney disease. Pediatr Nephrol. 2010;25(10):2049-59.

SECTION

10

Hypertension

CHAPTER

10.1

Epidemiology of Hypertension in Children

Girish C Bhatt, OP Mishra

INTRODUCTION

The prevalence of hypertension (HTN) in children and adolescents has been increasing over the past two decades, ranging from 1 to 5%.[1-3] About global prevalence of HTN in children, a meta-analysis reported 4% prevalence of HTN among normal-weight children and adolescents <19 years of age.[4] Recent studies and meta-analyses have shown increase in prevalence of HTN in children over the last decade due to increase in prevalence of obesity and sedentary lifestyle.[4,5] Childhood HTN has been correlated with high blood pressure (BP) later in adulthood as well as increased risk of cardiovascular disease (CVD).[6] Moreover, BP trajectory from childhood to young adult has been associated with target organ damage, especially left ventricular mass index (LVMI) and carotid intima-media thickness.[6,7] Also, HTN in childhood may contribute to premature atherosclerosis and subsequently lead to early development of CVD.[8]

DEFINITION AND CLASSIFICATION

Blood pressure classification in children depends upon a normative population distribution curve derived from National Health and Nutrition Examination Survey (NHANES) and other screening studies. The fourth report of normative BP tables was derived from approximately 70,000 healthy children including overweight and obese children, thus increasing the BP threshold upward.[9] The new American Academy of Pediatrics (AAP) normative BP tables are based on approximately 50,000 normal weight children.[10] Moreover, the AAP 2017 guideline has revised the categorization of BP in children and adolescents based on age as given in **Table 1**.

Further, the term "prehypertension" has been replaced by the new term "elevated BP" in new AAP guidelines to be consistent with adult guidelines and to convey importance of early lifestyle modifications to prevent development of HTN.[10]

MEASUREMENT OF BLOOD PRESSURE IN CHILDREN

Annual BP measurement is recommended for healthy children and adolescents ≥3 years of age. However, subgroups of children such as those with obesity, renal disease, diabetes, aortic arch obstruction, or coarctation of aorta and children taking medications known to cause HTN should undergo BP checking at each health facility visit or more frequently. Children <3 years of age with congenital heart disease, recurrent urinary tract infection, urological malformations, solid organ transplant, bone marrow transplant, malignancy, neurofibromatosis, tuberous sclerosis or sickle cell disease (SCD), small-for-gestational age newborns, premature (<32 weeks), very low birth weight babies, and neonates with umbilical arterial catheterization require regular BP monitoring.[10]

The standardized procedure for measurement of office BP in children is as follows:

- The first step is to select a proper sized cuff so that the cuff bladder length should cover 80–100% of the arm circumference. The width of the cuff should encompass at least 40% of the child's arm between acromion and

TABLE 1: Categorization of blood pressure (BP) in children and adolescents based on new American Academy of Pediatrics (AAP) guidelines.[10]

	Age 1 to <13 years	*Age ≥13 years*
Normal BP	Systolic and diastolic BP < 90th percentile	Systolic BP < 120 and diastolic BP < 80 mm Hg
Elevated BP	Systolic and diastolic BP ≥ 90th percentile to <95th percentile or 120/80 mm Hg to <95th percentile (whichever is lower)	Systolic BP 120–129 and diastolic BP < 80 mm Hg
Stage 1 HTN	Systolic and diastolic BP ≥ 95th to <95th percentile + 12 mm Hg, *or* 130/80–139/89 mm Hg (whichever is lower)	130/80–139/89 mm Hg
Stage 2 HTN	Systolic and diastolic BP ≥ 95th percentile + 12 mm Hg, *or* ≥140/90 mm Hg (whichever is lower)	≥140/90 mm Hg

(HTN: hypertension)

olecranon placed 2-3 cm above the antecubital fossa with the middle portion of the cuff at the brachial artery (**Figure 1**: Recommended cuff bladder length and cuff bladder width for measurement of BP in children).

- Child should be seated for 5 minutes in a quiet room with uncrossed legs and should not speak.
- BP should be measured in right arm at the level of heart with the child seating comfortably. Right arm is preferred for measurement of BP in children as normative reference data is generated from right arm and for consistency. In addition, the possibility of coarctation of the aorta would lead to falsely low BP readings in the left arm.
- For auscultatory BP, the cuff should be inflated 20-30 mm Hg above the point at which radial pulse disappears. The cuff should be deflated at a rate of 2-3 mm Hg and the first (Korotkoff phase I) and the last (phase V Korotkoff) audible sound should be taken as systolic BP and diastolic BP, respectively. In children, sometimes the Korotkoff sound phase V is heard at 0, repeat measurement is required with less pressure applied on the brachial artery, or the point where the muffling of sound has occurred is taken as diastolic BP.
- The documentation of BP readings should include the following: systolic BP, diastolic BP, location (e.g., right or left arm), status of the child (crying or calm), size of the cuff, and method of measurement (auscultatory or oscillometer).

The auscultatory method is the preferred method of BP measurement in children as the normative data being used were obtained by using a mercury sphygmomanometer.[10] As a mercury sphygmomanometer is no longer available, aneroid devices are appropriate substitute if they are calibrated regularly.[11] An oscillometric device may be used for the initial screening method due to its ease of use and decrease in observer bias. However, BP measured with the oscillometric device is usually higher than that obtained by auscultation.[12] Thus, any elevated BP recorded with an oscillometric device should be confirmed by auscultation. In such cases, two additional readings should be taken in the same visit and its average taken to categorize BP of child. HTN should be diagnosed based on the office readings on *three* separate visits. A BP device validated for pediatric population should be used for measurement purpose. The list of validated devices is available at: *http://www.dableducational.org/*.

CIRCADIAN BLOOD PRESSURE REGULATION

Both systolic and diastolic BP follow circadian rhythm, i.e., BP dips at night during rest, undergoes a steep increase in the morning (known as morning surge), and peaks in the late afternoon. In a healthy person, there is a nocturnal dip of 10-20% during night time [**Figure 2:** Normal nocturnal dipping (highlighted by solid arrow and gray shaded area)

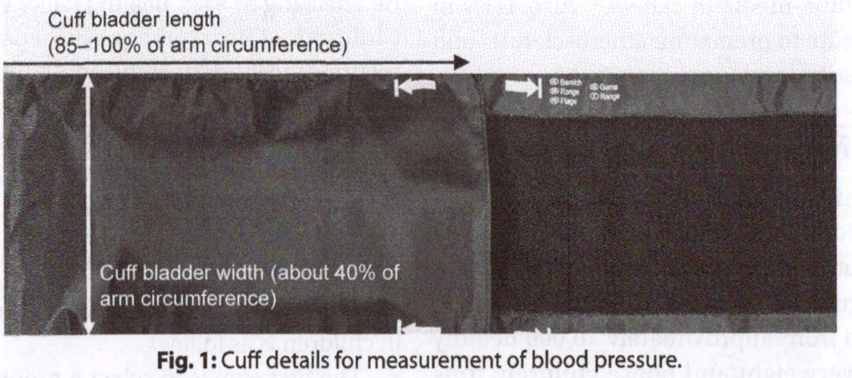

Fig. 1: Cuff details for measurement of blood pressure.

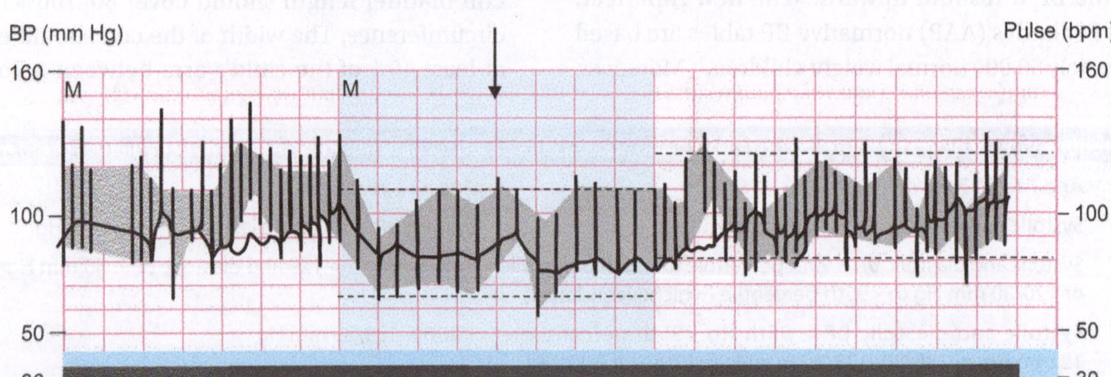

Fig. 2: Nocturnal dip depicted through ambulatory blood pressure monitoring.

in a child undergoing 24 hours ambulatory monitoring]. Nondippers are classified as having impaired dipping of <10% change in resting BP. The underlying mechanisms of nondipping are unknown, but intrinsic kidney defects, sleep apnea, and melatonin deficiency are implicated as contributory factors.[13] Nondipping may contribute to heart failure and other cardiovascular complications independent of the degree of HTN.[14]

EPIDEMIOLOGY

Primary HTN: In recent years, an increase in primary HTN in children and adolescents has been reported. The factors associated with essential childhood HTN are obesity, genetic predisposition, diet, gender, and academic stress.

The prevalence of childhood obesity has been increasing worldwide including middle- and low-income countries.[15] The prevalence of childhood obesity/overweight ranges from 4.3% to as high as 27% in India.[16] Obesity induces HTN by various mechanisms such as insulin resistance, activation of renin-angiotensin-aldosterone system (RAS), retention of salt, and consequent changes in vascular endothelial function.[17] Studies have shown that high BP in childhood is correlated with high BP and risk of CVD in adulthood and this relationship strengthens with age.[6] The prevalence of HTN in obesity ranges from 3.8% to as high as 25.5%.[10,18] Children with obesity also lack circadian variability of BP and half of these children have impaired BP dipping as determined by 24 hours ambulatory blood pressure monitoring (ABPM).[18,19] A study from India in obese children utilizing ABPM has shown 25.5% children as having ambulatory HTN and approximately 60% as having impaired dipping status.[18]

Genetic factor also plays an important role in the development of HTN. The estimated inheritability of BP is 50–60% in both children and adults. Data from large genome-wide association studies identified single nucleotide polymorphisms (SNPs) in adults of European ancestry and found that a genetic risk score (GRS) based on 29 loci had significant association with adult HTN.[20] Studies in children have shown that GRS of 13 SNPs were significantly associated with BP levels both in the longitudinal analysis from childhood to adulthood and in cross-sectional analysis. The GRS can explain 0.1–0.2% of the variation in BP, and its significant association with BP can be detected as early as age of 9 years for diastolic blood pressure (DBP) and age 24 years for systolic blood pressure (SBP).[21]

Excess consumption of sugar and salt has been associated with childhood HTN. Added sugars, especially fructose, can lead to excess weight gain and associated pathologies causing rise in systemic HTN.[22] Studies demonstrated that elevated fructose intake and, consequently, hyperuricemia induce inflammation in renal tubular epithelial cells leading to renal injury and development of HTN.[22] In addition, fructose increases the absorption of salt and water in small intestine, thus combining the synergistic action of both salt and fructose in the development of HTN. Further, a correlation between consumption of sugar-sweetened beverages (SSB) and higher levels of uric acid and BP was shown in the NHANES study population.[23]

Several epidemiological studies have shown a relationship between salt intake and HTN in children.[24-26] A study conducted in children aged 4–18 years under National Diet and Nutrition Survey for Young People program has shown that an increase in salt intake of 1 g increases systolic BP by 0.4 mm Hg.[24] Overweight children, children who are born preterm or small for gestational age, and African-American children are at increased risk of developing HTN due to high prevalence of salt sensitivity, defined as significant augmentation of arterial BP following increased salt intake.[24] Another study evaluating the effect of salt on normal weight and overweight children between 8 and 18 years of age found that for each gram intake of salt, the increase in SBP was 0.2, 1.3, and 1.5 mm Hg in normal, overweight, and obese children, respectively.[25] Similarly, another study in 298 children aged 8–9 years reported increase in daytime systolic BP (measured by ABPM) by 1.0 mm Hg per gram of dietary salt intake in overweight/obese children but not in normal weight boys or in girls.[26]

PREVALENCE OF HYPERTENSION AMONG CHILDREN WITH VARIOUS CHRONIC CONDITIONS

It is well evident that HTN is more commonly seen in children with chronic conditions such as sleep-disordered breathing (SDB), chronic kidney disease (CKD), SCD, diabetes, and children with history of prematurity.

The SDB is described as episodes of intermittent partial or complete upper airway obstruction during sleep, resulting from combination of increased upper airway resistant due to adenotonsillar hypertrophy and decreased pharyngeal dilator muscle tone while the child is asleep.[27] Various studies have identified association between childhood HTN and SDB,[28] while adult studies have shown association of SDB with resistant HTN.[29]

There is sufficient evidence showing high prevalence of HTN in children with CKD. In children with CKD, approximately 50% of the children are known to be hypertensive.[30,31] The Kidney Disease Outcome and Quality Initiative reported a prevalence of 70% in children with CKD which was as high as 80% in CKD-G4 and -G5.

A high prevalence of HTN has also been reported in children with SCD with prevalence of 13–35% through ABPM.[32,33] Recently, one study from central India reported ambulatory HTN in 13% of SCD children with 6.6% having masked HTN.[33] Similarly, the prevalence of HTN in children with type 1 diabetes was reported between 6 and 16%.[34]

Prematurity and low birth weight have been identified as a risk factor for HTN and other CVD in adults. One retrospective study showed 7.3% prevalence of HTN in children 3 years old who were born premature.[35] Impaired renal development in premature kidney, leading to reduction in the number of nephrons, has been implicated as a possible reason for HTN in this subgroup.[36]

CONCLUSION

Childhood HTN has been correlated with BP later in adulthood as well as increased risk of CVD. In recent years, an increase in primary HTN in children and adolescents has been reported due to lifestyle changes and increasing prevalence of obesity or overweight. Children with chronic conditions such as SDB, CKD, SCD, diabetes, and history of prematurity are at a higher risk for HTN.

KEY POINTS

- Hypertension is defined as SBP and DBP ≥ 95th percentile.
- Healthy children ≥3 years of age should undergo annual BP measurement.
- Subgroup of children at risk of HTN or on medications known to increase BP should undergo BP measurement at an earlier age with BP measured at each visit or more frequently.
- Validated BP instrument and appropriately sized cuff (cuff bladder length should cover 80–100% and width of cuff should encompass at least 40%) should be used for measurement of BP in children.
- Auscultatory method is the preferred method of BP measurement in children.
- Oscillometric devices may be used for initial screening method and any elevated BP should be confirmed by auscultatory method.

REFERENCES

1. Kearney PM, Whelton M, Reynolds K, Muntner P, Whelton PK, He J. Global burden of hypertension: analysis of worldwide data. Lancet. 2005;365(9455):217-23.
2. McNiece KL, Poffenbarger TS, Turner JL, Franco KD, Sorof JM, Portman RJ. Prevalence of hypertension and pre-hypertension among adolescents. J Pediatr. 2007;150(6):640-4,644.e1.
3. Sorof JM, Lai D, Turner J, Poffenbarger T, Portman RJ. Overweight, ethnicity, and the prevalence of hypertension in school-aged children. Pediatrics. 2004;113(3 Pt 1):475-82.
4. Song P, Zhang Y, Yu J, Zha M, Zhu Y, Rahimi K, et al. Global prevalence of hypertension in children: a systematic review and meta-analysis. JAMA Pediatr. 2019;173(12):1-10.
5. Din-Dzietham R, Liu Y, Bielo MV, Shamsa F. High blood pressure trends in children and adolescents in national surveys, 1963 to 2002. Circulation. 2007;116(13):1488-96.
6. Chen X, Wang Y. Tracking of blood pressure from childhood to adulthood: a systematic review and meta-regression analysis. Circulation. 2008;117(25):3171-80.
7. Brady TM, Fivush B, Flynn JT, Parekh R. Ability of blood pressure to predict left ventricular hypertrophy in children with primary hypertension. J Pediatr. 2008;152(1):73-8, 78.e1.
8. Berenson GS, Srinivasan SR, Bao W, Newman WP, Tracy RE, Wattigney WA. Association between multiple cardiovascular risk factors and atherosclerosis in children and young adults. The Bogalusa Heart Study. N Engl J Med. 1998;338(23):1650-6.
9. National High Blood Pressure Education Program Working Group on High Blood Pressure in Children and Adolescents. The fourth report on the diagnosis, evaluation, and treatment of high blood pressure in children and adolescents. Pediatrics. 2004;114(2 Suppl 4th Report):555-76.
10. Flynn JT, Kaelber DC, Baker-Smith CM, Blowey D, Carroll AE, Daniels SR, et al. Clinical practice guideline for screening and management of high blood pressure in children and adolescents. Pediatrics. 2017;40(3):e20171904.
11. Canzanello VJ, Jensen PL, Schwartz GL. Are aneroid sphygmomanometers accurate in hospital and clinic settings? Arch Intern Med. 2001;161(5):729-31.
12. Duncombe SL, Voss C, Harris KC. Oscillometric and auscultatory blood pressure measurement methods in children: a systematic review and meta-analysis. J Hypertens. 2017;35(2):213-24.
13. Fujii T, Uzu T, Nishimura M, Takeji M, Kuroda S, Nakamura S, et al. Circadian rhythm of natriuresis is disturbed in nondipper type of essential hypertension. Am J Kidney Dis. 1999;33(1): 29-35.
14. Fan HQ, Li Y, Thijs L, Hansen TW, Boggia J, Kikuya M, et al. Prognostic value of isolated nocturnal hypertension on ambulatory measurement in 8711 individuals from 10 populations. J Hypertens. 2010;28(10):2036-45.
15. Ranjani H, Mehreen TS, Pradeepa R, Anjana RM, Garg R, Anand K, et al. Epidemiology of childhood overweight and obesity in India: A systematic review. Indian J Med Res. 2016;143(2):160-74.
16. Khadilkar VV, Khadilkar AV, Cole TJ, Chiplonkar SA, Pandit D. Overweight and obesity prevalence and body mass index trends in Indian children. Int J Pediatr Obes. 2011;6:e216-24.
17. Kotchen TA. Obesity-related hypertension: epidemiology, pathophysiology, and clinical management. Am J Hypertens. 2010;23(11):1170-8.
18. Bhatt GC, Pakhare AP, Gogia P, Jain S, Gupta N, Goel SK, et al. Predictive model for ambulatory hypertension based on office blood pressure in obese children. Front Pediatr [Internet]. 2020;8:232.
19. Török K, Pálfi A, Szelényi Z, Molnár D. Circadian variability of blood pressure in obese children. Nutr Metab Cardiovasc Dis. 2008;18(6):429-35.
20. International Consortium for Blood Pressure Genome-Wide Association Studies, Ehret GB, Munroe PB, Rice KM, Bochud M, Johnson AD, et al. Genetic variants in novel pathways influence blood pressure and cardiovascular disease risk. Nature. 2011;478(7367):103-9.
21. Oikonen M, Tikkanen E, Juhola J, Tuovinen T, Seppälä I, Juonala M, et al. Genetic variants and blood pressure in a population-based cohort: the Cardiovascular Risk in Young Finns Study. Hypertension. 2011;58(6):1079-85.
22. Madero M, Perez-Pozo SE, Jalal D, Johnson RJ, Sánchez-Lozada LG. Dietary fructose and hypertension. Curr Hypertens Rep. 2011;13(1):29-35.
23. Nguyen S, Choi HK, Lustig RH, Hsu C. Sugar-sweetened beverages, serum uric acid, and blood pressure in adolescents. J Pediatr. 2009;154(6):807-13.
24. Lava SAG, Bianchetti MG, Simonetti GD. Salt intake in children and its consequences on blood pressure. Pediatr Nephrol. 2015;30(9):1389-96.
25. Yang Q, Zhang Z, Kuklina EV, Fang J, Ayala C, Hong Y, et al. Sodium intake and blood pressure among US children and adolescents. Pediatrics. 2012;130(4):611-9.

26. Correia-Costa L, Cosme D, Nogueira-Silva L, Morato M, Sousa T, Moura C, et al. Gender and obesity modify the impact of salt intake on blood pressure in children. Pediatr Nephrol. 2016;31(2):279-88.
27. Marcus CL, Brooks LJ, Draper KA, Gozal D, Halbower AC, Jones J, et al. Diagnosis and management of childhood obstructive sleep apnea syndrome. Pediatrics. 2012;130(3):e714-55.
28. Hartzell K, Avis K, Lozano D, Feig D. Obstructive sleep apnea and periodic limb movement disorder in a population of children with hypertension and/or nocturnal nondipping blood pressures. J Am Soc Hypertens. 2016;10(2):101-7.
29. Muxfeldt ES. Prevalence of obstructive sleep apnea in refractory hypertension. Hypertension. 2018;72(3):592-3.
30. Samuels J, Ng D, Flynn JT, Mitsnefes M, Poffenbarger T, Warady BA, et al. Ambulatory blood pressure patterns in children with chronic kidney disease. Hypertension. 2012;60(1): 43-50.
31. Flynn JT, Mitsnefes M, Pierce C, Cole SR, Parekh RS, Furth SL, et al. Blood pressure in children with chronic kidney disease: a report from the Chronic Kidney Disease in Children study. Hypertension. 2008;52(4):631-7.
32. Becker AM, Goldberg JH, Henson M, Ahn C, Tong L, Baum M, et al. Blood pressure abnormalities in children with sickle cell anemia. Pediatr Blood Cancer. 2014;61(3):518-22.
33. Dubey SRK, Shrivastava N, Sharma T, Bhatt GC, Dhingra B, Pakhare AP. et al. Abnormal ambulatory blood pressure and early renal dysfunction in sickle cell disease. Indian J Pediatr. 2021;88(6):562-7.
34. Downie ML, Ulrich EH, Noone DG. An update on hypertension in children with type 1 diabetes. Can J Diabetes. 2018;42(2): 199-204.
35. Mhanna MJ, Iqbal AM, Kaelber DC. Weight gain and hypertension at three years of age and older in extremely low birth weight infants. J Neonatal Perinatal Med. 2015;8(4):363-9.
36. Rodríguez MM, Gómez AH, Abitbol CL, Chandar JJ, Duara S, Zilleruelo GE. Histomorphometric analysis of postnatal glomerulogenesis in extremely preterm infants. Pediatr Dev Pathol. 2004;7(1):17-25.

CHAPTER

10.2 Etiopathogenesis of Hypertension

Shweta Priyadarshini, RW Thergaonkar

INTRODUCTION

This chapter is divided into four sections. The first section describes the mechanisms controlling blood pressure. The second, third, and fourth sections describe the pathogenesis of primary hypertension, secondary hypertension, and target organ damage consequent to hypertension in the pediatric age group.

REGULATION OF BLOOD PRESSURE

The regulation of systemic blood pressure (BP), a key determinant of tissue perfusion, is a vital function crucial to survival. BP regulation is a result of many intricate feedback mechanisms in different organ systems and their interaction that converges on the key determinants of blood pressure—cardiac output (CO) and systemic vascular resistance (SVR). BP may be represented by the formula:

$$BP \ \alpha \ CO \times SVR$$ [1]

Cardiac output is the volume of blood that is pumped out by the left ventricle each minute. CO is the product of the heart rate (HR) and the stroke volume (SV), i.e., the amount of blood that is pumped out by the left ventricle in each beat. This may be represented by the formula:

$$CO = HR \times SV$$

The SVR is the force required to maintain blood flow from the root of the aorta to the venous exit into the right atrium. Although blood from the left ventricle travels through the arteries, arterioles, capillaries, venules, and veins before returning to the right atrium, the key determinant of SVR is the vasomotor tone, i.e., the state of contraction of the vascular smooth muscle cells (VSMCs), inside the arteriolar bed.[1] The vasomotor tone is influenced by sympathetic nervous system (SNS) activity, humoral agents, and autacoid, i.e., paracrine substances.[2]

The role of the different physiological systems that control BP is described here.

Neural Control

The autonomic nervous system has important roles in short- and long-term control of BP. The SNS has preganglionic cholinergic neurons in the thoracic and lumbar spinal segments, ganglia in the sympathetic chain, and postganglionic adrenergic neurons in many organs. Relevant to BP regulation, the important postganglionic neurons synapse onto β1 receptors in the heart and α1 receptors in the arterioles; the responses to adrenergic stimulation therefore are tachycardia (increased CO) and vasoconstriction (increased SVR). In addition, some preganglionic neurons do not synapse in the sympathetic ganglia but terminate on the adrenal medulla where the cells are modified postganglionic neurons. Increased sympathetic tone leads to increase in circulating epinephrine and norepinephrine. The baseline level of activation of the SNS keeps the arterioles partially constricted and this, in a large way, contributes to the vasomotor tone. The chief parasympathetic regulator of BP is the vagus nerve, whose cholinergic action on the heart leads to bradycardia (reduced CO).[3] **Flowchart 1** schematically shows the neural regulation of BP including some important reflexes.

Flowchart 1: Neural control of blood pressure. Shapes and arrows in green represent stimulatory effects, while shapes and arrows in red represent inhibitory effect.

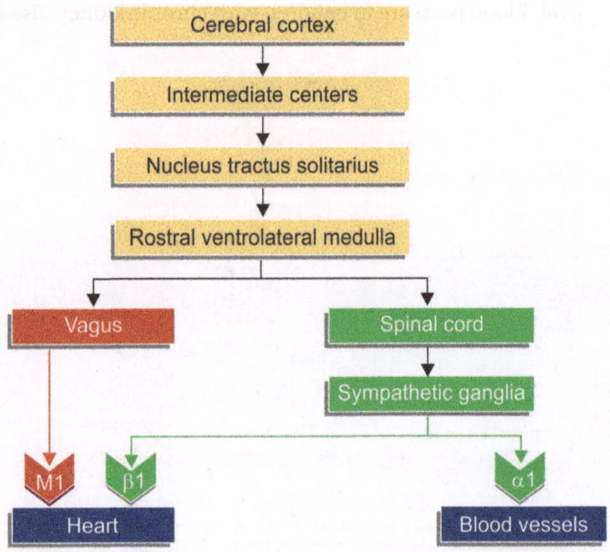

Humoral and Autacoidal Control

Renin–angiotensin–aldosterone System

The renin–angiotensin–aldosterone system (RAAS) is a key regulator of BP and sodium homeostasis in the body.

The classical RAAS pathway is responsible for fluid retention, vasoconstriction, and proinflammatory action while the opposite effects are noted for the more recently discovered noncanonical renin–angiotensin system.

Classical RAAS pathway: This is the first pathway that was discovered and is the dominant RAAS pathway.

The cascade begins with the secretion of angiotensinogen (Agt), an 118 amino acid globulin by the liver. Renin, a 340 amino acid aspartyl protease secreted by the juxtaglomerular apparatus, cleaves Agt into angiotensin I (Ang I), a decapeptide. Ang I is converted to angiotensin II (Ang II), an octapeptide, by angiotensin-converting enzyme (ACE), a zinc metalloprotease, by cleavage of two amino acids at the C-terminal end. The classical RAAS pathway describes the presence of ACE in the lungs; however, ACE is also present in the plasma, interstitium, and intracellular compartment in all major organ systems including the heart, vasculature, and kidneys. Ang II has the following actions—vasoconstriction, stimulation of secretion of aldosterone by the adrenal cortex, stimulation of adrenocorticotropic hormone (ACTH) secretion by the anterior pituitary, stimulation of thirst at the hypothalamus, and vasopressin secretion by the posterior pituitary gland. These are mediated by the angiotensin type 1 receptor (AT1R). The chief stimulants of the classical RAAS pathway are the secretion of renin by the renal juxtaglomerular apparatus in response to renal sympathetic activity, low intrarenal pressure, and low sodium level.[4]

Noncanonical RAAS pathways: Consequent to the discovery of the classical RAAS pathway, newer molecular pathways interacting with the classical pathway were discovered. These pathways seem to be active during organogenesis but are not canonical in later life. The effects of the stimulation of these pathways are somewhat opposite to those of stimulation of AT1R.[4] The classical and noncanonical RAAS pathways, also colloquially called the "YANG" and "YIN" pathways, need to be physiological harmony for the health of the individual.

The classical and noncanonical RAAS pathways are schematically shown in **Flowchart 2**.

Aldosterone

The aldosterone system is crucial for life in animals living on land because of its salt-retentive properties. Aldosterone is synthesized in the zona glomerulosa of the adrenal cortex by CYP11B2 in response to three signals—local and systemic Ang II levels, ACTH, and potassium concentration. The classical action of aldosterone, i.e., stimulation of sodium absorption in the distal convoluted tubule and collecting duct of the kidney, is mediated by the mineralocorticoid receptor (MR). Newer actions of aldosterone have been discovered in recent years. These include hypertrophy, inflammation and fibrosis of the VSMCs, endothelial dysfunction due to inhibition of nitric oxide (NO), and myocardial fibrosis.[4]

Endothelin-1

Endothelin-1 is secreted by endothelial cells. It acts chiefly on ET_A receptors that are located on the VSMCs to cause vasoconstriction and sodium retention via sympathetic stimulation.[4]

Nitric Oxide

Nitric oxide (NO) is synthesized in the endothelium from arginine by the endothelial enzyme NO synthetase. Nitric oxide causes vasodilatation via cyclic guanosine monophosphate (cGMP).[2] NO also exerts antiplatelet effects.[4]

Bradykinin

Bradykinin (BK) is formed by the cleavage of high-molecular-weight kininogen by kallikrein. BK through its receptors, B1R and B2R, causes (1) vasodilatation through increased production of NO, (2) natriuresis and diuresis, (3) release of inflammatory mediators, and (4) catecholamine release.[5]

Natriuretic Peptides

Atrial natriuretic peptide (ANP) and B-type natriuretic peptide (BNP) are secreted by the atrial and ventricular walls respectively in response to stretch. They act via the natriuretic peptide receptor-A (NPRA) to produce natriuresis and diuresis, vasorelaxation, increased endothelium permeability and antagonism of the renin-angiotensin system.[4]

Arginine Vasopressin

Arginine vasopressin (AVP) is secreted by the supraoptic and paraventricular nuclei of the hypothalamus in response to osmotic and pressure–volume stimuli. The chief action of AVP is reabsorption of water in renal tubules through the V2 receptor. In addition, AVP causes vasoconstriction through the V1 receptors.[4]

Dopamine

The direct vascular effects of dopamine in regulation of blood pressure in physiology is not significant. The kidneys have an intrinsic dopaminergic system. In the salt replete state, the chief role of this dopaminergic system is natriuresis via D1 receptors. When infused pharmacologically, dopamine acts on sympathetic α and β receptors over and above acting on the dopaminergic receptors.[4]

Thyroid Hormones

The thyroid hormones play a role in maintenance of cardiac metabolism, lipid profile, blood vessel dilatation, and endothelial health through genomic and nongenomic pathways.

Renal Control of BP

As discussed above, the kidneys play an important role in the regulation of BP by being the site for the initiation of the

Flowchart 2: Overview of the classical and non-canonical RAAS pathways. Peptides are shown in squares with rounded boxes. Enzymes are shown in hexagons. Red color indicates predominant action in classical RAAS. Blue color indicates predominant action in non-canonical RAAS.

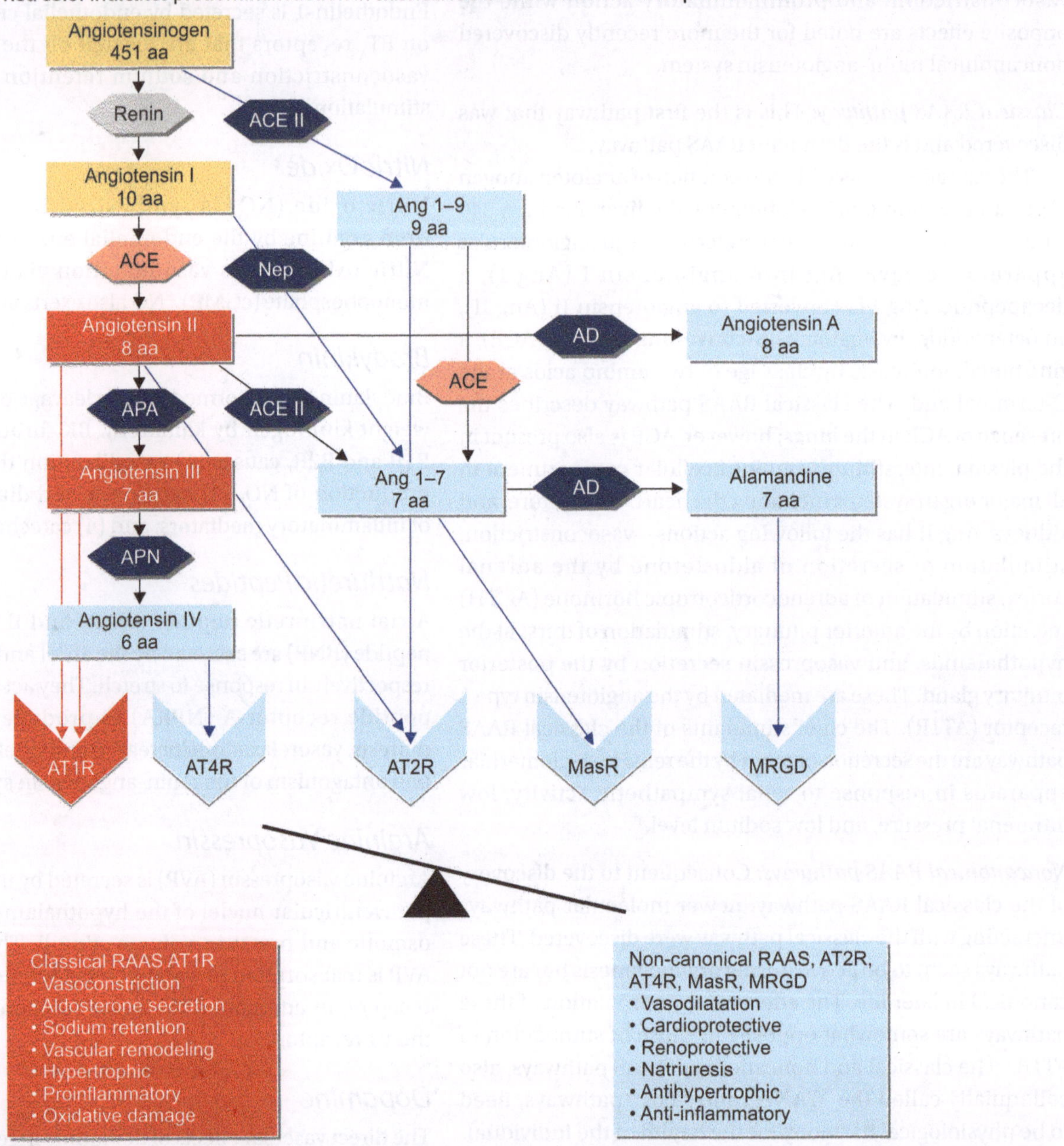

(ACE: angiotensin converting enzyme; ACE2: angiotensin converting enzyme type 2; AD: aspartate decarboxylase; APA: aminopeptidase A; APN: alanyl aminopeptidase N; AT1R: angiotensin receptor type 1; AT2R: angiotensin type 2 receptor; AT4R: angiotensin type 4 receptor; Mas R: Mas receptor; MRGD: Mas-related G protein-coupled receptor member D; Nep: neprilysin)

RAAS pathway as well as sodium and water homeostasis. The kidneys also possess intrinsic systems of RAS and dopamine that have a role in BP regulation. In addition, the kidney plays a regulatory role through two mechanisms—pressure natriuresis and tubular glomerular feedback.

Pressure Natriuresis

A series of animal experiments demonstrate that an increase in the intravascular volume results in natriuresis. This is most probably due to increase in the renal perfusion pressure and consequent increase in renal interstitial hydrostatic pressure (RIHP). An increase in RIHP can cause back leak of sodium from the interstitium into the renal tubules, stimulation of prostaglandin synthesis, and cytochrome P450 metabolites that may inhibit sodium reabsorption in the tubules or a direct inhibition of sodium pump activity in the renal tubules.[6]

Tubuloglomerular Feedback

The juxtaglomerular apparatus of the nephron consists of the macula densa cells (specialized cells in the thick ascending loop of Henle), extraglomerular mesangial cells that lie between the afferent and efferent glomerular arterioles and the VSMCs and renin-secreting cells in the afferent arteriolar media. The macula densa cells sense increase in

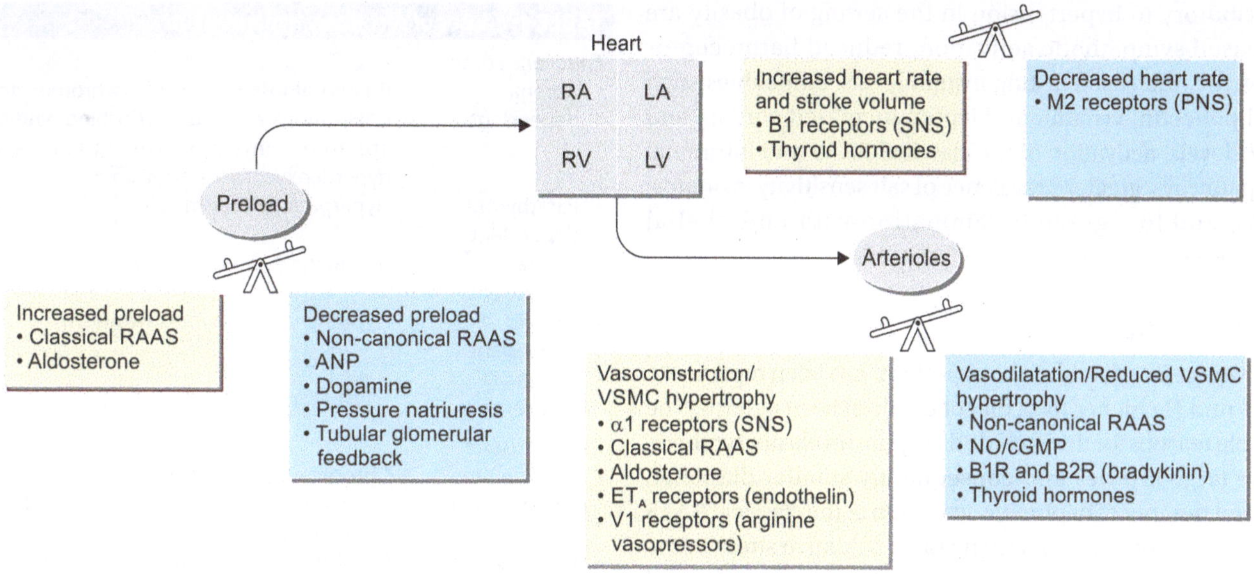

Fig. 1: Overview of control of blood pressure. (ANP: atrial natriuretic peptide; GPER: G-protein-coupled estrogen receptor-1; LA: left atrium; LV: left ventricle; MR: mineralocorticoid receptor; PNS: parasympathetic nervous system; RA: right atrium; RAAS: renin-angiotensin-aldosterone system; RV: right ventricle; SNS: sympathetic nervous system)

concentrations of sodium, potassium, and chloride using the NKCC2 cotransporter and send a signal to afferent arteriole via the mesangial cells to effect afferent arteriolar constriction and reduction in renin secretion. The mediator of this response is believed to be either adenosine or adenosine triphosphate (ATP) with Ang II and NO acting as modulators of this response.[7]

The mechanisms controlling BP are schematically summarized in **Figure 1**.

PRIMARY HYPERTENSION

Hypertension is considered primary when there is no clearly identified etiology. Genetic background and lifestyle are important factors leading to primary hypertension. Primary hypertension accounts for approximately 15% of childhood hypertension.[8] However, with rising incidence of obesity in pediatric population, the incidence of primary hypertension is increasing as well, thereby defining a close association between obesity and primary hypertension.[9]

A large number of factors have been implicated in the pathogenesis of primary hypertension. The important factors are discussed here.

Gender

Essential hypertension is more common among boys than girls; male:female ratio may be as high as 3:1.[10]

Genetic Factors

Genetic factors may play a role in primary hypertension in childhood. Association with polymorphisms in a large number of genes including those encoding RAAS pathway proteins, aldosterone synthase, NO synthetase, atrial natriuretic peptide (ANP), insulin receptor, β-adrenergic receptor, renin-binding protein, and angiotensinase C has been reported.[10]

Lifestyle

Increased salt intake and increased consumption of saturated and trans fatty acids, and reduced consumption of legumes, fruits, vegetables, and nuts are associated with hypertension across ages.[10]

Sympathetic Activity

Evidence of increased sympathetic activity such as increased levels of circulating norepinephrine and higher resting HR has been reported in children with primary hypertension.[11]

Salt Sensitivity

Salt sensitivity refers to the phenomenon of increased mean arterial pressure on ambulatory BP monitoring during periods of increased salt intake. This occurs due to reduced ability to excrete additional sodium loads. Salt sensitivity is reported in 51% hypertensive as compared to 26% normotensive individuals.[11]

Insulin Resistance

The cardiovascular effects of insulin resistance include blunted natriuresis, increased sympathetic activity, and attenuated vasodilatation.[12]

Specific Clinical Settings of Primary Hypertension

Obesity

Obesity is a growing problem in developing countries. As discussed above, the important factors that may be contributory to hypertension in the setting of obesity are increased sympathetic activation, reduced baroreceptor sensitivity, increased fasting insulin levels, adipokines such as adiponectin, visfatin, and leptin, increased cortisol and ACTH levels, activation of the classical RAAS and intrarenal RAS pathways, greater prevalence of salt sensitivity, oxidative stress, and low-grade inflammation with endothelial activation in the blood vessels.[13]

Preterm Birth

The average BP of children born preterm has been reported to be 2.5 mm Hg higher than that of children born at term. The possible reasons for this include disruption in elastin synthesis in the large arteries and consequently smaller diameter, reduced number of nephrons, activation of the classical RAAS pathway, increased sympathetic tone, oxidative stress in the setting of immature antioxidative mechanisms, accelerated vascular aging, and chronic low-grade inflammation.[14]

SECONDARY HYPERTENSION

Secondary hypertension is hypertension due to an identifiable underlying cause. Once the cause is identified, it is potentially correctable. In children, secondary hypertension is more common than primary hypertension with a reported prevalence of 75–85% according to various studies.[8]

Etiopathogenesis

It is important to try and establish the cause of secondary hypertension in view of its correctable nature. The index of suspicion for underlying secondary causes of hypertension should be higher in certain clinical situations such as sudden onset of refractory hypertension or a severe or accelerated course of hypertension.

The etiology of secondary hypertension varies according to the age of presentation. In children between birth and 18 years of age, the most common underlying causes are renal parenchymal disease and coarctation of aorta. In young adults between 19 and 39 years of age, thyroid dysfunction, fibromuscular dysplasia, and renal parenchymal disease are common and in middle-aged adults, the common causes are aldosteronism and thyroid dysfunction.[15] The important causes of secondary hypertension are summarized in **Table 1**.

TABLE 1: Causes of secondary hypertension.

Endocrine causes:	
• Adrenal dependent	Primary aldosteronism, pheochromocytoma, CAH, Chrousos syndrome, Cushing syndrome, apparent mineralocorticoid excess, and hyperdeoxycorticosteronism
• Parathyroid dependent	Hyperparathyroidism
• Pituitary dependent	Acromegaly, Cushing syndrome
• Thyroid dependent	Hypothyroidism, hyperthyroidism
• Vitamin D deficiency	
Renal causes:	
• Renal parenchymal	Chronic kidney disease, polycystic kidney disease, urinary tract obstruction, and renin-secreting tumor
• Renovascular	Renal artery stenosis, fibromuscular dysplasia
Vasculitis	Collagen vascular disease
Vascular causes	Coarctation of aorta
Neurogenic causes	Brain tumor, intracranial hypertension, autonomic dysfunction, and sleep apnea
Drugs and toxins	Alcohol, NSAIDs, cocaine, calcineurin inhibitors, caffeine, adrenergic medicines, erythropoietin, herbal medications containing heavy metals, and nicotine
Monogenic hypertension	Liddle syndrome, Gordon syndrome, congenital adrenal hyperplasia, Geller syndrome, syndrome of apparent mineralocorticoid excess, familial hypoaldosteronism type 1 and 2, hypertension and brachydactyly syndrome, and familial pheochromocytoma

(CAH: congenital adrenal hyperplasia; NSAIDs: nonsteroidal anti-inflammatory drugs)

MONOGENIC HYPERTENSION

Hypertension usually results due to interaction of genetic and environmental factors. However, various genetic mutations have been defined to cause hypertension. Monogenic hypertension is a term used to describe a group of specific genetic and usually single-gene disorders, which impede normal renal and/or adrenal BP regulation, leading to hypertension. DNA sequencing helps to provide insight into many of these conditions.

Volume expansion is the driving mechanism of hypertension in most forms of monogenic hypertension. The mechanisms causing volume expansion are (1) excessive reabsorption of sodium ions by hyperactive channels, (2) hyperstimulation of mineralocorticoid receptors, and (3) excess mineralocorticoid synthesis.[16,17] Some forms of monogenic hypertension may also have sympathetic or adrenergic excess as the underlying mechanism **(Table 2)**.

Liddle Syndrome

Liddle syndrome is a disease commonly seen in late childhood and adolescence. It is an autosomal dominant disease due to gain-of-function mutation of epithelial sodium channel (ENaC) in the collecting duct. It is characterized by severe hypertension, metabolic alkalosis, and hypokalemia along with low renin and aldosterone. Gain-of-function mutations in the genes encoding beta and gamma subunits, *SCNN1B* and *SCNN1G*, are usually responsible for constitutively active ENaC channels. This leads to increased sodium reabsorption and consequently volume expansion resulting

TABLE 2: Basic classification scheme for causes of monogenic hypertension.

Low renin level	Low aldosterone levels	Liddle syndrome Congenital adrenal hyperplasia Apparent mineralocorticoid excess Geller's syndrome
	Normal aldosterone levels	Gordon syndrome (pseudohypoaldosteronism type II)
	High aldosterone levels	Familial hyperaldosteronism type I (glucocorticoid-remediable aldosteronism) Familial hyperaldosteronism type II Familial hyperaldosteronism type III Familial hyperaldosteronism type IV
Adrenergic/sympathetic excess	High metanephrine and normetanephrine levels	Familial pheochromocytoma
Vascular smooth muscle proliferation		Hypertension and brachydactyly syndrome

in hypertension. This mechanism of sodium resorption is independent of aldosterone.

Gordon Syndrome

It is also called pseudohypoaldosteronism type 2. It is an autosomal dominant disease with characteristic hypertension, hyperkalemia, hyperchloremic metabolic acidosis, and normal glomerular filtration rate (GFR). Gordon syndrome is caused by mutations in the *WNK1* and *WNK4* genes found on chromosomes 12 and 17, respectively. Mutation leads to increased sodium reabsorption via activation of the ENaC and reduced inhibition of the Na/Cl cotransporter (NCC) channel, thereby leading to volume expansion and subsequent hypertension. Inhibition of renal outer medullary potassium (ROMK channel) leads to hyperkalemia.

Congenital Adrenal Hyperplasia

Congenital adrenal hyperplasia (CAH) variant due to deficiency of 21-hydroxylase is the most common form; however, CAH due to deficiency of 11-β-hydroxylase and 17-α-hydroxylase enzymes are associated with monogenic hypertension.

11-β-hydroxylase deficiency (CAH type IV) results in accumulation of deoxycortisone and deoxycortisol due to the prevention of their conversion into corticosterone and cortisol. This exerts significant mineralocorticoid activity leading to hypertension.

17-α-hydroxylase deficiency (CAH type V) manifests clinically as hypogonadism, hypokalemia, and hypertension. In this condition, the cortisol synthesis is impaired leading to stimulation of ACTH secretion. This overstimulation of ACTH secretion leads to increased levels of deoxycorticosterone and corticosterone, which ultimately manifest as low renin hypertension, hypokalemia, and metabolic acidosis. The products of 17-α-hydroxylase serve as substrate for production of dehydroepiandrosterone (DHEA) and androstenedione, which are the precursors for synthesis of androgen and estrogen. Thus, due to limited production of sex hormone, male patients may have ambiguous genitalia or female phenotype and females may have delay in sexual maturation and primary amenorrhea.

Syndrome of Apparent Mineralocorticoid Excess

It is an autosomal recessive condition presenting with hypertension and hypokalemia with metabolic alkalosis. The plasma renin activity is suppressed, and aldosterone is absent in circulation. There is an inactivating mutation in the gene encoding 11-β-hydroxysteroid dehydrogenase type 2 (*HSB11B2*). This mutation impairs the metabolism of cortisol to cortisone. The former is therefore available in excess to bind to MR, leading to manifestation similar to pseudohypoaldosteronism because there is excess mineralocorticoid activity despite low levels of aldosterone.[16]

Geller Syndrome

It is an autosomal dominant inherited gain-of-function mutation which results in activation of MR. The receptors remain active by the virtue of alterations in receptor sites. These alterations also lead to exaggerated response to steroid hormones including progesterone. Pregnancy being a high progesterone state can significantly accelerate the hypertension.[16]

Familial Hyperaldosteronism Type 1 (Glucocorticoid Remediable Hypertension)

It is an autosomal dominant condition presenting with early onset hypertension along with hypokalemia and normal or increased levels of aldosterone, even though the plasma renin activity is suppressed.[17] At the genetic level, there are alterations in *CYP11B1* and *CYP11B2* genes, which lie next to each other on chromosome 8.[16] A chimeric gene results due to unequal crossing over of both the genes. This chimeric gene is expressed in the zona fasciculata of the adrenal gland leading to the production of a protein with aldosterone synthase activity, which is regulated by ACTH rather than Ang II. Normally, aldosterone is produced by zona glomerulosa of adrenal gland. In this condition, however, it is ectopically produced by zona fasciculata.[16,17]

Flowchart 3: Renal parenchymal hypertension—mediators and mechanism.

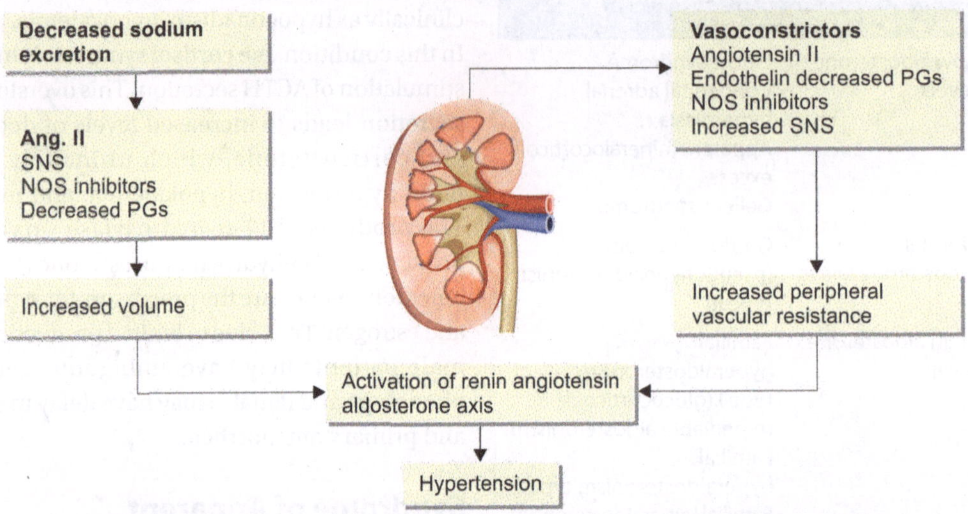

(NOS: nitric oxide synthase; PGs: prostaglandins; SNS: sympathetic nervous system)

Familial Hyperaldosteronism Type 2

As in familial hyperaldosteronism type 1, aldosterone is ectopically synthesized due to loss of negative feedback, which is exerted by physiological aldosterone secretion. However, this is not under the control of ACTH as in familial hyperaldosteronism type 1, and therefore mineralocorticoid secretion is not suppressible by dexamethasone. It is an autosomal dominant disorder with locus in chromosome 7p22.[16]

Other Forms of Monogenic Hypertension

Some forms of monogenic hypertension do not result from volume expansion.

Familial pheochromocytoma is caused by genetic mutations that lead to increased propensity to develop this tumor. Release of epinephrine and norepinephrine over and above the normal range leads to hypertension. Pheochromocytoma may present in an isolated manner or as a part of certain syndromes such as von Hippel–Lindau disease, multiple endocrine neoplasia type 2, and neurofibromatosis type 1.[17]

The mechanism of increased BP in autosomal dominant hypertension with brachydactyly is increased arteriogenesis and vasoconstriction.[17]

RENAL PARENCHYMAL DISEASE

The cause of hypertension in renal parenchymal disease varies. There may be impairment of salt and water excretion and/or reduced renal blood flow, excessive release of vasoconstrictors from the kidney such as Ang II and endothelin I, deficiency of NO which is a vasodilator, sympathetic activation, and endocrine and metabolic disturbances including calcium and phosphate disorders.[18]

HYPERTENSION IN CHRONIC KIDNEY DISEASE

The most common underlying cause of secondary hypertension in the pediatric age group is chronic kidney disease (CKD).[15] According to a study involving a cohort of children with CKD, an overall prevalence of hypertension was found to be 54%. It included all subjects with systolic or diastolic BP in the hypertensive range, or history of hypertension and hypertensive drug use.[19] Hypertension occurs early and is more severe in patients with renal parenchymal disease. It in turn accelerates the progression of renal parenchymal disease.[20]

The two major pathophysiological mechanisms causing hypertension in CKD are peripheral vasoconstriction and volume expansion **(Flowchart 3)**.[21] Both the above mechanisms cause activation of the classical renin angiotensin–aldosterone axis.

Other mechanisms include activation of the SNS, alterations in endothelial autacoids such as NO and endothelin, use of recombinant erythropoietin for treatment of anemia of CKD, prostaglandins, sleep apnea, and calcification of the arterial tree. These phenomena are exaggerated in patients on dialysis due to inadequate compliance with salt and fluid restriction, intermittent nature of dialytic therapies, and inadequate dialysis.[21] Hypertension can persist after renal transplantation because many of the factors contributing to hypertension in CKD are not reversible. In addition, factors such as the use of calcineurin inhibitors and arterial stenosis of the renal allograft may also be contributory.[18]

RENOVASCULAR HYPERTENSION

Hypertension resulting out of compromised renal blood supply is called renovascular hypertension.[22] The common causes for the above are renal artery stenosis mostly consequent to secondary atherosclerosis (RAS), fibromuscular dysplasia (FMD), arteritides such as Takayasu arteritis, antiphospholipid antibody (APLA), extrinsic renal artery compression, renal artery infarction, postradiation fibrosis, umbilical artery catheterization, trauma, congenital rubella syndrome, Marfan syndrome, and tuberous sclerosis. The pathophysiological mechanism of renovascular hypertension lies in decreased renal perfusion, which in turn stimulates the classical RAAS pathway.[23]

HYPERTENSION IN ENDOCRINE DISEASE

Hypertension may arise secondary to endocrine imbalances. Excess production of adrenal hormones, the mineralocorticoid, glucocorticoids and catecholamines, parathyroid hormone, thyroid hormone imbalance, growth hormone, diabetes mellitus, Cushing's disease, and vitamin D deficiency may cause hypertension. It is estimated that 5–10% of people with hypertension have endocrine disorders as a cause of secondary hypertension.[24]

Adrenal-dependent Causes

Primary Hyperaldosteronism

This condition was first reported by Conn as aldosterone-producing adenoma. There is unchecked production of aldosterone due to loss of regulation by the Ang II. This excess of aldosterone leads to absorption of sodium by the distal tubular ENaC channel, which in turn causes hypertension and suppression of the classical RAAS axis. Urinary loss of potassium and hydrogen ion in exchange for the sodium ion leads to hypokalemia and metabolic alkalosis.[18]

Pheochromocytoma

Pheochromocytoma a tumor of endocrine cells, which secretes epinephrine, norepinephrine, dopamine, and catecholamines, which in turn cause hypertension by their direct effect. The tumor of extra-adrenal chromaffin-secreting cells of the SNS is called paragangliomas. Both these tumors have similar manifestation. This tumor is commonly seen in adults between the age of 40 and 50 years but may also be seen in children. Hypertension is the most common presentation of pheochromocytoma, although the classic triad is sweating, tachycardia, and headache.[25]

Cushing Syndrome

Cushing syndrome or glucocorticoid excess causes hypertension by various mechanisms. Glucocorticoids lead to increased hepatic production of angiotensinogen, which in turn activates the classical RAAS axis causing hypertension. Other mechanisms include inhibition of the production of vasodilatory prostaglandins by inhibition of phospholipase A2, reduced activity of depressor kallikrein-kinin system, increased sensitivity to endogenous epinephrine and Ang II, and insulin resistance which lead to hypertension in Cushing syndrome.[18]

Congenital Adrenal Hyperplasia and Apparent Mineralocorticoid Excess

These entities have been described above in the section on monogenic hypertension.

Growth hormone excess or acromegaly is associated with hypertension in 35% of cases. Growth hormone causes retention of sodium that leads to volume expansion leading to hypertension.

Primary Hyperparathyroidism

Hyperparathyroidism accounts for approximately 0.3% of childhood hypertension.[24] The postulated mechanisms of hypertension in hyperparathyroidism are intracellular accumulation of calcium, presence of hypomagnesemia, raised renin activity, and abnormalities of glucose.[18]

Disorders of Thyroid Hormone

Hyperthyroidism is associated with activation of the classical RAAS axis and increased sensitivity to circulating catecholamines leading to hypertension.

Hypothyroidism is also associated with hypertension. Volume expansion and increased SVR form the basis of hypertension in these patients.[26]

Diabetes Mellitus

Hyperinsulinemia, volume expansion, sodium retention, and increased stiffness of the arteries are implicated in development of hypertension in patients with diabetes mellitus.[18]

CARDIOVASCULAR CAUSES OF HYPERTENSION

"Hypertension does not occur in the setting of primary cardiac illness." The exception to this dictum is coarctation of aorta. Palpation for radiofemoral delay and measurement of BP in all four limbs in children with hypertension are therefore important in a child with hypertension. Renal hypoperfusion activating the RAAS and sympathetic stimulation are the pathophysiological mechanisms causing hypertension.[18]

HYPERTENSION IN NEUROLOGICAL DISORDERS

The various neurological disorders associated with hypertension are hydrocephalus, neurotrauma, pseudotumor cerebri, Guillain–Barre syndrome (GBS), intracranial space occupying lesions, and seizure activity. The underlying mechanism in most cases is activation of SNS leading to peripheral vasoconstriction and sodium retention by the kidneys. Catecholamine levels are also found elevated in various conditions such as GBS and elevated intracranial pressure.[18]

HYPERTENSION AND OBSTRUCTIVE SLEEP APNEA

Usually, this is seen in patients with central obesity and with the rising prevalence of childhood obesity. Obstructive sleep apnea (OSA), an important cause of hypertension, is often seen in the setting of childhood obesity. Therefore, with increase

Flowchart 4: Pathophysiological mechanism of hypertension in obstructive sleep apnea (OSA).

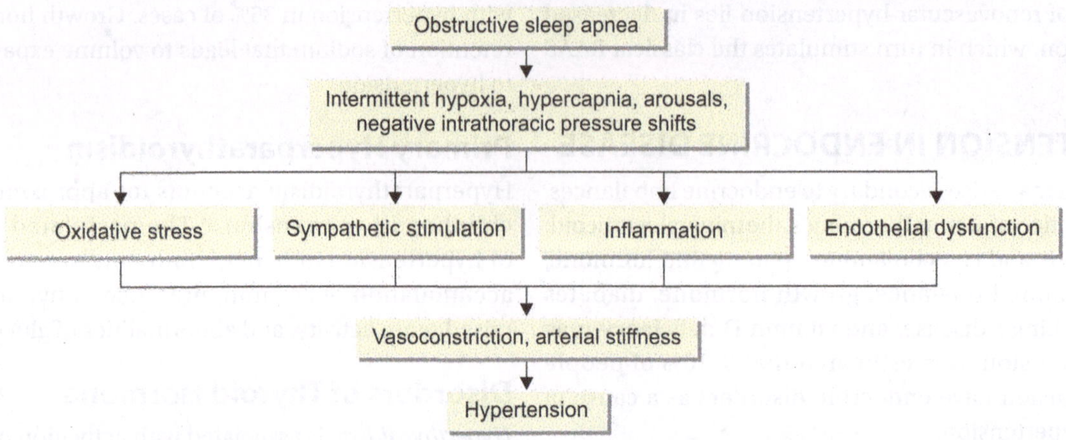

in the prevalence of obesity, assessment for OSA should be performed in children with obesity and hypertension. In OSA, there is episodic obstruction of upper airways, leading to hypoxia and hypercapnia. This in turn stimulates the chemoreceptors, which stimulate the SNS causing peripheral vasoconstriction and subsequent hypertension. This acute stimulation of the SNS may persist chronically into the awake phase causing hypertension. Plasma catecholamine levels have been found to be elevated in patients with OSA.[27]

Activation of the classical RAAS is also postulated to increase BP in patients with OSA. Studies have linked increased Ang II and aldosterone levels to OSA in patients.[27]

Repetitive deoxygenation and reoxygenation may lead to development of inflammation which leads to atherosclerosis and hypertension. Interleukin 6 (IL-6), tumor necrosis factor α (TNFα), and C-reactive protein (CRP) are found to be elevated in patients of OSA with hypertension.

Oxidative stress in OSA releases reactive oxygen species (ROS) and decreases NO in circulation. This leads to vasoconstriction and subsequent cardiovascular disease in patients with OSA.

Endothelial dysfunction causes increase in secretion of endothelin, which is known to cause vasoconstriction. The production of endothelin is possibly due to increased oxidative stress in patients with OSA. This endothelial dysfunction is postulated to play a fundamental role in promoting atherosclerosis and development of hypertension in patients with OSA. This event precedes the development of cardiovascular disease.[27] **Flowchart 4** schematically represents the pathophysiology of hypertension in OSA.

DRUGS AND HYPERTENSION

Certain therapeutic drugs, environmental toxins, illicit drugs, and herbal preparations may elevate hypertension and lead to refractory hypertension. Reviewing drug history in detail becomes important to avoid escalating the use of antihypertensives and to avoid unnecessary investigations.

The various drugs causing hypertension and the mechanism by which they do so are listed in **Table 3**.

Systemic corticosteroids such as dexamethasone, prednisolone, and fludrocortisone cause hypertension proportionate to their mineralocorticoid activity.[28]

Calcineurin inhibitors can cause hypertension due to renal vasoconstriction and hydrosodic (water and sodium) retention.[29]

Recombinant erythropoietin, despite having dramatically improved the care of patients with CKD, can cause hypertension by various mechanisms including increasing the hematocrit, increasing sensitivity to endogenous vasoconstrictors, and reduced production of endogenous vasodilators.[28]

Nonsteroidal anti-inflammatory drugs (NSAIDs), commonly used as over-the-counter preparation as pain killers, cause hypertension by increasing the secretion of endothelin and altering the metabolism of arachidonic acid.[28,29]

Substance abuse is also an important cause of hypertension. Alcohol, cocaine, amphetamines, and caffeine are known to cause elevation of BP.[28,29]

Antihypertensives of the diuretic and vasodilator subclass can cause paradoxical elevation of BP in patients who are in a volume-contracted, high-renin state. Central α-2 agonists such as clonidine may cause peripheral vasoconstriction. Abrupt clonidine withdrawal can cause rebound hypertension by rapid resumption of catecholamine production.[29]

Heavy metal such as lead exposure can also elevate BP both acutely and chronically.[29]

PATHOGENESIS OF HYPERTENSIVE END-ORGAN DAMAGE

Hypertension leads to various hormonal, biochemical, and hemodynamic changes that lead to organ damage involving the heart, vasculature—particularly in the retina, brain, and kidneys. The damage to these specific organs, consequently called the target organ damage, can result in cerebrovascular disease, retinopathy, renal failure, and atherosclerotic vascular disease.

TABLE 3: Drugs and their mechanism of action implicated in causing hypertension.

Drugs	Mechanism of action
Steroids	Increased sensitivity to catecholamines, stimulation of RAAS, sodium retention and blood volume expansion, increased plasma concentration of angiotensinogen
Oral contraceptives	Alteration in sodium and water balance
Cyclosporine	Renal vasoconstriction, volume expansion, SNS activation, ET-1 secretion
NSAIDs	Reduction in vasodilatory prostaglandins, salt and water retention, tubulointerstitial injury
Recombinant human erythropoietin	Reduction in NO-mediated vasodilatation, increased erythrocyte mass, direct vasopressor effect, arterial remodeling by production of vascular cell growth factor
Substances of abuse:	
• Alcohol	Sympathetic activity, impaired baroreceptor activity, cellular sodium metabolism alteration, increased intracellular calcium
• Cocaine	Stimulation of SNS, increased cardiac oxygen demand, glomerulosclerosis, direct vasoconstriction
• Caffeine	SNS stimulation, vasoconstriction, impaired baroreceptor activity
• Tobacco	SNS stimulation, increased arterial wall stiffness, decreased vasodilatation
Antidepressants	Increased half life of norepinephrine at sympathetic nerve endings
Antihypertensives:	
• Clonidine	Sudden resumption of catecholamine production that was blocked with clonidine
	Receptor upregulation
• Beta-blockers	RAAS stimulation
• Diuretics	
Anesthetics:	
• Ketamine	Increased sympathetic vascular resistance, sympathomimetic
• Desflurane	Increased intracellular calcium causing smooth muscle contraction
Ergot alkaloids:	Sympathomimetic
• Ginseng	Sympathomimetic, catecholamine release
• Ephedra	Sympathomimetic
• Glucagon	

(NO: nitric oxide; NSAIDs: nonsteroidal anti-inflammatory drugs; RAAS: renin–angiotensin–aldosterone system; SNS: sympathetic nervous system)

Many mechanisms are involved in the pathophysiology of end-organ damage. These include (1) endothelial activation related to decrease in NO activity, increase in endothelin activity, and increased plasmin activator inhibitor resulting in a procoagulant state and (2) impaired angiogenesis and imbalance between matrix metalloproteinase (MMPs) and their tissue inhibitors of metalloproteinases (TIMPs) leading to microvascular disease. The thrombotic complications of hypertension are paradoxically more common than the expected hemorrhagic complication of the high pressures exerted on the vessel wall in hypertension. This is called the "thrombotic paradox of hypertension" or the "Birmingham paradox."[30]

CONCLUSION

A mechanistic understanding of BP regulation is useful in evaluation and treatment of hypertension in children. While secondary hypertension is the predominant cause and should be sought in every child with hypertension, the prevalence of primary hypertension is on the rise.

KEY POINTS

- Neural mechanisms of BP control are:
  - Increased or decreased cardiac output through stimulation of β1 and M1 receptors respectively in the heart.
  - Vasoconstriction or vasodilatation on stimulation or inhibition of α1 and β2 receptors in the arteriolar bed.
- Humoral mechanisms of BP control are through the classical RAAS pathway and local autacoidal mechanisms.
- Renal mechanisms of BP control are pressure natriuresis and tubuloglomerular feedback.
- Primary hypertension accounts for a growing minority of the cases of hypertension, especially in the settings of premature birth and obesity.
- Genetic and lifestyle factors, insulin resistance, and salt sensitivity are contributory to primary hypertension.
- Secondary hypertension accounts for 75–80% of childhood hypertension.
- Important causes of secondary hypertension include renal parenchymal disease (usually CKD), renal vascular disease, endocrine disorders, neurological conditions, and OSA.
- Monogenic hypertension is usually caused by mutations that lead to water retention.

REFERENCES

1. Greene BA. Cardiac output and total peripheral resistance in anesthesiology: clinical applications. J Am Med Assoc. 1958;166(9):1003-10.
2. Patel P, Ali N. Mechanisms involved in regulation of systemic blood pressure. Arch Clin Hypertens. 2017;3(1):16-20.
3. McCorry LK. Physiology of the autonomic nervous system. Am J Pharm Educ. 2007;71(4):78.
4. Mannelli M, Rossi GP, Vanderriele PE, Parenti G. The endocrine regulation of blood pressure. In: Belfiore A, LeRoith D (Eds). Principles of Endocrinology and Hormone Action [Internet]. Cham: Springer International Publishing; 2018. pp. 611-25.
5. Ancion A, Tridetti J, Nguyen Trung ML, Oury C, Lancellotti P. A review of the role of bradykinin and nitric oxide in the cardioprotective action of angiotensin-converting enzyme inhibitors: Focus on perindopril. Cardiol Ther. 2019; 8(2):179-91.
6. Granger JP, Alexander BT, Llinas M. Mechanisms of pressure natriuresis. Curr Hypertens Rep. 2002;4(2):152-9.
7. Vallon V. Tubuloglomerular feedback and the control of glomerular filtration rate. Physiology. 2003;18(4):169-74.

8. Chrysaidou K, Chainoglou A, Karava V, Dotis J, Printza N, Stabouli S. Secondary hypertension in children and adolescents: Novel insights. Curr Hypertens Rev. 2020;16(1):37-44.
9. Falkner B. Recent clinical and translational advances in pediatric hypertension. Hypertens Dallas Tex 1979. 2015;65(5):926-31.
10. Sabri M, Gheissari A, Mansourian M, Mohammadifard N, Sarrafzadegan N. Essential hypertension in children, a growing worldwide problem. J Res Med Sci Off J Isfahan Univ Med Sci. 2019;24:109.
11. Raj M. Essential hypertension in adolescents and children: recent advances in causative mechanisms. Indian J Endocrinol metab. 2011;15(Suppl 4):S367-73.
12. Silva AA da, Carmo JM do, Li X, Wang Z, Mouton AJ, Hall JE. Role of hyperinsulinemia and insulin resistance in hypertension: Metabolic syndrome revisited. Can J Cardiol. 2020;36(5):671-82.
13. Wirix AJG, Kaspers PJ, Nauta J, Chinapaw MJM, Holthe JEK. Pathophysiology of hypertension in obese children: a systematic review. Obes Rev. 2015;16(10):831-42.
14. Sutherland Megan R, Mariane B, Marie-Amélie L, Fanny H, Catherine Y, Mai LT, et al. Preterm birth and hypertension risk. Hypertension. 2014;63(1):12-8.
15. Viera AJ, Neutze DM. Diagnosis of secondary hypertension: an age-based approach. Am Fam Physician. 2010;82(12):1471-8.
16. Garovic VD, Hilliard AA, Turner ST. Monogenic forms of low-renin hypertension. Nat Clin Pract Nephrol. 2006;2(11):624-30.
17. Simonetti GD, Mohaupt MG, Bianchetti MG. Monogenic forms of hypertension. Eur J Pediatr. 2012;171(10):1433-9.
18. Yamaguchi I, Flynn JT. Pathophysiology of hypertension. In: Pediatric Nephrology, 6th edition. Heidelberg: Springer-Verlag; 2009. pp. 1484-518.
19. Flynn JT, Mitsnefes M, Pierce C, Cole SR, Parekh RS, Furth SL, et al. Blood pressure in children with chronic kidney disease: a report from the Chronic Kidney Disease in Children Study. Hypertens Dallas Tex 1979. 2008;52(4):631-7.
20. Johnson JG, Hunt JC. Hypertension secondary to renal parenchymal disease. In: Amery A, Fagard R, Lijnen P, Staessen J (Eds). Hypertensive Cardiovascular Disease: Pathophysiology and Treatment Developments in Cardiovascular Medicine. Netherlands: Springer; 1982.
21. Mailloux LU, Levey AS. Hypertension in patients with chronic renal disease. Am J Kidney Dis Off J Natl Kidney Found. 1998; 32(5 Suppl 3):S120-141.
22. Textor SC. Renal arterial disease and hypertension. Med Clin North Am. 2017;101(1):65-79.
23. Tullus K, Brennan E, Hamilton G, Lord R, McLaren CA, Marks SD, et al. Renovascular hypertension in children. Lancet Lond Engl. 2008;371(9622):1453-63.
24. Velasco A, Vongpatanasin W. The evaluation and treatment of endocrine forms of hypertension. Curr Cardiol Rep. 2014; 16(9):528.
25. Thomas RM, Ruel E, Shantavasinkul PC, Corsino L. Endocrine hypertension: an overview on the current etiopathogenesis and management options. World J Hypertens. 2015;5(2):14-27.
26. Berta E, Lengyel I, Halmi S, Zrínyi M, Erdei A, Harangi M, et al. Hypertension in thyroid disorders. Front Endocrinol. 2019; 10:482.
27. Phillips CL, O'Driscoll DM. Hypertension and obstructive sleep apnea. Nat Sci Sleep. 2013;5:43-52.
28. Aronow WS. Drug-induced causes of secondary hypertension. Ann Transl Med. 2017;5(17):349.
29. Diaconu CC, Dediu GN, Iancu MA. Drug-induced arterial hypertension—a frequently ignored cause of secondary hypertension: a review. Acta Cardiol. 2018;73(6):511-7.
30. Nadar SK, Tayebjee MH, Messerli F, Lip GYH. Target organ damage in hypertension: pathophysiology and implications for drug therapy. Curr Pharm Des. 2006;12(13):1581-92.

CHAPTER 10.3

Renovascular Hypertension

Rajiv Sinha, Subhankar Sarkar

INTRODUCTION

Harry Goldblatt and his associates first demonstrated that reduction of blood flow to the kidneys can produce hypertension.[1] Renovascular hypertension (RVH) is defined as systemic hypertension caused by hormonal response secondary to the impaired blood flow to a part or all, of one or both kidneys. It is an uncommon but important cause of secondary hypertension in children. RVH is usually due to an occlusive lesion in the renal artery [renal artery stenosis (RAS)]. Significant RAS are usually defined as those where stenosis is >75% of the vessel lumen or at least 50% with poststenotic dilation. Early detection and management of RVH are critical to preventing ischemic nephropathy progressing on to chronic kidney disease (CKD) as well as other target organ damage secondary to hypertension.[2] Over the recent years, with major advances in vascular imaging technique and interventional radiology, RVH is often amenable to cure. In fact, after coarctation of the aorta, RVH is the second most common cause of correctable hypertension in children.

EPIDEMIOLOGY

With the epidemic of obesity, primary or essential hypertension has become the most common cause of childhood hypertension, particularly among older children. Secondary hypertension remains common among younger children. Among children with secondary hypertension, approximately 34–79% patients have renal parenchymal disorders and 5–25% have RVH.[3] Overall RVH comprises 5–10% of all cases of childhood hypertension.[4,5]

ETIOLOGY

Renovascular hypertension is a heterogeneous disease process that can be secondary to various etiologies **(Table 1)** including intrinsic lesions of the renal arteries, extrinsic compression by masses, and intraluminal occlusion by thrombosis. Commonly, it occurs in isolation as a result of fibromuscular dysplasia (FMD) of the renal arteries. It can also be a part of systemic vasculitis such as Takayasu's arteritis (TA) and polyarteritis nodosa (PAN) or as an extracranial manifestation of moyamoya disease (MMD). Although FMD is the most prevalent cause of RVH in western world, in countries such as India and South Africa, TA is reported in higher percentage (73–89%).[6-9] In contrast, MMD is more commonly reported as a cause of RVH in East Asia, Korea, and Japan. Among adults, atherosclerosis (90%) is the most common cause of RVH.[10]

TABLE 1: Etiologies of renovascular hypertension.

Fibrous and fibromuscular dysplasia[11]	• Medial fibroplasia • Perimedial fibroplasia • Intimal fibroplasia • Medial hyperplasia
Vasculitis	• Takayasu disease • Kawasaki disease • Moyamoya disease • Other systemic vasculitis
Vascular malformations	• Thromboembolism (e.g., prior history of umbilical catheterization, postangiography, post-trauma) • Arteriovenous malformation • Renal artery aneurysm
Inherited conditions	• Neurofibromatosis type 1 • Tuberous sclerosis • Williams' syndrome • Marfan's syndrome • Feuerstein–Mims syndrome • Tuberous sclerosis
Extrinsic compression	• Neuroblastoma • Wilms' tumor/other tumors • Congenital fibrous bands • Post-traumatic • Retroperitoneal fibrosis
Miscellaneous	• Radiation • Congenital rubella syndrome • Transplant renal artery stenosis

Fibromuscular Dysplasia

Typically, FMD affects the distal two-thirds of main renal arteries and its segmental branches, or both. McCormack and colleagues[11] developed a classification based on the layer of the vascular wall involvement **(Table 1)**. FMD most commonly involves the tunica media (80%) with or without aneurysm, but it may also involve other layers of arterial wall. Intimal lesion in FMD is characterized by circumferential or eccentric involvement, accumulation of loose fibrous matrix with a moderate number of cells without any inflammatory change, or lipid accumulation. The intimal media is often replaced by a collagenous fibrous matrix and degenerative elastic fibers, which displace and disorient smooth muscle cells leading to multiple stenotic lesions followed by poststenotic aneurysms, which can resemble a "string of beads" on angiogram.[12] Some patients with congenital rubella may also present with RVH secondary to FMD in renal arteries. Isolated FMD may have genetic association. About 11–60% of cases of RVH are familial with a pattern most consistent with autosomal dominant with variable penetrance.[13] Bofinger et al. noted a high frequency of angiotensin I-converting enzyme (ACE) allele among children with FMD, which often results in low-tissue concentration of angiotensin II. This can affect vascular muscles' development and explain the FMD.[14]

Genetic Syndromes

Neurofibromatosis 1 (NF1), Williams syndrome, Klippel-Trenaunay-Weber syndrome, and Feuerstein-Mims syndrome are some of the genetic syndromes associated with RVH. Renovascular lesions found in them are usually similar to intimal FMD. Among these genetic syndromes, NF1 is most common wherein lesions occur near the origin of the renal arteries unlike FMD, which affects more distally. Along with renal artery involvement, other arteries such as abdominal aorta, internal carotid, and vertebral arteries may also be involved in NF. Lesions in NF are varied and can be (1) pure intimal lesions, (2) advanced intimal lesions and medial changes, (3) nodular aneurysmal lesions with loss of media elements, (4) periarterial nodular abnormalities, and (5) epithelioid lesions with marked cellular proliferation.[15] Patients with tuberous sclerosis may develop RVH due to intra-renal cystic lipomatous lesions or occasionally arteriovenous malformations.[15]

Renal Artery Occlusion Secondary to Thrombus

Thrombus occluding the renal arteries is another important cause of RVH. It is more common among neonates and ranks among the top etiologies of neonatal acute hypertension[15] Umbilical arterial catheterization in premature or ill neonates causing trauma to endothelium leading to platelet aggregation and subsequent thrombus formation is a common predisposing factor. Renal artery thrombosis is rare in older children in whom blunt trauma of renal vessels resulting in thrombosis is more common.

Vasculitis

Vasculitis such as TA, MMD, sarcoidosis, and rarely Kawasaki disease can also cause RVH. A higher incidence of TA in Asian population contributing to RVH may be accounted for by the higher incidence of tuberculosis in the region.[6-9] A nonspecific inflammatory process in TA leads to stenosis and obliteration of the aorta and its primary branches causing renal ischemia and hypertension. TA usually involves bilateral renal artery and is frequently ostial/proximal, usually with coexistent stenosis of the perirenal aorta.

Middle Aortic Syndrome

Middle aortic syndrome (MAS) is rare in children and characterized by a severe narrowing of the distal thoracic and/or abdominal aorta. Most of them are idiopathic (64%), 15% are associated with Mendelian disorders, and 17% are related to inflammatory diseases.[16] Among the extra-aortic involvement, renal (70%), superior mesenteric (30%), and celiac (22%) arteries are common. In fact, a significant number of children with MAS present as RVH (66%) due to RAS. MAS usually involves both renal arteries (60%). A segmental narrowing of the renal artery is more commonly seen and the stenosis is restricted to the ostial region of the vessel.

Miscellaneous

Among children post kidney transplant, refractory hypertension should make us think of transplant RAS which is the most common vascular complication following renal transplant and may even contribute to transplant failure. Rarely, extrinsic compression can account for RVH wherein renovascular narrowing can be secondary to tumors (Wilms' tumor, neuroblastoma, pheochromocytoma, and lymphomas), congenital bands, neurofibromas, or post-traumatic hematomas.

PATHOPHYSIOLOGY

Pathophysiology of RVH is usually influenced by interaction of two factors:

1. Activation of renin–angiotensin–aldosterone system (RAAS) and
2. Presence of normal or abnormal contralateral kidney

Renal artery stenosiss (RAS) leads to renal ischemia and renin hypersecretion. Renin accelerates conversion of angiotensin I to angiotensin II and enhances adrenal release of aldosterone. Angiotensin II causes vasoconstriction, sodium retention, aldosterone secretion, sympathetic activation, and vessel changes and also has direct myocardial effects all of which augment hypertension **(Flowchart 1)**. Although angiotensin II causes vasoconstriction of both afferent and efferent arterioles, efferent arterioles vasoconstriction is more significant as the efferent arteriole has a smaller basal diameter. Angiotensin II mediates release of vasodilator prostaglandins and nitric oxide, which further minimizes the vasoconstriction effects on afferent arterioles. End result is increase in glomerular filtration pressure and consequent kidney damage. Also, angiotensin II mediates constriction of glomerular mesangium, which leads to a decreased surface area of filtration.

Flowchart 1: Mechanism of renin-mediated hypertension.

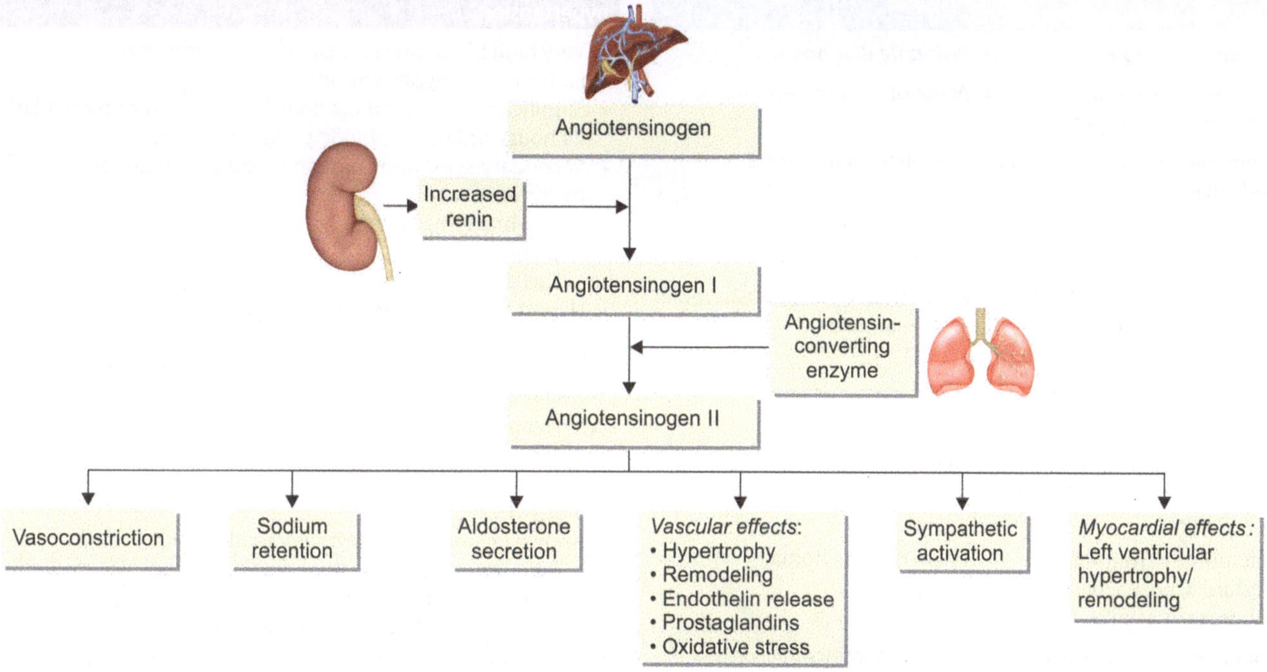

Three stages of development of RVH have been described:

1. *Renin-angiotensin-dependent phase:* In this initial phase, renal ischemia causes hyperreninemia, which leads to hypertension. Over days to week, intact contralateral kidney tries to compensate the altered homeostasis. This results in both kidneys opposing each other; the stenotic kidney avidly retains sodium and produces excess renin in response to renal ischemia, while the nonstenotic kidney excretes sodium and water to maintain euvolemia. In this phase, BP remains high along with a high renin level. Hence, the systemic hypertension seen in this phase is mediated by both renin and angiotensin.
2. *Phase of salt retention:* Herein sodium and water are retained to maintain perfusion pressure of ischemic kidney. As a result of hypervolemia, the renin level falls and hypertension becomes less dependent on angiotensin II and predominantly results from volume expansion. Perfusion pressure is restored at the expense of systemic hypertension and volume overload. Blood pressure returns to a normal level if blood flow to stenotic kidney is restored but in cases of persistent renal hypoperfusion, condition enters the third phase.
3. *Systemic renin-angiotensin independent phase:* In the third phase, hypertension is unremitting, persisting well even after the removal of the stenosis due to ischemic nephropathy in either or both kidneys.

Hyponatremic Hypertensive Syndrome

Unilateral RAS may present with severe hypertension along with hyponatremia secondary to natriuresis from the contralateral kidney, known as hyponatremic hypertensive syndrome (HHS). In unilateral RAS, decreased renal blood flow results in increased renin secretion, which increases the level of angiotensin II (AII) and level of aldosterone. AII causes arterial hypertension resulting in pressure diuresis and natriuresis from the contralateral normal kidney, clinically manifesting as polyuria and polydipsia. Both AII and aldosterone cause potassium loss, and resulting hypokalemia further stimulates renin secretion. Hyponatremia further increases aldosterone secretion, which also contributes to hypokalemia. Polyuria causes volume contraction and increasing thirst leads to antidiuretic hormone secretion, which also contributes to hyponatremia. So in HHS, activation of RAAS in presence of the hypertrophied contralateral kidney sets up a vicious cycle of natriuresis and hyponatremia along with the usual hypokalemia and metabolic alkalosis.[17]

CLINICAL SPECTRUM

Renin–angiotensin systems are usually bilateral (53–78%).[18-20] Intrarenal disease occurs in 44% and a combination of intrarenal disease and main artery stenosis occurs in 31%.[18] Although children without an associated comorbid condition usually have single focal branch stenosis, concomitant stenosis of other arteries is also not uncommon. Up to 70% of pediatric cases of RVH may be discovered as an incidental finding[18-22] Rest may present as severe symptoms secondary to target-organ damage, such as an acute cerebral incident, heart failure, or compromised kidney function presenting with fluid and electrolyte imbalance. Bell's palsy with facial nerve paralysis is another common presentation. Clinical findings may include asymmetric pulses, abdominal/neck bruit, weak femoral artery pulses, café-au-lait spots, and other neurocutaneous markers of conditions such as NF, tuberous sclerosis, etc. **(Table 2)**.

TABLE 2: Clinical clues which might help to identify underlying diagnosis in severe hypertension.

Signs and symptoms	*Probable diagnosis*
Hematuria, edema, and decreased urine output	Acute glomerulonephritis
Abdominal pain, vomiting, and bloody diarrhea	Hemolytic uremic syndrome
Sore throat or streptococcal skin infection	Poststreptococcal glomerulonephritis
History of umbilical catheterization in premature baby/abdominal or flank bruit	Renal artery thrombosis/renal artery stenosis
Recent use of serotonergic agents	Serotonin syndrome
Weight loss, tremor, heat intolerance, thyromegaly, and exophthalmos	Hyperthyroidism
Palpitation, intermittent tachycardia, headache, and diaphoresis	Pheochromocytoma
Bulging fontanelle and increased head circumference	Increased intracranial pressure
Ataxia, papilledema, visual field defect	Intracranial mass lesion
Neurocutaneous lesion such as café-au-lait spot, freckles, neurofibroma, and shagreen patches	Renal artery stenosis in neurofibromatosis or tuberous sclerosis
Abdominal mass	Renal artery stenosis secondary to Wilms' tumor, neuroblastoma, and polycystic kidney
Weak femoral pulse, discrepancy in four limbs, BP	Coarctation of aorta

DIAGNOSIS

Renovascular hypertension usually results in severe hypertension but paradoxically it is often diagnosed late as blood pressure is often not measured routinely in children. Measuring blood pressure in children needs some degree of expertise. A health professional should be aware of the importance of an appropriate cuff size (which may not be easily available) as well as age/height-appropriate blood pressure centile chart. Measuring blood pressure in infants is more challenging and Doppler devices may be useful.

A high index of suspicion is useful for early diagnosis of RVH and as given in **Box 1**, various clues can be useful from a good history and examination.

INVESTIGATIONS

Investigations for RVH are directed toward identifying any underlying cause and detecting any target organ damage **(Table 3)**.

Confirming suspected RAS among children is not easy and requires judicious use of noninvasive and invasive tests. In contrast to adults, noninvasive tests cannot reliably exclude all causes of potentially treatable RVH in children, and digital subtraction angiography (DSA) despite being invasive remains gold standard.[23] **Box 1** can be a useful guide wherein extensive evaluation beyond noninvasive investigations for RAS is merited.

BOX 1: When to have high index of suspicion for renovascular hypertension.

- Very high blood pressure (stage-2 hypertension)
- Early onset of hypertension
- Significantly elevated diastolic blood pressure particularly on 24 hours ambulatory blood pressure assessment
- Secondary symptoms of high blood pressure indicating severe hypertension:
  - Cerebral symptoms
  - Cardiac failure
  - Facial palsy
- Hypertension not controlled with two or more antihypertensive drugs
- Presence of underlying syndrome with a high risk of vascular disease:
  - Neurofibromatosis
  - Tuberous sclerosis
  - Williams syndrome
- Signs of vasculitis
- Known or suspected previous vascular insult:
  - Renal artery thrombosis or umbilical artery catheterization
  - Previous trauma or radiation
- Bruit heard over renal artery or arteries
- Transplanted kidneys
- Raised peripheral plasma renin
- Persistent moderate hypokalemia
- Asymmetric kidney size (e.g., unilateral small kidney)
- Rise in serum creatinine >30% after initiation of renin–angiotensin system inhibitor

TABLE 3: Basic investigation for suspected renovascular hypertension.

Evaluation for cause	• Four-limb blood pressure (BP) measurement • Ambulatory BP monitoring • Urinalysis • 24-hour urinary protein or spot protein to creatinine ratio • Hemogram • Blood urea, creatinine, and electrolytes • Fasting lipids, glucose, and uric acid • Renal ultrasonography and Doppler (for an older child)
Screen for target-organ damage	• Retinal fundus examination • *Urine*: Spot protein to creatinine ratio • Echocardiography

Noninvasive Investigations

As DSA remains the gold standard in pediatric practice, noninvasive investigations are usually restricted to those children with low suspicion of RAS, for follow-up evaluation, to exclude other possible causes of hypertension (such as pheochromocytoma), and for evaluating any target-organ damage [e.g., echocardiography for left ventricular hypertrophy (LVH)].

A basic renal profile includes urea, creatinine, and electrolytes (sodium, potassium, calcium, and phosphate), and urinalysis is usually routinely done. These tests will help in identifying any other causes of hypertension (such as CKD and hypercalcemia). Presence of proteinuria may be a clue to an underlying glomerular disorder. In the presence of RVH, proteinuria may also indicate renal end-organ damage and monitoring it with repeated quantification may give us some idea of any progression in kidney damage. Significant hypertension with low serum potassium is suspicious of increased renin and aldosterone activity, which is expected in children with RVH. Although plasma renin activity (PRA) is elevated in 50–80% of RVH, it has limited diagnostic utility as it may be suppressed by antihypertensive medicines, high-dietary sodium intake, volume expansion due to intrinsic renal disease, and bilateral RAS.

Noninvasive Imaging Tests

Duplex Doppler Ultrasonography

This is noninvasive, relatively inexpensive, and suitable for serial monitoring to determine the disease progression. It does give good visualization of abdominal aorta but proper visualization of renal arteries, particularly their intrarenal branches, can be challenging. To overcome this concern, various Doppler-derived parameters have been proposed as an indirect marker of RAS.[24,25] Among these, peak systolic velocity (PSV) and resistive index (RI = PSV minus end-diastolic velocity divided by PSV) are commonly used. Among adults, PSV has been reported to have 85% sensitivity and 92% specificity with a positive-predictive value of 84% and a false-positive rate of 8%.[26] In these studies, PSV > 300 cm/s has been found to be suggestive of hemodynamically important RAS.[27] Similarly for RI, adult data suggests sensitivity and specificity for detection of renovascular disease to be 80% and 54%, respectively.[28] RI > 80% is associated with a greater degree of intrinsic kidney damage or irreversible intrarenal vascular disease and less favorable outcome after revascularization. Most of these data are from adult studies, and pediatric literature is lacking. Disadvantages of using duplex Doppler ultrasonography are its technical difficulty making it operator dependent. A detailed examination of renal vessels is also quite time consuming. Obtaining good views of renal vessels and deriving correct Doppler-derived variables are challenging in young children as well as in obese patients. Thus, the American Academy of Pediatrics 2017 guideline suggests Doppler renal ultrasonography to be done in centers with appropriate expertise and to be restricted to normal-weight children and adolescents ≥8 years of age who are suspected of having RVH and who will cooperate with the procedure (grade C, moderate recommendation).[3]

Computed Tomographic Angiography

Computed tomographic angiography (CTA) **(Fig. 1)** is a useful noninvasive test with adult studies reporting sensitivity and specificity for detecting RAS at 94% and 93%, respectively.[3,29] It has to be remembered that most of these reports are from adult literature where atherosclerosis is the main etiopathogenesis. Its usefulness in children where FMD is more common needs further evaluation. In addition, most of the literatures are old and as CT technology has evolved significantly over the last decade, it may not be appropriate to come to a conclusion based on previously published data. Yield of multidetector CTA in diagnosing intrarenal stenosis, particularly in children, needs to be properly evaluated. The major disadvantage of CTA remains radiation exposure and chances of contrast nephropathy in a renal-compromised patient.

Magnetic Resonance Angiography

Magnetic resonance angiography (MRA) is a highly sensitive test for detecting proximal RAS. The sensitivity and specificity for the detection of RAS are 90% and 94%, respectively, for the pediatric group and up to 100% sensitivity has been reported in adult study.[3,29] However, MRA may miss accessory renal arteries and significant lesions in the intrarenal distal part of renal arteries. The main concern of MRA is gadolinium-associated nephrogenic systemic fibrosis among those with reduced renal function. With technical improvement such as imaging without gadolinium-based contrast or using breath-hold MRA with paramagnetic contrast such as gadopentetate dimeglumine, this modality may be increasingly used.

Luminal occlusion <60% rarely produces any significant hemodynamic effects.

Scintigraphy

Renal scintigraphy either with 99m-technetium-dimercapto-succinic acid (DMSA) or 99m-Tc-mercaptoacetyltriglycine (MAG3) along with angiotensin-converting enzyme inhibitor (ACEI) has been evaluated as a potentially useful noninvasive

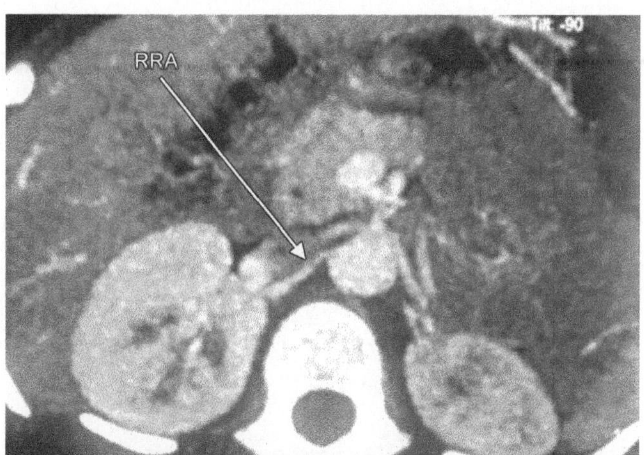

Fig. 1: Computed tomographic angiography of left renal artery stenosis. (RRA: right renal artery)

test. Among adults, the sensitivities and specificities for detecting RVH have been reported as 68–93% and 70–93%.[30] Unfortunately, pediatric studies have not been promising with reports of missing potentially treatable renovascular lesions.[31] The recently published AAP guideline did not support its use.[3]

Echocardiography and 24-hour Ambulatory Blood Pressure Monitoring

Echocardiography is important for evaluating the target organ damage on the heart. 24-hour ambulatory blood pressure monitoring (ABPM) is useful for monitoring treatment response in these children. In addition, significant hypertension, especially diastolic hypertension, detected by ABPM and loss of nocturnal dipping has been correlated with increased chances of having underlying secondary hypertension. Recent AAP guideline has strongly supported the use of both echocardiogram and 24-hour ABPM.

Invasive Test

Renal Vein Renin Sampling

Renal vein renin concentrations may be useful for localizing the site of significant lesion, particularly when RAS is bilateral, segmental, or both. Renin samples are taken from the infrarenal inferior vena cava and the main renal veins and their larger intrarenal tributaries through a femoral vein approach with the idea that the site with significant RAS will have higher renin activity.[32,33] This technique may help in not only localizing the kidney with RAS but may even localize the segment of the kidney being perfused by any stenosed tributaries of the main renal arteries. This will guide in segmental renal embolization for cases refractory to pharmacotherapy or not amenable to angioplasty.[34,35] The main limitation of renal vein renin sampling is obviously its invasiveness, which has resulted in, it not routinely been done in pediatric practice.

Diagnostic Angiography

Catheter-based DSA remains the most accurate technique for assessment of suspected renovascular disease in children and in presence of amenable stenosis, intervention can be carried out in the same setting **(Figs. 2A and B)**. Among a carefully selected cohort, it can have a diagnostic yield of 40%.[23,36] It can be done under local anesthesia in older children but usually needs general anesthesia for younger children (<10 years old). To established diagnosis, frontal and lateral oblique views are taken.[37] Sometime, delayed images are needed for complete renal artery occlusion to confirm patency of the distal renal artery by collateral perfusion.

Choosing the Diagnostic Test

Although noninvasive tests are initially preferred over invasive tests, the limitations of various noninvasive tests should be kept in mind, particularly in references to the challenges posed in pediatric practice. It has to be remembered that Doppler ultrasound is operator dependent, time consuming, and in children, it has been shown to miss significant RAS. CT/MRA can be done in younger children but it is more reliable for proximal RAS and may miss distal/intrarenal RAS. Hence, DSA remains the gold standard, particularly when one is having a high suspicion of RAS in a young child. Both DSA and CT angiography have the risk of contrast nephropathy and appropriate precautions should be followed.

MANAGEMENT

Treatment options for RVH include antihypertensive medication, endovascular intervention such as percutaneous transluminal angioplasty (PTA), and surgical interventions including revascularization surgery or unilateral nephrectomy. A tentative algorithm for management of children with RVH has been suggested in **Flowchart 2**.

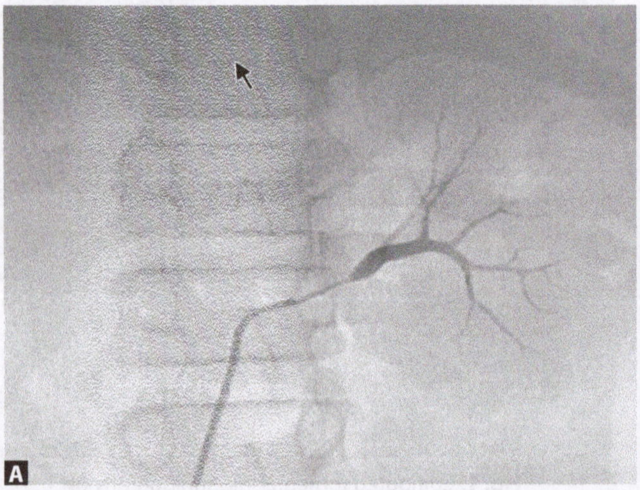
A

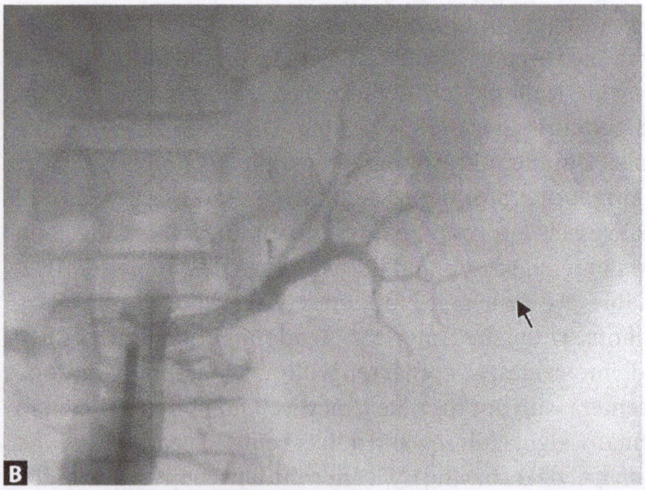
B

Figs. 2A and B: (A) Renal angiography shows left renal artery stenosis; (B) Left renal artery post-balloon angioplasty and stent.

Flowchart 2: Algorithmic approach for managing a child with renal artery stenosis.

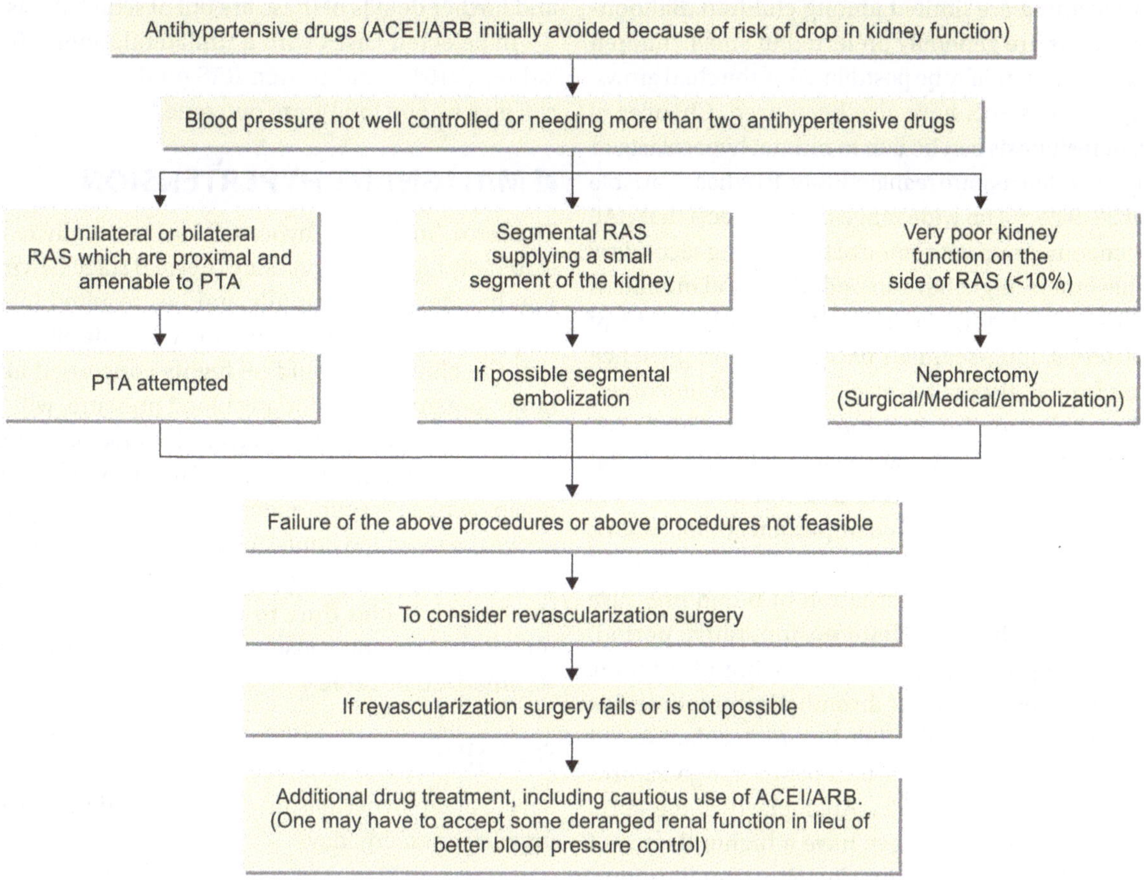

(ACEI: angiotensin-converting enzyme inhibitors; ARB: angiotensin receptor blocker; RAS: renal artery stenosis; PTA: percutaneous transluminal angioplasty)

Antihypertensive Medications

Most of the children with RVH require antihypertensive drugs at least initially. Initial medical therapy is usually started with either a calcium-channel blocker or a β-blocker, or both. Additional agents often required include prazosin, labetalol, clonidine, hydralazine, and/or minoxidil. Therapies with ACEI or angiotensin receptor blockers (ARBs) are avoided in patients with suspected or confirmed bilateral renovascular disease. ACEI and ARBs cause dilation of the glomerular efferent arteriole, which reduces the glomerular filtration pressure and can cause acute fall in GFR.[38] ACEI/ARBs may be used cautiously in those with unilateral RVH although in unilateral RAS, renal damage is difficult to monitor because it is often masked by a stable serum creatinine concentration courtesy the healthy contralateral kidney. In such a situation, DMSA scintigraphy is helpful for monitoring of renal function. In children on ACEI/ARBs, diuretics should be avoided. ACEI/ARB should be kept on hold in presence of volume depletion such as secondary to diarrhea and vomiting. ACEI/ARB may also be used as a last resort in severe RVH, which has been refractory to medical treatment and is not amiable to angioplasty or surgical intervention. These are usually those with bilateral diffuse long-segment RAS or multiple intrarenal RAS. Close monitoring of renal function including repeated nuclear scintigraphy is required to detect any significant fall in renal function although sometimes some compromise of renal function may have to be accepted in lieu of hypertension control.[39]

Endovascular Intervention

These are advocated when two or more antihypertensives are required for controlling blood pressure or when significant adverse effects are noted either from medications or from hypertension.[40]

Renal Angioplasty

Percutaneous transluminal angioplasty with or without stenting **(Figs. 2A and B)** has become well established even in pediatric practice.[41] Adult coronary angioplasty equipment are usually adequate and the approaches to the renal arteries are normally through the femoral. Diameter of the PTA balloon is normally equal to or less than the diameter of the artery proximal to the stenosis, which is determined from renal angiography. Renal artery stenting is an attractive option when immediate recoil to the original angiographic configuration takes place after angioplasty or after early recurrence of RAS after clinically successful PTA. Stenting is usually not required if postrecoil residual stenosis is <50%.[42] As the long-term outcome of these devices is unknown, indications for renal artery stenting are limited among children. Balloon-expandable stents are generally preferred in small children because they can potentially be postdilated as the child grows, but self-expanding stents have also been used. Chances of early in-stent restenosis can be due to intimal hyperplasia or thrombosis and often require reangioplasty. PTA has a variable cure rate of 28–94%.[43] The wide range likely reflects that RAS is a heterogeneous group with some of them being secondary to FMD while others might have an underlying inflammation such as those secondary to vasculitis. Involvement of nonrenal arteries, long-segment narrowing, and presence of diffuse intrarenal disease adversely affect PTA outcomes, and judicious selection for an appropriate candidate is a key to better outcome.[43] Arterial spasm including femoral artery spasm is the most common complication and is usually self-limiting. Other rare but important complications include dissection and arterial rupture with retroperitoneal extravasations of contrast. Fluctuation of blood pressure can happen during the immediate postoperative period, and hence close postoperative monitoring of vitals is recommended.[40] Possibilities of thrombotic complications require intraoperative use of either low-molecular-weight heparin or unfractionated heparin. Postdischarge aspirin is continued for at least 6 months. Angioplasty of the aorta for MAS is less successful, as they have a higher degree of immediate recoil as well as are prone to more complications. Despite these constraints, sometimes angioplasty is undertaken to buy time and delay surgery.

Ethanol Ablation

This is often useful for a segmental branch stenosis, which cannot be treated by angioplasty. This being less invasive may be preferred over partial nephrectomy although producing similar blood pressure control.[34,44] It is to be noted that coil embolization is not a good option as even after occlusion, the ischemic focus can recruit collaterals with persistent hypertension.[45]

Surgical Procedures

Surgery is indicated when medical treatment and angioplasty have failed for refractory hypertension. Options are usually revascularization surgery. The internal iliac artery is a useful conduit as is splenic artery on the left and hepatic and gastroduodenal arteries on the right, particularly if the celiac axis is unaffected. Saphenous vein is not used because of chances of aneurysmal degeneration. For smaller children, the preferred approach has been to maintain renal blood flow by endovascular means with a view to delaying the need for surgical revascularization until the child has reached puberty. The overall cure rate of hypertension is 36–70% by surgical revascularization.[39] Revascularization surgery is more frequently required for difficult RAS often with the aid of prosthetic graft. These are usually done in specialized centers, and further details of these are out of scope of this chapter.

In selected cases with a unilateral, poorly functioning kidney (<10%), and proven RAS on that side, nephrectomy can give a good long-term outcome.[37]

MALIGNANT HYPERTENSION

The term "malignant hypertension" is usually restricted for extremely high blood pressure (beyond stage II hypertension) that has developed rapidly and has resulted in some type of organ damage. The current AAP guideline advocates that the clinician should be highly concerned about acute target-organ damage for any blood pressure, which exceeds 30 mm Hg above the 95th percentile blood pressure target for the child's sex, age, and height.[3] The primary reason for end-organ damage is acute change in mean arterial pressure well above the tolerated limits. A child with chronic hypertension may also have very high BP but is often asymptomatic as the body has had time to adjust to the change in blood pressure. Common causes of severe acute hypertension are summarized in **Table 4**.

Definition

Severe acute hypertension can be classified as hypertensive urgency or emergency.

Hypertensive Emergency

These are defined when patients with stage-2 hypertension present with acute potentially life-threatening symptoms or features of target-organ damage involving central nervous system (encephalopathy, cerebral infarction, cerebral hemorrhage, and seizures), heart (pulmonary edema), kidneys (acute kidney injury), or eyes (papilledema and retinal hemorrhage). Among these, the most common presentation is hypertensive encephalopathy. Acute rise of blood pressure leads to loss of cerebrovascular autoregulation and endothelial damage causing vasogenic cerebral edema (**Fig. 3**). Children with hypertensive emergencies need rapid assessment and immediate initiation of hypertension management in a controlled setup.

TABLE 4: Some common causes of malignant hypertension.

Age groups	*Common causes of malignant hypertension*
Neonates	Renovascular disease such as renal artery thrombosis, congenital anomalies (such as autosomal-recessive polycystic kidney disease), coarctation of aorta, renal parenchymal disease, bronchopulmonary dysplasia, and congenital adrenal hyperplasia)
Children	Glomerulonephritis, endocrine disease, and renovascular causes
Adolescents	Glomerulonephritis, chronic kidney disease, and drugs intoxication

Hypertensive Urgencies

These are patients with stage-2 hypertension but without any evidence of target-organ damage. Symptoms are less and mild (e.g., headache and/or vomiting). These children, if not managed urgently, are at risk for progression to hypertensive emergencies.

It has to be emphasized that in defining hypertensive emergency/urgency, the presence or absence of life-threatening symptoms and/or target organ damage is more important than the absolute blood pressure level.

Pathophysiology and Clinical Features

Clinical features depend on etiology and age. Neonates may present with poor feeding irritability, vomiting, apnea, and cyanosis.[46,47] Older children present according to target-organ damage.

Neurological Manifestations

Cerebral blood flow is relatively constant over a wide range of systemic blood pressures because of autoregulation **(Fig. 3)**. Beyond a certain level of perfusion pressure, autoregulatory vasodilatation or vasoconstriction fails to work and may result in cerebral ischemia. This is particularly true for any acute significant change in blood pressure.

Hence, due to acute rise of blood pressure, cerebral autoregulation is lost leading to disruption of the blood-brain barrier and endothelial dysfunction resulting in imbalance in oxygen delivery, cerebral edema formation, and microhemorrhages.[48] Headache is the most common presentation along with other neurological signs and symptoms including seizures (25%), altered mental status or encephalopathy (25%), facial nerve palsy (12%), hemiplegia (8%), vomiting, signs of raised intracranial pressure, and/or focal neurological deficits.

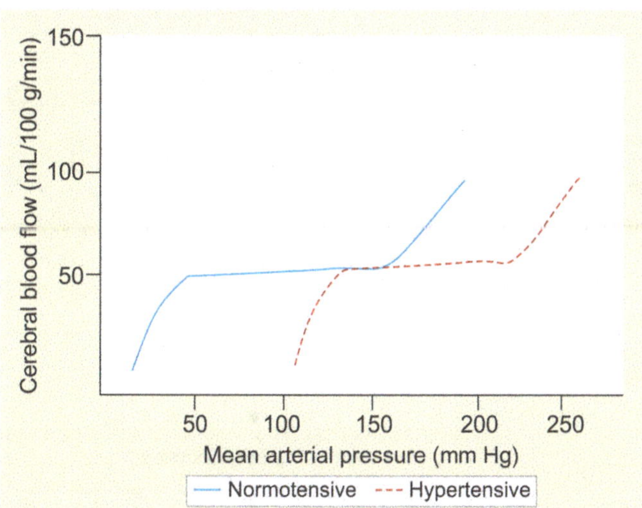

Fig. 3: Cerebral autoregulation. Cerebral blood flow (CBF) is relatively constant between 50 and 150 mm Hg of mean arterial pressure because of autoregulation but in chronically hypertensive patients, the autoregulation is shifted toward right. An abrupt change in blood pressure will not allow time for readjustment and can hence impair cerebral circulation.

Children with hypertensive encephalopathy often have features posterior reversible encephalopathy syndrome (PRES) wherein brain imaging shows lesions predominantly in the occipitoparietal white matter with occasional spread to basal ganglia, cerebellum, and brainstem. Other than hypertension, postchemotherapy, post-transplant, postinfectious, and autoimmune conditions may also cause PRES. PRES lesions as suggested by its nomenclature are usually reversible but rarely can have permanent sequel.

Cardiovascular Manifestations

Cardiac involvement may vary in the form of LVH, left ventricular failure, or left ventricular ischemia, depending on the duration and persistence of hypertension.[49,50] The incidence of LVH due to hypertension is up to 41% particularly in children with high body mass index (BMI).[51] Sudden acute increase in blood pressure may precipitate left ventricular failure, and the child may present with increased work of breathing, shortness of breath, chest pain, palpitations, decreased urine output, and poor appetite.

Renal Manifestations

Hypertension leads to loss of autoregulation of renal blood flow and results in kidney injury. Clinically, the child may present with hematuria, flank pain, and oliguria. Renal histopathology may demonstrate fibrinoid necrosis with thrombosis of intrarenal arteries.[52,53]

Ophthalmological Manifestations

Severe hypertension may lead to retinal bleeds, papilledema, loss of visual acuity, and cortical blindness.[54] The prevalence of hypertensive retinopathy in children with hypertension varies from 8.9% (assessed by direct fundoscopy) to 50% (assessed by retinal photographs).[11,55,56] Moderate-to-severe grades of retinopathy are relatively rare in children.

Evaluation

While controlling blood pressure to a safe level is an emergency priority, accurate diagnosis and evaluation of etiology of malignant hypertension are also important. Proper history and a thorough physical examination are essential. This will help in identifying conditions, which may require deviation from the usual algorithm of hypertensive emergency management. These include clinical conditions such as intracranial lesion, coarctation of aorta, pheochromocytoma, hypertension secondary to scorpion stings, or intake of recreational drugs. An extensive workup should be undertaken particularly in a young child who has extremely high pressure to rule out secondary causes of hypertension. Common investigations are summarized in **Table 5**.

Management

Severe hypertension has the potential to cause target-organ damage; hence, prompt recognition and treatment are of utmost importance. A child with hypertensive emergency

TABLE 5: Investigations for severe acute hypertension.

Initial workup	*Further workup*
• Complete blood count • Electrolytes (sodium, potassium, calcium, and chloride) • Serum urea and creatinine • Serum uric acid • Fasting lipid profile and blood glucose • Urine analysis • Echocardiography • Renal ultrasound with Doppler (older children)	• Thyroid-stimulating hormone, free T4, and free T3 • Serum cortisol and aldosterone • Plasma renin activity • 24-hour urinary catecholamine and metanephrine levels • Serum parathyroid hormone levels • Urine and serum toxicology screen • Urine pregnancy test • CT/MRI scan • DMSA/DTPA scan • MIBG scan • Antinuclear antibody/ erythrocyte sedimentation rate/C-reactive protein/ antidouble-stranded DNA/ anti-Smith/rheumatoid factor/antineutrophil cytoplasmic antibody (pANCA and cANCA)

(cANCA: cytoplasmic antineutrophil cytoplasmic antibody; DMSA: dimercaptosuccinic acid; DTPA: diethylenetriaminepentaacetate; MIBG: meta-iodobenzylguanidine; pANCA: perinuclear antineutrophil cytoplasmic antibody)

should preferably be admitted in the intensive care unit for close monitoring and prompt initiation of appropriate intravenous antihypertensive therapy. Initial management involves stabilization as per the standard emergency guideline focusing on ABC, i.e., airway, breathing, and circulation. Vascular access should be quickly established with preferably a dedicated vascular access for the antihypertensive agents, which are usually given intravenously in hypertensive emergencies. Oral antihypertensive agents may be tried in hypertensive urgencies provided the child is not vomiting and is tolerating oral intake. Seizures, if present, should be controlled with lorazepam. Blood pressure should be preferably monitored continuously by invasive intra-arterial line. Although intra-arterial blood pressure monitoring is desirable, treatment should not be delayed for lack of intra-arterial access. It should be initiated based on results of intermittent blood pressure measurement by noninvasive methods, which need to be done frequently, i.e., at least every 10–15 minutes. Target reduction of blood pressure is below 95th percentile for sex, age, and height (<130/80 for adolescent) over the initial 24–48 hours and thereafter target below the 90th percentile.[3] Blood pressure should not be lowered to >25% of the planned reduction over the first 8 hours with the aim to achieve 95th percentile target within 24–48 hours **Flowchart 3**. In patients with malignant hypertension and hypertensive encephalopathy, it is vital to lower the blood

Flowchart 3: Management algorithm of hypertension (HTN) emergency and urgency.

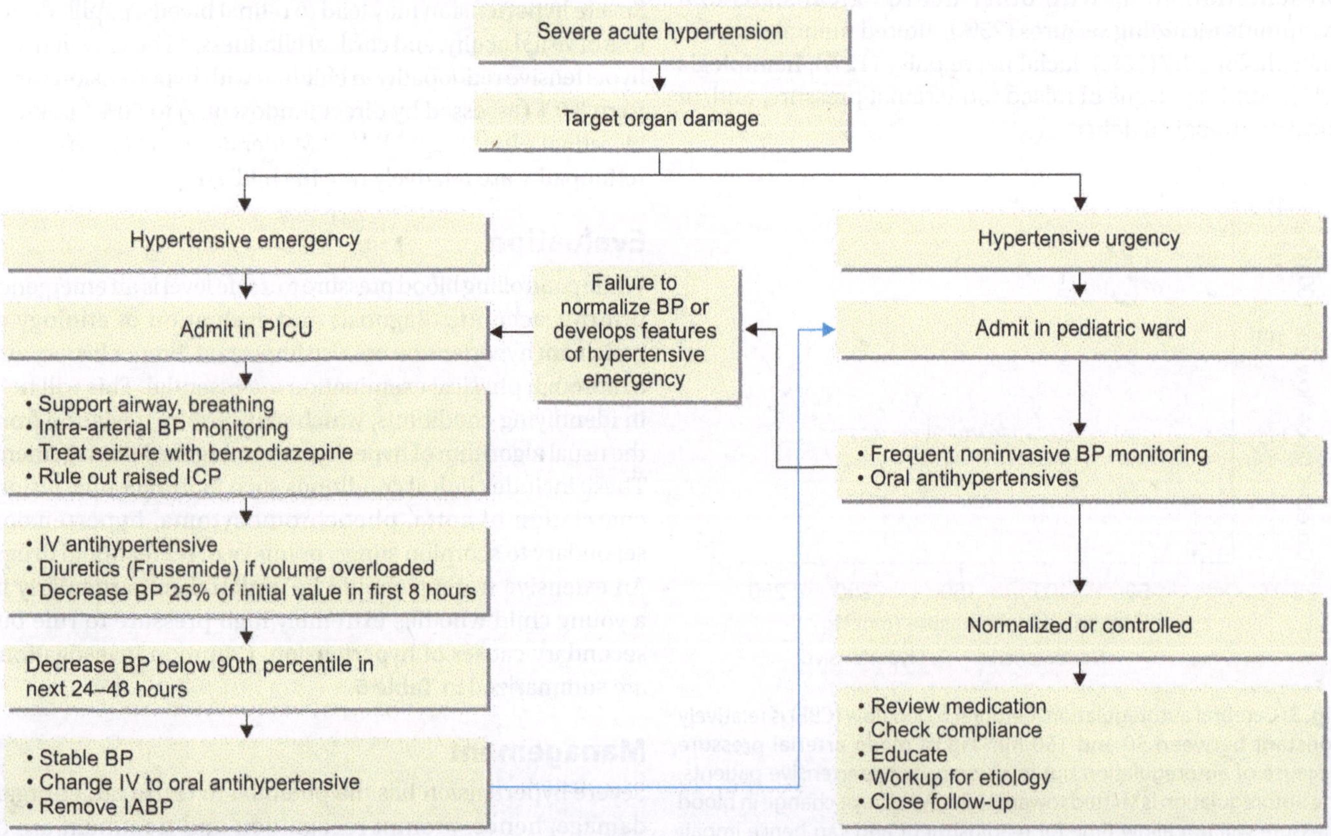

(BP: blood pressure; IABP: intra-aortic balloon pump; ICP: intracranial pressure; PICU: pediatric intensive care unit)

pressure, but it is equally important to do it in a controlled way, and much effort should be devoted to avoid precipitous fall in blood pressure in the early phase of treatment. When the blood pressure is lowered acutely, it may drop below the lower limit of autoregulation with a consequent fall in cerebral blood flow. Focal ischemia may be provoked if a significant stenosis is present on a larger cerebral resistance vessel.[48] A list of intravenous antihypertensive medicines with some salient points regarding their use is summarized in **Table 6**, and **Table 7** summarizes some special scenarios which might diktat modification of the standard approach to emergency blood pressure control.[47,57,]

TABLE 6: Antihypertensive agents for emergency use.[3,11,56,57]

Drugs	*Dose*	*Onset of action*	*Duration of action*	*Advantages*	*Caution*
Nifedipine	Oral or sublingual 0.25–0.50 mg/kg (maximum dose 20 mg)	15–20 minutes	2–5 hours	• Rapid onset • Orally active	Only useful in a conscious patient
Nicardipine	Continuous IV infusion 1–3 μg/kg/min (maximum 250 μg/min)	1–2 hours	2–4 hours	• Similar to nifedipine without the deleterious risk of depressing myocardial function • Promote natriuresis	• Elevation of intracranial pressure (ICP) (avoid in those at risk of raised ICP) • Tachycardia • Flushing • Headache • Hypotension • Peripheral edema • Gastrointestinal disturbance
Sodium nitroprusside	Continuous IV infusion 0.25–8.0 μg/kg/min Increase the dose by 25% every 5–10 minutes until desired BP control is obtained. If maximum dose is used for >10 minutes without good BP control, stop the drug because of toxicity risk	2 minutes	1–10 minutes		• Contraindicated: – Coarctation of aorta – Closed head injury – High intracranial pressure – Intracranial hemorrhage • Chronic use may cause cyanide and thiocyanate accumulation • Do thiocyanate levels if used >48 hours • Toxicity risk increased with decreased renal or liver function
Glyceryl trinitrate	Continuous IV infusion 1–10 μg/kg/min (maximum dose 400 μg/min)	At once	3–5 minutes	• Rapid onset and cessation • Relieves coronary spasm • Reduces preload and to a lesser extent afterload	• Bradycardia • Tachycardia • Headache • Vomiting • Methemoglobinemia
Furosemide	IV 1–5 mg/kg/dose 6 hourly Or continuous IV infusion 0.1–1.0 mg/kg/h	2–5 minutes	2 hours	Drug of choice in acute glomerulonephritis with fluid overload	• Hyponatremia • Hypokalemia
Labetalol	IV 0.2 mg/kg over 2 minutes If no response in 5–10 minutes, increase to 0.4–1.0 mg/kg (maximum	5 minutes	0.3–23 hours	• Favorable cardiac effect • Favorable CNS effect: • Use in patients with raised intracranial pressure	• Contraindicated in acute heart failure • Adverse effects: – Reactive airway disease – Heart failure

Contd...

Contd...

Drugs	Dose	Onset of action	Duration of action	Advantages	Caution
	bolus dose 20 mg) or continuous IV infusion 0.4–1.0 mg/kg/h (maximum dose 3 mg/kg/h)				– Heart block – Paradoxical hypertension – Postural hypotension – Hepatitis – Muscle weakness – Urinary retention – Scalp tingling – Burning in throat
Diazoxide	IV 1–3 mg/kg push, then 2–5 mg/kg/dose 6 hourly (maximum 150 mg)	15 minutes	4–24 hours	Does not raise intracranial pressure	• Tachycardia • Hyperlycemia • Profound hypotension if combined with other antihypertensives • Salt and water retention • Gastrointestinal disturbance • Hyperuricemia • Thrombocytopenia
Esmolol	IV 0.5 mg/kg over 1 minute, repeat every 5–10 minutes, if required IV infusion 1.5–18 mg/kg/h (undiluted 10 mg/mL)	1–2 minutes	10–20 minutes	• Useful during anesthesia to prevent postintubation hypertension and tachycardia • Useful in acute aortic dissection	• Hypotension • Nausea • Rarely given for >48 hours
Phentolamine	0.5–0.1 mg/kg stat (maximum dose 5 mg), then 5–50 µg/kg/min	1–2 minutes	3–10 hours	Drug of choice in catecholamine excess	Postural hypotension Tachycardia Cerebral vascular spasm Nausea

(CNS: central nervous system)

TABLE 7: Management of significant antihypertenisive in some special scenarios.[3,11,56,57]

Causes of malignant hypertension	Mechanism	Management
Pheochromocytoma	Due to excessive release of catecholamine	• Noncompetitive α2-blocker such as phenoxybenzamine is the medication of choice • For localized tumors, laparoscopic cortical-sparing adrenalectomy is the preferred surgery in children. Treatment options for invasive and metastatic tumors include embolization, systemic therapy with MIBG, or chemotherapy
Increased intracranial pressure	Neurogenic mediated	Priority should be given to managing the increased intracranial pressure. Significant reduction of blood pressure before controlling intracranial pressure might lead to compromise in cerebral perfusion
Advanced chronic kidney disease (CKD)	Volume overload is the most important factor leading to hypertension	• Maintaining dry weight by strict volume control and dialysis if indicated • Dietary salt restriction • Angiotensin-converting enzyme inhibitors (ACEI) and angiotensin receptor blocker (ARB) are considered as first choice in the treatment of hypertension in CKD for its nephroprotection by reducing proteinuria and suppression of cytokines and chemokine release. In advanced CKD, caution is advocated and many units avoid its use with glomerular filtration rate < 30 mL/min/1.73 m²

Contd...

Contd...

Causes of malignant hypertension	*Mechanism*	*Management*
		• Calcium channel blocker and β-blockers are other therapeutic options
Hypertension in thrombotic microangiopathies	Volume overload and endothelial damage	• Volume overload is an important factor and kidney replacement therapy is often required, particularly in oliguric stage • Hypertension in hemolytic-uremic syndrome and thrombotic thrombocytopenic purpura may be very difficult to control and may require multiple antihypertensive agents
Kidney transplant recipients	• Preexisting hypertension • Native kidney disease • Medications such as steroids, calcineurin inhibitors • Graft dysfunction • Renal artery stenosis • Thrombotic microangiopathy • Postbiopsy arteriovenous fistula	• Calcium-channel blockers decrease the vasoconstriction induced by the calcineurin inhibitors • Thiazide and loop diuretics, ACEI/ARB are also used for control of resistant hypertension • Minoxidil may be considered in patients with tacrolimus-induced alopecia
Medications or drugs	Sudden cessation of opiates, benzodiazepines, and clonidine cocaine toxicity	For cocaine toxicity, IV α-blocker such as phentolamine is the treatment of choice and β-blockers may be added if needed later in the treatment
	Monoamine oxidase inhibitors interact with food-containing tyramine and other medications such as dextromethorphan, methylene blue, selective serotonin reuptake inhibitors, and linezolid	α-blocker or sodium nitroprusside
	Amphetamine toxicity	• Decontamination, cooling, sedation, intravenous α-blockers, or sodium nitroprusside is the treatment of choice • Beta-blockers alone are absolutely contraindicated in all these toxidromes as they will worsen the hypertensive crisis due to unopposed action on α-receptors

CONCLUSION

Renovascular hypertension is an uncommon but distinctive form of secondary hypertension observed in children. This angiotensin-dependent hypertension commonly stems from FMD in children. Recognition of distinct types of renovascular disease manifesting with varying degrees of RAS is critical. Evaluation is based on imaging technologies and interventional strategies. Management of RVH demands multidisciplinary expertise comprising interventional radiologists or cardiologists or vascular surgeons.

KEY POINTS

- Renal angiography is the gold standard to diagnose renovascular hypertension.
- Medical management, angioplasty, and occasionally surgeries are indicated in the management.
- Control of hypertension may need more than four drugs.
- ACEI and ARBs are to be used with caution in unilateral cases and contraindicated in bilateral lesions.

REFERENCES

1. Goldblatt H, Lynch J, Hanzal RF, Summerville WW. Studies on experimental hypertension: I. The production of persistent elevation of systolic blood pressure by means of renal ischemia. J Exp Med. 1934;59(3):347-79.
2. Imanishi M, Akabane S, Takamiya M, Kawamura M, Matsushima Y, Kuramochi M, et al. Critical degree of renal arterial stenosis that causes hypertension in dogs. Angiology. 1992;43(10):833-42.
3. Flynn JT, Kaelber DC, Baker-Smith CM, Blowey D, Carroll AE, Daniels SR, et al. Clinical practice guideline for screening and management of high blood pressure in children and adolescents. Pediatrics. 2017;140(3):e20171904.
4. Gill DG, Mendes de Costa B, Cameron JS, Joseph MC, Ogg CS, Chantler C. Analysis of 100 children with severe and persistent hypertension. Arch Dis Child. 1976;51:951-6.
5. Wyszynska T, Cichocka E, Wieteska-Klimczak A, Jobs K, Januszewicz P. A single pediatric center experience with 1025 children with hypertension. Acta Paediatr. 1992;81:244-6.
6. Hari P, Bagga A, Srivastava RN. Sustained hypertension in children. Indian Pediatr. 2000;37:268-74.
7. Kumar P, Arora P, Kher V, Rai PK, Gulati S, Baijal SS, et al. Malignant hypertension in children in India. Nephrol Dial Transplant. 1996;11(7):1261-6.
8. McCulloch M, Andronikou S, Goddard E, Sinclair P, Lawrenson J, Mandelstam S, et al. Angiographic features of 26 children with Takayasu arteritis. Pediatr Radiol. 2003;33(4):230-5.
9. Tyagi S, Kaul UA, Satsangi DK, Arora R. Percutaneous transluminal angioplasty for renovascular hypertension in children: initial and long-term results. Pediatrics. 1997;99(1):44-9.

10. Plouin PF, Bax L. Diagnosis and treatment of renal artery stenosis. Nat Rev Nephrol. 2010;6(3):151-9.
11. Harrison EG Jr, McCormack LJ. Pathologic classification of renal arterial disease in renovascular hypertension. Mayo Clin Proc. 1971;46:161-7.
12. Slovut DP, Olin JW. Fibromuscular dysplasia. N Engl J Med. 2004;350:1862-71.
13. Rushton AR. The genetics of fibromuscular dysplasia. Arch Intern Med. 1980;140:233-6.
14. Bofinger A, Hawley C, Fisher P, Daunt N, Stowasser M, Gordon R. Polymorphisms of the renin-angiotensin system in patients with multifocal renal arterial fibromuscular dysplasia. J Hum Hypertens. 2001;15(3):185-90.
15. Ingelfinger JR. Renovascular disease in children. Kidney Int. 1993;43(2):493-505.
16. Rumman RK, Nickel C, Matsuda-Abedini M, Lorenzo AJ, Langlois V, Radhakrishnan S, et al. Disease beyond the arch: a systematic review of middle aortic syndrome in childhood. Am J Hypertens. 2015;28(7):833-46.
17. Mukherjee D, Sinha R, Akhtar MS, Saha AS. Hyponatremic hypertensive syndrome - a retrospective cohort study. World J Nephrol. 2017;6(1):41-4.
18. Deal JE, Snell MF, Barratt TM, Dillon MJ. Renovascular disease in childhood. J Pediatr.1992;121(3):378-84.
19. Daniels SR, Loggie JM, McEnery PT, Towbin RB. Clinical spectrum of intrinsic renovascular hypertension in children. Pediatrics. 1987;80:698-704.
20. McTaggart SJ, Gulati S, Walker RG, Powell HR, Jones CL, Gelati S. Evaluation and long-term outcome of pediatric renovascular hypertension. Pediatr Nephrol. 2000;14:1022-9.
21. Hiner LB, Falkner B. Renovascular hypertension in children. Pediatr Clin North Am. 1993;40(1):123-40.
22. Watson AR, Balfe JW, Hardy BE. Renovascular hypertension in childhood: a changing perspective in management. J Pediatr. 1985;106(3):366-72.
23. Vo NJ, Hammelman BD, Racadio JM, Strife CF, Johnson ND, Racadio JM. Anatomic distribution of renal artery stenosis in children: implications for imaging. Pediatr Radiol. 2006;36(10): 1032-36.
24. Brun P, Kchouk H, Mouchet B, Baudouin V, Raynaud A, Loirat C, et al. Value of Doppler ultrasound for the diagnosis of renal artery stenosis in children. Pediatr Nephrol. 1997;11(1):27-30.
25. Li JC, Wang L, Jiang YX, Dai Q, Cai S, Lv K, et al. Evaluation of renal artery stenosis with velocity parameters of Doppler sonography. J Ultrasound Med. 2006;25(6):735-42.
26. Williams GJ, Macaskill P, Chan SF. Comparative accuracy of renal duplex sonographic parameters in the diagnosis of renal artery stenosis: paired and unpaired analysis. AJR Am J Roentgenol. 2007;188(3):798-811.
27. Chi YW, White CJ, Thornton S, Milani RV. Ultrasound velocity criteria for renal in-stent restenosis. J Vasc Surg. 2009;50(1): 119-23.
28. Eklof H, Ahlstrom H, Magnusson A, Andersson LG, Andrén B, Hägg A, et al. A prospective comparison of duplex ultrasonography, captopril renography, MRA, and CTA in assessing renal artery stenosis. Acta Radiol. 2006;47(8):764-74.
29. Rountas C, Vlychou M, Vassiou K, Liakopoulos V, Kapsalaki E, Koukoulis G, et al. Imaging modalities for renal artery stenosis in suspected renovascular hypertension: prospective intra-individual comparison of color Doppler US, CT angiography, GD-enhanced MR angiography, and digital subtraction angiography. Ren Fail. 2007;29(3):295-302.
30. Fommei E, Ghione S, Hilson AJ, Mezzasalma L, Oei HY, Piepsz A, et al. Captopril radionuclide test in renovascular hypertension: a European multicentre study. Eur J Nucl Med. 1993;20:617-23.
31. Arora P, Kher V, Singhal MK, Kumar P, Gulati S, Baijal SS, et al. Renal artery stenosis in aortoarteritis: spectrum of disease in children and adults. Kidney Blood Press Res. 1997;20:285-9.
32. Dillon MJ, Ryness JM. Plasma renin activity and aldosterone concentration in children. Br Med J. 1975;4(5992):316-9.
33. Goonasekera CD, Shah V, Wade AM, Dillon MJ. The usefulness of renal vein renin studies in hypertensive children: a 25-year experience. Pediatr Nephrol. 2002;17(11):943-9.
34. Teigen CL, Mitchell SE, Venbrux AC, Christenson MJ, McLean RH. Segmental renal artery embolization for treatment of pediatric renovascular hypertension. J Vasc Interv Radiol. 1992;3:111-7.
35. Roebuck DJ. Interventional radiology in children. Imaging. 2001;13:302-20.
36. Shahdadpuri J, Frank R, Gauthier BG, Siegel DN, Trachtman H. Yield of renal arteriography in the evaluation of pediatric hypertension. Pediatr Nephrol. 2000;14:816-19.
37. Stanley JC, Criado E, Upchurch GR Jr, Brophy PD, Cho KJ, Rectenwald JE, et al. Pediatric renovascular hypertension: 132 primary and 30 secondary operations in 97 children. J Vasc Surg. 2006;44(6):1219-28.
38. Wong H, Hadi M, Khoury T, Geary D, Rubin B, Filler G. Management of severe hypertension in a child with tuberous sclerosis-related major vascular abnormalities. J Hypertens. 2006;24:597-99.
39. Tullus K, Brennan E, Hamilton G, Lord R, McLaren CA, Marks SD, et al. Renovascular hypertension in children. Lancet. 2008; 371(9622):1453-63.
40. Isobe N, Oki S, Sumida M, Kanou Y, Nabika S, Watanabe Y, et al. Internal carotid artery occlusion following correction of atypical aortic coarctation: case report. Neurol Med Chir (Tokyo). 2005;45:476-9.
41. Konig K, Gellermann J, Querfeld U, Schneider MB. Treatment of severe renal artery stenosis by percutaneous transluminal renal angioplasty and stent implantation: review of the pediatric experience—apropos of two cases. Pediatr Nephrol. 2006; 21(5):663-71.
42. Cura MA, Bugnone A, Becker GJ. Midaortic syndrome associated with fetal alcohol syndrome. J Vasc Interv Radiol. 2002;13(11):1167-70.
43. Shroff R, Roebuck DJ, Gordon I, Davies R, Stephens S, Marks S, et al. Angioplasty for renovascular hypertension in children: 20-year experience. Pediatrics. 2006;118:268-75.
44. Ishijima H, Ishizaka H, Sakurai M, Ito K, Endo K. Partial renal embolization for pediatric renovascular hypertension secondary to fibromuscular dysplasia. Cardiovasc Intervent Radiol. 1997;20(5):383-6.
45. Ognjanovic MV, Richardson D, de La Hunt M, Plant ND, Moghal NE, Lambert HJ, et al. Selective renal embolisation for renovascular hypertension? Arch Dis Child. 2002;86(2):127-9.
46. Flynn JT. Evaluation and management of hypertension in childhood. Prog Pediatr Cardiol. 2001;12(2):177-88.
47. Chandar J, Zilleruelo G. Hypertensive crisis in children. Pediatr Nephrol. 2012;27(5):741-51.
48. MacKenzie ET, Strandgaard S, Graham DI, Jones JV, Harper AM, Farrar JK. Effects of acutely induced hypertension in cats on pial arteriolar caliber, local cerebral blood flow, and the blood-brain barrier. Circ Res. 1976;39(1):33-41.

49. Chaversm BM, Herzog CA. The spectrum of cardiovascular disease in children with predialysis chronic kidney disease. Adv Chronic Kidney Dis. 2004;11(3):319-27.
50. Wilson AC, Mitsnefes MM. Cardiovascular disease in CKD in children: update on risk factors, risk assessment and management. Am J Kidney Dis. 2009;54(2):345-60.
51. Hanevold C, Waller J, Daniels S, Portman R, Sorof J. The effects of obesity, gender, and ethnic group on left ventricular hypertrophy and geometry in hypertensive children: a collaborative study of the international pediatric hypertension association. Pediatrics. 2004;113(2):328-33.
52. Shavit L, Reinus C, Slotki I. Severe renal failure and microangiopathic hemolysis induced by malignant hypertension—case series and review of literature. Clin Nephrol. 2010;73(2): 147-52.
53. Otsuka Y, Abe K, Sato Y. Malignant hypertension and microangiopathic hemolytic anemia. Jpn Heart J. 1976;17(2): 258-64.
54. Logan P, Eustace P, Robinson R. Hypertensive retinopathy: a cause of decreased visual acuity in children. J Pediatr Ophthalmol Strabismus. 1992;29(5):287-9.
55. Daniels SR, Lipman MJ, Burke MJ, Loggie JMH. The prevalence of retinal vascular abnormalities in children and adolescents with essential hypertension. Am J Ophthalmol. 1991;111(2):205-8.
56. Foster BJ, Ali H, Mamber S, Polomeno RC, MacKie AS. Prevalence and severity of hypertensive retinopathy in children. Clin Pediatr (Phila). 2009;48(9):926-30.
57. Rao G. Diagnosis, epidemiology, and management of hypertension in children. Pediatrics. 2016;138(2):e20153616.

CHAPTER

10.4

Ambulatory Blood Pressure Monitoring

Priya Pais

INTRODUCTION

Ambulatory blood pressure monitoring (ABPM) is an important method for the diagnosis and management of hypertension (HTN) in children. The ambulatory BP monitor consists of an inflatable cuff placed on the arm and connected by tubing to a wearable electronic device that measures BP (by oscillometry, most commonly, or auscultation) at regular programmed intervals, for a period of 24 hours. The ABPM procedure is performed outside of a clinical setting (ambulatory) while the child performs routine activities during the day (awake) and during the night (asleep). Thus, with ABPM, many BP measurements are obtained, which allow for assessment of mean daytime and nighttime BP values, the diurnal variation of BP, and nocturnal HTN.[1]

Advantages of ABPM:

- Better predictor of hypertensive target-organ damage [TOD; left ventricular hypertrophy (LVH), arterial stiffness, and elevated carotid intima-media thickness] than clinic BP. In the absence of data regarding cardiovascular (CV) outcomes of HTN in children, these measures of TOD are assumed to be surrogate outcomes of CV morbidity.[2]
- ABPM is the gold standard to diagnose white coat hypertension (WCH) and is a cost-effective approach to HTN management by avoiding unnecessary interventions.
- ABPM provides important data regarding the diurnal variation of BP, can detect the presence of masked HTN (MH), and indicates if BP control is truly effective.[3]

AMBULATORY BLOOD PRESSURE MONITORING DEVICE AND PROCEDURE

- *ABPM equipment:* It includes a battery-operated ABPM device along with ABPM cuffs of various sizes. The device is connected to the cuff with flexible tubing and placed in a protective pouch that is attached to the patient with a belt or shoulder strap.
- The ABPM device measures BP at preprogrammed intervals. The ideal ABPM device should be lightweight and allow for some patient movement while measuring BP. Multiple devices are available, usually measuring BP using oscillometry. Each device uses its own proprietary algorithm to derive the systolic BP (SBP) and diastolic BP (DBP) from a measured mean arterial pressure. Therefore, each device should undergo testing for validation and adhere to quality standards, such as the British Hypertension Society (BHS) or Association for Advancement of Medical Instrumentation (AAMI).
- *Clinic BP:* It is obtained using the standard recommended procedure.
- *ABPM procedure:* **Table 1** summarizes the steps to be followed for conducting ABPM in children. These adhere to the American Heart Association (AHA) scientific statement on ABPM in children and adolescents.[1]
- An ideal study would include at least one reading every hour including during sleep.

INTERPRETATION

Normative data: In adults, the threshold BP value, which defines HTN is based on BP values at or above, which adverse clinical outcomes occur. As these longitudinal data is lacking in children, statistical thresholds from normative datasets are used to define HTN (e.g., ≥ 95th percentile). The auscultatory normative data charts used for clinic BPs are not suitable for defining ambulatory HTN. The ambulatory normative data that is currently used has been derived by the German Working Group on Pediatric Hypertension. Data from 949 central European children, aged 5–20 years, was reanalyzed by the LMS method and is recommended for defining ambulatory HTN.[4] Although universally used, this normative data suffers from limitations—the data is not validated against CV outcomes and its validity for non-European children is unclear. The diastolic ambulatory BP values in the normative dataset have very little variation despite increasing heights. There is doubt about its generalizability. Also, data is not available for children <120 cm in height.[4]

IMPORTANT AMBULATORY BLOOD PRESSURE MONITORING MEASUREMENTS

Table 2 lists the BP measurements obtained from an ABPM study.

TABLE 1: Steps in performing an ambulatory blood pressure monitoring (ABPM) procedure.

ABPM placement	• Trained personnel are required to maintain and place the ABPM machine appropriately • The ABPM device should be programmed to obtain BP readings every 15–20 minutes during daytime and 20–30 minutes during sleep hours that can be set from 10 PM to 6 AM • An appropriate-sized cuff should be selected based on the mid-arm circumference (as per clinic BP measurement guidelines) and placed on the nondominant arm • The cuff should be connected via tubing to the device worn on a belt • Clinic BP should be measured and compared with ambulatory BP levels to ensure that the variation is within 5 mm Hg
Patient education	The child and family need to be instructed to: • Keep the arm still when a BP measurement is ongoing (indicated by a beep) and monitor for kinks in the tubing if BP readings are unsuccessful • Avoid vigorous activity, getting the monitor wet or other forms of damage • Avoid turning off or removing the monitor or cuff • Maintain a diary of sleep–wake times (essential for interpretation), daily activities, medication timings, discomfort during measurement, or symptoms related to high/low BP
Data interpretation	• The ABPM data is downloaded to proprietary software • Validity of the ABPM study is determined by the presence of at least one BP reading per hour and a total of 40–50 readings • Extreme outlier BP values may be programmed to be removed • Patient-reported sleep–wake times are used to manually define daytime and nighttime BPs • Threshold BP values are entered to define hypertension using the normative data tables • The analysis software calculates mean BP values, BP loads, and nocturnal dip for ABPM interpretation

TABLE 2: Ambulatory blood pressure monitoring (ABPM) parameters used for interpretation.[1]

ABPM parameter	*Definition*	*Relevance of parameter*	*Normal value*
Mean ambulatory BP	Mathematical mean SBP and DBP for the 24-hour, daytime (awake) and nighttime (asleep) periods	Is the mean BP elevated?	<95th percentile
BP load	Percentage of readings above the threshold (usually 95th percentile)	How often is the BP elevated?	<25%
Nocturnal dip	(mean daytime BP – mean nighttime BP) ÷ mean daytime BP × 100%	Is there a normal circadian fall in BP at night?	≥10%

(DBP: diastolic blood pressure; SBP: systolic blood pressure)

CLASSIFICATION OF AMBULATORY HYPERTENSION

The AHA scientific statement suggests the following classification of ambulatory SBP or DBP utilizing mean ambulatory BP and BP loads, as listed in **Table 3**.[5] The threshold for defining HTN is set at the 95th percentile of ambulatory normative data.

The European Society of Hypertension (ESH) recommends that adult threshold values of mean BP are used to define HTN, once the 95th percentile values exceed 135/85 mm Hg during the day and 125/75 mm Hg during the night. Also similar to adult ABPM guidelines, the ESH does not consider BP loads in the classification of ambulatory HTN.[6]

SIGNIFICANCE OF AMBULATORY BLOOD PRESSURE MONITORING DIAGNOSES

- *White coat HTN:* WCH refers to the phenomenon of elevated BP measured in clinical settings but normal BPs on ABPM (obtained outside the hospital). A confirmed diagnosis of WCH prevents unnecessary investigations and treatment of HTN. However, WCH in adults is associated with progression to sustained HTN and CV morbidity in adults. Although similar data in children is lacking, there is preliminary evidence that WCH in adolescents may track to sustained ambulatory HTN in adulthood.[7]
- *Masked HTN:* MH is the opposite of WCH, with normal clinic BPs but HTN present on ABPM. MH in adults is associated with the presence of TOD. MH in children on antihypertensive medications indicates uncontrolled HTN and is common in those with CKD and postrenal transplantation. Isolated nocturnal HTN occurs in children with obstructive sleep apnea.[8,9]
- *Sustained ambulatory HTN:* Patients with elevated clinic and ambulatory BP are at high risk for TOD. Sustained ambulatory HTN is a better predictor of LVH in children than clinic BPs. Ambulatory HTN is also associated with nocturnal HTN and a blunted nocturnal dip.

Patient management utilizing ABPM data depends on the ABPM diagnosis and whether the patient is already on antihypertensive medication or not. **Figure 1** describes an approach to managing a child who has completed an ABPM study.

TABLE 3: Classification of ambulatory blood pressure (BP).[5]

Classification	Clinic BP	Mean ambulatory SBP or DBP (awake or asleep or both)	SBP or DBP load
Normal	<90th percentile	<95th percentile	<25%
White coat HTN	≥95th percentile	<95th percentile	<25%
Pre-HTN	≥90th percentile or >120/80 mm Hg	<95th percentile	≥25%
Masked HTN	<95th percentile	>95th percentile	≥25%
Ambulatory (sustained) HTN	>95th percentile	>95th percentile	25%–50%
Severe ambulatory HTN	>95th percentile	>95th percentile	>50%

(AHA: American Heart Association; DBP: diastolic BP; HTN: hypertension; SBP: systolic BP)

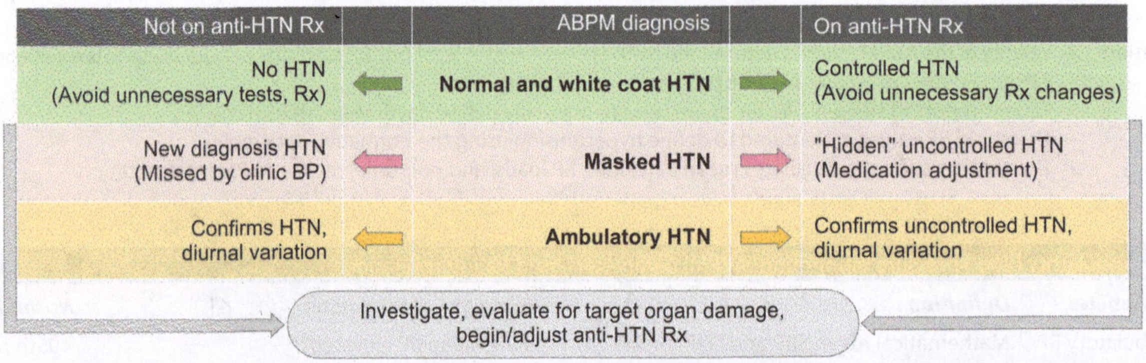

Fig. 1: Applying ambulatory blood pressure monitoring classification to patient care. (HTN: hypertension)

INDICATIONS FOR AMBULATORY BLOOD PRESSURE MONITORING

Table 4 lists clinical indications to perform ABPM and provides clinical examples of conditions, where ABPM is useful.

Pediatric ABPM in the literature:

- *Chronic kidney disease (CKD):* HTN is a known modifiable risk factor for CKD progression. In the ESCAPE trial, strict BP control by ABPM [mean arterial pressure (MAP) of 50th percentile] was associated with slower rate of progression in children with glomerular and nonglomerular CKD.[10] In the CKiD cohort, ABPM was shown to be a better predictor of TOD than clinic BP. Only 44% of the cohort had adequate BP control with high rates of MH.[11] The use of angiotensin-converting enzyme (ACE) inhibition was associated with better ambulatory BP control. In the 4C (Cardiovascular Comorbidity in Children with CKD) study, the prevalence of uncontrolled HTN was 26% with sustained ambulatory HTN being an independent predictor of LVH.[12]
- *Kidney transplant:* Uncontrolled HTN is a known risk factor for graft loss in adults. Multiple studies have shown that children postrenal transplantation have high rates of MH, isolated nocturnal HTN, and a blunted nocturnal dip. Introduction of ACE inhibitors has been demonstrated to improved nocturnal BP control.[13]
- *Obesity:* It is a frequent cause for secondary HTN in children. ABPM studies have shown that both daytime and nighttime ambulatory BPs are elevated in obesity with worsening ambulatory BP indices associated with higher BMI values. Obesity is also associated with disordered sleep breathing, a predictor of nocturnal HTN.[14]

TABLE 4: Summary of indications to perform ambulatory blood pressure monitoring (ABPM).

Indication	Clinical situations
Confirm suspected HTN	Elevated clinic BPs, suspected WCH
Screen for HTN in high-risk patients	• Structural kidney diseases, CKD, kidney transplant patients types I and II DM • Postcoarctation of aorta repair • Obesity • Genetic syndromes associated with HTN (e.g., neurofibromatosis) • History of prematurity, low birth weight
Assess effectiveness of antihypertensive therapy	Patients receiving antihypertensive therapy: • With target organ damage • Ensure strict BP control in CKD • To assist with adjustment of medication in those with elevated clinic BPs (? uncontrolled HTN) or hypotensive symptoms
Clinical research	• Clinical trials of antihypertensive medications • Determine prevalence of HTN in disease

(CKD: chronic kidney disease; DM: diabetes mellitus; HTN: hypertension; WCH: white coat hypertension)

LIMITATIONS OF ABPM

Although a critical tool in the management of pediatric HTN, challenges remain that limit the universal use of ABPM. The most important of these is the normative data set that lacks heterogeneity, as discussed above. Also, ABPM equipment is expensive, limiting its use to larger referral centers.

Ambulatory blood pressure monitoring cannot be used as a standard method of BP evaluation in very young children as they are unlikely to tolerate wearing the monitor for prolonged periods, and the absence of normative data.

CONCLUSION

Ambulatory blood pressure monitoring is a validated tool to improve the diagnosis and management of pediatric HTN. Due to numerous BP readings obtained in a nonclinical setting, ABPM can be used to diagnose WCH and MH and assess adequacy of BP control in those on antihypertensive medications. ABPM is indicated in children at high risk for HTN and in settings, where strict BP control is vital, such as CKD and after renal transplant. Despite its limitations of expensive equipment and limited availability, ABPM is now considered standard of care by several pediatric HTN guidelines.

KEY POINTS

- ABPM is an automated method of measuring BP in an ambulatory patient, outside of a hospital setting, for a period of 24 hours.
- ABPM has been found to be a better predictor of TOD than clinic BPs alone.
- ABPM is the gold standard for diagnosing WCH and MH and is used to confirm a diagnosis of HTN and to assess BP control in those on medications.
- Data obtained from a valid ABPM study include mean 24-hour, daytime, and nighttime SBP and DBP, BP loads, and the nocturnal dip.
- The pediatric normative data for ABPM is based on sex and height and does not include data for children <120 cm, a recognized shortcoming.

REFERENCES

1. Urbina E, Alpert B, Flynn J, Hayman L, Harshfield GA, Jacobson M, et al. Ambulatory blood pressure monitoring in children and adolescents: Recommendations for standard assessment: A scientific statement from the American Heart Association atherosclerosis, Hypertension, and Obesity in Youth Committee of the Council on Cardiovascular Disease in the Young and the Council for High Blood Pressure Research. Hypertension. 2008;52(3):433-51.
2. Flynn JT, Daniels SR, Hayman LL, Maahs DM, McCrindle BW, Mitsnefes M, et al. Update: Ambulatory Blood Pressure Monitoring in Children and Adolescents: A Scientific Statement From the American Heart Association. Hypertension. 2014; 63(5):1116-35.
3. Halbach SM, Hamman R, Yonekawa K, Hanevold C. Utility of ambulatory blood pressure monitoring in the evaluation of elevated clinic blood pressures in children. J Am Soc Hypertens. 2016;10(5):406-12.
4. Wühl E, Witte K, Soergel M, Mehls O, Schaefer F, German Working Group on Pediatric Hypertension. Distribution of 24-h ambulatory blood pressure in children: normalized reference values and role of body dimensions. J Hypertens. 2002;20(10):1995-2007.
5. Flynn JT, Kaelber DC, Baker-Smith CM, Blowey D, Carroll AE, Daniels SR, et al. Clinical practice guideline for screening and management of high blood pressure in children and adolescents. Pediatrics. 2017;140(3):e20171904.
6. Lurbe E, Agabiti-Rosei E, Cruickshank JK, Dominiczak A, Erdine S, Hirth A, et al. 2016 European Society of Hypertension guidelines for the management of high blood pressure in children and adolescents. J Hypertens. 2016;34(10):1887-920.
7. Westerståhl M, Forss M, Persson L, Bouma K, Gustavsson T, Wühl E, et al. Hypertension outcomes and cardiovascular status in young adults with childhood-diagnosed white coat hypertension. Arch Dis Child. 2018;103(1):113-4.
8. Stergiou GS, Asayama K, Thijs L, Kollias A, Niiranen TJ, Hozawa A, et al. Prognosis of White-Coat and Masked Hypertension. Hypertension. 2014;63(4):675-82.
9. Seeman T. Ambulatory blood pressure monitoring in pediatric renal transplantation. Curr Hypertens Rep. 2012;14(6):608-18.
10. Wühl E, Trivelli A, Picca S, Litwin M, Peco-Antic A, Zurowska A, et al. Strict Blood-Pressure Control and Progression of Renal Failure in Children. N Engl J Med. 2009;361(17):1639-50.
11. Wilson AC, Flynn JT. Blood pressure in children with chronic kidney disease: lessons learned from the Chronic Kidney Disease in Children Cohort Study. Pediatr Nephrol. 2020; 35(7):1203-9.
12. Schaefer F, Doyon A, Azukaitis K, Bayazit A, Canpolat N, Duzova A, et al. Cardiovascular phenotypes in children with CKD: The 4C study. Clin J Am Soc Nephrol. 2017;12(1):19-28.
13. Seeman T, Vondrák K, Dušek J. Effects of the strict control of blood pressure in pediatric renal transplant recipients—ESCORT trial. Pediatr Transplant. 2018;23(1):e13329.
14. Babinska K, Kovacs L, Janko V, Dallos T, Feber J. Association between obesity and the severity of ambulatory hypertension in children and adolescents. J Am Soc Hypertens. 2012;6(5):356-63.

CHAPTER

10.5 Management of Hypertension

Swathi Shiri, Priya Pais

INTRODUCTION

The broad goals of hypertension (HTN) management are as follows:

- Reduce the risk of development of HTN in those with risk factors such as obesity
- Treat symptomatic HTN
- Prevent and reverse target-organ damage (TOD) if present.

Reduce BP to <90th percentile or <130/80 mm Hg, whichever is lower, in all HTN patients.*[1]

Diagnose HTN early and ensure strict control of BP (ideally <50th percentile) in those with proteinuria and chronic kidney disease (CKD). Performing ambulatory blood pressure monitoring (ABPM) in CKD patients is recommended to diagnose and treat HTN adequately.[2]

Indications to initiate antihypertensive medications are:

- Persistent stage 1 HTN despite nonpharmacological therapy
- Stage 2 HTN without a reversible cause
- Any stage HTN with evidence of TOD [e.g., left ventricular hypertrophy (LVH)]
- Symptomatic HTN
- CKD with any stage of HTN
- Diabetes mellitus (type 1 or type 2) with any stage of HTN.

APPROACH TO INITIATING ANTIHYPERTENSIVE THERAPY

Although studies of antihypertensive agents in children have shown a reduction in blood pressure, there is no data to demonstrate effectiveness in lowering TOD or cardiovascular outcomes.[3] The choice of medication should be based on the pathophysiology of HTN and the presence of associated comorbidities. For example, renin–angiotensin–aldosterone inhibitors (RAASi) are the first-choice therapy for CKD, especially if proteinuria is present. Therapy with the drug of choice should be initiated (monotherapy) at the lowest therapeutic dose and gradually increased until BP is controlled or unwanted side effects occur. If BP remains uncontrolled or dosage of the first drug cannot be increased further due to side effects, a second drug with a different mechanism of action may be started. Long-acting medications, with once- or twice-daily dosing, would be ideal choices to encourage adherence. The dosing and common side effects of antihypertensive drugs used in children are summarized in **Table 1**.

MANAGEMENT OF HYPERTENSION ASSOCIATED WITH OBESITY

Confirm the diagnosis of HTN with ABPM if available to rule out white-coat HTN or masked HTN. Clinic BPs by auscultation should be obtained to confirm the presence of sustained HTN.

Nonpharmacologic Therapy

Weight Reduction

Weight loss is an important step in nonpharmacological HTN treatment.

Lifestyle Changes

In adults, an average weight loss of 5 kg was associated with a reduction of SBP and DBP of approximately 4 mm Hg, with benefits increasing with greater weight loss.[5]

DASH Diet

Dietary approach to stop hypertension (DASH): Eat more fruits, vegetables, whole grains, and lean meats. Eat less salt, saturated fats, and sweets. Avoid or limit intake of processed foods and fast foods.

Physical Activity

Increasing physical activity results in improvement in HTN.[6] The World Health Organization (WHO) recommends an

---

*AAP Guideline 2017 "the treatment goal with nonpharmacologic and pharmacologic therapy should be a reduction in systolic blood pressure (SBP) and diastolic blood pressure (DBP) to <90th percentile and <130/80 mm Hg in adolescents ≥13 years old."

European Society of Hypertension 2016 "treatment goal of hypertension is to aim BP below 90th percentile in <16 years and <130/85 mmHg in ≥16 years."[1,2]

TABLE 1: Oral antihypertensives used in children.[4]

Class	Drug	Initial dose	Maximum dose	Adverse effects
Calcium-channel blockers	Amlodipine	*1–5 years:* 0.1 mg/kg/day *≥6 years:* 2.5 mg/day	0.6 mg/kg/day (up to 5 mg/day) 10 mg/day	Flushing, pedal edema, dizziness
	Felodipine	2.5 mg/day	10 mg/day	
	Nifedipine (sustained release)	0.2–0.5 mg/kg/day	3 mg/kg/day (120 mg/day)	
ACE inhibitors	Captopril	*Infants:* 0.05 mg/kg/dose *Children:* 0.5 mg/kg/dose	6 mg/kg/day	Cough, hyperkalemia AKI, fetal toxicity
	Enalapril	0.08 mg/kg/day (5 mg/day)	0.6 mg/kg per day (40 mg/day)	
	Lisinopril	0.07 mg/kg/day (5 mg/day)	40 mg/day	
	Ramipril	1.6 mg/m²/day	6 mg/m²/day	
Angiotensin receptor blockers	Losartan	0.7 mg/kg/day (50 mg/day)	1.4 mg/kg/day (100 mg/day)	Headache Dizziness AKI
	Valsartan	1.3 mg/kg/day (up to 40 mg)	2.7 mg/kg/day (up to 160 mg)	
	Irbesartan	75 mg/day	150 mg/day	
	Candesartan	0.02 mg/kg/day (up to 4 mg/day)	0.4 mg/kg/day (up to 16 mg/day)	
Beta-blockers	Atenolol	0.5 mg/kg/day	1 mg/kg/day (50 mg/day)	Bronchial asthma, bradycardia, and hyperglycemia
	Metoprolol	1 mg/kg/day	2 mg/kg/day (200 mg/day)	
	Propranolol	1 mg/kg/day	8 mg/kg/day	
Alpha + beta-blockers	Labetalol	2–3 mg/kg/day	10–12 mg/kg/day	Hypotension
	Carvedilol	0.1 mg/kg/day	0.5 mg/kg/day (25 mg/day)	
Vasodilators	Hydralazine	0.25 mg/kg/day	7.5 mg/kg/day (200 mg/day)	Lupus-like syndrome, tachycardia, palpitations, headache
	Minoxidil	0.1 mg/kg/day	0.3 mg/kg/day (50 mg/day)	Dizziness
Alpha-blockers	Prazosin	0.5 mg/kg/day	20 mg/day	• Tachycardia palpitation • First dose hypotension
Central alpha-agonist	Clonidine	5 µg/kg/day	20 µg/kg/day (0.9 mg/day)	Drowsiness
Diuretics	Chlorthalidone	0.3 mg/kg/day	2 mg/kg/day (50 mg)	• Hypokalemia • Hyponatremia • Obstructive jaundice • Arrhythmias
	Hydrochlorothiazide	1 mg/kg/day	2 mg/kg/day (37.5 mg)	

(ACE: angiotensin-converting enzyme; AKI: acute kidney injury)

average of 60 minutes of moderate to vigorous physical activity daily for children and adolescents. Activity should be a combination of aerobic exercise and strength-building activities. Sedentary behavior (screen time) should be limited to a maximum of 2 hours/day.[7,8]

Pharmacologic Therapy

When HTN does not improve with nonpharmacological therapy or the child meets criteria for initiating antihypertensive medications, a long-acting agent (RAASi or calcium-channel blocker) may be initiated. Thiazide diuretics have been recommended by the guidelines but require regular monitoring for electrolyte abnormalities and hyperlipidemia.[9-11]

MANAGEMENT OF SECONDARY HYPERTENSION

Chronic Kidney Disease

Hypertension is an important modifiable risk factor for progression of pediatric CKD.[12,13] Strict control of hypertension has been shown to slow the progression of glomerular and nonglomerular CKD.

Goals of Therapy

The Evaluation Study of Congestive Heart Failure and Pulmonary Artery Catheterization Effectiveness (ESCAPE) trial demonstrated that mean arterial pressure (MAP) at or close to the 50th percentile was associated with lower risk of progression, especially in CKD associated with proteinuria. The approach to HTN in children with CKD is summarized in **Flowchart 1**.

Acute Glomerulonephritis

Acute glomerulonephritis is associated with HTN that results from salt and water retention.[14] Therefore, the medication of choice in managing HTN is a loop diuretic. Angiotensin-converting enzyme (ACE) inhibitors are not recommended for use in this setting. The approach to HTN in acute glomerulonephritis is summarized in **Flowchart 2**.

SPECIAL SITUATIONS

Hypertensive Emergencies

Hypertensive crises are defined as sudden and abrupt increases in blood pressure associated with rapid end-organ damage. Crises can be classified into hypertensive urgencies (HTN with mild symptoms or BPs elevated above stage II) or hypertensive emergencies, with severe symptoms with rapid end-organ damage in the form of hypertensive encephalopathy, HTN-associated congestive cardiac failure, or neuroretinopathy.[15] The American Academy of Pediatrics (AAP) 2017 clinical practice guideline for children and adolescents has replaced the terminology of hypertensive crisis, urgency, and emergency as acute symptomatic presentation of severe HTN (BP increase by 30 mm Hg or stage II HTN).[1]

The underlying etiology of acute severe HTN (summarized in **Table 2**) can be classified as follows:

- Secondary causes
- Primary HTN (rarely)

Clinical Approach and Management

The hypertensive emergencies can present in the following ways:

- *Hypertensive encephalopathy:* Severe stage II HTN with symptoms of headache and vomiting with seizures or focal neurological deficit with changes of posterior reversible encephalopathy syndrome on neuroimaging.
- *Congestive cardiac failure:* Severe stage II HTN with evidence of pulmonary edema (respiratory distress, orthopnea, basal crepitations in the basal lung fields). Raised jugular venous pressure and tender hepatomegaly can also occur, especially if HTN is associated with fluid overload.

Flowchart 1: Approach to hypertension in children with chronic kidney disease (CKD).

BP above 90th percentile: start oral medications

↓

Drug of choice are RAAS inhibitors*. Other medications are long acting calcium channel blockers and beta-blockers. Diuretics may be considered in oliguric patients with glomerular causes of CKD

↓

Target strict BP control (50th centile). ABPM is recommended to determine if masked HTN is present. If ABPM is unavailable, home BP monitoring may be considered, provided the device is regularly calibrated

↓

If on maintenance dialysis plan for adequate ultrafiltration and <1 kg of interdialytic weight gain

*RAAS inhibitors should be avoided when estimated glomerular filtration rate (eGFR) < 30 mL/min/1.73 m^2 in those patients not on dialysis due to risk of sudden irreversible decline in renal function and risk of hyperkalemia.

(ABPM: ambulatory blood pressure monitoring; HTN: hypertension; RAAS: renin–angiotensin–aldosterone system)

Flowchart 2: Approach to hypertension in glomerulonephritis.

History of edema, oliguria and cola-colored urine

↓

Examination:
CVS: Features of congestive cardiac failure
CNS: Seizures, focal neurological deficit
Fundus: Hypertensive retinopathy changes

↓

- IV Furosemide 1–2 mg/kg in 30 mL NS slow IV over 15 minutes and wait for diuretic response
- Re-examine the BP; if persists to be high and patient is symptomatic add nifedipine 0.25 mg/kg/dose sublingual 6th hourly.
- Fluid, sodium and potassium restriction.

↓

The mainstay of HTN therapy is loop diuretics, i.e., to promote salt and water diuresis. Add long acting antihypertensive amlodipine if BP persists to be high after 5 days

(CNS: central nervous system; CVS: cardiovascular system; HTN: hypertension; NS: normal saline)

Note: Although western guidelines do not recommend the use of nifedipine, in low-resource settings, the short-acting calcium-channel blocker nifedipine is easily available and inexpensive (compared with isradipine or nicardipine). In situations, where urgent blood pressure reduction is indicated, nifedipine may be used to initiate therapy cautiously, with continuous monitoring for sudden reductions in blood pressure and reflex tachycardia.

- *Neuroretinopathy:* Severe stage II HTN with visual disturbances including loss of vision (amaurosis fugax) with fundus changes of papilledema, hemorrhages, and cotton wool spots.

The approach to initial evaluation and management of acute severe HTN is summarized in **Flowchart 3**.

Section A: Rapid evaluation of a child with symptomatic HTN.

- Stage the HTN as per AAP 2017 recommendations
- Assessment of airway breathing and circulation
- If seizures present: Treat with anticonvulsants
- If the child is tachypneic, hypoxic with basal fine crepitations, fluid overload features, then give airway support by bi-level positive airway pressure (BiPAP)
- Do emergency laboratory tests such as arterial blood gas (ABG)/venous blood gas (VBG) to look at partial pressure of oxygen (PaO_2), serum potassium, serum bicarbonate, blood urea and serum creatinine levels.
- Ask history of preexisting diagnosis of HTN
- Ask history of preexisting diagnosis of kidney disease, current medications, underlying nature of illness, and recurrent urinary tract infection (UTI).

TABLE 2: Etiology of hypertensive emergencies in children.

Hypertension	*Etiology*
Secondary	
Renal parenchymal	• Glomerulonephritis, reflux nephropathy, polycystic kidney disease, congenital anomalies of kidney and urinary tract • Chronic kidney disease
Renovascular	• Renal artery stenosis • Thrombotic microangiopathy
Cardiovascular	Coarctation of aorta systemic vasculitis
Malignancies	Pheochromocytoma, neuroblastoma, and Wilms' tumor
Endocrinology	Cushing syndrome, congenital adrenal hyperplasia, thyrotoxicosis
Medications	Corticosteroids, calcineurin inhibitors, cocaine amphetamines
Monogenic hypertension	Liddle syndrome, Gordon syndrome, apparent mineralocorticoid excess, glucocorticoid remediable aldosteronism
Primary/essential hypertension	

Flowchart 3: Approach to initial evaluation and management of acute severe hypertension (HTN).

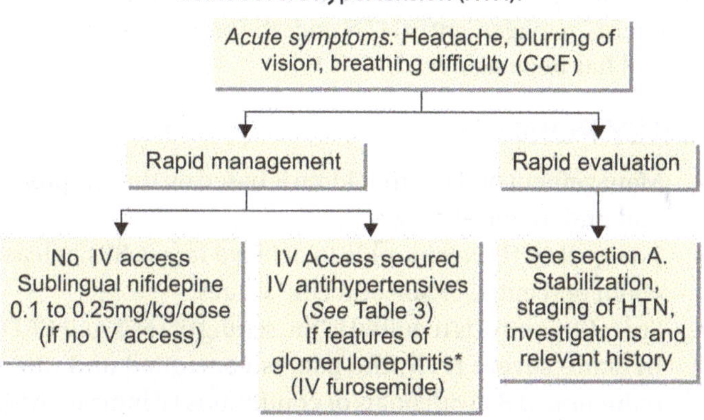

*Edema, oliguria, gross hematuria

APPROACH TO MANAGEMENT OF MONOGENIC HYPERTENSION

Monogenic HTN is one of the important inherited causes of HTN in childhood. Certain clinical features specific are family history of HTN with mild-to-moderate HTN that is difficult to treat with a conventional approach of antihypertensives. <5% can present as acute symptomatic hypertension. Apart from symptoms of HTN, they present with features of muscle weakness and paralytic ileus secondary to hypokalemia.[16]

A diagnostic approach to monogenic HTN is given in **Flowchart 4**.

Management

Apart from the general management of HTN with salt restriction and addition of antihypertensives, the treatment of monogenic HTN depends on underlying etiology:

- *Liddle syndrome:* Autosomal-dominant (AD) inherited disorder characterized by upregulation of epithelial sodium channel (ENaC) in aldosterone-sensitive distal nephron (ASDN). Treatment is ENaC channel inhibitor amiloride/triamterene.
- *Apparent mineralocorticoid excess:* Autosomal-recessive inherited disorder due to inactivation of the 11β-hydroxysteroid dehydrogenase (HSD) type 2 enzyme in ASDN resulting in uncontrolled binding of cortisol to mineralocorticoid receptor (MR). The treatment of choice is MR antagonist spironolactone or eplerenone.
- *Gordon syndrome:* AD disorder due to loss-of-function mutation with no lysine kinase 4 (WNK4) resulting in upregulated NCC (sodium chloride cotransporter) on the distal convoluted tubule (DCT). Treatment

Flowchart 4: Diagnostic algorithm of monogenic hypertension.[16]

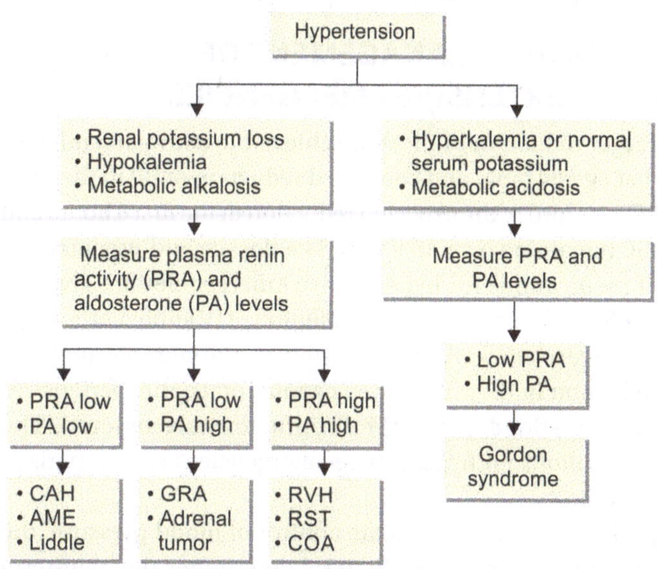

(AME: apparent mineralocorticoid excess; CAH: congenital adrenal hyperplasia; COA: coarctation of aorta; GRA: glucocorticoid remediable aldosteronism; RST: renin-secreting tumor; RVH: renovascular hypertension)

TABLE 3: Medications for hypertensive emergencies.[15]

Drug	*Class*	*Dose*	*Route*	*Adverse effect*
Intravenous				
*Sodium nitroprusside	Vasodilator	0.53–10 μg/kg/min	IV infusion	Cyanide and thiocyanate toxicity
*Labetalol	Alpha- + beta-blocker	*Bolus:* 0.2–1 mg/kg/dose to 40 mg/dose *Infusion:* 0.25–3 mg/kg/h	IV infusion	Caution in asthma and CCF
Hydralazine	Vasodilator	• 0.2–0.6 mg/kg bolus repeat after 4 hours • Maximum bolus 20 mg	• IV bolus • IM	• Reflex tachycardia headache • Fluid retention
Nicardipine	Calcium-channel blocker	*Bolus:* 30 μg/kg/dose up to 2 mg/dose *Infusion:* 0.5–4 μg/kg/min	• IV bolus • IV infusion	• Reflex tachycardia • Increased CNI drug levels
Esmolol	Beta-adrenergic blocker	100–500 μg/kg/min	IV infusion	Profound bradycardia
Fenoldopam	Dopamine receptor agonist	0.2–0.5 μg/kg/min up to 0.8 μg/kg/min	IV	Tachycardia
Oral				
Clonidine	Central alpha-agonist	2–5 μg/kg/dose up to 10 μg/kg/dose given every 6–8 hours	Oral	Dry mouth, drowsiness
Hydralazine	Direct vasodilator	0.25 mg/kg per dose up to 25 mg per dose given every 6–8 hours	Oral/IV	Genetically dependent acetylation rates
Isradipine	Calcium-channel blocker	0.05–0.1 mg/kg per dose up to 5 mg/dose given every 6–8 hours	Oral	Hypotension
Minoxidil	Direct vasodilator	0.1–0.2 mg/kg/dose up to 10 mg per dose given Q8–12 hours	Oral	Long-acting and potent vasodilator

*The details on preparation of labetalol and sodium nitroprusside infusions are mentioned in the last section of this book.

includes low-dose thiazide diuretics and hyperkalemia management.

- *Glucocorticoid remediable HTN:* AD characterized by duplication of 11β-hydroxylase gene resulting in adrenocorticotropic hormone (ACTH)-stimulated aldosterone production that is not dependent on renin levels. The treatment of choice is glucocorticoids to suppress ACTH along with MR antagonists.[16,17]

FURTHER MANAGEMENT OF HYPERTENSIVE EMERGENCIES

Target reduction of BP is to achieve the 95th percentile for that age by rapid and controlled reduction of BP in the form of one-third of the expected reduction in the first 8 hours and the remaining over 48 hours. The dosage and preparations of medications for hypertensive emergencies are given in **Table 3**. The preparation and dilution of IV antihypertensives are given below. After achieving an initial rapid targeted reduction in BP with IV medications, oral antihypertensives may be added, while the IV infusions are tapered. The medications for hypertensive emergencies are summarized in **Table 3**.

In addition to adequate control of blood pressure, the underlying etiology of the HTN determines the long-term prognosis. The main treatment strategy is to safely reduce the blood pressure to prevent the hypoperfusion of vital organs of which cerebral autoregulation is of utmost importance.[18,19]

CONCLUSION

The broad goal of management of HTN is to treat symptomatic HTN with prevention or reversal of TOD. The most common cause of HTN in children is secondary HTN; hence, the management of HTN depends on the cause and clinical situation. The target BP values, after achieving hypertensive symptoms control, depend on the underlying etiology of HTN. For example, strict BP control (<50th percentile, using ABPM) is targeted in those with CKD associated with proteinuria. In high-risk children with an underlying condition such as CKD, reflux nephropathy, or proteinuria, antihypertensives have to be initiated at the earliest. Nonpharmacological therapy alone is considered in children without severe or symptomatic HTN or in those with HTN associated with obesity. The principle of managing hypertensive crisis remains the same irrespective of the etiology, with evaluation for the underlying cause and long-term management of HTN once the target blood pressure control has been achieved.

KEY POINTS

- Management of HTN in children is based on the symptoms and underlying etiology.
- The goal of HTN control is to achieve target BPs at least <90th percentile of SBP and DBP values.
- Strict BP control is required in the setting of HTN and CKD.
- In acute severe HTN, the goal is controlled and rapid reduction of BP with bolus or continuous IV infusion with close monitoring.

REFERENCES

1. Flynn JT, Kaelber DC, Baker-Smith CM, Blowey D, Carroll AE, Daniels SR, et al. Clinical practice guideline for screening and management of high blood pressure in children and adolescents. Pediatrics. 2017;140(3):e20171904.
2. Lurbe E, Agabiti-Rosei E, Cruickshank JK, Dominiczak A, Erdine S, Hirth A, et al. 2016 European Society of Hypertension guidelines for the management of high blood pressure in children and adolescents. J Hypertens. 2016;34(10):1887-920.
3. Chaturvedi S, Lipszyc DH, Licht C, Craig JC, Parekh R. Pharmacological interventions for hypertension in children. Cochrane Database Syst Rev. 2014;(2):CD008117.
4. Lexicomp Paediatric Dosage Handbook, 27th edition. Philadelphia: Wolters Kluwer; 2021.
5. Neter JE, Stam BE, Kok FJ, Grobbee DE, Geleijnse JM. Influence of weight reduction on blood pressure: A meta-analysis of randomized controlled trials. Hypertension. 2003;42(5):878-84.
6. Casonatto J, Goessler KF, Cornelissen VA, Cardoso JR, Polito MD. The blood pressure-lowering effect of a single bout of resistance exercise: A systematic review and meta-analysis of randomised controlled trials. Eur J Prev Cardiol. 2016;23(16):1700-14.
7. World Health Organization. Cardiovascular diseases. SEARO; 2017.
8. Tran AH, Urbina EM. Hypertension in children. Curr Opin Cardiol. 2020;35(4):376-80.
9. Ferguson MA, Flynn JT. Rational use of antihypertensive medications in children. Pediatr Nephrol. 2014;29(6):979-88.
10. O'Brien E, Parati G, Stergiou G, Asmar R, Beilin L, Bilo G, et al. European Society of Hypertension Position Paper on Ambulatory Blood Pressure Monitoring. J Hypertens. 2013; 31(9):1731-68.
11. Halbach S, Flynn J. Treatment of hypertension in children with chronic kidney disease. Curr Hypertens Rep. 2015;17(1):503.
12. Wühl E, Trivelli A, Picca S, Litwin M, Peco-Antic A, Zurowska A, et al. Strict blood-pressure control and progression of renal failure in children. N Engl J Med. 2009;361(17):1639-50.
13. Barletta GM, Pierce C, Mitsnefes M, Samuels J, Warady BA, Furth S, et al. Is blood pressure improving in children with chronic kidney disease? A period analysis. Hypertension. 2018; 71(3):444-50.
14. Srivastava RN. Acute glomerulonephritis. Indian J Pediatr; 1999;66(2):199-205.
15. Seeman T, Hamdani G, Mitsnefes M. Hypertensive crisis in children and adolescents. Pediatr Nephrol. 2019;34(12):2523-37.
16. Simonetti GD, Mohaput MG, Bianchetti MG. Monogenic forms of hypertension. Eur J Pediatr. 2012;171(10):1433-9.
17. Aggarwal A, Rodriguez-Buritica D. Monogenic hypertension in children: A review with emphasis on genetics. Adv Chronic Kidney Dis. 2017;24(6):372-9.
18. Raina R, Mahajan Z, Sharma A, Chakraborty R, Mahajan S, Sethi SK, et al. Hypertensive crisis in pediatric patients: An overview. Front Pediatr. 2020;8:588911.
19. Chandar J, Zilleruelo G. Hypertensive crisis in children. Pediatr Nephrol. 2012;27(5):741-51.

SECTION

11

Acute Kidney Injury

CHAPTER

11.1 Definition, Diagnosis, and Staging

Christy Cathreen Thomas, Aditi Sinha

INTRODUCTION

Acute kidney injury (AKI) is defined as an abrupt deterioration in the kidney function resulting in sudden rapid decline of glomerular filtration rate (GFR), accumulation of waste products such as blood urea nitrogen and creatinine, and dysregulation of the homeostasis of fluid and electrolytes. AKI is characterized by decrease in kidney function over hours to weeks. It is a heterogeneous syndrome with varied etiology, severity, and outcome.[1] Patients may have asymptomatic elevation of serum creatinine or present with symptoms attributed to oligoanuric renal failure with fluid overload, dyselectrolytemia, and uremia. AKI may be present in isolation or be associated with other conditions. The term acute renal failure (ARF) was replaced by AKI as it did not recognize renal dysfunction as a continuum of events and overemphasized failure as a discrete event and to emphasize the importance of detecting even subtle drop in kidney function.

EPIDEMIOLOGY

The estimated incidence of AKI in children varies from 2 to 20 per million. Improved awareness about AKI has led to its increased recognition in the last three decades. The incidence of AKI varies based on the baseline risk factors and severity of ongoing illness, being highest in critically ill patients.[2] Information on incidence of AKI in different settings is based chiefly on unicentric retrospective series. AKI affected 14–53% of critically ill pediatric patients.[3-6] AKI is particularly common after cardiac surgery, affecting 20–60% infants postoperatively.[7] Sick neonates are also at high risk of AKI.[8] Epidemiologic estimates of community-based pediatric AKI indicate an annual incidence of ~1 per 1,000 patients.[9] A Norwegian national survey of hospitals providing specialized care in pediatric AKI estimated an average annual incidence rate of 3.3 cases per 100,000 patients.[10] Using electronic medical records of outpatient (n = 87,007) and inpatient (n = 57,879) data, the prevalence of community-acquired AKI in China was estimated at 4 per 1,000 outpatient visits and 17 per 1,000 hospital admissions; hospital-acquired AKI were observed in 9.7 per 1,000 hospital admissions.[11] The recent Assessment of Worldwide Acute Kidney Injury, Renal Angina, and Epidemiology (AWARE) study, a prospective multinational observational study, showed that AKI affected 30% of 4,683 critically ill pediatric patients, one-third of whom had severe AKI.[12]

DEFINITION AND STAGING OF ACUTE KIDNEY INJURY

A uniform definition and staging of AKI is essential to allow comparisons between populations and studies. Over the last few decades, various definitions and staging criteria were reported, chiefly differing in the degree of rise in serum creatinine, fall in estimated glomerular filtration rate (eGFR) from baseline, threshold values for urine output, and time interval over which the renal dysfunction was observed **(Tables 1 and 2)**. AKI is defined as a decrease in GFR over hours to weeks, which is manifested by a rise in serum creatinine from baseline, and/or a reduction in urine output.

The Acute Dialysis Quality Initiative (ADQI) group initially proposed the RIFLE criteria, an acronym for *r*isk of renal dysfunction, *i*njury to the kidneys, *f*ailure of kidney function, *l*oss of kidney function, and *e*nd-stage kidney disease, that had three grades of severity of AKI (risk, injury, and failure) and two outcome categories (loss of function and end-stage kidney disease).[13] This classification took into account timed urine output, rise in serum creatinine from baseline, and need for and duration of kidney replacement therapy (KRT). The pediatric RIFLE (pRIFLE) criteria, a modification of RIFLE for use in children, are based on creatinine clearance estimated from serum creatinine and height using the modified Schwartz formula [estimated creatinine clearance (eCrCl)].[14] The duration of oliguria was altered to 8, 16, and 24 hour in the risk, injury, and failure categories, respectively. Where baseline data was lacking, the pRIFLE criteria allowed for GFR to be imputed from age-appropriate values assuming normal kidney function. Further, an acute fall in eCrCl to <35 mL/min/1.73 m^2 was an additional criterion to classify as a failure category.

The AKI Network (AKIN) criteria, introduced in 2007, endorsed the RIFLE classification, but modified it to improve sensitivity to even small changes in serum creatinine

TABLE 1: Definition of acute kidney injury (AKI).

Risk injury failure loss end stage (RIFLE)	***Acute kidney injury network (AKIN)***	***Kidney disease improving global outcomes (KDIGO)***
Rise in serum creatinine to ≥1.5 times the baseline or decrease in GFR by >25% or fall in urine volume to <0.5 mL/kg per hour for 6 hours, over 1–7 days and persisting for >24 hours	Rise in serum creatinine by ≥0.3 mg/dL or to 1.5–2 times the baseline, over 48 hours, or fall in urine volume to <0.5 mL/kg per hour for >6 hours	Rise in serum creatinine by ≥0.3 mg/dL within 48 hours, or to ≥1.5 times the baseline, known or presumed to have occurred within 7 days, or fall in urine volume to <0.5 mL/kg per hour for >6 hours

(GFR: glomerular filtration rate)

TABLE 2: Staging of acute kidney injury (AKI).

Category or stage*	***Based on serum creatinine***				***Based on urine output***	
	RIFLE^	***pRIFLE***	***AKIN***	***KDIGO***	***RIFLE, AKIN, and KDIGO***	***pRIFLE***
Risk or stage 1	↑ to 1.5–2 times baseline, or ↓ in GFR by >25%, over <7 days	↓ in eGFR by ≥25%	↑ by ≥0.3 mg/dL or to 1.5–2 times baseline, in <48 hours	↑ to 1.5–1.9 times baseline, in <7 days, or by ≥0.3 mg/dL in <48 hours	<0.5 mL/kg per hour for 6–12 hours	<0.5 mL/kg/h × 8 hours
Injury or stage 2	↑ to 2–3 times baseline, or ↓ decrease in GFR by >50%	↓ in eGFR by ≥50%	↑ to more than 2–3 times baseline	↑ to 2–2.9 times baseline	<0.5 mL/kg/hour for ≥12 hours	<0.5 mL/kg/h × 16 h
Failure or stage 3	↑ to >3 times the baseline, or >4 mg/dL with an acute rise of >0.5 mg/dL, or ↓ in GFR by >75%	↓ in eGFR by ≥75% or eGFR <35 mL/min per 1.73 m²	↑ to >3 times baseline or, to ≥4 mg/dL with ↑ by ≥0.5 mg/dL, or initiation of KRT	↑ to ≥3 times baseline, or to ≥4 mg/dL, or initiation of KRT, OR (if <18-year-old) ↓ in eGFR to <35 mL/min per 1.73 m²	0.3 mL/kg/h for ≥24 hours or anuria for ≥12 hours	<0.5 mL/kg/h × 24 hours or anuria × 12 hours
Loss	Persistent acute renal failure for >4 weeks	Persistent acute renal failure for >4 weeks				
End stage	Failure for >3 months	Failure for >3 months				

*Category for risk injury failure loss or end stage (RIFLE) criteria and stage in acute kidney injury network (AKIN) and kidney disease improving global outcomes (KDIGO) classification
^AKI should be abrupt (1–7 days) and sustained (>24 hours)
(↑ increase; ↓ decrease; eGFR: estimated glomerular filtration rate calculated by Schwartz formula)

(>0.3 mg/dL or 50% increase from baseline), avoided estimation of GFR, and stringently specified a time span of 48 hours over which renal dysfunction had been observed.[15] The severity of AKI was specified as stages, with individuals requiring KRT being included in the most severe stage 3, and outcome variables were altogether omitted.

The 2012 classification of AKI, by the Kidney Disease Improving Global Outcomes (KDIGO), harmonizes RIFLE, AKIN, and pRIFLE criteria and is now the most widely used and accepted definition of AKI.[16] The KDIGO criteria retain a rise in serum creatinine by 0.3 mg/dL over 48 hours that were proposed by AKIN, while including a 50% increase in serum creatinine over 7 days as listed in RIFLE criteria. However, the threshold for acute change in serum creatinine is set by KDIGO as 0.5 mg/dL in patients with serum creatinine of 4 mg/dL who are classified as stage 3 AKI. The KDIGO criteria retained the pRIFLE criterion of an acute reduction in eGFR or eCrCl to <35 mL/min/1.73 m² as stage 3 AKI in pediatric patients. The urine output criteria of RIFLE and AKIN are maintained in KDIGO criteria.

The above criteria have been validated in several prospective and retrospective studies including adult and pediatric patients, wherein increasing severity or stages of AKI were associated with worse outcomes, including mortality, need for KRT, chronic kidney disease, and length of hospital stay.[17] In particular, the KDIGO criteria are demonstrated to show incremental risk for patient morbidity and mortality. However, the recent pediatric reference change value (RCV) optimized for AKI in children (pROCK) criteria, derived from a multicenter epidemiologic study on 100,081 hospitalized children in China, challenge the specificity of KDIGO criteria.[18] Based on the concept that only acute increase in serum creatinine above the upper limit (95th centile) of normal variability, termed as RCV, represents true renal dysfunction, pediatric AKI was defined as an increase in a serum creatinine by both ≥20 μmol/L (0.23 mg/dL) and ≥30% over the baseline within 7 days. While pROCK outperformed KDIGO in predicting mortality in two large multicenter studies from China, including one focusing on critically ill patients,[17,19] more studies are required worldwide to address its diagnostic utility versus the KDIGO criteria.

Limitations and Caveats

The chief determinants of AKI, namely serum creatinine or GFR and urine output, are both susceptible to many caveats. Rise in serum creatinine might take longer than 24–36 hours after AKI has set in. Further, serum creatinine may vary, based on the rate of its generation (that depends on muscle mass and liver function), its volume of distribution, and the method of estimation of creatinine. Agents interfering with tubular secretion of creatinine can increase its serum levels. In most acutely ill patients, prehospitalization values of creatinine are not available; while serum creatinine at baseline might have significant interindividual variability, even small changes in serum creatinine are associated with significant kidney injury. Further, critically ill children may not have stable levels of serum creatinine. Fluid overload might lead to dilution and underestimation of serum creatinine. Similarly, urine output is known to vary widely physiologically, and nonoliguric AKI is not uncommon in children. Further, the available classifications of AKI do not address the etiological factors determining AKI nor account for preexisting kidney disease. Hence, the KDIGO recommends exploring for the etiology, intrinsic susceptibility, and exposures in every patient with AKI.[15]

ACUTE KIDNEY DISEASE

Studies show that AKI lasting for <48 hours has better outcome than that which persists for longer.[20,21] Complete and sustained resolution in 48 hours of onset of AKI is called rapid reversal of, or transient AKI **(Table 3)**. Persistent AKI continues beyond 48 hours of onset and usually resolves by day 7. The term acute kidney disease (AKD) was introduced to categorize patients with renal dysfunction persisting for >7 days in whom a diagnosis CKD, conventionally diagnosed at 90 days or longer, is not yet met.[15] This definition also includes patients with impaired renal function that do not satisfy the definition of AKI, i.e., <50% increase in creatinine from baseline. Potential outcomes for patients with AKD include complete recovery, recurrence of AKI, progression to CKD, and/or death. A fair proportion of patients with persistent AKI evolve into AKD, of which several are subsequently labeled as CKD. Hence, the

TABLE 3: Nomenclature of renal dysfunction based on the duration after diagnosis.[19]

Nomenclature	*Duration of AKI*
Transient AKI	Reversal in 48 hours
Persistent or intrinsic AKI	48 hours to 7 days
Acute kidney disease	7–90 days
Chronic kidney disease	>90 days

TABLE 4: Risk factors for acute kidney injury (AKI).

Intrinsic factors	*Processes and exposure*
Chronic kidney disease	Nephrotoxic drugs; toxins
Chronic heart disease	Sepsis or shock
Diabetes mellitus	Volume depletion
Chronic liver disease	Cardiac surgery
Solid organ or hematopoietic stem cell transplant	Radiocontrast agents
Previous episodes of AKI	Mechanical ventilation
	Multi-organ dysfunction

terms persistent AKI, AKD, and CKD represent a continuum for patients with AKI stage 1 or greater lasting for longer than 1 week.

Diagnosis of Acute Kidney Injury

The symptoms and signs of AKI may vary from patient to patient based on the stage of AKI and underlying condition. A few children may present with established AKI, along with complications, such as fluid overload, encephalopathy, or those of electrolyte imbalance. Others may have no apparent symptoms, or symptoms due to the underlying condition leading to AKI. A high index of suspicion should be maintained in children at risk of AKI **(Table 4)**. The diagnosis of AKI should be made based on the urine output criteria or the creatinine-based criteria[13,15,16] and requires careful serial monitoring. Definition to be used in the diagnosis and staging of AKI are described in **Table 1**. While cystatin C-based eGFR equations exist, these have not yet found a place in the definition or classification of AKI.

Risk Stratification and Prediction of Severe Acute Kidney Injury

Since creatinine increases after AKI is already established, prevention of AKI requires identifying patients who are at risk, so that efforts to prevent AKI can be focused on these patients. Risk factors associated with AKI are classified as intrinsic factors, disease processes, and exposures **(Table 4)**. "At-risk" patients should be actively screened for AKI and preventive measures instituted *a priori* to prevent its occurrence. The success of one such measure was demonstrated by a quality improvement study called "nephrotoxic injury negated by just-in-time action (NINJA)" that found a decrease in the rate of AKI in neonates and noncritically ill children when a pharmacologist-based approach identified the use of nephrotoxic drugs, followed by interdisciplinary discussion to mitigate the exposure as well as identify AKI in a timely manner.[22] It is particularly important to predict occurrence of severe AKI, e.g., KDIGO stages 2–3 AKI, since it is associated with higher risk of adverse outcomes, including mortality. Tools to predict the occurrence of severe AKI and/or AKI risk stratification are discussed below.

Biomarkers

The delay in increase in serum creatinine in patients developing AKI led researchers to look for a "kidney troponin" that may enable early detection of AKI or identification of those at risk of severe AKI or progression to CKD. Based on pathophysiology, animal studies and limited reports, various biomarkers were proposed to fulfill the role, including neutrophil gelatinase-associated lipocalin (NGAL), kidney injury molecule 1 (KIM-1), interleukin-18, liver-type fatty acid-binding protein, angiotensinogen, tissue inhibitor of metalloproteinase-2 (TIMP-2), and insulin-like growth factor binding protein 7 (IGFBP7).[23] However, most of these biomarkers have not been validated consistently, and none of the markers convincingly mimicked a troponin-like performance in large studies like SAPPHIRE or TRIBE-AKI.[24,25] The first Food and Drug Administration (FDA)-approved biomarker-based test (NephroCheck®) is the product of two urinary biomarkers, TIMP-2 and IGFBP7, that predicts moderate-to-severe AKI in critically ill patients.[26] Biomarkers may show improved diagnostic utility when applied to specific clinical settings (e.g., after cardiopulmonary bypass),[27,28] if used in combination (e.g., NephroCheck®), or when coupled to other predictive tools, such as the renal angina index (RAI; discussed below). Serum and urine levels of cystatin C have been used as biomarkers in AKI. In a meta-analysis, including 1948 children in 24 studies, serum and urine cystatin C were useful in predicting AKI, with area under the curve of 0.83 and 0.85, respectively. Overall, serum cystatin C demonstrated better sensitivity and specificity than urine cystatin.[28]

Fluid Overload

Fluid overload in critically ill patients is multifactorial in origin, secondary to systemic inflammation leading to capillary leak, overzealous fluid administration, disordered fluid homeostasis, and/or AKI. Excessive fluid not only affects lung function but is also associated with AKI, potentially by increasing venous pressure in an encapsulated organ and/or through interstitial edema. Fluid overload is particularly common in pediatric intensive care units (ICUs) where early goal-directed therapy (EGDT) remains the cornerstone of management of septic and hypovolemic shock.[29] It remains the most common indication for the initiation of continuous kidney replacement therapy, and overload over 20% in such patients was linked to an eightfold increased risk of mortality.[30] The degree of fluid overload is estimated using either cumulative fluid balance or weight-based methods and is reported as cumulative or peak percent fluid overload, cumulative or peak percent weight change, net fluid balance relative to weight, and net fluid balance relative to body surface.[31] A meta-analysis of 44 studies, including 7,507 pediatric patients, established that percentage of fluid overload is associated with increased risk of mortality [odds ratio (OR), 4.3; 95% confidence interval (CI) 3.0–6.3], prolonged (>48 hours) mechanical ventilation (OR 2.2; 95% CI 1.3–3.7) and AKI (OR 2.4; 95% CI 1.3–4.4); based on adjusted analysis, there was a 6% increase in odds of mortality for every 1% increase in percentage fluid overload.[28]

Renal Angina Index

Renal angina index is a context-driven stratification system that identifies the risk of severe AKI according to the baseline clinical characteristics, alongside detecting signs of decreased kidney function.[32] The individual score, ranging from 1 to 40, is derived by multiplying the risk of AKI score, based on clinical characteristics, with the evidence of AKI score, based on the degree of fluid overload and change in serum creatinine from baseline, as shown in **Table 5**. A score of 8 or higher within 12 hours of admission, termed renal angina, is highly specific and sensitive for development of severe AKI on day 3 of admission to the ICU. Meta-analyses of 11 studies including 2,701 pediatric patients estimates that renal angina (an RAI of ≥8) is a reliable tool in predicting severe AKI in pediatric patients, with a diagnostic odds ratio of 20.[33] However, individual studies vary in the sensitivity, specificity, and negative predictive value of the test, and 8% of the patients have false-negative results.[23] Combining RAI to biomarkers, such as plasma NGAL and neutrophil elastase-2,[34]

TABLE 5: Renal angina index.

Risk or evidence of acute kidney injury		***Score***
Risk		
Admission to the pediatric intensive care unit		1
History of bone marrow or solid-organ transplantation		3
Mechanical ventilation or vasoactive support		5
Evidence of clinical injury		
Serum creatinine *versus* baseline	Fluid overload	
No change	<5%	1
1–1.49 times baseline value	5% to <10%	2
1.5–1.99 times baseline value	10% to <15%	4
≥2 times baseline value	≥15%	8

Renal angina index = Risk score × evidence scores; assessed 12 hours after admission; score ≥8 predicts severe AKI 72 hours later or conventional predictors of adverse outcome, such as serum lactate,[35] improved the diagnostic utility of the test.

Frusemide Stress Test

In early AKI, administration of a single intravenous dose of frusemide might provide a useful assessment of the integrity of tubular function.[36] Systematic review and meta-analysis of studies in adult patients indicate that a urine volume of <200 mL (100 mL/h) in the first 2 hours after administering furosemide has robust diagnostic accuracy in predicting progression of AKI, regardless of AKI criteria used or presence of underlying CKD (pooled diagnostic odds ratio 13.6; 95% CI 5.7–32.2).[37] Whether the frusemide stress test identifies pediatric patients at risk of severe and progressive AKI and the precise threshold urine output in children remains to be determined.

CONCLUSION

Timely identification of AKI is essential to institute measures to prevent its progression to severe stage and various deleterious consequences of AKI. Collaborative efforts have enabled consensus of definition of AKI and the stratification of its severity. Current research is focused on testing various tools to develop practical risk stratification strategies for the early recognition of AKI in at risk pediatric patients, using combinations of biomarkers and practical bedside tests and electronic medical record alerts that are applicable to routine clinical practice.[38]

KEY POINTS

- AKI has multiple causes, most commonly affecting renal perfusion.
- AKI may have varying severity and is defined and staged based on urine output and change in serum level of creatinine.
- Risk stratification of patients, to enable focusing early interventions on those most at risk of AKI, and/or prediction of severe AKI, includes use of biomarkers, determining percentage fluid overload, estimation of RAI and assessing response to frusemide stress test.

REFERENCES

1. Roy JP, Devarajan P. Acute kidney injury: diagnosis and management. Indian J Pediatr. 2020;87:600-07.
2. Waiker SS, Murray PT, Singh AK. Epidemiology and diagnosis. In: Waiker SS, Murray PT, Singh AK (Eds). Core Concepts in Acute Kidney Injury, 1st edition. New York: Springer; 2018. pp. 3-23.
3. Nawaz S, Afzal K. Pediatric acute kidney injury in North India: a prospective hospital-based study. Saudi J Kidney Dis Transpl. 2018;29:689-97.
4. Rustagi RS, Arora K, Das RR, Pooni PA, Singh D. Incidence, risk factors and outcome of acute kidney injury in critically ill children: a developing country perspective. Paediatr Int Child Health. 2017;37:35-41.
5. Mehta P, Sinha A, Sami A, Hari P, Kalaivani M, Gulati A, et al. Incidence of acute kidney injury in hospitalized children. Indian Pediatr. 2012;49:537-42.
6. Krishnamurthy S, Mondal N, Narayanan P, Biswal N, Srinivasan S, Soundravally R, et al. Incidence and etiology of acute kidney injury in southern India. Indian J Pediatr. 2013;80:183-9.
7. Li D, Niu Z, Huang Q, Sheng W, Wang T. A meta-analysis of the incidence rate of postoperative acute kidney injury in patients with congenital heart disease. BMC Nephrol. 2020;21:350.
8. Selewski DT, Charlton JR, Jetton JG, Guillet R, Mhanna MJ, Askenazi DJ, et al. Neonatal Acute Kidney Injury. Pediatrics. 2015;136:e463-73.
9. McGregor TL, Jones DP, Wang L, Danciu I, Bridges BC, Fleming GM, et al. Acute kidney injury incidence in noncritically ill hospitalized children, adolescents, and young adults: a retrospective observational study. Am J Kidney Dis. 2016;67:384-90.
10. Jenssen GR, Hovland E, Bangstad H, Nygård K, Vold L, Bjerre A. The incidence and aetiology of acute kidney injury in children in Norway between 1999 and 2008. Acta Paediatr. 2014;103:1192-97.
11. Hsu CN, Chen HL, Tain YL. Epidemiology and outcomes of community-acquired and hospital-acquired acute kidney injury in children and adolescents. Pediatr Res. 2018;83:622-9.
12. Lameire N, Van Biesen W, Vanholder R. Epidemiology of acute kidney injury in children worldwide including developing countries. Pediatr Nephrol. 2017;32:1301-14.
13. Bellomo R, Ronco C, Kellum JA, Mehta RL, Palevsky P, Acute Dialysis Quality Initiative workgroup. Acute renal failure—definition, outcome measures, animal models, fluid therapy and information technology needs: The second international consensus conference of the Acute Dialysis Quality Initiative (ADQI) Group. Crit Care. 2004;8:R204-12.
14. Akcan-Arikan A, Zappitelli M, Loftis LL, Washburn KK, Jefferson LS, Goldstein SL. Modified RIFLE criteria in critically ill children with acute kidney injury. Kidney Int. 2007;71:1028-35.
15. Mehta RL, Kellum JA, Shah SV, Molitoris BA, Ronco C, Warnock DG, et al. Acute Kidney Injury Network: report of an initiative to improve outcomes in acute kidney injury. Crit Care. 2007;11:R31.
16. KDIGO AKI Work Group. KDIGO clinical practice guideline for acute kidney injury. Kidney Int Suppl. 2012;2:1-138.
17. Sutherland SM, Byrnes JJ, Kothari M, Longhurst CA, Dutta S, Garcia P, et al. AKI in hospitalized children: comparing the pRIFLE, AKIN, and KDIGO definitions. Clin J Am Soc Nephrol. 2015;10:554-61.
18. Xu X, Nie S, Zhang A, Jianhua M, Liu H, Xia H, et al. A new criterion for pediatric AKI based on the reference change value of serum creatinine. J Am Soc Nephrol. 2018;29:2432-42.
19. Cui W, Gao H, Fang H, Xianhui Q, Danqun J, Haipeng L. Impact of and risk factors for pediatric acute kidney injury defined by the pROCK criteria in a Chinese PICU population. Pediatr Res. 2021;89(6):1485-91.
20. Chawla LS, Bellomo R, Bihorac A, Goldstein SL, Siew ED, Bagshaw SM, et al. Acute kidney disease and renal recovery: consensus report of the acute disease quality initiative (ADQI) 16 workgroup. Nat Rev Nephrol. 2017;13:241-57.
21. Kellum J, Sileanu F, Murugan R, Lucko N, Shaw AD, Clermont G, et al. Classifying AKI by urine output versus serum creatinine level. J Am Soc Nephrol. 2015;26:2231-8.
22. Goldstein SL, Dahale D, Kirkendall ES, Mottes T, Kaplan H, Muething S, et al. A prospective multi-center quality improvement initiative (NINJA) indicates a reduction in

nephrotoxic acute kidney injury in hospitalized children. Kidney Int. 2020;97:580-8.

23. Alge JL, Arthur JM. Biomarkers of AKI: a review of mechanistic relevance and potential therapeutic implications. Clin J Am Soc Nephrol. 2015;10:147-55.
24. Kashani K, Al-Khafaji A, Ardiles T, Artigas A, Bagshaw SM, Bell M, et al. Discovery and validation of cell cycle arrest biomarkers in human acute kidney injury. Crit Care. 2013;17:R25.
25. Parikh CR, Moledina DG, Coca SG, Thiessen-Philbrook HR, Garg AX. Application of new acute kidney injury biomarkers in human randomized controlled trials. Kidney Int. 2016;89:1372-9.
26. Fan W, Ankawi G, Zhang J, Digvijay K, Giavarina D, Yin Y, et al. Current understanding and future directions in the application of TIMP-2 and IGFBP7 in AKI clinical practice. Clin Chem Lab Med. 2019;57:567-76.
27. Greenberg JH, Zappitelli M, Jia Y, Thiessen-Philbrook HR, de Fontnouvelle CA, Wilson FP, et al. Biomarkers of AKI progression after pediatric cardiac surgery. J Am Soc Nephrol. 2018;29:1549-56.
28. Nakhjavan-Shahraki B, Yousefifard M, Ataei N, Baikpour M, Ataei F, Bazargani B, et al. Accuracy of cystatin C in prediction of acute kidney injury in children; serum or urine levels: which one works better? A systematic review and meta-analysis. BMC Nephrol. 2017;18:120.
29. Barbaro R, Fan E. In critically ill children, fluid overload is consistently associated with worse outcomes. BMJ Evid Based Med. 2019;24:41-2.
30. Sutherland SM, Zappitelli M, Alexander SR, Chua AN, Brophy PD, Bunchman TE, et al. Fluid overload and mortality in children receiving continuous renal replacement therapy: the prospective pediatric continuous renal replacement therapy registry. Am J Kidney Dis. 2010;55:316-25.
31. Alobaidi R, Morgan C, Basu RK, Stenson E, Featherstone R, Majumdar SR, et al. Association between fluid balance and outcomes in critically ill children: a systematic review and meta-analysis. JAMA Pediatr. 2018;172:257-68.
32. Basu RK, Zappitelli M, Brunner L, Wang Y, Wong HR, Chawla LS, et al. Derivation and validation of the renal angina index to improve the prediction of acute kidney injury in critically ill children. Kidney Int. 2014;85:659-67.
33. Abbasi A, Mehdipour Rabori P, Farajollahi R, Ali KM, Ataei N, Yousefifard M, et al. Discriminatory precision of renal angina index in predicting acute kidney injury in children; a systematic review and meta-analysis. Arch Acad Emerg Med. 2020;8:e39.
34. Basu RK, Wang Y, Wong HR, Chawla LS, Wheeler DS, Goldstein SL. Incorporation of biomarkers with the renal angina index for prediction of severe AKI in critically ill children. Clin J Am Soc Nephrol. 2014;9:654-62.
35. Huang L, Shi T, Quan W, Li W, Zhang L, Liu X, et al. Assessment of early renal angina index for prediction of subsequent severe acute kidney injury during septic shock in children. BMC Nephrol. 2020;21:358.
36. Chawla LS, Davison DL, Brasha-Mitchell E, Koyner JL, Arthur JM, Shaw AD, et al. Development and standardization of a furosemide stress test to predict the severity of acute kidney injury. Crit Care. 2013;17:R207.
37. Chen JJ, Chang CH, Huang YT, Kuo G. Furosemide stress test as a predictive marker of acute kidney injury progression or renal replacement therapy: a systematic review and meta-analysis. Crit Care. 2020;24:202.
38. Fuhrman D. The use of diagnostic tools for pediatric AKI: applying the current evidence to the bedside. Pediatr Nephrol. 2021;36(11):3529-37.

CHAPTER

11.2

Acute Kidney Injury in Children: Etiopathogenesis and Evaluation

Hamsa V Reddy, Priya Pais

INTRODUCTION

Acute kidney injury (AKI) is described as the sudden decline of kidney function associated with a reduction of glomerular filtration rate (GFR). Impairment of kidney function leads to retention of urea and other nitrogenous waste products and dysregulation of extracellular volume and electrolytes.[1] The surrogate measures of GFR in clinical practice are serum creatinine (SCr) and urine volume. Thus, clinical manifestations of AKI include a rise in SCr and a reduction of urine output. The severity of AKI can range from a mild elevation of SCr to complete anuria. The prevalence of AKI in critically ill children is especially high. AKI in children is associated with significant mortality and long-term renal sequelae.[2] The Assessment of Acute Kidney Injury, Renal Angina, and Epidemiology (AWARE), a multinational, prospective observational study on AKI incidence, outcomes, and risk stratification found the incidence of AKI to be 26.9% in 4,683 critically ill children, with an adjusted odds ratio of 1.77 for mortality with diagnosis of severe AKI. AKI is an independent risk factor for increased length of pediatric intensive care unit (PICU) stay, longer duration of mechanical ventilation, and increased mortality among critically ill children.[3] The severity of AKI is staged, based on the extent of SCr rise and/or duration of decreased urine output as per the Kidney Disease: Improving Global Outcomes (KDIGO) Staging of AKI.[4] Other recently developed criteria including pROCK criteria (pediatric reference change value optimized for AKI in children),[5] renal angina index,[6] and the utility of biomarkers are discussed in detail in the previous Chapter 11.1.

ETIOLOGY OF ACUTE KIDNEY INJURY IN CHILDREN

Traditionally, the causes of AKI can be classified based on the location of the insult—prerenal, intrinsic renal, or postrenal (obstructive). Examples of disease associated with each category are provided in **Table 1**.

Prerenal AKI occurs due to a reduced perfusion to the kidneys and results in a functional reduction in kidney

TABLE 1: Etiology of acute kidney injury (AKI) in children.

Prerenal causes	*Intrinsic causes*	*Postrenal causes*
Low intravascular volume • Hemorrhage/gastrointestinal losses • Postoperative, trauma, and severe dehydration • *Third-space losses:* Sepsis and capillary leak, burns, hypoalbuminemia (nephrotic syndrome/liver disease) *Decreased effective circulating volume* Congestive cardiac failure, sepsis, and cardiac tamponade	*Glomerular diseases* Acute glomerulonephritis secondary to any cause* *Tubular disease* • ATN—hypoxic/ischemic, toxin mediated** • Sepsis associated AKI, tumor lysis syndrome, and drug-related AKI *Interstitial disease* • Acute interstitial nephritis due to drugs, infections, and autoimmune disorders • Pyelonephritis *Vascular diseases* Hemolytic uremic syndrome renal vein/artery thrombosis, and large vessel vasculitis	*Obstruction* • Urethral obstruction and posterior urethral valves • Ureteral obstruction in solitary kidney • Bilateral ureteral obstruction—renal stones • External compression by mass

*Rapidly progressive glomerulonephritis (pauci-immune, immune-mediated, and Goodpasture's syndrome), immune-mediated diseases (lupus, IRGN, infectious, IgA nephropathy, MPGN, and vasculitis)

**Endogenous toxins—myoglobin and hemoglobin; exogenous toxins—metals, venom, illicit drugs (mushrooms), ethylene glycol, and methanol

(ATN: acute tubular necrosis; IgA: immunoglobulin A; IRGN: infection-related glomerulonephritis; MPGN: membranoproliferative glomerulonephritis)

function that is fluid responsive. The renal hypoperfusion results from either true volume loss or due to a reduced effective intravascular volume.

Intrinsic AKI results from diseases in the various compartments of the kidney—glomerulus, tubules, interstitium, or blood vessels.

Obstructive or postrenal AKI occurs when there is obstruction of the lower urinary tract.

Although a single cause of AKI is conceptually simple, AKI is often multifactorial, especially in the critical care setting. For example, a septic child in the PICU on inotropes and mechanical ventilation may have with AKI due to sepsis, reduced renal perfusion (shock), and use of nephrotoxic antibiotics.[2]

PATHOGENESIS OF ACUTE KIDNEY INJURY

In prerenal disease, the reduction in GFR is due to reduced renal blood flow. This is a functional impairment, not associated with structural damage. The renal tubular function remains preserved. In prerenal AKI, there is an increased reabsorption of sodium, with reduced urinary sodium excretion. This indicates "functional" tubules and forms the basis for the fractional excretion of sodium (FENa) test,[7] discussed later in the chapter. Thus, with restoration of renal blood flow the AKI is reversible. However, with prolonged or severe reduction in renal perfusion, ischemic acute tubular necrosis (ATN) occurs.

The pathogenesis of ischemic ATN will be described here. The pathogenesis of other intrinsic renal or obstructive causes of AKI will be dealt with in their respective chapters.

Pathogenesis of Acute Tubular Necrosis

Acute kidney injury due to ischemic ATN can be clinically divided into initiation, extension, maintenance, and recovery phases.[8] These clinical phases relate to cellular events occurring during the injury and recovery processes **(Fig. 1)**.

Initiation Phase

The renal blood flow decreases leading to severe cellular ATP depletion. Renal proximal tubule cells undergo a number of structural and functional alterations, the extent of which depends on the severity and duration of ischemia. There is a loss of proximal tubular cell brush border and polarity with severe depletion of ATP. Tubular cell death results from necrosis and apoptosis (programmed cell death). Dead cells detach from the basement membrane, fall into the tubular lumen, and cause obstruction. In addition, ischemic injury to vascular smooth muscle and endothelial cells during the early initiation phase induces a variety of chemokines and cytokines such as tumor necrosis factor (TNF)-alpha, heat shock proteins, and interleukin-6 (IL-6) initiating an inflammatory cascade. In ischemic ATN, normal tubular function is lost, with either oliguria due to reduced GFR or a reduced tubular reabsorptive capacity. This is confirmed by a high FENa.[7]

Extension Phase

This occurs during reperfusion and the resulting endothelial cell injury. There is an upregulation of adhesion molecules such as intracellular adhesion molecule 1 that recruit inflammatory cells. The hemodynamic imbalance between

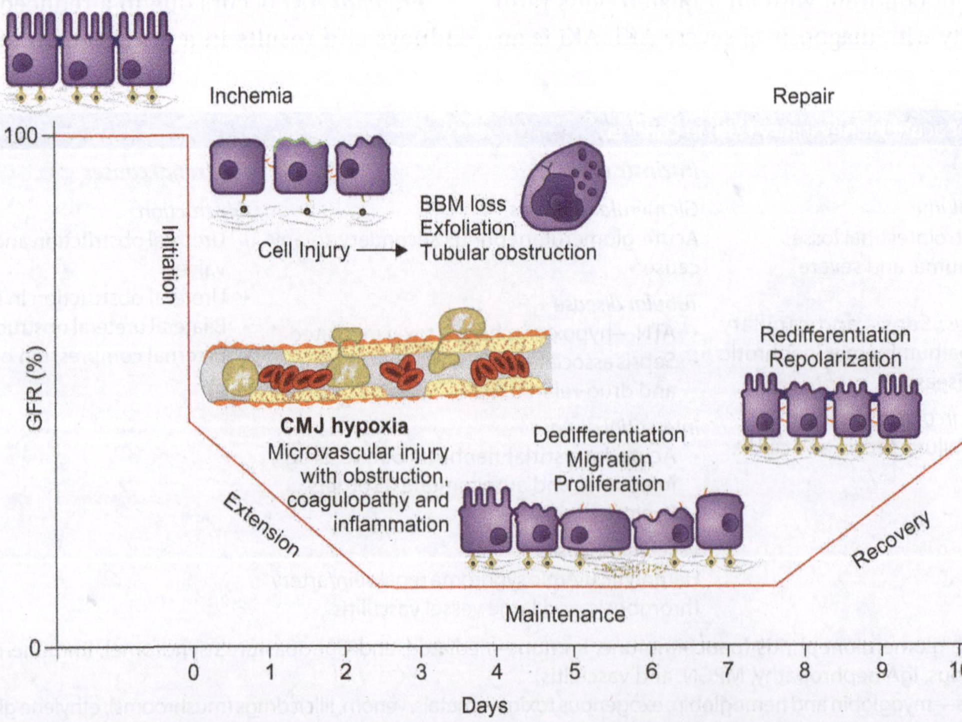

Fig. 1: Relationship of cellular to clinical phases of AKI.[8] (AKI: acute kidney injury; BBM: brush-border membrane; CMJ: corticomedullary junction; GFR: glomerular filtration rate)

vasoconstriction and vasodilation worsen the tubular ischemia. The GFR continues to fall as the cellular injury continues during this phase.

Maintenance Phase

In an attempt to restore cellular and tubule integrity, tubule cells undergo dedifferentiation, repair, migration, and proliferation. GFR is stable but remains substantially diminished. Renal blood flow returns toward normal and cellular homeostasis is restored.

The end result of the initiation and maintenance phase is severe renal tubular dysfunction with oliguria, loss of normal tubular reabsorptive capacity for electrolytes (e.g., sodium) and water.

Recovery Phase

Return of cellular differentiation, epithelial cell polarity, and normal cellular and organ function is achieved.

EVALUATION OF A CHILD WITH ACUTE KIDNEY INJURY

The evaluation of AKI aims to identify the cause for AKI to institute appropriate therapy. AKI is diagnosed when there is an elevation of SCr and/or oliguria and is staged based on the AKI criteria. KDIGO classification criteria are most often applied.

Challenges Associated with Serum Creatinine and Oliguria-based Acute Kidney Injury Staging

Serum creatinine is an insensitive functional marker of AKI because the value rises only after 25–50% of the kidney function has already been lost. Thus, the change in SCr is insensitive to small changes in GFR. In addition, several other factors affect SCr values including muscle mass, hydration status, age, gender, and method of measurement. Once dialysis has been initiated SCr cannot be used to assess renal function as it is dialyzable. Despite these limitations, it is the most widely used laboratory test for diagnosis of AKI as it can be easily measured.[4]

The KDIGO staging is based on a risen SCr from baseline. The lowest SCr measured in the last 6 months is considered the baseline. Most admitted children will not have a previous SCr value available. In previously healthy children, an SCr corresponding to an estimated GFR (eGFR) of 100–120 mL/m^2/min is presumed to be the baseline.[9]

Urine output is also an insensitive marker of GFR, confounded by hydration status, administration of fluids and diuretics and may be difficult to measure accurately. However, worsening degrees of oliguria indicate poor outcomes in AKI, and excluding oliguria as a diagnostic criteria is associated with substantial under diagnosis.[3] In resource-limited settings, oliguria should be used as an early indicator of AKI.[10]

New biomarkers that overcome the limitations of SCr have been studied. The ideal biomarker should be sensitive to early AKI, specific, noninvasive, and cost effective. Serum cystatin C, serum and urinary neutrophil gelatinase-associated lipocalin (NGAL), kidney injury molecule-1 (KIM-1), N-acetyl-β-D-glucosaminidase, interleukin-18, liver-type fatty acid binding protein, and cell cycle arrest markers (tissue inhibitor of metalloproteinases 2 and insulin-like growth factor binding protein) have been evaluated.[9] Though these biomarkers tend to detect AKI earlier than rise in SCr, their utility is mainly restricted to research purposes due to lack of standardized measurement. Also, validation has been achieved only in specific clinical settings such as after cardiac surgery.[11]

Awareness for the presence of risk factors for AKI enables close monitoring and early diagnosis. The patient may also present with the typical signs and symptoms associated with severe AKI—oliguria, fluid overload, and electrolyte abnormalities such as hyperkalemia and uremia. Other complications of AKI should be looked for including hyponatremia, hypocalcemia, hyperphosphatemia, and metabolic acidosis.[12]

Evaluation for the Cause of Acute Kidney Injury

Once AKI is diagnosed, a systematic evaluation for the cause is important. A thorough history, examination, and basic investigations are usually adequate to identify whether there is a prerenal, intrinsic renal or obstructive cause.

History and Examination

Prerenal Acute Kidney Injury

History of volume loss, ask for history suggestive of volume loss as hemorrhage, gastrointestinal, or renal loss. History of diarrhea or multiple episodes vomiting, large volume bleeds (melena, hematemesis, and long bone fractures), burns, or high-grade fever may give clues as to the underlying cause of AKI.[1,12]

History of edema, excessive fatigability, and exercise intolerance could be clinical features of secondary nephrotic syndrome, congestive cardiac failure, and liver failure, respectively.

Look for signs of dehydration, tachycardia, prolonged capillary refill time (CFT), tachypnea, hypotension, and/or severe pallor. The evolution and pattern of edema may give clue to nephrotic syndrome. Signs of congestive heart failure (pulmonary edema, tachycardia, and gallop on auscultation) or liver failure (jaundice, ascites, and hepatosplenomegaly) may point to specific etiology of AKI.

Intrinsic Renal Acute Kidney Injury

The clinical presentation will give clue as to the compartment of the kidney involved. Physical examination followed by appropriate investigations most often helps to reach a diagnosis in intrinsic AKI.

Glomerular Diseases

History of edema, oliguria, and gross hematuria points to glomerular involvement. Presence of pyoderma scars, systemic symptoms such as rash, oral ulcers, joint pains, prolonged fever, and unexplained weight loss are other clues for the underlying cause.

Symptoms of hypertension such as headache, vomiting, seizures, and blurred vision may sometimes be present.

Pyoderma scars suggest post-streptococcal glomerulonephritis (GN). Pallor, maculopapular rash with arthritis, and serositis could be the pointer towards a diagnosis of lupus nephritis, IgA, or antineutrophil cytoplasmic antibody (ANCA) vasculitis.[11]

Tubulointerstitial Disease

Acute tubular necrosis is the most common cause of intrinsic AKI. History prolonged dehydration and/or hypotension indicate ischemic ATN. Evidence of sepsis in a critically ill child indicates sepsis-associated AKI (SAKI). Acute tubulointerstitial nephritis is often nonoliguric and there may be history of fever, drug intake [nonsteroidal anti-inflammatory agents (NSAIDs), angiotensin-converting enzyme (ACE) inhibitors, and antibiotics], bites, or stings. High-grade fever with pyuria in AKI suggests the possibility of acute pyelonephritis. High-grade fever may sometimes be the only symptom in infants while older children will present with classic flank pain. Symptoms of urinary tract infection (UTI) may also be present in older children. A history of dribbling or poor stream and episodes of UTI in the past increase the likelihood of pyelonephritis.

History of sudden onset or progressive pallor along with hypertension, gross hematuria, and/or pain abdomen with or without preceding diarrheal illness points to the possibility of hemolytic uremic syndrome (HUS). Recent history of dysentery could be a pointer for *Shigella*/*Escherichia coli*-associated HUS.[12]

Postrenal (Obstructive) Acute Kidney Injury

History of sudden onset anuria indicates an acute obstructive cause in a child with single functioning kidney or bilateral obstruction with ureteral stones in children with an underlying predisposition. Gross hematuria and flank pain radiating to the groin (ureteric colic) occur with obstructing stones.

History of a poor urinary stream, straining while micturition, and recurrent UTI indicates that urinary obstruction is chronic (posterior urethral valve or neurogenic bladder). History of poor growth or chronic anemia should be elicited as an AKI that occur in the setting of chronic kidney disease in common in obstructive uropathies.

Abdominal examination for a palpable bladder or palpable kidneys indicates an underlying obstructive pathology such as posterior urethral valves. Neurogenic bladder must be suspected if there are the genital abnormalities, abnormal anal tone, obvious spinal defects or overlying tuft of hair, lipoma, or sacral agenesis. Examination of the lower extremity tone and gait is also important.

TABLE 2: Urine biochemistry to differentiate between prerenal and intrinsic acute kidney injury (AKI).

Laboratory parameter	*Prerenal AKI*	*Intrinsic AKI*
Fractional excretion of sodium (FENa)*	<1%	>1%
Fractional excretion of urea (FEUr)**	<35%	>35%
Urine sodium level (mEq/L)	<20	>40
Urine/plasma creatinine ratio	>40	<20
Urine osmolality (mOsm/kg)	>500	<400

*FENa% = $100 \times (S_{Cr} \times U_{Na})/(S_{Na} \times U_{Cr})$
**FEUr% = $100 \times (SCr \times U_{Urea})/(Serum_{Urea} \times U_{Cr})$

Laboratory Evaluation

Basic evaluation including a complete hemogram and urinalysis can help elucidate cause and severity of AKI. Urine biochemistry may help in differentiating between prerenal AKI and ATN **(Table 2)**. The laboratory investigations in a child with AKI **(Box 1)** should be guided by the history and physical examination.[13]

Urine biochemistry values indicate the reabsorptive capacity of renal tubules. Hence, these values help in differentiating between prerenal and intrinsic AKI. In the presence of reduced renal perfusion, if the tubular function is intact, tubular sodium reabsorption will be 99%. Enhanced proximal tubular reabsorption of sodium and water occurs as a response to hypovolemia. Hence, FENa is <1%. Whereas in conditions like ATN, with tubular damage FENa is >1%.[14] However, clinical use of FENa has limitations. FENa may be higher with the use of diuretic therapy in oliguric patients. FENa may be low in intrinsic AKI—myoglobinuria with ATN, contrast nephropathy, obstructive nephropathy, and acute GN.[15]

Fractional excretion of urea (FEUr) has been used to differentiate between prerenal and intrinsic AKI, especially when diuretics are used.[16] During hypovolemic states, urea is increasingly reabsorbed from the medullary collecting duct leading to decrease in FEUr and increase in serum blood urea nitrogen (BUN)/creatinine ratio. In conditions with osmotic diuresis, like diabetes mellitus or mannitol use, the proximal tubular reabsorption of salt and water is impaired, leading to high FEUr, even in states of hypoperfusion. Urine osmolality, a marker for urinary concentrating ability, is reduced in conditions associated with tubular injury. A value >500 mOsm/kg indicates that tubular function is still intact.[14]

CONCLUSION

Critically ill children are at high risk of AKI. The etiology of AKI is multifactorial. Identification of specific etiology by history and clinical examination, supported by relevant investigations helps in appropriate management of children with AKI.

BOX 1: Laboratory investigations in AKI to assess etiology.

Prerenal AKI
- *CBC:* Severe anemia may indicate possible blood loss or hemolysis; increased hematocrit suggests volume contraction
- *Coagulation profile:* Deranged with disseminated intravascular coagulation
- *Serum albumin:* Low with nephrotic syndrome or liver disease/hepatorenal syndrome
- Blood urea/serum creatinine ratio >40

Intrinsic renal AKI
- *Urine*
  - *Urine dipstick:* Positive nitrites or leukocyte esterase reaction—UTI; specific gravity ≤ 1.01—ATN or interstitial nephritis; proteinuria—ATN/AGN/ATIN
  - *Urine microscopy:* Dysmorphic RBCs, RBC casts—glomerulonephritis
  - Granular casts—ATN
  - *Hemogram:* Presence of schistocytes—microangiopathic hemolytic anemia (MAHA) and thrombocytopenia—HUS
  - Autoimmune hemolytic anemia and thrombocytopenia—SLE
  - *Electrolytes:* Hyperkalemia
  - *Creatinine kinase:* Elevated in rhabdomyolysis
  - *Autoimmune workup:* Antinuclear antibody, antinuclear cytoplasmic antibody, and complement factor C3 and C4 for evaluation of glomerulonephritis
- *Imaging*
  - *Renal ultrasound:* Increased renal echogenicity—ATN; glomerulomegaly with altered corticomedullary differentiation—AGN; dilated pelvicalyceal system with or without bladder changes—obstruction; also helps to determine the anatomy/rule out congenital abnormalities
  - *Renal biopsy:* Indications for renal biopsy in AKI are:
    - Absence of an obvious cause
    - Extrarenal manifestations compatible with a systemic disease, e.g., SLE
    - AKI > 3 weeks duration or prolonged anuria
    - Rapidly progressive renal failure

Postrenal AKI
- *Renal ultrasound:* To diagnose obstruction; may show dilatation of the pelvicalyceal system with/without ureteric dilatation, distended thickened bladder, and calculi
- *Computed tomography (CT) abdomen without contrast:* To detect renal calculi
- *Voiding cystourethrogram:* Diagnosis of PUV and VUR

(ACEI: angiotensin converting enzyme inhibitors; AGN: acute glomerulonephritis; AKI: acute kidney injury; AIN: acute interstitial nephritis; ATIN: acute tubulointerstitial nephritis; ATN: acute tubular necrosis; CBC: complete blood count; CCF: congestive cardiac failure; CFT: capillary refill time; HUS: hemolytic uremic syndrome; NSAIDs: nonsteroidal anti-inflammatory agents; PUV: posterior urethral valves; RBCs: red blood cells; SLE: systemic lupus nephritis; UTI: urinary tract infection; VUR: vesicoureteral reflux)

KEY POINTS

- AKI occurs in almost one-third of critically ill children and is associated with significant morbidity and mortality.
- Diagnosis of AKI is based most commonly on KDIGO criteria, which depends on changes in SCr and urine output from baseline.
- Etiology of pediatric AKI, especially in the ICU setting is multifactorial including prerenal and intrinsic renal causes.
- A focused history and clinical examination along with key relevant investigations will help in the timely diagnosis and appropriate management of the child with AKI.

REFERENCES

1. Goldstein SL, Zappitelli M. Evaluation and management of acute kidney injury in children In: Avner E, Harmon W, Niaudet P, Yoshikawa N, Emma F, Goldstein SL (Eds). Pediatric Nephrology, 7th edition. Heidelberg: Springer; 2016. pp. 2139-60.
2. Fortenberry JD, Paden ML, Goldstein SL. Acute kidney injury in children an update on diagnosis and treatment. Pediatr Clin N Am. 2013;60:669-88.
3. Kaddourah A, Basu RK, Bagshaw SM, Goldstein SL. Epidemiology of acute kidney injury in critically ill children and young adults. N Engl J Med. 2017;376(1):11-20.
4. Bunchman TE. Treatment of acute kidney injury in children: from conservative management to renal replacement therapy. Nat Clin Pract Nephrol. 2008;4(9):510-4.
5. Xu X, Nie S, Zhang A, Jianhua M, Liu HP, Xia H, et al. A new criterion for pediatric AKI based on the reference change value of serum creatinine. J Am Soc Nephrol. 2018;29(9):2432-42.
6. Goldstein SL. The renal angina index to predict acute kidney injury. Kidney Int Rep. 2018;3(3):516-8.
7. Miller TR, Anderson RJ, Linas SL, Henrich WL, Berns AS, Gabow PA, et al. Urinary diagnostic indices in acute renal failure. A prospective study. Ann Intern Med. 1978;89(1):47-50.
8. Basile DP, Anderson MD, Sutton TA. Pathophysiology of acute kidney injury. Compr Physiol. 2012;2:1303-53.
9. McCaffrey J, Dhakal AK, Milford DV, Webb NJA, Lennon R. Recent developments in the detection and management of acute kidney injury. Arch Dis Child. 2017;102(1):91-6.
10. Goldstein SL. Urine output assessment in acute kidney injury: The cheapest and most impactful biomarker. Front Pediatr. 2020;7:565.
11. Cho MH. Pediatric acute kidney injury: focusing on diagnosis and management. Child Kidney Dis. 2020;24:19-26.
12. Andreoli SP. Acute kidney injury in children. Pediatr Nephrol. 2009;24;253-63.
13. Hamsa V, Pais P. Oliguria and acute kidney injury. In: Hamsa V (Ed). Differential Diagnosis in Pediatrics, 1st edition. New Delhi: Jaypee Brothers Medical Publishers; 2019. pp. 19-23.
14. Lima C, Macedo E. Urinary biochemistry in the diagnosis of acute kidney injury. Dis Markers. 2018;2018:1-7.
15. Pahwa AK, Sperati CJ. Urinary fractional excretion indices in the evaluation of acute kidney injury. J Hosp Med. 2016;11(1):77-80.
16. Schrier RW, Poole B, Mitra A, Schrier RW, Wang W, Poole B, et al. Acute renal failure: definitions, diagnosis, pathogenesis, and therapy. J Clin Invest. 2004;114(1):5-14.

CHAPTER

11.3

Acute Kidney Injury in Pediatric Intensive Care Unit

Sasidaran Kandaswamy, S Thangavelu

INTRODUCTION

Acute kidney injury (AKI) is a clinical syndrome rather than a single disease entity and this had been elucidated well in recent literature. Incidence of AKI in critically ill children ranges from 16 to 51% in various studies.[1,2]

"Acute kidney injury" and "fluid overload (FO)" are very closely related. They are well-documented attributable risk factors for prolonged intensive care unit (ICU) stay, mechanical ventilation, and mortality in critically ill children and adults.[3] These observations in last two decades fueled the interest and development of "critical care nephrology" as a separate subspecialty in intensive care.

It is very important to understand that kidney dysfunction in ICU is bidirectional, it may either be a transient state of "augmented renal clearance (ARC)" in a child or adult with hyperdynamic cardiovascular status or a "classic AKI" with spectrum of different stages based on the magnitude of reduction in renal clearance.[4] The growing knowledge base on AKI resulting from surge in recent research interest help us to understand the different disease phenotypes, pathobiology, overlapping causes, natural history, and long-term outcome better. Unlike other disease conditions in critical care, AKI research in pediatrics has always kept pace with the adult counterpart and many of the seminal works in pediatric AKI has favorably improved the way we assess, understand, and treat AKI in children as well in adults in ICUs.

Acute kidney injury in pediatric intensive care unit (PICU) predominantly remains multifactorial, where the inciting event may be a primary renal disease or an acute onset systemic disease process or an acute illness on a preexisting renal disease. The outcome will be influenced by the medications received, host response pattern, other organ status, preexisting illness state, and fluid therapy.[5] Despite better understanding of the disease process, kidney replacement therapy (KRT) by intermittent or continuous dialytic methods either blood or peritoneal based remain the primary modality of therapy as there are no evidence-based targeted medical therapy for AKI currently available in clinical practice. "KRT" is the recent standardized nomenclature for commonly known "kidney replacement therapy (KRT)" and we preferably used this in all further discussions to maintain uniformity.

UNDERSTANDING THE DISEASE TRAJECTORY IN ACUTE KIDNEY INJURY

Acute kidney injury was traditionally considered as an acute illness without a link to subacute or chronic consequence. Once we started understanding the link between AKI and chronic kidney disease (CKD),[6,7] interest in exploring the "possible pathways to reverse AKI" and "preventing the risk of CKD in future" had gained momentum. KRT being the only available modality of therapy, the research edges towards finding the "time zone of best response to KRT" and "AKI reversibility" in the natural course of disease trajectory in critically ill children.

DEFINITION AND CLASSIFICATION OF ACUTE KIDNEY INJURY

A uniform interpretation and classification of a specific disease/syndrome is the first step in evolution of evidence-based understanding of disease biology and natural history. AKI being a heterogeneous syndrome, consensus definition is a mandate to ensure uniformity in interpretation. Until 2004, unavailability of consensus definition allowed huge variance in study definition of AKI in adult as well in pediatric population. Development of RIFLE criteria was the first step towards standardization of definition which paved path for development of pediatric specific pRIFLE criteria and Acute Kidney Injury Network (AKIN) criteria.[6,7,9] The most recent and currently well-accepted AKI diagnosis and staging criteria was developed by Kidney Disease: Improving Global Outcomes (KDIGO) workgroup.[10]

The KDIGO 2012 uniformed nomenclature defines kidney dysfunction as AKI/acute kidney impairment (AKI), acute kidney disease (AKD), CKD, and no kidney disease (NKD) **(Table 1)**. Apart from this, AKI severity is further classified to three stages based on urine output (UO) and creatinine based criteria **(Table 2)**. Most important inclusion in the KDIGO guideline is the timeline-based definition which helps us to understand better about disease trajectory in the index child

TABLE 1: Definitions of AKI, AKD, NKD, and CKD.[8]

Stage	*Functional criteria*	*Structural criteria*
AKI	Increase in creatinine by 50% within 7 days *Or* Increase in serum creatinine by 0.3 mg/dL within 2 days *Or* Urine volume <0.5 mL/kg/hour for 6 hours	None
CKD	GFR < 60 mL/min/1.73m^2 for >3 months	Kidney damage >3 months
AKD	AKI *Or* GFR <60 mL/min/1.73m^2 for <3 months *Or* Decrease in GFR >35% or Increase in serum creatinine >50% for <3 months	Kidney damage <3 months
NKD	GFR >60 mL/min/1.73m^2 Stable serum creatinine	No damage

(AKD: acute kidney disease; AKI: acute kidney injury; CKD: chronic kidney disease; GFR: glomerular filtration rate; NKD: no kidney disease)

TABLE 2: AKI Severity Grading–KDIGO 2012.

Stages	*Serum creatinine*	*Urine output*
1	1.5 to 1.9 times increase from baseline creatinine *Or* >0.3 mg/dL increase in creatinine	<0.5 mL/kg/hour for 6–12 hours
2	2 to 2.9 times increase from baseline creatinine *Or*	<0.5 mL/kg/hour for >12 hours
3	More than three times baseline creatinine *Or* Creatinine >4.0 mg/dL *Or* Initiation of kidney replacement therapy *Or* In patients <18 years age: eCrCl < 35 mL/min/1.73 m^2	<0.3 mL/kg for > 24 hours *Or* Anuria for >12 hours

Creatinine changes should have occurred within 7 days time period
Cause of AKI should be identified in each patient whenever possible
(AKI: acute kidney injury; eCrC: estimated creatinine clearance; KDIGO: Kidney Disease: Improving Global Outcomes)

and used as a tool for repeated assessment of kidney function status during the course of hospital stay.

APPLYING ACUTE KIDNEY INJURY DEFINITION IN CRITICALLY ILL CHILDREN: MERITS AND LIMITATIONS

Serum Creatinine in Staging of Acute Kidney Injury

Despite being a time-tested functional biomarker in identification and severity stratification of children with AKI, serum creatinine-based AKI staging has many inherent limitations. One of the major limitations is that significant creatinine rise is noted only 24–48 hours after the inciting insult[11,12] and any change to be depicted in creatinine needs 50% reduction in glomerular filtration rate (GFR).[13] Another component that deserves special mention in the KDIGO guideline is "baseline creatinine", but unavailability of a "previously measured creatinine value within 180 days (3–6 months) of current admission—baseline creatinine" is a usual scenario. There are many methods proposed to derive at "best assumption of baseline creatinine". As all those methods have their own demerits, we are still comfortable in considering "assumed baseline creatinine clearance as 120 mL/min/1.73 m^2—normal baseline renal function" while staging AKI in children wherever baseline creatinine value is not available. We should remember to apply "age-specific creatinine normal values" while classifying AKI in critically ill children.

Urine Output in Staging of Acute Kidney Injury

Urine flow rate may not be the best scientific marker in staging the AKI as there is always a probability of over-rating in a shorter observation period; still it remains as an easily quantifiable bedside measure in critical care unit. Many small children may not have indwelling Foley catheter in ICU and the "void count" may not be reflecting the urine volume clearly. Recently published Assessment of Worldwide Acute Kidney Injury, Renal Angina and Epidemiology in Critically Ill Children (AWARE) study emphasizes the importance of UO monitoring based on the observation that "absence of UO monitoring may need to underestimation of AKI incidence to the score of 30%".[14] Hence, UO monitoring and UO-based AKI staging is important in PICU. While using body weight-based hourly UO to classify AKI, we are not sure whether to use actual body weight (ABW) or ideal body weight (IBW) in children, especially in children with overweight or obesity. It is prudent to note that using ABW may improve the sensitivity of UO as functional marker, but using IBW may improve the specificity by removing false positives due to transient oliguria.[15] In such circumstances, it is advisable to use serum creatinine and UO to make therapeutic decision rather going by either of the measurements.

It is not uncommon to have discrepancies in the AKI stage by creatinine and UO estimates. In such cases, it is advisable to score the severity on the higher side (either based on serum creatinine or UO) to stage the AKI and continue to assess frequently for better understanding of disease trajectory in index child.

ACUTE KIDNEY INJURY INCIDENCE IN CRITICALLY ILL CHILDREN

Acute kidney injury is not an uncommon associate in critically ill children and the incidence is around 27% in the AWARE study. Most high-quality data on AKI epidemiology document the incidence between 16 and 51%[16-18] though it varies based on countries and pattern of patient mix in pediatric ICUs. High-FO% is also observed to be more associated with AKI in critically ill children though "FO%—a cause of AKI or effect of AKI", still remain unresolved. In a global perspective, understanding etiology and incidence of AKI in low and lower middle income country (LMIC) gains importance as KRT services remain inaccessible to at least 10% of children who are in need of KRT in these countries.[19-21]

APPROACH TO ACUTE KIDNEY INJURY IN CRITICALLY ILL CHILDREN

Stepwise approach includes:

- AKI risk stratification
  - "Risk screening checklist" to identify those on high risk of developing AKI
  - Risk categorization based on renal angina index (RAI) (RAI score ≥ 8—increased risk)
  - Biomarkers (uNGAL and/or pNGAL)-based risk stratification in special groups
- Investigative approach in AKI evaluation—cause identification
- Classify AKI based on **Figure 1** (A, B, C, D, or any combination, e.g., A + B or A + C + D)
- AKI severity staging based on KDIGO AKI staging **(Table 2)**
- Pre-KRT AKI support therapy and "frusemide stress test (FST)" wherever indicated
- Initiation of appropriate KRT and other organ support therapy.

Acute Kidney Injury "Risk Screening Checklist" and Risk Stratification in Pediatric Intensive Care Unit

"Acute kidney injury" and "FO" were identified to be important risk factors influencing long-term and short-term outcome of critically ill children. This had been reflected in clinical research studies by association of AKI with longer duration of ICU stay, mechanical ventilation, and around 6% absolute increase in risk of mortality.[20] This resulted in interest towards identifying the "risk factors" for AKI and "ways to predict AKI in critically ill children". **Table 3** provides an explicit list of relevant risk factors for daily use in PICU, but it is important to understand that the list is neither a validated one for independent risk factors nor a standardized scoring system. Still, similar checklists are used in most of the PICUs to understand a signal towards higher risk in an index child.

Studies observed that "AKI risk" is higher and it is proportionate to the "disease severity" in critically ill children. RAI is one of the standardized scoring system helps in predicting AKI in homogenous PICU population.[22] There are studies suggesting that biomarkers (uNGAL and pNGAL) combined with RAI may improve the prediction of AKI in heterogeneous PICU population[23] though the practical utility of these biomarkers is very limited.

Whenever we are evaluating a critically ill child in PICU, grading the risk by screening for following risk factors along with RAI **(Table 4)** and biomarkers **(Table 5)** based on availability may help in early identification of AKI and initiation of therapy. Enlisting medications used in children admitted in PICU and identifying the nephrotoxic medications **(Table 6)** is equally important in AKI preventive care directive.

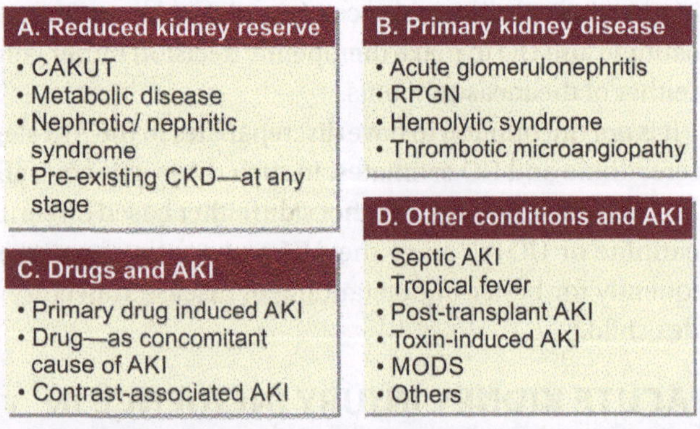

Fig. 1: Schematic diagram depicting therapy-directed AKI grouping in PICU. (AKI: acute kidney injury; CAKUT: congenital anomalies of kidney and urinary tract; CKD: chronic kidney disease; PICU: pediatric intensive care unit; RPGN: rapidly progressive glomerulonephritis; MODS: multiorgan dysfunction syndrome)

Investigative Approach in Acute Kidney Injury Evaluation (Table 7)

Etiology directed investigative workup is enlisted below. Investigative workup need to be individualized based on clinical presentation and the likelihood disease process. Some investigations such as pH, sodium, potassium, and serum creatinine level will be monitored frequently for the dynamic assessment of kidney function status.

TABLE 3: "Risk screening checklist" for assessing risk of acute kidney injury (AKI) in critically ill children.

Risk factor	*Response*
Age group <12 months	Yes/No
Sepsis/septic shock	Yes/No
Renal functional reserve	Likely normal/likely abnormal
>2 nephrotoxic medications (NTMx) exposure currently	Yes/No
>1 organ involvement	Yes/No
>1 vasoactive medication	Yes/No
Postoperative/trauma status	Yes/No
Burn injury/post-transplant	Yes/No
Possible volume depletion	Yes/No
Radiocontrast exposure <7 days	Yes/No
Obese/overweight	Yes/No

TABLE 4: Renal angina index.

Risk		Injury: Serum creatinine to baseline		Renal angina index
Intensive care unit admission	1	No change	1	Risk × Injury = 1–40 ≥8 = Positive
Stem cell/ solid-organ transplant	3	× 1–1.49 times increase	2	
Mechanical ventilation and/or inotrope use	5	× 1.5– 1.99 times increase	4	
		× ≥2 times increase	8	

TABLE 5: Renal biomarkers for identifying risk of acute kidney injury.

Biomarkers	Cut-off value
uNGAL on day 1 in children	>61.15 ng/mL
pNGAL on day 1 in children	>114.18 ng/mL

TABLE 6: Nephrotoxic medications (NTMx) causing acute kidney injury (AKI) in children.[24]

Acyclovir	Enalapril	Ioxilan	Polymyxin B
Amikacin	Enalaprilat	Ketorolac	Sirolimus
Amphotericin liposomal	Foscarnet	Lisinopril	Sulfasalazine
Amphotericin B	Ganciclovir	Lithium	Tacrolimus
Aspirin	Gentamicin	Losartan	Tenofovir
Captopril	Ibuprofen	Mesalamine	Ticarcillin–clavulanate
Carboplatin	Ifosfamide	Methotrexate	Tobramycin
Celecoxib	Indomethacin	Mitomycin	Topiramate
Cidofovir	Iodixanol	Nafcillin	Valacyclovir
Cisplatin	Iohexol	Naproxen	Valganciclovir
Cyclosporine	Iopamidol	Pamidronate	Valsartan
Colistimethate	Iopromide	Pentamidine	Vancomycin
Deferasirox	Ioversol	Piperacillin	Zoledronic acid
Diatrizoate meglumine	Ioxaglate meglumine	Piperacillin—tazobactum	Zonisamide
Diatrizoate sodium	Ioxaglate sodium		

*The given medication list is adopted from *NINJA* [*N*ephrotoxic *I*njury *N*egated by *J*ust in time *A*ction] study[24]
#Advisable to create unit specific list based on medications used in the specific hospital

Identification of Acute Kidney Injury Phenotypes for Therapeutic Decision Making

Acute kidney injury can be classified as primary or secondary based on etiology; prerenal, intrinsic renal, and postrenal based on mechanism of injury **(Table 8)**. Though this kind of classification would be providing better understanding of mechanism and pathophysiology, syndromic grouping may be of great help in approaching AKI in PICU. Unified approach to identify "syndromic categories" based on predisposition

TABLE 7: Laboratory evaluation of AKI.

Test	Value/inference	
Urine analysis	Prerenal	Intrinsic AKI
Specific gravity	>1.020	<1.010
Urine osmolality	>500 mOsm/kg	<350 mOsm/kg
FENa	<1%	>2%
FEUrea	<35%	>35%
BUN/Cr	>20	<20
Glycosuria	Tubular dysfunction/osmotic diuresis	
Red colored urine	RBC, myoglobin, free hemoglobin	
Proteinuria	Intrinsic AKI, nephrotic syndrome	
Eosinophils	Drug-induced acute interstitial nephritis (AIN)	
WBC, WBC cast	UTI, tubulointerstitial cause	
RBC, granular cast	Intrinsic AKI	
Blood		
Anemia	Dilutional, hemolytic—systemic lupus erythematosus (SLE), hemolytic uremic syndrome (HUS), renal vein thrombosis (RVT), malaria	
Leucopenia	SLE	
Thrombocytopenia	SLE, HUS, thrombotic microangiopathy (TMA), thrombocytopenia-associated multiple organ failure (TAMOF), RVT, disseminated intravascular coagulation	
Coagulopathy	HUS, snake bite	
Peripheral smear	Fragmented RBCs—HUS	
Biochemistry		
BUN, serum creatinine	Increased in AKI	
pH	Acidosis	
Serum K	>6.5—life threatening	
Hyponatremia	Dilutional, syndrome of inappropriate ADH secretion (SIADH)	
Hypocalcemia	Secondary to hyperphosphatemia	
Creatinine Kinase	Increased in tumor lysis syndrome (TLS)	
LFT	Abnormal in hepatorenal syndrome (HRS)	
Serology		
ANA	SLE	
Anti-GBM antibody	Goodpasture's disease	
ASO	Poststreptococcal or infective glomerulonephritis (PSGN) or (IRGN)	
C3 Complement	Low in SLE, PIGN, and MPGN	
Cultures	Relevant cultures to identify infectious etiology	
Radiology		
CXR	Cardiomegaly, pulmonary edema	
Ultrasound KUB	• Loss of corticomedullary differentiation, increased echogenicity, obstructive pathology, abscess, collection • Any structural issues related to upper or lower urinary tract	
CT/MRI	Renal size, structure, and vascularization	

(ADH: antidiuretic hormone; AKI: acute kidney injury; BUN: blood urea nitrogen; CXR: chest X-ray; KUB: kidney, ureter, and bladder; MPGN: membranoproliferative glomerulonephritis; PIGN: postinfectious glomerulonephritis; RBC: red blood cell; UTI: urinary tract infection; WBC: white blood cell)

TABLE 8: Conventional classification of acute kidney injury based on pathobiology.

Prerenal (hypoperfusion-related AKI)	*Renal (intrinsic renal injury)*	*Postrenal (obstructive AKI)*
Low intravascular volume • Hemorrhage • Severe dehydration • Third space loss • Sepsis • Capillary leak syndrome • Burns • Hypoalbuminemia *Decreased effective circulatory volume* • Primary cardiac dysfunction • Septic shock • Cardiac tamponade • Raised intra-abdominal pressure	*Glomerular* • Glomerulonephritis *Vascular* • Hemolytic uremic syndrome • Bilateral renal artery thrombosis • Renovascular injury • Malignant hypertension • Disseminated intravascular coagulation *Interstitial* • Acute interstitial nephritis • Pyelonephritis *Tubular* • Hypoxic/ischemic injury • Toxic injury – Endogenous toxins – Rhabdomyolysis – Tumor lysis syndrome • Exogenous toxins – Metals, venoms, mushrooms	• *Urethral obstruction* – Posterior urethral valve • *Obstruction at kidney and/or urinary tract* – Structural or stone disease • *Extrinsic obstruction by mass lesion/stones* • *Neurogenic bladder* • *Trauma*

status, current disease process, and drug exposure **(Fig. 1)** may help us to approach the pediatric AKI in critically ill children systematically and devise the methods of management better.

It is important to understand that delineation of a single specific cause for AKI in critically ill children may not be possible and denote an oversimplified approach. Hence, it is prudent to consider the possibility of more than one factor contributing to AKI and it would help in multipronged approach in managing such children.

Pre-Kidney Replacement Therapy and Acute Kidney Injury Support Therapy

Pre-KRT therapy optimization converges on multiple steps of preventive approach in AKI management. In view of poor access to KRT in LMIC countries, cautious application of preventive strategies plays an important role in improving AKI outcome in critically ill children.

Preventive step approach in AKI management includes the following:

- Effective circulatory volume and preload optimization
- Vasoactive medications to maintain mean arterial pressure (MAP) and renal perfusion pressure
- Correct hemoglobin to optimize oxygen carrying capacity
- Monitor and maintain electrolyte homeostasis
- Remove all nonessential/avoidable nephrotoxic medications
- Appropriate therapeutic drug dose modification and drug level monitoring
- Consider context specific interventions based on the primary disease
- Monitor and avoid FO (target FO% < 2%)
- Frusemide stress test only when indicated.

Preload Optimization in Critically Ill Children

Circulatory stabilization in critically ill children revolves around intravenous fluid therapy. In a critically ill child, total intravenous fluid is decided based on resuscitation fluid, maintenance fluid, and need for ongoing loss replacement.[25] In a child with circulatory shock, fluid resuscitation is targeted towards optimizing the preload status of the child and improving the stroke volume. As we know fluid responsiveness in a critically ill child is dependent on many other factors, such as fluid tolerability, cardiac functional status, ongoing capillary leak, and possibility of sustained fluid response, we need to be cautious while administering fluid for resuscitation.

In current intensive care practice, the focus is towards optimizing preload status of the child without compromising other organ functions status. In a child presenting with hypovolemic shock with prerenal AKI, circulatory optimization being the most important step in treating AKI, maintaining a delicate balance to avoid FO and pulmonary edema is equally important.

Vasoactive Medications and Maintaining Renal Perfusion Pressure

Wherever required, appropriate vasoactive medications need to be initiated on timely manner to achieve circulatory stabilization. Vasoactive (epinephrine/norepinephrine) initiation in fluid refractory shock is a standard practice to reach shock resolution targets. In the last decade, more emphasize is given in timely or early initiation of vasoactive medications avoiding multiple doses of fluid boluses in shock resuscitation.[26] As we know well, longer duration suboptimal MAP during resuscitation may reflect worse on the magnitude of organ injury.

Correcting Hemoglobin to Ensure Oxygen Carrying Capacity

Over years, transfusion thresholds have been defined better in pediatric critical care practice. Growing knowledge in transfusion medicine guides us towards "restrictive blood component therapy" and "indication-based blood component prescription". In an unstable critically ill child, trigger to transfuse packed red blood cell (PRBC) is kept at 9 g/dL with a target to maintain 10 g/dL; in case of stable critically ill children, the trigger is fixed at 7 g/dL to strictly follow restrictive strategy to avoid transfusion-related deleterious effects in critically ill children.[27] Though the number of organs involved or severity of kidney injury may not guide the trigger level to transfuse, in progressive AKI or in evolving multiorgan dysfunction syndrome (MODS) the "unstable critically ill child" trigger threshold are followed in decision making.

Monitor and Maintain Electrolyte Homeostasis

A child with AKI needs to be monitored for associated dyselectrolytemia (dysnatremia, hypo- or hyperkalemia, hypocalcemia, hypo- or hypermagnesemia, and acidosis) and be addressed adequately. Understanding the risk of "large quantity of isotonic saline in resuscitation and its effect on predisposing critically ill children and adults to hyperchloremic metabolic acidosis"[28,29] have led to increased use of "balanced crystalloids" in critical care setting. Current evidence suggests cautious administration of isotonic saline while using in large volumes and repeated bolus for shock resuscitation, at the same time does not mandate the complete transition from isotonic saline to balanced salt solutions in ICU. Dysnatremia in a child with established oliguric or anuric AKI may not be amenable to "fluid modification therapy" alone hence early initiation of KRT may need to be decided when and where needed.

Remove all Nonessential/Avoidable Nephrotoxins

Avoiding all nephrotoxic medications though desirable, not practically feasible in ICU environment. Hence, vigilant monitoring of treatment chart on daily basis by a designated person and therapeutic drug monitoring, dose modifications wherever needed would be the best possible approach in preventing nephrotoxic medications-induced AKI in critically ill children. The Nephrotoxic Injury Negated by Just in time Action (NINJA) project has provided some guidelines and principles which can be easily followed and we can avoid the occurrence of this subset of iatrogenic and avoidable AKI.

Basic steps to prevent nephrotoxic medication (NTMx)-induced AKI:

- Use appropriate diluents in indicated proportions when administering medications
- Check drug-drug interactions/additive side effects when prescribing polypharmacy
- Endorse the role of clinical pharmacist in PICU and daily pharmacist rounds
- Preoperative renal risk assessment before all complex surgeries in children
- Use NTMx medication list while screening for drug-induced AKI
- Try to avoid aminoglycosides when drug level monitoring is not available
- Try to avoid vancomycin if drug level monitoring is not feasible.

Context-specific Interventions based on Primary Cause of Acute Kidney Injury

Sepsis and AKI: Renal involvement in sepsis is multifactorial. Hypoperfusion may be the initiating factor and will further get complicated based on the infective organism, host immune response, duration of organ ischemia, circulatory shock, organ-organ cross talk, and secondary insult due to vasopressors.

Sepsis-associated AKI (SA-AKI) is defined as AKI along with sepsis, or the coexistence of sepsis and KDIGO AKI criteria. Common organisms causing septicemia are gram-positive organisms such as *Staphylococcus and Enterococcus* and gram-negative organisms such as *Klebsiella* and *Pseudomonas* and *Meningococcus.*

Decreased renal blood flow and tubular epithelial cell death leading to acute tubular necrosis (ATN) is the traditional hypothesis for SAKI. The latest pathophysiology theory of SA-AKI is unified theory, i.e., a triad of microvascular dysfunction, inflammation and immune-mediated oxidative stress, and adaptive response of tubules.[30]

- *Microvascular dysfunction:* At structural level due to sepsis there is endothelial dysfunction and altered glycocalyx. The altered relation between the endothelium and circulating cells results in activation of coagulation system resulting in formation of microthrombi. There is cessation of microvascular flow that results in intrarenal shunting affecting the GFR.

Inflammation and oxidative stress: Sepsis-related changes result in formation of microvesicles with endothelial cells, leukocytes, and coagulation factors. The microvascular dysfunction affects the S1 vertical portion of the proximal tubule. The pathogen-associated molecular patterns (PAMPs) and damage-associated molecular patterns (DAMPs) filtered through glomerular filtration barrier activates the toll-like receptor (TLR) 3 and 4. Cessation of the microvascular flow along with TLR activation results in release of tumor necrosis factor-alpha (TNF-α) which damages S2 and S3 segments of proximal tubule. Metabolic reprogramming mediated by mitochondria is also an important aspect in the pathophysiology.[31] High index of suspicion and early detection of AKI is very important for better management. Biomarkers such as tissue inhibitor of metalloproteinase (TIMP) and insulin-like growth factor binding protein 7 (IGFBP7) are particularly useful in SA-AKI.

Adaptive response of tubules: The tubular epithelium undergoes various stages of structural changes with initiation phase where brush border is affected, extension phase wherein the ischemic changes worsen with flattening of epithelium. These two phases are the adaptive and reversible changes of AKI. In longstanding AKI maintenance phase, there is dedifferentiation of the epithelium with sloughing of the cells; following which cells go into readaptation phase.[30]

Gut in SAKI: The gut dysbiosis is also an important pathophysiology of SA-AKI. Hypoperfusion, antibiotics, and uremia-related factors result in alteration of gut microbiota. This results in release of PAMPs, DAMPs that further perpetuates SA-AKI.

The key factor in management of AKI in systemic sepsis is making an early diagnosis and administration of appropriate antibiotics. Adequate fluid resuscitation and prompt use of inotropes are critical. Supportive care including careful use of nephrotoxic antibiotics is warranted. The modality of KRT depends on the available expertise, infrastructure, and patient-specific factors. Besides KRT and supportive therapy, targeted anti-infective therapy, source control, and other organ function optimization are of importance in salvaging kidney function in SA-AKI. The Acute Dialysis Quality Initiative (ADQI) highlights the importance for grading the recovery after AKI and the need for nephrology follow-up which is extremely important in the context of monitoring long-term outcomes.[7]

Fungal infections in PICU: Fungal infections of kidney and urinary tract are usually seen in patients who are immunosuppressed, with prolonged indwelling catheters, and in those with obstructive urologic abnormalities. The overall incidence of fungal infections in critically ill children is 5% and mortality of 50–60%.[32]

Candida and *Aspergillus* are common cause of invasive fungal infection in PICU. Invasive infections with *Candida* are five times more common than invasive infection with *Aspergillus*. Although fungal infections are seen in critically ill children, it is more common in neonatal age group. *Candida albicans* causes urinary tract infection (UTI) as a part of systemic candidiasis in immunocompromised patients. Children present with features of systemic sepsis which is characterized by hepatosplenomegaly, hyper- or hypoglycemia erythematous rash, and thrombocytopenia. The suspicion of diagnosis may arise by the presence of yeasts in the urine. *Candida* can affect literally any compartment of urinary tract ranging from glomeruli, tubules to urinary bladder. Microabscesses and fungal balls can be formed inside the renal parenchyma and fungal balls can cause obstruction in the urinary tract. Presence of indwelling catheters (which act as a focus for persistent infection) should be removed.[33] Invasive *Aspergillus* infection can also cause involve any organ commonly lungs followed by central nervous system. Fluconazole is the drug of choice in *Candida albicans* infections and non-albicans infections and *Aspergillus* usually need amphotericin B. Voriconazole and echinocandins are other options of treatment. In the presence of significant obstruction, percutaneous nephrostomy is also needed along with systemic antifungal therapy.[34]

Acute kidney injury after cardiopulmonary bypass: AKI after cardiopulmonary bypass (CPB) is predominantly caused by hemodynamic changes and unfavorable renal perfusion status due to nonpulsatile flow of CPB. Further, systemic inflammatory response syndrome (SIRS) is triggered by surgical trauma, contact with CPB surface and free hemoglobin. CPB-related rheological injury can be minimized by modified ultrafiltration methods. In case of anticipated postoperative AKI, peroperative insertion of peritoneal dialysis (PD) catheter or vascular catheter and early initiation of KRT may be of help.

Acute kidney injury in stem cell transplant: AKI in stem cell transplant (SCT) is usually a culmination of multiple risk factors such as prior reduced kidney reserve, chemotherapy, myeloablative medications used for conditioning, large volume of fluids and diluents used in therapy, sinusoidal obstruction syndrome, sepsis, and other nephrotoxic medications. Preventive approach may be more ideal in these circumstances, treating the primary cause of AKI by antibiotics or immunomodulatory medications may need to be decided simultaneously.

Hemolytic uremic syndrome and thrombotic microangiopathies: Targeted therapy towards the primary disease—steroids, immunoglobulin, and plasma exchange in combination with KRT may be needed based on primary etiology and disease trajectory assessment. Thrombotic microangiopathy and thrombocytopenia-associated multiorgan failure in children share common clinical features with hemolytic uremic syndrome (HUS) and most of the time targeted therapeutic pathway also need to be aligned similar to HUS. Detailed discussion on HUS is beyond the scope of this chapter and it is discussed elsewhere.

Pigment nephropathy: AKI induced by hemoglobinuria and/or myoglobinuria are classified as pigmenturia-associated nephropathy. This may be due to myriad of causes such as drug induced, traumatic muscle injury, hyperpyrexia, vascular occlusion, intravascular hemolysis, primary muscle disease, carbon monoxide poisoning, and prolonged seizure. Apart from early initiation of KRT, therapy targeting to stop the initiating process of hemoglobinuria or myoglobinuria becomes very important in successful renal recovery.

Hepatorenal syndrome (HRS): HRS is initiated by stress factors such as gastrointestinal (GI) bleed, sepsis, paracentesis, or surgical procedure in a patient with preexisting liver disease. Reduction in GFR occurs as a result of intense vasoconstriction. Usually systemic vascular resistance is low and intravascular volume is increased. Drug therapy for hepatorenal syndrome (HRS) to be initiated once it is confirmed.

Monitor and Manage Fluid Overload

Accurate measurement of fluid balance requires strict hourly intake-output monitoring in PICU. This need to include All ins and All outs as most of the parenteral fluid received in critically child may be in the form of obligatory fluids used in drug dilutions, vasoactive infusions, electrolyte corrections, or blood components. In this context, a standardized measurement and monitoring tool FO% had been introduced critical care monitoring and as a tool for fluid optimization. FO% = All Ins in L – All Outs in L expressed in percentage.

A FO% > 2% should be considered as signal to redial our fluid prescription and a progressive unavoidable FO% creeping >10% on any day of hospital stay in a critically ill child may indicate the need for KRT.[35]

Frusemide Stress Test

Frusemide stress test has limited role in critical care practice. Significant changes had happened in the practice of FST in an oligoanuric AKI over last two decades in children as well in adults.[36] Though the individualistic usage may be justifiable in few critically ill children with AKI, most circumstances it only allow us to buy time in preparing the KRT initiation.

We learnt over time that (1) FST response assessment is a "continuous process", a transient response need to be differentiated from sustained response, (2) administration of FST and response assessment will be based on "primary disease" in the index child and "anticipated disease trajectory", (3) frusemide is not intended to increase the kidney function rather it achieves only increase in UO, (4) FST can be attempted only in those with hyper/euvolemic by clinical assessment and serum albumin level >2 g/dL.

All the above mentioned principles need to be kept in mind while administering FST in a child admitted with AKI in PICU. UO response is assessed after 1 mg/kg frusemide bolus dose or 0.4 mg/kg frusemide bolus followed by 0.1–0.4 mg/kg/h infusion of 6–8 hours. Slow response pattern is possible with infusive dose hence the assessment period also proportionately prolonged to 6–8 hours instead of 2 hours in bolus frusemide administration. Though UO > 1 mL/kg/h is traditionally considered as response to FST, decision of avoiding KRT would rather be based on FO%, nature of AKI, amount of fluids/blood products to be given in next 12 hours, etc.

KIDNEY REPLACEMENT THERAPY IN PEDIATRIC INTENSIVE CARE UNIT

Indications for Kidney Replacement Therapy in Acute Kidney Injury

- Hyperkalemia—K > 6.5 mEq/L or rapidly rising or refractory to medical management
- Metabolic acidosis—pH < 7.15
- Symptomatic uremia
- Urine output <0.3 mL/kg/h for 24 hours or anuria > 12 hours
- Pulmonary edema not responding to diuretics defined by all of the following:
  - 10% fluid accumulation (FO% > 10%)
  - Urine output <0.5 mL/kg/h for 12 hours
  - Severely impaired oxygenation (P/F < 200)

Timing of Kidney Replacement Therapy Initiation in Pediatric Acute Kidney Injury

Peritoneal or blood based KRT is the only organ-directed treatment method available in the absence of a curative intent drug in clinical practice. Timely initiation of KRT believed to be improving the possibility of renal recovery in critically ill children. Identifying the appropriate timeline to initiate KRT remained controversial. Adult KRT studies intended to identify the efficacy of early versus late or conventional versus accelerated initiation of KRT failed to prove any therapeutic benefit in early or accelerated initiation. Despite creating clinical practice guidelines based on borrowed evidence from adult literature may not be appropriate, especially in AKI as the comorbid conditions and associated CKD status are very different in pediatric population. "Accelerated or conventional KRT initiation timeline" in pediatric AKI is currently predominantly based on the primary disease trajectory rather than kidney disease status alone. There is no proven superiority of blood-based dialysis over PD, hence either modality is chosen based on availability, expertise, unit comfort, size of the child, coagulation need, vascular cannulation skills, dose of dialysis needed, hemodynamic status of the child, etc.

Prescription and monitoring method for PD, hemodialysis, and continuous kidney replacement therapy (CKRT) are very much relevant to current critical care practice as the initiation, titration, and monitoring are decided and executed by critical care specialist. We are not discussing these in detail as these are dealt in dedicated topic on KRT for AKI.

ACUTE KIDNEY INJURY IN PEDIATRIC INTENSIVE CARE UNIT—OUTCOME AND PROGNOSIS

Recovery from functional AKI may be dramatic but not in the case of established AKI. Recovery from intrinsic or established AKI may pass through phases of high UO, poor tubular function, and poor urinary concentration. It is increasingly recognized that any developing AKI in PICU, especially those requiring KRT may need a long-term follow-up even if the creatinine values normalized at the time of discharge. Normal creatinine level in these children does not exclude partial recovery of AKI hence long-term follow-up becoming important. Long-term follow-up can be established by initiating prospective registry for those who developed significant AKI in PICU and particularly received KRT.

CONCLUSION

Acute kidney injury is a clinical syndrome rather than a single disease entity, where the clinical expression ranges from ARC to reduced or negligible renal clearance. The crucial part of AKI management is early diagnosis, preventive approach rather than upfront dialytic support in all children, at the same time it is equally important to decide on right time of starting kidney replacement support therapy to achieve best outcome. When children with AKI recover, they may transition to native kidney normal/near-normal function status or dialysis dependent state and long-term follow-up is important in either of the group.

KEY POINTS

- Monitoring renal function and FO% in PICU helps in early identification of AKI.
- Special effort to identify high-risk for AKI children may help improving outcome.
- Maintaining adequate effective circulatory volume is important to maintain renal perfusion.
- All fluid bolus administration to be preceded by test to predict preload responsiveness and followed by assessment of response.
- Overzealous fluid therapy leads to FO and worse AKI outcome.
- Avoid nephrotoxic medications to preserve functional kidney status in PICU children. Enlisting commonly used NTMx list as checklist has proven to reduce iatrogenic AKI.
- Dose modification of medications excreted by kidney and therapeutic drug monitoring of specific medications are helpful in preserving kidney function in critically ill.
- Time sensitive initiation of KRT based on disease trajectory is the best possible approach.
- When KRT is needed, decide either peritoneal or blood based dialysis based on the availability and expertise of the treating team.

REFERENCES

1. Selewski DT, Cornell TT, Heung M, Troost JP, Ehrmann BJ, Lombel RM, et al. Validation of the KDIGO acute kidney injury criteria in a pediatric critical care population. Intensive Care Med. 2014;40(10):1481-8.
2. Sutherland SM, Byrnes JJ, Kothari M, Longhurst CA, Dutta S, Garcia P, et al. AKI in hospitalized children: comparing the pRIFLE, AKIN, and KDIGO definitions. Clin J Am Soc Nephrol. 2015;10(4):554-61.
3. Sanchez-Pinto LN, Goldstein SL, Schneider JB, Khemani RG. Association between progression and improvement of acute kidney injury and mortality in critically Ill children. Pediatr Crit Care Med. 2015;16:703-10.
4. Heggan TVD, Dhont E, Peperstraete H, Delanghe JR, Walle JV, Paepe PD, et al. Augmented renal clearance: a common condition in critically ill children Pediatr Nephrol. 2019;34(6):1099-106.
5. Alobaidi R, Morgan C, Goldstein SL, Bagshaw S. Population-Based Epidemiology and Outcomes of Acute Kidney Injury in Critically Ill Children. Pediatr Crit Care Med. 2020;21(1):82-91.
6. Sigurjonsdottir VK, Chaturvedi S, Mammen C, Sutherland SM. Paediatric acute kidney injury and subsequent risk of CKD—is there a harm? Pediatr Nephrol. 2018;33(11):2047-55.
7. Chawla LS, Bellomo R, Bihorac A, Goldstein SL, Siew ED, Bagshaw SM, et al, Acute kidney disease and renal recovery: consensus report of the Acute Disease Quality Initiative (ADQI) 16 Workgroup. Nat Rev Nephrol. 2017;13(4):241-57.
8. Barry R, James MT. Guidelines for Classification of Acute Kidney Diseases and Disorders. Nephron. 2015;131:221-6.
9. Thomas ME, Blaine C, Dawney A, Devonald MAJ. The definition of acute kidney injury and its use in practice. Kidney Int. 2015;87(1):62-73.
10. Palevsky PM, Liu KD, Brophy PD, Chawla LS, Parikh CR, Thakar CV, et al. KDOQI US commentary on the 2012 KDIGO clinical practice guideline for acute kidney injury. Am J Kidney Dis. 2013;61(5):649-72.
11. Ostermann M, Bellomo R, Burdmann EA, Doi K, Endre ZH, Goldstein SL, et al. Controversies in acute kidney injury: conclusions from a Kidney Disease: Improving Global Outcomes (KDIGO) Conference. Kidney Int. 2020;98(2):294-309.
12. Moledina DG, Parikh CR. Phenotyping of acute kidney injury: Beyond serum creatinine. Semin Nephrol. 2018;38(1):3-11.
13. Malhotra R, Siew ED. Biomarkers for the early detection and prognosis of acute kidney injury. Clin J Am Soc Nephrol. 2017;12(1):149-73.
14. Kaddourah A, Basu RK, Bagshaw SM, Goldstein SL, AWARE Investigators. Epidemiology of Acute Kidney Injury in Critically Ill Children and Young Adults. N Engl J Med. 2017;376(1):11-20.
15. Thongprayoon C, Cheungpasitporn W, Akhoundi A, Ahmed AH, Kashani KB. Actual versus ideal body weight for acute kidney injury diagnosis and classification in critically ill patients. BMC Nephrol. 2014;15:176.
16. Ricci Z, Romagnoli S. Acute Kidney Injury: Diagnosis and Classification in Adults and Children. Contrib Nephrol. 2018;193:1-12.
17. Schneider J, Khemani R, Grushkin C, Bart R. Serum creatinine as stratified in the RIFLE score for acute kidney injury is associated with mortality and length of stay for children in the pediatric intensive care unit. Crit Care Med. 2010;38:933-9.
18. Alkandari O, Eddington KA, Hyder A, Gauvin F, Ducruet T, Gottesman R, et al. Acute kidney injury is an independent risk factor for pediatric intensive care unit mortality, longer length of stay and prolonged mechanical ventilation in critically ill children: A two-center retrospective cohort study. Crit Care. 2011;15:R146.
19. Soler YA, Nieves-Plaza M, Prieto M, García-De Jesús R, Suárez-Rivera M. Pediatric risk, injury, failure, loss, end-stage renal disease score identifies acute kidney injury and predicts mortality in critically ill children: A prospective study. Pediatr Crit Care Med. 2013;14:e189-95.
20. Mehta P, Sinha A, Sami A, Hari P, Kalaivani M, Gulati A, et al. Incidence of acute kidney injury in hospitalized children. Indian Pediatr. 2012;49:537-42.
21. Basu RK, Kaddourah A, Goldstein SL, AWARE Study Investigators. Assessment of a renal angina index for prediction of severe acute kidney injury in critically ill children: a multicentre, multinational, prospective observational study. Lancet Child Adolesc Health. 2018;2(2):112-20.
22. Abbasi A, Rabori PM, Farajollahi R, Ali KM, Ataei N, Yousefifard M, et al. Discriminatory Precision of Renal Angina Index in

Predicting Acute Kidney Injury in Children; a Systematic review and meta-analysis. Arch Acad Emerg Med. 2020;8(1):e39.
23. McGalliard RJ, McWilliam SJ, Magune S, Jones CA, Jennings RJ, Siner S, et al. Identifying critically ill children at high risk of acute kidney injury and renal replacement therapy. PLoS One. 2020;15(10):e0240360.
24. Uber AM, Rath MEM, Kwiatkowski DM, Krawczeski CD, Sutherland SM. Nephrotoxin exposure and acute kidney injury in critically ill children undergoing congenital cardiac surgery. Pediatr Nephrol. 2018;33(11):2193-9.
25. Langer T, Limuti R, Tommsino C, Regenmortel NV, Duval E, Caironi P, et al. Intravenous fluid therapy for hospitalized and critically ill children: rationale, available drugs and possible side effects. Anaesthesiol Intensive Ther. 2018;50(1):49-58.
26. Ismail J, Jayashree M. Advances in the Management of Pediatric Septic Shock: Old Questions, New Answers. Indian Pediatr. 2018;55(4):319-25.
27. Istaphanous GK, Wheeler DS, Lisco SJ, Shander A. Red blood cell transfusion in critically ill children: a narrative review. Pediatr Crit Care Med. 2011;12(2):174-83.
28. Brown RM, Wang L, Coston TD, Krishnan N, Casey JD, Wanderer JP, et al. Balanced Crystalloids versus Saline in Sepsis. A Secondary Analysis of the SMART Clinical Trial. Am J Respir Crit Care Med. 2019;200(12):1487-95.
29. Santi M, Lava SAG, Camozzi P, Giannini O, Milani GP, Simonetti GD, et al. The great fluid debate: saline or so-called "balanced" salt solutions? Ital J Pediatr. 2015;41:47.
30. Poston JT, Koyner JL. Sepsis associated acute kidney injury. BMJ. 2019;364:k4891.
31. Peerapornratana S, Manrique-Caballero CL, Gómez H, Kellum JA. Acute kidney injury from sepsis: current concepts, epidemiology, pathophysiology, prevention and treatment. Kidney Int. 2019;96(5):1083-99.
32. Brissaud O, Guichoux J, Harambat J, Tandonnet O, Zaoutis T. Invasive fungal disease in PICU: epidemiology and risk factors. Ann Intensive care. 2012;2:6.
33. Fisher JF, Sobel JD, Kauffman CA, Newman CA. Candida Urinary Tract Infections—Treatment. Clin Infect Dis. 2011;52(suppl_6): S457-66.
34. Joyce CL, Salvatore CM, Killinger JS. Diagnosis and Management of Fungal Infections in Pediatric Intensive Care Unit. Switzerland: Springer Nature Switzerland AG; 2019. pp. 257-67.
35. Alobaidi R, Morgan C, Basu RK, Stenson E, Featherstone R, Majumdar SR, et al. Association Between Fluid Balance and Outcomes in Critically Ill Children: A Systematic Review and Meta-analysis. JAMA Pediatr. 2018;172(3):257-68.
36. Chawla LS, Davison DL, Mitchell EB, Koyner JL, Arthur JM, Shaw AD, et al. Development and standardization of a furosemide stress test to predict the severity of acute kidney injury. Crit Care. 2013;17(5):R207.

CHAPTER

11.4

Conservative Management of Acute Kidney Injury

Richa Prakash, Alpana Ohri

INTRODUCTION

Acute kidney injury (AKI) is defined as an abrupt deterioration in the kidney function resulting in sudden rapid decline of glomerular filtration rate (GFR), accumulation of waste products such as blood urea nitrogen and creatinine, and dysregulation of the homeostasis of fluid and electrolytes.[1] The term acute renal failure (ARF), a former nomenclature, was replaced as it did not recognize renal dysfunction as a continuum of events and overemphasized failure as a discrete event.

The estimated incidence of AKI in children varies from 2 to 20 per million in children. Acute kidney injury constitutes about 1–5% of admissions in the hospitalized children, with incidence even up to 8% in the intensive care units.[2] The two large-scale multinational studies—AWARE [in the pediatric intensive care unit (PICU)] and AWAKEN [in the neonatal intensive care unit (NICU)]—detected an incidence of 26.9% and 29.9%, respectively.[3,4] In critically ill patients on mechanical life support or postcardiac surgery patients, the incidence is as high as 50–60%. Thus, the incidence of AKI depends on the degree of illness, population under study, and the definitions adopted for diagnosis [Kidney Disease: Improving Global Outcomes (KDIGO), Acute Kidney Injury Network (AKIN), pROCK, or cROCK] and the vigor of surveillance, i.e., the frequency of sampling.[5-9] Etiology of AKI has taken a dramatic turn in the last three decades, especially in the developed nations. In most, epidemiology has shifted from community-acquired to hospital-acquired [particularly the intensive care units (ICUs)]. Currently, most cases of AKI occur in ICUs and have multifactorial etiology with varying overlay of hypoxemic–ischemic injury with toxic nephropathy and sepsis. AKIs caused by primary renal diseases such as hemolytic–uremic syndrome (HUS) and immune-mediated kidney diseases contribute only to 7–10% of the hospitalized cases. But these causes merit specific attention as they may benefit from specific pharmacotherapies over and above the supportive therapy (which is the medical management possible in most cases of hospital-acquired AKI). **Table 1** depicts a summary of specific therapies for different conditions causing primary renal AKI.

MANAGEMENT OF ACUTE KIDNEY INJURY

Prevention of Acute Kidney Injury

The saying "Prevention is better than cure" holds great merit in the setting of AKI as most cases do not have specific therapy. Anticipation and close monitoring of serum creatinine as well as the urine output suffice an early diagnosis and hence timely intervention for reversing early AKI.

The most important strategy for prevention is risk stratification. AKI has been recognized now as an ongoing dynamic process with continuous developments and using an objective scoring system to stratify children at high risk. These high risk patients benefit from more vigorous monitoring and supportive care.

Risk Stratification and Early Diagnosis

Renal angina index (RAI) is a scoring system derived by multiplication of the *risk strata* (based on the need for intensive care as well as the treatment vigor required, which is determined by the clinical condition) and the *clinical injury score* [based on the creatinine values and the amount of fluid overload (FO)]. In the injury scores, either the decrease in creatinine clearance or the percentage fluid excess in the body, whichever is higher, is used.[10-12] It is a useful tool to identify and suspect the population at risk of developing AKI as illustrated in **Figure 1**.

FO is defined as the percent fluid excess (i.e., intake ? output) from the time of admission (i.e., based on the weight at admission).

$$\text{Percent fluid overload} = \frac{[(\text{Fluid input in liters}) - (\text{Fluid output in liters})]}{\text{Admission weight (kg)}} \times 100$$

Renal angina index is thus derived value computed by multiplication of these risk and injury scores. This value is calculated *on day 1* of PICU admission and predicts the risk of subsequent development of angina, i.e., severe stages of AKI (stages 2 and 3), in ensuing 3 days. Its negative predictive value is proposed to be 92–99%. The score values vary from *1 to 40*. Most studies postulate a composite score of 8 or more to indicate a state of renal angina. Few recent studies show that a score of >12 or >20 is more suggestive of AKI than conventional ≥8, in predicting any AKI on day 3 or a severe AKI on day 7, respectively.

TABLE 1: Summary of specific pharmacotherapies for different primary renal diseases.

Primary renal conditions	***Specific therapies***
HUS: Deficiency of complement regulators Acquired dysfunction of complement regulators (e.g., factor H antibody)	• Plasma infusions, anticomplement therapy • Plasma exchanges • *Immunosuppressives*: – Methylprednisolone/dexamethasone/prednisolone – Cyclophosphamide, MMF • Intravenous immunoglobulins • *Monoclonal antibodies*: Rituximab
Glomerulonephritis: Presenting as RPGN	• *Immunosuppressives*: – Methylprednisolone/dexamethasone/prednisolone – Cyclophosphamide, MMF • Plasma exchanges • Intravenous immunoglobulins • *Monoclonal antibodies*: Rituximab
Presenting as a chronic GN	• Immunosuppression with steroids, cyclophosphamide, MMF, and CNIs
Presenting as a CKD	• Immunosuppressives withdrawn. CKD management
Interstitial nephritis: Acute	• Oral steroids with/without MMF
Chronic	• Immunosuppressives withdrawn
Systemic vasculitis:	• As in RPGN

(CKD: chronic kidney disease; CNI: calcineurin inhibitor; HUS: hemolytic–uremic syndrome; GN: glomerulonephritis; MMF: mycophenolate mofetil; RPGN: rapidly progressive glomerulonephritis)

Renal angina index (1–40) = Risk score × Clinical injury score

Risk score

Patient type		
Sepsis or ICU admission	Moderate	1
Diabetes or SCT	High	3
Ventilation or Ionotropy	Very high	5

×

Clinical injury score

Decrease in eCrCl%	FO	
No change	≤ 5	1
0–24.9%	5–9.9	3
25–50%	10–14.9	5
≥ 50%	≥ 15	8

Fig. 1: Renal angina index. (ICU: intensive care unit; SCT: stem cell transplant)

Instituting Strategies for Prevention of Acute Kidney Injury

The pathway to prevent AKI can be achieved by multiple options—some have proved efficacy, some are awaiting further validation, and others are experimental as depicted in **Table 2**.

Hydration: In cases of suspected renal damage due to hemoglobinuria, myoglobinuria, tumor lysis syndrome, renal transplantation, and exposure to radiocontrast dye as well as nephrotoxic drugs and major surgical procedures, vigorous fluid administration has helped to prevent AKI. Studies in adults have shown significant reduction in occurrence of postoperative AKI by preoperative hydration with goal to optimize the fluid level.[13]

Fluid resuscitation: Timely and appropriate intravenous fluid therapy with normal saline improves the urine output (10–20 mL/kg over 30 minutes and repeated twice if necessary). If volume response does not occur, preservation of blood pressure and renal perfusion with inotropes will be of benefit.[14]

TABLE 2: Strategies for prevention of acute kidney injury.

Proven significance	***Speculative significance (needing validation)***
• Hydration • Fluid resuscitation • Avoiding nephrotoxins	• Fenoldopam • Loop diuretics • Theophylline • Dopamine (renal dose) • Rasburicase • N-acetyl cysteine • Natriuretic peptides • Mannitol

Nephrotoxin exposure: The nephrotoxic exposure has a direct dose and duration-dependent effect on the incidence of AKI. The nephrotoxic drugs are best avoided. But in situations when they are required as a life-saving measure, dosage should be modified in accordance with the creatinine clearance [estimated glomerular filtration rate (eGFR)]. A few recent studies initiated for detecting and avoiding nephrotoxic AKI by monitoring serial creatinine both in noncritically ill children and in NICU babies called NINJA (nephrotoxic injury negated by just in time action) and baby NINJA, respectively, have shown very promising results. The policy of medical stewardship reduced the risk of nephrotoxic medication (NTMx) exposure rate by 38–42% and incidence of nephrotoxin-associated AKI by 64–72%.[15-17] This was subsequently implemented across multiple centers in the states for reducing exposure to NTMx and associated AKI (NTMx-AKI) rates.[18]

Fenoldopam: It is a selective DA1 receptor agonist, reducing the systemic vascular resistance with increase in the renal blood flow. Adult studies have shown proven benefit in mortality, prevention, and treatment of AKI and reduced need for dialysis.[19] Only a single pediatric study has shown benefit by reducing the neutrophil gelatinase-associated lipocalin (NGAL) at the end of surgery and at 12 hours after ICU admission.[20]

Rasburicase: It is a recombinant urate oxidase, an enzyme that breaks down uric acid into more soluble allantoin. Accumulation of uric acid causes intratubular crystal deposition, which in turn causes renal vasoconstriction, endothelial damage, and oxidative stress via inhibition of nitric oxide synthase. Hobbs et al. and few other have reported definite benefit of using even a single dose of rasburicase in case of hyperuricemia in children and even neonates.[21-25]

Theophylline: It is a nonselective adenosine antagonist, which is known to have renoprotective effect in case of asphyxiated term neonates as well as preterm when given in a single dose of 5.5 mg/kg within the 1st hour of life, followed by 1.3 mg/kg every 12 hours.[26-29] Aminophylline has also shown similar beneficial effects with increase in the urine output and decrease in serum creatinine. But in case of hypothermic infants, dosing needs further trials due to altered pharmacodynamics with poor clearance.[30,31]

Loop diuretics: Furosemide is postulated to decrease injury by reducing energy consumption at a tubular level, by reducing active NaCl transport in the thick ascending limb of Henle's loop (TALH). Once the AKI sets in, furosemide challenge dose can help to predict progression to more severe stages and also convert an oliguric into a nonoliguric AKI. However, it has no prophylactic role for prevention of AKI.[32]

Natriuretic peptides: Small studies in children with cardiac failure have been done where nesiritide [brain natriuretic peptide (BNP)] has shown some benefit by improving the urine output and decreasing the serum creatinine.[33]

Dopamine: "Low-dose" dopamine (0.5–3 mg/kg/min) has renal vasodilatory and natriuretic effect but has not shown any beneficial effect in prevention of AKI. Instead, there are risks associated such as arrhythmia, myocardial ischemia, and intestinal ischemia.[34]

N-acetyl cysteine: Adult studies have shown benefit of using NAC as a prophylactic agent, especially after cardiac surgery and contrast nephropathy.[9,35] But the results for the pediatric age group are inconclusive.

Mannitol: It helps in increasing diuresis and also acts as a free radical scavenger. Hence, it can help by reducing the intratubular cast formation and free radical injury. But this action has not shown positive results in the clinical studies and on the contrary caused side effects including hyperosmolarity leading to hypervolemia and pulmonary edema. There are no recommendations for its use to prevent AKI.[32]

CONSERVATIVE MANAGEMENT OF ESTABLISHED ACUTE KIDNEY INJURY

Acute kidney injury due to primary renal diseases is amenable to specific therapy. Established AKI due to other causes requires only supportive treatment, which includes conservative management and timely kidney replacement. The conservative management includes removal of the inciting agent, optimizing the renal perfusion, correcting the fluid, acid–base and electrolyte imbalance along with providing appropriate nutrition, and monitoring the nephrotoxic load. But at any stage, deterioration of the kidney function and declining volume status involve readiness to administer any of the kidney replacement modality. Steps in the conservative management of AKI are given in **Table 3.**

Removal of the Inciting Agent or Correcting the Underlying Cause

Often children with intrinsic renal diseases, such as nephrotic syndrome, receiving certain offending agents such as calcineurin inhibitors or a combination with angiotensin converting enzyme, when challenged by a hypovolemic insult or a febrile illness, tend to develop AKI. Temporary cessation during such periods leads to prevention or rapid reversal of the insult.

TABLE 3: Steps in conservative management of acute kidney injury.

Fluid resuscitation	• Restore the end-organ perfusion • Goal to achieve CVP and PWP and adequate cardiac output
Maintenance of fluid balance	• Assess all the fluids needed on ongoing basis • Assess patients' output (urine, stool, and drains) • Assessment of heart rate, blood pressure, capillary refill, and skin turgor—key components of volume status
Fluid removal	• Fluid removal should be done fast enough to help in weaning but not fast enough to cause any ischemic insult

(CVP: central venous pressure; PWP: pulmonary wedge pressure)

Fluid Administration and Maintaining Renal Perfusion

Intravenous fluid resuscitation is the mainstay and first line of treatment for hypovolemia and hypotension. Fluid therapy in any hospitalized patient must be used judiciously, correcting hypovolemia and simultaneously being cautious of a net positive balance. Crystalloids have been preferred over the colloids for most conditions. The semisynthetic colloids are no longer recommended and have been detrimental for the kidney function with accumulation of colloid's low molecular fraction in proximal tubules and osmotic nephrosis.

Among crystalloids, balanced fluids are preferred rather than the chloride-rich fluids like 0.9% normal saline. This is to prevent the risk of developing hyperchloremic acidosis, due to overzealous correction, which may lead to coagulopathy and hyperkalemia. Balanced fluids contain metabolizable anions, which are incorporated to substitute bicarbonate. The sepsis campaign advocated initial fluid resuscitation (up to 30 mL/kg) within the first 6 hours of presentation. But after the initial resuscitation, persistent net positive fluid balance is not advised as the interstitial fluid overload and cumulative positive fluid balance have multiple adverse effects.[36]

Type of Fluid

Chloride-restrictive fluid when compared to normal saline has better prognosis, lower hospital mortality, and decreased incidence of AKI, with lesser alteration of cortical blood flow and oxygen delivery. The superphysiological high-chloride content in 0.9% saline activates the tubuloglomerular feedback and causes afferent arteriolar vasoconstriction. The venous congestion which occurs due to sudden fluid excess along with afferent arteriolar constriction causes further damage.[37,38]

Albumin infusions are useful in cases of hypovolemia in presence of hepatic failure, cirrhosis, or nephrotic syndrome. But they need to be used with overt caution because when used to recruit back the interstitial fluids, they may damage the endothelial barrier and leak into the interstitium. This may cause further increase in the interstitial oncotic pressure resulting in worsening edema and diminishing oxygen supply in kidneys.[39]

Kidneys are sensitive to both hypovolemia and fluid excess. Insufficient arterial blood flow or venous congestion can rapidly impair renal clearance. Venous congestion causes engorgement, known as intrarenal fluid retention, due to intracapsular pressure, reducing both venous and lymphatic outflow as well as arterial blood inflow. This leads to renal injury with ischemia and impaired oxygenation. On the contrary, conservative fluid administration and inotropes have led to reduced chance for development of AKI.[40]

Rate of Fluid Administration

Rapid infusion of fluid can lead to sudden atrial distension and release of atrial natriuretic peptide (ANP), which rapidly degrade the glycocalyx endothelial surface layer, compromising the barrier. Subsequently, the fluids enter the interstitial compartment, leading to increased intrarenal pressure and further increase the chance of developing microthrombosis, and hence sustained kidney dysfunction. Hence, fluid given slowly over an hour, instead of boluses, is recommended unless patients are in shock.

Vasopressors

Vasopressors are recommended in patients who fail to develop adequate urine output, i.e., inadequate renal perfusion despite the fluid resuscitation. This helps to improve kidney perfusion in adequately hydrated patients. Vasopressin and norepinephrine are the two preferred ones with favorable side effect profiles. The latter also has additional antidiuretic effect.[41] "Low-dose norepinephrine", also widely known as the "renal-dose norepinephrine", was proposed to improve renal and splanchnic blood flow and hence improve the urine output. It is used to provide benefit in avoiding/delaying kidney replacement procedures and is still used for neonates.[42] But both adult and pediatric ICUs have largely abandoned its use as systematic reviews failed to show any benefit.[43,44]

Diuretic Challenge

Diuretic challenge with a furosemide dosage (1–1.5 mg/kg IV) can be tried if establishment of intravascular volume, fails to produce urine. A single high-dose furosemide may help to convert the oliguric renal failure to a nonoliguric one but does not have an impact on the survival and renal recovery rate of patients with established ARF.[45] However, a better fluid balance may be of critical importance in certain subgroup of patients. These are patients with AKI with concomitant lung injury who are on mechanical ventilation by improving lung ventilation.[46]

Failure to produce adequate diuresis serves as a prognostic marker of higher grades of AKI and should strongly discourage its further use. Escape trial showed 3 times higher risk of death in patients with cardiorenal syndrome with insufficient response to diuretics.[47,48]

Though diuretics are useful in preventing fluid overload and help in resolution of positive fluid balance, its use must not be a reason to avoid or delay kidney replacement therapy (KRT) in indicated cases. It has not shown to avoid further AKI or has shown to improve patient outcomes. In a setting of >10% fluid overload, a KRT must be planned and in case of FO > 20%, one must definitely initiate KRT.[49,50]

Correcting the Electrolyte Abnormalities

Hyperkalemia, hyponatremia, hyperphosphatemia, and hypocalcemia are the commonly seen abnormalities in the setting of AKI. Medical management is the first line for these abnormalities, failing which KRT must be promptly initiated. Medical management of electrolyte dysfunction is given in **Table 4**.

All children must be maintained on a potassium and phosphorus-low or free diet, depending on symptoms and electrolyte levels, especially if not on KRT. Sodium restriction helps to prevent hypertension and fluid overload. If with

TABLE 4: Management of electrolyte dysfunction.

Electrolyte abnormality	*Treatment strategy*	*Time to action*	*Mode of action*
Hyperkalemia	Glucose (0.5 g/kg) and insulin (0.1 U/kg) over 30 minutes	30–120 minutes	Intracellular shift of potassium ions
	Sodium bicarbonate 1 mEq/kg IV over 10–30 minutes	15–30 minutes	Counteracts the intracellular acidosis
	Calcium gluconate 10%, 0.5–1 mL/kg IV over 5–15 minutes	Immediate	Stabilizes the cardiac membrane
	Albuterol—400 μg by nebulizer	30 minutes	Intracellular shift of potassium ions
	Sodium polystyrene sulfonate—1 g/kg orally	2–24 hours	Exchanges Na^+ for K^+ across the colonic mucosa
Hyponatremia	If hypovolemic, isotonic fluid replacement If fluid overloaded, fluid restriction and fluid removal with KRT For Na < 120 mEq/L, slow hypertonic saline infusion + free water restriction	NA	
Hyperphosphatemia	Dietary phosphate restriction *Phosphate binders:* Calcium-containing or noncalcium containing		

(KRT: kidney replacement therapy)

these restrictions nutrition is being compromised, parental nutrition must be started and kidney replacement initiated.

Acid–base Disturbances

Metabolic acidosis occurs due to renal dysfunction and is exacerbated by the worsening systemic disease. Severe acidosis with pH < 7.1 mandates immediate treatment with IV sodium bicarbonate, carefully avoiding the fluid overload. Those with refractory metabolic acidosis may require dialysis. The point to note is to monitor the ionic and total calcium levels prior to initiation of bicarbonate, to avoid symptomatic hypocalcemia as more calcium binds the protein with increasing pH, thereby decreasing ionized calcium.

Nutrition

Acute kidney injury is a highly catabolic state requiring optimal nutrition with adequate calories, proteins, and nutrients. Nutrition should be provided by the enteral route and if not accepting well, or if enteral supplements are not providing optimal nutrition, the parenteral route must be employed.

Proteins

Protein–energy wasting is widely observed in the patients with AKI, being directly associated with longer hospital stay and more complications.[51] Hence, recent evidence is to increase protein intake to 1.5–2 g/kg/day, especially for those on KRT associated with amino acid loss.[52]

Calories and Lipid

Critically ill children should receive 1–1.3 times their basal metabolic needs. High amount of calories is needed to prevent endogenous catabolism and to simultaneously promote protein synthesis. This can again be administered enterally or in the form of central or peripheral venous nutrition.[52,53]

TABLE 5: Drug dose modification in acute kidney injury.[63]

Loading dose	• Needs to be given for drugs where the volume of distribution is increased, or • Drug has a long half-life, or • Rapid steady-state levels are needed (e.g., hydrophilic antibiotics, including β-lactams, cephalosporins, and carbapenems, require 25–50% greater loading doses) *Patient's loading dose = Usual loading dose × [(Patient's V_D)/(Normal V_D)]*
Maintenance dose	To attain a single steady-state concentration, with similar peak, trough and AUC, general consensus is on prolonging the dosing interval while maintaining the same dose. This is because certain drugs such as vancomycin, imipenem, and ceftizoxime have preservation of nonrenal clearance and there is tendency toward positive fluid balance

(AUC: area under the curve)

Micronutrients

Patients with AKI, especially those with critical illness, are deficient in many vitamins including vitamin C and water-soluble vitamins. KRT increases the amount of vitamins and trace element loss along with small solute removal. Hence, appropriate supplementation is mandatory in children with AKI.[54]

MODIFICATION OF DRUG DOSAGE

During renal dysfunction (either chronic or acute), there is an alteration in the fluid status with resultant increased volume of distribution of the drug. The renal and nonrenal clearance of the drug is also affected. So, appropriate modifications in drug dosing as needed must be done. Modification of commonly used drugs in kidney failure is given in **Table 5**.

SPECIFIC CONDITIONS: CONTRAST-ASSOCIATED ACUTE KIDNEY INJURY

Contrast-induced AKI (CI-AKI or contrast-associated AKI) is a specific form of AKI defined as increase in serum creatinine concentration within a few hours to days of exposure to intravascular iodinated contrast. AKI is generally transient (temporary rise in creatinine with a self-limited course), but it may be associated with increased short- and long-term morbidity or mortality.

The reported incidence is around 4–10% in children with previously normal renal function.[55,56] The risk of developing CI-AKI depends on certain patient factors [underlying chronic kidney disease, diabetes, poor cardiac function, and use of nonsteroidal anti-inflammatory drugs (NSAIDs)] and procedural factors such as use of hyperosmolar contrast, high volume of contrast, intra-arterial procedure, and multiple exposures.[57-61]

Prevention is the key to management. Isotonic intravenous fluid administration reduces the risk, especially in those at elevated risk with typical regimens consisting of a 1 mL/kg/h infusion 12 hours before and 12 hours after contrast exposure,[62] or 3 mL/kg/hour 1 hour before and 1.5 mL/kg/h for 4–6 hours postprocedure. There has been no added benefit of intravenous sodium bicarbonate or N-acetylcysteine in preventing or reducing the risk of AKI as compared to placebo. Even hemodialysis after administration of contrast is ineffective for preventing CI-AKI.

RECENT ADVANCES

Biomarkers

As the change in serum creatinine and urine output occur late in AKI, generally 72 hours, RAI was considered more sensitive for predicting severe renal injury within 24 hours of admission. But the PERSEVERE biomarker study showed that the consortium of biomarkers was even more sensitive, specific, and had higher positive predictive value to detect AKI, especially for SAKI.[64,65] A recent study found NGAL, tissue inhibitor of metalloprotease-2 (TIMP2), insulin-like growth factor-binding protein 7 (IGFBP7), uromodulin, tumor necrosis factor-α (TNF-α), and interleukin-8 (IL-8) to predict AKI and the adverse clinical outcomes.[66]

Translational research found that the novel urinary proteins detected in the urine allowed early identification of tissue injury, even before the functions impaired and the treatment began. **Table 6** depicts the more commonly used biomarkers and their characteristics along with their time of appearance.[67]

However, the challenge with these biomarkers remains Food and Drug Administration (FDA) approval, their cost, and their availability. Studies on biomarkers have been heterogeneous with variable study settings, interobserver bias with markedly different results and also the concentrations of these biomarkers differ throughout childhood and also if concentration in reference to serum creatinine is used.

Cystatin C was found to be a predictor of AKI in critically ill patients and in patients with contrast-induced AKI. Its urinary levels predict AKI 1–2 days prior to rise in creatinine. The levels are not affected by age, gender, and muscle mass. The measurements are available as an automated standardized immunonephelometric assay. Though measurements are roughly five times more expensive than testing serum creatinine, it is considered a much better analyte.[68-70]

pRock

It is a new creatinine-based equation to predict AKI (better than consensus definitions of KDIGO and pRIFLE) recently proposed by a Chinese author.[6] It is based on a large multicentric epidemiologic study, which used experimentally derived reference curves of creatine to predict baseline Cr in hospitalized patients. AKI was defined as an absolute increase in SCr ≥20 *μmol/L and a relative increase of*≥30% at the same time within 7 days. Stages 2 and 3 AKI are defined as for *stage 2 serum creatinine increase >40 μmol/L or >60% and for stage 3*

TABLE 6: Biomarkers in diagnosis and prognosis of acute kidney injury.

Biomarker	*Source*	*Function*	*Biospecimen*	*Time of appearance*
NGAL	Proximal and distal tubules	Marker of renal parenchymal injury[74]	Urine	2–4 hours
KIM-1	Proximal tubules	Marker of tubular injury	Urine/blood	12–24 hours
IL-18	Proximal tubules	Marker of tubular injury	Urine	6–24 hours
IL-8[75,76]	Inflammatory cells	Marker of cell inflammation	Blood Urine	2–12 hours 12–24 hours
TNF-α[77]	Podocytes, PT, TAL, and CD	Markers of cell inflammation	Blood	6–24 hours
TIMP-2 × IGFBP7[78]	G-1 cell cycle arrest biomarkers	Markers of cell cycle arrest	Urine	12–24 hours
L-FABP	Proximal tubules	Marker of tubular injury	Urine	6 hours
Uromodulin[79]	TAL	Marker of tubular injury and loss of nephron mass	Urine	12–24 hours

(IGFBP7: insulin-like growth factor-binding protein 7; IL: interleukin; KIM-1: kidney injury model-1; L-FABP: liver fatty acid-binding protein; NGAL: neutrophil gelatinase-associated lipocalin; TIMP2: tissue inhibitor of metalloprotease-2; TNF: tumor necrosis factor) *serum creatinine ≥80 µmol/L or ≥ 120%*, respectively. pROCK was shown to be a better predictor of mortality risk and adverse outcomes, especially in children needing intensive care. This criterion looks very promising but is yet to be validated by other studies and in other patient populations.[6]

Furosemide Stress Test

A systematic review and meta-analysis conducted in 2020 validated it as a novel tool to help to identify volume-replete patients with stage 1 or 2 AKI who are likely to progress to more severe stages.[71] Furosemide stress test (FST) is to be used only after adequate volume repletion and under strict vital and urine output monitoring. In the standard protocol, furosemide is used in a dose of 1–1.5 mg/kg (lower dose in diuretic-naive vs. those who were exposed to furosemide within 7 days) and diuretic response adjudged in the ensuing 2 hours. A cutoff of 200-mL urine output at 2 hours signifies a good response and suggests less likelihood of progression to higher stages of AKI or need for kidney replacement therapy (KRT). It has been further suggested that diagnostic efficacy can be further enhanced by use of biomarkers.[72,73]

- *Cardiorenal and pulmonary renal cross-talk*: Mortality due to well-known complications of severe AKI such as fluid overload, hyperkalemia, severe acidosis, and hypocalcemia are well recognized. What was realized much later is that AKI is a proinflammatory state that has a direct negative effect on heart and lungs via upsurge of profibrotic and apoptotic factors. This partly explains the negative impact of AKI on mortality. This "uremic memory" enables one episode of AKI to leave an imprint on remote organs putting patients at risk for long-term morbidity and mortality not limited to kidneys.[80-82]
- *Concept of acute kidney disease*: AKI is a dynamic condition with a variable course ranging from a transient self-limited course to a persistent AKI. The implications of AKI which get reversed within 48 or 72 hours are markedly different from persistent AKI or AKD [now defined by Acute Disease Quality Initiative (ADQI)].[83] **Figure 2** shows the spectrum of AKI and **Table 7** defines the conditions associated with possible implications. The AKD period possibly represents the critical time window where therapeutic interventions might be initiated to alter the natural history of kidney disease.
- *Recognition of AKD-CKD nexus*: AKI and CKD are closely linked and likely promote one another. Underlying CKD is now recognized as a clear risk factor for AKI and AKI accelerates the progression of CKD. This association between AKI and CKD is amplified by pre-existing CKD, stage of AKI, and cumulative number of AKI episodes. Long-term follow-up studies have shown a 4.5–9-fold risk (in newborns and adults, respectively) of CKD in patients developing AKI. KDIGO guidelines currently recommend a 3-month postdischarge follow-up of patients who develop AKI. A layered approach of follow-up has been suggested where the intensity of surveillance is proportionate to the risk of future outcomes. Further concept of AKI clinics has been proposed for better management of graduates of AKD.[84-86]

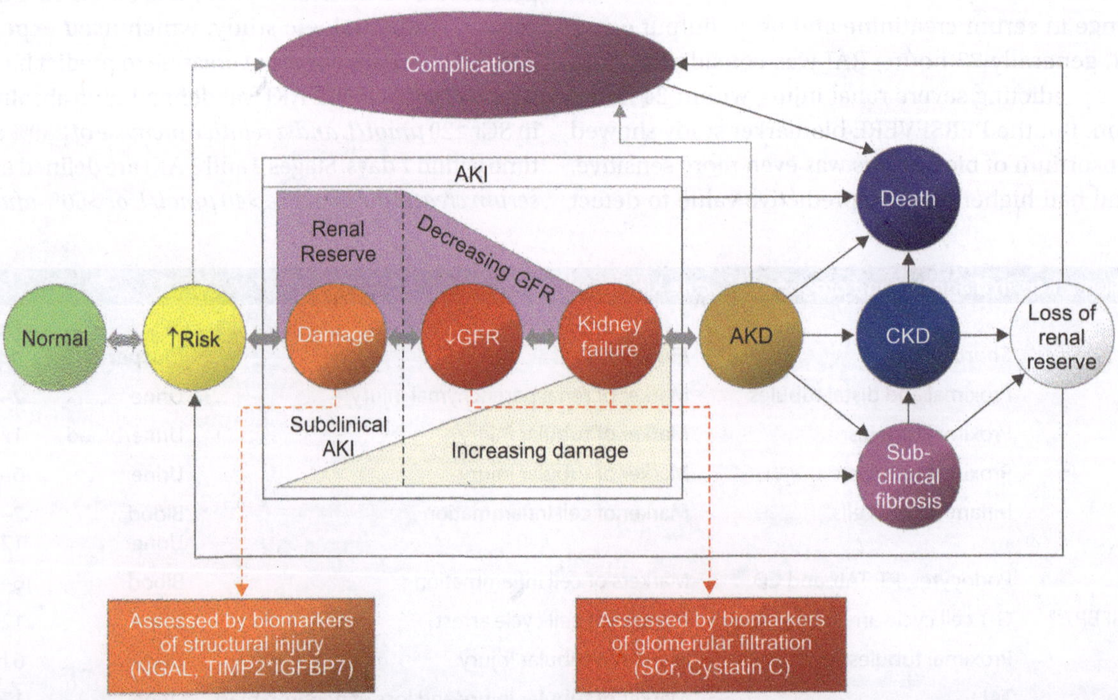

Fig. 2: Spectrum of acute kidney injury (AKI), acute kidney disease (AKD), and chronic kidney disease (CKD). (GFR: glomerular filtration rate; IGFBP7: insulin-like growth factor-binding protein 7; NGAL: neutrophil gelatinase-associated lipocalin; SCr: serum creatinine; TIMP2: tissue inhibitor of metalloprotease-2)

TABLE 7: Definitions relating to AKI.

Suspected AKI	All patients at high risk of developing AKI—premature, low birth weight, asphyxia, NICU and PICU graduates, underlying CKD, sepsis, nephrotoxic drug exposure, those undergoing surgery—cardiopulmonary bypass, stem cell transplant, etc.
Confirmed AKI	Abrupt decrease in kidney function over 7 days or less
Persistent AKI	Continuance of AKI by creatinine or urine output criteria beyond 48 hours of onset
Reversal of AKI	Recovery from AKI within 48 hours of the initiating event
AKD	Acute kidney disease is defined as a condition where AKI stage 1 or greater exists for ≥7 days after exposure and up to 90 days after exposure to an AKI initiating event
CKD	AKD persisting beyond 3 months or >90 days

(AKI: acute kidney injury; AKD: acute kidney disease; CKD: chronic kidney disease; NICU: neonatal intensive care unit; PICU: pediatric intensive care unit)

CONCLUSION

In conclusion, early recognition of AKI and/or AKI risk factors and thorough clinical assessment of fluid and volume status for adequate and prompt resuscitation with saline, removal of nephrotoxins, and optimization of nutrition remain the cornerstone for preventing and managing AKI.

KEY POINTS

- AKI in children is multifactorial, and preventive strategies should be instituted in all clinical settings.
- Timely management of hypovolemia with fluid resuscitation followed by maintenance of optimum hydration, providing inotropic support as needed, and avoidance of NTMxs helps to prevent AKI in children at high risk, especially in an ICU setting.
- Early diagnosis is possible with application of risk stratification strategies which are validated like renal angina index, especially in the critical care setting.
- In established AKI, the decision to continue with conservative management with KRT is based on the clinical setting, severity, and the etiology of AKI.
- Conservative management aims at maintaining internal milieu in a stable state till renal recovery avoiding fluid overload, electrolyte imbalance, acid-base imbalance, and uremic complications till renal recovery.
- Volume status is to be assessed daily and the fluid management should be optimized to maintain euvolemia as fluid overload is an independent risk factor for mortality, irrespective of severity of illness, especially in critically ill children.
- Maintaining electrolyte balance in AKI is important. Salt intake should be restricted to 2–3 mEq/kg/day to prevent sodium and fluid retention with resultant hypertension.
- Avoid intake of potassium or phosphorus in oligoanuric AKI unless there is significant hypokalemia or hypophosphatemia. Replacement therapy should be guided by close monitoring of plasma and urinary electrolytes.
- As AKI is associated with marked catabolism, aggressive nutritional management is needed to enhance the renal recovery. Maintaining adequate nutrition includes providing normal maintenance requirements and supplemental calories for ongoing catabolism.
- Dosage adjustment of drugs, especially antibiotics that are cleared by the kidney, should be done and drug levels should be monitored whenever feasible. NTMxs should be avoided.
- AKI-CKD transition may be a continuum bridged by AKD, and hence long-term follow-up is mandatory in all AKI survivors.

REFERENCES

1. Fragasso T, Ricci Z, Goldstein SL. Pediatric acute kidney injury. Contrib Nephrol. 2018;193:113-26.
2. Prowle JR. Acute kidney injury: an intensivist's perspective. Pediatr Nephrol. 2014;29(1):13-21.
3. Jetton JG, Boohaker LJ, Sethi SK, Wazir S, Rohatgi S, Soranno DE, et al. Incidence and outcomes of neonatal acute kidney injury (AWAKEN): a multicentre, multinational, observational cohort study. Lancet Child Adolesc Heal. 2017;1(3):184-94.
4. Kaddourah A, Basu RK, Bagshaw SM, Goldstein SL. Epidemiology of acute kidney injury in critically ill children and young adults. N Engl J Med. 2017;376(1):11-20.
5. Xu X, Wang L, Xiong M, Nie S, Liu Z, Feng Y, et al. New criterion to evaluate acute-on-chronic kidney injury based on the creatinine reference change. Am J Nephrol. 2020;51(6):453-62.
6. Xu X, Nie S, Zhang A, Jianhua M, Liu HP, Xia H, et al. A new criterion for pediatric AKI based on the reference change value of serum creatinine. J Am Soc Nephrol. 2018;29(9):2432-42.
7. Mehta RL, Kellum JA, Shah SV, Molitoris BA, Ronco C, Warnock DG, et al. Acute kidney injury network: Report of an initiative to improve outcomes in acute kidney injury. Crit Care. 2007; 11(2):R31.
8. Akcan-Arikan A, Zappitelli M, Loftis LL, Washburn KK, Jefferson LS, Goldstein SL. Modified RIFLE criteria in critically ill children with acute kidney injury. Kidney Int. 2007;71(10):1028-35.
9. Khwaja A. KDIGO clinical practice guidelines for acute kidney injury. Nephron Clin Pract. 2012;120(4):c179-184.
10. Basu RK, Kaddourah A, Terrell T, Mottes T, Arnold P, Jacobs J, et al. Assessment of worldwide acute kidney injury, renal angina and epidemiology in critically ill children (AWARE): study protocol for a prospective observational study. BMC Nephrol. 2015;16:24.
11. Basu RK, Zappitelli M, Brunner L, Wang Y, Wong HR, Chawla LS, et al. Derivation and validation of the renal angina index to improve the prediction of acute kidney injury in critically ill children. Kidney Int. 2014;85(3):659-67.
12. Basu RK, Kaddourah A, Goldstein SL, Akcan-Arikan A, Arnold M, Cruz C, et al. Assessment of a renal angina index for prediction of severe acute kidney injury in critically ill children:

a multicentre, multinational, prospective observational study. Lancet Child Adolesc Heal. 2018;2(2):112-20.
13. Brienza N, Giglio MT, Marucci M, Fiore T. Does perioperative hemodynamic optimization protect renal function in surgical patients? A meta-analytic study. Crit Care Med. 2009;37(6):2079-90.
14. Brierley J, Carcillo JA, Choong K, Cornell T, Decaen A, Deymann A, et al. Clinical practice parameters for hemodynamic support of pediatric and neonatal septic shock: 2007 update from the American College of Critical Care Medicine. Crit Care Med. 2009;37(2):666-88.
15. Goldstein SL, Mottes T, Simpson K, Barclay C, Muething S, Haslam DB, et al. A sustained quality improvement program reduces nephrotoxic medication-associated acute kidney injury. Kidney Int. 2016;90(1):212-21.
16. Goldstein SL, Kirkendall E, Nguyen H, Schaffzin JK, Bucuvalas J, Bracke T, et al. Electronic health record identification of nephrotoxin exposure and associated acute kidney injury. Pediatrics. 2013;132(3):e756-67.
17. Stoops C, Stone S, Evans E, Dill L, Henderson T, Griffin R, et al. Baby NINJA (Nephrotoxic Injury Negated by Just-in-Time Action): reduction in nephrotoxic medication-associated acute kidney injury in the neonatal intensive care unit HHS public access. J Pediatr. 2019;215:223-8.
18. Goldstein SL, Dahale D, Kirkendall ES, Mottes T, Kaplan H, Muething S, et al. A prospective multi-center quality improvement initiative (NINJA) indicates a reduction in nephrotoxic acute kidney injury in hospitalized children. Kidney Int. 2020;97(3):580-8.
19. Landoni G, Biondi-Zoccai GGL, Tumlin JA, Bove T, De Luca M, Calabrò MG, et al. Beneficial impact of fenoldopam in critically ill patients with or at risk for acute renal failure: a meta-analysis of randomized clinical trials. Am J Kidney Dis. 2007;49(1):56-68.
20. Ricci Z, Luciano R, Favia I, Garisto C, Muraca M, Morelli S, et al. High-dose fenoldopam reduces postoperative neutrophil gelatinase-associated lipocaline and cystatin C levels in pediatric cardiac surgery. Crit Care. 2011;15(3):R160.
21. Hobbs DJ, Steinke JM, Chung JY, Barletta GM, Bunchman TE. Rasburicase improves hyperuricemia in infants with acute kidney injury. Pediatr Nephrol. 2010;25(2):305-9.
22. Ghirardello S, Ardissino G, Mastrangelo A, Mosca F. Rasburicase in the treatment of hyperuricemia of newborns. Pediatr Nephrol. 2010;25(9):1775.
23. Acosta AA, Hogg RJ. Rasburicase for hyperuricemia in hemolytic uremic syndrome. Pediatr Nephrol. 2012;27(2):325-9.
24. Kennedy LD, Ajiboye VO. Rasburicase for the prevention and treatment of hyperuricemia in tumor lysis syndrome. J Oncol Pharm Pract. 2010;16(3):205-13.
25. Hooman N, Otukesh H. Single dose of rasburicase for treatment of hyperuricemia in acute kidney injury: a report of 3 cases. Iran J Kidney Dis. 2011;5(2):130-2.
26. Raina A, Pandita A, Harish R, Yachha M, Jamwal A. Treating perinatal asphyxia with theophylline at birth helps to reduce the severity of renal dysfunction in term neonates. Acta Paediatr. 2016;105(10):e448-51.
27. Jenik AG, Ceriani Cernadas JM, Gorenstein A, Ramirez JA, Vain N, Armadans M, et al. A randomized, double-blind, placebo-controlled trial of the effects of prophylactic theophylline on renal function in term neonates with perinatal asphyxia. Pediatrics. 2000;105(4):E45.
28. Bhat MA, Shah ZA, Makhdoomi MS, Mufti MH. Theophylline for renal function in term neonates with perinatal asphyxia: a randomized, placebo-controlled trial. J Pediatr. 2006;149(2):180-4.
29. Shafie MMA, Abdul-Shafy MS, Youssef DM. Role of theophylline on renal dysfunction of asphyxiated neonates. Ann Clin Lab Res. 2018;6(3):245.
30. Frymoyer A, Van Meurs KP, Drover DR, Klawitter J, Christians U, Chock VY. Theophylline dosing and pharmacokinetics for renal protection in neonates with hypoxic-ischemic encephalopathy undergoing therapeutic hypothermia. Pediatr Res. 2020;88(6):871-7.
31. Chock VY, Cho SH, Frymoyer A. Aminophylline for renal protection in neonatal hypoxic-ischemic encephalopathy in the era of therapeutic hypothermia. Pediatr Res. 2020;10:974-80.
32. Nigwekar SU, Waikar SS. Diuretics in acute kidney injury. Semin Nephrol. 2011;31(6):523-34.
33. Jefferies JL, Price JF, Denfield SW, Chang AC, Dreyer WJ, McMahon CJ, et al. Safety and efficacy of nesiritide in pediatric heart failure. J Card Fail. 2007;13(7):541-8.
34. Lauschke A, Teichgräber U, Frei U, Eckardt KU. "Low-dose" dopamine worsens renal perfusion in patients with acute renal failure. Kidney Int. 2006;69(9):1669-74.
35. Fishbane S. N-acetylcysteine in the prevention of contrast-induced nephropathy. Clin J Am Soc Nephrol. 2008;3(1):281-7.
36. Dellinger RP, Levy M, Rhodes A, Annane D, Gerlach H, Opal SM, et al. Surviving sepsis campaign: International guidelines for management of severe sepsis and septic shock: 2012. Crit Care Med. 2013;41(2):580-637.
37. Slattery J, Lobaz S. Fluid management. Surgery. 2019;37(8): 415-23.
38. Boer C, Bossers SM, Koning NJ. Choice of fluid type: physiological concepts and perioperative indications. Br J Anaesth. 2018;120(2):384-96.
39. Finfer S, Bellomo R, Boyce N, French J, Myburgh J, Norton R, et al. A comparison of albumin and saline for fluid resuscitation in the intensive care unit. N Engl J Med. 2004;350(22):2247-56.
40. Prowle JR, Chua HR, Bagshaw SM, Bellomo R. Clinical review: Volume of fluid resuscitation and the incidence of acute kidney injury - a systematic review. Crit Care. 2012;16(4):230.
41. Gordon AC, Russell JA, Walley KR, Singer J, Ayers D, Storms MM, et al. The effects of vasopressin on acute kidney injury in septic shock. Intensive Care Med. 2010;36(1):83-91.
42. Albanèse J, Leone M, Garnier F, Bourgoin A, Antonini F, Martin C. Renal effects of norepinephrine in septic and nonseptic patients. Chest. 2004;126(2):534-9.
43. Lauzier F, Lévy B, Lamarre P, Lesur O. Vasopressin or norepinephrine in early hyperdynamic septic shock: a randomized clinical trial. Intensive Care Med. 2006;32(11): 1782-9.
44. Chen Y-Y, Wu V-C, Huang W-C, Yeh Y-C, Wu M-S, Huang C-C, et al. Norepinephrine Administration is associated with higher mortality in dialysis requiring acute kidney injury patients with septic shock. J Clin Med. 2018;7(9):274.
45. Cantarovich F, Rangoonwala B, Lorenz H, Verho M, Esnault VLM. High-dose furosemide for established ARF: a prospective, randomized, double-blind, placebo-controlled, multicenter trial. Am J Kidney Dis. 2004;44(3):402-9.
46. Ho KM, Power BM. Benefits and risks of furosemide in acute kidney injury. Anaesthesia. 2010;65(3):283-93.
47. Ronco C, Haapio M, House AA, Anavekar N, Bellomo R. Cardiorenal syndrome. J Am Coll Cardiol. 2008;52(19)1527-39.
48. Kim MG. Cardiorenal syndrome. J Korean Med Assoc. 2020;63(1):20-9.
49. Grams ME, Estrella MM, Coresh J, Brower RG, Liu KD. Fluid balance, diuretic use, and mortality in acute kidney injury. Clin J Am Soc Nephrol. 2011;6(5):966-73.
50. Foland JA, Fortenberry JD, Warshaw BL, Pettignano R, Merritt RK, Heard ML, et al. Fluid overload before continuous hemofiltration and survival in critically ill children: a retrospective analysis. Crit Care Med. 2004;32(8):1771-6.
51. Fouque D, Kalantar-Zadeh K, Kopple J, Cano N, Chauveau P, Cuppari L, et al. A proposed nomenclature and diagnostic

criteria for protein-energy wasting in acute and chronic kidney disease. Kidney Int. 2008;73(4):391-8.
52. Cano N, Fiaccadori E, Tesinsky P, Toigo G, Druml W, Kuhlmann M, et al. ESPEN guidelines on enteral nutrition: adult renal failure. Clin Nutr. 2006;25(2):295-310.
53. Fiaccadori E, Maggiore U, Giacosa R, Rotelli C, Picetti E, Sagripanti S, et al. Enteral nutrition in patients with acute renal failure. Kidney Int. 2004;65(3):999-1008.
54. Nakamura AT, Btaiche IF, Pasko DA, Jain JC, Mueller BA. In vitro clearance of trace elements via continuous renal replacement therapy. J Ren Nutr. 2004;14(4):214-9.
55. Zo'o M, Hoermann M, Balassy C, Brunelle F, Azoulay R, Pariente D, et al. Renal safety in pediatric imaging: randomized, double-blind phase IV clinical trial of iobitridol 300 versus iodixanol 270 in multidetector CT. Pediatr Radiol. 2011;41(11):1393-400.
56. Windpessl M, Kronbichler A. Contrast-associated acute kidney injury (CA-AKI) in children: special considerations. Child Kidney Dis. 2019;23(2):77-85.
57. Verghese P. Contrast nephropathy in children. J Pediatr Intensive Care. 2015;3(2):45-52.
58. Barrett BJ, Carlisle EJ. Metaanalysis of the relative nephrotoxicity of high- and low-osmolality iodinated contrast media. Radiology. 1993;188(1):171-8.
59. Azzalini L, Vilca LM, Lombardo F, Poletti E, Laricchia A, Beneduce A, et al. Incidence of contrast-induced acute kidney injury in a large cohort of all-comers undergoing percutaneous coronary intervention: Comparison of five contrast media. Int J Cardiol. 2018;273:69-73.
60. Trout AT, Dillman JR, Ellis JH, Cohan RH, Strouse PJ. Patterns of intravenous contrast material use and corticosteroid premedication in children-a survey of Society of Chairs of Radiology in Children's Hospitals (SCORCH) member institutions. Pediatr Radiol. 2011;41(10):1272-83.
61. McDonald JS, Leake CB, McDonald RJ, Gulati R, Katzberg RW, Williamson EE, et al. Acute kidney injury after intravenous versus intra-arterial contrast material administration in a paired cohort. Invest Radiol. 2016;51(12):804-9.
62. Trivedi HS, Moore H, Nasr S, Aggarwal K, Agrawal A, Goel P, et al. A randomized prospective trial to assess the role of saline hydration on the development of contrast nephrotoxicity. Nephron Clin Pract. 2003;93(1):C29-34.
63. Matzke GR, Aronoff GR, Atkinson AJ, Bennett WM, Decker BS, Eckardt KU, et al. Drug dosing consideration in patients with acute and chronic kidney disease: a clinical update from Kidney Disease: Improving Global Outcomes (KDIGO). Kidney Int. 2011;80(11):1122-37.
64. Stanski NL, Stenson EK, Cvijanovich NZ, Weiss SL, Fitzgerald JC, Bigham MT, et al. PERSEVERE biomarkers predict severe acute kidney injury and renal recovery in pediatric septic shock. Am J Respir Crit Care Med. 2020;201(7):848-55.
65. Wong HR, Salisbury S, Xiao Q, Cvijanovich NZ, Hall M, Allen GL, et al. The pediatric sepsis biomarker risk model. Crit Care. 2012;16(5):R174.
66. Sandokji I, Greenberg JH. Novel biomarkers of acute kidney injury in children: an update on recent findings. Curr Opin Pediatr. 2020;32(2):354-9.
67. Greenberg JH, Parikh CR. Biomarkers for diagnosis and prognosis of AKI in children: one size does not fit all. Clin J Am Soc Nephrol. 2017;12(9):1551-7.
68. Pozzoli S, Simonini M, Manunta P. Predicting acute kidney injury: current status and future challenges. J Nephrol. 2018;31(2):209-23.
69. Griffin BR, Gist KM, Faubel S. Current status of novel biomarkers for the diagnosis of acute kidney injury: a historical perspective. J Intensive Care Med. 2020;35(5):415-24.
70. Alge JL, Arthur JM. Biomarkers of AKI: A review of mechanistic relevance and potential therapeutic implications. Clin J Am Soc Nephrol. 2015;10(1):147-55.
71. Chen JJ, Chang CH, Huang YT, Kuo G. Furosemide stress test as a predictive marker of acute kidney injury progression or renal replacement therapy: a systemic review and meta-analysis. Crit Care. 2020;24(1):202.
72. Clark Powell T, Warnock DG. The furosemide stress test and predicting AKI outcomes J Am Soc Nephrol. 2015;26(8):1762-4.
73. Koyner JL, Davison DL, Brasha-Mitchell E, Chalikonda DM, Arthur JM, Shaw AD, et al. Furosemide stress test and biomarkers for the prediction of AKI severity. J Am Soc Nephrol. 2015;26(8):2023-31.
74. Ghasemi K, Esteghamati M, Borzoo S, Parvaneh E, Borzoo S. Predictive accuracy of urinary neutrophil gelatinase associated lipocalin (NGAL) for renal parenchymal involvement in children with acute pyelonephritis. Electron Phys. 2016;8(2):1911-7.
75. Sirota JC, Walcher A, Faubel S, Jani A, McFann K, Devarajan P, et al. Urine IL-18, NGAL, IL-8 and serum IL-8 are biomarkers of acute kidney injury following liver transplantation. BMC Nephrol. 2013;14(1):17.
76. Liu KD, Altmann C, Smits G, Krawczeski CD, Edelstein CL, Devarajan P, et al. Serum Interleukin-6 and interleukin-8 are early biomarkers of acute kidney injury and predict prolonged mechanical ventilation in children undergoing cardiac surgery: a case-control study. Crit Care. 2009;13(4):R104.
77. de Fontnouvelle CA, Greenberg JH, Thiessen-Philbrook HR, Zappitelli M, Roth J, Kerr KF, et al. Interleukin-8 and tumor necrosis factor predict acute kidney injury after pediatric cardiac surgery. Ann Thorac Surg. 2017;104(6):2072-9.
78. Guzzi LM, Bergler T, Binnall B, Engelman DT, Forni L, Germain MJ, et al. Clinical use of [TIMP-2]•[IGFBP7] biomarker testing to assess risk of acute kidney injury in critical care: guidance from an expert panel. Crit Care. 2019;23(1):225.
79. Uwaezuoke S. Uromodulin and YKL-40 as biomarkers in pediatric acute kidney injury: a review of current evidence. J Integr Nephrol Androl. 2017;4(4):115-20.
80. Samoni S, Husain-Syed F, De Rosa S, Ronco C. Cardiopulmonary renal interactions. G Ital Nefrol. 2017;34(Suppl 69):162-77.
81. Husain-Syed F, Slutsky AS, Ronco C. Lung-kidney cross-talk in the critically ill patient. Am J Respir Crit Care Med. 2016;194(4):402-14.
82. Rangaswami J, Bhalla V, Blair JEA, Chang TI, Costa S, Lentine KL, et al. Cardiorenal syndrome: classification, pathophysiology, diagnosis, and treatment strategies: a scientific statement from the American Heart Association. Circulation. 2019;139(16):E840-78.
83. Chawla LS, Bellomo R, Bihorac A, Goldstein SL, Siew ED, Bagshaw SM, et al. Acute kidney disease and renal recovery: consensus report of the acute disease quality initiative (ADQI) 16 Workgroup. Nat Rev Nephrol. 2017;13(4):241-57.
84. Chawla LS, Eggers PW, Star RA, Kimmel PL. Acute kidney injury and chronic kidney disease as interconnected syndromes. N Engl J Med. 2014;371(1):58-66.
85. Gameiro J, Marques F, Lopes JA. Long-term consequences of acute kidney injury: a narrative review. Clin Kidney J. 2020; 14(3):789-804.
86. Bagshaw SM, George C, Bellomo R. Early acute kidney injury and sepsis: A multicentre evaluation. Crit Care. 2008;12(2):R47.

CHAPTER

11.5 Kidney Replacement Therapies

Ranjeet W Thergaonkar, Manish Kumar, Aditi Sinha

INTRODUCTION

Acute kidney injury (AKI), characterized by an abrupt decrease in kidney function over hours to weeks, is a heterogeneous syndrome with varied etiology and severity. While asymptomatic mild elevation of serum creatinine usually reverses with measures to avoid further nephrotoxic injury, patients presenting with oligoanuric AKI and fluid overload, dyselectrolytemia or uremia, require kidney replacement therapy (KRT). In KRT, the removal of extra fluid and nitrogenous waste products from the body relies on ultrafiltration (for fluid removal) and diffusion and convection (for solute clearance) across a semipermeable membrane. This chapter discusses the indications of KRT and choice of modality and outlines basic principles of each of the options of KRT used in children with AKI.

INDICATIONS FOR KIDNEY REPLACEMENT THERAPY

Kidney replacement therapy is indicated in critically ill patients with severe AKI [Kidney Disease Improving Global Outcomes (KDIGO) stages 2–3] who present with life-threatening and refractory hyperkalemia or metabolic acidosis, uremic encephalopathy, and pulmonary edema, as listed in **Box 1**.[1] In addition to severe AKI, acute KRT is also indicated in acute tumor lysis syndrome with refractory metabolic abnormalities, for removal of toxins, and in certain inborn errors of metabolism with severe or refractory hyperammonemia (urea cycle defects), metabolic acidosis (organic acidemia), or elevated leucine (maple syrup urine disease).[1]

TIMING OF KIDNEY REPLACEMENT THERAPY

The decision to institute dialysis is usually based on an overall assessment of the patient keeping in view the severity complications and likely course of AKI **(Box 1)**. However, the optimal timing of initiation of KRT in patients with severe AKI without complications, as listed in **Box 1**, remains controversial. There are arguments in favor of both early and delayed initiation of KRT. Early KRT prevents progressive fluid overload which is directly correlated with mortality, helps remove toxic solutes that contribute to an inflammatory milieu, and corrects metabolic acidosis that leads to hemodynamic instability. The rationale behind delaying KRT includes avoidance of procedure-related risk to a patient who might be managed conservatively until renal function improves spontaneously, rationing of resources, and avoidance of iatrogenic hypovolemia from excessive ultrafiltration.

Information on timing of dialysis initiation in children is limited. One observational study on 161 patients found that KRT was initiated earlier in patients that survived compared to those that succumbed (median 12.5 vs. 25.5 hours; p = 0.095).[2] Four recent trials have examined the timing of KRT in adult critically ill patients with AKI. ELAIN, a single-

BOX 1: Indications for kidney replacement therapy in acute illness.

Stage 2 or 3 AKI (as defined by KDIGO 2012)[1] with any of the following:
- Oliguria with fluid overload >10%
- Persistent or worsening metabolic acidosis: arterial pH <7.15 and $PaCO_2$ <35 or >50 mm Hg (pure or mixed metabolic acidosis)
- Refractory or severe hyperkalemia: serum potassium >5.5 mEq/L despite medical management or >6 mEq/L
- Hyponatremia (120 mEq/L, or symptomatic) or hypernatremia
- Anticipated fluid overload: requirement of large amounts of blood products/infusion
- Pulmonary edema, encephalopathy, and/or refractory hypertension

Acute tumor lysis syndrome, with refractory hyperphosphatemia, hypocalcemia, or hyperuricemia

Confirmed or suspected inborn error of metabolisms with any of the following:
- Hyperammonemia with rapidly worsening encephalopathy, or serum ammonia persistently >400 µmol/L despite medical management
- Organic acidemia with refractory metabolic acidosis
- Maple syrup urine disease: crisis with serum leucine >700 µmol/L

Acute poisoning: Alcohols (ethylene glycol, methanol, isopropyl alcohol, diethylene glycol, propylene glycol); aspirin; acetaminophen; metformin; lithium; antiepileptic drugs (valproic acid, phenytoin, barbiturates, carbamazepine); theophylline; paraquat; hair dye

(AKI: acute kidney injury; KDIGO: Kidney Disease Improving Global Outcomes)

center randomized controlled trial (RCT) that looked at a predominantly surgical cohort of 231 patients with KDIGO stage 3 AKI, found improved survival in patients with early initiation strategy (hazard ratio of death 0.66; 95% confidence interval 0.45–0.97; $p = 0.03$).[3] However, three larger multicenter RCTs (AKIKI, IDEAL-ICU, and STARRT-AKI) in critically ill adult patients failed to find any survival advantage with either early or delayed KRT initiation strategies.[4-6] An individual patient data meta-analysis on 2,083 patients with AKI included in 9 RCTs in the last decade (except the STARRT-AKI) shows that mortality does not differ significantly based on whether KRT was initiated early or delayed.[7] So in the absence of urgent indications such as a life-threatening metabolic complication, initiation of KRT can be safely postponed. Under close supervision, deliberately delaying KRT initiation till a clinical indication emerges seems acceptable with regard to both patient outcomes and economic utilization of resources.[7]

CHOICE OF MODALITY OF KIDNEY REPLACEMENT THERAPY

Available modalities for KRT for children with severe AKI include peritoneal dialysis (PD), intermittent hemodialysis (HD), sustained low-efficiency dialysis (SLED), and continuous KRT (CKRT), which includes hemofiltration and hemodiafiltration. Therapy may be intermittent (lasting <24 hours), such as intermittent HD or SLED, or continuous, such as PD or CKRT. A comparison of different KRT modalities is listed in **Table 1**. The choice of dialysis modality is influenced by several factors, including the goals of dialysis, the unique advantages and disadvantages of each modality, and institutional resources. The choice of modality is also influenced by the indication, age, weight, hemodynamic status, and parental choice.[8] While recent availability of newer KRT modalities, including SLED and CKRT, has allowed the therapy to be offered to sicker and hemodynamically unstable patients in the intensive care unit setting, studies to compare continuous versus intermittent therapies have not shown a beneficial effect on mortality.[8]

Peritoneal dialysis continues to remain a popular choice in the acute setting and is particularly useful in young infants and resource-limited settings.[9] A 2012 nationwide survey on the choice of dialysis modality in children with AKI in 26 centers across India indicated uniform availability of PD, making it the preferred KRT modality, particularly in children younger than 2 years of age. HD was available in 86% centers with pediatric nephrologist(s) and was preferred in children older than 7 years. Facilities for SLED and CKRT were available at less than one-fourth of the centers.[10]

An international survey of 650 pediatric and adult nephrologists across 223 centers revealed disparity in choices between developed and developing countries. While PD was available uniformly, HD was feasible at 85 versus 54% of centers in developed and developing world, respectively. CKRT was available at 60 versus 33% centers, respectively.[11] The practice of SLED was limited to 20–25% centers. For infant KRT, there was a clear preference for PD in developing countries (69%) and HD (72%) or CKRT (24%) in developed countries.

TABLE 1: Comparison of modalities of kidney replacement therapy for pediatric acute kidney injury.

Mode of therapy	*Peritoneal dialysis*	*Intermittent hemodialysis*	*Sustained low-efficiency dialysis*	*Continuous kidney replacement therapy*
Mechanism of clearance	Diffusion; convection	Diffusion; convection	Diffusion	Convection (CVVH, CVVHDF); diffusion (CVVHDF, CVVHD)
Duration of therapy	Continuous or intermittent	≤4 hours; on alternate days or daily	>6 hours; usually daily	Continuous
Access	Peritoneal catheter	Vascular; double-lumen catheter	Vascular; double-lumen catheter	Vascular; double-lumen catheter
Machines and equipment	Not necessary; automated cycler useful	HD machine, circuits, and dialyzer	HD machine, circuit, and dialyzer	CKRT machine, circuit, fluid bags, and dialyzers/filters
Blood flow rate	Not applicable	5–8 mL/kg/min	3–5 mL/kg/min	Infants 10–12 mL/kg/min; children 4–6 mL/kg/min; adolescents 2–4 mL/kg/min
Dialysate flow rate	20–30 mL/kg/cycle	Twice the BFR, or 500 mL/min	1.5–2 times the BFR	2 L/1.73 m^2/h (total of dialysate and/or replacement fluid)
Ultrafiltration control	Not possible	Possible	Possible	Possible
Suitability in patients with hemodynamic instability	Feasible	Risk of hypotension	Feasible	Feasible
Anticoagulation	Not needed	Usually required	Usually required	Usually required, continuously

(BFR: blood flow rate; CKRT: continuous kidney replacement therapy; CVVH: continuous venovenous hemofiltration; CVVHD: continuous venovenous hemodialysis; CVVHDF: continuous venovenous hemodiafiltration; HD: hemodialysis)

PERITONEAL DIALYSIS

Peritoneal dialysis is a form of KRT in which diffusive exchange of solutes and osmotic removal of fluid (ultrafiltration) occurs across the semipermeable peritoneal membrane. PD is technically simple and can be performed by personnel with limited training.[12] The procedure costs are approximately one-third to one-fifth of the extracorporeal blood-purifying therapies.[9] The slow and continuous nature of the exchange across fluid compartments makes it physiological. Selecting PD obviates the need for vascular access. Given the proportionately greater surface area of the peritoneal membrane in children, the procedure is expected to be efficient. Use of peritoneal membrane as the dialyzing surface is less proinflammatory than that in HD. The presence of large pores in the peritoneal membrane aids solute exchange and facilitates the removal of larger molecules, including toxic cytokines.[10,13] However, the need to access the peritoneal cavity to instill fluid requires an intact peritoneum. So PD is contraindicated in diaphragmatic hernia, gastroschisis, and omphalocele. PD can be associated with mechanical problems, such as worsening of shock due to reduced venous return or respiratory failure due to splinting of diaphragm in critically ill children. PD is associated with relatively slow and unpredictable rate of ultrafiltration and low clearance of small molecules, particularly in the presence of shock which causes visceral ischemia. In addition, PD can lead to metabolic disturbances such as protein loss, hyperglycemia, and hypernatremia.

Technique of Peritoneal Dialysis

Performance of PD requires an access to the peritoneum using a catheter, an appropriate dialysis fluid, preferably cycled in a closed system, and an appropriate prescription.

Peritoneal Access (Catheters)

The three main types of catheters that may be used are the stylet type or rigid (stiff) acute PD catheters, cuffed (soft) chronic PD catheters, and improvised catheters (**Figs. 1A to D**). Custom-made PD catheters have several openings on the side at the peritoneal end. While the 2020 guidelines of the International Society of Peritoneal Dialysis (ISPD) on acute PD for children recommend using cuffed catheters, they acknowledge the need for use of acute or improvised catheters when the former are not available in resource-limited settings.[14]

Figure 1B shows a rigid PD catheter, the most commonly available catheter in India. These catheters are stiff, uncuffed, inexpensive, can be placed at the bedside under local anesthesia, and require minimal expertise for insertion. The technique of insertion of a rigid PD catheter is described in **Box 2.**[15] Because acute catheters are uncuffed, there is fear of bacterial migration to the subcutaneous layers, and consequent peritonitis, after 48–72 hours; therefore, they should be removed or revised to soft-cuffed catheters if the need for KRT persists. Acute PD catheters also carry a high risk of injury or perforation of a hollow viscus during insertion. Cuffed PD (Tenckhoff) catheters are usually made of silicone

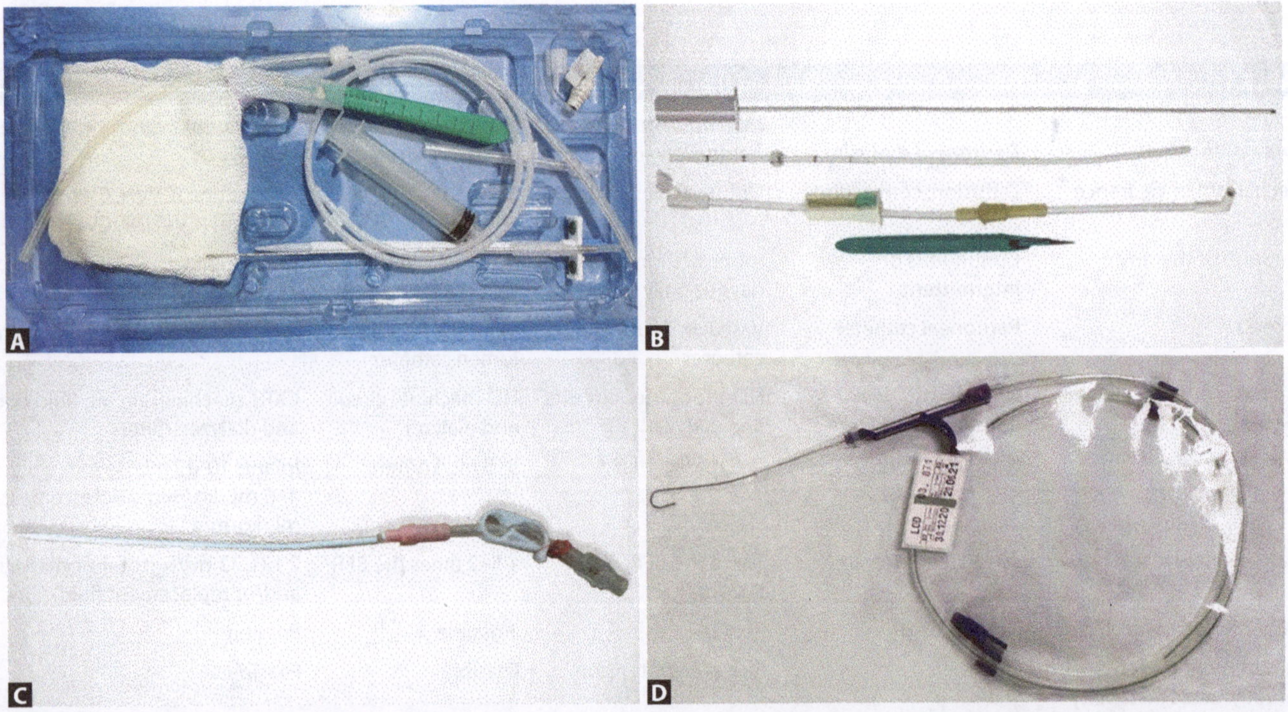

Figs. 1A to D: (A) Cuffed peritoneal dialysis (PD) catheter (Tenckhoff) with instruments for insertion; (B) Rigid PD catheter with stylet and instruments for insertion; (C) Single-lumen hemodialysis catheter (D) with guidewire; the latter (C and D) can be repurposed as a rigid PD catheter in neonates.
Courtesy: Dr Sumantra Raut, Siliguri.

BOX 2: Procedure for insertion of rigid (stiff) peritoneal dialysis catheter.

1. The urinary bladder is catheterized; if patient is constipated, bowels are emptied using an enema
2. The operators perform handwash and then dons sterile caps, masks, gowns, and gloves
3. The patient's abdomen is cleaned using chlorhexidine or isopropyl alcohol and povidone-iodine and then draped
4. Site for insertion of catheter is chosen in the midline in the mid-rectus abdominis sheath 1 inch below the umbilicus, or midpoint between the umbilicus and the anterior superior iliac spine. The inferior epigastric artery, which runs along lateral aspect of rectus abdominal sheath, should not be punctured using these landmarks
5. Local anesthesia should be administered at this point
6. Using a wide-bore IV cannula, approximately 30 mL/kg of normal saline as a "priming volume" is instilled into the abdomen until the flanks are slightly full. The fluid should flow readily and not cause subcutaneous swelling
7. The cannula is removed and a small nick is given in the skin to allow introduction of the catheter (but not so large that fluid leaks later); the catheter with stylet is introduced into the abdomen with a cork–screw movement
8. A "give way" is felt once the stylet enters the peritoneal cavity; the stylet is withdrawn slightly to prevent injury to the intra-abdominal structures, and the catheter is advanced into the abdominal cavity directing it into the pelvis at an angle of 45° or to the iliac fossa or to the para-colic gutter
9. The stylet is withdrawn and the upper end of the catheter is connected to the bottle of normal saline; free flow of the fluid is expected
10. A "test cycle" is run to assess for free in- and outflow of the fluid through the catheter; minor manipulation of the catheter position may be required to ensure this
11. The catheter is fixed to the abdomen using adhesive plaster in a "namaste" dressing to hold up the catheter at almost right angles to the abdominal wall
12. Using three-way and IV tubings, the catheter is connected to the PD fluid and drain bottle, bag or burette, or preferably, to the automated cycler device
13. PD is performed as per prescription

rubber or polyurethane and have cuffs made of Dacron.[10,14,16] These cuffs prevent migration of bacteria and can be used for prolonged time. **Figure 1A** shows a cuffed PD catheter commonly available in India, which can be placed surgically or percutaneously using a modified Seldinger technique using a peel-away sheath. The technique of insertion of a cuffed PD catheter are described in **Box 3**.[17] However, insertion of this catheter requires training.[18] Improvised devises include nasogastric tubes,[19] suprapubic catheters,[20] rubber catheters, intercostal drainage tubes, pigtail catheters, or single-lumen femoral catheters **(Figs. 1C and D)**.

Peritoneal Dialysis Delivery Systems

There are two types of PD delivery systems: automated cyclers and manual or gravity-based systems. Both automated and gravity-based systems may be closed systems that are commercially marketed or open systems that are set-up at the bedside. Closed manual systems that minimize the number of connections and therefore touch contamination[14] are not marketed in India. Therefore, open manual connections have to be improvised using IV tubings, burette sets and three-way connectors but carry risk of peritonitis through touch contamination. Automated cyclers have multiple programs that can be fed into the software to automate fluid cycling, thus reducing nursing workload as well as the risk of infections, since they minimize handling of catheter and connections. **Figure 2A** shows a child with AKI undergoing PD using an automated cycler. While cyclers require relatively expensive consumables, including bags and tubings, the overall cost of health care, including nursing costs and through reduced risk of peritonitis, are lower than that with manual connections.

BOX 3: Procedure for insertion of cuffed PD catheter.

Steps 1–5 are identical to those for introduction of a rigid PD catheter **(Box 2)**

6. A 0.035-inch guidewire is introduced into the abdomen through the introducer IV cannula. The introducer is now removed
7. A dilator with peel-away sheath is not placed inside the abdomen over the guidewire and the dilator removed
8. The cuffed PD catheter is now inserted into the peel-away sheath into the pelvis till a point where flow of fluid is free. The peel-away sheath is now removed. A "test-cycle" may be performed at this stage
9. The deep cuff (or only cuff is fixed in the case of single-cuff catheters) is fixed just outside the parietal peritoneum using suitable forceps
10. A tunnel is made from the site of insertion to the exit site. The exit site is usually lateral to the site of insertion and below the beltline. The superficial cuff (if present) is buried inside this tunnel approximately 2 cm away from the exit site
11. Suitable antisepsis is performed at the site of entry as per institutional protocol
12. The catheter is now connected to the PD delivery system and PD performed as per prescription

Prescription of Peritoneal Dialysis

The important components of PD prescription are described here, including (1) PD fluid composition (buffer; electrolytes), (2) dwell volume, (3) exchange and dwell time, (4) additives to dialysate, and (5) duration of PD therapy.

Peritoneal Dialysis Fluid

The dialysate for PD, termed PD fluid, consists of an osmotic agent (usually dextrose), a buffer (either lactate or bicarbonate), and electrolytes. PD fluids are marketed with glucose concentrations of 1.5, 2.5, or 4.25%.[21] Only the first two are easily available in the Indian market, in 2- and 5-L bags for chronic dialysis. PD fluids containing 1.7% dextrose are also available in 1-L plastic bottles. Patients who are euvolemic or with minimal fluid overload should undergo PD with lower dextrose strength fluids (1.5 and 1.7%). Higher dextrose strength fluid (2.5 and 4.25%) is reserved for use in fluid overload.

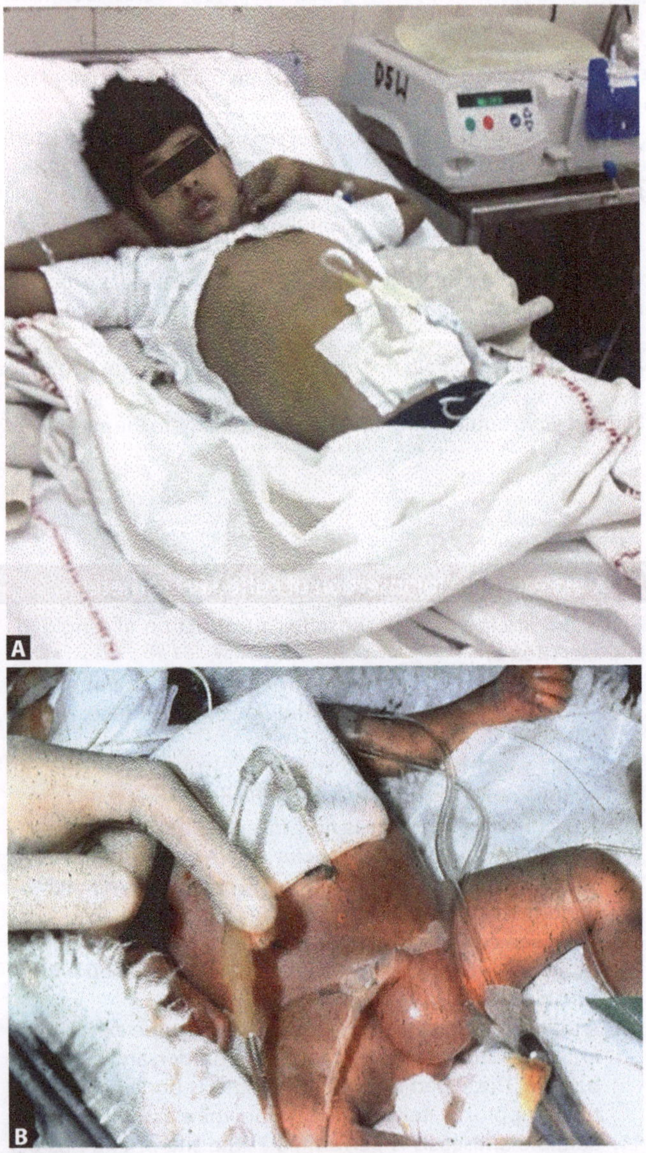

Figs. 2A and B: (A) A child undergoing acute peritoneal dialysis (PD) using an automated cycler; (B) Acute PD in a neonate with acute kidney injury (AKI).
Courtesy image A: Dr Sumantra Raut, Kolkata.
Courtesy image B: Dr Swati Bhardwaj, New Delhi.

Lactate is the usual buffer in PD fluids. It accepts a proton from carbonic acid to yield lactic acid and bicarbonate.[22] In situations of excess production of lactic acid, such as shock or in liver failure, and in neonates, bicarbonate-containing PD fluids are preferred.[14,23] If these are not available, lactate-containing fluids are used. While bicarbonate-containing fluid is associated with better correction of acidosis, meta-analysis of studies in adult and pediatric patients does not indicate any significant difference in mortality.[24] PD solutions usually contain sodium at 132–134 mEq/L, calcium 1–1.75 mmol/L, and magnesium 0.25–0.75 mmol/L.[14,21] While most PD fluids are devoid of potassium, some PD fluids marketed in India contain potassium at 2 mEq/L. In case PD fluid is not available commercially, it can be prepared within the hospital, preferably by the hospital pharmacy, or under careful sterile precautions in the ward.[14,21] Locally prepared PD solutions from IV fluid preparations have been used with success and acceptable safety.[25,26] Some methods for bedside preparation of PD solutions from IV fluids are given in **Table 2**. In using these locally prepared fluids, the following aspects are kept in mind: (1) the constitution of the fluid should be read carefully to avoid errors, (2) use of fewer constituents is preferred to lower the risk of infection and errors, (3) strict asepsis is necessary while mixing, and (4) bicarbonate and calcium should not be mixed in the same compartment.[14,21]

Dwell Volume

The dwell volume used in PD is usually kept at 25–40 mL/kg body weight or 800–1,100 mL/m² body surface area (BSA). While low volumes decrease dialysis efficacy, high dwell volumes are associated with mechanical complications of raised intraperitoneal pressure, such as pain, fluid leak, hernias, pleural effusion, and respiratory embarrassment; there may also be a drop in ultrafiltration due to lymphatic absorption. It is usual to start the session with low dwell volumes of 10–20 mL/kg (300–600 mL/m² BSA) and increase to an optimal volume of 30 mL/kg (800–900 mL/m² BSA). Larger volumes of 40–50 mL/kg (1,100–1,400 mL/m² BSA) may be attempted with cuffed PD catheter and cycler, if tolerated.[14,21]

TABLE 2: Locally prepared solutions that may be used if commercially available dialysate for peritoneal dialysis is not available.

Preparation	*Glucose, %*	*Na⁺*	*K⁺*	*Ca⁺⁺*	*Mg⁺⁺*	*Cl⁻*	*HCO_3^-*	*Lactate*
Normal saline 500 mL + 5% dextrose 440 mL + 7.5% $NaHCO_3$ 60 mL	2.2	126.5	–	–	–	72.5	54	–
N/2 saline in 5% dextrose 1,000 mL + 7.5% $NaHCO_3$ 40 mL + 3% NaCl 60 mL	2.4	138	–	–	–	103	35	–
Ringer lactate 1,000 mL + 50% dextrose 30 mL	1.45	127	3.8	1.36	–	107	–	27
PlasmaLyte B 1,000 mL + 50% dextrose 30 mL	1.45	126	3.8	–	1.45	108	27	–

Note: Except for glucose, the concentration of all constituents are in mmol/L.

TABLE 3: Regimens for prescribing peritoneal dialysis.

Regimen	Dwell time (min)	Session duration (h)	No. of sessions/week	Urea clearance (mL/min)	Weekly Kt/V
IPD	30–60	16–20	2–3	8–12	–
CEPD	240–300	8–12	7	12–15	1.80 ± 0.32
TPD	5–10	8–10	7	15	2.43 ± 0.87
HVPD	35–60	24	7	15–20	3.85 ± 0.62
CFPD	–	4–8	5–7	30–50	>5

(CEPD: continuous equilibrated peritoneal dialysis; CFPD: continuous flow peritoneal dialysis; HVPD: high-volume peritoneal dialysis; IPD: intermittent peritoneal dialysis; TPD: tidal peritoneal dialysis)

Peritoneal Dialysis Dwell and Exchange Time

The exchange time consists of inflow time, dwell time, and outflow time. The inflow time is the time required for the dwell volume to be instilled in the abdomen (usually under the effect of gravity). This time is usually 5–10 minutes, depending upon the dwell volume, height of the PD fluid bag, and resistance due to either kinking of the PD catheter or reduced gut motility. Outflow time is the time required for the dwell volume to drain out from the abdomen into the drain bag. This usually takes 20–30 minutes and is dependent upon the dwell volume, height difference between the patient and the drain bag, and resistance due to kinks in the catheter.[14,21,27] The dwell time is the period for which the dwell volume remains inside the abdomen. A minimum period of 20–30 minutes is required for ultrafiltration and solute exchange. Shorter dwell times are sufficient for small particles such as potassium ions, protons, and water; hence, rapid short cycles are used to correct hyperkalemia, metabolic acidosis, and fluid overload. However, longer periods are useful for the exchange of larger molecules, such as creatinine or phosphate.[14,21]

Additives to Peritoneal Dialysis Fluid

Heparin may be added to the PD fluid to prevent obstruction of the dialysis catheter by clots, particularly if catheter insertion was complicated by mild bleeding, or if fibrinous strands are seen in the effluent. Usually, 250–1,000 units of unfractionated heparin are added per liter of PD fluid.[14,21] In patients with hypokalemia, potassium is added at 3–4 mEq/L of PD fluid depending on the severity of hypokalemia. If patients on PF develop hyperglycemia, insulin may be added to the PD fluids in the dose of 4–5 U/L for 1.5% and 5–7 U/L for 2.5% dextrose-containing solutions, respectively.[28] In patients with hypernatremia, the concentration of sodium in PD fluid should be increased to within 15 mEq/L of the serum sodium concentration, so as to allow gradual and safe reduction in serum sodium.

Peritoneal Dialysis Exchange Regimens

Depending upon the dwell volume, dwell time, and duration of the therapy, there are many PD regimens, as described in **Table 3 and Figure 3.**[14,21] The regimen for a given patient with AKI could be selected from the above regimens or be tailored to the clinical status.

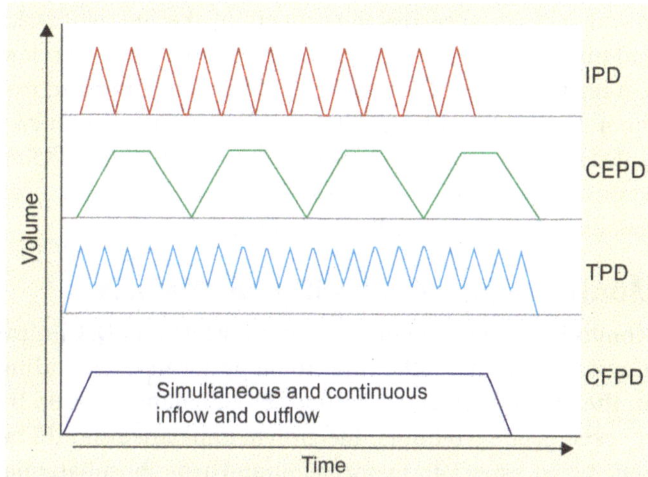

Fig. 3: Modalities of peritoneal dialysis. High-volume peritoneal dialysis (HVPD) can be represented in a manner similar to IPD but uses higher volumes and is repetitive. (CEPD: continuous equilibrated peritoneal dialysis; CFPD: continuous flow peritoneal dialysis; IPD: Intermittent peritoneal dialysis; TPD: tidal peritoneal dialysis)

Intermittent PD refers to a regimen with rapid cycles typically lasting 30–60 minutes, after which the PD fluid is drained out. This modality is useful early in the course of the session when the objectives are to remove fluid and exchange small molecules.[14,21] An old study reported satisfactory outcomes with early initiation of low-volume dialysis (10 mL/kg dwell volumes) with hourly exchanges in children with minor oliguria and fluid overload.[29] *Tidal PD* refers to a regimen where a small portion of the dwell volume (typically 25%) is retained in the peritoneum as the reserve volume, while the remaining part is drained out and replaced. This rationale behind this regimen is that time is not lost for inflow and outflow of fluids between cycles, there is better exchange of larger molecules, and the reserve volume keeps the PD catheter afloat.[30] A 2012 meta-analysis reported that the urea and creatinine clearance, phosphate and potassium removal, and ultrafiltration were similar for tidal PD as compared to continuous equilibrating PD.[29]

Continuous equilibrating PD is akin to chronic ambulatory PD (CAPD) with prolonged cycles lasting 3–6 hours. This modality is useful later in the course of AKI when the chief objective is to achieve removal of middle molecules.[21,29] *High-volume PD* is a high-dose regimen in which, using a cuffed PD catheter connected to an automated cycler, 18–22 cycles of high-volume (~1,200 mL/m² BSA) and short-duration dwells (50–60 minutes) are conducted over a session of 24 hours, and such sessions are conducted on all days.[31] This regimen was designed to overcome some of the traditional limitations of PD, such as peritonitis and inadequate metabolic control or clearances in catabolic state. An RCT of 120 adults reported urea clearance, mortality, and metabolic control similar to daily HD.[32] On the other hand, PD with high dwell volumes in young children carries the concern of altering right atrial and pulmonary artery pressures. *Continuous flow PD* refers to a regimen where high volumes of PD fluid enter and exit the peritoneal cavity simultaneously, either through two cuffed PD catheters or a three-way PD catheter, while keeping a constant volume inside. This regimen has excellent urea clearance but is technically challenging.[31]

Monitoring during Peritoneal Dialysis

Monitoring of the patient is important while on PD. Clinical monitoring of the patient has to be performed depending on the overall clinical condition. Fluid balance should be checked every 4–6 hours. Electrolyte imbalance should be anticipated, especially hypokalemia and hypophosphatemia. The patient should be weighed daily. Blood chemistries including urea, creatinine, electrolytes, pH, and bicarbonate should be tested daily.[14,21] Cytology of the PD effluent should be performed daily to rule out peritonitis. Poor dialysate outflow, severe abdominal pain, and change in color of PD effluent (especially, if cloudy or bloodstained) have to be detected and addressed.

Adequacy of Peritoneal Dialysis

There are three main objectives of PD in AKI: (1) fluid removal, (2) clearance of small solutes leading to correction of hyperkalemia and acidosis, and (3) clearance of middle molecules and cytokines.

Since water, potassium, urea, and bicarbonate move rapidly across the peritoneal membrane, fluid removal and correction of hyperkalemia and acidosis are usually achieved with rapid cycling over the first 24–48 hours of dialysis.[33] Similar to HD, small molecules clearance is quantified by urea kinetic modeling, using single-pool *Kt/V* to indicate the adequacy of PD. This parameter does not measure all aspects of adequacy of PD yet it is the only parameter that has been studied for adequacy of PD. The optimal *Kt/V* that ensures survival and good outcomes with minimal resources is not known. From a conceptual point of view, increasing doses of dialysis are incremental in improving survival till a particular limit is reached beyond which this benefit plateaus, and further increase in dose of dialysis is not beneficial.[14] The ISPD guidelines advocate that the optimal weekly *Kt/V* is >3.5 and recommend a weekly minimum *Kt/V* of 2.1 when comparing extracorporeal therapies.[14,34] It is important to keep in mind that targeting high clearances requires high volumes of PD fluid that may not be affordable in developing countries and may also be counterproductive because of the washout of immunoglobulins and opsonins, depletion of phagocytes, and reduced phagocytic function of macrophages.

Middle molecule clearance relies on convection as well as diffusion. Longer periods of contact between the PD fluid and peritoneum are also needed for the clearance of middle molecules. However, middle molecular clearance has not been quantified well. It is therefore recommended that, once life-threatening complications such as uremia, fluid overload, acidosis, and hyperkalemia have been dealt with, middle molecular clearance is addressed by either continuous equilibrated PD or tidal PD.[14,21,34]

Complications of Peritoneal Dialysis

Abdominal pain is a common complication of PD. It may result from abdominal distension, incorrect catheter position, or infection. *Leakage* around the point of insertion of the PD can occur, especially in the presence of comorbidities. Securing the catheter point of entry with a purse-string suture and use of fibrin glue are useful in controlling the leakage. *Perforation* of a hollow organ such as urinary bladder or intestine is uncommon (<1%) and can be avoided if adequate precautions are exercised. *Other mechanical complications* include displacement and obstruction of the catheter. Constipation can displace a PD catheter; bowel disimpaction is required to manage this. Omental wrapping of a PD catheter can cause obstruction to the outflow; surgical or laparoscopic revision is usually required.

Blood in the PD effluent can occur after rupture of abdominal vessels. This is usually not of concern and self-resolving except in case of rupture of a large vessel or if the patient has a bleeding diathesis. *Atelectasis and pneumonia* can occur due to raised intraperitoneal pressure. A block in the PD catheter can be the cause; if so, it should be relieved at the earliest.[4] *Hydrothorax* can rarely occur in the presence of a pleuroperitoneal fistula.[34]

Peritonitis is more common when using open PD delivery systems and when mixing of fluids is frequent. Use of cuffed catheter, closed systems, and automated cyclers reduces the risk of peritonitis considerably. Peritonitis should be prevented and managed as per ISPD guideline on PD peritonitis.[35] *Hypervolemia and hypovolemia* can occur due to inadequate or excessive ultrafiltration; close monitoring of fluid balance is therefore essential. *Dyselectrolytemia*, especially hypokalemia and hypophosphatemia, is common. *Hypoalbuminemia* is of concern in a setting of hypercatabolic states and malnutrition. Losses of up to 10–20 g/day have been noted; protein supplementation through oral or parenteral route is required in this situation. *Lactic acidosis* is uncommon, except in the setting of liver failure. *Hyperglycemia* might require administration of insulin, intraperitoneally or by subcutaneous route. *Hypothermia* may occur, especially in winter; it is uncommon with use of cyclers that warm the fluid.

Peritoneal Dialysis in Neonatal Acute Kidney Injury

Due to the difficulty in securing vascular access and the paucity of HD machines suited for extracorporeal therapies in infants, PD is often the only modality of KRT that is feasible in neonates.[36] Access into the peritoneal cavity is usually secured using a 31-cm single-cuff Tenckhoff catheter. Improvised access devices include single-lumen femoral catheters, intercostal drainage tubes, pigtail catheters, multifunctional catheters, and even wide-bore IV cannulae.[37,38] PD systems in the developing countries are usually open system. **Figure 2B** shows a preterm neonate undergoing PD.

HEMODIALYSIS

Hemodialysis is a technique of KRT that cleanses blood extracorporeally, using an HD machine and dialyzer, in an effective and rapid manner. The procedure requires placement of a double-lumen vascular access, a hemodynamically stable patient who will tolerate rapid fluxes in volumes and electrolytes, systemic anticoagulation, and technical expertise.[39] Several tertiary care centers in the country that offer HD to adult patients also manage HD in older pediatric patients; however, exclusive pediatric HD services are available only in a few centers.

Physiologic Principles of Hemodialysis

The basic principles of HD are similar to other KRT modalities. HD utilizes diffusion and convection for solute removal and ultrafiltration for excess fluid removal. The countercurrent flow of dialysate and blood across the dialyzer membrane maintains the maximum concentration gradient of the solutes between the two compartments in all parts of the dialyzer and increases the efficiency of the procedure. Ultrafiltration is conducted across a hydrostatic pressure gradient applied across the dialyzer by the machine. Along with the ultrafiltrated fluid, there is movement of toxins and waste molecules across the semipermeable membrane, irrespective of the concentration gradient by a process called convection or "solvent drag."[40]

Prerequisites for Pediatric Hemodialysis

Pediatric HD is technically more complex than HD in adult patients, and requires a multidisciplinary team approach, comprising pediatric nephrologist, dialysis nurse or technician, interventional radiologist, dietician, and clinical psychologist.[41] Following are the components of a pediatric HD unit and are discussed below: (1) HD machine, (2) water treatment unit, (3) dialyzer and tubings, (4) dialysate, and (5) vascular access.[40,42] The HD prescription is also discussed separately. The Indian Society of Nephrology has published guidelines on HD that provide guidance on setting up of HD units that can be applied to pediatric centers as well.[43]

Hemodialysis Machine

An HD machine has the following components, as shown in **Figure 4**: (1) blood circuit: comprising inflow circuit, a blood pump in the inflow circuit, a dialyzer, and an outflow circuit; (2) dialysate circuit, which has the admixture of the concentrated acid and bicarbonate solution/powder with the treated product water in a certain ratio, to form the

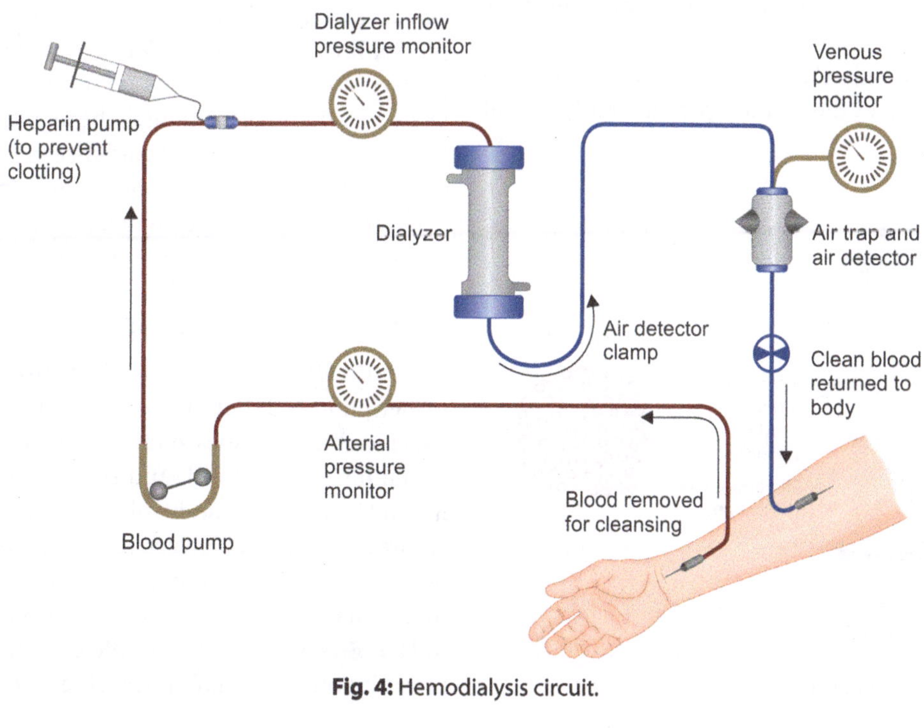

Fig. 4: Hemodialysis circuit.

final dialysate solution that is delivered to the dialyzer; (3) monitors, including arterial and venous pressure monitors, dialysate conductivity and temperature monitors, blood leak detector, and online *Kt/V* monitor; (4) ports, including the sampling port, saline infusion port, and heparin pump port. All recent HD machines are based on precise volumetrically controlled ultrafiltration control, allowing for a tight regulation of ultrafiltration, which is especially critical in small patients. Unfortunately, most of the available HD machines are not calibrated for use in children <20 kg.

Water Treatment Unit

As patients are exposed to large quantities of dialysate during each dialysis session, the chemical and microbiological purity of water used for dialysate preparation must be ensured.[44] Reverse osmosis is the most common water purification process used for HD. Product water and dialysis solution should meet the minimum standards of the Association for the Advancement of Medical Instrumentation (AAMI) criteria for purity of product water (bacterial colony count <100 CFU/mL and endotoxin <0.25 EU/mL).[45]

Dialyzer and Tubing

A dialyzer is a cylindrical shell packed with thousands of capillaries bound in a bundle. Blood passes through these capillaries from one end to the other end, and dialysate moves around these capillaries in the opposite direction **(Fig. 5)**. Selection of the dialyzer is based upon its membrane characteristics, surface area, ultrafiltration coefficient, and its urea clearance characteristics. Dialyzer membranes are usually made up of biocompatible synthetic materials, such as polysulfone or polymethylmethacrylate. The surface area of the chosen dialyzer should not exceed 70–100% of the patient's BSA. Dialyzers and bloodlines are available in different sizes for pediatric use.

The dialyzer and tubings together form the extracorporeal circuit. Ideally, volume of the extracorporeal circuit should not exceed 8–10% of the total blood volume of the child (80 mL/kg). If the volume of the circuit exceeds 10% of the total blood volume, it must be primed with normal saline, packed cells, or 5% human albumin to prevent sudden fall in blood pressure at the initiation of HD. HD machines, such as CARPEDIEM (CArdio Renal PEdiatric DIalysis Emergency Medicine) and NIDUS (Newcastle infant dialysis and ultrafiltration system), use smaller dialyzers (surface area 0.07–0.25 and 0.045 m^2, respectively) and tubings to enable dialysis in infants.

Based on the urea clearance rate, dialyzers are termed as high- or low-efficiency dialyzers. Most of the currently available dialyzers have high efficacy. High-flux dialyzers, on the other hand, have the capacity to remove bigger molecules up to the size of beta-2 microglobulin (MW 11,800) and water at higher rate because of the presence of larger pores in their membranes. *Ultrafiltration coefficient (KUf)* is a measure of flux and is defined as the volume of water filtered in mL/h/mm Hg of transmembrane pressure (TMP) gradient. *Mass transfer area coefficient (KoA)* is the efficiency of a given dialyzer in removing any solute at a given blood and dialysate flow rate. It can be defined as the maximum theoretical clearance of the dialyzer in milliliter per minute for a given solute at infinite blood and dialysis solution flow rate. Commonly used dialyzers have in vitro KoA values for urea ranging from 200 to 700 mL/min, whereas high-efficiency dialyzers have KoA >700 mL/min.[42,46]

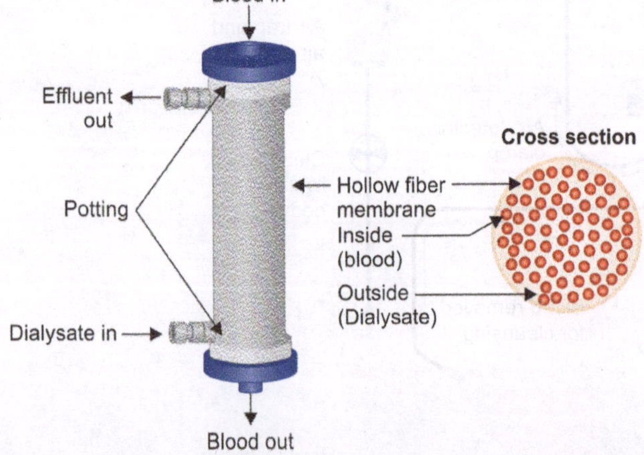

Fig. 5: Dialyzer.

Vascular Access

In children requiring acute HD, vascular access is obtained with a noncuffed, double-lumen central venous catheter (CVC). These catheters are available in sizes varying from 8 to 11.5 Fr, and the choice of the catheter depends upon the age and weight of the child. The catheter is inserted using the Seldinger technique. The right jugular vein is the most preferred vein followed by femoral and left jugular veins. Dialysis catheter placement in the jugular vein should always be made under ultrasound guidance to avoid inadvertent risk of arterial puncture. The subclavian vein should be avoided because of the increased chances of acute complications and higher risk of vascular stenosis later on.

Hemodialysis Prescription

An acute HD prescription differs from maintenance HD prescription and should be made in accordance with patient-specific characteristics such as age and weight of the child, initial blood urea level, and severity of fluid overload. An initial HD prescription involves the following components: (1) size and type of dialyzer, (2) blood flow rate, (3) dialysate flow rate, (4) dialysate composition, (5) target urea reduction, (6) ultrafiltration volume, (7) dose of heparin, and (8) duration of HD. **Box 4** gives an example outlining the principles of prescription for a child undergoing dialysis for AKI.

BOX 4: Model prescription of hemodialysis.

Case: A 7-year-old child, weighing 20 kg, is admitted with severe AKI secondary to hemolytic uremic syndrome. The child's weight is increased above his baseline weight by 1 kg (fluid overload of 1 L). Blood reports reveal urea of 200 mg/dL, creatinine 6.5 mg/dL, and serum potassium 6.5 mEq/L.

Example of a prescription for the first hemodialysis session:

- Dialyzer type (to avoid disequilibrium in first session): Low flux
- Dialyzer size (at less than or equal to body surface area): 0.7 m^2 (e.g., F4; fill volume 42 mL)
- *Blood tubings:* Pediatric blood lines (volume 52 mL)
- Priming fluid: Not required (total extracorporeal circuit volume, 42 + 58 mL=100 mL, represents ~6%, i.e., <10% of total blood volume)
- Blood flow rate (Q_b) (5–7 mL/min) = 100 mL/min
- Dialysate flow rate (Q_d) (two times Q_b; fixed at 300 or 500 mL) = 300 mL/min
- Ultrafiltration goal (not to exceed 5% body weight) = 500 mL
- *Anticoagulation:* Unfractionated heparin 1,000 IU (50 IU/kg) as loading dose, followed by 500 IU (25 IU/kg) bolus per hour to keep ACT) between 100 and 140 seconds
- *Duration of session:* Calculated to achieve not > 30% reduction on blood urea in the first hemodialysis session to avoid dialysis disequilibrium
  Desired postsession blood urea: 140 mg/dL
  Expected K of session: Based on type of dialyzer, its surface area, and blood flow rate: ~100 mL/min (see the manufacturer's website for estimates)
  T calculated based on the following equation for urea kinetic modeling:
  $Kt/V = -\ln C1/C0 = -\ln (1 - URR)$, where
  K is the dialyzer clearance rate for urea (100 mL/min)
  V is the urea distribution volume (equivalent to total body water, i.e., 0.6 × 20 = 12 L)
  –ln is natural logarithm
  C0 and C1 are pre- and postdialysis blood urea concentrations (140 and 100 mg/dL, respectively), URR = C1/C0 = 0.7
  $t = -\ln C1/C0 \times V/K = 43$ min
  So, the first hemodialysis session for this child should be planned for ~43 minutes

Changes in prescription for subsequent sessions:

- Target higher URR (40% for second session; 70% for third session)
- To achieve the higher URR, use longer session length (up to 4 hours), higher blood flow rate (up to 7 mL/kg/min), and/or high-flux dialyzer

(AKI: acute kidney injury; URR: urea reduction ratio)

Adequacy of Hemodialysis

Small solute clearance is currently the best measure for HD adequacy. Urea reduction ratio and Kt/V are the most commonly used parameters to assess the adequacy of HD. Kidney Disease Outcomes Quality Initiative (KDOQI) recommends a single-pool Kt/V (spKt/V) target of 1.4 per HD session for patients treated thrice weekly, with a minimum delivered spKt/V of 1.2.[46] Assessment of dialysis adequacy in the pediatric population goes beyond the biochemical targets and incorporates clinical goals such as growth, bone health, cardiac function, and quality of life.[39,42] KDIGO workgroup on AKI suggests maintaining Kt/V of ≥1.3 if the patient is maintained on thrice-weekly HD schedule. Increasing dialysis frequency to 6 days/week in hemodynamically stable patients with AKI may not improve clinical outcomes and may delay renal recovery in comparison to those maintained on thrice-weekly HD with targeted spKt/V_{urea} of 1.2–1.4.[46]

Complications of Hemodialysis

Complications associated with HD are related to either catheter insertion or HD session. Catheter insertion–related complications include arterial puncture, pneumo- or hemothorax, air embolism, arrhythmias, and brachial plexus injury. Late catheter-related complications may occur in the form of infections, central venous stenosis, thrombosis, or stricture.

Common complications during HD are hypotension, muscle cramps, nausea and vomiting, headache, backache, chest pain, itching, and fever with chills. Intradialytic hypotension is the most common complication and is caused by hypovolemia due to rapid removal of blood in the extracorporeal circuit or excessive ultrafiltration. Dialysis disequilibrium syndrome (DDS) is a set of systemic and neurological manifestations, characterized by headache, vomiting, irritability, seizure, altered sensorium, or even coma, which results from cerebral edema due to decrease in plasma osmolality secondary to rapid fall in blood urea level. Gradual decrease in blood urea with lesser dialysis time for initial few sessions may prevent this complication.

SUSTAINED LOW-EFFICIENCY DIALYSIS

Sustained low-efficiency dialysis is a form of prolonged intermittent kidney replacement therapy (PIKRT) that has recently emerged as a cost-effective and technically simple alternative to CKRT.[47] The therapy is delivered using the standard HD machines and connections, but the dialysis efficiency is lower and administered over a prolonged session of 6–12 hours.[39] The slow solute and fluid removal in the therapy reduce solute and hemodynamic disequilibrium. The prolonged duration of therapy grants adequate dose, and the intermittent nature of therapy offers convenience for care and procedures in between. This hybrid therapy combines the advantage of HD and continuous venovenous hemofiltration (CVVH). In a child with hemodynamic instability who satisfies indications for KRT, PIKRT/SLED can be offered. SLED is technically feasible at any center where HD facility is available and appears to be more cost effective compared to CKRT. However, pediatric data on SLED and the data on drug dosing during PIKRT are scarce.

The prescription of SLED differs slightly from HD.[47] A low-flux dialyzer of size similar to HD is used. The blood flow rate is lower than that with HD, at 3–5 mL/kg (<30 kg body weight) to a maximum of 150 mL/min.[47] The dialysate flow is preferred to be kept at 1.5–2 times the blood flow rate, but this is often limited by the minimum dialysate flow rates offered by the machines (200 or 300 mL/min).[47] The minimum duration prescribed for the session should be at least 6 hours, and the sessions of SLED are performed on 4–7 days a week. While heparin is the preferred anticoagulant, frequent saline flushes with adjustment in ultrafiltration target can be prescribed in children at risk of active bleeding, to avoid anticoagulation. Hemofiltration can be added to SLED, referred to as SLED-F. Key components of its prescription, in contrast to CKRT, are listed in **Table 4**. Complications of SLED are similar to that of HD and include hypotension, circuit clots, hypokalemia, and hypophosphatemia.

CONTINUOUS KIDNEY REPLACEMENT THERAPY

Continuous kidney replacement therapy is indicated in critically ill and hemodynamically unstable children with AKI in whom metabolic and fluid abnormalities necessitate KRT. This procedure uses diffusive and convective clearance, either alone or in combination (**Table 4**). Diffusive and convective clearances are equally effective at small molecule clearance, but larger molecules are more effectively cleared via convection. In hemofiltration, physiologic, sterile solution is introduced into the vascular space, either pre- or postmembrane in the CKRT circuit; further, across a pressure gradient, solvent flow is generated through the membrane.[48] Large amounts of fluid can thus be removed over an extended amount of time, allowing hemodynamic stability in critically ill children. Compared to HD, CKRT is slow and inefficient but allows more hemodynamic stability **(Box 1)**. Compared to PD, CKRT is a more effective and controlled technique. CKRT can be offered in patients on multiple inotropes or in those not tolerating HD, PD, or SLED. It can also be offered for hyperammonemia, organic acidemia and maple syrup urine disease, since it enables sustained removal of accumulated metabolites in various inborn errors of metabolism.[48,49]

The vascular access and the method of therapy decide the nomenclature of the procedure which includes CVVH, continuous venovenous hemodialysis (CVVHD), continuous venovenous hemodiafiltration (CVVHDF), and slow continuous ultrafiltration (SCUF) **(Table 4)**.[48–50] Hemofiltration provides convective clearance, while hemodiafiltration employs both dialysis and hemofiltration. The prospective pediatric CKRT (ppCKRT) registry reports that 21% of patients received CVVH, 48% received CVVHD, and 30% received CVVHDF.[49]

Continuous kidney replacement therapy requires the use of dedicated machines, filters, and replacement and dialysate fluids. Vascular access requires to be secured, similar to HD. It is suggested that access in the internal jugular vein is associated with better circuit life compared to femoral access.[51] The filters or dialyzers in the CKRT circuit are made of biocompatible membranes, such as polyarylethersulfone or polysulfone. The circuit of CKRT usually has a high extracorporeal volume relative to body size and requires priming, particularly in small children. The blood flow rate preferred in infants is 10–12 mL/kg/min, in children 4–6 mL/kg/min, and in adolescents 2–4 mL/kg/min. The replacement fluid used is bicarbonate based and also

TABLE 4: Comparison of modalities of continuous kidney replacement therapies and sustained low-efficiency dialysis.

Characteristic	*SLED*	*SCUF*	*CVVH*	*CVVHD*	*CVVHDF*
Solute transport mechanism	Diffusion	Convection	Convection	Diffusion	Diffusion and convection
Blood flow rate (Q_B)	3–5 mL/kg/min	10–12 mL/kg/min; children: 4–6 mL/kg/min; adolescents: 2–4 mL/kg/min			
Dialysate flow rate (Q_D)	1.5–2 times Q_B	0	0	2,000 mL/m²/h	+*
Substitution fluid rate (Q_S)	0	0	2,000 mL/m²/h	0	+*
Ultrafiltration rate (Q_{UF})	0.5–2 mL/kg/h	0.5–2 mL/kg/h or 1–3% of blood volume; $<20\%$ of Q_B			
Net ultrafiltration rate (Q_{net})	Q_{uf}	Q_{uf}	$Q_{ef}–Q_s$	Q_{uf}	$Q_{ef}–Q_s$
Effluent rate (Q_{ef})	Q_{uf}	Q_{uf}	$Q_{uf} = Q_s + Q_{net}$	$Q_d \pm Q_{net}$	$Q_{uf} + Q_d$

*Q_D and Q_S together form a total of 2,000 mL/m²/h in CVVHDF.
(CVVH: continuous venovenous hemofiltration; CVVHD: continuous venovenous hemodialysis; CVVHDF: continuous venovenous hemodiafiltration; Q_D: amount of dialysate fluid instilled into filter countercurrent to flow of blood; Q_S: substitution fluid instilled into vascular space pre- or postfilter to replace ultrafiltrate volume; Q_{UF}: plasma water removed from circulating blood into the effluent bag, includes the quantity of pre- and postdilution substitution fluids, Q_s plus the desired net fluid removal, Q_{net}; SCUF, slow continuous ultrafiltration; SLED: sustained low-efficiency dialysis)

contains sodium, potassium, chloride, glucose, phosphate, calcium, and magnesium. CKRT dose is calculated to ensure that the sum of the replacement fluid and the dialysate is approximately 2,000 mL/1.73 m^2/h. The ultrafiltration rate is determined based on the fluid status and volume of all fluids administered. Anticoagulation options available are heparin, citrate, prostacyclin, and no anticoagulation. Avoidance of anticoagulation is associated with markedly inferior circuit life span and a reduced ability to deliver CKRT. Frequent monitoring of ACT is required if heparin anticoagulation is used. The most commonly reported complications are hypothermia, hypotension, blood clotting in the circuit and filter, hypokalemia, and hypophosphatemia.[52]

Information from the Veterans Affairs/National Institutes of Health Acute Renal Failure Trial Network (VA/NIH ATN) and RENAL trials clearly indicates that high-dose CKRT has no apparent additive benefit compared to usual dose as a standard of care.[53,54] As a result, KDIGO and Acute Dialysis Quality Initiative (ADQI) recommend achieving a target CKRT effluent flow rate of 20–25 mL/kg/h.[47,48] However, using effluent volume to calculate delivered dose of dialysis might lead to overestimation of session efficiency since circuit malfunction and membrane fouling might lead to differences in calculated dose.[55] Use of replacement fluid prefilter decreases the risk of filter clotting, at the cost of increased need of replacement requirement and slower clearance.

OUTCOMES

The outcomes of KRT in childhood AKI are difficult to quantify because of the lack of prospective comparative studies, heterogeneity in clinical profile in retrospective studies, use of different regimens in PD, intermittent HD, and CKRT that make direct comparisons difficult. A retrospective study, in which 81 children received PD, 31 children received hemodiafiltration, and 18 children received intermittent HD, reported better survival with intermittent HD.[56] Another retrospective study of 118 children, of whom 82 received PD and 36 received HD, did not find significant difference in mortality between the two modalities.[10] An RCT on 125 adults in which 62 were randomized to receive CVVH and 63 to receive tidal PD reported better survival at 28 days in the tidal PD group as compared to the CVVH group (70 vs. 47%; $p < 0.01$).[57] Systematic reviews comparing adult patients with SLED versus CKRT demonstrated survival benefit in SLED in observational studies; however, this was not replicated in RCTs.[58] There was no difference in renal recovery, fluid removal, and length of ICU stay. Patient outcomes following the initiation of CKRT are largely dependent on the underlying disease state and comorbid conditions, the indication for initiation, and a range of clinical criteria. Large observational studies in adults indicate mortality of 50–80%.[59] Data in the ppCKRT registry indicates an overall mortality of 42% in pediatric patients.[49]

CONCLUSION

Kidney replacement therapy is often indicated in patients with severe AKI, particularly in intensive care units. Indications for AKI are fairly clear, and there seems to be no real advantage to early initiation of KRT. The optimal modality for KRT in children with AKI remains unclear, particularly in critically ill patients. Options of KRT include PD, intermittent HD, SLED, and CKRT. While PD and intermittent HD are most commonly utilized, hybrid modalities, such as SLED, a form of PIKRT, are fast emerging as feasible alternative to CKRT in critically ill children. Retrospective studies in children and multiple trials in adult patients suggest that the various modalities of KRT are associated with comparable outcomes.

KEY POINTS

- AKI is an independent predictor of morbidity and mortality in pediatric acute care settings.
- KRT is indicated in AKI associated with life-threatening complications as it will correct symptomatic uremia, metabolic and electrolyte imbalance, and severe fluid overload.
- KRT modalities for managing pediatric patients with AKI include PD, intermittent HD, and continuous KRT.
- The choice of KRT modality is based on patient factors such as underlying illness, size of the child, access available, local expertise, experience, and available resources.
- Patient outcomes are dependent on the underlying disease state and comorbid conditions.
- Risk factors for mortality include the severity of underlying disease, hypotension significant fluid overload at the start of KRT, use of inotropes during KRT, and infancy.
- The optimal modality for KRT in children with AKI remains unclear, particularly in critically ill patients, and different modalities of KRT are associated with comparable outcomes.

REFERENCES

1. Kidney Disease Improving Global Outcome. (2012). KDIGO clinical practice guideline for acute kidney injury 2012. [online]. Available from: http://kdigo.org/ home/guidelines/acute-kidney-injury/. [Last accessed September 26, 2020].
2. Cortina G, McRae R, Hoq M, Donath S, Chiletti R, Arvandi M, et al. Mortality of critically ill children requiring continuous renal replacement therapy: effect of fluid overload, underlying disease, and timing of initiation. Pediatr Crit Care Med. 2019;20:314-22.
3. Zarbock A, Kellum JA, Schmidt C, Van Aken H, Wempe C, Pavenstädt H, et al. Effect of early vs delayed initiation of renal replacement therapy on mortality in critically ill patients with acute kidney injury: the ELAIN randomized clinical trial. JAMA. 2016;315:2190-9.
4. Gaudry S, Hajage D, Schortgen F, Martin-Lefevre L, Tubach F, Pons B, et al. Comparison of two strategies for initiating renal replacement therapy in the intensive care unit: study protocol for a randomized controlled trial (AKIKI). Trials. 2015;16:170.

5. Barbar SD, Clere-Jehl R, Bourredjem A, Hernu R, Montini F, Bruyère R, et al. Timing of renal replacement therapy in patients with acute kidney injury and sepsis. N Engl J Med. 2018;379:1431-42.
6. STARRT-AKI Investigators; Canadian Critical Care Trials Group; Australian and New Zealand Intensive Care Society Clinical Trials Group; United Kingdom Critical Care Research Group; Canadian Nephrology Trials Network; Irish Critical Care Trials Group; Bagshaw SM, Wald R, Adhikari NKJ, Bellomo R, da Costa BR, Dreyfuss D, et al. Timing of initiation of renal-replacement therapy in acute kidney injury. N Engl J Med. 2020;383:240-51.
7. Gaudry S, Hajage D, Benichou N, Chaïbi K, Barbar S, Zarbock A, et al. Delayed versus early initiation of renal replacement therapy for severe acute kidney injury: a systematic review and individual patient data meta-analysis of randomised clinical trials. Lancet. 2020;395:1506-15.
8. Macedo E, Mehta RL. Continuous dialysis therapies: core curriculum 2016. Am J Kidney Dis. 2016;68:645-57.
9. Mishra OP, Gupta AK, Pooniya V, Prasad R, Tiwary NK, Schaefer F. Peritoneal dialysis in children with acute kidney injury: a developing country experience. Perit Dial Int. 2012;32:431-6.
10. Vasudevan A, Phadke K, Yap H-K. Peritoneal dialysis for the management of pediatric patients with acute kidney injury. Pediatr Nephrol. 2017;32:1145-56.
11. Raina R, Chauvin AM, Bunchman T, Askenazi D, Deep A, Ensley MJ, et al. Treatment of AKI in developing and developed countries: an international survey of pediatric dialysis modalities. PLoS One. 2017;12:e0178233.
12. Cullis B, Abdelraheem M, Abrahams G, Balbi A, Cruz DN, Frishberg Y, et al. Peritoneal dialysis for acute kidney injury. Perit Dial Int. 2014;34:494-517.
13. Mishra OP, Prasad R. Acute peritoneal dialysis in neonates with acute kidney injury. Indian Pediatr. 2020;57:399-400.
14. Nourse P, Cullis B, Finkelstein F, Numanoglu A, Warady B, Antwi S, et al. ISPD guidelines for peritoneal dialysis in acute kidney injury: 2020 update (paediatrics). Perit Dial Int. 2021;41:139-57.
15. Prabhu MV, Subhramanyam SV, Antony S, Nayak KS. Manual acute PD with rigid catheters: a relook. Open Urol Nephrol J. 2015;8:41-4.
16. Ash SR. Chronic peritoneal dialysis catheters: overview of design, placement, and removal procedures. Semin Dial. 2003;16:323-34.
17. Al-Hwiesh AK. Percutaneous peritoneal dialysis catheter insertion by a nephrologist: a new, simple, and safe technique. Perit Dial Int J Int Soc Perit Dial. 2014;34:204-11.
18. Peppelenbosch A, van Kuijk WHM, Bouvy ND, van der Sande FM, Tordoir JHM. Peritoneal dialysis catheter placement technique and complications. NDT Plus. 2008;1:Siv23-8.
19. Obiagwu PN, Gwarzo GD, Akhiwu H, Wada A. Managing acute kidney injury in a child with improvised peritoneal dialysis in Kano, Nigeria. Niger J Basic Clin Sci. 2012;9:84.
20. Fredrick F, Valentine G. Improvised peritoneal dialysis in an 18-month-old child with severe acute malnutrition (kwashiorkor) and acute kidney injury: a case report. J Med Case Reports. 2013;7:168.
21. Mahmood U, Cho Y, Johnson DW. (2016). Peritoneal dialysis solutions. In: Ekart R (Ed). Some Special Problems in Peritoneal Dialysis. [online]. InTech. Available from: http://www.intechopen.com/books/some-special-problems-in-peritoneal-dialysis/peritoneal-dialysis-solutions. [Last accessed March, 2022].
22. Ponce D, Balbi AL, Amerling R. Advances in peritoneal dialysis in acute kidney injury. Blood Purif. 2012;34:107-16.
23. Burdmann EA, Chakravarthi R. Peritoneal dialysis in acute kidney injury: lessons learned and applied. Semin Dial. 2011; 24:149-56.
24. Bai ZG, Yang K, Tian JH, Ma B, Liu Y, Jiang L, et al. Bicarbonate versus lactate solutions for acute peritoneal dialysis. Cochrane Database Syst Rev. 2014;7:CD007034.
25. Khomba MM, Munthali CK, Mulenga C, Bjornstad EC. Where there is no peritoneal dialysis fluid: a case series from Malawi. Perit Dial Int. 2019;39:392-3.
26. McCulloch MI, Nourse P, Argent AC. Use of locally prepared peritoneal dialysis (PD) fluid for acute PD in children and infants in Africa. Perit Dial Int. 2020;40:441-5.
27. Ansari N. Peritoneal dialysis in renal replacement therapy for patients with acute kidney injury. Int J Nephrol. 2011;2011:1-10.
28. Quellhorst E. Insulin therapy during peritoneal dialysis: pros and cons of various forms of administration. J Am Soc Nephrol. 2002;13(Suppl 1):S92-6.
29. Golej J, Kitzmueller E, Hermon M, Boigner H, Burda G, Trittenwein G. Low-volume peritoneal dialysis in 116 neonatal and paediatric critical care patients. Eur J Pediatr. 2002;161:385-9.
30. Jiang L, Zeng R, Yang K, Mi DH, Tian JH, Ma B, et al. Tidal versus other forms of peritoneal dialysis for acute kidney injury. Cochrane Database Syst Rev. 2012;6:CD007016.
31. Chionh CY, Ronco C, Finkelstein FO, Soni SS, Cruz DN. Acute peritoneal dialysis: what is the "adequate" dose for acute kidney injury? Nephrol Dial Transplant. 2010;25:3155-60.
32. Gabriel DP, Caramori JT, Martim LC, Barretti P, Balbi AL. High volume peritoneal dialysis vs daily hemodialysis: a randomized, controlled trial in patients with acute kidney injury. Kidney Int. 2008;73:S87-93.
33. Cullis B, Ponce D, Finkelstein F. What is the adequate DOSE for peritoneal dialysis in acute kidney injury: lower the bar or shift the goalposts? Perit Dial Int J. 2017;37:491-3.
34. Cullis B, Al-Hwiesh A, Kilonzo K, McCulloch M, Niang A, Nourse P, et al. ISPD guidelines for peritoneal dialysis in acute kidney injury: 2020 update (adults). Perit Dial Int. 2021;41:15-31.
35. Li PK-T, Szeto CC, Piraino B, de Arteaga J, Fan S, Figueiredo AE, et al. ISPD peritonitis recommendations: 2016 update on prevention and treatment. Perit Dial Int. 2016;36:481-508.
36. Lee MM, Chua AN, Yorgin PD. Neonatal peritoneal dialysis. NeoReviews. 2005;6:e384-91.
37. Okan MA, Topçuoglu S, Karadag NN, Ozalkaya E, Karatepe HO, Vardar G, et al. Acute peritoneal dialysis in premature infants. Indian Pediatr. 2020;57:420-2.
38. Rath B, Gopalan S, Gupta S, Puri RK, Talukdar B. Simpler tools for peritoneal dialysis of term newborns and young infants. Indian Pediatr. 1994;31:1131-2.
39. Fischbach M, Edefonti A, Schröder C, Watson A, The European Pediatric Dialysis Working Group. Hemodialysis in children: general practical guidelines. Pediatr Nephrol. 2005;20;1054-66.
40. Golper TA, Fissell R, Fissell WH, Hartle PM, Sanders ML, Schulman G. Hemodialysis: core curriculum 2014. Am J Kidney Dis. 2014;63:153-63.
41. Sethi SK, Bunchman T, Raina R, Kher V. Unique considerations in renal replacement therapy in children: core curriculum 2014. Am J Kidney Dis. 2014;63:329-45.
42. Daugirdas JT, Blake PG, Ing TS (Eds). Handbook of Dialysis, 5th edition. Philadelphia, PA: Wolters Kluwer Health; 2015.
43. Indian Society of Nephrology. (2012). The Indian Society of Nephrology guidelines for hemodialysis units. [online]. Available from: http://isn-india.org/images/Image/Docs/HD_GL.pdf. [Last accessed April 28, 2020].

44. Kawanishi H, Moriishi M, Takahashi N, Tsuchiya S. Preparation and quality management of fluids for hemodialysis. Contrib Nephrol. 2017;189:153-9.
45. Association for the Advancement of Medical Instrumentation. (2014). ANSI/AAMI 13959: water for hemodialysis and related therapies. [online]. Available from: ANSI/AAMI 13959 - Water For Hemodialysis and Related Therapies - Dialysis Water Solutions. [Last accessed April 28, 2020].
46. National Kidney Foundation. KDOQI clinical practice guideline for hemodialysis adequacy: 2015 update. Am J Kidney Dis. 2015;66:884-930.
47. Sethi SK, Mittal A, Nair N, Bagga A, Iyenger A, Ali U, et al. Pediatric continuous renal replacement therapy (PCRRT) expert committee recommendation on prescribing prolonged intermittent renal replacement therapy (PIRRT) in critically ill children. Hemodial Int. 2020;24:237-51.
48. Sutherland SM, Alexander SR. Continuous renal replacement therapy in children. Pediatr Nephrol. 2012;27:2007-16.
49. Symons JM, Chua AN, Somers MJG, Baum MA, Bunchman TE, Benfield MR, et al. Demographic characteristics of pediatric continuous renal replacement therapy: a report of the prospective pediatric continuous renal replacement therapy registry. Clin J Am Soc Nephrol. 2007;2:732-8.
50. Moore PK, Hsu RK, Liu KD. Management of acute kidney injury: core curriculum 2018. Am J Kidney Dis. 2018;72:136-48.
51. Hackbarth R, Bunchman TE, Chua AN, Somers MJ, Baum M, Symons JM, et al. The effect of vascular access location and size on circuit survival in pediatric continuous renal replacement therapy: a report from the PPCRRT registry. Int J Artif Organs. 2007;30:1116-21.
52. Ricci Z, Goldstein SL. Pediatric continuous renal replacement therapy. Contrib Nephrol. 2016;187:121-30.
53. Bellomo R, Cass A, Cole L, Finfer S, Gallagher M, Lo S, et al. Intensity of continuous renal-replacement therapy in critically ill patients. N Engl J Med. 2009;361:1627-38.
54. Palevsky P, Zhang J, O'Connor T, Chertow GM, Crowley ST, Choudhury D, et al. Intensity of renal support in critically ill patients with acute kidney injury. N Engl J Med. 2008;359:7-20.
55. Claure-Del Granado R, Macedo E, Chertow GM, Soroko S, Himmelfarb J, Ikizler TA, et al. Effluent volume in continuous renal replacement therapy overestimates the delivered dose of dialysis. Clin J Am Soc Nephrol. 2011;6:467-75.
56. Krause I, Herman N, Cleper R, Fraser A, Davidovits M. Impact of dialysis type on outcome of acute renal failure in children: a single-center experience. Isr Med Assoc J. 2011;13:4.
57. l-Hwiesh A, Abdul-Rahman I, Finkelstein F, Divino-Filho J, Qutub H, Al-Audah N, et al. Acute kidney injury in critically ill patients: a prospective randomized study of tidal peritoneal dialysis versus continuous renal replacement therapy. Ther Apher Dial. 2018;22:371-9.
58. Nash DM, Przech S, Wald R, O'Reilly D. Systematic review and meta-analysis of renal replacement therapy modalities for acute kidney injury in the intensive care unit. J Crit Care. 2017;41:138-44.
59. Iwagami M, Yasunaga H, Noiri E, Horiguchi H, Fushimi K, Matsubara T, et al. Current state of continuous renal replacement therapy for acute kidney injury in Japanese intensive care units in 2011: analysis of a national administrative database. Nephrol Dialysis Transplant. 2015;30:988-95.

CHAPTER

11.6 Oncology-related Acute Kidney Injury

Raji RP, Susan Uthup

INTRODUCTION

Acute kidney injury (AKI) is common in children with malignancies. There is growing concern regarding the burden of AKI in this group of patients in view of the high morbidity and mortality. The advancement in cancer diagnosis and treatment has significantly improved outcomes in the last two decades. Both traditional and nontraditional risk factors contribute to AKI. The diagnostic modalities using contrast agents as well as newer therapies have increased the risk of AKI.

ETIOLOGY AND CLASSIFICATION OF ACUTE KIDNEY INJURY IN MALIGNANCY

Acute kidney injury occurs in cancer patients due to prerenal, intrinsic renal, or postrenal factors. Causes of oncology-related AKI are given in **Box 1**. Several pathophysiological factors operate concurrently or develop subsequently in oncology-related AKI. The probability of developing AKI depends on the type and severity of malignancy as well as the therapy administered. AKI incidence in solid tumors is less than that of hematological malignancies.

Sepsis is very common in cancer patients who are immunocompromised due to cancer or anticancer treatment. In sepsis, combination of both hemodynamic and inflammatory factors contributes to the development of AKI. Anticancer treatment coupled with increased use of antibiotics leads to microbiome disruption and high risk of sepsis in oncology patients. Early diagnosis and prompt treatment of infections are important in AKI prevention. Optimizing fluid therapy, avoiding or stopping nephrotoxic drugs, and timely initiation of kidney replacement therapy (KRT) are crucial in managing sepsis-associated AKI (SAKI).[1] About 75% of hematopoietic stem-cell transplant patients who required intensive care unit (ICU) care developed AKI and mortality rate was 95% in those who received KRT.[2]

BOX 1: Causes of acute kidney injury in children with malignancies.

Prerenal causes:
- Renal hypoperfusion due to sepsis, ascites, and effusions
- Volume depletion (↓ oral intake, diarrhea, and overdiuresis)
- Impaired cardiac output
- Renal vein thrombosis
- Hepatic sinusoidal obstructive syndrome
- Hypercalcemia
- Non-chemo drugs (NSAIDs, ACEI/ARB, calcineurin inhibitors)
- Capillary leak syndrome (e.g., due to IL-2)

Intrinsic causes:
- Acute tubular necrosis due to:
  - Ischemia
  - Nephrotoxic agents, e.g., IV contrast, ifosfamide, cisplatin, and aminoglycoside
- Infiltration of the kidney (e.g., lymphoma)
- Cancer-associated glomerular diseases
- Acute interstitial nephritis
- Tumor lysis syndrome
- Graft versus host disease
- Thrombotic microangiopathy
- Calcineurin inhibitor toxicity

Postrenal causes:
Obstruction due to:
- Primary or metastatic abdominal or pelvic malignancy
- Retroperitoneal fibrosis
- Crystals (acyclovir, urate, and methotrexate)

(ACEI: angiotensin-converting enzyme inhibitor; ARB: angiotensin receptor blocker; IL: interleukin; IV: intravenous; NSAIDs: nonsteroidal anti-inflammatory drugs)

Prerenal Acute Kidney Injury

Renal hypoperfusion is the major mechanism in prerenal AKI. Both cancer-related and treatment-related factors may contribute to renal ischemia. Reduced food intake, malnutrition, cachexia, vomiting caused by chemotherapy, diarrhea, hypovolemia, and hypotension contribute to renal hypoperfusion. Hemorrhage, thrombosis in tumor, hepatorenal syndrome in liver cancer, paraneoplastic syndrome, hypercalcemia, and ischemic injury following nephrectomy may also lead to AKI.

Acute kidney injury is also common in the postsurgical period. Prolonged perioperative fasting and fluid loss can cause hypovolemia. Prolonged intensive thermal ablation intraoperatively causes reduction in intravascular volume, hyperviscosity, excessive destruction of blood cell components, and acid–base imbalance. There will be changes in glomerular filtration, microvascular endothelial cell damage, and urinary cast formation, finally culminating in oliguric AKI.

Treatment-related complications such as graft-versus-host disease (GVHD) occur after bone marrow transplantation (BMT) and hematopoietic stem cell transplantation (HSCT). Veno-occlusive disease (VOD) or sinusoidal obstruction syndrome and marrow infusion syndrome may lead to AKI. Capillary leak syndrome (CLS) caused by immunotherapeutic agents such as interleukin-2 (IL-2) also may cause renal hypoperfusion. Angiotensin-converting enzyme inhibitors, angiotensin receptor blockers, and diuretics are other prerenal risk factors.

Intrinsic Acute Kidney Injury

Intrinsic renal injury is the most important cause of AKI associated with malignancies. Glomerular, tubulointerstitial, and vascular damage as well as postrenal obstruction can occur due to malignancy-related and treatment-related factors. Renal infiltration by the tumor and nephrectomy reduces functional renal mass and leads to reduced function. Structural changes in renal tissue will also lead to reduced renal function.

Cancer-associated Glomerulonephritis

There is a recent increase in microvascular diseases and glomerulonephropathy in cancer patients. Glomerular injury is usually caused by paraneoplastic glomerular disorders. Chemotherapeutic drugs can also cause glomerular damage. Focal segmental glomerulosclerosis (FSGS) and minimal change disease (MCD) are sometimes seen associated with hematological malignancies. MCD, FSGS, membranoproliferative glomerulonephritis (MPGN), and immunoglobulin A (IgA) nephropathy are seen in association with Hodgkin's and non-Hodgkin's disease.[3] Membranous nephropathy and FSGS may occur in association with acute myeloid leukemia (AML). Wilms' tumor is associated with MPGN. Pheochromocytoma is associated with membranous nephropathy. HSCT is associated with membranous nephropathy and rarely MCD.

Prerenal AKI may occur in gastrointestinal GVHD. Proteinuria and glomerulonephritis are also seen in GVHD.[4] In GVHD, excessive release of proinflammatory cytokines such as transforming growth factor-β, tumor necrosis factor-α, and interleukin-6 (IL-6) induces renal damage.[5] Checkpoint inhibitors (CPIs) are novel biologic anticancer agents. They inhibit the regulatory interactions that limit T-cell cytotoxicity to tumors. The main targets of CPI are CTLA-4, PD-1, and its ligand, PD-L1. They may induce nephrotic syndrome with FSGS, MCD and membranous nephropathy, IgA nephropathy, lupus nephropathy, and pauci-immune glomerulonephritis. AKI due to these agents is, however, rare.[6]

Tubulointerstitial Acute Kidney Injury

The most common etiology of AKI in children with malignancy without renal infiltration or not undergoing nephrectomy is acute tubular necrosis (ATN). ATN may be due to ischemic or toxic injury. Drug-induced AKI is also common. Other causes include tumor infiltration of kidneys as in leukemia and lymphoma. Tumor lysis syndrome (TLS) is an important cause of malignancy-associated AKI and is one of the most common oncological emergencies. It occurs due to sudden release of the intracellular contents from dying cancer cells into the bloodstream. TLS may occur either spontaneously or in response to oncology treatment. Incidence of TLS may be as high as 26% as in high-grade B-cell acute lymphoblastic leukemia.[7] CPIs—such as anti-CTLA-4 monoclonal antibody ipilimumab, anti-PD-1 antibodies pembrolizumab and nivolumab and the anti-PD-L1 antibodies durvalumab and atezolizumab—are associated with TLS. These agents reactivate cytotoxic T cells and cause tumor cell lysis by blunting the braking mechanisms of the immune system.[8]

Acute tubulointerstitial nephritis (ATIN) is an important cause of oncology-related AKI. ATIN may be caused by targeted drugs or standard agents. Common drugs associated with TIN are antibiotics, proton-pump inhibitors, and CNIs. ATIN is also induced by immunotherapeutic agents such as CTLA-4 inhibitors and programmed death (PD)-1 inhibitors (nivolumab and pembrolizumab).[7,8]

Both BK virus and adenovirus are important in pediatric oncology. There is asymptomatic carriage of both these viruses. Immunosuppression as in HSCT recipients may reactivate these latent viruses causing hemorrhagic cystitis and sometimes acute interstitial nephritis (AIN).

Drug-induced Acute Kidney Injury

The common drugs causing ATN are listed in **Box 2.** Conventional cancer drugs may induce ATN. These drugs cause immediate toxic effects on the kidney and also on repeated administration, they reduce the renal functional reserve. This reduced reserve may increase renal susceptibility to further insults such as nephrotoxic targeted therapies or sepsis. Renin-angiotensin-aldosterone system (RAAS) antagonists may induce AKI when given in dehydrated, hypotensive children, especially in combination with other nephrotoxic medications such as nonsteroidal anti-inflammatory drugs (NSAIDs). There will be worsening of renal function in children with progressing AKI or advancing chronic kidney disease (CKD). There may also be the danger of life-threatening hyperkalemia in these situations.

Vascular Injury

The most common syndrome of vascular injury causing AKI in malignancy is thrombotic microangiopathy (TMA).[9] Kidneys are most often affected.[10] The usual causes of TMA are CNIs, interferon, mitomycin-C, gemcitabine, antivascular endothelial growth factor agents, tyrosine kinase inhibitors, and antiviral drugs for CMV and adenovirus. Acute GVHD, total body irradiation, or VOD/sinusoidal obstruction syndrome are

BOX 2: Commonly used cancer therapies associated with renal toxicity.

- *Tubular injury*
  - *Acute tubular injury:* Platinum, zoledronate, ifosfamide, mithramycin, pentostatin, imatinib, diaziquone, pemetrexed, zoledronate, vancomycin, aminoglycosides, ACEI/ARB, and contrast materials
- *Tubular syndromes*
  - *Renal tubular acidosis:* Ifosfamide, amphotericin, and calcineurin inhibitors
  - *Fanconi syndrome:* Cisplatin, ifosfamide, azacitidine, diaziquone, imatinib, and pemetrexed
  - *Salt wasting:* Cisplatin and azacitidine
  - *Magnesium wasting:* Cetuximab, cisplatin, and panitumumab
  - *Nephrogenic diabetes insipidus:* Cisplatin, ifosfamide, and pemetrexed
  - *Acute interstitial nephritis:* Sorafenib, sunitinib, and checkpoint inhibitors
  - *Crystalline nephropathy:* Methotrexate, acyclovir, and sulfa-based drugs
  - *Syndrome of inappropriate antidiuretic hormone:* Cyclophosphamide and vincristine
- *Glomerular injury*
  - *Focal segmental glomerulosclerosis:* Interferon (IFN) pamidronate, tyrosine kinase inhibitors
  - *Minimal change disease:* IFN, pamidronate
  - *Proteinuria:* Sorafenib, sunitinib, and axitinib
- *Renal vascular injury*
  - *Thrombotic microangiopathy:* Bevacizumab (anti-VEGF monoclonal antibody)
  - *Tyrosine kinase inhibitors:* Sorafenib, sunitinib, and imatinib
  - *Other agents:* Gemcitabine, mitomycin C, interferon-α, calcineurin inhibitors

(ACEI: angiotensin-converting enzyme inhibitor; ARB: angiotensin receptor blocker)

TABLE 1: Causes of acute kidney injury in relation to the timing of hematopoietic stem cell transplantation.

Time	*AKI etiology*
Before and hours after HSCT	• Tumor lysis syndrome from conditioning regimen (rare) • Systemic toxicity from conditioning regimen [e.g., volume depletion (common)] • DMSO (dimethylsulfoxide) toxicity from hemolysis, acidosis, and pigment nephropathy (rare)
Days to weeks after HSCT	• Prerenal AKI from volume depletion • AKI from neutropenic-sepsis • Drug toxicity (common) • AKI related to engraftment syndrome (rare)
Weeks to months after HSCT	• Sepsis • Volume depletion • Drug and radiocontrast toxicity (common) • AKI from sinusoidal obstruction syndrome of the liver • Graft versus host disease (GVHD) • Thrombotic microangiopathy • BK virus nephropathy (rare)
Months to years after HSCT	• CKD from previous AKIs • Calcineurin inhibitor toxicity especially with GVHD

(AKI: acute kidney injury; CKD: chronic kidney disease; HSCT: hematopoietic stem cell transplantation)

other causes of TMA. Another reason for AKI is disseminated intravascular coagulation (DIC) secondary to malignancy.

Acute Kidney Injury in Hematopoietic Stem Cell Transplantation

The incidence of AKI following HSCT ranges from 11 to 84%. Among these, 5–10% usually require KRT.[11,12] Prerenal AKI is very common after HSCT. Excessive diuresis related to treatment, chemotherapy-induced GI losses, and TLS, especially when there is failure of remission before conditioning, are the underlying causes.[2]

Other important complications in the early post-transplant period are engraftment syndrome and CLS.[13] Both are manifested by peripheral edema and diuretic-resistant effusions. These are mediated by proinflammatory cytokines.[14] In haploidentical HSCT, CLS is very important as a part of cardiorenal syndrome (CRS). Clinically significant renal failure occurs in 14% CRS. Steroids and anti-IL-6 therapies are used for treatment.[15]

Presentation of engraftment syndrome is almost similar to CLS but usually occurs during neutrophil regeneration. Engraftment syndrome usually presents with fever with rash and multiorgan dysfunction. Derangement in renal function occurs in 8% of allo-HSCT recipients[16] and in 27% of auto-HSCT recipients. Glucocorticoids, if started early, will show better results in engraftment syndrome.

One serious complication of HSCT is VOD/sinusoidal obstruction syndrome. The incidence of VOD is 14% in traditional myeloablative conditioning allo-HSCT and carries a high mortality rate of >80%.[17] The mechanism of renal injury in VOD is almost similar to that which occurs in hepatorenal syndrome. Endothelial damage and coagulation lead to obstruction of hepatic sinuses and portal hypertension.[18] There is renal hypoperfusion secondary to splanchnic vasodilatation and decreased effective arterial blood volume. No structural renal changes are identified.[19]

Managing fluid balance is of prime importance in patients receiving HSCT. Preoperative dehydration can contribute to postoperative AKI. Salt and fluid restriction combined with judicious use of diuretics is the cornerstone to prevent volume overload in VOD-associated AKI.[20] Judicious use of fluids and timely initiation of continuous kidney replacement therapy (CKRT) will be beneficial in critically ill patients with AKI. Early initiation of treatment with defibrotide will be useful in hepatic VOD/SOS with pulmonary/renal dysfunction.[21] The causes of AKI in relation to the timing of HSCT are given in **Table 1**.

Postrenal Acute Kidney Injury

The major cause of post-renal AKI is urinary tract obstruction (UTO). Urinary tract malignancies with enlarged lymph nodes and retroperitoneal fibrosis are important causes. Obstruction by clots from bleeding malignant tissues or drug-induced hemorrhagic cystitis can also lead to UTO. Imaging modalities such as X-ray, ultrasonography, computed tomography, or magnetic resonance imaging are required for confirming the diagnosis.

Another common complication after allogeneic HSCT is BK virus-associated hemorrhagic cystitis (BK-HC).[22] UTO and postrenal AKI develop following massive hematuria.[23] Viral copies can be quantitatively measured in plasma or urine. If viremia is detectable, asymptomatic BK virus carrier state is considered as a risk factor for AKI after HSCT.[24]

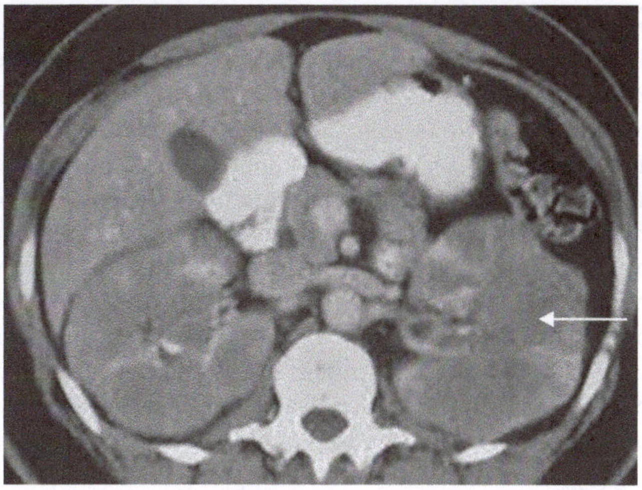

Fig. 1: Computed tomography (CT) scan demonstrating bilateral renomegaly due to infiltration of the renal parenchyma in a child with lymphoma and acute kidney injury (AKI).

ACUTE KIDNEY INJURY IN LEUKEMIA AND LYMPHOMA

Hypoperfusion, TLS, direct infiltration of malignant cells, and hemophagocytic syndrome are the common causes for AKI in hematological malignancies. Intrinsic renal causes such as ATN (especially from sepsis and nephrotoxic medications) or postrenal causes due to mechanical obstruction from lymphadenopathy or retroperitoneal fibrosis also contribute. Renal infiltrative disease is also a cause of AKI in leukemia or lymphoma. Leukemic or lymphomatous infiltration is suggested by renomegaly on imaging **(Fig. 1)**. Most often, renal infiltration is asymptomatic or subclinical. Urine analysis shows bland urine sediment and tubular proteinuria. AKI is thought to be due to tubular compression and increased interstitial pressure from the massive malignant cell infiltration. Renal histology often clinches the diagnosis **(Fig. 2)**.

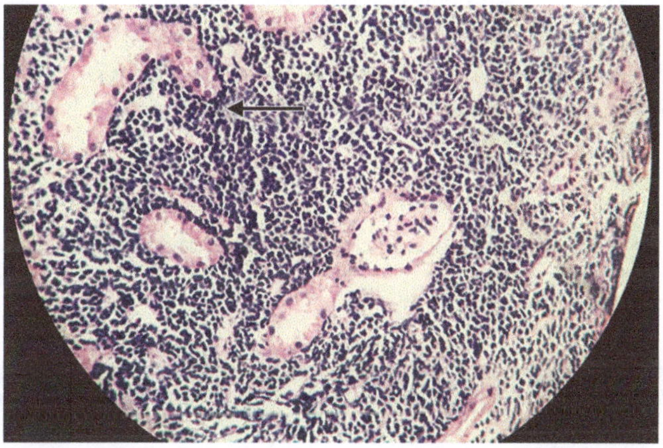

Fig. 2: Renal biopsy demonstrating B-cell lymphoma cells within the renal parenchyma (hematoxylin and eosin stain × 400) in a 4-year-old boy with renomegaly and acute kidney injury.

Lysozyme, a cationic protein that is easily filtered and reabsorbed in the renal proximal tubule, is produced in excess in these malignancies. Excess lysozyme in the tubules causes ATN and/or proximal tubular injury with full-blown Fanconi syndrome. Intrarenal leukostasis as in AML [white blood cell (WBC) count >100,000] is another cause of AKI. Renal leukostasis is associated with reduced renal perfusion and blast aggregation within the renal microvasculature. Endothelial damage is triggered by soluble cytokines. Emergent treatment with cytoreductive chemotherapy and leukopheresis is generally required.

TUMOR LYSIS SYNDROME AND ACUTE KIDNEY INJURY

Tumor lysis syndrome is caused by the massive and abrupt release of cellular components into the blood following rapid lysis of malignant cells. It is characterized by hyperuricemia, hyperkalemia, hyperphosphatemia, hypocalcemia, and uremia. After initiation of chemotherapy, massive release of nucleic acids, proteins, phosphorus, and potassium occurs from cancer cells. TLS commonly occurs in cancers with high proliferative rate, malignancies with large tumor burden, or tumors with high sensitivity to cytotoxic therapy. Uric acid or calcium phosphate crystalizes in renal tubules, which further leads to renal dysfunction. Precipitation of calcium leads to secondary hypocalcemia. TLS occurs most frequently in NHL, particularly Burkitt's lymphoma. TLS also occurs in other hematologic malignancies such as acute lymphocytic leukemia (ALL) and AML. Patients with elevated uric acid levels (8 mg/dL) and high phosphorus levels are at high risk for developing TLS. Symptoms of TLS may occur before the initiation of chemotherapy. Usually, symptoms occur within 12–72 hours after the initiation of treatment.[25] The clinical manifestations include lethargy, muscle cramps, tetany, nausea, vomiting, diarrhea, edema, hematuria, fluid overload, congestive heart failure, seizures, syncope, cardiac arrhythmias, and sudden death.

Classification of Tumor Lysis Syndrome

The children's oncology group currently uses the Cairo and Bishop Classification system **(Tables 2 and 3)**.[26] It is the most recent and preferred system that defines laboratory or clinical TLS (LTLS or CTLS). When two or more serum values of uric acid, potassium, and phosphate are more than normal or calcium is less than normal at presentation or if they change by 25% within 3 days before or 7 days after the initiation of treatment, LTLS is considered. For the diagnosis of CTLS, presence of LTLS in addition to one or more of the following significant clinical complications such as renal insufficiency, cardiac arrhythmias/sudden death, and/or seizures should be present. LTLS is diagnosed as either present or absent, and the maximal grade of clinical manifestation is used to define CTLS.[27]

TABLE 2: Cairo–Bishop definition of laboratory tumor lysis syndrome.

Element	*Value*	*Change from baseline*
Uric acid	≥476 µmol/L or 8 mg/dL	25% increase
Potassium	≥6.0 mmol/L or 6 mEq/L	25% increase
Phosphorus	≥2.1 mmol/L (6.5 mg/dL) for children or ≥1.45 mmol/L (4.5 mg/dL) for adults	25% increase
Calcium	≤1.75 mmol/L (7 mg/dL)	25% decrease

Note: Two or more laboratory changes within 3 days before or 7 days after cytotoxic therapy.

Prevention and Management of Tumor Lysis Syndrome

Identifying the risk factors, very close monitoring of high-risk patients, and timely interventions are the important measures to prevent or manage TLS. Risk factors for TLS are given in **Table 4.**

The key elements in the prevention and management of TLS are aggressive hydration and diuresis. Vigorous hydration and enhanced urine flow help in the excretion of uric acid and phosphate. Hydration should be done with caution in patients with renal failure or oliguria. Administer 2–3 L/m²/day IV or 200 mL/kg/day in <10 kg child. Urine output is to be maintained within 80–100 mL/m²/h (4–6 mL/kg/h if below 10 kg). Diuretics can be used to maintain output provided there is no hypovolemia or urinary obstruction. During initial hydration, potassium, calcium, and phosphate should be avoided from fluids. Monitor urine-specific gravity and keep it <1.010. Currently, alkalinization is not recommended routinely to promote uric acid excretion due to fear of calcium phosphate precipitation. So, sodium bicarbonate is given only for correction of metabolic acidosis if present.

Allopurinol is a xanthine analog, which in vivo is converted to oxypurinol which in turn competitively inhibits xanthine oxidase. The conversion of the purine metabolites xanthine

TABLE 3: Cairo–Bishop definition and grading of clinical tumor lysis syndrome.

	Grade					
Complication	***0***	***1***	***2***	***3***	***4***	***5***
Creatinine*	≤1.5 × ULN†	1.5 × ULN	>1.5–3 × ULN	>3.0–6.0 × ULN	>6.0 × ULN	Death
Cardiac arrhythmia*	None	Intervention not indicated	Nonurgent medical intervention indicated	Symptomatic and incompletely controlled medically or controlled with device (e.g., defibrillator)	Life-threatening (e.g., arrhythmia associated with HF, hypotension, syncope, and shock)	Death
Seizure*	None	–	One brief generalized seizure; seizure(s) well controlled by anticonvulsants or infrequent focal motor seizures not interfering with ADL	Seizure in which consciousness is altered; poorly controlled seizure disorder; with breakthrough generalized seizures despite medical intervention	Seizure of any kind which are prolonged, repetitive or difficult to control (e.g., status epilepticus, intractable epilepsy)	Death

Note: Clinical tumor lysis syndrome (CTLS) *requires one or more clinical manifestations* along with criteria for laboratory tumor lysis syndrome (LTLS). Maximal CTLS manifestation (renal, cardiac, and neuro) defines the grade.
*Not directly or probably attributable to therapeutic agent.
†If no institutional ULN is specified, age/sex ULN creatinine may be defined as follows >1 to <12 years both male and female, 0.69 mg/dL; 12 to <16 years both male and female, 0.99 mg/dL; ≥16 years female 1.19 mg/dL, male 1.29 mg/dL.
(ADL: activities of daily living; CHF: congestive heart failure; ULN: upper limit of normal)

and hypoxanthine to uric acid is blocked by allopurinol. So, allopurinol is used to decrease uric acid formation and hence renal failure due to crystal-induced obstruction. The dose of allopurinol is 50–100 mg/m^2 every 8 hours orally (maximum dose, 300 mg/m^2/day) or 10 mg/kg/day divided every 8 hours (maximum dose—800 mg/day). If unable to take orally, IV allopurinol at a dose of 200–400 mg/m^2/day in one to three divided doses (maximum dose—600 mg/day) is given. In intermediate-risk patients, allopurinol needs to be started 12–24 hours before the induction therapy. Allopurinol is to be continued until uric acid levels are normalized and tumor burden, WBC count, and other laboratory values are in the range for TLS risk and for up to 3–7 days afterward. In patients with renal failure, 50% dose reduction of allopurinol is required.

Allopurinol will not reduce uric acid produced before the treatment initiation but only prevents further uric acid formation. Allantoin is a uric acid metabolite, which is 5–10 times more soluble than uric acid in urine. Uric acid is converted into allantoin by the enzyme urate oxidase. Rasburicase is a recombinant form of urate oxidase that is useful for reducing uric acid in patients with severe hyperuricemia (>7.5 mg/dL). For the initial management of patients who are considered to be at high risk of developing TLS or with LTLS or CTLS, rasburicase is now recommended **(Tables 4 and 5)**. The intermediate-risk group patients are given rasburicase only if hyperuricemia develops even after prophylactic treatment with allopurinol. Glucose-6-phosphate dehydrogenase (G6PD) deficiency is a contraindication for the use of rasburicase and hence screening for G6PD deficiency is recommended before its use. The recommended dose is 0.15–0.2 mg/kg once daily in 50 mL of normal saline as an IV infusion over 30 minutes for five doses. Regular monitoring of the serum uric acid is required. Adverse drug reactions are rare with rasburicase. These include anaphylaxis, rash, respiratory distress, hemolysis, neutropenia, fever, sepsis, methemoglobinemia, and mucositis.

TABLE 4: Risk factors for tumor lysis syndrome.

Characteristic	*Risk factor*
Tumor type	• Burkitt's lymphoma, lymphoblastic lymphoma, diffuse large-cell lymphoma, ALL • Solid tumors with high proliferative rates and rapid response to therapy
Tumor burden/extent of disease	• Bulky disease (>10 cm) • Elevated LDH (>2 × ULN) • Elevated WBC (>25,000/μL)
Renal function	Preexisting renal failure/oliguria
Serum/plasma uric acid	Baseline uric acid >450 μmol/L (7.5 mg/dL)
Effective and rapid cytoreductive therapy	Disease-specific therapy, varies according to tumor type

(ALL: acute lymphoblastic leukemia; LDH: lactate dehydrogenase; WBC: white blood cell)

Asymptomatic hyperphosphatemia is treated by ensuring adequate hydration, avoiding phosphate from intravenous fluids, and the use of phosphate binders such as calcium carbonate and sevelamer hydroxide. Hemodialysis, peritoneal dialysis, or continuous venovenous hemofiltration may be used for severe hyperphosphatemia. However, phosphate clearance is more with hemodialysis when compared to other modalities.

Hyperkalemia is usually seen in TLS. All potassium sources (both oral and IV) should be eliminated. For asymptomatic hyperkalemia, sodium polystyrene sulfonate 1 g/kg can be used orally or rectally. The rectal route is avoided in those with neutropenia and in neonates. For symptomatic patients or if serum potassium is >7.0–7.5 mEq/L or the ECG shows changes such as widening of QRS complex, intravenous calcium gluconate and glucose insulin infusion are recommended.

After 4–6 hours of initial administration of chemotherapy, the laboratory and clinical TLS parameters need to be checked. These include uric acid, phosphate, potassium, calcium, creatinine, and lactate dehydrogenase (LDH). Fluid input and urine output should also be monitored. The uric acid level is to be rechecked after 4 hours of rasburicase administration and after that every 6–8 hours till TLS is resolved. Cytotoxic chemotherapy in high-risk patients should be administered

TABLE 5: Patient stratification by risk.

Type of cancer	*Risk*		
	High	Intermediate	Low
NHL	Burkitt's lymphoma lymphoblastic, B-ALL	Diffuse large B-cell lymphoma	Indolent NHL
ALL	WBC ≥ 100,000	WBC 50,000–100,000	WBC ≤ 50,000
AML	WBC 50,000, monoblastic	WBC 10,000–50,000	WBC ≤ 10,000
Hematologic malignancies and solid tumors		Rapid proliferation with expected rapid response to therapy	Remainder of patients

(ALL: acute lymphoblastic leukemia; AML: acute myeloid leukemia; NHL: non-Hodgkin lymphoma; WBC: white blood cell)

in a center with access to dialysis. After the introduction of rasburicase, the need for dialysis is reduced. Dialysis is indicated if urine output is progressively decreasing (oliguria or anuria) and there is high urea (>150 mg/dL) which is persisting, hyperphosphatemia (>10 mg/dL) or hyperkalemia (>7 mmol/L), or severe hypocalcemia which is life-threatening in spite of optimal conservative measures.

CANCER THERAPY AND ACUTE KIDNEY INJURY

Different anticancer treatments may predispose to AKI. Nephrectomy predisposes to chemotherapy-induced renal damage as there is reduction in total renal parenchyma. Commonly used cancer therapies associated with renal toxicity are given in **Box 2**. Renal injury caused by ifosfamide, cisplatin, and methotrexate (MTX) is briefly discussed here.

Ifosfamide-induced Nephrotoxicity

Ifosfamide is an alkylating, agent which is a cyclophosphamide analog.[28,29] Both cyclophosphamide and ifosfamide are associated with severe hemorrhagic cystitis. 2-mercapto-ethanesulfonate (MESNA) is used to prevent hemorrhagic cystitis. Ifosfamide causes renal epithelial cell damage and chronic nephrotoxicity due to formation of large amounts of chloroacetaldehyde.[30] This metabolite is not produced from cyclophosphamide.[31] Even though any of the nephron segments can be affected, the principal site affected is proximal renal tubule which manifests as proximal RTA and Fanconi's syndrome. The most common manifestation of ifosfamide nephrotoxicity is hypophosphatemia.[32,33] Hypophosphatemic rickets can develop. Distal tubule involvement leads to reduced urinary concentration, distal renal tubular acidosis (RTA), and rarely nephrogenic diabetes insipidus. Age, cumulative drug dose (total drug doses >60 g/m^2), concomitant use of cisplatin, preexisting kidney dysfunction, prior nephrectomy, or renal malformations such as Denys–Drash or WAGR appear to be important risk factors for ifosfamide nephrotoxicity. Children under the age of 5 years are more vulnerable to ifosfamide-induced proximal tubular damage. The primary event is tubular damage and can progress even several months after stopping the therapy. It subsequently leads to reduced glomerular function. Aminoaciduria is the first marker of nephrotoxicity. Avoid concurrent administration of other nephrotoxic drugs (e.g., cisplatin). The suspension of ifosfamide therapy and continuation with cyclophosphamide is considered if there is severe nephrotoxicity. Even after cessation of treatment, the children should be monitored for hypertension, electrolyte disturbances, proteinuria, and derangements of creatinine.

Cisplatin Nephrotoxicity

Cisplatin (CDDP—cis-diamminedichloroplatinum II) is a commonly used anticancer drug in pediatric oncology practice. There are three mechanisms for cisplatin toxicity: (1) cellular toxicity, (2) vasoconstriction, and (3) increased release of proinflammatory cytokines (caspases, tumor necrosis factor-α, IL-6, and interferon-γ).

Cellular toxicity: Cisplatin is highly protein-bound drug and only the unbound platinum has got anticancer properties.[34] Inside the cells, the low chloride concentration facilitates CDDP hydrolysis with generation of charged species. This hydrolysis product is the active form, which reacts with glutathione in the cytoplasm and DNA in the nucleus. Enhanced elimination of low-molecular-weight peptides and reduced excretion of Tamm–Horsfall protein contribute to renal damage.[35,36] The sulfhydryl groups bound to the platinum enter inside the tubule cells through an active transport mechanism with subsequent cellular distribution of the platinum metabolites.

The most common electrolyte disturbance with cisplatin therapy is hypomagnesemia. In severe cases, it leads to tetany or convulsions. Renal magnesium wasting is due to a defect in magnesium transport in juxtamedullary nephrons or collecting ducts.[37] Cumulative dose of cisplatin is the deciding element of incidence and severity of hypomagnesemia. Hypomagnesemia usually occurs when the cumulative doses are at least 300 mg/m^2.[38] So, during the interval between chemotherapy cycles, it is essential to monitor serum magnesium at least weekly. Hypokalemia in cisplatin toxicity is secondary to excessive loss of sodium, potassium, and water at the distal nephron. Hypomagnesemia also contributes to hypokalemia. Drug-induced vomiting can exacerbate hypokalemia. In the initial phases of cisplatin administration, there is tubular proteinuria. Later on, glomerular proteinuria begins with increased elimination of albumin and IgG.

Maintenance of good hydration prior to and during the drug administration and the infusion of mannitol along with the drug are the most important preventive measures to reduce cisplatin toxicity. This helps to reduce the urinary concentration of cisplatin and hence nephrotoxicity. Magnesium deficiency may enhance cisplatin nephrotoxicity. So, children receiving cisplatin-based chemotherapy should receive continuous magnesium supplementation. Carboplatin is a platinum analog that causes both glomerular impairment and hypomagnesemia but less commonly and to a lesser degree compared to cisplatin.

Methotrexate Nephrotoxicity

High-dose MTX is one of the most important chemotherapeutic drugs for the treatment of leukemias, lymphomas, and osteosarcoma. MTX is a structural analog of folic acid. Folate plays an important role in one carbon metabolism which is essential in replicating cells for methionine, adenine, purine, and deoxythymidylic acid biosynthesis. MTX acts as a folic acid antagonist. It mainly causes intestinal mucosal toxicity and bone marrow suppression. Kidney damage occurs with high-dose regimens.

Renal damage occurs due to the precipitation of MTX and its less soluble metabolites [7-OH-MTX and 2,4-diamino-N10-methylpteroic acid (DAMPA)] in acid urines.[39,40] It is manifested by rapid increase in urea and creatinine. Even before the raise of serum creatinine, renal toxicity can be understood by elevated urinary excretion of N-acetyl-beta-glucosamynidase (NAG). Renal failure further increases serum drug levels which aggravate systemic toxicity.[41-43]

Methotrexate-induced AKI is completely reversible. Application of hyperhydration and urinary alkalinization can prevent the precipitation of toxic metabolites. Prepare hydration fluid by adding 20 mL sodium bicarbonate and 10 mL KCl to 500 mL D5. Start hydration at the rate of 125 mL/m^2. Oral sodium bicarbonate 500 mg (6 mEq) is given three times daily. Urine pH is checked after 12 hours of hydration. If urine pH is >7, MTX can be started. If urine pH is <7, bolus infusion of 1 mEq/kg of sodium bicarbonate in 50 mL D5 over 15 minutes is to be given. High-dose MTX-induced AKI can be treated by glucarpidase. Glucarpidase is a recombinant form of bacterial carboxypeptidase (carboxypeptidase G2), which rapidly hydrolyzes MTX to inactive metabolites.[44]

CONCLUSION

While treating oncology-related AKI, comprehensive evaluation of the general condition and identification of all cancer and noncancer-related factors that affect renal function are mandatory. Frequent monitoring kidney function should be performed in those with hematological malignancies, urinary system cancers, and transplant recipients. Maintaining intravascular volume, hemodynamic stability, and infection-control measures are the most important steps to prevent AKI in children with malignancies. Identification of early symptoms and prompt initiation of appropriate therapy will help to improve the outcome. Renal impairment necessitates modification in diagnostic and treatment protocols and other supportive care. Treatment of AKI in oncology patients requires closer attention compared with the general population.

KEY POINTS

- Children with malignancy are at increased risk of AKI.
- The burden of AKI in this group of patients is of growing concern as it contributes to high morbidity and mortality.
- Acute kidney injury in malignancy may be due to prerenal, intrinsic renal, or postrenal factors.
- The most common cause of oncology-related AKI in children without renal infiltration or not undergoing nephrectomy is ATN.
- Tumor lysis syndrome is a common cause of AKI after cytoreductive chemotherapy in malignancies with high tumor burden.
- Fundamental steps in the prevention and management of TLS are aggressive hydration and diuresis.
- Drug-induced AKI is common in cancer patients. The immediate toxic effects on the renal parenchyma and the long-term reduction in renal functional reserve on repeated administration increase the susceptibility to further renal insults.
- Prevention of infection, maintaining good hydration, and hemodynamic stability are the most important factors that prevent AKI in children with malignancies undergoing therapy.

REFERENCES

1. Rosolem MM, Rabello LS, Lisboa T, Caruso P, Costa RT, Leal JV, et al. Critically ill patients with cancer and sepsis: clinical course and prognostic factors. J Crit Care. 2012;27:301-7.
2. Hingorani S. Renal complications of hematopoietic-cell transplantation. N Engl J Med. 2016;374:2256-67.
3. Silva WFD Junior, Pinho LLF, Farias CLG, Torres V, Costalonga EC, Filho GC, et al. Renal infiltration presenting as acute kidney injury in Hodgkin lymphoma - A case report and review of the literature. Leuk Res Rep. 2018;10:41-3.
4. Manohar S, Nasr SH, Leung N. Light chain cast nephropathy: practical considerations in the management of myeloma kidney—what we know and what the future may hold. Curr Hematol Malig Rep. 2018;13:220-6.
5. Michot JM, Bigenwald C, Champiat S, Collins M, Carbonnel F, Postel-Vinay S, et al. Immune-related adverse events with immune checkpoint blockade: a comprehensive review. Eur J Cancer. 2016;54:139-48.
6. Hochberg J, Cairo MS. Tumor lysis syndrome: current perspective. Haematologica. 2008;93:9-13.
7. Oki R, Hirakawa Y, Kimura H, Honda K, Hinata M, Abe H, et al. Renal effects after pembrolizumab treatment for non-small cell lung carcinoma. Intern Med. 2020;59:977-81.
8. Ornstein MC, Garcia JA. Toxicity of checkpoint inhibition in advanced RCC: a systematic review. Kidney Cancer. 2017;1:133-41.
9. de Nattes T, Moreau-Grangé L, Vezzosi D, Laurent C, Lemoine M, Dumont A, et al. Adrenocortical carcinoma complicated by renal thrombotic microangiopathy, a case-series. BMC Nephrol. 2020;21:35.
10. Arai Y, Yamashita K, Mizugishi K, Watanabe T, Sakamoto S, Kitano T, et al. Serum neutrophil extracellular trap levels predict thrombotic microangiopathy after allogeneic stem cell transplantation. Biol Blood Marrow Transplant. 2013;19:1683-9.
11. Raina R, Abusin GA, Vijayaraghavan P, Auletta JJ, Cabral L, Hashem H, et al. The role of continuous renal replacement therapy in the management of acute kidney injury associated with sinusoidal obstruction syndrome following hematopoietic cell transplantation. Pediatr Transplant. 2018;22:e13139.
12. Turki AT, Lamm W, Schmitt C, Bayraktar E, Alashkar F, Metzenmacher M, et al. Platelet number and graft function predict intensive care survival in allogeneic stem cell transplantation patients. Ann Hematol. 2019;98:491-500.
13. Siddall E, Khatri M, Radhakrishnan J. Capillary leak syndrome: etiologies, pathophysiology, and management. Kidney Int. 2017;92:37-46.
14. Shin JI, Lee KH, Lee IR, Oh JH, Kim DW, Shin JW, et al. Systemic capillary leak syndrome (Clarkson syndrome) in cancer patients: a systematic review. J Clin Med. 2018;7:418.
15. Abboud R, Keller J, Slade M, DiPersio JF, Westervelt P, Rettig MP, et al. Severe cytokine-release syndrome after T cell-replete

peripheral blood haploidentical donor transplantation is associated with poor survival and anti-IL-6 therapy is safe and well tolerated. Biol Blood Marrow Transplant. 2016;22:1851-60.
16. Chang L, Frame D, Braun T, Gatza E, Hanauer DA, Zhao S, et al. Engraftment syndrome after allogeneic hematopoietic cell transplantation predicts poor outcomes. Biol Blood Marrow Transplant. 2014;20:1407-17.
17. Coppell JA, Richardson PG, Soiffer R, Martin PL, Kernan NA, Chen A, et al. Hepatic veno-occlusive disease following stem cell transplantation: incidence, clinical course, and outcome. Biol Blood Marrow Transplant. 2010;16:157-68.
18. Mohty M, Malard F, Abecassis M, Aerts E, Alaskar AS, Aljurf M, et al. Sinusoidal obstruction syndrome/veno-occlusive disease: current situation and perspectives—a position statement from the European society for blood and marrow transplantation (EBMT). Bone Marrow Transplant. 2015;50:781-9.
19. Piano S, Tonon M, Angeli P. Management of ascites and hepatorenal syndrome. Hepatol Int. 2018;12:122-34.
20. Wallhult E, Kenyon M, Liptrott S, Mank A, Ní Chonghaile M, Babic A, et al. Management of veno-occlusive disease: the multidisciplinary approach to care. Eur J Haematol. 2017;98:322-9.
21. Richardson PG, Smith AR, Triplett BM, Kernan NA, Grupp SA, Antin JH, et al. Earlier defibrotide initiation post-diagnosis of veno-occlusive disease/sinusoidal obstruction syndrome improves day +100 survival following haematopoietic stem cell transplantation. Br J Haematol. 2017;178:112-8.
22. Coomes EA, Wolfe Jacques A, Michelis FV, Kim DDH, Thyagu S, Viswabandya A, et al. Efficacy of cidofovir in treatment of BK virus-induced hemorrhagic cystitis in post allogeneic hematopoietic cell transplant recipients. Biol Blood Marrow Transplant. 2018;24:1901-5.
23. Carreras E, Dufour C, Mohty N, Kröger N. The EBMT Handbook on Haematopoietic Stem Cell Transplantation and Cellular Therapies. Switzerland: Springer; 2019. pp. 388-90.
24. Höller K, Fabeni L, Herling M, Holtick U, Scheid C, Knops E, et al. Dynamics of BKPyV reactivation and risk of hemorrhagic cystitis after allogeneic hematopoietic stem cell transplantation. Eur J Haematol. 2017;99:133-40.
25. Rampello E, Fricia T, Malaguarnera M. The management of tumor lysis syndrome. Nat Clin Pract Oncol. 2006;3(8):438-47.
26. Cairo MS, Bishop M. Tumour lysis syndrome: new therapeutic strategies and classification. Br J Haematology. 2004;127:3.
27. Coiffier B, Altman A, Pui CH, Younes A, Cairo MS. Guidelines for the management of pediatric and adult tumor lysis syndrome: an evidence-based review. J Clin Oncol. 2008;26(16):2767-78.
28. Zalupski M, Baker LI-I. Ifosfamide. J Natl Cancer Inst. 1988;80: 556-66.
29. Schoenike SE, Dana WJ. Ifosfamide and MESNA. Clin Pharm. 1990;9:179-91.
30. Pratt CB, Meyer WH, Jenkins JJ, Avery L, McKay CP, Wyatt RT, et al. Ifosfamide, Fanconi's syndrome, and rickets. J Clin Onc. 1991;9:1495-9.
31. Caron HN, Abeling N, van Gennip A, de Kraker J, Voute PA. Hyperaminoaciduria identifies patients at risk of developing renal tubular toxicity associated with ifosfamide and platinate containing regimens. Med Pediatr Oncol. 1992;20:42-7.
32. Skinner R, Pearson AD, Price L, Coulthard MG, Craft AW. The influence of age on nephrotoxicity following chemotherapy in children. Br J Cancer. 1992;66:S30-5.
33. Sarosy G. Ifosfamide - pharmacologic overview. Semin Oncol. 1989;16:2-8.
34. Pinta AL, Lippard SI. Binding of the antitumor drug cis-diamminedichloroplatinum (II) (cisplatin) to DNA. Biochim Biophys Acta. 1985;780(3):167-88.
35. Jacobs C, Kalman SM, Tretton M, Weiner MW. Renal handling of cis-diammitzedichloroplatinurn (II). Cancer Treat Rep. 1980;64:1223-6.
36. Takeda M, Komeyama T, Tsutsui T, Mizusawa T, GoH, Hatano A, et al. Changes in urinary excretion of endothelin-I-like immunoreactivity in patients with testicular cancer receiving high-dose cisplatin therapy. Ara J Kidney Dis. 1994;24: 12-6.
37. Mavichak V, Wong NLM, Quarnme GA, Magil AB, Sutton RAL, Dirks JH. Studies on the pathogenesis of cisplatin-induced hypomagnesemia in rats. Kidney Int. 1985;28:914-21.
38. Quamme DA. Renal handling of magnesium: drugs and hormone interaction. Magnesium. 1986;5:248-72.
39. Ariceta G, Rodriguez-Soriano J, Vallo A, Navaja A. Acute and chronic effects of cisplatin therapy on renal magnesium homeostasis. Med Pediatr Oncol. 1997;28:35-40.
40. Jacobs SA, Stoller RG, Chabner BA, Johns DG. 7-Hydroxymethotrexate as a urinary metabolite in human subjects and rhesus monkeys receiving high-dose methotrexate. J Clin Invest. 1976;57:534-8.
41. Lankelma J, van der Klein E. The role of 7-hydroxymethotrexate during methotrexate anticancer chemotherapy. Cancer Lett. 1980;9:133-42.
42. Abelson HT, Fosburg MT, Beardsley GP, Goorin AM, Gorka C, Link M, et al. Methotrexate-induced renal impairment: clinical studies and rescue from systemic toxicity with high-dose leucovarin and thymidine. J Clin Oncol. 1983;1:208-16.
43. Pinedo HM, Zaharko DS, Bull JM, Chabner BA. The reversal of methotrexate cytotoxicity to mouse bone marrow cells by leucovorin and nucleosides. Cancer Res. 1976;36:4418-24.
44. Frei E 3rd, Blum RH, Pitman SW, Kirkwood JM, Henderson IC, Skarin AT, et al. High dose methotrexate with leucovorin rescue: rationale and spectrum of antitumor activity. Am J Med. 1980;68:370-6.

CHAPTER

11.7 Biomarkers in Acute Kidney Injury

Indira Agarwal, Nivedita Kamath

INTRODUCTION

Acute kidney injury (AKI) is characterized by a sudden reduction in kidney function. This may be triggered by various factors such as hypovolemia, hypotension, systemic or local renal infections, septic shock, or toxic insult. Reduction in urine output may be the first clinical clue while serum creatinine is currently the only test widely used to detect changes in kidney function. Unfortunately, serum creatinine is an unreliable indicator of acute changes in renal function for various reasons. Firstly, creatinine levels can vary widely with age, gender, lean muscle mass, muscle metabolism, and hydration status; these can vary widely, especially in children. Secondly, serum creatinine concentrations may not change until 50% of kidney function is lost. Thirdly, at lower rates of glomerular filtration, the amount of tubular secretion of creatinine results in overestimation of kidney function. Finally, when acute changes in glomerular filtration occur, serum creatinine takes time to reach a steady state of equilibrium, even up to several days and could take up to several days and hence does not accurately depict kidney function.[1]

Creatinine is retained in the serum for several hours before the level rises above normal value, by which time the kidney injury may extend and intensify. Efforts to diminish the effects and even aborting the injury process may be futile in spite of instituting therapeutic measures. In spite of best efforts, survivors may not regain renal function and progress to end-stage kidney disease (ESKD). Hence, there is the need for newer biomarkers, which will detect change in renal function as soon as exposure to a risk factor occurs.

DEFINITION

Biomarkers are defined as parameters or findings of a structural, biochemical, physiological, or genetic nature that indicate the presence of the pathological process of a disease, its severity, and progress.[2]

CONCEPT OF BIOMARKER

Cellular molecular modifications are initiated as soon as there is a renal insult. These gradually evolve into cellular damage and result in AKI. A clinical syndrome develops when markers of cell injury, which include certain biological cell metabolic products, are produced and the clinical syndrome develops. The biological clock (biomarker expression) always precedes the clinical clock and represents an earlier stage in the progression to the clinical syndrome. The detection of these biomarkers may provide the much-needed window of opportunity for effective therapeutic intervention to be effective and helps to prevent further injury. They may be considered as the troponin of the kidney. This may be of particular significance in pediatric intensive care units in patients where acute worsening of renal function is common in the setting of ischemia, toxins, or shock. Newer biomarkers of AKI can be components of serum, urine, imaging studies, or any other quantifiable parameter. It should be useful in facilitating early diagnosis, guiding targeted therapy, and helping to monitor disease progression. The desirable characteristics of an ideal biomarker are listed in **Box 1**.

BOX 1: Characteristics of an ideal biomarker for acute kidney injury (AKI).

- Undetectable whenever the disease is absent
- Capable of early detection
- Noninvasive
- Highly sensitive and specific for AKI
- Rapidly and reliably measurable
- Easily detectable in accessible samples such as serum or urine
- Able to give insight into etiology, nature, and duration of insult
- A marker of injury in addition to marker of function
- Predictor of AKI severity and reversibility
- Helpful in monitoring the course and the response to interventions
- Unaffected by other biological variables
- Inexpensive

EMERGING BIOMARKERS

The search is on for possible biomarkers for early diagnosis of AKI. In this regard, various urinary and serum proteins have been evaluated. Some of the emerging biomarkers have the ability to distinguish an early state of cell dysfunction from actual cell injury as well as are able to detect worsening in tubular epithelial cell injury.

Validation of these in different settings of AKI such as cardiac surgery and sepsis as well as in different clinical centers is being done. In the current scenario, various studies have shown that often a single biomarker may not suffice and a panel of biomarkers may be required to produce results that are more accurate.[3]

Urinary Tubular Enzymes

Box 2 lists urinary tubular enzymes that rise within 12 hours to 4 days earlier than a detectable rise in serum creatinine. These enzymes, which are released from the tubular epithelial cells, are useful in early detection of AKI. No validated cutoff points currently exist to distinguish prerenal failure from acute tubular necrosis (ATN).[4]

Urinary Low-molecular-weight Proteins

Box 3 lists proteins, which are freely filtered at the glomerulus and reabsorbed at the proximal tubule but not secreted. These are produced at different sites in the nephron. These biomarkers are promising and can differentiate prerenal from intrinsic causes of renal failure but cannot distinguish acute damage from persistent or irreversible damage as their levels may increase even after mild dysfunction.[5]

Cystatin C

Cystatin C is a cysteine protease inhibitor, which is freely filtered by the glomerulus, reabsorbed completely by the proximal convoluted tubules (PCTs) and not secreted. It is synthesized by all nucleated cells and has been found to be useful as both a serum and a urinary biomarker. It has the advantage that its levels are not affected by gender, age, race, or muscle mass unlike serum creatinine. The utility of cystatin C as a biomarker has been demonstrated by several studies. Using the RIFLE criteria to stratify the risk of developing AKI, a study by Herget-Rosenthal on 85 critically ill patients evaluated cystatin C as a biomarker to detect AKI. The study showed that cystatin C was able to detect AKI almost 2 days earlier than serum creatinine.[6]

Interleukin-18

Interleukin-18 (IL-18) is a proinflammatory cytokine that can be detected in urine following AKI. It is produced in the PCT and found to be an early predictor of AKI. It is particularly useful in patients with adult respiratory distress syndrome (ARDS) and been shown to be an independent predictor of mortality with an area under curve (AUC) of 0.73. Another study on postcardiac surgery patients demonstrated urinary IL-18 to increase 6 hours after cardiopulmonary bypass and peak at 12 hours in patients who later demonstrated a rise in serum creatine.[7] IL-18 has the advantage that it is more specific for ischemic AKI and its levels are not deranged in CKD, urinary tract infections, or nephrotoxic AKI.[5]

BOX 2: Tubular epithelial cell enzymes released into the urine after cell injury.

- Proximal renal tubular epithelial antigen (HRTE-1)
- Alpha-glutathione-S-transferase (α-GST)
- Pi-glutathione-S-transferase (pi-GST)
- Gamma-glutamyl transpeptidase (gamma-GT)
- Alanine aminopeptidase (AAP)
- Urinary lactate dehydrogenase (LDH)
- N-acetyl-beta-glucosaminidase (NAG)

BOX 3: Low-molecular-weight proteins released in urine in acute kidney injury (AKI).

- Alpha-1-microglobulin (α-1M)
- Beta-2-microglobulin (β2M)
- Retinol-binding protein (RBP)
- Adenosine deaminase-binding protein (ABP)

Alpha-1 Microglobulin

Alpha-1 microglobulin (α1M) is readily filtered by the glomerulus and reabsorbed by proximal tubule cells in its free form. It has been shown to be an early and sensitive biomarker for proximal tubular dysfunction even in the early phases of injury at a time when there is no observable evidence of histologic damage.[8]

Beta-2 Microglobulin

Beta-2 microglobulin (β2M) is a light chain protein filtered freely by the glomerulus and almost entirely reabsorbed and catabolized by the proximal tubular cells. This process may be impeded in the setting of AKI. Increased urinary β2M excretion has been observed to be an early marker of tubular injury in multiple situations such as postcardiac surgery and renal transplantation as well as after nephrotoxic exposure. It is known to rise as many as 4–5 days before a rise in serum creatinine is noted.[8]

Kidney Injury Molecule-1

Kidney injury molecule-1 (KIM-1) is a transmembrane protein, which was first studied in animal models and noted to be markedly overexpressed in the PCT in response to ischemic or toxic injury to the kidneys. Immunoassay of urine samples measures the ectoderm, which is shed from the cells in the PCT. Multiple cohort studies have demonstrated its usefulness in differentiating ischemic ATN from other forms of AKI and chronic kidney disease. A study of 38 patients showed that KIM-1 can be expressed in urine within 12 hours after the initial ischemic insult till regeneration of the epithelium occurs and can persist over time. Further studies are required to determine its usefulness in postischemic kidney.[9]

Neutrophil Gelatinase-associated Lipocalin

Neutrophil gelatinase-associated lipocalin (NGAL) is the most promising among all the emerging biomarkers. It is expressed in the PCT by neutrophils and other lining epithelial cells. Various human tissues including uterus, prostate, salivary gland, lung, trachea, stomach, colon, and kidney demonstrate *NGAL gene* expression. It is most abundantly expressed in the kidney where it is markedly upregulated in response to ischemia and acts by decreasing toxicity by reducing apoptosis and increasing the normal proliferation of kidney tubule cells.

It also helps to protect the kidney tubule cells by enhancing delivery of iron, thus upregulating heme oxygenase 1. It is measured in both urine (uNGAL) and plasma (pNGAL).

Plasma NGAL holds promise to be an important component of the "AKI panel" and likely to be the equivalent of "Troponin" of the kidney. NGAL has been tested in multiple settings through multiple studies in more than 4,000 patients who are at risk for AKI due to sepsis, cardiac surgery, exposure to contrast media, or after renal transplantation. The average sensitivity and specificity of NGAL measured in these studies 1–3 days prior to AKI diagnosis were 76% and 77%, respectively, for cardiac surgery patients and 73% and 80%, respectively, in patients admitted to intensive care units.[10]

Urinary NGAL was found to be one of the seven genes highly upregulated in renal ischemia reperfusion injury mouse models.[11] NGAL was detected in urine samples within 2 hours following ischemia and its levels correlated with the duration of ischemia. In a prospective study of 91 children with congenital heart disease undergoing elective cardiac catheterization with contrast administration, uNGAL and pNGAL were able to predict contrast-induced nephropathy within 2 hours of contrast administration.[12] However in another study on 143 critically ill children with systemic inflammatory response syndrome (SIRS) and septic shock, pNGAL was found to be highly sensitive (84%) but poorly specific (39%). The correlation with the severity of systemic disease was higher in children with septic shock than with SIRS.[13] Another study on 140 critically ill mechanically ventilated patients showed that uNGAL rose more than six times in levels and occurred 2 days earlier than the corresponding 50% increase in serum creatinine levels. Urinary NGAL was also noted to increase in a stepwise pattern with worsening RIFLE class.[14].

A recently published study from an emergency department showed uNGAL to be highly sensitive (90%) and specific (99%) in diagnosing AKI in the 635 children tested.[15] In a prospective study on a large group of 426 adult patients undergoing cardiac surgery, uNGAL correlated with cardiac pulmonary bypass time and aorta cross-clamping time, both indices of renal hypoperfusion and established risk factors for AKI occurrence.[16] In the setting of pediatric hemolytic uremic syndrome, however, pNGAL regardless of the cutoff values used was unable to reliably predict the need for kidney replacement therapy (KRT). At 5 days of hospitalization, uNGAL levels in these patients showed high sensitivity but continued to show low specificity in predicting the need for KRT.[17]

Studies have shown NGAL to be a useful tool in disease monitoring in other renal diseases, delayed graft function, lupus nephritis, immunoglobulin A (IgA) nephropathy, and polycystic kidney disease as well as for nonrenal conditions such as brain tumor, inflammatory bowel disease, and pre-eclampsia.

Retinol-binding Protein

Retinol-binding protein (RBP) is a protein that is synthesized in the liver and is responsible for transporting vitamin A from the liver to other tissues in the body. Like all other biomarkers, it is also freely filtered by the glomerulus, completely reabsorbed, and then catabolized by the proximal tubule. Urinary RBP is found to be a highly sensitive indicator of renal tubule dysfunction in AKI from various etiologies and is known to precede urinary N-acetyl-beta-glucuronidase (NAG) elevation, also a marker of ischemia reperfusion injury.[5]

NEWER BIOMARKERS

Insulin-like Growth Factor-binding Protein-7 and Tissue Inhibitor of Matrix Metalloproteinase

Insulin-like growth factor-binding protein-7 (IGFBP-7) and tissue inhibitor of matrix metalloproteinase (TIMP-2) are cell cycle arrest proteins that are expressed in the renal tubular cells during periods of cellular injury. TIMP-2 inhibits matrix metalloproteinase and has several effects on the cell cycle. It inhibits endothelial cell proliferation and angiogenesis. IGFBP-7 has several pleiotropic effects including cell cycle arrest in the G1 phase. Both these biomarkers have been shown to be upregulated in AKI. Several multicentric studies have validated the predictive role of the combination of IGFBP-7 and TIMP-2 in AKI.[2]

CLINICAL APPLICABILITY OF BIOMARKERS

Neutrophil Gelatinase-associated Lipocalin

One of the most widely studied biomarkers in AKI, NGAL has been used in the prediction of AKI in the setting of postcardiac surgery, critically ill patients, in the emergency setting, and following renal transplantation. Among all the new biomarkers, NGAL has been most widely studied. NGAL is expressed in a dose-dependent manner and correlates well with the severity of AKI. The reference normal range for NGAL has been established in the healthy adult population.

Neutrophil gelatinase-associated lipocalin is useful in differentiating prerenal AKI from intrinsic AKI. The AUC for determining intrinsic AKI ranged from 0.8 to 0.95. NGAL also predicted death or need for dialysis in the emergency room.[18] In a systematic review for the use of biomarkers to guide timing of initiation of KRT in AKI, NGAL was promising.[19] Plasma NGAL also has been found to be associated with nonrecovery of AKI (AUC—0.74).[20] Urinary NGAL levels were also correlated with mortality. In postrenal transplantation patients, higher NGAL levels were associated with a greater risk of poor graft function.

The disadvantage is that NGAL may be elevated in the setting of urinary tract infection and chronic kidney disease as well.

Kidney Injury Molecule-1

The KIM is a modest predictor of the onset of AKI. It is also a modest predictor of progression of AKI and need for dialysis.

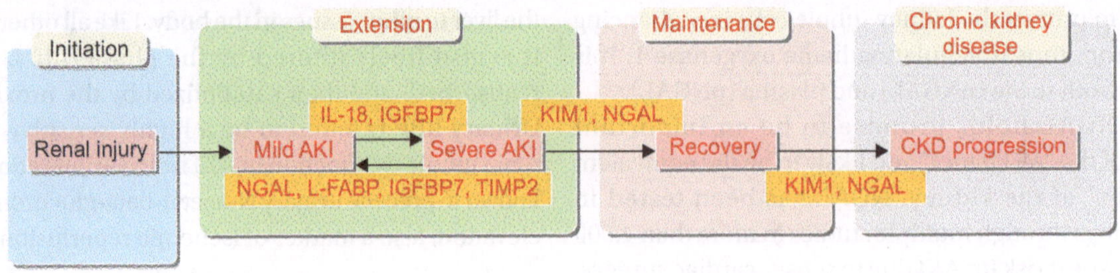

Fig. 1: Clinical application of various biomarkers in predicting the different stages of AKI. (AKI: acute kidney injury; CKD: chronic kidney disease; IGFBP7: insulin-like growth factor-binding protein-7; IL-18: interleukin-18; KIM1: kidney injury molecule-1; NGAL: neutrophil gelatinase-associated lipocalin; TIMP: tissue inhibitor of matrix metalloproteinase)
Source: Adapted from Schrezenmeier EV, Barasch J, Budde K, Westhoff T, Schmidt-Ott KM. Biomarkers in acute kidney injury—pathophysiological basis and clinical performance. Acta Physiol (Oxf). 2017;219(3):554-72.

In combination with IL-18, KIM-1 had a superior predictive ability for severe AKI.[2]

Interleukin-18

Interleukin-18 has been found to be a useful biomarker in predicting the risk of AKI. However, it is only a modest predictor of the severity of AKI. High levels of IL-18 have been associated with a risk of poor graft function in the postrenal transplantation period.[2]

Liver-type Fatty Acid-binding Protein

Liver-type fatty acid-binding protein (L-FABP) has a significant role in early prediction of AKI. Though L-FABP had a moderate correlation with severity of AKI, it was one of the biomarkers that correlated best with progression of AKI and need for dialysis.[2]

Insulin-like Growth Factor-binding Protein and Tissue Inhibitor of Matrix Metalloproteinase

Several large studies have shown that the combination of IGFBP and TIMP had the highest predictability for occurrence of AKI with a high sensitivity and negative predictive values. This biomarker has been approved for clinical use in adults with risk for developing AKI.[21] The role of various biomarkers in the different stages of AKI is depicted in **Figure 1**.

CONCLUSION

Biomarkers for AKI have mostly been validated in specific populations in various research studies. The lack of generalizability of these biomarkers for all causes of AKI and the absence of a simple, feasible, and reliable test have been major obstacles in the use of biomarkers as a point-of-care tool for diagnosis of AKI.

KEY POINTS

- AKI is characterized by a sudden reduction in kidney function. Serum creatinine is an unreliable indicator of acute changes in renal function.
- Efforts to diminish the effects and even aborting the injury process may be futile in spite of instituting therapeutic measures. So, there is a need for newer biomarkers, which will detect change in renal function as soon as exposure to a risk factor occurs.
- Biomarkers are defined as parameters or findings of a structural, biochemical, physiological, or genetic nature that indicate the presence of the pathological process of a disease, its severity, and progress.
- The detection of these biomarkers may provide the much-needed window of opportunity for effective therapeutic intervention to be effective and helps to prevent further injury. They may be considered as the troponin of the kidney.
- Newer biomarkers of AKI can be components of serum, urine, imaging studies, or any other quantifiable measure and have the ability to distinguish an early state of cell dysfunction from actual cell injury as well as are able to detect worsening in tubular epithelial cell injury.
- NGAL is the most promising among all the emerging biomarkers and has been used in the prediction of AKI in the setting of postcardiac surgery, critically ill patients, in the emergency setting, and following renal transplantation.
- Biomarkers for AKI have mostly been validated in specific populations in various research studies and translation to clinical management is lagging behind due to the absence of a simple, feasible, and reliable test.

REFERENCES

1. Nguyen MT, Devarajan P. Biomarkers for the early detection of acute kidney injury. Pediatr Nephrol. 2008;23(12):2151-7.
2. Alge JL, Arthur JM. Biomarkers of AKI: a review of mechanistic relevance and potential therapeutic implications. Clin J Am Soc Nephrol. 2015;10(1):147-55.
3. Bonventre JV. Diagnosis of acute kidney injury: from classic parameters to new bio-markers. Contrib Nephrol. 2007;156: 213-9.
4. Singh R, Dodkins J, Doyle JF, Forni LG. Acute kidney injury biomarkers: what do they tell us? Contrib Nephrol. 2018;193: 21-34.

5. Parikh CR, Devarajan P. New biomarkers of acute kidney injury. Crit Care Med. 2008;36(4):S159-65.
6. Herget-Rosenthal S, Marggraf G, Husing J, Göring F, Pietruck F, Janssen O, et al. Early detection of acute renal failure by serum cystatin C. Kidney Int. 2004;66(3):1115-22.
7. Parikh CR, Mishra J, Thiessen-Philbrook H, Dursun B, Ma Q, Kelly C, et al. Urinary IL-18 is an early predictive biomarker of acute kidney injury after cardiac surgery. Kidney Int. 2006;70(1): 199-203.
8. Han WK, Bailly V, Abichandani R, Thadhani R, Bonventre JV. Kidney injury molecule-1 (KIM-1): a novel biomarker for human renal proximal tubule injury. Kidney Int. 2002;62(1):237-44.
9. Wasung ME, Chawla LS, Madero M. Biomarkers of renal function, which and when? Clin Chim Acta. 2015;438:350-7.
10. Haase M, Haase-Fielitz A, Bellomo R, Mertens PR. Neutrophil gelatinase-associated lipocalin as a marker of acute renal disease. Curr Opin Hematol. 2011;18(1):11-8.
11. Mishra J, Ma Q Prada A, Mitsnefes M, Mitsnefes M, Zahedi K, Yang J, et al. Identification of neutrophil gelatinase-associated lipocalin as a novel early urinary biomarker for ischemic renal injury. J Am Soc Nephrol. 2003;14(10):2534-543.
12. Hirsch R, Dent C, Pfriem H, Allen J, Beekman RH 3rd, Ma Q, et al. NGAL is an early predictive biomarker of contrast-induced nephropathy in children. Pediatr Nephrol. 2007;22(12):2089-95.
13. Wheeler DS, Devarajan P, Ma Q, Harmon K, Monaco M, Cvijanovich N, et al. Serum neutrophil gelatinase-associated lipocalin (NGAL) as a marker of acute kidney injury in critically ill children with septic shock. Crit Care Med. 2008;36(4): 1297-303.
14. Zappitelli M, Washburn KK, Arikan AA, Loftis L, Ma Q, Devarajan P, et al. Urine neutrophil gelatinase associated lipocalin is an early marker of acute kidney injury in critically ill children: a prospective cohort study. Crit Care. 2007;11:R84.
15. Nickolas TL, O'Rourke MJ, Yang J, Sise ME, Canetta PA, Barasch N, et al. Sensitivity and specificity of a single emergency department measurement of urinary neutrophil gelatinase-associated lipocalin for diagnosing acute kidney injury. An Intern Med. 2008;148(3):810-19.
16. Wagener G, Gubitosa G, Wang S, Borregaard N, Kim M, Lee HT. Urinary neutrophil gelatinase-associated lipocalin and acute kidney injury after cardiac surgery. Am J Kidney Dis. 2008;52(3):425-33.
17. Trachtman H, Christen E, Cnaan A, Patrick J, Mai V, Mishra J, et al. Urinary neutrophil gelatinase-associated lipocalin in D+HUS: a novel marker of renal injury. Pediatr Nephrol. 2006;21(7): 989-94.
18. Schrezenmeier EV, Barasch J, Budde K, Westhoff T, Schmidt-Ott KM. Biomarkers in acute kidney injury—pathophysiological basis and clinical performance. Acta Physiol (Oxf). 2017;219(3): 554-72.
19. Klein SJ, Brandtner AK, Lehner GF, Ulmer H, Bagshaw SM, Wiedermann CJ, et al. Biomarkers for prediction of renal replacement therapy in acute kidney injury: a systematic review and meta-analysis. Intensive Care Med. 2018;44(3):323-36.
20. Srisawat N, Murugan R, Kellum JA. Repair or progression after AKI: a role for biomarkers? Nephron Clin Pract. 2014;127(1-4): 185-9.
21. Vijayan A, Faubel S, Askenazi DJ, Cerda J, Fissell WH, Heung M, et al.; American Society of Nephrology Acute Kidney Injury Advisory Group. Clinical use of the urine biomarker [TIMP-2] × [IGFBP7] for acute kidney injury risk assessment. Am J Kidney Dis. 2016;68(1):19-28.

CHAPTER

11.8

Outcome of Acute Kidney Injury: Evolution of Acute Kidney Injury to Chronic Kidney Disease

Subhankar Sarkar, Rajiv Sinha

INTRODUCTION

Acute kidney injury (AKI) is characterized by an abrupt fall in kidney function which is usually diagnosed by drop in urine output (UO) and/or rise in serum creatinine. Kidney Disease Improving Global Outcome (KDIGO) defined AKI as an increase in serum creatinine by at least 0.3 mg/dL within 48 hours or an increase of >1.5 times the baseline within prior 7 days or a decrease in UO to <0.5 mL/kg/h over 6 hours.[1] For long, the focus was on the acute event with assumption that if one survives the event, chances of long-term sequel are rare. With a drop in mortality during the acute phase, it has been increasingly recognized that AKI survivors are at higher risks for adverse long-term events including progression to chronic kidney disease (CKD).[2-5]

Development of standardized, multidimensional classification criteria for AKI and its application in numerous hospital-based cohort studies have helped to establish an indisputable strong association between development and severity of AKI and both short- and long-term morbidity/mortality. Future adverse events linked to AKI include recurrence of AKI episodes, development or progression of CKD, increased cardiovascular risks, increased need for hospital admission, reduced quality of life, and higher long-term risk of mortality.[6-10] Incidence of pediatric AKI (pAKI) has increased over the last 30 years likely secondary to shift in the epidemiology of AKI. A significant number of these children with AKI are at risk of progressing to CKD. Despite this fact, only minority of AKI gets regular nephrology follow-up after their discharge.[11,12]

EPIDEMIOLOGY

Estimated incidence of AKI ranges from 0.3 to 82% among critically ill children depending on the severity of illness as well as on the definition of AKI.[13-17] Even after standardization of AKI definition **(Table 1)**, studies have persistently shown a high percentage of children admitted in pediatric intensive care unit (PICU) developing AKI.[18] About 10% children admitted to PICU develop AKI which doubles if admitted for longer than 12 hours.[19,20] In a retrospective study of children surviving post AKI, Sinha et al. found that up to 25% of children were positive for at least one marker of kidney injury (abnormal creatinine, hypertension, hematuria, and proteinuria) at 10-year follow-up.[21] Mammen et al. reported CKD in up to 10% of post-AKI patients discharged from tertiary-care PICU in Canada at 1–3 years' follow-up.[22] Incidence may be higher in post-cardiac surgery patients wherein AKI has been reported among up to 36%[23-25] with nonrecovery in up to 28%.[24] Premature neonates with low birth weight and intrauterine growth restriction are also more prone to develop AKI and subsequent CKD. Studies of term and preterm infants in the neonatal intensive care unit (NICU) reported that 31% (range 9–83%) of neonatal AKI survivors may develop CKD.[26] Studies have also reported that premature infant even without AKI are at higher risk of progressing to CKD probably due to low nephron mass. Superadded incidence of AKI among this vulnerable group is likely to further hasten progression of CKD.

ACUTE KIDNEY INJURY TO CHRONIC KIDNEY DISEASE SPECTRUM

Recent epidemiologic studies from children and adults suggest that AKI can cause permanent long-term kidney damage, and survivors of AKI are at an increased risk of developing CKD as well as at an increased risk of mortality.[27-29] Data from adult studies showed that patients with AKI are at a ninefold increased risk of developing CKD, a threefold increased risk of developing kidney failure, and a twofold increased long-term mortality risk compared with patients without AKI.[30] A recent systematic review has shown pooled rate of CKD after AKI to vary from 10.17 to 25.8 per 100 person-years.[29,31] Kellum et al. described five phenotypes of renal recovery after AKI: early sustained AKI reversibility, late sustained AKI reversibility, relapse AKI and recovery, relapse AKI without recovery, and never recovered AKI **(Fig. 1)**.[5,32] As shown in **Figure 1**, in presence of pre-existing CKD, recovery could be further jeopardized by a current episode of AKI and change the patterns of outcome such as AKI to worsening CKD and AKI to initial recovery followed by worsening CKD.[33,34] The final outcome depends on underlying kidney reserves along with stage of AKI and time taken for the recovery of kidney function

TABLE 1: Defining acute kidney injury, acute kidney disease, and chronic kidney disease.

KDIGO definition of AKI	• Increase in serum creatinine by >0.3 mg/dL within 48 hours; or • Increase in serum creatinine to >1.5 times baseline, which is known or presumed to have occurred within the prior 7 days; or • Urine volume <0.5 mL/kg/h for 6 hours	
Transient AKI	Rapid reversal of AKI within 48 hours	
Persistent AKI	AKI persisting beyond 48 hours but reversal within 2–7 days	
AKD	AKI stage1 and above persisting beyond 7 days	
Stage of AKD	Stage 0	A: Absence of criteria for B or C
		B: Continued evidence of ongoing injury, repair, and/or regeneration or indicators of loss of renal glomerular or tubular reserve
		C: Serum creatinine level <1.5 times baseline but not back to baseline levels
		B/C: Serum creatinine level <1.5 times baseline but not back to baseline levels, and continued evidence of ongoing injury, repair and/or regeneration
	Stage 1	Serum creatinine level 1.5–1.9 times baseline
	Stage 2	Serum creatinine level 2.0–2.9 times baseline
	Stage 3	Serum creatinine level 3.0 times baseline or increase in serum creatinine to ≥353.6 μmol/L (≥4.0 mg/dL) or ongoing need for kidney replacement therapy
CKD	Abnormalities of kidney structure or function, present for ≥3 months, either GFR < 60 mL/min/1.73 m^2 or albuminuria (AER ≥ 30 mg/24 hours; ACR ≥30 mg/g), urine sediment abnormalities, electrolyte and other abnormalities due to tubular disorders, abnormalities detected by histology, structural abnormalities detected by imaging, history of kidney transplantation	

(ACR: albumin–creatinine ratio; AKD: acute kidney disease; AKI: acute kidney injury; CKD: chronic kidney disease; GFR: glomerular filtration rate; KDIGO: Kidney Disease Improving Global Outcome)

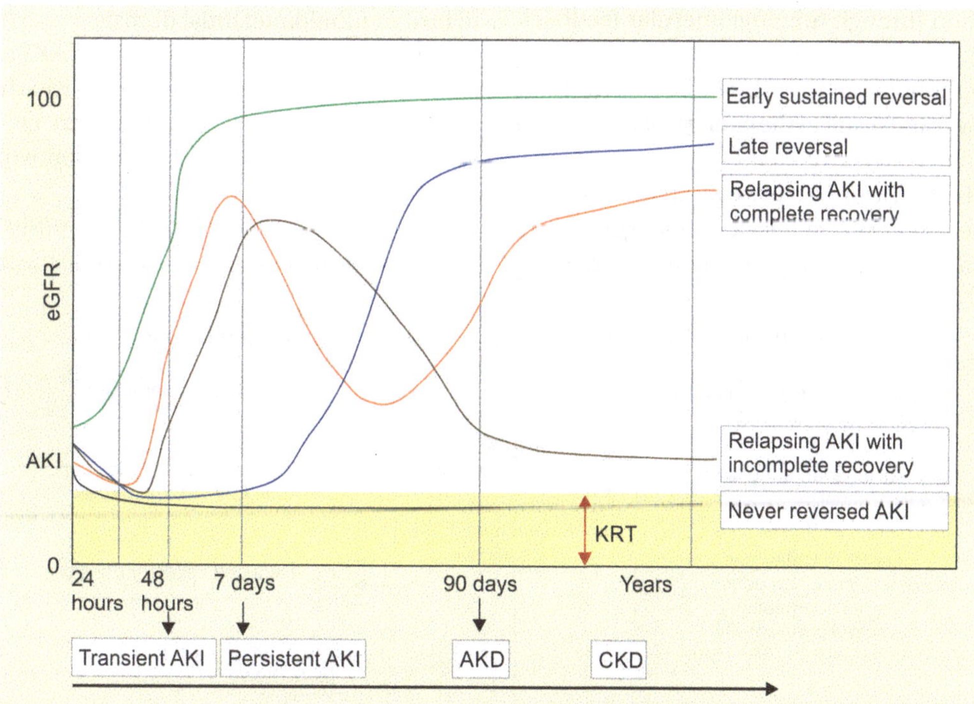

Fig. 1: AKI and kidney recovery: Spectrum of AKI–AKD–CKD. (AKD: acute kidney disease; AKI: acute kidney injury; CKD: chronic kidney disease; KRT: kidney replacement therapy)
Source: Modified from Acute Dialysis Quality Initiative 16

with early recovery having better short as well as long-term prognosis than late and nonrecovery. Several studies have shown that rapid recovery of AKI function carries better short-term prognosis and even among AKI Stage 1, it has been shown that resolution of AKI within 7 days has a better prognosis in contrast to those lasting beyond 7 days.[29,35-40] Appreciating the continuum of AKI to CKD and the prognostic importance of duration to recovery, KDIGO introduced the term acute kidney disease (AKD, persistence of AKI Stage 1 or greater for duration between 7 and 90 days) in 2012 and subsequently Acute Dialysis Quality Initiative (ADQI) introduced the concept of transient AKI (baseline renal function recovery within 48 hours) and persistent AKI (renal dysfunction lasting beyond 48 hours) **(Table 1 and Fig. 1)**.[1,35] Epidemiologic studies have shown that after episodes of AKI, 10–15% died in the course of the associated acute illness, 20–50% of survivors of AKI progressed to CKD, and 3–15% had permanent kidney failure.[33,34]

PATHOPHYSIOLOGY OF ACUTE KIDNEY INJURY RECOVERY AND/OR PROGRESSION TO CHRONIC KIDNEY DISEASE

Acute kidney injury among hospitalized children may be due to intrinsic renal disease, nephrotoxic drugs, or more commonly secondary to shock resulting from sepsis, major surgery, trauma, and/or cardiac dysfunction **(Table 1)**. An imbalance between demand and oxygenation at the microcirculation level is usually the cornerstone of AKI pathogenesis.[41-46] This imbalance can be secondary to hemodynamic instability, tubular cell injury, tubular obstruction, renal congestion, microvascular thrombi, endothelial dysfunction, and/or inflammation. Proximal tubular cells are most susceptible to injury which triggers a cascade of event such as afferent arteriole constriction through tubuloglomerular feedback, luminal obstruction, and back leak of filtrate through the damaged proximal tubular cells.[41] All of this contribute to glomerular shutdown and result in the clinical manifestations of AKI.

Kidney injury also results in the release of various vasoactive mediators promoting interstitial infiltrates and inflammation, which further aggravate renal damage. Inflammation plays an important role in AKI, and persistent inflammation secondary to maladaptive repair mechanism plays an important role in AKI–CKD continuum.[46-50] Maladaptive regeneration of damaged kidney tissue post AKI is considered to be the harbinger of CKD. Examples of maladaptive changes include impaired angiogenesis, reduced endothelial proliferation,[51] cell cycle arrest,[52] persistent fibrosis,[53] increased expression in kidney tissue microRNAs associated with renal fibrosis,[54] and ongoing inflammation.[55] In animal models, AKI has been shown to cause irreversible reduction in peritubular capillaries leading to hypoxia of renal parenchyma and chronic kidney damage.[56] AKI can also initiate a prolonged cellular inflammation triggered by a number of molecular pathways that can lead to fibrosis and long-term kidney dysfunction.[57,58] Depending on the site of injury and severity of inflammation, the phenotype of early chronic dysfunction may present in various combinations of proteinuria, hematuria, and hypertension with or without elevated creatinine. Severe and repeated injury in an inflammatory environment can aggravate maladaptive repair process and result in permanent reduction in kidney function. Renin–angiotensin–aldosterone axis (RAAS) activation also plays an important role in AKI to CKD transition and its inhibition may delay CKD progression. Another purported mechanism for AKI progressing to CKD is nephron loss secondary to AKI and consequent hypertrophy of the remaining nephrons and hyperfiltration, which leads to further tubulointerstitial fibrosis.

In summary, the progression of AKI to CKD is usually due to post-AKI regenerative mechanisms initiating a vicious maladaptive cycle through **(Flowchart 1)**:

- Interstitial immune cell infiltration which can augment fibrosis
- Peritubular capillary loss which results in renal hypoxia which again stimulates profibrotic mechanisms

Flowchart 1: Pathogenesis of acute kidney injury progressing to chronic kidney disease.

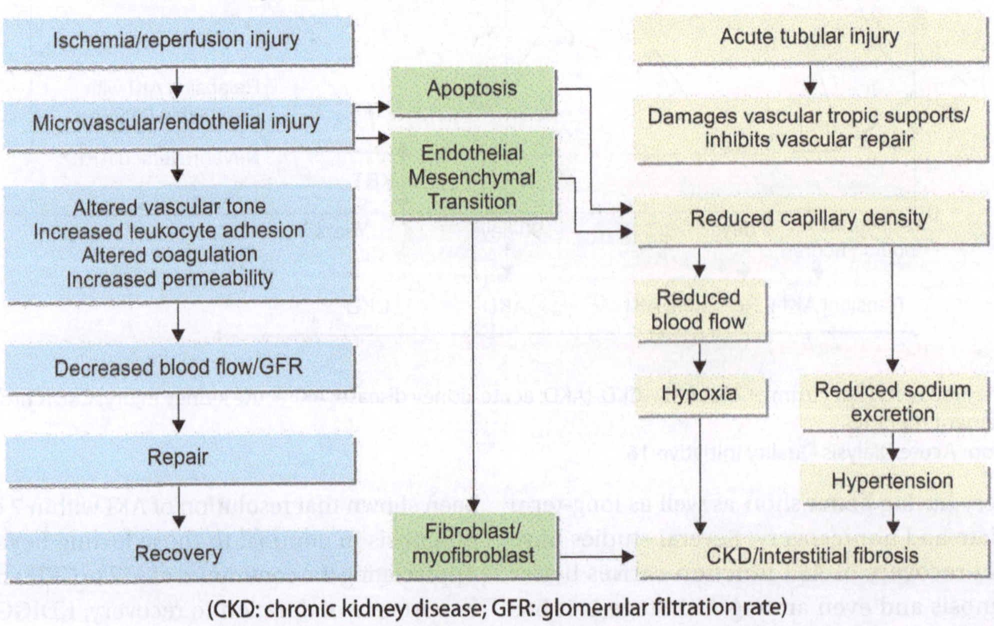

(CKD: chronic kidney disease; GFR: glomerular filtration rate)

- Injured renal tubular cells which can undergo a profibrotic phenotype change after cell cycle arrest, affecting other epithelial cells, pericytes, and the immune system
- Nephron loss leading to glomerular hyperfiltration and consequent renal injury.

Lower baseline kidney function, longer duration of AKI, higher severity of AKI, and repetitive kidney injury can all augment the profibrotic and proinflammatory arms of the regenerative pathways and precipitate adverse maladaptive consequences in the kidney leading to CKD.[59] The term AKD encompasses the time period of the pathophysiological process of renal recovery/maladaptive changes post AKI, bridging the AKI–CKD continuum. AKD can progress to CKD or may resolve.

RISK FACTORS FOR ACUTE KIDNEY INJURY AND FOR ACUTE KIDNEY INJURY PROGRESSION TO CHRONIC KIDNEY DISEASE

Major risk factors responsible for AKI include critically ill children on mechanical ventilation, need for vasopressor/ionotropic medications, nephrotoxic drugs, neonates with birth weight <1,500 g, perinatal asphyxia, and those who receive extracorporeal membrane oxygenation.[51,60] Kidney recovery from AKI is a complex mechanism and despite unraveling of new information, it remains ill understood. The ultimate outcome of the recovery process is dependent on multitude of interdependent factors including baseline kidney functions, etiology of AKI, severity of AKI, and duration of AKI. **Table 2** lists some of the important factors, which have been associated with failure of kidney to return to its baseline function post an AKI episode. Among children premature birth, intrauterine growth restriction and low-birth weight predispose to higher risk of CKD secondary to the associated reduced nephron mass and the risk can be accentuated with superadded AKI.

Patients with AKI are prone to have elevated blood pressure in long term, and high blood pressure is a known risk factor for progression to CKD.[2] Adult studies on long-term outcome of AKI have clearly shown increased incidence of hypertension and other related cardiovascular morbidities.[61,62] Higher stages of AKI have been shown to have increased cardiovascular morbidity and long-term mortality. AKI has increased propensity to recur, and repeated AKI is an established risk factor for CKD progression as well as increased mortality.[63-66] Prolonged requirement of kidney replacement therapy (KRT) also increases the risk of progression to CKD. Among AKI in postcardiac surgery, duration of AKI was a strong independent risk factor for subsequent CKD development. Coca et al. demonstrated that the longer the duration of AKI, the higher is the mortality across all stages of AKI (Scored as per AKI Network, i.e., AKIN criteria) in their diabetic cohort.[29] Transient AKI has been shown to have decreased mortality at 1 year [relative risk (RR) 3.77, 95% confidence interval (CI) 1.6–8.8] when compared to persistent AKI (RR 4.1, CI 1.8–9.5).[67]

Compared with non-AKI population, even transient AKI has higher long-term mortality.[67,68] Recovery from AKI has been shown to be an important negative risk factor for long-term mortality and morbidity.[69,70] Risk of end-stage kidney disease (ESKD) is higher for AKI superimposed on previous CKD than among AKI occurring in kidneys with normal baseline function.[71]

TABLE 2: Risks for AKI, AKI to CKD progression, long-term mortality, and cardiovascular morbidity.

AKI	*AKI nonrecovery*	*Development and progression of CKD*	*Long-term mortality*	*Cardiovascular outcome*
• Prematurity/low birth weight • Hypertension • Diabetes mellitus • CKD • CVD • Anemia • Hypoalbuminemia • Sepsis • Shock • Nephrotoxins • Surgery • Liver disease • Lung disease • HIV infection • COVID-19 Infection • Obesity • Hyperuricemia	• Severity of AKI Hemodynamic instability • KRT modality • Hypertension • Diabetes • CKD • CVD	• Prematurity/low birth weight • Severity of AKI • AKI relapses • Duration of AKI • Anemia • Illness severity • Need for KRT • Timing and type of AKI recovery • Albuminuria • Hypertension • Diabetes • CKD • CVD	• Prematurity/low birth weight • Severity of AKI • Duration of AKI • Hypoalbuminemia • Illness severity • Hypertension • Diabetes • CKD • CVD	• Severity of AKI Hypertension • CKD • CVD

(AKI: acute kidney injury; CKD: chronic kidney disease; CVD: cardiovascular disease)

BIOMARKERS OF ACUTE KIDNEY INJURY AND CHRONIC KIDNEY DISEASE PROGRESSION

Biomarkers are quick, noninvasive, and specific measurement tools which may help the clinician to monitor disease activity and detect early deterioration in organ function giving an opportunity for early intervention and prevention of significant organ dysfunction. Creatinine has well-known limitations as a biomarker of kidney dysfunction. Studies have demonstrated progression to CKD post AKI despite documentation of creatinine dropping to baseline at time of discharge.[72,73] Despite these limitations, creatinine remains the most commonly used biomarker for acute and chronic kidney injuries.

Higher stages of AKI, as defined by the estimated glomerular filtration rate (eGFR) based on serum creatinine and height, have correlated with higher risk of subsequent CKD. Albuminuria has been used as another biomarker of CKD progression as it has shown strong linear association with progression of CKD/end-stage kidney disease (ESKD) and all-cause mortality independent of eGFR. This has resulted in its inclusion in CKD staging in the 2012 KDIGO guideline.[1]

After insult, kidney tubular cells undergo a cascade of cellular responses that result in the production and accumulation of low-molecular-weight proteins in the urine and systemic circulation. As AKI and CKD share similar underlying mechanisms to functional and structural injury and exist on the same pathophysiologic continuum, biomarkers of AKI have also been explored for early prediction of CKD.[74,75] Neutrophils gelatinase-associated lipocalin (NGAL), liver-type fatty acid binding protein (L-FABP), kidney injury molecule-1 (KIM-1), hepatitis A virus cellular receptor 1 (HAVCR-1), tissue inhibitor of metalloproteinases-2 (TIMP-2), and insulin-like growth factor-binding protein 7 (IGFBP-7) are elevated in response to tubular injury. Cystatin C, α-microglobulin (α1M), B2-microglobulin (B2-M), L-type or liver-type fatty acid-binding protein (L-FABP), and uromodulin (UMOD) are small molecules that are filtered by the glomerulus and processed or reabsorbed by the proximal tubules. They serve as effective biomarkers of proximal tubular function.

In response to kidney injury, inflammatory mediators are raised and biomarkers such as interleukin-18 (IL-18), tumor necrosis factor-α (TNF-α), inducible nitric oxide synthase, macrophage inflammatory protein-2, monocyte chemoattractant protein-1 (MCP-1), and soluble TNF receptors (TNFR1 and TNFR2) can be useful. Repair and fibrosis may be captured by urinary biomarkers YKL-40 also known as chitinase 3-like protein 1 and BRP-39. Urinary procollagen type III N-terminal propeptide (PIIINP) is believed to be biomarker of early stages of kidney fibrosis. Urinary epidermal growth factor (EGF) has been shown to inversely correlate with interstitial fibrosis among patients with diabetic nephropathy, IgA nephropathy, adult polycystic kidney disease, and pediatric CKD. Most of the candidate biomarkers have not entered clinical practice. To date, only NGAL and TIMP-2 × IGFBP7 (tissue inhibitor of metalloproteinases-2 and insulin-like growth factor-binding protein 7 have been approved by the Food and Drug Administration (FDA) as biomarkers of kidney injury. TIMP-2 × IGFBP7 > 2 has been shown to predict mortality or need for dialysis at 9 months post AKI [hazard ratio (HR) = 2.16; 95% CI 1.32–3.53].[76] MicroRNAs (miRNAs) have selective expression by different organs, and the role of miRNA as biomarker of kidney injury has been undergoing evaluation.

FOLLOW-UP STRATEGIES FOR EARLY DETECTION OF CHRONIC KIDNEY DISEASE AND DELAYING CHRONIC KIDNEY DISEASE PROGRESSION

Chronic kidney disease is an independent risk factor for early onset cardiovascular disease (CVD) because of subclinical atherosclerosis, vessels calcification, endothelial dysfunction, hypertension, left ventricle hypertrophy, and microalbuminuria. Early detection of CKD and modification of CVD risk factors are paramount to prevent premature death and organ dysfunction. Despite accumulating evidence in favor of post-AKI patients having increased mortality/morbidity risk, very few of them get routine nephrology follow-up. The 2015 US Renal Data System annual report showed that only 19% post-AKI patients had nephrology follow-up at 1 year.[77] In another retrospective study reported by Siew et al., despite a high mortality rate of 22%, only 9% of post-AKI patients had nephrology follow-up during the study period.[78]

The KDIGO and the ADQI recommend all AKI to be followed by a nephrologist at least 3 months after an AKI episode.[1,35] As data among children are scant, currently we do not have a pediatric-specific recommendation. Askenazi et al. proposed that children post-AKI should be followed up within 1 month of hospital discharge, quarterly for two visits, and then annually for 2 years with treatment and additional monitoring if CKD or hypertension develops.[79]

One of the reasons for poor nephrology follow-up post-AKI discharge may be lack of strong evidence in favor of clinical benefits. Currently, evidence is limited to an adult retrospective study published by Harel et al. wherein they showed a 24% mortality reduction at 2 years among post AKI patients referred routinely for nephrology follow-up.[80] A randomized controlled trial (Fusion Trial) is comparing regular nephrology follow-up to the current practice and is expected to give more definite evidence regarding benefit if any of routine post-AKI follow-up with nephrologist.[81] The objective of follow-up in a nephrology clinic is to support steps aimed at improvement of kidney function to baseline if possible, preserve kidney function, and prevent its further deterioration. This can be achieved by controlling blood

TABLE 3: Follow-up care after episode of acute kidney injury.

Kidney related	*Cardiovascular related*	*Patient advocacy*
• Serum creatinine monitoring • Proteinuria monitoring • Anemia management • Metabolic control • Prevention of recurrent acute kidney injury • Dialysis preparation	• Use of preventive cardiovascular medication • Blood pressure control • Cholesterol monitoring • Volume management	• Patient education • Communication and education • Access to healthcare system • Medication reconciliation • Goal of care discussion

pressure, proteinuria, early detection, and treatment of any urinary tract infection and ensuring proper bladder drainage in children with bladder outlet obstruction. Educating family and the child regarding the need to avoid nephrotoxic drugs, hypovolemia, and encouraging them to adopt healthy lifestyles are other important objectives of the post-AKI follow-up clinic. Among medications which may be useful in interfering with this AKI–CKD continuum, the RAAS inhibitor may play an important role. Chou et al.[82] in a prospective study showed that RAAS inhibitors lower mortality risk at 2 years' follow-up of patients post AKI (26.6% vs. 42.2%, HR = 0.46, $p <$ 0.001). A larger retrospective study among post-AKI survivors (n = 46,253) also demonstrated a decreased mortality rate at 2 years (HR = 0.85, 95% CI 0.81–0.89) although a concern was the increased risk of hospitalization for renal cause.[83] Statins may be another drug which can be useful among post-AKI patients, but currently evidence is lacking in support of adopting its use in clinical practice. Future studies may show the benefit of sodium–glucose co-transporter-2 (SGLT2) inhibitors even in these populations of post-AKI patients as they have shown benefit among diabetic and nondiabetic CKD population.

Keeping the expected benefits of following up post-AKI patients in perspective some centers have started to establish outpatient care models dedicated to patients who survive an episode of AKI. Clinic visits consist of a standardized assessment by a nephrologist that highlights blood pressure and urine albumin control, review of core laboratory studies that are obtained quarterly (hemoglobin, electrolytes, serum creatinine, calcium, phosphate, and urine albumin to creatinine ratio), cardiovascular risk modification and management of CKD complications, medication reconciliation, and specialist referrals for comorbidity management **(Table 3)**. Medication review is particularly important to check newly prescribed medications, assess stopped medications, confirm appropriate kidney function dosing, and explore patient comprehension of their drug regimens.

CONCLUSION

Acute kidney injury can cause permanent long-term kidney damage. Survivors of AKI are at increased risk of developing CKD as well as at high risk of mortality. Appreciating the continuum of AKI to CKD, the term AKD has been introduced by KDIGO. Maladaptive regeneration of damaged kidney tissue post AKI is considered to be the harbinger of CKD. Epidemiologic studies have shown that after episodes of AKI, 10–15% died in the course of the associated acute illness, 20–50% of survivors of AKI progressed to CKD, and 3–15% had permanent kidney failure. The KDIGO and the ADQI recommend all AKI to be followed by a nephrologist at least 3 months after an AKI episode. Periodic assessment of blood pressure, eGFR, albuminuria, educating the family and the child regarding the need to avoid nephrotoxic drugs, hypovolemia, and encouraging them to adopt healthy lifestyles are the important objectives of the post-AKI follow-up clinics. Cardiovascular risk modification and management of CKD complications, medication reconciliation, and specialist referrals for comorbidity management are needed in all AKI survivors.

KEY POINTS

- AKI can cause permanent long-term kidney damage, and survivors of AKI are at increased risk of developing CKD as well as at increased risk of mortality.
- AKD can progress to CKD or may resolve. Persistence of AKI stage 1 or greater for duration between 7 and 90 days is AKD.
- AKI is transient if renal function recovers within 48 hours. Persistent AKI is renal dysfunction persisting beyond 48 hours.
- Persistent inflammation with maladaptive repair mechanism plays an important role in AKI–CKD continuum.
- Maladaptive changes include impaired angiogenesis, reduced endothelial proliferation, cell cycle arrest, persistent fibrosis, increased expression in kidney tissue microRNAs associated with renal fibrosis, and ongoing inflammation.
- Lower baseline kidney function, longer duration of AKI, higher severity of AKI, and repetitive kidney injury all influence the profibrotic and proinflammatory arms of the regenerative pathways and precipitate adverse maladaptive consequences leading to CKD.
- As AKI and CKD share similar underlying mechanisms of functional and structural injury and exist on the same pathophysiologic continuum, biomarkers of AKI may be useful for early prediction of CKD.
- Children post AKI should be followed up within 1 month of hospital discharge, quarterly for two visits, and then

annually for 2 years with treatment and additional monitoring if CKD or hypertension develops.

- Periodic assessment of blood pressure and quarterly assessment of hemoglobin, electrolytes, serum creatinine, calcium, phosphate, and urine albumin to creatinine ratio and sonographic assessment of kidneys annually should be planned in all AKI survivors.

REFERENCES

1. Kidney Disease Improving Global Outcomes (KDIGO). Acute Kidney Injury Work Group. KDIGO clinical practice guideline for acute kidney injury. Kidney Inter Suppl. 2012;2:1-138.
2. Hsu RK, McCulloch CE, Dudley RA, Lo LJ, Hsu C. Temporal changes in incidence of dialysis-requiring AKI. J Am Soc Nephrol. 2013;24:37-42.
3. Bagshaw SM, George C, Bellomo R, ANZICS Database Management Committee. Changes in the incidence and outcome for early acute kidney injury in a cohort of Australian intensive care units. Crit Care. 2007;11(3):R68.
4. Bellomo R. The epidemiology of acute renal failure: 1975 versus 2005. Curr Opin Crit Care. 2006;12(6):557-60.
5. Cruz DN, Ronco C. Acute kidney injury in the intensive care unit: current trends in incidence and outcome. Crit Care. 2007;11(4):149.
6. Chertow GM, Burdick E, Honour M, Bonventre JV, Bates DW. Acute kidney injury, mortality, length of stay, and costs in hospitalized patients. J Am Soc Nephrol. 2005;16(11):3365-70.
7. Kim J, Kim YJ, Ryoo S, Sohn CH, Seo DW, Ahn S, et al. One-year progression and risk factors for the development of chronic kidney disease in septic shock patients with acute kidney injury: a single-centre retrospective cohort study. J Clin Med. 2018;7(12):554.
8. Rubin S, Orieux A, Clouzeau B, Rigothier C, Combe C, Gruson D, et al. The incidence of chronic kidney disease three years after non-severe acute kidney injury in critically ill patients: a single-center cohort study. J Clin Med. 2019;8(12):2215.
9. Sawhney S, Mitchell M, Marks A, Fluck N, Black C. Long-term prognosis after acute kidney injury (AKI): what is the role of baseline kidney function and recovery? A systematic review. BMJ Open. 2015;5(1):e006497.
10. Chawla LS, Amdur RL, Shaw AD, Faselis C, Palant CE, Kimmel PL. Association between AKI and long-term renal and cardiovascular outcomes in United States veterans. Clin J Am Soc Nephrol. 2014;9(3):448-56.
11. Karsanji DJ, Pannu N, Manns BJ, Hemmelgarn BR, Tan Z, Jindal K, et al. Disparity between nephrologists' opinions and contemporary practices for community follow-up after AKI hospitalization. Clin J Am Soc Nephrol. 2017;12(11):1753-61.
12. Silver SA, Siew ED. Follow-up care in acute kidney injury: lost in transition. Adv Chronic Kidney Dis. 2017;24(4):246-52.
13. Soler YA, Nieves-Plaza M, Prieto M, García-De Jesús R, Suárez-Rivera M. Pediatric risk, injury, failure, loss, end-stage renal disease score identifies acute kidney injury and predicts mortality in critically ill children: a prospective study. Pediatr Crit Care Med. 2013;14(4):e189-95.
14. Uchino S, Kellum JA, Bellomo R, Doig GS, Morimatsu H, Morgera S, et al. Acute renal failure in critically ill patients: a multinational, multicenter study. JAMA. 2005;294(7):813-8.
15. Susantitaphong P, Cruz DN, Cerda J, Abulfaraj M, Alqahtani F, Koulouridis I, et al. World incidence of AKI: a meta-analysis. Clin J Am Soc Nephrol. 2013;8(9):1482-93.
16. Kaddourah A, Basu RK, Bagshaw SM, Goldstein SL; Investigators A. Epidemiology of acute kidney injury in critically ill children and young adults. N Engl J Med. 2017;376(1):11-20.
17. Mehta P, Sinha A, Sami A, Hari P, Kalaivani M, Gulati A, et al. Incidence of acute kidney injury in hospitalized children. Indian Pediatr. 2012;49(7):537-42.
18. Schneider J, Khemani R, Grushkin C, Bart R. Serum creatinine as stratified in the RIFLE score for acute kidney injury is associated with mortality and length of stay for children in the pediatric intensive care unit. Crit Care Med. 2010;38(3):933-9.
19. Alkandari O, Eddington KA, Hyder A, Gauvin F, Ducruet T, Gottesman R, et al. Acute kidney injury is an independent risk factor for pediatric intensive care unit mortality, longer length of stay and prolonged mechanical ventilation in critically ill children: a two-center retrospective cohort study. Crit Care. 2011;15(3):R146.
20. Akcan-Arikan A, Zappitelli M, Loftis LL, Washburn KK, Jefferson LS, Goldstein SL. Modified RIFLE criteria in critically ill children with acute kidney injury. Kidney Int. 2007;71(10):1028-35.
21. Sinha R, Nandi M, Tullus K, Marks SD, Taraphder A. Ten-year follow-up of children after acute renal failure from a developing country. Nephrol Dial Transplant. 2009;24(3):829-33.
22. Mammen C, Al Abbas A, Skippen P, Nadel H, Levine D, Collet JP, et al. Long-term risk of CKD in children surviving episodes of acute kidney injury in the intensive care unit: a prospective cohort study. Am J Kidney Dis. 2012;59(4):523-30.
23. Agus MS, Wypij D, Hirshberg EL, Srinivasan V, Faustino EV, Luckett PM, et al. HALF-PINT Study Investigators and the PALISI Network. Tight glycemic control in critically ill children. N Engl J Med. 2017;376(8):729-41.
24. Hollander SA, Montez-Rath ME, Axelrod DM, Krawczeski CD, May LJ, Maeda K, et al. Recovery from acute kidney injury and CKD following heart transplantation in children, adolescents, and young adults: a retrospective cohort study. Am J Kidney Dis. 2016;68(2):212-8.
25. Madsen NL, Goldstein SL, Froslev T, Christiansen CF, Olsen M. Cardiac surgery in patients with congenital heart disease is associated with acute kidney injury and the risk of chronic kidney disease. Kidney Int. 2017;92(3):751-6.
26. Perico N, Askenazi D, Cortinovis M, Remuzzi G. Maternal and environmental risk factors for neonatal AKI and its long-term consequences. Nat Rev Nephrol. 2018;14(11):688-703.
27. Wald R, Quinn RR, Luo J, Li P, Scales DC, Mamdani MM, et al. University of Toronto Acute Kidney Injury Research Group. Chronic dialysis and death among survivors of acute kidney injury requiring dialysis. JAMA. 2009;302(11):1179-85.
28. James MT, Hemmelgarn BR, Wiebe N, Pannu N, Manns BJ, Klarenbach SW, et al. Alberta Kidney Disease Network. Glomerular filtration rate, proteinuria, and the incidence and consequences of acute kidney injury: a cohort study. Lancet. 2010;376(9758):2096-103.
29. Coca SG, Singanamala S, Parikh CR. Chronic kidney disease after acute kidney injury: a systematic review and meta-analysis. Kidney Int. 2012;81(5):442-8.
30. Basile DP, Friedrich JL, Spahic J, Knipe N, Mang H, Leonard EC, et al. Impaired endothelial proliferation and mesenchymal transition contribute to vascular rarefaction following acute kidney injury. Am J Physiol Renal Physiol. 2011;300(3):F721-33.
31. See EJ, Jayasinghe K, Glassford N, Bailey M, Johnson DW, Polkinghorne KR, et al. Long-term risk of adverse outcomes after acute kidney injury: a systematic review and meta-analysis of cohort studies using consensus definitions of exposure. Kidney Int. 2019;95(1):160-72.

32. Kellum JA, Sileanu FE, Bihorac A, Hoste EA, Chawla LS. Recovery after acute kidney injury. Am J Respir Crit Care Med. 2017;195(6):784-91.
33. Amdur RL, Chawla LS, Amodeo S, Kimmel PL, Palant CE. Outcomes following diagnosis of acute renal failure in U.S. veterans: Focus on acute tubular necrosis. Kidney Int. 2009;76(10):1089-97.
34. Ponte B, Felipe C, Muriel A, Tenorio MT, Liano F. Long-term functional evolution after an acute kidney injury: A 10-year study. Nephrol Dial Transplant. 2008;23(12):3859-66.
35. Chawla LS, Bellomo R, Bihorac A, Goldstein SL, Siew ED, Bagshaw SM, et al.; on behalf of the Acute Disease Quality Initiative Workgroup 16. Acute kidney disease and renal recovery: consensus report of the Acute Disease Quality Initiative (ADQI) 16 work group. Nat Rev Nephrol. 2017;13(4):241-57.
36. Sood MM, Shafer LA, Ho J, Reslerova M, Martinka G, Keenan S, et al. Early reversible acute kidney injury is associated with improved survival in septic shock. J Crit Care. 2014;29(5):711-7.
37. Perinel S, Vincent F, Lautrette A, Dellamonica J, Mariat C, Zeni F, et al. Transient and persistent acute kidney injury and the risk of hospital mortality in critically ill patients. Crit Care Med. 2015;43(8):e269-75.
38. Fidalgo P, Ahmed M, Meyer SR, Lien D, Weinkauf J, Kapasi A, et al. Association between transient acute kidney injury and morbidity and mortality after lung transplantation: a retrospective cohort study. J Crit Care. 2014;29(6):1028-34.
39. Gameiro J, Duarte I, Marques F, Fonseca JA, Jorge S, Rosa R, et al. Transient and persistent AKI and outcomes in patients undergoing major abdominal surgery. Nephron. 2020;144(5):236-44.
40. Coelho S, Fonseca JN, Gameiro J, Jorge S, Velosa J, Lopes JA, et al. Transient and persistent acute kidney injury in acute liver failure. J Nephrol. 2019;32(2):289-96.
41. Ostermann M, Liu K. Pathophysiology of AKI. Best Pract Res Clin Anaesthesiol. 2017;31(3):305-14.
42. Case J, Khan S, Khalid R, Khan A. Epidemiology of acute kidney injury in the intensive care unit. Crit Care Res Pract. 2013;2013:1-9.
43. Akcay A, Nguyen Q, Edelstein CL. Mediators of inflammation in acute kidney injury. Mediators Inflamm. 2009;2009:1-12.
44. Basile DP, Anderson MD, Sutton TA. Pathophysiology of acute kidney injury. Compr Physiol. 2012;2(2):1303-53.
45. Devarajan P. Update on mechanisms of ischemic acute kidney injury. J Am Soc Nephrol. 2006;17(6):1503-20.
46. Sharfuddin AA, Molitoris BA. Pathophysiology of ischemic acute kidney injury. Nat Rev Nephrol. 2011;794:189-200.
47. Liu KD, Brakeman PR. Renal repair and recovery. Crit Care Med. 2008;36(4 Suppl):S187-192.
48. Bonventre JV. Pathophysiology of acute kidney injury: roles of potential inhibitors of inflammation. Contrib Nephrol. 2007;156:39-46.
49. Lee DW, Faubel S, Edelstein CL. Cytokines in acute kidney injury (AKI). Clin Nephrol. 2011;76(3):165-73.
50. Jang HR, Rabb H. Immune cells in experimental acute kidney injury. Nat Rev Nephrol. 2015;11(2):88-101.
51. Askenazi DJ, Feig DI, Graham NM, Hui-Stickle S, Goldstein SL. 3-5 year longitudinal follow-up of pediatric patients after acute renal failure. Kidney Int. 2006;69(1):184-9.
52. Wynn TA. Fibrosis under arrest. Nat Med. 2010;16(5):523-5.
53. Bechtel W, McGoohan S, Zeisberg EM, Müller GA, Kalbacher H, Salant DJ, et al. Methylation determines fibroblast activation and fibrogenesis in the kidney. Nat Med. 2010;16(5):544-50.
54. Ko GJ, Grigoryev DN, Linfert D, Jang HR, Watkins T, Cheadle C, et al. Transcriptional analysis of kidneys during repair from AKI reveals possible roles for NGAL and KIM-1 as biomarkers of AKI-to-CKD transition. Am J Physiol Renal Physiol. 2010;298(6):F1472-83.
55. Goldstein SL, Devarajan P. Acute kidney injury in childhood: Should we be worried about progression to CKD? Pediatr Nephrol. 2011;26(4):509-22.
56. Basile DP, Donohoe DL, Roethe K, Mattson DL. Chronic renal hypoxia after acute ischemic injury: effects of L-arginine on hypoxia and secondary damage. Am J Physiol Renal Physiol. 2003;284(2):F338-48.
57. Yang L, Besschetnova TY, Brooks CR, Shah JV, Bonventre JV. Epithelial cell cycle arrest in G2/M mediates kidney fibrosis after injury. Nature Med. 2010;16(5):535-43.
58. Lewers DT, Mathew TH, Maher JF, Schreiner GE. Long-term follow-up of renal function and histology after acute tubular necrosis. Ann Intern Med. 1970;73(4):523-9.
59. Yang L. How acute kidney injury contributes to renal fibrosis. Adv Exp Med Biol. 2019;1165:117-42.
60. Koralkar R, Ambalavanan N, Levitan EB, McGwin G, Goldstein S, Askenazi D. Acute kidney injury reduces survival in very low birth weight infant. Pediatr Res. 2011;69(4):354-8.
61. Legrand M, Rossignol P. Consequences of acute kidney injury. N Engl J Med. 2020;382(23):2238-47.
62. Odutayo A, Wong CX, Farkouh M, Altman DG, Hopewell S, Emdin CA, et al. AKI and long-term risk for cardiovascular events and mortality. J Am Soc Nephrol. 2017;28(1):377-87.
63. Siew ED, Parr SK, Abdel-Kader K, Eden SK, Peterson JF, Bansal N, et al. Predictors of recurrent AKI. J Am Soc Nephrol. 2016;27(4):1190-200.
64. Holmes J, Geen J, Williams JD, Phillips AO. Recurrent acute kidney injury: predictors and impact in a large population-based cohort. Nephrol Dial Transplant. 2019;35(8):1361-9.
65. Rodrigo E, Suberviola B, Santibáñez M, Belmar L, Castellanos Á, Heras M, et al. Association between recurrence of acute kidney injury and mortality in intensive care unit patients with severe sepsis. J Intensive Care. 2017;5:28.
66. Thakar CV, Christianson A, Himmelfarb J, Leonard AC. Acute kidney injury episodes and chronic kidney disease risk in diabetes mellitus. Clin J Am Soc Nephrol. 2011;6(11):2567-72.
67. Cheng W, Wu X, Liu Q, Wang HS, Zhang NY, Xiao YQ, Y et al. Post-contrast acute kidney injury in a hospitalized population: short-, mid-, and long-term outcome and risk factors for adverse events. Eur Radiol. 2020;30(6):3516-27.
68. Mizota T, Dong L, Takeda C, Shiraki A, Matsukawa S, Shimizu S, et al. Transient acute kidney injury after major abdominal surgery increases chronic kidney disease risk and 1-year mortality. J Crit Care. 2019;50:17-22.
69. Schiffl H, Lang SM, Fischer R. Long-term outcomes of survivors of ICU acute kidney injury requiring renal replacement therapy: a 10-year prospective cohort study. Clin Kidney J. 2012;5(4):297-302.
70. Fiorentino M, Tohme FA, Wang S, Murugan R, Angus DC, Kellum JA, et al. Long-term survival in patients with septic acute kidney injury is strongly influenced by renal recovery. PLoS One. 2018;13(6):e0198269.
71. Wu VC, Huang TM, Lai CF, Shiao CC, Lin YF, Chu TS, et al. Acute-on-chronic kidney injury at hospital discharge is associated with long-term dialysis and mortality. Kidney Int. 2011;80(11):1222-30.
72. Bucaloiu ID, Kirchner HL, Norfolk ER, Hartle JE 2nd, Perkins RM, et al. Increased risk of death and de novo chronic kidney

disease following reversible acute kidney injury. Kidney Int. 2012;81(5):477-85.

73. Heung M, Steffick DE, Zivin K, Gillespie BW, Banerjee T, Hsu CY, et al. Acute kidney injury recovery pattern and subsequent risk of CKD: an analysis of Veterans health administration data. Am J Kidney Dis. 2016;67(5):742-52.
74. Zhang WR, Parikh CR. Biomarkers of acute and chronic kidney disease. Annu Rev Physiol. 2019;81:309-33.
75. Lopez-Giacoman S, Madero M. Biomarkers in chronic kidney disease, from kidney function to kidney damage. World J Nephrol. 2015;4(1):57-73.
76. Koyner JL, Shaw AD, Chawla LS, Hoste EA, Bihorac A, Kashani K, et al. Tissue inhibitor metalloproteinase-2 (TIMP-2)_IGF-binding protein-7 (IGFBP7) levels are associated with adverse long-term outcomes in patients with AKI. J Am Soc Nephrol. 2015;26(7):1747-54.
77. Saran R, Li Y, Robinson B, Abbott KC, Agodoa LY, Ayanian J, et al. US renal data system 2015 annual data report: epidemiology of kidney disease in the United States. Am J Kidney Dis. 2016;67:A7-8.
78. Siew ED, Peterson JF, Eden SK, Hung AM, Speroff T, Ikizler TA, et al. Outpatient nephrology referral rates after acute kidney injury. J Am Soc Nephrol. 2012;23(2):305-12.
79. Askenazi DJ. Do children with acute kidney injury require long-term evaluation for CKD? Am J Kidney Dis. 2012;59 4):478-80.
80. Harel Z, Wald R, Bargman JM, Mamdani M, Etchells E, Garg AX, et al. Nephrologist follow-up improves all-cause mortality of severe acute kidney injury survivors. Kidney Int. 2013;83(5):901-8.
81. ClinicalTrials.gov. (2015). Nephrologist follow-up versus usual care after an acute kidney injury hospitalization (FUSION). [online] Available from: https://clinicaltrials.gov/ct2/show/NCT02483039. [Last accessed March, 2022].
82. Chou YH, Huang TM, Pan SY, Chang CH, Lai CF, Wu VC, et al. Renin-angiotensin system inhibitor is associated with lower risk of ensuing chronic kidney disease after functional recovery from. Sci Rep. 2017;7:46518.
83. Brar S, Ye F, James MT, Klarenbach S, Pannu N; Interdisciplinary Chronic Disease. Association of angiotensin converting enzyme inhibitor or angiotensin receptor blocker use with outcomes after acute kidney injury. JAMA Intern Med. 2018;178(12):1681-90.

CHAPTER

11.9 Extracorporeal Therapies

Dimpy Waghela, Kanav Anand

INTRODUCTION

Apheresis is an extracorporeal process in which peripheral blood is processed by a machine to separate it into different components. The selected component is later removed while the remainder is returned to the donor or the patient. As per the Greek language, apheresis means taking out or removal. The terms plasmapheresis, leukapheresis, erythrocytapheresis, and thrombocytapheresis describe the specific blood elements that are removed.

PLASMAPHERESIS

Plasmapheresis or plasma exchange is a technique for selective removal of plasma and replacing it with some other fluid such as colloid, crystalloid, or bank plasma. The basic principle of plasmapheresis is that by removing or decreasing levels of certain pathologic substances which are dissolved in the plasma, prevention of further damage or reversal of a pathologic process can be obtained.[1] The pathologic substance to be removed may be an immune complex, autoantibody, myeloma light chains, endotoxin, or cholesterol-containing lipoprotein.

Therapeutic plasma exchange (TPE) is considered as a rational therapeutic choice if at least one of the following conditions is present **(Box 1 and Fig. 1)**:

- Substance, which needs to be cleared, should have a long half-life so that extracorporeal removal is faster than endogenous clearance.
- Substance to be eliminated must be acutely toxic and/or resistant to conventional medical therapy.
- Substance to be removed should be large enough with a molecular weight >15,000 Dalton, so that it cannot be easily removed by conventional techniques such as hemofiltration or high-flux hemodialysis.

BOX 1: Ideal target molecule characteristics for therapeutic plasma exchange.

Identified etiologic agent or toxic substance with:
- High molecular mass (>15,000 D)
- Slow rate of formation
- Low turnover
- Low volume of distribution

Source: Adapted from Williams ME, Balogun RA. Principles of separation: indications and therapeutic targets for plasma exchange. Clin J Am Soc Nephrol. 2014;9(1):181-90.[2]

Indications

A comprehensive review of category-based indications for therapeutic apheresis **(Table 1)** based on current literature review is published periodically by the American Society for Apheresis (ASFA).[3]

The categories are defined as follows:

- *Category I:* Diseases for which apheresis is considered as a first-line therapy, either alone or as an addition to other modalities of treatment.
- *Category II:* Diseases for which apheresis is considered as a second-line therapy, either alone or as an addition to other modalities of treatment.
- *Category III:* Optimum role of apheresis treatment for that disease is not well established.
- *Category IV:* Diseases for which the published literature suggests apheresis to be ineffective or potentially harmful.

Common indications for plasmapheresis along with their details are discussed in **Box 2 and Table 2.**[4,5]

Nonrenal Indications

Plasma exchange is beneficial in many neurological disorders of autoimmune cause by aiding in the removal of inflammatory mediators, including autoantibodies, cytokines, and complement components. As per ASFA, plasmapheresis is considered as a first-line treatment for Guillain–Barré syndrome (GBS), chronic inflammatory demyelinating

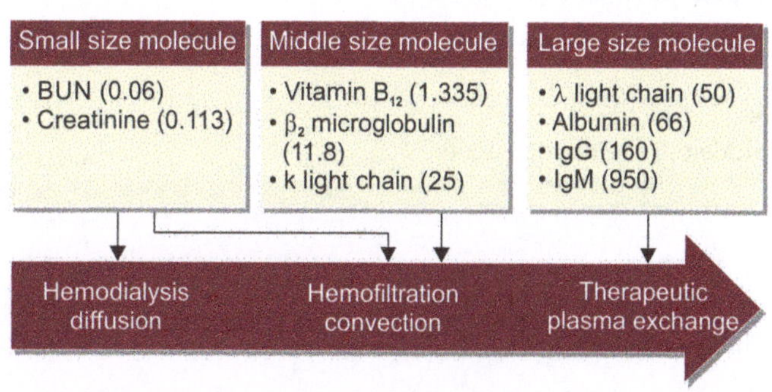

Fig. 1: Different extracorporeal therapies based on size of target substance. (Molecular masses are expressed in kilodalton.) (BUN: blood urea nitrogen; Ig: immunoglobulin)

TABLE 1: Category recommendations for therapeutic apheresis.

Disease	*Indication*	*Category*
Acute disseminated encephalomyelitis (ADEM)	Steroid refractory	II
Acute inflammatory demyelinating polyradiculopathy (GB syndrome)	Primary treatment	I
Acute liver failure		III
Anti-GBM disease (Goodpasture syndrome)	• Diffuse alveolar hemorrhage (DAH) • Dialysis independent • Dialysis dependent	I I III
Autoimmune hemolytic disease	Severe cold agglutinin disease	II
Chronic inflammatory demyelinating polyradiculopathy		I
Cutaneous T-cell lymphoma, Sezary syndrome	• Erythrodermic • Nonerythrodermic	I III
Familial hypercholesterolemia	• Homozygotes • Heterozygotes • Homozygotes/heterozygotes	I II II
Focal segmental glomerulosclerosis	• Recurrent in kidney transplant • Recurrent in kidney transplant/steroid resistant in native kidney • Steroid resistant in native kidney	I II III
Graft versus host disease	• Acute • Chronic	II II
Hereditary hemochromatosis		I
Hyperleukocytosis	• Symptomatic • Prophylactic/secondary	II III
Hyperviscosity in hypergammaglobulinemia	• Symptomatic • Prophylaxis for rituximab	I I
IgA disease (Berger disease)	• Crescentic • Chronic/progressive	III III
Lambert–Eaton myasthenic syndrome		II
Multiple sclerosis	• Acute attack/relapse • Chronic	II III
Myasthenia gravis	• Acute, short-term treatment • Long-term treatment	I II
NMDA receptor antibody encephalitis		I
Overdose, envenomation, and poisoning	• Mushroom poisoning • Envenomation • Drug poisoning	II III III
Pediatric autoimmune neuropsychiatric disorders associated with streptococcal infection (PANDAS)	PANDAS, exacerbation	II
Polycythemia vera; erythrocytosis	• Polycythemia vera • Secondary erythrocytosis	I III
Sepsis with multiorgan failure		III
Sickle cell anemia, acute	• Acute stroke • Acute chest syndrome • Other complications	I II III
Sickle cell anemia, non-acute	• Stroke prophylaxis • Pregnancy • Recurrent vaso-occlusive pain crises • Preoperative management	I II II III
Systemic lupus erythematosus	Severe complications	II
Thrombocytosis	• Symptomatic • Secondary, prophylactic	II III
Thrombotic microangiopathy, coagulation mediated	THBD, DGKE, and PLG mutations	III

Contd...

Contd...

Disease	Indication	Category
Thrombotic microangiopathy, coagulation mediated	• Factor H autoantibody • Complement factor gene mutation	I III
Thrombotic microangiopathy, drug associated	• Ticlopidine • Clopidogrel • Gemcitabine/quinine	I III IV
Thrombotic thrombocytopenic purpura (TTP)		I
ABO incompatible renal transplant	• Desensitization, living donor • Antibody-mediated rejection	II III
Wilson disease		I

(GB: Guillain–Barré; GBM: glomerular basement membrane; NMDA: N-methyl-D-aspartate; SRNS: steroid-resistant nephrotic syndrome)

BOX 2: Indications of plasmapheresis in kidney diseases.

Rapidly progressive glomerulonephritis:
- Pauci-immune GN
- Antiglomerular basement membrane GN
- IgA nephropathy
- Henoch–Schonlein purpura nephritis
- Cryoglobulinemia

Renal transplant recipient:
- *Pretransplant desensitization*: ABO-incompatible transplant
- Acute antibody-mediated rejection
- Post-transplant recurrence of FSGS

Others:
- Atypical hemolytic uremic syndrome
- TTP
- Multiorgan dysfunction
- Multiple myeloma with renal failure

(FSGS: focal segmental glomerulosclerosis; GN: glomerulonephritis; IgA: immunoglobulin A; TTP: thrombotic thrombocytopenia)
Source: Adapted from Ranganathan D, John GT. Therapeutic plasma exchange in renal disorders. Indian J Nephrol. 2019;29(3):151-9.

polyradiculoneuropathy, myasthenia gravis (moderate-severe crisis/preoperative), and N-methyl-D-aspartate receptor (NMDAR) antibody encephalitis.

Guillain–Barré Syndrome

In postpolio era, GBS is the most common cause of acute flaccid paralysis in healthy infants and children.[6] The paralysis usually follows a nonspecific gastrointestinal or respiratory infection, most commonly by *Campylobacter jejuni*. The disease results in symmetric weakness, paralysis, and distal paresthesia, which start with lower limbs and rapidly progress to proximal limbs and trunk over several days. CSF albumin-cytological dissociation (increased concentration of protein in the absence of pleocytosis) is diagnostic of GBS.

The main modalities of therapy for GBS are intravenous immune-globulin and plasma exchange **(Fig. 2)**.[7] Prompt initiation of treatment is preferred in case of progression of weakness, deteriorating respiratory status, especially if requiring mechanical ventilation, significant bulbar weakness, or inability to walk unaided. Earlier improvement in muscle strength, reduced need of mechanical ventilation, and better recovery have been demonstrated in children started on plasmapheresis.

Chronic Inflammatory Demyelinating Neuropathy

Chronic inflammatory demyelinating neuropathy is an immune-mediated acquired neuropathy affecting peripheral nerves and their nerve roots, hallmarked by relapsing or progressive course, glucocorticoid responsiveness, and pathological features of demyelination. In the classical form, chronic inflammatory demyelinating polyneuropathy (CIDP) results in symmetric, motor predominant neuropathy leading to both proximal and distal muscle weakness. TPE helps in removal of the circulating autoantibodies against various proteins and glycolipids of peripheral nerve.

Myasthenia Gravis

Myasthenia gravis is an autoimmune disorder of the neuromuscular junction, mediated by circulating autoantibodies against nicotinic acetylcholine receptor (AChR) resulting in fluctuating muscle weakness. The therapy for myasthenia gravis includes thymectomy, acetylcholine esterase inhibitors, corticosteroids, immunosuppressive drugs, TPE, and IVIG. TPE is presumed to eliminate circulating AChR antibodies and other humoral factors. TPE is indicated in cases requiring rapid clinical improvement, myasthenia crisis, impending crisis, preoperative stabilization, and children not responding to other forms of therapy.

Familial Hypercholesterolemia

Lipid apheresis is recommended as a cornerstone therapy for lipid lowering, especially when medical therapy with lipid-lowering drugs is ineffective. It is indicated in patients with homozygous familial hypercholesterolemia (HoFH) and severe heterozygous familial hypercholesterolemia (HeFH).

Toxins and Drugs

Therapeutic plasma exchange helps in removal of toxins, depending on the effective clearance, plasma protein

TABLE 2: Plasmapheresis for kidney disease in children: Indications and treatment guideline.

Disease	*Indication*	*Mechanism*	*TPE treatment*	*Replacement solution*
ANCA-associated rapidly progressive glomerulonephritis (RPGN)	• Dialysis dependent	ANCA autoantibody	1–1.5 total plasma volume (TPV) daily during rapidly progressive course then every alternate day, total 6–9 TPEs or until pulmonary hemorrhage is resolved	• Albumin or plasma
	• Diffuse alveolar hemorrhage (DAH) • Dialysis independent			• FFP is the first choice when DAH is present • For daily TPE, a mixture of albumin with FFP to prevent bleed
Anti-GBM glomerulonephritis	• DAH	Anti-GBM antibody	• 1–1.5 times TPV daily for a few days or for rapidly progressive period, then every other day	• Albumin or plasma
	• Dialysis dependent, no DAH • Dialysis independent, no RPGN		• 10–20 days until antibody level decreases • Continue until resolution of ongoing glomerular or pulmonary injury	• FFP is the first choice, if DAH is present • For daily TPE, mixture of albumin with FFP
Thrombotic microangiopathy (TMA)	• Hematopoietic stem cell transplantation	• Undefined	• 1–1.5 TPV daily, depending upon clinical or hematological response	Plasma
	• Factor H autoantibodies	• Anti-factor H	• 1–1.5 TPV daily, depending on patient condition and stable hematocrit and platelet count	Plasma
	• TTP	• Anti-ADAMTS autoantibody	• 1.5 TPV daily for a few days and then 1 TPV. Daily until the platelet count >150 × 10^9/L and LDH near normal for 2–3 consecutive days	Plasma
Sepsis with multiorgan failure		Inflammatory and anti-fibrinolytic factors	1–1.5 TPV daily for 2–14 days depending on improvement in organ function	Plasma
Kidney transplant	FSGS recurrence	Plasma factor of unknown origin	• 1–1.5 TPV daily or every alternate day • Acute recurrence: 9 TPEs over 2 weeks until proteinuria decreases/resolved • Maintenance TPE: Following initial daily TPEs, gradually taper as indicated, e.g., 3/week for the first 3 weeks, 2/week for 3 weeks, 1/week until month 3, and so on	• Albumin or plasma • Daily TPE with a mixture of albumin with plasma • Maintenance TPE—albumin
• Antibody mediated rejection (AMR)	• HLA antibodies		• For desensitization daily or every alternate day till negative crossmatch	• Albumin or plasma
• Pretransplant ABO incompatible (living donor)	• Isoagglutinin (Anti-A, Anti-B)		• Continue until antibody titer is less than critical threshold (<1:4) prior to transplant	• Albumin or plasma, use FFP that is compatible to both donor and recipient ABO type

(ANCA: antineutrophil cytoplasmic antibody; FFP: fresh frozen plasma; HLA: human leukocyte antigen; TPE: therapeutic plasma exchange)
Source: Adapted from Sethi SK, Raina R, McCulloch M, Bunchman TE. Critical Care Pediatric Nephrology and Dialysis: A Practical Handbook. New York City: Springer; 2019.

binding, and volume of distribution. TPE has been used to treat mushroom intoxication by *Amanita phalloides*. There is controversy about the proven beneficial effects of TPE in the treatment of life-threatening intoxications with tricyclic antidepressants, benzodiazepines, quinine, and phenytoin. Due to lack of supporting data from controlled studies, it is difficult to make recommendations for the treatment of poisonings and overdoses.

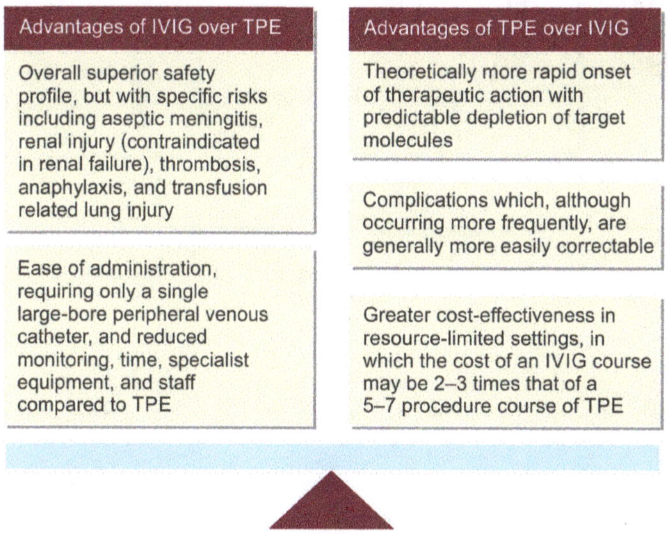

Fig. 2: Comparison of intravenous immunoglobulin (IVIG) and plasmapheresis in pediatric neurology. (TPE: therapeutic plasma exchange)
Source: Adapted from Eyre M, Hacohen Y, Barton C, Hemingway C, Lim M. Therapeutic plasma exchange in pediatric neurology: a critical review and proposed treatment algorithm. Dev Med Child Neurol. 2018;60(8):765-79.

Procedure of Plasma Exchange

Plasma exchange can be accomplished by two different techniques, namely:[8]

1. Centrifugation
2. Membrane filtration

Comparison of the two techniques is given in **Table 3**.

Prescription

Venous Access

Plasmapheresis can be performed using a wide range of vascular access such as central venous catheter (CVC), two large durable peripheral veins, arteriovenous (AV) fistula, AV graft, or CVC port. Appropriate size of CVC may be chosen according to the weight of the child **(Table 4)**.[9]

In an acute setting, temporary CVCs are preferred whereas, in chronic conditions, permanent external vascular access or AV fistulas can be used.

Exchange Volume

The goal is to exchange 1.0–1.5 plasma volume (PV) which is usually estimated by the formula: PV (in liters) is equal to the total blood volume (TBV) × (1 – Hct/100). In pediatrics, as the total body volume is variable (based on body weight and age of the child) **(Table 5)**, the dose of replacement fluid may also be calculated as 40–60 mL/kg/session. Single PV exchange clears 63% fraction; after the second session, it increases to 85%.

TABLE 3: Comparison of the plasmapheresis techniques.

Procedure	***Centrifugation TPE***	***Membrane TPE***
Mechanism	Separates plasma from cellular components based on density, molecular size, and weight **(Fig. 3A)**	Removal of substances occurs by sieving coefficient of membrane **(Fig. 3B)**
Apparatus	COMTEC (Fresenius Kabi)/Spectra Optia Apheresis system **(Fig. 4)**	Fresenius 4008/5008 machine with a plasmapheresis filter **(Fig. 5)**
Blood flow rate (mL/min)	10–150	150
Plasma extraction (%)	80	30
Anticoagulation	Citrate	Heparin
Blood volume in circuit (mL)	180	125
Replacement fluid	Fresh frozen plasma, albumin	Fresh frozen plasma, albumin
Sterilization	Gamma irradiation, ethylene oxide	Ethylene oxide

(TPE: therapeutic plasma exchange)

TABLE 4: Appropriate catheter size in children.[10]

Patient weight	***Catheter size***
Neonate/infant	Double-lumen 7 French
<20 kg	Double-lumen 8 French
20–30 kg	Double-lumen 10 French
>30 kg	Double-lumen 11.5 French

TABLE 5: Proposed formulas to estimate blood volume based on body weight and age.

Age and body weight	***Total blood volume***
Infant or <2 kg	80 mL/kg
Child or 20–50 kg	70 mL/kg
Adult or >50 kg	60 mL/kg

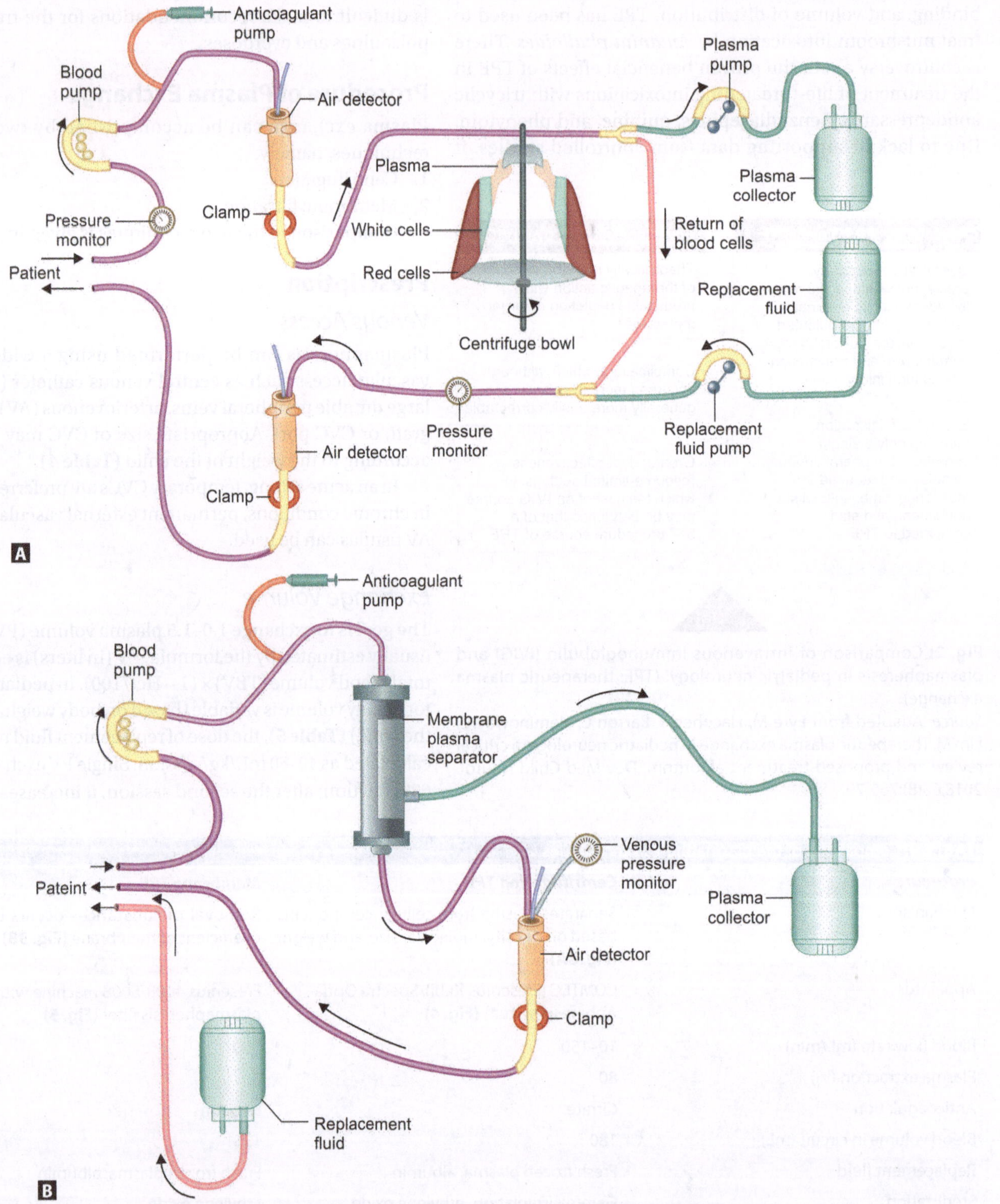

Figs. 3A and B: (A) Centrifugation: Blood is pumped into separate containers. As the centrifuge revolves, different blood components are separated into discrete layers, which can be harvested separately. Plasma is pumped out of the centrifuge into collection chamber. Red blood cells, leukocytes, and platelets are returned to the donor along with replacement fluid; (B) Membrane filtration separator for plasma exchange: Blood is pumped into biocompatible membrane that allows filtration of plasma while allowing return of cellular elements.
Source: Adapted from Madore F, Lazarus JM, Brady HR. Therapeutic plasma exchange in renal diseases. J Am Soc Nephrol. 2019;29(3):151-9.

Replacement Fluid

Fresh frozen plasma or 5% albumin or combination of both can be used as replacement fluid. FFP should be used in cases of derangements in coagulation factor or complements [as in atypical hemolytic-uremic (aHUS) syndrome] or ADAMTS-13 (thrombotic thrombocytopenic purpura). Patient fluid volume must be replaced to prevent marked volume depletion.

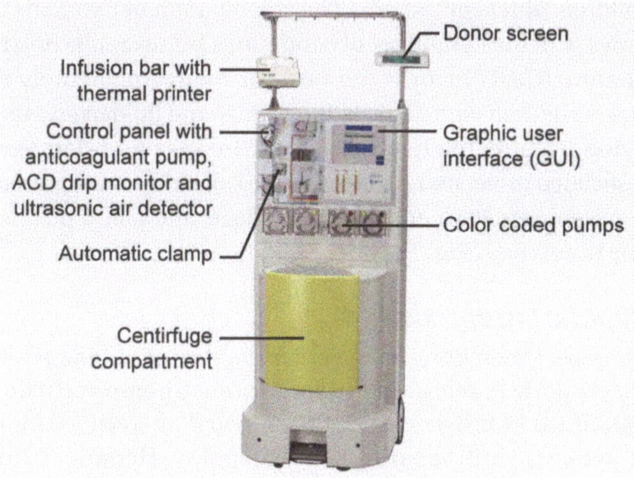

Fig. 4: Plasmapheresis centrifugation machine. (ACD: acid citrate dextrose)

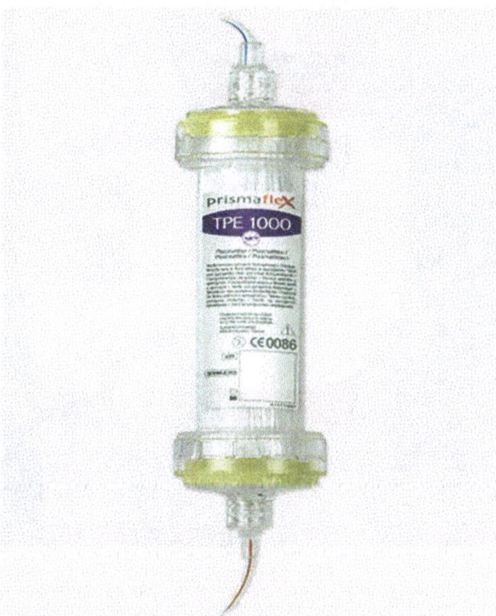

Fig. 5: Plasma filter.

Priming

Priming of circuit is done using normal saline or 5% albumin. Packed red blood cells may be used if extracorporeal circuit volume is >10% of total blood volume.

Anticoagulation

Apheresis requires anticoagulation to prevent clot formation in an extracorporeal circuit. Anticoagulation is chosen depending upon the technique of plasmapheresis used. Heparin is the choice of anticoagulant for membrane-based TPE whereas citrate is preferred for centrifugation-based TPE. Heparin is administered as an initial IV bolus of 40–60 IU/kg followed by a continuous infusion of 20 IU/kg/h so as to target a prothrombin time/partial thromboplastin time (PT/PTT) more than 1.5 times of the normal.

Components of the prescription for plasmapheresis are given in **Box 3**.

BOX 3: Prescription for plasmapheresis.

- *Access:* Secured access to venous line
- *Technique:* Centrifugation/membrane therapeutic plasma exchange
- *Blood flow rate:* 3–5 mL/kg/min and should not exceed 50 mL/kg/h
- *Replacement volume:* 40–60 mL/kg/session
- *Replacement fluid:* 5% albumin and/or FFP
- *Premedication:* Injection pheniramine, ondansetron, and paracetamol
- Injection calcium gluconate (10%) to be kept handy

Complications

- *Hypotension:* Various factors contribute to hypotension during the TPE procedure, such as volume loss (most common), hypocalcemia, or vasovagal reaction. It can be managed by administration of normal saline bolus or colloid solution. Hypotension can be avoided by careful management of intravascular volume shift and by priming of the circuit, especially if the circuit volume is more than 10% of the patient's blood volume.
- *Hypocalcemia:* Citrate-induced hypocalcemia is seen in 28.5% children undergoing TPE, as citrate binds to ionized calcium to form soluble calcium citrate reducing the ionized calcium concentration. Intravenous 10% calcium gluconate should be infused during the procedure to prevent hypocalcemia. The risk of citrate toxicity also increases with the use of large volume of blood component therapy containing citrate.
- *Citrate-induced metabolic alkalosis:* Citrate administration results in development of metabolic alkalosis, especially in patients with concurrent renal dysfunction. Metabolism of excess citrate generates bicarbonate, the excretion of which is limited in renal failure.
- *Inadvertent removal of medication:* Medications that are highly protein bound, small volume of distribution is substantially removed by TPE. Immunoglobulins, rituximab, and basiliximab are greatly removed by TPE. Calcineurin inhibitors (cyclosporine and tacrolimus) and corticosteroids are minimally removed by TPE.
- *Vascular catheter complication:* Potential complications of CVC include infection, pain, nerve damage, thrombosis, perforation, or AV fistula.
- *Anaphylactic reaction:* Anaphylactic reaction to plasma is a serious complication associated with TPE. Management of anaphylactic reaction includes antihistamines, epinephrine, glucocorticoids, or measures depending upon the severity of symptoms. It is advisable to premedicate the child prior to the procedure to prevent complication.
- *Hypokalemia:* Nonplasma replacement fluid can induce reduction in plasma K^+ concentration in the postapheresis period due to dilution. For at-risk individual, plasma K^+ should be monitored post-procedure and treated accordingly.

- *Hypothermia:* It is a frequent complication, which may occur due to circuit exposure, and so warmers must be used during the procedure.

HEMOPERFUSION

Hemoperfusion is an extracorporeal blood purification modality in which anticoagulated whole blood is passed through a device, usually a column that contains adsorbent particles. It is used for the removal of toxins in poisonings and has been used for removal of cytokines in septic patients. Hemoperfusion can remove substances up to 30 kDa depending on the characteristics of the sorbent material.

Indications

Poisoning

The use of extracorporeal therapies (ECTs) for any intoxication **(Table 6)** is justified if there are signs of severe toxicity, slow response to traditional therapy, and if it will remove the toxins by a rate which is 30% more than the endogenous excretion rate. Hemoperfusion is preferred over hemodialysis alone for paraquat poisoning. It provides early clearance of paraquat compared to high-flux hemodialysis. Hemodialysis possesses advantage over hemoperfusion in terms of increased availability, decreased cost, familiarity, and lower complication rate along with concurrent metabolic and acid-base correction.[11]

Sepsis

Hemoperfusion devices contain either the antibiotic polymyxin B or a polystyrene divinylbenzene copolymer. These help in removing cytokines or endotoxins from patients with sepsis. CytoSorb is a hemoadsorption cartridge column containing hemocompatible porous polymeric beads **(Fig. 6)**. It is effective in the removal of cytokines and other inflammatory mediators which fall in this range of 5–60 kDa. It has been well demonstrated that the levels of interleukin-6 (IL-6) and IL-10 significantly reduce after the therapy in children with septic shock. The combination of CytoSorb in series with the hemofilter of continuous kidney replacement therapy (CKRT) works the best for managing acutely ill septic children with acute kidney injury and fluid overload.[12] CytoSorb effectively eliminates cytokines and damage-associated molecular patterns (DAMPs), reduce vasopressor requirements, limit endothelial damage, and play a positive role in survival **(Fig. 7)**.

TABLE 6: Plasma drug extraction ratios with different therapies at BFR (blood flow rate) of 200 mL/min.[10]

Drug	*Hemodialysis*	*Hemoperfusion*
Acetaminophen	0.4	0.5–0.7
ASA	0.5	0.5
Digoxin	0.2	0.3–0.6
Glutethimide	0.16	0.65–0.8
Paraquat	0.5	0.6
Phenobarbital	0.3–0.7	0.5–0.85
Theophylline	0.5	0.7
Tricyclics	0.35	0.35

(ASA: acetylsalicylic acid or aspirin)

Hepatic Encephalopathy

Hemoperfusion done at an earlier stage results in increased survival and favorable outcomes. Post-hemoperfusion significant improvement has been noted in consciousness of patients with hepatic encephalopathy. Hepatic toxins

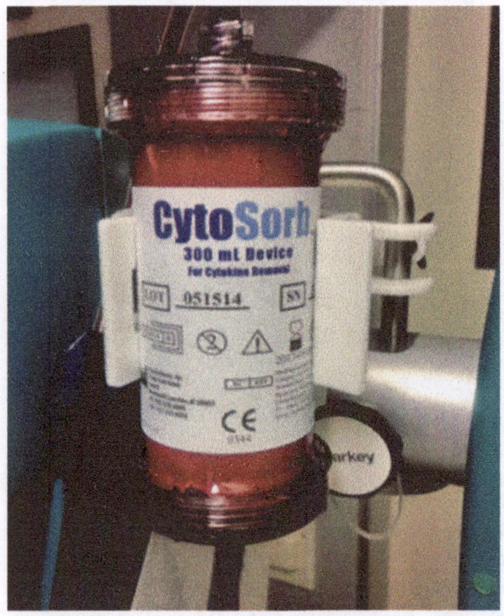

Fig. 6: CytoSorb.

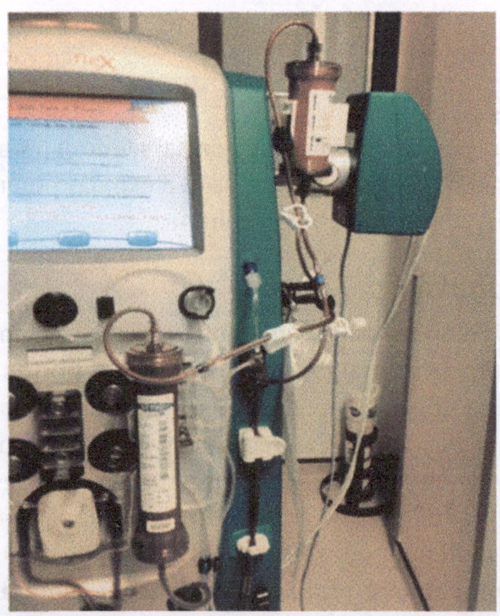

Fig. 7: CytoSorb column incorporated into return limb of continuous kidney replacement therapy circuit used for removal of cytokines in a child with sepsis.

TABLE 7: Substances relevant to hepatic failure removed with sorbent hemoperfusion.

Amino acids—aromatic > branched chain	Cytokines: IL (1, 6, 10, and 12)	Mercaptans
Bile acids	Dopamine	Norepinephrine
Bilirubin	Epinephrine	Octopamine
Coagulation factors	Fatty acids	Phenols
Protein-bound molecules	Middle molecules	

(Table 7) slowly equilibrate in the body, resulting in the need for the detoxification procedure on a periodic basis till the underlying disease improves.[13]

Others

Removal of pathogenic antibodies and antigen-antibody complexes in conditions such as systemic lupus erythematosus, vasculitis, antiglomerular basement membrane disease, atopic dermatitis, GBS, chronic inflammatory demyelinating polyneuropathy, myasthenia gravis, and multiple sclerosis and as a preconditioning protocol for ABO incompatible kidney transplant. Although standard of care is plasmapheresis or TPE, a possible advantage of hemoperfusion/immunoadsorption is more specific immune-modulation without the requirement of plasma product infusion.

Sorbent System

The sorbent device is made up of microbeads of activated carbons (charcoals), ion-exchange resins or nonionic resins, encased in a plastic case. This system has a high adsorptive capacity and low toxicity and is highly biocompatible.

Charcoal

Activated carbons can be obtained from various biological or nonbiological substances. The adsorptive capacity of the charcoal system depends on the surface area, porosity, and thickness of the membrane coating. Devices contain 70–300 g of activated charcoal. Complex physical forces (Van der Waals) trap the solutes in the charcoal pores **(Fig. 8)**. Charcoal hemoperfusion has been used for treating patients with theophylline, phenobarbitone, aspirin, and aluminum toxicity. It works well for molecules with a small volume of distribution and which are protein bound.

Exchange Resins

Ionic and nonionic resins **(Fig. 9)** are used as adsorptive materials for hemoperfusion. Ion exchange resins exchange one or more ions for another. Uncharged nonionic resins adsorb solutes with less energy. Resin-based hemoperfusion works most effectively for lipid-soluble substances such as glutethimide.

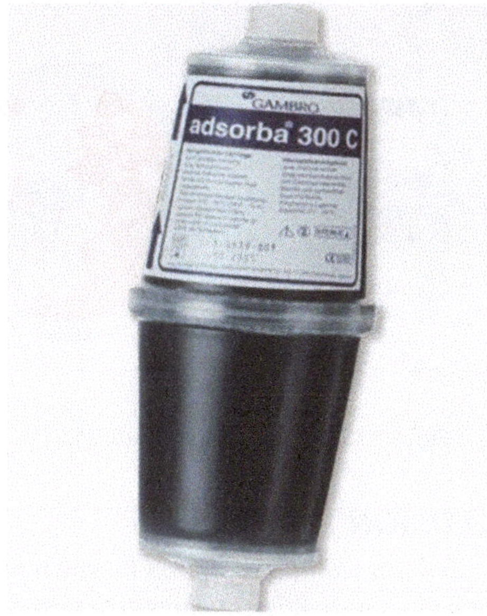

Fig. 8: Charcoal adsorber.

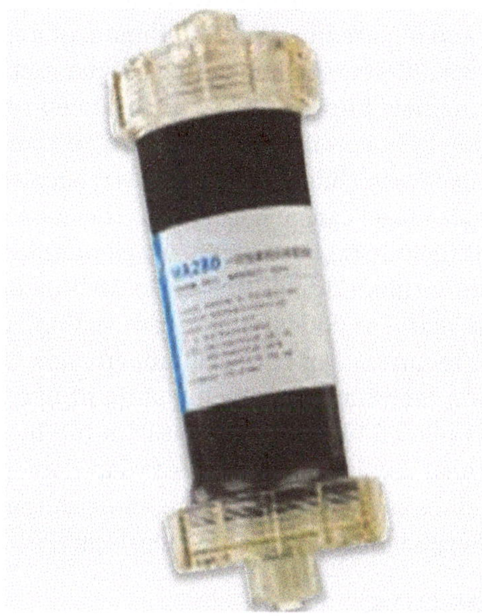

Fig. 9: Resin adsorber.

Mechanism

Adsorption: Molecules adhere to the surface of sorbent granules **(Fig. 10)**.

Complications

- *Thrombocytopenia:* Mild thrombocytopenia is caused by adsorption of platelets by activated charcoal. Platelet count usually recovers by 24–48 hours.
- *Transient leukopenia:* There occurs <10% decrease in total leukocyte count due to complement activation and migration of leukocytes.
- Fibrinogen and fibronectin are also reduced.
- Hypothermia.
- Hypoglycemia.
- Hypocalcemia.

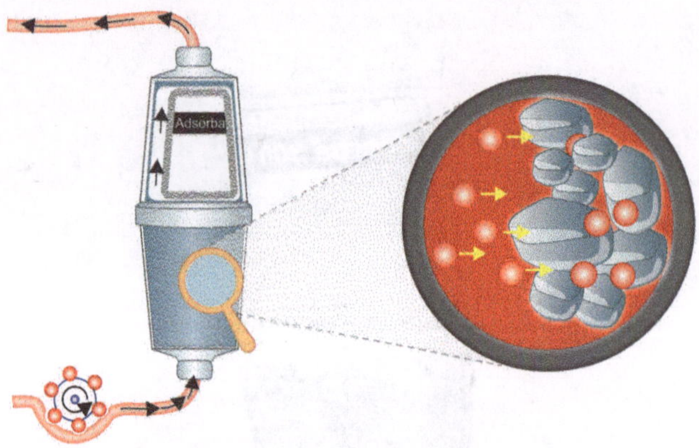

Fig. 10: Mechanism of hemoperfusion.

CONCLUSION

Apheresis is an extracorporeal process in which peripheral blood is separated into different components and selected component is removed while the remainder is returned. Plasmapheresis or TPE involves removal of a large volume of plasma and replacement with 5% albumin or fresh-frozen plasma. Two different techniques for plasma exchange are available, namely filtration by centrifugal cell separation and filtration by hollow fiber plasma filters. The procedure is safe and effective in children with various renal diseases but requires specialized care and expertise. The common renal indications include rapidly progressive glomerulonephritis, aHUS, pretransplant desensitization in ABO-incompatible transplant, acute antibody-mediated rejection, and post-transplant recurrence of FSGS. Hemoperfusion is a blood purification technique in which a sorbent like charcoal and resins placed in direct contact with the blood in an extracorporeal circuit helps to remove toxins. Hemoperfusion improves the outcome in many drug intoxications, sepsis, hepatic encephalopathy, and acute lung injury.

KEY POINTS

- Plasmapheresis or plasma exchange selectively removes pathologic substances which are dissolved in the plasma and replacement with plasma or albumin.
- The extracorporeal elimination efficiency of plasmapheresis for a given substance depends on the volume of distribution, protein binding, intercompartment equilibration, and exchange PV.
- Plasma exchange is done by either centrifugation or membrane filtration technique.
- Plasma exchange is beneficial in many renal autoimmune and neurological disorders and helps in the removal of inflammatory mediators, including autoantibodies, cytokines, and complement components.
- Hemoperfusion is an extracorporeal blood purification therapy using a column that contains adsorbent particles such as charcoal.
- Hemoperfusion is used in poisoning, sepsis, and hepatic encephalopathy.

REFERENCES

1. Daugirdas JT, Blake PG, Ing TS. Handbook of Dialysis. Philadelphia: Lippincott Williams & Wilkins; 2012.
2. Williams ME, Balogun RA. Principles of separation: indications and therapeutic targets for plasma exchange. Clin J Am Soc Nephrol. 2014;9(1):181-90.
3. Padmanabhan A, Connelly-Smith L, Aqui N, Balogun RA, Klingel R, Meyer E, et al. Guidelines on the use of therapeutic apheresis in clinical practice–evidence-based approach from the Writing Committee of the American Society for Apheresis: the eighth special issue. J Clin Apher. 2019;34(3):171-354.
4. Ranganathan D, John GT. Therapeutic plasma exchange in renal disorders. Indian J Nephrol. 2019;29(3):151.
5. Sethi SK, Raina R, McCulloch M, Bunchman TE. Critical Care Pediatric Nephrology and Dialysis: A Practical Handbook. Singapore: Springer Singapore; 2019.
6. Yu A, Chertow G, Luyckx V, Marsden P, Skorecki K, Taal M. Brenner and Rector's The Kidney, 2-Volume Set, 11th edition. Amsterdam: Elsevier; 2019.
7. Eyre M, Hacohen Y, Barton C, Hemingway C, Lim M. Therapeutic plasma exchange in pediatric neurology: a critical review and proposed treatment algorithm. Dev Med Child Neurol. 2018;60(8):765-79.
8. Madore F, Lazarus JM, Brady HR. Therapeutic plasma exchange in renal diseases. J Am Soc Nephrol. 1996;7(3):367-86.
9. Alhasan KA. Therapeutic plasma exchange for children with kidney disorders: definitions, prescription, indications, and complications. Saudi J Kidney Dis Transplant. 2019;30(2):291.
10. Hort WH, Koch KM, Lindsay RM, Ronco C, Winchester JF. Replacement of Renal Function by Dialysis, 5th edition. Dordrecht: Springer; 1989.
11. Gao Y, Chen YL, Zhong F, Li YJ, Ye H, Deng YM. Effect of hemoperfusion in treatment of children with acute poisoning. Zhonghua Er Ke Za Zhi. 2007;45(9):665-9.
12. Bottari G, Guzzo I, Marano M, Stoppa F, Ravà L, Di Nardo M, et al. Hemoperfusion with CytoSorb in pediatric patients with septic shock: a retrospective observational study. Int J Artif Organs. 2020;43(9):587-93.
13. Ash SR. Extracorporeal blood detoxification by sorbents in treatment of hepatic encephalopathy. Adv Ren Replace Ther. 2002;9(1):3-18.

SECTION

12

Chronic Kidney Disease

CHAPTER

12.1

Chronic Kidney Disease: Staging and Etiopathogenesis

Ranjeet W Thergaonkar

DEFINITION OF CHRONIC KIDNEY DISEASE

The Kidney Disease Improving Global Outcomes (KDIGO) 2012 clinical practice guideline for the evaluation and management of chronic kidney disease (CKD) document defines CKD as *"abnormalities of kidney structure or function, present for >3 months, with implications for health."*

The term "abnormalities of kidney structure" refers to any or more of the following:

- Significant albuminuria (or proteinuria in the case of children; **Table 1**)[1-3]
- Urine sediment abnormalities
- Electrolyte and other abnormalities due to tubular disorders[4-6]
- Abnormalities detected by histology
- Structural abnormalities detected by imaging
- History of kidney transplantation.

Abnormalities of function are defined by glomerular filtration rate (GFR) < 60 mL/min/1.73 m².[1] Decrease in GFR can be detected by estimated GFR using several validated equations. The equation commonly used for children in India is as follows:

$$GFR = 0.42 \times (height/serum\ creatinine)^{7}$$

However, if required, decreased GFR may be confirmed by measurement. The cutoff of 60 mL/min/1.73 m² does not apply to children aged <2 years where an age-appropriate value should be used[1,8] because the GFR has not reached the adult values. The criterion of duration of >3 months does not apply to infants aged <3 months if they otherwise meet the definition of structural abnormalities; GFR may even be normal for age.

TABLE 1: Significant proteinuria.

Age <6 months	*Age 6–24 months*	*Age >24 months*
>6–8 mg/m²/h	>4 mg/m²/h	>4 mg/m²/h
>240 mg/m²/day	>150 mg/m²/day	>150 mg/m²/day
	Up/Uc > 500 mg/g	Up/Uc > 200 mg/g

(Up/Uc: urine spot protein–creatinine ratio)

Rationale behind the Definition of Chronic Kidney Disease

Kidney disease is said to be acute if it lasts for less than 3 months and chronic if it lasts longer.[3] CKD is usually silent till the late course of the disease—even then, most clinical manifestations are not specific to the kidney. The diagnosis and estimation of the duration of renal disease, therefore, usually are reliant on laboratory values. It is likely that for this reason, there was no uniform definition of CKD for a long time.[9]

Keeping the burden of disease and benefits of early intervention in mind, the Kidney Disease Outcomes Quality Initiative (K/DOQI), an initiative by the National Kidney Foundation of USA, published a document in 2002 defining CKD in terms of kidney damage for at least 3 months as defined by structural and functional abnormalities with or without reduced GFR *or* GFR < 60 mL/min/1.73 m².[10]

The evidence review team from KDIGO reviewed this definition. They acknowledged that renal damage may occur in the form of albuminuria, abnormal urinary sediment, electrolyte abnormalities consequent to renal tubular disorders, abnormalities noted on histopathology after renal biopsy, and abnormal renal imaging. Renal transplantation was considered renal damage because of solitary kidney status as well as the common phenomenon of histopathological abnormalities detected even on routine renal biopsy.[11] The definition was, therefore, revised to the one described above.[1]

Limitations of the Definition

The KDIGO has acknowledged many limitations in the definition of CKD including the following:

- Chronicity, i.e., duration of disease ≥3 months, is not synonymous with irreversibility. Many conditions may show improvement.
- Glomerular filtration is not the only measure of kidney function.
- The use of a single cutoff for GFR irrespective of age, sex, and ethnicity for defining CKD can lead to misclassification.
- There may be clinical situations where the GFR declines but remains >60 mL/min/1.73 m² or there is an increase in albuminuria but less than the cutoffs for defining CKD.

Treating clinicians should be alert and keep such patients under close follow-up.[1]

Thus, the definition of CKD has certain limitations which need to be kept in mind while evaluating individual patients.

Other Considerations on Nomenclature

The KDIGO has acknowledged the need for clear communication with all stakeholders in patient care. Terms such as "renal" or "nephro" should preferably be avoided in general descriptions of kidney disease and function in such communication, especially with laypersons.

The term kidney replacement therapy (KRT) is used for the treatment modalities of dialysis or renal transplantation; the term "kidney replacement therapy" is to be avoided.

The term "kidney failure" refers to a situation with GFR < 15 mL/min/1.73 m^2 or treatment with dialysis. The term "end-stage kidney disease" is an administrative term used by Medicare of USA for patients with CKD requiring dialysis or renal transplantation and is to be avoided.[3]

STAGING OF CHRONIC KIDNEY DISEASE

Chronic kidney disease is classified based on cause, GFR category, and albuminuria (proteinuria) category (CGA).

The cause of CKD is classified whether it is a renal manifestation of systemic disease or a primary renal disease.

GFR categories are assigned as described in **Table 2.**

The GFR categories cannot be assigned to children aged <2 years where age-appropriate normative data and reference intervals may be used.

TABLE 2: Glomerular filtration rate (GFR) categories.

GFR category	*GFR (mL/min/1.73 m²)*	*Terms*
G1	≥90	Normal or high
G2	60–89	Mildly decreased*
G3a	45–59	Mildly to moderately decreased
G3b	30–44	Moderately to severely decreased
G4	15–29	Severely decreased
G5	<15	Kidney failure

*Relative to young adult level.

A commonly followed set of values are given in **Table 3.**[11]

Albuminuria/proteinuria categories are assigned in **Table 4.**[1,3]

Proteinuria exceeding 40 mg/m^2/h in a timed sample or 3 g/m^2/day is considered to be in the nephrotic range. Above the age of 24 months, albuminuria may be studied using cutoffs similar to those used in adults.[1]

Rationale behind the Staging of Chronic Kidney Disease

- The rationale behind including the cause of CKD is to highlight the fact that CKD is not a disease in itself—the cause requires identification and specific management.[1]
- The GFR categories were introduced because the risk of complications has been shown to increase with worsening in the category.[1,10]
- The albuminuria categories were introduced because many adverse patient outcomes were shown to increase with increasing proteinuria. Heavier albuminuria is associated with a faster trajectory to kidney failure. Proteinuria is used in children instead of albuminuria because of a greater role of tubular proteinuria in causing kidney damage and also because in this age group, it is more common to study proteinuria rather than albuminuria.[1]

Limitations of the Staging of Chronic Kidney Disease

- Although the location of disease is classified as systemic or renal, some conditions affect the kidney and other organs simultaneously, e.g., genetic conditions such as polycystic kidney disease.[1]

TABLE 3: Normal glomerular filtration rate (GFR) in children.

Age (sex)	*Mean GFR ± SD (mL/min/1.73 m²)*
1 week (males and females)	41 ± 15
2–8 weeks (males and females)	± 25
>8 weeks (males and females)	96 ± 22
2–12 years (males and females)	133 ± 27
13–21 years (males)	140 ± 30
13–21 years (females)	126 ± 22

TABLE 4: Albuminuria/proteinuria categories.

Category	*AER (mg/24 h)*	*ACR (mg/g)*	*PER (mg/24 h)*	*PCR (mg/g)*	*Terms*
A1	<30	<30	<150	<150	Normal to mildly increased
A2	30–300	30–300	150–500	150–500	Moderately increased*
A3	>300	>300	>500	>500	Severely increased†

*Relative to young adult level

†Including nephrotic range [albumin excretion usually >2,200 mg/24 h (ACR > 2,220 mg/g) protein excretion rate >3,500 mg/24 h (PCR > 3,500 mg/g)].

(AER: albumin excretion rate; ACR: albumin-to-creatinine ratio; PER: protein excretion rate; PCR: protein–creatinine ratio)

- There is no direct evidence of association of lower GFR with worse outcome in children; however, it is recommended that children with GFR lower than 1SD below mean for age be monitored carefully.[1]
- The highest category of albuminuria is considered too broad; the Canadian Society of Nephrology recommended addition of a category A4 for nephrotic range proteinuria.[12]
- The cutoffs used for proteinuria have inaccuracies. Normative values need adjustment for age, sex, race, puberty, and body size.[1]

The staging of CKD thus has certain limitations that need to be considered while assessing individual patients.

EPIDEMIOLOGY OF CHRONIC KIDNEY DISEASE

Incidence and Prevalence

The worldwide prevalence of CKD in adults is estimated at 11–13%.[13] An Indian study in apparently healthy central government employees reported 15.04% prevalence of early stages of CKD.[14] There is a paucity of epidemiological data on CKD in children because of lack of worldwide registry data and methodological limitations. The incidence and prevalence of CKD stages 3–5 among children in Europe have been estimated at 11–12 per million of the age-related population (pmarp).[15]

ETIOLOGY OF CHRONIC KIDNEY DISEASE IN CHILDREN

The most common causes of CKD in children are congenital anomalies of the kidney and urinary tract (CAKUT), neurogenic bladder, steroid-resistant nephrotic syndrome, chronic glomerulonephritis, and renal ciliopathies. The contributions of CAKUT and glomerular disease to CKD are higher in early and late childhood, respectively.[15,16] There are geographic and ethnic differences in the etiology of CKD in childhood. For instance, neurogenic bladder is more common in Asia (middle East) as compared to Western Europe while focal and segmental glomerulonephritis (FSGS) is more common in the Black population as compared to other populations in USA.[16]

An Indian study of 78 children in CKD stages II–IV from an urban tertiary care center reported etiology as follows: renal hypoplasia/dysplasia/aplasia: 20 (25.6%), obstructive uropathy: 12 (15.3%), neurogenic bladder: 13 (16.6%), reflux nephropathy: 5 (6.4%), cystinosis: 4 (5.1%), hemolytic uremic syndrome: 7 (8.9%), FSGS: 4 (5.1%), IgA nephropathy: 1 (1.2%), miscellaneous: 10 (12.8%), and unknown etiology: 2 (2.5%). The study also reported a high prevalence of comorbidities including short stature (65%), anemia (57%) including iron deficiency (56%), uncontrolled hypertension (66%), vitamin D deficiency (92%), hyperphosphatemia (32%), hyperparathyroidism (56%), proteinuria (94%), dyslipidemia (74%), and left ventricular hypertrophy (45%) suggesting a significant prevalence of preventable morbidity.[17] The Indian Society of Pediatric Nephrology has established a CKD registry with nearly 60 centers and more than 1,200 patients registered. Data from the registry is awaited.[18]

PATHOGENESIS

This section is divided into two parts: (1) pathogenesis of CKD—the cellular and molecular mechanisms that result in structural and functional kidney damage and (2) pathogenesis of the uremic syndrome—the clinical manifestation of CKD.

Pathogenesis of Chronic Kidney Disease

The progression of CKD can be understood to occur in three phases. In the first phase, an injury interferes with renal function. In the second phase, the response to injury results in scarring. In the third phase, loss of renal function occurs after maladaptive mechanisms attempt to cope with loss of nephrons. Initially, the decline in kidney function occurs at a variable pace depending on many factors, chiefly the cause of CKD. In later stages, the decline is more constant irrespective of cause.[19]

Phase I: Injury

The term "injury" refers to a variety of conditions that interfere with the functioning of the nephron or kidney including structural (e.g., cystic kidney disease), metabolic (e.g., diabetes), toxic (e.g., calcineurin inhibitor exposure), and systemic (e.g., systemic lupus erythematosus) diseases. The injurious processes act on different cells in the nephron and elicit certain common responses **(Table 5)**.[20-24]

Phase II: Inflammation and Scarring

The first response to injury in the nephron is inflammation. The outcome of inflammation could be either repair or fibrosis. Repair results in recovery of function while scar formation leads to tissue damage, maladaptive mechanisms, and loss of function.

Inflammation: The initial cellular inflammatory response to injury is by neutrophils, natural killer (NK) cells, and T helper cells that are rapidly replaced by macrophages. In recent times, it has been recognized that the overall macrophage response is important in determining whether the reparative or fibrogenesis route will be taken.

TABLE 5: Response of renal cells to injury.

Cell type	*Type of response*
Podocytes	Foot process effacement, loss of anchorage, apoptosis, podocyturia, and proliferation (rare)
Mesenchymal cells	Proliferation
Endothelial cells	Prothrombotic phenotype, proliferation
Tubular cells	Cyst formation, energy failure, toxic storage, necrosis, activation, and apoptosis

Macrophages have an important phagocytic function that is important to remove debris and facilitate repair. In addition, they synthesize and secrete different cytokines depending on their pattern of activation. There are different populations of macrophages. M1 macrophages with classic activation and M2 macrophages with alternate activation perform different roles in the renal microenvironment. M1 macrophages are essentially proinflammatory. M2 macrophages have various subtypes—M2a (profibrotic), M2b (immunoregulatory), and M2c (anti-inflammatory). The balance of macrophage population has an important role in deciding the overall renal response to injury.[25]

Fibrogenesis: Biochemically, scar formation involves deposition of the extracellular matrix (ECM) proteins but without the organized structure of functional tissue. The mesangial cells in the glomerulus and myofibroblasts in the tubulo-interstitium lay down the ECM. Myofibroblasts can be derived from the dedifferentiation of multiple cells including renal tubular epithelial cells, tubulointerstitial vascular pericytes, fibroblasts, fibrocytes, endothelial cells, and macrophages.[26]

Scarring is mediated by dyslipidemia, activation of the renin–angiotensin system, and reactive oxygen species (ROS). Repair is mediated by high-density lipoprotein (HDL) cholesterol and adiponectin, probably as compensatory responses.[19]

Changes at the intracellular level: Two important cellular processes determine the response of the nephron to injury: autophagy and endoplasmic reticulum (ER) stress. Autophagy refers to the breakdown or export of excess or misfolded proteins by cellular organelles. Reduced autophagy results in cellular hypertrophy while increased autophagy leads to apoptosis. Autophagy is believed to be a regulator of ECM accumulation and is itself controlled by factors such as starvation, available substrate, growth factors, oxidative stress, and lipids. ER stress refers to a phenomenon where cellular activation occurs if inappropriately folded or localized proteins are not removed by autophagy.[27]

Role of molecular mediators: A large number of substances secreted by different cells determine the overall response of the kidney. The balance between repair and fibrosis is controlled by these substances. Some important chemical mediators are summarized in **Table 6**.[28]

Changes at the level of the nephron: At the level of the nephron, there are two important responses to glomerular injury that lead to scarring and loss of function of the nephron.

The first response is misdirected filtration—a process by which due to synechiae formation, glomerular filtrate enters the periglomerular space and causes an inflammatory response followed by fibrosis and obstruction of the glomerulotubular junction.

TABLE 6: Some important molecular mediators of renal inflammation, repair, and scarring.

Proinflammatory/profibrotic			***Reparative/anti-inflammatory/antifibrotic***		
Substance	*Secreted by*	*Role*	*Substance*	*Secreted by*	*Role*
TNF-α	Renal epithelial cells, macrophages, and T cells	Proinflammatory	CSF-1	Tubular cells	Regenerative
TGF-β	Macrophages, lymphocytes, and tubule cells	Profibrotic	IL-10	NK cells, Th2 cells, T regulatory cells, macrophages, B-cells, mesangial cells, and endothelial cells	Anti-inflammatory and antifibrotic
IL-1β	Renal and inflammatory cells	Proinflammatory	IL-22	Innate lymphoid, Th-17, and Th-22 cells	Antiapoptotic, regenerative
MCP-1 /CCL2	Macrophages	Proinflammatory	S1P/S1PR	Renal endothelium and macrophages	Anti-inflammatory
CX3CL1	Tubular cells, macrophages	Proinflammatory, profibrotic	HMGB1	Tubular cells, macrophages	Cytotoxic, proinflammatory
Complement proteins	Tubular cells	Cytotoxic, proinflammatory	Heme oxygenase	Epithelial cells, macrophages	Antioxidant
CTGF	Most renal and inflammatory cells	Profibrotic	Ferritin	Epithelial cells and macrophages	Antioxidant
PDGF	Most renal and inflammatory cells	Profibrotic	EGF	Tubular cells	Antifibrotic
			BMP-7	Tubules, podocytes, and endothelium	Antifibrotic

(BMP-7: bone morphogenic protein-7; CCL2: chemokine (C-C motif) ligand 2; CSF-1: colony stimulating factor-1; CTGF: connective tissue growth factor; CXCL10: C-X-C motif chemokine 10; EGF: epidermal growth factor; HMGB-1: high-mobility group box-1; IL-1β: interleukin-1β; IL-10: interleukin-10; IL-22: interleukin-22; MCP-1: monocyte chemoattractant protein-1; PDGF: platelet-derived growth factor; S1P: sphingosine-1-phosphate; S1PR: sphingosine 1-phosphate receptor; TGF-β: transforming growth factor-β; TNF-α: tumor necrosis factor-α)
Source: Adapted from reference 28.

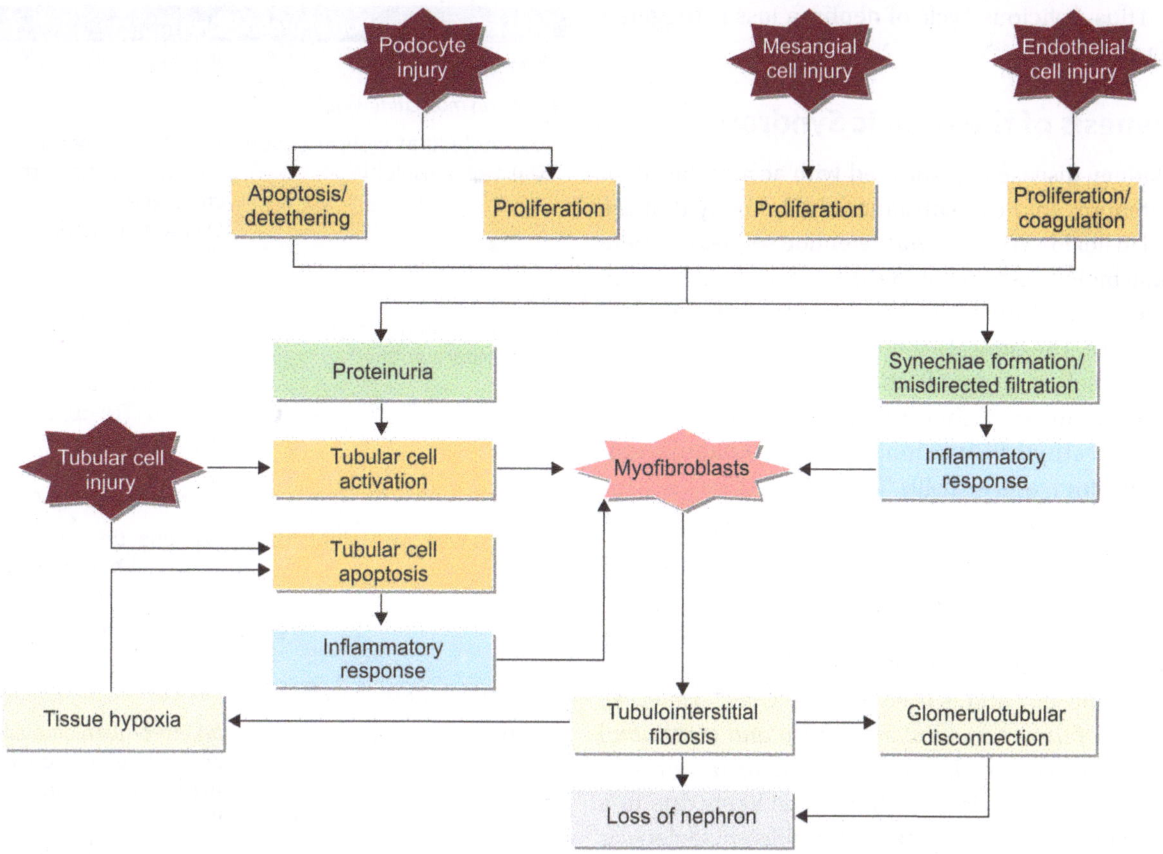

Fig. 1: Renal injury, inflammation, and scarring.

The second response is hyperfiltration because of which the renal tubules are exposed to high concentrations of filtered proteins, cytokines, and growth factors that activate the renal tubular epithelial cells and trigger an inflammatory response followed by fibrosis.[29]

The overall sequence of events related to renal injury followed by inflammation and fibrosis is summarized in **Figure 1**.

Phase III: Maladaptation, Progressive Nephron Loss, and Loss of Function

There are two important mechanisms that promote progressive loss of kidney function: the relatively hypoxic renal tubular microenvironment and maladaptive mechanisms of the surviving nephrons.

Although the kidney receives approximately 25% of the cardiac output, only 10–15% of this reaches the medulla. In addition, there is an arteriovenous shunting of oxygen because of countercurrent exchange of oxygen that reduces oxygen delivery to the renal tubules. The renal tubular cells have a high energy requirement, chiefly because of the need to reabsorb 99% of the filtered sodium. Consequently, even in health, the renal tubular *milieu* remains in a delicate balance of oxygen availability. With the renal damage, there is an increase in the single-nephron GFR (as discussed here)—this hyperfiltration poses increased oxygen requirement. In addition, glomerulosclerosis and tubulointerstitial fibrosis interrupt blood vessels and contribute to hypoxia.[30]

The response of the kidney to loss of nephrons is hyperperfusion and hyperfiltration (increased single nephron GFR) in the surviving nephrons. This is manifest by hypertrophy of the surviving nephrons. Hyperfiltration occurs through multiple mechanisms including activation of the renin-angiotensin-aldosterone system (RAAS) and increased intraglomerular pressure, stretching of glomerular basement membrane walls with increase in the pore size and loss of sieving function in the glomerular barrier, possibly through decreased expression of nephrin. This hyperfiltration results in loss of proteins including albumin, immunoglobulin G, complement factors, transferrin, transforming growth factor-β (TGF-β), insulin-like growth factor 1 (IGF-1), and angiotensin II. These proteins are absorbed by endocytosis by the proximal renal tubular cells (1) and upregulate the synthesis of proinflammatory and vasoactive substances such as endothelin-1, monocyte chemoattractant protein-1 (MCP-1), and regulated upon activation, normal T-cell expressed and secreted (RANTES) via the nuclear factor κB (NF-κB) transcription factor and (2) stimulate the dedifferentiation of the renal tubular cell into myofibroblasts.[31]

There is a mismatch between increased energy requirement and blood supply in the renal tubular cells which leads to hypoxia. This hypoxia results in generation of ROS, stimulation of the expression, and activity of hypoxia-inducible factors and acidosis due to anaerobic metabolism. All these events lead to fibrogenesis and ultimately loss of the nephron. Thus, a vicious cycle of nephron loss is triggered through hyperfiltration.[29]

Pathogenesis of the Uremic Syndrome

Chronic kidney disease is associated with accumulation of uremic retention solutes—substances in the body that are eliminated in health. When uremic retention solutes interfere with normal biological functioning, they are termed "uremic toxins." The uremic syndrome is the clinical manifestation of this interference. The clinical features of the uremic syndrome include atherosclerotic complications in the cardiovascular system, alterations in higher mental functions, anorexia and gastrointestinal ulceration, defective coagulation, immunodeficiency, and serositis.[32]

The term "uremic syndrome" stems from the fact that of the substances that are retained in the body in CKD, urea was the first to be described.[33] Measurement of serum urea forms the basis of urea kinetic modeling that measures the efficacy of dialysis.[34] Creatinine is also retained in the body, shown to have toxic effects,[35] and is used to study GFR.[36] *However, accumulation of these two substances (urea and creatinine) alone does not explain the pathogenesis of the uremic syndrome.*[32] The uremic syndrome is more likely due to a much larger number of uremic toxins with different molecular weights, water solubility, protein-binding capacity, and biological properties. Many uremic toxins have been cataloged by the European Uremic Toxin (EUTox) work group.[37]

There are many classifications of uremic toxins including those based on molecular weight and chemical structure as listed in **Table 7**.

TABLE 7: Classification of uremic toxins.

Type of toxin	*Example*
Based on molecular weight	
Low molecular weight (<500 kDa), water insoluble	ADMA (asymmetric dimethylarginine), creatine, creatinine SDMA (symmetric dimethylarginine), urea, and uric acid
Low molecular weight (<500 kDa), water soluble	Advanced glycation end products, cytokines, interleukins, tumor necrosis factor-α (TNF-α), indoxyl sulfate (IS), kynurenic acid, kynurenine, leptin, phenolic compounds, p-Cresyl sulfate (p-CS)
Middle molecular weight (>500 kDa)	Adiponectin, cystatin C, leptin, endothelin, ghrelin, prolactin, retinol-binding protein, β2-microglobulin, cholecystokinin and vasoactive intestinal peptide
Based on chemical structure	
Guanidine compounds	α-keto-δ-guanidinovaleric acid, α-N-acetylarginine, ADMA, argininic acid, β-guanidinopropionic acid, creatine, creatinine
Purine derivatives	Hypoxanthine, xanthine, and uric acid
Pyrimidine derivatives	Thymine, orotic acid, and uridine
Methylamine derivatives	Methylamine, dimethylamine, and trimethylamine
Phenyl derivatives	Phenol and p-Cresol
Indole derivatives	Kinurenine, indole-3-acetate, IS, and quinolinic acid

Source: Adapted from reference 34.

Advanced Glycation End-products

Advanced glycation end-products (AGEs) are a heterogeneous group of substances formed by the nonenzymatic glycation of carbohydrates, proteins, lipids, and nucleic acids. The toxic effects of accumulation of AGEs are oxidative stress and a proinflammatory phenotype. This is believed to be most marked in the vascular tree[38] as discussed here. The equilibrium between generation and detoxification of AGEs is disturbed in CKD.

Gut–Kidney Axis

In recent times, the gut-kidney axis has found importance in the understanding of the uremic syndrome. CKD is associated with a disturbance in the colonic barrier and alteration in the gut microbiota. The consequence is enhanced absorption of gut-derived toxins including indole and phenyl compounds. These substances have adverse effects on the functioning of the kidney itself as well as other organs including the brain, liver, and blood vessels. Interventions to reduce these adverse effects that are being studied include protein restriction in adult patients and use of probiotics and prebiotics.[39]

Two important mechanisms for the development of the uremic syndrome include the adverse effects on endothelium and establishment of an inflammatory process in the body.

Endothelial Dysfunction

Endothelial dysfunction results from inflammation, direct effects of the uremic toxins, and deficiency in α-Klotho and vitamin D and increase in fibroblast growth factor-23 (FGF-23). The clinical effects include (1) increased manifestations of atherosclerosis, (2) increased rigidity of blood vessels, (3) vascular calcification, and (4) abnormalities of vascular repair.[33,40]

Inflammation

Inflammation is an essential part of the uremic syndrome. A low-grade inflammatory state results from the increased synthesis and reduced breakdown of proinflammatory cytokines, oxidative stress and acidosis, recurrent and chronic infection, altered metabolism of adipose tissue, and intestinal dysbiosis. The clinical outcomes are early atherosclerosis and cardiovascular disease, protein–energy wasting, anemia with resistance to erythropoiesis-stimulating agents, and mineral bone disease. Not surprisingly, there is an overall increase in mortality.[41]

CONCLUSION

The definition and staging of chronic kidney are useful not only for epidemiology but also for early diagnosis and intervention in order to present long-term morbidity and mortality. CAKUT, obstructive uropathy, and neurogenic bladder are important causes of CKD in India. An insight into the pathogenesis of CKD as well as the uremic syndrome is useful in understanding the rationale behind treatment of CKD and dialytic strategies.

KEY POINTS

- CKD is defined as "abnormalities of kidney structure or function, present for >3 months, with implications for health."
- CKD is classified into using localization of disease, GFR, and albuminuria categories in order to ascertain severity of disease and predict the trajectory to kidney failure.
- CAKUT, obstructive uropathy, and neurogenic bladder are important causes of CKD in children.
- The pathogenesis of CKD involves renal injury, inflammation and scarring, and finally maladaptation leading to nephron loss.
- The uremic syndrome is caused by the retention of a large number of toxins that cause endothelial dysfunction and an inflammatory phenotype finally leading to morbidity and mortality.

REFERENCES

1. Levey AS, de Jong PE, Coresh J, El Nahas M, Astor BC, Matsushita K, et al. The definition, classification, and prognosis of chronic kidney disease: a KDIGO Controversies Conference report. Kidney Int. 2011;80:17-28.
2. Loghman-Adham M. Evaluating proteinuria in children. Am Fam Physician. 1998;58:1145.
3. Kidney Disease: Improving Global Outcomes (KDIGO) Glomerular Diseases Work Group. KDIGO 2021 Clinical Practice Guideline for the Management of Glomerular Diseases. Kidney Int. 2021;100:S1-S276.
4. Melkie M, Yigeremu M, Nigussie P, Teka T, Kinde S. Establishing reference intervals for electrolytes in newborns and infants using direct ISE analyzer. BMC Res Notes. 2013;6:199.
5. Adeli K, Higgins V, Nieuwesteeg M, Raizman JE, Chen Y, Wong SL, et al. Biochemical marker reference values across pediatric, adult, and geriatric ages: establishment of robust pediatric and adult reference intervals on the basis of the Canadian Health Measures Survey. Clin Chem. 2015;61(8):1049-62.
6. Zhu X, Wang K, Zhou Q, Guo W, Jia Y, Xu J. Age- and sex-specific pediatric reference intervals of serum electrolytes in Jilin Province of China Using the A Priori Approach. Am J Clin Pathol. 2020;154:708-20.
7. Hari P, Biswas B, Pandey R, Kalaivani M, Kumar R, Bagga A. Updated height- and creatinine-based equation and its validation for estimation of glomerular filtration rate in children from developing countries. Clin Exp Nephrol. 2012;16: 697-705.
8. Heilbron DC, Holliday MA, Al-Dahwi A, Kogan BA. Expressing glomerular filtration rate in children. Pediatr Nephrol. 1991;5:5-11.
9. Levey AS, Eckardt K-U, Tsukamoto Y, Levin A, Coresh J, Rossert J, et al. Definition and classification of chronic kidney disease: a position statement from Kidney Disease: Improving Global Outcomes (KDIGO). Kidney Int. 2005;67:2089-100.
10. National Kidney Foundation. K/DOQI clinical practice guidelines for chronic kidney disease: evaluation, classification, and stratification. Am J Kidney Dis. 2002;39:S1-266.
11. Hogg RJ, Furth S, Lemley KV, Portman R, Schwartz GJ, Coresh J, et al. National Kidney Foundation's Kidney Disease Outcomes Quality Initiative clinical practice guidelines for chronic kidney disease in children and adolescents: evaluation, classification, and stratification. Pediatrics. 2003;111:1416-21.
12. Akbari A, Clase CM, Acott P, Battistella M, Bello A, Feltmate P, et al. Canadian Society of Nephrology commentary on the KDIGO clinical practice guideline for CKD evaluation and management. Am J Kidney Dis Off J Natl Kidney Found. 2015;65:177-205.
13. Hill NR, Fatoba ST, Oke JL, Hirst JA, O'Callaghan CA, Lasserson DS, et al. Global prevalence of chronic kidney disease - a systematic review and meta-analysis. PLoS ONE [Internet]. 2016;11(7):e0158765.
14. Varma PP, Raman DK, Ramakrishnan TS, Singh P, Varma A. Prevalence of early stages of chronic kidney disease in apparently healthy central government employees in India. Nephrol Dial Transplant. 2010;25:3011-7.
15. Becherucci F, Roperto RM, Materassi M, Romagnani P. Chronic kidney disease in children. Clin Kidney J. 2016;9:583-91.
16. Harambat J, van Stralen KJ, Kim JJ, Tizard EJ. Epidemiology of chronic kidney disease in children. Pediatr Nephrol. 2012;27: 363-73.
17. Kamath N, Iyengar AA. Chronic kidney disease (CKD): an observational study of etiology, severity and burden of comorbidities. Indian J Pediatr. 2017;84:822-5.
18. Indian Society Of Pediatric Nephrology. (2021). Indian Society of Pediatric Nephrology CKD Registry [Internet]. [online] Available from: http://www.ispnregistry.com/. [Last accessed March, 2022].
19. Schnaper HW. Pathophysiology of progressive renal disease in children. In: Avner ED, Harmon WE, Niaudet P, Yoshikawa N, Emma F, Goldstein SL, (Eds). Pediatric Nephrology, 7th edition. Berlin Heidelberg: Springer-Verlag GmbH; 2016. pp. 2174-94.
20. Nagata M. Podocyte injury and its consequences. Kidney Int. 2016;89(6):1221-30.
21. Shankland SJ. The podocyte's response to injury: role in proteinuria and glomerulosclerosis. Kidney Int. 2006;69: 2131-47.
22. Kavanagh D, Goodship TH, Richards A. Atypical hemolytic uremic syndrome. Semin Nephrol. 2013;33:508-30.
23. Hodgkins KS, Schnaper HW. Tubulointerstitial injury and the progression of chronic kidney disease. Pediatr Nephrol. 2012;27:901-9.
24. Liu B-C, Tang T-T, Lv L-L, Lan H-Y. Renal tubule injury: a driving force toward chronic kidney disease. Kidney Int. 2018; 93:568-79.
25. Guiteras R, Flaquer M, Cruzado JM. Macrophage in chronic kidney disease. Clin Kidney J. 2016;9:765-71.

26. Black LM, Lever JM, Agarwal A. Renal inflammation and fibrosis: a double-edged sword. J Histochem Cytochem. 2019;67:663-81.
27. Cybulsky AV. The intersecting roles of endoplasmic reticulum stress, ubiquitin-proteasome system, and autophagy in the pathogenesis of proteinuric kidney disease. Kidney Int. 2013;84: 25-33
28. Genovese F, Manresa AA, Leeming DJ, Karsdal MA, Boor P. The extracellular matrix in the kidney: a source of novel non-invasive biomarkers of kidney fibrosis? Fibrogenesis Tissue Repair. 2014;7:4.
29. Schnaper HW. Remnant nephron physiology and the progression of chronic kidney disease. Pediatr Nephrol. 2014;29: 193-202.
30. Liu ZZ, Bullen A, Li Y, Singh P. Renal oxygenation in the pathophysiology of chronic kidney disease. Front Physiol. 2017; 8:385.
31. Ruggenenti P, Aros C, Remuzzi G. Renin-angiotensin system, proteinuria, and tubulointerstitial damage. In: Wolf G (Ed). Contributions to Nephrology [Internet]. Basel: Karger; 2001. pp. 187-99.
32. Lisowska-Myjak B. Uremic toxins and their effects on multiple organ systems. Nephron Clin Pract. 2014;128:303-11.
33. Meyer TW, Hostetter TH. Uremia. N Engl J Med. 2007;357: 1316-25.
34. Roa LM, Prado M. The role of urea kinetic modeling in assessing the adequacy of dialysis. Crit Rev Biomed Eng. 2004;32:461-539.
35. Varshney A, Rehan M, Subbarao N, Rabbani G, Khan RH. Elimination of endogenous toxin, creatinine from blood plasma depends on albumin conformation: site specific uremic toxicity & impaired drug binding. PLoS One. 201;6(2):e17230.
36. Kashani K, Rosner MH, Ostermann M. Creatinine: from physiology to clinical application. Eur J Intern Med. 2020; 72:9-14.
37. Vanholder R, De Smet R, Glorieux G, Argilés A, Baurmeister U, Brunet P, et al. Review on uremic toxins: classification, concentration, and interindividual variability. Kidney Int. 2003;63:1934-43.
38. Stinghen AEM, Massy ZA, Vlassara H, Striker GE, Boullier A. Uremic toxicity of advanced glycation end products in CKD. J Am Soc Nephrol. 2016;27:354-70.
39. Mafra D, Fouque D. Gut microbiota and inflammation in chronic kidney disease patients. Clin Kidney J. 2015;8:332-4.
40. Vila Cuenca M, Hordijk PL, Vervloet MG. Most exposed: the endothelium in chronic kidney disease. Nephrol Dial Transplant. 2020;35:1478-87.
41. Akchurin OM, Kaskel F. Update on inflammation in chronic kidney disease. Blood Purif. 2015;39:84-92.

CHAPTER

12.2 Chronic Kidney Disease: Clinical Approach and Evaluation

Rajiv Sinha, Subhankar Sarkar

INTRODUCTION

Chronic kidney disease (CKD) is associated with a progressive decline of renal function due to irreversible kidney damage. Estimates of the true burden of CKD are a challenge as there are several gaps across regions in the detection of disease and maintenance of national registries.[1,2] Based on the Kidney Disease Initiative Global Outcomes (KDIGO) classification of CKD, severity has been correlated with morbidity and mortality in children.[3-5]

Clinical manifestations of pediatric CKD (pCKD) and details of how to evaluate a child with CKD will be discussed in this chapter. Clinical presentation of a child with CKD is influenced by multiple factors. These include not only the underlying etiology and stage of CKD but also socioeconomic and health infrastructure prevalent in the region.[2,6] In areas with better health infrastructure and easier availability of health care, children with CKD tend to present earlier through urinalysis or imaging studies done either for unrelated cause or as part of routine health screening. In contrast, studies from India have shown that pCKD is detected late and children frequently present in medical emergency.[7-9]

CLINICAL MANIFESTATION AS PER UNDERLYING ETIOLOGY OF CHRONIC KIDNEY DISEASE

Table 1 summarizes the renal causes of CKD. In contrast to adults, nonglomerular pathologies are more common among children.[6-9] According to the North American Pediatric CKD registry (a large database with over 7,000 children with CKD), congenital anomalies of the kidney and urinary tract [CAKUT, which includes renal dysplasia, renal hypoplasia, as well as obstructive uropathies such as posterior urethral valves (57%)] and glomerular disease (17%) are the major causes of CKD in children.[6] CAKUT and glomerular disease were common among younger and older children, respectively. Because of routine antenatal fetal anomaly scan, most of the CAKUTs are detected antenatally whereas in emerging nations, CAKUT still presents in late stages of CKD. The higher percentage of glomerular disorders seen in Indian pediatric data likely reflects late detections of CAKUTs. Oliguria is common in adult CKD, but in children polyuria or normal urine output is common especially in dysplastic kidney, nephronophthisis, and tubulointerstitial disorders. Poorly concentrated urine leads to polyuria which usually is present even in the early stages. Apart from polyuria, growth failure is another unique presentation of pCKD. Children with underlying glomerular pathology present with more overt features including tea/cola color urine (indicating glomerular hematuria), proteinuria, edema, hypertension, and oliguria. Along with this, one may find features of underlying etiology of the glomerular pathology such as features of vasculitis seen in lupus or other vasculitic disorders such as Henoch-Schönlein purpura (HSP) and granulomatosis with polyangiitis (GPA).

TABLE 1: Etiology of pediatric chronic kidney disease.

Congenital	• Urinary tract malformations • Obstructive nephropathy (neurogenic/ posterior urethral valve), renal dysplasia/hypoplasia, reflux nephropathy	Congenital anomaly of kidney and urinary tract (CAKUT)
Hereditary/ metabolic	• Nephronophthisis • Cystinosis • Oxalosis • Alport syndrome • Polycystic kidney disease (autosomal recessive and dominant types)	
Glomerular disease	• Focal segmental glomerulosclerosis • Membranoproliferative glomerulonephritis (types I, II, and III)/C3 glomerulopathy • Congenital nephrotic syndrome • Finnish type, diffuse mesangial sclerosis IgA nephropathy (Buerger's disease) • Goodpasture (antiglomerular basement membrane) disease • Hemolytic-uremic syndrome • Henoch–Schönlein purpura • Systemic lupus erythematosus	
Others	Bilateral Wilms tumor (requiring bilateral nephrectomy)	

CLINICAL MANIFESTATION AS PER STAGES OF CHRONIC KIDNEY DISEASE

As CKD progresses, the kidney loses its physiological functions and various complications manifest **(Fig. 1)**. Infants with CKD commonly present with feeding problems and failure to thrive, whereas older children may present with short stature and fatigue. Generalized symptoms of CKD include malaise, anorexia, muscle cramps, pruritus, and poor cognition and school performance. CKD is associated with alterations of several endocrine axes on multiple levels, including somatotropic, gonadotropic, adrenal-corticotropic, thyrotropic, prolactin, hematopoietic, vitamin D, and carbohydrate/insulin metabolism.

In the early stages of CKD (G1 and G2), children are detected either because of a manifestation of their underlying structural kidney abnormalities/systemic disease or as an incidental finding on evaluation for some unrelated disorder. Features may include combinations of elevated creatinine, abnormal urinalysis (proteinuria, hematuria, or concentrating defect), or abnormal renal imaging.

Clinical manifestations of various complications of CKD **(Table 2)** start being apparent around CKD stage 3 and beyond. Herein apart from symptoms of their underlying disease, they start experiencing poor growth, metabolic acidosis, elevated blood pressure (BP), and alteration of biochemical parameters such as hyperkalemia as well as altered calcium phosphate metabolism typical of CKD-mineral bone disease (CKD-MBD). **Figure 1** illustrates the kidney functions that are impaired in CKD. These signs and symptoms become worse as CKD progresses, with anemia, acidosis, hypertension, hyperkalemia, CKD-MBD, and fluid overload becoming more common.[4,5] All of these complications may manifest as anorexia, nausea, vomiting, increased tiredness, respiratory distress, bone deformities, and failure to thrive.

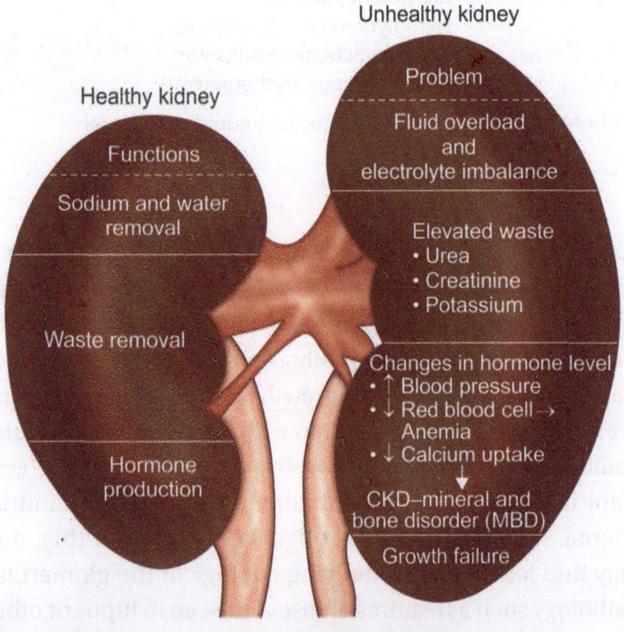

Fig. 1: Functions of a normal kidney and problems in chronic kidney disease (CKD).

CHILDREN AT RISK FOR CHRONIC KIDNEY DISEASE

Multiple risk factors have been identified for CKD and CKD progression **(Table 3)**. Many of the risk factors such as hypertension, proteinuria, anemia, and hyperphosphatemia are similar to the adult population.[10,11] In chronic kidney disease in children (CKiD) study, CKD progression was faster among glomerular disease and even among nonglomerular pathology proteinuria, and hypertension was linked to CKD progression.[12-14] Other factors such as male sex (more likely to have bladder outlet obstruction secondary to posterior

TABLE 2: Defining various complications common in pediatric chronic kidney disease as per Kidney Disease Improving Global Outcomes (KDIGO) Clinical Practice Guidelines

S. No.	Common complications of pediatric CKD		
1.	*Hypertension:* Auscultatory confirmed BP readings ≥95th percentile at 3 different visits is hypertension according to American Academy of Pediatrics (AAP) 2017 hypertension guideline. Children and adolescents with chronic kidney disease (CKD) and hypertension should have BP assessed by ambulatory blood pressure monitoring (ABPM) and hypertension should be treated to lower 24 hours mean arterial pressure <50th percentile as per KDIGO guideline 2020		
2.	*Anemia:* Hemoglobin concentration is <11.0 g/dL in children 0.5–5 years, <11.5 g/dL in children 5–12 years, and <12.0 g/dL in children 12–15 years, >15 years <13.0 g/dL in males and <12.0 g/dL in females (KDIGO 2012)		
3.	*Acidosis:* Bicarbonate <22 mmol/L among children >2 years of age <20 mmol/L among <2 years of age		
4.	*Albuminuria categories*		
		Albumin excretion rate (mg/24 h)	*Albumin creatinine ratio (mg/g)*
	Normal to mildly increased	<30	<30
	Moderately increased	30–300	30–300
	Severely increased	>300	>300
5.	*Hypo- or hypercalcemia:* Total calcium (mmol/L) not within age-appropriate range; 1–5 years = 2.3–2.6, 6–12 years = 2.33–2.58, 13–20 years = 2.2–2.3 *(mmol/L to mg/dL multiply by 4)*		
6.	*Hypo- or hyperphosphatemia:* Phosphate (mmol/L) not within age appropriate range; 1–5 years = 1.4–2.09, 6–12 years = 1.1–1.87, 13–20 years = 0.77–1.42 *(mmol/L to mg/dL multiply by 3.1)*		
7.	*Calcium phosphate product:* ≤12 years = ≤5.2 $mmol^2/L$, ≥12 years = ≤4.4 $mmol^2/L$		
8.	*High alkaline phosphatase:* Greater than the age appropriate range; 1–5 years = 100–350 U/L, 6–12 years = 60–450 U/L, 12–20 years = 40–180 U/L		
9.	*Hypo- or hyperparathyroidism:* Parathyroid hormone (pmol/L) not within CKD stage appropriate range stages 2 and 3 = 35–70 pg/mL, stage 4 = 70–110 pg/mL, stage 5 = 200–300 pg/mL		
10.	*Hypoalbuminemia:* Serum albumin <40 g/L		

TABLE 3: Risk factors for chronic kidney disease (CKD) and CKD progression.

General risk factors	*Pediatric specific*
• Hypertension • Acidosis • Proteinuria • Anemia • Hyperphosphatemia • Nephrotoxic agents • Recurrent urinary tract • History of acute kidney injury • History of recurrent urinary infections • Recurrent episodes of hypovolemia • High-risk genotype: APOL1	• Male sex • Congenital anomalies of kidney and urinary tract • Low nephron mass

urethral valve), low glomerular number (history of previous acute kidney injury, prematurity/low birth weight), and period of growth spurts during infancy/pubertal period (rapid increase in body mass puts higher pressure on residual glomerulus) are factors unique to children.[15-17] Ethnic variability in CKD progression has been identified though this area to a large extent is unexplored. Among the African ancestry, apolipoprotein L1 (APOL1) has been associated with CKD and faster CKD progression.[18]

EVALUATING A CHILD WITH CHRONIC KIDNEY DISEASE

Clinical evaluation of a child with CKD should consist of focused history, detailed physical examination, and comprehensive investigation targeted at identifying:

- Underlying etiology
- Any reversible factors
- Stage of CKD
- Complications associated with CKD
- Prognostic factors

History and Physical Examination

As detailed in **Table 4**, proper history and examination not only help in unraveling an underlying diagnosis but can also identify treatable causes and reversible factors such as bladder outlet obstruction, recurrent urinary tract infection, polyuria/polydipsia (which may predispose to hypovolemia and kidney injury), hypertension, pallor, and use of nephrotoxic drugs. Hypertension is a common complication among children with CKD (54–70%) and it could be also an initial manifestation.[19] Glomerular filtration rate (GFR) decline is associated with increased prevalence of hypertension.[4,20] Hypertension in CKD can have multiple etiologies including volume expansion, hyperreninemia, or due to adverse effects of medicine such as steroids or calcineurin inhibitors. With the use of ambulatory BP monitoring (ABPM), the detection rate for hypertension has increased. CKiD study not only

TABLE 4: History and physical examination.

History	*Physical*
• Family history of kidney disease • Family history of hypertension • Growth history, particularly poor linear growth • Polyuria, polydipsia, salt craving, or secondary enuresis (might suggest an underlying defect in urinary concentration as seen with dysplastic/hypoplastic kidneys and nephronophthisis) • Antenatal history (exposure to medicine like ACE inhibitor, viral fever, details of antenatal scan: liquor volume, renal anomalies) • Perinatal history (prematurity, umbilical artery catheterization, need for ventilation, nephrotoxic drug, history of AKI) • Urination/bladder and bowel history: Dribbling, wetting of pant, straining, hesitancy, urgency (may suggest underlying bladder outlet obstruction secondary to PUV or neurogenic bladder) • Bowel history (associated severe constipation can suggest a neurogenic cause) • Unexplained anemia and need for repeated blood transfusion • History of refractory rickets • Seizures • Fluid and electrolyte disorders • Detailed diet and nutrition history • Drug history (any intake of ACE inhibitor, NSAID, alternative medication such as ayurvedic or homeopathic) • Vaccination history including hepatitis B, pneumococcal and varicella	*General survey with special emphasis on:* • Anthropometry (weight, height and for children <3 years head circumference) for assessing growth parameters • Pallor • Edema • Blood pressure (including four limb blood pressure) • Peripheral pulses • Spinal deformity • Gait *Respiratory:* • Distress • Rales and crackles suggest pulmonary edema *Cardiovascular:* • Cardiac gallop • Cardiac rub, pericardial effusion *Abdominal:* • Any scars of previous urology operation or transplant • Bilateral renal lump palpable (suggests polycystic kidney disease) • Transplant kidney: tenderness, bruit • Tender hepatomegaly (along with features of overload supports the diagnosis of congestive cardiac failure) • Palpable bladder *Nervous system:* Assessment of lower limbs power and reflexes *Musculoskeletal:* Bony deformity (suggesting CKD–MBD)

(ACE inhibitor: angiotensin-converting enzyme inhibitor; CKD–MBD: chronic kidney disease–mineral bone disease; NSAID: nonsteroidal anti-inflammatory drug; PUV: posterior urethral valve)

confirmed hypertension in 18% (both elevated ambulatory and office BP) but interestingly masked hypertension (normal office but elevated ambulatory BP) was revealed in 34% of the cohort.[19] This has resulted in ABPM being advocated as a standard of care for children with CKD.

Physical examination may also give us clues regarding underlying etiology.

Anthropometric assessment is mandatory as growth retardation is an important complication of CKD. North

American data reveals that at the time of registration, children with CKD were on average 1.4 standard deviations (SD) below age and gender-adjusted normal mean height values and younger children were the most growth-retarded group of patients [e.g., <24 months: -1.81 standard deviation score (SDS), 2–5 years: -1.77 SDS and >12 years: -1.0 SDS) (NAPRTCS, 2006)].[6] It further showed that approximately 50% of children at dialysis initiation had heights <3rd percentile (SDS <-1.88) for chronological age (NAPRTCS, 2006). So younger the age of onset of CKD, more severe is the growth retardation.

Appropriate nutrition (calorie and protein) is important for all growing children; it is a crucial prerequisite for growth in early childhood, particularly around infancy as growth velocity is greatest during infancy and puberty. A thorough dietary nutritional history and anthropometric examination are vital not only for supporting growth but also for managing various CKD-related complications such as hypertension (salt intake), CKD-MBD (intake of phosphate, calcium, and vitamin D), and metabolic acidosis (type of protein intake, i.e., animal versus plant). In contrast to adult-onset CKD where salt usually has to be restricted, children with underlying salt-losing nephropathy may often require salt supplementation further underscoring the need for a proper dietary evaluation.

History should not miss exploring various aspects of quality of life including scholastic performance, performance in sports, and being able to cope with peer activities.[19,21] Proper evaluation of quality of life should include quality of sleep as sleep disturbances have been reported to happen in increased frequency among pCKD.[22]

Imaging

A judicious combination of various imaging modalities can give invaluable inputs in management planning.

Being noninvasive in nature and easily available, ultrasonography (US) is the most widely used imaging modality. It can be used to evaluate renal structure as well as the size of the kidneys. Sonographic data is available for normal kidney length to compare with the diseased kidney length. As children with CKD are short, it is always good to correlate the kidney length with respect to the body height to avoid overreporting of small kidneys.[23,24] Using US serial monitoring of renal length allows monitoring the growth of the kidney.[25,26]

Nuclear scans such as diethylenetriaminepentaacetic acid (DTPA), ethylene dicysteine (EC), and mercaptoacetyltriglycine (MAG3) provide information on any drainage problem and dimercaptosuccinic acid (DMSA) on scars as well as overall functions. DTPA/EC/MAG3 scan can also provide overall as well as individual approximate renal functions. It has to be remembered that nuclear scans are unlikely to be useful in advanced stages of CKD due to decreased uptake of the isotope by the poorly functioning kidneys.

Computed tomography and magnetic resonance imaging (MRI) studies are used less often and restricted to a scenario where US is unable to give adequate resolution/anatomical visualization. Micturating cystourethogram is useful for suspected vesicoureteric reflux or posterior urethral valves. While using imaging study needing ionic contrast agent, special precautions are needed to avoid contrast nephropathy in an already damaged kidney. The use of contrast agents based on gadolinium is usually avoided for advanced CKD as it may cause serious adverse effects such as nephrogenic fibrosing dermopathy and sometimes fatal nephrogenic fibrosis.[27,28]

An echocardiogram is useful to rule out left ventricular hypertrophy (LVH). Persistent hypertension can cause concentric LVH whereas eccentric LVH is due to volume overload and anemia in CKD. CKiD study reported LVH detected by echocardiography in 17% of cases (with 11% eccentric LVH and 6% concentric LVH). LVH is more common in presence of hypertension, either confirmed hypertension (34%) or masked hypertension (20%), when compared to those with normal BP (8%).[20]

Laboratory Testing

Blood test and urine analysis are frequently used to assess the underlying etiology of kidney disease, complication, and severity of CKD. Blood urea nitrogen (BUN) and serum creatinine are often used to estimate kidney function as it is easily available but have significant fallacies.[29,30] The BUN level depends on multiple factors including hydration status, amount of protein intake, use of steroids, and gastrointestinal tract bleeding. Although serum creatinine is commonly used for the estimation of GFR, it is not an ideal marker of GFR as it can be secreted by the kidneys, particularly when its level is elevated. Additionally, creatinine may be inappropriately low in case of malnutrition and major amputation and in these scenarios it will not reflect correct renal status. While interpreting creatinine values, it has to be remembered that it also varies with age and type of assay used in the laboratory. Despite this, in view of its low cost and easy availability creatinine continues to be widely used. The use of GFR estimating equations, i.e., estimated glomerular filtration rate (eGFR), is a more reliable way to use creatinine. In children, "Schwartz formula" is commonly used for eGFR calculation.[31,32] Presently used enzymatic method for the estimation of serum creatinine leads to lower value than the Jaffe method (older method) and can result in overestimating of GFR.[33] Modified Schwartz formula based upon serum creatinine derived from 349 children enrolled in CKiD study has been recently suggested to have a better correlation with the enzymatic method of creatinine estimation.[34] This formula is useful in the GFR range of 15–75 mL/min/1.73 m^2. As most of the eGFR formula continues to be dependent on serum creatinine value, they still run the risk of overestimating GFR in children with reduced muscle mass. CKiD study group has introduced another formula which along with creatinine also uses cystatin C.[34] Although this has been found to have a better correlation with the measured GFR, complexity of the formula has prevented its widespread acceptance in clinical use. Measuring GFR by the iohexol method (less cumbersome than inulin) or undertaking nuclear GFR estimation with radioactive tracers (e.g., iothalamate) are more accurate but not feasible in day-to-day clinical practice wherein repeated GFR estimation is required.

Easy availability of urine dipstick makes it a useful screening test for detecting proteinuria, urinary concentrating abnormalities, glycosuria, hematuria, and pyuria. Proteinuria is an important biomarker of CKD progression and can also be present in tubular dysfunction. Presence of hematuria with significant proteinuria indicates underlying glomerular pathology. Persistent high-grade proteinuria by dipstick should be checked either by calculation of urine protein and creatinine ratio or by 24 hours urine protein excretion for further evaluation for another marker of renal dysfunction.

Additional Laboratory Tests

Checking electrolytes including acid–base status helps in detecting important abnormalities such as sodium/potassium imbalance and metabolic acidosis. Metabolic acidosis usually manifests once GFR drop to below 40–50 mL/min/1.73 m^2 and it has been correlated with poor growth, CKD–MBD as well as CKD progression.[4,35] Pediatric CKD may often be secondary to salt-losing nephropathy, and hence urinary loss of salts should be evaluated as they can be an important cause of failure to thrive. Laboratory results can sometimes reveal a type IV renal tubular acidosis pathology which is common in children with obstructive nephropathy. Serum phosphate, calcium, 25-hydroxy vitamin D, and parathyroid hormone level are checked to evaluate bone mineral metabolism. The CKD–MBD or renal osteodystrophy have a variety of manifestation ranging from subtle biochemical manifestation (early stage 3a CKD) to overt rickets/osteomalacia in late CKD stages. Classical biochemical findings in CKD–MBD are low serum calcium and calcitriol levels and high phosphate and serum alkaline phosphatase level along with secondary or tertiary hyperparathyroidism.[36] Bone biopsies, particularly in adults, have thrown some insight into the spectrum of CKD–MBD. CKD–MBD can range from the high bone turnover states characterized by an increased number of osteoclasts, increased resorptive surface and fibrosis present in the trabeculae and bone marrow to the severe spectrum of low bone turnover state such as "adynamic bone disease" (ABD) characterized by both decreased osteoblast and osteoclast number and activity, with decreased osteoid formation and an absence of fibrosis. Excessive suppression of parathyroid hormone (PTH) has been associated with ABD, which is often described to be more dangerous than the high turnover type. Bone biopsies for CKD–MBD are usually not done regularly in pediatric practice. It is restricted to specialist centers with expertise in this subject and for difficult cases (such as recurrent fractures) wherein underlying pathology is not clear.

Anemia is the other major complication and can have multiple etiologies apart from reduced erythropoietin production secondary to kidney damage.[37,38] Anemia in children with CKD presents as easy fatigability, decreased attentiveness, increased somnolence, and poor exercise tolerance as well as left ventricular hypertrophy.[37-39] Anemia typically is present by the time the GFR has decreased to 20–35 mL/min/1.73 m^2. Complete blood count (CBC) along with reticulocyte count and peripheral smear to assess red cell characteristics are useful initial investigations. For microcytic hypochromic anemia, iron status should be checked. Always search for blood loss from any route, especially gastrointestinal tract and loss in dialysis.

Dyslipidemia is not uncommon among children with CKD and has been correlated with CKD progression in adults, so fasting lipid profile should be monitored.[40-42]

Chronic kidney disease states are often associated with "sick euthyroid syndrome" that is normal thyroid-stimulating hormone (TSH) level but low total and free T4 and T3 and normal or decreased thyroid hormone-binding globulin levels or thyrotropin-releasing hormone (TRH).

As CKD is a progressive disorder, regular monitoring of important hematological and biochemical parameters is warranted and KDIGO[3] has issued guidance regarding frequency of testing as per CKD staging **(Table 5)**. Small fluctuations in GFR are common and change of <25% in GFR may reflect physiologic variation rather than true progression (KDIGO, 2012).[3] Drop of GFR >25% from baseline is defined as a significant drop, which is associated with doubling the risk of all-cause mortality and a five-fold increase in the risk of kidney failure.[43,44] Steep fall of kidney function is associated with increased mortality and cardiovascular morbidity.[45-48] The fall of GFR is often nonlinear and is modified by the number of different factors such as intercurrent illness, medication, disease process, or combination of these factors.[49,50] Increasing albuminuria is significantly associated with kidney failure and/or doubling of serum creatinine.[51] Multiple risk factor influences CKD progression and some of the important factors include: etiology of CKD, GFR level, proteinuria, hypertension, diabetes, dyslipidemia, smoking, obesity, and exposure to nephrotoxic agents are important.[3] Kidney biopsy is rarely done and usually avoided in advanced stages of CKD. In advanced stages of CKD, it may not be useful as it usually shows fibrosis and sclerosis without giving any clues to underlying diagnosis and the procedure is associated with increased risk of bleeding. If done in early stage, biopsy can help in establishing the underlying diagnosis, severity, and potential of reversibility of the injuries. Ideally, light microscopy, immunofluorescence staining, and electron microscopy should be done in all biopsies as a combination of their findings may give a clue to the underlying pathology.

Keeping in mind that pCKD often has a genetic basis, next-generation sequencing (NGS) has opened new vistas in diagnosis and can be particularly useful in situations

TABLE 5: Minimum suggested frequency of monitoring in pediatric CKD as per Kidney Disease Improving Global Outcomes 2012 Clinical Practice Guideline.

Parameters	CKD stages						
	G1	***G2***	***G3a***	***G3b***	***G4***	***G5***	***G5d***
Nutritional assessment (weight, height, MAC, etc.)	Yearly	Yearly	6 monthly	3 monthly	Monthly	Monthly	Monthly
Blood pressure	Yearly	Yearly	3 monthly	Monthly	Monthly	Monthly	Monthly
Lipid profile	Baseline	Baseline	Yearly	3 monthly	3 monthly	3 monthly	Monthly
Calcium/phosphate*	Yearly	6–12 monthly			3–6 monthly	1–3 monthly	
iPTH*	Yearly	Based on baseline level and CKD progression			6–12 monthly	3–6 monthly	
Serum alkaline phosphatase*					12 monthly or more frequently if iPTH elevated		
25-OH vitamin D*	Baseline	Baseline and repeat if required					
Bicarbonate	Yearly	Yearly	6 monthly	3 monthly	3 monthly	Monthly	Monthly
Potassium	Yearly	Yearly	6 monthly	3 monthly	3 monthly	Monthly	Monthly
Hb — No anemia	Yearly				6 monthly		3 monthly
Hb — Anemia	Yearly		3 monthly				1–3 monthly
TSAT and ferritin	Yearly		3 monthly or				Monthly
Urinary protein	Yearly		4–6 monthly		3 monthly or more frequent		
Creatinine/eGFR	Yearly		4–6 monthly		3 monthly or more frequent		

*Increase frequency of monitoring if biochemical abnormalities are identified.
(eGFR: estimated glomerular filtration rate; G 5d: stage CKD on dialysis; G1 to G5: stages of CKD; Hb: hemoglobin; iPTH: intact parathyroid hormone; MAC: mid arm circumference; TSAT: transferrin saturation)

wherein biopsy results are unlikely to be helpful. Although not extensively explored in children, adult studies have thrown up interesting results on the use of NGS in CKD of unknown origin.[52]

CONCLUSION

Chronic kidney disease is a progressive disorder and the current focus is primarily on delaying CKD progression. Careful evaluation helps in management planning and may even enable one to identify any reversible factors.

KEY POINTS

- Proper evaluation through focused history, detailed clinical examination, and comprehensive investigations help in identifying underlying CKD etiology, any CKD-related complications, and importantly any treatable/reversible pathology.
- Children with nonglomerular disease are most often identified by imaging studies often as part of routine antenatal checkup. They can be asymptomatic or have subtle findings such as polyuria or poor growth.
- Glomerular disorder typically presents with more overt signs and symptoms. Apart from features of an underlying disorder such as of vasculitis, they commonly have proteinuria, edema, hematuria, and hypertension.
- As CKD progresses, clinical manifestations mirror the various complications of compromised kidney functions including fluid overload, hypertension, anemia, bone pain/bone deformity, electrolyte abnormalities including hyperkalemia and metabolic acidosis.
- Regular checking of hematological and biochemical parameters is important to monitor various complications of CKD. KDIGO has come up with guidelines regarding these tests including frequency of testing as per CKD stage.

REFERENCES

1. Harambat J, van Stralen KJ, Kim JJ, Tizard EJ. Epidemiology of chronic kidney disease in children. Pediatr Nephrol. 2012;27:363.
2. Ploos van Amstel S, Noordzij M, Warady BA, Cano F, Craig JC, Groothoff JW, et al. Renal replacement therapy for children throughout the world: the need for global registry. Pediatr Nephrol. 2018;33:863.
3. Kidney Disease Improving Global Outcomes. KDIGO 2012 clinical practice guideline for the evaluation and management of chronic kidney disease. Kidney Int Suppl. 2013;3:136.
4. Wong H, Mylrea K, Feber J, Drukker A, Filler G. Prevalence of complications in children with chronic kidney disease according to KDOQI. Kidney Int. 2006;70:585.
5. Furth SL, Abraham AG, Jerry-Fluker J, Schwartz GJ, Benfield M, Kaskel F, et al. Metabolic abnormalities, cardiovascular disease risk factors, and GFR decline in children with chronic kidney disease. Clin J Am Soc Nephrol. 2011;6:2132.
6. NAPRTCS 2008 Annual report. Rockville, MD, EMMES; 2008. Available from https://www.naprtcs.org/system/files/2008_Annual_CKD_Report.pdf https://web. [Last accessed January, 2021].

7. Gulati S, Mittal S, Sharma RK, Gupta A. Etiology and outcome of chronic renal failure in Indian children. Pediatr Nephrol. 1999;13(7):594-6.
8. Kamath N, Iyengar AA. Chronic kidney disease (CKD): an observational study of etiology, severity and burden of comorbidities. Indian J Pediatr. 2017;84(11):822-5.
9. Kanitkar M. Chronic Kidney Disease in Children: an Indian Perspective. Med J Armed Forces India. 2009;65(1):45-9.
10. Querfeld U, Anarat A, Bayazit AK, Bakkaloglu AS, Bilginer Y, Caliskan S, et al. The cardiovascular comorbidity in children with chronic kidney disease (4C) study: objectives, design, and methodology. Clin J Am Soc Nephrol. 2010;5(9):1642-8.
11. Staples AO, Greenbaum LA, Smith JM, Gipson DS, Filler G, Warady BA, et al. Association between clinical risk factors and progression of chronic kidney disease in children. Clin J Am Soc Nephrol. 2010;5(12):2172-9.
12. Warady BA, Abraham AG, Schwartz GJ, Wong CS, Muñoz A, Betoko A, et al. Predictors of rapid progression of glomerular and nonglomerular kidney disease in children and adolescents: the chronic kidney disease in children (CKiD) cohort. Am J Kidney Dis. 2015;65(6):878-88.
13. Fathallah-Shaykh SA, Flynn JT, Pierce CB, Abraham AG, Blydt-Hansen TD, Massengil SF et al. Progression of pediatric CKD of nonglomerular origin in the CKiD cohort. Clin J Am Soc Nephrol. 2015;10(4):571-7.
14. Fuhrman DY, Schneider MF, Dell KM, Blydt-Hansen TD, Mak R, Saland JM, et al. Albuminuria, proteinuria, and renal disease progression in children with CKD. Clin J Am Soc Nephrol. 2017;12(6):912-20.
15. Crump C, Sundquist J, Winkleby MA, Sundquist K. Preterm birth and risk of chronic kidney disease from childhood into mid-adulthood: national cohort study. BMJ. 2019;365:l1346.
16. Greenbaum LA, Muñoz A, Schneider MF, Kaskel FJ, Askenazi DJ, Jenkins R, et al. The association between abnormal birth history and growth in children with CKD. Clin J Am Soc Nephrol. 2011;6(1):14-21.
17. Ardissino G, Testa S, Daccò V, Paglialonga F, Viganò S, Felice-Civitillo C, et al. Puberty is associated with increased deterioration of renal function in patients with CKD: data from the ItalKid project. Arch Dis Child. 2012;97(10):885-8.
18. Friedman DJ, Pollak MR. APOL 1 nephropathy. From genetics to clinical application. Clin J Am Soc Nephrol. 2021;16(2):294-303. DOI: 10.2215/CJN.15161219.
19. Copelovitch L, Warady BA, Furth SL. Insights from the chronic kidney disease in children (CKiD) study. Clin J Am Soc Nephrol. 2011;6:2047-53.
20. Flynn JT, Mitsnefes M, Pierce C, Cole SR, Parekh RS, Furth SL, et al. Blood pressure in children with chronic kidney disease: a report from the chronic kidney disease in children study. Hypertension. 2008;52(4):631-7.
21. Wong CJ, Moxey-Mims M, Jerry-Fluker J, Warady BA, Furth SL. CKiD (CKD in children) prospective cohort study: a review of current findings. Am J Kidney Dis. 2012;60(6):1002-11.
22. Sinha R, Davis ID, Matsuda-Abedini M. Sleep disturbances in children and adolescents with non-dialysis-dependent chronic kidney disease. Arch Pediatr Adolesc Med. 2009;163(9):850-5.
23. Konuş OL, Ozdemir A, Akkaya A, Erbaş G, Celik H, Işik S. Normal liver, spleen, and kidney dimensions in neonates, infants, and children: evaluation with sonography. AJR Am J Roentgenol. 1998;171:1693.
24. Kadioglu A. Renal measurements, including length, parenchymal thickness, and medullary pyramid thickness, in healthy children: what are the normative ultrasound values? AJR Am J Roentgenol. 2010;194:509.
25. La Scola C, Ammenti A, Puccio G, Lega MV, De Mutiis C, Guiducci C, et al. Congenital solitary kidney in children: size matters. J Urol. 2016;196:1250.
26. Spira EM, Jacobi C, Frankenschmidt A, Pohl M, von Schnakenburg C. Sonographic long-term study: paediatric growth charts for single kidneys. Arch Dis Child. 2009;94:693.
27. Auron A, Shao L, Warady BA. Nephrogenic fibrosing dermopathy in children. Pediatr Nephrol. 2006;21:1307.
28. Grobner T, Prischl FC. Gadolinium and nephrogenic systemic fibrosis. Kidney Int. 2007;72:260.
29. Schmidt RL, Straseski JA, Raphael KL, Adams AH, Lehman CM. A risk assessment of the Jaffe vs enzymatic method for creatinine measurement in an outpatient population. PLoS One. 2015;10:e0143205.
30. Muhari-Stark E, Burckart GJ. Glomerular filtration rate estimation formulas for pediatric and neonatal use. J Pediatr Pharmacol Ther. 2018;23(6):424-31.
31. Schwartz GJ, Haycock GB, Edelmann Jr CM, Spitzer A. A simple estimate of glomerular filtration rate in children derived from body length and plasma creatinine. Pediatrics. 1976;58:259.
32. Counahan R, Chantler C, Ghazali S, Kirkwood B, Rose F, Barratt TM. Estimation of glomerular filtration rate from plasma creatinine concentration in children. Arch Dis Child. 1976; 51:875.
33. Schwartz GJ, Muñoz A, Schneider MF, Mak RH, Kaskel F, Warady BA, et al. New equations to estimate GFR in children with CKD. J Am Soc Nephrol. 2009;20:629.
34. Schwartz GJ, Schneider MF, Maier PS, Moxey-Mims M, Dharnidharka VR, Warady BA, et al. Improved equations estimating GFR in children with chronic kidney disease using an immunonephelometric determination of cystatin C. Kidney Int. 2012;82(4):445-53.
35. Madias NE. Metabolic acidosis and CKD progression. Clin J Am Soc Nephrol. 2021;16(2):310-2.
36. Ketteler M, Block GA, Evenepoel P, Fukagawa M, Herzog CA, McCann L, et al. Executive summary of the 2017 KDIGO chronic kidney disease-mineral and bone disorder (CKD-MBD) guideline update: what's changed and why it matters. Kidney Int. 2017;92(1):26-36.
37. Fadrowski JF, Pierce CB, Cole SR, Moxey-Mims MM, Warady BA, Furth SL. Hemoglobin decline in children with chronic kidney disease: baseline results from the chronic kidney disease in children prospective cohort study. Clin J Am Soc Nephrol. 2008;3(2):457-62.
38. Warady BA, Ho M. Morbidity and mortality in children with anemia at initiation of dialysis. Pediatr Nephrol. 2003;18(10): 1055-62.
39. Carlson J, Gerson AC, Matheson MB, Manne S, Warady BA, Hooper SR, et al. A longitudinal analysis of the effect of anemia on health-related quality of life in children with mild-to-moderate chronic kidney disease. Pediatr Nephrol. 2020;35(9): 1659-67.
40. Baek HS, Kim SH, Kang HG, Choi HJ, Cheong H, Ha IS, et al. Dyslipidemia in pediatric CKD patients: results from KNOW-PedCKD (KoreaN cohort study for Outcomes in patients With Pediatric CKD). Pediatric Nephrol. 2020;35:1455-61.
41. Kidney Disease Improving Global Outcome (KDIGO) Lipid Work Group. Assessment of lipid status in children with CKD. KDIGO Clinical Practice Guideline for Lipid Management in Chronic Kidney Disease. Kidney Int Suppl. 2013;3:280.
42. Saland JM, Kupferman JC, Pierce CB, Flynn JT, Mitsnefes MM, Warady BA, et al. Change in dyslipidemia with declining glomerular filtration rate and increasing proteinuria in children with CKD. Clin J Am Soc Nephrol. 2019;14(12):1711-8.

43. Turin TC, Coresh J, Tonelli M, Stevens PE, de Jong PE, Farmer CKT, et al. One-year change in kidney function is associated with an increased mortality risk. Am J Nephrol. 2012;36:41-9.
44. Turin TC, Coresh J, Tonelli M, Stevens PE, de Jong PE, Farmer CKT, et al. Short-term change in kidney function and risk of end-stage renal disease. Nephrol Dial Transplant. 2012;27:3835-43.
45. Al-Aly Z, Zeringue A, Fu J, Rauchman MI, McDonald JR, El-Achkar TM, et al. Rate of kidney function decline associates with mortality. J Am Soc Nephrol. 2010;21:1961-9.
46. Shlipak MG, Katz R, Kestenbaum B, Siscovick D, Fried L, Newman A, et al. Rapid decline of kidney function increases cardiovascular risk in the elderly. J Am Soc Nephrol. 2009;20:2625-30.
47. Cheng TY, Wen SF, Astor BC, Tao XG, Samet JM, Wen CP. Mortality risks for all causes and cardiovascular diseases and reduced GFR in a middle-aged working population in Taiwan. Am J Kidney Dis. 2008;52:1051-60.
48. Rifkin DE, Shlipak MG, Katz R, Fried LF, Siscovick D, Chonchol M, et al. Rapid kidney function decline and mortality risk in older adults. Arch Intern Med. 2008;168:2212-8.
49. Li L, Astor BC, Lewis J, Hu B, Appel LJ, Lipkowitz MS, et al. Longitudinal progression trajectory of GFR among patients with CKD. Am J Kidney Dis. 2012;59:504-12.
50. O'Hare AM, Batten A, Burrows NR, Pavkov ME, Taylor L, Gupta I, et al. Trajectories of kidney function decline in the 2 years before initiation of long-term dialysis. Am J Kidney Dis. 2012;59:513-22.
51. Schmieder RE, Mann JF, Schumacher H, Gao P, Mancia G, Weber MA, et al. Changes in albuminuria predict mortality and morbidity in patients with vascular disease. J Am Soc Nephrol. 2011;22:1353-64.
52. De Haan A, Eijgelsheim M, Vogt L, Knoers NVAM, de Borst MH. Diagnostic yield of next-generation sequencing in patients with chronic kidney disease of unknown etiology. Front Genet. 2019;10:1264.

CHAPTER

12.3 Conservative Management in Chronic Kidney Disease

Jyoti Sharma, Jyoti Singhal

INTRODUCTION

Chronic kidney disease (CKD) is an irreversible disorder, and progression to end-stage kidney disease (ESKD) occurs at a variable rate that depends upon the etiology. Signs and symptoms such as poor appetite, bone pains, growth failure, easy fatigability, volume overload, and hypertension (HTN) are insidious in onset and manifest late when the glomerular filtration rate (GFR) has decreased significantly. Appropriate, multidisciplinary management includes close monitoring of clinical, laboratory, and sometimes imaging parameters. Interventions are directed toward addressing biochemical abnormalities, alleviation of symptoms, and attempts to delay progression to ESKD.

GROWTH AND NUTRITION

In children with CKD, there is a negative impact on growth due to multiple reasons that include poor nutrition, altered endocrine milieu and abnormal hormone regulation, secretion and effect, hematological derangements, and mineral bone disease (MBD).[1] In addition to having a negative psychological impact, short stature and inadequate growth in children are associated, in the long-term, with poor outcome including death.

The Kidney Disease Outcomes Quality Initiative (KDOQI) guidelines and the Pediatric Renal Nutrition Taskforce (PRNT) recommend that for children with CKD stages 2 to 5 and 5D, dietary intake and nutritional status should be monitored periodically along with their growth parameters.[2,3] The latter include length or height, length velocity or height velocity, weight (dry, euvolemic), body mass index (BMI), and head circumference (for children <3 years) and these are compared with age and gender percentile or standard deviation score (SDS) should be calculated. The child's height should also be compared with the calculated gender-appropriate potential mid-parental height.[1,3-5] A child is considered to have short stature when her/his length/height *Z*-score < –1.88 or the length/height for age <3rd percentile; growth failure is defined as height velocity *Z*-score < –1.88 or a height velocity for age <3rd percentile that persists beyond 3 months. Management of growth failure is discussed in the section on endocrine disorders. The growth potential can be assessed by comparing a radiograph of left hand and wrist with the images of "standard" hand and wrist radiographs from children of different ages in the Greulich and Pyle skeletal age atlas. The Tanner staging scale of sexual maturity rating should be recorded to document age-appropriate pubertal development in children.

TABLE 1: Proposed criteria for protein energy wasting in patients with chronic kidney disease.

Criteria	*Description*
Dietary intake	Self-reported poor appetite
Growth	• Height-for-age and sex <3rd percentile, or a decrease in height-for-age and sex percentile • Low height velocity
Muscle mass	• Mid-upper arm circumference for height age and sex <5th percentile • Decrease in mid-arm muscle circumference
Body mass index (BMI)	• BMI-for-height-age and sex <5th percentile • Unintentional decrease in BMI-for-height-age and sex percentile
Biochemical parameters	• Serum albumin <3.8 g/dL • Serum transferrin <140 mg/dL • Total cholesterol <100 mg/dL • C-reactive protein >3 mg/L

Protein energy wasting (PEW) is a wasting syndrome characterized by anorexia and increased metabolic rate, seen in some patients with CKD. It occurs due to maladaptive responses and results in reduced muscle mass, while fat mass is preserved, or even increased **(Table 1)**.[6] Unlike malnutrition in other children, improvement in diet alone is inadequate to improve the child's status because of the complex metabolic contributing factors (metabolic acidosis, endocrine, metabolic bone disease) due to CKD.

Obesity

The prevalence of overweight and obesity has increased in children and adolescents all over the world, and this is applicable to children with CKD too.[1,7] Both extremes of BMI are associated with increased risk of mortality.[8]

Management

Children with any remaining natural kidney function have better growth than those who have none, even if they are on dialysis. Enhanced dialytic clearance [mean *Kt/V* of 2.0 per hemodialysis (HD) session] and control of hyperparathyroidism contribute to the improvement of growth in children and are covered in other sections. Aspects of nutrition and correction of metabolic acidosis are addressed here. The dietary intake should be assessed by an expert. The usual methods of performing this evaluation are by a diet diary maintained by a parent over 3 days or by recall of dietary intake over 3 days. Assessment of nutritional intake when combined with the measured growth parameters and growth velocity helps determine the role of diet in the poor growth of a particular child with CKD. The protein catabolic rate (PCR) normalized for the patient's weight provides a quantifiable parameter of dietary protein consumption of the child receiving maintenance HD and should be used to assess whether target protein intake is being achieved.[2]

The PRNT has provided clinical practice recommendations (CPRs) on energy and protein requirements in children based on the suggested dietary intake (SDI) **(Table 2)**.[9] For children with poor growth, it would be more appropriate to recommend the energy intake as per the *height for age* of the child rather than the chronological age and should be adjusted toward the upper limit of the SDI. In overweight and obese children, energy intake may be recommended at the lower end of the SDI, without compromising nutrition. Children on peritoneal dialysis (PD) receive extra calories (7.5 ± 7 to 9.08 ± 4.13 kcal/kg/day) from peritoneal fluid glucose absorption.[9] These may be considered as contributing toward their total calorie consumption, especially for children who are overweight or obese.

TABLE 2: Energy and protein requirements for infants, children, and adolescents with chronic kidney disease 2–5.[9,10]

SDI for energy and proteins (birth to 18 years)			
Age	***SDI for energy (kcal/kg/day)***	***SDI for protein (g/kg/day)***	
6–11 months	72–82	1.1–1.3	
12 months	72–120	0.9–1.14	
Years	*Male*	*Female*	*SDI for protein (g/kg/day)*
2	81–95	79–92	0.9–1.05
3	80–82	76–77	0.9–1.05
4–6	67–93	64–90	0.85–0.95
7–8	60–77	56–75	0.9–0.95
9–10	55–69	49–63	0.9–0.95
11–12	48–63	43–57	0.9–0.95
13–14	44–63	39–50	0.8–0.9
15–17	40–55	36–46	0.8–0.9

(SDI: suggested dietary intake)

Children on chronic PD lose protein via the peritoneal membrane so an additional protein intake of 0.15–0.3 g/kg/day, beyond SDI, is recommended for them. Those on maintenance HD need additional 0.1 g/kg/day of proteins to compensate for loss of amino acids.[1] In children with persistently high blood urea levels, high protein intake must be considered to be the cause when all other causes (e.g., occult gastrointestinal blood loss) have been excluded. In this situation, lowering the protein intake to the lower limit of SDI should be considered.

Other contributing factors for poor intake and undernutrition in children with CKD that need to be addressed are gastroesophageal reflux, vomiting, metabolic acidosis, and inadequate dialysis. Children on PD may develop early satiety because of fluid in the abdomen. When oral intake is inadequate to meet the nutritional requirements, enteral tube feeding or gastrostomy may be resorted to, especially in infants and toddlers. Rarely oral and/or enteral nutrition intake is insufficient, parenteral nutrition may be necessary, delivering concentrated solutions of amino acids, dextrose, and lipids when fluids are restricted.[2]

Vitamins

The current KDOQI guidelines recommend that children with CKD should receive at least 100% of the daily recommended intake (DRI) for water-soluble and fat-soluble vitamins, copper, and zinc. Children with CKD, not on dialysis, should receive *supplementation* only if they demonstrate clinical evidence of deficiency. All children receiving dialysis should be prescribed a water-soluble vitamin supplement because they are likely to lose vitamins during dialysis.

METABOLIC ACIDOSIS

Metabolic acidosis occurs because of increased protein breakdown, decreased albumin synthesis, and bone demineralization and usually becomes manifest when the GFR decreases to <50% of normal. In turn, metabolic acidosis causes poor appetite and malnutrition and is responsible for impaired linear growth in children by causing insensitivity to growth hormone (GH).

Current recommendations suggest that the serum bicarbonate level be maintained at at-least 22 mEq/L.[2] For children on maintenance HD, acidosis may be corrected by increasing the bicarbonate concentration of the dialysate. For the rest, oral supplements of sodium bicarbonate are usually initiated at a dose of 1–2 mEq/kg/day in three divided doses and titrated upward as required.

MANAGEMENT OF ANEMIA

The etiology of anemia in CKD is multifactorial and the common causes include erythropoietin (EPO) deficiency, iron deficiency, chronic inflammation, bone marrow suppression, hemolysis, and poor nutrition (vitamin B_{12} and folic acid deficiencies).

TABLE 3: Frequency of monitoring hemoglobin.[15]

Children without anemia	
CKD 3	Annually
CKD 4–5ND	Every 6 months
Children with anemia on oral iron	
CKD 3–5ND, CKD 5PD	Every 3 months
CKD 5HD	Every month
Children on ESA	
ESA therapy being initiated	Every month (along with iron studies)
ESA stable dose	Every 3 months
When ESA dose changed	Every 2 weeks

(CKD: chronic kidney disease; ESA: erythropoiesis-stimulating agents; HD: hemodialysis; ND: nondialysis; PD: peritoneal dialysis)

TABLE 4: Hemoglobin levels used to diagnose anemia.[15]

Age range	***Hemoglobin (g/dL)***
6 months–5 years	<11.0
5–12 years	<11.5
12–15 years	<12.0
>15 years	Females <12.5 Males <13.0

The importance of management of anemia lies in the fact that its correction in children with CKD is associated with improvement in subjective parameters such as better appetite and quality of life as well as enhanced exercise tolerance, improvement in intelligence testing scores, reduction of left ventricular mass, and left ventricular hypertrophy (LVH).[11-14] For appropriate and timely management, the Kidney Disease Improving Global Outcomes (KDIGO) has given guidance regarding frequency of monitoring of hemoglobin (Hb) and definition of anemia based on age **(Tables 3 and 4)**.[15] The initial evaluation of a child with CKD and anemia should include a complete blood count with red blood cell (RBC) indices, reticulocyte count, ferritin, serum iron, and total iron-binding capacity. Iron deficiency is characterized by microcytic hypochromic anemia, low ferritin (≤100 ng/mL), and low transferrin saturation [(TSAT) ≤20%; TSAT is serum iron divided by total iron-binding capacity multiplied by 100].[16] EPO deficiency typically manifests as normocytic normochromic anemia and a low reticulocyte count. Iron supplementation and the use of erythropoiesis-stimulating agents (ESAs) are the mainstay of management.

Iron Supplementation

Administration of oral iron (or IV iron in CKD HD patients) is recommended when there is demonstrable iron deficiency by laboratory parameters. Though ferritin levels <100 ng/mL and TSAT <20% qualify for a diagnosis of iron deficiency, there are a few caveats in patients with CKD. Firstly, ferritin is an acute phase reactant, and its levels may be high in patients with CKD because of the nonspecific inflammation. Secondly, when children with CKD and anemia are treated with iron and ESA, the rapid rate of RBC production decreases the circulating iron while iron stores remain adequate, resulting in a *functional iron deficiency*. A similar functional deficiency is seen in inflammatory states. Inflammation increases the production of hepcidin by the liver, and hepcidin decreases the bioavailability of iron for erythropoiesis by decreasing absorption in the duodenum, decreasing iron release from macrophages and from iron stores in hepatocytes. These children may have a normal ferritin, but a low TSAT. Iron therapy as *oral* elemental iron is 3–4 mg/kg/day (not to exceed 300 mg/day) for all patients other than those on HD.[17] Iron absorption is best when the stomach is empty so the supplement is advised an hour prior to or 2 hours post a meal; concomitant use of oral calcium and H2 receptor blockers should be avoided. *Intravenous iron* therapy is reserved for children receiving HD or if the child not on dialysis is either intolerant of oral iron or target Hb levels are not achieved with oral therapy. It is administered as an initial large (loading) dose to quickly correct the iron deficiency, followed by smaller weekly maintenance doses. The usual compound used is iron sucrose at a dose of 1.5 mg/kg/dose (not to exceed 125 mg/dose) given during the last hour of the HD session for eight consecutive sessions. This provides a total dose of 12 mg/kg (maximum dose of 1,000 mg). The recommended maintenance weekly dose is 1 mg/kg administered similarly.[17] Prior to parenteral iron administration, a test dose of 10 mg intravenously should be performed as per protocol. Once ESA therapy has been initiated, dosing is guided by monthly monitoring of Hb, TSAT, and serum ferritin levels till a stable dose of ESA has been reached. Following this, frequency of testing may be decreased to up to 3 months.[15] Intravenous iron should not be administered if TSAT exceeds 50%, serum ferritin is >500 ng/mL, and as in other children, if the patient acquires acute systemic infection. A caveat to remember is that TSAT is of limited value in children with low total iron-binding capacity (<200 µg/dL) as seen in children with severe proteinuria and malnutrition.

Treatment with ESAs should be initiated only once the child is iron replete. The most commonly used is the recombinant human EPO (rHuEPO). The dose depends on certain patient- and management-related factors, e.g., the following groups of children require higher doses: (1) children with higher stage of CKD, (2) children on HD (as compared to those not yet on dialysis or those on PD), (3) children younger in age, (4) children receiving ESA by intravenous route (vs. subcutaneous) **(Table 5)**.

The expected response to initiation of treatment or an increment in dose is a rise in Hb of 1–2 g/dL over 2–4 weeks. If the patient's Hb level does not increase despite receiving an adequate dose, the dose of EPO may be increased by 25%. The dose should be decreased by 25% if the rise of Hb

TABLE 5: Initial dose of recombinant erythropoietin.

Age	Predialysis or on peritoneal dialysis	On hemodialysis
<5 years	150 units/kg/week divided in two doses, subcutaneous route	200–300 units/kg/week divided in three doses, into dialysis circuit
>5 years	100 units/kg/week divided in two doses, subcutaneous route	150 units/kg/week divided in three doses into dialysis circuit

is >2.0 g/dL or exceeds 12.0 g/dL.[15] EPO use may cause or worsen HTN due to a rapid rise in red cell mass and due to a direct effect of the drug on blood vessels. A rare adverse effect is the development of *EPO resistance*. This occurs due to the development of antibodies against the recombinant forms of EPO and is characterized by low reticulocyte count even though the Hb progressively decreases.

Darbepoetin-alfa is another erythropoiesis-stimulating protein produced by DNA-recombinant technology. It has a longer half-life than rHuEPO and therefore can be administered at longer intervals. The dose recommended is 0.5 µg/kg/week. For patients converting from rHuEPO to darbepoetin-alfa, approximately 1.0 µg/kg/week darbepoetin-alfa should be prescribed for every 200 units/kg/week of rHuEPO. Once the target Hb has been achieved and a stable darbepoetin alfa dose is reached, the frequency of darbepoetin-alfa administration can be tapered from weekly to alternate weeks, and finally every 3–4 weeks, keeping the final total dose administered in a week unchanged.[17] The smallest available single-dose vial is 25 µg, and this may result in wasting of the drug when used for very small children. Darbepoetin is administered subcutaneously for patients not receiving dialysis or those on PD, while intravenous administration is used for children on HD through their vascular access.

A pegylated form of rHuEPO (methoxy polyethylene glycol-epoetin beta), also known as continuous erythropoiesis receptor activator (CERA), administered once a month, has been widely used in adults. It has been found useful in children on HD and for subcutaneous administration in children on PD.[18,19]

As mentioned earlier, for an ESA to be effective, a child should be in an iron-replete state. Other causes for an inadequate response to an adequate dose and compliance with ESA are an occult infection and chronic inflammation; rarer causes include carnitine and copper deficiency.

The use of *packed RBC transfusions* is minimized to avoid the inherent risks associated with them and the risk of allosensitization; however, they may be indicated acutely in case of hemorrhage or for perioperative use when emergency surgery is planned.

Roxadustat is an oral agent that increases endogenous EPO production. It is a hypoxia-inducible factor (HIF) stabilizer that competitively inhibits enzymes, which degrade HIF. In a recently concluded global phase 3 randomized study, roxadustat was found useful for correcting and maintaining Hb and was well tolerated in adults with CKD-related anemia not on dialysis.[20]

CHRONIC KIDNEY DISEASE–MINERAL BONE DISEASE

The term chronic kidney disease–mineral bone disease (CKD–MBD) refers to the disturbances of mineral and bone metabolism due to CKD that manifest as one or more of the following: (1) disturbances of calcium (Ca), phosphorus (P), parathormone (PTH), or vitamin D [25-hydroxyvitamin D (25(OH)D)] metabolism; (2) inadequate linear growth, recurrent fractures, or disturbed bone histology; and (3) vascular or other soft-tissue calcification.[21] Biochemical changes of bone mineral disease begin early in the course of CKD. Phosphate excretion declines and phosphate retention begins when the GFR decreases to <50 mL/min/1.73 m^2, and this is considered an initiating point in CKD–MBD. Circulating fibroblast growth factor-23 (FGF23) also increases early due to altered osteocyte function and decreased renal excretion. FGF, via its transmembrane receptor, Klotho, increases renal tubular phosphate excretion, decreases phosphate absorption from the gut, decreases circulating levels of 1,25-dihydroxyvitamin D, and causes progressive demineralization of bone. Increasing serum phosphate levels and declining calcitriol levels result in secondary hyperparathyroidism and high turnover bone disease. Elevated serum phosphate and FGF23 levels predispose patients to cardiovascular disease (CVD) and hence worsen morbidity and mortality. In advanced CKD, hyperphosphatemia increases PTH synthesis by gene transcription, and constant stimulation results in parathyroid cell proliferation and parathyroid gland hyperplasia. This monoclonal parathyroid cell proliferation is responsible for secondary hypoparathyroidism. The high serum phosphate levels further reduce renal 1,25 dihydroxyvitamin D [1,25$(OH)_2$D] synthesis, inhibit the negative feedback of 1,25$(OH)_2$D on PTH synthesis, and promote resistance of bone to PTH.[22] Metabolic acidosis, which is also present in CKD, causes calcium to efflux from bone as a result of suppression of osteoblasts and activation of osteoclasts. This is associated with impaired bone mineralization and an increased incidence of osteomalacia, which improves with correction of metabolic acidosis.

The term "renal osteodystrophy" refers to the histopathological changes in bone turnover, mineralization, and volume (TMV) in CKD. The type of renal osteodystrophy or changes seen would depend on the management interventions that have been instituted for the mineral bone alterations. Children who have been left untreated for CKD–MBD, histological signs of fibrosis, and demineralization will be seen, whereas overtreatment may result in adynamic bone disease associated with hypercalcemia, cardiovascular calcifications, and poor linear growth.[23]

Assessment of MBD is done by evaluating for growth, presence of bone pains, and bony deformities and by closely monitoring serum calcium, phosphorous, alkaline phosphatase (ALP), vitamin D, and PTH levels. Radiographs of the skeleton are not useful for routinely detecting renal bone disease. However, they may be performed to look for clinically important signs when severe persistent hyperparathyroidism is present. These are seen as subperiosteal resorption zones or acro-osteolysis at the end of phalanges and at the sites of ligament endings such as clavicles, ischium, pubes, femoral heads, and inner side of upper tibia diaphysis. Lesions of osteitis fibrosa (accumulation of fibrous tissue) are seen as widened radiolucent areas of the growth zones or as "brown tumors" at the metaphysis of long bones.

Measurements of bone mineral density is not routinely used in the monitoring of CKD-associated bone disease in children. Bone biopsy and micromorphometric analysis of the bone is the gold standard for characterization and quantification of renal bone disease but is limited to research studies.

Management of CKD-MBD focuses on three important aspects: (1) to maintain a normal *calcium-phosphate homeostasis* and *PTH levels* appropriate for CKD stage and hence maintain acceptable bone quality and prevent development of extraskeletal calcification, (2) to provide *optimal growth* in order to maximize the final height, and (3) to *correct all other metabolic and clinical abnormalities* that can worsen bone disease, growth, and CVD, i.e., metabolic acidosis, anemia, malnutrition, and 25(OH)D deficiency.[24]

The KDOQI 2005 guidelines provide details of frequency of monitoring of biochemical parameters of MBD and target values of PTH **(Table 6)**.[20,23] In children with CKD in whom biochemical abnormalities are identified or those who are being managed, the frequency of testing should be increased to monitor for trends and for evaluation of treatment efficacy. Changes in management should be based on *trends of serial results and persistent abnormalities* rather than a single result, and interpretation of results of serum Ca, P, PTH, ALP, and 25-vitamin D levels as a combination.[25] With increasing stage of CKD, resistance of the kidneys to PTH increases; therefore, an increasing PTH target level is considered acceptable **(Table 6)**. If plasma PTH levels are suppressed below the target range and serum calcium levels are high, vitamin D therapy and calcium-containing phosphate binders should be reduced or even discontinued, and a reduction in dialysate calcium concentration is advised.

Measurement of serum *total ALP*, a marker of osteoblast activity, can be helpful in predicting bone turnover in conjunction with PTH. Determination of serum $1,25(OH)_2D$ levels has no role when monitoring children with CKD-MBD.

Maintenance of Calcium–Phosphate Homeostasis

Growing infants and children need a positive calcium balance; hence, serum calcium must be maintained in the normal range **(Table 7)**. The calcium × phosphate product is no longer used in clinical practice. Frequent dietary assessment and appropriate advice is an important aspect of CKD-MBD treatment. Calcium-rich foods, such as dairy products, are also high in phosphorus; hence, increasing dietary consumption of calcium to meet daily needs is accompanied by an excessive intake of phosphorus. The extra phosphorous cannot be excreted in advanced CKD; hence, calcium supplementation as tablets is required to meet the age-appropriate daily recommended or SDI of calcium **(Table 8)**.[25] Thc total elemental calcium given orally as supplements (including

TABLE 6: Frequency of monitoring of biochemical parameters of chronic kidney disease–mineral bone disease by stage of chronic kidney disease and target parathormone levels.[19,23]

Stage	eGFR (mL/min/1.73 m²)	Calcium, phosphorous, bicarbonate	Alkaline phosphatase, PTH	Target PTH level (pg/mL)
2	60–89	At least yearly	At least yearly	35–70
3	30–59	At least every 6 months	At least every 6 months	35–70
4	15–29	At least every 3 months	At least every 3 months	70–110
5	<15 or dialysis	At least every month	At least every 3 months	200–300

(eGFR: estimated glomerular filtration rate; PTH: parathyroid hormone)

TABLE 7: Normal values for serum phosphorous, total calcium, ionized calcium (blood), and alkaline phosphatase.[25]

Age (years)	Serum phosphorous (mg/dL)	Serum total calcium (mg/dL)	Blood ionized calcium (mg/dL)	Alkaline phosphatase (IU/L)
0–0.25	4.8–7.4	8.8–11.3	4.89–5.61	
1–5	4.5–6.5	9.4–10.8	4.89–5.29	100–350
6–12	3.6–5.8	9.4–10.3	4.61–5.29	60–450
13–20	2.3–4.5	8.8–10.2	4.49–5.21	40–180

those given as phosphate binders) should not exceed up to twice (200%) SDI for calcium, and the total calcium intake including dietary calcium) should not exceed 2,500 mg/day.[2] In CKD stage 5, serum calcium levels should be maintained at the lower range of normal to avoid the risk of hypercalcemia and vascular calcification. In case hypercalcemia does occur, all calcium-containing phosphate binders must be withheld, vitamin D therapy should be stopped, and adjustments must be made to the dialysis solutions (PD fluid with 2.5 mEq/L calcium and lower dialysate calcium concentrations in HD patients). For those with low serum calcium levels, dialysate fluids with higher calcium concentrations are advisable.

Hyperphosphatemia is an independent risk factor for secondary hyperparathyroidism, renal osteodystrophy, and vascular calcifications; hence, the serum concentration of phosphate should be kept in the normal age-appropriate range **(Table 7)**. Dietary phosphate intake usually exceeds renal phosphate removal once GFR decreases to <40 mL/min/1.73 m^2. However, this threshold may be reached earlier if dietary phosphate intake is high. Counseling regarding dietary phosphate restriction to within the SDI should be performed when the patient has reached CKD stage II and may be sufficient for preventing hyperphosphatemia. Phosphate restrictions need to be more stringent, i.e., to the lower limit of the SDI in patients with advanced CKD and in those with persistent hyperphosphatemia or hyperparathyroidism.[2] However, strict adherence to dietary phosphate restriction is difficult for two reasons. Firstly, because low-phosphate diets are unpalatable. Secondly, phosphorous intake is directly linked to protein intake; 10–12 mg of phosphorus is present in each gram of protein; an adequate protein intake is critical in order to maximize growth in children. The recommended protein intake, depending on age, is 1–2.5 g/kg/day. The amount of phosphate removed by PD (300–400 mg/day) or HD (700–800 mg/treatment session) is not enough to maintain normal serum phosphate levels. Hence, patients treated with dialysis require phosphate-binding agents that reduce intestinal phosphate absorption by forming poorly soluble complexes with phosphorus in the intestinal tract.[21] A comparison between the two most commonly available phosphate binders, i.e., calcium carbonate and calcium acetate, shows that an equivalent dose of calcium acetate binds twice as much as phosphorus **(Table 9)**. Calcium-containing phosphate binders are best administered 10–15 minutes before or with meals to enhance phosphate absorption and between meals for absorption of calcium. The dose required to keep serum phosphate levels within the normal range may lead to hypercalcemia and can increase the risk of vascular calcification, especially in patients treated with 25(OH)D, when phosphate levels continue to be elevated and PTH levels are low (with likely adynamic bone disease). In such situations, calcium-free phosphate binders, e.g., sevelamer, are advised. Aluminum-containing phosphate binders, though very effective, are used in rare cases of severe hypophosphatemia (serum phosphate level exceeding 7.0 mEq/L), for 4–6 weeks, closely monitoring serum aluminum levels since these expose the patient to the risk of aluminum toxicity. A more effective method, though not always feasible, would be prolonged daily dialysis.

Vitamin D affects calcium homeostasis, regulates PTH levels, and may also play a role in the prevention of CVD, anemia, infectious and autoimmune conditions, renoprotection, glycemic control, and prevention of some common cancers.[26-28] Vitamin D deficiency is common in children with CKD. CPRs for native vitamin D therapy in children with CKD stages 2–5 and on dialysis recommend that vitamin D levels should be measured at 6–12-month intervals, depending on the CKD stage and after 3 months in those

TABLE 8: Summary of suggested dietary intake for calcium and phosphate in children with chronic kidney disease.[24]

Age	*SDI calcium (mg)*	*SDI phosphate (mg)*
0–<4 months	220	120
4–12 months	330–540	275–420
1–3 years	450–540	250–500
4–10 years	700–1,000	440–800
11–17 years	900–1,300	640–1,250

TABLE 9: Calcium supplements and phosphate binders.[24]

Name	*Calcium content (%)*	*Calcium absorbed (%)*	*Phosphate bound per gram of compound*	*Phosphate bound per milligram of calcium absorbed*	*Comment*
Calcium carbonate*	40	20–30	39 mg/g	~1 mg/8 mg	High Ca^{2+} Inexpensive
Calcium acetate*	25	22 (40% between meals)	45 mg/g	~1 mg/3 mg	Less Ca^{2+} load than $CaCO_3$ Inexpensive
Sevelamer carbonate†	0	0		~1 mg/2.3 mg	Calcium free Expensive

*Elemental calcium 50–75 mg/kg/day.
†Sevelamer 20–40 mg/kg/ day q8 hourly (maximum 1,600 mg/day).

on supplemental doses. If the levels are normal, vitamin D supplements should be given in maintenance doses and levels estimated 6 monthly. If levels are low, a course of intensive replacement therapy should be administered.[29]

Clinical practice recommendations for native vitamin D therapy in children with CKD stages 2–5 and on dialysis suggest that serum 25(OH)D concentrations should be maintained above >30 ng/mL (75 nmol/L) in children with CKD stages 2–5D and classify vitamin D status as follows: sufficiency >30 ng/mL (>75 nmol/L), insufficiency 20–30 ng/mL (50–75 nmol/L), deficiency 5–20 ng/mL (12–50 nmol/L), and severe deficiency <5 ng/mL (<12 nmol/L).[29] Vitamin D dosing regimens are mentioned in **Table 10**. Native vitamin D supplementation with cholecalciferol or ergocalciferol should be stopped when serum 25(OH)D concentration exceeds 48 ng/mL. Patients with CKD may have reduced urinary calcium excretion, hence if given large doses of vitamin D such as the stoss regime, these children are prone to developing hypercalciuria. The resulting nephrocalcinosis could worsen renal function. Hence, mega-dose vitamin D treatment regimens are not recommended.[29]

As kidney function decreases, synthesis of *active vitamin D [1,25 $(OH)_2D$]* declines due to decreased phosphate excretion, low serum 25(OH)D levels, and high serum FGF23. In turn, low serum 1,25$(OH)_2$D levels result in hypocalcemia and secondary hyperparathyroidism. If plasma PTH levels remain elevated despite normal serum 25(OH)D and phosphate levels, treatment with 1,25(OH)D (calcitriol) or 1-α hydroxyvitamin D (alpha-calcidiol) is indicated to compensate for reduced renal 1-α hydroxylase activity and to prevent and control secondary hyperparathyroidism. The recommended initial dose is 5–10 ng/kg/day and can be titrated upward to achieve target calcium and PTH concentrations, though the therapeutic window is very small. Treatment with these compounds increases intestinal phosphate absorption and may aggravate hyperphosphatemia-caused episodes of hypercalcemia and increases the risk of soft-tissue calcification. Prolonged treatment with active vitamin D is known to be associated with adynamic bone disease that results in a reduced growth rate. High 1,25$(OH)_2$D levels are also associated with increased FGF23 secretion, CVD, and mortality.[30]

Newer analogs of 1,25$(OH)_2$D, such as paricalcitol and doxercalciferol, are now available. They suppress PTH as effectively as calcitriol without increasing intestinal calcium and phosphorous absorption. However, these forms of active vitamin D are also associated with high serum levels of FGF23 and the associated detrimental effects on cardiac myocytes.

Calcimimetics are drugs that bind to the calcium-sensing receptor of the parathyroid gland. They increase its sensitivity to ionized calcium and in a dose-dependent manner can decrease plasma PTH levels by up to 80%. Their use should be considered in children who continue to have persistent hyperparathyroidism despite being vitamin D replete and who are compliant with dietary phosphate restriction and phosphate binders. The recommended starting dose of cinacalcet is 0.2 mg/kg/day. It may be increased by 0.2 mg/kg/day up to 2.5 mg/kg/day (Maximum dose 60 mg/day; available as 30, 60, and 90 mg tablets).[31]

Parathyroidectomy is indicated in patients who continue to suffer from persistent or recurrent hypercalcemia and hyperphosphatemia despite compliance with dietary advice and medication that includes cinacalcet or from debilitating bone disease and extraosseous calcifications.

In summary, CKD-MBD refers to biochemical abnormalities of Ca, P, ALP, PTH, FGF23, bone disease, growth retardation, and vascular and extravascular calcification. As kidney function decreases, phosphate excretion declines and levels in blood increase, FGF23 synthesis in bone increases, renal 1,25$(OH)_2$D synthesis is suppressed, and PTH secretion increases. In addition, there exist vitamin D deficiency, impaired intestinal calcium absorption, and hypocalcemia. Management is aimed at screening for hyperparathyroidism in CKD stage II, management of hyperphosphatemia with diet, addition of calcium-based phosphate binders and calcium-free phosphate binders in case of hypercalcemia. Additionally, hypocalcemia is managed with 25(OH)D in stages 2–3, active vitamin D in stages 4–5 and 5D, and by

TABLE 10: Doses of native vitamin D (cholecalciferol) for treatment of vitamin D deficiency in patients with chronic kidney disease 2–5D.

		Adapted from KDOQI guidelines*[2]	*Clinical practice recommendations*[28]
<1 year of age		–	*600 IU/day*
>1 year	*Serum 25 (OH) D levels*		
	<5	50,000 IU/week × 4 weeks, then twice/month × 2 months†	8,000 IU/day‡
	5–20	50,000 IU every 2 weeks × 3 months†	4,000 IU/day‡
	20–30	50,000 IU/ month × 3 months†	2,000 IU/day‡
	Maintenance	200–1,000 IU/day	<1 year: 400 IU/day >1 year: 1,000–2,000 IU/day based on CKD stage

*The commonly available preparation in India contains 60,000 IU/sachet.
†Measure serum 25(OH) D levels after 3 months.
‡Serum calcium and urinary calcium levels 1–3 monthly based on CKD stage and measure 25(OH) D levels: after 3 months.

increasing calcium content of dialysate. Calcimimetics like cinacalcet may be used for uncontrolled hyperparathyroidism and parathyroidectomy as a final measure.

ENDOCRINE DISORDERS

In children with CKD, disturbances in endocrine function usually occur either due to abnormalities in circulating hormone concentrations as a result of altered metabolism or due to a change at the site of action seen as resistance. Active management is feasible in a few select conditions.

Growth and Puberty

An important contributor to poor growth in children with CKD is resistance to GH and insulin-like growth factor 1 (IGF-1) that occurs due to uremia. Glucocorticoid treatment postrenal transplantation further contributes to this in children who have received an allograft. Administration of supraphysiological doses of recombinant human growth hormone (rhGH) increases levels of free IGF-1 enough to overcome the resistance significantly and improves height SDS and height velocity in children pre-dialysis, on dialysis, and postrenal transplantation. Thus, where financial constraints do not exist, rhGH therapy is the standard of care to optimize final height in children with CKD demonstrating growth failure that is persistent, defined as height below the third percentile and height velocity below the 25th percentile for more than 3 months in infants or more than 6 months in children once all *correctable factors have been taken care of*, i.e., the child is receiving adequate calories and proteins and does not have anemia or any metabolic abnormalities.[32] A daily dose of 4 IU/m^2 (0.04–0.05 mg/kg) is advised, to be administered subcutaneously in the evening, to synchronize with the endogenous GH secretion. Growth velocity due to therapy is the highest in prepubertal children and in the first year of treatment. Therapy is contraindicated in children with active malignancy, proliferative retinopathy, or who have a history of hypersensitivity to the drug or to any of the excipients. The growth response is considered to be adequate if the rate of growth during the first year of GH treatment is >2 cm/year over baseline. When therapy is initiated in the predialysis phase, it should be continued even when CKD progresses and the child becomes dependent on dialysis. Renal allograft recipients are expected to demonstrate catch-up growth if transplantation is performed prior to fusion of the epiphyses of the long bones. Hence, in children on rhGH therapy, who undergo transplantation, further therapy is withheld and the child is monitored for growth over 12 months. If growth during this period is inadequate, glucocorticoid withdrawal should be considered, followed by consideration of restarting rhGH if required.[7] Once the height that is the patient's genetic potential is achieved, treatment with rhGH may be omitted. While on rhGH, children need to be monitored for symptoms of headache and vomiting suggestive of raised intracranial HTN, glucose intolerance, and worsening of GFR.[32] GH therapy is discontinued if target height as predicted by mid parental height or 50th percentile for age is achieved or in patients who demonstrate an inadequate response, during 6 months of compliant therapy with GH or if there is closure of epiphyses.

However, the *onset* of puberty is usually delayed in children with CKD, genital development proceeds at a normal rate thereafter. In children with CKD stage 5, there exists a state of compensated *hypergonadotropic hypogonadism* characterized by increased plasma concentrations of luteinizing hormone (LH) and follicle-stimulating hormone (FSH), in combination with reduced release of hypothalamic gonadotropin-releasing hormone (GnRH). Males have low total and free testosterone (T) and dihydrotestosterone (DHT) levels. In girls, as GFR decreases, so do plasma estradiol levels. Reproductive function is permanently impaired and does not reverse even after transplantation. Males with CKD suffer from low libido and erectile dysfunction and women have difficulties in conception.[7] The anticipated surge in hormone levels that occurs during puberty is absent in patients on dialysis and is an important factor for the inadequate growth seen in these children. However, early renal transplantation before the onset of puberty prevents delay in pubertal development and improves adult height.[10]

Thyroid Disorders

The renal clearance of thyroid-releasing hormone (TRH) and thyroid-stimulating hormone (TSH) is decreased in CKD; hence, their circulating levels may be elevated. However, the response to these hormones is diminished. Serum-free and total thyroxine (T4) concentrations may be normal or slightly low due to impaired hormone binding to thyroid-binding globulin. Low serum free triiodothyronine (T3) is considered a compensatory response to the CKD state, minimizing further protein catabolism. Children with CKD should be diagnosed to have hypothyroidism when total and free T4 levels are significantly low, thyroid-binding globulin concentrations are normal, and basal TSH levels are elevated (>10 mU/L).

HYPERTENSION AND CARDIOVASCULAR DISEASE

Chronic kidney disease is a vasculopathic state and CVD is a cause of mortality of patients with CKD all over the world.[15,33] The prevalence of HTN in children and adolescents with CKD is as high as 50%.[33] It is an important contributor to progression of kidney disease. Blood pressure (BP) should be monitored at all clinic visits of children with CKD and once a year these children should undergo evaluation for masked or nocturnal HTN by ambulatory blood pressure monitoring (ABPM).[33] Management of HTN may slow the progression of or even reverse end-organ damage. The management goals for HTN are to achieve systolic and diastolic BP readings ≤50th percentile as per the normative data.

The KDIGO guidelines recommend that in children with CKD, treatment with angiotensin-converting enzyme inhibitors (ACE-I) or angiotensin receptor blockers (ARBs) be used as drugs of initial choice when BP is consistently >90th percentile for age, sex, and height. These drugs have been found useful since they additionally slow CKD progression, reduce renal sympathetic activity, and contribute to cardiac muscle remodeling.[15,16] However, they may cause an acute rise in serum potassium and a decline in GFR; therefore, they should be used carefully, if at all, once the GFR is <60 mL/min/1.73 m². Since the drug-induced decline in GFR occurs within the first few days after the treatment has been started, the serum creatinine and potassium concentrations should be remeasured within 7–10 days. A rise of creatinine >25% from the baseline value should prompt either omission or a decrease in the dose of the ACE-I/ARB.

A diuretic may be used for patients with HTN and edema. For patients in early stages of CKD [estimated GFR (eGFR) ≥ 45 mL/min/1.73 m²], a thiazide diuretic such as hydrochlorothiazide (1–3 mg/kg/day to a maximum of 50 mg/day) is useful, while for those with more advanced CKD, a loop diuretic is recommended (furosemide 1.0–2 mg/kg/day in one to two divided doses).

Beta-blockers are considered next in line as antihypertensive agents in children with CKD. Calcium channel blockers, alpha-adrenergic agents (prazosin, clonidine), and other vasodilators (hydralazine, minoxidil) may also be used when indicated.

Adjunctive therapy with lifestyle measures such as salt and sugar restriction; reduced fat; inclusion of more fruits, vegetables, and whole grains in diet; regular aerobic physical exercise; weight reduction for those who are obese; and avoidance of caffeine and energy drinks should also be advised. Children with CKD and HTN should undergo echocardiographic evaluation for LVH. Presence of concentric LVH is an indication for improvement in control of HTN.[33] Eccentric LVH is a consequence of persistent fluid overload and anemia, and avoidance of these can reduce the risk of its development.[34] Other cardiovascular abnormalities include left ventricular systolic and diastolic dysfunction, increased carotid intimal media thickness (cIMT), increased pulse wave velocity (PWV), and carotid artery calcification. Monitoring for, and early and vigorous management of HTN, dyslipidemia, bone and mineral metabolism abnormalities, anemia, attention to nutrition, adequate dialysis, and early renal transplantation may minimize the development of CVD.

DYSLIPIDEMIA

Lipid metabolism is abnormal in patients with CKD and contributes to the high risk for CVD seen in these patients.[35] The risk of dyslipidemia increases as the GFR decreases, being highest in those with ESKD and following kidney transplantation. Children more than 2 years of age with CKD should be screened for dyslipidemia annually.[15] Management consists of lifestyle changes with advice regarding limiting fat intake to <15% of total calories. Statins may be used in older children (males ≥10 years of age and postmenarchal female patients) in whom dyslipidemia remains severe (LDL > 130 mg/dL) despite dietary management.

Proteinuria, and more specifically albuminuria, is a marker for renal dysfunction and hence an essential criterion for the diagnosis of CKD.[15] It is often associated with HTN and a rapid decline in GFR.[33] Effective control of HTN and proteinuria delay the progression of CKD; hence, children with CKD should be monitored for proteinuria. The KDIGO guidelines recommend that testing for proteinuria should be performed on an early morning urine sample and expressed as an albumin:creatinine ratio (ACR, preferably) or as a protein:creatinine ratio. Children with an ACR ≥ 30 mg/g should be treated with ACE-I (usual doses are enalapril 0.2–0.6 mg/kg/once a day and ramipril 0.05 mg/kg/once a day up to 10 mg) with careful titration of dose and monitoring for hypotension, rise in serum creatinine, and hyperkalemia.

FLUID, SODIUM, AND POTASSIUM

The total sodium content of the body is directly linked to fluid balance. The requirement for sodium supplementation or restriction depends upon the primary cause of kidney disease and the residual urine output. Many children with CKD, e.g., those with renal hypodysplasia or obstructive uropathy, are polyuric with substantial sodium losses and infants on PD are at risk for hyponatremia due to sodium losses through the dialysate. Persistent sodium and water losses may result in chronic volume depletion and may impair linear growth. *Infants* with polyuric CKD may need supplementation with fluid volumes of 180–240 mL/kg/day and sodium intake of 2–4 mEq/100 mL of fluid.[36] As they are weaned to the family diet, dietary sodium intake increases and supplementation should be decreased accordingly.

Children with glomerular diseases and with oliguria need sodium and fluid restrictions to prevent enema and to control HTN. A lower salt intake also lowers albuminuria. As mentioned earlier, in early stages of CKD, use of hydrochlorothiazide and later loop diuretics may be used for the management of edema and HTN. The KDOQI guidelines recommend that in children with HTN, sodium intake should be limited to less than the dietary recommendation, i.e., 1,500 mg sodium per day for children 1–3 years old, 2,000–3,000 mg for older children.

Fluid intake should be adjusted depending on the residual urine volume, insensible losses, and the ultrafiltration that can be achieved. Children on HD should have a fluid intake only enough to limit weight gain to 5% of dry weight in the interdialytic period. Children on PD may require fewer restrictions as the dextrose concentration of dialysis fluid may be increased to increase the ultrafiltration volume. In order to decrease thirst and effectively restrict fluid intake, it is essential to restrict salt intake as mentioned above.

The risk of hyperkalemia increases as GFR decreases and predisposes the child to cardiac arrhythmias and arrest. Children with hyperkalemia are advised to restrict intake of high potassium-containing foods such as oranges, bananas, potatoes and potato products, tomatoes, legumes, lentils, yogurt, and chocolate. Dieticians recommend leaching of potassium from vegetables by soaking them in water before cooking. Diuretics may be used to manage hyperkalemia in children who are nonoliguric. Potassium-binding agents are nonabsorbable substances that exchange calcium for potassium when administered orally or rectally. Calcium polystyrene sulfonate is most commonly used, at a dose of 1–1.5 mg/kg/dose, three to four times a day. Patiromer, a potassium-binding polymer, has been studied in adults with CKD stage 3 or greater with hyperkalemia; however, approval for its use in children is awaited. Initiation of maintenance dialysis is indicated when hyperkalemia can no longer be controlled with low-potassium diet and the use of potassium-binding agents.

With CKD progression, certain clinical features develop, e.g., nausea, anorexia, and vomiting. Two complications that need specific management are platelet dysfunction and pericarditis. An increased tendency for bleeding is present due to abnormalities in platelet adhesion and aggregation. Desmopressin (DDAVP) may be given to children with uremia, prior to invasive procedures, at a dose of 0.3 μg/kg, intravenously or subcutaneously. Onset of action occurs within an hour of administration. In case of active bleeding due to any cause, cryoprecipitate (1–2 units/10 kg) may be used to manage the same.

Uremic pericarditis and pericardial effusion are late manifestations and respond to institution of dialysis.

IMMUNIZATION

Children with CKD are at increased risk for infections; hence, they should receive all childhood vaccinations. Unfortunately, they also have a reduced immunologic response to some vaccines and periodic evaluation of antibody titers and revaccination when required must be carried out, e.g., immune response to the hepatitis B (HB) vaccine can be poor and HB antibody titers wane quickly following vaccination; therefore, annual monitoring of anti-HB surface antigen–antibody titers is recommended. Certain special considerations for children with CKD are mentioned in **Table 11**. Live attenuated vaccines [varicella (VZV); measles, mumps, rubella (MMR); and live influenza vaccines] should not be administered to children on immunosuppressive medications; therefore, protection against these diseases should be documented or vaccines administered 4 weeks prior to kidney transplantation.[37,38]

TABLE 11: Special considerations for immunization of children with chronic kidney disease.

Hepatitis B vaccine	After the primary immunization is complete, antibody titers should be monitored. If protective antibody levels (>10 mIU/mL) are not achieved, up to three additional doses may be given antibody levels should be monitored annually and booster doses provided when levels fall below protective levels
Influenza	Annual immunization with killed vaccine
MMR	Antibody titers should be measured before transplant and a dose of vaccine to be administered if inadequate titers vaccination is avoided in children on immunosuppressive medications
Pneumococcal vaccine	• *In children <2 years:* PCV as per primary schedule followed by a dose of PPSV 2 years after the last dose of PCV • *In children >2 years:* Catch-up schedule as recommended by the Indian Academy of Pediatrics • In addition, all children require a dose of PPSV every 5 years up to a maximum of three doses
Varicella vaccine	Antibody titers should be measured before transplant in any patient without a history of wild-type infection. If positive antibody titers are absent, a dose of vaccine has to be administered. A second dose is required if titers are inadequate after first vaccination

(MMR: measles, mumps, rubella; PCV: pneumococcal conjugate vaccine; PPSV: pneumococcal polysaccharide vaccine)

COGNITIVE AND PSYCHOSOCIAL DEVELOPMENT

Children with CKD have some impairment of neurocognitive development and psychosocial adjustment attributed to a combination of exposure of the growing brain to uremia and other metabolites, medications as well as psychosocial factors such as missed school days, interrupted age-appropriate social and emotional experiences, and altered family dynamics.[39] They have been found to have lower scores for executive function, memory (verbal and visual), mathematics, reading, and spelling compared with their peers.[40] Those with a longer duration of illness and more severe disease are at greater risk. These children should undergo evaluation and early intervention when needed by experts in behavioral and developmental pediatrics to assess the cognitive and emotional abilities. Some may need individualized counseling and special educational facilities to optimize their functional potential. Close attention to nutrition and correction of anemia also improve developmental outcomes.[16]

PHYSICAL ACTIVITY

Children with CKD should be encouraged to participate in school and community sports and exercise programs.

PREPARATION FOR KIDNEY REPLACEMENT THERAPY

Kidney replacement therapy is usually required when the GFR decreases to <15 mL/min/1.73 m^2 (stage 5 CKD). Preparation should therefore begin when the GFR declines to <30 mL/min/ 1.73 m^2 (stage 4) by providing the family with information on the options available, i.e., kidney transplantation, PD, and HD. This process may require multiple counseling sessions with family members. In addition, certain precautions and preemptive management strategies are recommended, e.g., the nondominant arm is identified and efforts are made to protect it from proximal intravenous access, so that it will be available for vascular access when needed for HD; consultation with a vascular surgeon for the evaluation for fistula development before the actual need for dialysis; avoidance of unnecessary use of blood products in order to lower risk antigen exposure, and allosensitization.[16]

PALLIATIVE CARE

The care of children with CKD is characterized by high symptom distress for patients, functional limitations, and emotional and financial burden on caregivers. Palliative care is a specialized type of care focused on improving the quality of life for the patient and the family. A specialized team of doctors, nurses, and social workers provide an extra layer of physical, psychological, social, and spiritual support together with prescribed treatment or as management for those who choose to withdraw from advanced treatment, e.g., kidney replacement therapy.

Preventing progression and avoiding subsequent kidney injury is an important aspect of management of children with CKD.

CONCLUSION

Chronic kidney disease is a state of irreversible kidney damage and/or reduction of kidney function that is associated with progressive loss of kidney function over time. A progressive decrease in GFR manifests as a combination of various system involvement seen as growth retardation, anemia, HTN, endocrine dysfunction, MBD, proteinuria, and fluid and electrolyte abnormalities. Appropriate management entails early diagnosis, periodic assessment by clinical as well as laboratory parameters, and timely intervention following closely the evidence-based guidelines (e.g., KDIGO), KDOQI, PRNT) wherever available.

KEY POINTS

- CKD is a state of irreversible kidney damage often associated with a progressive loss of glomerular filtration rate.
- Symptoms arise when there is moderate-to-severe loss of kidney function and manifest chiefly as poor appetite, growth failure, anemia, HTN, features of fluid and electrolyte imbalance, and MBD.
- Management of CKD includes measures to delay progression and treatment of the biochemical, hematological, and endocrine abnormalities as they arise and eventually kidney replacement therapy when the disease progresses to ESKD. Simultaneous support of a team of social worker and psychologist/behavioral pediatrician for the child and caretakers is very useful.

REFERENCES

1. Haffner D, Rees L. Growth and puberty in chronic kidney disease. In: Geary DF, Schaefer F (Eds). Pediatric Kidney Disease, 2nd edition. Berlin, Heidelberg: Springer-Verlag; 2016. pp. 1425-54.
2. National Kidney Foundation. KDOQI clinical practice guideline for nutrition in children with CKD: 2008 update. Am J Kidney Dis. 2009;53(3):S11-104.
3. Nelms CL, Shaw V, Greenbaum LA, Anderson C, Desloovere A, Haffner D, et al. Assessment of nutritional status in children with kidney diseases—clinical practice recommendations from the Pediatric Renal Nutrition Taskforce. Pediatr Nephrol. 2021;36(4):995-1010.
4. Furth SL, Stablein D, Fine RN, Powe NR, Fivush BA. Adverse clinical outcomes associated with short stature at dialysis initiation: a report of the North American Pediatric Renal Transplant Cooperative Study. Pediatrics. 2002;109(5):909-13.
5. Furth SL, Hwang W, Yang C, Neu AM, Fivush BA, Powe NR. Growth failure, risk of hospitalization and death for children with end-stage renal disease. Pediatr Nephrol. 2002;17(6):450-5.
6. Foster B. Growth and development of the child with renal disease. In: Avner ED, Harmon WE, Niaudet P, Yoshikawa N, Emma F, Goldstein SL (Eds). Pediatric Nephrology, 7th edition. Berlin, Heidelberg: Springer-Verlag; 2016. pp. 637-66.
7. Schaefer F. Endocrine and growth abnormalities in chronic kidney disease. In: Avner ED, Harmon WE, Niaudet P, Yoshikawa N, Emma F, Goldstein SL (Eds). Pediatric Nephrology, 7th edition. Berlin, Heidelberg: Springer-Verlag; 2016. pp. 2295-349.
8. Wong CS, Gipson DS, Gillen DL, Emerson S, Koepsell T, Sherrard DJ, et al. Anthropometric measures and risk of death in children with end-stage renal disease. Am J Kidney Dis Off J Natl Kidney Found. 2000;36(4):811-9.
9. Shaw V, Polderman N, Renken-Terhaerdt J, Paglialonga F, Oosterveld M, Tuokkola J, et al. Energy and protein requirements for children with CKD stages 2-5 and on dialysis-clinical practice recommendations from the Pediatric Renal Nutrition Taskforce. Pediatr Nephrol. 2020;35(3):519-31.
10. Tainio J, Qvist E, Vehmas R, Jahnukainen K, Hölttä T, Valta H, et al. Pubertal development is normal in adolescents after renal transplantation in childhood. Transplantation. 2011;92(4): 404-9.
11. Burke JR. Low-dose subcutaneous recombinant erythropoietin in children with chronic renal failure. Australian and New Zealand Paediatric Nephrology Association. Pediatr Nephrol. 1995;9(5):558-61.
12. Morris KP, Skinner JR, Hunter S, Coulthard MG. Cardiovascular abnormalities in end stage renal failure: the effect of anaemia or uraemia? Arch Dis Child. 1994;71(2):119-22.
13. Gerson A, Hwang W, Fiorenza J, Barth K, Kaskel F, Weiss L, et al. Anemia and health-related quality of life in adolescents with chronic kidney disease. Am J Kidney Dis Off J Natl Kidney Found. 2004;44(6):1017-23.
14. Morris KP, Sharp J, Watson S, Coulthard MG. Non-cardiac benefits of human recombinant erythropoietin in end stage renal failure and anaemia. Arch Dis Child. 1993;69(5):580-6.
15. KDIGO clinical practice guideline for anemia in chronic kidney disease. Kidney Int. 2012;279-335.

16. VanDe Voorde RG, Wong C, Warady BA. Management of chronic kidney disease in children. In: Avner ED, Harmon WE, Niaudet P, Yoshikawa N, Emma F, Goldstein SL (Eds). Pediatric Nephrology, 7th edition. Berlin, Heidelberg: Springer-Verlag; 2016. pp. 2208-51.
17. Greenbaum L. Anemia in chronic renal disease. In: Geary DF, Schaefer F (Eds). Pediatric Kidney Disease, 2nd edition (2016 edition). Heidelberg: Springer; 2017. pp. 1507-32.
18. Cano F, Alarcon C, Azocar M, Lizama C, Maria Lillo A, Delucchi A, et al. Continuous EPO receptor activator therapy of anemia in children under peritoneal dialysis. Pediatr Nephrol Berl Ger. 2011;26(8):1303-10.
19. Fischbach M, Wühl E, Reigner SCM, Morgan Z, Schaefer F. Efficacy and long-term safety of C.E.R.A. maintenance in pediatric hemodialysis patients with anemia of CKD. Clin J Am Soc Nephrol CJASN. 2018;13(1):81-90.
20. Coyne DW, Roger SD, Shin SK, Kim SG, Cadena AA, Moustafa MA, et al. Roxadustat for chronic kidney disease-related anemia in non-dialysis patients. Kidney Int Rep. 2020;6(3):624-35.
21. Wesseling-Perry K, Salusky IB. Management of chronic kidney disease in children. In: Avner ED, Harmon WE, Niaudet P, Yoshikawa N, Emma F, Goldstein SL (Eds). Pediatric Nephrology, 7th edition. Berlin, Heidelberg: Springer-Verlag; 2016. pp. 2350-70.
22. Picton ML, Moore PR, Mawer EB, Houghton D, Freemont AJ, Hutchison AJ, et al. Down-regulation of human osteoblast PTH/PTHrP receptor mRNA in end-stage renal failure. Kidney Int. 2000;58(4):1440-9.
23. Wesseling-Perry K, Salusky IB. Chronic kidney disease: mineral and bone disorder in children. Semin Nephrol. 2013;33(2):169-79.
24. Schmitt CP, Shroff R. Disorders of bone mineral metabolism in chronic kidney disease. In: Geary DF, Schaefer F (Eds). Pediatric Kidney Disease, 2nd edition. Berlin, Heidelberg: Springer-Verlag; 2016. pp. 1533-66.
25. McAlister L, Pugh P, Greenbaum L, Haffner D, Rees L, Anderson C, et al. The dietary management of calcium and phosphate in children with CKD stages 2-5 and on dialysis—clinical practice recommendation from the Pediatric Renal Nutrition Taskforce. Pediatr Nephrol. 2020;35(3):501-18.
26. Li YC, Kong J, Wei M, Chen Z-F, Liu SQ, Cao L-P. 1,25-Dihydroxyvitamin D(3) is a negative endocrine regulator of the renin-angiotensin system. J Clin Invest. 2002;110(2):229-38.
27. Shroff R, Wan M, Gullett A, Ledermann S, Shute R, Knott C, et al. Ergocalciferol supplementation in children with CKD delays the onset of secondary hyperparathyroidism: a randomized trial. Clin J Am Soc Nephrol CJASN. 2012;7(2):216-23.
28. Shroff R, Aitkenhead H, Costa N, Trivelli A, Litwin M, Picca S, et al. Normal 25-hydroxyvitamin D levels are associated with less proteinuria and attenuate renal failure progression in children with CKD. J Am Soc Nephrol JASN. 2016;27(1):314-22.
29. Shroff R, Wan M, Nagler EV, Bakkaloğlu S, Fischer D-C, Bishop N, et al. Clinical practice recommendations for native vitamin D therapy in children with chronic kidney disease stages 2–5 and on dialysis. Nephrol Dial Transplant. 2017;32(7):1098-113.
30. Freedman BI, Bowden DW, Ziegler JT, Langefeld CD, Lehtinen AB, Rudock ME, et al. Bone morphogenetic protein 7 (BMP7) gene polymorphisms are associated with inverse relationships between vascular calcification and BMD: the Diabetes Heart Study. J Bone Miner Res Off J Am Soc Bone Miner Res. 2009;24(10):1719-27.
31. Bacchetta J, Schmitt CP, Ariceta G, Bakkaloglu SA, Groothoff J, Wan M, et al. Cinacalcet use in paediatric dialysis: a position statement from the European Society for Paediatric Nephrology and the Chronic Kidney Disease-Mineral and Bone Disorders Working Group of the ERA-EDTA. Nephrol Dial Transplant. 2020;35(1):47-64.
32. On behalf of the European Society for Paediatric Nephrology Chronic Kidney Disease Mineral and Bone Disorders, Dialysis, and Transplantation Working Groups, Drube J, Wan M, Bonthuis M, Wühl E, Bacchetta J, et al. Clinical practice recommendations for growth hormone treatment in children with chronic kidney disease. Nat Rev Nephrol. 2019;15(9):577-89.
33. Flynn JT, Kaelber DC, Baker-Smith CM, Blowey D, Carroll AE, Daniels SR, et al. Clinical practice guideline for screening and management of high blood pressure in children and adolescents. Pediatrics. 2017;140(3):e20171904.
34. Doyon A, Mitsnefes M. Cardiovascular disease in pediatric chronic kidney disease. In: Geary DF, Schaefer F (Eds). Pediatric Kidney Disease, 2nd edition. Heidelberg: Springer; 2017. pp. 1567-602.
35. Baek HS, Kim SH, Kang HG, Choi HJ, Cheong HI, Ha IS, et al. Dyslipidemia in pediatric CKD patients: results from KNOW-PedCKD (KoreaN cohort study for Outcomes in patients With Pediatric CKD). Pediatr Nephrol Berl Ger. 2020;35(8):1455-61.
36. Parekh RS, Flynn JT, Smoyer WE, Milne JL, Kershaw DB, Bunchman TE, et al. Improved growth in young children with severe chronic renal insufficiency who use specified nutritional therapy. J Am Soc Nephrol JASN. 2001;12(11):2418-26.
37. Esposito S, Mastrolia MV, Prada E, Pietrasanta C, Principi N. Vaccine administration in children with chronic kidney disease. Vaccine. 2014;32(49):6601-6.
38. Neu AM. Immunizations in children with chronic kidney disease. Pediatr Nephrol. 2012;27(8):1257-63.
39. Johnson RJ, Mendeley SR. Neurodevelopment in chronic renal disease. In: Geary DF, Schaefer F (Eds). Pediatric Kidney Disease, 2nd edition. Heidelberg: Springer; 2017. pp. 1455-76.
40. Chen K, Didsbury M, van Zwieten A, Howell M, Kim S, Tong A, et al. Neurocognitive and educational outcomes in children and adolescents with CKD: a systematic review and meta-analysis. Clin J Am Soc Nephrol CJASN. 2018;13(3):387-97.

CHAPTER

12.4 Progression of Chronic Kidney Disease

Nivedita Kamath

INTRODUCTION

Chronic kidney disease (CKD) in children is caused by diverse etiologies with a common factor of progressive decline of renal function over time. The prevalence of CKD has been reported to vary from 15 to 75 per million age-related population,[1] but this is probably an underestimate due to lack of uniform reporting across different regions. Though the triggering event for CKD ranges from a host of inherited and acquired diseases, the final pathway to end-stage kidney disease (ESKD) is the same. In this chapter, we discuss the various risk factors for progression of CKD, their pathogenetic mechanisms, and the preventive strategies to reduce the rate of progression in children with CKD.

DEFINITION

The rate of progression of CKD in children is heterogenous. Data from the North American Pediatric Renal Trials and Collaborative Studies (NAPRTCS) shows that 17% of children with CKD stages 2–4 progressed to ESKD in 1 year and 39% progressed by 3 years.[2] The data from chronic kidney disease in children (CKiD) showed that the average decline in glomerular filtration rate (GFR) was about 1.8 mL/year.[3] A prospective study from our center showed a higher rate of decline of GFR by 3.5 mL/year.[4] In the absence of a uniformly accepted or recommended definition for progression of CKD, studies have used various definitions. Progression has been defined as a >50% decline in GFR from baseline or initiation of dialysis.

PATHOGENESIS

The pathogenesis of progression of CKD has three major steps **(Flowchart 1)**:

1. *Primary injury/insult:* The primary insult may vary from an inherited abnormality like a hypodysplasia or an acquired condition such as focal segmental glomerulosclerosis.
2. Abnormal repair mechanisms.
3. *The final common pathway of progressive loss of remnant nephrons:* Once the damage to the kidney exceeds a certain threshold, the progression is irreversible and independent of the primary insult.[5]

Following an initial insult to the kidney, there may be a decrease in the number of functioning nephrons which results in a compensatory increase in single nephron glomerular filtration rate (snGFR), resulting in further injury. The initial insult results in injury to the tubulointerstitial compartment, eliciting an inflammatory and reparative response which induces fibrosis.

Change in glomerular function not only increases the snGFR of the remnant nephrons resulting in hypertrophy and

Flowchart 1: Pathophysiology of progression of chronic kidney disease.

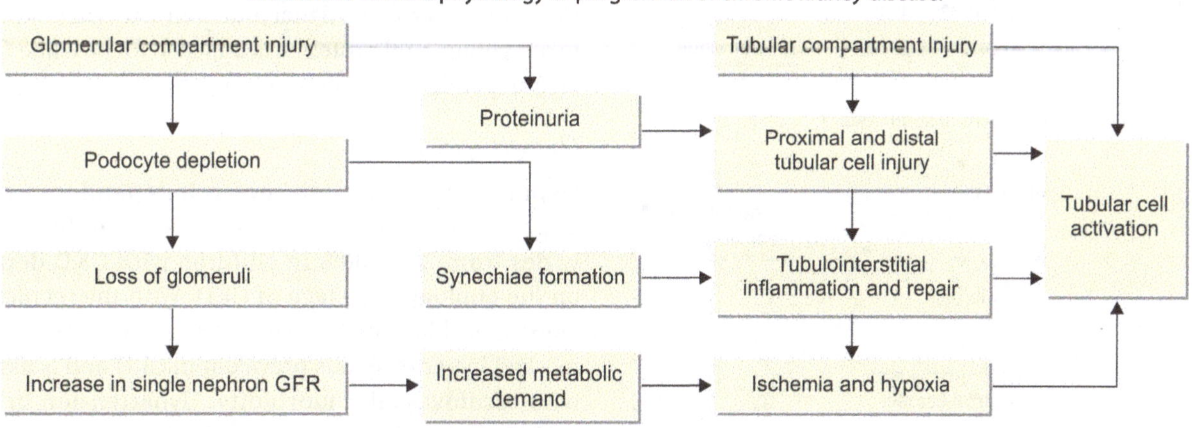

(CKD: chronic kidney disease; GFR: glomerular filtration rate)

Source: Adapted from Hodgkins KS, Schnaper W. Tubulointerstitial injury and the progression of chronic kidney disease. Pediatr Nephrol. 2012;27:901-9.

nephron overload but also causes misdirected filtration which enters into the periglomerular interstitium. In response to this, there is an inflammatory response which ultimately results in fibrosis. Obstruction to the flow of filtrate in tubules leads to tubular atrophy. Abnormality in the tubular reabsorption increases metabolic demands of the nephrons.

Activation of the tubular cell by various mechanisms results in enhanced cytokine production. The activated tubular cells act as antigen-presenting cells and incite various inflammatory pathways. The increase in metabolic demands results in hypoxia and apoptosis of the tubular cells resulting in tubular atrophy and interstitial fibrosis resulting in a vicious cycle of progressive tubulointerstitial damage. The myofibroblast derived from bone marrow or from dedifferentiated tubular cells by epithelial mesenchymal transition (EMT) is the key cell in the initiation and perpetuation of fibrosis. The renin angiotensin system plays an important role in the activation of transformation growth factor-β (TGF-β) which induces EMT and enhances fibrosis. Activation of renin–angiotensin–aldosterone system (RAAS) in the kidney injury elicits tubulointerstitial damage through various mechanisms. RAAS activation exacerbates hypoxia by causing efferent arteriolar constriction. RAAS activation is associated with endothelial cell damage and oxidative stress. It also induces the production of various cytokines and growth factors which are profibrogenic. Hypoxia induces the production of vascular endothelial growth factor and fibroblast growth factor which increases fibrogenesis **(Flowchart 2)**.[6]

RISK FACTORS

The risk factors for progression of CKD are classified as nonmodifiable and modifiable risk factors.

Flowchart 2: Consequences of tubular cell activation.

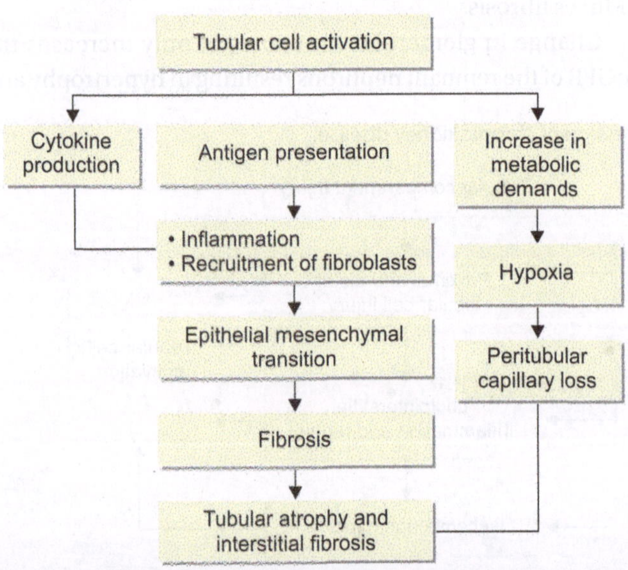

Source: Adapted from Hodgkins KS, Schnaper W. Tubulointerstitial injury and the progression of chronic kidney disease. Pediatr Nephrol. 2012;27:901-9.

Nonmodifiable Risk Factors

The potential nonmodifiable risk factors are the etiology of CKD, baseline GFR, acute kidney injury, and low nephron number. Glomerular diseases in children have a much faster progression to ESKD when compared to nonglomerular disease. The baseline GFR itself is an important risk factor. The progression of CKD is nonlinear; as the GFR declines, the rate of progression is more rapid. An episode of acute kidney injury in the past is also emerging as a risk factor. The presence of lower nephron number as seen in low birth weight or preterm babies is a potential risk factor for progression of CKD. Brenner's hypothesis suggests that a critical reduction in nephron number results in hyperfiltration in the remaining glomeruli, initiating a cascade of events resulting in progressive damage to the remnant nephrons.[7]

Modifiable Risk Factors

The most common potentially modifiable risk factors for progression of CKD are proteinuria and hypertension. These risk factors have been extensively studied in adults with CKD, and controlling these risk factors is associated with a significant reduction in the progression of CKD.

Proteinuria

Proteinuria is not only a consequence of CKD but also an early marker for the progression of CKD. Proteinuria induces interstitial inflammation, tubular cell apoptosis, increases production of TGF-β, proinflammatory, and fibrogenic cytokines. The CKiD study showed that the severity of proteinuria increased with the decline in GFR, irrespective of the etiology of CKD.[8] The study also showed that severe proteinuria (urine protein to creatinine ratio >2) was associated with 94% and 79% reduction in time to progression of CKD in children with glomerular and nonglomerular disease, respectively.[9] It also showed that proteinuria, even when in the non-nephrotic range, was associated with an increased risk of progression to CKD.[10] Similar results were also found from the Japanese National Registry for CKD in children.[10] The study from our center showed that proteinuria was highly prevalent in our cohort, and proteinuria adjusted for baseline GFR was an independent predictor of progression.[4]

Hypertension

Hypertension is a well-known independent predictor of progression of CKD. The prevalence of hypertension varies from 20 to 80% in children with CKD depending on the etiology and stage of CKD. With the regular use of ambulatory blood pressure monitoring, it has been found that masked hypertension is prevalent in CKD and is associated with cardiovascular morbidity. Hypertension in CKD is multifactorial, the common causes being activation of the RAAS, sympathetic system, vasoconstriction, and salt and water retention. The NAPRTCS data and the findings of the

CKiD study confirm that hypertension is an independent predictor of progression of CKD in children.[11]

Other Modifiable Risk Factors

- *Metabolic acidosis:* In children where tubulointerstitial diseases are common causes of CKD, metabolic acidosis is more severe and appears early in CKD. Recent studies in adults have shown that metabolic acidosis is an important risk factor for progression of CKD. Though the mechanism of progression is not clear, it is hypothesized that the residual nephrons increase ammoniagenesis to combat acidosis resulting in worsening tubulointerstitial damage. The 4C study is one of the first longitudinal studies in children which showed that metabolic acidosis was associated with progression of CKD.[12]
- *Dyslipidemia:* The CKiD study showed that dyslipidemia was present in children with glomerular and nonglomerular diseases. Dyslipidemia worsened with decline in GFR and with worsening proteinuria. In adults, dyslipidemia has been found to be associated with progression of CKD. However, in children, there is no data suggesting an association of dyslipidemia with progression of CKD.[13]
- *Anemia:* The NAPRTCS database showed that the prevalence of anemia varied from 19 to -68% in children with CKD stages 2–5. The CKiD study revealed that below a threshold GFR of 43 mL/min/1.73 m^2, the prevalence of anemia increases with the decline in GFR. Anemia has been associated with increased risk of progression of CKD in children and adults.[2]
- *Hyperuricemia:* Hyperuricemia defined as serum uric acid >7.5 mg% was associated with a significantly shorter time to progression of CKD.[14]
- *Others:* Other important risk factors for progression in clinical practice with some evidence in adult studies but little data from studies in children are dehydration, nephrotoxic medications, untreated obstruction to the urinary tract, and urinary tract infections. Most often, these result in acute kidney injury. Acute kidney injury is not only a risk factor for CKD but also for its progression.[15]

Dehydration, by increasing the levels of vasopressin, triggers progression of CKD.[16] The role of nephrotoxic medication in the progression of CKD has been studied in adults.[17] Identifying urinary tract obstruction and infection and early, appropriate management are important to prevent AKI and progression of CKD.

PREVENTIVE STRATEGIES

- *Control of proteinuria and hypertension:* There are several studies in adults which show that the control of proteinuria and hypertension is associated with a significant reduction in progression of CKD. In children, the ESCAPE trial showed that intensive control of blood pressure to <50th centile using angiotensin-converting enzyme (ACE) inhibitors was associated with a significant reduction in the progression of CKD. The effect of ACE inhibitor was more pronounced in those with more severe proteinuria and those with glomerular disease.[18] Though the ACE inhibitors initially reduced proteinuria, there was a rebound increase in proteinuria on follow-up. In children with Alport syndrome as well, ACE inhibitors are associated with a significant reduction in proteinuria. Though studies in adults have shown a significant effect of proteinuria reduction on the progression of CKD, there are no similar interventional studies in children.
  The RAAS inhibitors are the preferred drugs as they have a significant effect on both proteinuria and hypertension. The disadvantage of ACE inhibitors is hyperkalemia and a 25–30% rise in creatinine that may be seen upon initiation of these medications. β-blockers may also be used as they reduce the sympathetic activity. Metoprolol has been found to have a significant antiproteinuric effect.[7]
- *Control of other risk factors:* Though there is no evidence in children about the effectiveness of controlling other risk factors in reducing the progression of CKD, extrapolation of results from adult studies suggests that measures should be taken to control anemia, metabolic acidosis, dyslipidemia, cardiovascular disease, and hyperuricemia. Unlike adults where a low-protein diet has been found to be beneficial, restricting protein in the diet is not advisable in children with CKD.

Risk factors for progression and prevention of progression of CKD in adults: Progression of CKD, risk factors for progression, and prevention of progression of CKD have been extensively studied in adults. Several patterns of progression of CKD have been identified. The eGFR in adults may show a nonlinear progression, a linear progression, or remain stable over time.

Proteinuria, a modifiable risk factor for CKD, has been found to be the single most important risk factor for progression in diabetic and nondiabetic CKD in adults. Reduction of proteinuria by inhibition of the RAAS has shown to reduce CKD independent of blood pressure control.[19]

Hypertension is another important and modifiable risk factor for progression of CKD. However, the evidence for retarding progression with adequate blood pressure control and the target blood pressure to achieve control of progression of CKD is not well defined.

Genetics and family history are nonmodifiable risk factors for progression of CKD—mutations in apolipoprotein L1 contribute to a significant increase in risk of end-stage kidney disease (ESKD) in people of African origin.[20]

Prediction of progression: Predictive models for rate of progression of CKD such as the kidney failure risk equation have been studied.[21]

A time-centered approach to CKD shows that the time spent by a patient in each stage of CKD is variable, becomes shorter with advancing CKD, and is associated with risk factors such as poorly controlled diabetes, uncontrolled hypertension, and proteinuria. Addressing these risk factors in early stages of CKD provided great benefit in reducing the rate of progression.[22]

CONCLUSION

Chronic kidney disease in children progresses to ESKD over time. The important modifiable risk factors such as proteinuria and hypertension must be identified early and treated appropriately. Regular monitoring of all children with CKD is important to detect and treat the risk factors for progression.

KEY POINTS

- Progression of CKD over time results in ESKD and need for kidney replacement therapy.
- Important nonmodifiable risk factors are etiology of CKD, baseline GFR, and low nephron number.
- Important modifiable risk factors, the control of which has shown to retard progression of CKD, are proteinuria and hypertension.
- Other modifiable risk factors which have a potential role in retarding progression are metabolic acidosis, anemia, dyslipidemia, and preventable causes of AKI, i.e., dehydration, nephrotoxic medications, obstruction, and urinary tract infections.

REFERENCES

1. Harambat J, van Stralen KJ, Kim JJ, Tizard EJ. Epidemiology of chronic kidney disease in children. Pediatr Nephrol. 2012;27:363-73.
2. Staples A, Wong C. Risk factors for progression of chronic kidney disease. Curr Opin Pediatr. 2010;22:161-9.
3. Copelovitch L, Warady BA, Furth SL. Insights from the chronic kidney disease in children (CKiD) study. Clin J Am Soc Nephrol. 2011;6(8):2047-53.
4. Kamath N, Iyengar A, George N, Luyckx VA. Risk factors and rate of progression of CKD in children. Kidney Int Rep. 2019;4(10): 1472-7.
5. Hodgkins KS, Schnaper W. Tubulointerstitial injury and the progression of chronic kidney disease. Pediatr Nephrol. 2012; 27:901-9.
6. Oliveira EA, Mak RH. Progression of chronic kidney disease in children—role of glomerular hemodynamics and interstitial fibrosis. Curr Opin Pediatr. 2018;30(2):220-7.
7. Schaefer B, Wuhl E. Progression in chronic kidney disease and preventive strategies. Eur J Pediatr. 2012;171:1579-88.
8. Wong CS, Pierce CB, Cole SR, Warady BA, Mak RH, Benador NM, et al.; Chronic Kidney Disease in Children (CKiD) investigators. Association of proteinuria with race, cause of chronic kidney disease, and glomerular filtration rate in the chronic kidney disease in children study. Clin J Am Soc Nephrol. 2009;4(4): 812-9.
9. Warady BA, Abraham AG, Schwartz GJ, Wong CS, Muñoz A, Betoko A, et al. Predictors of rapid progression of glomerular and nonglomerular kidney disease in children and adolescents: The chronic kidney disease in children (CKiD) Cohort. Am J Kidney Dis. 2015;65(6):878-88.
10. Fathallah-Shaykh SA. Proteinuria and progression of pediatric chronic kidney disease: lessons from recent clinical studies. Pediatr Nephrol. 2017;32:743-51.
11. Vidi SR. Role of hypertension in progression of chronic kidney disease in children. Curr Opin Pediatr. 2018;30(2):247-51.
12. Harambat J, Kunzmann K, Azukaitis K, Bayazit AK, Canpolat N, Doyon A, et al.; 4C Study Consortium. Metabolic acidosis is common and associates with disease progression in children with chronic kidney disease. Kidney Int. 2017;92(6):1507-14.
13. Saland JM, Kupferman JC, Pierce CB, Flynn JT, Mitsnefes MM, Warady BA, et al. Change in dyslipidemia with declining glomerular filtration rate and increasing proteinuria in children with CKD. Clin J Am Soc Nephrol. 2019;14(12):1711-8.
14. Rodenbach KE, Schneider MF, Furth SL, Moxey-Mims MM, Mitsnefes MM, Weaver DJ, et al. Hyperuricemia and progression of CKD in children and adolescents: The chronic kidney disease in children (CKiD) cohort study. Am J Kidney Dis. 2015;66(6):984-92.
15. Macedo E, Mehta RL. Recurrent acute kidney injury: can we differentiate from nonrecovery and CKD progression? Am J Kidney Dis. 2019;73(2):150-2.
16. Roncal-Jimenez C, Lanaspa MA, Jensen T, Sanchez-Lozada LG, Johnson RJ. Mechanisms by which dehydration may lead to chronic kidney disease. Ann Nutr Metab. 2015;66(suppl 3):10-3.
17. Okoro RN, Farate VT. The use of nephrotoxic drugs in patients with chronic kidney disease. Int J Clin Pharm. 2019;41(3): 767-75.
18. Wühl E, Trivelli A, Picca S, Litwin M, Peco-Antic A, Zurowska A, et al. Strict blood pressure control and renal failure progression in children. The ESCAPE Trial Group. N Engl J Med. 2009;361: 1639-50.
19. Levey AS, de Jong PE, Coresh J, El Nahas M, Astor BC, Matsushita K, et al. The definition, classification, and prognosis of chronic kidney disease: a KDIGO controversies conference report. Kidney Int. 2011;80(1):17-28.
20. Collister D, Ferguson T, Komenda P, Tangri N. The patterns, risk factors, and prediction of progression in chronic kidney disease: a narrative review. Semin Nephrol. 2016;36(4):273-82.
21. Tangri N, Grams ME, Levey AS, Coresh J, Appel LJ, Astor BC, et al. Multinational assessment of accuracy of equations for predicting risk of kidney failure: a meta-analysis. JAMA. 2016;315(2):164-74.
22. Ku E, Johansen KL, McCulloch CE. Time-centered approach to understanding risk factors for the progression of CKD. Clin J Am Soc Nephrol. 2018;13(5):693-701.

CHAPTER

12.5

Kidney Replacement Therapy: Peritoneal Dialysis

Kanav Anand, Nivedita Kamath

INTRODUCTION

Dialysis is initiated in children once the glomerular filtration rate (GFR) falls to <15 mL/min/1.73 m^2 [chronic kidney disease (CKD) stage 5]. In some children, it may be started at an earlier stage in case they develop uremic symptoms, fluid overload, or metabolic abnormalities such as hyperkalemia, metabolic acidosis or hyperphosphatemia and growth failure, which are unresponsive to medical management. Rarely, children with refractory hypertension may also need an early initiation of dialysis. Dialysis also aids in providing space for the nutrition, especially in oliguric infants who are majorly on liquid diet.

CHOICE OF DIALYSIS

Chronic dialysis choices for children include peritoneal dialysis (PD) and hemodialysis (HD). The factors, which determine the choice of modality, are the age, ease of vascular access placement [arteriovenous (AV) fistula/central venous tunneled catheter], proximity to an HD center (travel time), recent or a planned intra-abdominal surgery, family support system, family preference, and cost of dialysis.[1,2] Abdominal defects such as omphalocele, gastroschisis, bladder exstrophy, and diaphragmatic hernia are a few contraindications for the initiation of PD. World over, PD is a preferred modality in younger children because of a number of advantages **(Fig. 1)**. In USA, PD is the most common initial modality of choice for children <9 years of age. A similar trend is seen in Europe too, where 47% of children with end-stage kidney disease (ESKD) are started on PD as compared to 33% with HD.[3]

In this chapter, we discuss the details of chronic PD in children. Chronic HD will be discussed in the next chapter.

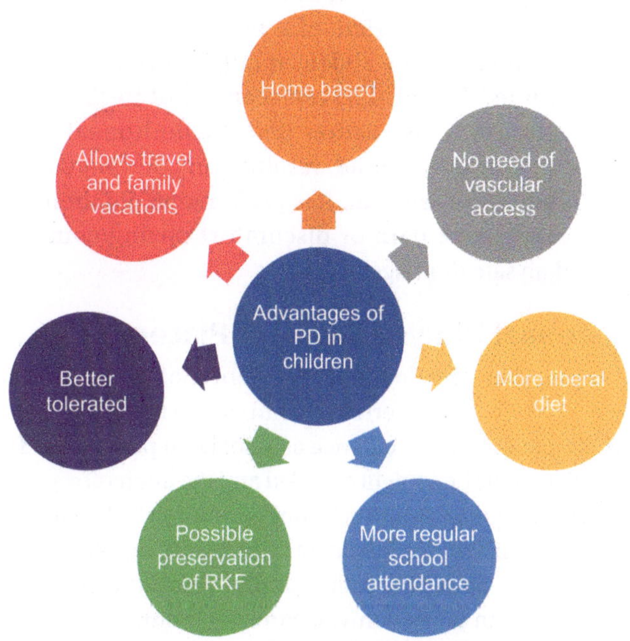

Fig. 1: Advantages of PD in children. (PD: peritoneal dialysis; RKF: residual kidney function)

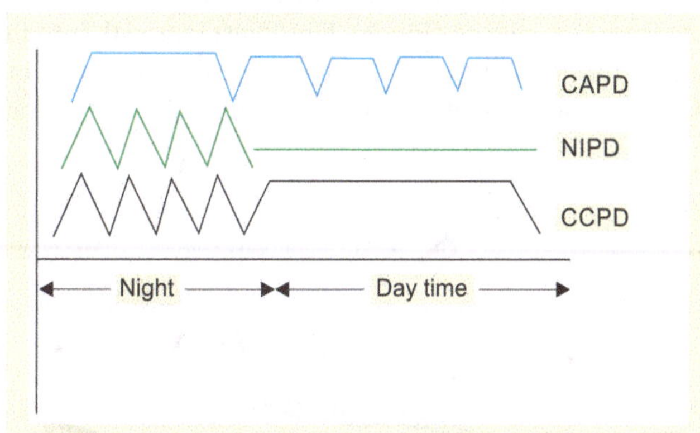

Fig. 2: The various modalities for peritoneal dialysis. (CAPD: continuous ambulatory peritoneal dialysis; CCPD: continuous cycling peritoneal dialysis; NIPD: night intermittent peritoneal dialysis)

PERITONEAL DIALYSIS

Peritoneal dialysis modalities:

The various modalities of PD are described in **Figure 2**.

- *Continuous ambulatory PD (CAPD):* In this manual form of PD, the caregiver attaches and instills a bag of sterile dialysate fluid into the peritoneal cavity through a surgically placed catheter, followed by drainage of the fluid through the same catheter after a stipulated amount of time (dwell time).
- *Automated PD (APD):* This form employs a cycler for doing the PD.[4,5] The advantage of this mode is that multiple exchanges of prewarmed fluid can be done at night with the help of the machine while the child is asleep without taxing the caregiver. This ensures enough free time during

the day so that the child can attend his school. Although a costly mode, it also has an option of remote monitoring which can decrease the patient's hospital visits. APD also has a lower risk of peritonitis.[6] There are three options for performing APD, namely:

1. *Night intermittent PD (NIPD):* Multiple exchanges are undertaken during the night with no dialysis during the day.
2. *Continuous cycling PD (CCPD):* Automated multiple night-time exchanges are followed by a prolonged day time exchange. This is a preferred option for children with very less residual renal function (RRF) as it ensures round-the-clock fluid and solute removal.
3. *Tidal PD (TPD):* Here, after initial infusion of dialysis solution into the abdomen only a partial amount is drained followed by replacement of fresh dialysis solution. This ensures that the peritoneal cavity is never free of fluid, resulting in continuous fluid and solute removal. It is preferred in children who experience pain or discomfort during complete dialysate drainage.[7]

Peritoneal Dialysis Catheter Placement

An appropriate-size double-cuffed Tenckhoff catheter made of silicon rubber is preferred in comparison to the single cuff variant due to lesser incidence of associated peritonitis. The catheter tip may be straight or coiled and the intercuff segment may be straight or swan nick configuration.[8-10] The catheter is surgically placed in the lateral abdominal or paramedian location after an atrial omentectomy. The catheter may be placed by open laparotomy, laparoscopic surgery, or using the Seldinger technique. The distal deep cuff is placed below (preperitoneal space) or within the rectus muscle, and the proximal superficial cuff is placed in the subcutaneous tunnel 2 cm from the exit site **(Fig. 3)**. Fibroblast ingrowth into the Dacron cuff not only helps in anchoring of the catheter but also acts like a seal to prevent leaks and infection. The exit site should be preferably downward or lateral facing, outside the diaper area and away from the colostomy or gastrostomy sites (if present).[8,9] The various sizes of catheters are mentioned in **Table 1**.

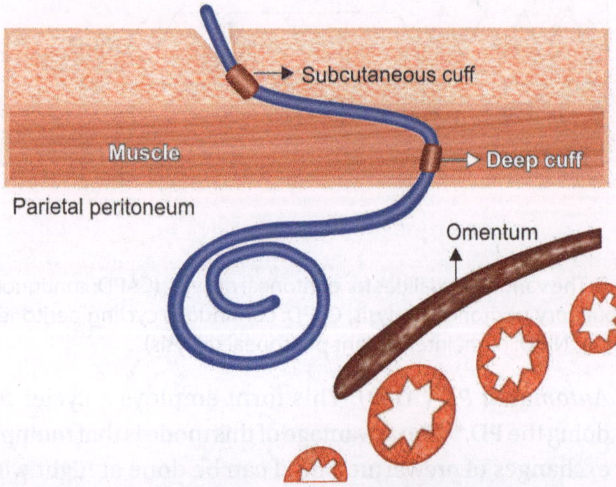

Fig. 3: Schematic diagram to demonstrate the peritoneal dialysis (PD) catheter position intraperitoneally.

The PD catheter is placed in the intraperitoneal space. The deep cuff lies in the abdominal muscle layer and the superficial cuff in the subcutaneous plane. The exit site is 1–2 cm lateral to the subcutaneous cuff.

Peritoneal Dialysis Prescription

- *Peritoneal dialysis solution:* The PD solution consists of water, electrolytes (sodium, calcium, chloride, and magnesium), buffers (acetate/lactate/bicarbonate), and osmotic agents (dextrose—in varying concentrations 1.5%, 2.5%, and 4.25%). Using a solution with increased osmolality enhances the ultrafiltration. More biocompatible, amino acid-based PD fluids are also commercially available. Icodextrin (higher molecular weight glucose polymer) containing fluid is used for long dwells for increasing the ultrafiltration, especially in children with high peritoneal membrane transport capacity.
- *Fill volume:* For manual PD, a fill volume of 900–1,100 mL/m² of body surface area (BSA) (35–45 mL/kg) is targeted, whereas for APD, a fill volume of 1,000–1,200 mL/m² is preferred in children >2 years of age and 600–800 mL/m² in children ≤2 years of age. Too small fill volumes will result in rapid solute equilibrium and inadequate ultrafiltration whereas too large volumes will cause discomfort, hernia, gastroesophageal reflux, and a reduced dialysis efficacy due to an increase in the intraperitoneal pressure resulting in increased lymphatic absorption.[11]
- *Dwell time:* In manual CAPD, the dwell time is kept as 4–6 hours, targeting around four dwells per day. A shorter dwell time of <4 hours may be kept for children who have high solute transport rates. In APD, shorter 1-hour dwell times are selected initially, which later can be modified depending on the goal. A longer dwell results in higher creatinine and phosphate clearance, whereas a shorter one increases the ultrafiltration and urea clearance.

A peritoneal equilibration test (PET) is done 4–8 weeks after initiation of PD to evaluate the transport characteristics of the peritoneal membrane, depending on which the PD prescription is modified to achieve the set goals.

Procedure for the PET: The standardized PET involves instillation of a dwell (1,100 mL/m²) of 2.5% dextrose

TABLE 1: Different sizes of catheters for children.

Tenckhoff catheter size (cm)	*Age group of patients*
31	Infants
37	Children
42	Adolescents
47	Adults

containing fluid overnight. This is drained in the morning and 2.5% fluid is instilled into the abdomen. Dialysate samples are drawn at 0, 2, and 4 hours and serum samples at 2 hours. The dialysate to plasma creatinine ratio (at 0, 2, and 4 hours) is plotted on the chart. The dialysate glucose to baseline glucose (D/D_o) is also plotted. Based on the nomogram curves, the peritoneal membrane characteristics are defined as high, high average, low average, and low transporters.

High transporters have rapid, complete equilibration. They achieve good solute clearance but may have poor ultrafiltration on long dwells. They do better with shorter dwell time. The low transporters in contrast have slow, incomplete equilibration. They usually have poor solute clearance but achieve good ultrafiltration. They require longer dwell time.[11]

Case Vignette 1

A 10-year-old boy with hypodysplastic kidneys is being initiated on chronic ambulatory PD. He weighs 30 kg and has a BSA of 1 m². A swan neck straight tip catheter has been inserted 2 days ago. The urine output in this child is 1 L/day. The blood pressure is 100/60 mm Hg on one antihypertensive drug. He is on erythropoietin, calcium supplements, and sodium bicarbonate supplements. His latest reports show a hemoglobin of 12 g/dL, serum calcium of 9.5 mg/dL, bicarbonate of 21 mEq/L, and serum phosphate of 4.5 mg/dL. When should PD be commenced in this patient? What will be the initial prescription for PD?

Peritoneal dialysis is usually initiated after 2 weeks of insertion of the PD catheter to allow complete healing of the exit site and tunnel. During this time, most centers avoid flushes, do a dressing of the exit site between 3 and 7 days, and thereafter only if there is soiling of leak. Earlier initiation could be considered in patients with fluid overload, uremic symptoms, or metabolic complications.

A PD prescription consists of the following components:

- *PD solution:* It is preferable to use a physiological PD solution of the lowest dextrose concentration. As bicarbonate-based fluids are not universally available, lactate-based solution with 1.5% dextrose is used.
- *Dwell volume:* The ideal dwell volume is 1,000–1,200 mL/m². In this child, this would amount to about 1 liter of dwell volume. While initiating PD, it is recommended to start lower fill volumes around 20 mL/kg and increase slowly over a few days to optimal dwell volume.
- *Dwell time:* A typical CAPD prescription consists of four dwells of 4 hours each with an overnight dwell. This may be modified based on the fluid status/ultrafiltration volume, RRF, and metabolic parameters.
- *Others:* Most centers prefer to add heparin to the dialysis solution. About 500–1,000 IU of unfractionated heparin can be added per liter of PD solution.

Modifications to the prescription: The PD prescription must be tailored to meet the needs of the child. If the ultrafiltration is not achieved, shorter dwells and higher dextrose concentration may be used. If clearance of urea and creatinine is suboptimal, the dwell time may need to be modified according to the transporter status of the patient.

Complications of Peritoneal Dialysis

- *Infectious complications:*
  - *Peritonitis:* It is the most common complication of PD resulting in morbidity and peritoneal membrane function loss.[12] Its rate is inversely proportional to the age of the patient. The annualized rate is 0.79 in children <1 year of age as compared to 0.57 in >12 years of age.[8] The most common manifestations of peritonitis are abdominal pain and turbid peritoneal effluent. Effluent fluid cell count, Gram stain, fungal stain, and culture aid to the diagnosis. If the cell count is >100 cells/mm³ with >50% neutrophils, it is strongly suggestive of peritonitis in a symptomatic child. Culture always remains the gold standard. Details of the treatment strategy are shown in **Figure 3** and **Flowcharts 1 and 2.**[13] Heparin in the dose of 500–1000 IU/L may be added to the PD fluid in order to prevent catheter blockage due to fibrin strands. The algorithms for management of infections are discussed in **Flowcharts 1 to 3.** The management of a child with peritonitis is discussed in the case vignette 1.
  - *Exit site and tunnel infections:* It is a significant cause of peritonitis in children on PD.[14-16] Simple aseptic care of the exit site like regular assessment and cleaning of the exit site with antiseptic and later applying antibiotic ointment like mupirocin shall not only reduce the incidence of exit site infections but also prolong the catheter life. An exit site scoring system has been elaborated in the International Society for Peritoneal

Flowchart 1: Initial management of peritonitis.

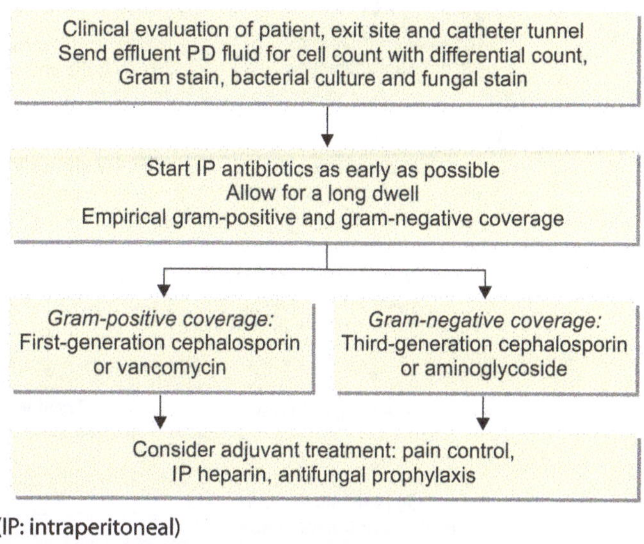

(IP: intraperitoneal)

Source: Adapted from Li PK, Szeto CC, Piraino B, de Arteaga J, Fan S, Figueiredo AE, et al. ISPD Peritonitis Recommendations: 2016 Update on Prevention and Treatment. Perit Dial Int. 2016;36(5):481-508.

Flowchart 2: Management algorithm for gram-positive cocci identified in dialysis effluent.

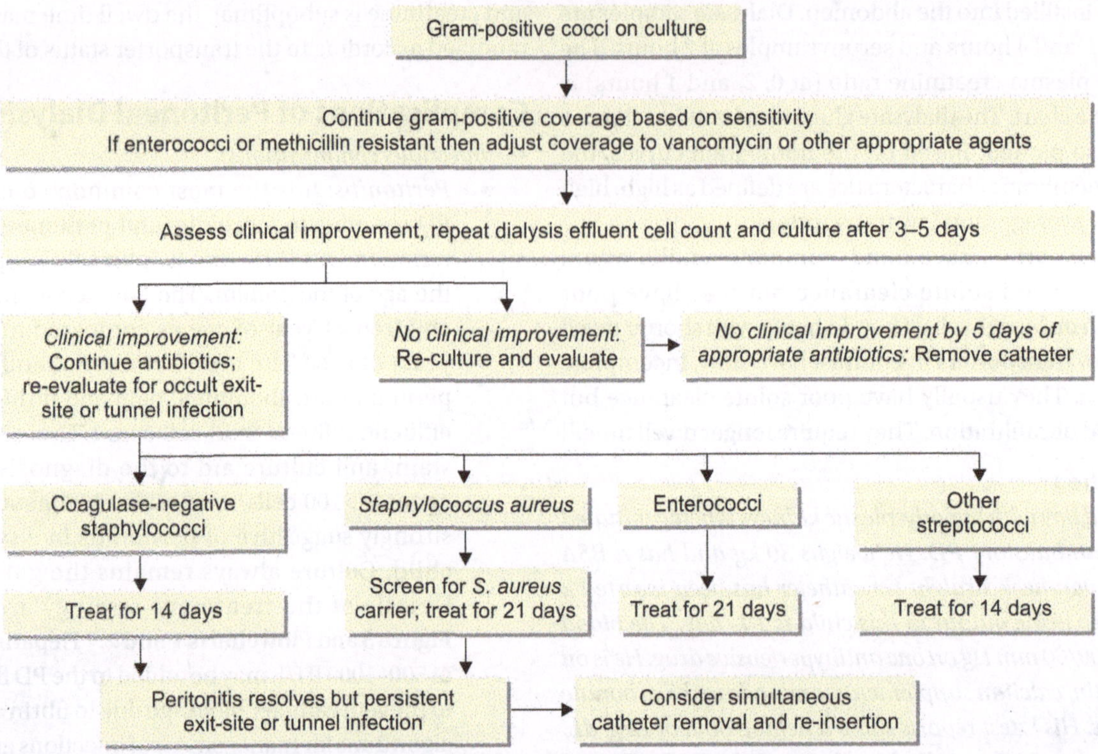

Source: Adapted from Li PK, Szeto CC, Piraino B, de Arteaga J, Fan S, Figueiredo AE, et al. ISPD Peritonitis Recommendations: 2016 Update on Prevention and Treatment. Perit Dial Int. 2016;36(5):481-508.

Flowchart 3: Management algorithm for gram-negative bacilli or mixed bacterial growth identified in dialysis effluent.

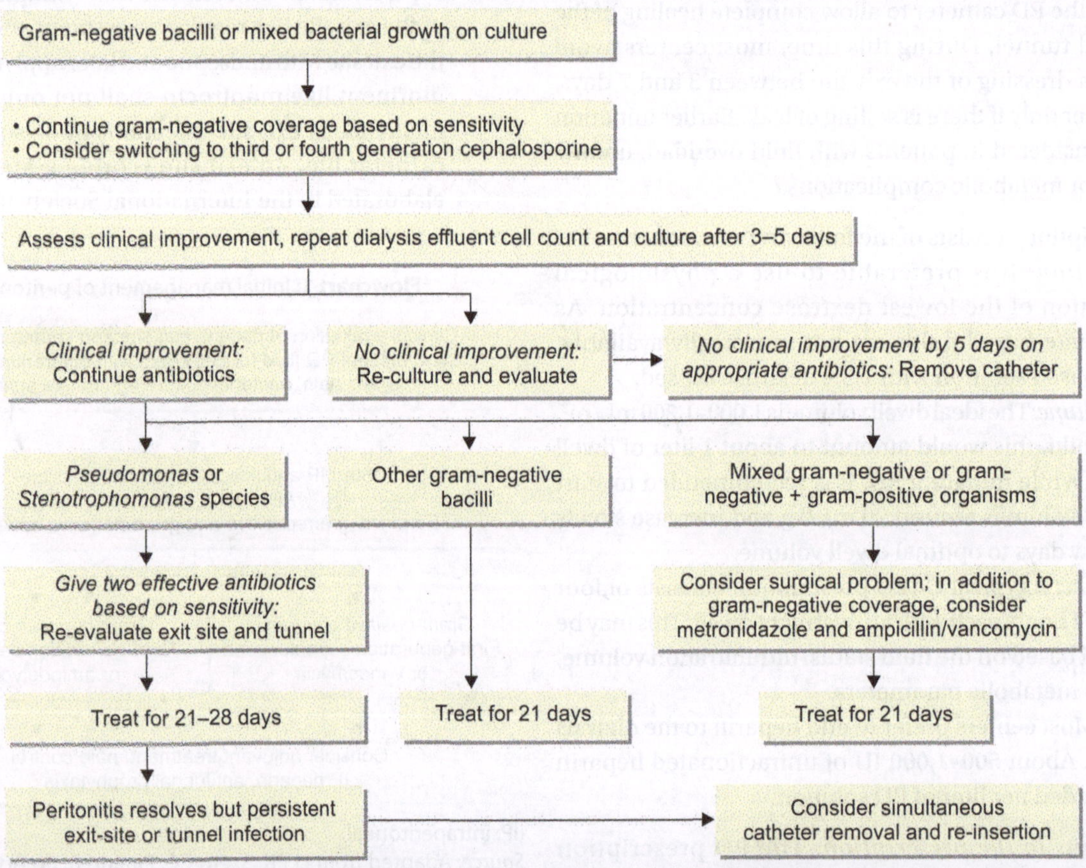

Source: Adapted from Li PK, Szeto CC, Piraino B, de Arteaga J, Fan S, Figueiredo AE, et al. ISPD Peritonitis Recommendations: 2016 Update on Prevention and Treatment. Perit Dial Int. 2016;36(5):481-508.

Dialysis (ISPD) guidelines which could be used to assess the severity of infection.[17]

Case Vignette 2

A 9-year-old girl with ESKD secondary to focal segmental glomerulosclerosis (FSGS) is on PD since the last 6 months. She is brough to the hospital with complaints of turbid fluid and abdominal pain. How will you manage this child with suspected peritonitis? What are the measures to prevent peritonitis in children on PD?

The diagnosis of peritonitis is made by the presence of two of the following:[13]

- Clinical features consistent with peritonitis
- >100 cells/mm^3 with >50% in the PD fluid effluent
- Positive culture.

The sample should be collected after an adequate dwell in the peritoneal cavity. At least 5–10 mL should be inoculated into blood culture or Bactec bottles.

The initial treatment of peritonitis involves the use of a broad-spectrum antibiotic. The ISPD guidelines recommend the use of either cefepime or a combination of a first-generation cephalosporin or vancomycin for gram-positive organisms and third-generation cephalosporin or aminoglycoside for gram-negative organisms. The route of administration is preferably intraperitoneal. Intraperitoneal antibiotics are given as continuous dosing or intermittent dosing. Intravenous antibiotics are recommended in children with systemic features of infection including sepsis.

Depending on the culture and sensitivity reports, antibiotics may be changed. Peritonitis by gram-positive organisms and culture-negative peritonitis are treated with antibiotics for 2 weeks. Peritonitis by gram-negative organisms and some gram-positive organisms such as *Staphylococcus aureus* and enterococci requires antibiotics for 3 weeks.

In addition to antibiotics, supportive therapy is required. Generally, the PD prescription is modified to perform cycles of shorter dwell time as the inflamed peritoneum may behave like a high transporter. Temporarily, the use of hypertonic dextrose solutions may be required to achieve adequate ultrafiltration. Heparin should be added to the PD fluid to prevent fibrin formation and catheter block. Pain relief may be required in the first few days of treatment. Fungal prophylaxis is recommended in all patients to prevent fugal peritonitis.[13]

It is important to understand the risk factors for peritonitis. Screening and treatment for nasal carriage in caregivers and patient are important. Risk factors such as constipation, breach in technique, and touch contamination require appropriate redressal.

Terminologies used in peritonitis:

- *Refractory peritonitis:* Failure of the effluent to clear after 5 days of appropriate therapy
- *Recurrent peritonitis:* Peritonitis that occurs within 4 weeks of treatment of an episode of infection but by a different organism
- *Relapsing peritonitis:* Peritonitis that occurs within 4 weeks of treatment of an episode of infection by the same organism
- *Repeat peritonitis:* Peritonitis that occurs after 4 weeks of treatment of an episode by the same organism.

Indications for catheter removal:[13]

- Refractory peritonitis
- Relapsing peritonitis
- Refractory exit site or tunnel infection
- Fungal peritonitis
- May be considered in repeat peritonitis and mycobacterial infection.

Prevention of peritonitis:[13] Prevention of peritonitis is an important goal in children on PD. There are several methods to be considered for prevention of peritonitis.

- Prophylactic antibiotic prior to catheter insertion
- Prophylactic antibiotics prior to invasive procedures such as coloscopy
- Detection of nasal carriage of *S. aureus* and treatment with mupirocin
- Use of Y connector, flush before fill technique
- Training—by trained nurse, end of training assessment, and retraining at periodic intervals and after episodes of peritonitis, home visits
- Prompt treatment of exit site and tunnel infection
- Fungal prophylaxis during treatment of peritonitis.

The Standardizing Care to Improve Outcomes in Pediatric Endstage Kidney Disease (SCOPE) collaborative introduced bundles of care for catheter insertion, training and follow-up care and found that adherence to these bundles reduced the rate of infection.[9]

Noninfectious Complications

- *Mechanical complications:* These result due to increased intraperitoneal pressure causing hernia (incisional, umbilical, and inguinal), pericatheter fluid leaks, and rarely hydrothorax.[18]
- *Technique-related complications:* Ultrafiltration failure (UFF) may result due to high peritoneal membrane solute transport capacity, aquaporin deficiency, repeated peritonitis episodes, iatrogenic small fill volumes, or encapsulating sclerosing peritonitis.[19]
- *Catheter-related complications:* Pericatheter leakage, catheter migration, superficial cuff extrusion at the exit site, and catheter outflow occlusion due to omental or intra-abdominal structure adhesions.[20,21]
- *Others:*
    - *Hemoperitoneum:* It is usually seen in the immediate postoperative period after insertion of the PD catheter. The catheter must be flushed with heparinized PD solution to prevent catheter block.
    - *Pain:* It can be due to peritonitis, overdistension of peritoneal cavity with fluid or irritation of the

peritoneum by the catheter or a cold jet of dialysis fluid. Rarely, malposition of catheter and introduction of air during the process of dialysis can also trigger abdominal pain.

- *Peritoneal membrane dysfunction and UFF:* UFF is defined as signs of fluid overload along with the inability to achieve ultrafiltration >400 mL with a modified PET (using 4.25%) after excluding catheter malfunction and leaks. Ultrafiltration failure is categorized into four types based on the peritoneal membrane characteristics. Type 1 UFF could be managed with hypertonic dextrose concentration. The other types of UFF are more difficult to manage.
- *Encapsulating peritoneal sclerosis:* It results from prolonged periods of PD, especially with hypertonic dialysis solutions. Recurrent peritonitis episodes can also result in this dreaded complication which leads to progressive loss in ultrafiltration capacity.[22]
- *Nutritional and metabolic issues:* Malnutrition can result from continuous protein loss in the dialysate. Dyselectrolytemias, especially hyponatremia and hypokalemia, are very common.

Management of Complications of End-stage Kidney Disease in Children on Peritoneal Dialysis

Anemia in Dialysis

Anemia in children on chronic PD can be multifactorial with the most common cause being decreased erythropoietin production by the failing kidneys. Other causes include concomitant iron and vitamin deficiencies, hyperparathyroidism, occult blood loss, chronic inflammation, rarely myelofibrosis, and pure red cell aplasia. The mainstay of treatment includes iron and vitamin (B_{12} and folic acid) supplementation. Erythropoietin-stimulating agents (ESAs) may be added to prevent Hb to fall below 9 g/dL. Keeping Hb level between 11 and 12 g/dL helps in improving the quality of life, decreases the load on the heart, decreases the risk of mortality, and alleviates the need for regular blood transfusions, thus preventing human leukocyte antigen (HLA) sensitization complicating the renal transplantation procedure in future.

Chronic Kidney Disease–Mineral Bone Disorder (CKD–MBD) in Dialysis

All patients on chronic dialysis should be monitored for evidence of bone disease either clinically, radiologically, or biochemically [serum calcium, phosphorus, alkaline phosphatase, bicarbonate, intact parathyroid hormone (PTH), and 25(OH)D3 levels]. Children need cholecalciferol supplementation if the level of 25(OH)D3 is <30 ng/mL. Adequate dietary calcium supplementation should be encouraged but ensuring that the total calcium intake from various sources (including calcium containing phosphate binders) should be within 100–200% of recommended dietary allowance (RDA). Nutritional phosphorus intake should be restricted to 100% of RDA in normophosphatemic dialysis patients and to 80% in hyperphosphatemic ones. Phosphate binders (calcium or noncalcium containing) may be started in patients with overtly high serum phosphate levels. PTH levels are targeted between 100 and 300 pg/mL as a lower value increases the chance of hypercalcemia and higher level increases the incidence of bone disease, thus affecting the linear growth. Supplementation of calcitriol and optimization of serum calcium and phosphorus levels help in achieving the target. Rarely, cinacalcet and subtotal parathyroidectomy may be employed for resistant cases.

Cardiovascular Health in Dialysis

Structural and functional abnormalities of the heart are more common in CKD patients on dialysis as compared to the ones not on dialysis. Uncontrolled hypertension in these children leads to left ventricular hypertrophy (LVH). Associated CKD-MBD increases the risk of LVH many folds due to induction of myocardial fibrosis. Regular blood pressure monitoring (manually as well as ambulatory blood pressure monitoring) should be undertaken so as to diagnose hypertension and to monitor the efficacy of the antihypertensive drugs. The mean 24 hours blood pressure should be maintained below the 95 percentile for the age, sex, and height of the child along with a physiological nocturnal pressure dip. Antihypertensive medications that need dose modification in children on dialysis, based on their dialysable property, are described in the last section of this book.

Adequacy of Peritoneal Dialysis

Peritoneal dialysis (PD) is an important modality of chronic dialysis in children.

Adequate treatment with PD is important to ensure the well-being of the child and reduce the risk of complications. Efficacy of small solute clearance is recommended for assessing the adequacy of dialysis. However, other parameters such as maintenance of normal volume status, acceptable levels of metabolic parameters, adequate control of anemia and metabolic acidosis, and normal growth and nutrition in a child are important parameters. Removal of middle molecules also has a significant bearing on long-term outcomes. Maintenance of the RRF is also an important goal in children on PD.[23,24]

Measurement of Adequacy of Peritoneal Dialysis

The conventional assessment of small solute clearance is done by measuring the peritoneal and renal clearance of small solutes such as urea and creatinine.

Measurement of PD adequacy using clearance of small solutes:[25]

Clearance of PD is measured as both *Kt/V* urea and creatinine clearance (CrCl/1.73 m^2). The measurement of clearance includes a peritoneal component and a renal component (in children with RRF).

Measurement of Kt/V:

$$Kt/V = \text{Peritoneal } Kt/V + \text{Renal } Kt/V$$

$$\text{Peritoneal } Kt/V = \frac{\text{24-hour dialysate urea nitrogen content}}{\text{Serum urea nitrogen}}$$

$$\text{Renal } Kt/V = \frac{\text{24-hour urine urea nitrogen}}{\text{Serum urea nitrogen}}$$

- *Calculation of V:* The KDOQI guidelines recommend the use of Mellits–Cheek formula for estimation of total body water:
  - Boys TBW (for height < 132.7 cm) = (–1.927) + 0.465 × weight + 0.045 × height
  - Boys TBW (for height > 132.7 cm) = (–21.993) + 0.406 × weight + 0.209 × height
  - Girls TBW (for height < 110.8 cm) = 0.076 + 0.507 × weight + 0.013 × height
  - Girls TBW (for height > 110.8 cm) = (–10.313) + 0.252 × weight + 0.154 × height
- Calculation of body surface area—using the Dubois/Mosteller formula

Creatinine clearance (CrCl):

$$\text{Total CrCl} = \text{Peritoneal CrCl} + \text{Renal CrCl (corrected for 1.73 m}^2\text{ BSA)}$$

$$\text{Peritoneal CrCl} = \frac{\text{24-hour dialysate creatinine}}{\text{Serum creatinine}}$$

Renal creatinine clearance

$$= \frac{0.5\,(\text{24-hour urine creatinine}}{\text{Serum creatinine}} + \frac{\text{24-hour urine urea nitrogen})}{\text{Serum urea nitrogen}}$$

For the measurement of *Kt/V*, the 24-hour dialysate will have to be sent to the laboratory for estimation of dialysate urea nitrogen and dialysate creatinine. The timing of measurement of serum urea nitrogen and creatinine in children on CAPD is not critical as it is relatively constant. However, in children on APD, the ideal time of measurement is in the middle of the noncycling duration. The daily *Kt/V* urea measured is multiplied by 7 to derive the weekly *Kt/V* value.

The CrCl is an average of the urinary urea and creatinine clearances as the creatinine clearance alone overestimates the true glomerular filtration rate. The daily total clearance is multiplied by 7 to derive the weekly CrCl. The high glucose level in the dialysate may erroneously elevate the measurement of creatinine when Jaffe's method is used to estimate creatinine. Every laboratory should derive its own correction factor for creatinine.

Determinants of clearance:

- *RRF:* It is well preserved in children on PD.
- *Peritoneal transport characteristics:* Low transporters have poor clearance of small solutes and do better with longer dwell time.
- *PD prescription:* The common measures used to achieve optimal clearance in children on PD are:
  - Optimize the dwell volume
  - Increase the number of cycles
  - Addition of a day dwell in children on APD.

Guideline recommendations for Kt/V: The KDOQI guidelines of 1997 recommended *Kt/V* > 2 based on cohort studies and the CANUSA study which predicted a better survival with high clearance. However, the ADEMEX and the Hong Kong study showed no significant difference with a lower clearance target. The benefit of higher *Kt/V* was attributed to the clearance achieved by the RRF. There is sufficient evidence to suggest that a *Kt/V* of <1.7 is associated with poor outcomes. Hence, the updated KDOQI guidelines (2006) recommend that the minimum total *Kt/V* target should be >1.7/week both in adults and in children. Routine measurement of the creatinine clearance for estimation of adequacy is not required.[26]

The KDOQI recommends the measurement of *Kt/V* within a month of initiating PD and every 4 months thereafter. Clearance should be assessed after every significant change in the PD prescription or patient's clinical status. Monitoring the nutritional status with markers such as serum albumin, nPNA (normalized protein equivalent of total nitrogen appearance) is recommended.

Fallacies of using Kt/V as a marker of adequacy of dialysis: In children, there are few studies on the correlation of *Kt/V* urea with long-term outcomes such as mortality. The optimum *Kt/V* in children on PD is extrapolated from studies in adults. Hence, the *Kt/V* recommended by the guidelines must be considered as a minimum standard to be achieved rather than as a marker of optimum PD.

Children, especially the younger children, have a larger total body water and the urea distribution based on total body water would imply that children require a lower dialysis dose to achieve the same *Kt/V* target. Since children have a higher metabolic rate and protein intake, it would be preferable to normalize the *Kt* to BSA.[27]

Irrespective of the *Kt/V*, the dose of dialysis may need to be increased if the child has clinical features of uremia, fluid overload, uncontrolled hypertension, hyperphosphatemia, or hyperkalemia.[26] *Kt/V* does not offer any information on middle molecule clearance. Hence, *Kt/V* urea is only a small component of assessment of dialysis adequacy.

Assessment of adequacy: Beyond small solute clearance: Due to the limitations of small solute clearance as an indicator of dialysis adequacy, several other markers have been studied. Some of these are peritoneal albumin clearance, protein equivalent of nitrogen appearance, sodium removal, and glucose absorption.

Preserving Residual Renal Function

Residual renal function (RRF) is defined as the ability of the native kidneys to eliminate water and uremic toxins. In clinical practice, the KDOQI guideline mentions RRF as urinary *Kt/V* urea of at least 0.1/week.

Residual renal function is better preserved in PD than in those on HD. RRF contributes significantly to the total clearance in patients on PD. Large studies such as the CANUSA and NECOSAD showed that the decline in RRF was significantly associated with an increase in mortality. The RRF contributes significantly to achieving good fluid control and clearance of middle molecules.[23] Preservation of RRF is also associated with a reduction in blood pressure, LVH, better clearance of middle molecules, better control of phosphate and acidosis, and improved quality of life.[28] Similar benefits have also been demonstrated in various studies in children. Improvement in nutrition and growth have also been demonstrated in children with adequate dialysis.[29]

Residual renal function is better preserved in patients on PD in comparison to HD. Avoiding nephrotoxic medications, prompt and adequate treatment of dehydration, and avoiding intradialytic hypotension are important aspects of preserving RRF. Prompt treatment of urinary tract infections is important for preservation of RRF. Though there is little evidence to support its use in children, diuretics may be used to maximize salt and water excretion. Use of angiotensin-converting enzyme inhibitors and biocompatible dialysate such as icodextrin has shown some promise in preserving RRF.[28]

Nutrition in Dialysis

Undernutrition is prevalent in children with CKD and those on dialysis. In contrast to malnutrition which is predominantly due to an inadequate nutritional intake, protein energy wasting is used to denote the state of decreased body protein mass and energy and is multifactorial in etiology.[30] Hence, protein energy wasting is a maladaptive response in CKD and is associated with an increased metabolic rate and low serum albumin levels.

Risk factors for protein energy wasting in ESKD:[30]

- *Hormonal imbalance:* Uremia results in a reduction in orexogenic hormones (acyl ghrelin) and increase in anorexogenic hormones (desacyl ghrelin, obestatin, and leptin) due to reduced renal clearance.
- *Decreased nutritional intake:* In addition to the reduced appetite caused by hormonal imbalance, several other factors influence nutritional intake. Studies have shown that the nutritional intake correlated significantly with the GFR. However, poor nutritional intake is seen even in early stages of CKD. Altered taste, nausea, and vomiting frequently seen in children are important factors influencing nutritional intake. Gastroesophageal reflux is a common problem in children with CKD.
- *RRF and dialysis adequacy:* Children with RRF have been found to have a significantly higher normalized protein catabolic rate (nPCR). In children on HD as well as in those on PD, the dialysis dose and clearance have been associated with better growth.
- *Inflammation:* Studies in adults have shown that inflammation is prevalent in CKD and is significantly associated with malnutrition resulting in the malnutrition-inflammation-atherosclerosis syndrome. Dialysis has been associated with higher inflammation when compared to nondialysis CKD.
- *Metabolic acidosis:* Metabolic acidosis has been associated with muscle wasting and low serum albumin.
- *Age at onset of CKD:* Growth in the first 2 years of life is rapid and is predominantly based on the nutritional status. Early onset CKD is associated with significant deficit in growth parameters. The deficit in growth is more in children with CKD who had low birth weight.
- *Other risk factors:* Other factors such as severe proteinuria, dialysis vintage, psychosocial problems, medications such as steroids, and presence of comorbidities are also determinants of nutritional status.

Assessment of the Nutritional Status

The assessment begins with history of appetite, symptoms such as nausea, vomiting, and constipation. Examination should focus on signs of malnutrition in the child.

- *Dietary assessment:* Dietary assessment is done by using a 3-day dietary diary or 3–24-hour dietary recalls (in older children). The intake of calories (carbohydrates and fats), proteins, vitamins, and minerals is calculated.[30,31]
- *Anthropometric parameters:* The recommended anthropometric parameters are—
  - Height/length for age percentile or standard deviation score (SDS)
  - Height/length velocity for age percentile or SDS
  - Weight for age percentile or SDS
  - BMI for height age percentile or SDS.

In children <3 years of age, head circumference for age percentile should be measured. In adolescents on HD, nPCR is suggested. Mid arm muscle circumference and skin fold thickness are not recommended as reliable measures of nutritional status in children with CKD.

Biochemical parameters: Though several biochemical parameters have been evaluated in studies, only serum creatinine and albumin have been used in clinical practice.

Other markers: Body composition monitoring using bioimpedance analysis and dual-energy X-ray absorptiometry have also been used in various studies but not translated into clinical practice.

nPCR (normalized protein catabolic rate): Protein catabolic rate is a measure of protein catabolism and can be calculated from nitrogen mass balance studies which are difficult to do in routine clinical practice. nPCR can be calculated by the urea generation rate measured by urea kinetic modeling in children on HD.[32]

The pediatric renal nutrition task force guidelines reiterate the KDOQI guidelines for assessment of nutritional status in children with CKD. In addition, they recommend the use of WHO growth chart for monitoring weight and height. They suggest assessing the growth potential using the mid-parental height.

The dietary assessment is done using a 3-day diet history or a 24-hour dietary recall.[33]

Management of Nutrition

- *Energy requirement:* The pediatric renal nutrition task force (PRNT) guidelines[34] endorse the KDOQI 2009 guidelines[31] which recommend that energy intake equal to the estimated energy requirement for age and further changes are made based on the weight gain.
- *Protein requirement:* The target protein intake should be at the upper end of the suggested dietary intake (SDI) for age. The protein intake in children on dialysis should be higher to account for dialytic protein losses. The KDOQI guidelines recommend a dietary protein intake, which is 100% of daily recommended intake (DRI) for ideal body weight plus an allowance of 0.15–0.3 g/kg in patients on PD and 0.1 g/kg in patients on HD.[31] The protein loss on PD is higher in younger children and infants. Protein losses are higher in high transporters and during an episode of peritonitis. The energy and protein requirements for children with CKD stages 2–5 is given in **Table 2**.
- In children on intensified HD of hemofiltration, dietary restrictions are minimal as these modalities allow good fluid and metabolic control.[34]
- *Calcium and phosphate requirement:* The assessment of calcium and phosphate in the diet can be done by a 3-day dietary intake assessment including supplements, dialysate, and medications including phosphate binders. The total calcium intake from diet and binders should be within the SDI and not exceed more than twice the SDI. The dietary phosphate intake should be within the SDI for age without compromising on the protein intake, especially in children with hyperphosphatemia.[35] The recommended calcium and phosphate requirements in children with CKD stages 2–5 are given in **Table 3**.
- *Vitamin and minerals:* The KDOQI guidelines recommend provision of at least 100% of DRI for B complex vitamins, vitamin E, C, K, folic acid, copper and zinc through the diet or through supplementation. Children on dialysis should receive water-soluble supplements.[31]
- *Vitamin D:* The PRNT guidelines recommend that the vitamin D levels be monitored at regular intervals and maintained at a level >75 nmol/L (30 ng/mL). Either vitamin D_2 or D_3 can be used and the regimen is based on the age and baseline vitamin D status of the child.[36]
- *Fluids and electrolytes:* Fluids are generally restricted in children on dialysis, especially in those with poor RRF. However, in children with polyuria, fluid supplementation may be required. Sodium supplementation should be considered in infants on PD as they have sodium losses in the dialysate.

TABLE 2: The energy and protein requirements for children with CKD stages 2–5 from birth to 18 years

SDI for energy and protein: birth to 18 years				
Month	***SDI energy (kcal/kg/day)***	***SDI protein (g/kg/day)***	***SDI protein (g/day)***	
0	93–107	1.52–2.5	8–12	
1	93–120	1.52–1.8	8–12	
2	93–120	1.4–1.52	8–12	
3	82–98	1.4–1.52	8–12	
4	82–98	1.3–1.52	9–13	
5	72–82	1.3–1.52	9–13	
6-9	72–82	1.1–1.3	9–14	
10–11	72–82	1.1–1.3	9–14	
12	72–120	0.9–1.14	11–14	
Year	***SDI energy (kcal/kg/day)***		***SDI protein (g/kg/day)***	***SDI protein (g/day)***
–	*Male*	*Female*		
2	81–95	79–92	0.9–1.05	11–15
3	80–82	76–77	0.9–1.05	13–15
4–6	67–93	64–90	0.85–0.95	16–22
7–8	60–77	56–75	0.9–0.95	19–28
9–10	55–69	49–63	0.9–0.95	26–40
11–12	48–63	43–57	0.9–0.95	34–42
13–14	44–63	39–50	0.8–0.9	34–50
15–17	40–55	36–46	0.8–0.9	Male: 52–65 Female: 45–49

Source: Adapted from Shaw V, Polderman N, Renken-Terhaerdt J, Paglialonga F, Oosterveld M, Tuokkola J, et al. Energy and protein requirements for children with CKD stages 2–5 and on dialysis-clinical practice recommendations from the Pediatric Renal Nutrition Taskforce. Pediatr Nephrol. 2020;35(3):519-31.

TABLE 3: Calcium and phosphate requirements in children with CKD stages 2–5

Age (years)	***SDI calcium (mg)***	***SDI phosphate (mg)***
0–<4 months	220	120
4–<12 months	330–540	275–420
1–3 years	450–700	250–500
4–10 years	700–1000	440–800
11–17 years	900–1300	640–1250

Source: Adapted from McAlister L, Pugh P, Greenbaum L, Haffner D, Rees L, Anderson C, et al. The dietary management of calcium and phosphate in children with CKD stages 2–5 and on dialysis-clinical practice recommendation from the Pediatric Renal Nutrition Taskforce. Pediatr Nephrol. 2020;35(3):501-18.

Feeding Practices

Breastfeeding is preferred in infants. When breastfeeding is not adequate, whey-based formula may be added. Both breast milk and formula may require to be fortified to provide the required calories and proteins. Solid food is added as part of the complementary feeding. Oral feeding is the preferred route for providing nutrition to infants and children. Supplemental enteral tube feeding is recommended in children who are unable to meet their nutritional requirements through oral feeding.

In children on PD, the presence of dialysate in the abdominal cavity may give a feeling of fullness and also be associated with a greater risk of gastroesophageal reflux. To mitigate this, continuous feeding may be required to reduce the volume of feed and increase the caloric density.

Enteral feeding: Enteral feeding may be supplemental or exclusive and is recommended in children who are unable to meet the nutritional requirements by oral feeding.

A nasogastric tube may be used as a short-term enteral feeding device, whereas a gastrostomy is the ideal long-term feeding device. Gastrostomy may be placed as a percutaneous endoscopic gastrostomy, radiologically inserted, open surgical or laparoscopic-assisted gastrostomy. In patients who are already on PD, an open gastrostomy or a laparoscopic procedure is recommended. Children who are likely to require PD may have the gastrostomy tube inserted percutaneously or radiologically, preferably before the insertion of the PD catheter. Broad-spectrum antibiotic prophylaxis and fungal prophylaxis must be given to all children on PD who undergo a gastrostomy. PD should be withheld for at least 24 hours after the gastrostomy placement if possible. Care of the exit site of the gastrostomy and PD catheter must be followed strictly to avoid infections.[37]

Special Aspects of Nutrition in Children on Dialysis

Children on dialysis may have higher protein losses and require an additional allowance of proteins. In those on PD, low transporter status ensures minimal loss of proteins and other essential nutrients. However, poor clearance of urea and creatinine may be associated with a lower appetite. High transporter status is associated with higher loss of protein and other essential nutrients. Children on thrice-weekly HD as well as those with low RRF require tight fluid control and this may hamper the provision of adequate nutrition, especially in infants who receive most of their nutrition in the form of fluids.[38]

Dialysate content of calcium should be included in the calculation of calcium intake and modified according to the serum calcium levels.

Intradialytic parenteral nutrition has been tried in children on HD by providing proteins and calories during HD. The carbohydrates provided prevent protein catabolism. This has been found to be useful in improving the nutritional status in a few pediatric studies.[32]

CONCLUSION

Dialysis is indicated in children with kidney failure (CKD stage 5) with clinical symptoms of uremia or metabolic and fluid-related complications. PD in children is a safe and effective modality of dialysis for children and infants. Peritonitis is an important complication that has a bearing on morbidity and mortality.

KEY POINTS

- Chronic PD is the modality of choice for kidney replacement therapy in children with end-stage kidney disease.
- Continuous ambulatory PD and APD are the important modalities of dialysis in children.
- The PD prescription should be tailored to the body size and metabolic profile of the child.
- Peritonitis is an important complication of PD which influences the technique survival.
- Adequacy of PD should include not just the Kt/V but also growth, nutrition, control of blood pressure, metabolic parameters, control of anemia, and mineral bone disease.
- Nutrition is an important aspect in the management of children with end-stage kidney disease.
- The KDIGO and PNRT guidelines emphasize on the need for adequate energy and protein intake provision of necessary vitamins and minerals in children with CKD.

REFERENCES

1. Sadowski RH, Harmon WE, Jabs K. Acute hemodialysis of infants weighing less than five kilograms. Kidney Int. 1994;45:903.
2. Carey WA, Talley LI, Sehring SA, Jaskula JM, Mathias RS. Outcomes of dialysis initiated during the neonatal period for treatment of end-stage renal disease: a North American Pediatric Renal Trials and Collaborative Studies special analysis. Pediatrics. 2007;119:e468.
3. Harambat J, Bonthuis M, Groothoff JW, Schaefer F, Tizard EJ, Verrina E, et al. Lessons learned from the ESPN/ERA-EDTA Registry. Pediatr Nephrol. 2016;31:2055.
4. Verrina E, Cappelli V, Perfumo F. Selection of modalities, prescription, and technical issues in children on peritoneal dialysis. Pediatr Nephrol. 2009;24:1453.
5. Fischbach M, Warady BA. Peritoneal dialysis prescription in children: bedside principles for optimal practice. Pediatr Nephrol. 2009;24:1633.
6. North American Pediatric Renal Trials and Cooperative Studies (NAPRTCS). 2008 Annual Report. Rockville: EMMES Corporation; 2008.
7. Hölttä T, Rönnholm K, Holmberg C. Adequacy of dialysis with tidal and continuous cycling peritoneal dialysis in children. Nephrol Dial Transplant. 2000;15:1438.
8. North American Pediatric Renal Trials and Collaborative Studies. (2011). NAPRTCS 2011 Annual Report: renal transplantation, dialysis, chronic renal insufficiency. [online] Available from: www.emmes.com/study/ped/annlrept/annualrept2011.pdf. [Last accessed March, 2022].
9. Sethna CB, Bryant K, Munshi R, Warady BA, Richardson T, Lawlor J, et al. Risk factors for and outcomes of catheter-associated peritonitis in children: the SCOPE Collaborative. Clin J Am Soc Nephrol. 2016;11:1590.
10. Crabtree JH, Shrestha BM, Chow KM, Figueiredo AE, Povlsen JV, Wilkie M, et al. Creating and maintaining optimal peritoneal

dialysis access in the adult patient: 2019 Update. Perit Dial Int. 2019;39:414.

11. Fischbach M, Terzic J, Menouer S, Bergere V, Ferjani L, Haraldsson B. Impact of fill volume changes on peritoneal dialysis tolerance and effectiveness in children. Adv Perit Dial. 2000;16:321.
12. Warady BA, Feneberg R, Verrina E, Flynn JT, Müller-Wiefel DE, Besbas N, et al. Peritonitis in children who receive long-term peritoneal dialysis: a prospective evaluation of therapeutic guidelines. J Am Soc Nephrol. 2007;18:2172.
13. Li PK, Szeto CC, Piraino B, de Arteaga J, Fan S, Figueiredo AE, et al. ISPD Peritonitis Recommendations: 2016 update on prevention and treatment. Perit Dial Int. 2016;36(5):481-508.
14. Swartz SJ, Neu A, Skversky Mason A, Richardson T, Rodean J, Lawlor J, et al. Exit site and tunnel infections in children on chronic peritoneal dialysis: findings from the Standardizing Care to Improve Outcomes in Pediatric End Stage Renal Disease (SCOPE) Collaborative. Pediatr Nephrol. 2018;33:1029.
15. Furth SL, Donaldson LA, Sullivan EK, Watkins SL. Peritoneal dialysis catheter infections and peritonitis in children: a report of the North American Pediatric Renal Transplant Cooperative Study. Pediatr Nephrol. 2000;15:179.
16. Aksu N, Yavascan O, Anil M, Kara OD, Erdogan H, Bal A. A ten-year single-centre experience in children on chronic peritoneal dialysis--significance of percutaneous placement of peritoneal dialysis catheters. Nephrol Dial Transplant. 2007;22:2045.
17. Pittet D, Allegranzi B, Boyce J, World Health Organization World Alliance for Patient Safety First Global Patient Safety Challenge Core Group of Experts. The World Health Organization Guidelines on Hand Hygiene in Health Care and their consensus recommendations. Infect Control Hosp Epidemiol. 2009;30:611.
18. Bargman JM. Complications of peritoneal dialysis related to increased intraabdominal pressure. Kidney Int Suppl. 1993;40:S75.
19. Harvey E. Non-infectious complications of peritoneal dialysis and hemodialysis. In: Warady BA, Schaefer F, Fine RN, Alexander SR (Eds). Pediatric Dialysis. Dordrecht; Kluwer Academic Publishers; 2004. p. 415.
20. Brandt M, Brewer E. Peritoneal dialysis access in children. Warady BA, Schaefer F, Fine RN, Alexander SR (Eds). Pediatric Dialysis. Dordrecht: Kluwer Academic Publishers; 2004. p.83.
21. Phan J, Stanford S, Zaritsky JJ, DeUgarte DA. Risk factors for morbidity and mortality in pediatric patients with peritoneal dialysis catheters. J Pediatr Surg. 2013;48:197.
22. Woodrow G, Fan SL, Reid C, Denning J, Pyrah AN. Renal Association Clinical Practice Guideline on peritoneal dialysis in adults and children. BMC Nephrol. 2017;18:333.
23. van den Wall Bake AWL, Kooman JP, Lange JM, Smit W. Adequacy of peritoneal dialysis and the importance of preserving residual renal function. Nephrol Dial Transplant. 2006;21:34-7.
24. Heimburger O. How should we measure peritoneal dialysis adequacy in the clinic. Contrib Nephrol. 2009;163:140-6.
25. Blake PG, Daugaridas JT. Adequacy of peritoneal dialysis and chronic peritoneal dialysis prescription. In: Daugirdas JT, Blake PG, Ing TS (eds). Handbook of Dialysis, 5th edition. Philadelphia: Wolters Kluwer Health; 2015. pp. 454-78.
26. National Kidney Foundation, KDOQI. (2006). Clinical Practice Guidelines for Peritoneal Adequacy, Update 2006. [online] Available from: https://www.kidney.org/sites/default/files/docs/12-50-0210_jag_dcp_guidelines-hd_oct06_sectiona_ofc.pdf. [Last accessed March, 2022].
27. Rees L. Assessment of dialysis adequacy: beyond urea kinetic measurements. Pediatr Nephrol. 2019;34(1):61-9.
28. Marrón B, Remón C, Pérez-Fontán M, Quirós P, Ortíz A. Benefits of preserving residual renal function in peritoneal dialysis. Kidney Int. 2008;(108):S42-51.
29. Roszkowska-Blaim M, Skrzypczyk P. Residual renal function in children treated with chronic peritoneal dialysis. Sci World J. 2013;2013.
30. Mastrangelo A, Paglialonga F, Edefonti A. Assessment of nutritional status in children with chronic kidney disease and on dialysis. Pediatr Nephrol. 2014;29(8):1349-58.
31. KDOQI Work Group. KDOQI Clinical Practice Guideline for Nutrition in Children with CKD: 2008 update. Executive summary. Am J Kidney Dis. 2009;53(3 Suppl 2):S11-104.
32. Srivaths PR, Wong C, Goldstein SL. Nutrition aspects in children receiving maintenance hemodialysis: impact on outcome. Pediatr Nephrol. 2009;24(5):951-7.
33. Nelms CL, Shaw V, Greenbaum LA, Anderson C, Desloovere A, Haffner D, et al. Assessment of nutritional status in children with kidney diseases—clinical practice recommendations from the Pediatric Renal Nutrition Taskforce. Pediatr Nephrol. 2021;36:995-10.
34. Shaw V, Polderman N, Renken-Terhaerdt J, Paglialonga F, Oosterveld M, Tuokkola J, et al. Energy and protein requirements for children with CKD stages 2-5 and on dialysis-clinical practice recommendations from the Pediatric Renal Nutrition Taskforce. Pediatr Nephrol. 2020;35(3):519-31.
35. McAlister L, Pugh P, Greenbaum L, Haffner D, Rees L, Anderson C, et al. The dietary management of calcium and phosphate in children with CKD stages 2-5 and on dialysis-clinical practice recommendation from the Pediatric Renal Nutrition Taskforce. Pediatr Nephrol. 2020;35(3):501-18.
36. Shroff R, Wan M, Nagler EV, Bakkaloglu S, Fischer DC, Bishop N, et al. European Society for Paediatric Nephrology Chronic Kidney Disease Mineral and Bone Disorders and Dialysis Working Groups. Clinical practice recommendations for native vitamin D therapy in children with chronic kidney disease Stages 2-5 and on dialysis. Nephrol Dial Transplant. 2017;32(7):1098-113.
37. Rees L, Shaw V, Qizalbash L, Anderson C, Desloovere A, Greenbaum L, et al. Pediatric Renal Nutrition Taskforce. Delivery of a nutritional prescription by enteral tube feeding in children with chronic kidney disease stages 2-5 and on dialysis-clinical practice recommendations from the Pediatric Renal Nutrition Taskforce. Pediatr Nephrol. 2021;36(1):187-204.
38. Nelms CL. Optimizing enteral nutrition for growth in pediatric chronic kidney disease (CKD). Front Pediatr. 2018;6:214.

CHAPTER

12.6 Kidney Replacement Therapy: Hemodialysis

Sriram Krishnamurthy, Nivedita Kamath

INTRODUCTION

Majority of the hemodialysis (HD) literature pertains to adults, with fewer data available in children. Theoretically, the principles of HD in adults have been extrapolated to children; however, modifications are required to take into consideration factors such as age, weight, and physiology that are specific to children. In this chapter, we discuss the principles of HD, vascular access for HD [with focus on arteriovenous (AV) fistula (AVF)], briefly about the HD apparatus, prescription for HD, common complications of HD, and finally a brief note on the assessment of adequacy of dialysis.

PRINCIPLES OF HEMODIALYSIS

Hemodialysis is a procedure in which the patient's blood passes against a semipermeable membrane (contained in an "artificial kidney" known as the dialyzer), with dialysis solution on another side. Two processes form the basis of HD in chronic kidney disease (CKD) to remove blood urea, uremic solutes (e.g., guanidinosuccinic acid, β2-microglobulin, myoinositol), excessive potassium in the blood, and other unwanted waste products that accumulate in the end-stage kidney disease (ESKD).

1. *Diffusion:* This is a process wherein there is movement of solutes from high- to low-concentration between the blood of the patient and the dialysis solution (dialysate). Uremic solutes and potassium diffuse into the dialysate solution, while other substances such as bicarbonate contained in the dialysate solution diffuse into the blood of the patient. Diffusion ceases once equilibrium is attained across both sides of the semipermeable membrane. The molecular weight is a determinant of the diffusion process. For example, low-molecular-weight solutes are easily diffusible and are able to easily move through the semipermeable membrane of the dialyzer. Large molecules diffuse through the membrane slowly since their movement is at lower velocity, and therefore they collide with the membrane less frequently.[1]
2. *Convective transport:* The other mechanism of solute transport across semipermeable membranes is ultrafiltration (convective transport). Since water molecules are small, they can move through semipermeable membranes. Hydrostatic or an osmotic force pushes water through the membrane, resulting in ultrafiltration. Through the membrane pores, those solutes that can move easily are removed along with water. This process is known as "solvent drag".

   Ultrafiltration results in excess fluid removed from the body through usage of a positive (blood) or negative (dialysate) gradient of pressure. The former form of ultrafiltration is known as hydrostatic ultrafiltration and is employed in HD, while the latter form known as osmotic ultrafiltration is used in continuous ambulatory peritoneal dialysis. Patients who are anuric or exhibit features of intravascular fluid overload or pulmonary edema require removal of large volumes of ultrafiltrate.[1]

HEMODIALYSIS: VASCULAR ACCESS INCLUDING ARTERIOVENOUS FISTULA

An ideal vascular access offers a flow rate optimal for the HD prescription, possesses a long half-life, and has a low complication rate (including infection, stenosis, thrombotic complications, aneurysm formation, and ischemia of the limb). AVF best fits into these characteristics.

A permanent vascular access, preferably an AVF, should be constructed before the first dialysis is initiated. Nevertheless, it is important to recognize that a large number of patients in developing countries present for HD without any access in place.[2] Hence, it is not always feasible to create an AVF in chronic HD patients, which is why temporary and permanent central venous catheters represent a practical alternative in some ESKD patients,[2] at least as a short-term measure. These catheters can be put to use soon after insertion. However, their usage must be weighed against the risk for thrombosis and infection.

For inserting temporary HD catheters (which may be required in emergency situations, e.g., pulmonary edema, uremic symptoms, refractory hyperkalemia, refractory metabolic acidosis) in the internal jugular vein, ultrasound-guided insertion technique is used.[2] The linear probe of the ultrasound is placed to visualize the position of the internal jugular vein horizontally in both the approaches—anterior and central. Once visualization of the carotid artery medially and the internal jugular laterally is done, vein compressibility and artery pulsatility are done. For femoral catheterizations, similar localization of femoral vein (which is medial to femoral artery) is done. Internal jugular vein puncture is avoided in patients with thrombocytopenia. The sizes of the double-lumen HD catheter recommended are as follows: body weight 6–15 kg, 8 Fr; 15–30 kg, 9 Fr; >30 kg, 10 Fr; >40 kg, 11.5 Fr. Once the vein is localized, catheterization is performed using the Seldinger technique. The insertion site skin is prepared with betadine and covered with a surgical cloth with the patient lying supine. After administration of local anesthesia, the internal jugular vein or femoral vein is punctured (using 18G/21G puncture needle) by ultrasound guidance. Thereafter, the guidewire is pushed through the puncture needle followed by the removal of the needle. Finally, the catheter is placed along the guidewire to the internal jugular vein or femoral vein after dilation with the dilators (Seldinger method). The procedure ends with flushing the catheters with normal saline, filling the lumens with heparin, and stabilizing the catheter with sutures and plaster bandages.

As far as permanent catheters are concerned, their insertion is more complex. The distance between the internal jugular vein puncture site and the tunnel end is measured using a guidewire. After the vein is punctured and the guidewire is inserted, a small incision of about 5 mm is given over the pectoral area followed by a tunnel formation to the site of guidewire entrance through the skin by a tunneling trocar, which is attached to the catheter end and moving the catheter within this tunnel. Once dilation of the soft tissues around the guidewire and insertion of the peel-away sheath are done, the catheter is inserted to the superior vena cava followed by peeling the sheath. After checking patency of the lumens, the lumens are saline flushed and filled with heparin and the catheter is fixed by sutures.

Kidney Disease Outcomes Quality Initiative (KDOQI) and the "Fistula First" initiative recommend creation of AVFs, advising at least 68% usage in prevalent patients on HD. In many Western countries, AVF rates have increased, leading to transformation of the slogan "fistula first" to "fistula first and catheter last".[3-7]

Beginning the Process of Establishing a Vascular Access

It is important to educate children with CKD stage 4, those with deteriorating kidney function, or those who need to be started on maintenance dialysis promptly about kidney failure and management options thereof, including venous preservation and modalities of kidney replacement therapy during their consultation with pediatric nephrology services. Up to 6 months might be required from the time of preoperative assessment till the time the fistula is made completely functional.

Vessel Preservation: Salient Features

- Superficial and deep veins of arms should be protected, since their use is expected for vascular access.
- Veins of dorsum of hands should be used, if necessary.
- Subclavian vein should not be cannulated due to the risk of central vein stenosis.
- Use of percutaneously inserted central catheter (PICC) lines should be minimized.
- Radial and brachial vessels should be protected.
- Emphasis on "Save Veins and No IV Draws".

Planning the Optimal Vascular Access in Children

Pediatric patients who require chronic HD should be managed with a functioning AVF wherever possible. AV grafts have many disadvantages in children **(Table 1)**. AVFs are superior in comparison to central venous lines (CVLs) in children. AVFs have higher rates of patency and access survival and need fewer interventions while the access is functional. Additionally, lower rates of infection, better adequacy of HD, and lower morbidity and mortality in comparison to CVLs are described.[4]

Preoperative Assessment for Arteriovenous Fistula Creation

Detailed history, clinical examination, ultrasound and Doppler examination of the upper limb vessels are advised in order to plan AVF formation **(Table 2)**. One should avoid AVF formation in the ipsilateral arm wherein central venous stenosis has occurred.

The usage of duplex ultrasound is commonly done for vascular access evaluation. A poor-quality vein is an important cause of fistula failure. A larger caliber vein paves the route for a technically feasible surgery and leads to lesser resistance, thus, allowing better flow and higher rates of AVF maturation.

TABLE 1: Permanent arteriovenous fistulas versus arteriovenous grafts: comparison (based on information from adult literature).

AV fistula	*AV grafts*
Lower infection rate	Higher infection rate
Lower thrombosis rate	Higher thrombosis rate/poor flow (neointimal hyperplasia in the segment downstream from the graft–vein anastomosis due to turbulence) as well as prolonged bleeding after needle removal
May take 3–6 months to mature	Usually able to use in few weeks
Primary failure rate is higher	Primary failure rate is lower
Secondary failure rates lower	Secondary failure rates higher

(AV: arteriovenous)

Deciding the Site of Arteriovenous Fistula Placement

It is ideal to place an AVF in the nondominant arm where feasible. Placing an AVF distally in the arm is suggested.

Practically, the decision on where to create an AVF is related to many factors requiring individualization on a case-to-case basis. Anatomy of the involved veins and arteries, prior access history, the individual's hand dominance, evaluation of the possibility of self-cannulation, body mass index (BMI), individual patient preferences, and skill of the surgeon creating the fistula; all should be taken into consideration.

TABLE 2: Preparing a child for arteriovenous fistula.

Parameter	Issues to be looked for suitability of AV fistula
Weight and age	• Child >1 year • Weight >10 kg
Identify and counsel when	CKD stage 4 (eGFR <30 mL/min/1.73 m²)
History	• Prior central venous catheter/PICC lines • Prior arterial cannulation • History of previous fistula • History of coagulation disorders • Symptoms of cardiac failure/heart disease (AV fistula in this situation may lead to complications) • Peripheral vascular disease/athero-sclerosis/diabetes (in adults)
Identify nondominant arm	• Avoid venipunctures in the forearm/arm • Avoid peripherally inserted central lines and CVC in this limb
Clinical examination	*Arterial:* • Allen's test • Examine peripheral pulses (axillary, brachial, radial, ulnar) • Measure BP in both upper limbs (systolic difference of >20 mm Hg suggests proximal artery disease) *Venous:* • Look for edema in limb • Compare arm sizes • Palpate for veins, sites of venipuncture for scars • Presence of collateral veins • Perform tourniquet test (5 mm above diastolic pressure to check for distension of veins) CVS systemic examination to be done
Ultrasound and Doppler	• Diameter of the artery should be ideally *2.0 mm* • Diameter of the vein should be ideally *2.5 mm* • Look for patency of veins, presence of branches, distension of veins on tourniquet application (>50%) (CT venogram not needed ordinarily)

Note: The minimum vein lumen diameter should be about 2.5 mm for successful surgical anastomosis and minimal arterial diameter should be 2.0 mm.

(AV: arteriovenous; BP: blood pressure; CKD: chronic kidney disease; CT: computed tomography; CVC: central venous catheter; CVS: cardiovascular system; eGFR: estimated glomerular filtration rate; PICC: peripherally inserted central catheter)

Radiocephalic AVFs have demonstrated improved patency rates in pediatric patients. Additionally, a distal fistula allows for proximal venous options for any fistula creation in the future.[4,5,8]

Preferred Sites for Arteriovenous Fistula Placements: In the Order of Preference

1. Radial artery and cephalic vein (radiocephalic)
2. Brachial artery and cephalic vein (brachiocephalic)
3. Brachial artery and basilic vein (brachiobasilic)
4. Ulnar artery and basilic vein
5. Femoral artery and saphenous vein

What is the Ideal Timing of Creation of Vascular Access?

Creating an AVF is recommended to be performed at least 3 months prior to its cannulation and usage. Pediatric literature describes a mean time for maturation of 8–10 weeks for most AVFs.[8,9]

Issues Regarding Creation and Maintenance of Arteriovenous Fistula

Creation of Arteriovenous Fistula: Points to Remember

- Site—distal vessels first, then move proximally
- Type of fistula—radiocephalic, followed by brachio-cephalic (**Fig. 1**) and brachiobasilic.
- Upper limb before lower limb (nondominant arm first)

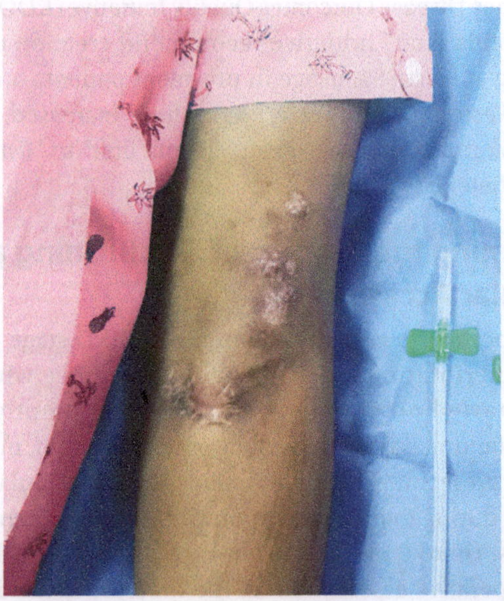

Fig. 1: Brachiocephalic arteriovenous fistula in the nondominant hand.

- Maintain blood pressure (BP) pre- and intraoperative procedure to avoid hypotension and increased thrombosis in fistula.
- Avoid dialysis on the day of surgery.
- Usually under general anesthesia in children.
- End-to-side anastomosis of a vein to an artery **(Fig. 2)** (prevents red hand syndrome than side to side anastomoses since distal vein is ligated off).
- Appearance of thrill immediately postsurgery indicates successful creation.

Maintenance: Postoperative Care

- One should elevate the limb to the level of heart to decrease any edema.
- Maintain BP.
- Check for the presence of thrill or bruit.
- Avoid compression of the fistula.
- Keep the next session of dialysis heparin free.
- Isometric hand exercises with tourniquet help to develop the fistula by increasing blood flow (e.g., squeezing rubber ball).
- Tight circumferential dressing should be avoided; do not use fistula for venipuncture.

How to do Assessment of Arteriovenous Fistula Maturation?

One should assess maturation 4–6 weeks after AVF creation by physical examination and duplex ultrasound so that we can plan the timing of AVF cannulation.[4,5]

Physical examination should focus on the presence of a thrill, bruit, quality of skin, potential needle sites, and mental preparedness of the patient requiring needling of AVF **(Fig. 3 and Table 3)**. Careful attention should be paid to avoid hypotension after AVF formation, especially after the first few days. BP measurements should not be performed on the AVF arm. One should avoid tight clothing since it might restrict

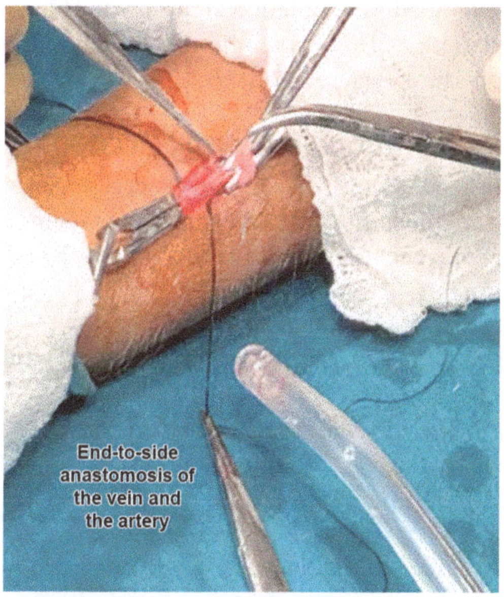

Fig. 2: Creation of an arteriovenous fistula.

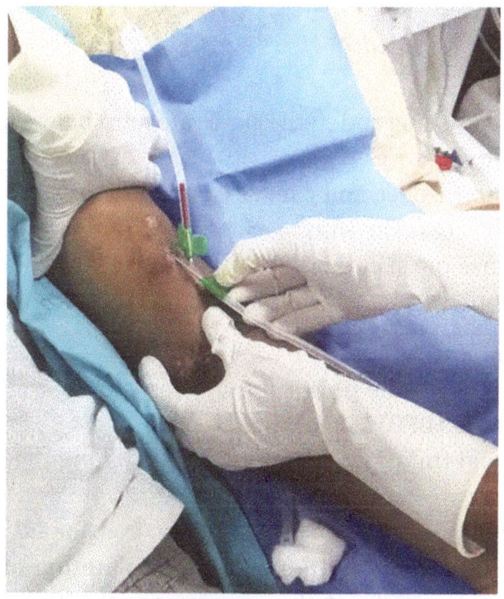

Fig. 3: Needling of the arteriovenous fistula.

TABLE 3: Fistula assessment: signs to be looked for.

Inspection (look)	*Palpation (feel)*	*Auscultation (listen)*
Normal—vein is easily seen, mature: • Collapsibility of vein when hand is over head *Abnormal*—vein is not easily seen, immature or deep: • Presence of accessory veins, aneurysms • Distal collapse with proximal dilation—stenosis • Edema—central venous stenosis • Color of limb—bluish (steal syndrome) • Signs of infection	*Normal*—thrill at anastomosis and entire outflow part which is easily compressible: • Augmentation—occlusion of juxta anastomotic segment: Thrill disappears, pulse is felt *Abnormal:* • Weak/absent thrill—thrombosis/immature vein • Poor augmentation—poor arterial flow or stenosis of juxta-anastomotic site • If thrill is present despite occlusion—accessory vein • Induration—infection • Cold limb—steal syndrome • Prominent fistula, pulsatile thrill, thickened wall stenosis	*Normal*—normal bruit, continuous, systolic–diastolic *Abnormal*—high-pitched systolic bruit with minimal diastolic component (stenosis)

flow through the veins. It is also important to continue with physical activity. Nevertheless, one should avoid activities that might lead to direct trauma to the AVF.[4,10]

How to Assess if Fistula is Ready for Use?

- Maturation of AVF may take 6–8 weeks to mature; it can take up to 6 months in children.
- Prior to first needling, ensure (rule of sixes) through duplex ultrasound that:
  - The vein is >6 mm diameter.
  - Fistula is <6 mm from skin surface.
  - Blood flow is >600 mL/min.
  - At least a segment of 6 cm is available for needling.
  - Generally, 6 weeks after surgery.

Arteriovenous Fistula Cannulation

One should be cannulating an AVF after optimal maturation. It is recommended to use an aseptic technique for AVF cannulation, by either rope ladder or buttonhole technique.

Needling a Fistula

Skin preparation:

- Hand washing and sterile gloves are must before handling fistula.
- Locate, inspect, and palpate cannulation site.
- Wash access site with soap and needle.
- Cleanse the skin thoroughly with 2% chlorhexidine/70% alcohol with 10% povidone iodine.

Cannulation:

- Use 17G needle [this is the smallest size; permits blood flow rate (BFR) 250 mL/min].
- Arterial (inlet) needle: anterograde (along the flow) or retrograde (against the flow)
- Arterial needle should be 3–5 cm away from the anastomosis
- Venous needle (outlet) should be anterograde, 5 cm downstream from the arterial needle (to minimize recirculation).
- Apply tourniquet; pull the skin in opposite direction to make it taut.
- Stabilize the vein and hold the needle at 25° angle with bevel up.
- Once the vein is punctured, hold the needle parallel to the skin and advance.
- Fix needle to the skin and confirm the position by flushing and aspirating using a 10 cc syringe filled with normal saline.
- Once the position is confirmed, insert the second needle.

Cannulation techniques ***(Fig. 2)****:*

- Buttonhole technique—AVF is cannulated at the same spot, at the same angle as well as depth of penetration at each time. A scar tissue tunnel track forms. This permits the use of buttonhole (blunt) fistula needle.
- Rope ladder technique—One rotates sites of needle placement for each session of dialysis, selecting sites at a predefined distance from the previous sites of puncture. Use is limited by the number of sites, but there is a lower risk of aneurysms.

Removal of needles:

- After dialysis session is over, remove the needle at the same angle as insertion.
- After removing, apply pressure for 10 minutes.

Arteriovenous Fistula Surveillance

Duplex ultrasound must be performed three to six times monthly for routine surveillance of AVFs. The case must be referred to a vascular access surgeon in case the AVF is not functioning or if complications (see below) are identified.[4,9]

An "ABCD" approach can be adopted for the clinical care of AVFs: *A*, Fistula assessment through clinical examination; *B*, Blood flow and changes in flow from baseline—volume flow assessment by duplex ultrasound; *C*, Clinical problems, e.g., problems in needle cannulation, or protracted bleeding after decannulation; *D*, Dialysis monitoring (adequacy, trends of venous pressure, recirculation).[4,11]

Pulse Augmentation and Arm Elevation Tests

These are used to quickly examine AV access:

- *Pulse augmentation test:* To check inflow segment. When one occludes the AV access outflow by the examining finger:
  a. Thrill is expected to disappear.
  b. The part of access upstream should become hyperpulsatile (augment).

  If (a) and (b) do not happen, there is an accessory pathway.
- *Arm elevation test:* To check outflow tract (to look for downstream stenosis).

How to Assess Fistula on Ongoing Basis?

Physical examination of fistula should be during every dialysis.

- Recognize "at-risk fistula" difficulty in needling the fistula.
- Any fistula "at risk" should be evaluated clinically by a vascular expert for signs—edema, collaterals, altered thrill.
- Surveillance of "at-risk" fistula.
- Direct flow measurement, duplex ultrasound 6 monthly.

Prevention of Arteriovenous Fistula Thrombosis

Antiplatelet drugs, e.g., aspirin, clopidogrel, or ticlopidine, are often given in the first few months following AVF formation and reduce the chances of AVF thrombosis.[4]

Monitoring for Complications of Arteriovenous Fistula

These include aneurysms, pseudoaneurysms, infection, thrombosis, bleeding, infiltration (hematoma), stenosis, and steal syndrome. These need to be looked for during every dialysis session.

HEMODIALYSIS APPARATUS

The HD apparatus consists of the blood circuit and the dialysis circuit that combine at the dialyzer. The blood circuit starts from the vascular access. The arterial limb of the circuit takes the blood from the vascular access to the dialyzer. The blood from the dialyzer is then returned to the patient via the venous limb. The dialysate circuit consists of the dialysate supply system. This system creates the dialysate by mixing concentrated dialysate mix with purified water in a predetermined proportion. The dialysate thus prepared is then pumped through the dialysate compartment of the dialyzer. The dialyzer is separated from the blood compartment by a semipermeable membrane.

The blood circuit and the dialysate circuit have several pressure monitors and detectors to ensure that the dialysis is done safely:

- *Blood circuit:* The blood from the vascular access is brought into the dialyzer using the arterial limb of the circuit which consists of the tubing (pre-pump, pump, and post-pump segments, respectively) and the roller pump. A pictorial representation of the blood circuit is given in **Figure 4**. The roller pump is a self-occluding pump that rotates and flattens the tubing to allow the forward flow of blood. The BFR is dependent on the rotation rate of the pump and the volume of the pump segment.

  BFR = rotations per minute × pump segment volume ($\pi r^2 l$). The pre-pump segment has a sampling port and a saline infusion port. This is the part of the circuit that has the highest negative pressure and air can quickly enter the blood line. It is advisable to have a pre-pump pressure monitor in this segment. The post-pump segment has a heparin infusion port and a post-pump monitor.[12]

  The venous line has a drip chamber to allow for easy removal of any air that has managed to enter the circuit before returning the blood to the patient. The line also has an air detector which detects the microbubbles in the circuit. Clotting also occurs first in the drip chamber of the venous line. The venous pressure is monitored by a pressure pump and a rise in venous pressure indicates a propensity for clotting.
- *Dialysate circuit:* It consists of—
  - *Water purification system:* Purifies raw water through a series of devices including the reverse osmosis system to provide water suitable for dialysis.
  - *Proportioning system:* The proportioning systems mix the electrolyte solutions/powder with purified water to prepare the final dialysate. The dialysate should then be delivered to the dialyzer at appropriate temperature and free of dissolved air.
  - *Heating and degassing:* The dialysate is heated to a temperature of 35–38°C and during this process the dissolved gases bubble out and are removed.
  - *Monitors and safety alarms:* There are several monitors in the dialysate circuit, which ensure that the dialysate is delivered in a safe manner.[12]
- *Conductivity:* The conductivity of the dialysate is dependent on the degree of concentration of electrolytes in the dialysate and is measured as millisiemens per centimeter (mS/cm). The normal conductivity is in the range of 12–16 mS/cm. If the conductivity of the dialysate exceeds the upper set limit, the bypass valve is opened and the dialysate is diverted to the drain.
- *Temperature:* Low dialysate temperature can cause hypothermia and high dialysate temperature can cause hemolysis. The temperature monitor checks the temperature of the dialysate and if it exceeds the upper set limit, the dialysate is diverted to the drain.
- *Blood leak detector:* This monitoring device looks for blood in the spent dialysate which indicates a leak across the dialyzer membrane and activates an alarm and stops blood flow through the dialyzer.

  A pictorial representation of the dialysate circuit is given in **Figure 5**.

HEMODIALYSIS PRESCRIPTION

Illustrative Case Scenario 1

A 7-year-old boy, a case of CKD stage 5 secondary to focal segmental glomerulosclerosis (FSGS), presents with breathing difficulty for 1 day associated with poor urine output. On examination, he is severely pale, edematous, and has stage 2 hypertension (BP 160/110 mm Hg). He is afebrile. The heart rate is 130/min, respiratory rate is 60/min, and oxygen saturation is 88% on room air. He has signs of

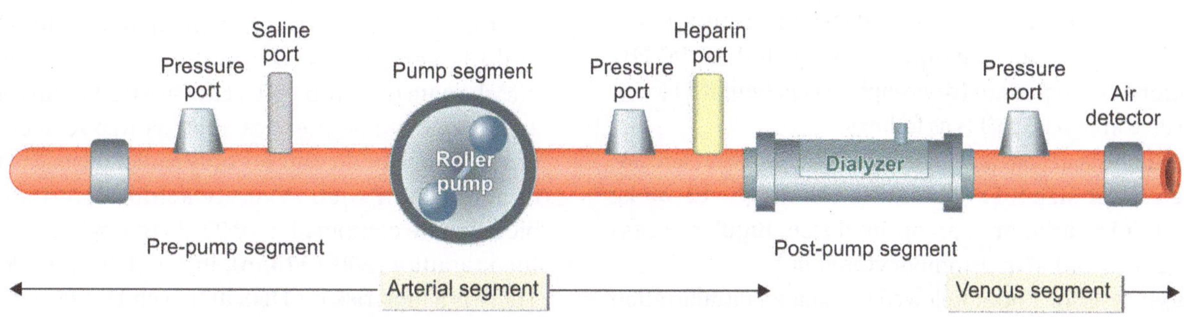

Fig. 4: A pictorial representation of the blood circuit.

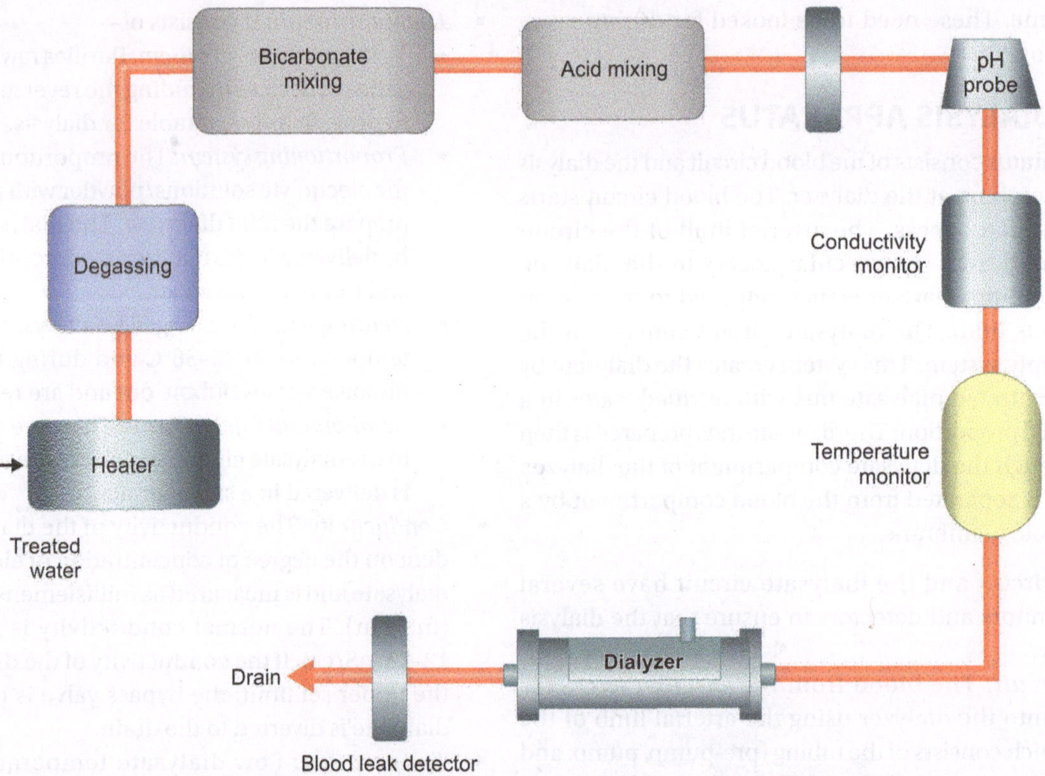

Fig. 5: Pictorial representation of the dialysate circuit.

intravascular fluid overload [gallop rhythm, elevated jugular venous pressure (JVP), basal crepitations, and orthopnea]. His weight at admission is 26 kg (previous documented weight 1 month ago was 23 kg) and height is 115 cm. The laboratory values are as follows: blood urea 250 mg/dL, serum creatinine 4.5 mg/dL, serum potassium 5.6 mEq/L, sodium 131 mEq/L, bicarbonate 9.2 mmol/L, serum albumin 2.2 g/dL, hemoglobin 5.6 g/dL, total leukocyte count 14,000/mm^3, and platelet count 5.2 lakh/mm^3. Prothrombin time is normal. He is immediately administered oxygen by mask. Medical management for hyperkalemia and hypertension is initiated. Echocardiogram shows severe concentric left ventricular hypertrophy (LVH) and ophthalmological evaluation reveals grade 3 hypertensive retinopathy. How should an initial HD prescription be written for this patient?

Answer:

The child described in the above case scenario is a case of CKD stage 5 (native kidney disease FSGS) who has presented with pulmonary edema and is oliguric. He has stage 2 hypertension leading to concentric LVH and hypertensive retinopathy. He is hyperkalemic and acidotic. A suggested initial HD prescription for the patient (dry weight 23 kg, height 115 cm, body surface area 0.85 m^2) is as follows:

- Hemodialysis access—right internal jugular vein access: HD catheter size 9 Fr (Remarks: For weight 15-30 kg weight, 9 Fr catheter is an optimal size. Jugular access should be avoided in thrombocytopenia.)
- Hemodialysis for 1 hour followed by isolated ultrafiltration for 3 hours. [*Remarks:* Initial sessions of HD should be restricted to 1 hour to avoid dialysis disequilibrium syndrome (DDS). The extremely high levels of blood urea in this child with CKD indicate high risk of DDS, mandating restriction of HD to 1 hour. However, since he is in pulmonary edema, more fluid is required and hence, isolated ultrafiltration for 3 additional hours would be optimal.]
- Dialyzer size—F4 dialyzer [*Remarks:* Dialyzer size should be 80–100% of the body surface area. It is better to choose a smaller size dialyzer to prevent DDS. In this case, F4 corresponds to 0.7 sq. m body surface area (BSA).]
- BFR—115 mL/min (*Remarks:* 5 mL/kg/min)
- Dialysate flow rate—230 mL/min (*Remarks:* 10 mL/kg/min)
- Ultrafiltration rate—2 L ultrafiltrate removal over 4 hours (*Remarks:* The child is in pulmonary edema and requires large volume of fluid removal. He is documented to be 3 kg above his original weight. As an initial measure, removal of 2 L fluid over 4 hours is expected to relieve the pulmonary symptoms.)
- Dialysate fluid composition—Sodium 135 mEq/L, potassium 2 mEq/L, glucose 100 mg/dL, bicarbonate 25 mmol/L (*Remarks:* The bicarbonate level of the child is very low, <10 mmol/L. Using a "standard" bicarbonate of 35 mmol/L is not advised in this situation as adverse consequences such as hypocalcemia may ensue. One should aim for only initial partial correction of acidosis in such severely acidotic patients using bicarbonate composition of 25–28 mmol/L.)
- Inj. mannitol (20%) 115 mL in the first hour (*Remarks:* There is a high risk for DDS in this child. Mannitol would be helpful in decreasing the risk of DDS.)

- Inj. heparin 460 U in the first hour followed by 230 U/h till the last hour (*Remarks:* If thrombocytopenia, heparin should be avoided and saline dialysis should be used.)
- *Additives:* Packed red blood cells 250 mL (1 U) during dialysis. (*Remarks:* This volume can be added to the set ultrafiltrate volume.)

The goals of HD are to clear solutes, such as uremic solutes and potassium, and to remove excess fluid. For optimal attainment of these objectives, one must estimate adequate clearance. It is also important to estimate the patient's dry weight. Thereafter, one should select the BFR, dialyzer, examine the characteristics of the extracorporeal circuit, and decide regarding dialysate fluid composition and the feasibility of anticoagulation.[13]

Estimation of Dry Weight

Ultrafiltration should be planned to attain a "dry weight". Dry weight is defined as the post-HD weight at which the patient is as close to euvolemic state and asymptomatic. Overestimation of the dry weight poses a risk of developing a hypervolemic state. Underestimation of the dry weight increases the risk of intradialytic hypotension (IDH).[13] It is important to regularly re-evaluate the dry weight in children since growth and changes in lean body mass are the usual norm. Clinical examination for the detection of volume status (e.g., BP, signs of fluid overload) is of paramount importance to ensure an uneventful session of HD.

Vascular Access

The vascular access for HD could be right internal jugular venous (IJV) access or femoral venous access. The right internal jugular vein is an optimal site since the venous pathway to the right atrium is quite straight. The subclavian vein must be avoided in general since its cannulation is associated with a greater incidence of insertion-associated complications including pneumothorax, hemothorax, perforation of the vessel, injury to the brachial plexus as well as central venous stenosis. If an AVF has been created and has matured, it can be used for access.

The chances of uncuffed catheters getting infected increase significantly after the first week of insertion. Consequently, the KDOQI 2006 vascular access guidelines[4] recommend insertion of a cuffed catheter if the HD is expected to be used for more than a week. These guidelines also mention that femoral catheters in bed-ridden patients should not be used for >5 days. These recommendations may be too difficult to implement in practice.

The sizes of the double-lumen HD catheter recommended are as follows: body weight 6–15 kg, 8 Fr; 15–30 kg, 9 Fr; >30 kg, 10 Fr; >40 kg, 11.5 Fr. The bigger the catheter, the better the blood flow during dialysis, thereby increasing the efficiency of dialysis. IJV access should be avoided in a thrombocytopenic patient.[13] Insertion of the HD catheter is done using a modified Seldinger technique, with the usage of a 21G/18G micropuncture needle, guidewire, and dilator, under strict aseptic procedures and sedation with monitoring of vital signs. The temporary catheter is ultimately advanced over the guidewire into position. Thereafter, a chest roentgenogram should be taken to check the position of the catheter.

Extracorporeal Circuit

The extracorporeal circuit is made up of the arterial (inflow) and venous (outflow) lines (tubing) and the dialyzer. A child can tolerate up to a maximum of 10% of his or her total blood volume in the extracorporeal circuit, and a safe volume of the circuit is targeted at 8% of total blood volume of the child. As an example, the upper safe limit for a child who weighs 10 kg (total blood volume of 800 mL) would be 64–80 mL.[14]

Choice of Dialyzer

As a thumb rule, the dialyzer membrane surface area should be close to 80–100% of the child's body surface area. Most centers have dialyzers with surface areas ranging from 0.4 up to 1.3 m^2 and above **(Table 4)**.

Every dialyzer has an ultrafiltration coefficient (KUf), which reflects its capacity to remove fluid. KUf is related to the surface area of the dialyzer and the dialyzer membrane characteristics. Dialyzers with KUfs <10 mL/h are known as low flux, and those with a rate of 15–60 mL/h/mm Hg are termed high flux. High-flux dialyzers offer improved permeability for middle and larger molecules. They are particularly needed for hemodialfiltration.[14]

Mass transfer area coefficient (KoA) is the highest possible clearance of a given dialyzer at infinite BFRs and dialysate flow rates. The KoA is the product of two quantities: *Ko*,

TABLE 4: Surface area, KUf, KoA, and urea clearance (at a blood flow rate of 200 mL/min) of various dialyzers available in India.

Dialyzer type	*Surface area M^2*	*KUf (mL/h/mm Hg)*	*KoA (mL/min)*	*Urea clearance QB 200 mL/min*
F4	0.7	8	494	170
F5	1	10	604	179
F6	1.3	13	731	186
Fx 40	0.6	20	494	170
Fx 50	1	33	809	189
Fx 60	1.4	46	955	193

the permeability coefficient of the dialyzer membrane for a particular solute, and *A*, total effective surface area of membrane in the dialyzer. The higher the KoA, the more permeable is the dialyzer.

Blood Flow Rate

Blood flow rate is the speed at which the blood is pumped out of the patient and around the circuit. It is an important determinant of the solute clearance. Although higher BFRs augment solute clearance by optimization of diffusion and convection, excessive BFRs can compromise cardiovascular stability. Typically, BFRs are set at 5 mL/kg/min (range 3–8 mL/kg/min). Lower BFRs usually mandate the use of heparin to prevent coagulation of blood in the extracorporeal circuit.[15]

Dialysate Flow Rate

The dialysate fluid rate is typically set at double the BFR. Dialysate flow rates of 200–500 mL/min are typically used based on the child's weight.

Ultrafiltration Rate/Fluid Removal

The amount of fluid removal per session is dependent on the difference between the predialytic weight and the optimal weight of the patient, whether the child has residual renal function (native urine output) and the presence of a fluid overload state. Although the amount of fluid removal per hour that a child will be able to tolerate is quite variable, a generally safe starting point is approximately 10 mL/kg/h.

Dialysate Fluid Composition

Modern HD machines make up the dialysis fluid as per the prescription from two canisters containing acid and base along with electrolytes (**Table 5**).

Sodium

Patients are typically dialyzed against dialysate fluid sodium ranging from 135 to 145 mEq/L. Hyponatremic dialysis leads to dialysis disequilibrium and hypotension. Hypernatremic dialysis leads to increased thirst. It also promotes increased interdialytic weight gain and may worsen hypertension. Altering the dialysate sodium concentration throughout dialysis, termed sodium profiling, uses a sodium concentration that falls in a step, linear, or exponential manner. This might confer a therapeutic advantage in some cases.[13]

Potassium

Usually, a potassium bath of 1–2 mmol/L is used. In severe hyperkalemia, a lower dialysate potassium concentration of 0–1 mmol/L is often needed (for the initial 1–2 hours). If serum potassium levels are normal prior to HD, a potassium bath of 3–4 mmol/L may be used.

Bicarbonate

Dialysis corrects the metabolic acidosis of ESKD by removing organic anions and rectifying the bicarbonate deficit. Standard dialysate has bicarbonate concentrations of 35 mmol/L and is generally appropriate for usage. However, if the predialysis plasma bicarbonate level is 28 mmol/L or higher, or if the patient has respiratory alkalosis, a customized dialysis solution adjusting to a lower bicarbonate level (e.g., 20–28 mM) should be preferred.[13]

Calcium

Usual calcium concentration in dialysate fluid can range from 1.25 to 3 mmol/L. To avoid hypercalcemia and calcium deposition in the extraskeletal tissues, it is suggested to maintain serum calcium levels in the lower side of normal reference values.

Glucose

The dialysate glucose concentration generally is around 100–200 mg/dL (6–11 mmol/L). This concentration is expected to keep patients normoglycemic.

Dialysate Temperature

Usually, this is maintained at 35–37°C. Patients susceptible to hypotension might benefit from maintaining a lower dialysate temperature.[15]

Anticoagulation

Anticoagulation (with heparin) of the extracorporeal circuit is a usual practice. Nonetheless, one should evaluate the risk of bleeding in an individualized manner versus clotting of the circuit which would lead to blood loss. Standard regimens

TABLE 5: Dialysis fluid composition.

Constituent	*Acid (mmol/L)*	*Base (mmol/L)*	*Overall (approx.)*
Sodium	99–110	27–40	140 (Range 135–145)
Potassium	0–3	0	2 or 2.5 (range 0–4)
Calcium	1.25–2.0	0	1.25–3
Magnesium	0.75	0	0.5–0.75
Chloride	99–110	0	99–124
Bicarbonate	0	27–40	30–40
Glucose	5.5 (or 200 mg/dL)	–	100–200 mg/dL

consist of a bolus dose of 20 units/kg of unfractionated heparin at the beginning of dialysis followed by a continuous infusion of 10 units/kg/h. Low-dose ("tight") heparin or heparin-free dialysis using intermittent saline flushes should be performed in children with higher risk of bleeding. In saline dialysis, the dialyzer and tubing are flushed with saline (100 mL in <20 kg, 150 mL in >20 kg) every 15–30 minutes.[15] Saline dialysis is advised after recent surgery, coagulopathy, thrombocytopenia, and 12 hours before biopsy or proposed surgery.

Length of Dialysis Session

The length of the first dialysis session should not exceed 1–2 hours in CKD to avoid a urea reduction ratio (URR) > 40%. This will ensure prevention of DDS.

Additives

These include the following:

- Intravenous 20% mannitol (if blood urea >150 mg/dL)—especially during first dialysis (dose 5 mL/kg in the first hour)
- Normal saline intravenous boluses—if hypotension
- Intravenous dextrose (if hypoglycemia) in young children
- Intravenous hydrocortisone and adrenaline if anaphylaxis during dialysis

Hemodialysis Adequacy

In children, it has been proposed that dialysis adequacy be defined as >1.2 for *Kt/V* and >65% for URR. This is usually attainable with a thrice-weekly dialysis lasting 4 hours (for each session of dialysis).[15]

Table 6 depicts a model HD prescription highlighting the various components of the prescription.

Illustrative Case Scenario 2

A 10-year-old girl, a case of CKD stage 5 secondary to nephronophthisis, presents with lethargy and recurrent vomiting. On examination, she is severely pale and has bony deformities. BP is 90/60 mm Hg. There is no edema. Peripheries are warm. The urine output the previous day as quantified by the mother is 1.7 L. She is afebrile. The heart rate is 110/min, respiratory rate is 26/min (acidotic breathing), and oxygen saturation is 96% on room air. There are no signs of intravascular fluid overload or dehydration. Her weight at admission is 28 kg and height is 110 cm. The laboratory values are as follows: blood urea 208 mg/dL, serum creatinine 8.3 mg/dL, serum potassium 8.5 mEq/L, sodium 125 mEq/L, bicarbonate 8.3 mmol/L, serum calcium 9.8 mg/dL, serum albumin 3.3 g/dL, hemoglobin 3.5 g/dL, total leukocyte count 12,000/mm^3, and platelet count 3.2 lakh/mm^3. Prothrombin time is normal. ECG shows tall T waves. Treatment with intravenous calcium gluconate and salbutamol nebulization is commenced. Intravenous sodium bicarbonate (in view of hyperkalemia with metabolic acidosis) followed by insulin-dextrose is also started. However, the repeat serum potassium thereafter is 6.7 mEq/L and serum bicarbonate is 9 mmol/L, with serum sodium 126 mEq/L. How should an initial HD prescription be written for this patient?

Answer:

The child described in the above case scenario is a case of CKD stage 5 (native kidney disease—nephronophthisis)

TABLE 6: Model dialysis prescription.

Name of the child/hospital no.	*Value*
Body weight	____kg
Ultrafiltrate volume (L)	____L (according to intradialytic weight gain and volume status) Initial UF 8–10 mL/kg/h
• Dialyzer (sq. m) • F3-0.4, F4-0.7, F5-0.9, F6-1.3	____ (0.8 × BSA)
Priming solution (blood/5% albumin solution circuit priming in <10 kg patients)/tubings	______Neonate 25 mL Pediatric 75 mL
Extracorporeal blood volume	______mL
Blood flow rate (QB)	_____3–8 mL/kg/min (generally 5 mL/kg/min)
Dialysate flow rate (QD)	200–500 mL/min *(two times the blood flow rate)*
Treatment rate (h)	• First HD 1–2 hours • Subsequent 3–4 hours
Heparin dosing	• Saline dialysis—if deranged coagulation/12 hours before biopsy • Bolus heparin—20 U/kg stat followed by 10 U/kg/h (if platelet <50,000 rigid/tight heparin protocol)
Sodium modeling (135/145) Potassium (1.5/3.5)	• Avoid difference >10 mEq/L with serum sodium • If hyperkalemia 1.5 mEq/L; others 3.5 mEq/L
Additives	Inj. mannitol (20%) 5 mL/kg in the first hour (during first dialysis in a CKD patient)

(BSA: body surface area; CKD: chronic kidney disease; HD: hemodialysis) who has presented with uremic symptoms. She has persistent hyperkalemia and refractory metabolic acidosis with hyponatremia. The indications for HD in this case are uremia, refractory metabolic acidosis, and persistent hyperkalemia. A suggested initial HD prescription for the patient (dry weight 28 kg, height 110 cm, body surface area 0.92 m^2) is as follows:

- *Hemodialysis access*—right internal jugular vein access—HD catheter size 9 Fr (*Remarks:* For weight 15–30 kg 9 Fr catheter is an optimal size.)
- Hemodialysis for 1 hour [prior blood priming (75 mL) is recommended in this case as she is severely pale and might become hypotensive at the commencement of dialysis. Moreover, BP is normal 90/60 mm Hg.] (*Remarks:* The initial session of HD should be restricted to 1 hour to avoid DDS. Additional fluid removal in the form of isolated ultrafiltration for additional ultrafiltration is not required in this case as she is not having signs of intravascular fluid overload.)
- *Dialyzer size*—F4 dialyzer (*Remarks:* Dialyzer size should be 80–100% of the body surface area. It is better to choose a smaller size dialyzer to prevent DDS. In this case, F4 corresponds to 0.7 sq. m BSA.)
- *BFR*—140 mL/min (*Remarks:* 5 mL/kg/min)
- *Dialysate flow rate*—280 mL/min (*Remarks*: 10 mL/kg/min)
- *Ultrafiltration rate*—200 mL over 1 hour (*Remarks:* Minimal ultrafiltration is required as she has no signs of intravascular fluid overload.)
- *Dialysate fluid composition*—sodium 135 mEq/L, potassium 2 mEq/L, glucose 100 mg/dL, bicarbonate 25 mmol/L (*Remarks:* The child has hyponatremia. The dialysate sodium should be within 10 mEq/L of the serum sodium. Potassium is easily diffusible and hyperkalemia is expected to resolve after 1 hour of dialysis. The bicarbonate level of the child is very low, <10 mmol/L. One should aim for only initial partial correction of acidosis in such severely acidotic patients using bicarbonate composition of 25–28 mmol/L.)
- Injection mannitol (20%) 140 mL in the first hour (*Remarks:* Mannitol would be helpful in decreasing the risk of DDS.)
- Injection heparin 560 U in the first hour
- Additives: Packed red blood cells 250 mL (1 unit) during dialysis

COMPLICATIONS OF HEMODIALYSIS AND MONITORING

Dialysis Disequilibrium Syndrome

The brain adapts to the high osmolarity in the blood (resulting from the accumulating uremic solutes in CKD) by generating idiogenic osmoles. Upon commencement of HD in a patient with CKD, the uremic solutes are removed, thereby leading to reduction in blood osmolarity in relation to the brain. This leads to fluid shift from the intravascular compartment to the cerebral tissue, culminating in cerebral edema.[13,16,17]

Dialysis disequilibrium manifesting during or immediately after HD is very often a self-limiting entity, but sometimes serious life-threatening complications might ensue. Headache, blurred vision, vomiting, and convulsions are the most common symptoms of DDS.

Dialysis disequilibrium syndrome can be prevented by reducing the URR, by following the measures mentioned below:[13,16,17]

- Using a smaller dialyzer (not exceeding BSA of the child)
- Decreasing the blood and/or dialysate flow rate
- First session of HD not exceeding 1–2 hours
- Usage of mannitol (20%) during the first session of HD—a maximal intradialytic dose of 3–5 mL/kg is recommended.

Management of DDS entails the usage of anticerebral edema measures, including usage of antiepileptic drugs (if the patient has seizures), and might require an ICU setting for this purpose.

Intradialytic Hypotension

Intradialytic hypotension has been associated with poor short-term (higher mortality, myocardial stunning, etc.) as well as long-term outcomes. The prevalence of IDH is greatest in patients with low predialysis BP, which could be a pointer toward an underlying cardiac disease.[13]

Causes of IDH are as follows[16]:

- *Volume-related:*
    - Excessive weight gain (high ultrafiltration rate)
    - Shorter weekly dialysis time (high ultrafiltration rate)
    - Too low target ("dry") weight
- *Inadequate vasoconstriction:*
    - High dialysis solution temperature
    - Autonomic neuropathy
    - Antihypertensive medications
    - Eating during treatment
    - Anemia
- *Cardiac factors:*
    - Diastolic dysfunction
- *Uncommon etiologies:*
    - Pericardial tamponade
    - Occult hemorrhage
    - Sepsis
    - Dialyzer reaction
    - Hemolysis

Intradialytic hypotension can be prevented by the following measures[13,16]:

- Prevent excessive interdialytic weight gains by emphasizing salt and fluid restriction.
- Increasing weekly treatment time—four hours of dialysis therapy should be administered for all patients dialyzed on a thrice-weekly schedule, irrespective of the weight.
- Choose target weight carefully—a patient's target weight or "dry weight" is decided based on BP, features of

intravascular fluid overload, presence of edema, and tolerance of ultrafiltration. Try increasing the dry weight estimate.
- Use an appropriate dialysis solution sodium level—high dialysis fluid sodium levels might lead to more interdialytic weight gain and increased thirst.
- Lower dialysis solution temperature—levels of 35.5–36.0°C are appropriate initial choices and can be modified based on factors such as tolerance (chills in the patient) and efficacy (BP).
- Avoid the intake of food during dialysis in patients prone to hypotension—this might occur due to splanchnic vasodilatation in some patients.

Management of Intradialytic Hypotension

- An intravenous bolus of 0.9% saline should be administered.
- The ultrafiltration rate must be decreased to as near to zero as possible, under constant monitoring. Ultrafiltration can be restarted at a lower rate once stabilization of vital signs is documented.
- Reduction of the BFR to treat IDH is not likely to benefit much with current dialysis practice. In refractory cases, blood pump rates may be transiently reduced. It should be recognized that lower BFRs are at the expense of ineffective solute clearance.

Muscle Cramps

Muscle cramps may occur due to hypotension, hypovolemia (patient below dry weight), high ultrafiltration rate, and use of low-sodium dialysis solution. These lead to hypoperfusion of muscles and consequent impairment of muscle relaxation. In addition, hypocalcemia, hypokalemia, and hypomagnesemia should be looked for.[13,16]

If related to hypotension, management with 0.9% saline might be beneficial. Forced stretching of the muscle involved might provide some benefit. Prevention of hypotensive episodes (by correct estimation of dry weight) will eliminate most cramping.

Nausea and Vomiting

Nausea and vomiting might occur in up to 10% of dialysis sessions.[16] Causes described include hypotension, disequilibrium syndrome, dialyzer reactions, gastroparesis, and contaminated or incorrectly formulated dialysis solutions. Treatment should be directed toward hypotension management. Antiemetics can provide significant relief.

Headache

Although quite common, its cause is largely unknown. It may be a subtle manifestation of the disequilibrium syndrome. If there is severe headache, a neurologic cause (e.g., intracranial bleed precipitated by anticoagulation) should be investigated for. Paracetamol can be given during dialysis to treat headache.[13,16]

Itching

Itching is reported in dialysis patients. It may be related to hypersensitivity to dialyzer or components of the blood circuit. Signs of viral (or drug induced) hepatitis and scabies should also be looked for. Emollients and antihistaminics are beneficial. Adequacy of dialysis should be ensured. If related to disturbances in serum calcium, phosphorus, and parathormone (PTH) levels, these should be corrected. Gabapentin has been used successfully in some cases.

Dialyzer Reactions

Dialyzer reactions is of two types:

1. *Type A (anaphylactic type):* Dyspnea and a feeling of warmth at the fistula site or throughout the body are common presenting symptoms of a type A reaction.[13] Some cases may have milder symptoms such as itching, urticaria, cough, sneezing, coryza, abdominal cramping, or diarrhea. Most patients have symptoms within few minutes of initiation of HD, but occasionally these might be delayed up to half an hour. In the past, hypersensitivity reactions to ethylene oxide, used to sterilize dialyzers, was the dominant cause. Another described cause is AN69 (acrylonitrile-sodium methallyl sulfonate) dialysate membrane in patients receiving angiotensin-converting enzyme (ACE) inhibitors, due to activation of the bradykinin system. Dialysis solution contamination with bacteria and endotoxin, or anaphylaxis to heparin are also well described as causes of type A dialyzer reaction.

   If type A dialyzer reaction is suspected, one should stop dialysis immediately. Blood lines should be clamped and the dialyzer/blood lines should be discarded without returning the blood contained therein. Resuscitation may be required. Management with antihistamines, steroids, or epinephrine is recommended. If there is a history of anaphylaxis to an ethylene oxide–sterilized dialyzer, the dialyzer should be changed to a γ-irradiated, steam-sterilized, or electron beam–sterilized dialyzer.
2. *Nonspecific type B dialyzer reactions:* Chest pain, sometimes accompanied by back pain, is reported in this type of dialyzer reaction. These symptoms usually occur 20–40 minutes after the initiation of dialysis. They are much milder than type A reactions.[13,16]

   Complement activation might be involved in the pathogenesis of type B dialyzer reaction. Supportive management including oxygen administration should be provided. Dialysis can be continued, as symptoms are likely to subside after the initial hour. One can try a different dialyzer if problems persist.

Air Embolism

Air embolism is a life-threatening complication and should be identified early. It may manifest with altered sensorium, convulsions, dyspnea, cough, and chest pain or tightness or arrhythmias. Air entry can occur through the arterial needle, the pre-pump arterial tubing segment, and an inadvertently opened end of a central venous catheter.

For management, one should clamp the venous blood line and stop the blood pump. The patient should be immediately placed in a recumbent position on the left side with the chest and head tilted downward. Cardiorespiratory support including oxygenation should be provided. Cardiac catheterization or aspiration of air from the atrium or ventricle by trained specialists might be required in some cases.

Hemolysis

Acute hemolysis during dialysis may pose management challenges. Symptoms include back pain, pallor, chest tightness, and breathlessness. Port wine color of blood in the venous blood line might be noticed. A decrease in hemoglobin and hyperkalemia (due to release of potassium from red blood cells) can occur. Identifiable etiologies of acute hemolysis include:[13,16] (1) an obstruction or narrowing in the blood line, catheter, or needle; (2) overheated or hypotonic dialysis solution or contamination with formaldehyde, bleach, chloramine, copper, fluoride, nitrates, and fluorides; and (3) underlying disease, e.g., G6PD deficiency.

For management, the blood pump must be immediately stopped and clamping of the blood lines should be done. The hemolyzed blood is hyperkalemic and must not be returned to the patient. Hyperkalemia and drop in hematocrit should be managed appropriately. A complete blood count, methemoglobin level, reticulocyte count, and lactate dehydrogenase (LDH) should be obtained. Quality of the water used to prepare dialysate solution (chloramine, nitrates, metals) and the characteristics of the dialyzer should be additionally investigated.

Intradialytic or Paradoxical Hypertension

Intradialytic hypertension is rarely reported. The pathogenesis of intradialytic hypertension is complex. Reasons include the following:[16]

- Osmotic agents, e.g., sodium, mannitol, or concentrated albumin solutions, or high dialysate fluid sodium: These iatrogenically mobilize extracellular fluid.
- Failure to attain an optimal dry weight—excessive ultrafiltration might activate the renin-angiotensin system leading to vasoconstriction.
- Increased endothelin I production during HD in hypertensive patients has been noted. This has led to the theory of paradoxical hypertension resulting from an imbalance in nitric oxide and endothelin I production.
- Many antihypertensive drugs are removed by dialysis. For example, beta blockers, ACE inhibitors, minoxidil, nitroprusside, and diazoxide are removed during dialysis.

Intradialytic hypertension should be managed by further salt and fluid restriction, trying to decrease dialysate fluid sodium, using calcium channel blockers (that are not dialyzable) and renin-angiotensin system blockade with angiotensin receptor blockers (ARBs).

Other Complications

Other complications include LVH, myocardial stunning, endothelial dysfunction, atherosclerosis, arteriosclerosis, calcification, inflammation, malnutrition, dialysis-related carnitine disorder, and hyperhomocysteinemia.

- *Catheter-related bloodstream infections (CRBSIs):* These should be considered as an etiology of fever in febrile children with CKD having an HD catheter in situ. Patients with CRBSI clinically present with fever and rigors most commonly. Rarely, they may present with malaise, hypotension/shock, or exit site drainage. Inflammatory markers such as serum C-reactive protein and procalcitonin, along with other evidences such as neutrophilic leukocytosis, may be useful supportive evidence to support the diagnosis when CRBSI is suspected. When CRBSI is suspected, central and peripheral line blood cultures are taken. When both show growth of the same microorganism, CRBSI is confirmed. Majority of CRBSIs are due to a gram-positive organism, including coagulase-negative *Staphylococcus aureus* [including methicillin-resistant *S. aureus* (MRSA)] and *Enterococcus*. A significant proportion of CRBSIs are also accounted for by gram-negative bacteria. When CRBSI is suspected, broad-spectrum empirical antibiotic coverage for both gram-positive and gram-negative organisms (with drugs, e.g., vancomycin and ceftazidime/cefoperazone-sulbactam, based on institutional sensitivity patterns) should be started promptly after taking blood cultures.

Catheter-related blood stream infections can be classified into complicated and uncomplicated CRBSIs:

- A complicated CRBSI is defined as: (1) a CRBSI with hypotension, (2) persistent fever or positive blood culture results for >48 hours after initiation of appropriate antibiotics, (3) a CRBSI associated with thromboembolic events, and (4) a tunnel infection or port abscess.
- For uncomplicated CRBSI, treatment with sensitive antibiotics for appropriate duration (based on the microorganism isolated, e.g., *S. aureus* 4–6 weeks; gram-negative bacilli, *Candida*, *Enterococcus*—up to 2 weeks) is recommended and it is possible to retain and salvage the catheter. For complicated CRBSI (e.g., in situations such as shock, suppurative thrombophlebitis, endocarditis, osteomyelitis, or possible metastatic seeding), removal of the catheter along with sensitive antibiotics for appropriate duration (based on the microorganism isolated, as mentioned above) is advised.

SUPPORTIVE TREATMENT DURING HEMODIALYSIS

Management of Anemia

Anemia in CKD is defined as hemoglobin < 11 g/dL in children between 6 months and 5 years, <11.5 g/dL between 5 and 12 years, and <12 g/dL between 12 and 15 years. Between 15 and 18 years, anemia is defined as hemoglobin < 13 g/dL for males and <12 g/dL for females.[18] Erythropoietin deficiency and iron deficiency are the major causes of anemia in ESKD. Iron deficiency is also encountered in patients on HD due to blood loss from repeated sampling for laboratory investigations, blood loss through usage of dialyzers and dialysis tubings, B12 and folate deficiency, and an overall shortened lifespan of the red blood cells due to secondary carnitine deficiency. For the management of anemia, children on chronic HD require subcutaneous erythropoietin at doses ranging from 250 to 350 U/kg/week along with elemental iron (doses up to 6 mg/kg/day) orally (using formulations such as ferrous fumarate and colloidal iron) to maintain levels of serum ferritin at >100 ng/mL and transferrin saturation at >20%.[18]

Parenteral iron therapy is indicated if there is no improvement in the hemoglobin levels despite oral iron administration for 1 month in optimal doses, intolerance to oral iron therapy, need to rapidly increase iron levels on erythropoietin-stimulating agents (ESAs), and poor response to ESA with inadequate transferrin saturation (TSAT) levels despite adequate treatment with ESA and oral iron and exclusion of confounding factors (e.g., ongoing inflammation due to uremia, fluid overload, hyperparathyroidism leading to myelofibrosis).

Parenteral iron therapy is contraindicated in the presence of acute or chronic infection, known hypersensitivity, clinical or biochemical evidence of liver damage, and serum ferritin >500 ng/mL or TSAT > 50%. The dose of parenteral iron to be calculated (the iron deficit) is done using Ganzoni's formula [total dose of iron = body weight in kg × (target hemoglobin – actual hemoglobin) × 2.4 + iron stores]. The iron stores are assumed to be 15 mg/kg for children <35 kg, while children it is 500 mg in children >35 kg. The target hemoglobin is assumed to be 12 g/dL for calculation purposes generally. Iron sucrose is a commonly used preparation for parenteral iron therapy. It is diluted in normal saline to achieve a concentration of 1 mg/mL and thereafter infused slowly intravenously (at the calculated iron deficit dose) over 1 hour (during the last hour of HD through the venous limb of the HD circuit) under careful monitoring for anaphylactic reactions (which might occur most commonly over the first 15 minutes by which 25% of the calculated dose would have been infused). Iron dextran is not used commonly for parenteral iron therapy due to increased anaphylactic reactions, as a result of which iron sucrose and ferric gluconate are more commonly used.[18]

Management of Chronic Kidney Disease–Mineral Bone Disorder

For patients on chronic HD, management of CKD-mineral bone disorder (MBD) should be decided based on serial measurements of serum calcium, phosphate, and PTH levels considered together.[2,19] Serum 25-hydroxycholecalciferol levels should be measured annually.

Elevated phosphorus levels must be lowered toward the normal range by reducing dietary phosphorus (usage of the dietary "phosphorus pyramid" could be a useful approach to reduce dietary phosphorus intake), using phosphorus binders (e.g., calcium carbonate, calcium acetate, or sevelamer with food), and ensuring adequacy of dialysis. Patients on chronic HD should be managed with adequate dialysis to manage hyperphosphatemia, which could be ensured through increased time (4 hours per session) and frequency of dialysis (thrice a week). This would more effectively lower the serum phosphorus toward the normal range.

Calcitriol, vitamin D analogs, and calcium supplements (e.g., in the form of calcium carbonate) should be used to maintain serum calcium levels within the age-appropriate normal range. In patients on chronic HD, PTH levels should be maintained in the range of approximately two to nine times the upper normal of the reference range of the assay.[19]

Care should be taken to avoid hypercalcemia during therapy in children on chronic HD. The doses of calcium carbonate, calcitriol, or vitamin D analogs should be carefully titrated to avoid any hypercalcemia (serum calcium >11 mg/dL). In the event of hypercalcemia, calcium supplements, vitamin D analogs, calcitriol, and calcium-based potassium binders (e.g., calcium polystyrene sulfonate) should be temporarily withheld and the child can be dialyzed against low calcium dialysate (1.25 mmol/L) as against the usual practice of standard calcium dialysate (1.75 mmol/L). Calcitonin can be used as a temporary measure to lower serum calcium levels in this situation.

Tertiary hyperparathyroidism is an autonomous and advanced form of secondary hyperparathyroidism that is noted in patients with ESKD on long-term dialysis and can be managed with cinacalcet for parathyroidectomy.

Nutrition

Daily protein intake in CKD5D should be 100% of the dietary reference intake plus an allowance for dialytic protein and amino acid losses.[20] For children on HD, following protein intake is advised:

Up to 6 months—1.6 g/kg/day*
6–12 months—1.3 g/kg/day*
1–3 years—1.15 g/kg/day*
4–13 years—1.05 g/kg/day*
14–18 years—0.95 g/kg/day*
(*Plus 0.1 g/kg/day to compensate for dialytic losses)

Energy requirements should be 100% of the estimated energy requirements for chronological age, individually adjusted for BMI:

- Up to 6 months—108 kcal/kg/day
- 6 months to 1 year—98 kcal/kg/day
- 1-3 years—1,240 kcal/day
- 4-6 years—1,690 kcal/day
- 7-9 years—1,950 kcal/day

- 10–12 years (boys)—2,190 kcal/day; (girls)—1,970 kcal/day
- 13–15 years (boys)—2,450 kcal/day; (girls)—2,060 kcal/day
- 16–18 years (boys)—2,640 kcal/day; (girls)—2,060 kcal/day

Patients on HD are advised to take high-quality protein because it produces less uremic solutes for removal during dialysis. High-quality protein comes from meat, poultry, fish, and eggs. Patients on HD can be managed by usage of the dietary "phosphorus pyramid" which could be a useful approach to reduce dietary phosphorus intake. Avoiding processed meats, junk foods, colas, and canned foods, which have high amounts of sodium and phosphorus, is advised.[20] Restriction of potassium-rich foods, e.g., fruit juices, coconut water, bananas, is rational.

HEMODIALYSIS ADEQUACY

Clearance of small solutes is currently considered the recommended standard for the assessment of dialysis adequacy despite all its limitations. Small solute clearance has two perspectives—clearance from the perspective of the dialyzer and clearance from the perspective of the patient. The recommended indices of adequacy like *Kt/V* are patient perspectives of small solute clearance. Urea clearance is the standard measure for small solute clearance because urea, a small solute, is easily removed through conventional dialysis. It is easily measured and its levels correlate fairly with clinical symptoms.

Definition of Clearance

Clearance is defined as the extent to which the plasma is completely cleared of a particular solute during its passage through the dialyzer.[1] The reduction of any solute as it passes through the dialyzer (extraction ratio) is influenced by the BFR. The slower the BFR, the higher the contact time with the dialyzer and greater the extraction of the solute. For example, when the serum urea nitrogen (SUN) at the inlet is 200 mg/dL and at the outlet is 80 mg/dL, then the extraction ratio would be (200 – 80)/200 = 60%. The clearance achieved by the dialyzer could then be measured using the formula:

Dialyzer clearance (Kd) = BFR × extraction ratio/100

The clearance achieved by a particular dialyzer is influenced by the:

- BFR
- Dialyzer flow rate
- Hematocrit
- KoA of the dialyzer (mass transfer area coefficient)
- Efficiency and flux of the dialyzer
- Molecular weight of the solute

Measurement of Urea Removal

Mathematic modeling of the pre- and postdialysis urea concentration gives the best estimate of the average clearance during the dialysis session.[1,21] The predialysis sample is drawn before using saline, heparin, or any other potential diluents. The postdialysis urea measurement is done by a slow blood flow method or a stop-dialysate flow method. The slow-blood flow method involves slowing the blood flow to about 100 mL/min for 10–20 seconds at the end of the dialysis session when the postdialysis urea sample can be drawn. Alternately, the stop dialysate flow which consists of stopping the dialysate flow for about 3 minutes at the end of the dialysis session can be used.

Indices for Measurement of Urea Removal

Urea reduction ratio (URR):

URR = Predialysis SUN – postdialysis SUN

Predialysis serum urea nitrogen (SUN): For example, the predialysis SUN is 80 mg/dL and the postdialysis SUN is 20 mg/dL; then the URR is 0.75 or 75% if expressed as a percentage.

Although the URR is a simplistic method of estimation of the urea removal, it is quite erroneous in providing an accurate estimate of the urea clearance as it does not take two important factors into consideration—the volume of distribution and the urea generation rate.

Kt/V: This was introduced in the National Cooperative Dialysis Study (NCDS), which showed that a *Kt/V* urea of <0.8 was associated with high mortality.[21] *Kt/V* is a dimensionless value which represents the ratio of volume of urea cleared over a period of time (*Kt*) to the volume of distribution of urea.

As only a portion of the volume of distribution of urea is cleared at a given point in time and returned to the main pool, there is dilution of the urea in the pool. Also, a single pass through the dialyzer does not completely remove urea. Hence with time, lesser urea is removed with each subsequent pass through the dialyzer.

Also, urea is constantly being generated in the body and added to the pool, and this would influence the amount of urea during the dialysis session.

The calculation of *Kt/V* is typically based on the postdialysis calculation of *V*. However, the ultrafiltrate removed also contains urea and invariably the postdialysis *V* is less than the predialysis *V*. This component also should be considered in the calculation of solute clearance.

So, in reality, a *Kt/V* of 1 corresponds to a URR of 0.63. Taking the urea generation and ultrafiltration rate into account, the formula for assessment of *Kt/V* is

$$Kt/V = -\ln(R - 0.008 \times t) + (4 - 3.5 \times R) \times 0.55\ UF/V$$

where R is the ratio of postdialysis to predialysis SUN, t the length of the session in hours, UF the volume of fluid removed during the dialysis session (liters), and V the postdialysis urea distribution volume (liters). The term 0.008 × t adjusts for the urea generation.

Single-pool Kt/V: The single-pool *Kt/V* assumes that urea in the body is in a single compartment. However, urea is sequestered in tissues such as muscle, hence resulting in a relatively larger drop in urea from the smaller apparent volume of distribution in the early phase of dialysis. This is called urea inbound. Following dialysis, there is a rebound of urea from the tissues into the vascular space resulting in a urea rebound.

Equilibrated Kt/V: The equilibrated *Kt/V* accounts for the urea rebound. Equilibrated URR can be calculated by measuring the postdialysis urea after 30–60 minutes.

The equilibrated Kt/V can be measured using the formula:

$$eKt/V = spKt/V \times T_d/(T_d + 30.7), \text{ where } T_d \text{ is the dialysis time in minutes.}$$

The *Kt/V* is also modified by access recirculation. The impact of access recirculation on *Kt/V* can be reduced by slowing the BFR to 100 mL/min for 10–20 seconds. The dialysate flow can be stopped for 3 minutes to reduce the impact of access recirculation.

Case Vignette

A 7-year-old girl is on maintenance HD—4-hour sessions thrice a week. Her postdialysis weight is 19 kg and height is 119 cm. The predialysis SUN is 96 mg/dL and the postdialysis SUN is 16 mg/dL. The total ultrafiltration volume is 1.8 L. What is her *Kt/V*?

The volume of distribution (V) is calculated using Watson's formula:

Total body water (in males) = 2.447 − 0.09516 × age + 0.1074 × height + 0.3362 × weight

Total body water (in females) = 0 − 2.097 + 0.1069 × height + 0.2466 × weight

The total body water = 15.4 L

Single pool *Kt/V* = −ln (R − 0.008 × t) + (4 − 3.5 × R) × 0.55 UF/*V*

In this child, the URR = 96 − 16/96 = 83.3%

Sp*Kt/V* = *1.1*

Recommendations for Kt/V: The KDOQI guidelines (2015) recommend the ideal *Kt/V* urea of 1.4/session of HD and a minimum of 1.2/session in patients on thrice-weekly HD.[22] The URR is recommended to be maintained at >65%. In those with residual renal function (Kru), the dose of dialysis could be reduced to achieve a combined *Kt/V*; however, the Kru must be measured regularly.

The correlation of *Kt/V* urea with mortality has been shown in many observational studies and one controlled study. Although there is little evidence to show that a higher *Kt/V* is associated with better outcomes, the evidence for higher mortality associated with lower *Kt/V* is significant.

Drawbacks of Kt/V as a measure of adequacy:[23] Dialysis adequacy should be a comprehensive measure of the level of fluid control, BP control, control of metabolic parameters, and improvement in growth, nutrition, and quality of life. *Kt/V* alone is a poor indicator of dialysis adequacy. In addition, *Kt/V* may be influenced by the volume of distribution, and this will underestimate the *Kt/V* in children. The *Kt/V* urea measurement does not take into account the clearance of other uremic toxins and middle molecules. With the availability of newer modalities for dialysis like frequent dialysis and hemodiafiltration, the concept of *Kt/V* has become redundant.

Other measures of measuring clearance are as follows:

- Changes in dialysate conductance
- UV absorbance of spent dialysate

Kt/V in children:[24] There are several drawbacks in extrapolating these formulae and recommended levels to children. The optimum *Kt/V* target in children is not known. The volume of distribution is different in children; hence, normalizing to body surface area may provide a better measure of adequacy. The volume of distribution also varies with age. The protein intake and metabolic activity are not taken into account in the measurement of urea clearance.

There is little data on the *Kt/V* in children on HD. The NAPRTCS data showed that the target *Kt/V* was achieved in 75% of sessions. About 85% had an average *Kt/V* of >1.2 and URR > 65%. *Kt/V* was lower than the recommended level in infants, blacks, children in the early phase of dialysis and in those with higher BMI scores.[25]

Potential Measures to Achieve Adequate Dialysis

In the presence of a low Sp*Kt/V* or other measures of dialysis adequacy, the potential measures that can be undertaken to improve the adequacy of dialysis are as follows:

- *Increasing the duration of dialysis:* Increase in duration of dialysis increases middle molecule clearance and enhances fluid removal.
- Increase in frequency of dialysis
- Incremental dialysis
- Preservation of residual renal function

CONCLUSION

Hemodialysis is an important modality of dialysis in children with end-stage kidney disease. Obtaining a good vascular access, providing the optimal prescription for dialysis, and being equipped to manage the complications of HD are important for a successful dialysis program.

KEY POINTS

- HD is an important modality of kidney replacement therapy in children with end-stage kidney disease.
- AVF is the vascular access of choice even in children. However, temporary catheters and permcaths continue to be used as short-term access and in younger children.
- The prescription for pediatric dialysis is based on the size and weight of the child.
- Comprehensive management of a child on HD includes not only the dialysis prescription but also the management

of associated complications such as anemia, mineral bone disease, and nutrition.

- Adequacy on HD is measured not only by a *Kt/V* value but also fluid management, nutrition, growth, control of metabolic parameters, and quality of life.

REFERENCES

1. Daugirdas JT. Physiologic principles and urea kinetic modeling. In: Daugirdas JT, Blake PG, Ing TS (Eds). Handbook of Dialysis, 5th edition. Philadelphia, PA: Wolters Kluwer Health; 2015. pp. 34-65.
2. Indian Society of Nephrology guidelines for hemodialysis units. Indian J Nephrol. 2012;22(Suppl):S1-S46.
3. Chand DH, Valentini RP, Kamil ES. Hemodialysis vascular access options in pediatrics: considerations for patients and practitioners. Pediatr Nephrol. 2009;24:1121-28.
4. Shroff R, Calder F, Bakkaloğlu S, Nagler EV, Stuart S, Stronach L, et al.; European Society for Paediatric Nephrology Dialysis Working Group. Vascular access in children requiring maintenance haemodialysis: a consensus document by the European Society for Paediatric Nephrology Dialysis Working Group. Nephrol Dial Transplant. 2019;34(10):1746-65.
5. National Kidney Foundation. 2006 NKF-K/DOQI clinical practice guidelines for vascular access: update 2006. Am J Kidney Dis. 2006;48(Suppl 1):S177-S277.
6. American Nephrology Nurses' Association. "Save the Vein" project. [online]. Available from http://www.annanurse.org/resources/save-the-vein-campaign. [Last accessed March, 2022].
7. Fistula First Initiative. Available from http://www.fistulafirst.org. [Last accessed September, 2020].
8. Kim SM, Min SK, Ahn S, Min SI, Ha J. Outcomes of arteriovenous fistula for hemodialysis in pediatric and adolescent patients. Vasc Specialist Int. 2016;32:113-8.
9. Shroff R, Sterenborg RB, Kuchta A, Arnold A, Thomas N, Stronach L, et al. A dedicated vascular access clinic for children on haemodialysis: two years' experience. Pediatr Nephrol. 2016;31:2337-44.
10. Kaspar CD, Bholah R, Bunchman TE. A review of pediatric chronic kidney disease. Blood Purif. 2016;41(1-3):211-7.
11. Chan CT, Blankestijn PJ, Dember LM, Gallieni M, Harris DCH, Lok CE, et al.; Conference Participants. Dialysis initiation, modality choice, access, and prescription: conclusions from a Kidney Disease: Improving Global Outcomes (KDIGO) Controversies Conference. Kidney Int. 2019;96(1):37-47.
12. Ahmad S, Misra M, Hoenich N, Daugirdas JT. Hemodialysis apparatus. In: Daugirdas JT, Blake PG, Ing TS (Eds). Handbook of Dialysis, 5th edition. Philadelphia, PA: Wolters Kluwer Health; 2015. pp. 82-98.
13. Hothi DK, Laskin B, Geary DF. Pediatric hemodialysis prescription, complications, and future directions. In: Geary DF, Schaefer F (Eds). Pediatric Kidney Disease. Berlin, Heidelberg: Springer-Verlag; 2016. pp. 1725-65.
14. Rees L. Hemodialysis in children. In: Avner ED, Harmon WE, Niaudet P, Yoshikawa N, Emma F, Goldstein SL (Eds). Pediatric Nephrology, 7th edition. Berlin, Heidelberg: Springer-Verlag; 2016. pp. 2433-56.
15. Ross EA, Nissenson AR, Daugirdas JT. Acute hemodialysis prescription. In: Daugirdas JT, Blake PG, Ing TS (Eds). Handbook of Dialysis, 5th edition. Philadelphia, PA: Wolters Kluwer Health; 2015. pp. 172-91.
16. Sherman RA, Daugirdas JT, Ing TS. Complications during hemodialysis. In: Daugirdas JT, Blake PG, Ing TS (Eds). Handbook of Dialysis, 5th edition. Philadelphia, PA: Wolters Kluwer Health; 2015. pp. 215-36.
17. Jörres A, John S, Lewington A, ter Wee PM, Vanholder R, Biesen WV, et al.; The Ad-hoc Working Group of ERBP. A European Renal Best Practice (ERBP) position statement on the Kidney Disease Improving Global Outcomes (KDIGO) clinical practice guidelines on acute kidney injury: part 2: renal replacement therapy. Nephrol Dial Transplant. 2013;28:2940-5.
18. KDIGO Anemia Work Group. KDIGO clinical practice guideline for anemia in chronic kidney disease. Kidney Int Suppl. 2012;2(4):279-335.
19. Kidney Disease: Improving Global Outcomes (KDIGO) CKD-MBD Update Work Group. KDIGO 2017 clinical practice guideline update for the diagnosis, evaluation, prevention, and treatment of chronic kidney disease-mineral and bone disorder (CKD-MBD). Kidney Int Suppl. 2017;7:1-59.
20. Ikizler TA, Burrowes JD, Byham-Gray LD, Campbell KL, Carrero JJ, Chan W, et al.; KDOQI Nutrition in CKD Guideline Work Group. KDOQI clinical practice guideline for nutrition in CKD: 2020 update. Am J Kidney Dis. 2020;76(3 Suppl 1):S1-S107.
21. Daugirdas JT. Kt/V (and especially its modifications) remains a useful measure of hemodialysis dose. Kidney Int. 2015;88(3): 466-73.
22. National Kidney Foundation. KDOQI clinical practice guideline for hemodialysis adequacy: 2015 update. Am J Kidney Dis. 2015;66(5):884-930. [Erratum in: Am J Kidney Dis. 2016; 67(3): 534.]
23. Vanholder R, Van Biesen W, Lameire N. A swan song for Kt/Vurea. Semin Dial. 2019;32(5):424-37.
24. Rees L. Assessment of dialysis adequacy: beyond urea kinetic measurements. Pediatr Nephrol. 2019;34(1):61-9.
25. Perl J, Dember LM, Bargman JM, Browne T, Charytan DM, Flythe JE, et al.; American Society of Nephrology Dialysis Advisory Group. The use of a multidimensional measure of dialysis adequacy-moving beyond small solute kinetics. Clin J Am Soc Nephrol. 2017;12(5):839-47.

CHAPTER

12.7

Kidney Replacement Therapy: Transplantation

Arpana A Iyengar, Arvind Bagga

INTRODUCTION

Renal transplantation is the therapy of choice for children with end-stage kidney disease (ESKD). A successful renal transplantation provides better quality of life and a lower risk of morbidity and mortality compared to dialysis therapy. Patient and graft survival have significantly improved over the decades with changes in immunosuppressive protocols, operative techniques, and strategies for infection prophylaxis and monitoring. This chapter provides a description of indications, immunobiology, evaluation, monitoring, complications, management, and outcomes of transplantation in children.

CAUSES OF END-STAGE KIDNEY DISEASE AND INDICATIONS FOR TRANSPLANTATION

Congenital abnormalities of the kidney and urinary tract account for 40% children who need transplantation followed by chronic glomerulonephritis and focal segmental glomerulosclerosis (FSGS). Polycystic kidney diseases, nephronophthisis, Alport syndrome, congenital nephrotic syndrome, cystinosis, and oxalosis make up for the rest of the causes of ESKD.[1,2] A study from a tertiary care center in India found a high prevalence of neurogenic bladder among patients with chronic kidney disease (CKD).[3]

The pediatric committee of the American Society of Transplant Physicians defines the indications for kidney transplantation in children as follows:[4]

- Symptoms of uremia not responsive to standard therapy
- Failure to thrive because of limited caloric intake
- Delayed psychomotor development, and poor control of comorbidities, including hypervolemia, hyperkalemia, and metabolic bone disease.

Contraindications include the presence of untreated malignancy, active infections, chronic infection with human immunodeficiency virus (HIV) or hepatitis B or C, and progressive neurological disease. A multidisciplinary team should carefully evaluate the option of transplantation in children with multiple congenital anomalies and severe mental retardation, with consent from ethicists and informed inputs from parents. Socioeconomic factors should be considered carefully before preparing infants and children for transplantation.[5] In preemptive transplantation, renal transplantation is undertaken without initiation of dialysis and is an ideal treatment option in children with good long-term outcomes. Dialysis vintage of 12–18 months has a higher risk of allograft failure and mortality compared to those undergoing preemptive kidney transplantation.[6]

TRANSPLANT IMMUNOBIOLOGY

Three types of immunity are activated during transplantation **(Flowchart 1)**. Innate immunity (type I immunity) is the first line of defense that includes the activation of cells such as dendritic cells and macrophages along with vascular endothelial cells. Mediators such as interleukin-1 (IL-1) and IL-6 and tumor necrosis factor-α (TNF-α) come into play, and specific receptors such as damage-associated molecular patterns (DAMP) and pathogen-associated molecular patterns (PAMP) are expressed as a part of innate immunity. Adaptive immunity (type II immunity) includes activation of major histocompatibility complex (MHC) class I or II based on the type of antigen protein that leads to T-cell activation with

Flowchart 1: Immunity in transplantation.

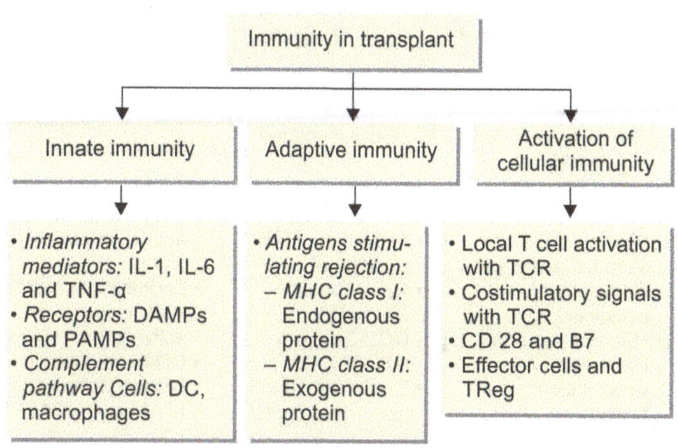

(CD: cluster of differentiation; DAMP: damage-associated molecular patterns; DC: dendritic cells; IL-1: interleukin-1; IL-6: interleukin-6; MHC: major histocompatibility complex; PAMP: pathogen-associated molecular patterns; TCR: T-cell receptor; TNF: tumor necrosis factor; TReg: T regulatory cell)

T-cell receptor. Costimulatory signals CD28 and B7 activate effector cells Th1, Th2 and T-regulatory cells. After the initial trauma and placement of the graft, there is activation of antigen-presenting cells (direct or indirect presentation) followed by activation of T cell by T-cell receptor. All three types of T-cell immunity get activated (Th1, Th2, and Th17). The stages of immune activation are illustrated in **Flowchart 2**. Unchecked migration of activated T cells can result in graft rejection.[7-9]

As depicted in **Flowchart 3**, in T cell-mediated rejection, based on endogenous or exogenous protein activation of MHC class I or II, respectively, the T-cell receptor gets activated by CTL-CD8 resulting in the generation of CCL-3, CCL-5, and CX3CL1 chemokines (type III immunity). These recruit T cells that release mediators such as interferon gamma, IL-17, and TNF-α or -β. In antibody-mediated rejection (ABMR), based on the circulating donor-specific antibody or in vivo antibody, binding to endothelial antigen results in activation of complement pathways and infiltration of macrophages and neutrophils that predispose to thrombus formation. Vascular rejection is also mediated by MHC class I or II, which results in interactions between the endothelium and polymorphonuclear neutrophils resulting in intimal or transmural arteritis.[10-12]

Flowchart 2: Stages of immunity activation in transplantation: After the initial trauma and placement of the graft, there is activation of antigen-presenting cells (direct or indirect presentation) followed by activation of T cell by T-cell receptor. Three types of T cell immunity will be activated (T1, T2, and Th17). Unchecked migration of activated T cells can result in graft rejection.

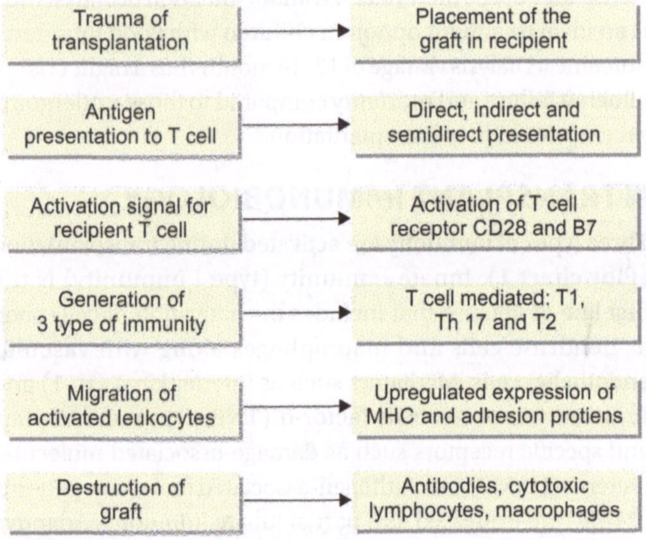

(CD: cluster of differentiation; MHC: major histocompatibility complex; Th: T helper cell)
Source: Adapted from reference 12.

Flowchart 3: Immune system activation in various types of rejection.

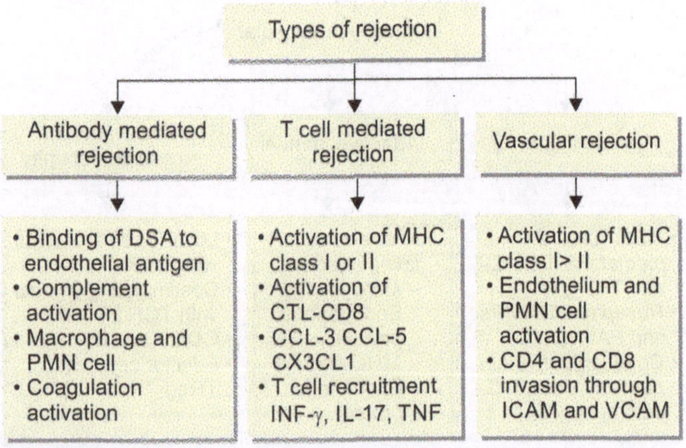

(CCL: CC chemokine ligand; CD: cluster of differentiation; CTL: cytotoxic T cell; CX3CL: chemokine with C-X3-C motif; ICAM: intercellular adhesion molecule; IL: interleukin; INF: interferon; MHC: major histocompatibility complex; PMN: polymorphonuclear cell; TCR: T-cell receptor; TNF: tumor necrosis factor; VCAM: vascular cell adhesion)

PRETRANSPLANT EVALUATION

The challenge of late detection of CKD and its comorbidities still exists as studies have observed one-third of children presenting for the first time to the nephrologist in stages III/IV with 25% already being in stage V. This is a barrier to optimal pretransplant preparation.[3,13] Pretransplant evaluation is performed to make sure that the child can bear the surgical stress and identify any contraindications to transplantation. Evaluation includes immune evaluation with human leukocyte antigen (HLA) and cross-matching, and optimization of anemia, cardiac function, bone disease, and nutritional status.

After clinical examination, a number of tests are performed, including blood group, HLA typing (A, B, and DR), and preformed cytotoxic antibodies. The absolute requirements for a transplant are a compatible blood group and a negative cytotoxic cross-match. Serology for hepatitis (B and C) virus, HIV, cytomegalovirus (CMV), Epstein-Barr virus (EBV), varicella, and syphilis is mandatory. A chest X-ray film, electrocardiogram, and echocardiogram are obtained to rule out tuberculosis and cardiac lesions.

Urological Interventions

Evaluation of the lower urinary tract is required in patients with congenital anomalies of the kidney and urinary tract with or without obstruction. A renal ultrasound and voiding cystourethrography are mandatory to assess the lower urinary tract. When indicated, bladder evaluation requires cystoscopy and urodynamic studies. Children with small bladder capacity benefit with use of medications that result in relaxation of the detrusor muscle. Many patients require clean intermittent catheterization (CIC) of native bladders before and following transplantation. Bladder capacity is increased by its augmentation with segments of ileum, stomach, or appendix and creation of a permanent cutaneous conduit (Mitrofanoff) that enables the child to be continent with timely drainage through CIC.

Vesicoureteral reflux (VUR) post-transplant may contribute to urinary tract infections (UTIs), especially when associated with voiding dysfunction. However, in the post-transplant period, the presence of reflux per se without voiding dysfunction does not correlate with subsequent graft function, hypertension, or rejection. In patients with VUR, evaluation of the bladder for obstruction, spasticity, and function is required. If the native ureters have not been reimplanted, both native dilated ureters can serve as vascularized patch grafts for augmentation cystoplasty. Transplant outcomes in patients with high-grade reflux may be disappointing due to postoperative UTIs. Reimplantation prior to transplant can cause perivesical changes that could complicate the planned transplant surgery.[14]

Indications for pretransplant nephrectomy include the need for space to place the allograft (polycystic enlarged kidneys, small child receiving an adult kidney), massive proteinuria (congenital nephrotic syndrome), uncontrolled hypertension, recurrent pyelonephritis, severe polyuria (better volume control immediately post-transplant), and malignancy.

Vaccination

Potential recipients should receive all age-appropriate immunizations, including hepatitis A and B, pneumococcal, and varicella vaccinations.[15,16] Live vaccines should be given at least 4 weeks prior to transplantation. Inactivated or killed vaccines can be administered 3–6 months post-transplantation.

Human Leukocyte Antigens Typing and Cross-matching

The ABO blood group and HLA are important for the survival of the transplanted grafts. ABO blood group antigens are expressed on the endothelial cells. In the presence of ABO incompatibility, naturally present antibodies to these antigens may attach to antigens on the graft endothelium to cause hyperacute rejection and irreversible graft loss. Genetic differences between individuals are determined by differences in the composition of the MHC, also known as HLA. Since HLA class I (A, B, and C) antigens are present on all nucleated cells, red cells lack these antigens. HLA class II (DR, DQ, and DP) antigens are present on macrophages, dendritic cells, B cells, activated T lymphocytes, and tubular epithelial and endothelial cells. These antigens are expressed codominantly, with each individual inheriting one haplotype from each parent. HLA mismatches refer to a number of nonshared HLA antigens between the donor and recipient. Children are one-haplotype matched with their parents, while siblings can be completely matched, one-haplotype matched, or completely mismatched, depending upon haplotype recombination.

There are three main types of cross-match tests that are important for pretransplant preparation: complement-dependent cytotoxicity (CDC), CDC-antihuman globulin HLA, and flow cytometry. The details of these investigations, including the risk of rejection, are given in **Table 1**.[17,18] The immunological risk of transplant is considered as "high risk" when the cross-match is positive by all three methods, "intermediate risk" when flow cytometry and Luminex single antigen bead (SAB) cross-match are positive, and "standard risk" when only Luminex SAB is positive. Least risk is considered when all the methods are negative.

The three methods of cross-match for donor-specific antibodies are CDC, CDC antihuman globulin, and flow cytometry. The type of antibody detected by each of this method has been depicted in **Table 1**. In addition, the immunological risk of transplant based on cross-match methods is highlighted.

Human Leukocyte Antigens and ABO Incompatibility

Human leukocyte antigen-DR, HLA-A, and HLA-B are important factors that influence post-transplant outcomes. Children may be sensitized (positive flow cytometry cross-match or positive complement-dependent cytotoxic cross-match) as a consequence of repeated blood transfusions, infections, and previous event of renal transplantation. Rh matching is usually not a requirement for successful

TABLE 1: Types of cross-matching and immunological risk of transplant.

Parameters measured	*Complement-dependent cytotoxicity (CDC)*	*CDC-antihuman globulin*	*Flow cytometry*
HLA antibodies	Yes	Yes	Yes
Non-HLA antibodies	Yes	Yes	Yes
IgM antibodies	Yes	Yes	No
Antibody titer detected	Moderate to high	Moderate to low	Low
Low antibody titers detected	No	Some extent	Yes
Risk of rejection: • *High* • *Intermediate* • *Standard* • *Least risk*	 + – – –	 + – – –	 + + – (Luminex+) –

(HLA: human leukocyte antigen)

transplantation. While ABO compatibility between donor and recipient is considered a prerequisite for successful transplantation, ABO-incompatible transplantations are often performed following desensitization with plasmapheresis, and therapy with intravenous immunoglobulin (IVIg) and anti-CD20 monoclonal antibodies.[19,20]

Pretransplant Counseling

Families of recipients and donors need to be counseled regarding the risks of surgery and the need for lifelong follow-up. Patients are counseled regarding the risks of graft dysfunction, infections, and importance of adherence to medications.

Diseases such as FSGS and atypical hemolytic uremic syndrome may recur post-transplantation. Cardiac, pulmonary, dental, and psychological evaluation may be required depending upon comorbidities. Growth and nutrition should be optimized as both malnutrition and obesity predispose to post-transplant complications. Clinical practice guidelines on the process of transplant evaluation are provided by Kidney Disease: Improving Global Outcomes (KDIGO).[21,22]

Intra- and Perioperative Issues

In infants and young children, the allograft is placed intra-abdominally. The renal artery is anastomosed to the aorta and renal vein to the inferior vena cava **(Fig. 1)**. In children weighing more than 30 kg, the graft is placed in the iliac fossa and renal artery and vein are connected to the common or external iliac artery and vein, respectively.[10] Meticulous attention to the technique of vascular anastomosis has decreased allograft loss secondary to renal arterial and venous thrombosis. The ureter is anastomosed to the bladder using ureteroneocystostomy. Attention should be paid to preserve the arterial supply to the lower segment of the ureter that originates from the iliac vessels; interruption of blood supply results in ischemia of this segment and causes ureteral obstruction or urinary leaks.

Children need attention with regard to maintenance of hemodynamic stability during the intraoperative and perioperative periods.[11,12] Intraoperative medical management includes close attention to fluid therapy, administration of immunosuppressive medication, diuretics, and antibiotics. Central venous pressure should be maintained at 10–15 cm of water before the aortic cross-clamps are removed to ensure good blood flow to the allograft. The adult kidney can contain up to 250 mL of blood, which may represent a large percentage of total blood volume in an infant or a small child. A low circulatory state can promote thrombosis of the allograft. Mannitol 20% (0.5–1 g/kg) and 1–2 mg/kg of furosemide may be given if there is a need to induce osmotic diuresis.

POSTOPERATIVE MANAGEMENT

Postoperative management includes close monitoring of fluid and electrolytes, immunosuppressive therapy, and anti-infective prophylaxis. In living-related transplants, the allograft kidney begins making urine almost immediately. Fluid and electrolyte management includes replacement of insensible losses with 5% dextrose and urine output with a fluid comparable in electrolyte composition to that of urine. Generally, normal saline is a good replacement fluid. Close monitoring of serum electrolytes every 8 hourly/12 hourly is mandatory for further adjustments. Central venous pressure should be kept at 5–10 cm of water. A urinary catheter is left in place for 4–5 days. Antibiotic prophylaxis is given for 48–96 hours. A summary of the medical and surgical perioperative protocol is given in **Box 1**.

Immunosuppression

The aim of immunosuppressive therapy in transplant recipients is to prevent or reduce sensitization to the allograft. This must be accomplished with constant attention to maintaining a balance in immunosuppression. Excess therapy results in increased risk of infection and malignancy, while inadequate immunosuppression results in allograft rejection. Immunosuppression is initiated at the time of transplant

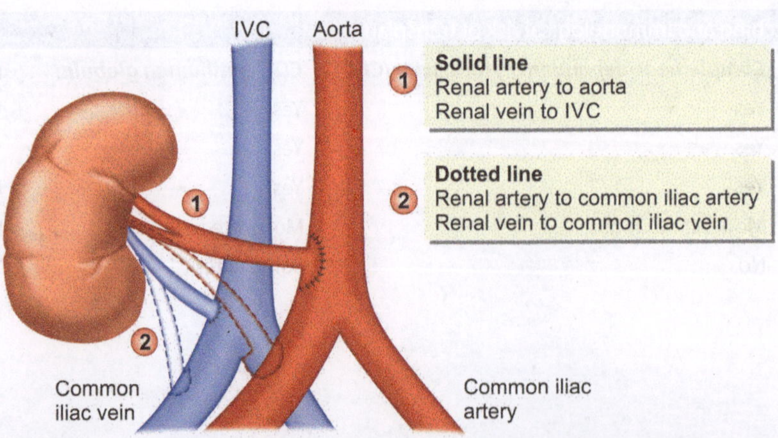

Fig. 1: Vascular anastomoses in young children and infants (1) and in older children (2). (IVC: inferior vena cava).

BOX 1: Intraoperative medical and surgical details during transplantation.

Medical

Intraoperative

Before release of clamps:

- Maintain central venous pressure (CVP) 13–15 cm; mean arterial pressure >60 mm Hg
- Close monitoring of hemoglobin, pH, bicarbonate, and electrolytes
- Administer packed cells (with leukoreduction filter); bicarbonate infusion and dobutamine as required
- *Administer fluids:* Normal saline or Ringer lactate to maintain blood pressure, CVP
- Flush kidney with normal saline
- IV Furosemide 1 mg/kg just before release of clamp (if risk for delayed graft function)

After release of clamps:

- Hemodynamic status maintained by fluids and inotropes (rarely required, unless complicated)
- Fluids to match urine output
- IV heparin infusion 5 U/kg/h; maintain activated clotting time ~150–200 seconds

Postoperative

- Fluid replacement (Type of fluid: normal saline; General protocol: if urine output is <100 mL/h-replacement fluid is urine output + 100 mL; if urine output is between 100 and 500 mL/h, replacement fluid is equal to urine output and if urine output is >100 mL/h, replacement fluid is urine output – 100 mL) is based on urine output
- Maintain blood pressure in the higher range of normal for adequate perfusion of allograft
- Triple immunosuppression with calcineurin inhibitor, mycophenolate mofetil, and corticosteroids

Surgical

- Intraperitoneal approach; midline incision
- Native kidney nephrectomy (specific indications; usually not necessary)
- *Vascular anastomosis:* Donor renal artery and vein, to patient aorta and vena cava/common iliac vein
- Transplant ureter implanted by submucosal tunnel technique (avoids distal ureteric necrosis)
- Closure of abdomen with fascia to avoid compression on adult kidney

surgery (induction) and continues through the life of the allograft. The mechanism of action of various medications is shown in **Figure 2.**[23] The immunosuppressive protocols as summarized in **Table 2** are discussed here.[9,24]

Induction Therapy

Induction therapy is used to deplete or modulate T-cell responses at the time of antigen presentation; decrease incidence, frequency, and severity of acute rejection; improve survival of the allograft; and perhaps reduce subsequent immunosuppression. The initial immunosuppression should be appropriate enough to avoid rejection, particularly in patients at high risk. Induction agents include antithymocyte globulin (ATG) and interleukin-2 receptor (IL2R) antibodies.

Interleukin-2 receptor antagonists (basiliximab) are nonlymphocyte depleting agents that inhibit proliferation

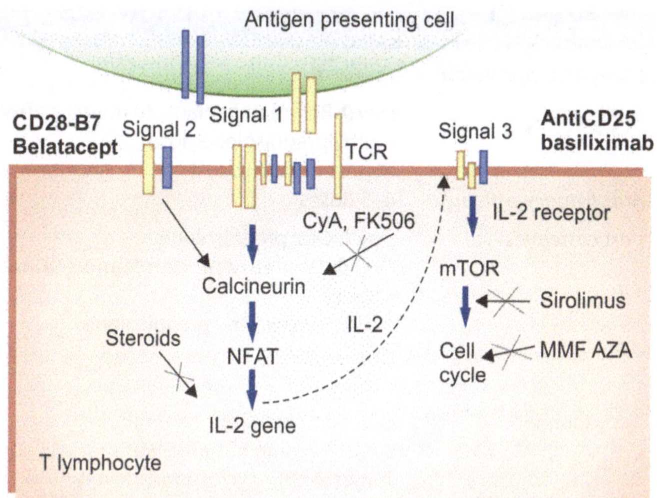

Fig. 2: T-cell activation and mechanism of action of immunosuppressive medications. Alloantigen, presented by the recipient antigen-presenting cells, is recognized by the T-cell receptor (TCR). Three signals are necessary for alloantigen-mediated activation of T cells. CyA (cyclosporine) and FK506 (tacrolimus) inhibit calcium-activated calcineurin, blocking activation of nuclear factor of activated T cells (NFAT) and synthesis of IL-2 (interleukin-2) (signal 1 blockade). Steroids directly inhibit IL-2 synthesis and also have inhibitory action on antigen-presenting cell function. Basiliximab inhibits binding of IL-2 to its receptor (IL-2R) (signal 3 blockade). Rapamycin binds to mammalian target of rapamycin (mTOR) and blocks the cell cycle after IL-2 binds to IL-2R. Mycophenolate mofetil (MMF) and azathioprine (AZA) inhibit purine synthesis, which is necessary for cell division.
Source: Adapted from reference 23.

of activated T and B lymphocytes. Hypersensitivity reactions need to be monitored. Antithymocyte thymoglobulin (thymoglobulin, rabbit; ATGAM, horse) is a polyclonal lymphocyte-depleting agent that targets the HLA and other immune cell receptors resulting in cellular inactivation and depletion. Infusion-related reactions, leukopenia, and thrombocytopenia are common side effects. Alemtuzumab (Campath-1H) is a monoclonal agent targeting CD52 receptors, resulting in depletion of T and B cells.

Infants and young children have relatively strong immune reactions, show rapid clearance of medications, and might benefit from induction therapies. In low-risk individuals (first transplant, unsensitized recipients), most centers prefer to use either no induction or IL2R antibodies (basiliximab). Induction with basiliximab is extended in steroid avoidance protocols. Polyclonal antibody (thymoglobulin, ATG) is used in high-risk recipients, such as highly sensitized patients, retransplants, and patients with delayed graft function. These agents, including alemtuzumab, are also part of steroid withdrawal and immunosuppression-minimization protocols.

Steroid Avoidance

Long-term adverse effects of steroids have resulted in steroid-avoidance trials, especially in children. The KDIGO guidelines recommended that steroids can be discontinued in the 1st week of transplant in those with low risk and if the induction therapy was administered.[25] However, there is wide

TABLE 2: Immunosuppressant protocol.

Immunosuppression	Protocol	Dose
Basiliximab	*Day 0:* Before transplant; 30 minutes after methylprednisolone dose Repeat dose on day 4	12 mg/m²; IV infusion over 30 minutes <30 kg: 10 mg; >30 kg: 20 mg
Antithymocyte globulin	4–5 doses	1.5 mg/kg
Corticosteroids	*Day 1:* Oral prednisolone *Day 0:* IV methylprednisolone ~90 minutes before surgery *Day 1 onward:* Oral prednisolone	60 mg/m² 10 mg/kg 60–30 mg/m²/day till day 30 30–15 mg/m² till day 60 15–7.5 mg/m² till 6 months, taper
*Cyclosporine**	*Day 1 onward:* Oral *Day 0:* Evening of transplant Target 2-hour cyclosporine levels *0–3 months:* 1,000–1,200 ng/mL *3–12 months:* 800–1000 ng/mL *>12 months:* 600–800 ng/mL	6–8 mg/kg/day in two divided doses Dose titrated to 2-hour drug levels
Tacrolimus†	*Day 1 onward:* Oral *Day 0:* Evening of transplant Target trough tacrolimus levels *0–3 months:* 10–12 ng/mL *3–12 months:* 8–10 ng/mL *>12 months:* 5–8 ng/mL	0.1–0.15 mg/kg/dose twice a day Dose titrated to trough levels
Mycophenolate mofetil	Day 1 onward: Oral	600 mg/m²/dose Reduced by 50% if receiving tacrolimus

*C-2 level: First month: 1,500–2,000 ng/mL, 1–3 months: 1,300–1,500 ng/mL; 4–6 months: 1,100 ng/mL; 7–12 months: 900 ng/mL; later 800 ng/mL.
†Tacrolimus 12-hour trough level: First 2 months: 10–12 ng/mL; 3–6 months: 8–10 ng/mL; later 4–7 ng/mL.

variability in the use of such protocols across centers.[26] Early steroid withdrawal or avoidance is generally used following the induction therapy with mono- or polyclonal antibodies, while late steroid withdrawal is undertaken when no induction therapy was used. Protocols of steroid minimization show growth-related benefit only in prepubertal patients.[27] Steroid avoidance in pediatric kidney transplanted children is effective in terms of graft outcomes during the 1st year following transplantation with limited adverse effects.[28]

POST-TRANSPLANT COMPLICATIONS

Delayed Graft Function

Delayed graft function is empirically defined as the need for dialysis in the first 7 days following transplantation; the condition is more common in deceased donor compared to live donor transplants.[29] Delayed graft function has detrimental consequences on the graft, including the risk of acute rejection and lower graft survival. Intradialytic hypotension and thrombosis can potentially affect graft survival.[30] The overall incidence of delayed graft function in live-related transplantation is 1-4%, while it is 5-50% in deceased donor transplantation.[31]

The underlying pathophysiology of delayed graft function is due to ischemia (before or during organ procurement), which is aggravated by the reperfusion injury during implantation of the harvested organ in the recipient. There is tissue injury due to stimulation of various factors, for example, inducible nitric oxide synthase, anaerobic metabolism with depletion of adenosine triphosphate (ATP) that results in the generation of reactive oxygen species resulting in the tissue injury.[32] There is inflammatory cell infiltration that releases mediators, which further aggravates the injury. The consequences are detrimental and can result in acute rejection to compromised long-term graft survival.

Surgical Complications

These include lymphocele, perirenal serous fluid collection, hematoma, urinary leaks, and ureterovesical junction obstruction. Usually, no therapy is needed. If perirenal fluid collection is massive or causing pressure on the transplant kidney, percutaneous aspiration may be needed. Ureteral stents are used for the prevention and treatment of ureterovesical junction obstruction. Vascular complications include renal arterial and venous thrombosis, which are particularly common in infants and small children because of the small size of the vessels. Attention to technical details and prevention of postoperative dehydration helps prevent these complications.

Acute Rejection

Acute deterioration in kidney allograft function is associated with specific pathologic changes in the graft. Acute rejection is of two types: ABMR and T-cell mediated rejection (TCMR). Features of ABMR, TCMR, and vascular rejection are illustrated in **Flowchart 3**. Hyperacute rejection could happen within minutes after the transplant due to preformed antibody or ABO incompatibility. Presence of circulating donor-specific alloantibodies, inflammation of glomeruli (glomerulitis), or peritubular capillary (peritubular capillaritis) are hallmarks of ABMR. Lymphocytic infiltration of the tubules, interstitium, and occasionally the arterial intima is characteristic of TCMR.[33]

Screening for rejection is done by conventional methods of measuring serum creatinine, estimated glomerular filtration rate (eGFR), and quantification of protein excretion. Periodic screening for polyomavirus and EBV is indicated. Renal biopsy is undertaken in the event of a rise of serum creatinine. Post-transplant HLA alloantibody screening is used to characterize the type of acute rejection.

Recently, noninvasive biomarkers for diagnosis of rejection have emerged that include—omics technologies, detection of cell-free DNA, urinary chemokines, C3 gene polymorphism for ABMR, ATP generation by CD4 lymphocytes, peripheral blood and leukocyte gene expression, and micro-RNA assays.[34]

The Banff classification for rejection includes six categories of diagnosis:[35,36] (1) normal biopsy or nonspecific changes, (2) antibody-mediated changes, (3) borderline acute TCMR, (4) TCMR, (5) interstitial fibrosis and tubular atrophy, and (6) other nonrejection changes.

Banff classification for ABMR:

- *Active ABMR morphology:* Microvascular inflammation, intimal arteritis; *Immunology*: Linear C4d staining in peritubular capillaries; *Serology*: Donor-specific antibodies **(Figs. 3A and B)**.
- *Chronic active ABMR morphology:* Transplant glomerulopathy, peritubular capillary basement membrane multilayering, and intimal fibrosis; *Immunology:* Linear C4d staining in peritubular capillaries; *Serology:* Donor-specific antibodies **(Fig. 3B)**.
- *Chronic ABMR morphology:* Transplant glomerulopathy, peritubular capillary basement membrane multilayering, and intimal fibrosis; *Immunology:* Prior diagnosis of active or chronic active ABMR; *Serology:* Donor-specific antibodies.

BANFF CLASSIFICATION FOR T CELL-MEDIATED REJECTION

Active TCMR 1A—moderate tubulitis with interstitial inflammation; 1B—severe tubulitis with interstitial inflammation; 2A—mild-to-moderate intimal arteritis; 2B—severe intimal arteritis; 3 transmural arteritis with/without fibrinoid necrosis **(Fig. 4)**.

Chronic active TCMR 1A—moderate tubulitis with cortical inflammation; 1B—severe tubulitis with cortical inflammation; 2—arterial intimal fibrosis with mononuclear cell inflammation **(Fig. 4)**.

The reader is directed to recent reviews for details on management of acute rejection. A summary of therapies is given in **Table 3**.[37,38]

Chronic Rejection

This is defined as impaired graft function of at least 3 months after transplant that is independent of acute rejection, drug toxicity, and recurrence of disease. Chronic rejection results in a progressive decline in glomerular filtration rate (GFR) in the presence of hypertension and proteinuria.[39] Histopathological features range from transplant glomerulopathy to arteriosclerosis, chronic interstitial fibrosis, and tubular atrophy. Chronic rejection is one of the chief causes of graft loss, accounting for 4% graft loss per year.[40] Theories proposed for the pathophysiology of chronic allograft nephropathy include chronic antibody-mediated rejection, senescence theory of

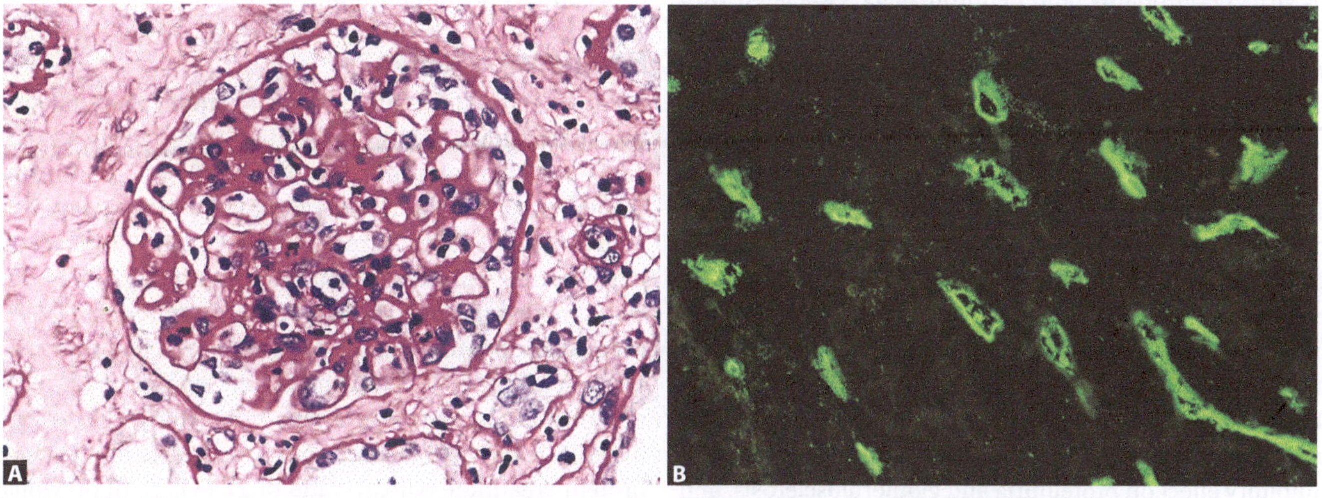

Figs. 3A and B: (A) Transplant glomerulitis in active antibody-mediated rejection: Periodic acid–Schiff (PAS) stain highlights the glomerular capillaries which are dilated and partially obliterated by mononuclear and swollen endothelial cells; (B) C4d by immunofluorescence in a patient with acute antibody-mediated rejection. There is widespread circumferential staining of the peritubular capillaries.
Courtesy: Dr Anila Abraham, Renopath Laboratory, Chennai.

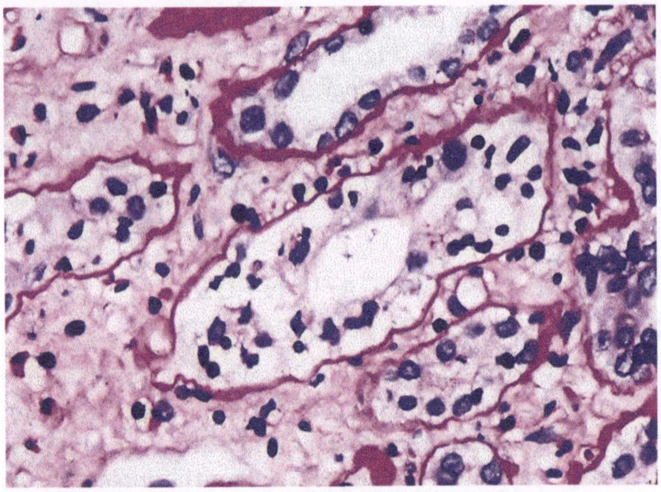

Fig. 4: Severe tubulitis in a patient with acute cell mediated rejection. Periodic acid–Schiff (PAS) stain delineates the tubular basement membrane, allowing identification and counting of lymphocytes within the tubule.
Courtesy: Dr Anila Abraham, Renopath Laboratory, Chennai.

TABLE 3: Therapeutic options in management of antibody-mediated rejection and T cell-mediated rejection.

Antibody-mediated rejection	*T cell-mediated rejection*
• Pulse corticosteroids • Thymoglobulin • Plasma exchange • Rituximab • Bortezomib • Eculizumab	• Pulse corticosteroids, oral steroids • Thymoglobulin • Optimize immunosuppression • Alemtuzumab

input stress model, cumulative damage due to progressive decrease in the number of nephrons, and oxidative stress due to reactive oxygen species.[41] Risk factors include the presence of donor-specific antibodies, recurrent acute rejection, inadequate immunosuppression, and nonimmune factors such as deceased donor transplantation, recurrent infections, BK virus nephropathy, and nephrotoxicity associated with calcineurin inhibitors (CNI). The management is supportive, with change to non-CNI-based therapy in those with histological features of CNI toxicity.

Hypertension

Hypertension in the early post-transplant period is related to fluid overload and due to the use of corticosteroids and CNI. Later, hypertension is seen in a majority of patients and may be related to disease of native kidneys, and side effect of immunosuppressive medications. Hypertension is managed with a low-sodium diet and medications, usually calcium channel or β-adrenergic blockers. Angiotensin-converting enzyme inhibitors (ACEIs) are considered useful due to their inhibitory effect on proteinuria and glomerulosclerosis, and cardioprotection. A combination of both calcium channel blockers and ACEI is satisfactory therapy in those with severe hypertension.[42] Monitoring by ABPM helps in diagnosis of masked and nocturnal hypertension, both of which may contribute to cardiovascular morbidity.[43]

Side Effects of Medications

Cosmetic side effects may be the reason for noncompliance and delayed acute rejection, particularly in adolescents. Tacrolimus is associated with nephrotoxicity, tremors, and diabetes mellitus; cyclosporine can cause nephrotoxicity, hypertension, tremors, hirsutism, and gum hyperplasia. Diarrhea, vomiting, and myelosuppression are common with MMF; patients receiving AZA need monitoring for myelosuppression, pancreatitis, and hepatotoxicity.

Metabolic and Hematological Complications

Metabolic complications following transplantation include hypomagnesemia (due to CNI), hypophosphatemia (secondary hyperparathyroidism, elevated levels of fibroblast growth factor, vitamin D deficiency), hyperkalemia, and renal tubular acidosis (CNI, ACEI, acute rejection). Dyslipidemia is a complication of therapy with steroids, sirolimus, and CNI. Children receiving tacrolimus are at risk of hyperglycemia, with ~5% developing new-onset diabetes after transplantation (NODAT) on the long-term. Nevertheless, tacrolimus-based immunosuppression is an acceptable and safe option with optimized prescription.[44] Other risk factors for NODAT include the use of high-dose steroids and family history of diabetes. Strict control of diabetes is essential for long-term patient and graft survival.

Hematological complications include anemia, erythrocytosis, and thrombocytopenia. Anemia may be related to bone marrow suppression due to therapy with MMF, azathioprine, or tacrolimus. Aplastic anemia can occur due to parvovirus B19 and CMV infection, and hemolytic anemia due to recurrent hemolytic uremic syndrome. Neutropenia and thrombocytopenia might be due to underlying viral infection or secondary to immunosuppressive medication(s).

Recurrent Disease

Disease recurrence is an important complication following transplantation. Patient morbidity and graft loss can be prevented while preparing the patient for renal transplantation.[45] In children undergoing kidney transplant, 7–8% graft loss is secondary to recurrence of which 70–80% is due to glomerulonephritis.[46] Recurrence of primary disease may result in high risk of graft loss (>30–50%) in FSGS (14–50%), membranoproliferative GN (30–100%), membranous nephropathy (50%), hemolytic uremic syndrome (20–60%), and primary hyperoxaluria type I (80–100%). Recurrence in FSGS is defined as persistent proteinuria of urine spot protein creatinine (UPCR) ratio of ≥1 in case of previously anuric patient or increase of UPCR by ≥1 in patients with proteinuria at the time of transplantation. While preparing for renal transplantation, genetic testing is important as the risk of recurrence is lower in patients with pathogenic or likely pathogenic variants. Risk factors that predict recurrence include late steroid resistance (>80%), time to end-stage kidney disease <48 months (>55%), and sclerosis at the time of renal biopsy. The donor should undergo genetic evaluation (heterozygous carrier of recessive *SRNS* gene and variant of unknown significance can be considered for transplantation after explaining the risk of recurrence).[47,48]

Strategies to prevent recurrent FSGS include prophylactic plasmapheresis or immunoadsorption, lipid apheresis, and perioperative rituximab in addition to induction treatment.[47] Confirmation of proteinuria and renal biopsy is indicated. Therapy for recurrent diseases includes the use of IV methylprednisolone pulses, plasmapheresis, rituximab, and increasing dose of CNI. In the absence of complete remission, ACEI can be considered if graft function is stable.[45]

Urological Disorders

Patients with urological problems have a higher rate of infections and urological procedures post-transplant. A study from India showed that of 44 patients with abnormal bladder who underwent renal transplantation, graft survival at 1 and 2 years was 72.7% and 59%, respectively.[14]

Infections

Infections are a major morbidity following transplantation. Rubin's timetable projects the occurrence of common infectious agents in the post-transplant period.[49] While bacterial infections are most commonly observed in the 1st month of transplantation, fungal and viral infections occur at 1–6 months post-transplant. UTIs are important, especially in patients with congenital abnormalities of the urinary tract, neurogenic bladder, and bladder dysfunction.

A retrospective study in adult transplant recipients from India showed that CMV, tuberculosis, and fungal infections had a prevalence of 21.8%, 10.6%, and 23%, respectively. Pulmonary infections due to *Pneumocystis jirovecii* need early recognition and therapy. Cotrimoxazole prophylaxis, up to 6 months following transplantation, is strongly recommended. Tuberculosis can rarely develop in the 1st year following transplantation and that requires intensive therapy for 3 months, followed by a less-intensive schedule for the next 9 months. The use of rifampicin is restricted due to its interactions with CNI. Systemic mycoses due to *Aspergillus*, *Candida*, and *Cryptococcus* may rarely occur.

With limited access to molecular diagnostic tests, regular monitoring for CMV, EBV, and BK virus is a challenge **(Table 4)**. For details, the reader is directed to the KDIGO guidelines on hepatitis C infection in transplantation and a recent review on viral infections in pediatric transplantation.[50,51]

Highly Sensitized Patient

Primary goal in transplantation of a highly sensitized recipient is to find the donor-recipient pair with least incompatibility. Patients who are broadly sensitized to HLA with high strength of reactivity have low rates of transplantation or long waiting times on the decease donor waiting list. Sensitization with regard to deceased organ donation is defined as panel reactive

TABLE 4: Common viral infections following renal transplantation.

Virus	*Clinical features*	*Diagnosis*	*Treatment*
Cytomegalovirus	• Fever, malaise • *Invasive disease:* Organ dysfunction	• Pancytopenia, elevated transaminases • PCR • Biopsy shows viral inclusions	Valganciclovir daily till PCR negative, followed by prophylaxis for 180 days
Epstein–Barr virus	• Infectious mononucleosis-like syndrome • Lymphoproliferative disease	• PCR for RNA load • Viral capsid or nuclear antigen • *Biopsy:* Nuclear inclusions	• Reduce immunosuppression • Rituximab • Chemotherapy
Hepatitis C virus	• Asymptomatic • Weight loss, jaundice • Isolated elevated tacrolimus trough levels	• Nucleic acid testing positive • Abnormal liver function tests • *Renal biopsy:* Membranous or membranoproliferative glomerulonephritis	• GFR > 30 mL/min: • *Genotype 1,4:* S+L • 2,3,5,6: G+P • GFR < 30 mL/min/1.73 m^2 • 1,4: Gr/G+ P/E • 2,3,5,6:G+P
BK virus	• Preclinical latent phase • *Clinical:* Graft dysfunction 1st year • Sterile pyuria • Hemorrhagic cystitis • Ureteric stenosis	• *Blood PCR:* BK virus >4 log copies/mL • *Urine PCR:* >1 × 10^7 copies/mL • mRNA >6log copies/ng total urine RNA • *Urine:* Decoy cells • *Renal biopsy:* Tubulointerstitial fibrosis Electron microscopy:: Haufen cells??	• Reduce immunosuppression >10,000 copies/mL • CNI-sparing regimen • Cidofovir leflunomide??

(CNI: calcineurin inhibitors; Hepatitis C viral treatment: S + L: Sofosbuvir + ledipasvir; G + P: glecapravir + pibrentsavir; Gr +E: grazoprevir + elbasvir; PCR: polymerase chain reaction)

antibodies >80%.[52] Based on cross-match tests, transplantation is contraindicated if the CDC cross-match is positive. If CDC cross-match is negative with flow cross-match being positive, then further testing with SAB assay and the mean fluorescence intensity are undertaken (negative if <1,000, and positive if >2,000).[53] Irrespective of deceased donor or living donor, desensitization protocol, to reduce antibody strength to an acceptable level that allows a successful transplantation, is undertaken with intravenous immunoglobulin and rituximab along with plasmapheresis. Other protocols with bortezomib and eculizumab are under study.[54]

Growth and Nutrition

Growth failure or short stature impedes the quality of life and has an important effect on psychological development.[55] Majority of pediatric allograft recipients do not achieve a normal adult height even with good graft function. Post-transplant growth is more likely to be affected in young children than in older children and adolescents. Efforts to improve nutritional intake, correct metabolic acidosis, and minimize corticosteroid therapy are necessary. Growth hormone therapy would be indicated for those with persistent short stature in the event of poor response to steroid avoidance therapy with good renal function or in those with impaired renal function.[56-58]

Malignancy

The risk of malignancy is increased with the intensity and duration of immunosuppression. The chief malignancy in children is a post-transplant lymphoproliferative disorder, noted in 1–10% transplant recipients, particularly in seronegative recipients of EBV-positive donors. Increased risk of post-transplant lymphoproliferative disorder is seen in younger children and can manifest as early as the 1st year of transplant or later in the 2nd or 3rd year. The severity ranges from infectious mononucleosis-like illness to a lymphoma-like illness. The key strategy for management includes the use of less immunosuppression while intravenous immunoglobulin has a limited role.[58,59]

ADULT VERSUS PEDIATRIC RENAL TRANSPLANTATION

There are many differences between adult and pediatric renal transplantation, listed in **Table 5**.[60,61] The distinguishing features are the spectrum of native kidney disease, pharmacokinetics of transplant-related medications, risk of infection, issues related to growth, quality of life, and immunological basis for better graft survival. Maintaining long-term graft function is critical since the projected patient survival is several decades longer than in adults. Multidisciplinary inputs from the pediatric nephrologist, transplant surgeon, urologist, anesthetist, immunologist, dietitian, and social worker are vital in providing optimum care to children.

Transplant Outcomes

Data from the North American Pediatric Renal Transplant Registry (NAPRTCS) shows graft survival rates at 1, 3, and 5 years as 99.5%, 97.2%, and 94.9% in living-donor transplants, and 97.6%, 94.4%, and 90.1%, respectively, in deceased-donor transplants.[1] Pre-emptive transplantation is associated with improved patient and graft survival.[1,6] Though the 1-year allograft survival rates of transplants across centers in India are quite similar to the NAPRTCS report, the outcomes at 5 years are less satisfactory.[62-68] Several factors might contribute to the disparities in transplant outcomes between the developed and

TABLE 5: Differences between adult and pediatric renal transplantation.

Characteristics	*Adult*	*Children*
Common native kidney disease	Diabetes, hypertension	Congenital anomalies of kidneys and urinary tract, chronic glomerulonephritis
Immunological function	• Thymic atrophy • High expression of CD40L on T cells	• Good thymic activity • Low expression of CD40L on T cells • Decreased mature macrophages, dendritic and HLA-alloreactive B cells
Pretransplant evaluation	Urological preparation not a common need	Need urological evaluation and preparation in selected cases
Vascular anastomoses	Mainly the external iliac vessels	Involve the distal aorta and vena cava just cephalad to the bifurcation in infants; common iliac vessels in young children; external iliac vessels in adolescents
Drug pharmacokinetics	Well-established drug response and toxicity profiles	• Need higher dose immunosuppression (mg/kg) to maintain therapeutic levels • Higher drug metabolism • Varied adverse effects and toxicity profile • Need for special formulations
Physical growth	Not a relevant parameter	Important determinant of well-being
Infection	Seropositive to viral infections	Seronegative to most viral infections
Graft survival	Reduces with age	• Best in children <5-year-old • Adolescents are a high-risk group

the developing world. These include biological, immune and genetic factors; associated comorbidities; time on dialysis; donor and organ characteristics; socioeconomic status; medication adherence; access to care; and public health policies.[69,70]

Deceased organ transplantation programs are active only in a few states in our country, and there is a need to focus on prioritized allocation criteria for children. A dedicated website (*www.notto.gov.in*) has been launched by the National Organ Transplant Program for providing information on organ and tissue donation, organ and tissue pledging, networking of hospitals, and establishing the national registry of organ and tissue transplantation and donation. The two important amendments made with regard to kidney transplantation under the Transplantation of Human Organs and Tissue Act (THOTA) include expansion of the definition of near relative to include grandparents and provision of swap donation.

In children, the outcomes of graft survival are comparable between deceased organ and living donor transplantation.[71,72] An Indian study on 37 children, who received kidneys from adult deceased donors, showed 1-, 3-, 5-, and 10-year death-censored graft survival to be 90.4%, 86.4%, 73.3%, and 73.3%, respectively.[72]

CONCLUSION

Kidney transplantation is the most effective form of kidney replacement therapy in children. With advances in immunobiology and immunosuppressants, both allograft and patient outcomes continue to improve. Main morbidities following transplantation are related to bacterial and viral infections, growth, and medication-related toxicities. Young children weighing <10 kg and those with congenital or functional disorders of the lower urinary tract pose significant medical and surgical challenges.

KEY POINTS

- Kidney transplantation is the ideal modality of kidney replacement therapy in children that demands extensive evaluation of both the recipient and the donor.
- Preemptive renal transplantation in children has better graft and patient survival compared to those with a dialysis vintage of 12–18 months.
- Kidney transplant surgery can be technically challenging in low-body-weight children and infants.
- In developing countries, though the 5-year allograft survival is excellent, long-term graft survival poses challenges.
- While adherence to medications is a critical issue relevant to adolescents, growth and susceptibility to infections need special attention in post-transplant care.

REFERENCES

1. Chua A, Cramer C, Moudgil A, Martz K, Smith J, Blydt-Hansen T, et al. Kidney transplant practice patterns and outcome benchmarks over 30 years: the 2018 report of the NAPRTCS. Pediatr Transplant. 2019;23(8):e13597.
2. North American Pediatric Renal Trials and Collaborative Studies. (2014). NAPRTCS 2014 Annual Transplant Report. [online] Available from: https://naprtcs.org/system/files/2014_Annual_Transplant_Report.pdf. [Last accessed March, 2022].
3. Kamath N, Iyengar AA. Chronic kidney disease (CKD): an observational study of etiology, severity and burden of comorbidities. Indian J Pediatr. 2017;84(11):822-5.
4. Davis ID, Bunchman TE, Grimm PC, Benfield MR, Briscoe DM, Harmon WE, et al. Pediatric renal transplantation: indications and special considerations. A position paper from the Pediatric Committee of the American Society of Transplant Physicians. Pediatr Transplant. 1998;2(2):117-29.
5. Iyengar A, Lewin S, Lantos JD. Considering family resources when making medical recommendations. Pediatrics 2018; 141(1):e20171198.
6. Amaral S, Sayed BA, Kutner N, Patzer RE. Preemptive kidney transplantation is associated with survival benefits among pediatric patients with end-stage renal disease. Kidney Int. 2016;90:1100-8.
7. Chan-On C, Liberto JM, Sarwal MM. Mechanisms and biomarkers of immune quiescence in kidney transplantation. Human Immunol. 2018;79(5):356-61.
8. Morozumi K, Takeda A, Otsuka Y, Horike K, Gotoh N, Narumi S, et al. Reviewing the pathogenesis of antibody-mediated rejection and renal graft pathology after kidney transplantation. Nephrology (Carlton). 2016;21(Suppl 1):4-8.
9. Morris PJ, Knechtle SJ. Immunology of graft rejection. In: Kidney Transplantation, 7th edition. Edinburgh: Elsevier Saunders; 2014. pp. 10-30.
10. Salvatierra Jr O, Millan M, Concepcion W. Pediatric renal transplantation with considerations for successful outcomes. Semin Pediatr Surg. 2006;15(3):208-17.
11. Salvatierra Jr O, Singh T, Shifrin R, Conley S, Alexander S, Tanney D, et al. Successful transplantation of adult-sized kidneys into infants requires maintenance of high aortic blood flow. Transplantation. 1998;66(7):819-23.
12. Ghane Sharbaf F, Bitzan M, Szymanski KM, Bell LE, Gupta I, Tchervenkov J, et al. Native nephrectomy prior to pediatric kidney transplantation: biological and clinical aspects. Pediatr Nephrol. 2012;27(7):1179-88.
13. Hari P, Singla IK, Mantan M, Kanitkar M, Batra B, Bagga A. Chronic renal failure in children. Indian Pediatr. 2003;40:1035-42.
14. Mishra SK, Muthu V, Rajapurkar MM, Desai MR. Kidney transplantation in abnormal bladder. Indian J Urol. 2007;23(3):299-304.
15. Kroger AT, Duchin J, Vázquez M. (2017). ACIP General Best Practice Guidelines for Immunization | Recommendations | CDC. [online] Available from: https://www.cdc.gov/vaccines/hcp/acip-recs/general-recs/index.html [Last accessed February, 2018].
16. Banerjee S, Dissanayake PV, Abeyagunawardena AS. Vaccinations in children on immunosuppressive medications for renal disease. Pediatr Nephrol. 2016;31(9):1437-48.
17. Althaf MM, El Kossi M, Jin JK, Sharma A, Halawa AM. Human leucocyte antigen typing and crossmatch: a comprehensive review. World J Transplant. 2017;7(6):339-48.
18. South AM, Grimm PC. Transplant immuno-diagnostics: crossmatch and antigen detection. Pediatr Nephrol. 2016;31:897-905.
19. Jha PK, Bansal SB, Sethi SK, Jain M, Sharma R, Nandwani A, et al. ABO-incompatible renal transplantation in developing world - crossing the immunological (and mental) barrier. Indian J Nephrol. 2016;26(2):113-8.

20. Sethi SK, Bansal SB, Wadhwani N, Tiwari A, Arora D, Sharma R, et al. Pediatric ABO-incompatible kidney transplantation: evolving with the advancing apheresis technology: a single-center experience. Pediatr Transplant. 2018;22(3):e13138.
21. Lentine KL, Kasiske BL, Levey AS, Adams PL, Alberú J, Bakr MA, et al. KDIGO clinical practice guideline on the evaluation and care of living kidney donors. Transplantation. 2017;101(8S Suppl 1):S1-09.
22. Chadban SJ, Ahn C, Axelrod DA, Foster BJ, Kasiske BL, Kher V, et al. KDIGO clinical practice guideline on the evaluation and management of candidates for kidney transplantation. Transplantation. 2020;104:S103.
23. Wiseman AC. Immunosuppressive medications. Clin J Am Soc Nephrol. 2016;11(2):332-43.
24. Danovitch GM. Immunosuppression medications and protocols for kidney transplantation. Handbook of Kidney Transplantation, 5th edition. Philadelphia: Lippincott Williams and Wilkins; 2010. pp. 77-125.
25. Kidney Disease: Improving Global Outcomes (KDIGO) Transplant Work Group. KDIGO clinical practice guideline for the care of kidney transplant recipients. Am J Transplant. 2009;9(Suppl 3):S1.
26. Nehus E, Liu C, Hooper DK, Macaluso M, Kim MO. Clinical practice of steroid avoidance in pediatric kidney transplantation. Am J Transplant. 2015;15(8):2203-10.
27. Grenda R, Watson A, Trompeter R, Tönshoff B, Jaray J, Fitzpatrick M, et al. A randomized trial to assess the impact of early steroid withdrawal on growth in pediatric renal transplantation: the TWIST study. Am J Transplant. 2010;10(4):828-36.
28. Puliyanda DP, Pizzo H, Rodig N, Somers MJG. Early outcomes comparing induction with antithymocyte globulin vs alemtuzumab in two steroid-avoidance protocols in pediatric renal transplantation. Pediatr Transplant. 2020;24(3):e13685.
29. Organ Procurement and Transplantation Network (OPTN) and Scientific Registry of Transplant Recipients (SRTR) OPTN/SRTR 2012 Annual Data Report. Rockville, MD: Department of Health and Human Services, Health Resources and Services Administration, Healthcare Systems Bureau, Division of Transplantation; 2014. pp. 11-44.
30. Schröppel B, Legendre C. Delayed kidney graft function: from mechanism to translation. Kidney Int. 2014;86:251-8.
31. Grenda R. Delayed graft function and its management in children. Pediatr Nephrol. 2017;32(7):1157-67.
32. Siedlecki A, Irish W, Brennan DC. Delayed graft function in the kidney transplant. Am J Transplant. 2011;11(11):2279-96.
33. Naik RH, Shawar SH. Renal Transplantation Rejection. In: StatPearls [Internet]. Treasure Island (FL): StatPearls Publishing; 2020.
34. Singh N, Samant H, Hawxby A, Samaniego MD. Biomarkers of rejection in kidney transplantation. Curr Opin Organ Transplant. 2019;24(1):103-10.
35. Jeong HJ. Diagnosis of renal transplant rejection: Banff classification and beyond. Kidney Res Clin Pract. 2020;39(1):17-31.
36. Roufosse C, Simmonds N, Clahsen-van Groningen M, Haas M, Henriksen KJ, Horsfield C, et al. A 2018 reference guide to the Banff classification of renal allograft pathology. Transplantation. 2018;102:1795-1814.
37. Djamali A, Kaufman DB, Ellis TM, Zhong W, Matas A, Samaniego M. Diagnosis and management of antibody-mediated rejection: current status and novel approaches. Am J Transplant. 2014;14(2):255-71.
38. Leblanc J, Subrt P, Paré M, Hartell D, Sénécal L, Blydt-Hansen T, et al. Practice patterns in the treatment and monitoring of acute T cell-mediated kidney graft rejection in Canada. Can J Kidney Health Dis. 2018;5:2054358117753616.
39. Shreshta B, Haylor J. Evolution of the concept and pathogenesis of chronic renal allograft injury: an updated review. Exp Clin Transplant. 2016;6:596-605.
40. Nankivell BJ, Alexander SI. Rejection of the kidney allograft. N Engl J Med. 2010;363:1451-62.
41. Cornell LD, Neal Smith R, Colvin RB. Kidney transplantation: mechanisms of rejection and acceptance. Annu Rev Pathol Mech Dis. 2008;3:189-220.
42. Seeman T, Feber J. Should ACE inhibitors or calcium channel blockers be used for post-transplant hypertension? Pediatr Nephrol. 2021;36:539-49.
43. Pais P, Dello Strologo L, Iyengar A, Velusamy V, Greenbaum LA. Nocturnal hypertension and left ventricular hypertrophy in pediatric renal transplant recipients in South India. Pediatr Transplant. 2020;24(4):e13710.
44. Jouve T, Noble J, Rostaing L, Malvezzi P. An update on the safety of tacrolimus in kidney transplant recipients, with a focus on tacrolimus minimization. Expert Opin Drug Saf. 2019;18(4):285-94.
45. Lim WH, Shingde M, Wong G. Recurrent and de novo glomerulonephritis after kidney transplantation. Front Immunol. 2019;10:1944.
46. Cosio FG, Cattran DC. Recent advances in our understanding of recurrent primary glomerulonephritis after kidney transplantation. Kidney Int. 2016;91(2):304-314.
47. Cochat P, Fargue S, Mestrallet G, Jungraithmayr T, Koch-Nogueira P, Ranchin B, et al. Disease recurrence in paediatric renal transplantation. Pediatr Nephrol. 2009;24:2097-108.
48. Trautmann A, Vivarelli M, Samuel S, Gipson D, Sinha A, Schaefer F, et al. IPNA clinical practice recommendations for the diagnosis and management of children with steroid-resistant nephrotic syndrome. Pediatr Nephrol. 2020;35(8):1529-61.
49. Fishman JA. Rubin RH. Infection in organ-transplant recipients. N Engl J Med. 1998;24:1743.
50. Kidney Disease: Improving Global Outcomes (KDIGO) Hepatitis C Work Group. KDIGO 2018 clinical practice guideline for the prevention, diagnosis, evaluation, and treatment of hepatitis C in chronic kidney disease. Kidney Int Suppl. 2018;8:91-165.
51. Scaggs Huang FA, Danziger-Isakov L. Infectious disease risks in pediatric renal transplantation. Pediatr Nephrol. 2019;34(7):1155-66.
52. Keith DS, Vranic GM. Approach to the highly sensitized kidney transplant candidate. Clin J Am Soc Nephrol. 2016;11:684-93.
53. Salazar E, Eagar TN, Land GA. LBP33: Defining a clinically relevant cutoff for the identification of HLA antibodies using the single antigen bead assay. Human Immunol 2015;76:210-38.
54. Akalin E. A new treatment option for highly sensitized patients awaiting kidney transplantation. Am J Kidney Dis. 2018;71:458-60.
55. Harambat J, Cochat P. Growth after renal transplantation. Pediatr Nephrol. 2009;24(7):1297-1306.
56. Mehls O, Fine RN. Growth hormone treatment after renal transplantation: a promising but underused chance to improve growth. Pediatr Nephrol. 2013;28:1-4.
57. Ingulli EG, Mak RH. Growth in children with chronic kidney disease: role of nutrition, growth hormone, dialysis, and steroids. Curr Opin Pediatr. 2014;26(2):187-92.

58. Martinez OM. Biomarkers for PTLD diagnosis and therapies. Pediatr Nephrol. 2020;35(7):1173-81.
59. Mynarek M, Schober T, Behrends U, Maecker-Kolhoff B. Posttransplant lymphoproliferative disease after pediatric solid organ transplantation. Clin Dev Immunol. 2013;2013:814973.
60. Dharnidharka VR, Fiorina P, Harmon WE. Kidney transplantation in children. New Engl J Med. 2014;371(6):549-58.
61. Medeiros M, Castañeda-Hernández G, Ross CJD, Carleton BC. Use of pharmacogenomics in pediatric renal transplant recipients. Front Genet. 2015;6:41.
62. Chacko B, Rajamanickam T, Neelakantan N, Tamilarasi V, John GT. Pediatric renal transplantation—a single center experience of 15 yr from India. Pediatr Transplant. 2007;11(8):844-9.
63. Vasudevan A, Iyengar A, Jose B, Phadke K. Pediatric renal transplantation: a single-center experience. Transplant Proc. 2008;40(4):1095-98.
64. Sinha A, Hari P, Guleria S, Gulati A, Dinda AK, Mehra NK, et al. Outcome of pediatric renal transplantation in north India. Pediatr Transplant. 2010;14(7):836-43.
65. Meena J, Sinha A, Hari P, Dinda AK, Khandelwal P, Goswami S, et al. Pediatric kidney transplantation: experience over two decades. Asian J Pediatr Nephrol. 2018;1:22-8.
66. Srivastava A, Prabhakaran S, Sureka SK, Kapoor R, Kumar A, Sharma RK, et al. The challenges and outcomes of living donor kidney transplantation in pediatric and adolescent age group in a developing country: A critical analysis from a single center of north India. Indian J Urol. 2015;31(1): 33-7.
67. Phadke K, Iyengar A, Karthik S, Kumar A, Olakkengil S. Pediatric renal transplantation: the Bangalore experience. Indian Pediatr. 2006;43(1):44-8.
68. Bijalwan P, Sanjeevan KV, Mathew A, Nair TB. Outcome and complications of living donor pediatric renal transplantation: experience from a tertiary care center. Ind J Urol. 2017;33(3): 221-5.
69. Gordon EJ, Ladner DP, Caicedo JC, Franklin J. Disparities in kidney transplant outcomes: a review. Semin Nephrol. 2010;30(1):81-9.
70. Odetunde OI, Okafor HU, Uwaezuoke SN, Ezeonwu BU, Ukoha OM. Renal replacement therapy in children in the developing world: challenges and outcome in a tertiary hospital in southeast Nigeria. Sci World J. 2014;2014:903151.
71. Chantarogh S, Tangnararatchakit K, Tirapanich W, Viseshsindh W, Saisawat P, Pirojsakul P. Clinical outcomes in pediatric renal transplant recipients who received steroid-based immunosuppressive regimen. Transplant Proc. 2017;49(5):971-6.
72. Kute VB, Trivedi HL, Vanikar AV, Shah PR, Gumber MR, Patel HV, et al. Long-term outcome of deceased donor renal transplantation in pediatric recipients: a single-center experience from a developing country. Pediatr Transplant. 2012;16(6):651-7.

SECTION

13

Pediatric Urology

CHAPTER

13.1

Genetic Basis of Congenital Anomalies of the Kidney and Urinary Tract

Prajnya Ranganath

INTRODUCTION

Congenital anomalies of the kidney and urinary tract (CAKUT) encompass a diverse group of structural malformations that result from abnormal morphogenesis of the kidney and urinary tract. CAKUT are among the most common birth defects constituting approximately 20–30% of all anomalies identified in the prenatal period and have an estimated worldwide incidence of around 3–6 per 1,000 live births.[1,2] They account for a significant proportion, i.e., almost 30–50% of cases of chronic kidney disease (CKD) and end-stage kidney disease (ESKD) in the pediatric age group.[3,4]

The wide spectrum of anomalies included under the umbrella term of CAKUT vary greatly in their age of presentation, severity, and outcome. CAKUT may be unilateral or bilateral, may involve one or more segments of the urinary tract, and may occur in isolation or along with extrarenal manifestations as part of a syndrome.

The pathogenesis of renal and urinary tract malformations is a complex process involving a complex interplay of genetic, environmental, and epigenetic factors.[5,6] Both syndromic and nonsyndromic forms of CAKUT result from disruption of the cellular, molecular, and morphogenetic mechanisms which regulate normal development of the renal system.[6] Conventionally, genetic studies of syndromic and familial forms of CAKUT and functional studies based on cell lines and animal models have provided valuable insights into the genetic basis of these congenital malformations. Recently, however, with the availability of high throughput techniques such as next-generation sequencing (NGS)-based whole exome or whole genome sequencing, it has become possible to perform genome-wide screening for candidate genes/potential pathogenic gene variants in large cohorts of patients with not only the syndromic and familial forms of CAKUT but also isolated CAKUT, and the underlying genetic etiology is being identified in an increasing proportion of cases.[7,8] Yet, even though approximately 40 different genes have been identified, to date, to be associated with monogenic causes of CAKUT, together these account for only around 10–20% of patients with CAKUT.[9] In addition to this, approximately 10–15% of cases have been reported to have chromosomal copy number variations (CNVs).[10] The challenges related to identification of specific genetic causes of CAKUT include the significant heterogeneity, variable expressivity, and incomplete penetrance of these disorders.[9]

This chapter provides an overview of the molecular etiopathogenesis of CAKUT and briefly summarizes the current understanding about the genetic basis of syndromic as well as nonsyndromic forms of CAKUT.

NORMAL DEVELOPMENT OF THE KIDNEY AND URINARY TRACT

Normal development of the kidney and lower urinary tract involves a combination of complex cellular processes including mitosis, cell differentiation, morphogenesis, and apoptosis, which are driven by diverse molecules, such as growth factors and cell adhesion molecules. The expression of these regulatory molecules is, in turn, controlled by transcription factors.[11]

The mammalian kidney is a complex organ containing more than 25 distinct functional cell types, which arise from one of two intermediate mesoderm-derived cell populations, the metanephric mesenchyme and the ureteric bud. Broadly, the development of the kidney and urinary tract can be categorized into the following stages, which are graphically depicted in **Figures 1A to E**:[11-15]

- *Ureteric bud induction:* The nephrogenic cords develop from the intermediate mesoderm at about 3 weeks of gestation in humans and give rise to three sets of nephric structures: pronephros, mesonephros, and metanephros. The cranial-most part, the pronephros, regresses by 4 weeks of gestation. The mesonephros includes the mesonephric mesenchyme and an epithelial tube called the Wolffian duct (WD). The mesonephric mesenchyme degenerates, while the WD inserts into the cloaca and a bulge on the lower part of the WD develops into the primary ureteric bud that grows toward the metanephric mesenchyme.
- *Mesenchymal-to-epithelial transition (MET):* The invasion of the ureteric bud into the metanephric mesenchyme induces the metanephric mesenchymal

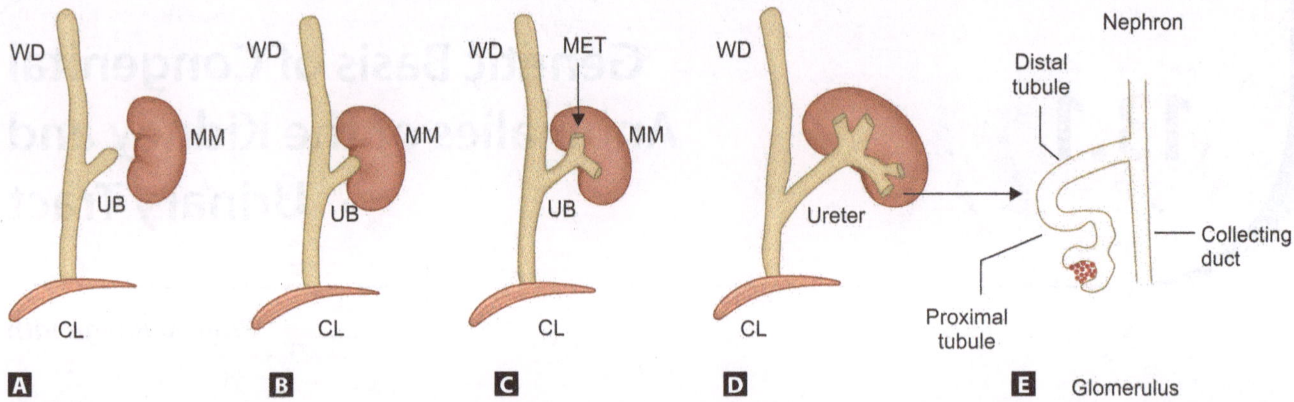

Figs. 1A to E: Stages of nephrogenesis; (A) Ureteric bud induction; (B and C) Mesenchymal condensation and mesenchymal-to-epithelial transition; (D) Renal branching morphogenesis; (E) Nephron patterning and elongation. (CL: cloaca; MET: mesenchymal-to-epithelial transition; MM: metanephric mesenchyme; UB: ureteric bud; WD: Wolffian duct)

cells to condense around the tip of the ureteric bud to form the cap mesenchyme. When the primary ureteric bud tip branches, the metanephric mesenchymal cells coalesce around the branched tips, which lead to polarization of the mesenchyme to generate epithelial cells of the nephron. This process is called mesenchymal-to-epithelial transition (MET).

- *Renal branching morphogenesis:* The primary ureteric bud undergoes proliferation and serial branching to give rise to around 15 generations of branches. The first few branches develop into the major and minor calyces, while the successive branches develop into the collecting ducts. Nephrons develop at the tip of each branching bud.
- *Nephron patterning and elongation:* The condensed metanephric mesenchymal cells near the tips of the branching ureteric buds develop into the nephrons. Each nephron progenitor differentiates into the glomerulus, proximal tubules, descending and ascending loops of Henle, distal tubules, and connecting tubules. The endothelial progenitor cells and stromal cells develop into the glomerular capillaries and mesangial cells, respectively. The process of nephrogenesis gets completed before birth in humans.
- *Ascent and rotation:* In the initial stages, the kidneys grow in a posterior direction but as embryonic development progresses, they rotate anteromedially and ascend upward. They reach their final position in the retroperitoneal region of the abdomen by 9 weeks of gestation. Blood supply of the developing kidneys is derived from the descending aorta, from its caudal branches in the initial stages, and after ascent, from its cranial branches. Defects in ascent and rotation of the kidneys can result in fusion of the kidneys or ectopic kidneys.
- *Development and maturation of the ureters:* While the tip of the primary ureteric bud gets encompassed by the metanephric mesenchyme and progresses to branch and develop into the major and minor calyces and the nephrons, the stalk of the primary ureteric bud remains outside the metanephric mesenchyme, elongates, and develops into the ureter. The ureter separates from the WD through a process of remodeling and gets inserted into the bladder. The distal portion of the WD develops into the epididymis, vas deferens, ejaculatory duct, and seminal vesicle in males, while in females, it undergoes degeneration.
- *Development of the bladder:* During week 4 of gestation, the urogenital septum divides the cloaca (which is derived from the endoderm) into the urogenital sinus anteriorly and the rectum posteriorly. The upper portion of the urogenital sinus develops into the bladder, while its lower end develops into the urethra. A part of the mesonephric duct fuses with the cloaca, gets incorporated into the posterior wall of the bladder, and forms the trigone region.

GENES AND SIGNALING PATHWAYS INVOLVED IN NEPHROGENESIS

The processes involved in each of the developmental stages mentioned above are controlled by a large number of genes and signaling pathways.[13] In the past few years, with the advent of new technologies such as high throughput expression analysis techniques, NGS, and transgenic mice, there have been significant advances in our understanding of the molecular basis of renal development. Since embryonic development of the kidney and urinary tract is highly conserved anatomically and molecularly in the mammalian species, studies into the genetic and cellular mechanisms of renal system organogenesis in model organisms such as the mouse and rat have helped to provide valuable insights into the developmental processes of the human renal system.[11] The genes that are postulated to be involved in the different stages of nephrogenesis are listed in **Table 1.**[13]

The renin-angiotensin system plays a crucial role in the normal development of the urinary tract. Mouse models genetically engineered to lack the angiotensin II types 1A and 1B receptor gene (*AGTR1*) or the angiotensinogen gene (*AGT*) have been documented to have abnormal development

TABLE 1: Genes postulated to be involved in different stages of nephrogenesis.

Stages of nephrogenesis	*Genes involved*
Ureteric bud induction	*Genes involved in the GDNF-RET signaling pathway:* • *RET* (rearranged during transfection proto-oncogene) • *GDNF* (glial cell line-derived neurotrophic factor) • *PAX2* (paired box gene 2) • *EYA1* (homolog of drosophila "eyes absent" transcriptional coactivator and phosphatase 1) • *SALL1* (Sal-like 1) • *BMP4* (bone morphogenetic protein 4)
Mesenchymal-to-epithelial transition	*Genes involved in the WNT signaling pathway and genes encoding some members of FGF family of proteins:* • *WNT9B* (wingless-type integration site family member 9B) • *WNT4* (wingless-type integration site family member 4) • *SIX2* (homolog of drosophila "sine oculis homeobox" 2) • *FGF8* (fibroblast growth factor 8) • *FGF9* (fibroblast growth factor 9) • *FGF20* (fibroblast growth factor 20)
Renal branching morphogenesis	*Genes encoding components of the renin–angiotensin system:* • *AGT* (angiotensinogen) • *REN* (renin) • *ACE* (angiotensin-converting enzyme) • *AGTR1* (angiotensin II receptor type 1) • *AGTR2* (angiotensin II receptor type 2)
Nephron patterning and elongation	*UMOD* (uromodulin)
Exact developmental stage not ascertained	• *HNF1B* (hepatocyte nuclear factor 1 beta)—expressed in the Wolffian duct from a very early developmental stage • *DSTYK* (dual serine/threonine and tyrosine protein kinase)

of the renal medulla and delayed glomerular maturation. Mice with null mutations in the angiotensin II type 2 receptor gene (*AGTR2*) have been found to develop a spectrum of urinary tract malformations including renal dysplasia, renal hypoplasia, hydronephrosis, and vesicoureteral malformations. These malformations are believed to occur because of the delayed apoptosis of the mesenchymal cells in the fetal kidney and lower urinary tract, due to the genetic mutations. Neonatal renal failure associated with maternal intake of angiotensin-converting enzyme inhibitors (ACE inhibitors) during pregnancy has been postulated to occur because of hemodynamic mechanisms as well as a renal tubular dysgenesis-like pathology, which results from disruption of the renin–angiotensin axis in the fetus.[13,14]

The WNT and Notch signaling pathways have been documented to be involved in the developmental processes that lead to specialization of the different functional segments of the nephron. Wnt4 and Wnt9b have been shown to play an important role in the process of MET and Notch2 has been found to be involved in proximal tubule specification. Members of the SHH (sonic hedgehog)-GLI (glioma-associated oncogene), BMP (bone morphogenetic protein), and FGF (fibroblast growth factor) family of proteins have also been reported to be involved in morphogenesis of the kidney and urinary tract.[13,14]

Thus, normal morphogenesis of the kidney and lower urinary tract involve complex interactions between the developmental genes and signaling pathways expressed in the mesenchyme, stroma, ureteric bud, and cloaca, at multiple developmental stages. Mutations in these renal developmental genes and disruption of the molecular pathways that direct these processes disturb normal nephrogenesis and thereby result in different forms of CAKUT.

ROLE OF EPIGENETIC AND ENVIRONMENTAL FACTORS IN THE PATHOGENESIS OF CAKUT

Even though alterations in renal developmental genes play a very important role in the etiopathogenesis of CAKUT, as mentioned above, monogenic causes and chromosomal CNVs together account for only around 20–30% of all CAKUT cases.[9,10] In a larger proportion of cases, CAKUT is of multifactorial origin and results from a complex interplay of genetic mutations, modifier genes, epigenetic factors, and in utero environmental influences.[6,16]

Modifier Genes

The expression and thereby actual phenotypic manifestation of a particular mutation in a renal developmental gene are modified to a significant extent by the influence of modifier genes as well as epigenetic factors. The interactions between different modifier genes and the disease-causing genetic mutation, which influence the phenotypic expression, are called "epistatic" gene interactions. For instance, the wide spectrum of urinary tract malformations associated with *HNF1B* and *UMOD* (uromodulin) mutations is most likely the result of the modifying influences of modifier genes.

Epigenetic Factors

Epigenetic regulation or epigenetic programming is another important influence on gene expression and disease causation. The major mechanisms in epigenetic control of gene regulation are DNA methylation and histone (chromatin protein) acetylation. DNA methylation and histone acetylation recruit additional proteins that can modify histones to form compact, inactive heterochromatin or opened, active euchromatin and alter the transcription of renal developmental genes. Pax2, a transcription factor critical for normal kidney development, has been found to be an important determinant of epigenetic regulation during metanephric organogenesis.[6]

Assisted reproductive technologies (ARTs), such as in vitro fertilization (IVF), have been found to be associated with an increased risk of birth defects including CAKUT. This is believed to be due to alteration of the normal epigenetic regulation that occurs during early embryonic development and the resultant inappropriate silencing or activation of developmental genes.[16]

Environmental Factors

Some environmental factors are clearly established to be associated with CAKUT, while the role of many others is not yet clearly defined. Maternal malnutrition, uteroplacental insufficiency, low birth weight, and premature delivery have been found to be associated with a lower number of nephrons. Maternal diabetes is known to increase the risk of renal anomalies as well as outflow tract abnormalities in the fetus. Vitamin A deficiency in the mother and maternal substance abuse (especially with alcohol and cocaine) have been reported to be associated with an increased risk of renal hypoplasia, renal dysplasia, and vesicoureteral reflux (VUR) in the baby. Intake of drugs such as ACE inhibitors and angiotensin receptor blockers by the mother, especially in the second or third trimesters of pregnancy, leads to acute renal injury and renal hypoplasia in the baby.[16] The other environmental factors that are believed to contribute to the causation of CAKUT include maternal obesity, low-protein diet, folic acid deficiency, and maternal smoking.[6]

SPECTRUM OF CONGENITAL ANOMALIES OF THE KIDNEY AND URINARY TRACT

The CAKUT disorders are phenotypically diverse. Based on the nature of the anomaly and the anatomical region involved, they can be categorized as listed in **Table 2.**[16]

With increasing use of high-resolution fetal ultrasonography, a significant proportion of CAKUT are being identified in the antenatal period. For the more serious anomalies, early diagnosis in the antenatal period allows consideration of termination or active therapeutic intervention.[17] More severe bilateral malformations such as renal agenesis and dysplasia may be associated with oligoanuria, oligohydramnios, fetal compressive effects, and lung hypoplasia termed the "Potter sequence."

TABLE 2: Spectrum of congenital anomalies of the kidney and urinary tract (CAKUT).

Anomaly	*Description*
Abnormality of kidney number	
Renal agenesis	Unilateral or bilateral absence of kidney and outflow tract
Abnormality of kidney size and morphology	
Renal hypoplasia	Kidney contains formed but significantly fewer than normal nephrons
Renal dysplasia	Kidney shape and tissue differentiation are abnormal
Multicystic dysplastic kidney	Kidney is dysplastic, has an abnormal shape, and is distended with multiple cysts
Duplex kidney	Kidney is separated into two parts: the upper part is often dysplastic and attached to an obstructed ureter and the lower part is usually attached to a refluxing ureter
Hydronephrosis	Renal pelvis is distended and the renal parenchyma may be dysplastic or hypoplastic; may occur secondary to reflux or urinary tract obstruction
Abnormality of kidney position	
Horseshoe kidney	Both kidneys become fused posteriorly during development and may include dysplastic components
Ectopic kidney	Kidney is in an abnormal ectopic location, away from its usual retroperitoneal position in the abdomen, more commonly in the pelvis
Abnormalities of the urinary outflow tract	
Ureteropelvic junction obstruction	Junction between the kidney and the ureter is obstructed, resulting in blockage of outflow of urine from the renal pelvis to the ureter; usually results in hydronephrosis
Megaureter	Distended and widened ureter which can result from an intrinsic abnormality of the ureter itself (primary) or due to backflow of urine due to lower urinary tract obstruction (secondary)
Duplex collecting system	Duplication of ureter and renal pelvis, which may be associated with duplication of the kidney, may be associated with obstruction or reflux
Vesicoureteral reflux	Urine flows in a retrograde direction from the bladder to the ureter, pelvis, and medullary collecting ducts of the kidney
Posterior urethral valves	Urinary outflow from the bladder is anatomically obstructed by a posterior urethral membrane, almost exclusively occurs in males, and is usually associated with bilateral hydroureteronephrosis

GENETICS OF NONSYNDROMIC CONGENITAL ANOMALIES OF THE KIDNEY AND URINARY TRACT

The occurrence of familial cases of nonsyndromic renal and urinary tract anomalies such as renal agenesis, renal hypoplasia, renal dysplasia, renal tubular dysgenesis, multicystic dysplastic kidney, or VUR supports the fact that even nonsyndromic CAKUT have a genetic basis. Apart from this, the observations that diverse forms of CAKUT occur in the same family suggest that specific genetic mutations can potentially lead to CAKUT, but the final renal phenotype depends on the influence of other modifier genes or environmental factors. However, in most of the studies so far, mutations in potential CAKUT-causing renal developmental genes have been documented in only around 10–20% of patients with CAKUT.[7,18,19] **Table 3** lists the genes which have been found to be associated with nonsyndromic CAKUT. Mutations in many of these genes can also cause syndromic CAKUT.[6,20]

GENETICS OF SYNDROMIC CAKUT

Renal tract malformations can occur as a component of multiorgan syndromes. Some important genetic syndromes associated with CAKUT are listed in **Table 4.**[6,20]

As mentioned in the previous section, some of the genes associated with syndromic CAKUT have also been reported to be mutated in isolated nonsyndromic CAKUT. For instance, *HNF1B*, the gene that encodes the developmentally expressed transcription factor hepatocyte nuclear factor 1, is associated with the RCAD (renal cysts and diabetes) syndrome, but mutations in the gene have also been reported in cases with nonsyndromic renal tract malformations including multicystic dysplastic kidney, hypoplastic kidney, and glomerulocystic kidney.

In addition to monogenic conditions, chromosomal anomalies (gross numerical or structural anomalies as well as submicroscopic CNVs, i.e., microdeletions or microduplications) that encompass genes, which are critical to normal nephrogenesis, have been reported to account for around 10–15% of patients with CAKUT.[6,10,16,21] **Table 5** lists some of the chromosomal anomalies which are known to be associated with CAKUT.[6,10,21,22]

In addition to the CNVs listed in **Table 5** which are more commonly reported in association with CAKUT, many other CNVs involving other chromosomal loci have been reported in different studies.[10]

GENETIC TESTING IN THE CLINIC

Identification of the underlying genetic etiology through appropriate genetic testing helps in better prognostication, appropriate management, accurate genetic counseling, and early intervention in the proband. Even when one is confident of the clinical diagnosis, confirmation by relevant genetic testing is essential, because there can be significant overlap in the clinical features of different genetic conditions, and many disorders are genetically heterogeneous (i.e., the same phenotype can be caused by mutation(s) in any one of many different genes). Further, for severe CAKUT conditions with a poor prognosis, birth of further similarly affected babies in the family can be prevented through accurate carrier testing and prenatal genetic testing through targeted mutation testing, which also require the exact genetic mutation(s) to be identified in the index case.

If the clinical features are suggestive of a syndrome or a specific genetic condition, targeted genetic testing can be done for confirmation of the same. If a specific syndrome caused by a gross chromosomal anomaly (e.g., Down syndrome) is being considered clinically, karyotyping would be the test of choice. For clinically suspected chromosomal microdeletion syndromes (e.g., Williams–Beuren syndrome, DiGeorge syndrome), confirmation can be done through targeted CNV testing through the fluorescence in situ hybridization (FISH) or multiplex ligation-dependent probe amplification (MLPA) test. If a specific single-gene disorder is suspected, sequencing of the associated gene can be done through Sanger sequencing (for a small single gene or a specific known mutation) or through NGS (if the gene is large). For patients where more than one monogenic condition is being considered in the differential diagnosis and for genetically heterogeneous conditions, NGS-based multigene panel testing or clinical exome sequencing is the preferred testing modality. However, when the clinical and laboratory evaluation does not point to any specific etiology, especially for nonsyndromic CAKUT, whole exome sequencing may be done to look for sequence variants related to monogenic conditions, and/or chromosomal microarray to look for genome-wide chromosomal CNVs. Whole genome sequencing is also being increasingly used in the clinic as it helps to screen the entire genome for sequence variants in both the exonic and the intronic regions of genes, as well as for CNVs, throughout the genome, but the cost and the issues related to interpretation of the huge number of variants detected are the limiting factors.

GENETIC COUNSELING

The patterns of inheritance vary for different monogenic causes of CAKUT (as listed in **Tables 3 and 4**), and accordingly the risk of recurrence of the condition in subsequent offspring also varies. Confirmation of the genetic basis through the evaluation approach outlined above is the first and most essential step toward providing accurate genetic counseling for the affected patient and family. Genetic counseling by an appropriately trained clinical geneticist or genetic counselor should help the affected individual/family to comprehend the medical facts about the disorder including the genetic basis, prognosis and the available management, understand the risk of recurrence in other family members, understand the alternatives for dealing with the risk of recurrence, choose a course of action which seems appropriate to them in view of their risk, family values, and ethical standards, and thereby help them to cope in the best possible manner to the condition.

However, exact genotype-phenotype correlation for accurate prognostication for an identified genetic mutation may not always be possible, because of the modifying influences of modifier genes, epigenetic factors and environmental factors, which lead to intra- and interfamilial variable expressivity, as discussed above.

TABLE 3: Genes associated with nonsyndromic congenital anomalies of the kidney and urinary tract (CAKUT).

Gene	OMIM number and pattern of inheritance†	Gene locus	Renal pathology	Extrarenal manifestations
AGT (angiotensinogen)	*106150 AR	1q42	Reduced number of proximal tubules, short proximal tubules without brush border, atrophic loops of Henle and collecting ducts, closely packed glomeruli, marked thickening and disorganization of interlobular and preglomerular arteries	Potter facies, limb-positioning defects, arthrogryposis, lung hypoplasia, skull ossification defects
AGTR1 (angiotensin II receptor, type 1)	*106165 AR	3q24	Renal tubular dysgenesis similar to *AGT* phenotype, PUV	Similar to *AGT* phenotype
AGTR2 (angiotensin II receptor, type 2)	*300034	Xq23	PUJ obstruction, megaureter, multicystic dysplastic kidney, hydronephrosis, PUV (possible association)	–
ACE (angiotensin I converting enzyme)	*106180 AR	17q23	Renal tubular dysgenesis similar to *AGT* phenotype, renal hypodysplasia, PUV	Similar to *AGT* phenotype
BICC1 (bicaudal C1, homolog)	*614295 AD	10q21	Multicystic dysplastic kidney	–
BMP4 (bone morphogenetic protein 4)	*112262 AD	14q22	Renal hypodysplasia	Cleft lip, microphthalmia (syndromic microphthalmia)
DSTYK (dual serine/threonine and tyrosine protein kinase)	*612666 AD	1q32	Renal hypodysplasia, PUJ obstruction, solitary kidney, VUR	
EYA1 (eyes absent homolog 1)	*601653 AD	8q13	Unilateral or bilateral renal agenesis, renal hypodysplasia, VUR	Deafness, ear malformations, branchial cysts (branchiootorenal syndrome)
FRAS1 (Fraser syndrome 1 gene)	*607830 AR	4q21	Renal agenesis, renal hypodysplasia	Ear and heart defects, syndactyly cryptophthalmos (Fraser syndrome)
FREM2 (Fras1-related extra-cellular matrix protein 2)	*608945 AR	13q13	Renal agenesis, renal hypodysplasia	Ear and heart defects, syndactyly, cryptophthalmos (Fraser syndrome)
GATA3 (glutamyl-tRNA amidotransferase subunit A binding protein 3)	*131320 AD	10p14	Renal dysplasia	Hypoparathyroidism, sensorineural deafness (Barakat syndrome)
HNF1B (hepatocyte nuclear factor 1 homeobox B)	*189907 AD	17q12	Renal hypodysplasia, cysts	Diabetes
ITGA8 (integrin alpha 8)	*604063 AR	10p13	Renal hypodysplasia, renal aplasia	–
PAX2 (paired box 2)	*167409 AD	10q24	Renal hypoplasia, VUR	Optic nerve coloboma, branchial cysts
REN (renin)	*179820 AR	1q32	Renal tubular dysgenesis similar to *AGT* phenotype	Similar to *AGT* phenotype
RET (rearranged during transfection protooncogene)	*164761 AD	10q11	Renal agenesis	Hirschsprung disease
ROBO2 (roundabout homolog 2)	* 602431 AD	3p12	Renal hypoplasia, duplex renal system, VUR	–
SIX2 (sine oculis-related homeobox 2 homolog)	*604994	2p21	Renal hypodysplasia (possible association)	–
SLIT2 (Slit homolog 2)	*603746	4p15	Renal agenesis, multicystic dysplastic kidney (possible association)	–
SOX17 [sex-determining region (SRY)-box 17]	*610928 AD	8q11	VUR	–
UMOD (uromodulin)	*191845 AD	16p12	Cysts in distal tubules and collecting ducts, renal dysplasia	–

Contd...

Contd...

Gene	OMIM number and pattern of inheritance†	Gene locus	Renal pathology	Extrarenal manifestations
UPK3A (Uroplakin 3A)	*611559	22q13	Renal agenesis, renal hypodysplasia (possible association)	–
USF2 (upstream transcription factor 2)	*600390	19q13	Multicystic kidney dysplasia, PUJ obstruction (possible association)	–

†Pattern of inheritance is mentioned only for the genes where the associated phenotype is clearly listed with a phenotype number in OMIM; it is not mentioned for the genes which have a possible but not clearly established CAKUT phenotype in humans.
(AD: autosomal dominant inheritance; AR: autosomal recessive inheritance; OMIM: online Mendelian inheritance in man database; PUJ: pelviureteric junction; PUV: posterior urethral valve; XL: X-linked inheritance; VUR: vesicoureteral reflux)

TABLE 4: Syndromes associated with congenital anomalies of the kidney and urinary tract (CAKUT).

Syndrome (OMIM number)	Gene	Systemic manifestations	Renal pathology
Autosomal dominant			
Alagille syndrome-1 (#118450) Alagille syndrome-2 (#610205)	*JAG1* (Jagged 1) *NOTCH2* (Notch receptor 2)	Facial dysmorphism, cholestasis, cardiac anomalies, vertebral segmentation defects, ocular abnormalities	Renal hypoplasia, renal dysplasia, renal cysts, vesicoureteral reflux (Other associated renal anomalies apart from CAKUT—renal tubular acidosis, renal mesangiolipidosis)
Branchio-otorenal syndrome-1 (#113650) Branchio-otorenal syndrome-2 (#610896)	*EYA1* (Eyes absent homolog1) *SIX5* (Sine oculis-related homeobox 2 homolog)	Sensorineural/conductive/mixed hearing loss, structural defects of ear, branchial fistulas or cysts	Renal abnormalities ranging from mild hypoplasia to complete absence
Branchio-oculofacial syndrome (#113620)	*TFAP2A* (transcription factor activating enhancer-binding protein 2 alpha)	Branchial cleft sinus defects, ocular anomalies, facial dysmorphism, cleft or pseudocleft of lip/palate	Renal agenesis, renal cysts
Hypoparathyroidism, sensorineural deafness and renal disease (Barakat syndrome) (#146255)	*GATA3* (glutamyl-tRNA amidotransferase subunit A binding protein 3)	Hypoparathyroidism and sensorineural deafness	Renal dysplasia
Mullerian aplasia and hyperandrogenism (#158330)	*WNT4* (Wingless-type integration site family member 4)	Aplasia or hypoplasia of Mullerian duct derivatives, hyperandrogenism	Renal hypodysplasia, unilateral renal aplasia
Pallister–Hall syndrome (#146510)	*GLI3* (Gli–Kruppel family member 3)	Hypothalamic hamartoma, pituitary dysfunction, central polydactyly, imperforate anus, visceral malformations	Ectopic kidney, renal dysplasia
Renal coloboma (papillorenal) syndrome (#120330)	*PAX2* (Paired box 2)	Ocular anomalies including optic nerve coloboma, hearing loss, central nervous system anomalies, genital anomalies	Renal hypodysplasia, oligomeganephronia, and vesicoureteral reflux
Renal cysts and diabetes (#137920)	*HNF1B* (Hepatocyte nuclear factor 1 homeobox B)	Diabetes, gout, abnormalities of genital tract	Renal cysts, glomerular tufts, enlarged renal pelvis, abnormal calyces, small kidney, oligomeganephronia, single kidney, and horseshoe kidney
Townes–Brocks syndrome (#107480)	*SALL1* (Sal-like protein1)	Imperforate anus, triphalangeal thumbs, anomalies of hands and feet, and sensorineural deafness	Renal malrotation, ectopic kidney, horseshoe kidney, renal hypoplasia, polycystic kidneys, and vesicoureteral reflux

Contd...

Contd...

Syndrome (OMIM number)	Gene	Systemic manifestations	Renal pathology
Autosomal recessive			
Bifid nose with or without renal agenesis and anorectal malformations (# 608980)	*FREM1* (Fras1-related extracellular matrix protein 1)	Median nose cleft, wide bulbous nasal tip, anorectal malformations	Unilateral or bilateral renal agenesis
Cenani–Lenz syndactyly syndrome (#212780)	*LRP4* (low-density lipoprotein receptor-related protein 4)	Facial dysmorphism, syndactyly of hands and feet, anomalies of forearm bones	Renal aplasia, renal hypoplasia
Fraser syndrome-1 (#219000) Fraser syndrome-2 (#617666) Fraser syndrome-3 (#617667)	*FRAS1* (Fraser syndrome1 gene) *FREM2* (Fras1-related extracellular matrix protein 2) *GRIP1* (Glutamate receptor-interacting protein 1)	Cryptophthalmos, ear malformations, syndactyly, genital tract malformations, laryngeal anomalies	Unilateral or bilateral renal agenesis with/without ureteral agenesis, hypoplastic or absent bladder, cystic dysplasia of kidneys
Prune belly (Eagle–Barrett) syndrome (#100100)	*CHRM3* (Cholinergic receptor, muscarinic 3)	Thin abdominal musculature with overlying lax skin, cryptorchidism	Megacystis, megaureter, and bilateral hydronephrosis
Robinow syndrome—autosomal-recessive type (#268310)	*ROR2* (receptor tyrosine kinase-like orphan receptor 2)	Facial dysmorphism, short stature, mesomelic or acromesomelic limb shortening, vertebral segmentation defects, and genital abnormalities	Hydronephrosis and renal duplication
Urofacial syndrome-1 (#236730) Urofacial syndrome-2 (#615112)	*HPSE2* (Heparanase 2) *LRIG2* (Leucine-rich repeats and immunoglobulin-like domains-containing protein 2)	Peculiar facies with grimace-like facial expression, constipation, and cryptorchidism	Hydroureteronephrosis, urethral obstruction, and vesicoureteral reflux
X-linked			
Kallmann syndrome 1 (#308700)	*KAL1* (Kallmann syndrome 1 gene)	Anosmia and hypogonadotropic hypogonadism	Unilateral renal agenesis
Simpson–Golabi–Behmel syndrome (#312870)	*GPC3* (glypican 3)	Somatic overgrowth, coarse facies, congenital heart defects, and tumors	Large dysplastic kidneys, hydronephrosis
STAR (syndactyly, telecanthus, and anogenital and renal malformations) syndrome (#300707)	*FAM58A* (Family with sequence similarity 58, member A)	Pre- and postnatal growth retardation, facial dysmorphism, toe syndactyly, cardiac anomalies, and anogenital malformations	Solitary kidney, ectopic kidney, hydronephrosis, vesicoureteral reflux, and small unstable bladder
Genetic basis uncertain			
Mayer–Rokintansky–Kuster–Hauser syndrome (%277000)	Believed to have female-limited autosomal dominant inheritance	Anomalies of the female genital tract (ranging from upper vaginal atresia to total Mullerian agenesis)	Unilateral or bilateral renal agenesis
VACTERL association (%192350)	–	Vertebral defects, anal atresia, cardiac defects, tracheoesophageal fistula, radial dysplasia, limb defects	Renal agenesis and renal dysplasia

(OMIM: online Mendelian inheritance in man database)

CONCLUSION

Thus, even though a large proportion of patients with congenital anomalies of the renal tract have a multifactorial etiology, monogenic or chromosomal causes may be seen in as many as 20–30% of patients with CAKUT. A specific genetic cause is more likely to be identified for syndromic and familial forms of CAKUT. Identification of the exact genetic basis in an affected individual helps not only in appropriate management and prognostication of the index patient but also in appropriate genetic counseling of the family.

KEY POINTS

- CAKUT are among the most common birth defects and account for almost 30–50% of cases of CKD and ESKD in the pediatric age group.

TABLE 5: Chromosomal anomalies associated with congenital anomalies of the kidney and urinary tract (CAKUT).

Chromosomal anomaly	***Associated CAKUT***
Gross chromosomal anomalies (detectable through karyotyping)	
Trisomy 21 (Down syndrome)	Renal anomalies found in around 5–10% of patients. Reported anomalies include: renal agenesis or hypoplasia, horseshoe kidney, hydroureteronephrosis, pelviureteric junction obstruction, hypoplastic bladder, posterior urethral valve, and urethral stenosis
Trisomy 13 (Patau syndrome)	Renal anomalies present in around 50–60% of patients. Reported anomalies include: cystic kidneys (most common), hydroureteronephrosis, duplication of the kidney and urinary tract, fetal lobulation of the kidneys, megacystis, bladder neck stenosis, vesicoureteral obstruction, horseshoe kidney, and unilateral renal agenesis
Trisomy 18 (Edward syndrome)	Renal anomalies present in around 30–70% of patients. Reported anomalies include: duplication of the urinary tract, horseshoe kidney, cystic kidneys, hydroureteronephrosis, ectopic kidney, renal agenesis or hypoplasia, unilateral renal hyperplasia, renal hamartoma, fetal lobulation, rotational anomalies, and renal dysplasia
Monosomy X (Turner syndrome)	Renal anomalies present in around 30–40% of patients. Reported anomalies include: horseshoe kidney (most common), duplication of the urinary tract, ureteropelvic obstruction, hydronephrosis, ectopic kidney, aplastic or hypoplastic kidney, and urethral meatal stenosis
Mosaic trisomy 8	Renal anomalies present in around 70–80% of patients. Reported anomalies include: hydronephrosis, bifid pelvis, horseshoe kidney, and vesicoureteral reflex
Partial tetrasomy 22 (Cat eye syndrome)	Renal anomalies present in 60–80% of patients. Reported anomalies include: renal agenesis, hypoplasia, cystic dysplasia, horseshoe kidney, pelvic kidney, ureteropelvic junction obstruction, urethral stenosis, and vesicoureteral reflux
5p deletion (Cri-du-chat syndrome)	Renal anomalies reported in some patients. Reported anomalies include: horseshoe kidney, duplication of the urinary tract, and solitary kidney
Submicroscopic chromosomal copy number variations	
1q21.1 deletion 1q21.1 duplication	Renal hypodysplasia Vesicoureteral reflux
4p16.3 deletion (Wolf–Hirschhorn syndrome)	Renal agenesis or hypoplasia, vesicoureteral reflux
7q11.23 deletion (Williams–Beuren syndrome)	Renal hypoplasia, solitary kidney, pelvic kidney, vesicoureteral reflux, bladder diverticula, and urethral stenosis
16p11.2 deletion 16p11.2 duplication	Renal hypodysplasia, obstructive uropathy Renal hypodysplasia
17q12 deletion 17q12 duplication (17q12 includes *HNF1B* gene which is associated with renal cysts and diabetes syndrome)	Renal hypodysplasia, cystic dysplasia, obstructive uropathy Renal hypodysplasia
22q11.2 deletion (DiGeorge syndrome) 22q11.2 duplication	Hydronephrosis, renal agenesis, multicystic dysplastic kidney Renal hypodysplasia

- Monogenic causes are identified in around 10–20% and chromosomal CNVs in around 10–15% of patients with CAKUT.
- A specific genetic etiology is more often identified in syndromic and/or familial forms of CAKUT.
- If the clinical features suggest a specific syndromic entity, the relevant cytogenetic or molecular genetic test can be done for confirmation of the same.
- Whole exome sequencing for pathogenic variants related to monogenic causes and chromosomal microarray for chromosomal CNVs are the currently preferred modalities for genetic testing of nonsyndromic CAKUT.

REFERENCES

1. Livera LN, Brookfield DS, Egginton JA, Hawnaur JM. Antenatal ultrasonography to detect fetal renal abnormalities: a prospective screening programme. BMJ. 1989;298(6685):1421-3.
2. Loane M, Dolk H, Kelly A, Teljeur C, Greenlees R, Densem J, EUROCAT Working Group. Paper 4: EUROCAT statistical monitoring: identification and investigation of ten year trends of congenital anomalies in Europe. Birth Defects Res A Clin Mol Teratol. 2011;91(Suppl 1):S31-43.
3. Ardissino G, Daccò V, Testa S, Bonaudo R, Claris-Appiani A, Taioli E, et al. Epidemiology of chronic renal failure in children: Data from the ItalKid project. Pediatrics. 2003;111:382-7.
4. Sanna-Cherchi S, Ravani P, Corbani V, Parodi S, Haupt R, Piaggio G, et al. Renal outcome in patients with congenital anomalies of the kidney and urinary tract. Kidney Int. 2009;76:528-33.

5. Sanna-Cherchi S, Caridi G, Weng P, Scolari F, Perfumo F, et al. Genetic approaches to human renal agenesis/hypoplasia and dysplasia. Pediatr Nephrol. 2007;22:1675-84.
6. Nicolaou N, Renkema KY, Bongers EM, Giles RH, Knoers NV. Genetic, environmental, and epigenetic factors involved in CAKUT. Nat Rev Nephrol. 2015;11:720-31.
7. van der Ven AT, Connaughton DM, Ityel H, Mann N, Nakayama M, Chen J, et al. Whole-exome sequencing identifies causative mutations in families with congenital anomalies of the kidney and urinary Tract. J Am Soc Nephrol. 2018;29:2348-61.
8. Nigam A, Knoers NVAM, Renkema KY. Impact of next generation sequencing on our understanding of CAKUT. Semin Cell Dev Biol. 2019;91:104-10.
9. van der Ven AT, Vivante A, Hildebrandt F. Novel insights into the pathogenesis of monogenic congenital anomalies of the kidney and urinary tract. J Am Soc Nephrol. 2018;29:36-50.
10. Sanna-Cherchi S, Kiryluk K, Burgess KE, Bodria M, Sampson MG, Hadley D, et al. Copy-number disorders are a common cause of congenital kidney malformations. Am J Hum Genet. 2012;91:987-97.
11. Schedl A. Renal abnormalities and their developmental origin. Nat Rev Genet. 2007;8:791-802.
12. Jain S, Chen F. Developmental pathology of congenital kidney and urinary tract anomalies. Clin Kidney J. 2019;12:382-99.
13. Vivante A, Kohl S, Hwang DY, Dworschak DC, Hildebrandt F. Single-gene causes of congenital anomalies of the kidney and urinary tract (CAKUT) in humans. Pediatr Nephrol. 2014;29:695-704.
14. Reidy KJ, Rosenblum ND. Cell and molecular biology of kidney development. Semin Nephrol. 2009;29:321-37.
15. Shah MM, Sampogna RV, Sakurai H, Bush KT, Nigam SK. Branching morphogenesis and kidney disease. Development. 2004;131:1449-62.
16. Murugapoopathy V, Gupta IR. A primer on congenital anomalies of the kidneys and urinary tracts. Clin J Am Soc Nephrol. 2020;15:723-731.
17. Talati AN, Webster CM, Vora NL. Prenatal genetic considerations of congenital anomalies of the kidney and urinary tract (CAKUT). Prenat Diagn. 2019;39:679-92.
18. Lei T-Y, Fu F, Li R, Wang D, Wang R-Y, Jing X-Y, et al. Whole-exome sequencing for prenatal diagnosis of fetuses with congenital anomalies of the kidney and urinary tract. Nephrol Dial Transplant. 2017;32:1665-75.
19. Bekheirnia MR, Bekheirnia N, Bainbridge MN, Gu S, Coban Akdemir ZH, Gambin T, et al. Whole-exome sequencing in the molecular diagnosis of individuals with congenital anomalies of the kidney and urinary tract and identification of a new causative gene. Genet Med. 2017;19:412-20.
20. Adalat S, Bockenhauer D, Ledermann SE, Hennekam RC, Woolf AS. Renal malformations associated with mutations of developmental genes: messages from the clinic. Pediatr Nephrol. 2010;25:2247-55.
21. Sanna-Cherchi S, Westland R, Ghiggeri GM, Gharavi AG. Genetic basis of human congenital anomalies of the kidney and urinary tract. J Clin Invest. 2018;128:4-15.
22. Barakat AY, Butler MG. Renal and urinary tract abnormalities associated with chromosome aberrations. Int J Pediatr Nephrol. 1987;8:215-26.

CHAPTER

13.2

Antenatal Hydronephrosis and Postnatal Outcomes

Sushmita Banerjee, Subhasis Saha

INTRODUCTION

Modern-day obstetrics includes the performance of ultrasound scans (USS) regularly during the intrapartum period in pregnant women. Abnormalities of the fetus, amniotic fluid, and placenta may thus become evident at an early stage enabling optimum planning for therapy and timing of delivery. The kidney formation starts from the 5th week postconception. Renal abnormalities may be detected by ultrasound from the 9th to 12th week of gestation. The amniotic fluid volume is dependent on fetal urine production; thus, oligohydramnios may be due to severe bilateral fetal renal disease.[1]

Accumulation of fluid within the renal collecting system causing dilatation of the renal pelvis ± calyces is termed as "hydronephrosis (HDN)." It may be physiological, causing no harm to the developing kidney. However, it may also indicate congenital obstruction which will result in progressive renal damage and/or other complications such as urinary tract infection (UTI), stones, renal dysfunction, and even renal failure, if not treated effectively. Congenital renal obstruction is defined as "impaired urinary drainage, which, if uncorrected, will limit the ultimate functional potential of the developing kidney."[2] To date, no single imaging study exists which can definitively prove or disprove the presence of renal obstruction at this early stage and hence the controversy surrounding management.[3] The challenge is to select patients who have such damaging pathologies and investigate and treat them early and aggressively, while avoiding overinvestigating those that will have a benign course. Having a prognosis-based follow-up protocol also helps in counseling the parents about the implications of the antenatal finding on ultrasonography. This necessitates the formulation of a universally acceptable classification system which may give us a prognostic as well as a therapeutic guideline as to how to proceed with these cases. Various descriptive terminologies are in use such as "pelvicaliectasis," "pelviectasis," "HDN," "pelvic fullness," which adds to the confusion. So, it makes sense for all the concerned specialties (fetal medicine specialists, obstetricians, pediatricians, radiologists, and pediatric surgeons) to speak in a common language using a common set of descriptive terms.

EPIDEMIOLOGY

Hydronephrosis is the most commonly detected antenatal fetal anomaly. The epidemiology of antenatal HDN (ANHDN) reported in different studies varies according to defining criteria and timing of the study, with a prevalence between 0.6 and 5%; of these, 17–54% occurring bilaterally.[4,5] Following the criteria of renal pelvic diameter ≥4 mm in the second trimester and ≥7 mm in the third trimester, a prospective study from New Delhi reported ANHDN in 0.83% of 32,443 fetuses.[6] In the same study, over 70% of second-trimester HDN had resolved postnatally, while >85% of third-trimester HDN with renal pelvic diameter >10 mm resulted in postnatal congenital anomalies of the kidney and urinary tract (CAKUT).

ETIOLOGY AND PATHOLOGY

The large proportion of HDN detected antenatally is transient (i.e., resolves prenatally), while some reduce or resolve over months to years after birth and do not cause progressive renal damage or other complications. However, HDN that is severe, progressive, and requires follow-up, monitoring, and interventions may be due to the following underlying abnormalities:[7]

- Obstruction at the pelviureteric junction obstruction (PUJO)
- Structural or functional obstruction at the ureteric level:
    - Ureteric stricture
    - Vesicoureteric junction obstruction (VUJO)
    - Ureterocele/ectopic ureteric opening
    - Congenital megaureter
    - Prune belly syndrome
- Vesicoureteric reflux (VUR)
- Structural or functional obstruction at the level of the lower urinary tract (LUTO):
    - Posterior urethral valves (PUV)
    - Anterior urethral valves
    - Urethral stricture/atresia
    - Cloacal anomaly/urogenital sinus
    - Detrusor-sphincter dyssynergia

Of these, the most frequently occurring defect is PUJO followed by VUR and then VUJO. Among LUTO, the most common pathology is PUV.[8]

Rarely, the renal abnormality is part of a syndrome involving other organs,[9] and may be associated with major cardiovascular or neurological abnormality. Several genetic etiologies of ANHDN have been detected and genes involving the renin-angiotensin system have been implicated. The molecular pathways of renal damage after producing experimental obstruction have been described. Interested readers are recommended to read other sources for detailed information, which is beyond the scope of this chapter.[10-12]

In case of obstructive uropathies, urinary drainage is impaired to an extent that causes increased back pressure and stasis within the proximal renal tract. The intrinsic compliance of the renal pelvicalyceal system may initially compensate, causing dilatation without damage to the renal parenchyma. Extrarenal pelvis has greater compliance than intrarenal pelvis while calyces have the least compliance.[13] Persistent and severe obstruction will lead to parenchymal compression with thinning, poor growth, and eventually reduced renal function. Patients with conditions such as PUV, VUR, and prune belly syndrome may have elements of coexisting renal dysplasia which can also add to renal functional compromise. Infection associated with VUR is associated with a higher risk of developing renal parenchymal scars.

In all such cases, the aim is to relieve obstruction, normalize intrarenal pressure, and prevent urinary tract infections (UTIs) so as to optimally preserve renal function.

SYMPTOMATOLOGY

Antenatal HDN is usually an incidental finding on a routine pregnancy ultrasound. The finding of associated oligohydramnios is indicative of possible severe and bilateral renal involvement. Gross oligohydramnios may cause hypoplastic lungs, intrauterine growth retardation, and intrauterine death.

Postnatal isolated HDN may also be completely asymptomatic. However, urinary stasis increases the risk of UTIs, which is the most common complication. Severe HDN may be associated with a palpable renal mass. Older children may complain of flank pain, which is seen in progressive severe HDN or when there is twisting of the renal pedicle. LUTO may present with a poor urinary stream and a palpable urinary bladder. Associated undescended testes and a deficient abdominal wall musculature indicate prune belly syndrome. A prolapsed ureterocele may present as a cystic mass at the introitus. Patients may have hypertension or delayed growth, anemia, bone changes, or acidosis due to chronic kidney disease (CKD) when both kidneys have significant damage. Hematuria may occur due to sudden decompression, as following catheterization in the posterior urethral valve (to prevent this nongravitational drainage is preferred, keeping the Urobag in the same horizontal plane or slightly lower than the bladder for the first 24 hours, enabling slow decompression).

EVALUATION FOR DIAGNOSIS

Diagnosis is made by the finding of a dilated renal pelvis ± calyceal system on antenatal ultrasound. Calyceal dilatation is associated with a greater risk of renal parenchymal damage than pelvic dilatation alone. Measurements are required for definition, to track changes, and also serve as an indication of severity and prognosis. Several grading systems exist; the anteroposterior diameter (APD), Society of Fetal Urology (SFU), and urinary tract dilatation (UTD) systems are described below. In situations where ultrasound findings are ill defined (e.g., maternal obesity), magnetic resonance imaging (MRI) may be resorted to.

Anteroposterior Diameter Grading System

A renal anteroposterior diameter (APD) of ≥4 mm in the second trimester and ≥7 mm in third trimester is generally taken as the cutoffs for the diagnosis of ANHDN[13] **(Table 1)**. The largest anteroposterior (AP) diameter is considered; however, measurements are observer dependent and subject to variability depending on the state of hydration and bladder filling. HDN is classified as mild, moderate, and severe depending on the measurement obtained and the time of gestation. This system does not factor in the presence of calyceal dilatation, an extrarenal pelvis, or parenchymal characteristics. In the postnatal period, renal pelvic APD >7 mm in a neonate and >1 cm in an older child is considered abnormal and an indication for further investigation and follow-up.

Society of Fetal Urology Grading

The SFU grading takes into account the renal pelvic dilatation as above, plus calyceal dilatation and parenchymal thinning,[8] and classifies HDN into grades 1–4 **(Fig. 1)**. However, interobserver variability remains an issue. Additionally, only fetal urinary tract dilatation is assessed. It is difficult to corroborate this grading system with postnatal urinary tract dilatation.

In addition to measurements of pelvicalyceal dilatation, it is also important, in fact having a greater bearing on prognosis, to measure renal cortical/parenchymal thickness, particularly in the follow-up of HDN in the postnatal period. The measurements of cortical thickness are less variable than the measurements of dilatation, as they are not influenced by hydration, position, and bladder-filling status. They are also less operator dependent.[13] Cortical thinning is associated with renal functional damage and loss of nephrons. In infants, normal cortical thickness is >3 mm, and measurements <1.5 mm are associated with irreversible damage.

TABLE 1: Gradation by pelvic anteroposterior diameter.

Classification of hydronephrosis	*Renal pelvic anteroposterior diameter*	
	Second trimester	*Third trimester*
Mild	4–6 mm	7–9 mm
Moderate	7–10 mm	10–15 mm
Severe	>10 mm	>15 mm

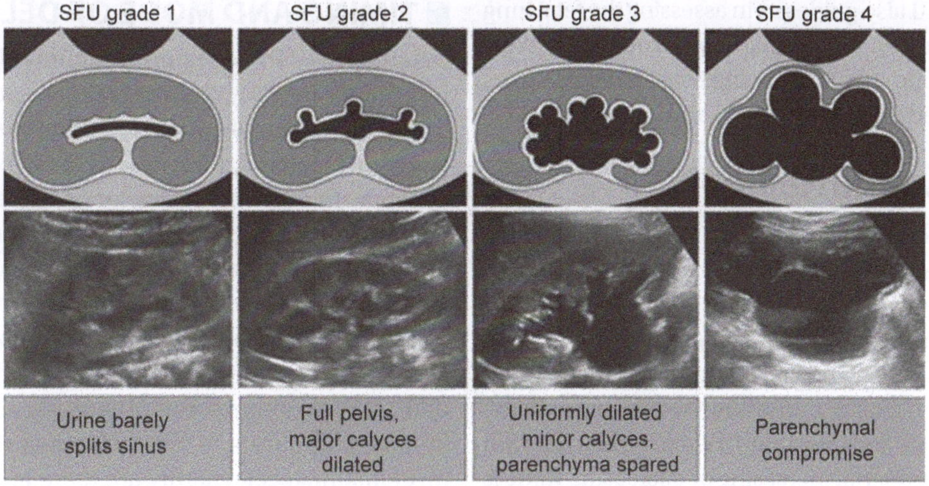

Fig. 1: Society of Fetal Urology (SFU) grading.

TABLE 2: Ultrasonography (USG) parameters included in the urinary tract dilatation (UTD) classification.

US parameters	*Measurement/findings*	*Note*
Anteroposterior renal pelvic diameter (APRPD)	mm	Measured on transverse image at the maximal diameter of intrarenal pelvis
Calyceal dilation • Central (major calyces) • Peripheral (minor calyces)	 Yes/No Yes/No	
Parenchymal thickness	Normal/Abnormal	Subjective assessment
Parenchymal appearance	Normal/Abnormal	Evaluate echogenicity, corticomedullary differentiation, and for cortical cysts
Ureter	Normal/Abnormal	Dilation of ureter is considered abnormal; however, transient visualization of the ureter is considered normal postnatally
Bladder	Normal/Abnormal	Evaluate wall thickness, for the presence of ureterocele, and for a dilated posterior urethra

Increased echogenicity of the renal parenchyma, cystic changes, and loss of corticomedullary differentiation are bad prognostic factors for renal function.[14]

The USS evaluation should also involve details of any ureteric dilatation, bladder filling and emptying, amniotic fluid volume and bladder wall thickness, and/or presence of any diverticula in the bladder. Ureteric dilatation is associated with VUR, congenital megaureter, ureteric stricture, ureterocele, and VUJO. The finding of bilateral HDNU regardless of the degree with associated thick bladder wall and poor bladder emptying, or presence of urinoma, indicates LUTO. The presence of oligohydramnios indicates severe LUTO and/or renal functional compromise and is a major warning sign.

Urinary Tract Dilatation Classification

This is the only classification system that includes all the above parameters and correlates antenatal with postnatal dilatation of the urinary tract **(Tables 2 to 4; Flowcharts 1 and 2)**. This classification was proposed by a consensus meeting convened on March 14–15, 2014 in Linthicum, Maryland, USA. Fetal medicine specialists, radiologists, pediatric nephrologists, and pediatric urologists came together to suggest a seamless guideline to follow these babies up from antenatal life to postnatally.[14] It is important that all the parameters mentioned in **Table 2** are assessed during antenatal or postnatal ultrasonography; normal values are given in **Table 3**. The consensus panel recommended avoiding the use of nonspecific terms (e.g., HDN, pelvicaliectasis, and pelvic fullness) and consistently use the term "UT dilatation," besides the specific sonographic findings mentioned in **Table 2**. During any USS of the renal system, pelvic APD exceeding 1 cm is considered significant and involves added risk at any time of the pregnancy. Renal parenchymal echogenicity is compared to that of the surrounding viscera (liver and spleen) and that of the vertebra.

This single unified system can accommodate all cases who have been graded antenatally even by a different grading system. For example, SFU grades 1 and 2 would be equivalent to UTD P1, SFU grade 3 to UTD P2, and SFU grade 4 to UTD P3 **(Table 4)**.

Role of Antenatal MRI

Fetuses with ANHDN can be further assessed with fetal MRI in a few select cases (complex anomalies, single kidney, and bilateral HDN).[15] MRI also guides us in assessing the fetal lung volume, when fetal interventions such as fetoscopic cystoscopy and/or vesicoamniotic shunts are being considered in babies with underdeveloped lungs between 28 and 32 weeks.

ANTENATAL MONITORING

In the antenatal period, follow-up of HDN is by USS performed every 4–6 weeks. However, suspicion of LUTO, particularly in the presence of oligohydramnios, increases the requirement of monitoring frequency.[4] Biochemical examination of fetal urine to assess the severity of renal compromise is an option in centers where such facilities exist but is associated with the risk of premature labor and infection.[16] When the biochemical examination is done, a serial increasing or decreasing value is more informative than a single value, which, being invasive, is not usually resorted to.

TABLE 3: Normal values for the urinary tract dilatation (UTD) classification.

Ultrasound findings	*Time at presentation*		
	16–27 weeks	***≥28 weeks***	***Postnatal (>48 hours)***
Anteroposterior • Renal pelvis • Diameter (APRPD)	<4 mm	<7 mm	<10 mm
Calyceal dilation • Central • Peripheral	 No No	 No No	 No No
Parenchymal thickness	Normal	Normal	Normal
Parenchymal appearance	Normal	Normal	Normal
Ureter (s)	Normal	Normal	Normal
Bladder	Normal	Normal	Normal
Unexplained oligohydramnios	No	No	NA

TIMING AND MODE OF DELIVERY

Usually, ANHDN does not preclude delivery near term. Indications for early delivery are rare, and mentioned below, however, even in such cases, attempt should be made to continue pregnancy till at least 34–36 weeks. Preterm delivery comes with its own baggage of possible morbidity such as necrotizing enterocolitis and bronchopulmonary dysplasia. Premature infants and neonatal intensive care unit (NICU) graduates have been seen to have increased incidences of learning disabilities, speech delay, and behavioral disorders as well. Smaller babies also have the added disadvantage of difficult cystoscopic access. The mode of delivery is dictated by maternal indications. Except for cloacal exstrophy and large myelomeningocele, hardly are there indications of elective lower uterine segment cesarean section (LUCS) just for the presence of HDN.

POSTNATAL INVESTIGATIONS AND FOLLOW-UP

In all patients with a dilated renal system, a postnatal USS must be performed to confirm findings. In a patient with mild unilateral HDN, this is better performed after 48 hours and before the end of the first week to have a normal hydration state, since early neonatal life may be associated with a relatively dehydrated state with poor urinary output, and mild HDN may not be evident. If postnatal USS is normal, a repeat at 4–6 weeks is advised for confirmation.[4,17]

The most vital issue again is to exclude LUTO. If there is LUTO suspicion from antenatal workups, or clinically the baby has a poor urinary stream, urosepsis, or a distended palpable poorly emptying bladder, then a USS should be performed urgently, and investigations for infection and renal function performed. In suspected LUTO, a micturating cystourethrogram (MCU) is required, but undertaken after ensuring adequate bladder drainage, sterile urine, and

TABLE 4: Prognostication and guidance to management based on urinary tract dilatation (UTD) classification (with reference to Flowcharts 1 and 2).

Antenatal and initial postnatal assessment	*Postnatal follow-up*
UTD A1 (low risk): • If diagnosed <32 weeks—a repeat USG scan after 32 weeks • If USG beyond 32 weeks shows resolved renal architecture—no further follow-up antenatally • If USG shows UTD A1—postnatal USG at >48 hours but <1 month and 6 months later *UTD A 2-3 (higher risk):* • Monthly USG assessment • Prenatal counseling session with pediatric nephrologist/urologist • Postnatal USG > 48 hours but <1 month (except bilateral lesions and evidence of bladder outlet obstruction where assessment has to be <48 hours after birth or earlier)	• *UTD P1:* Follow-up USG in 1–6 months. Recommendations for VCUG and CAP are left to the treating physician as management of asymptomatic VUR varies greatly across the globe • *UTD P2:* Follow-up USG in 1–3 months. Need for VCUG, CAP, and functional scans are left to the treating physician's discretion • *UTD P3:* Follow-up USG is recommended in a month. VCUG and CAP are recommended. Need for functional scans is left to the discretion of the treating physicians

(CAP: continuous antibiotic prophylaxis; USG: ultrasonography; UTD: urinary tract dilatation; VCUG: voiding cystourethrogram; VUR: vesicoureteric reflux)

metabolic equilibrium. The main reason is to diagnose the precise cause of LUTO and initiate early management.

After postnatal confirmation of HDN and in the absence of LUTO, subsequent management depends on the findings on initial postnatal USS and clinical findings. An MCU is also indicated if there is ureteral dilatation (to differentiate ureteral obstruction from bladder pathologies, ureteroceles, and VUR) and if there is gross bladder dilatation and/or bladder wall thickening suggesting LUTO.

Flowchart 1: Antenatal assessment of risk by urinary tract dilatation (UTD) classification.

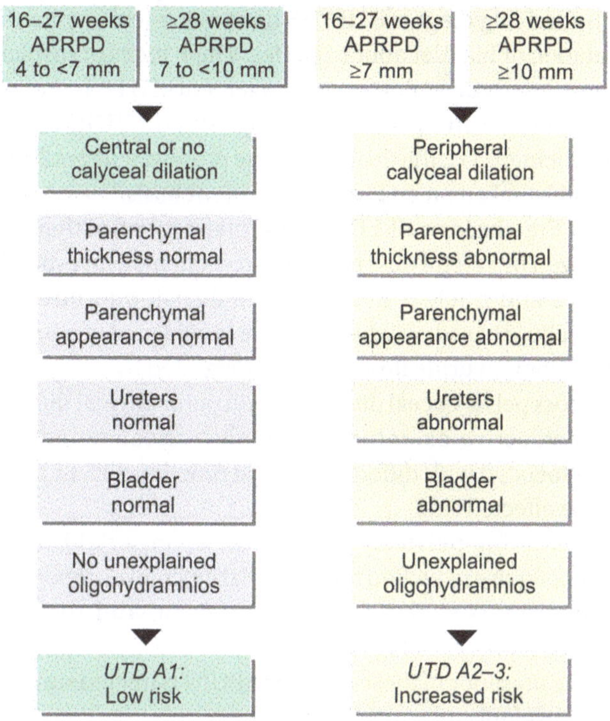

(APRPD: anteroposterior renal pelvic diameter)

A diethylenetriaminepentaacetic acid (DTPA), ethylene dicysteine (EC), or mercaptoacetyltriglycine (MAG3) scan is indicated when there is significant HDN and we want to look at the excretory pattern as well as differential renal function. It is preferably performed at least after 6–8 weeks of age in unilateral pelvicalyceal dilatation to allow for some degree of maturation of neonatal cortical function. Furosemide is administered to differentiate obstruction from "reservoir effect." Obstruction is indicated when one-half of the administered isotope (T1/2) is not excreted by 20 minutes.

Dimercaptosuccinic acid (DMSA) scan is occasionally performed to detect renal functioning parenchyma, differential function, and scarring.

In some patients, magnetic resonance urography (MRU) may be indicated in the postnatal period to exclude ureteric stricture or VUJO. It is also useful for diagnosing ectopic ureteral opening, duplex renal systems, and delineating complex congenital malformations. The presence of an aberrant blood vessel causing external obstruction may also be detected by this technique. MRU gives a clear anatomical picture of the urinary tract and some software even allows a 3D reconstruction, which prevents the need for an intravenous urography (IVU). The cost and need for sedation/anesthesia are significant drawbacks.

Intravenous urography is rarely used nowadays because of the radiation burden it carries. Rarely it is used for anatomical and functional investigation of complex anomalies

Flowchart 2: Postnatal assessment of risk by urinary tract dilatation (UTD) classification.

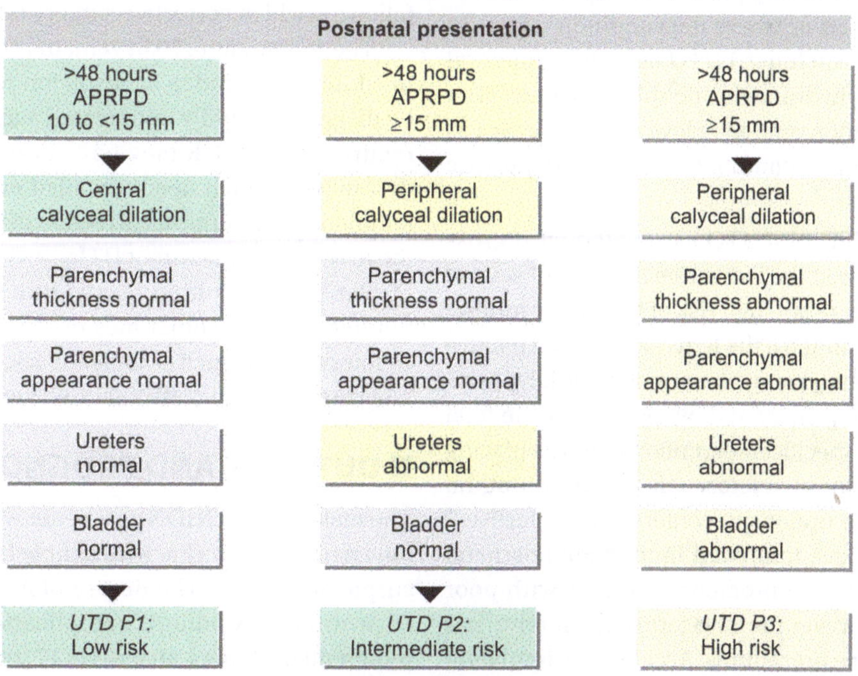

(APRPD: anteroposterior renal pelvic diameter)

(ureteral stricture, ectopic ureteric opening, etc.) where other modalities are unavailable or have failed to provide information adequately. Dynamic contrast MRU is replacing IVU or contrast-enhanced computed tomography (CECT) wherever facilities are available. It diminishes the overall radiation exposure.

Several biomarkers are under investigation[18] for the differentiation of HDN which will result in renal damage without interventions, from those that will not. Till date, these have not reached significant relevance in clinical practice.

DIFFERENTIAL DIAGNOSIS

When HDN is detected in the antenatal period, the workup both in the antenatal period and extending onto the postnatal period involves differentiation between the various causes as listed previously. A multicystic dysplastic kidney may be mistaken for HDN but is differentiated by the presence of noncommunicating cysts with the absence of normal renal parenchyma, and nonfunction demonstrated by nuclear imaging postnatally.

When the condition is missed in the antenatal period, it may present postnatally during workup after a UTI, in case of urinary symptoms or with abdominal pain. In such cases, the disease has to be differentiated from other postnatal causes of urinary tract obstruction, such as stones and tumors. Patients with neurogenic bladder, detrusor-sphincter dyssynergia, and other bowel-bladder malfunctions can develop progressive HDN which needs to be differentiated from the etiologies listed previously.

THERAPY

It is most important to identify pathologies in which both kidneys may be damaged or where the condition occurs in a solitary kidney. This includes LUTO as well as bilateral severe PUJO/VUR or a hydronephrotic solitary kidney. The threshold for surgical intervention is lower in such cases as they do not have a healthy contralateral kidney to provide functional reserve.

In the antenatal period, LUTO associated with gross oligohydramnios has been the indication for trials of several interventions. When there is a high risk of fetal compromise, early delivery can be planned if the fetus has reached relative maturity. Intrauterine infusions with normal saline have been used to prolong the pregnancy and allow time for the fetal lungs to mature. More specific interventions such as placing a fetal vesicoamniotic shunt or fetoscopic posterior urethral valve ablations are also options in centers with expertise.[19] Generally, the latter have improved immediate postnatal survival and ventilation requirement in fetuses with poor prognostic features; however, the long-term renal survival has not improved with these procedures. Accidental stimulation of labor and infection are the associated risks.[20]

In the postnatal period, LUTO has to be treated on an urgent basis. A urethral catheter is placed to allow bladder drainage. Urinary infection and metabolic derangements, if any, are corrected. The baseline renal function is recorded. Once the baby is medically stable, a specific intervention is performed. Most commonly, this involves the fulguration of PUV.

Prophylactic antibiotics for the prevention of UTIs are a controversial issue. The main reason for prescribing them, until investigations are complete, is the possibility of VUR as an underlying diagnosis. If USS does not reveal any ureteric dilatation or bladder abnormalities, a high index of suspicion aimed at early detection and management of UTIs is probably sufficient. In the presence of high-grade VUR, or after documented UTI, the decision to use prophylactic antibiotics should be taken on an individual patient basis.[21]

In the absence of LUTO, the majority of patients are managed by careful observation and sequential investigation by USS and nuclear imaging. The decision to intervene surgically is based on whether there is evidence of structural obstruction to urine flow.[22] This is suggested by:

- Gross pelvicalyceal dilatation with parenchymal thinning, obstructive excretory curve on nuclear renography associated with differential renal function 10% or less on the affected side
- Increasing pelvicalyceal dilatation on serial USS and progressive reduction in differential function on renography
- Symptoms such as pain, hematuria, and recurrent infections

The presence of these criteria in PUJO is treated surgically with a pyeloplasty.

These may also occur in VUJO or in ureteric stenosis, where the ureter will also be dilated. Making the differentiation may require an MRU to locate the exact site of obstruction following which corrective surgery may be planned.

The treatment of VUR remains controversial. There is a need for a high index of suspicion for UTIs which need to be diagnosed rapidly and treated aggressively. Patients with recurrent UTI/VUR may have underlying bowel bladder dysfunction which needs detailed evaluation. Prophylactic antibiotics and surgical correction of VUR are the choices for those who have persistent UTIs.

Patients with bladder dysfunction require detailed noninvasive and sometimes urodynamic studies, followed by interventions such as biofeedback, anticholinergics, alpha blockers, CIC, and rarely bladder augmentation.

OUTCOME AND PROGNOSIS

The majority of ANHDN gets better with no intervention and only needs monitoring with simple USS and a high index of suspicion for UTI. The degree of ANHDN predicts the risk of postnatal pathology, complications, and intervention requirement. A meta-analysis of 17 studies found that this risk was 11.9% for mild, 45.1% for moderate, and 88.3% for severe

ANHDN. However, the risk of postnatal VUR did not vary with the degree of ANHDN.[7]

Long-term follow-up for proteinuria, hypertension, and renal function is indicated in all persistent cases.

CONCLUSION

Antenatal HDN is the most common fetal anomaly detected on pregnancy USS. Transient and benign forms are the most common and have to be differentiated from conditions that will cause renal damage or other complications. Having a consensus classification of grading and terminologies helps a seamless transfer of radiological information from the obstetrician or fetal medicine specialists to the pediatric nephrologists/pediatric surgeons. Urinary tract dilatation classification provides a comprehensive assessment of all aspects needed for diagnosis as well as prognostication. The presence of oligohydramnios and other features of LUTO needs to be picked up early and monitored closely. LUTO requires early postnatal intervention in a center that has all the appropriate neonatal and nephrourology facilities. Postnatal monitoring and investigations are required to diagnose conditions that are progressive and require intervention.

KEY POINTS

- The majority of antenatal HDN is transient and benign.
- However, we need to correctly select patients who have significant underlying disease and require interventions to avoid progressive kidney damage.
- The presence of features of lower urinary tract obstruction requires close monitoring and delivery in a unit with NICU and nephrourology setup.
- Obstructed renal systems will have signs of severe/progressive dilatation and deterioration of function and require early detection and intervention.
- A standardized system of classification and nomenclature will help in early prognostication and planning of follow-up.

REFERENCES

1. Hindryckx A, De Catte L. Prenatal diagnosis of congenital renal and urinary tract malformations. Facts Views Vis Obgyn. 2011;3(3):165-74.
2. Peters CA. Urinary tract obstruction in children. J Urol. 1995;154:1874-83.
3. Capolicchio JP, Braga LH, Szymanski KM. Canadian Urological Association/Pediatric Urologists of Canada guideline on the investigation and management of antenatally detected hydronephrosis. Can Urol Assoc J. 2018;12:85-92.
4. Sinha A, Bagga A, Krishna A, Bajpai M, Srinivas M, Uppal R, et al. Revised guidelines on management of antenatal hydronephrosis. Indian Pediatr. 2013;50(2):215-31.
5. Dos Santos J, Parekh RS, Piscione TD, Hassouna T, Figueroa V, Gonima P, et al. A new grading system for the management of antenatal hydronephrosis. Clin J Am Soc Nephrol. 2015;10(10): 1783-90.
6. Arora M, Prasad A, Kulshreshtha R, Baijal A. Significance of third trimester ultrasound in detecting congenital abnormalities of kidney and urinary tract—a prospective study. J Pediatr Urol. 2019;15(4):334-40.
7. Lee RS, Cendron M, Kinnamon DD, Nguyen HT. Antenatal hydronephrosis as a predictor of postnatal outcome: a meta-analysis. Pediatrics. 2006;118(2):586-93.
8. Nguyen HT, Herndon CD, Cooper C, Gatti J, Kirsch A, Kokorowski P, et al. The Society for Fetal Urology consensus statement on the evaluation and management of antenatal hydronephrosis. J Pediatr Urol. 2010;6(3):212-31.
9. Pal A, Reidy KJ. Genetic syndromes affecting kidney development. Results Probl Cell Differ. 2017;60:257-79.
10. van der Ven AT, Connaughton DM, Ityel H, Mann N, Nakayama M, Chen J, et al. Whole-exome sequencing identifies causative mutations in families with congenital anomalies of the kidney and urinary tract. J Am Soc Nephrol. 2018;29(9):2348-61.
11. Avner ED, Harmon WE, Niaudet P, Yoshikawa N, Emma F, Goldstein SL. Pediatric Nephrology, 7th edition. Berlin: Springer-Verlag; 2016. pp. 1749-71.
12. Jackson L, Woodward M, Coward RJ. The molecular biology of pelvi-ureteric junction obstruction. Pediatr Nephrol. 2018;33(4):553-71.
13. Onen A. Grading of hydronephrosis: an ongoing challenge. Front Pediatr. 2020;8:458.
14. Nguyen HT, Benson CB, Bromley B, Campbell JB, Chow J, Coleman B, et al. Multidisciplinary consensus of the classification of prenatal and postnatal urinary tract dilatation (UTD classification system). J Pediatr Urol. 2014;10:982-98.
15. Chalmers DJ, Meyers ML, Brodie KE, Palmer C, Campbell JB. Inter-rater reliability of the APD, SFU and UTD grading systems in fetal sonography and MRI. J Pediatr Urol. 2016;12(5):305.e1-5.
16. Beksac MS, Beksac AT, Tanacan A, Mumusoglu S, Katlan D, Celik HT. Antenatal hydronephrosis and fetal urine sampling. Congenit Anom (Kyoto). 2020;60(1):4-9.
17. Davenport MT, Merguerian PA, Koyle M. Antenatally diagnosed hydronephrosis: current postnatal management. Pediatr Surg Int. 2013;29(3):207-14.
18. Paraboschi I, Mantica G, Dalton NR, Turner C, Garriboli M. Urinary biomarkers in pelvic-ureteric junction obstruction: a systematic review. Transl Androl Urol. 2020;9(2):722-42.
19. Smith-Harrison LI, Hougen HY, Timberlake MD, Corbett ST. Current applications of in utero intervention for lower urinary tract obstruction. J Pediatr Urol. 2015;11(6):341-7.
20. Salam MA. Posterior urethral valve: outcome of antenatal intervention. Int J Urol. 2006;13(10):1317-22.
21. Storm DW, Braga LH, Cooper CS. Continuous antibiotic prophylaxis in pediatric urology. Urol Clin North Am. 2018;45(4):525-38.
22. Kıllı I, Avlan D, Taşkınlar H, Kara PP, Apaydın FD, Delibaş A, et al. Effective predictors for surgical decision in antenatal hydronephrosis: a prospective multiparameter analysis. Turk J Urol. 2017;43(3):361-5.

CHAPTER

13.3

Congenital Anomalies of the Kidney and Urinary Tract and Fetal Interventions

Shubha AM, G Nandhini, N Prasad

INTRODUCTION

Congenital anomalies of the kidney and urinary tract (CAKUT) occur in around 1 in 500 newborns[1] and constitute approximately 20–30% of all anomalies identified in the prenatal period.[2] They account for 30–60% cases of chronic kidney disease (CKD) and end-stage kidney disease (ESKD) in the pediatric age group.[3] While most cases of CAKUT are sporadic and isolated to the urinary tract, some have a syndromic or familial association. The pathogenesis of renal and urinary tract malformations is a complex process involving a composite interplay of many factors. Both syndromic and nonsyndromic forms of CAKUT result from disruption of the cellular, molecular, and morphogenetic mechanisms, which regulate normal development of the renal system. Genetic studies of syndromic forms and animal models of CAKUT are providing valuable insights into the molecular pathogenesis of these congenital malformations.

MOLECULAR MECHANISMS IN NORMAL KIDNEY AND URINARY TRACT DEVELOPMENT

With the advent of new technologies such as high throughput expression analysis techniques, next-generation sequencing, and transgenic mice models, there have been significant advances in the understanding of the molecular basis of renal development. Studies into the genetic and cellular mechanisms of renal system organogenesis in model organisms such as the mouse and rat have helped to provide valuable insights into the developmental processes of the human renal system.[4]

During the fourth week of gestation, the ureteric bud (UB) arises from the mesonephric duct and invades the metanephric blastema; a series of reciprocal interactions between the two result in the development of the renal system. As the UB grows into the metanephric mesenchyme, it undergoes serial dichotomous branching to give rise to the ureter, pelvicalyceal system, calyces, and collecting ducts. The stromal and epithelial components of the kidney are derived from the metanephric mesenchyme.

MOLECULAR GENETICS

Glial-derived neurotrophic factor (GDNF) secreted by the metanephric mesenchyme interacts with RET (rearranged during transfection) receptor tyrosine kinase expressed on the UB to induce branching of the UB. The GDNF-RET pathway (**Fig. 1**) is influenced by multiple regulatory transcription and growth factors, which determine the local expression and activity of GDNF in the metanephric mesenchyme.[5]

Molecular mediators such as Eya1, Pax2, WT1, Six1, 2, and 4 stimulate GDNF expression in the metanephric mesenchyme,[6] whereas SLIT2 and ROBO2 signaling pathways have a negative regulation of GDNF-RET pathway and prevent development and propagation of more than one UBs.[7] Similarly, SPRY1 expression reduces the sensitivity of the mesonephric duct to GDNF, thereby preventing outgrowth of multiple UBs that result in the development of duplex kidneys. WNT proteins WNT9b and WNT4 and FGF8 are also the key mediators of mesenchymal and epithelial interactions.

The renin-angiotensin system plays a crucial role in the normal development of the urinary tract. Mouse models genetically engineered to lack the angiotensin II types 1A and 1B receptor gene (*AGTR1*) or the angiotensinogen gene (*AGT*) have been documented to have abnormal development

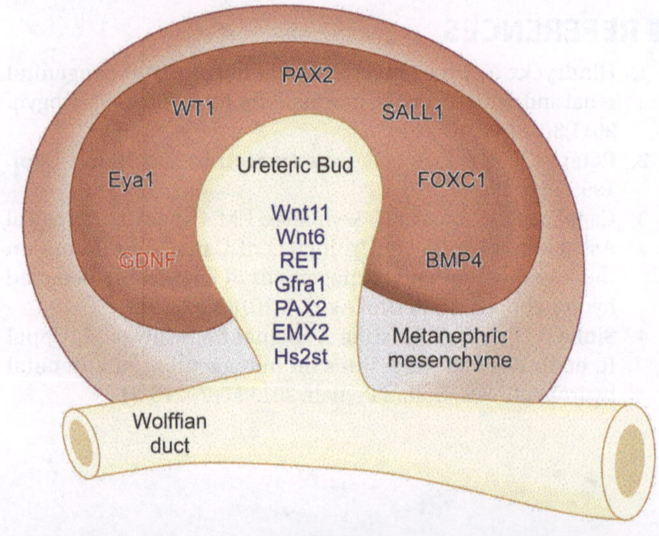

Fig. 1: GDNF-RET pathway. (GDNF: glial-derived neurotrophic factor; RET: rearranged during transfection).

of the renal medulla and delayed glomerular maturation. Mice with null mutations in the angiotensin II type 2 receptor gene (*AGTR2*) have been found to develop a spectrum of urinary tract malformations including renal dysplasia, renal hypoplasia, hydronephrosis, and vesicoureteric malformations. These malformations are believed to occur because of the delayed apoptosis of the mesenchymal cells in the fetal kidney and lower urinary tract, due to the genetic mutations. Neonatal renal failure associated with maternal intake of angiotensin-converting enzyme (ACE) inhibitors during pregnancy has been postulated to occur because of hemodynamic mechanisms as well as a renal tubular dysgenesis-like pathology, which results from disruption of the renin-angiotensin axis in the fetus.[1]

The WNT (wingless-type mouse mammary tumor virus integration site family) and Notch signaling pathways have been documented to be involved in the developmental processes that lead to specialization of the different functional segments of the nephron. Wnt4 and Wnt9b have been shown to play an important role in the process of mesenchymal-to-epithelial transition and Notch2 has been found to be involved in proximal tubule specification. Members of the SHH (Sonic hedgehog) and GLI, bone morphogenetic protein (BMP), and fibroblast growth factor (FGF) family of proteins have also been reported to be involved in morphogenesis of the kidney and urinary tract.[8]

SPECTRUM OF CAKUT

The pathogenesis of CAKUT is a complex process that depends on the interplay of many factors including genetic factors [single-gene mutations, modifier genes, epigenetic factors, and microribonucleic acids (micro-RNAs)] and in utero environmental factors (chemical and pharmacological teratogens, impairment of fetal urinary flow, and maternal malnutrition) **(Table 1)**.

Studies have indicated that environmental factors may produce secondary alterations in gene activity or act in concert with single-gene mutations to cause CAKUT. The nutritional, chemical, and pharmacological agents to which exposure during pregnancy is implicated to cause urinary tract malformations in the fetus include low-protein diet, high- or low-sodium intake, hyperglycemia, vitamin A deficiency, cocaine, alcohol, glucocorticoids, renin-angiotensin blockers, antiepileptic drugs, cyclophosphamide, and mycophenolate mofetil.[9]

TABLE 1: Spectrum of congenital anomalies of the kidney and urinary tract (CAKUT).

Anomaly	*Description*
Upper urinary tract	
Renal agenesis	Kidney is totally absent
Renal hypoplasia	Kidney contains formed but significantly fewer than normal nephrons; if nephrons are large in size—termed oligomeganephronia
Renal dysplasia	Kidney contains undifferentiated tissues. In renal aplasia, the kidney is very small in size; in cystic and multicystic dysplastic conditions, the kidney is distended by cysts
Duplex kidney	Kidney is separated into two parts: upper part is often dysplastic and attached to an obstructed ureter and lower part is usually attached to a refluxing ureter
Horseshoe kidney	Both kidneys become fused during development and may include dysplastic components
Hydronephrosis	Renal pelvis is distended and renal parenchyma may be dysplastic or hypoplastic and may occur secondary to reflux or urinary tract obstruction
Lower urinary tract	
Agenesis	Ureter and bladder trigone are absent
Duplication of ureter	It may occur in association with a duplex kidney
Vesicoureteral reflux	Urine flows in a retrograde direction from the bladder to the ureter, pelvis, and medullary collecting ducts of the kidney
Posterior urethral valves	Urinary outflow from the bladder is anatomically obstructed

ANATOMICAL PRESENTATION OF CAKUT

CAKUT are a family of diseases with a diverse anatomical spectrum which can present as single or multiple defects **(Fig. 2)**. The specific embryonal defects or events of the CAKUT spectrum can be divided into four broad categories—renal parenchymal, ureteric, bladder, and urethral anomalies as below. Ureteric defects contribute maximum to this spectrum.

It contains a wide spectrum of intrinsic renal anomalies from metanephric blastema dysmorphogenesis such as agenesis, aplasia, hypoplasia, dysplasia, and multicystic dysplastic kidneys (MCDKs). Extrarenal parts of the spectrum arising from the UB dysmorphogenesis encompass the ureteric anomalies such as megaureter, ureteropelvic junction obstruction, ureterovesical junction (UVJ) obstruction, or incompetence. Anomalies of the bladder and urethra arise from the defects in the urogenital sinus development. Miscellaneous conditions such as ectopic kidneys, crossed fused ectopia, horseshoe kidneys (where ascent of kidney is disturbed), and duplex kidneys/ureters (abnormal or double ureteric budding) occur. Most anomalies are often concurrent such as posterior urethral valve (PUV) or vesicoureteric reflux (VUR) associated with dysplasia, hypoplasia of the ipsilateral, or contralateral kidney. These have a familial pattern showing incomplete and variable penetrance.

ONTOGENY OF CAKUT

A wide spectrum of anomalies are explained by different theories such as:

- Physical stress on the kidney and the ureter because of a urinary outflow obstruction

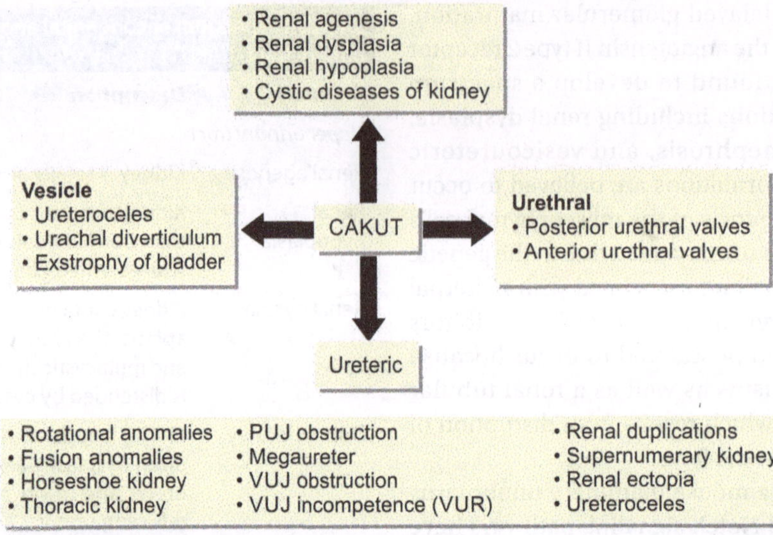

Fig. 2: Anatomical presentation of CAKUT. (CAKUT: congenital anomalies of the kidney and urinary tract; PUJ: pelviureteric junction; VUJ: vesicoureteric junction).

- Physical stress secondary to bladder dysfunction or vesicoureteral junction obstruction
- Ectopia of the initial budding of the ureter from the Wolffian duct
- A primary defect in the interaction at the cellular level between the metanephric mesenchyme and the UB. This theory seems more promising as shown by various genetic and molecular studies

Peters et al. in 1992 created complete obstruction at various anatomical levels along the urinary tract of fetal sheep at 55–66 days of gestation (comparable to 14–16 weeks of human gestation). They noted that the most remarkable consequence of fetal obstructive uropathy was its effect on renal parenchymal growth in terms of cystic or dysplastic changes.[10] However, other investigators such as Stephens et al. in 1996 questioned the lack of correlation between the degree of obstruction and the severity of renal parenchymal abnormality.

With the recent advances in genetic analysis and molecular biosignaling theories in embryology, >30% of the CAKUT spectrum is shown to result from a genetic aberration. Maternal hypothyroidism, drugs, and teratogen exposure of the fetus have impacted regular nephrogenesis. For example, ACE inhibitors and receptor blockers used to treat maternal hypertension can cause neonatal renal failure from a combination of hemodynamic compromise and renal tubular dysgenesis. Similarly, retinoic acid, a natural metabolite of vitamin A, impacts nephrogenesis if the levels are not normal.

Maternal diet has been contemplated to have impact in the CAKUT spectrum by *Barker's hypothesis*[11] or FOAD (Fetal Origin of Adult Disease). Dr David Barker first popularized the concept of FOAD by studies conducted with European birth registries. The FOAD hypothesis states that insulting events early in the development of fetus have a profound impact on one's risk for development of future adult disease. Low birth weight, a surrogate marker of poor fetal growth and nutrition, is linked to coronary artery disease, hypertension, renal failure, obesity, and insulin resistance. Implications of the FOAD extend beyond the low birth weight population and include babies exposed to stress, both nutritional and non-nutritional, during different critical periods of development, which ultimately result in a disease state.

High glucose levels in diabetic mothers have proven etiology in the CAKUT spectrum. A Canadian study suggests that diabetes mellitus (DM) in the first 20 weeks of pregnancy is associated with CAKUT in exposed infants. The association between CAKUT and LGA suggests that poor glycemic control impacts normal nephrogenesis.[12]

Antenatal steroids given to stimulate lung development in preterm babies induce CAKUT—hypoplasia. There is experimental animal evidence that high-dose corticosteroids halt or seriously retard nephrogenesis reducing the number of nephrons.

Physical stress in the form of obstruction to the urinary outflow in conditions such as ectopic ureters in single or duplex moieties, ectopic ureteroceles, VUJ obstruction, and PUVs contributes significantly to renal dysplasia by impacting the nephrogenesis, either unilateral or bilateral.

CAKUT: INTRINSIC RENAL ANOMALIES

Renal Agenesis/Aplasia

- Agenesis is a primary defect with aberrant initiation of the pronephros-mesonephros sequence and/or failure of UB outgrowth. In contrast, renal aplasia occurs when kidneys were initially induced but failed to progress through nephrogenesis and then involuted. Interestingly, the left kidney is more often missing; the reason is unknown but there is slightly different timing of nephrogenesis on each side which may be important and causative for more left renal anomalies.

- Absence of both kidneys is rare at 1:7,000 to 1:10,000 births with a slight male preponderance. These babies usually die at birth with the Potter sequence of anhydramnios, lung hypoplasia along with limb, and face deformities.

Renal Dysplasia

- Dysplasia can occur as an isolated anomaly or as a part of multiorgan syndrome. Unilateral dysplasia is more common than bilateral and coexists with anatomical abnormalities of the urinary tract in 50–75% of patients, such as horseshoe kidney, duplex moieties, obstructive megaureters, PUJ obstruction, and VUR. Prognosis is poor for bilateral dysplasias as they have an intrinsic nephron deficit, with severity ranging from the lethal Potter's sequence to hypodysplasia causing neonatal renal failure which progresses to CKD rapidly.
- Multicystic dysplastic kidney occurs when the metanephros development is disrupted by any of the causes stated above. The dysplastic kidney can be either larger or smaller with multiple noncommunicating cyst and no discernible parenchyma. Characteristic features include disrupted organization of normal nephrons, abundance of undifferentiated cells, metaplastic cartilage, and primitive, poorly branched ducts. Such kidneys are often attached to an atretic ureter, raising the possibility of early pathology at the time of bud outgrowth and ureteric development.

Renal Hypoplasia

- Hypoplastic kidneys are defined as ones weighing <50% of the normal size for age and lacking any primary histological abnormality—they may contain significantly fewer nephrons, but the formed nephrons appear normal and there are no undifferentiated tissues.
- In one variant, oligomeganephronia—both glomeruli and tubules—are significantly enlarged. Hypoplasia may be isolated or part of a wider malformation syndrome such as the renal coloboma syndrome associated with low birth weight and prematurity, which are linked to low nephron number and increased risk of hypertension, proteinuria, and kidney disease in later life supporting Barker's hypothesis.

Bilateral Renal Agenesis (Potter Syndrome)/ BRAHD

Complete absence of both kidneys (Potter's syndrome) is one of the most severe congenital renal anomalies that had been recognized since the 18th century. It was Dr Edith Potter who described bilateral renal agenesis in 1946 stating the role of fetal kidneys in maintaining normal amniotic fluid volume. She also documented the association of abnormal facies and hypoplasia of lungs with renal agenesis.

It is now widely recognized that the so-called Potter's face with folds under the eyes, flat nose, receding chin, and low-set ears as well as pulmonary hypoplasia, wide hands, and rocker-bottom feet are mechanical deformities produced by oligohydramnios.

Recessive mutations of the integrin-α8 (ITGA8) encoding gene in two families (one of them consanguineous) are identified to play a crucial role in renal development and it is expressed in the metanephric mesenchyme surrounding the UB, concluding the fact that bilateral renal agenesis can be an autosomal recessive disorder.

Bilateral renal agenesis/hypoplasia/dysplasia (BRAHD) are malformations of the renal parenchyma that are usually lethal. Translocation breakpoint mapping has identified *ESRRG* as a plausible candidate gene for BRAHD. The EUROCAT registry (a European network of population-based registries for the epidemiologic surveillance of congenital anomalies) reports an incidence of 1.3/10,000 live births, fetal deaths/still births, and terminations of pregnancy for fetal anomaly. BRAHD shows a male preponderance with a male:female ratio of 2.5:1. The most commonly reported BRAHD-associated single gene disorders are Fraser syndrome and branchiootorenal syndrome. In addition to genetic factors, there is a strong association between BRAHD and maternal insulin-dependent diabetes mellitus (IDDM). This appears to be the result of a direct teratogenic effect of hyperglycemia on specific tissues within the embryo. The cases with extrarenal malformations were further characterized by whether they had any component of three well-known malformation associations considered to overlap with BRAHD, namely VACTERL association (vertebral malformation, anal atresia, cardiovascular anomalies, tracheoesophageal fistula, esophageal atresia, renal anomalies, and limb malformations), Müllerian duct anomalies (MURCS association, Mayer-Rokitansky-Küster-Hauser syndrome) or—"craniofacial anomalies, hemifacial microsomia/Goldenhar syndrome/ Oculoauriculovertebral spectrum."[13]

CAKUT: URETERAL ANOMALIES

Development of the excretory system from the UB plays the key role in both ends—the nephrogenesis at the cranial side (from metanephric blastema) and the bladder-urethra development at the caudal side (from urogenital sinus). The abnormal site and timing of ureteric budding create a combination of CAKUT from both ends like renal hypodysplasia along with ectopic insertions/duplications in the lower urinary tract.

It is very important to understand the normal ureteric budding and the two main embryological theories (Mackie-Stephens theory and Weigert-Meyer principle) on abnormal ureteric budding which explain multitude of CAKUT anomalies.[14]

Renal anomalies are often associated with the abnormalities of the distal urinary tract. It is found that both severity of renal dysmorphism and lack of mature glomeruli (oligonephronia) correlate closely with the location of the ureteral orifice within the bladder, specifically the degree of deviation from the normal site. This latter feature led Mackie and Stephens to propose the "bud theory" of kidney and urinary tract abnormalities.

The bud theory stems from two kinds of morphologic correlations:

1. Between the location of the ureteral orifice versus the degree of kidney dysplasia or hypoplasia (ectopic ureter, duplex collecting systems)
2. Between the location of the ureteral orifice versus the abnormalities of the ureter (i.e., VUR and primary megaureter)

As per Mackie-Stephens hypothesis, abnormalities in both the kidney and the ureter are derived from a single common mechanism at a very early stage of development, specifically at the first stage of ureteral budding from the Wolffian duct. The ureteral orifice is transposed from its original budding site on the Wolffian duct into the bladder at point "b" **(Fig. 3)**. This transposition is engendered by expansion of the terminal part of the duct with the budding ureter attached and its incorporation into the base of the bladder as the hemitrigone. If the bud arises more caudally on the duct, (A) the orifice of the ureteral bud becomes incorporated onto an elongated cornu of the hemitrigone [lateral displacement as in point a **(Fig. 3)**]. The ectopic situation of the orifice means that the length of the submucosal tunnel is abnormally short, the valve mechanism is defective, and VUR ensues. If the bud arises more cranial to the normal site, it results in more medial insertion at point c **(Fig. 3)** of the ureteric orifice resulting in an obstructive pattern in the ureter.

Another consequence of distal budding from the Wolffian duct is the effect on the developing metanephros. Alongside the distal end of the Wolffian duct lies the metanephros, which is heaped beside the normally located bud leading to development of the normal kidney. However, if the bud arises distal or proximal to the normal site, it projects into sparsely populated caudal or cranial nephrogenic mesoderm leading to oligonephronia and potentially dysplasia.

Alternatively, bud ectopia can lead to overexpansion of the distal end of the Wolffian duct and the ureteral bud leading to enlargement of the hemitrigone, enlargement of the ureteral orifice, shortening of the submucosal tunnel, and megamodeling of the ureter. In this context, two different clinical abnormalities (i.e., VUR and renal dysplasia/hypoplasia) are derived from one abnormal embryologic event (i.e., abnormal ureteral budding).

Similarly, the duplex system in kidney is explained by primitive division of UB before it reaches the metanephric mesenchyme to induce renal development. These have a spectrum of lesions from complete duplication, Y duplication, and bifid pelvis. This in addition has another error of ectopia explained by a principle formulated by Weigert in 1877. The Weigert-Meyer principle predicts that in a duplex kidney, the upper kidney mass drains into the orifice within the bladder at a site lower than the orifice to which the lower kidney mass drains **(Fig. 4)**. The upper moiety mostly ends in ureterocele and presents with obstruction and the lower moiety ends in lateral insertion than the normal site and presents with VUR. Hence, the anomalies in three different tissues constituting CAKUT (i.e., abnormal UVJ, abnormalities of the ureter, and dysmorphic kidney) can be derived from a single abnormal embryonic event, the ectopic ureteral budding.[15]

The most common ureteric anomalies encountered are PUJ obstruction, VUJ obstruction, ureterocele, and VUR. The

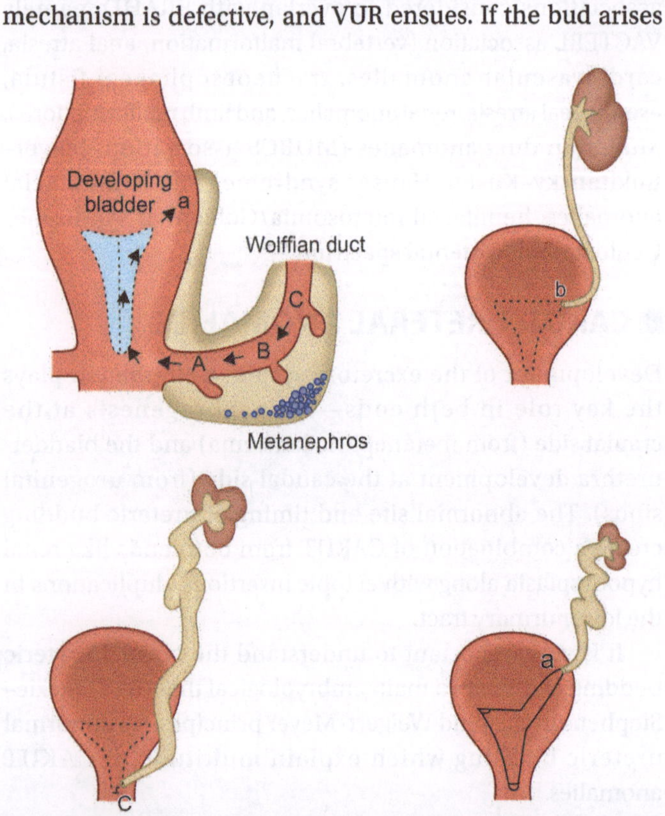

Fig. 3: Normal ureteric budding at site B inducing normal renal genesis and abnormal budding at sites A and C resulting in urinary and renal anomalies (Mackie–Stephens theory).

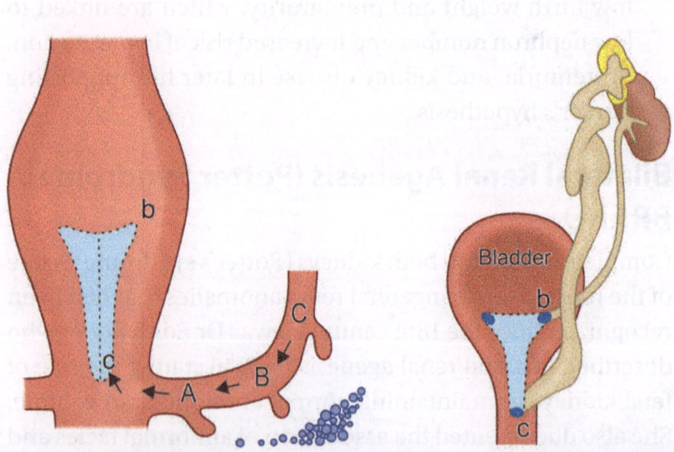

Fig. 4: Ureteric budding in duplex system with the upper moiety entering in a more caudal position in the bladder—Weigert–Meyer principle.

most accepted hypothesis for the embryological defects is discussed below:

- *Hydronephrosis:*
  - Pelvicalyceal dilatation—unilateral or bilateral—is the most common anomaly detected in the prenatal scans. During embryogenesis, from 28 to 35 days of development, the ureter is a patent diverticulum from the mesonephric duct. Mesonephros producing urine fills the ureteric tube from 37 to 40 days of developing ureter and loses its lumen. At 40 days of development, the ureter recanalizes—starting at the midpoint and progressing in both directions toward the developing kidney and the urogenital sinus, the lumen of the ureter reforms. The last segments of the ureter to gain a lumen are at either ends (kidney or urogenital sinus).
  - If this is delayed or partly disrupted at the pelviureteric junction, hydronephrosis **(Fig. 5)** will occur. As the lumen fully opens, there will be no residual obstruction.
  - Another hypothesis is that high urine flow causes hydronephrosis in adult patients with diabetes insipidus. Similar theory is proposed to be a cause of prenatal hydronephrosis as renal tubular reabsorption is not fully developed in a fetus and urine output on a per kilogram basis is high. This explains prenatal pelviectasis which resolves spontaneously on follow-up.
  - Maternal progesterone relaxes the maternal bladder and ureteral musculature. It has shown that progesterone has the same effect in the fetus causing delay on drainage of urine from kidney, resulting in prenatal hydronephrosis.

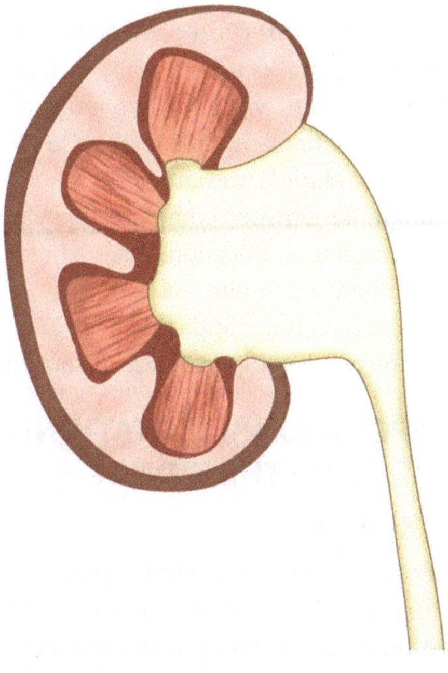

Fig. 5: Pelviureteric junction obstruction.

- *UVJ obstruction:*
  - This anomaly has got rare incidence in children and presents as obstructive megaureter clinically. Embryologically, defective absorption of the mesonephric duct into the urogenital sinus to create a separate insertion of the ureter in bladder development is the causative factor for UVJ obstruction.
  - Pathophysiology is identified to be a segment of ureter just outside the bladder that has only circular muscle developed and no longitudinal muscle. This then causes the ureter to close as it contracts, inhibiting peristalsis.
  - Fascinating fluoroscopic studies show that the peristaltic wave arising from the renal calyces goes down the ureter normally and to the aperistaltic segment at the UVJ. At UVJ, the ureter closes on itself and the peristalsis reverses, heading back up to the renal calyces. This leads to the classic appearance of obstructive megaureter with a dolphin nose deformity at the UVJ during surgery.
- *Ureterocele:*
  - A ureterocele **(Fig. 6)** is defined as a cystic dilatation of the distal ureter at the UV junction. The most accepted embryological explanation is the persistence or incomplete dissolution of Chwalla membrane (ureter recanalization defect at UVJ), which transiently obstructs the ureteric orifice at its insertion in the urogenital sinus at 37 weeks of gestation.
  - Another theory explains the ballooning of the distal ureter by a deficiency or absence of muscle layers, shown in 90% of the specimens in a clinical study.
  - Renal dysplasia is hypothesized to occur in cases where the UB interacts with the metanephric blastema at more polar locations, as Mackie and Stephens demonstrated, whereas the middle of the blastema is most conductive to normal nephron formation.
  - Orthotopic ureteroceles do well clinically whereas ectopic ureteroceles are always associated with renal dysplasia.
- *Vesicoureteric reflux:*
  - Primary VUR **(Fig. 7)** is caused by failure of vesicoureteric junction to develop properly. The UB when arises more caudally on the mesonephric duct by the Mackie-Stephens principle, the orifice of the ureteral bud becomes incorporated into an elongated cornu of the hemitrigone (lateral displacement of UVJ). The ectopic UVJ orifice means that the length of the submucosal tunnel is abnormally short, the valve mechanism is defective, and VUR ensues.
  - The ratio of the length of the ureter within the bladder wall to its diameter should be 5:1 by Pacquain rule (which is reduced in refluxing units). This occurs early during embryonic development of the ureter at 6 weeks of gestation.

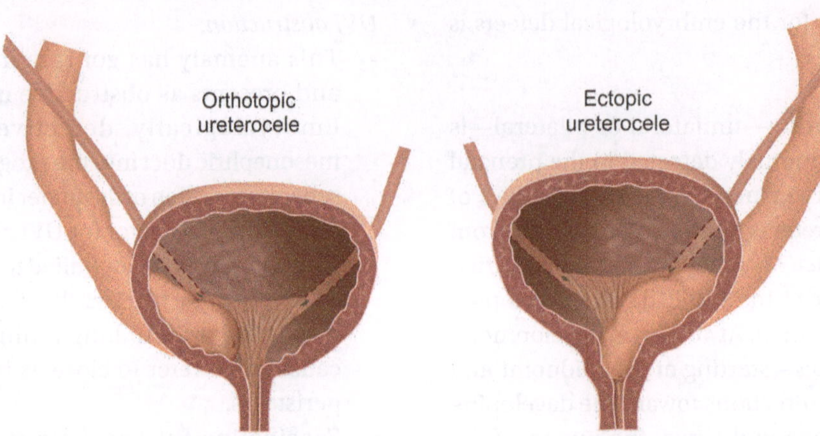

Fig. 6: Orthotopic/ectopic ureterocele.

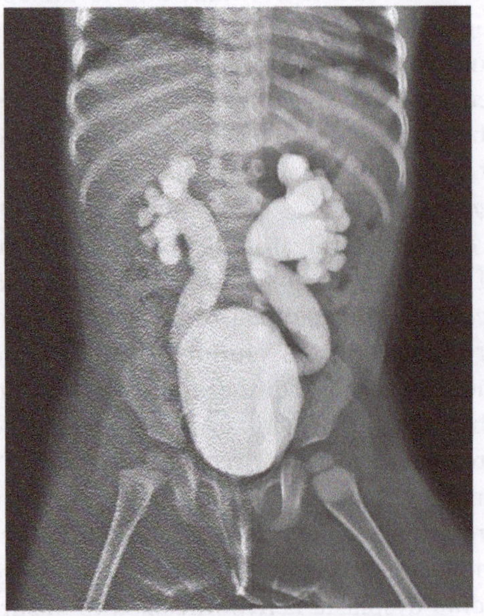

Fig. 7: Primary vesicoureteric reflux in a female child.

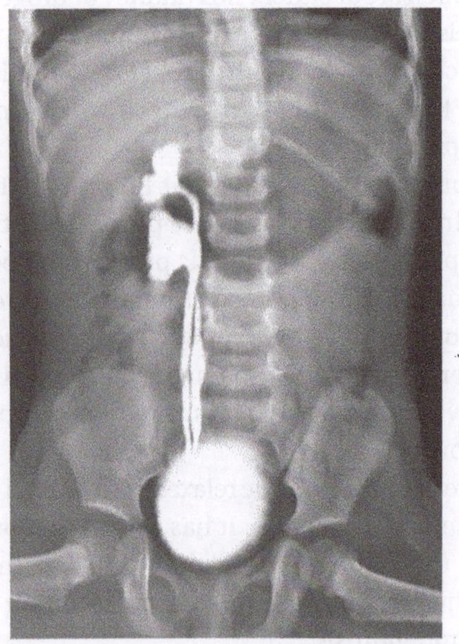

Fig. 8: Complete right renal duplication in a female child.

- *Duplex kidneys:*
  - The Weigert-Meyer principle predicts that in a duplex kidney, the upper moiety drains into an orifice at a site lower than the orifice to which the lower moiety drains. The upper moiety mostly ends in ureterocele (medial and obstructive) and the lower moiety ends in laterally and presents with VUR (lateral and refluxing).
  - These CAKUT anomalies show dysmorphogenesis in three different tissues constituting abnormal UVJ, abnormalities of the ureter, and dysmorphic kidney—derived from a single abnormal embryonic event, the ectopic ureteral budding.
  - The ectopic medial site insertion of the upper moiety can happen outside the bladder, following the path of Wolffian duct structures in males. Urinary incontinence does not ensue in males because the ureter inserts into structures proximal to the external urinary sphincter, such as the bladder neck or posterior urethra, the seminal vesicle, the utricle, the ejaculatory duct, or the vas.
  - But in females, insertion can occur in the urethra, vestibule, vagina, cervix, uterus, or Gartner's duct (a Wolffian duct remnant), bypassing the external sphincter mechanism, thus leading to incontinence as the major clinical presentation.
  - The difference between complete duplication **(Fig. 8)** and incomplete duplication arises when a single UB branches early on or late.
  - Renal dysplasia is a mandated coexisting anomaly in all the units with ectopic ureteric insertions.

CAKUT: POSITIONAL/ROTATIONAL ANOMALIES OF THE KIDNEY

Ascent of Kidney

- The developing metanephric kidney originates within the pelvis. During its development, the kidney ascends to its final location in the retroperitoneum at a vertebral level of approximately T12–L3. Renal ascent is completed by the eighth week of gestation. During the process of ascent, the kidney rotates medially 90° gaining an anteromedial lie. The ascending kidney has a dynamic vascular supply during the course of its ascent, which derives from the adjacent common iliac vessel which later derives from the aortic segment directly.

- Ascent of kidney is prevented by the developing inferior mesenteric artery; both the kidneys have medial fusion and form horseshoe kidney as depicted in **Figures 9A to C**.
- If unascended, it leads on to a pelvic kidney.
- If it crosses the lumbar position, it forms a thoracic kidney.
- Similarly, the crossed renal ectopia to the opposite side may or may not be with fusion as shown in **Figures 10A to D**.
- All of them are clinically not detectable unless symptomatic. They can present with renal pelviectasis, either by obstruction or by reflux. Prenatal detection by ultrasonography (USG) can be done by its anatomical position.

CAKUT: URETHRAL AND BLADDER ANOMALIES

- *Posterior urethral valves:*
  - The normal male urethra contains a pair of lateral, small folds called plicae colliculi that arise at the distal lateral edge of the verumontanum and continue distally onto the lateral walls of the urethra for a short distance. Stephens postulated that these folds represent the integration of the mesonephric duct into the cloaca.
  - Stephens et al. proposed that PUV results from the mesonephric duct integrating at a more anterior position (anterior fusion of leaflets), a lack of posteromedial migration resulting in PUV.
  - It is hypothesized that type I PUVs result when the mesonephric duct enters the cloaca in a more anterior portion than normal and type III valves result from incomplete dissolution of the urogenital portion of the cloacal membrane.
  - Dewan et al. postulated that all PUVs **(Figs. 11A and B)** are not true valves but rather are a single obstructive membrane with a small posterior midline opening. They proposed using the term "congenital obstructing posterior urethral membrane (COPUM)" for this entity.
  - Partial bladder obstruction induces detrusor muscle hypertrophy with replacement of smooth muscle tissue with fibrotic connective tissue. Numerous studies over the past few decades have shown

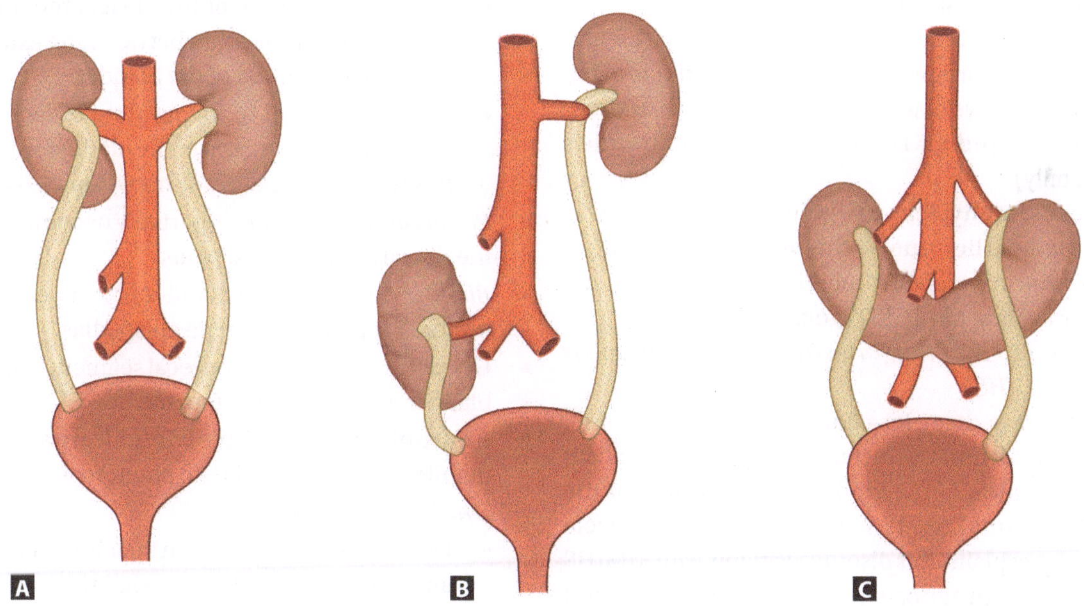

Figs. 9A to C: Anatomical malformation in kidneys. (A) Normal kidney; (B) Right pelvic kidney; (C) Horseshoe kidney.

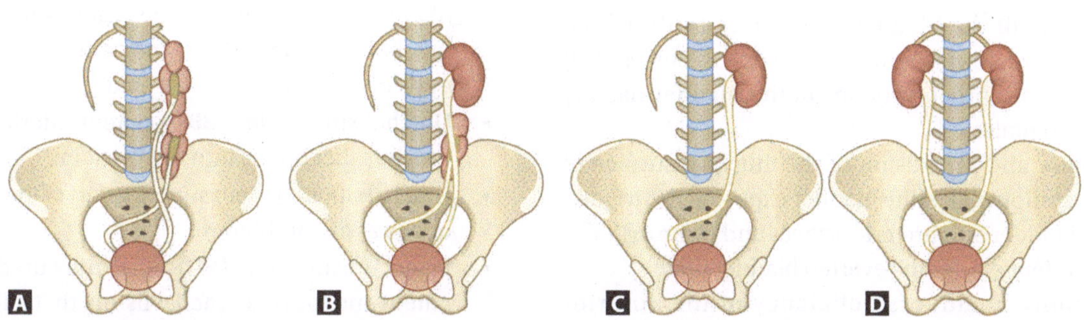

Figs. 10A to D: Crossed renal ectopia. (A) With fusion; (B) Without fusion; (C) Solitary; (D) Bilateral.

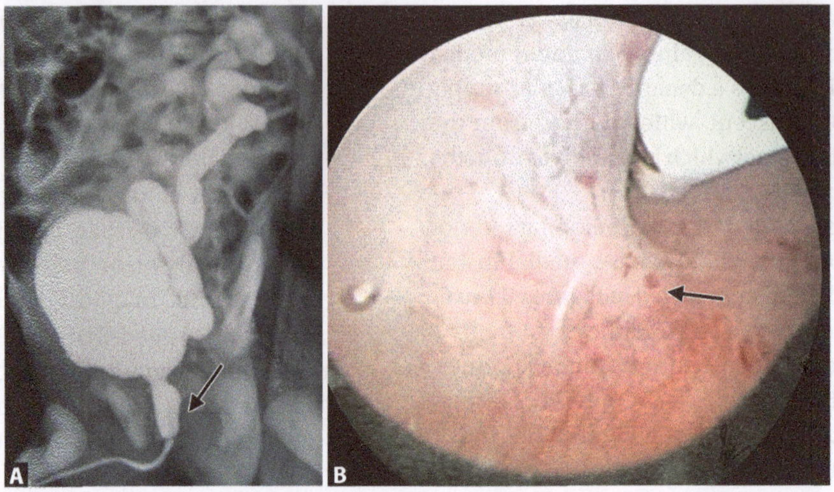

Figs. 11A and B: (A) Posterior urethral valve with unilateral reflux by micturating cystourethrogram (MCU); (B) Right valve leaflet cut by energy device.

that many other factors also play a role in bladder changes from obstruction including diminished blood flow to the developing bladder, diminished mitochondrial enzyme activity, reduced nerve density with decreased autonomic detrusor innervation, changes in collage-type ratios, and downregulation of bladder angiotensin-II receptors.
 - The significant bladder changes occurring in early weeks of gestation are irreversible and contribute to the entity called valve bladder (a noncompliant bladder—culprit of rapid CKD progression if unattended postnatally).
 - This causes physical stress in nephrogenesis as discussed earlier due to the obstruction to urine outflow and in turn causes renal hypodysplasia in these kidneys leading onto CKD progression later.
- *Megacystis-microcolon-intestinal-hypoperistalsis syndrome (MMIHS):*
 - This is a rare disorder characterized by a grossly distended but nonobstructed bladder with significant hypoperistalsis of the bladder and portions of the gastrointestinal tract. A systemic smooth muscle myopathy explains this disorder. Patients with MMIHS have dismal prognosis and most patients do not survive past the first year of life.
- *Exstrophy bladder:*
 - Exstrophy of the bladder, a very rare birth defect, occurs approximately once in every 10,000–40,000 births. Exstrophy (eversion) of the bladder usually occurs in males.
 - Exposure and protrusion of the mucosal surface of the posterior wall of the bladder exposing the trigone of the bladder and ureteric orifices and urine dribbles intermittently from the everted bladder plate.
 - Exstrophy bladder is deficiency of the anterior abdominal wall and the anterior wall of the urinary bladder. The defect results from the failure of mesoderm to migrate between the ectoderm and endoderm of the abdominal wall. This results in the deficiency of rectus muscles and external and internal oblique and transversus abdominis muscles along with the anterior bladder wall.
 - Preemptive rupture of the cloacal membrane results in wide communication between the exterior and the mucous membrane of the bladder.
 - All of these lead to incomplete bladder filling and cycling and hypoplasia of the bladder wall. Prenatally, this will show a poorly or nonvisualized bladder.
- *Epispadias:* The urethra is partially or completely open on the dorsal surface of the penis.
- *Bladder exstrophy:* The bladder is an open plate and the urethra is open as complete epispadias.
- *Cloacal exstrophy:* The ileocecal segment of the bowel and bladder are exstrophied together.
- Exstrophy variants involving alternative or partial manifestations of the classic phenotypes
- *Urachal anomalies:*
 - Developing bladder has an attachment to the allantois and later regresses as a urachal remnant obliterating the lumen. In approximately 50% of cases, the lumen is continuous with the cavity of the bladder. Remnants of the epithelial lining of the urachus may give rise to urachal cysts **(Fig. 12A)**. They are symptomatic if the cysts become infected and enlarged.
 - Urachal sinus **(Fig. 12B)**—patent inferior end of the urachus that opens into the bladder.
 - Urachal sinus—patent superior part of the urachus that opens at the umbilicus.
 - Patent urachus **(Fig. 12C)**—the entire urachus remains patent and forms a urachal fistula that allows urine to escape from the umbilical orifice.[16]

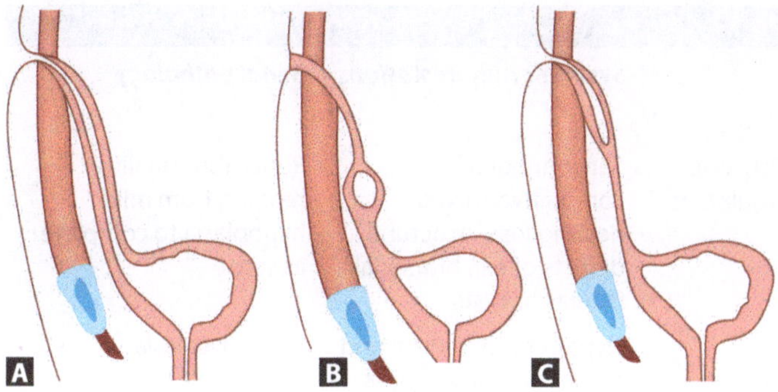

Figs. 12A to C: (A) Patent urachus; (B) Urachal cyst; (C) Urachal sinus.

GENETICS IN NONSYNDROMIC CAKUT

Anomalies such as renal agenesis, renal hypoplasia, renal dysplasia, renal-tubular dysgenesis, MCDK, or vesicoureteral reflux are often nonsyndromic but can be familial suggesting a role of specific genetic mutations leading to their occurrence. The final CAKUT phenotype seems to result from the complex interaction of various modifier genes and environmental factors. However, presence of mutations in potential CAKUT causing renal developmental genes (RDGs) has been documented in only 1.9–20% of patients with nonsyndromic CAKUT.

GENETICS IN SYNDROMIC CAKUT

Renal tract malformations can occur as a component of multiorgan syndromes. Some important genetic syndromes associated with CAKUT are listed in **Table 2**.

The cause of human CAKUT and studies on a variety of mutant strains of mice have identified more than 30 RDGs to be essential for kidney development till date. As mentioned in the previous section, some of the genes associated with syndromic CAKUT have also been reported to be mutated in isolated nonsyndromic CAKUT. For instance, *HNF1B*, the gene that encodes the developmentally expressed transcription factor—hepatocyte nuclear factor 1, is associated with the renal cysts and diabetes (RCAD) syndrome, but mutations in the gene have also been reported in cases with nonsyndromic renal tract malformations including MCDK, hypoplastic kidney, and glomerulocystic kidney.

The expression and thereby actual phenotypic manifestation of a particular mutation in a renal developmental gene are modified to a significant extent by the influence of modifier genes as well as epigenetic factors. The interactions between different modifier genes and the disease-causing genetic mutation, which influence the phenotypic expression, are called "epistatic gene interactions." For instance, the wide spectrum of urinary tract malformations associated with *HNF1*β and uromodulin (*UMOD*) mutations is most likely the result of the influences of modifier genes.

Epigenetic regulation or epigenetic programming is another important influence on gene expression and disease causation. The major mechanisms in epigenetic control of gene regulation are deoxyribonucleic acid (DNA) or chromatin protein methylation and acetylation. Chromatin methylation and acetylation recruit additional proteins that can modify histones to form an important determinant of epigenetic regulation during metanephric organogenesis.[17]

PRENATAL DIAGNOSIS OF CAKUT

Prenatal diagnosis of CAKUT requires a meticulous detailed examination of the entire urinary tract by ultrasound for the kidney size, architecture, position, ureters, bladder, amniotic index, and its variations. Any urinary tract anomaly should be screened for associated anomalies, along with a detailed family history, especially in a fetus with polycystic kidney disease, bilateral renal agenesis, or dysgenesis, etc. Genetic testing and counseling will be beneficial in syndromic variants as the nonsyndromic gene mutations are secondary to environmental factors inducing disruptions in biomolecular signaling **(Flowchart 1)**.

GENETIC TESTING IN THE CLINICAL SETTING

Genetic testing is useful for confirmation of clinical diagnosis, better prognostication, appropriate management, accurate genetic counseling, and early intervention in the proband. Identification of the disease causing genetic mutation would also be useful to the family for prenatal diagnosis and carrier testing. For syndromic CAKUT, testing of the one or two known associated genes can be done. However, for nonsyndromic CAKUT, genetic testing may not always be feasible or cost effective, in view of the high level of genetic heterogeneity. Likewise, accurate prediction of the exact phenotype of a prenatally detected genetic mutation also may not be possible, because of the modifying influences of modifier genes, epigenetic factors, and environmental factors, as discussed above. Therefore, appropriate pretest and post-test counseling by a qualified genetic counselor is very important. For diagnostic purposes, genetic testing is most often done through sequence analysis of the known, causative gene(s).

GENOMIC TECHNOLOGIES FOR RESEARCH

The newer genomic technologies, which are being used for studying the genetic basis of CAKUT, include high throughput expression analysis techniques such as chromosomal microarray (CMA) and genome-wide association studies (GWAS), wherein genetic markers [usually single nucleotide polymorphisms (SNPs)] spanning the entire genome are studied, to identify genomic loci potentially linked to/associated with a disease. Whole exome sequencing (sequence analysis of the whole exome, i.e., of all exons or coding portions of the genome) and whole genome sequencing (sequence analysis of the entire genome) using massively parallelized next-generation sequencing techniques are the recently developed, emerging technologies that have

TABLE 2: Syndromes associated with renal tract malformations.

Syndrome	OMIM number	Gene	Systemic manifestations	Renal pathology
Autosomal dominant				
Branchiootorenal syndrome types 1 and 2	113650 and 610896	*EYA1* and *SIX5* (encode transcription regulation proteins)	Sensorineural/ conductive/mixed hearing loss, structural defects of ear, branchial fistulas or cysts	Renal abnormalities ranging from mild hypoplasia to complete absence
Hypoparathyroidism, sensorineural deafness and renal disease (Barakat syndrome)	146255	*GATA3* (encodes a transcription factor)	Hypoparathyroidism and sensorineural deafness	Renal dysplasia
Renal-coloboma (papillorenal) syndrome	120330	*PAX2* (encodes a transcription factor)	Ocular anomalies including optic nerve coloboma, hearing loss, central nervous system (CNS) anomalies, genital anomalies	Renal hypodysplasia, oligomeganephronia, and VUR
Renal cysts and diabetes	137920	*HNF1B* (encodes a transcription factor)	Diabetes, gout, abnormalities of genital tract	Renal cysts, glomerular tufts, enlarged renal pelvis, abnormal calyces, small kidney, oligomeganephronia, single kidney, horseshoe kidney
Townes–Brocks syndrome	107480	*SALL1* (encodes a transcription factor)	Imperforate anus, triphalangeal thumbs, anomalies of hands and feet, sensorineural deafness	Renal malrotation, ectopic kidney, horseshoe kidney, renal hypoplasia, polycystic kidneys, vesicoureteral reflux
Autosomal recessive				
Fraser syndrome	219000	*FRAS1* and *FREM2* (encode basement membrane-associated proteins)	Cryptophthalmos, ear malformations, syndactyly, genital tract malformations, laryngeal anomalies	Unilateral or bilateral renal agenesis with/ without ureteral agenesis, hypoplastic or absent bladder, cystic dysplasia of kidneys
Prune belly (Eagle–Barrett syndrome)	100100	Cholinergic receptor, muscarinic 3 (*CHRM3*) (encodes a transmembrane receptor)	Thin abdominal musculature with overlying lax skin, cryptorchidism	Megacystis, megaureter, bilateral hydronephrosis
X-linked				
Kallmann syndrome	308700	*KAL1* (encodes a cell adhesion molecule)	Anosmia and hypogonadotropic hypogonadism	Renal agenesis
Simpson–Golabi–Behmel syndrome	312870	*GPC3* (encodes an extracellular matrix-associated protein)	Somatic overgrowth, coarse facies, congenital heart defects, and tumors	Large dysplastic kidneys, hydronephrosis
Genetic basis uncertain				
Mayer–Rokitansky–Kuster–Hauser syndrome	277000	Believed to have female-limited autosomal dominant inheritance	Anomalies of the female genital tract (ranging from upper vaginal atresia to total Müllerian agenesis)	Unilateral or bilateral renal agenesis

Contd...

Contd...

Syndrome	*OMIM number*	*Gene*	*Systemic manifestations*	*Renal pathology*
VACTERL association	192350	–	Vertebral defects, anal atresia, cardiac defects, tracheoesophageal fistula, radial dysplasia, limb defects	Renal agenesis, renal dysplasia
Meckel–Gruber syndrome	249000	Basal body proteome (MKS1; 609883) on chromosome 17q22	Occipital encephalocele, cleft palate, polydactyly	Large cystic kidneys
Joubert syndrome	213300	Homozygous mutation in the *INPP5E* gene (613037) on chromosome 9q34 Autosomal recessive	Hypoplasia of the cerebellar vermis, intellectual disability, retinal dystrophy, ocular coloboma, rotatory nystagmus, polydactyly, and congenital hepatic fibrosis	Cystic renal dysplasia
Bardet–Moon–Biedl syndrome	209900	*BBS1* gene on chromosome 11q13	Retinitis pigmentosa, obesity, polydactyly, learning disability, and hypogenitalism	Renal dysplasia
Zellweger spectrum and peroxisomal disorder	601498	HGNC-approved gene symbols: *PEX1, PEX2, PEX3, PEX5, PEX6, PEX10, PEX12, PEX13, PEX14, PEX16, PEX19*, or *PEX26* genes	Leukodystrophies craniofacial abnormalities hepatomegaly, chondrodysplasia punctata, eye abnormalities	Cystic renal dysplasia

Flowchart 1: Protocol for prenatal workup of congenital anomalies of the kidney and urinary tract (CAKUT).

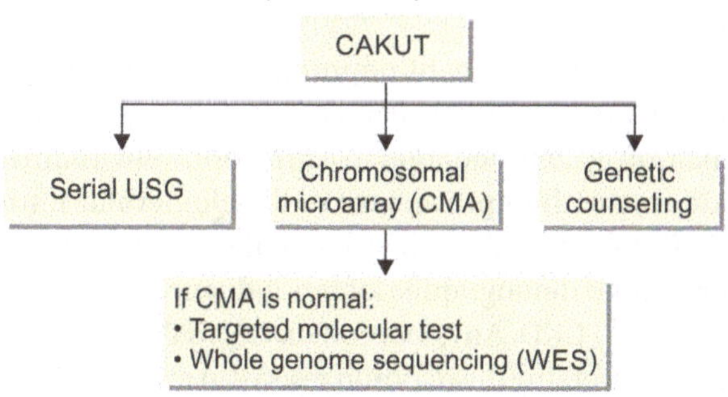

revolutionized genetic testing and can serve as powerful tools for identifying pathogenic mutations in all forms of CAKUT.

FETAL UROSONOGRAPHY (EXTENDED)

Serial USG assessment of the fetal kidneys can be done from 12 weeks of gestation with high-frequency transducers in coronal, longitudinal, and axial planes. Kidneys will appear bean shaped on either side of the spine with slit-like fluid-filled renal pelvis. In the second trimester, kidneys appear echo poor and in the third trimester, the corticomedullary differentiation can be clearly delineated. Urinary bladder is seen as lower midline fusiform echo poor cystic structure with two umbilical arteries skirting on either side of it. The bladder is visualized from the 12th week of gestation once fetal urine production starts. Demonstration of bladder cycling, i.e., serial filling and emptying of bladder due to fetal micturition, is a key indicator of a normal lower urinary tract. Hence, a persistent, overdistended bladder denotes bladder outflow obstruction and needs a thorough review of the rest of the urinary tract along with amniotic fluid volume and index at regular intervals to confirm the diagnosis and monitor progress. If the bladder outlet obstruction (BOO) is suspected, sonographic fetal MCU (SFMCUG) can be done using color Doppler imaging. This is a sonographic demonstration of the bladder emptying, urethral dilatation along with the urine outflow from the meatus.

Amniotic fluid index, pelvicalyceal dilatation, and cystic renal diseases are the key points to be observed in the extended fetal urosonography.

Amniotic Fluid and CAKUT

Amniotic fluid is contributed majorly by fetal urine by 16–18 weeks of gestation. CAKUT and amniotic fluid are closely associated and amniotic fluid volume is a prime indicator of the presence of CAKUT.

- *Polyhydramnios:* Barter's syndrome, fetal anemia, and twin-twin transfusion syndrome
- Oligohydramnios may result from BOO/bilateral renal diseases

- *Protocol for oligohydramnios:* PROM should be ruled out.
- Overdistended bladder indicates BOO.
- If UB is not seen persistently, renal fossae should be scanned for cystic diseases or agenesis.
- Bladder may appear small persistently in unilateral agenesis; small kidneys with less urine output will be evident by 20–24 weeks of gestation.
- If UB/kidney is normal, placenta should be looked for hypermaturity and placental dysfunction with features of fetal growth restriction. Color Doppler will add value to the study.

Urinary Tract Dilatation and CAKUT

Urinary tract dilatation (UTD) is the most common antenatal anomaly identified in 1–2% of the fetuses. It may be transient and physiologic in >50–70% of the cases and may resolve spontaneously. Most common anomalies identified are pelviureteric obstruction, vesicoureteric reflux, PUV, and primary obstructive megaureter. Other less common anomalies in the spectrum identified are duplex kidneys, rotational anomalies, ectopic ureter, prune belly syndrome, or urethral atresia. Nguyen et al. published a classification on prenatal and postnatal UTD with multidisciplinary consensus for a standardized terminology and protocol for perinatal evaluation of UTD. The statement gives directions for a standard term UTD with measurement of the anteroposterior renal pelvic diameter (APRPD) and its measurement technique with spine at 6 or 12'O clock positions.[18]

The other renal parameters to be evaluated are (1) calyceal dilatation, (2) renal parenchymal thickness, (3) parenchymal features—corticomedullary differentiation/echogenicity/cortical cyst if any, (4) ureteric dilatation, (5) bladder wall thickness/distension/ureterocele/key hole sign with urethral dilatation, and (6) amniotic index for oligohydramnios. The APRPD values >4 mm at <28 weeks/>7 mm at >28 weeks/>10 mm postnatally are considered abnormal and diagnosed as UTD. UTD is further classified into low- and high-risk groups to predict an increased risk for postnatal uropathy.

Cystic Renal Diseases

Multiple cysts and renal hyperechogenicity are the two main sonographic features. Parents need to be checked for familial diseases [corticomedullary differentiation (CMD)/calcifications/pelvic congestion syndrome (PCS) dilatation].[19]

- Obstructive dysplasia—unilateral or bilateral—hyperechoic cortex with or without cyst/PCS dilated
- MCDK—multiple cysts noncommunicating with little parenchyma. It can be in single, duplex moieties or in ectopic ureteric insertions of kidneys.
- Simple renal cyst—well-defined anechoic cystic lesion with clear fluid
- Polycystic renal diseases—familial/isolated/part of malformations. Fetal, infantile, and juvenile variants are seen. Fetal type presents in the second trimester with oligohydramnios/no CMD/enlarged echogenic kidneys occupying the entire abdomen/with or without cysts. UB is not seen. Infantile type—same findings with hyperechogenic medullary pyramids. Juvenile type—less severe—reversed CMD/normal UB and amniotic fluid.
- Glomerular cystic renal disease—autosomal dominant/same pattern as ARPKD/show enlarged hyperechoic kidneys with loss of CMD with cortical and subcapsular cysts.
- ADPKD affects the kidneys, liver, pancreas, and macro-vessels.
- Nephronophthisis—hyperechoic without CMD differentiation—autosomal recessive
- Polymalformative syndromes—Bardet-Biedl, Meckel-Gruber, Ivemark syndrome II, JATD, Ellis-van Crevald syndrome
- Differential diagnosis of echogenic kidneys—cytomegalovirus (CMV) infection/nephrotic syndrome/medullary nephrocalcinosis/trisomy/transient.

NEONATAL MARKERS AND RISK FACTORS FOR CHRONIC KIDNEY DISEASE IN CAKUT

The CAKUT spectrum is the most common congenital cause of ESKD and accounts for >50–70% of those children requiring kidney replacement therapy (KRT). Majority of them are detected antenatally or present within the first year of life. The most challenging factor is the early management of CAKUT with timely surgical intervention to arrest the CKD progression.

The natural history of nephrogenesis in the perinatal period with or without insults is not completely understood. The natural accommodation to extrauterine environment of the kidneys with improvement in the glomerular filtration rate (GFR) from birth till 2 years of life is consistent. Many biological and demographic factors influence severe CAKUT to progress to CKD. Any decision on CAKUT management is aimed at preserving the nephron reserve to maintain the renal parameters normal.

Katsaufis et al. analyzed a birth cohort to identify neonatal markers for severe CAKUT and formulated the points below:

- <36 weeks preterm male child has high propensity for CKD progression in severe CAKUT.
- Neonatal cystatin C levels >3.0 mg/L have the highest sensitivity and specificity to predict early CKD.
- A serum creatinine >0.6 mg/L is an early predictor to progression of CKD to ESKD.
- Associated genetic anomalies such as VACTERL syndrome, association of pulmonary hypoplasia or pulmonary hypertension by oligohydramnios, any infective complications in the urinary tract, and hormonal and metabolic complications in renal dysfunction are factors that contribute for early progression of CKD toward ESKD.[20]

Hypoplasia/Dysplasia Scale

To quantify the hypoplasia and dysplasia, the hypodysplasia (HD) scale was devised from glomerular counts, dysplasia scores, and the ratio of normal nephrons to dysplastic structures. Fetal or neonatal renal biopsy may indicate the severity of CAKUT and future renal development.

A radial glomerular count means the average number of glomeruli arrayed alongside a straight medullary ray cut in section from calyx to capsule and perpendicular to the capsule of the kidney. The dysplasia score is the total number of points allotted to any one kidney according to the types of abnormal structures present that met the criteria of dysplasia. The ratio of normal to abnormal structures is judged from low power microscopy surveys of areas of renal tissue expressed as a percentage of nephrons. The average normal radial glomerular count is of 8 ± 0.5 in kidneys. Hypoplasia is labeled when the radial glomerular count is <7 in number.

The degree of dysplasia is assessed by characteristics of five histological features:

1. Primitive ducts
2. Ductules with low cuboidal epithelium and mesenchymal collars
3. Cartilage
4. Loose mesenchymal fibrous tissues
5. Cyst and heterotopic erythropoiesis

Each criterion with accentuated importance can give a point score up to maximum 22 dysplasia score. Both the scores have been studied in infants less than 3 months of age to study the pathogenesis of hypodysplasia before the urodynamic effects of the obstruction and reflux with inflammation had destroyed the renal morphology. The degree of hypodysplasia seems to correlate with the degree of lateral ectopia of the ureteric orifice.

Complete obstruction of the ureter in ureteral atresia increases the HD scale along with ischemic changes and cystic changes in the nephrons leading on to MCDKs—a nonfunctioning renal tissue. A disordered expression of diverse growth factors, cell survival genes, and transcription factor genes correlate with disordered cell turnover and maturation, resulting in excessive growth followed by apoptotic involution. Upregulated proliferation of dysplastic epithelium results in cystic changes, and subsequent excess apoptosis in the adjacent mesenchyme causes involution of dysplastic kidneys as is commonly noted in MCDK.

Approach to Diagnosis and Evaluation of Renal Hypodysplasia

Renal hypoplasia is defined as abnormally small kidneys (<2 SD below the expected mean when correlated with age or parameters of somatic growth) with normal morphology and reduced nephron number. But this definition is a misnomer as majority of congenitally small kidneys also exhibit evidence of tissue maldifferentiation, defined as renal dysplasia. Hence, the exact incidence of pure renal hypoplasia (without dysplasia) is difficult to estimate. By definition ~2.2% of the population exhibit renal hypoplasia, whereas epidemiologic studies suggest an estimated incidence of 1 in 400 births.[2,21]

Both hypoplasia and dysplasia are histologic diagnosis, with a *hypoplastic* kidney being nephron deficient whereas a *dysplastic* kidney being composed, in whole or in part, of undifferentiated and metaplastic tissues. Since definitive histology is seldom available, kidneys are called "hypoplastic" when they are significantly shorter than normal but retain a normal shape and some function and "dysplastic" when they are smaller to larger than normal in size with either reduced or no excretory function. They have loss of corticomedullary differentiation on USG and contain cysts that may cause renomegaly. However, as there is no definite confirmatory evidence to label either, the term hypodysplasia is in vogue.[22,23]

Renal hypoplasia/dysplasia is the leading cause of childhood ESKD. When bilateral, it leads to significant impairment of intrauterine renal function causing the oligohydramnios sequence, incompatible with life. On the other hand, mild bilateral renal hypoplasia is associated with the development of adult-onset hypertension and chronic renal failure.[24,25]

Genetic Basis of Renal Hypoplasia

Kidney development involves a complex, reciprocal inductive interaction between the ureteric cell lineage and the metanephric mesenchyme (MM) cell lineage.

Ureteric Cell Lineage Contribution to Renal Hypoplasia

Multiple processes are required within the UB for development before it stimulates the metanephric blastema to initiate nephrogenesis. These include induction, growth, branching, survival, and differentiation. These processes are primarily regulated by receptor tyrosine kinase signaling pathways and transcription factors expressed in the UB.

Genes involved in Induction, Growth, and Branching

The interactions between the UB tip-specific receptor RET and its ligand GDNF are crucial for the initial UB induction from the Wolffian duct. Loss of these interactions leads to renal agenesis.[26] Maintenance of GDNF and RET expression is controlled by an autoregulatory feedback loop with Wnt11.[27] UB development and branching are regulated by FGF signaling via the FGFR2 receptor, MET, Egfr, and transcription factor Lim1. Mutations in *PAX2* gene are for ureteric growth, branching, and survival.

*Hnf1*β-regulated gene transcription is critical to the UB and MM interplay as it exhibits in vivo binding to noncoding regulatory DNA sequences of PAX2, Lim1, and Wnt9b.[28-30]

Ureteric Cell Differentiation

The transcriptional control of UB differentiation, especially of the tip domain, is essential for UB development and proper nephron formation. Ectopic overexpression of nuclear phosphoprotein p53 in the UB results in defective differentiation of the UB and a secondary survival defect in the MM leading to a 50% decrease in both kidney size and nephron number.[31] Hedgehog signaling effectors also regulate the differentiation of the UB tip domain. HH activity is normally restricted to the medullary domain of the kidney.

Metanephric Mesenchyme Cell Lineage Contribution to Renal Hypoplasia

As nephron formation is dependent on inductive signals from the ureteric tip, the number of ureteric tips is considered a strong determinant of nephron endowment. GDNF, the ligand for RET (and GFRα1), in GDNF/RET pathway is expressed in the MM and is critical for ureteric branching morphogenesis. The renal stroma contributes to nephron endowment, via retinoic acid-signaling axis. Retinoic acid is the active form of dietary vitamin A synthesized by enzyme Raldh2, and signals through retinoic acid receptors (Rar). Genetic elimination of Raldh2 hence causes renal hypoplasia.[32]

Members of the Myc family of genes mediate cell growth, proliferation, and apoptosis. During metanephric development, expression of c-myc is restricted to early uninduced mesenchyme and n-myc to early mesenchymal aggregates. Targeted deletion of c-myc to the MM lineage or n-myc deficiency results in renal hypoplasia due to a significant decrease in mesenchymal proliferation, independent of changes in apoptosis.[33] Six2 is exclusively expressed in the cap mesenchyme, marking the nephron progenitor population. Genetic elimination of Six2 results in severe renal hypoplasia, characterized by premature and ectopic differentiation of nephrogenic tubules and a rapid depletion of the nephrogenic progenitor population.[34]

Principal Genes associated with Renal Agenesis, Hypoplasia, and Dysplasia

Principal genes associated with renal agenesis, hypoplasia, and dysplasia are given in **Table 3**.

Environmental Factors and Renal Hypoplasia

Several in utero environmental factors play a role in the pathogenesis of renal hypoplasia. Maternal undernutrition and uteroplacental insufficiency are known to cause significant reduction in nephron endowment and predispose to hypoplasia. Maternal vitamin A deficiency hampers genetic signaling and results in hypoplasia.[35]

Maternal diabetes, exposure to alcohol, and drugs such as dexamethasone and thalidomide have been implicated in nephron loss and hence deficit **(Table 4)**.

TABLE 3: Principal genes associated with renal agenesis, hypoplasia, and dysplasia.

Gene	*Kidney phenotype*
FOXD1	Small, fused, undifferentiated kidney
EYA1	Absent kidneys
EMX2	Absent kidneys
HOXA11/HOXD11	Small or absent kidneys
LHX1	Absent kidneys
PAX2	Small or absent kidneys
WT1	Absent kidneys
AGTR2	Multiple urinary tract malformations
BMP4	Altered ureteric bud (UB) branching
BMP7	Disrupted nephrogenesis
WNT4	Undifferentiated kidneys
RET	Absent kidneys, severe dysgenesis
GDNF	Absent kidneys, severe dysgenesis
SIX1	Absent kidneys
SIX2	Small kidneys
SALL1	Absent kidneys
FGFR1/FGFR2	Absent kidneys
SLIT3	Small or absent kidneys
PBX1	Small or absent kidneys
FGF8	Small kidneys
RARA/RARB2	Small kidneys
LIM1	Absent kidneys

TABLE 4: Nutritional factors impact on congenital anomalies of the kidney and urinary tract (CAKUT).

Fetal exposure to	*Renal phenotype*
Uteroplacental insufficiency	Hypoplasia
Vitamin A deficiency	Hypoplasia, hydronephrosis/ureter
Low protein diet	Hypoplasia
Hyperglycemia	Agenesis, ectopic/horseshoe, cystic/dysplasia, hypoplasia, hydronephrosis/ureter
Cocaine	Agenesis, hypoplasia, hydronephrosis/ureter
Alcohol	Agenesis, ectopia/horseshoe, cystic dysplasia, hypoplasia, hydronephrosis/ureter
Dexamethasone/corticosterone	Hypoplasia
Thalidomide	Agenesis, ectopic/horseshoe, cystic dysplasia, hypoplasia, hydronephrosis/ureter

Management of Renal Hypodysplasia

The principal aim once the diagnosis is established is to identify the entity and prevent ongoing damage to the remaining nephrons.

Evaluation

Regular blood pressure (BP) monitoring is to be done for early detection and treatment of hypertension. Genetics assessment is to be done to establish the pathogenesis, specially if associated with syndromic features. This will also aid in future genetic counseling.

In unilateral cases, serum creatinine and urea concentrations would be normal. In severe cases, renal function should be assessed with baseline GFR for calculation for CKD staging. Serum electrolytes are to be assessed for hyponatremia, especially in the presence of polyuria which may require sodium chloride supplementation. Hyperkalemia due to reduced glomerular filtration, reduced tubular secretion, and associated metabolic acidosis can be life-threatening.[36,37]

Imaging

Antenatal ultrasound would guide preemptively with findings of absent or small kidney. Any antenatal detection of anatomical renal anomalies warrants postnatal USG to confirm the same. Postnatal scan is taken as the baseline to document the hydronephrosis or hydroureteronephrosis in unilateral or bilateral systems which facilitates timely and prompt follow-up. Dimercaptosuccinic acid (DMSA) nuclear imaging is preferred in cases of renal ectopia to identify a functioning renal parenchyma. CT or MR urogram is ideal in cases of complex anatomical anomalies. Vesicoureteral reflux is common, and hence a voiding cystourethrogram (VCUG) to rule out reflux in the contralateral kidney is useful.

Medical or surgical intervention is decided based on the need for anatomical corrections and to protect the functioning renal parenchyma avoiding/delaying progression to chronic renal failure.

FETAL INTERVENTION: HISTORY AND EVOLUTION

Advances in antenatal ultrasound have revolutionized prenatal diagnosis and intervention of various congenital anomalies. In experienced hands, the sensitivity of two-dimensional ultrasound is around 50% in the first trimester, increasing to 90% by 22–24 weeks of gestation.

Fetal intervention aims to address diseases that progress with gestation and create significant end-organ damage. Posterior urethral valve is the most common anomaly requiring early intervention to avoid perinatal mortality and morbidity due to pulmonary hypoplasia and progressive renal failure.[38]

Fetoscopy was introduced in the early 1970s for diagnostic purposes; later, with the advent of technical improvements as in smaller endoscopes, better optics, availability of laser, mini and microcatheters, it has been increasingly used for therapeutic interventions.

Initially, fetoscopy was carried out only in amniotic fluid medium, using a single port, an endoscope with a working channel for a laser fiber, balloon insertion, or small bipolar forceps. The fluid medium posed limitations for surgeries requiring dissection and suturing, allowed fluctuating fetal positions and led to lower quality of the acquired images, more so in the presence of bleeding that hindered completion of the procedure. Hence, an aerial medium was developed to allow further advances in fetal surgery. Partial amniotic carbon dioxide insufflation (PACI) is utilized to overcome these problems and has been successfully tested in sheep and thereafter in human fetoscopic surgical procedures. However, further assessment of its risks, safety margins, and management issues still remains to be addressed.[39]

Open fetal surgery by maternal hysterotomy and open fetal vesicostomy was first advocated by Harrison et al. in the 1980s. Fetal intervention for obstructive uropathy was first performed at the University of California, San Francisco, in 1981. It was concluded that fetal surgery for obstructive uropathy should be performed only in patients with severe oligohydramnios and normal-appearing kidneys.

FETAL INTERVENTION FOR UROLOGIC DISORDERS

Infravesical obstructive uropathy appears to be the only indication for antenatal intervention, the common causes being PUVs and urethral atresia.

Keyhole sign (dilated bladder and urethra) is the classical image of the PUV on USG. Unilateral or bilateral hydronephrosis, amniotic fluid index, multiple renal cortical cyst, loss of corticomedullary differentiation, and cortical echogenicity are other key points to be noted. Features of renal hypodysplasia, unfavorable urinary indices, and early detection before 24 weeks of gestation have poor prognostication.

The options for intervention include bladder drainage by serial vesicocentesis, a continuous drainage into the amniotic cavity by placing a vesicoamniotic shunt, and fetal endoscopic laser ablation of valves **(Fig. 13)**. Open procedures include vesicostomy and ureterostomy.

Basis for Fetal Intervention

The basis for fetal intervention is prenatal vesicoamniotic shunting attempts to reduce or avoid renal parenchymal damage and chronic oligohydramnios that can adversely affect pulmonary development and hence increase survival in the postnatal period and subsequently overcome progression to CKD.

Vesicoamniotic Shunting

Fetal intervention may be offered if indicated and available between 24 and 34 weeks of gestation. Double reversed pigtail catheters with stylets for puncture are used percutaneously under ultrasound guidance to achieve vesicoamniotic shunting. Fetal complications include frequent dislodgement

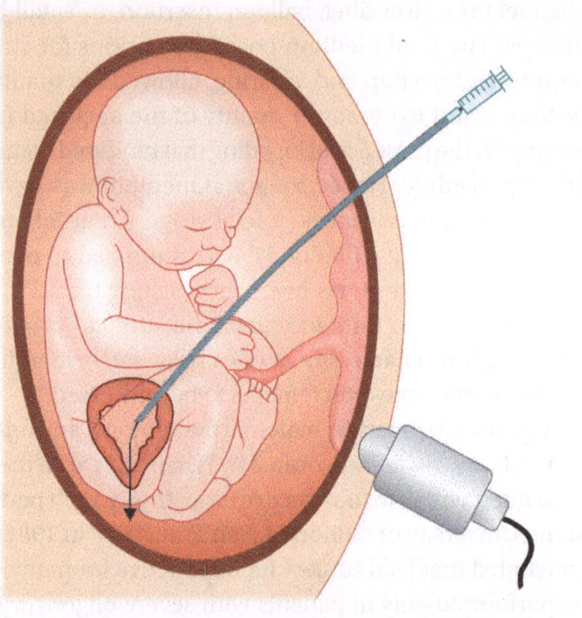

Fig. 13: Fetal cystoscope, ultrasonography (USG) guided for vesicoamniotic (VA) shunt or valve fulguration/double-J (DJ) stenting across urethra.

of the vesicoamniotic stents (after the bladder shrinks from distended contour) in >50%, blockage of shunt, and migration of shunt creating fetoperitoneal drainage. Expandable wire mesh stents inserted into vesicocutaneous fistulas created endoscopically have been tried to reduce stent-migration rates. Maternal complications include chorioamnionitis and maternal amnioperitoneal leaks.[40]

The PLUTO (percutaneous vesicoamniotic shunting for lower urinary tract obstruction) trial was conducted by the University of Birmingham as a prospective randomized multicenter trial. 21 fetal medicine centers in England, Scotland, Ireland, and the Netherlands participated in the study, seven of which (from England, Scotland, and the Netherlands) recruited women in the trial. Inclusion criteria were consenting pregnant women who had a singleton male fetus with an ultrasound diagnosis of LUTO (diagnosed on the basis of the visualization of an enlarged bladder and dilated proximal urethra, bilateral or unilateral hydronephrosis, and cystic parenchymal renal disease). Fetuses with additional major structural or chromosomal anomalies and female fetuses were excluded from the trial.

Pregnancies were allocated to placement of vesicoamniotic shunt or conservative management. Vesicoamniotic shunting was done under sedation and prophylactic antibiotics were given 2 hours before the procedure. The fetus and fetal bladder were visualized continuously by high-quality, high-resolution, real-time 2D ultrasound. With a sterile, minimum-touch technique, a vesicoamniotic pigtail catheter was inserted percutaneously with either the King's College/Rocket introducer or the Harrison shunting set, according to the clinician preference. Optimum placement of the stent (with the distal end in the fetal bladder and the proximal end in the amniotic cavity) and fetal viability were confirmed immediately and at several hours postprocedure. The scheduled follow-up was continued postnatally and the results were analyzed.

The observational evidence suggested that vesicoamniotic shunting improved overall perinatal survival, but the long-term outcome for these babies was poor, with high mortality and morbidity. The findings of the trial were limited by the small number of participants recruited and high proportion of women who did not receive their allocated treatment. This crossover occurred either because of clinician choice or because of changing clinical features as the pregnancy progressed. Serious adverse events to the rate of 45% were documented and included pregnancy loss before 24 weeks, premature rupture of membranes, chorioamnionitis, damage to maternal uterus or other organs, damage to fetal organs, and migration of stent/block.[41]

FETAL ENDOSCOPIC VALVE ABLATION

For almost a decade, the vesicoamniotic shunt was the only fetal intervention available for PUVs. Quintero et al., in 1995, introduced fetal cystoscopy and ablation of PUVs. It has been tried by various study groups with limited success and is sought with a lot of complications.[42] Endoscopic fetal urethrotomy for anterior urethral valves has also been described.[43] Several technical modifications have been advocated to overcome access to the proximal urethra from physiologic angulation of the bladder neck and improvised for antegrade vision of the posterior urethra.

Fetal valve ablation is usually done by laser coagulation for its precise cutting. But the technical difficulty in an antegrade introduction of fetoscope to have direct visualization of PUVs (by angle of the urethra) resulted in collateral damage to the surrounding tissues or inadequacy in valve fulguration. Considering the risks involved, judicious case selection is therefore advised.[44] Fetuses with poor renal indices (suggesting renal hypodysplasia) are not candidates for intervention. Only those with bilateral hydroureteronephrosis and good renal indices who develop oligohydramnios need fulguration to avoid pulmonary hypoplasia whereas the ones with good amniotic index and bilateral hydroureteronephrosis can be managed postnatally. In patients with severe oligohydramnios, amnioinfusion is considered to continue pregnancy and ensure fetal lung maturity.

Ruano et al. suggest percutaneous early fetal cystoscopy and laser (Nd-YAG) valve fulguration for severe first-trimester megacystis using specially designed microcannula and conclude that it prevents deterioration of renal and bladder function and improves postnatal follow-up.[45]

The controversy in the serial analysis of fetal urine sample with USG guidance is that the urine sample taken from the bladder is a static urine which is not cycled and may not reflect

Bladder Outlet Obstruction (BOO)/Posterior Urethral Valves (PUV)

Total Number of Evaluations		
460	Fetoscopic intervention	25
	Amnioport for Serial Amnioinfusions Performed as adjunct therapy for BOO/PUV and other GU anomalies including renal agenesis	26
	Vesicoamniotic shunting is also a surgical option offered by out team	

Fig. 14: Annual report from Cincinnati Fetal Center (2019)—stating fetoscopic intervention and amnioinfusions as the lead procedures. (GU: genitourinary)

the actual urinary indices at that point in time. Hence, other parameters to improve the fetal selection in earlier gestation need to be researched upon **(Fig. 14)**.

More recently, fetoscope is used to insert a guidewire and double-J stent across the urethra simulating a vesicoamniotic shunt—to improve the urinary drainage from the bladder. This process of fetal catheterization promises to overcome the complications of shunt displacement encountered in vesicoamniotic shunting.

OPEN FETAL SURGERY

Open fetal surgery comprises maternal laparotomy, followed by hysterotomy with direct exposure of the fetus. Fetal vesicostomies and ureterostomies have been performed with limited success. The risk of early fetal loss and chorioamnionitis is high. The delivery has to be done 4 weeks after hysterotomy, to avoid uterine dehiscence. Hence, the purpose of urinary diversion may not help much in the renal dysmorphogenesis. Instead, amnioinfusions can serve the purpose of holding the amniotic index supporting lung maturity.

INDIAN SCENARIO

The Division of Fetal Medicine, All India Institute of Medical Sciences, New Delhi, India, performs around four to five shunts per year. Few centers in Kerala, Chennai, and Bengaluru do occasional shunting procedures. Delayed diagnosis, technical factors, costs involved, and imbalance in the risks and benefits have been major deterrents toward widespread acceptance of fetal interventions in India.[46,47]

RUMINATING POINTS

- Fetal interventions can limit the hypoplasia occurrence in the last trimester by increasing the nephron numbers (improvement in urine drainage, removing the back-pressure effect in kidney when nephron numbers are increasing).
- Renal dysplasia cannot be remodeled by any kind of fetal intervention.
- Technical feasibility of a particular procedure has to be case-to-case guided.
- There is a need for a multidisciplinary team comprising obstetricians, neonatologist, fetal medicine specialist, pediatric surgeons, and a genetic counselor to dictate case-selected treatment options.
- Parents need to be counseled in detail regarding the nature of procedure and its impact on the growing kidneys. They must be prepared for an adverse event of fetal loss during the course of treatment.
- A structured training program in fetal intervention with the latest updates across the globe, a multidisciplinary team, and official ethical board supervision are mandatory to have a periodical information and introspection of fetal intervention procedures.
- The high risk of infection, fetal loss, prematurity, and above all the high costs involved outweigh the benefit of fetal intervention in our country. An official body to obtain ethical and legal clearance for fetal intervention procedures is yet to be formulated.
- Appropriate fetal selection, ideal surgical techniques, and postnatal management accompanied by the development of sophisticated devices are yet to be protocolized without compromise on the quality and outcomes.
- Thus far, early identification of renal hypodysplasia and timely surgical interventions for anatomical abnormalities remain the key player in the management of CAKUT.

CONCLUSION

Awareness about CAKUT and its etiopathogenesis helps in its early detection. Early detection, timely surgical intervention often delays the progression of CKD to ESKD.

KEY POINTS

- CAKUT contributes significantly to ESKD in children.
- CAKUT presents as a wide anatomical spectrum, either isolated or associated with diverse extrarenal manifestations.

- Research on genetic mutations is ongoing and nearly 30 genes have been identified as causative factors in CAKUT.
- Routine use of prenatal ultrasound has resulted in its early detection.
- Advances adopted in fetal interventions aim to reduce ongoing renal damage. This reduces the aftermath on pulmonary development contributing to overall increase in postnatal survival.

REFERENCES

1. Song R, Yosypiv IV. Genetics of congenital anomalies of the kidney and urinary tract. Pediatr Nephrol. 2011;26:353-64.
2. Schedl A. Renal abnormalities and their developmental origin. Nat Rev Genet. 2007;8(10):791-802.
3. Harambat J, van Stralen KJ, Kim JJ, Tizard EJ. Epidemiology of chronic kidney disease in children. Pediatr Nephrol. 2012;27:363-73.
4. Yosypiv IV. Congenital anomalies of the kidney and urinary tract: a genetic disorder? Int J Nephrol. 2012;2012:909083.
5. Costantini F, Shakya R. GDNF/Ret signaling and the development of the kidney. Bioessays. 2006;28:117-27.
6. Weber S, Moriniere V, Knuppel T, Charbit M, Dusek J, Ghiggeri GM, et al. Prevalence of mutations in renal developmental genes in children with renal hypodysplasia: results of the ESCAPE study. J Am Soc Nephrol. 2006;17:2864.
7. Grieshammer U, Le M, Plump AS, Wang F, Tessier-Lavigne M, Martin GR. SLIT2-mediated ROBO2 signaling restricts kidney induction to a single site. Dev Cell. 2004;6:709-17.
8. Hahn H. Genetics of kidney development: pathogenesis of renal anomalies. Korean J Pediatr. 2010;53:729-34.
9. Woolf AS. A molecular and genetic view of human renal and urinary tract malformations. Kidney Int. 2000;58(2):500-1.
10. Peters CA, Carr MC, Lais A, Retik AB, Mandell J. The response of the fetal kidney to obstruction. J Urol. 1992;148(2 Pt 2):503-9.
11. Dover GJ. The Barker hypothesis: how pediatricians will diagnose and prevent common adult-onset diseases. Trans Am Clin Climatol Assoc. 2009;120:199-207.
12. Dart AB, Ruth CA, Sellers EA, Au W, Dean HJ. Maternal diabetes mellitus and congenital anomalies of the kidney and urinary tract (CAKUT) in the child. Am J Kidney Dis. 2015;65(5):684-91.
13. Harewood L, Liu M, Keeling J, Howatson A, Whiteford M, Branney P, et al. Bilateral renal agenesis/hypoplasia/dysplasia (BRAHD): postmortem analysis of 45 cases with breakpoint mapping of two de novo translocations. PLoS One. 2010;5(8): e12375.
14. Moore KL, Persaud TV, Torchia MG. Chapter 12 urogenital system. The Developing Human: Clinically Oriented Embryology. Edinburgh: Saunders; 2016. pp. 241-80.
15. Barakat AJ, Rushton HG. Chapter 8: Duplication Anomalies of the Kidney and Ureters. Congenital Anomalies of the Kidney and Urinary Tract Clinical Implications in Children. Cham: Springer International Publishing; 2016. pp. 155-73.
16. Sadler TW. Urogenital system. Langman's Medical Embryology. Philadelphia: Walters Kluwer; 2019. pp. 256-83 (Chapter 16).
17. Nakanishi K, Yoshikawa N. Genetic disorders of human congenital anomalies of the kidney and urinary tract (CAKUT). Pediatr Int. 2003;45(5):610-16.
18. Nguyen HT, Benson CB, Bromley B, Campbell JB, Chow J, Coleman B, et al. Multidisciplinary consensus on the classification of prenatal and postnatal urinary tract dilation (UTD classification system). J Pediatr Urol. 2014;10(6):982-98.
19. Avni FE, Garel C, Cassart M, D'Haene N, Hall M, Riccabona M. Imaging and classification of congenital cystic renal diseases. Am J Roentgenol. 2012;198:1004-10.
20. Katsoufis CP, DeFreitas MJ, Infante JC, Castellan M, Cano T, Safina Vaccaro D, et al. Risk assessment of severe congenital anomalies of the kidney and urinary tract (CAKUT): a birth cohort. Front Pediatr. 2019;7:182.
21. Hiraoka M, Tsukahara H, Ohshima Y, Kasuga K, Ishihara Y, Mayumi M. Renal aplasia is the predominant cause of congenital solitary kidneys. Kidney Int. 2002;61:1840-4.
22. Woolf AS, Price KL, Scambler PJ, Winyard PJ. Evolving concepts in human renal dysplasia. J Am Soc Nephrol. 2004;15:998-1007.
23. Rosenbaum DM, Korngold E, Teele RL. Sonographic assessment of renal length in normal children. AJR Am J Roentgenol. 1984;142:467-9.
24. Brenner BM, Chertow GM. Congenital oligonephropathy and the etiology of adult hypertension and progressive renal injury. Am J Kidney Dis. 1994;23:171-5.
25. Keller G, Zimmer G, Mall G, Ritz E, Amann K. Nephron number in patients with primary hypertension. N Engl J Med. 2003;348:101-8.
26. Zhang Z, Quinlan J, Hoy W, Hughson MD, Lemire M, Hudson T, et al. A common RET variant is associated with reduced newborn kidney size and function. J Am Soc Nephrol. 2008;19:2027-34.
27. Majumdar A, Vainio S, Kispert A, McMahon J, McMahon AP. Wnt11 and Ret/Gdnf pathways cooperate in regulating ureteric branching during metanephric kidney development. Development. 2003;130:3175-85.
28. Ishibe S, Karihaloo A, Ma H, Zhang J, Marlier A, Mitobe M, et al. Met and the epidermal growth factor receptor act cooperatively to regulate final nephron number and maintain collecting duct morphology. Development. 2009;136:337-45.
29. Kobayashi A, Kwan KM, Carroll TJ, McMahon AP, Mendelsohn CL, Behringer RR. Distinct and sequential tissue-specific activities of the LIM-class homeobox gene Lim1 for tubular morphogenesis during kidney development. Development. 2005;132:2809-23.
30. Quinlan J, Lemire M, Hudson T, Qu H, Benjamin A, Roy A, et al. A common variant of the PAX2 gene is associated with reduced newborn kidney size. J Am Soc Nephrol. 2007;18:1915-21.
31. Godley LA, Kopp JB, Eckhaus M, Paglino JJ, Owens J, Varmus HE. Wild-type p53 transgenic mice exhibit altered differentiation of the ureteric bud and possess small kidneys. Genes Dev. 1996;10:836-50.
32. Rosselot C, Spraggon L, Chia I, Batourina E, Riccio P, Lu B, et al. Non-cell-autonomous retinoid signaling is crucial for renal development. Development. 2010;137:283-92.
33. Bates CM, Kharzai S, Erwin T, Rossant J, Parada LF. Role of N-myc in the developing mouse kidney. Dev Biol. 2000;222:317-25.
34. Self M, Lagutin OV, Bowling B, Hendrix J, Cai Y, Dressler GR, et al. Six2 is required for suppression of nephrogenesis and progenitor renewal in the developing kidney. EMBO J. 2006;25:5214-28.
35. Cain J, Di Giovanni V, Smeeton J, et al. Genetics of renal hypoplasia: insights into the mechanisms controlling nephron endowment. Pediatr Res. 2010;68:91-8.
36. La Scola C, Hewitt I, Pasini A. Postnatal management of congenital bilateral renal hypodysplasia. J Matern Fetal Neonatal Med. 2010;23:97-100.

37. Winyard P, Chitty LS. Dysplastic kidneys. Semin Fetal Neonatal Med. 2008;13:142-51.
38. Kohl T. Minimally invasive fetoscopic interventions: an overview in 2010. Surg Endosc. 2010;24:2056-67.
39. Kohl T, Tchatcheva K, Weinbach J, Hering R, Kozlowski P, Stressig R, et al. Partial amniotic carbon dioxide insufflation (PACI) during minimally invasive fetoscopic surgery: early clinical experience in humans. Surg Endosc. 2010;24(2):432-44.
40. Clark TJ, Divakaran TG, Divakaran TG, Whittle MJ, Kilby MD, Khan KS. Prenatal bladder drainage in the management of fetal lower urinary tract obstruction: a systematic review and meta-analysis. Obstet Gynecol. 2003;102:367-82.
41. Morris RK, Malin GL, Quinlan-Jones E, Middleton LJ, Hemming K, Burke D, et al. for the Percutaneous vesicoamniotic shunting in Lower Urinary Tract Obstruction (PLUTO) Collaborative Group. Percutaneous vesicoamniotic shunting versus conservative management for fetal lower urinary tract obstruction (PLUTO): a randomised trial. Lancet. 2013; 382(9903):1496-506.
42. Quintero RA, Hume R, Smith C, Johnson MP, Cotton DB, Romero R, et al. Percutaneous fetal cystoscopy and endoscopic fulguration of posterior urethral valves. Am J Obstet Gynecol. 1995;172:206.
43. Sago H, Hayashi S, Chiba T, Ueoka K, Matsuoka K, Nakagawa A, et al. Endoscopic fetal urethrotomy for anterior urethral valves: a preliminary report. Fetal Diagn Ther. 2008;24:92-5.
44. Welsh A, Agarwal S, Kumar S, Smith RP, Fisk NM. Fetal cystoscopy in the management of fetal obstructive uropathy: experience in a single European center. Prenat Diagn. 2003;23: 1033-41.
45. Ruano R, Yoshisaki CT, Salustiano EMA, Giron AM, Srougi M, Zugaib M. Early fetal cystoscopy for first-trimester severe megacystis. Ultrasound Obstet Gynecol. 2011;37(6):696-701.
46. Menon P, Rao KL. Current status of fetal surgery. Indian J Pediatr. 2005;72(5):433-6.
47. Sharma S. Progress in fetal surgery: a buoyant start or watchful reluctance? Perspectives for India. J Indian Assoc Pediatr Surg. 2019;24(1):1-3.

CHAPTER

13.4

Urinary Tract Infection

Jitendra Meena, Pankaj Hari

INTRODUCTION

Urinary tract infection (UTI) is one of the most common bacterial infections in childhood and an important diagnosis in febrile infants presenting to hospital. In infancy, prevalence of UTI is higher in boys than girls; however beyond infancy and during prepubertal age, UTI is more prevalent in girls compared to their counterparts.[1,2] Of those who develop a febrile UTI in childhood, a significant proportion develop recurrence of UTI in the next 6–12 months.[3] Apart from anomalies of the urinary tract, bladder-bowel dysfunction and circumcision status are also considered as important risk factors for recurrence of UTI.

The significance of UTI lies in the risk of recurrence and acute febrile illness caused by it rather than long-term consequences such as proteinuria, hypertension, and end-stage kidney disease (ESKD) as was understood previously. Earlier investigators found a significant relationship between UTI, vesicoureteric reflux (VUR), and kidney damage, also called reflux nephropathy. Hence, a great deal of emphasis was put on identifying VUR by voiding cystourethrogram (VCUG). However, as understanding about reflux nephropathy has evolved, it is considered that kidney damage resulting in chronic kidney disease (CKD) is caused chiefly by congenital dysplasia rather than scarring acquired secondary to UTI. This is also supported by lack of decline in kidney scarring and ESKD following surgical correction of VUR. 30–40% of children presenting with UTI have VUR. Overall, the risk of ESKD in all children with VUR is considered very low. This paradigm shift in understanding about reflux nephropathy has resulted in a significant change in practices for the evaluation and management of children with UTI.

DEFINITION

Urinary tract infection refers to the growth of pathogenic microorganism within the urinary tract. UTI can be divided into two types. Infection limited to urinary bladder is cystitis (lower UTI). Cystitis usually presents with lower urinary tract symptoms such as dysuria and increased frequency of urination, with or without low-grade fever. Pyelonephritis (upper UTI) occurs when a pathogenic microorganism infects the kidney parenchyma either through the ascending route or as a result of blood-borne infection. Acute pyelonephritis typically presents with high-grade fever with or without other symptoms such as abdominal or loin pain. Asymptomatic presence of bacteria in urine without any evidence of inflammation is referred to as asymptomatic bacteriuria. Classification of UTI as pyelonephritis versus cystitis is based on clinical symptoms and may be difficult in infants. Any febrile UTI in an infant or young child is considered as pyelonephritis. Differentiation between cystitis and pyelonephritis is important as it helps in determining the treatment and prognosis.

EPIDEMIOLOGY

Urinary tract infection is a common bacterial infection in childhood affecting 1.7% boys and 8.4% girls within the first 7 years of life. Among febrile children aged less than 5 years, prevalence of UTI was 3.4%.[4] The pooled prevalence of UTI was 7% in febrile children less than 24 months and 7.8% in older children. The incidence of UTI depends on age and sex. It is highest during the first year of life. In boys, UTI is most common during the initial 6 months; afterward incidences drop as they grow older, unlike girls in whom incidence does not change significantly. A systematic review reported the prevalence of febrile UTIs in girls aged 0–3 months to be 7.5% as compared to 8.4% in boys.[1] Prevalence is significantly higher in uncircumcised boys (20.1%) as compared to circumcised boys (2.4%).[1] A considerable proportion of children (10–30%) with febrile UTI develop recurrence with the first year of the initial episode.[3,5] Bladder-bowel dysfunction, VUR, female sex, and circumcision status in boys are the chief risk factors reported for recurrence of UTI in children.[3,5,6]

Escherichia coli is the most common (80–90%) causative organism reported in childhood across the globe.[7-11] Most of the pathogens causing UTI in children arise from fecal flora. Apart from *E. coli*, other common gram-negative bacteria causing UTI are *Klebsiella, Pseudomonas, Proteus, Enterobacter*, and *Citrobacter* spp. Some gram-positive organism have also been reported to cause UTI such as *Staphylococcus saprophyticus, Enterococcus* spp, and (rarely)

Staphylococcus aureus. In immunocompromised host and children with indwelling catheters, *Candida* can cause UTI.[12]

PATHOGENESIS

Urinary tract infection results from an imbalance between host defense mechanism and bacterial virulence. The urinary tract has several mechanisms to prevent the invasion of uropathogenic bacteria such as the antegrade unidirectional flow of urine from the kidney to the bladder and intermittent complete emptying of the bladder. This washout process clears most of the uropathogens from the urinary tract.[13] Urine also has many antimicrobial properties including low pH, neutrophils, and Tamm–Horsfall protein glycoprotein (uromodulin), which prevent bacterial adhesion to uroepithelium.[14] UTI occurs if failure of the above mechanism results in the introduction of uropathogen in the urinary tract followed by its adhesion to uroepithelium that supports its colonization and finally microbial multiplication.

Most of the urinary tract is sterile with exception of the distal-most part of the urethra. In the physiological state, the periurethral area contains fecal bacteria, chiefly gram-negative organisms. While *E. coli* is the most common bacterium in girls but after initial 6 months of life, *Proteus mirabilis* predominates in boys in the periurethral area.[15] Older children do not have bowel flora in the periurethral area, but it has been reported that UTI is preceded by colonization of gram-negative uropathogens.[16] Some factors such as use of broad-spectrum antibiotic therapy and anatomical abnormalities increase the risk of bacterial colonization. Apart from the ascending route of infection where gut bacteria reach the urinary tract after traveling through the perineum, another route is hematogenous spread. The later route is chiefly reported in the neonatal period. Uropathogens that cause UTI in otherwise healthy children often possess specific properties to overcome the defense machinery of the host in the urinary tract. Since uropathogenic *E. coli* is the most common bacterium accounting for 80–90% infection, its pathogenesis has been studied in detail. In uropathogenic serotypes of *E. coli*, bacterial adhesion to uroepithelium is mediated by different types of fimbriae present on the surface of bacteria. These different fimbriae bind to different types of oligosaccharide receptors present on uroepithelium.[17-19] While S fimbriae bind to receptors on sialylated glycoproteins and glycolipids, type 1 fimbriae bind to glycoproteins such as secretory IgA. P fimbriae recognize Galα1-4Galβ epitopes in the glycolipids; this antigen is linked to the P blood group system. Expression of P fimbriae is closely related to the virulence of bacteria as reflected by the fact that almost 80% patients infected by such strain of *E. coli* develop acute pyelonephritis. Other virulence factors are lipopolysaccharide, capsular polysaccharide, hemolysins, and flagella-mediated motility. Glycosylated polysaccharide capsule of *E. coli* interferes with phagocytosis and complement-mediated damage; hence, it acts as a defensive mechanism. Aerobactin, a high-affinity iron-binding protein, is produced by most of the uropathogenic *E. coli* strain that causes acute pyelonephritis. Aerobactin supports the bacterial survival as it is able to compete with the host cell for micronutrient such as iron.[20] Strain of *E. coli* detected in children with asymptomatic bacteria usually lacks these virulence factors.

The uroepithelium is the first-line defense mechanism against uropathogens. The uroepithelium secretes inflammatory cytokines as well as protective glycoproteins such as uroplakin and uromodulin. Uroplakins are the important structural component of uroepithelium; hence, patients with deficiency of uroplakins are at increased risk of recurrent UTI as it compromises the uroepithelial permeability barrier.[21] Patients with recurrent UTI have been shown to have a lower urinary level of uromodulin.[22] Recent evidence suggests that uromodulin interacts with uropathogens and resulting uromodulin-pathogen complex prevents bacterial adhesion to glycoprotein on uroepithelium, hence promoting their clearance during micturition.[23,24] Response of host to UTI chiefly depends on the innate immune system more so during the acute phase. Immune response is triggered by activation of toll-like receptors (TLRs) through binding of P fimbriae to glycolipid receptors. TLR activation results in release of transcription factors which subsequently trigger production of cytokine and recruitment of the neutrophil to kill bacteria. The role of TLR is also highlighted by the fact that children with asymptomatic bacteriuria usually have lower TLR4 expression due to genetic variation. This inflammatory process and cytokine production lead to signs and symptoms of UTI. Interleukin-6 (IL-6) secreted by uroepithelium apart from acting as pyrogen also stimulates C-reactive protein production by liver as well as mucosal IgA production. Similarly, IL-8 increases neutrophil migration and activation at the site of infection.

DIAGNOSIS

Diagnosis of UTI is confirmed based on growth of uropathogen in urine culture in a patient with clinically suspected UTI. Other findings on urine examination such as leukocyturia and positive nitrite test are used as supportive evidence for UTI.

CLINICAL FEATURES

Symptoms and signs in childhood UTI are remarkably nonspecific, especially in infants. While fever is most common in children diagnosed with UTI, other clinical features vary depending on age. Infants younger than 3 months usually present with vague symptoms such as failure to thrive, lethargy, irritability, refusal to feed, sepsis, diarrhea, jaundice, oliguria, or polyuria. Foul-smelling urine can also be a symptom of UTI in younger children.[25] A combination of these clinical features is usually more useful than individual clinical finding.[26] In older children younger than 24 months, fever, vomiting, anorexia, and failure to thrive are the typical symptoms.[27] Abdominal pain, back pain, new-onset incontinence, dysuria, and frequency are more common in children older than 5 years. Adolescent girls usually manifest with typical clinical features suggestive of cystitis such as dysuria, urgency, frequency, cloudy urine, hematuria, and lower abdominal discomfort. Findings of physical examination can be nonspecific but should include examination of the sacral region for dimple, pits, or sacral fat pad, which are suggestive of neurogenic bladder. Abdominal palpation may reveal a mass secondary to enlarged kidney or tenderness in flank region.

URINALYSIS

Initial urinalysis is useful in making presumptive diagnosis of UTI and facilitates initiation of empirical antibiotic therapy. However, confirmation of diagnosis through urine culture is obligatory. The first step in urinalysis is to obtain an uncontaminated urine sample. Commonly employed techniques for urine collection in children are clean-catch, bag, bladder catheterization, and suprapubic aspiration. While clean-catch is the most commonly used method, invasiveness, contamination rates, and acceptability to parents vary across these four methods. Plastic bag specimens are easier to obtain but have unacceptably high contamination rates (26–88%) even with thorough perineal area cleaning; hence, they are not recommended. Similarly, pad and nappy specimens are also not recommended.[28] Among noninvasive methods, clean-catch has a lower rate of contamination (5–38%) and is most commonly employed in toilet-trained children. Studies have reported that bladder-stimulation technique such as finger tapping and cold saline may improve the urine-collection success rate in precontinent children.[29] Catheterization specimen is reliable provided that the initial few drops of urine are discarded. This method is used in nontoilet-trained children where collection of urine through clean-catch is not feasible. Catheterization is less invasive than suprapubic aspiration and has good diagnostic performance (sensitivity 95% and specificity 99%) when compared to specimen collected through suprapubic aspiration. Suprapubic aspiration is an invasive and painful procedure, considered the best method to avoid contamination of urine specimen. It can be performed inserting a 21-22-G needle, 1–2 cm above pubic symphysis, through the abdominal wall into the bladder. Using ultrasound guidance significantly improves the success rate of obtaining a urine specimen.[28] A large study reported a very low complication rate (0.22%) with suprapubic aspiration.[30] In children with indwelling catheter, the specimen should be collected using a sterile needle and syringe from catheter and collecting urine from bags should be avoided. The collected urine specimen should be transported to the laboratory as soon as possible; if not feasible, it can be stored in a refrigerator at 4°C for up to 72 hours before plating to avoid growth of contaminating pathogens.

Leukocyturia (five white cells/high-power field in centrifuged urine) is detected in almost 90% children with UTI. Presence of white cells in urine is not an obligatory criterion for diagnosis of UTI as a considerable proportion of children do not have leukocyturia. On the contrary, many children with fever and infection outside the urinary tract may have leukocyturia.[31,32] Hence, it cannot be used as a confirmatory test for UTI. Presence of white cell cast in children with suspected UTI is highly suggestive of acute pyelonephritis. Dipstick testing of urine for leukocyte esterase, an enzyme present in granules of neutrophils, is a surrogate marker for the presence of white cell. It is more accurate than microscopy in detecting the presence of white cells because enzyme activity is still retained despite disintegration of leukocytes.[33] Gram stain examination of urine for bacteria has better diagnostic performance (sensitivity—91%, specificity—96%) than leukocyturia and microscopic examination of unstained urine for bacteria.[34] Many gram-negative uropathogens convert urinary nitrate to nitrite by enzyme nitrate reductase which is detected by urine dipstick. Not all bacteria causing UTI produce nitrite and it requires urine to stay for some time in the bladder, hence leading to less accurate tests in infants who void very frequently. Due to these shortcomings, this test is not used in isolation for diagnosis of UTI despite having high specificity.[25] Thus, neither nitrite test nor leukocyte esterase is sensitive or specific enough to be used for diagnosis of UTI; however, it can be used as a screening test. Positivity of either leukocyte esterase or nitrite provides the best discriminatory value with sensitivity of 88% and specificity of 79% **(Table 1)**.

Growth of a single uropathogen in urine culture remains the gold standard for diagnosis of UTI in children. However, detection of bacteriuria is fraught with problems in children. First, contamination of specimen with vaginal and preputial flora is a significant problem.[35] Second, although most guidelines use a cutoff of 10^5 colony-forming unit (CFU)/mL for differentiating between contamination and infection, almost 20% children with UTI have lower colony counts than 10^5 CFU/mL.[36,37] Hence, using this single cutoff might underdiagnose UTI in many children. In clinical practice,

TABLE 1: Diagnostic accuracy of rapid and dipstick tests for urinary tract infection in children.

Parameters	*Sensitivity (95% CI)*	*Specificity (95% CI)*
Leukocyturia	74 (67–80)	86 (82–90)
Bacteria	88 (75–94)	92 (83–96)
Gram stain	91 (80–96)	96 (92–98)
Leukocyte esterase	79 (73–84)	87 (80–92)
Nitrite	49 (41–57)	98 (96–99)
Leukocyte esterase or nitrite	88 (82–91)	79 (69–87)
Leukocyte esterase and nitrite	45 (30–61)	98 (96–99)

(CI: confidence interval)

TABLE 2: Cutoff for a significant colony count in urine for diagnosis of UTI.

Method	*Indian Society of Pediatric Nephrology, 2011 (CFU/mL)*	*AAP, 2016*	*Italian Society of Pediatric Nephrology, 2020 (CFU/mL)*
Suprapubic aspiration	Any number	5×10^4	10^4
Catheter	$>5 \times 10^4$	5×10^4	10^4
Clean-catch	10^5	NR	5×10^4
Bag	NR	NR	10^5

(AAP: American Academy of Pediatrics; NR: not recommended; UTI: urinary tract infection)

one needs to keep in mind while discarding lower CFU as contamination that CFU quantification is a semiquantitative method and depends on a technician in a microbiology laboratory to differentiate 10 and 100 CFUs on an agar plate. Therefore, the clinician should also take into account clinical symptoms of the patient rather just relying on the colony count on urine culture. While most guidelines agree that any bacterial growth on a suprapubic specimen indicates UTI, for catheter specimen and clean catch, the colony count varies from 10^4 to 10^5 CFU/mL **(Table 2)**.[38-41]

OTHER INVESTIGATIONS

Other investigations in a child with UTI include blood urea, creatinine, and markers of inflammation such as leukocyte count, C-reactive protein, and procalcitonin. Some of these investigations are done with the aim to differentiate acute pyelonephritis from acute cystitis, as this would influence the route and duration of antimicrobial therapy. While the photopenic area on acute phase ^{99}Tc dimercaptosuccinic acid (DMSA) scan is considered as the reference standard for the diagnosis of acute pyelonephritis, it is used uncommonly due to high cost, inconvenience, and radiation exposure. A recent Cochrane review showed that an elevated procalcitonin (>0.5 ng/mL) level has better probability of detecting acute pyelonephritis with pooled sensitivity of 81% and specificity of 76%. On the other hand, a low C-reactive protein value (<20 mg/L) is useful in excluding acute pyelonephritis with sensitivity of 93% and specificity of 37%. However, these tests are not routinely recommended in clinical practice to differentiate acute pyelonephritis from acute cystitis.[42]

TREATMENT

The aim of therapy in children with UTI is to prevent renal scarring and associated complications. Delayed initiation of antimicrobial therapy in children with febrile UTI had been reported as one of the risk factors for the development of renal scarring. Delaying initiation of antibiotic beyond 48 hours or more increases the odds of kidney scarring.[43] Hence, antibiotic should be started promptly after collecting urine specimen for culture. The duration and route of antimicrobial therapy should be determined based on age, severity, clinical symptoms, and location of UTI. Since urine culture takes 24–48 hours before any growth of uropathogen is detected, hence the initial antibiotic should be selected based on the most common organism and its local susceptibility pattern.

TABLE 3: Antibiotics for empirical therapy in UTI.

Oral antibiotics	*Dose (mg/kg/day)*
Co-amoxiclav	30–40 of amoxicillin, in two divided doses
Cefixime	8–10, in two divided doses
Cefuroxime axetil	8–10, in two divided doses
Cephalexin	40–60, in two to three divided doses
Ciprofloxacin	10–20, in two divided doses
Ofloxacin	15–20, in two divided doses
Parenteral antibiotic	
Ceftriaxone	75–100, in one to two divided doses IV
Cefotaxime	100–150, in two to three divided doses IV
Amikacin	10–15, single dose IV, IM
Gentamicin	5–6, single dose IV, IM
Co-amoxiclav	60–100 of amoxicillin, in two divided doses IV

(IM: intramuscular; IV: intravenous; UTI: urinary tract infection)

Acute Pyelonephritis

Children with acute pyelonephritis are febrile and usually ill-appearing; hence, they should promptly be started on antimicrobial therapy after ensuring that urine for culture has been obtained. A Cochrane meta-analysis showed that the risk of kidney damage as assessed by DMSA 6–12 months after UTI did not differ between children treated with intravenous antibiotics for 3–4 days followed by oral antibiotic and those children treated with oral antibiotics for 10–14 days. In another meta-analysis, the risk of kidney scarring on DMSA scan 3–12 months after UTI was similar in children treated with intravenous antibiotic 3–4 days followed by oral antibiotic as compared to those treated with 7–14 days of oral antibiotic therapy. Hence, considering these findings, majority of children with acute pyelonephritis can be managed with oral antibiotic therapy.[44] Although observation from these studies are not applicable for some specific group of children including those with sepsis, young infants aged less than 3 months and children with poor oral intake. These latter groups of children, specifically neonates with acute pyelonephritis, should be hospitalized and initiated on intravenous antibiotic therapy for longer duration (10–14 days).[45] Children with community-acquired febrile UTI should receive broad-spectrum antibiotic therapy targeted against common uropathogens such as third-generation cephalosporin **(Table 3)**. These patients should preferably be initiated on a single broad-spectrum antibiotic. Few specific groups of children may need to be initiated on a broader spectrum of antibiotics including those with malformation of the urinary tract, immunocompromised, and hospital-acquired UTI. Children who are on low-dose antibiotic prophylaxis may have UTI caused by an organism resistant to that drug; hence, they should be started on a different antibiotic accordingly.

Acute Cystitis

Children with chiefly lower tract symptoms can be managed with a short course (3–5 days) of antibiotic therapy. Cystitis is mostly diagnosed in adolescents as it is difficult to differentiate acute pyelonephritis from acute cystitis in younger children. A Cochrane review meta-analyzed data from seven clinical trials comparing short course of antibiotic (2–4 days) to long course (7–10 days) did not find any difference in the bacteriological cure rate between the two groups.[46] When a single dose of antibiotic was compared with 10 days of oral antibiotic therapy, the former was less effective in bacterial clearance.[47]

Patients should be evaluated 48–72 hours after initiation of antibiotic therapy. If a patient's clinical features do not begin to improve within 72 hours, it might indicate failure of therapy. Treatment failure might occur due to poor compliance, incorrect diagnosis, multi-resistant organism, renal abscess, and malformation of the urinary tract. Routinely, a repeat urine culture to document response to therapy is not necessary and should be repeated only if the patient fails to respond to the therapy.

IMAGING FOLLOWING FIRST FEBRILE URINARY TRACT INFECTION

The basic rationale for evaluating a child following a febrile UTI is to identify malformation of the genitourinary tract that increases the risk of recurrent UTI and kidney scarring. Previous guideline used to recommend aggressive imaging following the first episode of UTI, but now the current understanding suggests that most children with complication either can be recognized on ultrasound scan or have recurrent UTI. Hence, recent guideline puts emphasis on less aggressive imaging following initial UTI. Ultrasound scan, voiding cystourethrogram (VCUG), and DMSA scan are the modalities commonly used to assess the structural and functional integrity of the urinary tract.[48]

Ultrasound Scan

Ultrasound scan of kidney, ureter, and bladder is noninvasive, relatively inexpensive, and appropriate first-line investigation with the limitation being investigator dependence. Ultrasound scan provides information on size and shape of kidneys as well as can identify dilated pelvis, ureter, ureterocele, and bladder thickness. Thus, it can provide a clue related to high-grade VUR or obstructive uropathy, if present. However, it is not a very sensitive investigation to detect low-grade VUR, acute pyelonephritis, or kidney scarring. An ultrasound scan should preferably be done after resolution of acute symptoms in order to avoid the false-positive findings due to acute inflammation. It can also identify complication of UTI such as renal abscess; hence, those children who failed to respond to antibiotic therapy within 72 hours of initiation should also undergo ultrasound scan.

Contrast-enhanced voiding urosonography (CeVUS) is a newer dynamic imaging modality for the urinary tract. CeVUS involves administration of contrast agent via transurethral catheter into the bladder. The main advantage of CeVUS is that it provides high-quality diagnostic images without exposing children to ionizing radiation.[49] A systematic review observed that CeVUS has excellent diagnostic accuracy for detection VUR as compared to VCUG.[50] However some drawbacks of CeVUS such as higher cost of contrast agent, high operator dependence, and lack of widespread availability prevent its routine use in clinical practice.

Voiding Cystourethrogram

In VCUG, the bladder is catheterized and radiopaque contrast material is filled and child is asked to void. This entire process is monitored under fluoroscopy; hence, any abnormality in bladder filling, emptying, and reflux into ureters can be identified. The sensitivity of VCUG can be increased by cyclic procedures, i.e., filling the bladder and having the child void two or more times. However, cyclic VCUG involves unacceptably high radiation burden. While VCUG is considered the gold standard for detecting and grading severity of VUR, it also exposes children to radiation and is an invasive procedure.

^{99}Tc Dimercaptosuccinic Acid Scintigraphy

^{99}Tc DMSA scan is a nuclear isotope uptake scan in which DMSA is injected intravenously. Renal cortical imaging with DMSA is sensitive and specific for the diagnosis of acute pyelonephritis. It is characterized by the photopenic area due to decreased tracer uptake in the area of cortical ischemia and acute tubular necrosis during UTI. Decrease uptake on DMSA scan can also be suggestive of kidney scarring. Early DMSA scan (within 2 weeks of UTI) is used for detection of acute pyelonephritis and late DMSA scan (≥4 months after UTI) is used for identification of kidney scarring. While DMSA is not widely available in resource-limited setting such as ours, it is also expensive, invasive, and associated with radiation exposure.

Various international guidelines[38,41,51] differ on recommendation related to the use of ultrasound scan following UTI **(Table 4)**. The American Academy of Pediatrics (AAP) guideline recommends routine ultrasound in all children aged less than 2 years while the National Institute for Health and Care Excellence (NICE) guideline recommends it in infants less than 6 months only. The guideline from the Indian Society of Pediatric Nephrology (ISPN) recommends ultrasound in every child following an episode of febrile UTI. While the AAP guideline advises performing VCUG only after second febrile UTI or if the initial ultrasound scan is abnormal, the NICE guideline recommends VCUG in infants with recurrent UTI or children up to 3 years of age with atypical UTI defined by sepsis, infection with an organism other than *E. coli*,

TABLE 4: Imaging protocols following first febrile UTI in various international guidelines.

	Ultrasound	***VCUG***	***DMSA scan***
Indian Society of Pediatric Nephrology, 2011	All	<1 year >1 year*	<5 years
American Academy of Pediatrics, 2016†	<2 years	<2 years‡	Not recommended
National Institute for Health and Care Excellence, 2017	<6 months	<3 years‡	1–7 years
Italian Society of Pediatric Nephrology, 2020	All	<3 years§	Only in VUR grade IV and V

Perform all (US, VCUG, and DMSA) if any of the above tests is abnormal.
*Only if abnormal ultrasound or DMSA.
†Recommendations for <2-year-old only.
‡Atypical or recurrent UTI.
§Only if abnormal ultrasound, atypical, or recurrent UTI.
(DMSA: dimercaptosuccinic acid; UTI: urinary tract infection; VCUG: voiding cystourethrogram)

and failure to respond to antibiotics within 48 hours. The ISPN guideline recommends VCUG in all children below 1 year and only if ultrasound or DMSA is abnormal in older children. All children with recurrent UTI should undergo VCUG irrespective of the age of the child. While AAP does not recommend routine use of late DMSA scan for detection of kidney scarring, the NICE guideline states that late DMSA (4–12 months after UTI) should be done in all children with recurrent UTI and following the first atypical UTI in children younger than 3 years. The ISPN guideline recommends DMSA in all children with recurrent UTI and after the first UTI in infants. For older children, DMSA following UTI is recommended only if they have abnormality on ultrasound. A suggested algorithm for imaging following febrile UTI in children is depicted in **Figure 1**. This approach is based on the fact that UTI is common in young children and majority of them do not have an abnormal urinary tract; hence, VCUG in every child would unnecessarily expose him/her to investigations without much benefit. VCUG may be considered in infants with atypical UTI younger than 6 months or if there is a suspicion of previous undiagnosed UTI.

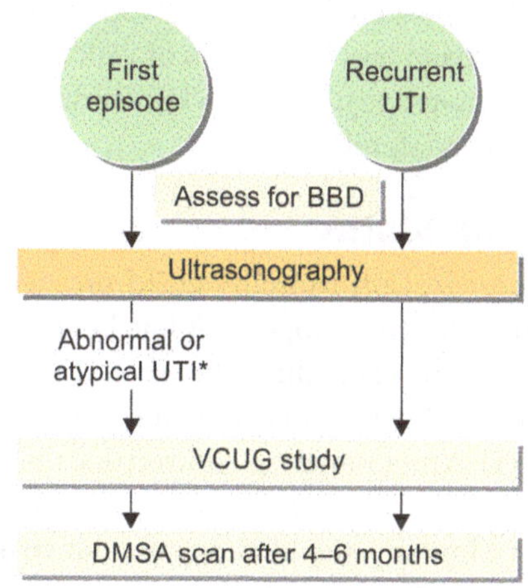

Fig. 1: Approach to imaging following febrile urinary tract infection (UTI).

***Atypical UTI:**
- Septicemia
- Poor urine flow, abdominal mass
- Raised creatinine
- No response within 48 hours
- Non-*E. coli* infection

RECURRENT URINARY TRACT INFECTION

Recurrent UTI is defined by occurrence of ≥2 discrete episodes of acute pyelonephritis or ≥3 episodes of acute cystitis.[51] Recurrence is observed in 10–30% children within 12 months following the first febrile UTI.[3,52] While *E. coli* is still the most common organism in recurrent UTI, recurrence is more frequent in children with index UTI caused by other organisms such as *Klebsiella*, *Proteus*, and *Enterococcus*. Similarly, recurrence is higher in children with index febrile UTI caused by drug-resistance uropathogens. Bladder–bowel dysfunction, VUR, circumcision status in boys, and young age are considered important risk factors for recurrence of UTI.[3,6,52,53] In adolescents, history about sexual exposure should be elicited to diagnose postcoital UTI.

Bladder-bowel Dysfunction

Bladder-bowel dysfunction is a broad term used to describe a wide spectrum of lower urinary tract symptoms accompanied by bowel dysfunction such as constipation or encopresis. Diagnosis of bladder-bowel dysfunction is made in children without any structural or neurological abnormalities. Screening for bladder-bowel dysfunction can be done easily through a questionnaire-based available tool.[54] Bladder-bowel dysfunction in most children can be detected based on history and physical examination and rarely requires invasive diagnostic studies such as urodynamics. Prevalence of bladder-bowel dysfunction is significantly higher in children presenting with UTI. A systematic review by authors showed that prevalence of bladder-bowel dysfunction ranges from 41 to 49% in patients with UTI and/or primary VUR.[6] Presence of bladder-bowel dysfunction in children with primary VUR increases the risk of UTI recurrence by twofold and also delays resolution of VUR. Most children with bladder-bowel dysfunction can be managed with urotherapy (frequent, double voiding) and aggressive treatment of constipation, and only a small proportion of patients require pharmacotherapy.

Primary Vesicoureteric Reflux

Vesicoureteric reflux is retrograde flow of urine from bladder to ureters. It increases urinary stasis; therefore, it increases risk of colonization with uropathogens. VUR also increases risk of infection to kidney parenchyma by allowing ascent of uropathogens. Presence of primary VUR, particularly high-grade VUR, is considered as an important risk factor for recurrence of UTI. Children with VUR have a 1.6-fold higher risk of recurrence of febrile UTI as compared to those without VUR.[3] Primary VUR is detected in almost 30% children with first febrile UTI. Presence of primary also associates with kidney scarring. In most cases, it is just merely associated with congenital dysplasia but only a small proportion of cases develop post-UTI kidney scars in children with primary VUR.[25] Primary VUR in most children resolves spontaneously years after the initial diagnosis. Resolution of VUR is much rapid in children with low-grade unilateral VUR as compared to those with high-grade bilateral VUR.

Circumcision Status

Urinary tract infection in many children is preceded by colonization with uropathogens. It has been reported that uropathogens accumulate under the prepuce and in urethra of uncircumcised boys; hence, they are at increased risk of developing UTI. A meta-analysis showed that the risk of UTI is 10-fold higher in uncircumcised infants as compared to their counterparts. Similarly, the lifetime cumulative incidence of UTI is significantly higher in uncircumcised males (32%) than circumcised males (8.8%).

PREVENTION OF RECURRENCE OF URINARY TRACT INFECTION

Low-dose Antibiotic Prophylaxis

The previous guideline by ISPN in 2011 recommends antibiotic prophylaxis for prevention of recurrence of UTI in children with recurrent UTI and normal urinary tract. Since then, emergence of newer scientific literature showed that antibiotic prophylaxis may not be a useful strategy for prevention of febrile UTI as it also increases the risk of antimicrobial resistance. A recent Cochrane review showed that low-dose antibiotic prophylaxis has little or no effect on prevention of repeat UTI when compared with placebo or no treatment.[55] Long-term, low-dose antibiotic prophylaxis increases the risk of UTI with organism resistance to prophylactic drug by 2.4 times. Considering the evidence, it can be concluded that antibiotic prophylaxis should not be used for prevention of UTI in children with a normal urinary tract. However, low-dose antibiotic prophylaxis may be beneficial in children with primary VUR as observed in two large clinical trials.[56,57] However, a study from India showed contradictory findings that antibiotic prophylaxis may even increase the risk of UTI recurrence.[58] Findings from a meta-analysis in patients with primary VUR showed that antibiotic prophylaxis has doubtful efficacy in preventing repeat UTI.[59] However, reduction in risk of repeat UTI was more significant in children with high-grade VUR as compared to those with low-grade VUR. Considering the fact that patients with high-grade VUR are at a higher risk of recurrence of UTI, antibiotic prophylaxis can be beneficial for this cohort of children. A cost-effective analysis of a previous clinical trial also found that antibiotic prophylaxis is cost effective only in children with high-grade VUR (III–IV).[60] Antibiotics with narrow spectrum such as nitrofurantoin and co-trimoxazole are commonly used for long-term prophylaxis. These antibiotics are relatively cheap and do not alter gut microflora. While cotrimoxazole is less efficacious than nitrofurantoin in preventing repeat UTI compliance to therapy is poor to later due to its gastrointestinal side effects. A large randomized trial observed that most of the repeat UTIs develop within 6 month of index febrile UTI.[56] While there is dearth of studies evaluating the duration of antibiotic prophylaxis, most observation studies suggest that it can be discontinued in children who are toilet trained and did not have febrile UTI in last 12 months.

Circumcision

Circumcised boys are at a significantly lower risk of developing UTI as compared to their counterparts. While the risk of developing UTI in healthy uncircumcised boys is ~1–2% and the rate of complication following circumcision is that of 0.3–0.5%, it can be as high as 1.5–2%.[61] Complication rates also depend on the person performing the circumcision and age of the child. Since the UTI recurrence rate (10–15%) is significantly higher in children at risk of UTI recurrence such as those with primary VUR, hence they outweigh the complications associated with circumcision. Based on this evidence, it can be suggested that circumcision may be beneficial for children who are at risk of developing UTI recurrence.

Nonantibiotic Prophylactic Interventions

As concerns related to safety (antimicrobial resistance) and efficacy of antibiotic prophylaxis for preventing repeat UTI are growing, the clinician and researcher have explored some of the nonantibiotic intervention such as cranberry and probiotics. While cranberry prevents bacterial adhesion to uroepithelium, probiotic prevents bacterial colonization, thus reducing the risk of UTI recurrence.[62] Proanthocyanidins are the chief antiadhesive agent present in cranberry and they act by inhibiting P-fimbriae-mediated attachment of uropathogenic *E. coli* to uroepithelium. A minimum of 36–72 mg of proanthocyanidins need to be ingested to achieve an adequate concentration in the urinary tract in order to prevent bacterial adhesion.[63,64] There is relative paucity of pediatrics literature on cranberry products for preventing UTI recurrence. While the cranberry extract is effective in reducing the risk of recurrence in children with a normal urinary tract, its efficacy is not proven in those with an abnormal urinary tract. Two small clinical trials found promising results with probiotic therapy but its efficacy is still doubtful; hence, it cannot be recommended for use in clinical practice.[65,66] While there is an ongoing effort to develop vaccine to prevent repeat febrile UTI, no vaccines have been evaluated in children till date. However, two vaccines Urovac® and Uro-Vaxom® had shown promising results in preventing recurrence of UTI in adult population.[67]

LONG-TERM CONSEQUENCES

Most of the children with acute pyelonephritis do not develop long-term sequalae. Risk of developing ESKD in a child with UTI is very low; 1 ESKD in 10,000 children with UTI. This is also supported by the findings that incidence of ESKD attributed to reflux nephropathy has not altered despite the intervention for reducing the risk of UTI in children.[68,69] Kidney scarring associated with UTI is of two types. Small focal defects can develop following UTI and is referred to as post-UTI scarring. The other form of renal damage is generalized impairment of kidney function with small kidney size, also known as congenital kidney dysplasia. A systematic review found that 18% [95% confidence interval (CI): 14–23%] children develop kidney scarring following' the first UTI.[70] Earlier studies reported kidney scarring in higher proportion of patients as compared to latter. As the physician's understanding about prompt initiation of antibiotic is improving, the incidence of focal post-UTI scarring may decrease. A study from United Kingdom showed that the children treated in 2000s were less likely to develop post-UTI scars as compared to those managed in 1990s.[71]

Systematic reviews of cohort studies reported that <0.4% children develop CKD or end-stage kidney damage or hypertension on long-term following UTI in children without kidney damage at presentation.[72,73] A study investigated 193 young people from a cohort of 1,161 children evaluated for their first febrile UTI. These patients were followed up and those with obstruction and congenital dysplasia were excluded. After 6–17 years, 15% children who underwent ultrasound had kidney damage or reduced kidney size but estimated glomerular filtration rate (eGFR) and blood pressure were within the normal range for all the patients.[74]

CONCLUSION

Urinary tract infection, a common bacterial infection in children, requires a high index of clinical suspicion. The diagnosis should be confirmed by culture of an appropriately collected urine sample. Timely initiation of sensitive antibiotics is recommended. Imaging of the urinary tract is necessary in high-risk groups to identify urinary tract malformation, which may increase the risk of scarring and recurrent infections.

KEY POINTS

- The significance of UTI lies in its risk for recurrence and morbidity associated with an acute febrile illness.
- Malformations of the urinary tract and bowel bladder dysfunction are risk factors for recurrent UTI.
- The newer guidelines recommend a more conservative approach to imaging of the urinary tract, reserving invasive procedures only to high-risk groups.
- The long-term consequences of UTI such as CKD and hypertension are uncommon.

REFERENCES

1. Shaikh N, Morone NE, Bost JE, Farrell MH. Prevalence of urinary tract infection in childhood: a meta-analysis. Pediatr Infect Dis J. 2008;27(4):302-8.
2. Zorc JJ, Levine DA, Platt SL, Dayan PS, Macias CG, Krief W, et al. Clinical and demographic factors associated with urinary tract infection in young febrile infants. Pediatrics. 2005;116(3):644-8.
3. Keren R, Shaikh N, Pohl H, Gravens-Mueller L, Ivanova A, Zaoutis L, et al. Risk factors for recurrent urinary tract infection and renal scarring. Pediatrics. 2015;136(1):e13-21.
4. Craig JC, Williams GJ, Jones M, Codarini M, Macaskill P, Hayen A, et al. The accuracy of clinical symptoms and signs for the diagnosis of serious bacterial infection in young febrile children: prospective cohort study of 15 781 febrile illnesses. BMJ. 2010;340:c1594.
5. Conway PH, Cnaan A, Zaoutis T, Henry BV, Grundmeier RW, Keren R. Recurrent urinary tract infections in children: risk factors and association with prophylactic antimicrobials. JAMA. 2007;298(2):179.
6. Meena J, Mathew G, Hari P, Sinha A, Bagga A. Prevalence of bladder and bowel dysfunction in toilet-trained children with urinary tract infection and/or primary vesicoureteral reflux: a systematic review and meta-analysis. Front Pediatr. 2020;8:84.
7. Sorlózano-Puerto A, Gómez-Luque JM, Luna-Del-Castillo J de D, Navarro-Marí JM, Gutiérrez-Fernández J. Etiological and resistance profile of bacteria involved in urinary tract infections in young children. Bio Med Res Int. 2017;2017:4909452.
8. Badhan R, Singh DV, Badhan LR, Kaur A. Evaluation of bacteriological profile and antibiotic sensitivity patterns in children with urinary tract infection: A prospective study from a tertiary care center. Indian J Urol Soc India. 2016;32(1):50-6.
9. Shrestha LB, Baral R, Poudel P, Khanal B. Clinical, etiological and antimicrobial susceptibility profile of pediatric urinary tract infections in a tertiary care hospital of Nepal. BMC Pediatr. 2019;19(1):36.
10. Tullus K. Vesicoureteric reflux in children. Lancet. 2015; 385(9965):371-9. doi: 10.1016/S0140-6736(14)60383-4. Epub 2014 Aug 24. PMID: 25164069.
11. Edlin RS, Shapiro DJ, Hersh AL, Copp HL. Antibiotic resistance patterns of outpatient pediatric urinary tract infections. J Urol. 2013;190(1):222-7.
12. Phillips JR, Karlowicz MG. Prevalence of *Candida* species in hospital-acquired urinary tract infections in a neonatal intensive care unit. Pediatr Infect Dis J. 1997;16(2):190-4.
13. Cox CE, Hinman F. Experiments with induced bacteriuria, vesical emptying and bacterial growth on the mechanism of bladder defense to infection. J Urol. 1961;86:739-48.
14. Sobel JD. Pathogenesis of urinary tract infection. Role of host defenses. Infect Dis Clin North Am. 1997;11(3):531-49.

15. Bollgren I, Winberg J. The periurethral aerobic flora in girls highly susceptible to urinary infections. Acta Paediatr Scand. 1976;65(1):81-7.
16. Hansson S, Jodal U, Norén L, Bjure J. Untreated bacteriuria in asymptomatic girls with renal scarring. Pediatrics. 1989;84(6):964-8.
17. Johnson JR. Microbial virulence determinants and the pathogenesis of urinary tract infection. Infect Dis Clin North Am. 2003;17(2):261-78, viii.
18. Bower JM, Eto DS, Mulvey MA. Covert operations of uropathogenic *Escherichia coli* within the urinary tract. Traffic Cph Den. 2005;6(1):18-31.
19. Wullt B, Bergsten G, Connell H, Röllano P, Gebretsadik N, Hull R, et al. P fimbriae enhance the early establishment of Escherichia coli in the human urinary tract. Mol Microbiol. 2000;38(3):456-64.
20. Russo TA, Carlino UB, Johnson JR. Identification of a new iron-regulated virulence gene, ireA, in an extraintestinal pathogenic isolate of *Escherichia coli*. Infect Immun. 2001;69(10):6209-16.
21. Wu X-R, Kong X-P, Pellicer A, Kreibich G, Sun T-T. Uroplakins in urothelial biology, function, and disease. Kidney Int. 2009;75(11):1153-65.
22. Garimella PS, Bartz TM, Ix JH, Chonchol M, Shlipak MG, Devarajan P, et al. Urinary uromodulin and risk of urinary tract infections: the cardiovascular health study. Am J Kidney Dis Off J Natl Kidney Found. 2017;69(6):744-51.
23. Weiss GL, Stanisich JJ, Sauer MM, Lin C-W, Eras J, Zyla DS, et al. Architecture and function of human uromodulin filaments in urinary tract infections. Science. 2020;369(6506):1005-10.
24. Devuyst O, Olinger E, Rampoldi L. Uromodulin: from physiology to rare and complex kidney disorders. Nat Rev Nephrol. 2017;13(9):525-44.
25. Tullus K, Shaikh N. Urinary tract infections in children. Lancet Lond Engl. 2020;395(10237):1659-68.
26. Shaikh N, Morone NE, Lopez J, Chianese J, Sangvai S, D'Amico F, et al. Does this child have a urinary tract infection? JAMA. 2007;298(24):2895-904.
27. Smellie JM, Hodson CJ, Edwards D, Normand IC. Clinical and radiological features of urinary infection in childhood. Br Med J. 1964;2(5419):1222-6.
28. Diviney J, Jaswon MS. Urine collection methods and dipstick testing in non-toilet-trained children. Pediatr Nephrol. 2021;36(7):1697-1708.
29. Chandy M, Dewey A, Fogg C, Pilkington K. Non-invasive techniques for stimulating urine production in non-toilet trained children: a systematic review. Emerg Med J. 2020;37(3):162-9.
30. Hildebrand WL, Schreiner RL, Stevens DC, Gosling CG, Sternecker CL. Suprapubic bladder aspiration in infants. Am Fam Physician. 1981;23(5):115-8.
31. Shaikh N, Shope TR, Hoberman A, Vigliotti A, Kurs-Lasky M, Martin JM. Association between uropathogen and pyuria. Pediatrics. 2016;138(1):e20160087.
32. Turner GM, Coulthard MG. Fever can cause pyuria in children. BMJ. 1995;311(7010):924.
33. Williams GJ, Macaskill P, Chan SF, Turner RM, Hodson E, Craig JC. Absolute and relative accuracy of rapid urine tests for urinary tract infection in children: a meta-analysis. Lancet Infect Dis. 2010;10(4):240-50.
34. Boon HA, Struyf T, Bullens D, Van den Bruel A, Verbakel JY. Diagnostic value of biomarkers for paediatric urinary tract infections in primary care: systematic review and meta-analysis. BMC Fam Pract. 2021;22(1):193.
35. Tullus K, Hooman N, Easty M. Flushing of the vagina and the prepuce-a cause for contaminated urine cultures in children. Pediatr Nephrol Berl Ger. 2017;32(1):107-11.
36. Swerkersson S, Jodal U, Åhrén C, Sixt R, Stokland E, Hansson S. Urinary tract infection in infants: the significance of low bacterial count. Pediatr Nephrol Berl Ger. 2016;31(2):239-45.
37. Roberts KB, Wald ER. The diagnosis of UTI: Colony count criteria revisited. Pediatrics. 2018;141(2):e20173239.
38. Indian Society of Pediatric Nephrology, Vijayakumar M, Kanitkar M, Nammalwar BR, Bagga A. Revised statement on management of urinary tract infections. Indian Pediatr. 2011;48(9):709-17.
39. Ammenti A, Alberici I, Brugnara M, Chimenz R, Guarino S, La Manna A, et al. Updated Italian recommendations for the diagnosis, treatment and follow-up of the first febrile urinary tract infection in young children. Acta Paediatr Oslo Nor 1992. 2020;109(2):236-47.
40. 't Hoen LA, Bogaert G, Radmayr C, Dogan HS, Nijman RJM, Quaedackers J, et al. Update of the EAU/ESPU guidelines on urinary tract infections in children. J Pediatr Urol. 2021;17(2):200-7.
41. AAP Subcommittee on Urinary Tract Infection. Reaffirmation of AAP Clinical Practice Guideline: The diagnosis and management of the initial urinary tract infection in febrile infants and young children 2–24 months of age. Pediatrics. 2016;138(6):e20163026.
42. Shaikh KJ, Osio VA, Leeflang MM, Shaikh N. Procalcitonin, C-reactive protein, and erythrocyte sedimentation rate for the diagnosis of acute pyelonephritis in children. Cochrane Database Syst Rev. 2020;9:CD009185.
43. Shaikh N, Mattoo TK, Keren R, Ivanova A, Cui G, Moxey-Mims M, et al. Early antibiotic treatment for pediatric febrile urinary tract infection and renal scarring. JAMA Pediatr. 2016;170(9):848-54.
44. Strohmeier Y, Hodson EM, Willis NS, Webster AC, Craig JC. Antibiotics for acute pyelonephritis in children. Cochrane Database Syst Rev. 2014;(7):CD003772.
45. Shaikh N, Craig JC, Rovers MM, Da Dalt L, Gardikis S, Hoberman A, et al. Identification of children and adolescents at risk for renal scarring after a first urinary tract infection: a meta-analysis with individual patient data. JAMA Pediatr. 2014;168(10):893-900.
46. Michael M, Hodson EM, Craig JC, Martin S, Moyer VA. Short versus standard duration oral antibiotic therapy for acute urinary tract infection in children. Cochrane Database Syst Rev. 2003;(1):CD003966.
47. Fitzgerald A, Mori R, Lakhanpaul M, Tullus K. Antibiotics for treating lower urinary tract infection in children. Cochrane Database Syst Rev. 2012;(8):CD006857.
48. Kaufman J, Temple-Smith M, Sanci L. Urinary tract infections in children: an overview of diagnosis and management. BMJ Paediatr Open [Internet]. 2019;3:e000487.
49. Duran C, Beltrán VP, González A, Gómez C, Riego JD. Contrast-enhanced voiding urosonography for vesicoureteral reflux diagnosis in children. Radiogr Rev Publ Radiol Soc N Am Inc. 2017;37(6):1854-69.
50. Chua ME, Kim JK, Mendoza JS, Fernandez N, Ming JM, Marson A, et al. The evaluation of vesicoureteral reflux among children using contrast-enhanced ultrasound: a literature review. J Pediatr Urol. 2019;15(1):12-7.
51. National Institute for Health and Care Excellence. (2018). Urinary tract infection (recurrent): antimicrobial prescribing. [online] Available from https://www.nice.org.uk/guidance/

ng112/resources/urinary-tract-infection-recurrent-antimicrobial-prescribing-pdf-66141595059397#%5B%7B%22num%22%3A24%2C%22gen%22%3A0%7D%2C%7B%22name%22%3A%22XYZ%22%7D%2C0%2C770%2C0%5D. [Last accessed May, 2022]
52. Shaikh N, Hoberman A, Keren R, Gotman N, Docimo S, Mathews R, et al. Recurrent urinary tract infections in children with bladder and bowel dysfunction. Pediatrics. 2016;137(1): e20152982.
53. Morris BJ, Wiswell TE. Circumcision and lifetime risk of urinary tract infection: a systematic review and meta-analysis. J Urol. 2013;189(6):2118-24.
54. Farhat W, Bägli DJ, Capolicchio G, O'Reilly S, Merguerian PA, Khoury A, et al. The dysfunctional voiding scoring system: quantitative standardization of dysfunctional voiding symptoms in children. J Urol. 2000;164(3 Pt 2):1011-5.
55. Williams G, Craig JC. Long-term antibiotics for preventing recurrent urinary tract infection in children. Cochrane Database Syst Rev. 2019;(4):CD001534.
56. Craig JC, Simpson JM, Williams GJ, Lowe A, Reynolds GJ, McTaggart SJ, et al. Antibiotic prophylaxis and recurrent urinary tract infection in children. N Engl J Med. 2009;361(18):1748-59.
57. RIVUR Trial Investigators, Hoberman A, Greenfield SP, Mattoo TK, Keren R, Mathews R, et al. Antimicrobial prophylaxis for children with vesicoureteral reflux. N Engl J Med. 2014;370(25): 2367-76.
58. Hari P, Hari S, Sinha A, Kumar R, Kapil A, Pandey RM, et al. Antibiotic prophylaxis in the management of vesicoureteric reflux: a randomized double-blind placebo-controlled trial. Pediatr Nephrol Berl Ger. 2015;30(3):479-86.
59. Williams G, Hodson EM, Craig JC. Interventions for primary vesicoureteric reflux. Cochrane Database Syst Rev. 2019;(2): CD001532.
60. Shaikh N, Rajakumar V, Peterson CG, Gorski J, Ivanova A, Gravens Muller L, et al. Cost-utility of antimicrobial prophylaxis for treatment of children with vesicoureteral reflux. Front Pediatr. 2019;7:530.
61. Weiss HA, Larke N, Halperin D, Schenker I. Complications of circumcision in male neonates, infants and children: a systematic review. BMC Urol. 2010;10:2.
62. Tewary K, Narchi H. Recurrent urinary tract infections in children: Preventive interventions other than prophylactic antibiotics. World J Methodol. 2015;5(2):13-9.
63. Goldman RD. Cranberry juice for urinary tract infection in children. Can Fam Physician Med Fam Can. 2012;58(4):398-401.
64. Howell AB, Botto H, Combescure C, Blanc-Potard A-B, Gausa L, Matsumoto T, et al. Dosage effect on uropathogenic *Escherichia coli* anti-adhesion activity in urine following consumption of cranberry powder standardized for proanthocyanidin content: a multicentric randomized double blind study. BMC Infect Dis. 2010;10:94.
65. Sadeghi-Bojd S, Naghshizadian R, Mazaheri M, Ghane Sharbaf F, Assadi F. Efficacy of probiotic prophylaxis after the first febrile urinary tract infection in children with normal urinary tracts. J Pediatr Infect Dis Soc. 2020;9(3):305-10.
66. Lee SJ, Lee JW. Probiotics prophylaxis in infants with primary vesicoureteral reflux. Pediatr Nephrol Berl Ger. 2015;30(4): 609-13.
67. Meena J, Thomas CC, Kumar J, Raut S, Hari P. Non-antibiotic interventions for prevention of urinary tract infections in children: a systematic review and meta-analysis of randomized controlled trials. Eur J Pediatr. 2021;180(12):3535-45.
68. Craig JC, Williams GJ. Denominators do matter: it's a myth—urinary tract infection does not cause chronic kidney disease. Pediatrics. 2011;128(5):984-5. doi: 10.1542/peds.2011-2631.
69. Craig JC, Irwig LM, Knight JF, Roy LP. Does treatment of vesicoureteric reflux in childhood prevent end-stage renal disease attributable to reflux nephropathy? Pediatrics. 2000; 105(6):1236-41.
70. Shaikh N. Acute urinary tract infection in infants and young children. CMAJ Can Med Assoc J Assoc Medicale Can. 2010; 182(8):800-1.
71. Coulthard MG, Lambert HJ, Vernon SJ, Hunter EW, Keir MJ, Matthews JNS. Does prompt treatment of urinary tract infection in preschool children prevent renal scarring: mixed retrospective and prospective audits. Arch Dis Child. 2014; 99(4):342-7.
72. Salo J, Ikäheimo R, Tapiainen T, Uhari M. Childhood urinary tract infections as a cause of chronic kidney disease. Pediatrics. 2011;128(5):840-7.
73. Toffolo A, Ammenti A, Montini G. Long-term clinical consequences of urinary tract infections during childhood: a review. Acta Paediatr Oslo Nor 1992. 2012;101(10):1018-31.
74. Hannula A, Perhomaa M, Venhola M, Pokka T, Renko M, Uhari M. Long-term follow-up of patients after childhood urinary tract infection. Arch Pediatr Adolesc Med. 2012;166(12):1117-22.

CHAPTER

13.5

Vesicoureteric Reflux

Beena SV

INTRODUCTION

Vesicoureteric reflux (VUR), defined as retrograde flow of urine from the bladder into the ureters and upper urinary tract, is a common clinical entity. Affecting up to 30% of all children with a urinary tract infection (UTI) and 17% without UTI,[1] VUR has also been detected following investigation for hypertension, proteinuria, voiding dysfunction, and chronic renal insufficiency. Male to female prevalence ratio of VUR can be as high as 3:1 at 0–6 months of age but shifts to approximately 1:1 by 21–24 months.[2] The introduction of endoscopic management with injectable biodegradable crosslinked polysaccharide dextranomer and stabilized hyaluronic acid, reexamination of the need for continuous antibiotic prophylaxis (CAP), and management of bowel-bladder dysfunction (BBD) all have initiated an introception of virtually all aspects of reflux.

ETIOLOGY AND PATHOLOGY

Anatomy of Antireflux Mechanism

The primary defense mechanism for VUR prevention is the neuromuscular peristaltic activity of the ureter which acts as a dynamic conduit for onward propulsion of urine. The anatomic design of vesicoureteric junction (VUJ) is the second key defense mechanism in reflux prevention. The intramural ureter that travels within the detrusor muscle is the main component of this unique mechanism.[3] At the extravesical bladder hiatus, the muscle layers of the ureter separate. The outer muscle layer merges with the outer detrusor muscle to form Waldeyer's sheath, which contributes to the formation of deep trigone. The inner muscle layer contributes to the formation of the superficial trigone. The intramural ureter due to its oblique course remains passively compressed by the layers of the bladder wall during bladder filling, preventing urine from entering the ureter. Paquin's early dissections of the VUJ in children revealed that in nonrefluxing junctions approximately 5:1 ratio of tunnel length to ureteral diameter is seen while in refluxing junctions it is only in the range of 1.4:1.[4] Opening of VUJ is achieved by active contraction of longitudinal muscles within the tunnel which draws the inner meatal opening outward and the outer hiatal opening inward shortening and widening the tunnel and allows passage of urine bolus into the bladder. Configuration of ureteric orifice (UO) is also important just like the intramural ureter length[5] in determining VUJ competence. The orifice configuration, tunnel length, ureteral collapsing pressures, and their relation with reflux all have been extensively studied by computer modeling.[6] The neurophysiologic studies of VUJ have pointed that there are fine afferent and efferent neuromuscular coordinations that take place between VUJ and periureteric bladder wall.[7] The architectural and anatomical deficiency of tunnel length and abnormalities in smooth muscle, extracellular matrix, and neural composition of VUJ all contribute in different ways to promote reflux.[6,8]

CAUSES OF VESICOURETERIC REFLUX

Primary Reflux

Here, reflux occurs due to an inherent abnormality in the structure and function of VUJ in spite of a low pressure storage of urine. Here intramural ureteral tunnel length as well as the ratio of tunnel length and ureteric diameter is always seen abnormal[4] **(Fig. 1)**.

Secondary Reflux

Here, bladder pathology creates a hostile environment, which overpowers a normal antireflux mechanism. Such pathologies can be secondary to increased bladder pressure or bladder

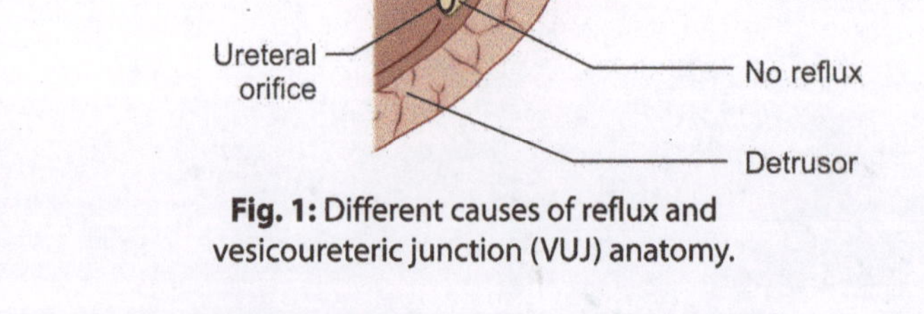

Fig. 1: Different causes of reflux and vesicoureteric junction (VUJ) anatomy.

outlet pressure. Increased bladder pressure could be due to anatomical causes in outlet or functional causes in outlet. The most common cause for anatomical abnormality in boys causing reflux is posterior urethral valve (PUV). Reflux is present in 48–70% of patients with PUV.[9-11] Adequate valve ablation and relief of obstruction are known to effectively bring down reflux in 3–6 months' time.[11] The initial report of McGuire et al.[12] suggested that pressures in excess of 40 cm of water measured at full capacity are associated with reflux and upper tract deterioration. Treatments to maintain pressures below this value resulted in significant reflux resolution.

In girls, anatomical bladder neck obstruction is rare. Among these a prolapsing ureterocele, which causes bladder neck obstruction and reflux in the contralateral orifice due to pressure effect, tops the list. Here also reflux subsides with relief of obstruction. Generally if relief of the obstruction results in rapid reflux resolution, the reflux was likely secondary.

Neurogenic bladder associated with spina bifida or occult spinal dysraphism is a common cause for elevated bladder pressure of neurofunctional etiology.[13] The features of occult spinal dysraphism such as sacral dimple or hairy patch, gluteal cleft abnormality, diminished rectal tone, significant constipation, or encopresis should be carefully looked for in any child with a neurogenic bladder.

Secondary reflux could be due to raised bladder pressures. In male infants, urodynamic evaluations have shown that there is elevated bladder pressure and high voiding pressure due to inadequate sphincter relaxation.[14] Uninhibited detrusor activity has also been observed, again predominantly in male infants.[15] VUR resolution has been achieved in such dysfunctional voiders by timed voiding, biofeedback, anticholinergics, and alpha-blockers.[16]

Bowel–bladder dysfunction is a behavioral abnormality which presents as VUR in the older child. Although the precise cause is not known, it is said to evolve during toilet-training months by volitional contraction of external sphincter to overcome the detrusor contractions.[17] Once this behavior becomes intensified, bladder pressure increases and continence is achieved by incomplete emptying resulting in secondary reflux and higher UTI risk. The American Urological Association (AUA) panel on VUR guidelines now suggests that BBD is by far one of the most critical and modifiable variables that affect VUR management and attendant UTIs.[18] An older child presenting with VUR should be carefully evaluated for symptoms of dribbling, urgency, incontinence, curtsying behavior in girls, and squeezing the penis in boys in an attempt to suppress bladder contractions. The frequent association of constipation and encopresis with reflux and UTI is often ascribed to the close proximity of the bladder and anal outlets which leads to sympathetic contraction of the anal sphincter.[19-22] Thus, treatment of constipation forms an integral part of reflux management.

Multiple studies have documented a significant risk of VUR in family members of patients with reflux. The reported risk of sibling reflux ranges from 27 to 34%,[23] while as many as 66% of the offspring of women with reflux also have VUR. Because of these studies, it has been suggested that siblings, especially those below 2 years, should be screened for an associated reflux.

PATHOGENESIS AND CLINICAL MANIFESTATIONS

Reflux paves way for a hydrodynamic mechanism that facilitates the ascent of microorganisms from the bladder to the kidneys. It may be considered that reflux accelerates renal tissue infection, following bacterial colonization of the bladder.[24] The frequency of scarring itself appears to be directly proportional to the grade of reflux with which it is associated.[25,26] In children with reflux-associated hydroureter and hydronephrosis, the dilated system acts as a reservoir for pathogenic organisms from the bladder, where they colonize and retrograde recycling occurs and sterilizing the urinary tract may prove difficult in such cases.[27] Similarly, ureteral atony secondary to the presence of endotoxin adds to the stasis and aggravates the condition.[28]

Scarring is always a consequence of injury and its subsequent healing and in kidney it indicates fibrous contracted regions that have been destroyed by infection. Areas of scar tissue appear hyperechoic and shrunken in sonography and are seen as photopenic areas in scintigraphy. Scarring should be differentiated from congenital dysplasia/ dysmorphism, which is a nonpreventable developmental sequela of the urinary tract.[29]

Renal dysplasia is associated with reflux [VURD (valves, unilateral reflux, and renal dysplasia)]. The association of renal maldevelopment with high grades of reflux is described by the theory of Mackie and Stephens,[30] which suggests that a suboptimal interaction of an abnormally originating ureteric bud with the metanephric blastema leads to a dysplastic kidney. Dysplastic kidneys are usually seen in male infants and reflux is usually of grade 4 or 5.[31] Several studies have confirmed the association between high-grade VUR and a smaller than normal ipsilateral kidney, an overall reduced relative renal function, and global[32,33] or focal[34] areas of poor uptake by scintigraphy. Boys are usually spared reflux-associated acquired renal scarring as compared to dysplastic scarring.[2]

Factors affecting scarring are as follows:

- *Age:* The risk of postpyelonephritic scarring decreases with increasing age of the child. This is a factor of prime importance in reflux diagnosis and choice of therapy. Patients younger than 4 years are more prone to developing scarring after a single UTI than older children,[35] though scarring may still occur beyond 5 years of age.[35,36] But the greatest risk for postinfectious renal scarring is during the first year of life[2,37] (Big Bang Theory by Ransley and Risdon[38]), though there are suggestions against it.

- *Papillary anatomy:* The configuration of the renal papillae and the alignment of ductal opening are other factors which decide renal scarring. Compound papillae have a concave architecture and have their ducts at right angles, whereas more convex simple papillae possess ducts that end obliquely, producing a valvular effect that guards against backflow of urine into the medullary collecting ducts (**Fig. 2**). Compound papillae are preferentially seen in both renal poles compared to the middle region. The former are more commonly the site of intrarenal reflux (reflux into the ducts) and are the prime regions of susceptibility for scarring. It has also been shown that reflux into compound papillae occurs at lower pressures (with as little as 2 mm Hg pressure in neonates) than into simple papillae. In an infant, this pressure required is increased 10-fold and helps to explain the relative infrequency of intrarenal reflux in older children.[39]
- *Bacterial virulence:* Pathogenic virulent bacteria have the ability to adhere to uroepithelium and are mediated by interaction between specific molecules or ligands located on bacterial fimbriae and specific receptors on host uroepithelial cells. Bacterial response to facilitate their survival and proliferation, as well as to inhibit host defenses, is by release of endotoxin and reduction of ureteral peristalsis, which may further reduce antegrade flow of urine and aggravate stasis.
- *Host susceptibility and response:* Periurethral organisms and vaginal organisms are the ones which access the urinary tract nonhematogenously. Thus, the type and number of these will determine individual propensity for bladder colonization. The great majority of UTIs in both sexes younger than 6 months old is confined to uncircumcised boys[40] and is consistent with the observation that *Escherichia coli* colonization is dense in infant boys but sparse in girls.[41] Local factors such as hygiene and bowel habits will also influence the bacterial load presented to the perineal surface from the intestinal tract. All factors put together, the greatest risk factor in promoting UTI susceptibility is urinary dwell time. The postvoid urine volume has traditionally been considered as providing sanctuary for ascending urethral organisms. In a bladder that is not emptied for several hours, *E. coli* whose multiplying time is in minutes can easily incubate exponentially. Institution of antimicrobial therapy in a timely fashion, usually within 24–48 hours, is the single-most effective pharmacologic strategy till date to limit the scarring consequence.[42]
- *Hypertension:* Although the precise pathophysiology is not clear, derangements in the renin–angiotensin system and sodium–potassium adenosine triphosphatase activity[43] have been ascribed as causative mechanisms of VUR-associated hypertension. But it remains unclear whether it is the nephropathy associated with postinfection scarring, reflux-associated congenital dysplasia, or a combination of both that predisposes to hypertension.[44] Successful correction of reflux alone is not seen to ameliorate blood pressure.[45] At times, nephrectomy of a small unilateral congenitally dysmorphic or globally scarred and shrunken kidney is also seen to correct renovascular hypertension.[46,47]
- *Renal growth:* Although renal growth retardation is seen associated with reflux, correction of reflux is not associated with renal growth, especially in unilateral VUR.[48,49] This is because a significant factor governing the growth of an ipsilateral kidney is the function of its contralateral mate. Although preventing infection in the presence of VUR will maintain the normal renal growth in most cases,[50] the compensatory hypertrophy of the contralateral kidney will magnify the perceived impact of infection on renal growth on the ipsilateral VUR-affected kidney.

Renal Failure and Somatic Growth

Renal failure due to primary VUR is now a rarity and is largely due to the advances in reflux management championed by Smellie and colleagues during their pivotal studies of reflux and infection in children during the 1970s and 1980s. Chronic pyelonephritis as a primary cause of end-stage kidney disease has fallen from 25 to 15%[51] to <2%.[52,53] Reflux nephropathy which was the second-most common medical renal disease[54] and associated with renal scarring can be due to hyperfiltration, concentrating defects, proteinuria, microalbuminuria,[55] renal tubular acidosis,[56] and increased

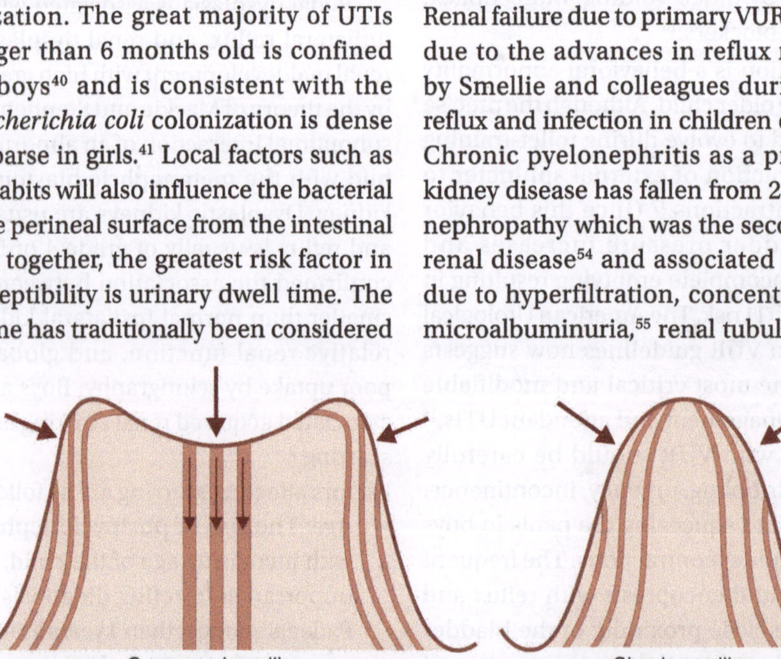

Fig. 2: Compound papillae and simple papillae with the arrangement of collecting ducts showing ease of intrarenal reflux in compound papillae.

fractional excretion of sodium and magnesium. The concentrating defect is proportional to reflux grade and improves following reflux cessation. Apart from renal dysplasia and the impact of infection, the relative obstruction caused by retrograde urine flow may also contribute to nephropathy.

The age-adjusted growth curve falls below normal in many children with VUR, particularly those with bilateral reflux and some degree of renal damage. But surgical correction of reflux itself as well as successful suppression of pyelonephritis by medical management can result in catch-up growth, both for height and for weight.[57,58]

DIAGNOSIS AND EVALUATION OF VESICOURETERAL REFLUX

Details on the confirmation of UTI have been dealt with in Chapter 13.4.

EVALUATION AND GRADING OF VESICOURETERIC REFLUX

The probability of finding VUR in children with a UTI is 29–50%.[1] Radiographic investigation for VUR has generally been directed to all children with a febrile UTI and younger than 5-year-old and in any male with a UTI regardless of age or fever, unless sexually active. The advent of prenatal ultrasound further increased the detection of asymptomatic reflux in newborns, as a result of workup for persistent postnatal hydronephrosis. Indeed, there is little correlation between the degree of antenatal hydronephrosis and the existence of reflux.[59] As a corollary, a normal postnatal ultrasound was seen in 25% of the patients with VUR and antenatal hydronephrosis.[60] The workup and evaluation of UTI have evolved from an aggressive manner of detecting each and every case of VUR to a child-friendly mode aimed at detecting more of complicated and high-grade VUR.

The American Academy of Pediatrics (AAP) recommends ultrasonography in children younger than 2 years of age with a first febrile UTI as the initial diagnostic test and delays a voiding cystourethrogram (VCUG) unless there are significant findings on ultrasonography.[61]

ASSESSMENT OF LOWER TRACT

Cystographic Imaging

To detect the reflux, the retrograde passage of an imaging contrast material from bladder to ureter and proximal collecting system should be documented. The two approaches are the direct cystogram and indirect cystogram depending on the contrast entering the bladder directly after urethral catheterization or indirectly following excretory urography. Indirect cystography though noninvasive is prone to false-positive interpretation due to contrast that does not originate from the bladder but retained in the ureter or pelvis after filtration and false-negative results in lower grades of reflux.[62] The VCUG and radionuclide cystogram (RNC), therefore, are the two common forms of direct cystography and constitute the present-day gold standard approaches to reflux detection.

In VCUG though done under fluoroscopic control, demonstration of reflux is dependent on factors such as bladder contraction during voiding, the fluid volume instilled into the bladder, and inflammation of the VUJ mucosa. Reflux should be looked for both during filling and during voiding (high bladder pressure occurs). Consequently, if a patient is unable to void in the artificial setting of the radiography suite, false-negative results may ensue. More importantly, even during voiding, reflux may not be demonstrated on a single filling-voiding cycle. A roughly 12–20% greater detection rate for VUR is seen if a cyclic study is performed.[63-65]

A cyclic VCUG involves a second or third cycle of bladder filling and emptying under fluoroscopic observation. Reflux during filling, or passive reflux, is generally considered a poor prognostic sign for reflux resolution and suggests the presence of a fixed decompensation of the VUJ since the reflux occurs with very low intravesical pressure. This is commonly seen in patients with acquired or neurogenic voiding dysfunction, wherein high-resistance voiding has led to remodeling of the bladder wall and VUJ, leading to complete failure of the antireflux mechanism, and immediate reflux during the filling phase.[66] This is in contrast to the reflux that occurs during the high-pressure voiding phase. The ratio of instilled volume-to-bladder capacity [(age in years + 2) × 30 mL] during the radiographic technique can lead to variations in rates of reflux detection. If the bladder is overfilled or underfilled for a given degree of progressive VUJ incompetency, reflux may be overdetected or underdetected, respectively. After a UTI, the general consensus has been to delay the voiding study for at least a week or longer to allow for adequate recovery from the acute infection episode.[67] Only in children with a history of recurrent pyelonephritis and repeatedly negative voiding studies in the intercurrent periods should cystography during UTI be considered though there are studies suggesting that clinical improvement from UTI alone is needed before a VCUG and a sterile urine culture is not a must before VCUG.[68]

Findings noted are bladder contour abnormalities, presence of diverticula or ureteroceles, grade of reflux, configuration and blunting of calyces, intrarenal reflux, filling phase or voiding phase reflux, bladder neck anatomy, funneling or dilatation of urethra, urethral patency, and the presence of post-void residual (PVR) urine. A PVR of >10% of bladder volume is considered significant. A suspected obstructed system study will be complete only by taking delayed films where a retained contrast in renal pelvis may be seen in concomitant pelviureteric junction (PUJ) obstruction.

Radionuclide Cystography

This could also be done in a direct manner or as an indirect nuclear cystogram. The biggest advantage of RNC is its low risk of radiation. It requires only approximately 1% radiation exposure generated by the VCUG.[69,70] Presently, the reduced radiation requirements of modern digital techniques have significantly narrowed the difference between VCUG and RNC. In contrast to the VCUG, the instilled bladder contrast material, usually technetium Tc-99m pertechnetate, is itself the radiation source. Reflux is detected on scintigraphic gamma camera images. Although the delineation of anatomic detail by the RNC is poor, it is ideal both as a screening modality and for monitoring the natural history or surgical follow-up of reflux. Detection of grades 2–5 reflux is more with RNC, while the detection rate of grade 1 reflux is poor due to anatomical overlap. In toilet-trained children, when an invasive procedure has to be avoided, indirect RNC is done.

Another modality gaining attention is ultrasonic cystography to detect reflux. Modern transducers along with the use of echo-enhancing contrast agents can image reflux well in the older children,[65,71,72] but the technique remains of limited use in neonates.[73] Furthermore, while radiation exposure is eliminated, the invasiveness of bladder catheterization is still there.[74]

Grading

In 1981, the International Reflux Study Committee proposed a system of five grades of reflux that remains in current use even today.[9,75] Five grades of reflux are currently used to depict the appearance of the ureter, renal pelvis, and calyces as seen on the radiographic contrast images generated by the VCUG. Grading standardizes the description of the degree of reflux and it is the initial grade of reflux in the primary cystogram, the most significant parameter associated with prediction of reflux resolution. Despite the widespread use of the five-point grading system, several shortcomings exist. For example, there is often significant interobserver variability when images are read and grades are assigned,[76] especially for grades II–IV, although there was reasonable concordance at extremes of grading.[77]

Grading of Vesicoureteral Reflux (Fig. 3)

1. Into a nondilated ureter
2. Into the pelvis and calyces without dilatation
3. Mild-to-moderate dilatation of the ureter, renal pelvis, and calyces with minimal blunting of the fornices
4. Moderate ureteral tortuosity and dilatation of the pelvis and calyces
5. Gross dilatation of the ureter, pelvis, and calyces; loss of papillary impressions; and ureteral tortuosity.

Intrarenal reflux is the retrograde flow of urine from calyces into the collecting ducts and tubules of nephrons, and this is ultimately responsible for infection and scarring **(Figs. 4 and 5)**.[78]

RNC Grading

When compared to VCUG images, RNC images are not discrete and hence reflux grading is difficult. Grade 1 reflux is not identifiable due to overlap with the bladder. By collapsing grades 2 and 3, as well as grades 4 and 5, into low-grade and high-grade reflux, respectively **(Fig. 6)**, grading is simplified but the efficacy is questionable.

The available grading systems do not take into account the variables that affect reflux such as the degree of bladder filling, the voiding cycle, the number of filling cycles during the contrast cystogram, and whether the reflux occurs during filling or only during voiding. One study utilizing the data from Randomized Intervention for Children with Vesicoureteral Reflux (RIVUR) study found that among radiologists though there was agreement on bladder shape and bladder abnormalities, there was dispute in VUR grading, especially grades 2–4. But there was reasonable agreement when extreme grades were considered.[76,77]

Uroflowmetry

Because of its invasive nature, a uroflowmetry is done only when dysfunctional voiding and BBD are suspected. A lack of smoothness of the flow-velocity curve suggests incomplete relaxation of the bladder outlet during voiding and indicates relatively higher pressures during voiding, which could delay the resolution of reflux.

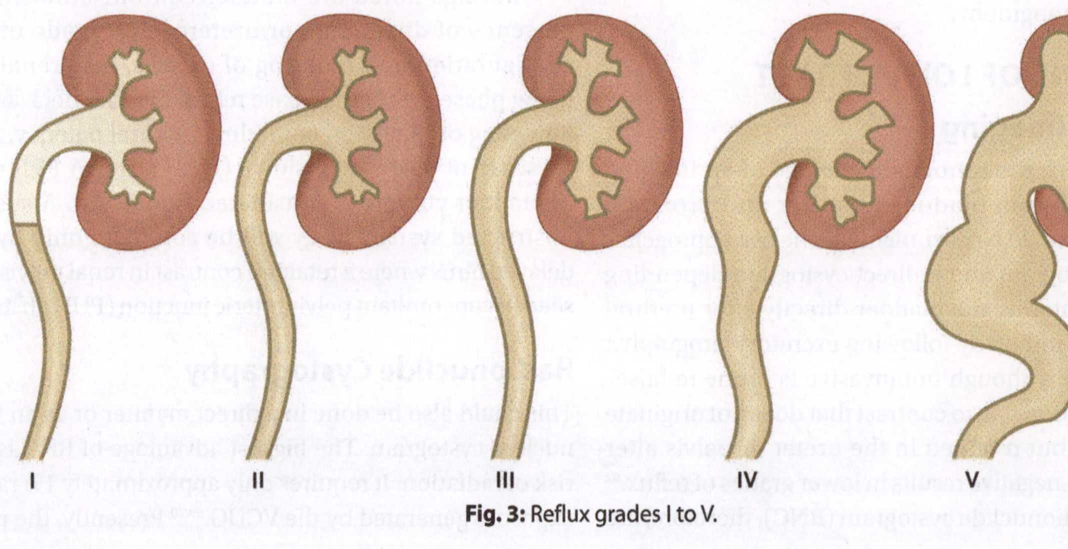

Fig. 3: Reflux grades I to V.

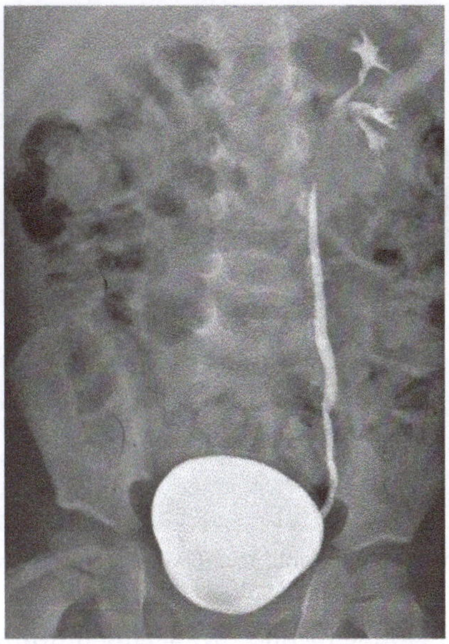

Fig. 4: Grade 2 reflux in a 7-year-old female child.

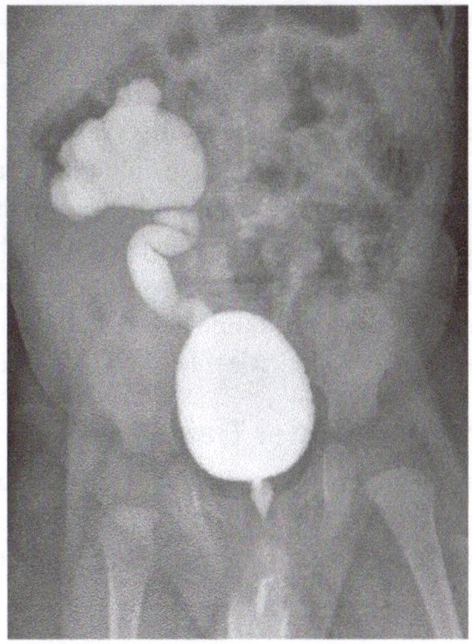

Fig. 5: Grade 4 vesicoureteric reflux (VUR) with minimal posterior urethral dilatation in an infant.

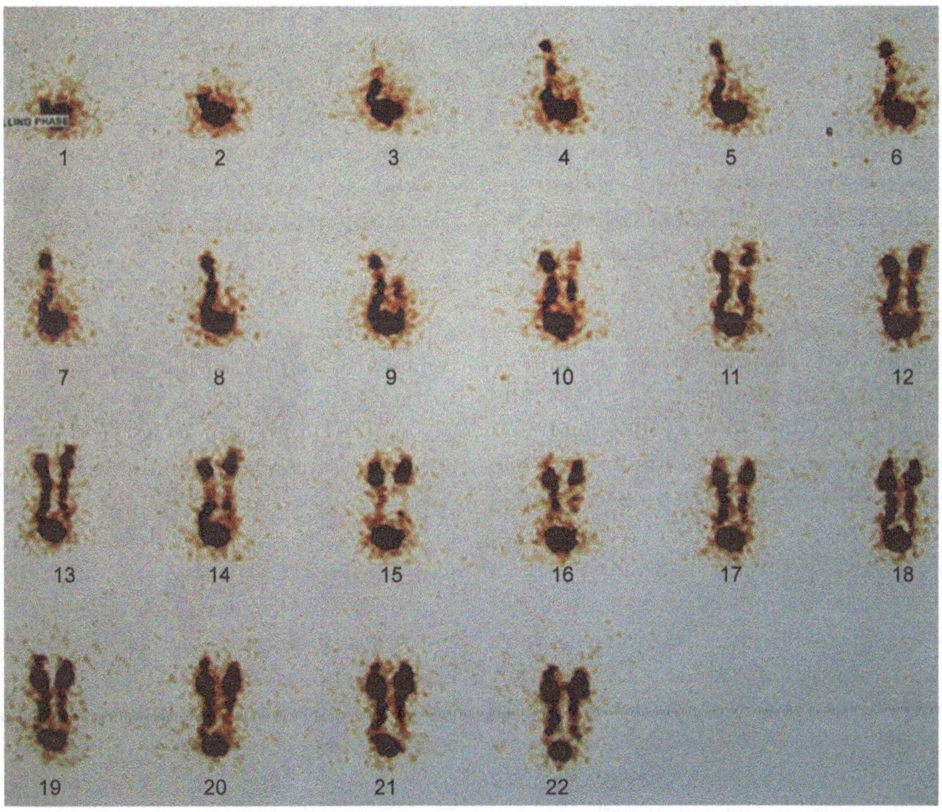

Fig. 6: Radionuclide cystogram (RNC) image showing bilateral high-grade reflux.

Cystoscopy and the Positional Installation of Contrast Cystogram

Current management of reflux does not include routine cystoscopy. The appearance and configuration of the ureteric orifices and intramural tunnel length that are looked for in cystoscopy and once considered useful parameters have over time provided little correlation with either the diagnosis or the grade of reflux.[79] Cystoscopy is a must before open surgery to confirm the position and number of orifice and the proximity of diverticula if any to the orifice, and clarify urethral patency and has no role in initial conservative management.

The positional instillation of contrast (PIC) technique (PIC at the UO) appears to detect reflux under general anesthesia in patients with a history of febrile UTIs but a normal VCUG and uncovers borderline refluxes. With the bladder empty, the cystoscope beak is positioned close to and facing the UO and contrast is instilled at the UO using the irrigation port of the cystoscope from a height of 1 m above the bladder. PIC-VUR is confirmed by fluoroscopy if retrograde flow of contrast into the ureter or renal pelvis is observed. The drawback is that it may at times create iatrogenic reflux rather than unmasking relevant, physiologically borderline reflux. Several studies have shown occult reflux unveiled by PIC study and a reduction in UTI rate after successful medical or surgical management.[80,81] But until randomized studies of PIC-VUR management are available, the role of PIC is limited.

Assessment of Upper Tracts

Upper tract assessment is a must in VUR not only to detect the hydronephrosis associated with the higher grades of reflux but also to assess the associated renal dysplasia or medical renal disease.

Renal Sonography

The primary investigation in all cases of suspected VUR is renal bladder ultrasonography (RBUS). Its easy availability, nonionizing, and noninvasive imaging nature as well as its ability to assess renal vasculature make it ideal for serial follow-up of renal growth and development which can be done quantitatively.[82,83] Apart from renal growth assessment, loss of corticomedullary differentiation and an increase in the overall echogenicity of the kidney are all associated with some degree of renal functional impairment.[84] A relatively smaller ipsilateral kidney, loss of corticomedullary differentiation, or increased echogenicity suggests a degree of intrinsic renal dysplasia, which is inherently associated with high-grade VUR. Just as serial documentation of height, weight, and blood pressure is the basic component of most pediatric clinic reviews, serial sonography every 6–24 months should be a routine in the follow-up of reflux, and it confirms normal renal growth.

Although the presence of postnatal hydronephrosis on sonography can point to the presence of particularly higher grades of reflux, there is no significant correlation between a normal ultrasound and the absence of reflux.[59,85] Sonography is better suited to pick large cortical defects or renal size asymmetry.[86] Renal resistive index of interlobar and arcuate arteries is significantly increased in higher grades of reflux and correlate positively with recurrent pyelonephritis.[87]

Renal Scintigraphy

Functioning renal parenchyma is best imaged by scintigraphy using 99mTc-labeled dimercaptosuccinic acid (DMSA). The radiotracer is taken up only by functioning proximal tubular cells where it binds for several hours. The uptake of DMSA provides a good proportional representation of glomerular filtration as well.[88] Because pyelonephritis impairs tubular uptake of radiotracer, these will appear as photopenic areas in resultant renal cortical images. Although many such affected areas in the kidney resolve, especially if prompt medical treatment is given,[89] persistence of such defects indicates scarring **(Fig. 7)**.[90]

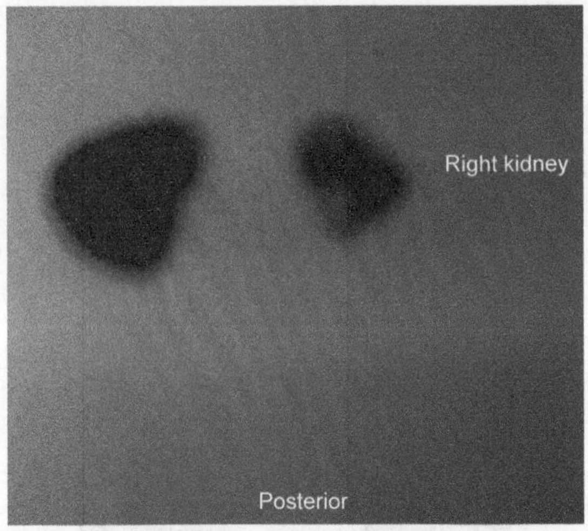

Fig. 7: Dimercaptosuccinic acid (DMSA) image showing small contracted scarred right kidney.

Single-photon emission computed tomography (SPECT) imaging approach reconstructs three-dimensional images of the renal cortical architecture, which can be viewed in any aspect in 360° of rotation. SPECT images provide slightly higher sensitivity for the detection of cortical defects, but they do not add appreciably to decision-making in the clinical management of reflux.[91]

Top–Down Approach

This approach is based on the notion that only reflux with the potential to cause renal injury is worthy of uncovering. During workup of UTI, a DMSA) renal scan is obtained following a febrile UTI and cystography is reserved for patients with abnormal scintigraphy. Children with a negative DMSA do not require further evaluation unless they develop recurrent UTI, in which case a VCUG should be obtained. Thus, all children with significant VUR who are at risk for renal scarring are detected while those who are not at risk are not subjected to invasive evaluation and unnecessary treatment.[92]

Acute-phase and delayed-phase DMSA scan has been advised as part of the top–down approach (TDA); one study showed little clinical utility in the acute-phase scan as most irregularities of significance were seen on the delayed scan. They advised against an acute-phase DMSA scan during infection since similar rates of febrile UTIs were found in patients with or without defects on the acute-phase DMSA scan (5%).[93]

Although the TDA approach can decrease the number of VCUGs and detect more significant VUR, recent studies have shown that the TDA performs poorly at detecting high-grade VUR with a sensitivity and specificity of only 79 and 53%, respectively.[94] In the most recent Cochrane review on the subject,[95] the authors concluded that DMSA scans lack the specificity to detect any VUR, even high-grade VUR. They also found that children with a normal DMSA scan have a <1% probability of having high-grade VUR.[95] But the reverse is not true because 70% of children with febrile UTIs would have positive findings on DMSA even if they do not have reflux. TDA should be used on a risk-stratified basis and more efforts need to be directed to early and reliable identification of UTI, institution of effective treatment, addressing BBD, as well as any other risk factors.[96] TDA should aid in determining which patients with a history of UTI show enough evidence to support further evaluation with a VCUG.

Guidelines for Workup

The National Institutes for Clinical Excellence (NICE) in the United Kingdom proposed a set of guidelines for the investigation and treatment of children with UTI aiming at reducing morbidity, antibiotic usage, and cost of medical management.[97,98] In infants younger than 6 months of age, investigations are limited to RBUS, with cystography and DMSA reserved for those with "atypical" or recurrent UTIs.

In patients older than 6 months but less than 3 years of age, a VCUG is recommended if the child has "atypical" or recurrent UTIs, which includes dilation on ultrasonography, poor urine stream, infection with non-*E. coli* bacteria, or family history of VUR. If a child in this age group responds well to treatment in 48 hours, no VCUG is indicated.

Children older than 3 years of age undergo only an RBUS after a UTI, no routine VCUG or DMSA unless they have an abnormal RBUS. The major criticism to this approach lies in the poor correlation between the appearance of the kidneys on ultrasonography and the presence of renal parenchymal changes or the presence and grade of VUR.[95,99]

As per the revised guidelines of AAP, in children 2–24 months of age[61] the following are recommended:

- To establish the diagnosis, stricter criteria for the diagnosis of infection were suggested, including a lowered threshold for urine culture colony-forming units per milliliter (50,000 to 100,000) and the additional requirement of an abnormal urinalysis.
- Oral and parenteral antibiotic treatments are now considered equally effective.
- RBUS to be done for all cases for screening.
- To forgo VCUG after the first febrile UTI unless indicated by any abnormal RBUS findings or after a subsequent febrile UTI. If hydronephrosis or findings suggestive of renal scarring/dysplasia or obstructive uropathy are present, a VCUG should be obtained. Similarly, any complex or clinically atypical scenario supports obtaining a VCUG after the first febrile UTI.

These recommendations attempt to balance the risk for missing clinically significant VUR after a first febrile UTI in infants, against the invasiveness, radiation exposure, and patient and family anxiety surrounding VCUG. Some of the critical issues regarding these guidelines are related to inclusion of data from underpowered studies, nonuniform urine-collection techniques, not accounting for either the role of BBD or the link between VUR and renal scarring, and last, assuming that presenting infection was truly the first clinically significant infection.[100] Undoubtedly the AAP recommendations have resulted in a significant reduction in the number of children undergoing VCUG; however, the guidelines fail to address the need for an individualized, risk-based approach to treating children with suspected VUR.

The key points recommended by the Indian guidelines are as follows:

- The importance of urine culture on a correctly collected specimen is reemphasized. The diagnosis of UTI must be based on a positive urine culture.
- Patients with UTI should be evaluated for the presence of complications, underlying anomalies, or voiding dysfunction.
- Recommendations on imaging following the first episode of UTI are revised. Detailed investigations are done in infants. In older children, micturating cystourethrography is done in those who show abnormalities on ultrasonography and DMSA scintigraphy.
- Patients with recurrent UTI and/or VUR should be evaluated for BBD.
- Patients with grades I and II reflux should receive antibiotic prophylaxis till they are 1 year old. Those with higher grades of reflux are given prophylaxis till 5 years of age, or longer in case of BBD or breakthrough UTI.

Associated Anomalies and Conditions

Ureteropelvic Junction Obstruction

Vesicoureteric reflux and ureteropelvic junction (UPJ) obstruction are often seen associated and range from 9 to 18%.[27,101] It has been speculated that a developmental ureteral bud anomaly may be responsible for the imperfect formation of both the VUJ and the UPJ.[102] Causes ascribed for secondary ureteropelvic junction obstruction (UPJO) are (1) high-grade reflux causing kinking of the pelviureteric junction, (2) the chronic effects of reflux resulting in an atonic renal pelvis which is unable to propel urine through the UPJ, and (3) UTI propagated to the upper tracts by reflux, inflammation, and ureteritis also contribute to transient or chronic obstruction at the UPJ. Coexistence of PUJ and vesicoureteric junction (VUJ) is suggested by three radiological signs. A dilated ureter with no contrast in pelvis shows nonentry of dye into the pelvis or contrast that does enter the pelvis but poorly visualized due to dilution in a large pelvis. Finally, a large pelvis that retains contrast in delayed films is also suggestive of UPJO.

Both primary UPJO with incidental low-grade reflux and secondary UPJO from high-grade reflux represent true anatomic obstruction for which pyeloplasty is recommended. Another group which presents as significant dilation of the upper tracts but without obstruction, confirmed by documenting good drainage by imaging,[101] needs only management of reflux.

Ureteral Duplication

Vesicoureteric reflux is the most common abnormality associated with complete ureteral duplications. The studies of Weigert and Meyer,[103] who documented the more lateral and proximal insertion of the lower pole ureter associated with a shorter intramural ureter, has also documented reflux into the lower pole ureter **(Fig. 8)**. The incidence of reflux is increased in patients with complete ureteral duplication.[104] Even low-grade reflux present in duplication may take longer to resolve than single-system reflux.[105] Duplication per se does not carry an increased risk of high-grade reflux, breakthrough infection, or scarring,[106] and hence conservative management is the primary option. Females with high-grade reflux are at the risk of breakthrough UTI and scarring, and hence aggressive management[105,107] is indicated.

Bladder Diverticula

The outpouching of mucosa between detrusor muscle bundles, which lacks any true muscle backing, is a bladder diverticulum. The configuration of the diverticulum could compromise the antireflux configuration of the VUJ resulting in reflux. A large paraureteral diverticulum could expand within Waldeyer fascia to cause ureteral obstruction or project forward into the bladder to obstruct the bladder outlet like a ureterocele and cause secondary reflux. Reflux associated with paraureteral diverticula resolves at rates similar to primary reflux and should be managed according to the prevailing indications for the reflux itself, irrespective of the diverticulum.[108] However, when a refluxing ureter enters a diverticulum, it is no longer paraureteral and with no muscular support to the VUJ, reflux is not expected to resolve.

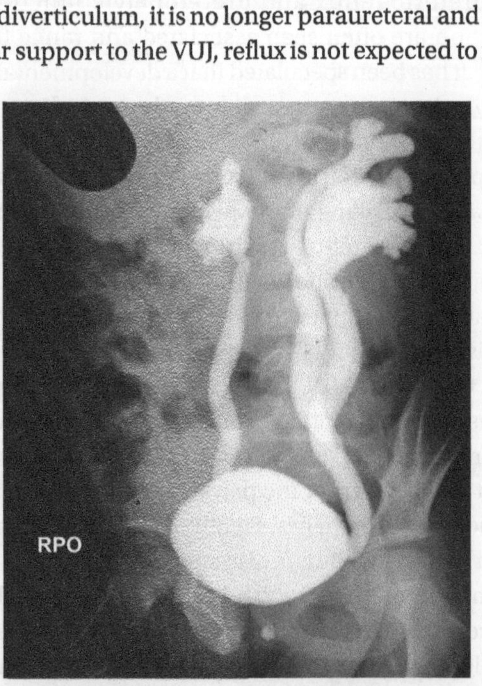

Fig. 8: Bilateral grade 3 reflux with incomplete duplication on the left. (RPO: right posterior oblique)

Megacystis–Megaureter Association

Here, there is massive bilateral VUR that can cause a gradual remodeling of the entire upper urinary tract and an inefficient bladder as the refluxed urine returns to the bladder. This perpetuates marked ureteral dilation leading to the radiographic appearance of massive hydroureter and a thin-walled enlarged bladder.[109] This is a nonobstructive condition similar to cardiac dilatation by regurgitation from incompetent valves. Unlike in PUV and prune belly, the posterior urethra is open in this and the persistent large residual urine is a risk factor for recurrent UTI. Surgical correction of reflux is indicated and it should be followed by a period of bladder rehabilitation[110] during which the bladder regains its contractile behavior and normal capacity.

Natural History and Management

Spontaneous Resolution

This is the cornerstone of reflux management and is the one, which creates confusion in study designs. At birth, the probability of spontaneous resolution of primary reflux is roughly inversely proportional to the initial grade. Reflux resolves spontaneously due to remodeling of the VUJ over time. The progressive elongation of the intravesical ureter consolidates the antireflux mechanism, and stabilization of bladder dynamics with growth of child also adds to the resolution. Conversely, failure of bladder dynamics likely accounts for reflux persistence beyond the expected norms in many patients.

Resolution by Grade

Most cases of low-grade reflux (grades 1 and 2) will resolve. Several studies have documented this high rate of spontaneous resolution, but the reported resolution rates were seen variable in different studies ranging from 63 to 85%. This variation in different studies shows that lower urinary tract dynamics may also play a role in reflux resolution. Grade 3 reflux will resolve in approximately 50% of cases.[79,111] Very few cases of higher grade reflux (grades 4 and 5, and bilateral grade 3) will resolve spontaneously and the resolution rates range from 25%[25] to as little as 9%.[112]

Vesicoureteral reflux index (VURI) is a validated prediction tool that incorporates timing of reflux, presence of associated anomalies, sex, and VUR grade to predict complete or partial resolution of reflux by at least two grades. It has been validated for children younger than and older than 24 months of age.[113,114]

Apart from the above indices, ratio of ureteric diameter, normalized to the L1–L3, vertebral body distance was also used as a predictive tool. They found that the ratio correlated with VUR grade and that the higher the ureteral diameter ratio, the lower the likelihood of spontaneous resolution.[115,116] The volume at which VUR occurs on cystography was also found to be a useful predictor of reflux resolution. When reflux occurred at >75% of the predicted bladder capacity, it was significantly more likely to resolve spontaneously than if VUR occurred at lower volumes.[117]

Resolution by Age

The 1997 AUA guidelines data provided a reasonable statistical estimate of resolution rates segregated by age and grade.[118] Interpretation of more recent follow-up study[119] suggests that diagnosis at the age of 5 years, as well as in infancy, is associated with a similar resolution rate (20% per year), regardless of age. Clearly then, what constitutes reflux resolution depends on the period over which resolution is sought. High-grade reflux showed no difference in resolution rates between subjects younger and older than 1 year of age and may reflect the generally poor resolution rate of high-grade reflux even in infancy.[111] A few recent studies have shown that even for children with high-grade reflux, when diagnosed early on, there is spontaneous resolution in more than one third of patients, and this should at least warrant consideration for primary conservative therapy irrespective of reflux grade.[120,121]

These principles likely underlie the observation that when reflux resolves, it often does so within the first few years of life. The study by Skoog et al. observed that 30–35% of subjects resolved their reflux each year. Younger patients with grade 3 required slightly more time than grade 2 to resolve (1.56 vs. 1.97 years, $P < 0.04$). The traditional period of observation for resolution is 5 years, probably because the greatest proportion of growth and anatomic remodeling of the VUJ is complete by this time. In McLorie et al.'s study, 92% of grade 3 reflux resolution occurred within 4 years.[111] Recent studies have shown an unusually high rate of spontaneous resolution, with a cumulative resolution rate over a 5-year period for grades I, II, III, IV, and V of 92.9, 94.9, 85, 74.4, and 64.4%, respectively.[122]

Principles of Management

Reflux correction is not indicated merely because it can be corrected easily and reliably. As stated earlier, almost 80% of low-grade and half of grade 3 reflux will resolve spontaneously. Walker (1994) summarized the essential tenants of reflux management as follows: (1) Spontaneous resolution of reflux is very common; (2) high-grade reflux is less likely to resolve spontaneously, especially in an older child; (3) sterile reflux is benign; (4) extended use of prophylactic antibiotics is benign; (5) prevention of UTI is more important than VUR correction; and (6) although the success of surgical correction is very high, there is a role for medical management in all reflux cases and is still relevant.

In the face of the paradigm shift after the 2011 AAP recommendation to limit the initial investigation of UTI to RBUS,[61] an ultimate reduction in cystography and associated diagnosis of VUR has occurred[123] and clinical practices have evolved to refocus management into a risk-based fashion.

Age at presentation and grade are the predictive factors on which resolution is likely to occur. In patients diagnosed after one or more episodes of pyelonephritis, the presence of scarring on renal scintigraphy may promote an early intervention, particularly if there are extensive scars, high-grade reflux, globally depressed renal function, or dysplasia of one or both kidneys. In newborns, it is reasonable to wait till 5 years if no significant breakthrough infection is occurring.

Boys with asymptomatic reflux will require little or no formal follow-up after 5 years but the need for lifelong attention to good bladder habits is reinforced, and they are counseled to seek prompt medical attention as well as reassessment of their reflux status if a pyelonephritis were to occur in the future. It is still controversial whether to correct asymptomatic bilateral high-grade reflux with normal renal parenchyma and function in an older boy. In girls even for asymptomatic reflux that fails to resolve by the age of 5 years, surgical correction is advised on the premise that it will reduce maternal and fetal morbidity during a future pregnancy.[101,124]

Endoscopic indications have a wider theoretic potential than open surgery. The potential of endoscopic treatment though temporary can be utilized in the prime age up to 5 years where the risk of pyelonephritic scarring is maximum. Beyond 5 years, postinjection recurrence of asymptomatic reflux in males, were it to occur, would be of little clinical consequence. Regardless of the substance injected and the uneven durability reported to date compared with open reflux correction, the endoscopic approach to reflux management has gained favor over the past several years all over the world.

Medical Management: Watchful Waiting

Medical management is more accurately described as watchful waiting since by judicious use of single daily low-dose antimicrobial prophylaxis, urinary sterility is maintained and an occurrence of UTI is being watched. Antibiotics are given as oral suspensions once daily preferably at night. The rationale of nighttime dosing is to allow antibiotic concentration in the bladder urine over the longest period of expected physiologic retention, when infection is most likely to develop. For children younger than 2 months of age, the most commonly used medications are trimethoprim and amoxicillin. The relative hepatic immaturity and inability to clear sulfamethoxazole efficiently make it contraindicated before 2 months and amoxicillin more recommended. After 2 months of age, the antibiotic of choice becomes trimethoprim-sulfamethoxazole (TSX, Septran, Bactrim).

The other most commonly used drug is nitrofurantoin. Nitrofurantoin may minimize the development of resistance to fecal organisms, which acts as common causative agents of urine infectivity. The known side effects are pulmonary fibrosis and, rarely, interstitial pneumonia. However, its poor taste and gastrointestinal symptoms makes it less favorable compared to TSX.

Currently, there is a growing literature on the use of probiotics (live microorganisms such as strains of *Lactobacillus*, which may displace and suppress the growth of uropathogenic bacteria) in UTI prophylaxis in children. The mechanisms that underlie the demonstrated benefit of probiotic use are only emerging.[125,126] Further studies will be required to define the use of this attractive approach in the medical treatment of patients with reflux.

Breakthrough febrile UTI (BUTI) while on antibiotic prophylaxis is considered an indication for termination of medical management. Although the interaction between host defenses and bacterial virulence factors is what determines breakthrough infection, causes ascribed for breakthrough infection are as follows: (1) If the organism is sensitive to the prescribed prophylactic antibiotic, the child or parent has likely not been compliant or the dose is too low; (2) if the organism is resistant to the prescribed antibiotic, either the residual bladder volume is too high too often or the dose is too high.[127]

Additionally, several risk calculators have been devised that incorporate current, known modifiers of risk profile for breakthrough UTI.[128] Some of these factors include grade and laterality of reflux, age of child, presence of BBD, number of infections, presenting symptoms, bladder volume at the time of reflux, associated anomalies, and presence of renal scarring.[128,129] It was concluded that children at greatest risk for BUTIs were females, infants, those who had high-grade VUR, bilateral VUR, BBD, scars, and those that presented initially with UTI. Patients were stratified into low-risk and high-risk groups based on these variables, thus tailoring management for each child, while providing guidance to the individualized approach to each child's care.[130] The clinician can use this risk stratification and decide upon the management options.

Once the radiographic resolution of reflux has been documented, antibiotic prophylaxis is terminated, usually a few days after the cystogram. However, while the child is being discharged from regular follow-up, a lifelong adoption of good toileting and bladder behaviors should be reinforced.

One major landmark study addressing the controversies in reflux management is termed the RIVUR study, which was a multicenter, double-blind, randomized, placebo-controlled trial designed to evaluate the effectiveness of antimicrobial prophylaxis in children found to have reflux after an initial UTI. One significant conclusion was that antimicrobial prophylaxis was associated with a substantially reduced risk of recurrence of UTI but not of renal scarring.[131-133]

Certain controversial conclusions of the recent studies are as follows: (1) Antibiotic prophylaxis appears to provide little benefit for those with grade II or lower VUR, particularly in the absence of BBD.[134,135] (2) Conversely, antibiotic prophylaxis does appear to be beneficial for those with grade III or higher VUR, at least among girls.[136] (3) Approximately 15% of children with VUR will have a recurrent febrile UTI within 2 years, and about 15% of these children will develop a renal scar.[137] (4) Bowel and/or bladder dysfunction is a major risk factor for recurrent UTIs on or off antibiotics, which will occur in about 45% of children with BBD, as opposed to 15% of those without BBD.[18] (5) A higher grade of VUR is associated with an increased risk for both pyelonephritis and new renal damage.[138] (6) The effect of age on the risk for renal damage is not well defined, although many believe that younger children are more susceptible to renal damage from pyelonephritis.

Where low-dose antibiotic prophylaxis may be of questionable value in low-grade reflux, the effectiveness of appropriate full-dose antibiotic treatment of UTI by eliminating fever and symptoms of acute illness, as well as eradicating the infection, is well approved. Therefore, one alternative for reflux management is close observation for UTI symptoms without prophylaxis, coupled with precise treatment of culture-proven UTI.

Medical management is destined to fail without adequate teaching and periodic review of perineal hygiene techniques, timely bladder emptying habits, and anticonstipation measures. Similarly, family compliance with the antibiotic administration and follow-up visits for imaging may vary widely. Careful open discussion should take place to assess whether watchful waiting is appropriate in each case. In carefully selected patients, options of alternative regimens such as alternate-day dosing of prophylactic antibiotics, or early aggressive treatment of UTI with full-dose antibiotics with no prophylaxis otherwise, may be chosen. If families or patients are willing but unable to maintain all the elements of a watchful waiting treatment regimen, then consideration for open or endoscopic correction of VUR may be relatively indicated.

Surgical Management

While the decision to perform antireflux surgery must be carefully individualized, absolute indications for operative correction of VUR include (1) progressive renal injury, (2) documented failure of renal growth, (3) breakthrough pyelonephritis, and (4) intolerance or noncompliance with antibiotic suppression. Other relative indications for correction of VUR are high-grade (IV–V) reflux in young children after a year of conservative follow-up, pubertal age with nephropathy at diagnosis, parental preference, and failure to spontaneously resolve with watchful waiting.

Surgical Principles of Reflux Correction

The principles to be followed are as follows:

- Exclude causes of secondary VUR
- Adequate mobilization of the distal ureter without tension or damage to its delicate blood supply
- Creation of a submucosal tunnel of generous caliber and satisfying the 5:1 ratio of length to width recommended by Paquin

- Attention to the entry point of the ureter into the bladder (hiatus), the direction of the submucosal tunnel, and the ureteromucosal anastomosis to prevent stenosis, angulation, or twisting of the ureter
- Attention to the muscular backing of the ureter to achieve an effective antireflux mechanism
- Gentle handling of the bladder to reduce postoperative hematuria and bladder spasms.

These goals can be attained by a variety of procedures, most commonly via an open Pfannenstiel approach but also laparoscopically and robotically assisted. There are important differences between these operative procedures. Variables include (1) presence or absence of a ureteral anastomosis, (2) need for detrusor closure, (3) transgression of the urothelium, and (4) whether the neohiatus is fashioned by an appropriately sized detrusor incision or by the closure of the detrusor around the ureter. Performance of a ureteral anastomosis increases the risk of postoperative obstruction, whereas the need for detrusor closure increases the risk of diverticula. In general, excellent results are nearly uniformly attained in all open procedures.

Cystoscopy

Historically, a prognostic cystoscopy was done in many centers following the diagnosis of VUR, since it was used for predictive assessment of the likelihood of spontaneous resolution of VUR. Parameters such as shape (except for the golf hole orifice associated with high-grade reflux), location of the ureteral orifice, and the submucosal tunnel length were subsequently found not to have a predictive value.[75] Currently, cystoscopy is done prior to surgical repair or for endoscopic treatment and to confirm or manage anomalies found on other imaging modalities.

Postoperative Evaluation

In expert hands, the success rate for ureteroneocystostomy in patients with low-grade primary VUR approaches 100%. Most agree that an ultrasound is necessary at 6–12 weeks postoperatively. Following ureteroneocystostomy, the presence of minimal ureteral dilatation and low-grade hydronephrosis on early postoperative ultrasound is not unusual.[102] Indeed, this common finding should argue against performing such studies too early after surgery. On the other hand, persistence of this dilatation beyond 3 months or its progression should be further investigated. Additionally, the development of new renal scars on late follow-up ultrasound, a discrepancy in renal growth, or recurrent UTIs may warrant complete radiologic re-evaluation of the patient.

Complications of Ureteral Reimplantation

Early Complications

Persistent reflux: Early reflux following ureteroneocystostomy is usually not a significant clinical problem and commonly resolves by 1 year on repeat cystography.

Contralateral reflux: Recommendations for management of contralateral reflux range from observation in the majority of cases to intervention for the control of clinical pyelonephritis episodes. In asymptomatic children, younger than 4–5 years of age, prophylactic antibiotics are warranted for postoperative contralateral reflux, particularly if one is to be consistent with the medical therapy for the previous ipsilateral reflux. If the child remains asymptomatic and infection free, repeat VCUGs may not be necessary because contralateral reflux usually resolves.

Obstruction: It is not unusual to detect a mild-to-moderate degree of hydronephrosis in the early postoperative period by ultrasound. This should resolve spontaneously with time. Progressive, significant obstructions usually become apparent in the first 2 weeks after surgery. The children typically present with symptoms of acute ureteral obstruction including acute abdominal pain, nausea, and vomiting. In the more significant cases, drainage of the system either by retrograde insertion of a double-J stent or a percutaneous nephrostomy tube may be necessary. Many of these cases resolve without requiring additional surgery.

Endoscopic Treatment of Vesicoureteral Reflux

Matouschek (1981) first described the injection of polytetrafluoroethylene (PTFE) paste at the ureteral orifice to correct VUR. It was O'Donnell and Puri (1986) who popularized this and coined the term STING (Subureteric Teflon Injection). Although the procedure became popular in many countries due to concerns regarding the potential migration of PTFE particles, FDA approval was not given in United States. The ability to correct reflux in a large proportion of patients with success rates approaching 90% after one injection of dextranomer/hyaluronic acid (Dx/HA deflux), especially in low-grade primary reflux, revolutionized endoscopic treatment. They further modified the technique with the addition of a second injection inside the orifice and named it the double hydrodistention implantation technique (double HIT), resulting in further improvement in results.

Endoscopic Deflux is a low-risk procedure. The most commonly occurring serious side effect is ureteral obstruction which has been documented to occur in 0.6% of injected ureters. This obstruction is usually transient and can be successfully managed with temporary ureteral stenting. Several studies have reported late-onset ureteral obstruction with Dx/HA.[139-141] The introduction of the double HIT by the Atlanta group has resulted in higher reflux resolution rates of 90%.[142] Although concern has been raised regarding the cost effectiveness of Deflux injection therapy (the cost of a 1-mL vial of Deflux is INR 40,000), it remains a reasonable alternative particularly suited for children with mild-to-moderate low-grade VUR without concomitant BBD or anatomic bladder anomalies whose parents desire to avoid more invasive forms of surgical correction. It should be used only with the informed consent of its variable success.

Follow-up

The child is continued on antibiotics for 3 months. An early USG at 2–4 weeks is done to rule out obstruction. After 3 months, a follow-up ultrasound and VCUG are obtained. If reflux is persistent, a repeat injection can be considered at 6 months after the initial injection. If there is still no resolution, then open/laparoscopic/robotic surgery is advised. At open surgery, the injected material if seen is found well encapsulated but in an incorrect plane either inside or outside the bladder.

Minimally Invasive Surgical Procedures

Even though both laparoscopic and robotic-assisted antireflux surgery apply the same surgical principles as those of open surgery, early reports failed to reproduce the high success rates reported by classical open surgeons of 95.9% and the resolution rates were around 83–92%. Complications that were unusual after open procedures such as ureteral injury, obstruction, and urinary leakage were seen especially after the intravesical vesicoscopic procedures.[143-146] More recent multi-institutional reviews have also documented success rates that continue to fall short of the gold standard approach of open reconstruction and higher complication rates.[147] With laparoscopic ureteral reimplantation procedures confined to few centers, robotic-assisted ureteral reimplants appear to have overtaken the field.[148] Due to inherent problems with creating and maintaining pneumovesicum, in addition to the very confined working space for the articulating instruments of the robot inside the bladder, extravesical methods are more popular with robotic surgeons.[149-153]

CONCLUSION

Vesicoureteric reflux is a commonly encountered condition in children, particularly after an evaluation for a UTI. The natural history varies from a benign self-limiting condition to one that can cause severe nephropathy and renal insufficiency. Although CAP is the cornerstone of reflux management operative intervention when warranted, excellent outcomes can be achieved with a low risk of complications.

KEY POINTS

- The younger the child with UTI, the greater is the likelihood of VUR.
- Integrity of antireflux mechanism depends on many anatomical and physiological mechanisms.
- Reflux may be due to anatomic or functional abnormalities of VUJ, bladder outlet, or bladder.
- Parental perceptions must be considered when treating a child with reflux.
- Resolution of VUR is inversely proportional to grade.
- Cornerstone of reflux management is maintaining urinary sterility.
- CAP reduces UTI but does not reduce scar.
- CAP is more beneficial for those with high-grade reflux, BBD, or those presenting with febrile UTI.
- Open reimplantation procedures have 100% success rate and endoscopic procedures are helpful in buying time, especially in young children.

REFERENCES

1. Sargent MA. What is the normal prevalence of vesicoureteral reflux? Pediatr Radiol. 2000;30(9):587-93.
2. Capozza N, Gulia C, Heidari Bateni Z, Zangari A, Gigli S, Briganti V, et al. Vesicoureteral reflux in infants: what do we know about the gender prevalence by age? Eur Rev Med Pharmacol Sci. 2017;21(23):5321-9.
3. Elbadawi A. Anatomy and function of the ureteral sheath. J Urol. 1972;107(2):224-9.
4. Paquin AJ. Ureterovesical anastomosis: the description and evaluation of a technique. J Urol. 1959;82:573-83.
5. Lyon RP, Marshall S, Tanagho EA. The ureteral orifice: its configuration and competency. J Urol. 1969;102(4):504-9.
6. Villanueva CA, Nelson CA, Stolle C. Intravesical tunnel length to ureteral diameter ratio insufficiently explains ureterovesical junction competence: a parametric simulation study. J Pediatr Urol. 2015;11(3):144.e1-e5.
7. Shafik A. Electroureterogram in the obstructed ureter and vesicoureteral reflux. J Surg Res. 1996;65(2):145-8.
8. Oswald J, Schwentner C, Brenner E, Deibl M, Fritsch H, Bartsch G, et al. Extracellular matrix degradation and reduced nerve supply in refluxing ureteral endings. J Urol. 2004;172(3):1099-102.
9. Lebowitz RL, Olbing H, Parkkulainen KV, Smellie JM, Tamminen-Möbius TE. International system of radiographic grading of vesicoureteric reflux. International Reflux Study in Children. Pediatr Radiol. 1985;15:105-9.
10. Puri P, Kumar R. Endoscopic correction of vesicoureteral reflux secondary to posterior urethral valves. J Urol. 1996;156:680.
11. Priti K, Rao KLN, Menon P, Singh N, Mittal BR, Bhattacharya A, et al. Posterior urethral valves: Incidence and progress of vesicoureteric reflux after primary fulguration. Pediatr Surg Int. 2004;20(2):136-9.
12. McGuire EJ, Woodside JR, Borden TA, Weiss RM. Prognostic value of urodynamic testing in myelodysplastic patients. J Urol. 1981;126:205-9.
13. Bauer SB, Colodny AH, Retik AB. The management of vesicoureteral reflux in children with myelodysplasia. J Urol. 1982;128(1):102-5.
14. Chandra M, Maddix H, McVicar M. Transient urodynamic dysfunction of infancy: relationship to urinary tract infections and vesicoureteral reflux. J Urol. 1996;155(2):673-7.
15. Yeung CK, Godley ML, Dhillon HK, Duffy PG, Ransley PG. Urodynamic patterns in infants with normal lower urinary tracts or primary vesico-ureteric reflux. Br J Urol. 1998;81(3):461-7.
16. Fast AM, Nees SN, Van Batavia JP, Combs AJ, Glassberg KI. Outcomes of targeted treatment for vesicoureteral reflux in children with nonneurogenic lower urinary tract dysfunction. J Urol. 2013;190(3):1028-32.
17. Allen TD. Vesicoureteral reflux and the unstable bladder. J Urol. 1985;134(6):1180.

18. Peters CA, Skoog SJ, Arant BS Jr, Copp HL, Elder JS, Hudson RG, et al. Summary of the AUA guideline on management of primary vesicoureteral reflux in children. J Urol. 2010;184(3):1134-44.
19. O'Regan S, Yazbeck S. Constipation: a cause of enuresis, urinary tract infection and vesico-ureteral reflux in children. Med Hypotheses. 1985;17(4):409-413.
20. O'Regan S, Schick E, Hamburger B, Yazbeck S. Constipation associated with vesicoureteral reflux. Urology. 1986;28(5):394-6.
21. Chase JW, Homsy Y, Siggaard C, Sit F, Bower WF. Functional constipation in children. J Urol. 2004;171(6 Pt 2):2641-3.
22. Grundy L, Brierley SM. Cross-organ sensitization between the colon and bladder: to pee or not to pee? Am J Physiol Gastrointest Liver Physiol. 2018;314(3):G301-8.
23. Chertin B, Puri P. Familial vesicoureteral reflux. J Urol. 2003;169:1804-8.
24. Majd M, Rushton HG, Jantausch B, Wiedermann BL. Relationship among vesicoureteral reflux, P-fimbriated *Escherichia coli,* and acute pyelonephritis in children with febrile urinary tract infection. J Pediatr. 1991;119(4):578-85.
25. Winter AL, Hardy BE, Alton DJ, Arbus GS, Churchill BM. Acquired renal scars in children. J Urol. 1983;129:1190-4.
26. Weiss R, Duckett J, Spitzer A. Results of a randomized clinical trial of medical versus surgical management of infants and children with grades III and IV primary vesicoureteral reflux (United States). The International Reflux Study in Children. J Urol. 1992;148(5 Pt 2):1667-73.
27. Lebowitz RL, Blickman JG. The coexistence of ureteropelvic junction obstruction and reflux. AJR Am J Roentgenol. 1983;140:231-8.
28. Roberts JA. Vesicoureteral reflux and pyelonephritis in the monkey: a review. J Urol. 1992;148(5 Pt 2):1721-5.
29. Gobet R, Cisek LJ, Zotti P, Peters CA. Experimental vesicoureteral reflux in the fetus depends on bladder function and causes renal fibrosis. J Urol. 1998;160(3 Pt 2):1058-62, discussion 1079.
30. Mackie GG, Stephens FD. Duplex kidneys: a correlation of renal dysplasia with position of the ureteral orifice. J Urol. 1975;114:274-80.
31. Marra G, Barbieri G, Dell'Agnola CA, Caccamo ML, Castellani MR, Assael BM. Congenital renal damage associated with primary vesicoureteral reflux detected prenatally in male infants. J Pediatr. 1994;124(5 Pt 1):726-30.
32. Najmaldin A, Burge DM, Atwell JD. Reflux nephropathy secondary to intrauterine vesicoureteric reflux. J Pediatr Surg. 1990;25:387-90.
33. Burge DM, Griffiths MD, Malone PS, Atwell JD. Fetal vesicoureteral reflux: outcome following conservative postnatal management. J Urol. 1992;148:1743-5.
34. Risdon RA. The small scarred kidney in childhood. Pediatr Nephrol. 1993;7(4):361-4.
35. Smellie JM, Normand IC. Urinary infections in children. Postgrad Med J. 1985;61(720):895-905.
36. Benador D, Benador N, Slosman D, Mermillod B, Girardin E. Are younger children at highest risk of renal sequelae after pyelonephritis? Lancet. 1997;349(9044):17-9.
37. Winberg J. Commentary: progressive renal damage from infection with or without reflux. J Urol. 1992;148(5 Pt 2):1733-4.
38. Ransley PG, Risdon RA. The pathogenesis of reflux nephropathy. Contrib Nephrol. 1979;16:90-7.
39. Funston MR, Cremin BJ. Intrarenal reflux: papillary morphology and pressure relationships in children's necropsy kidneys. Br J Radiol. 1978;51(609):665-70.
40. Rushton HG, Majd M. Pyelonephritis in male infants: how important is the foreskin? J Urol. 1992;48(2 Pt 2):733-6, discussion 737-8.
41. Bollgren I, Winberg J. The periurethral aerobic bacterial flora in healthy boys and girls. Acta Paediatr Scand. 1976;65(1):74-80.
42. Ransley PG, Risdon RA. Reflux nephropathy: effects of antimicrobial therapy on the evolution of the early pyelonephritic scar. Kidney Int. 1981;20(6):733-42.
43. Goonasekera CD, Dillon MJ. Reflux nephropathy and hypertension. J Hum Hypertens. 1998;12(8):497-504.
44. Wolfish NM, Delbrouck NF, Shanon A, Matzinger MA, Stenstrom R, McLaine PN. Prevalence of hypertension in children with primary vesicoureteral reflux. J Pediatr. 1993;123(4):559-63.
45. Wallace DMA, Rothwell DL, Williams DI. The long-term follow-up of surgically treated vesicoureteric reflux. BJU Int. 1978;50(7):479-84.
46. Dillon MJ, Smellie JM. Peripheral plasma renin activity, hypertension and renal scarring in children. Contrib Nephrol. 1984;39:68-80.
47. Schlomer BJ, Smith PJ, Barber TD, Baker LA. Nephrectomy for hypertension in pediatric patients with a unilateral poorly functioning kidney: a contemporary cohort. J Pediatr Urol. 2011;7(3):373-7.
48. Hagberg S, Hjälmås K, Jacobsson B, Sillén U. Renal growth after antireflux surgery in infants. Z Kinderchir. 1984;39(1):52-4.
49. Shimada K, Matsui T, Arima M, Ikoma F. Clinical analysis of the small kidney associated with VUR. Int Urol Nephrol. 1988;20(3):231-8.
50. Smellie JM, Normand IC, Katz G. Children with urinary infection: a comparison of those with and those without vesicoureteric reflux. Kidney Int. 1981;20(6):717-22.
51. Advisory Committee to the Renal Transplant Registry. The 12th report of the human renal transplant registry. Prepared by the Advisory Committee to the Renal Transplant Registry. JAMA. 1975;233(7):787-96.
52. Meiland R, Stolk RP, Geerlings SE, Peeters PHM, Grobbee DE, Coenjaerts FEJ, et al. Association between *Escherichia coli* bacteriuria and renal function in women: long-term follow-up. Arch Intern Med. 2007;167(3):253-7.
53. Geerlings SE. Clinical presentations and epidemiology of urinary tract infections. Microbiol Spectr. 2016;4(5).
54. Hinchliffe SA, Kreczy A, Ciftci AO, Chan YF, Judd BA, Van Velzen D. Focal and segmental glomerulosclerosis in children with reflux nephropathy. Pediatr Pathol. 1994;14(2):327-38.
55. Lama G, Salsano ME, Pedulla M, Grassia C, Ruocco G. Angiotensin converting enzyme inhibitors and reflux nephropathy: 2-year follow-up. Pediatr Nephrol. 1997;11:714-18.
56. Guizar JM, Kornhauser C, Malacara JM, Sanchez G, Zamora J. Renal tubular acidosis in children with vesicoureteral reflux. J Urol. 1996;156(1):193-5.
57. Polito C, La Manna A, Capacchione A. Height and weight in children with vesicoureteric reflux and renal scarring. Pediatr Nephrol. 1996;10(5):564-7.
58. Polito C, Marte A, Zamparelli M, Papale MR, Rocco CE, La Manna A, et al. Catch-up growth in children with vesico-ureteric reflux. Pediatr Nephrol. 1997;11(2):164-8.
59. Farhat W, McLorie G, Geary D, Capolicchio G, Bägli D, Merguerian P, et al. The natural history of neonatal vesicoureteral reflux associated with antenatal hydronephrosis. J Urol. 2000;164:1057-60.
60. Lebowitz RL. Neonatal vesicoureteral reflux: what do we know? Radiology. 1993;187:17.
61. AAP Subcommittee on Urinary Tract Infection. Reaffirmation of AAP clinical practice guideline: the diagnosis and management of the initial urinary tract infection in febrile infants and young children 2–24 months of age. Pediatrics. 2016;138(6):e20163026.

62. Conway JJ, Belman AB, King LR, Filmer RB. Direct and indirect radionuclide cystography. J Urol. 1975;113(5):689-93.
63. Paltiel HJ, Rupich RC, Kiruluta HG. Enhanced detection of vesicoureteral reflux in infants and children with use of cyclic voiding cystourethrography. Radiology. 1992;184(3):753-5.
64. Papadopoulou F, Efremidis SC, Oiconomou A, Badouraki M, Panteleli M, Papachristou F, et al. Cyclic voiding cystourethrography: is vesicoureteral reflux missed with standard voiding cystourethrography? Eur Radiol. 2002;12(3): 666-70.
65. Novljan G, Kenig A, Rus R, Kenda RB. Cyclic voiding urosonography in detecting vesicoureteral reflux in children. Pediatr Nephrol. 2003;18:992-5.
66. Koff SA. Relationship between dysfunctional voiding and reflux. J Urol. 1992;148:1703-5.
67. Craig JC, Knight JF, Sureshkumar P, Lam A, Onikul E, Roy LP. Vesicoureteric reflux and timing of micturating cystourethrography after urinary tract infection. Arch Dis Child. 1997;76: 275-7.
68. Golmakani H, Sharbaf FG, Esmaeili M, Alamdaran Ali, Soltani S, Ahmadzadeh-saani T, et al. Comparison of the voiding cystourethrogram results one and three weeks after the first urinary tract infection in 1-month to 15-year-old children. J Pediatr Nephrol. 2016;4(3):97-101.
69. Blaufox MD, Gruskin A, Sandler P, Goldman H, Ogwo JE, Edelmann CM. Radionuclide scintigraphy for detection of vesicoureteral reflux in children. J Pediatr. 1971;79(2):239-46.
70. Diamond DA, Kleinman PK, Spevak M, Nimkin K, Belanger P, Karellas A. The tailored low dose fluoroscopic voiding cystogram for familial reflux screening. J Urol. 1996;155:681-2.
71. Riccabona M, Ring E, Maurer U. Scintigraphy and sonography in reflux nephropathy: a comparison. Nucl Med Commun. 1993;14(4):339-342.
72. Galia M, Midiri M, Pennisi F, Farina R, Bartolotta TV, De Maria M, et al. Vesicoureteral reflux in young patients: comparison of voiding color Doppler US with echo enhancement versus voiding cystourethrography for diagnosis or exclusion. Abdom Imaging. 2004;29:303-8.
73. McEwing RL, Anderson NG, Hellewell S, Mitchell J. Comparison of echo-enhanced ultrasound with fluoroscopic MCU for the detection of vesicoureteral reflux in neonates. Pediatr Radiol. 2002;32(12):853-8.
74. Kuzmanovska D, Risteski A, Kambovska M, Trpcevski T, Sahpazova E, Petrovski M. Voiding urosonography with second-generation ultrasound contrast agent for diagnosis of vesicoureteric reflux: first local pilot study. Open Access Maced J Med Sci. 2017;5(2):215-21.
75. Duckett JW, Bellinger MF. A plea for standardized grading of vesicoureteral reflux. Eur Urol. 1982;8:74-7.
76. Schaeffer AJ, Greenfield SP, Ivanova A, Cui G, Zerin JM, Chow JS, et al. Reliability of grading of vesicoureteral reflux and other findings on voiding cystourethrography. J Pediatr Urol. 2017;13(2):192-8.
77. O'Neil BB, Cartwright PC, Maves C, Hoeg K, Presson AP, Wallis MC. Reliability of voiding cystourethrogram for the grading of vesicoureteral reflux. J Pediatr Urol. 2014;10(1):107-11.
78. Hodson CJ, Maling TM, McManamon PJ, Lewis MG. The pathogenesis of reflux nephropathy (chronic atrophic pyelonephritis). Br J Radiol. 1975;(Suppl 13):1-26.
79. Duckett JW. Vesicoureteral reflux: a "conservative" analysis. Am J Kidney Dis. 1983;3(2):139-44.
80. Palmer BW, Hemphill M, Wettengel K, Kropp BP, Frimberger D. The value of PIC cystography in detecting de novo and residual vesicoureteral reflux after dextranomer/ hyaluronic acid copolymer injection. Int J Nephrol. 2011;2011:276308.
81. Matsumoto F, Shimada K, Matsui F, Itesako T. Positioning the instillation of contrast at the ureteral orifice cystography can be useful to predict postoperative contralateral reflux in children with unilateral vesicoureteral reflux. Int J Urol. 2011;18(1):80-2.
82. Rodriguez LV, Lock J, Kennedy WA, Shortliffe LM. Evaluation of sonographic renal parenchymal area in the management of hydronephrosis. J Urol. 2001;165(2):548-51.
83. Chen JJ, Pugach J, Patel M, Luisiri A, Steinhardt GF. The renal length nomogram: multivariable approach. J Urol. 2002;168(5):2149-52.
84. Chi T, Feldstein VA, Nguyen HT. Increased echogenicity as a predictor of poor renal function in children with grade 3 to 4 hydronephrosis. J Urol. 2006;175(5):1898-901.
85. Zamir G, Sakran W, Horowitz Y, Korean A, Miron D. Urinary tract infection: is there a need for routine renal ultrasonography? Arch Dis Child. 2004;89(5):466-8.
86. Merguerian PA, Jamal MA, Agarwal SK. Utility of SPECT DMSA renal scanning in the evaluation of children with primary vesicoureteral reflux. Urology. 1999;53(5):1024-8.
87. Ozçelik G, Polat TB, Aktas S, Cetinkaya F. Resistive index in febrile urinary tract infections: predictive value of renal outcome. Pediatr Nephrol. 2004;19(2):148-52.
88. Taylor CM, Corkery JJ, White RH. Micturition symptoms and unstable bladder activity in girls with primary vesicoureteric reflux. Br J Urol. 1982;54(5):494-8.
89. Fernández-Menéndez JM, Málaga S, Matesanz JL, Solís G, Alonso S, Pérez-Méndez C. Risk factors in the development of early technetium-99m dimercaptosuccinic acid renal scintigraphy lesions during first urinary tract infection in children. Acta Paediatr. 2003;92(1):21-6.
90. Rushton HG, Majd M, Jantausch B, Wiedermann BL, Belman AB. Renal scarring following reflux and nonreflux pyelonephritis in children: evaluation with 99m technetium dimercaptosuccinic acid scintigraphy. J Urol. 1992;147(5):1327-32.
91. Majd M, Rushton HG, Chandra R, Andrich MP, Tardif CP, Rashti F. Technetium-99m-DMSA renal cortical scintigraphy to detect experimental acute pyelonephritis in piglets: comparison of planar (pinhole) and SPECT imaging. J Nucl Med. 1996;37(10): 1731-4.
92. Hansson S, Dhamey M, Sigström O, Sixt R, Stokland E, Wennerström M, et al. Dimercapto-succinic acid scintigraphy instead of voiding cystourethrography for infants with urinary tract infection. J Urol. 2004;172(3):1071-3, discussion 1073-4.
93. Kawai S, Kanai T, Hyuga T, Nakamura S, Aoyagi J, Ito T, et al. Top-down approach is possible strategy for predicting breakthrough fUTIs and renal scars in infants. Pediatr Int. 2017;59(7):781-5.
94. Mantadakis E, Vouloumanou EK, Georgantzi GG, Tsalkidis A, Chatzimichael A, Falagas ME. Acute Tc-99m DMSA scan for identifying dilating vesicoureteral reflux in children: a meta-analysis. Pediatrics. 2011;128(1):e169-e179.
95. Shaikh N, Spingarn RB, Hum SW. Dimercaptosuccinic acid scan or ultrasound in screening for vesicoureteral reflux among children with urinary tract infections. Cochrane Database Syst Rev. 2016;(7):CD010657.
96. Abdelhalim A, Khoury AE. Critical appraisal of the top-down approach for vesicoureteral reflux. Investig Clin Urol. 2017;58(Suppl 1):S14-S22.
97. Urinary Tract Infection in Under 16s: Diagnosis and Management. London: The National Institute for Health and Care Excellence; 2018. pp. 1-24.
98. Baumer JH, Jones RWA. Urinary tract infection in children, National Institute for Health and Clinical Excellence. Arch Dis Child Educ Pract Ed. 2007;92(6):189-92.

99. Hung TW, Tsai JD, Liao PF, Sheu JN. Role of renal ultrasonography in predicting vesicoureteral reflux and renal scarring in children hospitalized with a first febrile urinary tract infection. Pediatr Neonatol. 2016;57(2):113-119.
100. Wan J, Skoog SJ, Hulbert WC, Casale AJ, Greenfield SP, Cheng EY, et al. Section on Urology response to new Guidelines for the diagnosis and management of UTI. Pediatrics. 2012; 129(4):e1051-3.
101. Hollowell JG, Altman HG, Snyder HM 3rd, Duckett JW. Coexisting ureteropelvic junction obstruction and vesicoureteral reflux: diagnostic and therapeutic implications. J Urol. 1989;142(2 Pt 2):490-3, discussion 501.
102. Bomalaski MD, Hirschl RB, Bloom DA. Vesicoureteral reflux and ureteropelvic junction obstruction: association, treatment options and outcome. J Urol. 1997;157(3):969-74.
103. Meyer R. Normal and abnormal development of the ureter in the human embryo: a mechanistic consideration. Anat Rec. 1946;96(4):355-71.
104. Privett JT, Jeans WD, Roylance J. The incidence and importance of renal duplication. Clin Radiol. 1976;27(4):521-30.
105. Estrada CR, Passerotti CC, Graham DA, Peters CA, Bauer SB, Diamond DA, et al. Nomograms for predicting annual resolution rate of primary vesicoureteral reflux: results from 2,462 children. J Urol. 2009;182(4):1535-41.
106. Husmann DA, Allen TD. Resolution of vesicoureteral reflux in completely duplicated systems: fact or fiction? J Urol. 1991;145:1022-3.
107. Afshar K, Papanikolaou F, Malek R, Bagli D, Pippi-Salle JL, Khoury A. Vesicoureteral reflux and complete ureteral duplication. Conservative or surgical management? J Urol. 2005;173(5):1725-7.
108. Afshar K, Malek R, Bakhshi M, Papanikolaou F, Farhat W, Bagli D, et al. Should the presence of congenital para-ureteral diverticulum affect the management of vesicoureteral reflux? J Urol. 2005;174(4):1590-3.
109. Burbige KA, Lebowitz RL, Colodny AH, Bauer SB, Retik AB. The megacystis-megaureter syndrome. J Urol. 1984;131:1133-6.
110. Koefoot Jr RB, Webster GD, Anderson EE, Glenn JF. The primary megacystis syndrome. J Urol. 1981;125:232-4.
111. McLorie GA, McKenna PH, Jumper BM, Churchill BM, Gilmour RF, Khoury AE. High grade vesicoureteral reflux: analysis of observational therapy. J Urol. 1990;144:537-40; discussion 545.
112. Skoog SJ, Belman AB, Majd M. A nonsurgical approach to the management of primary vesicoureteral reflux. J Urol. 1987;138(4 Pt 2):941-6.
113. Kirsch AJ, Arlen AM, Leong T, Merriman LS, Herrel LA, Scherz HC, et al. Vesicoureteral reflux index (VURx): a novel tool to predict primary reflux improvement and resolution in children less than 2 years of age. J Pediatr Urol. 2014;10(6):1249-54.
114. Garcia-Roig M, Ridley DE, McCracken C, Arlen AM, Cooper CS, Kirsch AJ. Vesicoureteral reflux index: predicting primary vesicoureteral reflux resolution in children diagnosed after age 24 months. J Urol. 2017;197(4):1150-7.
115. Cooper CS, Alexander SE, Kieran K, Storm DW. Utility of the distal ureteral diameter on VCUG for grading VUR. J Pediatr Urol. 2015;11(4):183.e1-e6.
116. Arlen AM, Kirsch AJ, Leong T, Cooper CS. Validation of the ureteral diameter ratio for predicting early spontaneous resolution of primary vesicoureteral reflux. J Pediatr Urol. 2017; 13(4):383.e1-e6.
117. McMillan ZM, Austin JC, Knudson MJ, Hawtrey CE, Coope CS. Bladder volume at onset of reflux on initial cystogram predicts spontaneous resolution. J Urol. 2006;176(4 Pt 2):1838-41.
118. Elder JS, Peters CA, Arant BS Jr, Ewalt DH, Hawtrey CE, Hurwitz RS, et al. Pediatric vesicoureteral reflux guidelines panel summary report on the management of primary vesicoureteral reflux in children. J Urol. 1997;157(5):1846-51.
119. Connolly LP, Zurakowski D, Connolly SA, Peters CA, Drubach LA, Cilento Jr BG, et al. Natural history of vesicoureteral reflux in girls after age 5 years. J Urol. 2001;166(6):2359-63.
120. Wildbrett P, Schwebs M, Abel JR, Lode H, Barthlen W. Spontaneous vesicoureteral reflux resolution in children: a ten-year single-centre experience. Afr J Paediatr Surg. 2013; 10(1):9-12.
121. Nordenström J, Sjöström S, Sillén U, Sixt R, Brandström P. The Swedish infant high-grade reflux trial: UTI and renal damage. J Pediatr Urol. 2017;13(2):146-54.
122. Cha J, Lee SJ. High spontaneous resolution rates of severe primary vesicoureteral reflux and minimal development of new renal scars. Child Kidney Dis. 2016;20(1):18-22.
123. Lee T, Ellimoottil C, Marchetti KA, Banerjee T, Ivančić V3, Kraft KH, et al. Impact of clinical guidelines on voiding cystourethrogram use and vesicoureteral reflux incidence. J Urol. 2017;199(3):831-6.
124. Roihuvuo-Leskinen HM, Vainio MI, Niskanen KM, Lahdes-Vasama TT. Pregnancies in women with childhood vesicoureteral reflux. Acta Obstet Gynecol Scand. 2015;94(8):847-51.
125. Reid G, Bruce AW. Probiotics to prevent urinary tract infections: the rationale and evidence. World J Urol. 2006;24(1):28-32.
126. Storm DW, Patel AS, Koff SA, Justice SS. Novel management of urinary tract infections. Curr Opin Urol. 2011;21(4):328-33.
127. Smellie JM. Reflections on 30 years of treating children with urinary tract infections. J Urol. 1991;146(2 Pt 2):665-8.
128. Baquerizo BV, Peters CA. Antibiotic prophylaxis and reflux: critical review and assessment. F1000Prime Rep. 2014;6(104): 104.
129. Cooper CS. Individualizing management of vesicoureteral reflux. Nephrourol Mon. 2012;4(3):530-4.
130. Hidas G, Billimek J, Nam A, Soltani T, Kelly MS, Selby B, et al. Predicting the risk of breakthrough urinary tract infections: primary vesicoureteral reflux. J Urol. 2015;194(5):1396-401.
131. Chesney RW, Carpenter MA, Moxey-Mims M, Nyberg L, Greenfield SP, Hoberman A, et al. Randomized intervention for children with vesicoureteral reflux (RIVUR): background commentary of RIVUR investigators. Pediatrics. 2008;122(Suppl 5):S233-9.
132. Greenfield SP, Chesney RW, Carpenter M, Moxey-Mims M, Nyberg L, Hoberman A, et al. Vesicoureteral reflux: the RIVUR study and the way forward. J Urol. 2008;179(2):405-.
133. Keren R, Carpenter M, Greenfield S, Hoberman A, Mathews R, Mattoo T, et al. Is antibiotic prophylaxis in children with vesicoureteral reflux effective in preventing pyelonephritis and renal scars? A randomized, controlled trial. Pediatrics. 2008;122(6):1409-10, author reply 1410-1.
134. Wang ZT, Wehbi E, Alam Y, Khoury A. A reanalysis of the RIVUR trial using a risk classification system. J Urol. 2018;199(6): 1608-14.
135. Garcia-Roig M, Travers C, McCracken CE, Kirsch AJ. National trends in the management of primary vesicoureteral reflux in children. J Urol. 2018;199(1):287-93.
136. Holmdahl G, Brandström P, Läckgren G, Sillén U, Stokland E, Jodal U, et al. The Swedish reflux trial in children: II. Vesicoureteral reflux outcome. J Urol. 2010;184(1):280-5.
137. Shaikh N, Ewing AL, Bhatnagar S, Hoberman A. Risk of renal scarring in children with a first urinary tract infection: a systematic review. Pediatrics. 2010;126(6):1084-91.

138. Alsaywid BS, Saleh H, Deshpande A, Howman-Giles R, Smith GHH. High grade primary vesicoureteral reflux in boys: long-term results of a prospective cohort study. J Urol. 2010;184(4 Suppl):1598-603.
139. Rubenwolf PC, Ebert AK, Ruemmele P, Rösch WH. Delayed-onset ureteral obstruction after endoscopic dextranomer/hyaluronic acid copolymer (Deflux) injection for treatment of vesicoureteral reflux in children: a case series. Urology. 2013;81(3):659-62.
140. Christen S, Mendoza M, Gobet R, Bode P, Weber D. Late ureteral obstruction after injection of dextranomer/hyaluronic acid copolymer. Urology. 2014;83(4):920-2.
141. Papagiannopoulos D, Rosoklija I, Cheng E, Yerkes E. Delayed obstruction with asymptomatic loss of renal function after dextranomer/hyaluronic acid copolymer (deflux) injection for vesicoureteral reflux: a close look at a disturbing outcome. Urology. 2017;101:63-6.
142. Kalisvaart JF, Scherz HC, Cuda S, Kaye JD, Kirsch AJ. Intermediate to long-term follow-up indicates low risk of recurrence after double HIT endoscopic treatment for primary vesico-ureteral reflux. J Pediatr Urol. 2012;8(4):359-65.
143. Peters CA, Woo R. Intravesical robotically assisted bilateral ureteral reimplantation. J Endourol. 2005;19(6):618-21, discussion 612-621.
144. Kutikov A, Guzzo TJ, Canter DJ, Casale P. Initial experience with laparoscopic transvesical ureteral reimplantation at the Children's Hospital of Philadelphia. J Urol. 2006;176(5):2222-5, discussion 2225-6.
145. Canon SJ, Jayanthi VR, Lowe GJ. Which is better—retroperitoneoscopic or laparoscopic dismembered pyeloplasty in children? J Urol. 2007;178(4 Pt 2):1791-5, discussion 1795.
146. Kurtz MP, Leow JJ, Varda BK, Logvinenko T, Yu RN, Nelson CP, et al. Robotic versus open pediatric ureteral reimplantation: costs and complications from a nationwide sample. J Pediatr Urol. 2016;12(6):408.e1-e6.
147. Grimsby GM, Dwyer ME, Jacobs MA, Ost MC, Schneck FX, Cannon GM, et al. Multi-institutional review of outcomes of robot-assisted laparoscopic extravesical ureteral reimplantation. J Urol. 2015;193(5 Suppl):1791-95.
148. Bowen DK, Faasse MA, Liu DB, Gong EM, Lindgren BW, Johnson EK. Use of pediatric open, laparoscopic and robot-assisted laparoscopic ureteral reimplantation in the United States: 2000 to 2012. J Urol. 2016;196(1):207-12.
149. Smith RP, Oliver JL, Peters CA. Pediatric robotic extravesical ureteral reimplantation: comparison with open surgery. J Urol. 2011;185(5):1876-81.
150. Akhavan A, Avery D, Lendvay TS. Robot-assisted extravesical ureteral reimplantation: outcomes and conclusions from 78 ureters. J Pediatr Urol. 2014;10(5):864-8.
151. Schomburg JL, Haberman K, Willihnganz-Lawson KH, et al: Robot-assisted laparoscopic ureteral reimplantation: a single surgeon comparison to open surgery. J Pediatr Urol. 2014;10(5):875-9.
152. Gundeti MS, Boysen WR, Shah A. Robot-assisted laparoscopic extravesical ureteral reimplantation: technique modifications contribute to optimized outcomes. Eur Urol. 2016;70(5):818-23.
153. Boysen WR, Akhavan A, Ko J, Ellison JS, Lendvay TS, Huang J, et al. Prospective multicenter study on robot-assisted laparoscopic extravesical ureteral reimplantation (RALUREV): outcomes and complications. J Pediatr Urol. 2018;14(3):262e1-e6.

CHAPTER

13.6 Ureteropelvic Junction Obstruction

Sethunath S, Shinaz Sadiq

INTRODUCTION AND DEFINITION

Ureteropelvic junction obstruction (UPJO) is the most common cause of neonatal hydronephrosis. It is defined as the impaired flow of urine from the renal pelvis into the proximal ureter, causing dilatation of the collecting system and possible renal damage. The natural history of hydronephrosis due to UPJO varies. In high-grade and chronic obstructions, the raised intrapelvic pressure and poor outflow of urine can cause irreversible renal damage whereas in low-grade obstructions, the developing kidneys can remain in a homeostatic state and often show temporal growth and improvement.

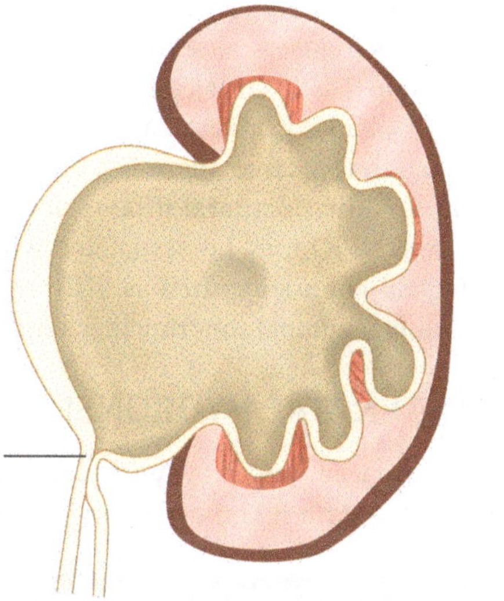

Fig. 1: Intrinsic ureteropelvic junction obstruction (UPJO).

INCIDENCE AND ETIOPATHOGENESIS

The overall incidence of UPJO is 1 in 1,250 births[1,2] with a male to female ratio of 2:1 and with left-sided obstructions occurring in 60%. Bilateral UPJO occurs in 10–36% of patients, with the highest percentage occurring in the younger age group.[3]

Historically, the embryopathogenesis of UPJO has been attributed to developmental arrest and incomplete recanalization of the ureter.[4] The exact cause is still unknown. Other postulates include abnormal innervations of ureteropelvic junction (UPJ), delayed maturation affecting segmental peristalsis, abnormalities in the local renin-angiotensin mechanism, and absence of angiotensin receptors. The ureteric bud, which interacts with mesonephros and metanephric blastema, has a bidirectional inductive role in normal nephrogenesis. UPJO is thought to be due to imprecision in the complex cellular "crosstalk" and abnormalities in the bidirectional induction.

Two types of UPJO have been described by Koff:[5,6] (1) intrinsic and (2) extrinsic. The intrinsic type is the most common type, which is classically known as an adynamic narrow segment, which is poorly distensible and interferes with normal peristalsis **(Fig. 1)**. Deficient and dysmorphic circular muscle fibers, along with increased collagen deposition and fibrosis, are the histologic features seen in UPJO.[7,8]

Mechanical factors can cause an extrinsic type of UPJO by kinking or compressing the UPJ by creating an abrupt angulation at the site. An aberrant, accessory, or early branching lower pole vessel is the most common cause of extrinsic UPJO **(Fig. 2)**. In most cases, the aberrant vessel is a covariable that exists along with the intrinsic type of UPJO.[9] Other causes of extrinsic obstruction include adhesive bands, arteriovenous malformations, and ureteral folds (Östling folds). Other than these two types of UPJO, there are intraluminal causes such as valvular mucosal folds and benign fibroepithelial polyps. Secondary UPJO can occur in 0.75–3.5% of vesicoureteral reflux (VUR) (especially in higher grades)

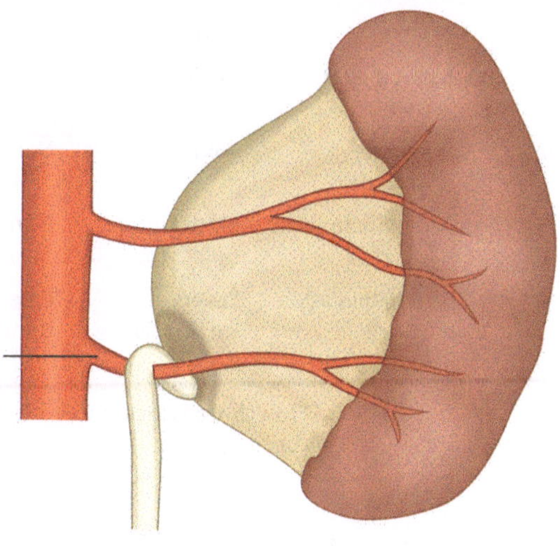

Fig. 2: Crossing lower pole vessel causing extrinsic ureteropelvic junction obstruction (UPJO).

due to kinking of the dilated upper ureter and UPJ, atonicity and inability to propel urine through the UPJ in a chronically stretched pelvis, and inflammation due to urinary stasis.

CLINICAL FEATURES

Routine prenatal sonography has enabled the antenatal detection of fetal hydronephrosis and early postnatal diagnosis of UPJO in these infants,[10] who are otherwise asymptomatic. Older children may present with a palpable abdominal mass, episodic flank or upper abdominal pain, urinary tract infection, hematuria,[3] nephrolithiasis, failure to thrive, feeding intolerance, and rarely hypertension. The paroxysms of colicky pain may be associated with a tender flank mass, nausea, and vomiting related to intermittent obstruction (Dietl's crisis), attributed to acute hydronephrosis caused by kinking or vascular obstruction of the ureter of a floating kidney. Thus, there is a bimodal age distribution: asymptomatic postnatal infants and symptomatic older children. UPJO may be associated with other congenital urological anomalies such as VUR, renal dysplasia, renal fusion and rotational abnormalities, renal duplex, and ectopia.

ANTENATAL HYDRONEPHROSIS

Fetal urine is produced by the mesonephros by the 8th week of gestation and it is the primary source of amniotic fluid by the 16th week of gestation. Maternal-fetal sonography should initially be performed between 16 and 20 weeks of gestation, even though markedly dilated collecting systems can be identified as early as 12–14 weeks. Sonographic detection of antenatal hydronephrosis is reported in 0.2–5% of all pregnancies,[11] but differentiation between true obstructive uropathy and transient hydronephrosis of the neonate is difficult. Sonographic features in favor of UPJO include (1) unilateral or, less frequently, bilateral pelviectasis, (2) normal amniotic fluid volume, (3) no evidence of ipsilateral ureteral dilation, and (4) normal thickness of the bladder wall and normal cycling of the bladder.[12] The Society of Fetal Urology (SFU) has suggested a grading system[11] for antenatal hydronephrosis that is discussed in detail in the chapter on "Antenatal Hydronephrosis" **(Table 1)**. Ngyuen et al. defined antenatal hydronephrosis[11] as when the anterior-posterior diameter of the renal pelvis is ≥4 mm in the 2nd trimester or ≥7 mm in the 3rd trimester. Classification of hydronephrosis based on the anterior-posterior diameter of the pelvis is described in the chapter on antenatal hydronephrosis. The higher the degrees of pelvicalyceal dilatation, the less are the chances of spontaneous postnatal resolution.[13] Adequate prenatal counseling is mandatory for postnatal evaluation to track progression or resolution of hydronephrosis as well as to establish the management principles with the family **(Flowchart 1)**.

TABLE 1: The Society of Fetal Urology (SFU) grading of hydronephrosis.

Grade	*Renal pelvis*	*Calyces*	*Parenchyma*	*Description*	*Postnatal resolution rates*
0	Normal	Normal	Normal	–	–
1	Slight dilatation	Normal	Normal	Slight splitting of the central renal complex without calyceal involvement	50%
2	Moderate dilatation	Mild caliectasis	Normal	Splitting of the central renal complex with extension to nondilated calyces	36%
3	Large dilatation	Moderate caliectasis	Normal	Wide splitting of the renal pelvis, dilated outside the renal border, calyces uniformly dilated	16%
4	Severe dilatation	Severe caliectasis	Parenchymal thinning	Large, dilated calyces (may appear convex); parenchymal thinning to 50% of the normal kidney	3%

Flowchart 1: Incidence of antenatal hydronephrosis, results of postnatal studies, and causes.

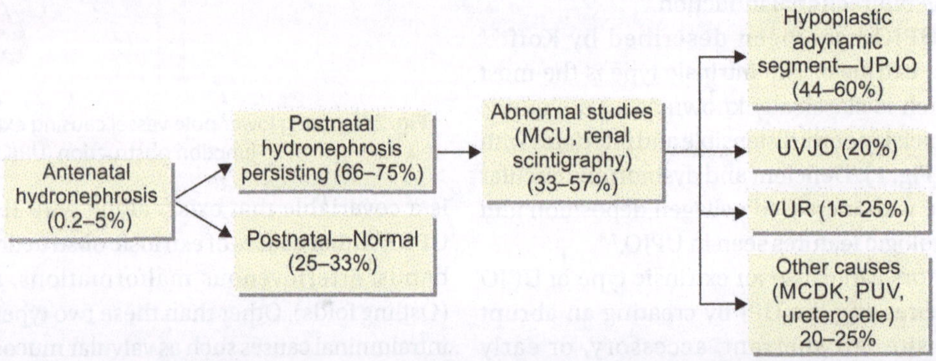

(MCU: micturating cystourethrogram; MCDK: multicystic dysplastic kidney; PUV: posterior urethral valves; UPJO: ureteropelvic junction obstruction; UVJO: ureterovesical junction obstruction; VUR: vesicoureteral reflux)

DIAGNOSIS

Although the detection of hydronephrosis is easy, it is difficult to prove obstruction and no single investigation can always prove whether the obstruction is significant enough to cause progressive renal damage and loss of renal function. Hence, sequential radiographic studies are required for this purpose.

Renal Ultrasound Scan

Renal ultrasound scan (USS) has become the standard method for identifying prenatal and postnatal hydronephrosis. It is accurate, easily available, relatively inexpensive, noninvasive, and safe with no radiation exposure. USS findings of UPJO include (1) pelviectasis and caliectasis **(Fig. 3)**, (2) no ipsilateral ureteric dilatation, and (3) normal urinary bladder wall thickness and cycling. Sonographic findings of increased renal echotexture, absent corticomedullary differentiation, parenchymal thinning on the affected side, and compensatory renal hypertrophy on the opposite side are seen in severe cases. The ratio of renal parenchyma to pelvicalyceal system and the calculation of renal resistive index can also be used to assess the severity of obstruction.

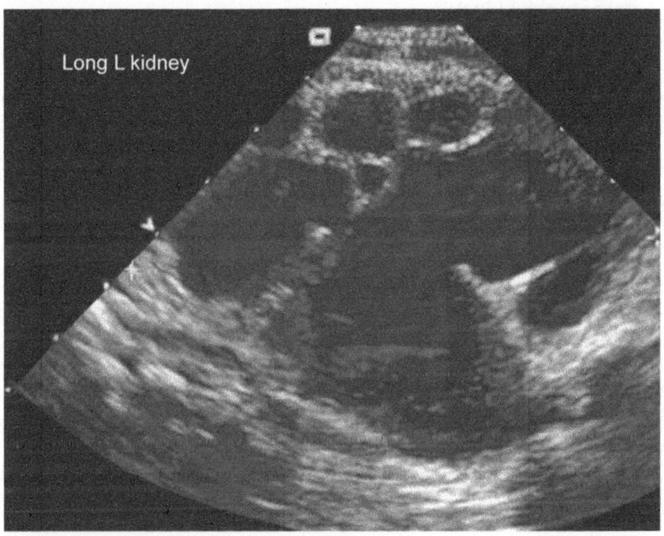

Fig. 3: Severe dilatation of the pelvis and calyces in ureteropelvic junction obstruction (UPJO), with the characteristic "bear paw" sign.

Intravenous Urogram

Intravenous urogram (IVU) used to be the investigation of choice in the past as it provided anatomic and qualitative information regarding renal function. IVU has now been replaced by sonography and renal scintigraphy. IVU is still useful in: (1) cases with discordant findings in usual investigations, (2) when there are other associated renal anomalies such as duplex or VUR, (3) urolithiasis, and (4) recurrent UPJO. IVU findings of UPJO include delayed or negative nephrogram, retention of contrast with delay in drainage, dilution of contrast medium, or uniform cortical loss **(Figs. 4A to C)**.

Micturating Cystourethrogram

Approximately 9–14% of children with UPJO have vesicoureteral reflux (VUR). Several investigators have challenged the routine practice of using micturating cystourethrogram (MCU) for the evaluation of all cases of prenatal hydronephrosis. Majority of the VURs coexisting with UPJO are of low grade and resolve spontaneously. Most of the higher grades of VUR could be easily detected by sonography. MCU is indicated in cases where sonography reveals a dilated ureter and for children with a history of urinary tract infection. It is also used in cases of bilateral hydronephrosis, other congenital anomalies such as multicystic dysplastic kidneys, renal duplex.

Renal Scintigraphy/ Diuretic Nuclear Renogram

Technetium 99m renal scintigraphy is the investigation of choice to estimate the overall and differential renal function (DRF). DRF is an important parameter in defining significant obstruction and the need for surgical correction. The radiotracers used are technetium 99m-diethylene-

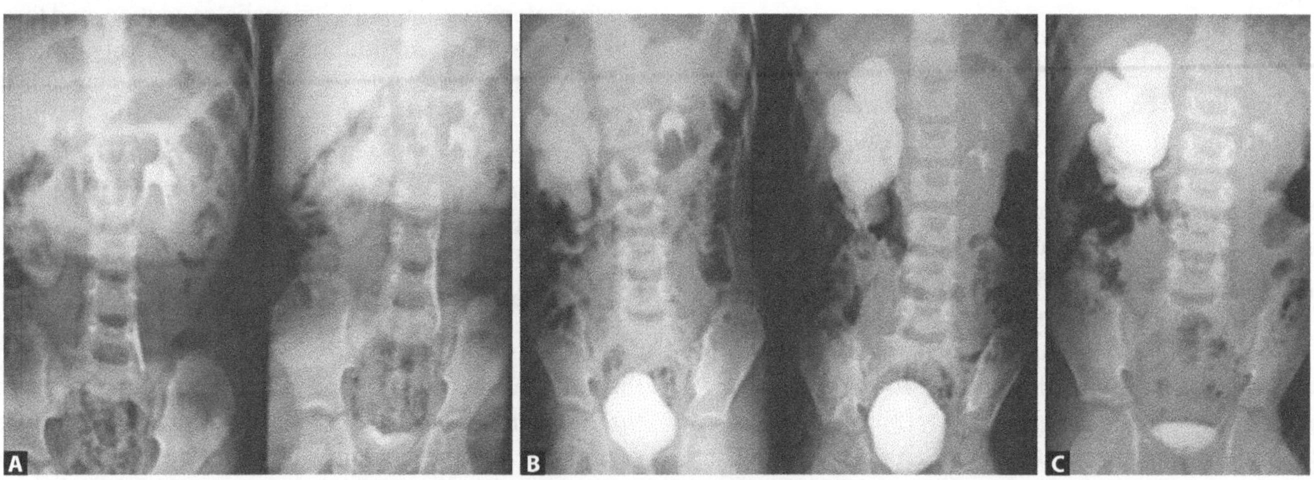

Figs. 4A to C: Intravenous urogram (IVU) images in a case of right-sided ureteropelvic junction obstruction (UPJO) showing delayed nephrogram and contrast retention even in late films.

triaminepentaacetic acid (99mTc-DTPA), technetium 99m-mercaptoacetyltriglycine (99mTc-MAG-3), and technetium 99m-ethylene dicysteine (99mTc-EC). Since they are preferentially concentrated by the kidney and have a near-complete renal excretion, they can be used to estimate DRF and urinary drainage.

Diethylenetriaminepentaacetic acid (DTPA) is neither secreted nor reabsorbed by the renal tubules, whereas mercaptoacetyltriglycine (MAG-3) is secreted by the tubules. DTPA renogram helps to indirectly measure the glomerular filtration rate (GFR) as it is excreted only by the glomerular route. MAG-3 has a higher extraction fraction of about 50% in the mature kidneys, whereas DTPA has only a 20% extraction fraction. MAG-3 remains essentially within the intravascular space. This provides a high target-to-background ratio, good image quality, and more accurate numerical values, particularly when the kidney function is low or immature.[14,15] Ethylene dicysteine (EC) has the advantage of its simplicity in preparation, lower hepatobiliary uptake, better renal extraction, and clearance in immature kidneys which makes it useful in infants <3 months of age.

The procedure should be done in a well-hydrated child with normal oral feeding before and during the procedure. After intravenous injection of the radioactive isotope and diuretic (furosemide), information is gathered in a numerical form about the kidney's ability to extract the isotope; transit across the UPJ is noted and the time taken for it to be completely excreted is assessed. The concept of a standardized "well-tempered" diuretic renogram was suggested by a consortium of members of the Society for Fetal Urology and the Pediatric Nuclear Medicine Council.[15] Here, the infants should be prehydrated with 10-15 mL/kg of saline and the urinary bladder has to be catheterized. There is no correct time to give a diuretic. Some institutions prefer the diuretic prior to tracer (usually 15 minutes, F -15), some with the tracer (times 0 or 2-3 minutes, F 0), and other institutions give the diuretic when the renal pelvis is full of tracer (15-20 minutes, F +20).

The nuclear renogram is one test that can assess the drainage pattern and define whether obstruction exists. Along with the clinical context, the following parameters are used to interpret the renogram: (1) DRF, (2) GFR in DTPA renogram [effective renal plasma flow (ERPF) in EC renogram], (3) time-activity curve, (4) renogram images, (5) Tmax = time interval between injection and peak of curve, (6) clearance half time ($t_{1/2}$) = time for half the radiotracer to clear.

A kidney that shows symmetric uptake and good washout is by definition not obstructed. Such a kidney would then have a renogram with the normal three phases in the time-activity curve: (1) rapid uptake, (2) a sharp peak, and (3) a falling third phase **(Fig. 5)**. In an obstructed system, there is slow or no tracer drainage into the ureter and tracer retention in the delayed renogram images **(Figs. 6 and 7)**.

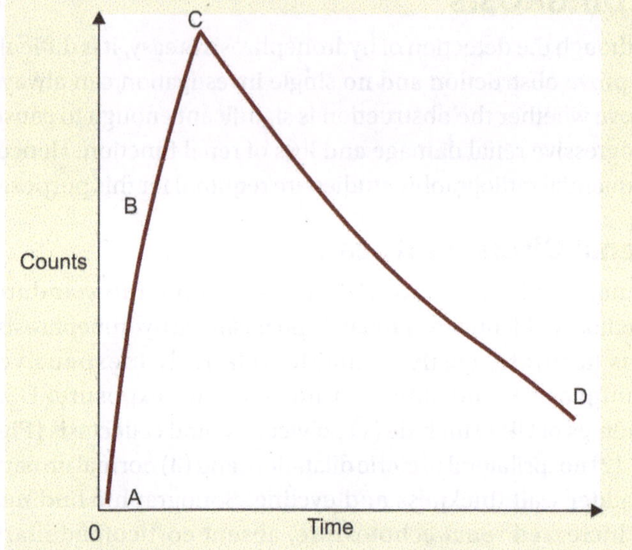

Fig. 5: Time-activity curve in a nonobstructed system peaks within a few minutes after injection of the tracer and then falls.
- The initial steep rising part (AB) = The delivery of the circulating tracer to the kidney
- BC = Accumulation of tracer within the nephrons
- AC = Intrarenal transit time
- CD = Excretory phase; exponential fall in tracer activity in a nonobstructed system, whereas in an obstructed system the fall is flatter or the curve plateaus (Fig. 8)

A nonobstructed system will have a $t_{1/2}$ < 10 minutes (after diuretic administration). $t_{1/2}$ > 20 minutes is associated with obstruction. $t_{1/2}$ between 10 and 20 minutes is considered indeterminate.

Magnetic Resonance Urography

Recently, several investigators have reported gadolinium-enhanced magnetic resonance urography (Gd-MRU) to be superior to USS and nuclear renogram in assessing the urinary tract anatomy and excretion, to detect obstruction if present, and also to calculate the DRF.[17] Moreover, magnetic resonance urography (MRU) has the added advantage of being nonionizing, unparalleled spatial resolution, and three-dimensional views. Additionally, the renal transit time (RTT) can be calculated in MRU, which is analogous to the half-life ($t_{1/2}$) that is calculated for nuclear scintigraphy studies **(Table 2)**. The limitations of MRU include higher expense, need for sedation, and higher frequency of adverse reactions to the contrast agent.

Retrograde Pyelography

Retrograde pyelography (RGP) is not routinely used in the initial workup for UPJO. But it can provide information on the anatomy of the UPJ, identify obstruction, and also exclude the presence of another distal obstruction. In cases of suspected recurrent UPJO following pyeloplasty, RGP can differentiate actual obstruction from residual hydronephrosis.

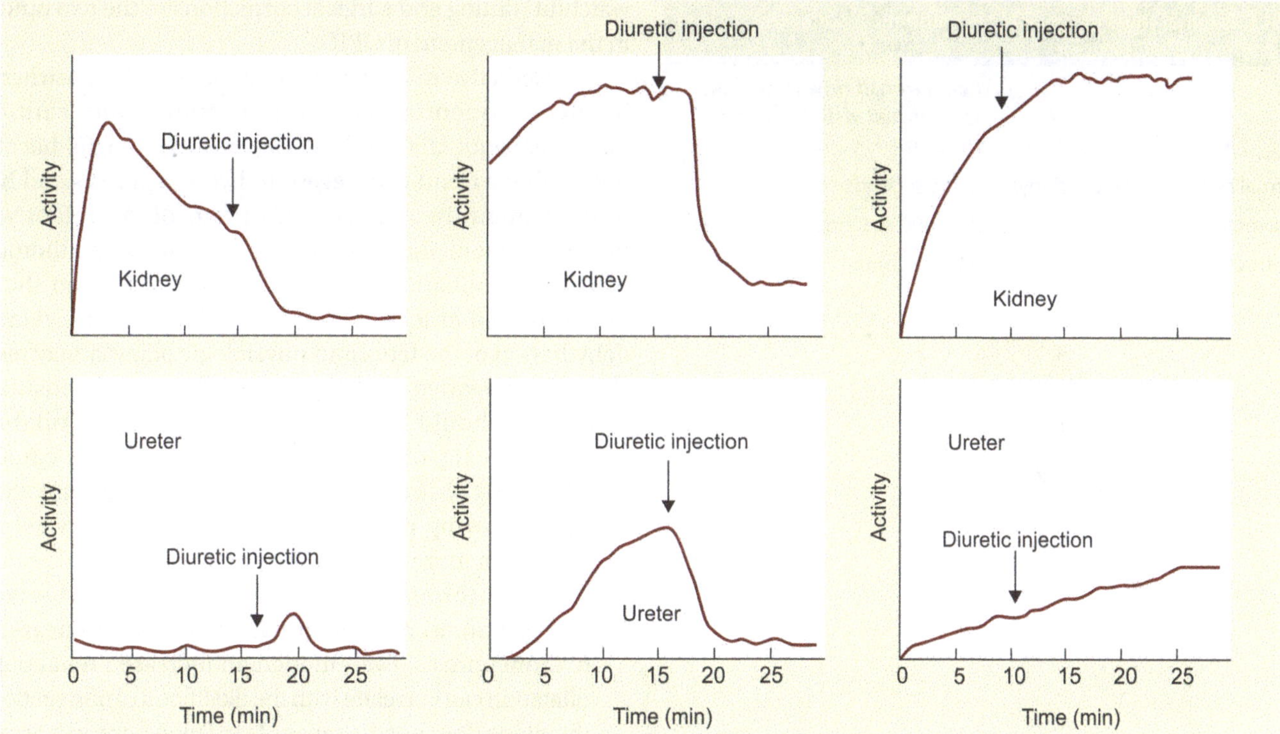

Fig. 6: Diuretic renogram, classic patterns: normal, dilated nonobstructed, and obstructed.[16]

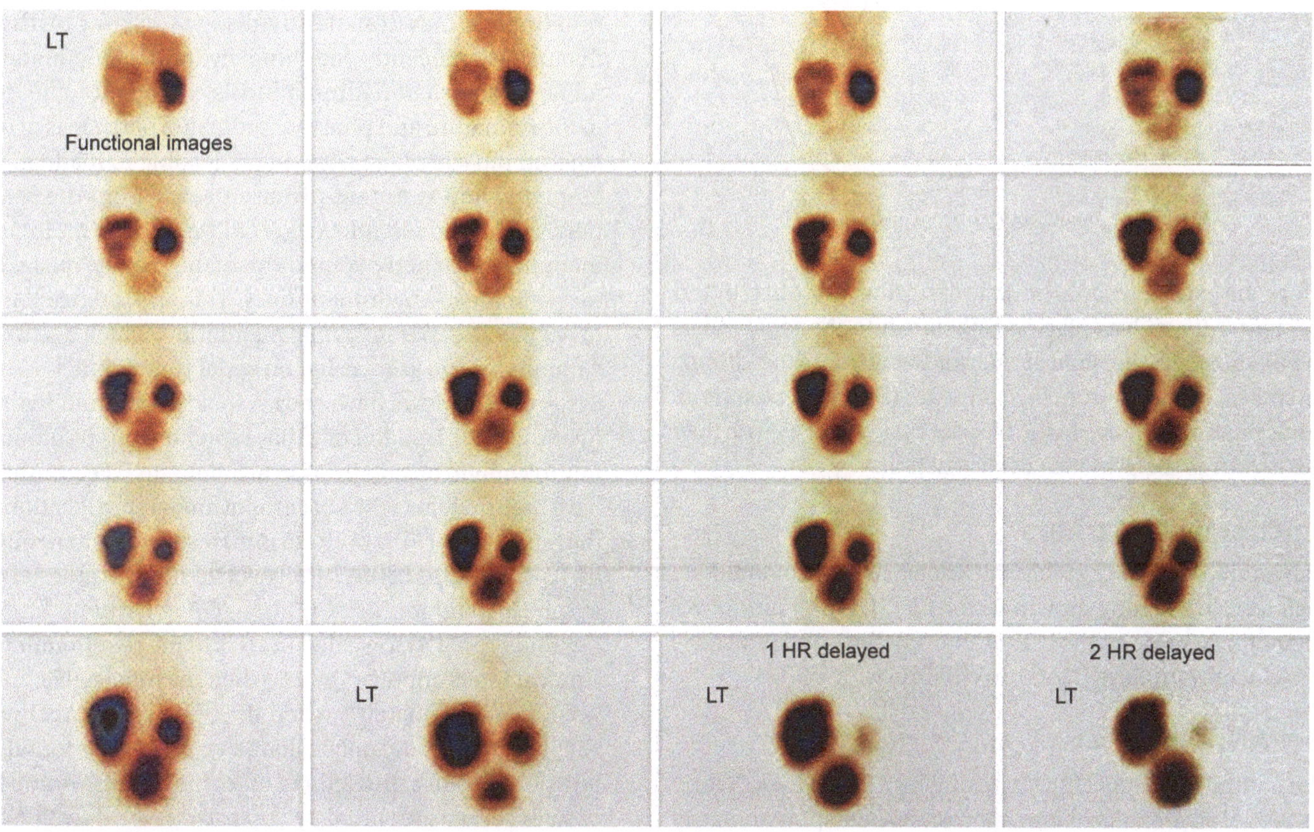

Fig. 7: Diuretic renogram images showing a hydronephrotic left kidney with slow tracer uptake and significant tracer retention even at 2 hours, suggestive of left ureteropelvic junction obstruction (UPJO). There is prompt tracer uptake and excretion in the nonobstructed right kidney.

Pressure Flow Study

The pressure flow study was introduced by Backlund and popularized by Whitaker. The test is invasive, prone to technical errors, requires general anesthesia, has radiation exposure, and hence done rarely now. But this study is unaffected by the kidney's GFR and its antegrade pyelography

TABLE 2: Renal transit time (RTT) in magnetic resonance urography (MRU).

	Renal transit time (time taken for contrast visualization in the ureter)
Normal nonobstructed kidneys	≤245 seconds
Equivocal cases	245–490 seconds
Obstructed	>490 seconds

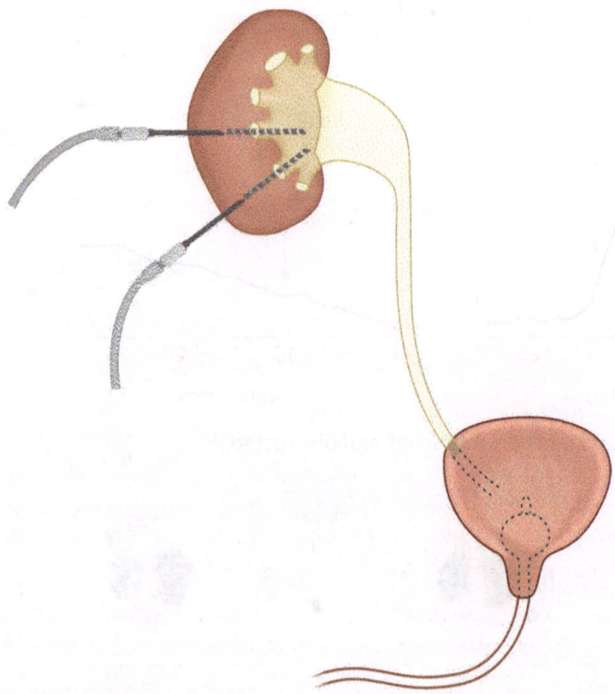

Fig. 8: Pressure flow study.

offers an excellent anatomic location of the obstructed segment.[18] It involves placing catheters into the renal pelvis and bladder, infusing fluid at a rate of 10 mL/s into the kidney, and measuring the intrapelvic pressure **(Fig. 8)**. A high renal pelvic pressure relative to the bladder pressure at a given flow rate confirms the presence of obstruction.

Biochemical Markers

A few studies have found elevated urinary levels of biomarkers such as transforming growth factor-β1 (TGF-β1), monocyte chemotactic protein-1 (MCP-1), endothelin-1 and *N*-acetyl-β-D-glucosaminidase (NAG), in children with UPJO.[19]

MANAGEMENT

The natural history of UPJO is not uniform in all cases. Nearly 40–80% of all prenatal hydronephrosis resolve spontaneously with postnatal follow-up.[11] Nevertheless, many cases develop progressive hydronephrosis and renal deterioration. Most surgeons consider urinary stasis (infection, calculi, hypertension, and pain), worsening renal function, and UPJO presenting with abdominal mass as definite indications for surgical correction. Currently, conservative management with watchful waiting and surgical correction are the two options in the management of UPJO.

Conservative management of unilateral UPJ obstruction involves sequential radiographic studies and cautious patience. Sequential studies[11] become meaningful because they define a trend with regard to hydronephrosis and help to implement the management protocol. An infant with prenatal hydronephrosis should be evaluated with a thorough physical examination initially. Postnatal sonogram should be performed at least 4 days after birth because relative dehydration of the fetus and physiologic oliguria may result in a false-negative study after birth.[20] An early postnatal sonogram should be taken in cases of severe bilateral hydronephrosis, oligamnios, and in conditions causing bladder outlet obstruction such as posterior urethral valve.

The following parameters in sequential USS help in guiding the management protocol:

- *Renal pelvic anteroposterior diameter (APD):* This is the most common parameter used to assess the degree of hydronephrosis. Even though an increased renal pelvic dilatation can correlate with the likelihood of obstruction,[13] this alone does not diagnose obstruction nor can it answer whether the hydronephrosis will improve or worsen. In many neonates, the hydronephrosis in a highly compliant renal pelvis may transiently disappear after birth or fluctuate significantly with time, hydration, and bladder fullness. Transient hydronephrosis is thought to be due to the immature and poorly coordinated peristalsis of the smooth muscle of the renal pelvis leading to inadequate emptying and resultant urinary stasis within the renal pelvis.[21] Moreover, an extrarenal pelvis or sonolucent medullary area and pyramids of infancy can be mistaken for pathological hydronephrosis. This appearance tends to resolve after parenchymal maturation, which occurs at 3 months of age as revealed on serial sonograms.
  Systematic reviews have shown that 98% of mild hydronephrosis (SFU grade 1 or 2) have spontaneous resolution, improvement, or stabilization at follow-up.[22] Few authors have reported that >90% of cases of moderate dilatation of the renal pelvis (APD of 10–15 mm) resolve spontaneously by 12–14 months of life.[23] Prospective studies undertaken at the Hospital for Sick Children, Great Ormond Street, London **(Table 3)**, revealed the risk of the requirement of surgical intervention to be 2% when the renal pelvic APD was <15 mm and 100% when the renal pelvic APD was >50 mm.[24] But renal pelvic diameter, alone, was found to be a poor positive predictor of outcome because only 34% of such patients required pyeloplasty.
- *Renal growth:* Sequential studies help in assessing axial growth of the kidneys in addition to the progression of hydronephrosis on the affected side. Compensatory hypertrophy of the contralateral normal kidney may be indicative of progressive obstruction and a greater risk of functional deterioration in the hydronephrotic kidney.

TABLE 3: Findings derived from prospective studies undertaken at the Hospital for Sick Children, Great Ormond Street, London.

Maximum pelvic APD (mm)	*Risk of requirement of surgical intervention*
<15	2
15–20	7
20–30	29
30–40	61
40–50	67
>50	100

(APD: anteroposterior diameter)

- Increasing renal echotexture and loss of corticomedullary differentiation suggest progression of hydronephrosis and worsening of the renal function on the affected side.
- The ratio of renal parenchyma to the pelvicalyceal system of <1.6 correlates well with an obstructive process and need for pyeloplasty, whereas patients with a ratio >1.6 can be safely observed.
- *Resistive index (RI) on renal Doppler scan:* It is defined as the peak systolic velocity minus the lowest diastolic velocity divided by the peak systolic velocity. Though not specific for UPJO, RI > 0.7 and an RI difference of >0.10 between kidneys in children are suggestive of renal obstruction, while RI < 0.70 generally indicates nonobstructive dilation.[25]

Renal sonogram suggesting UPJO should be followed by additional diagnostic studies to confirm or exclude the obstruction, to rule out other possible causes of hydronephrosis, and to detect other associated urological anomalies.

Renograms should be interpreted on the basis of clinical context, drainage pattern, and curve analysis in addition to the DRF. Most studies have shown that cases of severe hydronephrosis (SFU grades 3 and 4) demonstrate obstruction on diuretic renogram. Based on these studies, an arbitrary DRF of 35% is considered as the pivotal function around which intervention or observation is determined.[26] If the DRF > 35%, the neonate may be monitored conservatively by renal ultrasound every 3 months. If the DRF < 35% on the initial study or if there is a decrease in function of 10% by repeat renogram, consideration should be given to surgical intervention. A DRF < 35% and renal pelvic APD > 20 mm can be taken as an indication for surgery **(Flowchart 2)**.

In cases of bilateral UPJO, the side with severe obstruction and poor function is operated first. Most often, the relatively less obstructed side shows improvement following surgery of the severely obstructed kidney. Ipsilateral UPJO and VUR cause a management dilemma as to which condition to be treated first. Conventionally, it has been advocated that pyeloplasty should be done first as: (1) chances of VUR resolving with time are higher whereas proven obstructed UPJ worsens with time,[27] (2) high chance of failure of a "dry" ureteric reimplantation if it is done prior to correction of the obstructed UPJ, (3) higher chance of renal damage if infected urine refluxes into the pelvicalyceal system of a kidney with UPJO.

The use of prophylactic antibiotics in infants with postnatal hydronephrosis in the absence of VUR continues to be controversial.[28]

Surgical Repair

The aim of surgery is to preserve renal function by ensuring unobstructed drainage of urine from the renal pelvis to the ureter. Open pyeloplasty is considered to be the gold standard in the treatment of UPJO, with a success rate of 90–100%.

Open Pyeloplasty

Different techniques have been described. The dismembered pyeloplasty (Anderson–Hynes) is the most popular procedure done **(Fig. 9)**. The usual approach in children is anterior subcostal. Other options are posterior prone or the lateral flank approach. Here, the obstructed UPJ and the hypoplastic ureteral segment are excised and the normal ureter is widely spatulated. The large pelvis is trimmed and a water-tight pelviureteric anastomosis is done in a dependent fashion. The principal reasons for the universal acceptance of the dismembered pyeloplasty are: (1) broad applicability, including preservation of anomalous vessels; (2) excision of the pathologic UPJ and appropriate repositioning; and (3) successful reduction pyeloplasty. UPJO associated with an aberrant lower pole vessel requires the performance of a standard dismembered pyeloplasty after transposing the neo-UPJ anterior to the crossing vessel in a dependent nonobstructed position. Other types of pyeloplasties are described in **Table 4**.

Minimally Invasive Pyeloplasty

Recent studies have reported that pyeloplasties performed by laparoscopy and robotic surgery have almost similar success rate to open pyeloplasty.[31,32] The approach can be transperitoneal or retroperitoneal. The former is used most often in children because it allows increased working space along with easy identification of crossing vessels and readily identifiable anatomic landmarks. The usual procedure done is a dismembered pyeloplasty.

Endourologic procedures include balloon dilatation, percutaneous antegrade endopyelotomy, ureteroscopic retrograde endopyelotomy, and retrograde cutting-wire balloon endopyelotomy. These procedures are of limited use in children because (1) low success rate of 70%[33] which decreases to 39–44% when a crossing vessel is present, (2) risk of bleeding when a crossing vessel is present, and (3) lack of availability of smaller endourologic equipment for children less than 2 years of age.

Flowchart 2: Algorithm followed in SAT Hospital for evaluation and treatment of antenatal hydronephrosis. Mild HN: SFU grade 1; Moderate HN: SFU grade 2; Severe HN: SFU grades 3 and 4.

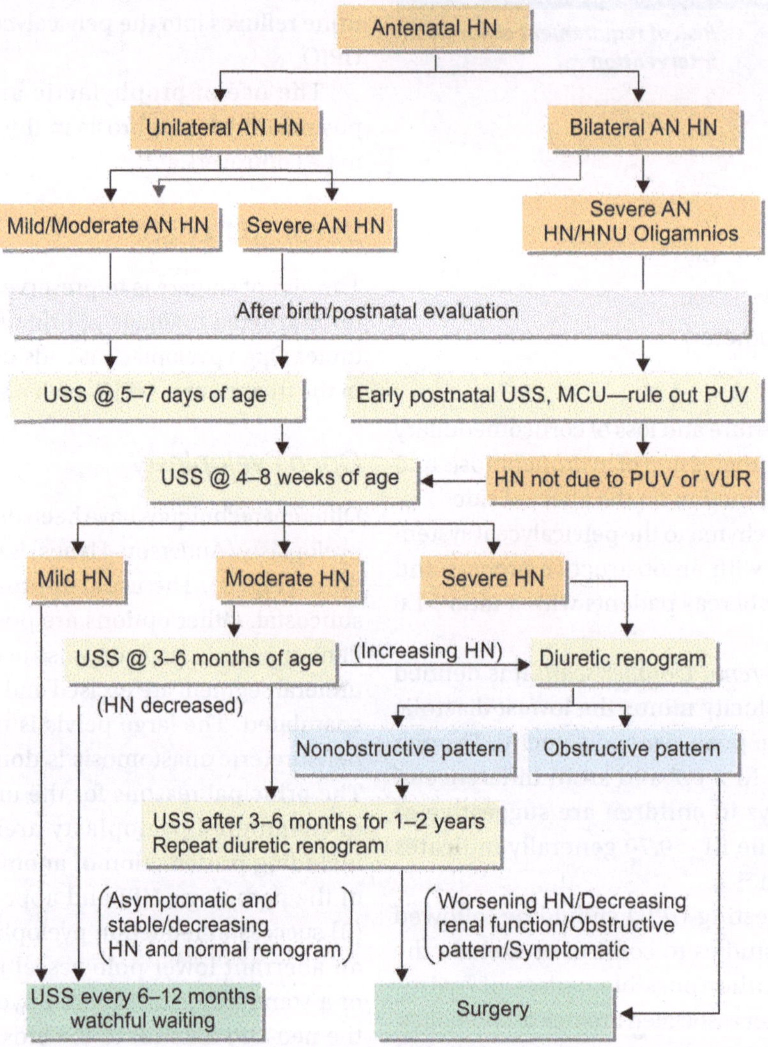

(AN: antenatal; HN: hydronephrosis; HNU: hydroureteronephrosis; MCU: micturating cystourethrogram; PUV: posterior urethral valve; USS: ultrasound scan; VUR: vesicoureteral reflux)

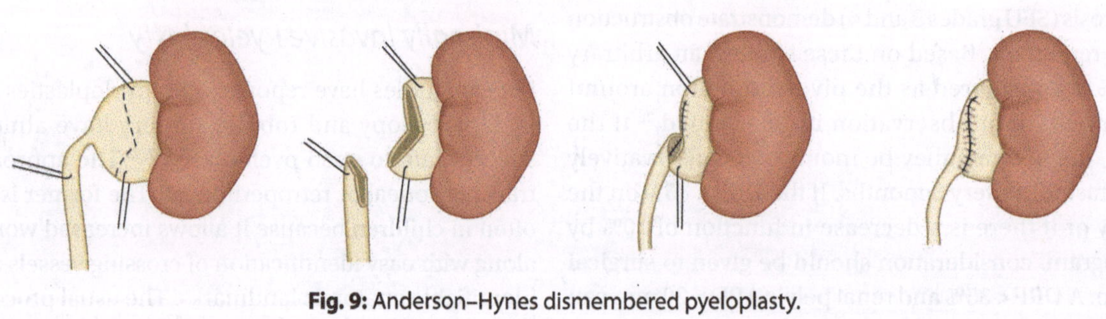

Fig. 9: Anderson–Hynes dismembered pyeloplasty.

OUTCOME

The success of surgical correction is monitored with a sonogram and renal scintigraphy as evidenced by an improvement in the hydronephrosis, gradual increase in the renal parenchymal thickness, improved axial growth of the affected kidney, adequate urinary drainage, and an improvement in the DRF. Meticulous attention to surgical principles—use of proper pediatric instruments, atraumatic tissue handling, careful tissue dissection, adequate excision of the diseased segment, and a dependent tension-free watertight ureteropelvic anastomosis—has resulted in a success rate as high as 98%. Recovery in a very poorly functioning kidney is often noted but cannot be guaranteed, even after unobstructed flow is ensured following surgery. Secondary obstruction or failure of primary procedure causing recurrent UPJO occurs in 1-2%. This occurs due to scarring or fibrosis,

TABLE 4: Other types of pyeloplasties.[29,30]

Type		*Indications/advantages*	*Disadvantages*
Flap type	Foley Y-V plasty	Useful for correction of UPJO with high ureteral insertion	• Cannot be used in cases with a lower polar crossing vessel • No significant reduction of the renal pelvic size
	Culp and DeWeerd's spiral flap	Indicated for relatively long areas of proximal ureteral obstruction when the UPJ is already in a dependent position	
	Scardino and Prince vertical flap	Useful when a dependent UPJ is situated at the medial margin of a large, box-shaped extrarenal pelvis	
Incisional intubated	Davis intubated ureterotomy	It is applicable when multiple or extensive strictures of the proximal ureter are present but cannot be bridged by a pelvic flap	Depends on secondary epithelialization from the incised ureter

a nondependent anastomosis, ureteral angulation secondary to renal malrotation, or ureteral narrowing distal to the anastomosis. We recommend a renal sonogram 3 months after surgery and a diuretic renogram after 12 months. In the absence of symptoms, subsequent renal ultrasounds are performed annually at least for 3 years.

CONCLUSION

Ureteropelvic junction obstruction is an important cause of antenatal and neonatal hydronephrosis and has the potential to result in a progressive deterioration in kidney function. Prenatal ultrasound and postnatal renograms have contributed to the early detection of UPJO. The main goals of management are relief of symptoms and improving kidney function.

KEY POINTS

- UPJO can be intrinsic or extrinsic, partial, or complete.
- UPJO can be asymptomatic or present as a palpable abdominal mass in younger children or manifest with symptoms such as abdominal pain, hematuria, vomiting, and urinary infection in older children.
- Renal scintigraphy is the mainstay of confirming the diagnosis and MRU has appreciable advantages over renograms.
- While a good proportion of UPJOs have a potential to resolve spontaneously, in general, a DRF of 35% and an anterior-posterior diameter of >20 mm are considered the indications for surgery.

REFERENCES

1. Hubert KC, Palmer JS. Current diagnosis and management of fetal genitourinary abnormalities. Urol Clin North Am. 2007;34:89-101.
2. Capello SA, Kogan BA, Giorgi LJ, Kaufman RP. Prenatal ultrasound has led to earlier detection and repair of ureteropelvic junction obstruction. J Urol. 2005;174:1425-8.
3. Carr MC, El-Ghoneimi A. Anomalies and surgery of the ureteropelvic junction in children. In: Wein AJ, Kavoussi LR, Novick AC (Eds). Campbell-Walsh Urology, 9th edition. Philadelphia: WB Saunders; 2007. pp. 3359-82.
4. Ruano-Gil D, Coca-Payeras A, Tejedo-Mateu A. Obstruction and normal recanalization of the ureter in the human embryo. Its relation to congenital ureteric obstruction. Eur Urol. 1975;1:287-93.
5. Koff SA. Postnatal management of antenatal hydronephrosis using an observational approach. Urology. 2000;55:609-11.
6. Koff SA, Campbell KD. The nonoperative management of unilateral neonatal hydronephrosis: Natural history of poorly functioning kidneys. J Urol. 1994;152:593-5.
7. Hanna MK, Jeffs RD, Sturgess JM, Barkin M. Ureteral structure and ultrastructure. Part II. Congenital ureteropelvic junction obstruction and primary obstructive megaureter. J Urol. 1976;116:725-30.
8. Djurhuus JC, Nerstrom B, Gyrd-Hansen N, Rask-Andersen H. Experimental hydronephrosis. An electrophysiologic investigation before and after release of obstruction. Acta Chir Scand Suppl. 1976;472:17-28.
9. Starr NT, Maizels M, Chou P, Brannigan R, Shapiro E. Microanatomy and morphometry of the hydronephrotic "obstructed" renal pelvis in asymptomatic infants. J Urol. 1992; 148:519-24.
10. Wiener JS, Emmert GK, Mesrobian HG, Whitehurst AW, Smith LR, King LR. Are modern imaging techniques over diagnosing ureteropelvic junction obstruction? J Urol. 1995;154:659-61.
11. Nguyen HT, Herndon CD, Cooper C, Gatti J, Kirsch A, Kokorowski P, et al. The Society for Fetal Urology consensus statement on the evaluation and management of antenatal hydronephrosis. J Pediatr Urol. 2010;6:212-31.
12. Siegel MJ. Urinary tract. In: Siegel MJ (Ed). Pediatric Sonography. Philadelphia: Lippincott Williams & Wilkins; 2011. pp. 384-460.
13. Coelho GM, Bouzada MC, Pereira AK, Figueiredo BF, Leite MR, Oliveira DS, et al. Outcome of isolated antenatal hydronephrosis: a prospective cohort study. Pediatr Nephrol. 2007;22:1727-34.
14. Chung S, Majd M, Rushton HG, Belman AB. Diuretic renography in the evaluation of neonatal hydronephrosis: is it reliable? J Urol. 1993;150:765-8.
15. Conway JJ. "Well-tempered" diuresis renography: its historical development, physiological and technical pitfalls, and standardized technique protocol. Semin Nucl Med. 1992;22:74-84.
16. Fung LCT, Lakshmanan Y. Anomalies of the renal collecting system: ureteropelvic junction obstruction [pyelocalyectasis]

and infundibular stenosis. In: Belman AB, King LR, Kramer SA (Eds). Clinical Pediatric Urology, 4th edition. London: Martin Dunitz; 2002. p. 594.

17. Grattan-Smith JD, Little SB, Jones RA. MR urography evaluation of obstructive uropathy. Pediatr Radiol. 2008;38(Suppl 1):S49-69.
18. Veenboer PW, de Jong TP. Antegrade pressure measurement as a diagnostic tool in modern pediatric urology. World J Urol. 2011;29:737-41.
19. Shokeir AA. Role of urinary biomarkers in the diagnosis of congenital upper urinary tract obstruction. Indian J Urol. 2008;24(3):313-9.
20. Wiener JS, O'Hara SM. Optimal timing of initial postnatal ultrasonography in newborns with prenatal hydronephrosis. J Urol. 2002;168(4 Pt 2):1826-9.
21. Sharma G, Sharma A. Postnatal management of antenatally detected hydronephrosis. World J Clin Urol. 2014;3:283-94.
22. Sidhu G, Beyene J, Rosenblum ND. Outcome of isolated antenatal hydronephrosis: a systematic review and meta-analysis. Pediatr Nephrol. 2006;21:218-24.
23. Mami C, Paolata A, Palmara A, Marrone T, Berte LF, Marseglia L, et al. Outcome and management of isolated moderate renal pelvis dilatation detected at postnatal screening. Pediatr Nephrol. 2009;24:2005-8.
24. Wen JG, Frøkiær J, Jørgensen TM, Djurhuus JC. Obstructive nephropathy: an update of the experimental research. Urol Res. 1999;27:29-39.
25. Tublin ME, Bude RO, Platt JF. Review. The resistive index in renal Doppler sonography: where do we stand? AJR Am J Roentgenol. 2003;180:885-92.
26. Ulman I, Jayanthi VR, Koff SA. The long-term followup of newborns with severe unilateral hydronephrosis initially treated nonoperatively. J Urol. 2000;164:1101-5.
27. Lebowitz RL, Blickman JG. The coexistence of ureteropelvic junction obstruction and reflux. AJR Am J Roentgenol. 1983;140:231-8.
28. Islek A, Güven AG, Koyun M, Akman S, Alimoglu E. Probability of urinary tract infection in infants with ureteropelvic junction obstruction: is antibacterial prophylaxis really needed? Pediatr Nephrol. 2011;(26):1837-41.
29. Foley FE. A new plastic operation for stricture at the uretero-pelvic junction: report of 20 operations. J Urol. 1937;38:643.
30. Culp OS, DeWeerd JH. Pelvic flap operation for certain types of ureteropelvic obstruction. Mayo Clin Proc. 1951;26:483-8.
31. Minnillo BJ, Cruz JA, Sayao RH, Passerotti CC, Houck CS, Meier PM, et al. Long-term experience and outcomes of robotic assisted laparoscopic pyeloplasty in children and young adults. J Urol. 2011;185:1455-60.
32. Lam PN, Wong C, Mulholland TL, Campbell JB, Kropp BP. Pediatric laparoscopic pyeloplasty: 4-year experience. J Endourol. 2007;21:1467-71.
33. Kim EH, Tanagho YS, Traxel EJ, Austin PF, Figenshau RS, Coplen DE. Endopyelotomy for pediatric ureteropelvic junction obstruction: a review of our 25-year experience. J Urol. 2012;188:1628-33.

CHAPTER

13.7 Posterior Urethral Valves

Binu MK, Asok Kumar GM

INTRODUCTION

Posterior urethral valves (PUVs) are the most common cause of urethral obstruction in male neonates with an incidence of 1 in 5,000–8,000 live births. They account for about 10% of urinary obstructions diagnosed prenatally.[1] Most of the patients with PUV are diagnosed antenatally. However, they may present later in life or even in adulthood. The symptoms depend on the age of presentation and the severely affected often present earlier than those with lesser degree of obstruction. The clinical presentations have a wide spectrum that can vary from neonates presenting with life-threatening renal impairment to older children with minor voiding symptoms. The patients need prompt treatment and lifelong follow-up as PUVs are the most common cause of end-stage kidney disease (ESKD) in boys.

ETIOLOGY OF POSTERIOR URETHRAL VALVES

Hugh Hampton Young in 1919 described the clinical entity and coined the term posterior urethral valve. Based on the anatomy, he classified the valves into three types.

Type I: They (95%) are obstructing membranes coursing anteriorly and distally from verumontanum toward the membranous urethra. They fuse in the midline with an opening close to the posterior urethral wall. Type I valve is thought to result from abnormal anterior insertion of mesonephric ducts preventing their normal migration.

Type II: Its valves are prominent folds from the membranous urethra toward the bladder neck. They are nonobstructive and have no clinical relevance.

Type III: Its valve (5% in incidence) is a complete membrane distal to verumontanum with a central hole and is believed to result from incomplete dissolution of the urogenital membrane.[2]

Both types I and III may be a congenital obstructing posterior urethral membrane (COPUM) which develop their characteristic appearance following instrumentation (iatrogenic).[1,3]

PATHOPHYSIOLOGY

The bladder outlet obstruction from PUV affects the entire urinary tract from the proximal urethra to the kidneys. The prostatic urethra dilates, elongates, and becomes thin walled and with increasing voiding pressure it may appear more dilated than the bladder.[4] Fetal bladder develops hypertrophy and hyperplasia and an increase in connective tissue. The bladder becomes thick walled, rigid, and less compliant. The storage pressure of the bladder rises and is transmitted to the ureters and kidneys. The vesicoureteral junction may be abnormal and the resultant vesicoureteral reflux (VUR) further increases the ureteral dilation and the severity of renal damage. The renal injury associated with PUV has two components.[4] The first one is the injury due to high pressure which affects both glomerular and tubular function. The glomerular injury results in deranged renal function and a fall in glomerular filtration rate (GFR). The tubular injury leads to decreased ability to concentrate and acidify urine resulting in high urine output (nephrogenic diabetes insipidus). The obstructive uropathy though progressive is potentially reversible with relief of obstruction. The second component is renal dysplasia (RD) which is not reversible with treatment. The pathogenesis of RD is not clear as to whether it results from the impact of high pressure on the developing kidneys or from an abnormal embryological process. The diagnosis of dysplasia is primarily histological, but ultrasound findings of hyperechoic kidneys and renal cortical cysts strongly suggest RD.

The fetal urine output may be decreased due to renal injury and the resultant oligohydramnios affects lung development. It may also lead to musculoskeletal abnormalities and Potter syndrome.

CLINICAL PRESENTATION

Antenatal ultrasound evaluation with fetal anomaly scan is an integral part of standard obstetric care; hence, the diagnosis of PUV is made in utero in most of the patients. However, in one-third of the patients, the diagnosis is made postnatally.

ANTENATAL DIAGNOSIS

Posterior urethral valve in fetus is suggested by bilateral hydroureteronephrosis (HUN) along with distended and thick-walled bladder with poor emptying over 30-minute scan.[5] Presence of oligohydramnios is an associated grave sign. The distended thick-walled bladder with dilated prostatic urethra resembles a keyhole ("keyhole sign"). Hyperechoic

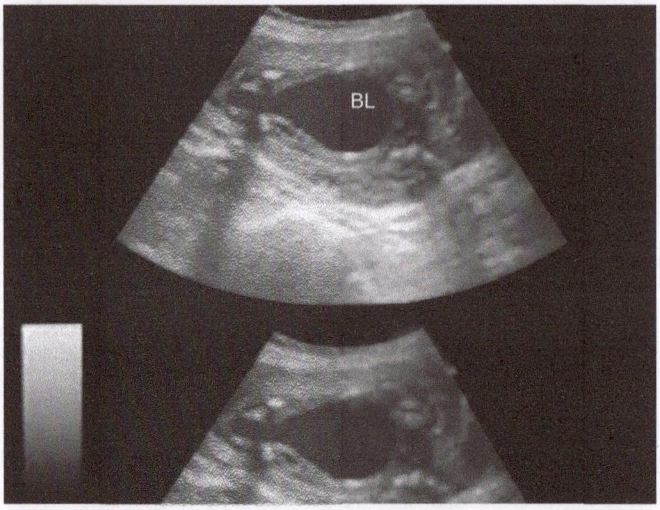

Fig. 1: Antenatal ultrasound scan showing dilated bladder and posterior urethra. (BL: bladder).

BOX 1: Biochemical parameters of fetal urine suggesting good renal function (18–30 weeks).

- Sodium <100 mEq/L
- Chloride <90 mEq/L
- Osmolality <210 mOsm/L
- β_2-microglobulin <6 mg/L
- Total protein <40 mg/dL

kidneys with cortical cysts suggest RD. A distended bladder with bilateral HUN is not specific to PUV. Prune-belly syndrome, high-grade bilateral VUR, and urethral atresia can also have the same findings **(Fig. 1)**. RD associated with PUV suggests poor outcome and fetal intervention is contraindicated. Biochemical parameters of fetal urine are reliable predictors of fetal renal function **(Box 1)**.

ANTENATAL MANAGEMENT

Antenatal management includes diagnosis, counseling, and therapy. The sonological findings for prenatal diagnosis have already been discussed.

Antenatal Counseling

Posterior urethral valve has no specific fetal sonological findings. The sensitivity and specificity of the antenatal diagnosis of PUV have been reported as 94% and 43%, respectively.[5] RD associated with obstructive uropathy may occur early in fetal development and is not reversed with relief of obstruction. The long-term outcome of PUV despite advances in fetal therapy is far from satisfactory. When followed up to adolescence, a significant number will have chronic renal failure (54%), hypertension (37%), lower urinary tract symptoms (29%), and ESKD (21%).[5]

In India, medical termination of pregnancy is allowed but fetal sex determination is prohibited. These facts should be borne in mind while counseling the parents.

Sharma et al. have elaborated the various options for managing fetus diagnosed to have lower urinary tract obstruction and posterior urethral valve **(Table 1)**.[5]

TABLE 1: Antenatal counseling—options.[5]

Gestational age	*Indicators of poor prognosis*	*Antenatal advice*
Before 20 weeks	Early gestational age	Medical termination of pregnancy (MTP)
20–24 weeks	None Oligohydramnios	Continue to term MTP/watchful waiting
24–34 weeks	None Oligohydramnios	Continue to term Fetal intervention if facilities available
Beyond 34 weeks	None Oligohydramnios	Continue to term Early induction/ C-section

FETAL INTERVENTION IN POSTERIOR URETHRAL VALVES

Fetal intervention aims at relieving urethral obstruction and its sequelae of oligohydramnios and pulmonary hypoplasia. All procedures are technically challenging with a fetal mortality rate of 43% and are therefore carried out only in selected centers.[6] Fetal urine sampling with an assay of biochemical parameters is helpful in predicting renal function **(Box 1)**. Elevated biochemical parameters of fetal urine suggest poor function, and RD and fetal intervention are not recommended. The fetal intervention for PUV includes early vesicoamniotic shunting (VAS), percutaneous fetal cystoscopy, and open fetal surgery. Both fetal cystoscopy and VAS improve the 6-month survival rates, but only fetal cystoscopy prevents impairment of renal function.[7] However, it is important to note that none of the procedures currently in practice can reverse or correct RD in fetuses with PUV.[2]

POSTNATAL EVALUATION

Neonates

A newborn male with antenatal bilateral HUN needs clinical and radiological evaluation for PUV. This holds true even if the observed urinary stream is normal.[3] An infant with PUV classically has a poor urinary stream with a palpable thick bladder.

The abdomen may be distended due to a large bladder, enlarged kidneys, or urinary ascites. A neonate with antenatal oligohydramnios may present postnatally with respiratory distress due to pulmonary hypoplasia or pneumothorax and needs respiratory support. Renal insufficiency in the newborn is evidenced by the presence of intrauterine growth restriction (IUGR), poor activity, and muscle tone.

Older Children

Older children present with a variety of symptoms related to UTI or voiding dysfunction or a combination of both.

POSTNATAL MANAGEMENT

Initial Stabilization

Clinical assessment of the general condition of the newborn is done. An infant with respiratory difficulties or with features of uremia or electrolyte imbalance is managed in neonatal intensive care units under the direct supervision of the neonatologist. The newborn with uremia or metabolic acidosis needs immediate bladder drainage with fluid and electrolyte therapy including bicarbonate supplements. Prophylactic antibiotics are started in all patients in addition to obtaining blood sample for assaying biochemical parameters of renal function.

Radiographic Evaluation

Postnatal Ultrasonography

All male neonates with antenatal bilateral hydronephrosis or other antenatal scan findings suggesting PUV are to undergo postnatal ultrasound scan to assess the kidneys, ureters, bladder, and proximal urethra [kidney, ureter, and bladder (KUB) scan]. This is done prior to bladder catheterization and whenever possible within the first 48 hours so that prompt treatment can be offered without delay. Kidneys are assessed for parenchymal thickness, echotexture, corticomedullary differentiation (CMD), cortical cysts, and pelvicalyceal dilation. The ureters are assessed for their size and extent of dilation. The bladder is assessed for size, wall thickness, and presence of diverticulum. A dilated posterior urethra is diagnostic of PUV.

Voiding Cystourethrogram

A voiding cystourethrogram (VCUG) is the gold standard investigation for the postnatal diagnosis of PUV and is undertaken once the baby is stable. It is preferably done under fluoroscopy by a trained radiologist in the presence of a pediatric surgeon. Classically, the posterior urethra is dilated and elongated with a high bladder neck in voiding films. Cystogram shows a bladder irregular in outline with multiple diverticula. Vesicoureteral reflux if present will also be demonstrated **(Figs. 2 and 3)**.

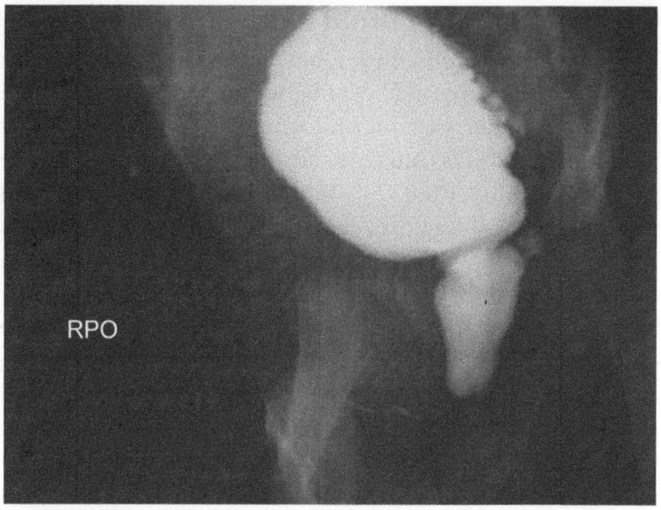

Fig. 2: Voiding cystourethrogram (VUCG) showing posterior urethral dilation with irregular bladder in posterior urethral valves. (RPO: right posterior oblique).

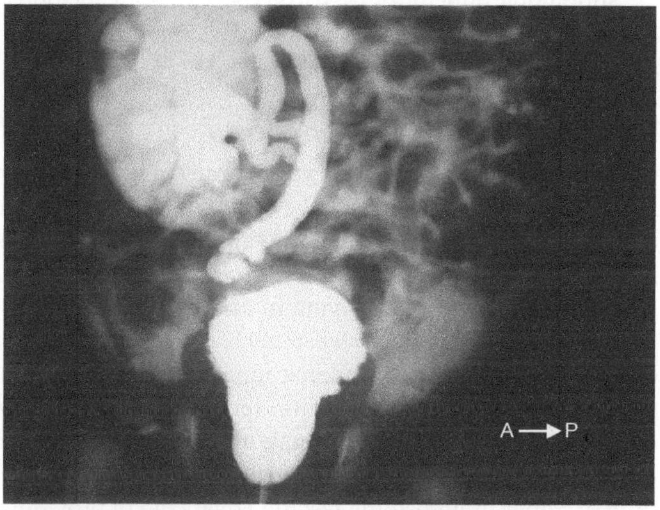

Fig. 3: Voiding cystourethrogram (VUCG) showing vesicoureteral reflux with posterior urethral dilatation and irregular bladder.

Nuclear Scans

Nuclear scans do not serve any diagnostic purpose in the initial workup. However, they are essential components of long-term management. Tc-99m DMSA scan is undertaken in the presence of VUR or cortical changes to detect the site and extent of renal scarring. They also provide the differential renal function. A diuretic renogram with Tc-99m DTPA (or EC or MAG3) is carried out to assess the location and severity of obstruction and for estimating GFR. The timing of nuclear scan is decided based on clinical and radiological findings and is generally not undertaken before 6–8 weeks after birth in view of immature renal function in the early days of life.

INITIAL SURGICAL MANAGEMENT

Initial treatment starts with bladder catheterization, particularly if the neonate has a deranged renal function, urinary dribbling, or a palpable thick bladder. Infant feeding tubes are preferred to Foley catheter as the balloon often causes bladder spasm, which interferes with urine drainage or may slip into the dilated posterior urethra. The tip of the feeding tube should be positioned in the bladder as it can coil in the posterior urethra (can be confirmed with bladder ultrasound scan) and still drain urine.[2] The newborn may develop postobstructive diuresis after catheterization with the need of aggressive fluid and electrolyte therapy.

Serial monitoring of serum creatinine is done on a daily basis until stable. The values in the first 48 hours reflect maternal serum creatinine levels. The fall of serum creatinine to 0.3–0.4 mg/dL indicates good renal function and the neonate undergoes primary valve ablation.[1] Even if the creatinine levels do not fall to normal levels, primary valve ablation can still be offered to a clinically stable patient. If the neonate has rising creatinine levels or develops features of uremia, urinary diversion in the form of vesicostomy or ureterostomy is considered.

Cystoscopy and Primary Valve Ablation

Primary valve ablation is undertaken in a term neonate with 8–9.5-Fr cystoscope and 3-Fr Bugbee electrode or cold knife preferably under video monitoring. Preterm or small for gestational age (SGA) infants need a smaller 6.5-Fr cystoscope for valve ablation. Cold knife is preferred to Bugbee to avoid thermal injury. Resectoscopes with hook electrode can also be used for valve ablation. The presence of valve is suggested by roomy posterior urethra with the valves displayed distally from verumontanum and trabeculated bladder. The valve ablation is carried out by incising the valve with a cutting current or cold knife at 5, 7, and 12 o'clock under normal saline or glycine infusion. The valve ablation is successful in >90% of the patients and the most common complication is incomplete ablation with residual obstruction in which case a repeat cystoscopy with ablation of residual valve is carried out. Stricture urethra can occur if large caliber cystoscopes are forced into the bladder for valve ablation **(Figs. 4 and 5)**.

Suprapubic puncture is used to access valves for ablation if a cystoscope of suitable size is not available. This is particularly applicable to preterm or SGA babies with PUV.

Temporary Urinary Diversion

Urinary diversion in the form of vesicostomy or ureterostomy is undertaken as an alternative to valve ablation when a small-sized cystoscope is not available or when there is a deterioration of renal function after valve ablation. Ureterostomy may be lifesaving in an infant with uremia or urosepsis. The aim of vesicostomy is to keep the bladder empty without catheter to optimize renal function. Blocksom vesicostomy is the most common technique practiced in patients with PUV. Loop ureterostomy and Sober ureterostomy are the techniques widely practiced for upper tract diversion in PUV. Sober ureterostomy has the advantage of providing good upper tract drainage along with bladder cycling (a part of the urine enters the bladder). In cases with bilateral VUR, ureterostomy can be limited to one side so that the urine from the contralateral kidney enters the bladder allowing its growth while the distal limb of the ureterostomy acts as a pop-off mechanism.[5] However, studies show that ureterostomy does not confer any long-term protection from ESKD.[5]

Urinary Ascites and Urinoma

Urinary ascites or urinoma is seen in 5–15% of neonates with PUV.[1] Urinary extravasation along with VURD (posterior urethral Valve, Unilateral vesicoureteral reflux, Renal Dysplasia) syndrome and bladder diverticula is considered as a pressure pop-off mechanism, which decreases the intraluminal pressure and protects the developing kidneys. As intraluminal pressure rises, the calyces rupture and the urine is forced across the renal fornix to form urinoma in the retroperitoneum. When the extravasated urine enters the peritoneal cavity as transudate, it forms urinary ascites. The solutes in the urine are absorbed by the large surface of the peritoneum and the urine aspirated from the peritoneal cavity will have the same electrolyte and creatinine values *as those of serum*. Recent studies dispute the projected beneficial effects of urinary extravasation. Bilateral urinomas are associated with good renal function whereas in unilateral urinoma and urinary ascites, the affected kidneys show deranged function.[4]

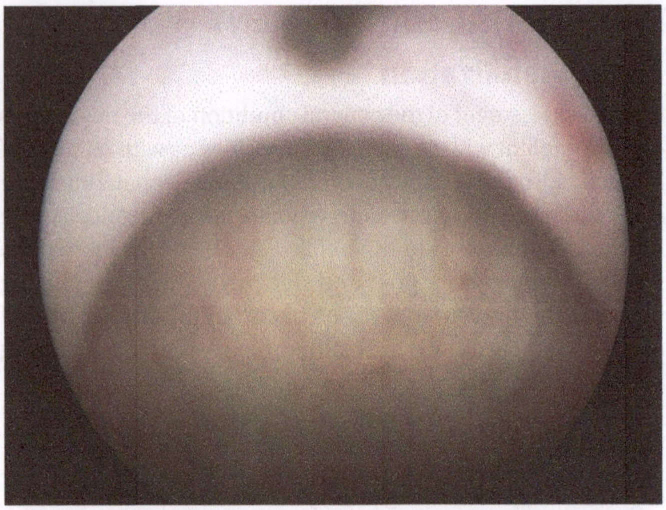

Fig. 4: Cystoscopy showing posterior urethral valve (PUV).

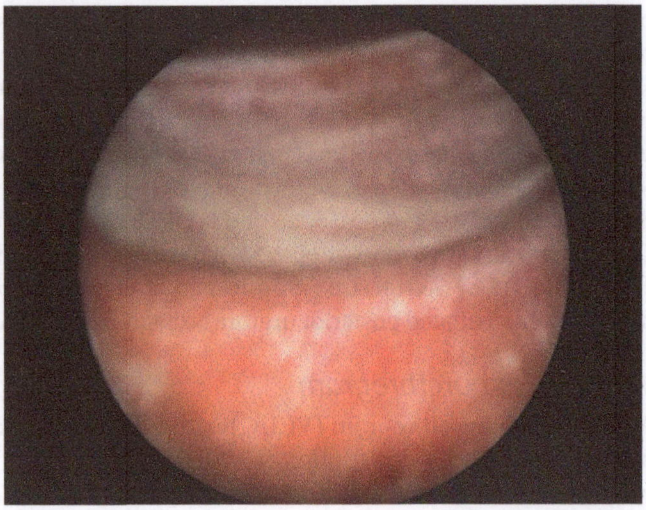

Fig. 5: Posterior urethral valve (PUV) with bladder trabeculation.

The neonate with urinary extravasation can present with electrolyte abnormalities or significant abdominal distension, which may embarrass respiratory function. The treatment includes placement of bladder catheter, which often relieves the pressure in the urinary tract and controls the extravasation. Percutaneous drainage or nephrostomy is considered if extravasation persists and/or serum creatinine continues to rise.[1]

MANAGEMENT AFTER INITIAL SURGICAL THERAPY

The infants need close urologic follow-up through childhood to puberty. Antibiotic prophylaxis is continued till the upper tract dilation resolves. If the urinary stream is not satisfactory, cystoscopy is repeated with ablation of any residual valve.

The common clinical problems encountered after valve ablation are polyuria, metabolic acidosis, hypertension, hypocalcemia, and hyperphosphatemia. The follow-up is undertaken with the support of a pediatric nephrologist aiming at optimizing renal and bladder function and preventing recurrent urinary infection.

Patients with good somatic growth are followed up with periodic ultrasound KUB, renal function tests (RFT), electrolyte assay, urinalysis, and blood pressure monitoring. Bicarbonate supplementation for managing acidosis and vitamin D_3 therapy for hypocalcemia are also considered.[1]

MANAGEMENT AFTER INITIAL URINARY DIVERSION

Undiversion vesicostomy or ureterostomy depends largely on the status of renal function and also the indication for which the procedure was initially undertaken. The diversion may have to be continued in a patient with severe renal impairment till transplantation is underway.

PROGNOSIS AFTER INITIAL THERAPY

Long-term prognosis for renal function in PUV after primary valve ablation depends on several factors. Serum creatinine is the single-most important factor predicting prognosis. Serum creatinine value <0.8 mg/dL at 1 month and 1 year after initial therapy is found to be an indicator of good prognosis. If the nadir creatinine (lowest serum creatinine) is <0.4 mg/dL the risk for ESKD is low whereas if it is >0.8 the risk for renal failure is high. The creatinine values in between carry an intermediate risk for chronic kidney disease (CKD).[1] Pop-off mechanisms such as unilateral high-grade VUR (VURD), large bladder diverticula, and urinary extravasation are considered to lower pressure and protect kidneys from damage. Lack of CMD, echogenic kidneys, and renal cortical cysts (RD) suggest a poor prognosis. Bilateral VUR, bilateral hydronephrosis, recurrent febrile UTI, proteinuria, and failure to achieve daytime bladder control by 5 years of age are factors predicting poor renal outcome.[1]

VESICOURETERAL REFLUX IN POSTERIOR URETHRAL VALVES

Vesicoureteral reflux is seen in 30–50% of the patients with PUV.[1,5] Unilateral and bilateral reflux is present in an equal distribution. VUR resolves over time in about 50% of the patients with primary valve treatment alone if there is no bladder dysfunction. Higher grades of reflux do not resolve. Surgical intervention is considered for persistent reflux in the form of endoscopic injection of dextranomer/hyaluronidase or reimplantation of ureters.

HYDRONEPHROSIS IN POSTERIOR URETHRAL VALVES

Hydroureteronephrosis is a constant finding in almost all children with PUV.[8] The ureters may remain dilated even in the absence of VUR for many years after valve ablation. Often, there is no obstruction at VUJ or bladder outlet.[4] These nonreflexing and nonobstructing hydroureters improve over time and surgical treatment is usually not indicated.

BLADDER DYSFUNCTION

In patients with PUV, bladder function may remain abnormal even after the relief of obstruction. The term valve bladder syndrome (Mitchel 1986) is often used to describe a noncompliant thick-walled bladder, with persistent upper tract dilatation, incontinence, and nephrogenic diabetes insipidus.[1,9,10] Poor urinary stream, incontinence, and recurrent urinary tract infection are common complaints after valve ablation. Daytime incontinence is seen in about 50% of the boys with PUV.[1] The incontinence, which was earlier attributed to sphincteric incompetence, is now considered to be due to abnormal detrusor function that persists after valve ablation.[11,12] The polyuria due to impaired tubular function, detrusor sphincter dyssynergia, and high-pressure voiding due to incomplete valve ablation also contribute to incontinence.[1,9,10]

Urodynamic studies show that the pattern of bladder abnormalities after valve ablation changes with the age of the child but with considerable overlap during childhood and through adolescence.[1,13,14] Hypertonic small capacity bladder with poor compliance, hyper-reflexic bladder with uninhibited contractions, and myogenic failure with Valsalva voiding and overflow incontinence are the three common patterns seen in PUV.[12,15] Hypercontractility is seen in young children after fulguration and this progresses to hypocontractility and myogenic failure. Older boys and adolescents have large capacity bladder with poor contractility and incomplete emptying.[1] The bladder dysfunction in PUV needs active intervention and the management strategy is planned in accordance with the urodynamic findings and the clinical situation. The primary goal is to achieve proper bladder emptying. Anticholinergics such as oxybutynin are used to control uninhibited bladder contractions and alpha blockers (terazosin) to overcome bladder neck obstruction. Measures such as behavioral modification, timed voiding, clean intermittent catheterization (CIC), and overnight bladder drainage are employed to keep the bladder empty. If the conservative measures fail, bladder augmentation with enterocystoplasty or ureterocystoplasty is undertaken **(Table 2)**.

END-STAGE KIDNEY DISEASE AND RENAL TRANSPLANTATION

In spite of optimal treatment, 15–20% of patients with PUV develop ESKD.[5] The prognostic factors predicting poor renal outcome have already been discussed. Renal transplantation is safe and effective, and the graft survival is similar to that of children with nonobstructive causes of renal failure. However, if the bladder dysfunction is not corrected, it can contribute to transplant graft dysfunction.[16,17]

SEXUAL FUNCTION AND FERTILITY

Posterior urethral dilatation, open bladder neck, and the possibility of vasal reflux raise concern toward normal

TABLE 2: Bladder dysfunction (Valve Bladder Syndrome)—management strategy.

Management options	*Benefits*
Anticholinergics (oxybutynin 0.2 mg/kg/day in 2–4 divided doses)	Control detrusor overactivity
Alpha blockers (terazosin 0.25–2 mg)	Improves bladder emptying
• Timed voiding • CIC • Nocturnal bladder drainage	Keeps the bladder empty and stabilize function
Surgical options • Mitrofanoff appendicovesicostomy • Bladder augmentation – Enterocystoplasty – Ureterocystoplasty	• Makes CIC easier • Improve bladder storage function

(CIC: clean intermittent catheterization)

sexual function in adults treated for PUV during childhood. Retrograde ejaculation, decreased libido associated with renal failure, and association of cryptorchidism are other contributing factors.[11] Available data suggest that erectile dysfunction and paternity rates in PUV are similar to those of the general population.[18] Total semen counts and motility are found to be compatible with paternity in most patients.[19]

CONCLUSION

Posterior urethral valve is the most common obstructive urological disorder leading to end-stage kidney disease in boys. Though antenatal diagnosis of hydronephrosis is an important finding that prompts postnatal exclusion of PUV, late detection and improper bladder management, pose major long-term challenges.

KEY POINTS

- Characteristic antenatal ultrasonographic signs such as hydronephrosis, oligohydramnios, megacystitis, thickened bladder, and keyhole appearance help in the identification of PUV.
- Differential diagnosis to PUV includes anterior urethral valves and urethral atresia.
- Neonates can present with urinary obstruction, kidney dysfunction, metabolic acidosis, dyselectrolytemia, and urinary infection.
- Bladder dysfunction can persist even after relief of obstruction and needs evaluation and medical management and rarely surgical intervention.
- Valve ablation and urinary diversion procedures are the mainstay surgical interventions.
- Associated RD, nadir creatinine < 0.8 mg/dL at 1 year of age, and bladder dysfunction have an impact on the long-term outcomes of PUV.

REFERENCES

1. Elder JS, Shapiro E. Posterior urethral valves. Holcomb and Ashcraft's Pediatric Surgery, 7th edition. Philadelphia: Elsevier; 2020. pp. 884-96.
2. Patrick Murphy J, Gatti JM. Abnormalities of urethra, penis, and scrotum. In: Coran AG (Ed). Pediatric Surgery, 7th edition. 2012. Philadelphia: Elsevier; pp. 1555-7.
3. Hodges SJ, Patel B, McLorie G, Atala A. Posterior urethral valves. Sci World J. 2009;9:1119-26.
4. Casale AJ. Posterior urethral valves. In: Campbell-Walsh Urology, 10th edition. Philadelphia: Saunders; 2011. pp. 3389-406.
5. Sharma S, Joshi M, Gupta DK, Abraham M, Mathur P, Mahajan JK, et al. Consensus on the management of posterior urethral valves from antenatal period to puberty. J Indian Assoc Pediatr Surg. 2019;24:4-14.
6. Holmes N, Harrison MR, Baskin LS. Fetal surgery for posterior urethral valves: long-term postnatal outcomes. Pediatrics. 2001;108(1):E7. s
7. Luks FI. Re: Fetal intervention for severe lower urinary tract obstruction: a multicenter case-control study comparing fetal cystoscopy with vesicoamniotic shunting. Runano R, Sananes N, Sangi-Haghpeykar H, Hernandez-Ruano S, Moog R, Becmeur F, et al. Ultrasound Obstet Gynecol. 2015;45:452-8. Ultrasound Obstet Gynecol. 2015;45(4):375-6.
8. Churchill BM, McLorie GA, Khoury AE, Merguerian PA, Houle AM. Emergency treatment and long-term follow-up of posterior urethral valves. Urol Clin North Am. 1990;17(2):343-60.
9. Glassberg KI. The valve bladder syndrome: 20 years later. J Urol. 2001;166(4):1406-14.
10. Koff SA, Mutabagani KH, Jayanthi VR. The valve bladder syndrome: pathophysiology and treatment with nocturnal bladder emptying. J Urol. 2002;167(1):291-7.
11. Parkhouse HF, Woodhouse CR. Long-term status of patients with posterior urethral valves. Urol Clin North Am. 1990;17(2):373-8.
12. Peters CA, Bauer SB. Evaluation and management of urinary incontinence after surgery for posterior urethral valves. Urol Clin North Am. 1990;17(2):379-87.
13. Wani SA, Jadhav V, Munianjana NB. Urodynamic changes with age in boys with posterior urethral valves. Med Surg Urol. 2020;9(4).
14. Polak-Jonkisz D, Rehan LR, Fornalczyk K, Hackemer P, Zwolińska D. Valve bladder syndrome in children: on the trail of the best strategies to prevent chronic kidney disease. Adv Clin Exp Med. 2017;26(8):1293-300.
15. Thomas J. Etiopathogenesis and management of bladder dysfunction in patients with posterior urethral valves. Indian J Urol. 2010;26:480-9.
16. Otukesh H, Basiri A, Simfroosh N, Hoseini R, Fereshtehnejad SM, Chalian M. Kidney transplantation in children with posterior urethral valves. Pediatr Transplant. 2008;12(5):516-9.
17. DeFoor W, Tackett L, Minevich E, McEnery P, Kitchens D, Reeves D, et al. Successful renal transplantation in children with posterior urethral valves. J Urol. 2003;170(6 Pt 1):2402-4.
18. Taskinen S, Heikkilä J, Santtila P, Rintala R. Posterior urethral valves and adult sexual function. BJU Int. 2012;110(8 Pt B):E392-6.
19. López Pereira P, Miguel M, Martínez Urrutia MJ, Moreno JA, Marcos M, Lobato R, et al. Long-term bladder function, fertility and sexual function in patients with posterior urethral valves treated in infancy. J Pediatr Urol. 2013;9(1):38-41.

CHAPTER

13.8 Neurogenic Bladder

Sukanya Govindan, Saravanan M, Sripathi V

INTRODUCTION

The term "neurogenic bladder" refers to a condition where the bladder cannot store urine at low pressures nor can it empty completely. Myelomeningocele (MMC) and sacral anomalies are the most common causes.[1,2] However, occult spinal conditions, which cause tethering of the cord during growth, should be kept in mind. Pelvic surgery in a child can result in lasting injury to the sacral outflow (anorectal malformation correction, pull through for Hirschsprung's disease, and surgery for cloaca). Posterior urethral valve disease, ectopic ureterocele, or any form of bladder outlet obstruction (including voiding dysfunction) can ultimately lead to "neurogenic bladder." The term "non-neurogenic neurogenic" refers to a child presenting with a neurogenic bladder but without any spinal abnormality or urethral obstruction. This was formerly called "Hinman's syndrome."[3]

PRESENTATION

Recurrent urinary tract infections (UTIs), wetting, and encopresis are the usual presenting features. Sustained high bladder pressures [with or without vesicoureteral reflux (VUR)] often result in severe renal scarring, chronic kidney disease (CKD), and ultimately end-stage kidney disease (ESKD). Early identification of lower urinary tract (LUT) dysfunction and initiation of treatment are essential. 60–80% of the children with neurogenic bladder develop recurrent UTIs and renal damage within the first years of life. Without treatment, <5% achieve dryness.[3]

EVALUATION OF A CHILD WITH NEUROGENIC BLADDER

The key element in evaluation is the identification of abnormal urinary tract function. Significant changes to the degree and type of LUT dysfunction can occur during the first 6 years of life and at puberty, as rapid linear growth causes tethering of the cord and traction on the sacral nerves. The currently available tools for assessment include history, clinical examination, renal and bladder ultrasound (RBUS), voiding cystourethrogram (VCUG), urodynamics, and renal function assessment including isotope scans.

History

A comprehensive history of bowel and bladder habits is essential and can give useful information on the type of LUT dysfunction (graphically seen in a bladder diary). The International Children's Continence Society (ICCS) published an update on the standardization of terminology for defining LUT symptoms, and both doctors and parents/caretakers should use this to define and quantify symptoms.[4]

History should include *assessment of LUT symptoms* such as frequency, urgency, intermittency, incontinence, or any UTI; *assessment of completeness of bladder evacuation* with each void (postvoid residue measurement); and *assessment of stooling history* such as frequency and consistency of stool and stool accidents (encopresis). Bowel dysfunction influences bladder function, hence the term "bladder–bowel dysfunction" (BBD). *Review of antenatal records* including the growth of the head, renal growth, and amniotic fluid index is important. *Review of milestones* including motor, adaptive, language, and social behavior should be part of the assessment.

Clinical Examination

A thorough clinical examination with specific focus on motor power, tone, and reflexes in combination with history can often give clues to the level of spinal lesion and status of the bladder. Postnatally, the first assessment should include the movement of lower limbs, voiding, and defecation. Examination for neurocutaneous markers must be done. These include midline hemangioma, sinus tracts, sacral pits, and tufts of hair. All these signs (including ammoniacal dermatitis due to wetting) might indicate an underlying "spina bifida occulta". Note should also be made of fontanelle widening, splitting of cranial sutures, and dysmorphic features.

The following signs should be looked for in a child with neurological disorders at the first visit and changes or new signs should be sought in subsequent visits: height, weight, head circumference, and gait. Examination of the abdomen will indicate fecal loading (palpable sigmoid), urinary retention (palpable bladder), and leak of urine with abdominal pressure (indicating a lax urethral sphincter). Examination of the musculoskeletal system will show muscle atrophy, limb contractures, hemihypertrophy, muscle tenderness, pes cavus, clubfoot, and trophic ulcers (at pressure points). Palpation for missing sacral segments should be done. The appearance of external genitalia, gluteal fold symmetry, and anal tone should be noted.

Renal and Bladder Ultrasound

An RBUS is done at diagnosis or at birth and thereafter is recommended every 6 months for the first 2 years and yearly thereafter.[3,5] A detailed scan should include kidney size, renal parenchymal thickness (upper, middle, and lower poles), pelvic, and ureteric dilatation. The shape of the bladder, wall thickness, presence of trabeculations, and amount of postvoid residual should be noted.

Asymmetry of kidney size (>1 cm) is suggestive of renal scarring due to recurrent UTIs. Parenchymal thinning is also an indirect measure of nephron loss. Increased bladder wall thickness and trabeculations suggest that the bladder is working against increased "outlet resistance." A "fir tree-like appearance" of the bladder is pathognomonic of the neurogenic bladder **(Fig. 1)**. Large postvoid residue indicates incomplete emptying due to either myogenic failure of the detrusor muscle or detrusor-sphincter dyssynergia (DSD). Any worsening of hydronephrosis or renal asymmetry from baseline warrants repeating investigations such as urodynamics (UDS), VCUG, and functional renal imaging.[3,5]

Voiding Cystourethrogram

A VCUG under fluoroscopy guidance can give information on the presence (and timing) of VUR, presence of trabeculations and sacculation, bladder capacity, bladder outlet, stream, and postvoid residue. In addition, a lateral X-ray of the spine will show if all sacral segments are present. A VCUG should always be done at birth or at diagnosis and then should be done whenever there is a worsening in the status of the urinary tract or when there are new-onset symptoms or signs.[3,5]

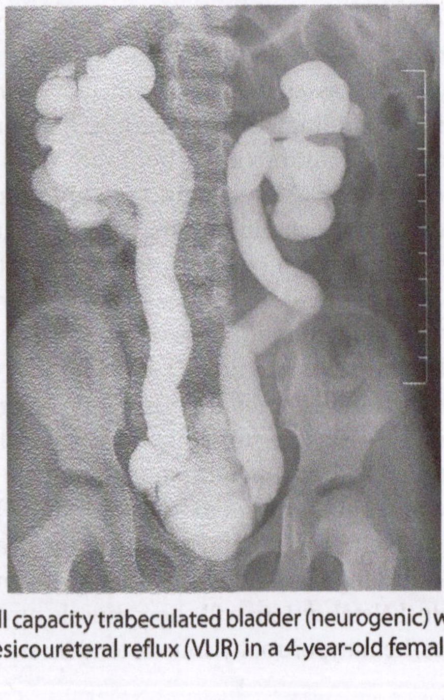

Fig. 1: Small capacity trabeculated bladder (neurogenic) with massive bilateral vesicoureteral reflux (VUR) in a 4-year-old female child.

Urodynamics

The type and level of neurological lesion correlate poorly with LUT dysfunction. The study of bladder pressure during filling and voiding (UDS) helps to clarify the specific LUT dysfunction and leads to appropriate management. Four different combinations of detrusor and sphincter dysfunction can be present: (1) overactive sphincter/overactive detrusor—dangerous to the kidneys, (2) overactive sphincter/underactive detrusor—dangerous to the kidneys, (3) underactive sphincter/overactive detrusor, and (4) underactive sphincter/underactive detrusor.

A UDS should be performed preferably within 6–12 months of age and repeated whenever there is a worsening in the status of the urinary tract as assessed by RBUS or in the presence of new-onset symptoms (such as gait changes, weakness, wetting, urgency, and encopresis).[3,5]

Renal Function Assessment

Renal function is typically assessed by measuring serum creatinine. Recently, cystatin C has been proposed as a better marker of glomerular filtration rate (GFR)[3] as in children with MMC with low muscle mass, serum creatinine will overestimate GFR. Technetium dimercaptosuccinic acid (DMSA) renal scan is the best available functional imaging modality to detect renal scars due to VUR and recurrent UTIs. RBUS is not a sensitive test to detect cortical scars. Progressive renal scarring leads to hypertension, proteinuria, and finally ESKD if left unchecked.

TREATMENT

The care of a child with neurogenic bladder starts right after the closure of MMC. There are two different approaches to bladder management (in newborns and infants): expectant versus proactive. The ICCS recommends *expectant management* wherein patients undergo RBUS every 6 months until 2 years of age. The child is offered clean intermittent catheterization (CIC) or UDS only if there is a clinical deterioration such as worsening hydronephrosis or VUR, increasing postvoid residual volumes, worsening renal function, or recurrent UTIs.[6] The *proactive approach* supports initiating CIC early in the neonatal period and anticholinergics if necessary. UDS is performed after recovery from the neurosurgical closure and annually thereafter.

Whatever be the approach, the goals of treatment include: (1) renal preservation, prevention of UTI, and urinary tract deterioration; (2) achieving bowel and bladder control; (3) normal sexual function and fertility; and (4) normal childhood (with dryness enabling play and interaction with peers).

Medical Management

The main goal is to reduce bladder pressures during filling and eliminate residue after voiding. This can be achieved by initiating anticholinergic therapy to relax the detrusor and starting CIC when emptying is incomplete. In the majority of children with neurogenic bladder, dryness can be obtained with these two measures alone.

Clean Intermittent Catheterization and Nighttime Drainage

Emptying the bladder at regular intervals prevents renal deterioration by lowering pressures and preventing UTIs. CIC is advised every 3 hours and an indwelling catheter is left to drain the bladder overnight [nighttime drainage (NTD)]. These two techniques form the cornerstone of the management of the neurogenic bladder.[1,6]

Anticholinergic Medication

This group of drugs decreases detrusor overactivity and improves bladder compliance by lowering intravesical pressure.[3,6,7] Early use of anticholinergics reduces new-onset renal scarring and may eliminate the need for bladder augmentation.

Muscarinic (M) Blockers—Nonselective and Selective M3 Receptor Blockers

The proposed mechanism of action involves blocking the M3 receptor subtype, which mediates detrusor contraction. The most commonly used anticholinergic agent is *oxybutynin*, which is a nonselective agent blocking both M1 and M3 receptor subtypes. The extended-release preparation is given as a single daily dose of 5 mg (children aged 5 years or more). In younger children, short-acting preparation is given at a dose of 0.2 mg/kg per dose three times a day (or approximately 1 mg/yr of age per dose). Due to its nonselective muscarinic blockade, the following side effects are observed—new-onset constipation, dry mouth, flushing, heat intolerance, and neuropsychiatric effects.

Solifenacin, tolterodine, and *darifenacin* are selective M3 blocking agents. Only solifenacin is approved for usage in children with an overactive bladder (OAB) whereas other agents are not approved in children. Solifenacin is started at a dose of 2 mg/day and increased by 5–10 mg/day depending on the response to therapy.

β3-adrenoceptor Agonists

β3-adrenoreceptor activation results in relaxation of the detrusor smooth muscle during the urine storage phase, thus increasing the bladder capacity.[3,7] β3-agonist mirabegron is commonly used in adults and the usage in children is expanding now. It is reserved for children with OAB which is refractory to treatment with anticholinergics. The starting dosage of mirabegron is 12.5 mg/day and can be increased to 25–50 mg/day depending on the response to therapy. The common side effects are mild-to-moderate dry mouth and gastrointestinal disturbances.

α-adrenergic Agonists

These agents facilitate bladder emptying by relaxing the bladder neck and proximal urethra, thereby facilitating complete emptying and reducing postvoid residuals.[3,8,9] Doxazosin (0.5–2 mg oral daily) and tamsulosin (0.2–0.4 mg oral daily) are commonly used agents.

Biofeedback and Pelvic Floor Muscle Training

Biofeedback therapy teaches children how to identify and control the muscle groups (pelvic floor muscle) involved in voiding.[7] The visual or auditory feedback from noninvasive urodynamic monitoring allows the child to become aware of and gain control over their bladder function. The child is taught how to voluntarily relax (or contract) the urethral sphincter and pelvic diaphragm.

Generally, biofeedback is reserved for children with wetting or constipation (due to BBD) that is resistant to conservative management.

Electrical Stimulation Therapy (Neuromodulation)

In children with OAB refractory to anticholinergics (and behavioral modification), neuromodulation can be tried.[7] This involves noninvasive stimulation of sacral nerves or the posterior tibial nerve. Electrical impulses stimulate spinal inhibitory pathways to relax the detrusor.

Botulinum Toxin (Botox)

Botulinum toxin A is a neurotoxin, which inhibits calcium-mediated release of acetylcholine from nerve terminals.[1,10] This results in a temporary reduction in muscle contraction and muscle atrophy. When injected into the detrusor or the external sphincter, spastic overactivity is abolished. The effect of Botox is temporary and lasts for approximately 3–6 months. The use of Botox injection in children with refractory overactivity or detrusor-sphincter dyssynergia is well established.

OTHER ASPECTS OF MEDICAL MANAGEMENT

Bowel Dysfunction

Treatment options (for refractory constipation) include rectal suppositories or enemas, long-term oral laxatives, and use of the malone antegrade continence enema (MACE) procedure.[3,11] The MACE procedure enables antegrade washouts of fecal matter from the entire colon and rectum.

Urinary Tract Infection

Asymptomatic bacteriuria is seen in many children on CIC and does not warrant treatment. Febrile UTIs should be promptly treated and recurrent UTIs in infancy may warrant long-term uroprophylaxis to reduce scarring.

Sexuality and Fertility

Counseling adolescents with neurogenic bladder should be an integral part of management. Females with neurogenic

TABLE 1: Therapeutic strategies for children with neurogenic bladder.

Overactive bladder	*Underactive bladder*
Lifestyle changes: • Delayed voiding • Scheduled voiding • Pelvic floor exercises • Bladder diary • Dietary changes	*Lifestyle changes:* • Scheduled voiding • Double voiding • Bladder diary • Dietary changes
Drugs: • Anticholinergic agents • Oxybutynin (nonselective) • Solifenacin, tolterodine, darifenacin (M3 blockers) • β-3 agonists—mirabegron	*Drugs:* • Avoid anticholinergics • If urine retention—alpha blocker—tamsulosin, doxazosin
Neuromodulation: • Sacral nerve • Peripheral tibial nerve	*Catheters:* • CIC—clean intermittent catheterization • Continuous
Botulinum toxin A	*Surgery:* Appendix Mitrofanoff for painless catheterization
Non-neurogenic dysfunctional voiding: • Pelvic floor relaxation exercises • Biofeedback • Drug—α antagonist	

bladder have a higher risk of precocious puberty. Women with spinal dysraphism (SD) have 1–5% chance of having a child with SD and need to be on folic acid and vitamin B_{12} supplements before planning pregnancy. Pregnant women with SD have a higher risk of premature labor, uterine prolapse, etc.

Table 1 summarizes the therapeutic strategies for children with neurogenic bladder.

Surgery

In children with a neurogenic bladder, surgery is commonly used to alter the urinary tract for safe storage of urine and/or to achieve continence. Bladder augmentation is done in children with high bladder pressures, which are deleterious to the upper tracts. Bladder capacity is increased by adding an isolated segment of bowel to the bladder (augmentation cystoplasty). Artificial sphincter/bladder neck tightening is done in those children who leak at low filling pressures.[1,12]

In those children who find it impossible to do CIC due to a sensate urethra, an appendix Mitrofanoff channel can be created to allow painless access to the bladder.[12]

CONCLUSION

Neurogenic bladder is a complex disorder and should be managed by a multidisciplinary team of urologists, nephrologists, and pediatricians. A thorough clinical and radiological assessment is essential to identify and treat LUT dysfunction. Antimuscarinic drugs and CIC should be used early to reduce detrusor overactivity. Intravesical injection of Botox and bladder augmentation surgery is required by a small subset of patients who fail to respond to conservative measures.

KEY POINTS

- Early identification of LUT dysfunction and initiation of treatment are essential to prevent the risk of UTI and upper tract damage.
- The goals of therapy include achieving urinary continence, preventing renal damage, and minimizing the risk of UTI.
- Clean intermittent catheterization and drugs to reduce bladder pressure and increase compliance such as anticholinergic agents are the mainstay of treatment.

REFERENCES

1. Sripathi V, Mitra A. Management of neurogenic bladder. Indian J Pediatr. 2017;84(7):545-54.
2. Le H, Cardona-Grau D, Chiang G. Evaluation and long-term management of neurogenic bladder in spinal dysraphism. NeoReviews. 2019;20(12):e711-24.
3. Stein R, Bogaert G, Dogan H, Hoen L, Kocvara R, Nijman R, et al. EAU/ESPU guidelines on the management of neurogenic bladder in children and adolescent part I diagnostics and conservative treatment. Neurourol Urodyn. 2020;39(1):45-57.
4. Austin PF, Bauer SB, Bower W, Chase J, Franco I, Hoebeke P, et al. The standardization of terminology of lower urinary tract function in children and adolescents: update report from the standardization committee of the International Children's Continence Society. Neurourol Urodyn. 2016;35(4):471-81.
5. Bauer SB, Austin PF, Rawashdeh YF, de Jong TP, Franco I, Siggard C, et al. International Children's Continence Society's recommendations for initial diagnostic evaluation and follow-up in congenital neuropathic bladder and bowel dysfunction in children. Neurourol Urodyn. 2012;31(5):610-4.
6. Rawashdeh YF, Austin P, Siggaard C, Bauer SB, Franco I, de Jong TP, et al. International Children's Continence Society's recommendations for therapeutic intervention in congenital neuropathic bladder and bowel dysfunction in children. Neurourol Urodyn. 2012;31(5):615-20.
7. Yang S, Chua ME, Bauer S, Wright A, Brandström P, Hoebeke P, et al. Diagnosis and management of bladder bowel dysfunction in children with urinary tract infections: a position statement from the International Children's Continence Society. Pediatr Nephrol. 2018;33(12):2207-19.
8. Cain MP, Wu SD, Austin PF, Herndon CD, Rink RC. Alpha blocker therapy for children with dysfunctional voiding and urinary retention. J Urol. 2003;170:1514-5.
9. Santos JD, Lopes RI, Koyle MA. Bladder and bowel dysfunction in children: an update on the diagnosis and treatment of a common, but underdiagnosed pediatric problem. Can Urol Assoc J. 2017;11(1-2 Suppl1):S64-72.
10. Cooley LF, Kielb S. A review of botulinum toxin A for the treatment of neurogenic bladder. PM R. 2019;11(2):192-200.
11. Sripathi V. Voiding dysfunction - a review. J Indian Assoc Pediatr Surg. 2005;10(4):229.
12. Stein R, Bogaert G, Dogan HS, Hoen L, Kocvara R, Nijman RJM, et al. EAU/ESPU guidelines on the management of neurogenic bladder in children and adolescent part II operative management. Neurourol Urodyn. 2020;39(2):498-506.

CHAPTER

13.9 Nephrolithiasis

Mehul A Shah

INTRODUCTION

Renal stone disease has been reported since several centuries, including from ancient India, based on archeological findings and ancient medical literature.[1] It was well-perceived to be an adult health care concern in the previous century with children accounting for 1% of total patients. The incidence is lower in children likely due to the higher concentration of citrate and magnesium that are natural inhibitors of crystal formation in urine. However, it is now recognized that pediatric nephrolithiasis is an increasing entity with a three-fold increase in the past three decades and now accounting for ~4% of total patients.[2] The incidence in children increases with age and risk is highest amongst the adolescents. As with adults, there are stone-endemic areas in the world like the Afro-Asian stone belt that includes Sudan, Egypt, Saudi Arabia, UAE, Iran, Pakistan, India, Myanmar, Thailand, Indonesia, and Philippines. Dry arid climate, dietary habits, malnutrition, and infections are the major factors associated with endemicity of urolithiasis. In India, certain states such as Maharashtra, Gujarat, Rajasthan, Punjab, Haryana, Delhi, Madhya Pradesh, Bihar, and West Bengal are known to have a higher incidence of renal stone disease.[3] There are few studies that have evaluated pediatric stone disease in India. In one recent study from central India, 1,341 children with kidney stones were identified over a 10-year period.[4]

Multiple factors have contributed to the increased incidence of pediatric nephrolithiasis including increased intake of salt, animal protein, and processed foods; global warming (factors related to urbanization); and reduced intake of water and fruits as well as advances in imaging techniques. The most important factor is the three- to six-fold increase in salt intake, especially in urban children. In children, positive family history of nephrolithiasis, underlying metabolic abnormality in 20–90%, and anatomical abnormalities in 10–18% children (below 2 years) are noted.[5,6] Recurrence of stones in up to 50% of children has been reported, especially those with an underlying metabolic abnormality.[5] Pediatric nephrolithiasis contributes to significant morbidity (severe pain, hospital visits, acute pyelonephritis, acute kidney injury, requirement of procedures, economic burden) and chronic kidney disease (CKD). Hence, it is important to evaluate a child with nephrolithiasis for appropriate dietary modification, targeted therapy, counseling, and reducing risk of recurrence as well as CKD.

PATHOGENESIS

The three main factors responsible for precipitation of salts in urine include the following:

1. Increased excretion of various solutes that *promote* stone formation (calcium, oxalate, uric acid, cystine, and xanthine)
2. Decreased urinary excretion of *crystal inhibitors* such as citrate, magnesium, pyrophosphate, and macromolecules (Tamm-Horsfall protein and osteopontin)
3. *Low urinary water excretion* (mainly due to decreased water intake)

The most common risk factors include low urinary flow rate (<1 mL/kg/h), hypercalciuria, and hypocitraturia. In addition, anatomic abnormalities of the urinary tract that result in obstruction, stasis, and infection [pelviureteric junction obstruction (PUJO), ureterovesical junction obstruction (UVJO) obstruction, neurogenic bladder post-augmentation cystoplasty, or vesicoureteric reflux (VUR)] as well as certain medications can predispose to stone formation. Often, there are multiple factors contributing to renal stone disease. Conversely, adequate water intake to maintain a dilute urine reducing concentrations of salt-forming solutes and adequate crystal inhibitors in urine would reduce the risk of stone formation. In children, calcium-based stones are more common and uric acid stones less common than in the adult population.[7] This is likely related to the higher urinary pH within a pediatric population compared to in adults.

The basic pathophysiology in stone formation is a change from solubility to supersaturation where the dissolved salts condense into solids. Supersaturation is the point at which the salts crystallize, and precipitate out of the solution, whereas solubility is the opposite where the solute stays dissolved in the solution. When calcium oxalate supersaturation is higher than its solubility, the dissolved calcium oxalate can form nuclei of its solid phase, a process called as nucleation. Nuclei usually form on an existing surface such as Randall's plaques (calcium phosphate deposits) at renal papillae, cell debris, bacterial debris, urinary casts, and other crystals.

Randall's plaque formation depends on calcium phosphate supersaturation at the tip of the renal papilla and precede the development of kidney stones. Hence, stone formation requires the formation of a nidus in the urinary tract. When this nidus gets trapped, then a large crystal structure is formed on it. The main determinants of calcium oxalate supersaturation are urine volume and urine calcium & oxalate concentration. For calcium phosphate supersaturation, urine volume, urine calcium concentration, and urine pH are the determining factors, whereas urinary pH is the main determinant of uric acid supersaturation.

Although there is a risk of stone formation in humans due to the chemical constituents, there are natural inhibitors of crystal formation that prevent stone formation.[8] The most important inhibitor is urinary citrate. *Citrate* is a natural inhibitor of stone formation. This occurs due to its chelating effect on calcium-forming calcium citrate that is several fold more soluble in urine than calcium oxalate. Similarly, *pyrophosphate*, a polyvalent anion with a high affinity for polyvalent cations like Ca^{2+} inhibits both calcium oxalate and calcium phosphate crystallization. It is a naturally occurring substance found in nuts, legumes, poultry, eggs, and fish. Pyrophosphates are also widely used during food processing and in canned foods to maintain color and freshness. *Phytate*, a natural compound in plant-derived foods, acts as an inhibitor of calcium crystallization in the urine. *Magnesium* is another important inhibitor of stone formation. Magnesium binds to intestinal oxalate and reduces intestinal oxalate absorption. It also reduces urinary oxalate concentration by binding to oxalate in urinary lumen forming magnesium oxalate complexes that are 100 times more soluble than calcium. Magnesium also corrects intracellular acidosis that reduces proximal tubular citrate reabsorption and increases tubular citrate excretion. Other inhibitors of calcium-based stone formation which have been described are the *urinary macromolecules* such as osteopontin, calgranulin, Tamm-Horsfall glycoprotein, albumin, and glycosaminoglycans. All these substances have in common long stretches of polyanion chains that can bond with surface calcium atoms and prevent crystal growth.

The pathophysiology of *endemic calculi*, noted in malnourished children, is related to imbalance in dietary factors. They have almost disappeared from the western world about a century ago and decreased in developing countries with improvement in nutrition. The main factors contributing to the formation of bladder calculi are high intake of cereals (whole wheat, millets, and pulses), high intake of oxalate through green leafy vegetables (promoters), and low intake of animal protein/milk (reduced calcium and phosphate intake) as well as deficient magnesium and citrate intake (inhibitors). This carbohydrate-rich diet is acidogenic and low in phosphate resulting in increased urinary ammonium excretion as there is now limited urinary phosphate available as a buffer. Also, due to rapid growth, urinary uric acid excretion is higher in younger children. Dehydration secondary to recurrent infectious diarrhea related to unsafe drinking water and hot weather conditions leads to decreased urinary volume, metabolic acidosis, increased urinary ammonium excretion and reduced urinary citrate excretion (in response to acidemia), and increased urine pH. Combination of higher ammonium, urate, and oxalate in a concentrated urine with higher pH leads to precipitation, crystallization, and stone formation in the bladder (ammonium urate oxalate stone). In summary, higher concentration of promoting factors, reduced inhibitor concentration, and reduced urine volumes are responsible for bladder calculi in developing countries.[9]

ETIOLOGY

The etiological factors can be broadly divided into four main groups:

1. Metabolic causes in 20–90% (most common)
2. Anatomic abnormalities—PUJO, UVJO, VUR, neurogenic bladder, in up to 15%, especially in children younger than 2 years
3. Medications—frusemide, ceftriaxone, sulfa drugs, vitamin C, indinavir, allopurinol
4. Endemic calculi (mostly bladder stones)

Metabolic Causes

Metabolic causes are the most common factors and can be identified in 20–90% cases depending upon how aggressively they are looked for.[7,10,11] These include hypercalciuria, hyperoxaluria (primary and secondary), hyperuricosuria, cystinuria, xanthinuria, and hypocitraturia. An underlying metabolic abnormality often leads to bilateral stone disease, more severe presentation, and is also a risk factor for recurrent stone disease.

Specific metabolic findings and their frequency in children with an identifiable metabolic abnormality include the following:

- Hypercalciuria—45–75%
- Hyperoxaluria—10–20%
- Hyperuricosuria—2–8%
- Cystinuria—5%
- Hypocitraturia—10%

Normocalcemic Hypercalciuria

Normocalcemic hypercalciuria is the most common metabolic abnormality and accounts for 45–75% of metabolic causes of pediatric nephrolithiasis. It is defined as urinary calcium excretion of >4 mg/kg/day or random urine calcium creatinine ratio >0.20 (in children >2 years of age) **(Table 1)**. The etiology of hypercalciuria is usually idiopathic and is most commonly due to increased gastrointestinal absorption of calcium (absorptive hypercalciuria). Other causes include distal renal tubular acidosis (RTA), familial hypomagnesemic hypercalciuric nephrocalcinosis (FHHNC), Dent disease, medications (furosemide, vitamin D, corticosteroids), etc.

TABLE 1: Reference urinary values of solutes in 24-hour and random urine samples.[12,13]

Solute	*Normal urine value in 24-hour urine collection*	*Random urine sample for solute and creatinine in mg/dL*
Calcium	<4 mg/kg/day	Infants <6 months; <0.8 6 months to 2 years; <0.5 >2 years; <0.20
Oxalate	<50 mg/1.73 m²/day	<0.06
Cystine	<60 mg/1.73 m²/day	• All ages; <0.02 • Screening test with cyanide + nitroprusside = purple color
Citrate	>400 mg/g creatinine	
Uric acid	• <11.5 mg/kg/day (<3 years) • <10 mg/kg/day (>3 years)	• >3 years; <0.56 mg/dL glomerular filtration rate • [Urine uric acid/urine creatinine] × serum creatinine <0.56 mg/dL in >2 years • Urine creatinine

Hypercalcemia is an extremely rare cause of hypercalciuria in children. Often, microscopic hematuria or lower urinary tract infection (UTI) due to hypercalciuria precedes the development of renal stones.

Hyperoxaluria

Hyperoxaluria is the second common metabolic abnormality, noted in 10–20% children, and is defined as urinary oxalate >50 mg/1.73 m²/day. Oxalate is an end product of glycine, serine, and hydroxyproline metabolism and is excreted through the kidney. The toxicity of oxalate in humans results from the extreme insolubility of its calcium salt, calcium oxalate, which may precipitate in the renal parenchyma or renal tract, causing either nephrocalcinosis or stones. Hyperoxaluria could be primary or secondary. Primary hyperoxaluria (PH) results from increased synthesis in liver and is related to the deficiency of hepatic enzyme involved in oxalate metabolism. PH is of three types—type 1, due to defect in alanine-glyoxylate aminotransferase (AGT) enzyme; type 2, due to defect in glyoxylate reductase/hydroxypyruvate reductase (GR/HPR); and type 3, due to defect in hydroxy-2-oxoglutarate aldolase (HOGA).[14] Secondary hyperoxaluria, uncommon in children, is caused by gastrointestinal malabsorption, inflammatory bowel disease, pancreatitis, cystic fibrosis [all resulting in increased gastrointestinal (GI) absorption of oxalate], and excess vitamin C ingestion (increased hepatic production). Rarely, ethylene glycol (present in antifreeze solution) poisoning can cause hyperoxaluria.

Primary hyperoxaluria type 1 is caused by a deficiency of the liver-specific peroxisomal enzyme AGT that requires pyridoxal phosphate as a cofactor and catalyzes the transamination of glyoxylate to glycine. In PH type 1, AGT deficiency allows the glyoxylate to diffuse through the peroxisomal membrane into the cytosol where it is oxidized to oxalate catalyzed by lactate dehydrogenase and subsequently excreted in urine. Patients who have the Gly170Arg or Phe152Ile mutation have a better overall outcome than other patients with type 1 disease, partly because of their sensitivity to pyridoxine. The exact mechanism of pyridoxine is unknown but may be related to increase in expression, activity, and peroxisomal targeting of AGT enzyme.[11] PH1 accounts for 70–80% of all PH cases. One subtype of PH type 1 is infantile hyperoxaluria that results in rapid progression to end-stage kidney disease (ESKD), especially after an episode of dehydration. About 70–80% of nonpyridoxine-sensitive patients with PH type 1 progress to ESKD within the first two decades. Renal damage is caused by a combination of tubular toxicity from oxalate, nephrocalcinosis (with both intratubular and interstitial deposits of calcium oxalate), and renal obstruction by stones, often with superimposed infection. With progressive decrease in glomerular filtration rate (GFR), oxalate excretion is reduced with increase in blood oxalate level. When the plasma oxalate level increases above 50 µmol/L, its solubility in plasma is exceeded with subsequent deposition of oxalate in tissues including skeleton, eyes, myocardium, and arteries (systemic oxalosis). PH type 2 is also associated with renal stone disease and nephrocalcinosis but with a delayed presentation in the first decade. PH type 2, initially thought to have more favorable prognosis than type 1, is also associated with progressive CKD and ESKD. In comparison, PH type 3 can be asymptomatic in 20% and has a benign course relative to other two types with only recurrent stone disease noted in adults.

Hyperuricosuria

Hyperuricosuria is defined as uric acid excretion of greater than 11.5 mg/kg in children less than 3 years and >10 mg/kg in children more than 3 years age. The urinary uric acid excretion is fairly constant after 2 years of age. It is observed in 2–8% of children with nephrolithiasis, and could be primary related to reduced reabsorption of urate in renal tubules (hyperuricosuric hypouricemia) or increased production (lymphoreticular malignancy, Lesch-Nyhan syndrome). The primary sources of uric acid are endogenous breakdown of purine and from dietary ingestion of purines present in animal proteins. Uric acid crystallization occurs in acidic urine pH and concentrated urine. In young children with acute gastroenteritis-associated dehydration, uric acid gravel in both ureters can cause anuric acute kidney injury. The only clue could be mild hydroureteronephrosis in the above clinical settling. Uric acid stones are radiolucent due to the absence of sulfur content.

Inherited Xanthinuria

Inherited xanthinuria is a rare autosomal recessive disorder of purine metabolism leading to the accumulation of xanthine and hypoxanthine. There are two types—type 1 due to the deficiency of only xanthine oxidase enzyme that converts hypoxanthine to xanthine and xanthine to uric acid and type 2, xanthine oxidase combined with aldehyde oxidase deficiency (required for the conversion of allopurinol to oxypurinol). Very rarely, it may be caused due to the defect of a molybdenum-containing cofactor. Children will present with orange-to-brown discoloration of urine, recurrent stones, and very low blood uric acid level (<2 mg/dL). Xanthine stones, such as uric acid stones, develop in acidic urine and are radiolucent. Acquired xanthinuria is due to allopurinol treatment in patients with tumor lysis syndrome, administered to block uric acid production, and can rarely cause xanthine crystal nephropathy [acute kidney injury (AKI)].

Cystinuria

Cystinuria is a rare and only pure genetic cause of metabolic renal stone disease, noted in <5% children. Cystinuria is caused by mutations in the *SLC3A1* and *SLC7A9* genes resulting in defective basic amino acid transport protein (rBAT). This prevents proximal tubular reabsorption of dibasic or positively charged amino acids: cystine, ornithine, arginine, and lysine. Only cystine precipitates in acidic urine causing cystine calculi. The cystine transporter defect is also present in intestinal cells but does not contribute to the pathology. Cystinuria is diagnosed by identifying hexagonal-shaped cystine crystals in urine, 24 hours' urine cystine >60 mg/1.73 m^2/day or random urine cystine creatinine ratio of >0.02, stone analysis, and mutation analysis **(Figs. 1A to E)**.

Hypocitraturia

Hypocitraturia is noted in 10–50% of children with renal calculi and is defined as urine citrate to creatinine <0.4. Etiology includes polygenetic, high animal protein intake; chronic metabolic academia including distal RTA; and hypokalemia. Citrate is partly produced in Krebs cycle and partly introduced

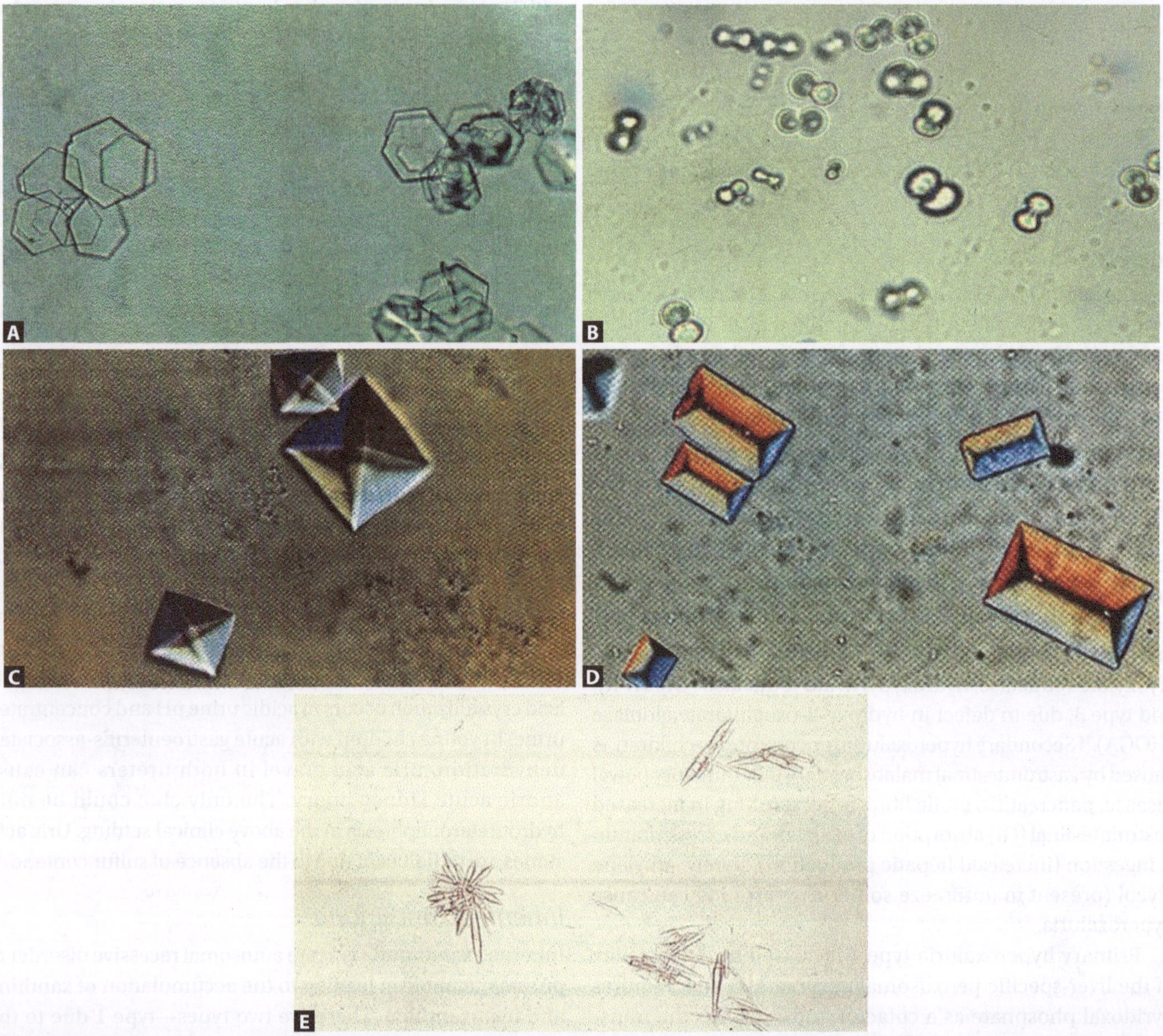

Figs. 1A to E: Various urinary crystals that provide clue to the etiology of nephrolithiasis. (A) Hexagonal crystals in cystinuria; (B) Dumbbell crystals of calcium carbonate stone; (C) Envelop-shaped crystals in hyperoxaluria; (D) Coffin-lid crystals of struvite stones; (E) Rosette/pointed fingers crystals of calcium phosphate stones.

by consumption of citric foods such as lemons, oranges, and grapefruit.[15] Hypocitraturia can be isolated or associated with other metabolic conditions such as hypercalciuria or hyperoxaluria. Urinary citrate deficiency can be corrected by reducing protein intake or by the exogenous supplementation of potassium citrate. A dosage of 0.25–1 mEq/kg is considered safe and does not expose the patient to risk of hyperkalemia or any other adverse events, such as stomach pain, which can disrupt the treatment adherence.

Ketogenic Diet

Ketogenic diet is high in proteins and hence contributes to hypercalciuria, hyperuricosuria, and hypocitraturia.

Cystic Fibrosis

Cystic fibrosis can be associated with calcium oxalate stones, mostly due to enhanced enteric oxalate absorption. Lipid malabsorption from pancreatic insufficiency results in binding of intestinal calcium by free fatty acids and hence, less calcium is available to bind to intestinal oxalate.

Melamine

Melamine is a synthetic product used to form resins with formaldehyde and is found in a variety of products in which resin-based coatings are used. It is also found in melamine tableware. This risk was highlighted by the 2008 melamine-tainted baby formula scandal in China that resulted in over 50,000 affected infants, including 13,000 who were hospitalized, ~15,000 with acute renal failure (ARF), and 6 deaths. The scandal involved milk and infant formula along with other food materials and components being adulterated with melamine. The chemical was used to increase the nitrogen content of diluted milk, giving it the appearance of higher protein content in order to pass quality control testing. Children exposed to high-melamine formula were 7.0 times as likely to have stones as those exposed to no-melamine formula.[16] Unlike typical urinary tract stones, most of the melamine-associated stones are not radio-opaque, did not have shadowing on ultrasonography (USG), and were composed primarily of uric acid and melamine. Melamine stones could be easily treated with hydration and alkalinization, consistent with urate component of the stones. Rarely, surgery may be required.

Other Causes of Hereditary Renal Stone Disease and Chronic Kidney Disease

Besides PH type 1, and cystinuria, there are other causes of inherited renal stone disease that can progress to ESKD if not identified early and treated.

Familial Hypomagnesemia with Hypercalciuria and Nephrocalcinosis

Familial hypomagnesemia with hypercalciuria and nephrocalcinosis (HMHNC) is an autosomal recessive disorder due to mutations in genes (*CLDN16* and *CLDN19*) encoding claudin-16 and claudin-19 proteins, respectively, that are present in tight junctions of the thick ascending limb of loop of Henle. It results in increased urinary magnesium and calcium excretion. The condition is characterized by hypomagnesemia, hypercalciuric nephrocalcinosis, and normal to low blood calcium level. Claudin-19 protein is also present in eyes, and children with mutations in *CLDN19* gene can have nystagmus, coloboma, myopia, and pigmentary retinitis. Treatment includes measures to reduce hypercalciuria including thiazide diuretics and oral magnesium oxide supplementation besides the usual dietary modification.

Dent Disease

This X-linked recessive genetic condition is due to mutations in *CLCN5* or *OCRL* genes that result in proximal renal tubular dysfunction and partial renal Fanconi syndrome. It is characterized by low-molecular-weight proteinuria, hematuria, hypercalciuria, renal stone disease, nephrocalcinosis, and, in some patients, hypophosphatemic rickets, hypokalemia, and ESKD by third to fourth decade. Treatment is aimed at correcting hypercalciuria by dietary measures & thiazides and associated metabolic abnormalities of Fanconi syndrome, if present.

2,8-Dihydroxyadenine Urolithiasis and Dihydroxyadenine Nephropathy

It is caused by adenine phosphoribosyltransferase (APRT) deficiency and inherited as an autosomal recessive disorder. The APRT enzyme is required to convert adenine to adenine monophosphate (AMP). In APRT deficiency, adenine is catabolized by xanthine dehydrogenase to 2,8-dihydroxyadenine (2,8-DHA), a highly insoluble metabolite resulting in urinary stone formation, and nephrocalcinosis. Like uric acid and xanthine stones, 2,8-DHA stones are also radiolucent and can be detected by USG. Presentation can be from infancy to adult life with ~20% patients being asymptomatic. Infants may have red-brown crystals in diaper (2,8-DHA) and older children present with recurrent stones. Up to 70% of the affected patients have red hair or relatives with this hair color. A high index of suspicion in children with recurrent, radiolucent stones, and nephrocalcinosis is necessary for diagnosis as the usual blood and urine biochemical tests are not helpful. Diagnosis is suggested by reddish-brown 2,8-DHA crystals on microscopic examination, stone analysis, or genetic mutation analysis. Therapy includes high intake of water, low salt, vegetarian diet, avoiding animal protein (purine) intake, and use of allopurinol or febuxostat (a xanthine dehydrogenase inhibitor, which makes adenine the major urinary component).[17]

Struvite Stones

Struvite stones are also called infective stones, since >90% of children will have infected urine at the time of diagnosis. They are more frequently observed in children younger than 5 years of age and with anatomical abnormalities such as PUJO, vesicoureteric reflux, and neurogenic bladder that predispose them to urine infection. The incidence of struvite stones has reduced from earlier 10–15% to <5% over the past few decades mainly due to early evaluation, and management of anatomical abnormalities, as well as prompt treatment of UTI.

The struvite stones are composed of triple phosphate (ammonium magnesium phosphate) and form in the presence of infection by urease-secreting bacteria such as *Proteus* species, *Morganella morganii, Klebsiella, Enterobacter*, and *Ureaplasma urealyticum*. These bacteria secrete urease that metabolize urea into ammonia and carbon dioxide. Ammonia neutralizes H^+ and makes urine pH more alkaline. This leads to deprotonation of phosphate into PO_4^{3-} and subsequent precipitation of magnesium ammonium phosphate and calcium phosphate carbonate (calcium apatite) stones. In addition, infections may also produce a soft radiolucent mucoid substance called "matrix concretion" that may calcify readily and account for the rapid formation of some infection-related calculi.

The stones are often located in the renal pelvis, grow rapidly into the calyces, taking staghorn shape, and require prompt surgery since the infection is resistant to medical therapy unless the stone is removed. The stone fragments are soft and often passed as a paste in urine. Diagnosis is suggested by the staghorn appearance on imaging as well as detection of coffin-lid crystals on urine microscopy **(Figs. 1A to E)**.

Drugs and Renal Stones

There are several medications that can cause renal stones through mechanisms including increase in promoter excretion, alteration of urine pH, and crystallization of primary drug itself due to low solubility at normal pH.[18] Common medications such as ceftriaxone, ciprofloxacin, sulfonamides, indinavir, and triamterene can form crystalline aggregates in urine. While ceftriaxone and triamterene stones contain calcium and hence are radiopaque, ciprofloxacin and sulfonamide stones are radiolucent. Magnesium trisilicate, an antacid when used in excess, can produce silicate stones. Other agents that are implicated in renal stone formation include furosemide, glucocorticoids, vitamin D (all of them increase urinary calcium excretion), and vitamin C by increasing oxalate production and excretion in urine. Acetazolamide and topiramate inhibit carbonic anhydrase resulting in reduction in proximal renal tubular bicarbonate reabsorption, increase in urine pH, and increase in the risk of calcium phosphate and calcium oxalate stone formation.

CLINICAL MANIFESTATIONS

Pediatric nephrolithiasis is often asymptomatic in up to 45% cases and is identified during ultrasound screening for nonurinary complaints. This is especially seen when the stones are small and in the pelvicalyceal region. Symptoms are observed when the stone breaks away from the renal papillae and moves down the urinary tract. It is likely to get stuck at three areas of anatomical narrowing—pelviureteric junction, the crossing site of iliac vessels (junction of mid and lower one-third of the ureter), and ureterovesical junction. The following symptoms can be observed:[19,20]

- Acute colicky pain, vomiting in 30–50% (ureteric calculi)
- Gross hematuria in 20–50% (uniformly red or painful, terminal)
- Dysuria, frequency of urination in ~10%
- Fever in 10–35% (due to associated UTI)
- Rarely, with anuric acute kidney injury in <2% (due to obstructing urethral calculus or bilateral ureteric calculi or uric acid crystals)

Evaluation of Pediatric Nephrolithiasis

Before proceeding to evaluation of the child, some general points need to be ascertained.

History specific to

- Current symptoms and associated features of UTI, sepsis, dehydration
- Failure to thrive, polyuria, polydipsia (distal RTA, Bartter syndrome)
- Recurrent urinary tract infections (underlying PUJO, UVJO, bladder abnormality)
- Gastrointestinal pathology (pancreatitis, cystic fibrosis)
- Medication intake (frusemide, ceftriaxone, sulfa drugs, vitamin C, indinavir, allopurinol, calcium) and vitamin D therapy
- Detailed dietary history of animal protein & salt intake by the family and water & milk products consumed by the child is important.
- History of nephrolithiasis in family members would provide clue toward a possible metabolic risk factor as well as dietary habits.

Physical examination should focus on:

- Growth parameters
- Blood pressure
- Hydration status
- Flank mass
- Palpable bladder

Evaluation of a child with suspected renal stone disease can be divided into the following aspects **(Table 2)**:

- Confirm renal stone
- Assess for associated urine infection and renal function in a sick child
- Evaluate for underlying metabolic risk factors
- Evaluate for anatomical abnormalities

Ultrasonography

Ultrasonography should be the initial radiological method of confirming renal stones. Although the sensitivity of USG for renal stones is only up to 80%, especially for calculi >3 mm and

TABLE 2: Stepwise evaluation of a child with suspected renal or ureteric calculus.

Steps	*Why?*	*When?*
Assess severity of colic, hydration status	Oral or parenteral analgesia + IV fluid based on clinical status	At presentation
Complete urine examination	Treat for UTI only if plenty of pus cells, febrile, or sick child	At presentation
USG abdomen	Confirm diagnosis of renal stone, location, and number, as well as hydroureteronephrosis	At presentation
CT scan KUB	Only if high index of suspicion and USG is not confirmatory + prior to surgery	At presentation (only in select cases)
Blood renal function tests, biochemistry	If suspicion of AKI, bilateral ureteric calculi, sepsis	At presentation (in select cases)
Venous blood gas, serum electrolytes, calcium, phosphorus, magnesium, uric acid	If failure to thrive, polyuria, polydipsia, or nephrocalcinosis	At presentation (in select cases)
Metabolic evaluation	24-hour urine or random urine sample (often has to be repeated two to three times)	3–4 weeks after stone extruded or removed and when on usual diet at home (not on modified diet)
Mutation analysis	Nephrocalcinosis, recurrent calculi, Suspicion of hyperoxaluria/cystinuria/Dent disease/FHMHNC	Any time
Stone analysis	Definitive metabolic abnormality	To send stone for analysis on multiple occasions as the composition may change
MCU/DTPA renal scan/IVP	Suspecting anatomical abnormality, especially in children below 3 years of age	After stone has extruded or removed and USG shows persistent hydronephrosis or hydroureteronephrosis

(AKI: acute kidney injury; CT: computed tomography; DTPA: diethylenetriamine pentaacetic acid; FHMHNC: familial hypomagnesemic hypercalciuric nephrocalcinosis; KUB: kidney ureter bladder; MCU: micturating cystourethrogram; UTI: urinary tract infection; USG: ultrasonography)

specificity of 97%, it is easily available, economical, and free of radiation exposure. The sensitivity of USG for ureteric calculi is even lower at ~40%, partly due to the overlying gas-filled intestines.[21] Using the stone-triggered artifact (called twinkling artifact) on color Doppler mode increases the sensitivity of ultrasound. The twinkling artifact is a mixture of rapidly alternating red and blue pixels behind a strongly reflective object (e.g., calculus) resembling turbulent blood flow.

Plain computed tomography (CT) scan of kidney ureter bladder (KUB) is almost 100% sensitive in detecting small calculi. It helps to quantify the number, size, and location of calculi, especially in the ureter. Due to the radiation exposure, it should not be used as a first-line radiological tool. CT scan should be considered in patients with high suspicion of renal stone disease when USG does not confirm renal/ureteric calculi as well as prior to urological procedures. Both the American Urological Association and European Society of Pediatric Radiology recommend ultrasound as the initial imaging modality. Similarly, there is a very limited role of plain X-ray in diagnosing calculi. Plain X-ray can show radio-opaque calculi but will be negative for radiolucent stones due to uric acid.

Complete Urine Examination

Complete urine examination may demonstrate concentrated urine (due to dehydration or decreased water intake), microscopic hematuria (in ~60–90%), crystals, and pus cells **(Figs. 1A to E)**. Pyuria is often noted in 20% of children with renal stone disease and should not be treated with antimicrobial agents assuming urine infection. Associated urine infection should be considered only if the child has fever, features of sepsis, plenty of pus cells in urine, or debris in the pelvicalyceal system. Here, antimicrobial therapy should be initiated after sending urine for culture.

A sick child presenting with vomiting, signs of dehydration or sepsis, or oligoanuric state will need measurement of serum electrolytes, blood urea, blood creatinine, complete blood picture, and additional biochemistry tests.

Evaluation of Metabolic Risk Factors

- A *complete urine examination* is the first step toward evaluating metabolic risk factors. Urine-specific gravity gives a clue to the state of hydration with concentrated urine suggestive of reduced water intake. Urine pH of >6.5 (in absence of UTI) is suggestive of adequate intake of citrate-rich foods commonly observed when vegetarian diet is consumed. Often uric acid, calcium oxalate, and calcium phosphate crystals are noted in urine of healthy children and may not be significant. However, in the presence of renal stone disease, these crystals give a clue to the possible underlying metabolic risk factor.

Cystine crystals are always pathological and even a single hexagonal cystine crystal should be considered significant.

- A more *detailed metabolic evaluation* including excretion of solutes such as calcium, oxalate, uric acid, cystine, citrate, magnesium, and sodium, should take place after the acute episode has resolved and the child is on regular diet. A minimum of 3–4 weeks is recommended between stone expulsion or removal and 24-hour urine collection since the concentration of substances can be underestimated when a stone is present within the urinary tract. Also, the state of dehydration, use of intravenous fluids, and reduced oral intake during an acute episode will influence the urinary concentration of various solutes. Dietary modification should be deferred until the evaluation as these may obscure some diagnoses (e.g., hypercalciuria, hyperuricosuria). Either a 24-hour urine collection (repeated two to three times) can be obtained for more detailed evaluation or a random urine solute to creatinine ratio can be utilized. In many laboratories, two or three separate collections are required to obtain all the necessary measurements because different solutes will need to be collected and tested in separate solutions. For example, uric acid is measured in an alkaline solution, calcium and oxalate in hydrochloric or nitric acid, and citrate in an acidified solution. The reference values for urinary solute excretion are mentioned in **Table 1.** These values are obtained in children from western countries where there is higher intake of animal protein. There are few studies evaluating solute excretion in Indian children. One study from north India found that the urinary excretion of calcium, magnesium, phosphate, uric acid, oxalate, and creatinine was lower compared to children in western countries likely related to less than recommended dietary intake of calcium, proteins, and other nutrients.[22] Hence, regional differences in solute excretion and its normative values should be considered when evaluating the results.

Spot urine samples are an alternative sampling method, especially when 24-hour urine collection is difficult in nontoilet-trained children. Spot urine studies normally link the excretion rates to creatinine. Because the results may vary with collection time and patients' sex, body weight, and age, the value of spot urine studies is limited. Often, there is a disagreement between 24-hour and spot urine value results, believed to be mainly due to the time-to-time variations in the urinary solute concentrations (urinary volume) that vary according to the body hydration status, diurnal circadian rhythm, meal intake, and dietary patterns affecting oxalate excretion.[23] In the study by Christer Ahlstrand, the highest concentration of calcium was observed before noon, and between 7 and 11 PM, whereas oxalate concentration was highest between 6 and 10 AM. Consequently, the highest levels of supersaturation were recorded between 6 and 10 AM, and 6 and 10 PM.[23] The inhibition index was at the highest level during the first morning hours and could be important in counteracting crystal growth at that time. In a more recent study, Paccaud et al. found a relatively strong correlation between the evening and first morning calcium/creatinine ratio on a single spot urine sample and 24-hour urinary calcium excretion in healthy children.[24]

Specific analysis for urine glycolate in PH type 1, L-glycerate in PH type 2, and 4-hydroxyglutamate in PH type 3 may be helpful to differentiate the type of PH. Observation of birefringent oxalate crystals under polarized light on a kidney biopsy tissue and enzyme assays in liver biopsy tissues were done previously for the diagnosis of hyperoxaluria. With genetic studies now affordable and increasingly available, such studies may not be required.

- *Chemical analysis of the renal stone* or fragments by infrared spectroscopy or radiograph diffraction should always be performed. Stone analysis should be performed in recurrent stone formers during each stone episode, even if the initial stone composition is known, because changes in stone content have been reported in recurrent stone formers.
- *Biochemical investigations* including blood gas, serum electrolytes, calcium, phosphorus, uric acid, magnesium, and creatinine should be obtained, especially in children with renal stones and failure to thrive, polyuria, polydipsia, and nephrocalcinosis. In an otherwise healthy well-grown child, we do not see any major abnormalities in these blood parameters.

Molecular genetic testing for mutations with improved sensitivity and reduced cost is now readily available and can be used to evaluate various inherited conditions such as PH, cystinuria, 2-3 DHA crystalluria, Dent disease, FHHNC, and distal RTA. It helps not only in the confirmation of diagnosis with targeted therapy but also in counseling parents during subsequent pregnancy.

Evaluation for Underlying Anatomical Abnormalities

Evaluation for underlying anatomical abnormalities such as PUJO, UVJO, and VUR should be completed in children with persistent hydronephrosis and hydroureter after the extrusion of ureteric calculus. Such abnormalities are more common in children less than 2 years of age and are associated with stasis and urine infections and would require MCU, DTPA renal scan, and, occasionally, intravenous pyelogram (IVP)/magnetic resonance (MR) urography.

Summary of evaluation of a child with suspected renal or ureteric calculus:

- Assess severity of pain and hydration status as well as presence of febrile UTI.
- Obtain complete urine examination and USG abdomen.
- Obtain plain CT scan KUB only if USG abdomen is not confirmatory and suspicion of ureteric stone is high.

- Further evaluation for renal stone disease once the stone has extruded or acute symptoms subsided and the child is on regular, nonmodified diet at home.

MEDICAL MANAGEMENT

The objectives of management of pediatric nephrolithiasis are outlined in **Box 1**. The following management issues need to be considered:

- Emergency management of acute renal colic
- Indications for hospitalization
- Antibiotic therapy
- Intravenous hydration
- Active medical expulsive therapy (MET)
- Surgical interventions
- Evaluation for etiology
- Dietary modification—decreases risk of recurrence
- Specific therapy for metabolic abnormality

Pain Control

Children with calculi in the pelvicalyceal system do not have pain, and the acute renal colic is due to ureteric calculi. For children without vomiting, oral paracetamol, mefenamic acid, and dicyclomine + simethicone (Cyclopam) can be used. If the pain is associated with severe vomiting, intramuscular/intravenous dicyclomine (Cyclopam) or tramadol can be considered along with Ondansetron. Potent nonsteroidal anti-inflammatory drugs (NSAIDs) should be avoided, especially if the child is dehydrated. There are reports of use of intranasal desmopressin (DDAVP) at 5–10 µg in children who have severe pain and cannot be given narcotics. DDAVP works by direct relaxation of ureteric musculature and possibly due to release of hypothalamic beta-endorphins. Different antiemetic agents that have been used include metoclopramide, promethazine, and ondansetron.

Indications for Admission

Indications for admission are based on clinical parameters such as ineffective oral analgesics, persistent vomiting or dehydration, associated febrile UTI, sepsis or pyonephrosis, and acute kidney injury due to bilateral obstructing ureteric calculi or urethral calculus. About 20% of children with renal stone disease require admission in western countries.

BOX 1: Objectives of management of pediatric nephrolithiasis.

- Control pain and vomiting
- Preserve renal function by removing obstructing ureteric calculi
  - MET for ureteric calculi 4–10 mm
  - Surgical therapy for calculi >10 mm, AKI, no response to MET
- Prevent increase in size of renal calculi by the use of potassium citrate and other medicines if required
- Metabolic evaluation when on regular diet and not on any medicine
- Reduce risk of recurrence by increased water intake by the child and dietary modification for family + medications in select conditions

(AKI: acute kidney injury; MET: medical expulsive therapy)

Antibiotic Therapy

Pyuria is common in children with renal stone disease and does not indicate urine infection. Irrational use of antibiotics should be discouraged. Antibiotics are to be considered after sending urine for culture if the child has fever, sepsis, and has plenty of pus cells.

Intravenous Hydration

Intravenous hydration in the presence of renal colic is controversial since although it may hasten stone passage, it is more likely to increase colic due to increased hydrostatic pressure created by diuresis. In a study of 43 adult patients in the emergency room, there was no statistical difference in pain score or rate of spontaneous stone passage in those receiving normal saline (NS) 2 L over 2 hours versus those on NS 20 mL/h. Intravenous hydration should be limited to children with dehydration, sepsis, or prior to contrast procedure (IVP). Fluids should be given to maintain euvolemia and not to increase urine volume.[25]

Medical Expulsive Therapy

About 20% of renal stones are in the ureter. The likelihood for a ureteric calculus to pass through the vesicoureteric junction (VUJ) depends mainly upon its size. Ureteric calculi >10 mm in size are unlikely to pass out spontaneously. Other reasons for ureteric calculi not passing out spontaneously include muscle spasm, mucosal edema, local infection, or ureteric narrowing (anatomical). Ureteric calculi <3 mm have >90% chance to pass out spontaneously, whereas the stone size >4 mm would likely need intervention. Ureteric stones <3 mm can be managed with analgesics and observation up to 6 weeks. The management of obstructing ureteric calculi in children depends upon the size, location, associated infection or acute kidney injury, edema, available infrastructure, and expertise as well as physician and family preference. Surgical options include open surgery, percutaneous nephrolithotomy (PCNL), extra shock wave lithotripsy (ESWL), and ureterorenoscopic lithotripsy (URSL). Although improvement in endourological procedures has resulted in >95% success, they are costly and are associated with complications. Also, with high risk of stone recurrence, some children may need multiple procedures. Thus, if ureteric stones of >4 mm can be expelled with medical pharmacotherapy, surgical procedures with its costs and complications could be avoided.

Medical expulsive therapy using smooth muscle relaxants such as tamsulosin (alpha-1 adrenergic receptor blocker) & nifedipine (calcium channel blocker), and deflazacort (anti-inflammatory) have been used in adults with ureteric calculi.[26] The ureter is lined by smooth muscle cells. An increase in calcium levels causes ureteric muscle contraction, while a decrease determines relaxation.[27] The ureteric smooth muscles are supplied with alpha-adrenergic receptors, with increased density in the distal third of the ureter. Calculi may induce ureteric spasms that interfere with calculi expulsion; thus, muscle relaxation with maintenance of normal antegrade peristaltic activity may facilitate passage. Both tamsulosin and nifedipine inhibit basal smooth muscle tone and uncoordinated activity without any effect on tonic propulsive contractions. Several studies in adults have shown the benefit of MET in reducing the pain, increasing frequency of stone passage, and reducing the need for surgery. The European Association of Urology (EAU) guidelines of 2016 recommend MET with alpha-blockers in adults with distal ureteral stones >5 mm, and not in urgent need for urologic intervention (well-controlled pain, good renal function, and no infection).[28] Tamsulosin and nifedipine have been used for 2–4 weeks and Deflazacort for 10–14 days in adults. Minimal side effects of headache and abdominal pain are reported, more with nifedipine than with tamsulosin.

Expectedly, there are limited studies on MET in children with most studies reporting use of tamsulosin. In a meta-analysis of 5 trials including 406 pediatric patients, Tian et al. showed that there was a higher stone expulsion rate with adrenergic alpha-antagonist [odds ratio (OR) = 2.70] and few adverse effects (dizziness, drowsiness, nausea).[29] Pediatric patients with radiopaque lower ureteral stones of <10–12 mm or smaller have received the following doses: tamsulosin 0.4 mg PO at bedtime for children older than 4 years and 0.2 mg PO at bedtime for children 4 years or younger (pdr. net). We could not find any studies on nifedipine as MET in children with ureteric calculi. There is a wide experience in the use of nifedipine over the past four decades in children with hypertension. Besides cardiovascular indications, nifedipine has been used in normotensive adult patients with Raynaud's phenomenon, preterm labor, and obstructing ureteric calculi.[30]

In our own experience (unpublished), we used nifedipine as MET in 29 euvolemic children between 3 and 16 years of age with ureteral stone (mean size 6.59 ± 2.25 mm). Mean nifedipine dose was 1.14 ± 0.27 mg/kg/day (range 15–40 mg) and duration 18.34 ± 6.11 days (range 4 days–4 weeks). In all children treated with nifedipine, the colicky pain resolved within maximum 3 days, 90% had spontaneous passage of stone, and only 2 of 29 (6.25%) had headache. There was no significant drop in blood pressure, and none required parenteral analgesic therapy. Additionally, all 6 out of 29 children with proximal or midureteric calculi responded to nifedipine with expulsion of calculi.

Stones <3 mm size have >85% chance of spontaneous passage and hence, MET is not indicated. MET is most useful in euvolemic children with acute distal ureteric stones 4–10 mm in size and without the evidence of dehydration, infection, or acute kidney injury. Stones that have been present for more than 1–2 weeks are less likely to respond to MET due to the possible impaction and mucosal edema.

Water Intake

One of the most important contributing factors to nephrolithiasis is inadequate water intake by the child. Partly, it is related to preoccupation with gadgets and activities, and partly related to reducing urine volume so as not to use the washroom. Physiologically, we drink water when we are thirsty. Children with kidney stone disease should have water as their medicine and consume even when not thirsty. Water therapy reduces the solute concentration in urine, thereby reducing the risk of new stone formation, prevents an increase in size of stones in situ, and may assist in expulsion. Children need to be encouraged to drink at least 2 L water/m^2/day and even higher volume during summer months. Ensuring that the urine transparency is similar to that of water is a practical way to confirm adequate water intake. Certainly, maintaining compliance with hydration is difficult in children. Positive reinforcement and some dietary indiscretion are permitted with the intake of few additional glasses of water when ingesting salty foods or chocolates. Children should be encouraged to consume more water or oral rehydrating solution during intercurrent viral infections and gastroenteritis—conditions associated with dehydration and the risk of stone formation.

Dietary Modification

The dietary modification should be for the entire family and not for the child alone. This ensures better compliance, creates a positive mental state in the child, and reduces the risk of stone recurrence. The following measures are recommended for all children with nephrolithiasis **(Table 3)**:

- Low salt intake is the first step toward dietary modification. Approximately 75% of filtered sodium chloride and water are reabsorbed in renal proximal tubules. This results in higher intraluminal calcium concentration that drives passive calcium reabsorption across the paracellular channel down its concentration gradient. Almost 70%

TABLE 3: Dietary management of pediatric nephrolithiasis.

To be increased	*To be reduced*
Water intake >2 L/m^2/day (additional 25% during summer months and when having salty foods or chocolates)	Low salt intake for family (reduce salt to 3–5 g/day)
Daily intake of fruits and vegetables (source of citrate, phytate, and pyrophosphate)	Avoid animal protein intake for family (is a source of purine and acid through metabolism of sulfur-containing amino acids)
300 mL milk and milk products (to provide RDA of calcium)	Reduce oxalate-rich foods (spinach, beans, nuts, rhubarb, chocolates, tea, coffee)
Can have eggs and sea food if desired	Reduce the intake of salty foods, canned foods (has high salt content)

(RDA: recommended dietary allowance)

of filtered calcium is reabsorbed in this manner. Now, higher salt intake results in mild volume expansion, higher filtered load of NaCl, and reduced proximal NaCl reabsorption due to inhibition of angiotensin II. Hence, there is decreased proximal tubular calcium and uric acid reabsorption. Thus, reducing salt intake to ~3–4 g/day (and this is the physiological requirement against 12–20 g of salt intake in most countries) will allow proximal tubular NaCl and also calcium & uric acid reabsorption, decreasing the tubular fluid calcium and uric acid concentration and excretion, both major stone-producing solutes.

- Increased intake of fruits and vegetables will provide citrate that is a natural chelator of calcium in urine.
- Daily recommended allowance of calcium through milk, milk products, and eggs should be continued. Calcium intake is necessary for a child's growth as well as to bind oxalate in the intestinal lumen. Restriction in calcium intake will allow increased absorption of oxalate contributing to increased urinary oxalate excretion. Certainly, excess intake of milk or calcium supplementation is discouraged.
- Animal protein intake should be avoided since these are a direct source of uric acid through purine content and also acid production through metabolism of sulfur-containing amino acids (cysteine, methionine). While the carbonate ion of calcium carbonate released from bone will buffer the acid produced, calcium is excreted in the urine contributing to hypercalciuria. In adults, dietary restriction of animal protein is associated with a lower risk of calcium oxalate stone recurrence.
- Reduction in oxalate-rich foods is also important in families, especially those with hyperoxaluria. High content of oxalate is found in spinach, rhubarb, beetroot, beans, nuts, chocolates, tea, and coffee.

Citrate Supplementation

Citrate supplementation is often provided to most children with nephrolithiasis. Potassium citrate is preferred to sodium citrate to reduce the sodium load. Citrate helps in increasing urine pH to 6–7 and prevents crystallization of uric acid, cystine, and calcium oxalate. Overzealous use of potassium citrate can increase urine pH to >7 and induce calcium phosphate stone formation.

Specific Therapy for Metabolic Risk Factor

Hypercalciuria

The first step in treatment is increased water intake and dietary modification as outlined above. Despite these measures, if hypercalciuria persists, then potassium citrate should be added followed by thiazide diuretics in the third step. The dietary modification should be continued lifelong, whereas potassium citrate supplementation can be given for 3–6 months or more depending upon the symptoms and compliance with diet. Excess calcium and vitamin D_3 therapy should be avoided as vitamin D_3 not only increases gastrointestinal absorption of calcium (absorptive hypercalciuria) but also inhibits parathormone (PTH) secretion that in turn reduces distal nephron calcium reabsorption and, combined together, contributes to hypercalciuria. If the child has recurrent nephrolithiasis or hypercalciuria persists despite the above dietary modification measures, and potassium citrate therapy for 3–6 months' period, then thiazide diuretic should be initiated to reduce hypercalciuria. In most children, a low dose of hydrochlorothiazide at 0.5–1.0 mg/kg/day in two divided doses is sufficient to reduce urinary calcium excretion.[31]

Hyperoxaluria

Treatment of hyperoxaluria includes the following measures:

- Decrease intake of oxalate-rich foods such as beetroot, beans, spinach, rhubarb, sweet potato, nuts, tea, and coffee
- Reduce gastrointestinal absorption of oxalate by ensuring adequate calcium intake, citrate intake, and low-fat diet (so that fatty acids do not bind to calcium and reduce its availability for binding oxalate). Commercial preparation of *Oxalobacter formigenes*, an organism present in the intestinal lumen that metabolizes oxalate, can also be used to degrade oxalate and reduce absorption.
- Reduce commercial vitamin C intake since vitamin C is metabolized to oxalate in liver.
- Pyridoxine (vitamin B_6) is a cofactor for hepatic AGXT enzyme that converts glyoxylate to glycine and reduces hepatic oxalate production by enzyme induction. It is used at 5–10 mg/kg/day and is effective in ~40% patients with hyperoxaluria type I but not in other forms of PH.[32]
- Increase solubility of oxalate in urine by increasing water intake to at least 2–2.5 L/m^2/day.
- Use of potassium citrate as a chelating agent
- Finally, in children with type 1 PH who progress to ESKD, combined liver and kidney transplant is the definitive therapy. Kidney transplantation alone will lead to oxalate deposition in the graft with subsequent graft failure. Simultaneous or sequential liver transplantation will provide the deficient AGXT enzyme and prevent oxalate production.

Hyperuricosuria

Avoidance of animal protein and reduction in salt intake are the initial measures in the treatment of hyperuricosuria. Since uric acid crystals precipitate in acidic urine, use of alkali to increase urinary pH to 6.5 that increases solubility of uric acid is an effective therapy. Uric acid stones are the only type of renal stones that can be dissolved by urinary alkalinization, a process called chemolysis. Various alkali preparations include sodium bicarbonate, potassium citrate, and magnesium citrate. These agents, besides alkalinizing the urine, also provide citrate that prevents aggregation of calcium oxalate crystals. Occasionally, allopurinol at 5–10 mg/kg/day may be added if the plasma uric acid level remains high despite dietary modification or in children with tumor lysis syndrome. Recently, with use of rasburicase (recombinant urate oxidase enzyme that converts uric acid to allantoin, a highly soluble molecule in urine) in hematopoietic malignancy, there is a reduced need for allopurinol in this setting. It is important to note that allopurinol, a xanthine oxidase inhibitor, will not be effective in children with renal hyperuricosuria (hypouricemic) and xanthinuria (xanthine oxidase deficiency); both conditions are associated with a decreased blood uric acid level.

Cystinuria

Cystinuria is a long-term medical disease and maintaining urine-free cystine level <100 Umol/mmol creatinine is thus important to prevent cystine crystal formation. The most important management of cystinuria is high fluid therapy targeted to reduce urinary cystine concentration below 250 mg/dL and has to be continued both during day and night. Cystine crystals are more soluble in alkaline urine pH of ~7.0–7.5, and this can be attempted by vegetarian diet and use of potassium citrate. Both these measures may not be achieved despite maximal efforts and often lead to nonadherence. Medical therapy of cystinuria is challenging and often disappointing as children tend to develop recurrent stone disease. Combined cystine-binding drug therapy with tiopronin (mercaptopropionyl glycine) and D-penicillamine that bind cystine forming highly soluble complexes can be successfully used in children resistant to supportive therapy. Side effects of these drugs are common and include proteinuria, fever, rash, bone marrow suppression, and arthropathy. Discontinuation of drugs due to side effects or compliance leads to recurrence of cystine stones. Surgery is frequently required in children with cystine stones.[33]

Hypocitraturia

This can be corrected by increased intake of fruits and vegetables, reduction in animal protein intake, and often supplementation by potassium citrate at 0.5–1.0 mEq/kg/day. This dose minimizes gastrointestinal upset and does not lead to hyperkalemia unless if GFR is <30 mL/min/1.73 m^2. Citrate forms a highly soluble complex with calcium and reduces availability of calcium to bind to phosphate and oxalate.[34]

MEDICATIONS USED IN PEDIATRIC RENAL STONE DISEASE (TABLE 4)

- Urinary alkalinization using potassium citrate, magnesium citrate, and sodium-potassium citrate not only is useful for uric acid and cystine stones but also chelates calcium preventing calcium oxalate precipitation. Urine pH should be targeted at 6.5–7.0 except in cystinuria where pH of 7–8 is desirable. At higher urine pH, there is risk of calcium phosphate crystallization. Potassium citrate can be used at 0.5–1.0 mEq/kg/day in three divided doses. Sodium citrate may be used in place of potassium citrate, if GFR is decreased and serum potassium is increased.
- *Thiazide diuretics* reduce urinary calcium excretion by increasing both proximal and distal renal tubular calcium reabsorption. Low dose of 0.5–1.0 mg/kg/day in two divided doses is usually effective in treating hypercalciuria. Sodium restriction is important when using thiazide diuretics, otherwise excess sodium intake will promote calcium excretion. Hypokalemia is a common side effect

TABLE 4: Common medications used in nephrolithiasis.

Medicines	*Indication*	*Dose*	*Duration*	*Target*	*Common side effects*
Potassium citrate	All types of renal stone disease	0.5–1.0 mEq of K$^+$/kg/day in three divided doses	3–6 months or longer, if required	• Normal urine calcium/creatinine ratio • Urine pH 6.5–7.0 • Urine pH > 7 in cystinuria • No recurrence of stones	• Bloating, nausea • Hyperkalemia (in CKD)
Hydrochloro-thiazide	Hypercalciuria	0.5–1.0 mg/kg/day in two divided doses	3–6 months or longer, if required	Normal urine calcium/creatinine ratio	• Hypokalemia • Hypomagnesemia • Weakness, dizziness, cramps • Hyperglycemia • Skin rash
Pyridoxine	Primary hyperoxaluria type 1	5–10 mg/kg/day in two to three divided doses	Long term	24-hour urinary oxalate should decrease by 30%	• Numbness • Paresthesias (sensory neuropathy) • Nausea, headache
Allopurinol	Hyperuricemic hyperuricosuria and 2,8-DHA stones	5–10 mg/kg/day in two to three divided doses	• 3–6 months • Long term in 2,8-DHA stones	Plasma uric acid less than 5 mg/dL	• Rash • GI irritation • Leucopenia • Neuritis

(CKD: chronic kidney disease; 2,8-DHA: 2,8-dihydroxyadenine; GI: gastrointestinal) of thiazide diuretic and hence, the serum potassium level needs to be monitored.

- *Allopurinol*, a xanthine oxidase inhibitor, reduces the serum uric acid level and is hence used in patients with a high blood uric acid level despite dietary modification. The dose is 5–10 mg/kg/day in two to three divided doses. It is not effective in children with hypouricemic hyperuricosuria and xanthinuria.
- *Pyridoxine* at 5–10 mg/kg/day in two to three divided dose is effective in ~40% children with type I PH but not types 2 and 3. The recommended starting dose is 5 mg/kg/day, increasing by 5 mg/kg steps to a maximum of 20 mg/kg/day. Responsiveness is currently defined by a >30% decrease in urinary oxalate excretion after a test period of a minimum of 3 months at maximum dose. Side effects are rarely seen and sensory neurotoxicity is unusual (paresthesias, numbness). A subset of patients carrying one or two copies of p.Gly170Arg or p.Phe152Ile mutation are more likely to respond to pharmacological doses of pyridoxine.[35]

FOLLOW-UP

At follow-up, questions concerning symptoms related to kidney stone disease, water intake, and dietary modification for family are enquired. Specific gravity and pH on complete urine examination will provide information on compliance with water intake (adequate will show dilute urine whereas concentrated urine would indicate inadequate water intake) and diet/medication intake (high urine pH reflects intake of fruits and vegetables as well as potassium citrate if the child is taking). In most cases, ultrasound at 2–3 months' interval would be sufficient. In children with recurrent renal stone disease, repeated 24-hour urine collection would be indicated to look for change in metabolic parameters as well as dietary sodium and water intake reflected in urine volume. Finally, blood tests to look for medication side effects should be performed periodically, especially serum electrolytes when on thiazide diuretic.

OUTCOME

In children and adolescents, renal stones recur frequently, especially those who have an underlying metabolic abnormality. In a large case series of 221 children from the Mayo Clinic, ~65% had recurrence at a mean follow-up of 59 months.[36] Other centers have reported a lower but still substantial recurrence rate of ~30%.[37]

Children with renal stone disease are more likely to have AKI compared to adults. In a recent study by Farris et al., 23% of children with nephrolithiasis had AKI and the major contributing factors were dehydration due to vomiting and use of NSAIDs. Febrile urinary tract infections and ureteral obstruction by calculi or uric acid gravel in single functioning kidney or both ureters could also contribute to AKI.[38]

Children with recurrent renal stone disease, associated nephrocalcinosis, infections, and AKI are at risk for CKD including ESKD. Certain inherited types of nephrolithiasis such as PH type 1, Dent disease, FHHNC, and 2,8-DHA urolithiasis are more likely to have progressive CKD. Hence, prompt treatment of dehydration, febrile urinary tract infection, avoidance of NSAIDs, reinforcement of dietary modification for family plus extra water intake by the child, and targeted pharmacological therapy in selected children plays an important role in reducing the morbidity associated with these nephrolithiasis.

CONCLUSION

In conclusion, the incidence of pediatric nephrolithiasis has increased over the past three decades. Increase in salt and animal protein intake along with reduced water intake are the major contributing factors. A metabolic factor is usually identified in majority of children that predisposes them to recurrent stone disease. Evaluation for underlying metabolic factor through urinary solute excretion tests 3–4 weeks after the stone has extruded or removed, and more recently, genetic mutation analysis would allow for targeted therapy. In general, increased intake of water, reduction in salt intake, and avoidance of animal protein should be incorporated in every child with nephrolithiasis. Additionally, supplementation with potassium citrate, thiazide diuretic, pyridoxine, and allopurinol can be used in specific conditions. MET has been shown to be effective and safe in select children with obstructing ureteric calculi of 4–10 mm. Advances in miniature surgical procedures allow removal of large calculi. Renal stone disease is associated with significant morbidity including pain, infections, acute kidney disease, increased medical costs, and CKD requiring kidney replacement therapy.

KEY POINTS

- Incidence of pediatric nephrolithiasis has increased over the past few decades.
- A metabolic factor is usually found in up to 90% children, with hypercalciuria being the most common abnormality.
- USG should be the first modality of investigation.
- MET with tamsulosin is an effective and safe option in euvolemic children with 4–10 mm obstructing ureteric calculi and without AKI.
- Increased water intake and dietary modification for the family are the initial steps in reducing the risk of recurrence followed by addition of potassium citrate and medications.
- There is associated significant morbidity including ESKD.

REFERENCES

1. López M, Hoppe B. History, epidemiology and regional diversities of urolithiasis. Pediatr Nephrol. 2010;25:49-59.
2. Ward JB, Feinstein L, Pierce C, Lim J, Abbott KC, Bavendam T, et al. Pediatric urinary stone disease in the United States: the Urologic Diseases in America Project. Urology. 2019;129:180-7.

3. Ganesamoni, R. Epidemiology of stone disease in Northern India. In: Singh SK (Ed). Urolithiasis. London: Springer; 2012. pp. 39-46.
4. Kulshrestha SS. Epidemiology of pediatric renal stone disease in Bundelkhand region of India. Global J Res Anal. 2020;9:52-4.
5. Chang Kit L, Filler G, Pike J, Leonard MP. Pediatric urolithiasis: experience at a tertiary care pediatric hospital. Can Urol Assoc J. 2008;2(4):381-6.
6. Kumar AJ, Mandhani A, Srivastava A, Ansari MS. Pediatric urolithiasis: experience from a tertiary referral center. J Pediatr Urol. 2013;6:825-30.
7. Defoor W, Asplin J, Jackson E, Jackson C, Reddy P, Sheldon C, et al. Results of a prospective trial to compare normal urine supersaturation in children and adults. J Urol. 2005;174(4): 1708-10.
8. Ratkalkar VN, Kleinman JG. Mechanisms of stone formation. Clin Rev Bone Miner Metab. 2011;9(3-4):187-97.
9. Soliman NA, Rizvi SA. Endemic bladder calculi in children. Pediatr Nephrol. 2017;32:1489-99.
10. Penido MG, Srivastava T, Alon US. Pediatric primary urolithiasis: 12-year experience at a Midwestern Children's Hospital. J Urol. 2013;189(4):1493-7.
11. Peres LA, Langer SS, Schmidt RC, Nacke RA, Francescon PV, Almeida RC, et al. Nephrolithiasis in pediatric patients: metabolic and anatomical investigation. J Bras Nefrol. 2011;33(1):34-8.
12. De Santo NG, Di Iorio B, Capasso G, Paduano C, Stamler R, Langman CB, et al. Population based data on urinary excretion of calcium, magnesium, oxalate, phosphate and uric acid in children from Cimitile (southern Italy). Pediatr Nephrol. 1992; 6(2):149-57.
13. Marra G, Taroni F, Berrettini A, Montanari E, Manzoni G, Montini G. Pediatric nephrolithiasis: a systematic approach from diagnosis to treatment. J Nephrol. 2019;32:199-210.
14. Cochat P, Rumsby G. Primary hyperoxaluria. N Engl J Med. 2013;369:649-58.
15. Tekin A, Tekgul S, Atsu N, Sahin A, Ozen H, Bakkaloglu M. A study of the etiology of idiopathic calcium urolithiasis in children: hypocituria is the most important risk factor. J Urol. 2000;164(1):162-5.
16. Guan N, Fan Q, Ding J, Zhao Y, Lu J, Ai Y, et al. Melamine-contaminated powdered formula and urolithiasis in young children. N Engl J Med. 2009;360(11):1067-74.
17. Harambat J, Bollée G, Daudon M, Ceballos-Picot I, Bensman A, APRT Study Group. Adenine phosphoribosyltransferase deficiency in children. Pediatr Nephrol. 2012;27(4):571-9.
18. Viljoen A, Chaudhry R, Bycroft J. Renal stones. Ann Clin Biochem. 2019;56(1):15-27.
19. Coward RJ, Peters CJ, Duffy PG, Corry D, Kellet MJ, Choong S, et al. Epidemiology of pediatric renal stone disease in the UK. Arch Dis Child. 2003;88:962-5.
20. Edvardsson V, Elidottir H, Indridason OS, Palsson R. High incidence of kidney stones in Icelandic children. Pediatr Nephrol. 2005;20(7):940-4.
21. Roberson NP, Dillman JR, O'Hara SM, Defoor DR, Reddy PP, Giordano RM, et al. Comparison of ultrasound versus computed tomography for the detection of kidney stones in the pediatric population: a clinical effectiveness study. Pediatr Radiol. 2018;48(7):962-72.
22. Sweid HA, Bagga A, Meera Vaswani M, Vasudev V, Ahuja RK, Srivastava RN. Urinary excretion of minerals, oxalate, and uric acid in north Indian children. Pediatr Nephrol. 1997;11:189-92.
23. Ahlstrand C, Larsson L, Tiselius HG. Variations in urine composition during the day in patients with calcium oxalate stone disease. J Urol. 1984;131:77-81.
24. Paccaud Y, Rios-Leyvraz M, Bochud M, Tabin R, Genin B, Russo M, et al. Spot urine samples to estimate 24-hour urinary calcium excretion in school-age children. Eur J Pediatr. 2020;179(11):1673-81.
25. Springhart WP, Marguet CG, Sur RL, Norris RD, Delvecchio FC, Young MD, et al. Forced versus minimal intravenous hydration in the management of acute renal colic: a randomized trial. J Endourol. 2006;20(10):713-6.
26. Davenport k, Timoney A, Keeley F. Effect of smooth muscle relaxant drugs on proximal human ureteric activity in vivo: a pilot study. Urol Res. 2007;35:207-13.
27. Andersson KE, Forman A. Effects of calcium channel blockers on urinary tract smooth muscle. Acta Pharmacol Toxicol. 1986;58:193-200.
28. Turk C, Knoll T, Seitz C, Skolarikos A, Chapple C, McClinton S. Medical expulsive therapy for ureterolithiasis: the EAU recommendations in 2016. Eur Urol. 2017;71:504-7.
29. Tian D, Li N, Huang W, Zong H, Zhang Y. The efficacy and safety of adrenergic alpha-antagonists in treatment of distal ureteral stones in pediatric patients: a systematic review and meta-analysis. J Pediatr Surg. 2017;52:360-5.
30. Lederballe PO, Christensen NJ, Rämsch, KD. Comparison on acute effects of Nifedipine on normotensive and hypertensive man. J Cardiovasc Pharmacol. 1980;2:357-66.
31. Choi JN, Lee JS, Shin JI. Low-dose thiazide diuretics in children with idiopathic renal hypercalciuria. Acta Paediatr. 2011; 100(8):e71-4.
32. Hoyer-Kuhn H, Kohbrok S, Volland R, Franklin J, Hero B, Beck BB, et al. Vitamin B6 in primary hyperoxaluria I: first prospective trial after 40 years of practice. CJASN. 2014;9(3):468-77.
33. Dello Strologo L, Laurenzi C, Legato A, Pastore A. Cystinuria in children and young adults: success of monitoring free-cystine urine levels. Pediatr Nephrol. 2007;22(11):1869-973.
34. Caudarella R, Vescini F. Urinary citrate and renal stone disease: the preventive role of alkali citrate treatment. Arch Ital Urol Androl. 2009;81:182-7.
35. Cochat P, Hulton SA, Acquaviva C, Danpure CJ, Daudon M, De Marchi M, et al. Primary hyperoxaluria type 1: indications for screening and guidance for diagnosis and treatment. Nephrol Dial Transplant. 2012;27:1729-36.
36. Milliner DS, Murphy ME. Urolithiasis in pediatric patients. Mayo Clin Proc. 1993;68(3):241-8.
37. Tasian GE, Kabarriti AE, Kalmus A, Furth SL. Kidney stone recurrence among children and adolescents. J Urol. 2017; 197(1):246-52.
38. Farris N, Raina R, Tibrewal A, Brown M, Colvis M, Schwaderer A, et al. Acute kidney injury associated with urinary stone disease in children and young adults presenting to a pediatric emergency department. Front Pediatr. 2020;8:1-9.

CHAPTER

13.10

Lower Urinary Tract Dysfunction in Childhood

Vivek Parameswara Sarma, CS Aravind

INTRODUCTION

The concepts in the diagnosis and management of lower urinary tract dysfunction (LUTD) in children have evolved significantly over the past few decades. The widely prevalent confusion regarding terminologies, diagnostic guidelines, and role of various therapeutic options has been sorted to a great extent in recent years. A greater understanding of the underlying factors associated with voiding disorders and advances in functional assessment of the lower urinary tract (LUT) has enabled clearer demarcation of these variegated, but occasionally, overlapping disorders.

The normal function of LUT depends on the normal development of bladder and urethral sphincter mechanism and also the neural/voluntary control over bladder and sphincter function. In most children, voiding control is usually established by 4–5 years of age. When *lower urinary tract symptoms* (*LUTS*) occur beyond that age, the condition is referred to as *LUTD*. Any functional disturbance (abnormal holding and/or voiding pattern) in voiding that occurs beyond the expected age of completion of toilet training, in the absence of anatomical or neurological causes, is considered a *voiding disorder*.[1,2]

Functional disorders of the LUT constitute abnormalities in the filling and/or emptying phases of the bladder, with no obvious neurological or anatomical abnormality, associated with variable etiology and prognosis. These include a broad spectrum of clinical entities that may originate from behavioral factors that affect toilet training and inhibit the development of normal urinary control. The term *LUTD* includes a wide spectrum of disorders with variable pathophysiology and symptomatology **(Box 1)**. LUTD can lead to vesicoureteral reflux (VUR) and recurrent urinary tract infections (UTIs) with a significant risk of progressive renal scarring. LUTD is often associated with constipation and emotional/behavioral disorders such as anxiety, depression, aggressiveness, and social isolation. But the cause and the consequence relationship between these factors have not been clearly established.

The nomenclature previously used for description in LUTD had been rife with interchangeable terms that were even vague and inaccurate. This resulted in uncertainty and made it difficult to compare research and study outcomes among different groups. The standardization of the nomenclature for pediatric and adolescent LUT function has been critical in the optimal understanding and management of LUTD and more effective interaction among the healthcare workers.[3,4]

BOX 1: Classical characteristics of lower urinary tract dysfunction (LUTD).

LUTD includes a group of functional disorders of the LUT characterized by the following features:
- Abnormalities in the filling and/or emptying phases of the bladder
- Absence of a definite etiologic anatomical abnormality
- Absence of a definite etiologic neurological lesion
- Daytime urinary incontinence is usually a predominant voiding symptom
- Association with obstruction, UTI, and VUR
- Association with constipation/bowel dysfunction
- Association with behavioral disorders/psychosocial issues
- Alterations in urinary control that requires functional assessment for diagnosis
- Potential for long-term urinary tract and renal injury

(LUT: lower urinary tract; LUTD: lower urinary tract dysfunction; UTI: urinary tract infection; VUR: vesicoureteral reflux)

NORMAL URINARY CONTROL

Achievement of an adult pattern of urinary control depends on the outcome of three events in the development of bladder form and function:

1. Increase in bladder capacity to serve as an adequate reservoir
2. Voluntary control over the periurethral striated muscle sphincter
3. Direct, volitional control over the spinal reflex that controls the detrusor smooth muscle, which is the most complex phase of the function.

The last two events are critical to the ability of voluntary initiation and termination of voiding. Urodynamic studies demonstrate that detrusor contraction will not occur even at bladder capacity unless voluntarily initiated. The striated sphincter muscles are activated reflexively during bladder filling, thus preventing incontinence. The voluntary initiation of detrusor contraction with simultaneous reflex relaxation of sphincter enables low-pressure voiding. The final phase of micturition control is when the *sacral micturition reflex arc* is brought under cortical control. This signifies that the cerebral cortex can control the detrusor, by initiating or inhibiting a contraction, at any given bladder volume. Normally, even infants have a certain degree of cortical control over bladder emptying, enabling them to be dry between voiding episodes. The adult pattern of urinary control is also characterized by an absence of uninhibited detrusor contractions during bladder filling. This is usually achieved by 4 years of age in most children, though there can be significant variability in attaining this milestone. The number of voiding episodes in continent children is generally between three and seven times daily. The usual capacity of the neonatal bladder is 30–60 mL and bladder capacity increases by about 30 mL/year each year till puberty. The *expected bladder capacity* (*EBC*) in childhood can be estimated by *Koff's formula*: *Capacity in mL = (Age in years + 2) × 30*. In age < 1 year, EBC in mL = 7 × Weight in kg.

Proper urinary continence involves both external striated sphincter (under voluntary control via the pudendal nerve) and internal sphincter mechanisms of the bladder neck and proximal urethra (under sympathetic control via the α-adrenergic receptors). α-adrenergic receptor inhibition decreases the outlet resistance. Muscarinic receptors are found in the human detrusor muscle, and bladder contractions are initiated by stimulation of these receptors with the release of acetylcholine (ACh) from cholinergic nerves. The main action of anticholinergics is on the M1 and M3 receptor subtypes, which are thought to be responsible for the pathogenesis of detrusor hyperactivity.[2-4]

CLASSIFICATION OF LOWER URINARY TRACT DYSFUNCTION

Previously, a multitude of terms was used in the classification and description of the vaguely titled *"dysfunctional voiding disorders."* These include *unstable bladder, small capacity bladder, detrusor hyperreflexia, "Lazy" bladder syndrome, dysfunctional elimination syndromes* (*DES*), and the classical *non-neurogenic neurogenic bladder* (*NNNGB/Hinman syndrome*). Though the symptom complexes thus described are clinically apparent in many cases, the diagnosis is based on individual interpretation and hence subjective in many instances. The lack of proper characterization and uniform scientific terminology resulted in vagueness of description and diagnostic confusion. Hence, the new standardization of nomenclature has been proposed by the *International Children's Continence Society* (*ICCS*)[1,2,4,5] **(Box 2)**. Of particular relevance is the age of the child when applying terminology to describe pediatric LUT function. The reference point used by the ICCS is 5 years of age or older (4 years of age for bowel dysfunction) because this age is used scientifically to characterize urinary incontinence disorders. The classification of conditions with *daytime incontinence* as a central symptom is complicated by the following considerations:

- There is considerable overlap between the conditions.
- Borderline cases are very common.

BOX 2: The International Children's Continence Society (ICCS), classification of LUTD.

- Bladder and bowel dysfunction (BBD)
- Overactive bladder (OAB)
- Voiding postponement
- Underactive bladder
- Dysfunctional voiding
- Bladder outlet obstruction
- Stress incontinence
- Vaginal reflux
- Giggle incontinence
- Extraordinary daytime urinary frequency (EDUF)
- Bladder neck dysfunction

- The rationale for grouping symptom complexes into specific conditions is often not fully evidence based.
- The symptom complexes often evolve with time (e.g., a child may have urge incontinence to begin with, continue to have symptoms of voiding dysfunction and voiding postponement, and finally have features of underactive bladder).

The ICCS advises researchers studying these children to assess and document four parameters, for greater clinical relevance:[1,4,5]

1. Incontinence (presence or absence and symptom frequency)
2. Voiding frequency
3. Voided volumes
4. Fluid intake.

EPIDEMIOLOGY OF LOWER URINARY TRACT DYSFUNCTION

Lower urinary tract dysfunction is commonly encountered in daily practice, accounting for up to 40% of pediatric urology clinic visits annually. This condition has been reported to affect 5–20% of children. Overactive bladder (OAB), characterized by urgency, is the most commonly encountered LUTD in children and has a peak incidence between 5 and 7 years of age. Daytime incontinence varies with both age and gender. Studies on the prevalence of voiding disorders in school-age children indicate that daytime urinary incontinence is up to five times more common in girls. Various studies have proven an association between body mass index (BMI) and LUT or bladder and bowel dysfunction (BBD) in school-age children. There is also significant negative impact of the LUTS on the self-esteem of the child and quality of life.[2,4,6]

SYMPTOMATOLOGY IN LOWER URINARY TRACT DYSFUNCTION

The symptoms of LUTD can be classified based on their relation to the voiding and/or storage phase of bladder function.[1,2,4,6]

Symptoms Related to Storage Function of Urinary Bladder

- *Voiding frequency: Increased or decreased*—if the child consistently voids eight or more times daily, after the age of 5 years or attainment of bladder control, it indicates *increased daytime frequency*. Three or fewer voidings daily denote *decreased daytime frequency*. Bladder diary (BD) is an important aid to assess this and related parameters.
- *Incontinence: Urinary incontinence* means uncontrollable leakage of urine, which can be continuous or intermittent. *Continuous incontinence* means constant leakage of urine, which is usually associated with congenital malformations (such as ectopic ureter) or iatrogenic damage to the external urethral sphincter. This term has replaced that of *total incontinence*. *Intermittent incontinence* means urinary leakage in discrete amounts, which can occur at day and/or night. *Enuresis* means intermittent incontinence while sleeping. The symptom of bedwetting is called enuresis (also called *nocturnal enuresis*) or (*intermittent*) *nocturnal incontinence* regardless of the presence or absence of concomitant daytime symptoms. This is both a symptom and a condition. Children with enuresis with concomitant LUTS differ clinically and therapeutically from those without. Hence, they are classified based on these grounds into monosymptomatic and nonmonosymptomatic enuresis.[1,2,7,8] Enuresis in children *without* any other LUTS (nocturia excluded) and *without* a history of LUTD is defined as *monosymptomatic enuresis*. Children with enuresis associated with any other LUTS are diagnosed as *nonmonosymptomatic enuresis*. *LUTS* relevant to this definition are *increased/decreased voiding frequency, daytime incontinence, urgency, hesitancy, straining, weak stream, intermittency, holding maneuvers, a feeling of incomplete emptying, postmicturition dribble, and genital/LUT pain* (bedwetting in a child with concomitant daytime incontinence is still called enuresis, of the nonmonosymptomatic variety). Based on the onset of symptoms, the term *secondary enuresis* is used for children who have had a previous dry period of at least 6 months. Otherwise, the term *primary enuresis* should be used.[1,4,7,8] *Daytime incontinence* refers to incontinence that is confined only during the day. Some children with both significant daytime incontinence and enuresis should have dual diagnoses. The conditions characterized by daytime incontinence and other LUTS are significantly variegated with considerable overlap **(Box 3)**.
- *Urgency:* This is defined as the sudden and unexpected experience of an immediate need to void. The term is applicable only after the age of 5 years or attainment of bladder control, whichever is earlier.
- *Nocturia:* This is defined as the need for the child, >5 years, to awaken at night to void. This is a common symptom and not necessarily indicative of LUTD.

BOX 3: Definitions of incontinence in children based on the terminology of the International Children's Continence Society (ICCS), 2016.

- *Primary incontinence:* Involuntary urination in children >5 years who have never been dry
- *Secondary incontinence:* Involuntary urination in children who have previously been dry for >6 months
- *Continuous incontinence:* Constant leakage of urine day and night
- *Daytime incontinence:* Involuntary urination during the day
- *Enuresis:* Involuntary urination during sleep in children >5 years
- *Primary enuresis:* Involuntary urination during sleep in children >5 years who have never been dry
- *Secondary enuresis:* Involuntary urination during sleep in children >5 years who have previously been dry for >6 months
- *Monosymptomatic enuresis:* Involuntary urination during sleep without daytime urinary tract symptoms
- *Nonmonosymptomatic enuresis:* Involuntary urination during sleep and daytime urinary tract symptoms

Symptoms Related to Voiding

These symptoms may not be specifically reported by the child or observed by the parent but have to be categorically elicited in clinical history.

- *Hesitancy:* This denotes difficulty in the initiation of voiding or the presence of a significant waiting period before the start of voiding.
- *Straining:* This denotes the application of abdominal pressure by the child to initiate and maintain voiding.
- *Weak stream:* This denotes observed weak force of ejection of urinary stream.
- *Intermittency:* This denotes the occurrence of micturition in several discrete spurts rather than in a continuous stream. This may be physiological up to 3 years of age.

Other Symptoms

- *Holding maneuvers:* These denote observable strategies to postpone voiding or suppress urgency. They include standing on tiptoe, the classical "*Vincent's curtsy*," forceful crossing of the legs, or squatting with heel pressed into the perineum.
- *Feeling of incomplete emptying:* This is a significant complaint in older children and adolescents.
- *Postmicturition dribble:* This denotes involuntary leakage of urine immediately after voiding has finished.
- *Genital and LUT pain:* It is usually nonspecific and difficult to localize.

COMMON COMORBIDITIES ASSOCIATED WITH LOWER URINARY TRACT DYSFUNCTION

Urinary Tract Infection

Various studies have repeatedly demonstrated a clear and consistent relationship between LUTD and UTI. UTI occurs not only as an effect of LUTD but can also precipitate the development of LUTD, specifically OAB. The incidence of UTI is significantly higher in girls with LUTD (especially with underactive bladder) than in boys. The association between UTI and LUTD was most often noted for LUTD which is associated with urinary stasis.

Vesicoureteric Reflux

Voiding against a closed sphincter increases intravesical pressure and contributes to the development and persistence of VUR. The incomplete bladder emptying in children with LUTD leads to urinary stasis with subsequent UTI, causing inflammatory changes in the bladder wall that stimulate hypertrophy and overactivity. This is characteristic in older children who present with febrile UTI after toilet training. It is postulated that detrusor hypertrophy can alter the closure mechanism at the ureterovesical junction, leading to VUR. Dilating reflux and female sex have been implicated as risk factors for the development of LUTD. Significant association has been noted between recurrent UTI and LUTD, and the prevalence of LUTD is lower in children with spontaneous resolution of VUR. The association between LUTD and treatment failure after surgical correction of VUR has been observed in multiple studies. It has also been demonstrated that targeted treatment for LUTD improves the spontaneous resolution rates for VUR. Studies have proven that patients with combined BBD and VUR are at higher risk for developing recurrent UTI than children with BBD or VUR alone.[2,3,9]

Behavioral Disorders/ Psychological Associations

In the present era, there is increasing awareness of the significant association between behavioral disorders and LUTD in children. Functional causes of LUTD have been postulated to originate from behavioral issues that evolve from personal stressors and/or adverse events that occurred around the time of toilet training. Environmental factors, including personal and familial interactions, are seen to have an important effect on the continence of school-age children. Considering the fact that between 20 and 40% of children with LUTD have associated behavioral disorders, it has been recommended that screening for psychosocial comorbidities should be an integral part of the evaluation of pediatric LUTD. A major epidemiological study revealed a significantly increased rate of psychological problems [attention-deficit hyperactivity disorder (ADHD), conduct disorders, oppositional behavior, etc.] among children with LUTD compared with those who were dry. Clinicians should be aware of the association with disorders such as ADHD in children with daytime wetting, because this is likely to interfere with treatment success.[1,2,4,10]

Constipation/Bowel Dysfunction

When constipation and LUTD are both present, the condition is referred to as *BBD*, which will be described in detail here. Children with constipation are up to eight times more likely to have LUTD, compared to children with normal bowel function. LUTS are seen in approximately 30% of children who present with constipation. It has been reported that nearly 50% of patients presenting with LUTS also had evidence of functional constipation. Various theories attribute the functional abnormalities of the bladder in LUTD to the secondary effects of chronic rectal distension or chronic contraction of pelvic musculature in constipation. The relationship between abnormal bowel and bladder activity is presently termed *BBD* and is part of an entity originally described previously as *the DES* (Koff et al. 1998). They recommended that each LUTD be treated specifically while addressing any concomitant bowel dysfunction, ideally before treatment of the LUTD.[1,2,4,10]

DESCRIPTION OF THE DIFFERENT TYPES OF LOWER URINARY TRACT DYSFUNCTION IN CHILDREN

Bladder and Bowel Dysfunction

Bladder and bowel dysfunction is a broad term used to describe children who present a constellation of LUTS associated with constipation and/or encopresis. In this clinical condition, bladder symptoms such as urgency, frequency, and incontinence are caused by problems in emptying and/or storage. The loaded rectum compresses the bladder and decreases the bladder capacity, leading to urgency and frequency. The fecal mass in the rectum may cause chronic pelvic spasms, which result in incomplete bladder emptying and significant postvoid residual urine. Children who voluntarily hold urine for longer periods will gradually present decreased sensation/urge to evacuate establishing the BBD cycle pattern. BBD is a more representative term for a spectrum of disorders, commonly referred to previously as *dysfunctional voiding* and/or *DES*. It is the secondary symptoms of wetting, constipation, or UTI that usually prompts further evaluation of these children.[10-13]

Overactive Bladder

This common group of LUTD is characterized by frequent episodes of an urgent need to void, countered by contraction of the pelvic floor muscles and holding maneuvers. The typical symptom is *urinary urgency* associated with increased voiding frequency and incontinence, in the absence of infection or other pathology. OAB often presents in association with other types of LUTD, such as voiding postponement and dysfunctional voiding. *"The hallmark of OAB is urgency and, thus, children with this symptom can be said to have an OAB"* (ICCS standardization of LUTS terminology document, J Urol, 2006). Patients with OAB usually have incontinence secondary to *detrusor overactivity*, which has to be documented by a urodynamic study. The term OAB has replaced the previous nomenclature of *bladder instability*.[1,6,10,13]

Voiding Postponement

This is characterized by low daytime voiding frequency (≤3 times/day) but is not associated with any postvoid residual urine. The child performs *holding maneuvers* to postpone voiding. It is often associated with a feeling of urgency due to a full bladder. Some children restrict fluid intake to increase voiding intervals and decrease incontinence. There is a high incidence of psychological comorbidity or behavioral disorders.[1,4,10]

Dysfunctional Voiding

A child with dysfunctional voiding (this phrase is preferred over *voiding dysfunction*) habitually contracts the urethral sphincter during voiding. The term is applied only if verified by an invasive urodynamic study or repeated uroflow studies show curves with *staccato pattern.* The characteristic feature is discordant bladder and perineal activity, with or without postvoid residual urine. The child fails to relax the bladder neck at the time of voiding. It may also be associated with storage symptoms such as incontinence. The use of this term to denote any kind of LUTD is strongly discouraged.[1,6,10]

Hinman syndrome (Hinman-Allen syndrome/non-neurogenic neurogenic bladder—NNNB): Though this nomenclature is not included in the current classification, it is important to recognize this entity as a particular type of dysfunctional voiding. *Hinman syndrome* is the most severe form of dysfunctional voiding, with varied clinical presentation. The secondary obstructive sequelae may resemble those associated with structural (PUV) or neurological abnormalities (neurogenic bladder). It is characterized by functional bladder outlet obstruction in the absence of anatomical or neurological deficits. These children try to inhibit urination by voluntarily contracting the external sphincter **(Figs. 1A and B).** These voluntary contractions lead to an obstruction of the urinary tract, characterized by an intermittent stream, increased residual urine, and increased intravesical pressure. The resultant changes of the urinary tract resemble true neurogenic bladder. Patients may present with a wide array of symptoms including urgency with incontinence, infrequent voiding, intermittency, straining, enuresis, UTI, and abdominal pain. This is probably due to acquired behavioral and psychosocial disorders manifested as bladder dysfunction mimicking neurologic disease. It can be differentiated from neurogenic bladder by five criteria: (1) intact perineal sensation and anal tone, (2) normal anatomy and function of the lower extremities, (3) absence of skin lesions overlying the sacrum, (4) normal lumbosacral spine at plain radiography, and (5) normal spinal cord on imaging. The diagnosis of Hinman syndrome is based on clinical and radiological manifestations of neurogenic bladder in the absence of an underlying neurological abnormality or an obstructive lesion. It can result in a trabeculated bladder, ureterovesical obstruction, hydronephrosis, and even chronic renal failure can occur in the most extreme cases.[2]

Underactive Bladder

Underactive bladder describes a child who is required to raise intra-abdominal pressure to initiate, maintain, and complete voiding (straining). The terminology of "*Lazy bladder*" has been replaced by the nomenclature of an underactive bladder. This is typically associated with low voiding frequency during the day (≤3 times/day) associated with high postvoid residual urine. Detrusor function is abnormal (*detrusor underactivity*) on urodynamic assessment. An *interrupted pattern* on uroflow measurement is characteristic. This clinical situation is a primary indication for urodynamic study as part of the initial workup. The primary approach is with timed voiding and double voiding to more efficiently empty the bladder and lower the ultimate postvoid residual volume of urine. If this treatment strategy fails to achieve the desired effect, it is recommended to start clean intermittent catheterization (CIC) with frequency dependent on symptom severity.[1,10]

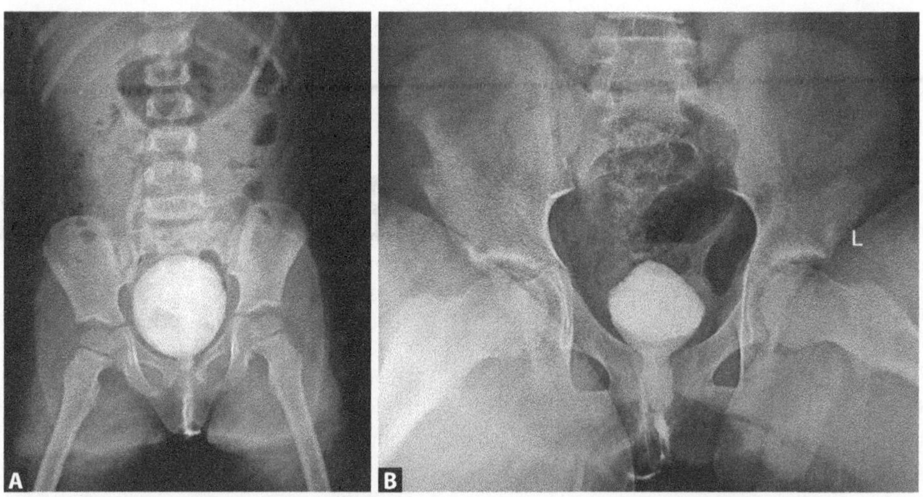

Figs. 1A and B: (A) A micturating cystourethrogram (MCU) showing hyperactive sphincter and right vesicoureteral reflux (VUR) in a female child; (B) MCU of another female child with significant posterior urethral dilatation secondary to hyperactive sphincter during voiding.

Giggle Incontinence (Enuresis Risoria)

This uncommon disorder is characterized by apparently complete voiding that occurs specifically during or immediately after laughing. Bladder function is otherwise normal. This is classically seen in school-age females. The accepted theory is that of a central nervous system inactivation (i.e., cataplexy) in association with laughter resulting in urinary incontinence. Giggle incontinence is not a form of stress incontinence nor is it due to weakness of the sphincter. This has to be distinguished from more common situations of sudden episodes of incontinence associated with OAB, voiding postponement, or underactive bladder. It is a diagnosis of exclusion, and it is usually established on history and supplemented by the absence of other voiding symptoms or abnormal findings on investigations. There is a high incidence of daytime voiding symptoms reported in patients with giggle incontinence, suggesting detrusor instability. Currently, available treatment strategies include biofeedback or methylphenidate.[1,2,4,5]

Vaginal Reflux (Vaginal Entrapment and Vaginal Voiding)

Vaginal reflux is characterized by incontinence after normal voiding in the absence of other LUTS. Prepubertal, toilet-trained girls with moderate incontinence episodes, consistently occurring within 10 minutes after normal voiding, are considered to have vaginal reflux, due to vaginal entrapment of urine. This occurs due to the position adopted by some girls, particularly overweight girls, while voiding. As the girl gets up, urine dribbles from the vagina. It can be associated with labial adhesions as a result of chronic irritation and inflammation from skin exposure to urine. Reassurance and postural modification to ensure complete vaginal emptying is the only treatment required.[1,2,4]

Extraordinary Daytime—Only Urinary Frequency/Pollakiuria

This term is applied to children who void frequently and with small volumes (average voided volumes are <50% of bladder capacity or even lesser) during daytime only. This is typically associated with a sudden increase in daytime voiding frequency (at least once hourly) unrelated to either urgency or incontinence. Unlike virtually all other categories of voiding dysfunction where females predominate over males by a 5:1 ratio, children with extraordinary daytime only urinary frequency (EDOUF) are predominantly male. Nocturnal bladder habits are usually normal for the age of the child. The term can be applied from the age of daytime bladder control or 3 years. A characteristic feature, which differentiates it from OAB, is that the symptoms are limited only to the daytime. It is seen in early childhood (4–6 years of age) and associated with a history of recent death or life-threatening event in the family. It usually runs a benign, self-limited course over a period of approximately 6 months.[1,2,4]

Bladder–Neck Dysfunction

Internal sphincter/primary bladder–neck dysfunction (PBND) is a non-neurogenic entity characterized by failure of the bladder neck to relax and permit flow, causing functional obstruction at the bladder neck. This requires video urodynamics for documentation. The presentation is with LUTS, which are typical of other more common LUTD. PBND is characterized by the constellation of prolonged bladder neck opening time, incomplete bladder neck funneling, quiet pelvic floor electromyography (EMG) during voiding, and obstructive pressure flow parameters. Though uncommon, this is a significant and commonly overlooked cause of LUTD in children.[1-3]

DIAGNOSIS OF LOWER URINARY TRACT DYSFUNCTION

Diagnosis of LUTD is essentially based on clinical history, physical examination, BD, symptoms score such as the dysfunctional voiding score system (DVSS), associated with uroflowmetry (UFM) and bladder ultrasonography to measure postvoid residual urine volume.[2,5,14]

Clinical History

The diagnosis of LUTD is essentially based on detailed evaluation of the clinical history. Urinary frequency, hesitancy, daytime incontinence, enuresis, urgency, urge incontinence, pelvic pain, and urine flow patterns are common LUTS. The presence of any of these symptoms in children over 5 years of age should alert to the possibility of LUTD. Bladder storage, voiding symptoms, and constipation should also be assessed. It is vital to consider all diagnostic possibilities in children who present with significant LUTS (**Box 4**). Many of the children with LUTD perform *holding maneuvers* to avoid involuntary urine loss. In girls, crossing their legs, with one knee over the other, pressing their genitals, walking on tiptoe, and squatting are classical holding maneuvers. This includes the characteristically described position of *Vincent's curtsy*. More than 70% of children with LUTD perform holding maneuvers.[2,3] Constipation is characterized by symptoms such as excessive straining during defecation, hard stools, a feeling of incomplete evacuation or

BOX 4: Differential diagnosis of pediatric urinary incontinence: The "ABCs."

- *Anatomic:* Ectopic ureter, posterior urethral valves, epispadias, labial adhesions
- *Behavioral:* Voiding postponement
- CNS, neurogenic bladder
- Developmental
- Endocrine, renal
- Functional (Hinman syndrome)
- Genetic (neuromuscular disorders)
- Habitual

(CNS: central nervous system)

anorectal blockage, the use of manual evacuation maneuvers to facilitate defecation or the occurrence of fewer than three spontaneous evacuations per week. The characteristics of the stools should be documented. Recognition and management of BBD are critical, since constipation should be treated together with voiding problems. Treatment of constipation usually reduces urinary symptoms and decreases the risk of UTI.[11-13] Psychological development of the child, particularly with regard to stressful events, the presence of anxiety, and excessive shyness or aggressiveness should be evaluated. If an emotional disorder is suggested, the child should be referred for psychological evaluation.

Clinical History in Evaluation of Lower Urinary Tract Dysfunction: Cardinal Points

- Antenatal history (maternal disease/fetal anomaly/fetal hydronephrosis)[2,3]
- Developmental milestones
- *Wetting history*:
  - Toilet training
  - Voiding pattern/habits
  - Voiding frequency and intervals
  - Age at onset of symptoms; duration and frequency of episodes
  - Urgency ± incontinence
  - Incontinence episodes and intervals (diurnal/nocturnal, giggle/stress, awareness, need for a protective pad, associated urge to void)
  - Fluid intake/thirst
  - Bowel habits (frequency, consistency as described by Bristol scale, associated rectal or abdominal pain)
  - Posturing (leg-crossing, squatting, dancing, and wiggling when needed to void, Vincent's curtsy)
- Behavioral disorders (ADHD, obsessive-compulsive disorder, mania, or depression)
- *Psychosocial history:* Social and family history of pertinent risk factors (family strife, school stress, and recent deaths in family)
- Medical history
  - *Urinary tract infection:* Number of episodes, details of therapy
  - Neurological disease (spinal dysraphism, hydrocephalus, seizure disorder, and sleep apnea)
  - Systemic disease (renal disease, diabetes mellitus, and diabetes insipidus)
  - *Medications (with recognized urinary adverse effects):* Antidepressants, antihistamines, diuretics, antiepileptics, lithium, and anticholinergics
- *Surgical history:*
  - Urological (UTI, VUR, PUV, duplex system, anorectal malformations)
  - *History of previous operative procedure (genitourinary/abdominal/pelvic/spine):* Endoscopic therapy or surgery for PUV/VUR/duplex system, hypospadias repair, oncological surgery, rectal pull through
  - Trauma
- Family history of voiding dysfunction
- Response of the child and family to the problem.

Physical Examination

- Distended bladder
- Presence of a palpable fecal mass in the abdomen
- Fecal impaction in the rectal ampulla
- The cremasteric and anal sphincter reflexes are tested.
- *Weight and height:* Evaluated with respect to growth charts and previous measurements
- Blood pressure
- *Perineum:* Look for labial adhesion, phimosis, meatal stenosis, anal pathology such as fissure-in-ano and signs of fecal incontinence
- *Sacral region:* Look for signs of occult spina bifida; sacral dimple, hairy patch of skin, altered pigmentation, asymmetry, swelling/lipoma
- Neurology sensitivity in the anogenital area, reflexes and strength in the lower extremities.

Documentation of Clinical Data

- *Voiding diary:* Time of voiding episodes, volume voided, and leakages (for at least 2 days)
- Voiding frequency *(normally four to seven times per day)*
- *Bladder capacity (maximum voided volume):* The highest volume excluding the first morning voided volume
- Expected bladder capacity [*30 mL* + (*age in years* × *30*)]
- Reduced bladder capacity [*<65% of EBC*]
- *Fluid intake:* Time, volume, and type of drinks (for at least 2 days) *(fluid intake: recommended 25–30 mL/kg/day or 1,200–1,500 mL/day for schoolchildren).*

Bladder Diary

- Record urine output and frequency
- Fluid intake
- Any occurrence of urgency or involuntary urine loss
- Bladder diary maintained over a 2–3-day period
- The color of the urine helps assess the state of hydration
- *Nocturnal BD:* Nappy weight, nocturnal urine volume, and morning urine volume for at least 7 days (must use nappy when sleeping)
- *Nocturnal urine production:* Sum of nappy weight, morning urine volume, and nocturnal urine volume, if applicable (*nocturnal polyuria*: *Nocturnal urine production >130% of EBC*).

A possible bias must be considered, on account of BD use, which may lead to a bladder training effect, and nights during recording have evidenced relevant variations in the frequency of nocturnal voids. Despite that, it continues to be one of the most important and simplest tools to access LUTS, setting more confidence to the diagnosis commonly overestimated by DVSS.[5,6,14]

SYMPTOMS SCORE SYSTEMS IN LOWER URINARY TRACT DYSFUNCTION

Specific questionnaires have been developed for use in the investigation of LUTS, including the *DVSS*, the *dysfunctional voiding and incontinence score system* (*DVISS*), and the *incontinence symptoms index-pediatric* (*ISI-P*). These scores may not have great relevance in clinical practice, but constitute important tools in clinical investigation, particularly with respect to standardizing the terms used and as a guide for professionals with less experience.[14,15] They are complementary tools to BD, in order to evaluate not only the actual voiding but also the self-reported behavior, a direct reflection of how LUTD impacts. Due to the significant association between constipation and LUTD, this condition should also be assessed through the use of questionnaires such as the *Rome IV diagnostic criteria* and the *Bristol stool scale*. The pathology may not be diagnosed correctly, if not properly evaluated.

INVESTIGATIVE MODALITIES IN LOWER URINARY TRACT DYSFUNCTION

The primary tools for assessment of LUTD in children are elaborate clinical history, observation and systematic, thorough physical examination. BD, urine flow measurements, and invasive urodynamic techniques are central to the diagnostic process.[9,10,16]

Bladder Diary

The systematic documentation of voiding and bladder-related symptoms at home under normal conditions is vital in the assessment of LUTD in children.

Urine Flow Measurements (Uroflowmetry)

The most commonly performed diagnostic procedure in pediatric urodynamic practice is the measurement of urine flow and residual urine with ultrasound scan, as a standalone examination. *UFM* is an indispensable test for children with LUTD. It is simple to perform, noninvasive, and fast and provides important data such as voided volume, voiding time, maximum flow, curve pattern, and rate of flow. UFM results showing a voided volume of at least 50 mL or 50% of the EBC for age [(age in years + 1) × 30] are considered adequate. This helps to decide on the need for invasive urodynamic studies. Flow measurement is a cornerstone of diagnosis in LUTD. The addition of pelvic floor EMG recordings to this can increase the diagnostic value.[16-18]

- *Maximum flow rate (Qmax):* This is the most relevant variable in assessing bladder outflow **(Fig. 2)**.
- *Flow curve shape:* This is determined by detrusor contractility, abdominal straining, and the bladder outlet.
  - The normal curve is smooth and *bell*-shaped.
  - OAB is characterized by a high amplitude curve of short duration (*tower*-shaped curve).
  - Organic outlet obstruction is characterized by a *plateau*-shaped curve.
  - Sphincter overactivity during voiding is typically associated with an irregular/*staccato* flow curve.
  - Underactive bladder with acontractile detrusor is associated with an *interrupted* or *fractionated* flow curve.

  Interpreting UFM curves can be subjective. The *flow index* (*FI*) is a new parameter calculated by dividing the actual Qmax by the estimated Qmax **(Table 1)**.
- *Uroflowmetry with electromyography (uroflow—EMG)*: This is a noninvasive evaluation method that provides information on the functionality of the pelvic floor and external sphincter. The procedure consists of attaching electrodes in the perineal area at the 3 and 9 o'clock positions. Simultaneous use of EMG during UFM adds relevant data during micturition, including coordination or lack of coordination in the relaxation of the sphincter. It provides the *EMG lag time*, i.e., the time required for the pelvic floor to relax once micturition is initiated (normally, 2–6 seconds). Thus, EMG lag time is the time duration after the external sphincter relaxes and the flow of urine. The time taken by the pelvic floor to relax prior to detrusor contraction and the beginning of voiding is longer in patients with LUTD. No pelvic floor activity is

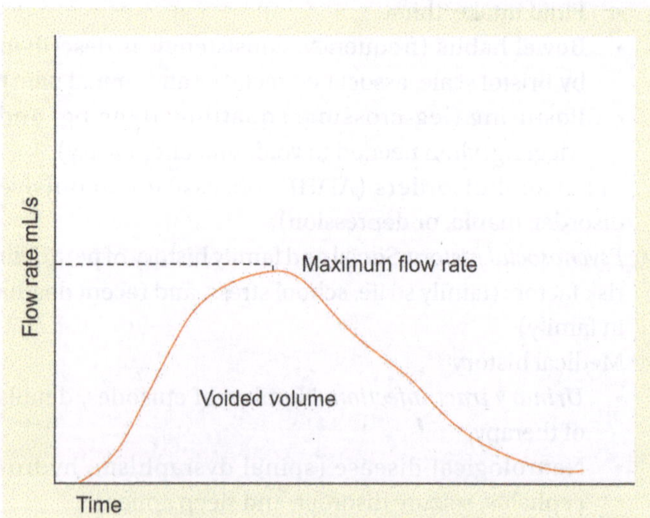

Fig. 2: Normal bell-shaped uroflow curve. Maximum flow rate corresponds to peak of the curve.

TABLE 1: Correlation of uroflowmetry curve with flow index in males and females.

Uroflowmetry curve	*Flow index: Males*	*Flow index: Females*
Flat curve	<0.70	<0.68
Bell-shaped curve	0.71–1.25	0.69–1.1
Tower-shaped curve	>1.25	>1.1

expected during voiding in patients with genuine OAB. Conversely, patients with dysfunctional voiding will have a tonic contraction of the sphincter during voiding (sharp peaks on the EMG).[16-18]

- *Measurement of postvoid residual urine volume:*
  - Bladder volume should be between 50 and 115% of the expected capacity for age, for reliable data to be obtained.
  - Postvoid residual urine volume should be measured in the first 5 minutes after micturition.
  - Value <5 mL is normal, 5–20 mL is indeterminate and needs repetition, and >20 mL is indicative of abnormal emptying.
  - Bladder wall thickness, measured on an empty bladder, should be <3 mm.
  - Measuring the rectal diameter is also helpful in constipated children, with measurements >3 cm being clinically significant.

Dynamic bladder ultrasonography is useful in evaluating pelvic floor contraction when involuntary contractions are present in cases of OAB.

Biomarkers

Nerve growth factor (NGF) and brain-derived neurotrophic factor (BDNF) are messengers emitted from the uroepithelial bladder smooth muscle aiming to differentiate neuronal cell in the peripheral nervous system. These biomarkers are believed to be increased in the urine of patients with OAB. Studies have already observed decreased urine levels during treatment as well as an increase after quitting the treatment, inciting questions about the role of the biomarker in the pathophysiology.[2,3,9]

Urodynamic Testing

Urodynamic studies investigate the filling and emptying phase of bladder function.[2,15,17,18] Urodynamic testing in children with LUTD and no neurological abnormalities is only recommended in the following situations:

- Persistently failure of therapy
- Underactive bladder
- *Significant bilateral dilation of the upper urinary tract:* In such situations, videourodynamics is useful to identify VUR and differentiate between bladder neck and bladder sphincter discoordination. The term *cystometry* denotes urodynamic investigation during the filling phase of micturition cycle. The technique of choice in pediatric urodynamics is *natural fill (ambulatory) cystometry*. If this is not feasible, a *filling rate* of 5–10% of *EBC*, expressed in mL per minute, is used.

  Bladder storage function should be described in terms of bladder sensation, detrusor activity, bladder compliance, and bladder capacity during filling cystometry.[15,19]
  - *Bladder sensation during filling cystometry:* This is only applicable to older children and adolescents.[1,7] *Underactive detrusor* is associated with *decreased or absent (no) sensation* throughout bladder filling. The lack of sensation when filling exceeds EBC is referred to as *reduced bladder sensation.*
  - *Detrusor function during filling cystometry:* Normal detrusor function allows bladder filling with little or no change in pressure and without involuntary phasic contractions. Any detrusor activity observed prior to voiding is considered pathological. *Detrusor overactivity* denotes involuntary contractions during the filling phase, with an increase in pressure of >15 cmH_2O above baseline. This can be classified as *neurogenic* or *idiopathic* based on etiology. This term replaces the previously used ones of *detrusor instability* and *detrusor hyperreflexia.*
  - *Bladder capacity and compliance during filling cystometry: Bladder compliance* describes the relationship between change in bladder volume and change in detrusor pressure. *Detrusor pressure* of 10 cmH_2O or less at EBC for age is acceptable. As compliance normally changes according to bladder volume and age, it should always be related to bladder capacity.
- *Urethral function during filling cystometry:* Urethral function in children is assessed by pelvic floor EMG. *Urethral relaxation incontinence* (earlier referred to as urethral instability) is defined as leakage due to urethral relaxation in the absence of increased abdominal pressure or detrusor overactivity.[15,18] *Urodynamic stress incontinence* is defined as involuntary urine leakage during increased abdominal pressure, in the absence of a detrusor contraction. *Abdominal leak point pressure* (previously referred to as *Valsalva leak point pressure*) is the intravesical pressure at which urine leakage occurs in the absence of a detrusor contraction, due to increased abdominal pressure. *Detrusor leak point pressure* is the intravesical pressure at which urine leakage occurs due to detrusor contraction, excluding any abdominal component. High leak point pressure signifies risk of upper urinary tract damage.[15,19]
- *Pressure flow studies: Cystometric evaluation during voiding phase*—this has low clinical relevance in infants and children. In infants, high detrusor pressures during voiding can be normal. *Detrusor underactivity* is a contraction of decreased strength and/or duration, causing prolonged/incomplete bladder emptying within a normal time span **(Fig. 3)**. This finding and that of an *acontractile detrusor* constitute an *underactive bladder* in the clinical setting.[15,18]

Dysfunctional voiding is a urodynamic entity characterized by an intermittent and/or fluctuating uroflow rate, due to involuntary intermittent contractions of the striated muscle of the external urethral sphincter or pelvic floor, during voiding in neurologically normal

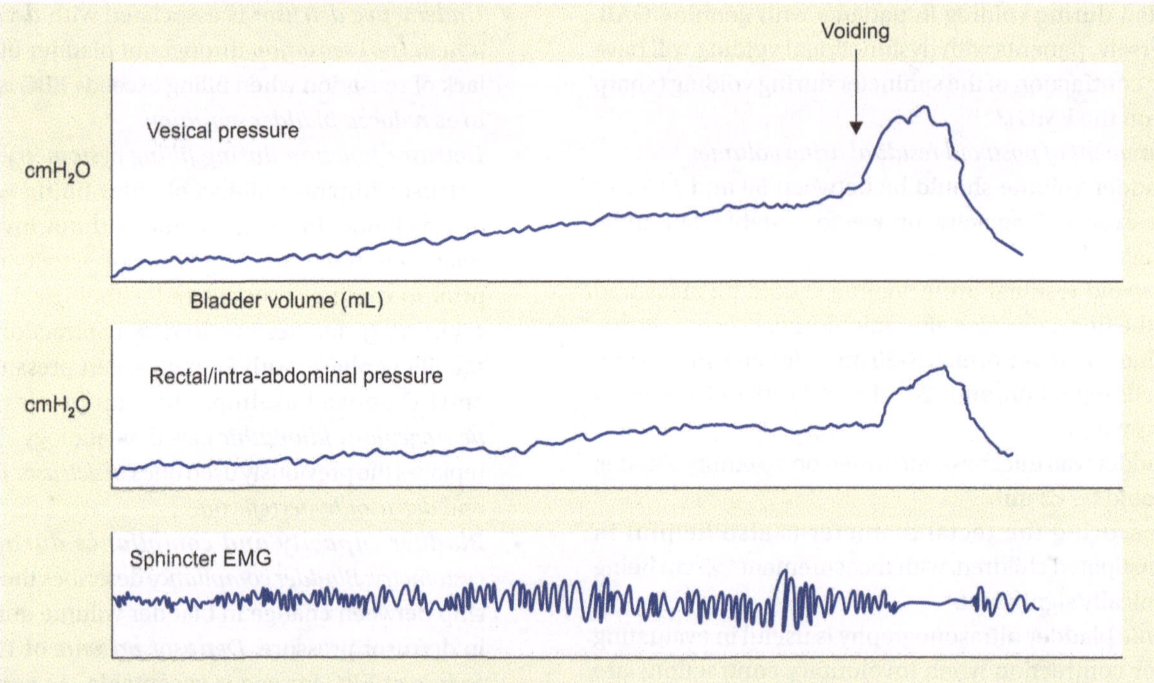

Fig. 3: Diagrammatic representation of cystometry in an underactive bladder. There is no significant rise of bladder pressure even with large volume of urine and child voids by straining represented by increased rectal pressure. Note the sphincter relaxes during voiding. Voiding is also incomplete.

individuals **(Fig. 4)** (*use of the nonspecific and general term voiding dysfunction, especially to denote any type of LUTD, should be avoided*).

Detrusor-sphincter dyssynergia is the cystometric observation of a detrusor voiding contraction concurrent with an involuntary contraction of the urethra and/or periurethral striated muscle and is common in patients with neurogenic bladder disturbance.[1,2,15,18]

- *4-hour voiding observation:* This is a scientifically validated technique used to evaluate bladder function in infancy. It implies continuous observation of a freely moving infant with frequent sonological assessment of bladder filling, measurement of voided volumes, and residual urine after each voiding.[1,19]
- *Signs related to voided volume*: The ICS and ICCS recommend that *voided volume* should replace the term *functional bladder capacity. EBC* is estimated by the formula [30 + (age in years × 30)] in mL. It is useful up to 12 years, after which EBC is around 390 mL. *Maximum voided volume* (with addition of residual urine) is considered less or more if found to be <65% or >150% of EBC.[1,15,19]
- *Residual urine:* This is the volume of urine present in the bladder immediately after voiding. This parameter is useful at all ages.
- *Signs related to urine output:* The predicted maximum rate of urine production by the kidneys is calculated by body weight (in kg) divided by 4 and expressed in *mL per minute. Polyuria* should be defined as a 24-hour urine output of >2 L/m² body surface area, in children of all ages.

Urological Evaluation in Lower Urinary Tract Dysfunction

The children who are detected to have hydronephrosis on sonology should undergo the standard evaluation including selective use of voiding cystourethrogram (VCUG), intravenous urogram (IVU), and isotope renal studies. VCUG demonstrates the presence and grade of VUR, bladder morphology (capacity, shape, postvoid residue, and presence of wall irregularities/trabeculations), and configuration of urethra (persistent or intermittent narrowing in the region of external sphincter) **(Figs. 3 and 4)**. VCUG also helps to rule out the presence of structural anomalies, such as PUV in male children. IVU can be helpful in precise definition of the anatomy of urinary tract, ruling out anomalies such as duplex system and ectopic ureter and assessment of bladder. Isotope renal scans aid to rule out obstruction and assess relative renal function, while renal cortical scintigraphy helps to detect renal scarring, in the presence of VUR. In the presence of significant findings, VCUG and isotope renal scans can be repeated during follow-up to assess progression and response to therapy.

TREATMENT OF LOWER URINARY TRACT DYSFUNCTION

Principles of Therapy

- Identify and target the underlying cause of symptoms
- Symptomatic relief (of incontinence, constipation, UTI)
- Recognize and manage comorbidities

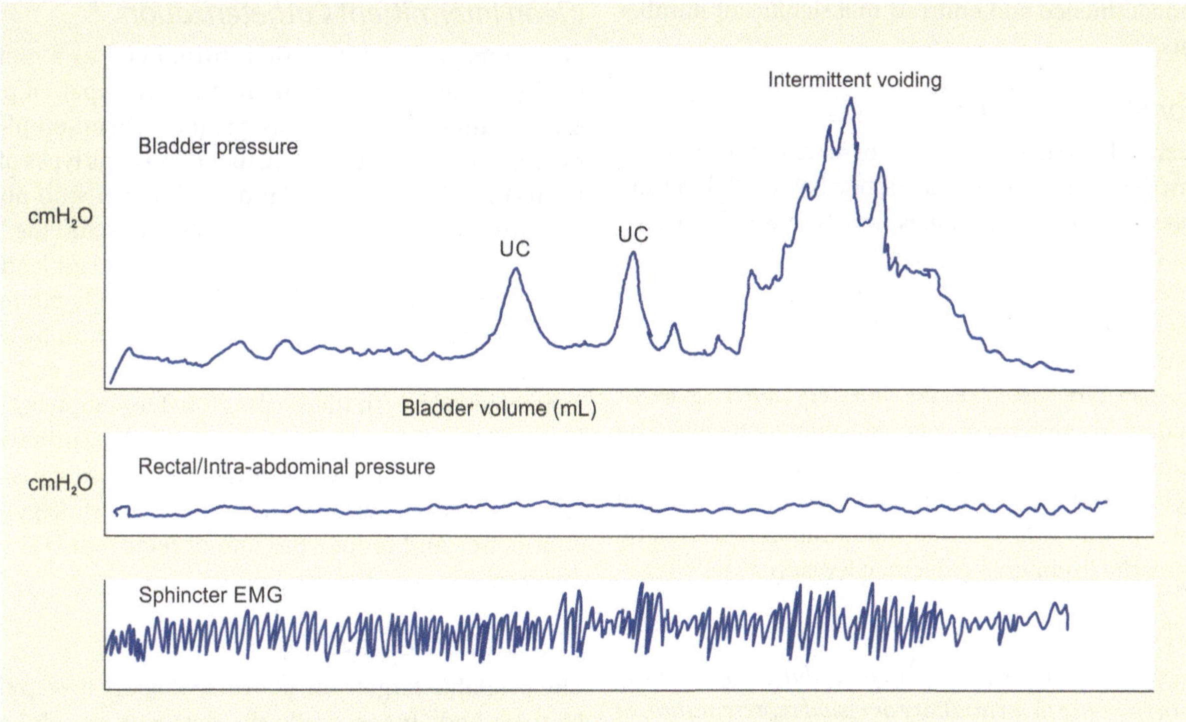

Fig. 4: Diagrammatic representation of cystometry in dysfunctional voiding. Note the hyperactive external sphincter even during voiding which is intermittent. There are uninhibited bladder contractions (UC) also.

- Protection of upper tracts from progressive damage
- Stepwise approach from the least invasive to more invasive therapies.

The treatment of LUTD is discussed separately under the following headings, though the actual clinical management involves the apt sequential and selective use of multiple modalities and a continuum between different therapies, depending on the specific problems in a particular child. Hence, these broad guidelines require a great degree of individualization, which is critical to a successful outcome.

- Urotherapy
- Constipation and bowel management
- Behavior modification
- Biofeedback therapy
- Clean intermittent catheterization
- Pharmacotherapy (anticholinergics, α-blockers)
- Botulinum toxin
- Neuromodulation.

Urotherapy

This conservative mode of treatment aims to rehabilitate the LUT and involves multiple healthcare professionals. It involves combination of education, behavior modification, treatment of constipation, and cataloging of voiding patterns, and is termed *standard urotherapy*. It should be the first step in management. Urotherapy can be divided into *standard therapy* and *specific interventions*.[20-22] *Standard urotherapy* includes the following:

- *Education* regarding the basic anatomy and physiology helps to clarify LUT function for the child and parents. It is helpful to explain how the particular child deviates from normal.
- *Instruction* on how to resolve LUTD (i.e., *behavior modification, timed voiding schemes, bowel management/* treatment of constipation).
- *Lifestyle advice:* It includes balanced fluid intake and diet modification, regular bladder and bowel emptying patterns, avoidance of holding postures, proper hygiene, and review of optimal posture during voiding.
- *Documentation* of symptoms and voiding habits, using *bladder diaries* or frequency–volume charts and evolving use of mobile applications.
- *Support* and encouragement by regular follow-up with the caregiver.

Specific interventions of urotherapy include various forms of pelvic floor muscle retraining (biofeedback), neuromodulation, and intermittent catheterization.[23-26]

Constipation and Bowel Management

The preliminary step is to identify the frequently associated bowel dysfunction with LUTD, based on clinical history and examination. A bowel regimen of high-fiber diet and concurrently increased fluid intake is initiated. The rule of thumb for daily fiber intake is age in years plus 15–20 for the total number of grams to be taken daily. The bowel regimen should be continued throughout the treatment course to maximize therapeutic efficacy for the LUTD component and counteract the constipation caused by anticholinergic medications, if administered. Relief of constipation can result in disappearance of symptoms such as daytime urinary incontinence and enuresis in a significant number of patients.[27-29]

Behavior Modification

The objective of any structured behavior modification program is to return the child to normal micturition habits. Children are encouraged to urinate before they have a sense of urgency, ensure complete bladder emptying, and avoid abdominal straining. An individualized voiding regimen is set to establish a consistent voiding routine. The classic regimen involves *timed voiding* with frequent voids scheduled every 2 hours during the day. Wristwatch alarms/vibratory watch can assist older children to comply with a timed voiding schedule. The establishment of a reward system/positive reinforcement with a voiding diary can significantly improve the self-esteem, and compliance of the child behavior modification is seen to be more successful in children older than 8 years of age.[30-32]

Biofeedback

The concept of biofeedback is the *modulation of a bodily function in response to an auditory or visual representation of that function.* It is a treatment modality that uses electronic or mechanical instruments to relay perceptual evidence to assist a person in gaining control over a physiologic process or function. It employs noninvasive urodynamic instrumentation to measure, record, and provide direct, instantaneous information to the child about voiding function. Real-time UFM allows the patient to observe the urine flow rate, while concurrent placement of adhesive pads on the perineum measures sphincter and/or pelvic floor activity. Abdominal EMG also can be performed simultaneously. The visual and auditory feedback (sometimes with interactive video games, called *animated biofeedback*) allows the child to become aware of and gain control over LUT function by teaching them how to voluntarily relax their sphincter and pelvic floor musculature during voiding. EMG activity is translated into an animated sequence that can be controlled by the child on contraction/relaxation of the external urinary sphincter. Upon isolating the sphincter, the child uses the games to learn to modulate the sphincter and thus repeat this modulation while voiding. Children with dysfunctional voiding have a better improvement of symptoms than children with OAB with biofeedback, although this is an effective treatment in both groups. In patients with dysfunctional voiding and VUR, biofeedback expedited the resolution of VUR or lowered the grade of VUR and created a bladder environment more favorable for surgical treatment, where required. It has also been helpful in the treatment of giggle incontinence to increase external urethral sphincter awareness and recruitment. The concept of *voiding school* has been proposed (Hoebeke et al.) where children are reeducated on voiding and fluid intake, and individualized voiding diaries, pelvic floor biofeedback training, UFM, alarm therapy, cognitive therapy, and psychological support are employed.[32-34]

Clean Intermittent Catheterization

The concept of CIC was first introduced as a method of emptying the bladder in neurologically impaired patients. This treatment strategy has gradually been employed in neurologically intact individuals with various types of LUTD. In dysfunctional voiding and in children who postpone micturition, the detrusor muscle stretches and the bladder becomes chronically overdistended. This can lead to two types of changes of the detrusor muscle: (1) *bladder wall thickening* caused by hyperplasia and hypertrophy resulting in OAB or (2) an *underactive bladder* with the end result of myogenic failure. In these cases, bladder emptying is often incomplete, resulting in large postvoid residual urine volumes, urinary incontinence, and recurrent UTIs from stasis. CIC is a safe, effective, and well-tolerated treatment strategy to attain continence and reduce the rate of recurrent UTI in these children.[20-23]

Pharmacotherapy

The available targets for pharmacological therapy are the bladder body (specifically the detrusor muscle) and the bladder outlet (specifically the bladder neck and proximal urethra). Pharmacological agents that target the detrusor muscle include bladder relaxants and anticholinergic therapies that facilitate storage by relaxing the detrusor smooth muscle. The other aim is to promote bladder emptying by targeting the bladder outlet using α-adrenergic antagonists (α-blockers). Thus, anticholinergic agents and α-adrenergic receptor antagonists (i.e., α-blockers) are used to enhance bladder filling and emptying, respectively. One or both of these medications are generally initiated once all other conservative measures have been exhausted. α-blockers are started concomitantly with biofeedback in some instances.[21-23]

- *Anticholinergic agents:* Anticholinergics (i.e., antimuscarinics) are the current gold standard in the treatment of patients with symptoms referable to OAB. The main action of anticholinergics is on the M1 and M3 receptor subtypes, which are thought to be responsible for the pathogenesis of detrusor overactivity. They act by reducing the frequency and intensity of uninhibited detrusor contractions during the filling phase of the bladder, resulting in an increase in functional bladder capacity and compliance. *Oxybutynin* was among the first generation of modern antimuscarinic medications available for treating incontinence in children. The currently employed anticholinergic agents for the treatment of OAB include *darifenacin, oxybutynin, solifenacin, tolterodine,* and *trospium.* Oxybutynin has antimuscarinic, antispasmodic, and analgesic properties. It causes the antispasmodic effect by acting as a calcium channel blocker. The main side effects include constipation, dry mouth, blurred vision, reduced sweating, flushing, and altered behavior and cognition. Other methods of delivery of oxybutynin are intravesical and transdermal. The ideal patient for treatment of OAB with anticholinergics is the low capacity OAB with complete emptying. In children with significant postvoid residual urine and incomplete emptying, anticholinergic treatment for OAB is not as efficacious, and therapy should be aimed at improving emptying and avoidance of overdistension that may be responsible for the OAB symptoms.[21,23,35-37]

- *α-adrenergic receptor antagonists:* α-adrenoreceptors have been demonstrated in the LUT, with a large concentration located at the bladder neck and urethra. α-adrenergic blockade results in smooth muscle relaxation and decreased bladder outlet resistance. Limitations of early α-adrenergic receptor antagonists (α-blockers) included their side effect profile with hypotension and dizziness. With subsequent development of more "selective" α-blockers that targeted α1A-adrenergic receptors rather than both α1A- and α1B-adrenergic receptors, these side effects were reduced. Examples of selective α-blockers include *alfuzosin, doxazosin, prazosin, silodosin, tamsulosin,* and *terazosin.* α-blocker treatment selection of children with LUTD is done through a comprehensive treatment program that involves an *escalating treatment paradigm* or identifying patients with characteristic uroflow abnormalities. The uroflow finding of a prolonged "EMG lag time" is associated with bladder neck and internal urethral sphincter discoordination and may be used to select patients for α-blocker therapy. A prolonged EMG lag time of greater than 6 seconds is suggested as a reliable indicator of tailoring LUTD treatment with α-blocker therapy.[23,38-40]

Botulinum Toxin

In refractory cases of LUTD, a relatively recent investigational pharmacologic approach is the *reversible chemical denervation* using *botulinum neurotoxin type A (BoNTA)*. BoNTA is directly injected into the detrusor muscle (in patients with OAB) or external urinary sphincter (in patients with dysfunctional voiding) under cystoscopic guidance. It acts by inhibiting ACh release at the presynaptic neuromuscular junction. Inhibited ACh release results in regionally decreased muscle contractility and atrophy at the injection site. Preliminary studies suggest that repeated BoNTA injections are safe in children and do not induce additional fibrosis in the bladder wall. The duration of treatment effect peaks at 6 weeks and usually lasts between 3 and 12 months. The need for retreatment, due to the reversible nature of the chemical denervation secondary to synaptic terminal resprouting within 6 months of injection, is a main drawback.[41;42]

Neuromodulation

In neuromodulation, electrical stimuli are exerted in a noninvasive manner to alter the existent neural transmission pattern and modulate detrusor activity. The proposed mechanism involves acting centrally by rebalancing excitatory and inhibitory information and returning the neural drive toward a more neutral status. The aim of neuromodulation in LUTD is to block the afferent limb of the sacral reflex arc leading to inhibition of detrusor contraction. *Cutaneous* (presacral area) and *percutaneous* approaches (implantable device at the posterior S3 foramen) via peripheral nerves have been used. The options include *sacral neuromodulation with implanted electrode* (SNM), *pudendal nerve stimulation,* and *percutaneous tibial nerve stimulation* (PTNS). *Presacral transcutaneous electrical neurostimulation (*TENS) has been successfully used for refractory OAB. SNM has been approved for use for urinary urgency/frequency, urge incontinence, pelvic floor dysfunction, and nonobstructive urinary retention.[29,32,43]

ASSESSMENT OF OUTCOME IN LOWER URINARY TRACT DYSFUNCTION

The affected child and the family are the ones who determine the criteria for success of treatment in the clinical situation. In the research setting, uniform standards are necessary for comparison and analysis. According to the ICCS, researchers and/or clinicians should recognize three basic principles of treatment outcomes: (1) The *symptom frequency during baseline and after treatment* each should be documented. (2) The *assessment of treatment response* must be based on *pretreatment baseline* registration symptom frequency. This enables grouping into *responders* and *nonresponders.* (3) The *response during treatment* should be noted, as well as the *response after cessation of treatment* for a specified period; and these two responses may not be the same.[3,5,10,29,43] This has been outlined as follows:

- *Initial success (based on symptom frequency):*
  - *No response:* <50% reduction
  - *Partial response:* 50–99% reduction
  - *Complete response:* 100% reduction
- *Long-term success:*
  - *Relapse:* More than one symptom recurrence per month
  - *Continued success:* No relapse in 6 months after cessation of treatment
  - *Complete success:* No relapse in 2 years after cessation of treatment.

CONCLUSION

A greater understanding of the etiopathologic factors, clarity in nomenclature, better definition of diagnostic guidelines, and advancements in functional assessment have revolutionized the concepts in LUTD in children. This has been supplemented by the recognition of the need for escalating therapeutic regimens, involving various treatment modalities and multiple healthcare professionals. As the concepts in diagnosis and treatment continue to evolve, the management aims to be holistic and comprehensive.

KEY POINTS

- Lower urinary tract dysfunction in children constitutes a variegated group of disorders with no underlying anatomical or neurological defect.
- The characteristic features in these children include the symptom of daytime incontinence, association with bowel dysfunction, and psychosocial issues.
- Lower urinary tract dysfunction is associated with VUR, UTI, and the risk of progressive renal scarring in severe cases.
- The standardization of nomenclature has enabled greater clarity in diagnosis of the wide spectrum of disorders.
- Functional assessment of bladder by uroflowmetry and urodynamic study provides better understanding of the pathophysiology in LUTD.
- A comprehensive treatment regimen that recognizes the need for comorbidities is central to therapy and involves an escalating treatment protocol, from least invasive to more invasive options.
- Proper outcome analysis, continued support, and long-term follow-up are critical to the success of therapy.

REFERENCES

1. Nevéus T, von Gontard A, Hoebeke P, Hjälmås K, Bauer S, Bower W, et al. The standardization of terminology of lower urinary tract function in children and adolescents: report from the Standardisation Committee of the International Children's Continence Society. J Urol. 2006;176:314-24.
2. Austin PF, Seth A. Functional disorders of the lower urinary tract in children. Chapter 35. Campbell Walsh Wein Urology, 12th edition. Amsterdam: Elsevier; 2020. pp. 652-66.
3. Palmer LS. Evaluation and targeted therapy of voiding dysfunction in children. Urology. 2016;92:87-94.
4. Austin PF, Bauer SB, Bower W, Chase J, Franco I, Hoebeke P, et al. The standardization of terminology of lower urinary tract function in children and adolescents: update report from the Standardization Committee of the International Children's Continence Society. J Urol. 2014;91(6):1863-5.
5. Chase J, Austin P, Hoebeke P, McKenna P, International Children's Continence Society. The management of dysfunctional voiding in children: a report from the standardisation committee of the International Children's Continence Society. J Urol. 2010;183(4):1296-302.
6. Sureshkumar P, Jones M, Cumming R, Craig J. A population-based study of 2,856 school-age children with urinary incontinence. J Urol. 2009;181:808-15.
7. Franco I, von Gontard A, De Gennaro M, International Childrens's Continence Society. Evaluation and treatment of nonmonosymptomatic nocturnal enuresis: a standardization document from the International Children's Continence Society. J Pediatr Urol. 2013;9(2):234-43.
8. Nevéus T, Eggert P, Evans J, Macedo A, Rittig S, Tekgül S, et al. Evaluation of and treatment for monosymptomatic enuresis: a standardization document from the International Children's Continence Society. J Urol. 2010;183(2):441-7.
9. Hoebeke P, Bower W, Combs A, De Jong T, Yang S. Diagnostic evaluation of children with daytime incontinence. J Urol. 2012;183(2):699-703.
10. Bauer SB, Nijman RJ, Drzewiecki BA, Sillen U, Hoebeke P, International Children's Continence Society Standardization Subcommittee. International Children's Continence Society standardization report on urodynamic studies of the lower urinary tract in children. Neurourol Urodyn. 2015;34(7):640-7.
11. Santos J, Varghese A, Williams K, Koyle MA. Recommendations for the management of bladder bowel dysfunction in children. Pediatr Ther. 2014;4:191.
12. Yang S, Chua ME, Bauer S, Wright A, Brandström P, Hoebeke P, et al. Diagnosis and management of bladder bowel dysfunction in children with urinary tract infections: a position statement from the International Children's Continence Society. Pediatr Nephrol. 2018;33(12):2207-19.
13. Burgers RE, Mugie SM, Chase J, Cooper CS, von Gontard A, Rittig CS, et al. Management of functional constipation in children with lower urinary tract symptoms: report from the Standardization Committee of the International Children's Continence Society. J Urol. 2013;190(1):29-36.
14. Farhat W, Bägli D, Capolicchio G, O'Reilly S, Merguerian PA, Khoury A, et al. The dysfunctional voiding scoring system: quantitative standardization of dysfunctional voiding symptoms in children. J Urol. 2000;164:1011.
15. Akbal C, Genc Y, Burgu B, Ozden E, Tekgul S. Dysfunctional voiding and incontinence scoring system: quantitative evaluation of incontinence symptoms in pediatric population. J Urol. 2005;173(3):969-73.
16. Schewe J, Brands FH, Pannek J. Voiding dysfunction in children: role of urodynamic studies. Urol Int. 2002;69(4):297-301.
17. Hjalmas K, Hoebeke PB, de Paepe H. Lower urinary tract dysfunction and urodynamics in children. Eur Urol. 2000;38(5):655-65.
18. Rakowska M, Jobs K, Paruszkiewicz G, Jung A. Interpretation of uroflowmetry in the paediatric population. Pediatr Med Rodz. 2017;13:40-52.
19. Hoebeke P, Van Laecke E, Van Camp C, Raes A, Van De Walle J. One thousand video-urodynamic studies in children with non-neurogenic bladder sphincter dysfunction. BJU Int. 2001;87(6):575-80.
20. Tekgul S, Stein R, Bogaert G, Undre S, Nijman RJM, Quaedackers J, et al. EAU-ESPU guidelines recommendations for daytime lower urinary tract conditions in children. Eur J Pediatr. 2020;179:1069-77.
21. Fuentes M, Magalhães J, Barroso Jr. U. Diagnosis and management of bladder dysfunction in neurologically normal children. Front Pediatr. 2019;7:298.
22. Chang SJ, Van Laecke E, Bauer SB, von Gontard A, Bagli D, Bower WF, et al. Treatment of daytime urinary incontinence: a standardization document from the International Children's Continence Society. Neurourol Urodyn. 2017;36:43-50.
23. Thom M, Campigotto M, Vemulakonda V, Coplen D, Austin PF. Management of lower urinary tract dysfunction: a stepwise approach. J Pediatr Urol. 2011;8(1):20-4.
24. Hellstrom AL. Urotherapy in children with dysfunctional bladder. Scand J Urol Nephrol Suppl. 1992;141:106-7.
25. Hoebeke P. Twenty years of urotherapy in children: what have we learned? Eur Urol. 2006;49:426-8.
26. Brownrigg N, Braga LH, Rickard M, Farrokhyar F, Easterbrook B, Dekirmendjian A, et al. The impact of a bladder training video versus standard urotherapy on quality of life of children with bladder and bowel dysfunction: a randomized controlled trial. J Pediatr Urol. 2017;13(4):374.e1-8.

27. Sampaio C, Sousa AS, Fraga LG, Veiga ML, Bastos Netto JM, Barroso Jr. U. Constipation and lower urinary tract dysfunction in children and adolescents: a population-based study. Front Pediatr. 2016;4:101.
28. Malykhina AP, Brodie KE, Wilcox DT. Genitourinary and gastrointestinal co-morbidities in children: the role of neural circuits in regulation of visceral function. J Pediatr Urol. 2017;13: 177-82.
29. Feldman AS, Bauer SB. Diagnosis and management of dysfunctional voiding. Curr Opin Pediatr. 2006;18:139-47.
30. Özen MA, Mutluer T, Necef I, Shabsog M, Taşdemir M, Bilge I, et al. The overlooked association between lower urinary tract dysfunction and psychiatric disorders: a short screening test for clinical practice. J Pediatr Urol. 2019;15(4):332.e1-5.
31. Wiener JS, Scales MT, Hampton J, King LR, Surwit R, Edwards CL. Long-term efficacy of simple behavioral therapy for daytime wetting in children. J Urol. 2000;164:786.
32. Barroso Jr. U, Lordêlo P, Lopes AA, Andrade J, Macedo Jr A, Ortiz V. Nonpharmacological treatment of lower urinary tract dysfunction using biofeedback and transcutaneous electrical stimulation: a pilot study. BJU Int. 2006;98:166-71.
33. Khen-Dunlop N, Van Egroo A, Bouteiller C, Biserte J, Besson R. Biofeedback therapy in the treatment of bladder overactivity, vesicoureteral reflux and urinary tract infection. J Pediatr Urol. 2006;2:424-9.
34. Combs AJ, Glassberg AD, Gerdes D, Horowitz M. Biofeedback therapy for children with dysfunctional voiding. Urology. 1998;52:312-5.
35. Marcelissen T, Rashid T, Antunes Lopes T, Delongchamps NB, Geavlete B, Rieken M, et al. Oral pharmacologic management of overactive bladder syndrome: where do we stand? Eur Urol Focus. 2018;5(6):1112-9.
36. Chapple CR, Khullar V, Gabriel Z, Muston D, Bitoun CE, Weinstein D. The effects of antimuscarinic treatments in overactive bladder: an update of a systematic review and meta-analysis. Eur Urol. 2008;54:543-62.
37. Ko Y, Malone DC, Armstrong EP. Pharmacoeconomic evaluation of antimuscarinic agents for the treatment of overactive bladder. Pharmacotherapy. 2006;26:1694-702.
38. Cain MP, Wu SD, Austin PF, Herndon CD, Rink RC. Alpha blocker therapy for children with dysfunctional voiding and urinary retention. J Urol. 2003;170(4 Pt 2):1514-5.
39. Kramer SA, Rathbun SR, Elkins D, Karnes RJ, Husmann DA. Double-blind placebo controlled study of alpha-adrenergic receptor antagonists (doxazosin) for treatment of voiding dysfunction in the pediatric population. J Urol. 2005;173(6): 2121-24.
40. Yucel S, Akkaya E, Guntekin E, Kukul E, Akman S, Melikoglu M, et al. Can alpha-blocker therapy be an alternative to biofeedback for dysfunctional voiding and urinary retention? A prospective study. J Urol. 2005;174(4 Pt 2):1612-5.
41. Uçar M, Akgül AK, Parlak A, Yücel C, Kiliç N, Balkan E. Noninvasive evaluation of botulinum-A toxin treatment efficacy in children with refractory overactive bladder. Int Urol Nephrol. 2018;50:1367-73.
42. Petronijevic V, Lazovic M, Vlajkovic M, Slavkovic A, Golubovic E, Miljkovic P. Botulinum toxin type A in combination with standard urotherapy for children with dysfunctional voiding. J Urol. 2007;178:2599-602.
43. Chancellor MB. Neuromodulation treatment of underactive bladder. In: Chancellor MB, Diokno AC (Eds). The Underactive Bladder. Cham: Springer; 2016. pp. 115-34.

CHAPTER

13.11 Enuresis

Madhuri Kanitkar, Saroj Kumar Patnaik

INTRODUCTION

Enuresis or bedwetting is the most common voiding complaint among children.[1] The characteristic feature is intermittent urinary incontinence combined with an inability to awaken from sleep despite a full bladder with or without detrusor overactivity.[2,3] Ability to continue to sleep in a wet bed is an attribute of enuresis. It often remains mismanaged.[4] Hitherto considered as a benign disorder, current evidence suggests that there are long-term psychosocial, emotional, and pathophysiological consequences for the affected child and the family.[5] The pathobiology of enuresis requires better characterization and understanding.

TERMINOLOGY AND DEFINITION

The International Children's Continence Society (ICCS) (2020) document defines enuresis as bedwetting above *5 years of age* irrespective of underlying pathogenesis or daytime symptoms.[2,3] Enuresis is an intermittent nonvolitional urinary incontinence during sleep and needs to be differentiated from other causes of urinary incontinence **(Table 1)**. The symptoms must occur *two or more times per week for at least 3 months to be termed enuresis.*[4,5] Previously used terminology of diurnal enuresis for daytime incontinence is no longer in vogue.[2,3]

EPIDEMIOLOGY

Reported prevalence of enuresis depends upon the setting, age group, tools for assessment, gender, family history, and various comorbidities encountered.[2,3,5,6] The prevalence of enuresis decreases from 15–20% under 5 years to 1–2% by adolescence. A small percentage of these may continue into adult life. Enuresis is two to three times more common among boys and increases by 44–77% if either or both parents had enuresis.[7,8]

Community-based studies primarily designed to estimate the occurrence of enuresis are scanty. Few children remain affected after the age of 16 years and gender difference decreases in the second decade of life.[2] Many hospital-based studies, especially from India, report the prevalence of enuresis during assessment of psychological morbidity in schoolgoing children.[8] Approximately 20–30% of patients

TABLE 1: Urinary incontinence in children.

Urinary incontinence	Continuous	Continuous dribbling	*Anatomic:* Urethral obstruction, ectopic ureter
			Neurologic: Spina bifida, spinal trauma, etc.
	Intermittent	Discrete involuntary voiding interspersed with periods of dryness	*Only night-time bedwetting:* Monosymptomatic nocturnal enuresis (MNE)
			With daytime symptoms/LUTS/recurrent urinary tract infection/bowel dysfunction:* Nonmonosymptomatic nocturnal enuresis (NMNE)

**LUTS (lower urinary tract symptoms): Presence of any of the following:* Daytime incontinence, urgency, voiding difficulties such as poor stream, hesitancy, need to strain to void. Voiding <4 or >7 times per day is abnormal

Terminology for enuresis

Primary enuresis: Child has never been dry for >6 months
Secondary enuresis: Enuresis after child having remained dry for at least 6 months
Frequent enuresis: Episodes occur more than thrice in a week
Voided volume: Volume of urine passed in a single episode of micturition
Maximum voided volume (MVV): Derived as the maximum voided volume in the daytime over a period of 3–4 days after exclusion of the first morning voided volume
Expected storage capacity of bladder for age (EBC): Calculated urinary bladder capacity calculated as EBC (mL) = 30 + Age (years) × 30; adult capacity is constant 400 mL
Nocturnal polyuria: Nocturnal urine production on a night with enuresis of at least 130% of the EBC for the child's age. Derived as (weight of urine in sheet covers/diapers + first morning void) in mL or >20 × (Age + 9) mL + volume of the first void in the morning
Normal bladder reservoir function: Maximum voided volume >65% of EBC

with enuresis also suffer from a psychological, behavioral, or psychiatric disorder such as attention-deficit/hyperactivity disorder (ADHD), autism, oppositional defiant disorder, or mood disorder and these are twice as common as in the general population.[9-11] Increased incidence of delayed language and slowed motor performances are noted with enuresis.[12] The effects that enuresis may have on the child are poor self-esteem, social avoidance, poor academic performance, and susceptibility for abuse. Parental stress adds to the woes of the child. These are more often associated with nonmonosymptomatic nocturnal enuresis (NMNE). Sleep disorders, especially obstructive sleep apnea, are more often associated with monosymptomatic nocturnal enuresis (MNE) and a significant set of these children benefit from adenotonsillectomy.[13]

ETIOPATHOGENESIS

Micturition is a complex function controlled centrally and ultimately executed by spinal-myoneural axis involving bladder and its sphincters innervated by the autonomic and somatic nerves. Developmental maturation of the nervous system pertaining to bladder-bowel function is preprogrammed in utero. After birth, learning and behavioral aspects get superimposed and refine volitional control of voiding in a psychosocial context to achieve bowel-bladder continence. Fecal continence is achieved first followed by daytime urinary continence and finally nocturnal continence by 5 years of age.[14-16] Bladder capacity at birth is around 60 mL and thereafter increases with age. Antidiuretic hormone (ADH) secretion is thought to be stimulated with bladder distension and the feedback loop helps in regulating nocturnal urine output. Variation of the bladder compliance is by modulation of the detrusor and sphincter activity in response to sensation of bladder filling during sleep.[17] Arousal to ensure a volitional void after a particular threshold of filling is an individualized complex interplay of the sensorimotor cortex, autonomic system, and brainstem. Neural networks around the locus coeruleus and a noradrenergic neuron group in the upper pons are important.[6] Interference in the age-related progressive maturation in bladder capacity, stability, and awareness of fullness as well as the inability to suppress the onset of bladder contraction during sleep results in enuresis.[17]

Precise etiopathogenesis of enuresis remains unknown.[6,17-20] *Enuretic children do not wake up to void.* Nocturnal polyuria and altered bladder urodynamics alone are not sufficient to result in enuresis in presence of an intact bladder sensory feedback, voluntary sphincter control, and arousal mechanisms. A consistent alteration in the pelvic tilt and posture of children with MNE has been noted suggesting an alteration in integration of the neuromuscular system for balance and voiding.[12] Higher prevalence of motor clumsiness, perceptual dysfunction, and speech disturbances in children with enuresis is described. A defective signal processing associated with maturational sensorimotor delay, altered bladder function, and a disturbed circadian sleep diuresis rhythm is postulated.

Occurrence in families suggests a genetic loading for enuresis.[21] There is as yet no single gene implicated for enuresis and current studies reveal a poor genotype-phenotype correlation. Family history though an important association is poorly predictive of genetic susceptibility.

A schematic depiction of the pathophysiology of enuresis is presented in **Figure 1**. Nocturnal polyuria is more common in MNE, whereas NMNE is more likely to be associated with decreased bladder storage capacity. Maturational delay of bladder control is a contributory factor. *Instead of viewing MNE and NMNE as separate disorders, perhaps it may be more appropriate to view them as a spectrum disorder.* Sleep quality of enuretic children is often impaired in the face of a poor arousal.[16] Obesity, constipation, and obstructive airway disease superimpose poor sleep.[22]

EVALUATION

All pediatric healthcare providers should proactively enquire about bedwetting in children beyond 5 years during routine visits to the clinic.[23] This will facilitate parents to seek timely professional help even if they are not aware of medical help being available.

Detailed history and physical examination form the cornerstone of diagnosis and optimal management of enuresis. A history of constipation is sought in every child. The same can be further verified using the Bristol Stool Chart.[2] Various validated questionnaire tools such as clinical management tool for screening in outpatient department (OPD) setting are available.[2,3,23] The aim is to identify any symptoms or signs suggestive of a possible underlying voiding disorder that points to an NMNE as depicted in **Tables 2 and 3**. It is emphasized that the pediatrician must talk to the parents *as well as the child*.[24] It is important to address all the behavioral problems the child may have and offer appropriate professional referral. A good clinical examination, especially of the external genitalia and the sacral region to rule out neuroanatomical etiology, is important and some clinical pointers are depicted in **Table 3**. Physical examination is mostly unremarkable in children with MNE.[3]

This should be followed by a voiding diary review as described subsequently. It is important to identify comorbidities and treat them first. In event of NMNE or a nonresponse after 3 months of initial behavioral therapy for MNE, the child should be referred to a specialist.

There is no role of routine laboratory tests.[25-28] A routine urinalysis is sufficient. Urine culture is not required in the absence of symptoms of urinary tract infection (UTI) or daytime lower urinary tract symptoms (LUTS) of recent onset. Blood tests are indicated only if there is glucosuria, polyuria, or features suggesting renal failure.

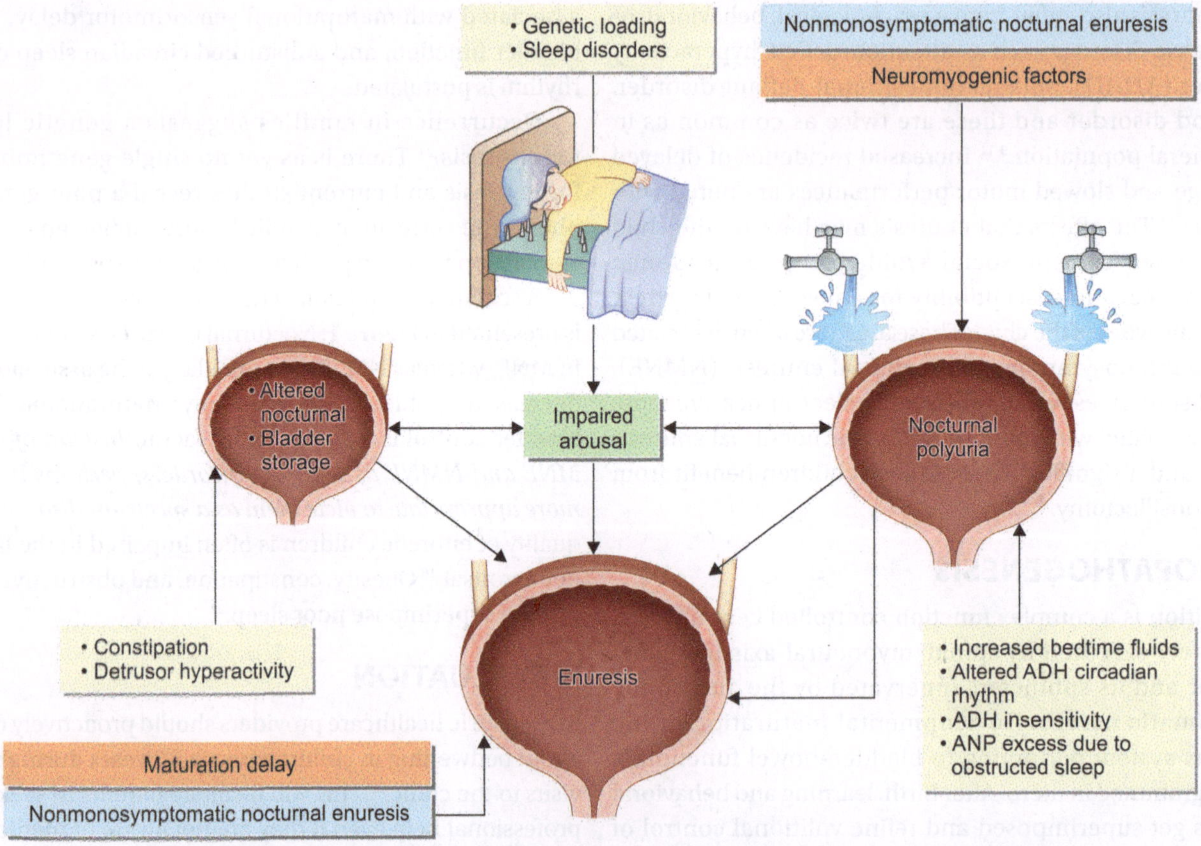

Fig. 1: Pathobiology of enuresis. (ADH: antidiuretic hormone; ANP: atrial natriuretic peptide)

TABLE 2: Key points for evaluation.

History *Onset:* Primary versus secondary *Pattern:* • Number of episodes per night and per week • *Volume per episode:* Large suggestive of nocturnal polyuria and small associated with small capacity or overactive bladder • Any daytime symptoms of LUTS including squatting maneuvers • *Any proven UTI** *Daytime symptoms:* • *Wetting during day** • *Voids <3 or >8 times a day** • *Prolong voiding time or need to strain** *Intake:* Fluid, caffeine, food, drugs • *Drink lots of fluid?** *Family history:* Either or both parents enuretic *Treatment history:* • Past medical help for bedwetting* *Associations:* • *Constipation or fecal soiling** • *Developmental delay or poor school performance* • *Snoring or sleep disordered breathing** • *Behavioral problem socially** • *Social disruptions: Anxiety, stress, abuse, bullying, and punishment in individual and family* • *Punishment for bedwetting*	*Physical examination* *Anthropometry:* Failure to thrive suggests systemic disease *Dysmorphism:* Facies, nasal obstruction, abnormal facial phenotype, and high-arched palate *Blood pressure* *Throat:* Adenotonsillar hypertrophy *Genitals:* • Phallic/meatal anomalies (boys) • Labial adhesions/urethral anomalies (girls) • Perianal excoriation/vulvovaginitis • Wet undergarments *Lumbosacral region:* • Occult spinal dysraphism • Pelvic tilt *Abdomen:* Tone, divarication recti, distended bladder, palpable thecoma *Neurological:* Abnormal muscle tone, sensation, or reflexes *Rectal examination:* Fecal impaction

*Screening checklist in OPD for daytime incontinence, NMNE, or secondary causes. (LUTS: lower urinary tract symptoms; UTI: urinary tract infection)

TABLE 3: Red flag signs with enuresis.

Sign	*Pointers toward etiology*	*Further evaluation*
Secondary NE of recent onset	Urinary tract infection, diabetes mellitus, chronic kidney disease, neurological lesion	Clinical examination with blood pressure, blood biochemistry, and urine neuroimaging if indicated
Weight loss, growth retardation	Diabetes mellitus, chronic kidney disease	
Polydipsia, especially nocturnal	Diabetes mellitus, diabetes insipidus, chronic kidney disease	Blood and urine with specific gravity and osmolality, fluid intake output charting
LUTS, squatting maneuvers, constipation	NMNE urological or spinal abnormality	Voiding diary, uroflowmetry, USS for urinary bladder wall thickness and pre- and postvoid residual urine
Recurrent UTI	Bowel–bladder dysfunction	Above plus imaging
Snoring, sleep apnea, or adenoid facies Daytime sleepiness	Obstructive sleep apnea Sleep disorder	ENT evaluation, sleep evaluation
Poor academic performance or behavioral disturbances	Mental retardation, ADHD, learning disabilities	Psychometric evaluation

(ADHD: attention-deficit/hyperactivity disorder; ENT: ear, nose, and throat; LUTS: lower urinary tract symptoms; NMNE: nonmonosymptomatic nocturnal enuresis; NE: nocturnal enuresis; USS: ultrasound scan; UTI: urinary tract infection)

An abdominal skiagram or neuroimaging in absence of red flag signs suggestive of occult spinal dysraphism is not indicated. If performed for some other reason, it may be helpful in demonstrating severe constipation. Routine ultrasonography and uroflowmetry are not required in children with nocturnal enuresis. Indications for an ultrasound abdomen are a high index of suspicion for NMNE or MNE with lack of response to therapy. When performed, the following need to be specifically sought, namely postvoid residual volume, bladder capacity, and bladder wall thickness. A transversal rectal diameter behind the bladder in excess of 30 mm is suggestive of rectal impaction in children with severe constipation.[3,5] Voiding cystourethrogram can be useful in children with significant daytime complaints or history of recurrent urinary tract infection.

VOIDING DIARY

The 48-hour fluid intake and urine voided volume charts complemented with at least 1-week assessment of day and night incontinence along with nocturnal urine output are recommended in the initial evaluation of all children with enuresis.[2,3,23,25] Voiding charts reveal relevant data regarding adequacy and timing of fluid intake, renal, and lower urinary tract function including daytime urinary frequency **(Table 4)**. Nocturnal polyuria is defined as urine output through the night including first morning void >130% of expected bladder capacity for age.[2] A voiding diary helps to improve the awareness of the child and family regarding bladder function. Maintaining the voiding diary itself can help to improve the motivation and, at times, the enuresis. It serves as a baseline record to assess the efficacy of subsequent intervention and treatment adherence on follow-up. Parents need motivation to initiate and maintain the voiding diary for at least 3–4 days. The same if done over weekends and holidays allays concerns about school absenteeism.

Daytime diary is used for determining the maximum voided volume (MVV) at each void excluding the first morning void. This is combined with the total fluid intake during the day. A diary maintained over 7–14 days may be more reliable to diagnose nocturnal polyuria (NP), constipation, and severity of enuresis.[3] To obtain the night-voided volume, the child is asked to sleep wearing a diaper. The sum of the diaper's weight and the volume of the first morning void will give the nocturnal urine output.

MANAGEMENT

When do we treat enuresis?

Treatment can be initiated in any child above 5 years or earlier if the child or parent seeks attention and the motivation of the child to participate in treatment seems high. The presence of adverse psychosocial consequences or the presence of daytime symptoms in a child mandates the initiation of therapy early.[3,6]

Who can treat?

Monosymptomatic nocturnal enuresis usually can be managed effectively by the primary care provider.[4-6] However, NMNE is best managed by an interprofessional team consisting of the primary care provider, along with nursing staff, pediatric nephrologist, urologist, and mental health professionals as required.[6] The first step is to treat constipation and provide good general advice for all children. Thereafter, dry-bed training or basic urotherapy is explained to every child as depicted in **Box 1**. Behavioral intervention and urotherapy form the cornerstone for initial treatment of enuresis along with the treatment of constipation. It needs to be initiated as the initial step even when other therapeutic modalities are offered. Used alone urotherapy may be effective in <20% of cases but can improve the effect of other modalities in the long term when used in conjunction. *Urotherapy*

TABLE 4: Voiding diary.

		Voiding episodes		Leakage	
Time	Fluid intake (mL)	Amount (mL)	Associated with urge to void?	Circumstance (stress, urge, or unaware)	Amount

BOX 1: Advice for treatment of enuresis.

General measures

- Talk to the child as well as the parents and reassure the availability of therapy
- Make families see it as a medical condition rather than a disciplinary issue
- Inform the natural history to reduce guilt of child, provide hope, and prevent any punitive response or control struggle
- Remove any misconceptions about enuresis resulting from poor parenting skills and reassure that the kidneys are not failing
- Child needs to be motivated to participate actively in therapy and encouraged to keep a dry bed chart and change the wet bed by himself or herself
- Reward for positive behaviors rather than dry nights
- Caregivers informed about different therapeutic options
- Talk about regulating fluid intake and adequate fluids during daytime to remain well hydrated while decreasing caffeinated beverages before bedtime
- Advice on measures to mitigate the impact of bedwetting with bed protection and disposable products, room deodorizers, and emollients to prevent chafing
- Discourage unsuccessful strategies and inappropriate interventions for enuresis such as abusing the child, restricting fluid intake, and compulsory diapers

Dry bed therapy and basic urotherapy

- Establish regular voiding habits at regular intervals at least six times per day
- Avoid holding urine after a desire to void including adopting maneuvers
- Ensure regular bowel habits and treat constipation
- Void prior to going to bed and make a bedtime resolution
- Adopt a good voiding posture on the toilet to promote relaxation of the pelvic floor with an appropriate-sized seat, footrest, forward bending of the torso and thighs well supported or the relaxed squatting position on the Indian style toilet
- Stress on normal not increased fluid intake during day, especially in the mornings and early afternoon and reducing fluid intake before sleep. Fluid requirements in children are approximately 30–40 mL/kg body weight
- Avoid caffeine, citric fruit juices, and excess salt at night
- Support and encouragement through regular follow-up with the child and caregiver, providing positive reinforcement. *One of the commonly used methods is Star Charts: a star for every dry night, and a reward after a number of stars have been earned*

should be continued for 4–12 weeks prior to evaluating the response and offering other therapeutic options. Daytime LUTS, if present, need to be evaluated and treated. This is followed by first-line monotherapy consisting of the alarm, desmopressin (DDAVP), or anticholinergic medications as shown in **Flowchart 1**. Second- and third-line therapy is available for the nonresponders.[3-6,23,25]

What are the goals of treatment?

Reduction of number of wet nights is the basic measurable parameter; however, the expectation of the family must be identified to manage the perception of treatment outcome. The outcomes are measured as follows:[4,5]

- *Complete response:* 100% of the symptoms are resolved
- *Partial response:* Improvement of 50–99% of the symptoms

Flowchart 1: Management algorithm for enuresis.

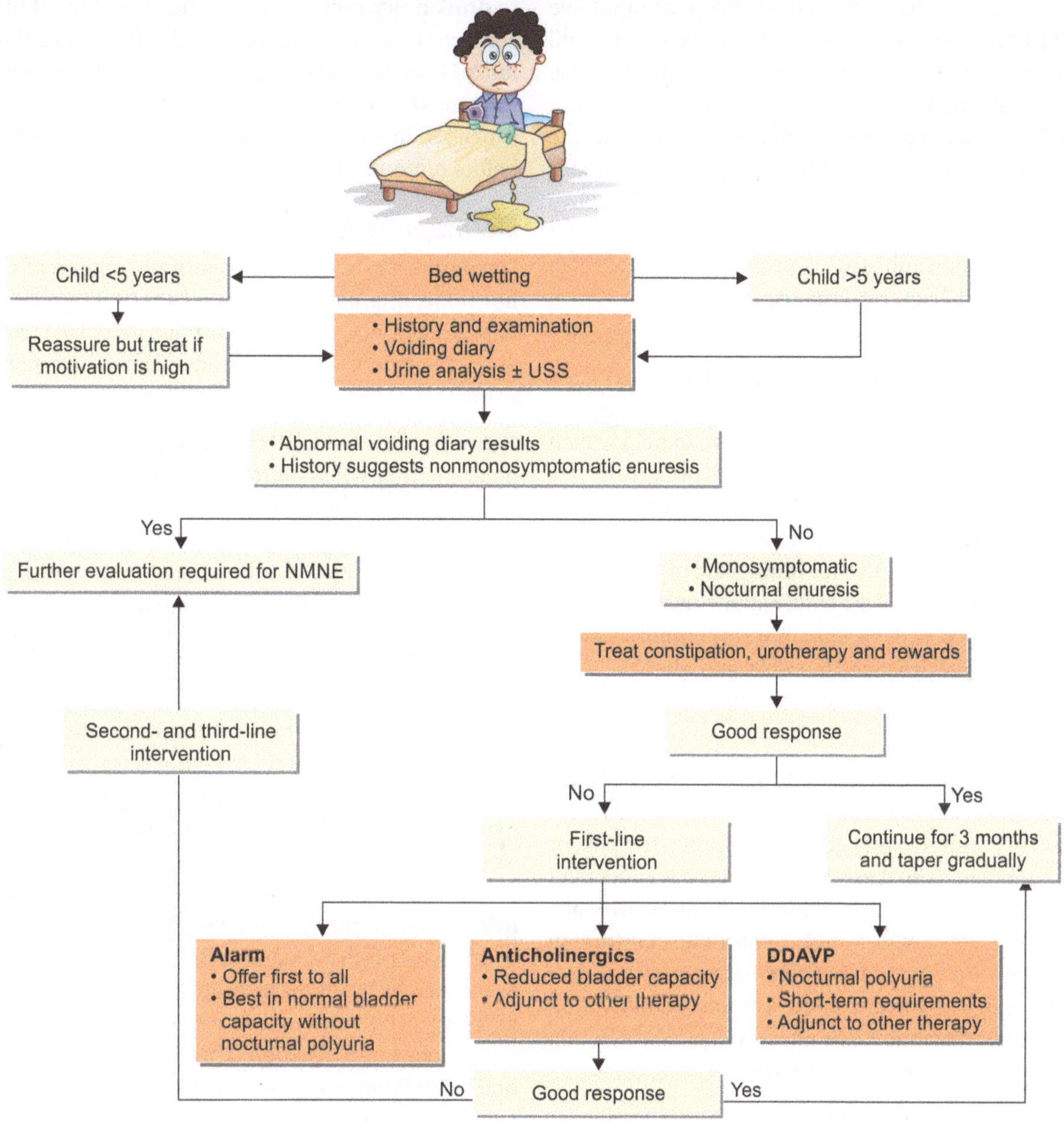

(DDAVP: desmopressin; NMNE: nonmonosymptomatic nocturnal enuresis; USS: ultrasound scan)

- *No response:* <50% improvements of the symptoms
- *Relapse:* More than one episode occurs per month after a response
- *Continuous success:* Absence of relapse in 6 months
- *Complete success:* No relapses over 2 years

First-line Therapy

The choice of the first-line therapy is planned after reviewing the voiding diary and discussing with the parents and child. The level of motivation is very important for the alarm to be used as an initial therapy for best long-term outcomes. The voiding diary may help to determine if the child has NP or reduced daytime MVV.[3,4] This can be used to help provide the appropriate option for initial therapy as follows:

- No NP + Low MVV : Enuresis alarm first
- NP + Normal MVV : DDAVP first
- No NP and normal MVV : Enuresis alarm or DDAVP
- NP + Low MVV : Enuresis alarm and DDAVP

Conditioning Therapy: Enuresis Alarm

This relies on a device which gives a strong arousal stimulus to the child, usually acoustic and/or vibratory, the moment urine activates a humidity detector located in the child's bed or clothing. There are two types of alarm—the body-worn alarm and the bed pad alarm; while children prefer the former, evidence for superiority of any type is lacking.

Mechanism: The alarm wakes the child up during the enuretic episode and makes him or her go to the toilet to complete micturition. It acts as a conditioning mechanism designed to change the cycle of light sleep, deep sleep, or rapid eye movement (REM) sleep to arousal around the time of the full bladder. Initially, if the child does not wake with the noise or vibration, it is important for parents to wake him or her up. Gradually, the child awakens progressively earlier in the course of the enuretic episode until the sensation of bladder fullness causes the child to awaken before wetting. The alarm may also increase nocturnal functional bladder capacity and vasopressin production and lead to a positive behavioral effect indirectly through the central nervous system.

Indication: First-line therapy for any child >5 years age with a normal bladder capacity. It works best in a child who is highly motivated and mature enough to accept and understand the treatment. The parents need to be supportive to help waken the child and constipation needs to be treated prior to the use of the alarm. In case parents or the child have reservations or are averse to the use of alarm, it is unlikely to be useful. Alarm may not be the best alternative for immediate or short-term results as the conditioning of the child happens over time. The alarm should be used with caution in warm humid weather conditions as it may get triggered by sweat, and when the child is at risk for getting shamed or bullied while sleeping in the same room with others.

Duration: The alarm is used continuously every night without interruption till at least 14 consecutive dry nights achieved. It may take 2–3 months to achieve this. Failure in the past or a relapse after previous success does not preclude successful repeat treatment with the alarm. While on the alarm therapy, rewarding the success with a sticker chart and reinforcing positive change are critical. Lack of parental support or winter season may contribute toward failure. Increasing motivation of the child and parents should be attempted prior to offering other modalities for better long-term results.

Outcomes: Enuresis alarms are by far the most effective for long-term results. About 62–75% achieve success by 3 months; 45% get cured even after stopping treatment with a relapse rate of 15–30% during long-term follow-up.[3-6] It is important to know that 30–50% may discontinue using the alarm due to lack of motivation. Alternate modalities may then be offered or combination of the alarm with DDAVP.

Use of alarm when combined with "overlearning" increases chance for long-term remission.[6] After 14 consecutive dry nights, the child is offered a couple of extra glasses of water to drink every evening. The same is continued till the child achieves a fresh 14 consecutive dry nights despite the extra fluid. Desmopressin is contraindicated during this phase to prevent severe hyponatremia. Intermittent reinforcement is needed in which the child uses the alarm every other day before discontinuing it.

Desmopressin

Desmopressin acetate is a synthetic analog of the natural hormone, arginine vasopressin.[2-4,6,8] Its effect is to decrease nocturnal urine production through increased reabsorption. Thus, the volume of urine produced can be accommodated within the bladder capacity.

Indication: MNE with NP and normal daytime voided volumes, older children, when short-term quick success for dry nights is the goal, such as an overnight stay, or an adolescent girl during her periods are the indications. Children in whom the alarm cannot be used may also be offered desmopressin. It is best avoided in children with habitual polydipsia.

Preparation: Oral tablets (0.2 mg), oral quick-melting lyophilizate (120 µg), and intranasal spray (10 µg per puff).

Dosage: 0.2–0.6 mg oral tablet per night or 120–360 µg lyophilizate. Alternately, 10–40 g nasal sprays are given. Medication needs to be administered in the evening 1 hour prior to bedtime. The child and the parents need to be informed specifically to avoid free fluid intake at least 1 hour prior to the medication and subsequent 8 hours to reduce hyponatremia and water intoxication. It is appropriate to start with 0.1–0.2 mg to a maximum of 0.6 mg per night regardless of age or weight. Lyophilizate preparation is easier to administer in younger children as it does not require water to swallow and has a quick onset of action. The spray is not recommended if oral formulation is available, in order to reduce the chance of overdose during self-administration **(Table 5)**.

Precautions: Restrict fluid intake during the last hour before bedtime and during the night. Children who are dehydrated or thirsty due to intense exercise or sweating can quench their thirst with water during the earlier part and still take desmopressin later.

Duration: The initial treatment should be continued for 2–4 weeks in order to obtain maximum effect. The dose is increased

TABLE 5: Pharmacotherapy for enuresis.

Medication	*Dose*	*Age*	*Side effects*
Desmopressin	Oral tablet 0.2–0.6 mg/day Nasal spray 10–40 g/day Oral lyophilizate 120–360 µg/day	Any	Hyponatremia Nasal stuffiness, headache, epistaxis
Oxybutynin Tolterodine	2.5–10 mg/day in divided doses 2–4 mg/day an hour before bed	>6 years	Dryness of mouth, facial flushing, blurring of vision, constipation, and increase in postvoid residue
Imipramine	25–50 mg/day an hour before bedtime	>7 years	Anxiety, mood disturbances palpitations, cardiac toxicity

gradually and titrated to achieve a decrease in the nocturnal urine output. Thereafter, the medication is continued for at least 12 weeks and tapered down gradually in order to reduce the risk of relapse.[29-32] In case of a suboptimal response, the nocturnal urine output and voiding diary record need to be reassessed. In case of worsening of symptoms or a poor response, DDAVP is discontinued. If used for a longer duration beyond 3 months, a drug holiday is recommended every 3 months and then it can be used without major risks or side effects.

Outcome: 33% become dry as long as they are on medication, 33% show partial response, and 33% show no response to DDAVP.[3,5,29-31] The long-term efficacy is 10–65% with 65–80% relapsing on stopping the medication, especially when the drug is withdrawn rapidly. A higher plasma copeptin level predicts better desmopressin response.

Anticholinergics

Anticholinergic medications reduce detrusor overactivity and thereby increase the functional bladder capacity. Detrusor overactivity is more often seen in NMNE.

Indication: It may be used as a first line in a child with increased voiding frequency and a low <65% bladder capacity for age. Typically, the child may wet the bed soon after bedtime or multiple times during a single night. It can be used in combination with the alarm or desmopressin.

Dose: Oxybutynin 2.5–10 mg daily and tolterodine 2–4 mg daily can be used in older children. Medication is taken in the evening 1 hour before bedtime, to be started with the lowest dose and increased every alternate week till dryness is achieved or maximum dose given whichever is earlier. The same is then continued for 6–8 weeks of continued dry nights and thereafter weaned off gradually. Newer anticholinergics such as fesoterodine and solifenacin have not yet been approved for use in children.

Precautions: Anticholinergics are contraindicated with underlying constipation or significant postvoid residual urine, as the same can be aggravated with medication. Dryness of mouth and rarely psychiatric effects such as mood swings may be noted with oxybutynin. All side effects wane as medication is discontinued. An ultrasonography to measure postvoid residue may be warranted in a child with previous UTI or unexplained fever and constipation needs treatment prior to using an anticholinergic.

Outcome: It is not very effective as monotherapy in MNE; 40% of therapy-resistant enuresis may respond to a combination with desmopressin.[33] Higher doses up to 10 mg oxybutynin may be required in such cases.

Second-line Therapy

If the first-line monotherapy fails, then the child may switch to an alternative monotherapy. If two monotherapies fail, a combination of two first-line therapies may be tried for 6–8 weeks. Combining desmopressin and alarm can lead to response rates close to 100%. Therapy-resistant enuresis is defined as inability to achieve at least a partial response in symptoms after an adequate trial of treatment even with a combination of options for 12 weeks.[3-6] In this setting, referral to a team which specializes in the management of bedwetting is warranted. Factors related to poor therapeutic response such as motivation of the family, fluid intake, underlying psychological conditions, or constipation should be carefully re-evaluated prior to considering a child resistant to treatment. A relook at daytime symptoms is important. The child may need evaluation for sleep disorders including restless leg syndrome. If there is no improvement despite successful treatment of constipation and other comorbidities, the child possibly has desmopressin-resistant enuresis and a repeat record of the voiding diary may unmask NP.[33]

Third-line Therapy

Tricyclic antidepressant imipramine[3,4,6] has a combination of noradrenergic, serotoninergic, and anticholinergic action on the bladder, urine production, and arousal mechanisms. It decreases the amount of time spent in REM sleep, stimulates vasopressin secretion, and relaxes the detrusor muscle.

Indication: Failure of first- and second-line therapy or in an older patient who cannot afford other therapeutic options or is diagnosed to have underlying psychological comorbidities.

Dose: The initial dose is 10 mg and gradually increased up to 25 mg in children below 9 years of age and up to 50 mg in those above 9 years of age after 1 week. The dose is continued for 4 weeks prior to the assessment of response.

Precautions: An ECG is suggested in the presence of history of syncope, palpitations, or family history of sudden cardiac death prior to starting this medication as it can cause fatal cardiotoxicity, especially unstable arrhythmia with long QT interval in higher doses. The medication needs to be discontinued for 2 weeks by gradual tapering to give a drug holiday every 3 months if used for a longer duration as it can cause mood swings, nausea, and tolerance with time.

Response: About 30–50% may benefit from imipramine. Initially, the child may show some reduction in wet nights per week. However, in the long term, majority relapse on discontinuation and barely 25% of initial responders remain dry. Abrupt withdrawal increases the chance of relapse.

Newer medications such as reboxetine, an antidepressant with noradrenergic action, and mirabegron, a noradrenergic agent, have been approved for adults with detrusor overactivity.

Extratherapy-resistant Children

This is a vexing issue and merits a thorough reinvestigation to identify any missed comorbidities and anatomical or functional causes of enuresis.[34,35] These children have continued bedwetting despite an adequate and correct trial of first-, second-, and third-line therapy and form an extremely difficult-to-treat subset. Anecdotal therapeutic options such as peripheral electrical stimulation or botulinum toxin injections into the detrusor, hypnotherapy, acupuncture, and chiropractic therapy have been described. Bladder-stretching exercises, retention control training by delaying urination for extended periods of time during the day to increase functional bladder capacity, and stop-start training which teaches children to interrupt their stream of urine in order to strengthen their pelvic floor muscles have no consistent evidence for being effective and can be unpleasant.

NONMONOSYMPTOMATIC ENURESIS

Presence of diurnal symptoms associated with enuresis occurs in about a third of all children with enuresis.[2,3] An increased risk of UTI, greater association with constipation, and emotional disorders are noted. Apart from historical assessment for LUTS, voiding diary, evaluation of the postvoid urinary residue by ultrasound, and uroflowmetry are important for a correct diagnosis and treatment.[6] Assessment of bowel function with Rome IV criteria and Bristol Stool Scale is important.

CONCLUSION

Enuresis is a multifactorial condition with a complex pathophysiology. While secondary causes need to be identified and treated, primary enuresis needs structured evaluation of bladder, bowel, neurological, and sleep functions. A quartet of maturational delay in control of bladder-bowel functions, altered neuroendocrine control of diuresis, perturbed bladder capacity, and a disturbed sleep arousal network underly enuresis.

KEY POINTS

- Monosymptomatic enuresis without any red flag signs, needs a psycho-behavioral, urine production, bladder capacity, and sleep arousal approach to evaluation and management.
- While an age-related resolution of primary monosymptomatic enuresis is common, a proactive management is important to prevent secondary stressful consequences for the child and the family.
- Children with refractory nocturnal enuresis may benefit from referral to a healthcare professional who specializes in the management of recurrent or refractory enuresis.
- Additional indications for referral include nonmonosymptomatic enuresis; developmental, attention, or learning difficulties; behavioral or emotional problems; and known or suspected physical or neurologic problems.

REFERENCES

1. Rakowska-Silska M, Jobs K, Paturej A, Kalicki B. Voiding disorders in pediatrician's practice. Clin Med Insights Pediatr. 2020;14:1179556520975035. doi: 10.1177/1179556520975035. eCollection 2020.
2. Austin PF, Bauer SB, Bower W, Chase J, Franco I, Hoebeke P, et al. The standardization of terminology of lower urinary tract function in children and adolescents: update report from the standardization committee of the International Children's Continence Society. Neurourol Urodyn. 2016;35:471-81.
3. Nevéus T, Fonseca E, Franco I, Kawauchi A, Kovacevic L, Nieuwhof-Leppink A, et al. Management and treatment of nocturnal enuresis—an updated standardization document from the International Children's Continence Society. J Pediatr Urol. 2020;16(1):10-9.
4. Bogaert G, Stein R, Undre S, Nijman RJM, Quadackers J, 't Hoen L, et al. Practical recommendations of the EAU-ESPU guidelines committee for monosymptomatic enuresis—bedwetting. Neurourol Urodyn. 2020;39(2):489-97.
5. Netto JMB, Rondon AV, de Lima GRM, Filho MZ, Schneider-Monteiro ED, Molina CAF, et al. Brazilian consensus in enuresis—recommendations for clinical practice. Int Braz J Urol. 2019;45(5):889-900.
6. Sinha R, Raut S. Management of nocturnal enuresis—myths and facts. World J Nephrol. 2016;5:328-38.
7. Wright AJ. The epidemiology of childhood incontinence. Pediatric Incontinence, Evaluation and Clinical Management. Hoboken: John Wiley & Sons, Ltd; 2015. pp. 37-60.
8. Kanitkar M, Ramamurthy HR. Bed wetting-silent suffering: an approach to enuresis and voiding disorders in children. Indian J Pediatr. 2013;80:750-3.
9. Feehan M, McGee R, Stanton W, Silva PA. A 6 year follow-up of childhood enuresis: prevalence in adolescence and consequences for mental health. J Paediatr Child Health. 1990;26:75-9.
10. Hellström AL, Hanson E, Hansson S, Hjälmås K, Jodal U. Micturition habits and incontinence in 7-year-old Swedish school entrants. Eur J Pediatr. 1990;149:434-7.
11. Maternik M. Understanding of and misconceptions around monosymptomatic nocturnal enuresis: findings from patient and physician surveys. J Pediatr Urol. 2019;15(1):37.e1-8.
12. Pavione Rodrigues Pereira R, Nascimento Fagundes S, Surry Lebl A, Azevedo Soster L, Machado MG, Koch VH, et al. Children with nocturnal enuresis have posture and balance disorders. J Pediatr Urol. 2016;12(4):216.e1-6.
13. National Institute for Health and Clinical Excellence. NICE Clinical Guideline CG111. London: NICE; 2010. Nocturnal enuresis: the management of bedwetting in children and young people. [online] Available from http://guidance.nice.org.uk/CG111 [Last accessed June, 2022].
14. Vasconcelos MMA, East P, Blanco E, Lukacz ES, Caballero G, Lozoff B, et al. Early behavioral risks of childhood and adolescent daytime urinary incontinence and nocturnal enuresis. J Dev Behav Pediatr. 2017;38(9):736-42.
15. Ece A, Coşkun S, Şahin C, Tan I, Karabel D, Çim A. BDNF and NGF gene polymorphisms and urine BDNF-NGF levels in children with primary monosymptomatic nocturnal enuresis. J Pediatr Urol. 2019;15(3):255.e1-e7.
16. Dossche L, Walle JV, Van Herzeele C. The pathophysiology of monosymptomatic nocturnal enuresis with special emphasis on the circadian rhythm of renal physiology. Eur J Pediatr. 2016;175(6):747-54.
17. Nevéus T. Pathogenesis of enuresis: towards a new understanding. Int J Urol. 2017;24(3):174-82.
18. Yu B, Sun H, Ma H, Peng M, Kong F, Meng F, et al. Aberrant whole-brain functional connectivity and intelligence structure in children with primary nocturnal enuresis. PLoS One. 2013;8(1):e51924.
19. Lei D, Ma J, Du X, Shen G, Tian M, Li G. Altered brain activation during response inhibition in children with primary nocturnal enuresis: an fMRI study. Hum Brain Mapp. 2012;33(12):2913-9.

20. von Gontard A, Schmelzer D, Seifen S, Pukrop R. Central nervous system involvement in nocturnal enuresis: evidence of general neuromotor delay and specific brainstem dysfunction. J Urol. 2001;166(6):2448-51.
21. von Gontard A, Schaumburg H, Hollmann E, Eiberg H, Rittig S. The genetics of enuresis: a review. J Urol. 2001;166:2438-43.
22. Hodgkinson B, Josephs K, Hegney D. Best practice in the management of primary nocturnal enuresis in children: a systematic review. JBI Libr Syst Rev. 2010;8(5):173-254.
23. Trajanovska M, King S, Goldfeld S, Gibb S. A novel method of rapid appraisal of clinical practice guidelines for children with enuresis. J Pediatr Urol. 2019;15(4):333.e1-9.
24. Brown ML, Pope AW, Brown EJ. Treatment of primary nocturnal enuresis in children: a review. Child Care Health Dev. 2011;37:153-60.
25. Neveus T, Eggert P, Evans J, Macedo A, Rittig S, Tekgul S, et al. Evaluation of and treatment for monosymptomatic enuresis: a standardization document from the International Children's Continence Society. J Urol. 2010;183:441-7.
26. van Dyk JC, Duvenhage F, Coetzee LJ, Segone AM, Fockema M, Smart D, et al. South African guidelines for the management of nocturnal enuresis. S Afr Med J. 2003;93(5):338-40.
27. Vande Walle J, Rittig S, Bauer S, Eggert P, Marschall-Kehrel D, Tekgul S, et al. Practical consensus guidelines for the management of enuresis. Eur J Pediatr. 2012;171:971-83.
28. Bayne AP, Skoog SJ. Nocturnal enuresis: an approach to assessment and treatment. Pediatr Rev. 2014;35:327-34.
29. Caldwell PH, Deshpande AV, Von Gontard A. Management of nocturnal enuresis. BMJ. 2013;347:f6259.
30. Fagundes SN, Lebl AS, Azevedo Soster L, Sousa E Silva GJ, Silvares EF, Koch VH. Monosymptomatic nocturnal enuresis in pediatric patients: multidisciplinary assessment and effects of therapeutic intervention. Pediatr Nephrol. 2017;32(5):843-51.
31. Kuwertz-Bröking E, von Gontard A. Clinical management of nocturnal enuresis. Pediatr Nephrol. 2018;33(7):1145-54.
32. Houts AC, Peterson JK, Whelan JP. Prevention of relapse in full-spectrum home training for primary enuresis: a component analysis. Behav Ther. 1986;17:462-9.
33. De Guchtenaere A, Vande Walle C, Van Sintjan P, Donckerwolcke R, Raes A, Dehoorne J, et al. Desmopressin resistant nocturnal polyuria may benefit from furosemide therapy administered in the morning. J Urol. 2007;178(6):2635-9.
34. Ohtomo Y. Atomoxetine ameliorates nocturnal enuresis with subclinical attention-deficit/hyperactivity disorder. Pediatr Int. 2017;59(2):181-4.
35. Van Hoecke E, Baeyens D, Vanden Bossche H, Hoebeke P, Vande Walle J. Early detection of psychological problems in a population of children with enuresis: construction and validation of the short screening instrument for psychological problems in enuresis. J Urol. 2007;178(6):2611-5.

CHAPTER

13.12

Common Renal Tumors

G Nandhini, Anoop Subash

INTRODUCTION

Wilms' tumor (WT) or nephroblastoma, an embryonal malignancy of the kidney, is the most common renal tumor of childhood, which accounts for 6–7% of all childhood cancers. It typically affects young children (median age 3.5 years), although older children and occasionally even adults can be affected. The disease occurs equally in girls and boys worldwide. Its incidence is 7.6 cases for every million children <15 years of age or 1 case per 10,000 infants. Its frequency varies by race; it is rarer in East Asian populations than in Caucasians, but more frequent in Africa and African-American children.

WILMS' TUMOR

Presentation

Wilms' tumor usually presents as an abdominal mass in an otherwise apparently healthy child. Older children present with abdominal pain, gross hematuria, and fever. Occasionally, a child will present with an acute abdomen due to tumor rupture, with hemorrhage into the peritoneal cavity, extension of the tumor into the renal vein, and inferior vena cava (IVC). Varicocele, hepatomegaly due to hepatic vein obstruction, ascites, and congestive heart failure are found in fewer than 10% of patients with intracaval or atrial tumor extension. Hypertension is present in 25% of cases and has been attributed to elevated plasma-renin levels. Renin production by tumor, renal ischemia by tumor compression on renal artery or intrarenal AV fistula are the contemplated causes of the hypertension. Macroscopic hematuria at the initial presentation is seen in 10% of children with WT. WT has the potential for both local and distant spread. The tumors have a propensity to invade the renal vein and to form thrombi in the inferior vena cava, sometimes progressing into the heart. Local and distant lymph node involvement can also occur. The most common sites of distant metastasis are the lungs and liver, with rare instances of spread to bone and brain. Approximately, 5–10% of children with WT have bilateral or multicentric tumors. The average age at presentation is 42–47 months for children with unilateral WT and 30–33 months for those with bilateral WT.

ETIOLOGY

Current models of WT development propose that a genetic mutation predisposes to nephrogenic rests, benign foci of embryonal kidney cells that persist abnormally into postnatal life. Nephrogenic rests are found in approximately 1% of newborn kidneys and usually regress or differentiate by early childhood (Beckwith et al. 1990). Some nephrogenic rests persist into childhood. These rests are considered to be WT precursors;[1] nephrogenic rests that sustain additional mutations transform into a WT.[2] Nephrogenic rests are characterized as intralobar or perilobar.

Immature nephroblasts develop in proximity to the ureteric bud and migrate to the periphery of the developing renal lobe as they mature. WT1 mutations, decreased WT1 expression, and 11p loss of heterozygosity (LOH) interfere with maturation and lead to intralobar nephrogenic rest (ILNR)-like WT derived from pluripotent nephroblasts, accounting for the presence of heterotypic elements, such as muscle and cartilage. In contrast, loss of imprinting of the insulin-like growth factor-2 (*IGF2*) gene in mature nephroblasts leads to increased IGF2 expression, a failure of proliferation arrest and the development of perilobar nephrogenic rest (PLNR) like tumors at the periphery of the renal lobe.

The location of ILNRs within the renal lobe and of PLNR at the periphery of the renal lobe indicates that ILNR and PLNR occur early and late in the kidney development, respectively. The ILNR includes a mesenchymal stem cell, as ILNR-derived WTs differentiate into both the nephrogenic (Epi) and the ectopic mesenchymal lineages (Mes). On the other hand, PLNR contains a more mature precursor cell[3] (a putative nephrogenic stem cell) than ILNR, because the histology of PLNR-derived WTs shows a restricted differentiation that recapitulates kidney epithelial development (Epi WT) without ectopic mesenchymal differentiation. WNT signaling is activated only in WT from the mesenchymal lineage (Mes WT) **(Figs. 1A and B)**.

Intralobar rests are usually solitary and randomly distributed throughout the kidney, although they tend to be situated centrally within the renal lobe. Intralobar rests are associated with two syndromes related to WT1 mutations:

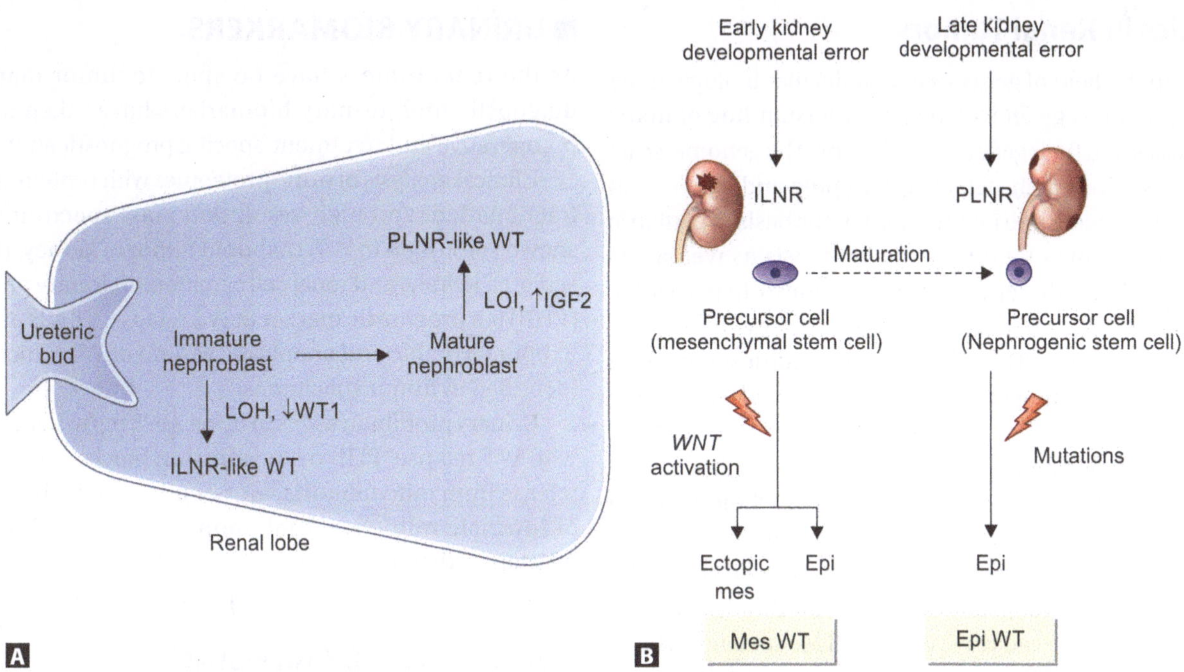

Figs. 1A and B: Molecular model for the divergent pathogenesis of Wilms' tumor (WT).

Wilms' tumor-aniridia-genital anomalies-retardation (WAGR) syndrome and Denys-Drash syndrome (male pseudohermaphroditism, renal mesangial sclerosis, and nephroblastoma).[4]

Perilobar rests tend to be located at the periphery of the kidney and are often multiple. Perilobar rests are associated with Beckwith-Wiedemann syndrome (BWS)[4] (macroglossia, macrosomia, hemihypertrophy, omphalocele) (Breslow et al., 2006).

The term nephroblastomatosis is used to describe the presence of multiple nephrogenic rests. Nephroblastomatosis[5] may manifest as a diffuse overgrowth of rests, producing a rim that enlarges the kidney, or as multiple distinct rests[3] (Perlman et al., 2006). It is sometimes challenging to distinguish nephrogenic rests from WT, even with biopsies. Although nephrogenic rests are considered benign, chemotherapy has been advocated if the rests are growing or if a child becomes symptomatic. Some evidence indicates that chemotherapy may decrease the risk of subsequent WT development in children with nephrogenic rests[2] (Coppes et al., 1999). However, the association between type of nephrogenic rest and predisposition syndrome is not absolute.

GENETIC ORIGIN

A germline mutation is thought to be the cause of about 10–15% of WT. WT1 germline mutations give rise to WAGR syndrome, DDS, Frasier syndrome, and isolated WT (i.e., WT with no evidence of an underlying syndrome). The majority of WT have genetic alterations at chromosome 11p13. Germline WT1 mutations are associated with genitourinary anomalies. No increased risk of mutation is found in patients with nephrogenic rests, bilateral WT, or a family history of WT.

A second potential *WT* gene, WT2, has been identified on chromosome 11p15, based on the observation of loss of heterozygosity at this site, but the actual gene responsible remains to be determined. Epigenetic and genomic alterations of chromosome 11p15 give rise to BWS. Recent studies suggest that abnormal expression of embryonal growth factor encoded by the *IGF2* gene is involved in the pathophysiology of BWS. Approximately, 1–2% of individuals with WT have at least one relative also diagnosed with WT; however, the underlying genetic mechanisms are usually not known. Linkage analysis has mapped WT predisposition genes to 17q (locus name FWT1) and 19q (locus name FWT2). Because in some families the WT phenotype does not show linkage to WT1, FWT1, or FWT2, the existence of one or more other genes in which mutations cause familial WT is likely.

A genetic referral is recommended for all children with WT who have a positive family history of cancer, bilateral kidney involvement, or presence of syndrome-specific features. Investigators in Canada have developed the McGill Interactive Pediatric OncoGenetic Guidelines (MiPOGG)[6] to assist in determining whether a child with WT should undergo a genetics referral.

The MiPOGG algorithm consists of five criteria including:

1. Diagnosis before 2 years of age
2. Bilateral or multifocal tumors
3. Stromal-predominant histology
4. Presence of nephrogenic rests
5. Overgrowth features

These criteria should be taken into consideration along with the family history and presence of congenital anomalies and/or dysmorphic features.

Genetics in Renal Tumors

Progress in the field of genetics and molecular biology in the last few years has given us a better understanding of many tumor basics and their genetic correlations. The genome-scale analyses—such as high-density genotyping and exome and genome sequencing—to identify the genetic basis of pediatric tumors have shown light to many diagnosis as well as its response to chemotherapy or its resistance also. In particular, exome sequencing has contributed to the evidence that about a significant 10% of children and adolescents with tumors have germline genetic variants associated with cancer predisposition.

We need to be familiar with large-scale genomic analyses such as whole-exome sequencing (WES) or whole-genome sequencing (WGS).[7] These can identify even uncommon and moderate penetrant variants. Since WES investigates only the coding regions of the genome, it has proved very useful in detecting most of the causative variants of Mendelian diseases and more complex diseases. On the other hand, WGS can capture nearly all known genetic variations, including those falling in regulatory elements, with much more uniform coverage of the genome, but it does not allow to detect mosaic variants with low clonality or variations causing DNA repetitions.

The detection of cancer predisposition leads to dual clinical benefits for patients, both for the genetic alteration detection and to refine the therapeutic choices in resistant mutations.

The spectrum of somatic genetic alterations in WT is quite broad, with classical genetic changes involving *WT1*, the *IGF2* locus, the WNT pathway, *MYCN*, and *TP53* but also driver mutations in several additional cancer genes including epigenetic remodelers, miRNA processing genes, and transcription factors essential for nephrogenesis.

Two recent WGS and WES studies have identified new pathologic germline variants in CHEK2 and PALB2 in children with sporadic WT involved in DNA repair pathways. The vast majority of studies are based on a "candidate-gene" approach, which means they focus on specific subsets of genes already known to play a key role in cancer predisposition and tumorigenesis.

Genetic Counseling

If a proband has syndromic WT, genetic counseling for the specific syndrome is appropriate. Nonsyndromic WT most frequently occurs as a simplex case (i.e., a single occurrence in a family). Empiric risks to the siblings of a proband who is a simplex case are unknown, but likely to be low. Prenatal diagnosis for pregnancies at 50% risk of inheriting a WT1 or 11p15 genomic alteration from a parent is possible when the mutation and/or genetic mechanism in the family are known.

URINARY BIOMARKERS

As the renal tumors have no specific tumor markers as diagnostic tool, urinary biomarkers have taken a lead in preoperative and treatment-specific prognostication.

Clinical analysis of urine proteomes with protein isolation, fractionation, and high-resolution mass spectrometry has shown some light in WT, rhabdoid tumor of kidney, clear cell sarcoma kidney, and renal cell carcinoma. Urinary prohibitin[8] (PHB) is a prognostic marker in WT relapse. This is expressed in both favorable and anaplastic variant of WT which can be identified in tumor specimens.

Urinary prohibitin levels in urine > 998 ng/mL is associated with WT relapse. PHB overexpression blocks cytochrome C release from mitochondria, an essential step in the initiation of intrinsic mitochondrial apoptosis, causing apoptosis resistance, thereby promoting chemotherapy resistance and WT therapy failure can be prognosticated earlier.

DIAGNOSIS BY IMAGING

Apart from the baseline blood evaluation, no specific serum tumor markers are available in WT. The workup of a child with suspected WT begins with appropriate diagnostic imaging studies. Ultrasonography is the recommended first-line test, because it provides a panoramic view of the abdomen. Enlarged lymph nodes, intra-abdominal metastasis (mainly liver) and thrombus in renal vein, IVC, or right atrium must be looked for. X-ray chest is done to see for pulmonary metastasis with incidence in 15–20% of WT patients. Splaying of calyces may be seen in IVP as space-occupying lesion.

Computed tomography (CT) with IV contrast visualizes pelvic and abdominal structures, as well as lymph nodes crucial for clinical staging of the disease and detection of distant metastasis. Magnetic resonance imaging (MRI) may facilitate the distinction between WT and nephrogenic rests. Nuclear scan of bone is required in clear cell sarcoma and MRI brain in rhabdoid tumor to diagnose brain metastasis. New techniques such as 18F-fluorodeoxyglucose-positron emission tomography (FDG-PET), CT, and diffusion-weighted imaging (DWI) with MRI are being evaluated for their potential value in the imaging strategy of malignant renal tumors in adults and children. The definitive diagnosis of WT can be made only by surgical resection or biopsy (staging) and the histopathology for the favorable or unfavorable prognostication **(Figs. 2A and B)**.

STAGING AND MANAGEMENT

The type of management entirely depends on the clinical staging and the histopathology of the specimen. Macroscopically, WT usually compresses the adjacent normal renal parenchyma, forming a pseudocapsule composed of compressed, atrophic renal tissues. This intrarenal pseudocapsule can be helpful to distinguish WT from other renal tumors. Microscopically, the classic triphasic pattern includes varying proportions of three

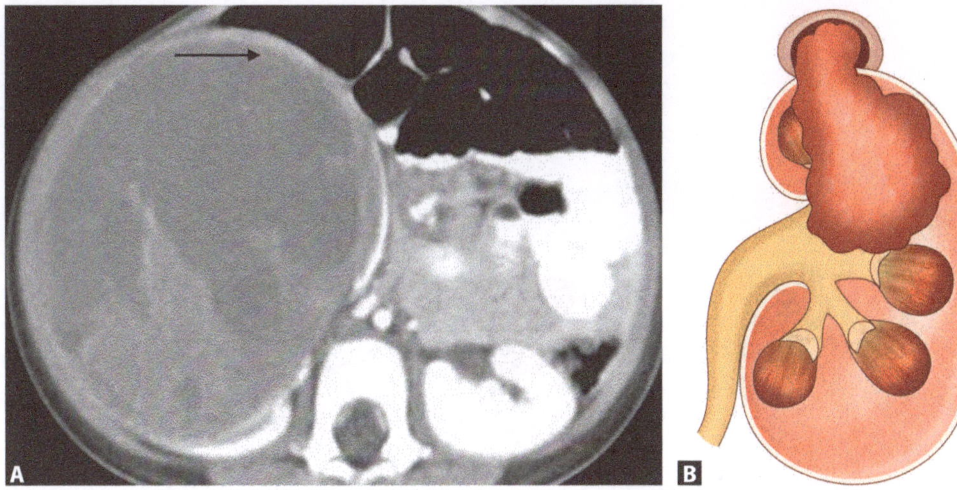

Figs. 2A and B: Tumor arising from the renal parenchyma within the capsule and the computed tomography (CT) scan showing compressed normal renal tissue as ring enhancement.

cell types—blastemal, stromal, and epithelial. The proportion of each of these components varies.

Anaplasia[9] is defined by the presence of gigantic polyploid nuclei within the tumor sample. It is rare in the first 2 years of life, but the incidence increases to 13% in children ≥5-year-old. Anaplasia is a feature of WT that is clearly associated with resistance to chemotherapy. Anaplasia has been further divided into focal and diffuse patterns to reflect the different prognosis of anaplasia that is present throughout the kidney or in an extrarenal location **(Figs. 3 and 4)**.

Focal anaplasia requires that cells with anaplastic nuclear changes be confined to sharply restricted foci within the primary tumor. Diffuse anaplasia is diagnosed when anaplasia is present in more than one portion of the tumor or is found in any extrarenal or metastatic site. When the anaplastic component is completely removed (stage I), the outcome is generally excellent. When anaplastic changes are not present, the tumor is referred to as being of favorable histology (FH), because of the generally good outcome for these patients. Unfavorable histologic features were associated with increased rates of relapse and death.

Staging **(Fig. 5)** and management of WT require a special mention on the various study trial groups namely NWTSG, SIOP, and COG which have come out with standardized protocols on the management of WT and had increased the survival rates worldwide dramatically.

National Wilms' Tumor Study Group

Three cooperative groups, the Children's Cancer Study Group (CCSG), the Cancer and Leukemia Group B (CALGB), and the Southwest Oncology Group (SWOG) combined to form a intergroup known as National WT Study (NWTS) in 1969 to gather a statistically significant number of tumor patients to study.[10] Many oncology centers over 250 in United States, Canada, and other countries joined this group and enrolled

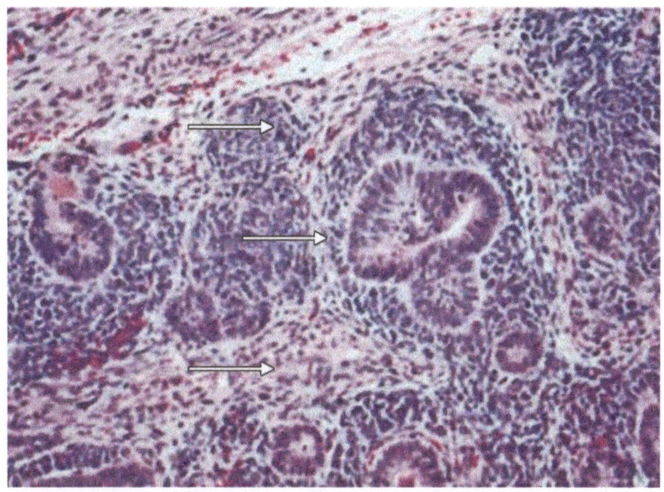

Fig. 3: Triphasic differentiation with blastemal, epithelial, and stromal and tubular elements in varying amounts.

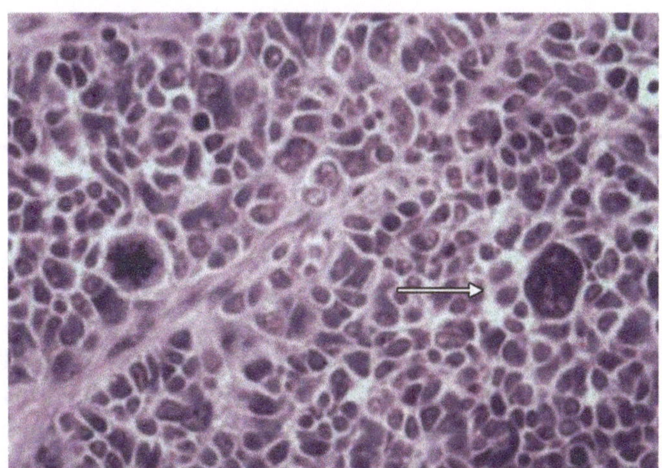

Fig. 4: Two histologic criteria for anaplasia, namely multipolar polyploid mitotic figures and marked nuclear enlargement with hyperchromasia. Confined to one area of kidney is focal anaplasia and if generalized, it is diffuse anaplasia as in the figure.

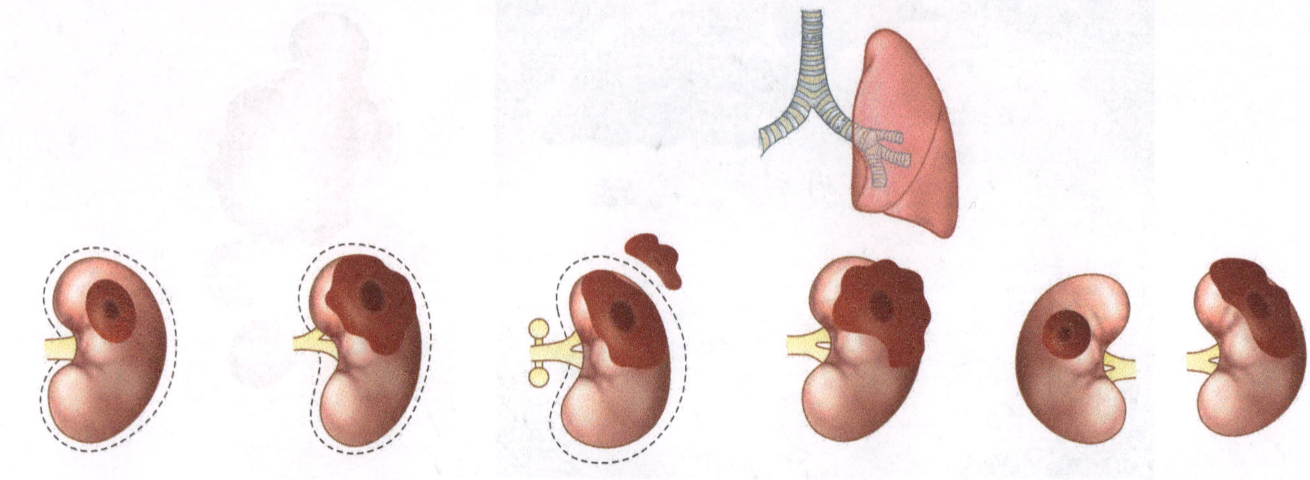

Fig. 5: Staging of Wilms' tumor from stage 1 to 5.

more than 70–80% of patients with WT in the country. NWTS ran five clinical trials—NWTS-1 to NWTS-5. The first four were randomized trials, whereas the NWTS-5, which was completed in 2003, was a clinical trial designed to look primarily at the biological prognostic factors and was not randomized.

Purpose of Study

- NWTS 1—to determine the effect of surgical technique on the results of the treatment
- NWTS 2—to study the prognosis of patients with WT
- NWTS 3—to reduce the treatment for low-risk patients and find better chemotherapy for high-risk patients for relapse
- NWTS 4—to reduce the efficacy, toxicity, and cost of different chemoregimens for the treatment
- NWTS 5—to identify the biologic prognostic factors

In 2001, NWTS merged with various other pediatric oncology groups to create the "Children's Oncology Group" (COG). But till date, the NWTSG is actively involved in its long-term follow-up of previously enrolled patients (LATE) **(Table 1)**.

TABLE 1: Wilms tumor—staging.

Stage	*Description*
I	• Tumor limited to kidney and completely excised • No penetration of the renal capsule or involvement of renal • sinus vessels
II	• Tumor extending beyond the kidney, but completely excised • No residual tumor apparent at or beyond the margins of excision • Tumor thrombus in vessels outside the kidney is stage II, if the thrombus is removed en bloc with the tumor
III	Gross or microscopic residual tumor remaining post-operatively, including: • Inoperable tumor • Positive surgical margins • Diffuse tumor spillage or biopsy • Regional lymph node metastasis • Transected tumor thrombus
IV	Hematogenous metastasis (lung, liver, bone, and brain) or lymph node metastasis outside the abdominal or pelvic cavities
V	Bilateral renal tumors at diagnosis

Note: Tumor biopsy or local spillage confined to the flank was considered stage II by the NWTSG in the past; such events are considered stage III on current COG studies.

Societe Internationale D'oncologie Pediatrique

Societe Internationale D'oncologie Pediatrique (SIOP) is another European group formed in 1971 for studies on WT.[10] The concept of SIOP is to reduce the risk of tumor rupture during upfront surgery by initially giving radiotherapy and later chemotherapy to shrink the tumor. SIOP conducted trials in which children received prenephrectomy chemotherapy or abdominal radiation therapy. The trials and their conclusions are given here:

- *SIOP 1-(09/71):* Preoperative radiotherapy significantly prevents tumor rupture. Additional actinomycin D (6×) does not improve outcome in diffuse or focal anaplasia.
- *SIOP 2-(10/74):* SIOP 1+ postoperative chemotherapy for 6 months is as good as 15 months. Hence, postoperative chemotherapy following nephrectomy should be given only for 6 months.
- *SIOP 5-(01/77):* Preoperative two drug chemotherapy is as effective as preoperative radiation therapy.
- *SIOP 9-(12/87): Stages I, II, and III*—8 weeks preoperative treatment does not produce favorable stage distribution compared to 4 weeks in stage 2 patients with negative

lymph nodes; the rate of relapse was reduced by epirubicin without radiation therapy.

- *SIOP 93-01-(12/93):* Reduction of postoperative chemotherapy for intermediate risk and anaplastic WT to four doses of vincristine (VCR) and one dose of dactinomycin was not less effective than standard postoperative chemotherapy according to histologic features.

Hence, now both the staging systems have proven valuable in predicting the outcomes with upfront surgery-based NWTSG and upfront chemotherapy-based system SIOP.

UMBRELLA SIOP-RTSG, 2016 (UMBRELLA Protocol)

Wilms' tumor outcomes have dramatically improved to 90% EFS (event-free survival) across the globe in the past decade. But, certain specific subgroups of patients with relapse, anaplastic histology, and bilateral or unilateral high-risk tumors continue to have poor EFS and are at risk for significant late effects from both abdominal radiotherapy and toxic high-dose chemotherapy. Post-treatment effects occur as chronic health conditions in more than 25% of survivors of WT which include renal failure, infertility, cardiac toxicity, pulmonary hypertension and fibrosis, and the development of secondary malignancies.

The Renal Tumor Study Group of the International Society of Paediatric Oncology (SIOP-RTSG)[11] has developed a new standardized protocol for the diagnosis and treatment of childhood renal tumors, the UMBRELLA SIOP-RTSG 2016 (the UMBRELLA protocol) **(Fig. 6)**. On the basis of the results of previous national and international trials and studies, AREN03B2—UMBRELLA of four therapeutic clinical trials (AREN 0532, AREN 0533, AREN 032, and AREN 0534) as shown in **Table 2**, SIOP-RTGS formulated the results as protocol retrospecting both COG and SIOP results.

The UMBRELLA protocol[11] should promote international collaboration across 50 countries and already five countries (UK, Germany, the Netherlands, France, and Italy) are enrolled in the centralized data collection of the renal neoplasms and research and serve as the SIOP-RTSG best available treatment standard across the globe.

This protocol addresses both Wilms' tumor and non-Wilms' tumor. These recommendations were established by a multidisciplinary panel of leading experts on renal tumors within the SIOP-RTSG, which include pediatric oncologists, surgeons, radiologists, pathologists, radiation oncologists, statisticians, and scientists involved in basic research. Thorough communications were undertaken with colleagues with similar expertise involved in the Children's Oncology Group (COG), to ensure all relevant evidence was applied when deciding how to implement the results of the SIOP-2001 randomized trial, which investigated the safety of omitting doxorubicin in treating stage II-III intermediate-risk Wilms' tumors, and to refine recommendations for patients with Wilms' tumor.

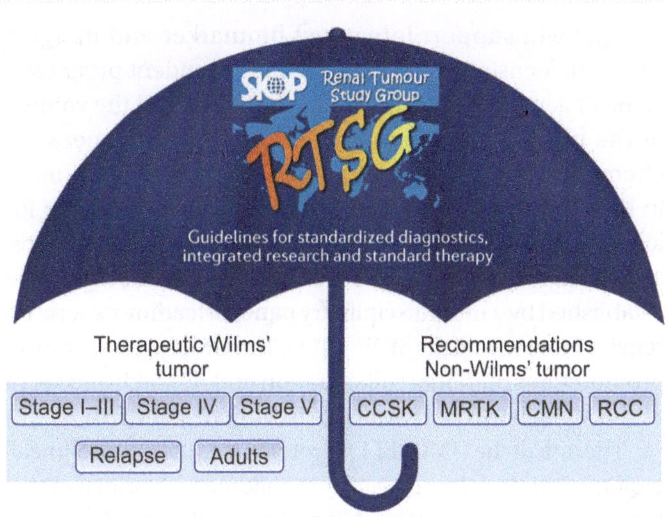

Fig. 6: UMBRELLA SIOP-RTSG logo. (CCSK: clear cell sarcoma of the kidney; CMN: congenital mesoblastic nephroma; RCC: renal cell carcinoma; MRTK: malignant rhabdoid tumor of the kidney)
Source: Consensus statement of RTGS

TABLE 2: AREN03B2—UMBRELLA of four therapeutic clinical trials (AREN 0532, AREN 0533, AREN 032, and AREN 0534).

AREN03B2—eligibility criteria	Imaging, histology, stage, age, tumor weight, response to therapy, and biological markers [e.g., loss of heterozygosity (LOH) of 1p and 16q; 1q gain]
AREN 0532	• Studied very-low-risk, low-risk, and standard-risk favorable histology Wilms tumor (FHWT) • To demonstrate excellent outcomes for patients <2 years of age with small, stage I FHWT after treatment with nephrectomy alone • Additional objective was to correlate relapse with known biomarkers LOH 1p and 16q, and 1q gain
AREN 0533	• Examined COG-enrolled patients with higher-risk FHWT • Stratified therapy for patients with unilateral FHWT and pulmonary metastases based on the response of the metastases to initial chemotherapy
AREN 0321	• Intensified therapy for patients with anaplastic WT using the revised UH-1 regimen • Future trials will investigate novel agents for treatment of these high-risk groups with the goal of improving outcomes and minimizing toxicity • Surgical resection for this high-risk group remains an important component of therapy • Advances in imaging such as 3-D computer reformatting and printing models
AREN 0534	• First cooperative group trial dedicated to children with BWT and unilateral high-risk patients • The primary aims related to patients with BWT were to improve 4-year EFS to 73% • To prevent complete removal of at least one kidney in 50% of patients by using a pre-nephrectomy three-drug chemotherapy regimen [vincristine, dactinomycin, and doxorubicin (VAD)] • To perform definitive surgical treatment in 75% of children with BWT by 12 weeks after initiation of chemotherapy

This will support integrated biomarker and imaging research, focusing on assessing the independent prognostic value of genomic changes within the tumor and the volume of the blastemal component that survives preoperative chemotherapy. Treatment guidelines for Wilms' tumors in the UMBRELLA protocol include recommendations for localized, metastatic, and bilateral disease, for all age groups, and for relapsed disease. These recommendations have been established by a multidisciplinary panel of leading experts on renal tumors within the SIOP-RTSG. The UMBRELLA protocol promotes international collaboration and research and serve as the SIOP-RTSG best available treatment standard.

The aim of the UMBRELLA protocol is to collect all clinical, biological, and outcomes data from children with primary renal tumors in a comprehensive data registry, with central review of diagnostics (radiology, pathology, and surgery), standardized biobanking, and precise treatment recommendations for the most common pediatric renal tumors. Molecular biology research within the protocol is primarily focused on the validation of the prognostic value of 1q gain, which might lead to a more personalized treatment approach. Consequently, short-term and long-term outcomes might be improved for all children with renal tumors by increasing survival, but also by reducing high-dose treatment in specific subgroups, resulting in diminished direct and late adverse effects. Timely genetic analysis and step-wise extension to additional targets such as *TP53* or several of the newly identified driver candidates for stratification and inclusion of liquid biopsies (circulating tumor DNA) in blood might help to reach this goal.

Staging Criteria in the SIOP UMBRELLA Protocol

Stage I

- Tumor is limited to the kidney
- Tumor is present in the perirenal fat but is surrounded by a fibrous (pseudo) capsule. The (pseudo) capsule might be infiltrated by viable tumor, which does not reach the outer surface
- Tumor might show protruding (botryoid) growth into the renal pelvis or the ureter but does not infiltrate their walls
- The vessels or the soft tissues of the renal sinus are not involved by tumor. Intrarenal vessel involvement might be present[11]

Stage II

- Viable tumor is present in the perirenal fat and is not covered by a (pseudo) capsule, but is completely resected (resection margins are clear)
- Viable tumor infiltrates the soft tissues of the renal sinus
- Viable tumor infiltrates blood and/or lymphatic vessels of the renal sinus or of the perirenal tissue, but it is completely resected
- Viable tumor infiltrates the wall of the renal pelvis or of the ureter
- Viable tumor infiltrates the vena cava or adjacent organs (except the adrenal gland) but is completely resected

Stage III

- Viable tumor is present at a resection margin. Nonviable tumor or chemotherapy-induced changes present at a resection margin are not regarded as stage III
- Abdominal lymph node involvement is present by either viable or nonviable tumor
- Preoperative or intraoperative tumor rupture, if confirmed by microscopic examination (viable tumor at the surface of the specimen at the area of the rupture)
- Viable or nonviable tumor thrombus is present at resection margins of ureter, renal vein, or vena cava inferior (always discuss resection margins with the surgeon)
- Viable or nonviable tumor thrombus, which is attached to the inferior vena cava wall, is removed piecemeal by a surgeon
- Wedge or open tumor biopsy before preoperative chemotherapy or surgery
- Tumor implants (viable or nonviable) are found anywhere in the abdomen
- Tumor (viable or nonviable) has penetrated through the peritoneal surface

Stage IV

Hematogenous metastases (for example, lung, liver, bone, and brain) or lymph node metastases outside the abdominopelvic region

Stage V

Bilateral renal tumors at diagnosis, each side should be substaged according to the above criteria

SIOP-RTSG UMBRELLA, 2016 Protocol–Pathology Panel

Pathology aims

To optimize pathological diagnostics by rapid central review in order to:

- Classify and stage tumors accurately in order to optimize treatment and avoid undertreatment or overtreatment
- Monitor and give appropriate feedback on local pathological diagnosis and stage
- Accurately assess the blastema in postchemotherapy specimens
- Correlate blastema volume and biomarkers with event-free and overall survival[11]

Biobanking aims

- To store biological material from all participating centers
- To show the feasibility of storing serial blood and urine samples and tumor and germline material at diagnosis and at specific time points during treatment for international collaborative studies
- To establish national biobanks (if not yet present) and generate a study-wide virtual biobank for translational research
- To test the feasibility of returning biomarker results to treatment centers within a clinically relevant time frame

Molecular biology aims

- To assess genomic 1q gain as a prognostic marker in Wilms' tumor
- To analyze biomarkers with potential prognostic relevance (simultaneous loss of 1p and 16q, *MYCN* gain and 17p loss encompassing the *TP53* locus)
- To assess molecular characteristics of blastemal-type Wilms' tumors
- To explore whether aberrations in *WT1, CTNNB1, AMER1, TP53, MYCN, FBXW7, GPC3, MLLT1, DIS3L2, DICER1, DROSHA, DGCR8, SIX1*, or *SIX2* considerably affect event-free or overall survival
- To explore circulating biomarkers (micro-RNA and DNA) in blood, and/or plasma, and/or urine and to support research
- On epigenetics, tumor cell culture, and/or organoids and xenografts

Goals and recommendations of SIOP-RTGS UMBRELLA protocol are:

- Aim of validating 1q gain as a prognostic marker
- Assessment of the independent prognostic value of the absolute volume of the blastemal component that survives preoperative chemotherapy.
- The SIOP-RTSG agreed that the blastemal volume threshold at which the risk of relapse rises dramatically needs to be established before its implementation as a prognostic factor.
- Histological classification after preoperative chemotherapy defines three major subgroups of Wilms' tumors—low-risk (completely necrotic Wilms' tumor), high-risk (blastemal type and diffuse anaplasia), and intermediate-risk tumors (all other types).
- Pretreatment biopsy is not routinely recommended.
- Percutaneous Trucut biopsy can be considered in young children with stage IV disease and in children >10 years of age, as the frequency of non-Wilms' tumors [rhabdoid tumor of the kidney (RTK) and renal cell carcinoma, respectively] is increased in these age groups.
- Percutaneous needle biopsies do not upstage tumor.
- Biopsies are not advised in children <6 months of age and in fully cystic tumors; immediate surgery is recommended in these children.
- Open wedge biopsy upstages tumors to stage III, irrespective of other findings, and regarded as capsule breach.
- In the UMBRELLA protocol, institutional pathologists will not be required to calculate the volume of blastema in tumors, the estimated percentages of the nonviable, and viable components (especially blastema) will be recorded.
- Blastemal volume will be calculated in the centralized protocol database. This calculation will be based on both pathological and imaging measurements of the tumor.
- To diagnose anaplasia, all three criteria need to be present: large atypical tripolar and/or multipolar mitotic figures; marked nuclear enlargement, with nuclear diameters at least three times those of adjacent cells; and hyperchromatic tumor cell nuclei. It can be focal or diffuse anaplasia.
- By consensus of the SIOP-RTSG pathology panel, the size of the anaplastic focus does not exceed 15 mm (which was previously undefined).
- Wilms' tumor with focal anaplasia is regarded as an intermediate-risk tumor in the UMBRELLA protocol. If focal anaplasia is present in blastemal-type Wilms' tumor, it is regarded as a high-risk tumor.
- Accumulation of the TP53 protein in WT specimens has been associated with unfavorable histology and treatment resistance.

Two primary practical aims of UMBRELLA protocol are biobanking and biomarker analysis.

- Biobanking aim is to demonstrate the feasibility to store the serial blood and urine samples as well as tumor and germline material, at diagnosis and at specific points during treatment for international collaborative studies. Biobanks will be instrumental to reach the aims of study, evaluation of novel genomic driver candidates, informative microRNA patterns, epigenome analysis, and panel sequencing that will be performed in national laboratories. For baseline diagnostics, EDTA blood samples and tumor tissue together with healthy kidney tissue, if available, will be collected from primary tumors and relapses and stored at –80°. Additional materials—blood for miRNA analysis and liquid biopsy of circulating tumor dNA, urine for proteomic analysis should be collected at multiple points. This will help in parallel and future translational research activities.
- Biobanking of frozen materials will be complemented by surplus formalin-fixed, paraffin-embedded (FFPE) blocks that are also a valuable resource for research, including the molecular analysis of microdissected nephrogenic rests, tumor subcompartments, and anaplastic foci. Sample collection in this virtual biobank, including medical records, informed consent for biobanking by parents and (if applicable) children will be documented in the web-based SIOP UMBRELLA database.
- *Biomarker analysis:* Children's Oncology Group (COG) protocols in the USA already include molecular markers in clinical decision making. The two primary biomarkers under study—blastemal volume and 1q gain—must be considered in the context of any co-dependencies with existing risk factors (tumor stage and histology) and the treatment given to prove their additional value for clinical decision making.

Successful implementation of the UMBRELLA protocol will have the potential to shape future therapeutic approaches and to improve outcomes by biomarker analysis. Standardization of biobanking across the globe for uniform data collection will be feasible. The UMBRELLA protocol provides guidelines for clinical practice and will hopefully stimulate further international collaboration with harmonization of treatment protocols and research. The UMBRELLA study will provide increased patient cohorts, rapid central pathology review, the standardization of specimen handling, improved collection of biological samples by pathologists will provide large numbers of specimens with increased homogeneity compared with other studies collected prospectively.

Prognostic Staging

National Wilms' Tumor Study Group classification is either favorable or unfavorable histology based on histological features of the biopsied specimen—the biphasic/triphasic pattern with or without anaplasia (focal or diffuse anaplasia). The SIOP classification is based on cell differentiation including chemotherapy-induced "regressive" changes. As it is proven already, the anaplastic features are not altered by chemotherapy. Hence, the histologic classification of SIOP provides adequate risk stratification. The three groups proposed by the revised SIOP histologic classification are as follows:

1. Low risk—completely necrotic nephroblastoma or cystic partially differentiated nephroblastoma
2. Intermediate risk—regressive, epithelial, stromal, mixed, or focal anaplastic nephroblastoma
3. High risk—blastemal or diffuse anaplastic nephroblastoma

MANAGEMENT

Management of WT[12] as per NWTS protocol 5 **(Table 3)**, management of WT as per SIOP protocol **(Box 1)** and regime of postoperative therapy as per SIOP protocol **(Box 2)** should be noted.

Concerns in Both Protocols

Societe Internationale D'oncologic Pediatrique protocol has the disadvantages of:[10]

- Benign lesions being given chemotherapy as prechemotherapy tissue confirmation is not mandatory
- Chemotherapy administration may differ in a different histological type of malignancy
- Modification of tumor histology by the preoperative chemotherapy
- Loss of staging information

But the prenephrectomy chemotherapy has a major advantage in tumor reduction in size, which prevents spillage intraoperatively and opens a possibility of nephron sparing surgery with size reduction.

The NWTS protocol on the other hand has concerns as:

- Tumor spillage intraoperatively, which increases risk of local relapse and poor outcome.
- Failure to sample nodes leads to downstaging and undertreatment of the disease.

Both the protocols have large series of patient trials. Both the treatment approaches yield almost equivalent clinical outcomes though a valid debate continues about the relative merits of each approach **(Table 4)**.

Indian Council of Medical Research Guideline for Workup

Indian Council of Medical Research (ICMR)[13] has proposed guidelines on approach and investigations in a suspected case of WT (Adapted from ICMR guidelines[12] for developing countries with limited resources) **(Flowchart 1)**.

TABLE 3: Treatment scheme used in National Wilms' Tumor Study-5.

Stages and details	*Radiotherapy*	*Chemotherapy**
Stage I and II, favorable histology	None	Regimen EE-4A
Stage I focal or diffuse anaplasia	None	Regimen EE-4A
Stage I, favorable histology, age <2 year, tumor weight <550 g	None	Regimen EE-4A
Stage III and IV, favorable histology	Yes	Regimen DD-4A
Stage II–IV, focal anaplasia	Yes	Regimen I
Stage II–IV, diffuse anaplasia	Yes	Regimen I
Stage I–IV clear cell sarcoma of the kidney	Yes	Regimen RTK
Stage I–IV rhabdoid tumor of the kidney	Yes	Regimen RTK

*1998 modification to original protocol

- *Regimen EE-4A:* Pulse-intensive dactinomycin, vincristine (18 weeks)
- *Regimen DD-4A:* Pulse-intensive dactinomycin, vincristine, doxorubicin (24 weeks)
- *Regimen I:* Dactinomycin, vincristine, doxorubicin, cyclophosphamide, and etoposide (24 weeks)
- *Regimen RTK:* Carboplatin, etoposide, and cyclophosphamide (24 weeks)
- Stage IV/FH patients are given radiation based on the local tumor stage.

BOX 1: Management of Wilms' tumor as per SIOP protocol.

- *Localized lesion:* 4 weeks of dactinomycin/vincristine—followed by surgical staging
- *Metastatic lesion:* 6 weeks of dactinomycin/vincristine/epirubicin and proceed to histological diagnosis

BOX 2: Regime of postoperative therapy as per SIOP protocol.

Stage 1/low grade:	None
Stage 1/intermediate grade + anaplasia:	18 weeks dactinomycin/ vincristine
Stage 2 (no lymph nodes):	28 weeks dactinomycin/ vincristine/epirubicin
Stage 2 + 3:	28 weeks dactinomycin/ vincristine/epirubicin + radiotherapy tumor bed
High grade:	34 weeks epirubicin/ifosfamide/ VP-16/carboplatin + radiotherapy
Metastatic grade 4:	As per local stage for tumor + treatment of metastasis—radiotherapy and/or excision

TABLE 4: Wilms' tumor (favorable histology) 5-year survival rates.

Stage	*5-year survival (%)*
I/II	90%
III	80–85%
IV	60–80%
V (bilateral)	70–80%

Flowchart 1: Indian Council of Medical Research (ICMR) guideline for treatment plan.[13]

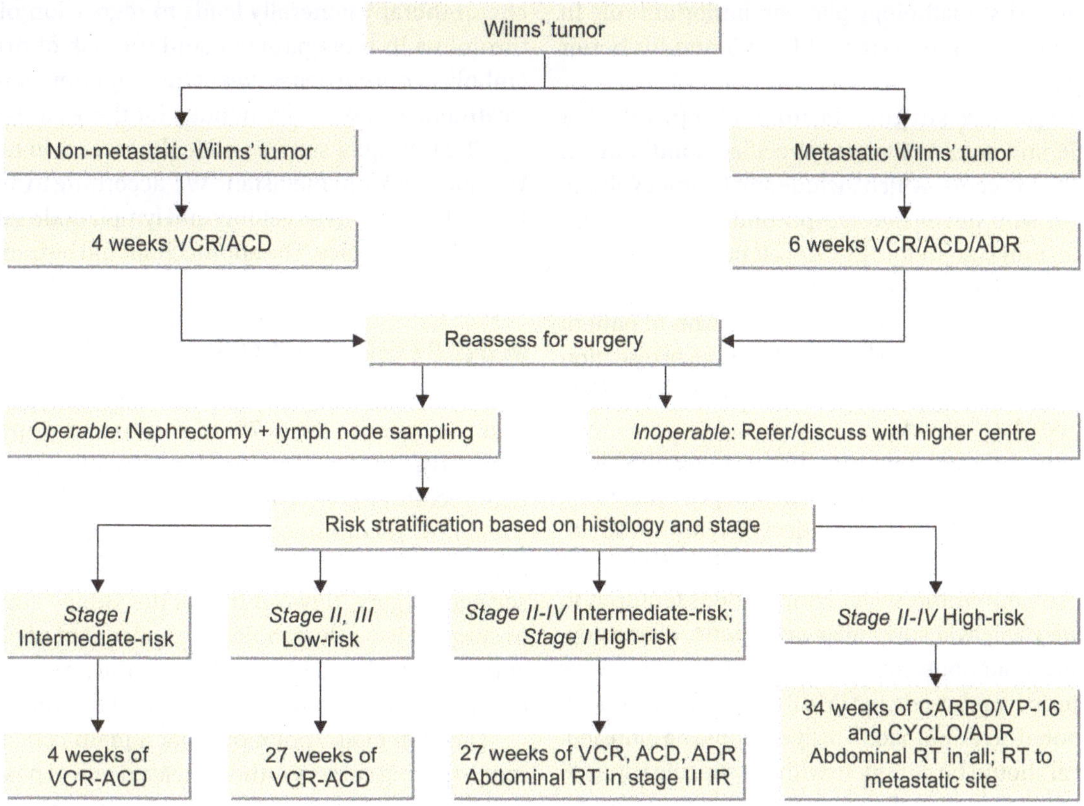

Baseline Investigations and Evaluation

Physical Examination

- Nutritional status
- Side and size of the tumor
- Size of the liver
- Blood pressure
- Suspected lymph nodes or other masses
- Congenital anomalies and syndromic features, if any

Laboratory investigations and imaging:

- Complete hemogram
- *Biochemistry:* Liver and renal function tests
- Contrast-enhanced CT scan of chest, abdomen, and pelvis
- *Optional:* Fine-needle aspiration cytology or Trucut biopsy of the tumor
- May be done as per the individual institutional practice

Needle biopsy should be from a retroperitoneal approach without more than 2–3 attempts, and image guided when possible. Biopsy is not recommended in bilateral tumors if radiological picture is consistent.

Needle biopsy is to be considered in following situations:

- *Inoperable renal mass*—pre-chemotherapy—since 5–10% of renal masses may be non-Wilms' tumor.
- *Unusual clinical presentations:* Age >5–6 years
- Urinary infection, septicemia, and Psoas inflammation
- *Unusual findings by imaging:* Calcification, voluminous adenopathies, and renal parenchyma not visible or almost totally extrarenal process

Abdominal radiology should mention the following points:

- Size of tumor in maximum dimension
- Laterality with a comment on contralateral kidney
- Presence of thrombus
- Lymph node status
- *Liver nodules:* Number, size, and site
- *Relationship with aorta and inferior vena cava:* Pushed, engulfed, and none
- *Origin of tumor:* Upper pole, lower pole, or hilum

Chest radiology should mention the following points:

Contrast enanced CT:

- Metastasis—present/absent
- Unilateral/bilateral
- *Number on each side:* Up to five or more than five
  - CT scan of chest is recommended for detection of pulmonary metastasis.
  - If chest radiograph is showing a doubtful lesion, then a CT chest would be desirable.

Surgery in Wilms' Tumor

In surgical options for WT, nephron-sparing surgery (NSS) in selective patients helps to preserve functional renal units and long-term renal function, without compromising overall survival and event-free survival. NSS has been advocated, if tumor is resectable in polar regions or if enucleation is possible. Bilateral WT is the ideal candidates for NSS[14]—now, it is extended even to unilateral WT depending on the resectability by contrast-enhanced computed tomography (CECT) imaging. Histopathology plays an important role in identifying the tumor-free margin at least 5 mm for better prognostication.

Nephron-sparing surgery is now acceptable for nonsyndromic unilateral WT under specified conditions in the UMBRELLA protocol,[11] which include small tumor volume (<300 mL) and who never had lymph node involvement. A new classification system for NSS, developed by a group of surgeons and pathologists from SIOP–RTSG, was adopted in the UMBRELLA protocol to optimize comparison of patient outcomes. This classification includes SRM (surgical resection margin), PRM (pathological resection margin), and RRM (remaining renal parenchyma).

Operative notes should mention whether done outside or within the Gerota's fascia (as per the institutional practice). Sampling and histological examination of lymph nodes[15] should be done, even when not enlarged on clinical evaluation or radiology. The minimum seven lymph nodes required to be sampled are paracaval suprahilar node/infra-hilar node, paraaortic supra-hilar node/infra-hilar node, both iliac nodes and a mesenteric lymph node in UMBRELLA SIOP protocol. Any nodules noted on examination of liver should be biopsied. Tumor removal should be complete without capsule rupture. Comment on spillage, even if absent, and on the presence/absence of renal vein or inferior vena caval thrombus and whether thrombus is adherent or nonadherent. These are data required for the uniform standardization of centralized data across the globe.

Minimally invasive surgical techniques[16] are safe in experienced hands. These are commonly advocated in adults with fear of tumor spillage and port-site metastasis. Technology is catching up in pediatric oncology nowadays. This gives the advantage to look at the opposite side kidney in unilateral WT, unilateral nephrectomy and contralateral NSS, lymph node sampling, and liver nodule resection if any, through smaller ports thereby reducing the pain and recovery time for the children.

Contralateral exploration is not advocated in UMBRELLA SIOP as highly sensitive and specific cross-sectional imaging by MRI/CECT gives adequate information on metastasis. Even adrenals adjacent to the WT kidney can be preserved with a clear margin. Node sampling of minimum 7–10 is warranted for staging purposes.

Pulmonary nodules by contrast imaging do not necessarily need a radioablation, as it leads to pulmonary hypertension and fibrosis in the long term. Adjuvant chemotherapy is good enough to tackle these nodule. Metastasectomy[15] provides good survival outcomes negating the need for whole-lung radiotherapy in patients with nodules that do not respond to chemotherapy.

The NWTS retrospective analyses have shown that adherent IVC tumor thrombus up to the level of the hepatic veins increases the risk of massive intraoperative hemorrhage and is a now a contraindication to upfront resection. Upfront chemotherapy generally leads to regression of caval/atrial thrombus in most patients, and the risk of progression or embolism during neoadjuvant therapy is low, so neoadjuvant treatment is now recommended for these cases presurgery.

The timing of surgery is ideally week 5 in nonmetastatic WT and week 7 in metastatic WT according to SIOP protocol. Radical nephroureterectomy and lymph node sampling is the procedure of choice. The approach should be transabdominal/transperitoneal.

BILATERAL WILMS' TUMOR

Bilateral Wilms' tumor can be synchronous or metachronous and it accounts for 6–7% of the tumor population. The surgical management in initial days was a radical surgery with nephrectomy followed by dialysis and renal transplant. NWTS trials now recommend conservative approach of bilateral biopsy followed by preoperative chemotherapy and then renal salvage surgery. If two-thirds of the kidney could be spared in surgery, it is salvageable. The concept of nephron-sparing surgery has taken a big lead in both the protocols depending on the individual staging of a bilateral tumor.

Davidoff et al.[14] point out that a main concern regarding renal-sparing surgery is the increased rate of positive margins and thus, the increased risk of local recurrence. One problem in patients with bilateral tumors is trying to determine, whether new tumors are the result of residual disease or *de novo* tumors that have developed from other sites. These patients have multifocal disease and a high incidence of nephrogenic rests. Not all of these rests are eradicated with chemotherapy and late occurrence of new tumors has been observed in this patient population.

ANAPLASTIC WILMS' TUMOR

The unresponsive nature of anaplastic tumor to chemotherapy has led to increase in trials and modification of chemoregimen in anaplasia. NWTS-5 has formulated the treatment plans as here:

Stage 2/3/4 with diffuse anaplasia received abdominal irradiation and a novel chemoregimen of VCR, doxorubicin, and dactinomycin alternating with cyclophosphamide and etoposide. Patients with stage 2/3/4 and focal anaplasia were treated with abdominal irradiation, VCR, doxorubicin, and dactinomycin. The 4-year event-free survival for patients with diffuse and focal anaplasia was 55.1% and 74.9%, respectively.

The NWTSG has recommended preoperative chemotherapy under certain circumstances, including the occurrence of WT in a solitary kidney, bilateral WT, tumor in a horseshoe kidney, tumor thrombus in the inferior vena cava above the level of the hepatic veins, and respiratory distress resulting from the presence of extensive metastatic tumor.

In the current SIOP protocol, a special clause is made for patients with lung lesions detected on chest CT and not on CXR. These lesions are called CT-only lung metastasis. The

SIOP protocol prescribes that these lesions should be ignored and the patients with CT-only nodules should be treated as if without lung metastasis (double agent instead of three-drug chemotherapy and no lung irradiation). One of the aims of the study is to evaluate the outcome of these patients with CT-only metastasis.[17]

CHIEF INDICATIONS OF RADIOTHERAPY

The following are the chief indications for radiotherapy: Abdominal RT (1,000 cGy + booster as indicated) is preferred for the following indications, all stage III tumors, stage IV, all anaplastic tumors beyond stage I, all clear cell sarcomas of kidney and abdominal relapse. Chest RT (1,200 cGy) is given for lung metastasis.

For UMBRELLA protocol, the radiotherapy guidelines used in SIOP–2001 were refined based on the experience from a 2017 SIOP–2001 analysis and prior COG–NWTS trials.

The dosage of whole-lung irradiation was decreased from 15 to 12 Gy in the UMBRELLA protocol, to be in line with previous NWTS experience demonstrating high relapse-free and overall survival (72% and 78%, respectively) for favorable—histology tumors after treatment with doxorubicin, actinomycin-D, VCR, and 12 Gy to the lungs.

The SIOP-RTSG board[18] radiology panel with ten collaborating pediatric radiation oncologists has conducted four live international consensus meetings formulating—regional radiotherapy in children. This is to avoid the entire abdominal radiotherapy causing long-term fibrosis of the adjacent normal viscera in growing children.

The final guideline includes eight chronological steps to generate the tumor bed and clinical, internal, and planning target volumes, and it describes the optional use of surgical clips to optimize treatment planning. This guideline will be added into the radiotherapy guideline of the UMBRELLA SIOP-RTSG protocol for pediatric renal tumors to improve international consistency of highly conformal flank target-volume delineation.

- Radiation oncologists affiliated to SIOP-RTSG adapted the conventional approach of flank irradiation into a guideline for highly conformal flank target-volume delineation.
- The tumor bed is defined as the contact zone of the primary tumor after preoperative chemotherapy with subtraction of all uninvolved organs at risk, therefore taking into account the postoperative changes in anatomy
- Surgeons and radiation oncologists are encouraged to closely collaborate, since the use of a superior clip can personalize motion of the target volume, whereas a lateral clip can define the lateral tumor extension in patients with a tumor volume expanding into the anterior part of the abdomen.
- The role of surgical clips in the era of 3D-guided and 4D-guided radiotherapy was discussed.

On the basis of preoperative MRI scans and postoperative CT and MRI scans in radiotherapy treatment position, participants outlined the gross tumor volume (GTV), tumor bed, and clinical target volume (CTV) for three series of two patients with pediatric renal tumors.

- *Step 1 (optional): Surgical clip placement*—the use of lateral clips on the interior abdominal wall, close to the paracolic peritoneal reflection where the retroperitoneal surgical dissection has been done (near to the white line of Toldt), demarcates the anterolateral extension of the postoperative resection margin and is therefore of value to guide radiation fields after nephrectomy.
- *Step 2: Imaging in radiotherapy position* to do a 4D-CT scan to estimate motion of the target volume.
- *Step 3: Image co-registration*—optimal co-registration of the postoperative CT scan in radiotherapy position, with the MRI (or CT) scan done after preoperative chemotherapy and before surgery, is essential for obtaining maximum benefit from the delineation guideline.
- *Step 4: Delineation of the organs at risk:* Pelvic region, delineation of the bladder, testicles, uterus, and ovaries is needed, and ovarian transposition or tissue cryopreservation, or both, should be considered.
- *Step 5: Delineation of the tumor bed with or without lymph nodes*—GTV-Tpost or GTV-Npost need to include the contact zone of the primary tumor with the involved organ.
- *Step 6:* Delineation of the CTV
- *Step 7:* Delineation of the internal target volume
- *Step 8:* Delineation of the planning target volume

Indications for flank irradiation have remained roughly unchanged compared with the SIOP-2001 protocol. In brief, patients with Wilms' tumor stage II (diffuse anaplastic subtype), Wilms' tumor stage III (intermediate-risk and all high-risk histologies), as well as all malignant rhabdoid tumors of the kidney and clear cell sarcomas of the kidney stage II–III will receive adjuvant locoregional radiotherapy with risk-adapted doses.

FOLLOW-UP IMAGING

Follow-up imaging studies in children with WT without metastasis at the time of diagnosis is important and the recommendations are given in **Table 5**.

OTHER RENAL TUMORS OF CHILDHOOD

Introduction

Other renal neoplasms of childhood may resemble multilocular cystic renal tumors:[5] WT with cyst formation as a result of hemorrhage and necrosis, clear cell sarcoma, cystic mesoblastic nephroma, cystic partially differentiated nephroblastoma (CPDN), RTK, and renal cell carcinoma. Similarly, multicystic dysplastic kidney, especially the segmental form, may be mistaken for multilocular cystic renal mass.

Multicystic dysplastic kidney may mimic the imaging characteristics of multilocular cystic renal tumor. Usually,

TABLE 5: Recommended follow-up imaging studies in children with Wilms' tumor without metastasis at diagnosis*.

Stage and type of Wilms' tumor	*Imaging studies*	*Off-treatment schedule*
Stages I, II, and III with favorable histology; stages I, II, and III with anaplastic histology	Chest radiography	6 weeks and 3 months after surgery, then every 3 months (5 times), then every 6 months (3 times), then yearly (2 times)
All stages in patients aged <48 month at diagnosis with nephrogenic rests	Abdominal ultrasonography	Every 3 months for 6 years
All stages in patients aged >48 month at diagnosis with nephrogenic rests	Abdominal ultrasonography	Every 3 months for 4 years
Stages I and II with favorable histology	Abdominal ultrasonography	Yearly (6 times)
Stage III with favorable histology	Abdominal ultrasonography	6 weeks and 3 months after surgery, then every 3 month (5 times), then every 6 months (3 times), then yearly (2 times)
All stages with unfavorable histology	Abdominal ultrasonography	Every 3 months (4 times), then every 6 months (4 times)

*Subsequent imaging studies should be performed as clinically indicated.

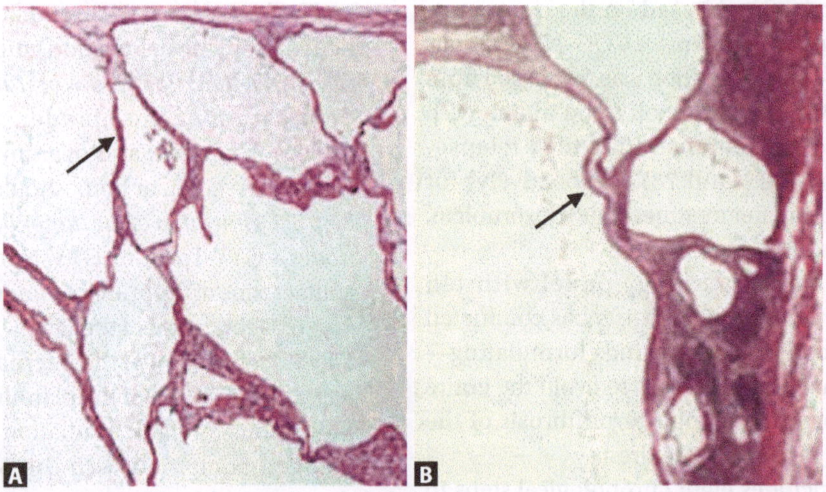

Figs. 7A and B: Cystic nephroma represents an encapsulated mass composed entirely of cystic spaces separated by septa containing only mature elements and without solid nodules. The identification of immature nephroblastic elements within the septa (arrow mark) distinguishes cystic partially differentiated nephroblastoma from cystic nephroma. The presence of any solid nodules indicates the diagnosis of cystic Wilms" tumor and excludes the diagnosis of cystic, partially differentiated nephroblastoma or cystic nephroma.

the differential diagnosis poses no difficulty because, unlike unilocular cystic renal tumors, the cysts of multicystic dysplastic kidney fill the entire kidney. Furthermore, no cases of cystic nephroma or CPDN have been detected antenatally or in the newborn period, when multicystic dysplastic kidney is usually detected. Nevertheless, differentiation of multicystic dysplastic kidney from cystic nephroma or CPDN is important, since the trend in treatment of the former is conservative follow-up rather than surgery.

Cystic Nephroma and Cystic Partially Differentiated Nephroblastoma

Multilocular cystic renal tumor is a term that encompasses two histologically distinct, but grossly indistinguishable lesions: cystic nephroma and cystic partially differentiated nephroblastoma (CPDN). Cystic nephroma is a segmental, purely cystic mass characterized by multiple septations composed entirely of differentiated tissues, without blastemal elements. CPDN is also a multiloculated lesion without nodular solid components, but its septa contain embryonal cells **(Figs. 7A and B)**. Multilocular cystic tumors primarily affect boys during early childhood, with a substantial number of the lesions containing blastema (CPDN) and adult women, with lesions that more commonly lack septal blastema (cystic nephroma). As a rule, nephrectomy is curative and the clinical course is benign, but CPDN may recur locally. Although cystic nephroma and CPDN cannot be distinguished radiologically, failure to do so has no practical impact on management, since all of these tumors are surgically removed.

An attractive concept has been proposed in which cystic nephroma, CPDN, and solid WT represent benign and malignant ends of a spectrum, analogous to the continuum in which ganglioneuroma, ganglioneuroblastoma, and neuroblastoma rebate to each other.

Congenital Mesoblastic Nephroma

Congenital mesoblastic nephroma (CMN) is the most common renal tumor in neonates and infants, with a mean age at diagnosis of 3.5 months. This is also called tumor of Bolande, as it was first reported by Bolande et al. in 1967. The typical presentation is a newborn with an abdominal mass, but in recent years, a number of cases have been recognized prenatally, with polyhydramnios a frequent prenatal finding. Tumor induction is postulated to occur at a time when the multipotent blastema is predominately stromagenic. The neoplasm is distinct from WT and has three histologic subtypes: classic, cellular, and mixed (showing areas of both classical and cellular). The classic subtype, 24% of cases, is characterized by interlacing sheets of bland spindle cells. Classic CMN resembles infantile fibromatosis. The cellular variant, 66% of cases, has a solid sheet-like growth pattern and cells with little cytoplasm and frequent mitoses. The cellular variant is virtually identical histologically to congenital fibrosarcoma. Molecular studies have found a similar translocation in both tumors that fuses the *ETV6 (TEL)* gene from chromosome 12p13 with the chromosome 15q25 neurotrophin-3 receptor gene, *NTRK3*.

Imaging studies cannot reliably distinguish CMN from other renal mass lesions. Abdominal CT shows a heterogeneous solid mass arising from the kidney. Complete excision is curative for most patients with CMN. Local recurrence and metastasis can occur, particularly with the cellular variant of CMN. The pathology specimen will often identify extension of tumor into the hilar or perirenal soft tissue; therefore, complete surgical resection is important. The risk of recurrence is thought to be less in children under 3 months of age at diagnosis, but metastasis has been reported in a few infants. Neither chemotherapy nor radiation therapy is routinely recommended, but consideration for adjuvant treatment should be given to patients with cellular variants that are incompletely resected. There are reports demonstrating response of both inoperable and recurrent tumors to chemotherapy.

Clear Cell Sarcoma of the Kidney

Clear cell sarcoma of the kidney (CCSK) tumor is also known as the "bone-metastasizing renal tumor of childhood" because of its predilection for these sites. There are also an increased number of brain metastasis with this entity. CCSK accounts for 3% of renal tumors reported to the NWTSG. Unlike anaplastic WT, even stage I CCSK lesions are associated with increased rates of relapse. There are no reports of children with bilateral CCSK.

Histologically, CCSK exhibits diverse morphologic patterns mimicking other cystic neoplasms, often leading to misdiagnosis. Recent immunohistochemical and molecular genetic tests support the diagnosis by identifying the internal tandem duplications in BCL-6 coreceptor (BCOR) and a translocation t(10;17) creating the fusion gene *YWHAE-NUTM2B/E*.

Immunohistochemistry for BCOR[19] is both a sensitive and specific marker for CCSK. Positive expression of CD99 and absence of the *SYT-SSX* fusion gene by polymerase chain reaction differentiate clear cell sarcoma of the kidney (CCSK) from synovial sarcoma.

The most common sites of metastases at presentation are regional lymph nodes, bone, lung, and liver. Histology shows nests or cords of cells that are separated by regularly spaced fibrovascular septae—"chicken-wire" appearance, or more robust and cellular, which is a characteristic feature of CCSK. CCSK shows nonspecific positivity for vimentin, nerve growth factor (NGFR), cyclin D1, negative for epithelial, neural, vascular, and muscle markers.

Diffuse strong nuclear staining with a commercially available BCL-6 coreceptor (BCOR) antibody has been shown to be highly sensitive and specific for the diagnosis of CCSK in pediatric age groups.

Improved intensive chemotherapy regimens have influenced the clinical course of the disease, with late relapses now being less frequent. In the current SIOP protocol, preoperative chemotherapy with actinomycin and VCR is indicated for stages I to III disease, with the addition of doxorubicin for stage IV disease. Following initial surgical resection, postoperative chemotherapy comprises etoposide, carboplatin, and ifosfamide, alternating with cyclophosphamide and doxorubicin. Abdominal radiotherapy is added for stages II to IV disease.

Studies have demonstrated that the use of doxorubicin (DOX) is associated with a significant improvement in outcome for these children. Patients with CCSK were treated on NWTS-5 with a regimen combining VCR, DOX, cyclophosphamide, and etoposide in an attempt to further improve the survival of this high-grade tumor. All patients with CCSK require irradiation to the tumor bed.

Rhabdoid Tumor of the Kidney

Rhabdoid tumor of the kidney was first identified by NWTSG pathologists in 1978. This is a highly malignant tumor of the kidney and accounts for 2% of renal tumors registered to the NWTSG. The tumor derives its name from the resemblance to rhabdomyoblasts, but it is not derived from myogenic cells; the cell of origin is unknown. This tumor is typically seen in infants and very young children, with a median age of 13 months. Infants with RTK often have concurrent brain tumors. It is difficult to ascertain if these are metastasis or two distinct primary tumors. Recent studies suggest that there is a common genetic basis for renal and extrarenal rhabdoid tumors in infants. There is a deletion or mutation in the tumor suppressor gene *INI-1* on chromosome 22 that predisposes to the development of this tumor. Staining for the products of the *INI-1* gene can be useful, as RTK is consistently negative. The prognosis of patients with rhabdoid tumor remains dismal with conventional chemotherapeutic regimens, with over 80% of children dying within 1 year of diagnosis. In NWTS-5, children with all stages of rhabdoid tumor were treated with carboplatin, cyclophosphamide, and etoposide; they also received abdominal irradiation, but results of that trial are pending.

Renal Cell Carcinoma

Only 5% of renal cell carcinomas occur in children. These patients generally present after age 5 years and it is the most common renal malignancy in the second decade of life. Survival of children with renal cell carcinoma is dependent on the staging and complete resectability of the tumor. Overall event-free survival is about 50%. Age is also a prognostic factor, with improved survival in children <11 years. Renal cell carcinomas in children differ in their morphology and molecular characterization than adults.

The most common translocations identified in pediatric RCC[20] involve the *TFE3* gene (transcription factor micro E3), which is located at the p11.2 locus of the X chromosome. TFE3 expression is a useful marker of the probability of lymph node metastasis and of overall prognosis, but its absence may also be a useful screening tool to rule out translocation. Histopathology of Xp11.2 translocation tumors show Psammoma bodies characteristically.

The second common translocation involves the gene *TFEB*, which is found at the p21 locus of chromosome 6. Histologically, this tumor type demonstrates epithelioid cells with clear cytoplasm mimicking standard clear-cell RCC.

Children with Von Hippel Lindau syndrome typically develop clear-cell tumors, and often are multifocal or bilateral. Their kidneys often contain renal cysts or angiomyolipomas together.

Robson's staging and classification of RCC are based on the relationship to Gerota's fascia, involvement of renal vein, and regional nodes. *Robson's staging* of renal cell carcinoma is simple and is now been replaced by the TNM staging. For simple practical purposes, Robson's staging can be used **(Box 3)**.

Selection criteria to undergo partial nephrectomy included tumor size of <4 cm, location amenable to partial resection (polar regions), and Robson stage 1 or 2 lesions. For this group, 5-year event-free overall survival was 100% with mean follow-up of 61 months (12–127 months).

Studies reveal use of adjuvant and neoadjuvant chemotherapy, radiotherapy, and immunotherapy (interleukin-2, interferon alfa-2a, or 13-cis-retinoic acid) have not shown any significant reduction in tumor volume.

Stage-specific 5-year survival has been reported to range between 92.4 and 96% for stage 1 (disease confined to renal capsule), 84.6 and 86% for stage 2 (disease between renal capsule and Gerota's fascia), 72.7 and 77% for stage 3 (involvement of renal vein, inferior vena cava, or regional lymph nodes) and 9 and 13.9% for stage 4 (metastatic disease). These tumors do not appear responsive to chemotherapy or radiation therapy and are often poorly prognosticated.

BOX 3: Robson's staging.

- *Stage I:* Limited to kidney
- *Stage II:* Involvement of perinephric fat but remains limited to *Gerota's fascia*
- *Stage III:*
  - *IIIa:* Renal vein involvement
  - *IIIb:* Nodal involvement
  - *IIIc:* Both IIIa and IIIb
- *Stage IV:*
  - *IVa:* Direct invasion of adjacent organs/structures
  - *IVb:* Distant metastases

CONCLUSION

Wilms' tumor has evolved exponentially over 70 years with better understanding of the occurrence, nephrogenic rests, molecular basics, genetic mutations, familial and syndromic variants by extensive research by several clinical trials. Two clinical groups NWTS (COG) and SIOP have standardized the workup/treatment and follow-up protocols for WT. The multidisciplinary team or tumor board consisting (pediatric nephrologist/pediatric surgeon/pediatric oncologist/discuss on individual cases, staging and decide on the availability of the resources.

UMBRELLA SIOP-RTGS is giant leap in the research forum of WT in developed countries which is recruiting countries to join their group. In developing countries with limited resources, it will take a long time to join the race of biomarkers, gene sequencing, molecular studies, biobanking, and central standardization. To improve the clinical outcomes of the individual cases, at least institutional or regional standardization of the workup/surgery/pathology/treatment/follow-up protocols need to be ratified.

KEY POINTS

- Wilms' tumor protocol—either NWTS (COG) or SIOP needs to be followed by the institution of practice with a multidisciplinary team of tumor board.
- Essential to ask for genome/exome sequencing for genetic mutation identification/prognostication in WT at least in familial or syndromic children.
- To add up the urinary biomarker, prohibitin in the workup to identify the relapse cases.
- Contrast-enhanced CT scan plays a crucial role in preoperative tumor volume identification/nodal status/vascular thrombus/distant metastasis, and postoperative target volume estimation in case of children needing radiotherapy.
- Advances in surgery—nephron-sparing tumor excision even in unilateral cases/minimally invasive surgery for faster postoperative recovery.
- Pathology along with immunohistochemistry plays a vital role in the current staging with type of tumor and prognostication of relapse. It is the main scale in follow-up of treatment with chemotherapy and radiotherapy.
- Follow-up protocol is essential to be discussed well ahead to the parents to ensure a disease-free or event-free survival in children.

REFERENCES

1. Gylys-Morin V, Hoffer FA, Kozakewich H, Shamberger RC. Wilms tumor and nephroblastomatosis: imaging characteristics at gadolinium-enhanced MR imaging. Radiology. 1993;188:517-21.
2. Dome JS, Coppes MJ. Recent advances in Wilms tumor genetics. Curr Opin Pediatr. 2002;14:5-11.
3. Perlman EJ, Faria P, Soares A, Hoffer F, Sredni S, Ritchey M, et al. Hyperplastic perilobar nephroblastomatosis: long-term survival of 52 patients. Pediatr Blood Cancer. 2006;46:203-21.
4. Breslow NE, Beckwith JB, Perlman EJ, Reeve AE. Age distributions, birth weights, nephrogenic rests and heterogeneity int he pathogenesis of Wilms tumor. Pediatr Blood Cancer. 2006;47:260-7.
5. Agrons GA, Wagner BJ, Davidson AJ, Suarez ES. Multilocular cystic renal tumor in children: radiologic-pathologic correlation. Radiographics. 1995;15:653-69.
6. Goudie C, Coltin H, Witkowski L, Mourad S, Malkin D, Foulkes WD. The McGill Interactive Pediatric OncoGenetic Guidelines: An approach to identifying pediatric oncology patients most likely to benefit from a genetic evaluation. Pediatr Blood Cancer. 2017;64(8):Epub 2017 Jan 18.
7. Capasso M, Montella A, Tirelli M, Maiorino T, Cantalupo S, Iolascon A. Genetic predisposition to solid pediatric cancers. Front Oncol. 2020;10:590033.
8. Ortiz MV, Ahmed S, Burns M, Henssen AG, Hollmann TJ, MacArthur I, et al. Prohibitin is a prognostic marker and therapeutic target to block chemotherapy resistance in Wilms' tumor. (n.d.). JCI Insight. 2019;4(15):e127098.
9. Docimo SG, Canning DA, Khoury AE. The Kelalis–King–Belman: Textbook of Clinical Pediatric Urology, 5th edition. London: Informa Healthcare UK Ltd; 2007. Chapters 32-33, pp. 497-528.
10. Bhatnagar S. Management of Wilms' tumor: NWTS vs SIOP. J Indian Assoc Pediatr Surg. 2009;14(1):6-14.
11. Van den Heuvel-Eibrink MM, Hol JA, Pritchard-Jones K, van Tinteren H, Furtwängler R, Verschuur AC, et al. Position paper: Rationale for the treatment of Wilms tumor in the UMBRELLA SIOP-RTSG 2016 protocol. Nat Rev Urol. 2017;14(12):743-52.
12. Metzger ML, Dome JS. Current therapy for Wilms' tumor. Oncologist. 2005;10:815-26.
13. Prasad M, Vora T, Agarwala S, Laskar S, Arora B, Bansal D, et al. Management of Wilms Tumor: ICMR Consensus Document. Indian J Pediatr. 2017;84(6):437-45.
14. Davidoff AM, Giel DW, Jones DP, Jenkins JJ, Krasin MJ, Hoffer FA, et al. The feasibility and outcome of nephron-sparing surgery for children with bilateral Wilms' tumor. The St Jude Children's Research Hospital Experience: 1999–2006. Cancer. 2008;112:2060-70.
15. Shamberger RC. Renal tumors. In: Carachi R, Grosfeld JL, Amir F Azmy (Eds). The Surgery of Childhood Tumors, 2nd edition. Berlin Heidelberg: Springer-Verlag; 2008. Chapter 10, pp. 171-200.
16. Rauth TP, Slone J, Crane G. Laparoscopic nephron-sparing resection of synchronous Wilms' tumors in a case of hyperplastic perilobar nephroblastomatosis. J Pediatr Surg. 2011;46(5): 983-8.
17. Smets AM, de Kraker J. Malignant tumors of the kidney: imaging strategy. Pediatr Radiol. 2010;40:1010-18.
18. Janssens GO, Melchior P, Mul J, Saunders D, Bolle S, Cameron AL, et al. The SIOP-Renal Tumor Study Group consensus statement on flank target volume delineation for highly conformal radiotherapy. The Lancet Child Adolescent Health. 2020;4(11):846-52.
19. Aldera AP, Pillay K. Clear Cell Sarcoma of the Kidney. Arch Pathol Lab Med. 2020;144(1):119-23.
20. Young EE, Brown CT, Merguerian PA, Akhavan A. Pediatric and adolescent renal cell carcinoma. Urol Oncol. 2016;34(1):42-9.

SECTION

14

Assorted Themes

CHAPTER

14.1 Immunization in Kidney Disease

Sushmita Banerjee

INTRODUCTION

The advent of mass vaccination programs has dramatically reduced the prevalence of several infective diseases in the world. Immunization is one of the most cost-effective preventive health methods available and every child has the right to be protected against vaccine-preventable diseases (VPDs). It is also important to note that high rates of vaccination uptake in healthy children indirectly provide benefits of herd immunity to children who are unable to take specific vaccinations or respond to them optimally.[1]

Children with kidney disease already have significant underlying morbidities and complications due to their condition. It is, therefore, even more important to ensure that they are immunized optimally so that illness due to VPD is prevented. Because of underlying issues that may affect immune responses, the vaccination schedules and doses may need to be altered. This chapter reviews this need and the recommendations available.

THE PATIENTS

A major cause for mortality and morbidity in kidney disease is associated infection. Despite this, studies indicate that patients with chronic kidney disease (CKD) or those approaching kidney replacement therapies (KRTs) are often inadequately immunized.[2] Kidney patients may be at higher risk for VPDs due to several reasons. CKD is an immunosuppressed (IS) state with documented impairment of innate and adaptive immunity.[3] The presence of edema, uremia, and malnutrition further increases infection risks. Dialysis access involves a break in the body's cutaneous barriers and abnormal exposure of tissues to potential infections. Hepatitis B virus (HBV) infection is considered a particular risk in patients on hemodialysis (HD) or in those receiving blood products. Children with complement deficiencies or those receiving eculizumab have increased risk of meningococcal infection.[4]

The presence of proteinuria causes loss of immunoglobulins, complement factors, and other proteins involved with the body's defense mechanisms. Children with nephrotic syndrome (NS) have increased risk of infection, particularly due to *Streptococcus pneumoniae*. Viral infections such as influenza are common causes of NS relapse while varicella infections may be very severe in NS and in IS patients.[5]

Patients with glomerulopathies and kidney transplant (KT) patients are treated with immunosuppressive drugs (ISDs), increasing VPD risks. In KT patients, infection may precipitate rejection. KT patients have significantly higher risk of malignancies in the long-term and human papillomavirus (HPV) vaccine can prevent cervical and anal cancers.[6]

THE VACCINES

The available pediatric vaccines are either made of killed cell components or toxoids or are live attenuated forms of the organism. Live-attenuated vaccines (LAVs) stimulate the most robust immune response in the host. Among inactivated vaccines (IAVs), the immune reaction elicited by protein vaccines is better than that caused by polysaccharides. The immunogenicity of polysaccharide vaccines can be enhanced by conjugating them with proteins.[7]

- *Inactivated vaccines:* IAVs contain killed cell components or toxoids of the organism. These vaccines can be given safely in all patients with kidney disease. Examples are tetanus, diphtheria, pertussis, *Haemophilus influenzae*, hepatitis A and B, *Meningococcus*, typhoid, Salk polio (IPV), Japanese encephalitis, rabies, and papillomavirus vaccines. In addition, influenza and pneumococcal vaccines are particularly recommended in the IS and HBV vaccine in patients on HD or receiving blood products. Conjugate vaccines are preferred. *Pneumococcus* vaccine is available as both conjugated and unconjugated forms and a combination is recommended in kidney patients **(Table 1)**.
- *Live attenuated vaccines:* Examples are BCG, Rotavirus, Measles, Mumps, Rubella, oral Sabin Polio, and Varicella vaccines. In patients receiving high-dose steroids or other ISD, LAV may lose their attenuated status and cause vaccine-derived disease which can have severe consequences and are, therefore, contraindicated in these groups.

TABLE 1: Supplemental vaccines for patients with kidney disease.

Vaccine	Age and doses	Comments
Inactivated vaccines		
Influenza	*>6 months to <8 years:* Two doses 4 weeks apart in first year, then an annual dose *>8 years:* Annual dose	
Pneumococcal conjugate* 10/13 valent	*6 weeks–6 months:* Three doses >4 weeks apart and booster at 12–15 months *7–11 months:* Two doses >4 weeks apart and booster in 2nd year *12–23 months:* Two doses >8 weeks apart *2–6 years:* Two doses >8 weeks apart *>6 years:* One dose	(One dose if previously immunized)
Pneumococcal polysaccharide 23 valent	*>2 years:* Single dose 8 weeks post- PCV, repeated once after 5 years	
Hepatitis B	Two doses 4–6 weeks apart, and third dose at 6 months *Accelerated dose schedule:* Three doses 4 weeks apart with booster at 1 year. Double doses and adjuvants used in trials and in adults.	If previously immunized, check titers and maintain >10 mIU/mL with boosters
Quadrivalent *Meningococcus* conjugate	*9 months–24 months:* Two doses 3 months apart *2–7 years:* Two doses 8–12 weeks apart and booster after 3 years and then 5 yearly *>7 years:* Two doses 8–12 weeks apart and booster 5 yearly	Close household contacts can be given a single dose
Human papillomavirus	*>9 years:* Two doses 1–2 months apart and third dose at 6 months	Second dose timing depends on brand
Live-attenuated vaccines		
Varicella	*>15 months:* Two doses 2–3 months apart	Avoid in immunosuppressed, and within 1 month of kidney transplant (KT)
Measles, mumps, rubella	*>9 months:* Two doses >4 weeks apart	

*Pneumosil not recommended above 2 years.
Note: COVID-19 vaccine recommendations as per current Government of India guidelines for children.
Source: Adapted from References 4 and 7.

Several vaccines are available in both inactivated and live attenuated forms; the former are preferred in IS patients (e.g., polio, influenza, Japanese encephalitis, and typhoid vaccines).

IMMUNIZATION IN SPECIFIC PATIENT GROUPS

- *Patients with nephrotic syndrome who receive steroids:* Nephrotic syndrome in itself is a condition, which predisposes to infection; conversely, infection can cause NS relapse. Treatment with steroids further increases infection risk and also increases the risk of reduced vaccine response.[5] To avoid the latter, it is best to give vaccines in remission, when the child is off or on minimal steroid dose. However, all IAVs may safely be given at any time. Pneumococcal infections are most common; fortunately, responses to pneumococcal vaccines have been reported to be adequate even in relapse while on steroids.[8,9] However, vaccines such as HBV may require additional doses to provide adequate antibody titers.[10,11] Viral infections are common causes of relapse and annual influenza vaccine should be administered to all.
  A patient on steroids is defined to be IS when she is on prednisolone 2 mg/kg/day (or 20 mg/day in patients >10 kg) for >14 days. Such patients should receive LAV only after being off steroids for >1 month.[3,4] Two doses of varicella vaccine have been shown to provide adequate seroconversion and are, therefore, recommended 4 weeks apart when the child is in remission, off steroids, or on the lowest possible dose.[12,13]
  Although some vaccines have been associated with risk of relapse, this should not be seen as a deterrent, as relapses are easily treated in steroid-sensitive NS and benefit is considered to outweigh the risk.[14-16]
- *Patients on other IS (cyclophosphamide, azathioprine, mycophenolate mofetil, calcineurin inhibitors, and rituximab):* Patients with glomerulopathies and vasculopathies are treated with ISD for long periods of time. Diseases such as systemic lupus erythematosus (SLE) are in themselves considered to be immunosuppressive. Live vaccines are contraindicated but IAV may be given, ideally targeting the time periods when the lowest ISD doses are being used. Since immune responses may be reduced, it would be ideal to check titers and deliver

booster doses as required.[17,18] An annual influenza vaccine is recommended in all patients with stable disease and in SLE to those with low or moderate disease activity.[19] These high-risk groups should also be vaccinated against HBV and *Pneumococcus*. Patients receiving eculizumab are at a particular risk of meningococcal infections and should receive vaccination at least 2 weeks prior to treatment if time permits. After rituximab therapy, vaccines should not be given for 6–12 months.[4,20]

The time interval between stopping these ISD and administering an LAV may be about 3 months according to reports from rheumatology literature; however, this evidence is of low quality.[19] The administration of live vaccines such as MMR (measles, mumps, rubella) and varicella should be delayed in patients who have received immunoglobulins and blood products by at least 6 months, as these may contain neutralizing antibodies to the vaccine organism.[20]

- *Patients with CKD on conservative treatment, on or starting dialysis, or approaching KT:* Patients with CKD generally have better antibody responses if vaccinated prior to starting KRT.[2] Therefore, while there is time at hand, it is important to examine documentation of all vaccines received, check antibody titers, and catch up on immunizations as indicated. In previously immunized patients, hepatitis B surface antibody (HBsAb) titers prior to initiation, and on an annual basis, with appropriate boosting to maintain levels >10 mIU/mL is particularly indicated in patients on HD.[2,5] Although double doses have been used in trials and adjuvant-added vaccines are used in adults, there are no specific guidelines for such use in children. After completion of a vaccination course or administration of a booster dose, antibody titers should be checked after 4 weeks. Leading up to dialysis or KT, accelerated vaccine schedules may be used for those who are unimmunized.[5] In potential KT recipients, it is particularly important to protect with LAV such as MMR and varicella, up to 1 month prior to the procedure, as these are avoided post-KT.
- *Kidney transplant recipients:* During work-up for KT, protection against VPDs should be optimized as has been mentioned above. Accelerated dose schedules may be considered to ensure maximum protection.[1,5] Post-KT patients may lose immunological memory to some prior vaccines and require boosters or revaccination for high-risk VDPs as for cancer patients, but specific recommendations are lacking.

Vaccines are usually not given in the first 6 months after KT, for fear of inciting rejection, and because the high ISD doses during this time may not enable an immune response. Similarly, they are avoided after periods of intensified ISD such as after treatment of rejection episode.[1,6]

Thereafter, IAV may be given (the influenza vaccine appears to be safe and effective even if given earlier and should be given annually), but booster doses may be required to achieve adequate antibody levels. Similar to patients on dialysis, recommendations are to monitor HbsAb titers and revaccinate to maintain protective levels. Pneumococcal vaccination is recommended as in **Table 1**. Meningococcal vaccine is advised in high-risk patients. The risk of malignancies in the long-term indicates use of HPV in addition to HBV vaccination for the prevention of these infection-related malignancies.[1,4]

Note: The *coronavirus disease 2019 (COVID-19)* pandemic poses a further challenge to IS and KT patients in whom high rates of AKI and mortality are reported, particularly in the elderly.[21] Current evidence indicates a better outcome in IS children.[22] With several COVID-19 vaccines becoming available, this will be one more vaccine that should be given early to patients with kidney disease.

GENERAL IMMUNIZATION RECOMMENDATIONS

- *Vaccinate healthy children early according to normal schedules:* The response to vaccines appears to be more robust in children than in adults. The majority of pediatric vaccinations are given in the first few years of life and, in most cases, should have been received prior to the onset of the kidney disease. A better immune response after early routine vaccination compared to patients vaccinated after the kidney diagnosis or after initiation of KRT has been shown.[10,23] This stresses the ideal of delivering pediatric vaccines to all at the appropriate time as per the routine country schedule. The latest IAP schedule for pediatric and adolescent vaccinations is given in Kasi et al.[7] In the current COVID-19 pandemic state, the advisory committee on immunizations of IAP recommends that all routine vaccination is continued at the earliest opportunity and provides guidelines for vaccination in COVID-suspected or COVID-positive patients.[24]
- *Catch-up/supplement vaccines at the earliest opportunity in high-risk patients:* Children on dialysis have better seroconversion rates after vaccination than adults on dialysis.[5] If routine vaccines have been missed previously, the earliest opportunity should be used to provide these.[2,3] In addition, patients with kidney disease should receive supplemental vaccines as described in **Table 1**. The underlying kidney disease should be in a stable state at the time of vaccination and ISD should be minimal.
- *In high-risk groups, test vaccine response and provide booster doses as necessary:* In patients with CKD, patients on dialysis, patients receiving ISD, or patients approaching KT, the immunity to previously received vaccines may have waned. The response to fresh vaccination vaccine may be inadequate.[3,5] Thus for high risk VPDs (e.g., HBV and varicella), it is important to check antibody levels and provide boosters as indicated.

- *Avoid live vaccines in IS patients:* In primary immunodeficiencies, LAVs are recommended only in children with ≥500 CD4 cells/μL, ≥200 CD8 cells/μL, and a normal mitogen response or those with CD4 cells/μL ≥25%.[25] Although there are several studies examining the safety of LAV in IS and KT patients,[3] these are under similar stringent preconditions and monitoring, in the absence of which adverse effects may occur, so they are generally to be avoided.
- *Immunize family and close contacts optimally:* The immunization of close contacts and siblings reduces exposure to VPDs. Live vaccines such as MMR and varicella are advised for close contacts; however, vaccinees who develop rash should be isolated from KT patients. Oral polio and rotavirus vaccines are contraindicated as they may be shed in the stool and transmitted to the IS family member. However, if inadvertently received, these family members should be segregated from the index patient.

CONCLUSION

The challenge of a chronic disease tends to veer attention away from the issue of immunization, which is often neglected. The pediatric nephrologist and pediatrician should work in concert to ensure that optimal vaccine protection is given at the times when they are safe and best likely to produce robust response. Patients at particular risk, such as those treated with ISD and on KRT, should ideally be immunized optimally prior to commencement of these therapies. In addition to all routine vaccination, supplemental vaccination with influenza, *Pneumococcus*, *Meningococcus*, HBV, varicella, and HPV vaccine is advised in specific risk groups.

KEY POINTS

- Patients with kidney diseases have increased risk of VPDs and should be immunized optimally against them.
- In addition to all routine vaccines, supplemental immunization with influenza, *Pneumococcus*, hepatitis B, varicella, *Meningococcus*, and HPV vaccines is advised in specific risk groups.
- While all IAVs can be given safely, LAVs are avoided in those on high-dose steroids or other immunosuppressive medications.
- The earliest opportunity to vaccinate should be taken, once the underlying disease is in a stable state. This is particularly important in those approaching KRT when accelerated schedules may be used.
- Vaccine responses may be suboptimal, and protective antibody levels may wane faster than in healthy children; therefore, checking of titers and booster doses are needed to maintain protection.
- Household contacts/siblings should receive standard immunizations including nontransmissible live vaccines.

ACKNOWLEDGMENT

I would like to thank Dr Pallab Chatterjee, Member of Indian Academy of Pediatrics (IAP) Advisory Committee on Vaccines and Immunisation Practices 2018–2019, for reviewing this manuscript and his important suggestions.

REFERENCES

1. Fox TG, Nailescu C. Vaccinations in pediatric kidney transplant recipients. Pediatr Nephrol. 2019;34(4):579-91.
2. Neu AM. Immunizations in children with chronic kidney disease. Pediatr Nephrol. 2012;27(8):1257-63.
3. Esposito S, Mastrolia MV, Prada E, Pietrasanta C, Principi N. Vaccine administration in children with chronic kidney disease. Vaccine. 2014;32(49):6601-6.
4. ACIP. (2020). Altered Immunocompetence Guidelines for Immunizations, November 18. [online] Available from: https://www.cdc.gov/vaccines/hcp/acip-recs/general-recs/immunocompetence.html. [Last accessed March, 2022].
5. Banerjee S, Dissanayake PV, Abeyagunawardena AS. Vaccinations in children on immunosuppressive medications for renal disease. Pediatr Nephrol. 2016;31(9):1437-48.
6. Arora S, Kipp G, Bhanot N, Sureshkumar KK. Vaccinations in kidney transplant recipients: clearing the muddy waters. World J Transplant. 2019;9(1):1-13.
7. Kasi SG, Shivananda S, Marathe S, Pemde HK, Balasubramanian S, Agarwalla S, et al. Indian Academy of Pediatrics (IAP) Advisory Committee on Vaccines and Immunization Practices (ACVIP): Recommended Immunization Schedule (2020-21) and Update on Immunization for Children Aged 0 Through 18 Years. Indian Pediatr. 2021;58(1):44-53.
8. Ulinski T, Leroy S, Dubrel M, Danon S, Bensman A. High serological response to pneumococcal vaccine in nephrotic children at disease onset on high-dose prednisone. Pediatr Nephrol. 2008;23:1107-13.
9. Goonewardene ST, Tang C, Tan LT, Chan KG, Lingham P, Lee LH, et al. Safety and efficacy of pneumococcal vaccination in pediatric nephrotic syndrome. Front Pediatr. 2019;7:339.
10. Mantan M, Pandharikar N, Yadav S, Chakravarti A, Sethi GR. Seroprotection for hepatitis B in children with nephrotic syndrome. Pediatr Nephrol. 2013;28:2125-30.
11. Neupane N, Krishnamurthy S, Jagadisan B, Dhodapkar R. Hepatitis B seroprotection in pediatric nephrotic syndrome. Indian Pediatr. 2019;56(8):659-62.
12. Furth SL, Arbus GS, Hogg R, Tarver J, Chan C, Fivush BA, Southwest Pediatric Nephrology Study Group. Varicella vaccination in children with nephrotic syndrome: a report of the Southwest Pediatric Nephrology Study Group. J Pediatr. 2003;142:145-8.
13. Kamei K, Miyairi I, Ishikura K, Ogura M, Shoji K, Funaki T, et al. Prospective study of live attenuated vaccines for patients with nephrotic syndrome receiving immunosuppressive agents. J Pediatr. 2018;196:217-222.e1.
14. Boyer O, Baudouin V, Bérard É, Biebuyck-Gougé N, Dossier C, Guigonis V, et al. Vaccine recommendations for children with idiopathic nephrotic syndrome. Nephrol Ther. 2020;16(3):177-83.
15. Andrews N, Stowe J, Miller E. Nephrotic syndrome in infants and toddlers before and after introduction of the meningococcal B vaccine programme in England: an ecological study. Vaccine. 2020;38(31):4816-9.

16. Ishimori S, Kamei K, Ando T, Yoshikawa T, Kano Y, Nagata H, et al. Influenza virus vaccination in children with nephrotic syndrome: insignificant risk of relapse. Clin Exp Nephrol. 2020;24(11):1069-76.
17. Battafarano DF, Battafarano NJ, Larsen L, Dyer PD, Older SA, Muehlbauer S, et al. Antigen-specific antibody responses in lupus patients following immunization. Arthritis Rheum 1998;41:1828-34.
18. Liao Z, Tang H, Xu X, Liang Y, Xiong Y, Ni J. Immunogenicity and safety of influenza vaccination in systemic lupus erythematosus patients compared with healthy controls: a meta-analysis. PLoS One. 2016;11(2):e0147856.
19. Rahier JF, Moutschen M, Van Gompel A, Van Ranst M, Louis E, Segaert S, et al. Vaccinations in patients with immune-mediated inflammatory diseases. Rheumatology (Oxford). 2010;49:1815-27.
20. American Academy of Pediatrics. Committee on Infectious Diseases. Red book: report of the Committee on Infectious Diseases, 30th edition. Elk Grove Village, IL: American Academy of Pediatrics; 2015. pp. 38-40.
21. Merhi B, Gohh R. Kidney transplantation and COVID-19. R I Med J. 2020;103(8):34-37.
22. Marlais M, Wlodkowski T, Al-Akash S, Ananin P, Bandi VK, Baudouin V, et al. COVID-19 in children treated with immunosuppressive medication for kidney diseases. Arch Dis Child. 2020;106:798-801.
23. Sheth RD, Peskin MF, Du XL. The duration of hepatitis B vaccine immunity in pediatric dialysis patients. Pediatr Nephrol. 2014;29(10):2029-37.
24. Kasi SG, Dhir SK, Verma S, Pemde HK, Balasubramanian S, Agarwalla S, et al.; Advisory Committee on Vaccines and Immunization Practices (ACVIP), 2020-21, Indian Academy of Pediatrics, India. Immunization During the COVID-19 Pandemic: Recommendations from Indian Academy of Pediatrics Advisory Committee on Vaccines and Immunization Practices. Indian Pediatr. 2020;57(12):1147-52.
25. Principi N, Esposito S. Vaccine use in primary immunodeficiency disorders. Vaccine. 2014;32:3725-31.

CHAPTER

14.2 Nephropharmacology

Jyoti Singhal, Jyoti Sharma

INTRODUCTION

Nephropharmacology deals with pharmacologic considerations in kidney disease, including estimation of kidney function for drug dosing, safety principles of medication, and common drug nephrotoxicities.

There is limited data on drug therapy in general, in the pediatric age group, and more so in children with kidney disorders. Appropriate drug-dose modifications need to be made in patients with kidney diseases, to avoid underdosing as well as drug toxicity as these can affect patient outcomes in terms of increased morbidity, prolonged hospital admissions, and, sometimes, death. This is feasible based on information of pharmacokinetics and pharmacodynamics of drugs since this information is helpful in predicting actions of drugs as well as in a rational application and modification of their doses.

PHARMACOKINETICS

Pharmacokinetics: It refers to alteration of the drug by the body and can be divided into *a*bsorption, *d*istribution, *m*etabolism, and *e*xcretion (*acronym*: ADME) **(Fig. 1)**. Presence of renal disease can affect these processes altering the therapeutic effects of drugs in these patients.

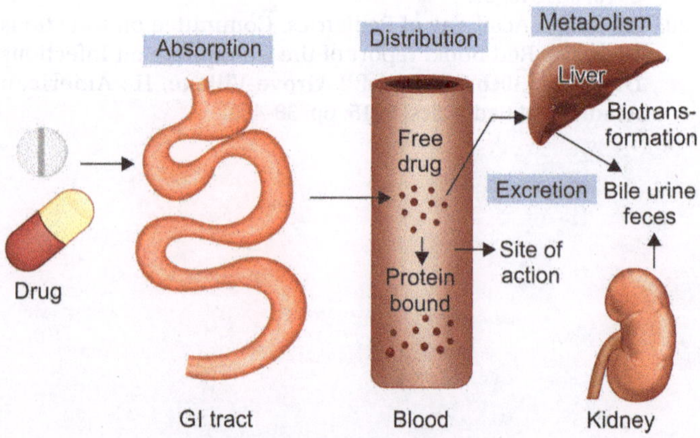

Fig. 1: Pharmacokinetics processes.

Absorption

Bioavailability is the rate and the extent of drug absorption from a particular dosage formulation. For a drug administered intravenously, bioavailability is 100% except for some drugs that are administered as prodrugs, e.g., fosphenytoin. For those administered orally, it can be calculated based on the area under the curve.

The total drug exposure of tissues across time is expressed **(Fig. 2)** in the form of maximum concentration in plasma (C_{max}) and/or the area under the concentration–time curve (AUC). This profile can be optimized in children with renal disorders once we understand the pharmacokinetics of the drug.

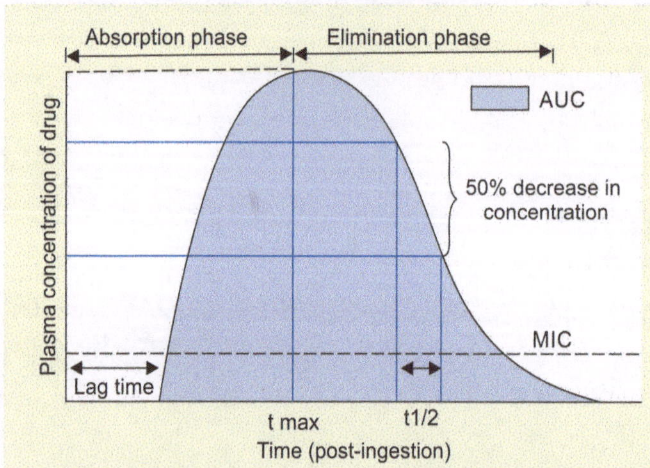

Fig. 2: Concentration time curve of a drug. (AUC: area under curve; MIC: minimum inhibitory concentration)

Drugs that are taken per oral are absorbed across the intestinal epithelium and some of them undergo a first-pass metabolism in the liver or intestinal epithelia cells before reaching the systemic circulation and onward to excretion. In children with renal disease, bioavailability of an orally administered drug can be affected in different ways:

- *Altered gastric pH:* In uremic patients, high urea gets converted to ammonia by gastric urease. The ammonia buffers the gastric acid and increases the gastric pH. This alkaline pH decreases absorption of drugs such as iron salts and ketoconazole.[1]
- *Edema of gastrointestinal (GI) tract:* Decreases absorption usually; may increase in some cases, if the expression of P-glycoprotein is decreased or this efflux transporter has reduced function.
- *Delayed gastric emptying time:* Decreases drug absorption
- *Impaired gut mucosal integrity:* Increases absorption
- Drug interaction, e.g., oral iron absorption may be inhibited by concomitant use of H_2 receptor blockers

(antacids) or calcium-containing phosphate binders in children with chronic kidney disease (CKD).

Distribution

After drugs enter the systemic circulation, most of them get distributed to tissues, organs, and other fluid spaces. The plasma concentration of a drug is dependent on the total amount of drug absorbed and its volume of distribution (V_d). This V_d can be calculated by formula:

$$V_d \text{ (liters/kg)} = \frac{\text{Concentration of drug in body}}{\text{Concentration of drug in plasma}}$$

During dialysis, knowledge about the V_d of a drug provides some understanding about the amount of drug that is likely to be removed during a session of hemodialysis (HD). For example, drugs that have a high V_d because of extensive tissue binding (e.g., digoxin and tricyclic antidepressants) will not be dialyzed easily, thereby leading to inadequate removal from the body. Many patient and drug factors affect V_d **(Table 1)**.[2-4]

When the usual dose of a drug is used in a patient with a high V_d, e.g., in a patient with sepsis or with nephrotic syndrome, in whom there is an increased interstitial fluid accumulation, the concentration of the drug in plasma is inadequate. In these patients, and where achieving a minimum inhibitory concentration is essential, a *loading dose* of the drug is utilized to achieve the desired plasma level quickly.

Protein Binding

Albumin and α_1-acid glycoprotein (AAG) are the predominant proteins in plasma which bind acidic drugs (e.g., penicillins, cephalosporins, furosemide, and phenytoin), and alkaline drugs respectively and transport them to their site of action. Patients who have proteinuric illness and those who have poor nutrition secondary to chronic kidney disease have low serum albumin. Additionally, in patients with CKD, the ability of proteins to binds to drugs also decreases. This results in an increase in the V_d of the alkaline drugs and a decrease in their availability at the site of action. When levels of organic acids, e.g., hippuric acid, indoxyl sulfate, and 3-carboxy-4-methyl-5-propyl-2-furanpropionic acid (CMPF), are increased in patients with advanced CKD, they compete with acidic drugs in binding to proteins.[5] In some situations, this may result in an increased concentration of the active drug in the extravascular tissues and places the patient at risk of toxicity.

TABLE 1: Factors affecting volume of distribution.

Patient	
Factors	***Effect***
Age	*Neonates*: 70–80% of body weight is water *Children*: 60% of body weight *(High V_d in neonates as compared to older children)*
Obesity	Increased fat mass increases V_d
Disease state	
CKD/AKI Hypoalbuminemia Fluid overload	Increased V_d
Dehydration Muscle wasting	Decreased V_d
Drug	
Protein binding	Highly protein-bound drug: Decreased V_d
Hydrophilic drug	Decreased V_d as confined to intravascular space
Lipophilic drug	Increased V_d as diffuses into tissues

(AKI: acute kidney injury; CKD: chronic kidney disease; V_d: volume of distribution)

Metabolism (Biotransformation)

It is an important mechanism for drug elimination and the primary site is liver, others being kidney, intestine, lungs, and plasma. The processes of metabolism are oxidation, hydrolysis, reduction, conjugation, etc., which may either form an inactive metabolite, convert an inactive drug to active compound or form active metabolite from an active drug. Impaired renal function can modify these processes, thereby affecting drug elimination.[5] Many of the active metabolic by products of drugs [e.g., angiotensin-converting enzyme (ACE) inhibitors, β-blockers, azathioprine, cephalosporins, metronidazole, etc.] are removed from the body by the kidneys, so in the face of deteriorating renal function, they can accumulate and have adverse effects when the kidney function decreases. Cytochrome P450 enzymes (CYP enzymes) are essential for the metabolism of many drugs. The activity of CYP enzymes and drug transporters can also be inhibited by uremic toxins.[6]

Excretion

Drug clearance is defined as the volume of plasma that is entirely cleared of the drug in unit time. Drugs are removed from the body through renal, biliary, salivary, mammary, sweat, lung, and intestinal pathways. Many uptake and efflux transporters in liver, intestine, and renal tubules are responsible for the disposition of drugs **(Figs. 3A to C)**. Kidneys are generally the most important in drug elimination so drug clearance can get affected in children with poor renal function.

Nonrenal Clearance

Both chronic kidney disease and acute kidney injury (AKI) are known to decrease nonrenal clearance as well. As mentioned earlier, this may happen because the activity of certain enzymes and transporters (e.g., hepatic drug metabolism by CYP450 and transporter-mediated biliary drug clearance) may be suppressed by uremic toxins that accumulates in these patients.[7,8]

Renal Clearance (L/h or mL/min)

It is the combined effect of glomerular filtration, tubular secretion, and tubular reabsorption.

- *Glomerular filtration:* Certain drugs and drug metabolites are primarily eliminated by glomerular filtration. The rate of their elimination equals the creatinine clearance or the glomerular filtration rate (GFR). As the GFR decreases, these drugs will accumulate if drug doses are not appropriately

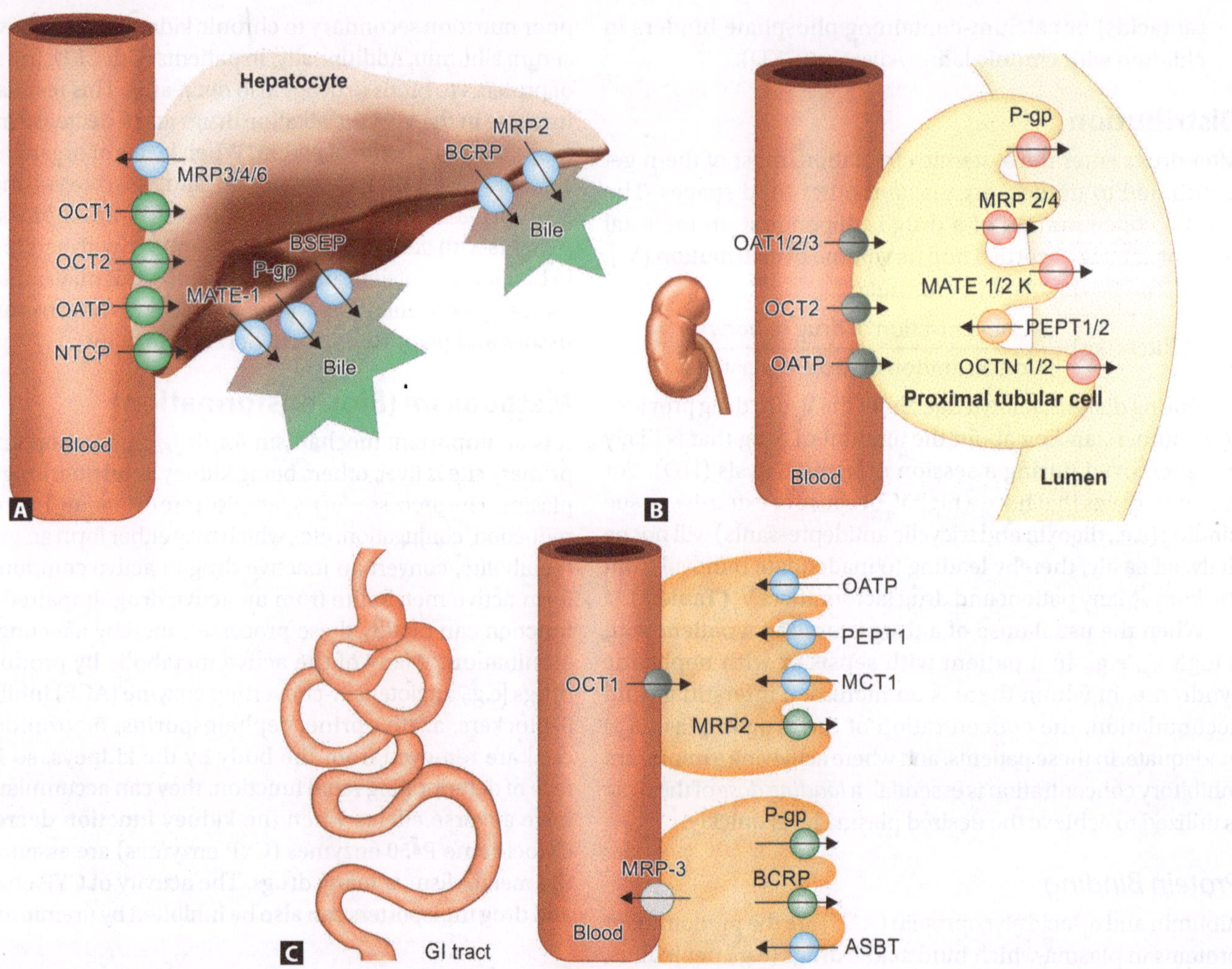

Figs. 3A to C: Uptake and efflux transporters involved in drug disposition. (A) Liver; (B) Renal tubules; (C) Intestine. (OCT: organic cation transporter; OCTN-2: organic cation/carnitine transporter 2; OAT: organic anion transporter; OATP: organic anion transporting polypeptide; BCRP: breast cancer resistant protein; BSEP: bile salt export pump; MATE-1: multidrug and toxin extrusion proteins; MRP: multidrug-resistant protein; NTCP: sodium taurocholate co-transporting polypeptide; P-gp: P-glycoprotein; PEPT: oligopeptide transporter; MCT: monocarboxylate transporter; ASBT: apical sodium-dependent bile acid transporter)

adjusted. The glomerular filtration of drugs depends on their molecular size and protein binding. Although the filtration of a protein-bound drug decreases with a decline in GFR, the amount secreted by the renal tubule may be relatively increased and must be accounted for.

- *Tubular secretion*: Some drugs and drug metabolites are secreted by relatively nonspecific anionic and cationic transport systems in the proximal tubule **(Fig. 3B)**, and this contributes to renal clearance. This is the more significant mode of elimination for certain drugs such as metformin, meropenem, amoxycillin, and cephalexin. These drugs require a larger reduction in the dose in patients with tubular injury as compared to those with a similar GFR due to a primary glomerular injury.

  Competition may occur between simultaneously administered drugs, which are substrates of these transporters, e.g., probenecid inhibits secretion of penicillin by the tubules. Creatinine secretion can be inhibited by triamterene, spironolactone, amiloride, and trimethoprim, causing increase in its blood levels.

  In patients with CKD, organic acids accumulate and compete with acidic drugs (e.g., methotrexate, sulfonylureas, penicillins, and cephalosporins) at OAT1 and OAT3 for tubular transport and secretion into the urinary space. Appropriately lower doses, adjusted to the kidney function, should be used so that excess plasma levels and adverse reactions can be avoided.

- *Tubular reabsorption:* Reabsorption of a drug depends on its pKa (or how acidic it is) and urine pH. Basic urine (urine pH > 7.5) will increase reabsorption of basic drugs as it favors nonionized form and vice versa. This can be clinically utilized in cases of barbiturate and salicylate poisoning when urine alkalinization can enhance their excretion.

DRUG DOSING IN CHRONIC KIDNEY DISEASE

Drug dosing in CKD can be modified by aiming at a therapeutic target or depending on the severity of renal dysfunction.

Based on a Therapeutic Target

- This can be achieved by therapeutic drug monitoring (TDM), especially for those with a *narrow therapeutic index,* such as the aminoglycosides or vancomycin.
- Measuring the clinical effect, e.g., dose of oral hypoglycemic agents, can be titrated to target blood glucose concentration as well as the effect on hemoglobin A1c.

For some drugs, it would be rational to begin prescribing a dosage regimen so as to aim at achieving the mean or median drug concentration that has been found effective in clinical trials.[9]

Based on the Severity of Renal Dysfunction and Amount of Drug Cleared

Dose adjustment for a particular drug is usually not required when <30% of the administered dose is eliminated by the kidneys.[10] As kidney function decreases and hence drug clearance is reduced, drug toxicity has to be prevented by either decreasing the maintenance dose or increasing the interval between doses.[9]

The maintenance dose is the dose required to achieve the target plasma concentration of a drug at a steady state and is determined by its clearance rate.[10]

$$\text{Dose} \times \text{F/interval} = \text{Concentration (steady state)} \times \text{Clearance (F = bioavailability)}$$

Drug toxicity can be avoided in children with impaired clearance by dose modifications in the form of either increasing the dosing interval or decreasing the dose administered. For drugs whose clearance *only* is affected by diminished renal function while protein binding, distribution, and metabolism remaining unchanged, a dosing adjustment factor *Q* can be estimated using the following equation:

$$Q = \frac{1 - [\text{Fractional renal elimination} \times (1 - \text{Child's creatinine clearance})]}{\text{Normal creatinine clearance}}$$

Adjusted drug dose = Q × Normal dose

Adjusted dosing interval = Normal dosing interval + Q

This factor accounts for the change occurring in patients with decreased renal function but not for any additional clearance by dialysis.

In general, *increasing the dosing interval* will be helpful for drugs with a long half-life and a broad therapeutic index, whose effects are concentration dependent (e.g., aminoglycosides), as it will increase the variation between peak and trough blood concentration. In contrast, decreasing the dosing amount would be required for drugs with a short half-life and requiring a relatively stable blood concentration, such as cephalosporins or antihypertensives.

Loading dose: It is needed for drugs to achieve a steady-state concentration rapidly and in condition with increased V_d (nephrotic syndrome and sepsis), so decreased renal clearance does not affect the dose.

For practical purposes, drug doses in renal failure can be adjusted according to the references available as described under the last section of this book.

DRUG DOSING IN CHILDREN WITH ACUTE KIDNEY INJURY

Children with AKI are usually critically ill. As V_d is usually increased, the initial dose should be increased and administered as a loading dose to achieve a prompt response, especially for hydrophilic antibiotics, such as penicillins.[9] AKI reduces renal clearance of a drug, so the maintenance dose needs to be decreased. In these patients, there occurs a wide variation in the clearance and distribution of the drug over hours or days and it is practically difficult to assess GFR accurately. Thus, formulation of the correct approach to drug dosing in children with AKI is a challenge. Critically ill children with AKI also have altered bowel, hepatic, and kidney perfusion, thereby affecting drug absorption and elimination.

Therapeutic Drug Monitoring

Therapeutic drug monitoring overcomes interindividual variation in pharmacokinetics and helps in individualizing drug dosing in each patient. Where facilities are available, drug levels should be monitored to check for attainment of the therapeutic levels and avoid nephrotoxicity. This becomes especially important in conditions when it is difficult to measure the therapeutic endpoint, for example in patients with a seizure disorder, to document the nonoccurrence of epileptic seizures. TDM is now an accepted standard of care especially to assess the appropriate dosing of antibiotics.[11]

IMPACT OF DIALYSIS

Hemodialysis

Drug removal is considered clinically significant when >25% of the administered dose is removed by HD.[12] Various drug characteristics and factors associated with dialysis determine its dialyzability **(Table 2)**. The usual maintenance dose of a drug should be administered after the dialysis session. In children on maintenance HD, it is recommended that a supplemental dose of a drug (partial or entire dose) is administered after the HD session in order to restore the amount which was removed by dialysis. For antibiotics with concentration-dependent killing (e.g., aminoglycosides and fluoroquinolones), a large dose (2–2.5 times the normal dose) can be given predialysis for achieving maximum concentration and clearance by dialysis prevents toxic effects.[9]

Peritoneal Dialysis

Peritoneal dialysis (PD) is less efficient in drug removal than HD. As the dialysate may remove many antibiotics at a low rate when administered intraperitoneally, it helps in the adequate treatment of peritonitis. If a drug is known to be removed via PD, an increase in the dosing amount or frequency would be recommended. Patients on PD usually retain residual kidney function for a longer duration than patients on HD. Therefore, it is recommended that drug dosing in children can be adapted from the dosing recommendations for patients with estimated glomerular filtration rate (eGFR) <15 mL/min.[13]

TABLE 2: Factors determining dialyzability of a drug.

	Characteristic	Effect
Drug related	Molecular weight	*>500 Dalton:* Not dialyzed
	Protein binding	*>90% bound:* Not dialyzed
	Small V_d (<0.7 L/kg)	Easily dialyzable
Factors associated with hemodialysis	Blood flow rate (Qb)	Increased removal of low molecular weight drugs can be achieved by increasing Qb, Qd, and by using dialyzer with a larger surface area
	Dialysate flow rate (Qd)	
	Dialyzer surface area	
	High flux membrane	Can remove drugs with molecular weight of up to 40,000 Da by convection (e.g., vancomycin, carbamazepine, cisplatin, and daptomycin)

TABLE 3: Examples of drugs causing acute kidney injury (AKI).

Type of AKI	Pathophysiology	Drugs
Prerenal	Afferent arteriole vasoconstriction	• Calcineurin inhibitors (cyclosporin and tacrolimus) • Vasopressors • Osmotic radiocontrast dyes
	Altered intraglomerular renal perfusion	• ACE inhibitors • Angiotensin receptor blockers • NSAIDs
Renal	Direct tubular cell injury (Acute tubular necrosis) Usually, dose dependent	• Aminoglycosides • Cidofovir • Amphotericin • Quinolones
	Endothelial injury (producing picture like thrombotic microangiopathy)	• Calcineurin inhibitors (tacrolimus cyclosporine) • Clopidogrel • Interferon
	Acute tubulointerstitial nephritis (immunologically mediated, dose independent)	• Penicillin • Sulfonamides • Thiazides • NSAIDs • Pantoprazole/ omeprazole • Ciprofloxacin
	Intratubular obstruction (crystalluria)	• Acyclovir • Methotrexate • Triamterene • Indinavir • Foscarnet

(ACE: angiotensin-converting enzyme; NSAIDs: nonsteroidal anti-inflammatory drugs)

Continuous Kidney Replacement Therapy

Continuous kidney replacement therapy (CKRT) is performed in the pediatric critical care setting for AKI and sepsis. Drug removal by CKRT is mainly affected by the V_d of the drug. Clearance of a drug can be increased by diffusion in CKRT by increasing the dialysate flow rate and through convection by increasing the ultrafiltration rate. For any given blood flow rate, drug clearance of CKRT modalities decreases in the following order: CVVHF (continuous venovenous hemofiltration; mostly convective clearance) > CVVHDF (continuous venovenous hemodiafiltration; combination of diffusive and convective clearance), > CVVHD (continuous venovenous HD CVVHD; mostly diffusive clearance).[3]

If the drug clearance by CKRT is <25% of the total body clearance by other routes, dosing adjustment for CKRT is usually not required. Otherwise, a typical initial loading dose would be given, and maintenance doses would be similar to those given to a patient with a creatinine clearance of 30–50 mL/min/1.73 m^2. Apart from this, other factors related to this mode of dialysis, as discussed before, need to be considered while prescribing drugs.[5]

Of the three modes of dialysis, HD has the greatest efficacy for drug removal and PD is least efficacious, though the total amount of drug removal may be similar because CKRT and PD are continuous modes performed over a longer period.

NEPHROTOXICITY

Drug-induced nephrotoxicity may present as mild kidney injury or, at the other end of the spectrum, with severe injury. Early recognition and removal of the offending drug can reverse the injury.

Nephrotoxicity can present clinically as:

- Acute kidney injury
- Glomerular dysfunction
- Tubular dysfunction
- Electrolyte imbalance
- Chronic renal injury

Some commonly used drugs and their nephrotoxicity are mentioned in the following examples:[3,14]

- *Acute kidney injury:* Various drugs can lead to either pre-renal or intrinsic renal AKI **(Table 3)** and close monitoring is required as the renal failure may be nonoliguric and be missed.
- *Glomerular dysfunction:* Drugs such as penicillamine, gold, nonsteroidal anti-inflammatory drug (NSAID), and captopril can cause nephrotic syndrome. The most common form is membranous nephropathy.
- *Tubular dysfunction:*
    - *Proximal tubule:* Fanconi-like syndrome can occur because of drugs such as amphotericin B, calcineurin inhibitors, cisplatin, methotrexate, and pentamidine.
    - *Distal tubule:* Drugs such as lithium, foscarnet, ifosfamide, and amphotericin B can cause distal tubular acidosis. Lithium, demeclocycline, vincristine, and foscarnet can sometimes lead to nephrogenic diabetes insipidus.

- *Electrolyte imbalance:*
  - *Excessive use of diuretics:* Hyponatremia and hypokalemia
  - NSAID, potassium-sparing diuretics, ACE inhibitors, β-blockers, and calcineurin inhibitors: Hyperkalemia
  - *Amphotericin B:* Potassium and magnesium loss
- *Chronic renal injury:*
  - *Chronic interstitial fibrosis:* NSAIDs, aspirin, lithium, acyclovir, and calcineurin inhibitors
  - *Ureteral obstruction secondary to retroperitoneal fibrosis:* Methyldopa, hydralazine, atenolol, and methysergide

PREVENTION AND MANAGEMENT OF NEPHROTOXICITY

Avoid using nephrotoxic drugs when alternatives are available, especially in high-risk conditions, such as critically ill children, high-risk surgical patients, chronic kidney disease, and sepsis.[3]

Examples:

- Using lipid formulation of amphotericin B instead of conventional formulation.
- Aztreonam can be used instead of aminoglycosides in children and low-birth-weight infants with gram-negative infections.
- In cephalosporin group, ceftazidime is the safest to use in children with reduced renal function.
- Pretreatment hydration can help in reducing nephrotoxicity of drugs such as amphotericin B, NSAIDs, aminoglycosides, and radiocontrast agents. Care should be taken to avoid fluid overload at the same time.
- Always ensure correct dosing adjusted eGFR and wherever possible utilize TDM (e.g., vancomycin and aminoglycosides).
- Avoid using concomitant nephrotoxic drugs (e.g., avoid using ACE inhibitor and diuretics together) and limit the duration of treatment to as short as feasible.
- Monitor renal function closely while the child is on nephrotoxic medications to detect early damage and prevent its progression by timely omission of the drug.
- Modify drug doses and intervals in children with low GFR.

CONCLUSION

It is of utmost importance to apply the knowledge of pharmacokinetics and pharmacodynamics when using drugs in children with kidney diseases. This serves a dual purpose of achieving therapeutic targets and avoiding nephrotoxicity.

KEY POINTS

- Alteration in processes of drug absorption, distribution, and metabolism in the liver, gut, and kidneys can occur in patients suffering from chronic kidney disease.
- Improper modifications in drug doses may lead to sub- or supratherapeutic concentrations in plasma, thereby causing either a therapeutic failure or adverse drug reactions.
- Drug dosing can be optimized after being familiar with the fundamental concepts of pharmacokinetics and therapeutic drug monitoring, especially for drugs with a narrow therapeutic index.
- While prescribing nephrotoxic drugs, always consider an alternative, limit the duration of therapy, closely monitor renal function, avoid concomitant use of two or more nephrotoxic drugs, and stop the drug(s) at the earliest sign of renal injury.

REFERENCES

1. Tett SE, Kirkpatrick CMJ, Gross AS, McLachlan AJ. Principles and clinical application of assessing alterations in renal elimination pathways. Clin Pharmacokinet. 2003;42(14):1193-211.
2. Filler G, Kirpalani A, Urquhart B. Handling of drugs in children with abnormal renal function. In: Avner ED, Harmon WE, Niaudet P, Yoshikawa N, Emma F, Goldstein SL (Eds). Pediatric Nephrology, 7th edition. Berlin: Springer; 2015. pp. 2268-90.
3. Schwab M, Billing H, Morike K. Drug use, dosing, and toxicity in renal disease. In: Geary DF, Schaefer F (Eds). Pediatric Kidney Disease, 2nd edition. New York: Springer; 2017. pp. 1927-47.
4. Perazella MA, Parikh C. Pharmacology. Am J Kidney Dis. 2005;46(6):1129-39.
5. McIntyre C, Shaw S, Eldehni M. Prescribing drugs in kidney disease. In: Taal MW, Brenner B, Chertow G, Marsden P, Skorecki K, Y ASU (Eds). Brenner and Rector's The Kidney, 9th edition. Philadelphia, PA: Elsevier Health Sciences; 2011. pp. 2258-91.
6. Jansen J, Jankowski J, Gajjala PR, Wetzels JFM, Masereeuw R. Disposition and clinical implications of protein-bound uremic toxins. Clin Sci (Lond). 2017;131(14):1631-47.
7. Naud J, Michaud J, Leblond FA, Lefrancois S, Bonnardeaux A, Pichette V. Effects of chronic renal failure on liver drug transporters. Drug Metab Dispos Biol Fate Chem. 2008;36(1): 124-8.
8. Yeung CK, Shen DD, Thummel KE, Himmelfarb J. Effects of chronic kidney disease and uremia on hepatic drug metabolism and transport. Kidney Int. 2014;85(3):522-8.
9. Roberts DM, Sevastos J, Carland JE, Stocker SL, Lea-Henry TN. Clinical pharmacokinetics in kidney disease: application to rational design of dosing regimens. Clin J Am Soc Nephrol. 2018;13(8):1254-63.
10. Lea-Henry TN, Carland JE, Stocker SL, Sevastos J, Roberts DM. Clinical pharmacokinetics in kidney disease: fundamental principles. Clin J Am Soc Nephrol. 2018;13(7):1085-95.
11. Schuts EC, Hulscher MEJL, Mouton JW, Verduin CM, Stuart JWTC, Overdiek HWPM, et al. Current evidence on hospital antimicrobial stewardship objectives: a systematic review and meta-analysis. Lancet Infect Dis. 2016;16(7):847-56.
12. Levy G. Pharmacokinetics in renal disease. Am J Med. 1977;62(4):461-5.
13. Matzke GR, Aronoff GR, Atkinson AJ, Bennett WM, Decker BS, Eckardt K-U, et al. Drug dosing consideration in patients with acute and chronic kidney disease—a clinical update from Kidney Disease: Improving Global Outcomes (KDIGO). Kidney Int. 2011;80(11):1122-37.
14. Choudhury D, Ahmed Z. Drug-associated renal dysfunction and injury. Nat Clin Pract Nephrol. 2006;2(2):80-91.

CHAPTER

14.3 Vitamin D in Health and Disease

Indira Agarwal

INTRODUCTION

Vitamin D is a fat-soluble prohormone discovered from the antirachitic effect of cod liver oil in the early part of the 20th century. It is an essential micronutrient that has generated great interest in recent years due to recognition of its nonskeletal functions. Vitamin D deficiency is relatively common in the healthy population and almost 1 billion people worldwide are estimated to be vitamin D deficient. The role of vitamin D in skeletal and nonskeletal biological function in both normal healthy individuals and those with chronic diseases such as chronic kidney disease (CKD), cystic fibrosis, and Crohn disease has been reanalyzed.[1,2]

NORMAL PHYSIOLOGY OF VITAMIN D

Sources of Vitamin

Vitamin D is a secosteroid, which can be either endogenously synthesized in skin or ingested from both plant and animal food sources. Vitamin D_2 (ergocalciferol) and vitamin D_3 (cholecalciferol) are from plant and animal sources, respectively, and differ in a double bond between C22 and C23 and a methyl group on C24. The function or metabolism is not affected by this minor structural difference and both forms are handled similarly by the body. These two forms of vitamin D have equivalent bioefficiency, although there is a suggestion that cholecalciferol may be more potent in raising and maintaining serum 25-hydroxyvitamin D, i.e., 25(OH)D, concentrations compared with ergocalciferol. During exposure to solar ultraviolet B radiation (290–315 nm), 7-dehydrocholesterol in the skin is converted to previtamin D_3, which then undergoes isomerization to form vitamin D_3. Exposure of face, arms, and legs for 5–30 minutes (depending on time of day, season, latitude, and skin pigmentation) between the hours of 10 AM and 3 PM twice a week is often adequate to synthesize vitamin D. The cutaneous production of vitamin D is affected by the melanin level of the skin, age, latitude, time of the day, and season. Melanin competes with 7-dehydrocholesterol for the ultraviolet B light, and thus people with darker skin pigment require longer exposure to sunlight to make an equivalent amount of vitamin D compared to light-skinned individuals. Older adults make almost 30% less vitamin D compared to young adults when exposed to the same sunlight. Casual exposure to the sunlight in spring and summer provides 80–100% of vitamin D, which is stored in fat to be used in winter. Children and adults who always wear sun protection or apply sunscreen are at risk of vitamin D deficiency.[3]

The new recommendations from the Institute of Medicine (IOM) for Dietary Reference Intakes (DRIs) for vitamin D in infants are 400 units (10 µg) per day and in children are 600 units (15 µg) per day.[4]

25(OH)D is the major circulating form of vitamin D and is used to determine vitamin D status. The earlier cutoffs for sufficiency, insufficiency, mild deficiency, and severe deficiency were >30, 16–30, 5–15, and <5 ng/mL, respectively, but the IOM 2011 report has changed these cutoffs to more than 20, 12–20, 8–12, and <8 ng/mL, respectively. The skeletal and nonskeletal physiological functions of vitamin D may have different cutoffs for sufficiency, insufficiency, and deficiency.[5]

ACTIVATION OF VITAMIN D

Vitamin D from the skin or gastrointestinal tract enters the circulation, where it is bound to vitamin D-binding protein (DBP) for transport to the liver. In the liver, one or more of cytochrome P450 enzyme (CYP27A1, CYP3A4, CYP2R1, and CYP2J3) vitamin D25-hydroxylase adds a hydroxyl group on carbon 25 to form 25(OH)D. There is a high affinity and low capacity enzyme in the microsome and low affinity and high capacity in the mitochondria. The enzymatic step of 25-hydroxylation is not tightly regulated and is not under a negative or positive feedback loop. It is substrate dependent and thus serum levels of 25(OH)D reflect nutritional status. Serum 25(OH)D has a half-life of 3–4 weeks. Its catabolism is enhanced by antiseizure medications, glucocorticoids, and rifampicin that may further contribute to vitamin D deficiency.

25(OH)D is then transported to the kidney bound to vitamin D-binding protein where it is freely filtered. It is then transported into the proximal renal tubule cells by megalin protein, which is critical for reuptake of low molecular weight proteins (e.g., DBP bound to 25-OHD) from the ultrafiltrate. This step is relevant in children with Donnai–Barrow syndrome and Dent disease, where the megalin-mediated transport is disrupted due to mutation in the *LRP2* and *CLCN5* genes, respectively. The mitochondrial P450 enzyme

25(OH)D-1α-hydroxylase (CYP27B1) adds a hydroxyl group to C1 to form the active metabolite, 1,25(OH)D. The enzyme 25(OH)D-1α-hydroxylase is present in a wide variety of tissues, e.g., macrophages, osteoblasts, keratinocytes, prostate, and breast, where $1,25(OH)_2D$ is also produced. The extrarenal enzyme does not contribute significantly to the serum level and has an important role in the nonskeletal functions of $1,25(OH)_2D$ such as cell growth, apoptosis, angiogenesis, and regulation of the immune system. This is relevant in diseases such as chronic granulomatous disease, sarcoidosis, malignancy, subcutaneous fat necrosis, where excessive synthesis contributes to hypercalcemia. Excess $1,25(OH)_2D$ inhibits 25(OH)D-1α-hydroxylase and stimulates 25(OH)D-24-hydroxylase (CYP24), which results in the formation of inactive water-soluble calcitroic acid **(Fig. 1)**. This enzymatic activity is tightly regulated by parathyroid hormone (PTH), calcitonin, fibroblast growth factor-23 (FGF23), calcium, phosphorus, and $1,25(OH)_2D$. The regulation of functional vitamin D is complex given interplay between organs, namely parathyroid gland, gastrointestinal tract, bone, and kidney, which is further orchestrated by multiple hormones. 25(OH)D-1α-hydroxylase enzyme activity is upregulated by low serum phosphorus, PTH, and calcitonin and is inhibited by FGF23 and $1,25(OH)_2D$.[6]

Vitamin D-binding Receptor

The biological actions of $1,25(OH)_2D$ are mediated by vitamin D receptor (VDR), a member of the steroid-thyroid-retinoid receptor gene superfamily of nuclear transcription factors. The VDR is composed of an N-terminal DNA-binding domain that mediates binding and specificity of VDR–DNA interactions and a C-terminal ligand-binding domain that binds to $1,25(OH)_2D$. The ligand-binding site also contains the binding sites for coactivator and corepressor proteins. The VDR heterodimerizes with the retinoid X receptor (RXR) and the complex then binds to vitamin D response elements (VDREs) in target gene promoters. Mutations have been identified in the VDR that disrupts ligand binding, DNA binding, RXR heterodimerization and co-activator binding.

CALCIUM AND PHOSPHORUS REGULATION IN THE GASTROINTESTINAL TRACT, KIDNEY, AND BONE

Calcium absorption in the gastrointestinal tract is a sum of two transport processes, a saturable transcellular absorption that is physiologically regulated by vitamin D and a nonsaturable

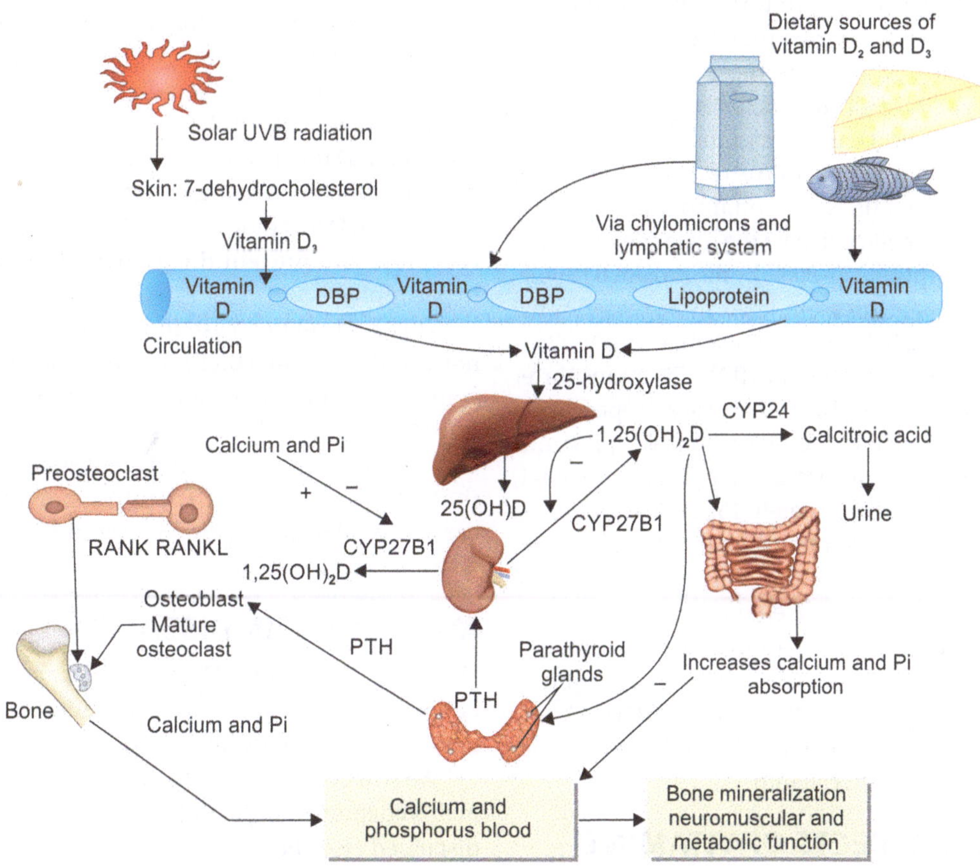

Fig. 1: The production, metabolism, and biologic effects of vitamin D. Vitamin D is produced in the skin by exposure to sunlight or is ingested in the diet. Vitamin D (D_2 and D_3) is converted by the vitamin D25-hydroxylase (CYP27A1, CYP3A4, CYP2R1, and CYP2J3) in the liver to 25(OH)D. 25(OH)D is converted in the kidneys by CYP27B1 to $1,25(OH)_2D$. $1,25(OH)_2D$ enhances intestinal calcium and phosphorus absorption and stimulates the expression of RANKL on the osteoblasts to interact with its receptor RANK on preosteoclasts to induce differentiation into mature osteoclasts, which release calcium and phosphorus into serum. In addition, $1,25(OH)_2D$ inhibits the renal CYP27B1 and stimulates the expression of the renal 25(OH)D-24-hydroxylase (CYP24). The induction of CYP24 results in metabolism of $1,25(OH)_2D$ into a water-soluble inactive metabolite calcitroic acid. (DBP: D-binding protein; PTH: parathyroid hormone; UVB: ultraviolet B)

paracellular absorption that is dependent on the calcium concentration within the lumen. The nonsaturable paracellular pathway is thought to predominate when the diet is replete in calcium, while the saturable vitamin D-dependent transcellular pathway becomes critical when the dietary calcium is limited. In contrast to intestine, calcium transport in the distal tubule is regulated by both PTH and $1,25(OH)_2D$. The active transcellular absorption is mediated by epithelial calcium channels' transient receptor potential TRPV5 (epithelial Ca channel: ECaCl) and TRPV6 (CaT1 or ECaC2), which are under the regulation of $1,25(OH)_2D$. TRPV5 and TRPV6 are coexpressed in the intestine and kidney. TRPV6 is the major calcium channel in the intestine. TRPV6 is expressed from the esophagus down to the jejunum, while TRPV5 is restricted to the duodenum and jejunum. In contrast TRPV5 is abundantly expressed in the renal distal convoluted duct and connecting tubule, while limited expression of TRPV6 is observed in these tubular segments. TRPV5 and TRPV6 colocalize with calbindin D, Na^+/Ca^{2+} exchanger and Ca^{2+}-ATPase. Calbindin D acts as the principal calcium shuttle from the apical to the basolateral surface. The subsequent basolateral calcium transport occurs via both Na^+/Ca^{2+} and Ca^{2+}-ATPase, which are estimated to transport 70% and 30% of calcium, respectively. There are three types of sodium-phosphate (Na/Pi) cotransporter that are present in the renal proximal tubule (type I, type IIa, and type III Na/Pi cotransporters). Type I Na/Pi cotransporter is not regulated under normal physiological conditions and is not believed to be a major determinant of phosphorus reabsorption by the proximal tubule. The type IIa Na/Pi cotransporter (Npt2a) is highly expressed and is believed to be the major determinant of phosphorus reabsorption (70–80%) by the proximal tubule. Absence of renal Npt2a expression leads to increased renal phosphate loss resulting in hypophosphatemia. The Npt2a is inhibited by PTH and FGF23. The type III Na/Pi cotransporter (Glvr-1 and Ram-1) is expressed at the basolateral aspect of the proximal tubule and is believed to play a housekeeping role. In maintaining cellular Pi concentration, Npt1, Npt2, Glvr-1, and Ram-1 account for approximately 15, 84, 0.5, and 0.5%, respectively, of the total Na^+/Pi cotransporter mRNA in kidney.

The effect of $1,25(OH)_2D$ on the bone depends on the calcium intake. $1,25(OH)_2D$, while eating a normal-calcium diet in healthy subjects, leads to an increase in intestinal calcium absorption and an increase in urinary calcium excretion. On a calcium-restricted diet, $1,25(OH)_2D$ acts on osteoblasts to induce osteoclast formation and bone resorption to maintain serum calcium.

EXTRARENAL EFFECTS OF VITAMIN D

Vitamin D has pleiotropic effects on the immune, cardiovascular, and neurological systems and has antineoplastic activity. Extrarenal organs possess the enzymatic activity to convert 25(OH)D to $1,25(OH)_2D$. Despite many unanswered questions, much data support the use of vitamin D in renal patients.

In patients suffering from chronic kidney disease, the prevalence of cardiovascular disease is much more common than in the general population. Abnormalities of calcium, phosphorus, vitamin D, and PTH are associated with occurrence of cardiovascular disease in CKD. Some studies indicate a relationship of vitamin D with hypertension, insulin resistance, diabetes, and dyslipidemia.[7] Vitamin D decreases the cardiovascular risk due to multiorgan protective effects. The influence of vitamin D on mortality may be related to several mechanisms including the downregulation of the renin and angiotensin system, protection of proper endothelial cell function, modulation of inflammatory processes including the activation of proinflammatory cytokines as interleukin-8 (IL-8), tumor necrosis factor-α (TNF-α), and oxidative stress. Hindering vascular smooth muscle proliferation, inhibition of myocardial cell hypertrophy, proliferation, and finally improvement of insulin secretion and sensitivity may be other protective factors.

EFFECTS OF VITAMIN D ON ENDOTHELIAL DYSFUNCTION

Vitamin D deficiency has been independently associated with the incidence of both acute myocardial infarction and heart failure, suggesting a role for vitamin D in cardiac function.[8,9] It has also been associated with increased ventricular mass due to myocardial collagen deposition, cardiomegaly, and decreased contractility of the myocardium.[10,11] Clinical studies on vitamin D therapy have proved to improve left ventricular diastolic function as compared to placebo.[12]

Vitamin D receptors present in the myocardium stimulate receptors and prevent the growth of myocardium and its hypertrophy.[13]

This leads to decrease in the secretion of cardiac brain natriuretic peptide (BNP) in the myocyte of atria and the ventricles. Vitamin D supplementation was also found to improve flow-mediated vasodilatation in children with CKD. Collectively, there is sufficient evidence to hypothesize that adequate vitamin D status may directly decrease cardiovascular dysfunction or act indirectly by decreasing systemic inflammation.

VITAMIN D IN DISEASES

Deficiency of vitamin D as well as defective activation or action due to receptor abnormalities may cause serious adverse effects on health.[1]

We will be discussing the impact of vitamin D deficiency in this chapter. Abnormalities of activation and action will be discussed elsewhere. The newer vitamin D analogs will also be discussed briefly.

Nutritional Rickets/Osteomalacia

The vitamin D endocrine system plays an important role in calcium and phosphorus metabolism. Normal bone growth and mineralization require an optimal level of calcium and phosphate, which is tightly regulated by PTH, FGF23, and vitamin D. Rickets is characterized by delay or failure of mineralization of the growth plates at the end of long bones that results in bone deformities, while osteomalacia is poor mineralization of the osteoid formed at sites of bone turnover. Rickets/osteomalacia can occur from nutritional deficiencies of vitamin D, calcium, and/or phosphorus. Vitamin D-deficiency rickets was a common disorder in the early 20th century, which was nearly eliminated with adequate supplementation of breastfed infants and fortification of infant formulas with vitamin D.[14,15]

The incidence of vitamin D deficiency rickets in children peaks between 3 and 18 months of age. During the first 3 months of age, infants are protected due to maternal transfer of 25(OH)D from the mother to the fetus. Congenital rickets has been described in neonates born to mothers who are severely 25(OH)D deficient.

There are three stages of nutritional rickets which are as follows:

Stage I is characterized by hypocalcemia, normal serum phosphorus, normal urinary phosphate and amino acid excretion and minimal or no findings of rickets on X-rays. Stage I is transient and is rarely symptomatic and lasts for days to weeks of vitamin D deficiency. Vitamin D deficiency prevents the efficient absorption of dietary calcium and phosphorus (only 10–15% of dietary calcium and 50–60% of dietary phosphorus are absorbed). A low serum ionized calcium level is recognized by the calcium sensor in parathyroid glands, which results in an increase in the expression, synthesis, and secretion of PTH. In the past, prior to refinement of serum assays for PTH, this stage was attributed to decreased vitamin D level and lack of development of secondary hyperparathyroidism, which is not true as PTH is definitely elevated in stage I.[16] The sustained hypocalcemia, normal serum phosphorus, and normal urinary phosphate excretion are from end-organ resistance to PTH that occurs at a point beyond renal adenylate cyclase activation in the presence of vitamin D depletion. This resistance is subsequently overcome by higher serum PTH levels in stage II.

Stage II is associated with normocalcemia, hypophosphatemia, phosphaturia, aminoaciduria, and mild-to-moderate rickets on X-rays, attributed to the development of secondary hyperparathyroidism, which maintains normocalcemia. The biochemical and radiological findings of nutritional rickets can be explained by the secondary hyperparathyroidism. PTH increases tubular reabsorption of calcium in both the proximal and the distal convoluted tubules and enhances the production of mature osteoclasts through its action on osteoblasts to mobilize calcium from bone. The increased bone turnover is associated with an increase in serum alkaline phosphatase and breakdown of bone matrix. PTH also decreases phosphorus reabsorption in the proximal tubule by upregulating expression of Npt2a in the kidney. Thus, in stage II, the child will have normal serum calcium, low serum phosphorus, elevated PTH, low 25(OH)D, and variable $1,25(OH)_2D$ blood levels. $1,25(OH)_2D$ measurement is of no value in determining nutritional rickets and is often misleading. The bone is now unable to mineralize the osteoid laid down by osteoblasts (with inadequate calcium and phosphorus product) and appears as frayed zone of nonrigid tissue ("rachitic metaphysis") **(Fig. 2)**. On clinical examination, the patient has flaring of ends of bones and the "rachitic rosary."

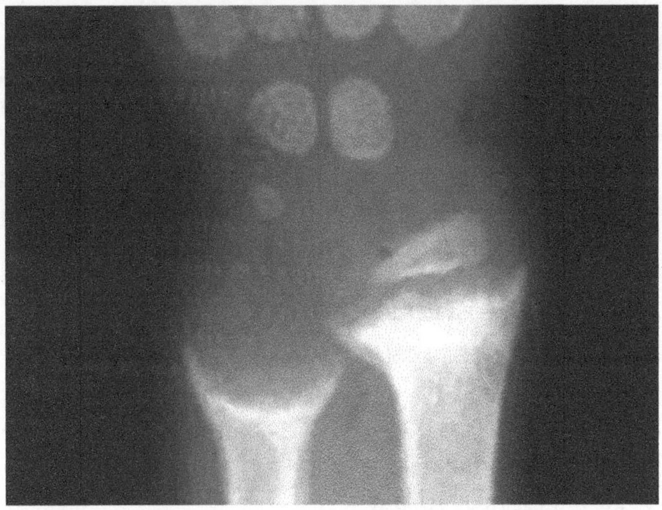

Fig. 2: X-ray of the wrist shows generalized osteopenia, widening of unmineralized epiphyseal growth plates, and fraying of the metaphyseal region (rachitic metaphyseal).

Stage III is similar to stage II but is associated with hypocalcemia and advanced rickets. The natural history of the disease is to progress in time from one stage to the next until an intervention is made. Severe calcium deficiency also can lead to rickets in a similar manner to vitamin D deficiency.

The formation of vitamin D can be compromised by use of sunscreens and inadequate exposure to sunlight as in immobilized/institutionalized children or increased catabolism of vitamin D by the anticonvulsant class of drugs in children with seizure disorder. The phosphorus absorption can be affected by drugs such as cholestyramine and aluminum-containing antacids or increased urinary phosphorus loss from chemotherapy drugs such as ifosfamide and cisplatinum or diseases leading to renal Fanconi syndrome.

There are various inherited and acquired disorders that can disrupt calcium and phosphorus metabolism and result in defective mineralization of the skeleton leading to rickets/osteomalacia. The studies of these rare genetic disorders discussed below have allowed us to better understand the complex physiology of mineral metabolism. $1,25(OH)_2D$ is critically important for normal mineralization of bone and plays a key role in calcium and phosphorus absorption in intestine and kidney. A discussion on inherited disorders that affect mineral metabolism and bone mineralization prior to 1α-hydroxylation, at 1α-hydroxylation, and following 1α-hydroxylation is given in Chapter 8.6.

TREATMENT OF VITAMIN D DEFICIENCY RICKETS

Vitamin D deficiency rickets is treated with inactive vitamin D (cholecalciferol or ergocalciferol) to correct the clinical, biochemical, and radiological abnormalities and to restore vitamin D reserve. Different treatment regimens are available now and two most commonly used ones are given below:

Low-dosage and Long-term Vitamin D Therapy

Depending on the age of the child, vitamin D is given at a dose of 1,000–10,000 IU/day for 2–3 months.[17] The dosage guidelines are as follows:

- *Neonates:* 1,000 IU/day
- *1–12 months:* 1,000–5,000 IU/day
- *Beyond infancy:* 5,000 IU/day

Levels of Ca and P are normalized in 6–10 days of starting treatment and it takes 1–2 months for PTH to normalize. Depending on the severity of the disease, it may take 3 months for serum ALP to become normal and the radiological findings to disappear. Once deficiency is corrected, a maintenance dose of 400 IU/day is continued.

Stoss Therapy

A high dose of vitamin D can be given orally or intramuscularly as a single dose of 100,000–600,000 IU after the first month of life in those with poor compliance. This regimen induces a rapid clinical response with biochemical recovery in a few days and radiological recovery in 2 weeks.

In symptomatic hypocalcemia, parenteral calcium is given as Ca gluconate (1–2 mL/kg of 10% Ca gluconate, providing 10–20 mg/kg of elemental Ca). It is administered intravenously and slowly, over 5–10 minutes. If there are no symptoms of hypocalcemia, calcium is given orally for 1–2 weeks.[17] Vitamin D deficiency in the population can be prevented by improving awareness in the society and ensuring that pregnant and lactating mothers as well as children are sufficiently exposed to sunlight and eat a balanced diet rich in calcium and vitamin D.

Newer Vitamin D Receptor Analogs of Vitamin D

Kidney Disease Outcomes Quality Initiative (KDOQI) and Kidney Disease Improving Global Outcomes (KDIGO) experts have recognized that vitamin D insufficiency and deficiency should be avoided in CKD and dialysis patients by using supplementation to avoid secondary hyperparathyroidism (SHPT). Many vitamin D supplementation regimens using ergocalciferol or cholecalciferol daily, weekly or monthly, have been reported. There are studies which report that vitamin D receptor activator (VDRA) use is associated with better outcomes and is more efficient in reducing PTH levels.[18]

Abnormal vitamin D metabolism plays a major role in the development of SHPT in CKD. As calcitriol levels progressively decrease, the negative feedback normally exerted on the parathyroid glands becomes ineffective, promoting the development of SHPT. Phosphate retention, hyperphosphatemia, and ensuing hypocalcemia are the other major factors contributing to the development of SHPT. The dose-dependent development of hypercalcemia and hyperphosphatemia with possible consequent soft tissue and vascular calcifications as well as concerns for the development of a dynamic bone disease prompted the development of calcitriol analogs for PTH suppression with less calcemic activity. Vitamin D analogs activate the VDR differently when compared with calcitriol.[19]

Prohormones

- *Alfacalcidol* or 1-α-hydroxy-vitamin D_3 is a prohormone, which requires 25-hydroxylation in the liver in order to become active, 25-$(OH)_2D_3$ and stimulate the VDR. It is available in oral and intravenous formulations. Oral alfacalcidol significantly improves bone histology in patients with abnormal bone turnover. In dialysis patients, both oral and parenteral forms suppress PTH having activity similar to calcitriol.
- *Doxercalciferol* or 1-α hydroxyvitamin D_2 is also a prohormone which requires 25-hydroxylation in the liver to become active 1,25$(OH)_2D_2$. Both oral and intravenous forms suppress PTH with low rates of hypercalcemia and hyperphosphatemia.

Direct Vitamin D Receptor Activators

Paricalcitol or 19-nor-1α, 25-hydroxyvitamin D_2 is an analog of 125$(OH)_2D_2$ obtained by the elimination of the methylene group from carbon 10. In an experimental model of CKD, paricalcitol had one-third the potency of the calcitriol in decreasing PTH and one-tenth the potency of calcitriol in increasing serum calcium and phosphorus. This makes paricalcitol threefold more selective of PTH suppression than calcitriol.

Maxacalcitol or 22-oxa-1α, 25-dihydroxyvitamin D_3 is similar to calcitriol but has an oxygen between C21 and C25 with equal efficacy and safety.

Falecalcitriol or 26,27-hexafluoro-1α, 25-dihydroxyvitamin D_3 is a hexafluoro derivative of 1,25$(OH)_2D_3$. The oral form is effective in decreasing PTH in dialysis patients. The approval of paricalcitol and doxercalciferol for clinical use represented a new paradigm shift in the treatment of SHPT, where the use of calcitriol, which was limited by the development of hypercalcemia and hyperphosphatemia, is now replaced by new vitamin D analogs with a wider therapeutic window. Noncalcitriol VDR activator (VDRA) can be used at higher doses to treat SHPT in humans, with little or no effects on calcium and phosphorus.[19]

VITAMIN D AND COVID-19 INFECTION

Vitamin D plays a role in immune function and inflammation. There has been an ongoing debate regarding the role of vitamin D supplementation in the prevention and treatment of COVID-19 infection. A recent systematic review and meta-analysis concluded that the role of vitamin D supplementation based on observational studies has not found a robust link to prevention or treatment of COVID infection.[20,21] We need to monitor for emerging evidence on the efficacy, safety, and dose schedule of vitamin D in relation to COVID disease.

CONCLUSION

Vitamin D is an important prohormone that regulates calcium and phosphate homeostasis. It has numerous extraskeletal effects, especially on the immune mechanisms, cardiovascular system, central nervous system (CNS), endocrine functions, cell differentiation, cell growth, and repair. Vitamin D produced in the skin by exposure to sunlight or ingested in the diet is converted by 25-hydroxylase (CYP27A1, CYP3A4, CYP2R1, and CYP2J3) in the liver to 25(OH)D. 25(OH)D is converted in the kidneys by CYP27B1 to 1,25$(OH)_2$D. 1,25$(OH)_2$D enhances intestinal calcium and phosphorus absorption. Active vitamin D exerts pleotropic effects on skeletal system, cardiac, endocrine, CNS, and immune functions. Vitamin D inadequacy is a global problem. Though recommendations of daily vitamin D intake have been provided, higher levels may be required for real preventive or treatment effects.

KEY POINTS

- The vitamin D endocrine system plays an important role in calcium and phosphorus metabolism.
- It has generated great interest in recent years due to recognition of its nonskeletal functions.
- Normal bone growth and mineralization require an optimal level of calcium and phosphate, which is tightly regulated by PTH, FGF23, and vitamin D.
- The skeletal and nonskeletal physiological functions of vitamin D may have different cutoffs for sufficiency, insufficiency, and deficiency.
- The new recommendations from the Institute of Medicine (IOM) for dietary reference intakes (DRIs) for vitamin D in infants are 400 units (10 μg) per day and in children are 600 units (15 μg) per day.
- Vitamin D deficiency has been independently associated with incidence of heart failure, suggesting a role for vitamin D in cardiac function.
- Abnormal vitamin D metabolism plays a major role in the development of SHPT in CKD.

REFERENCES

1. Holick M. Vitamin D for health and in chronic kidney disease. Semin Dial. 2005;18:266-75.
2. Rosen C, Compston, Lian J. Primer on the metabolic bone diseases and disorders of mineral metabolism, 7th edition. Washington, DC: Wiley; 2008.
3. Joiner TA, Foster C, Shope T. The many faces of vitamin D deficiency rickets. Ped In Rev. 2000;21(9):296-302.
4. Ross AC, Taylor CL, Yaktine AL, Del Valle HB. Institute of Medicine (US) Committee to Review Dietary Reference Intakes for Vitamin D and Calcium; Dietary Reference Intakes for Calcium and Vitamin D. Washington, DC: National Academies Press; 2011.
5. Srivastava T, Garg U, Ruiz M, Dai H, Alon US. Serum 25(OH)-vitamin D level in children: Is there a need to change the reference range based on 2011 Institute of Medicine Report? Clin Pediatr (Phila). 2013;52(2):178-82.
6. Glorieux F, Pettifor J, Juppner H. Pediatric Bone Biology and Diseases, 2nd edition. San Diego, CA: Academic Press; 2011.
7. Gluba-Brzozka A, Franczyk B, Cialkowska-Rysz A, Olszewski R, Rysz J. Impact of vitamin D on the cardiovascular system in advanced chronic kidney disease (CKD) and dialysis patients. Nutrients. 2017;9(4):374.
8. Giovannucci E, Liu Y, Hollis BW, Rimm EB. 25-hydroxyvitamin D and risk of myocardial infarction in men: a prospective study. Arch Intern Med. 2008;168(11):1174-80.
9. Zittermann A, Schleithoff SS, Tenderich G, Berthold HK, Korfer R, Stehle P. Low vitamin D status: a contributing factor in the pathogenesis of congestive heart failure? J Am Coll Cardiol. 2003;41(1):105-12.
10. Weishaar RE, Kim SN, Saunders DE, Simpson RU. Involvement of vitamin D3 with cardiovascular function. III. Effects on physical and morphological properties. Am J Physiol. 1990;258(1 Pt 1):E134-42.
11. Weishaar RE, Simpson RU. Involvement of vitamin D3 with cardiovascular function. II. Direct and indirect effects. Am J Physiol. 1987;253(6 Pt 1):E675-83.
12. Singh NP, Sahni V, Garg D, Nair M. Effect of pharmacological suppression of secondary hyperparathyroidism on cardio-vascular hemodynamics in predialysis CKD patients: A preliminary observation. Hemodial Int. 2007;11(4):417-23.
13. Aytac MB, Deveci M, Bek K, Kayabey O, Ekinci Z. Effect of cholecalciferol on local arterial stiffness and endothelial dysfunction in children with chronic kidney disease. Pediatr Nephrol. 2016;31(2):267-77.
14. Holick M. Resurrection of vitamin D deficiency and rickets. J Clin Invest. 2006;116:2062-72.
15. Nield L, Mahajan P, Joshi A, Kamat D. Rickets: not a disease of the past. Am Fam Physician. 2006;74(4):619-26, 629-30.
16. Srivastava T, Alon US. Stage I vitamin D-deficiency rickets mimicking pseudohypoparathyroidism type II. Clin Pediatr (Phila). 2002;41(4):263-8.
17. Misra M, Pacaud D, Petryk A, Solberg FC, Kappy M. Vitamin D deficiency in children and its management: Review of current knowledge and recommendations. Pediatrics. 2008;122: 398-417.
18. Jean G, Souberbielle JC, Chazot C. Vitamin D in chronic kidney disease and dialysis patients. Nutrients. 2017;9:328.
19. Negrea L. Active vitamin D in chronic kidney disease: getting right back where we started from? Kidney Dis. 2019;5:59-68.
20. Bassatne A, Basbous M, Chakhtoura M, El Zein O, Rahme M, El-Hajj Fuleihan G. The link between COVID-19 and vitamin D (VIVID): A systematic review and meta-analysis. Metabolism. 2021;119:154753.
21. Liu N, Sun J, Wang X, Zhang T, Zhao M, Li H. Low vitamin D status is associated with coronavirus disease 2019 outcomes: a systematic review and meta-analysis. Int J Infect Dis. 2021;104:58-64.

CHAPTER

14.4

COVID-19 and the Kidney

Urmila Anandh, Arpana A Iyengar

INTRODUCTION

With the first description of the severe acute respiratory syndrome (SARS) following a new coronavirus in 2019,[1] the world has been grappling with a pandemic impacting 220 countries and territories worldwide. The virus has been designated as COVID-19 by the World Health Organization (WHO) and it has as of now affected approximately 186 million people with more than 4 million dying of this infection. The American Academy of Pediatrics has reported more than 4 million children infected with COVID-19. The numbers in children are rising in India as reported during the second wave. In a report from China, of the total infections, 2.4% were found in children.[2] The data from the United States of America had shown an incidence of 1.7% infections in children.[3] COVID-19 infection in children is less severe, but some manifest with a severe form of an inflammatory response 4–6 weeks following the initial infection.[4]

Coronaviruses causing respiratory symptoms have been known to mankind for many years. The precursor of the current virus responsible for SARS was first identified in 2003.[5] The current virus (SARS-CoV-2) is considered to be more transmissible but responsible for a less-severe form of infection. COVID-19 infection can range from subclinical manifestations to severe multiorgan dysfunction. This is because of the virus interaction with angiotensin-converting enzyme 2 (ACE-2) receptor present in many organs. The virus also has the ability to engender a cytokine storm which is primarily responsible for multiorgan failure seen in a small proportion of patients.

This chapter summarizes the clinical impact of the virus on the kidney.

PATHOBIOLOGY OF THE VIRUS

Coronaviruses belong to the family Coronaviridae of the order Nidovirales. Structurally, they are characterized by an unusually large RNA genome and club-like glycoprotein spikes that project from the surface of its envelope. These spikes give the virus an appearance similar to the solar corona, hence the name.[6]

The spike protein on the viral surface has receptors that bind with ACE-2 on the host cell surface. Furin or another enzyme transmembrane protease, serine 2 (TMPRSS2) on the outer surface of the host cell membrane cleaves the spike protein exposing fusion peptides. These small amino acid chains fuse the viral membrane with the host cell membrane and gain entry into the host cell. Upon entry, the viral mRNA hacks the host cell's replication apparatus and multiplies. At exit, furin may prime the spike proteins facilitating their entry into other cells.[7] The virus predominantly infects organs which have cell surface ACE-2 receptors. This not only includes pneumocytes and the tubular epithelial cells of the kidney but also many other cells in organs such as heart, testes, brainstem, small intestines, stomach, liver, blood vessels, and nasal and oral mucosa.[8] This explains the multiorgan involvement of SARS-CoV-2, in direct contrast to its predecessors.[9]

PATHOPHYSIOLOGY OF RENAL INVOLVEMENT

The renal involvement in kidneys is considered to be because of:

- Direct cytopathic involvement of the COVID-19 virus
- Local/systemic inflammatory response

Direct Cytopathic Involvement

Angiotensin-converting enzyme 2 receptors have been shown to be present on podocytes and the tubular epithelium. A direct injury of the renal cells is postulated by the virus—ACE-2 receptor interaction.[10] This renal tropism of SARS-CoV-2 in contrast to SARS-CoV is because of increased affinity to ACE-2 receptors. Postmortem analyses of the kidneys have shown the presence of viral nucleocapsid in renal tubules.[11] Another autopsy study revealed the presence of viral particle in tubular epithelial cells and podocytes by electron microscopy. The electron microscopic images showed podocyte effacement, vacuolation, and detachment of podocytes from the glomerular basement membrane.[12,13] Another report from our center revealed the presence of tubuloreticular inclusions and viral particles (**Fig. 1**) in the biopsy of a transplant recipient with COVID-19 infection.[14] Certain authors have questioned the validity of ultrastructural presence of virions in the kidney but with increasing evidence it is believed that the electron

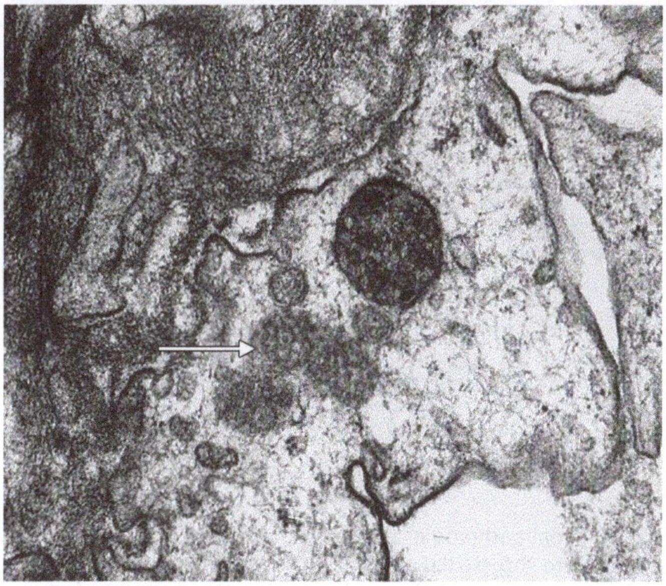

Fig. 1: Electron microscopic image of an allograft biopsy showing the presence of COVID-19 virions (arrow).
Courtesy: Dr Urmila Anandh and Dr Alok Sharma.

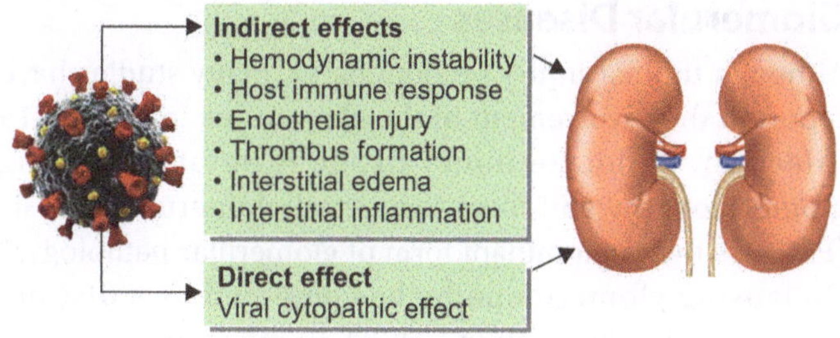

Fig. 2: Pathophysiologic mechanisms in COVID-19-induced renal injury.

microscopy images are in fact COVID-19 virus and not multivesicular bodies (MVBs) as suggested.

Besides autopsy studies, various other studies have provided evidence about the direct infection of COVID-19 virus. They are as follows:

- Reverse transcription-polymerase chain reaction (RT-PCR) and or in situ hybridization detection of viral mRNA in kidneys infected by COVID-19[15]
- Immunocytochemistry evidence showing the presence of viral proteins[16]
- Recovery of live virus[15]

These findings along with the consensual role of ACE-2 in renal physiology lead us to believe that COVID-19 infection is responsible for a complex multifactorial pathophysiology leading to direct cytopathic effect of the virus and subsequent local disruption in renin-angiotensin-aldosterone homeostasis in the kidney.

COVID-19-associated Cytokine Release Syndrome

High levels of cytokines, especially interleukin 1β (IL-1β), IL-8, interferon γ, and tumor necrosis factor α (TNF-α), have been reported in critically sick COVID-19-infected patients with acute kidney injury (AKI).[17] COVID-19 tropism to monocytes and lymphocytes can contribute to the cytokine storm.[18]

Excessive cytokine release impacts the kidney by multiple mechanisms. Hypotension, ischemia reperfusion injury, inflammatory damage, coagulation abnormalities, and apoptosis contribute to kidney injury. This is similar to the pathophysiology of AKI in sepsis.[19]

Virus-infected cells are usually destroyed by CD8+ T cells; however, in COVID-19 infection, the T cells are depleted.[20] This results in insufficient cytotoxic killing of the virus. Lymphopenia stimulates the overproduction of cytokines leading to organ damage. NK cells are overactivated further aggravating the tissue injury. Collective immunologic disturbances in COVID-19 infection are responsible for this cytokine storm.[21] The hyperinflammation in COVID-19 is similar to that of macrophage activation syndrome.[22]

The combination of the imbalance in renin-angiotensin-aldosterone system (RAAS; which also promotes a proinflammatory phenotype) and the virus-mediated cytokine release is responsible for a multifaceted kidney dysfunction (**Fig. 2**).[23]

RENAL SYNDROMES IN COVID-19: PATHOLOGY

The kidney is affected in COVID-19 in various ways. The most common manifestation of renal involvement in COVID-19 infection is mild proteinuria which is seen in early stage of infection.[24] However, the most important clinical syndrome in patients is AKI. Besides AKI, prerenal azotemia, acute interstitial nephritis, glomerulonephritis, and thrombotic microangiopathy (TMA) are also reported in literature.

Acute Kidney Injury

Acute kidney injury is increasingly recognized as an important complication of COVID-19 infection and may affect the overall prognosis in these patients.[25,26] Majority of AKI biopsies reveal acute tubular necrosis (ATN). ATN occurs because of both ischemic (volume depletion, relative intravascular volume deficit in cytokine storm) and nephrotoxic (therapy of COVID-19 infection) insults. Most of the biopsies record significant tubular injury with loss of brush border and presence of nonisometric vacuolation. Occasional protein and pigment casts are noted intraluminally. Erythrocyte aggregation and congestion are also seen in peritubular capillaries. Interstitium is edematous with prominent lymphocytic infiltrate. The changes are most prominent in the proximal tubular cells.[27,28] Presence of myoglobin casts in patients with rhabdomyolysis has also been reported.[29] Besides, excessive intake of vitamin C leads to the development of intratubular oxalate crystals and acute tubular injury.[30] In children, there are reports of AKI but rarely there was any necessity for a renal biopsy.[31]

Glomerular Diseases

Although tubular injury predominates, many studies have reported the involvement of the glomerulus in COVID-19 infection. Podocyte injury in the form of collapsing glomerulopathy and focal segmental glomerulosclerosis (FSGS) is the predominant form of glomerular pathology.[32] Collapsing glomerulopathy has emerged as a distinct pathological entity seen in COVID-19 infection. It is often seen in patients with African ancestry.[33,34] Other glomerular diseases reported with COVID-19 infection are minimal change disease, antineutrophil cytoplasmic antibody (ANCA)-associated vasculitis, antiglomerular basement membrane disease, membranous nephropathy, and immunoglobulin A vasculitis.[35] These pathological manifestations suggest that immune complex deposition also played an important role in the development of renal diseases in COVID-19. In children who present with nephrotic syndrome and COVID-19 infection, renal biopsies have not been done in most of the cases.[36,37]

Thrombotic Microangiopathy

Endothelial injury and coagulation abnormalities have been implicated in COVID-19-mediated renal injury. Endothelial damage and subsequent complement activation are an important underlying pathomechanism in COVID-19 infection.[38] Renal biopsies documenting TMA as a primary phenomenon or associated with other glomerular diseases have been reported in the literature.[39] Jhaveri et al. have described extensive cortical necrosis and glomerular thrombi in a patient with COVID-19 infection with alternate complement pathway defects.[40] Renal biopsy in a child with a clinical presentation of multisystem inflammatory syndrome and TMA revealed evidence of globally sclerotic glomeruli, papillary tuft necrosis, and endotheliosis compatible with TMA.[41]

Mixed/Miscellaneous Lesions

Case reports of lupus nephritis and membranous nephropathy have been reported. Some biopsies show a combination of lesions such as acute tubular injury, collapsing glomerulopathy, and interstitial nephritis.

The myriad pathological lesions reported in the literature are depicted in **Figure 3**.

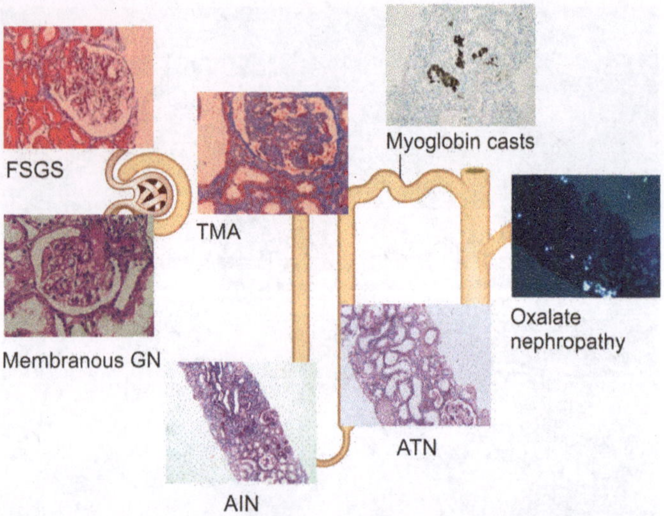

Fig. 3: Renal pathologic changes reported in COVID-19 biopsies. (AIN: acute interstitial nephritis; ATN: acute tubular necrosis; FSGS: focal segmental glomerulosclerosis; GN: glomerulonephritis; TMA: thrombotic microangiopathy)
Courtesy: Dr Urmila Anandh and Dr Swarnalata Gowrishankar.

TABLE 1: Clinical signs and symptoms of SARS-CoV-2 infection in children.[42]

Clinical characteristics	*Incidence (%)*
Cough	48.5
Pharyngeal erythema	46.2
Fever	41.5
Diarrhea	8.8
Fatigue	7.6
Vomiting	6.4
Rhinorrhea	7.6
Nasal congestion	5.3

CLINICAL FEATURES

Although most children infected with SARS-CoV-2 have either mild disease, severe illness is not rare. The incubation period is similar to that of adults. The most common clinical signs and symptoms of SARS-CoV-2 infection in children are given in **Table 1**. Some children may present with a rash.[42] Besides the respiratory tract involvement, extrapulmonary involvement is also common **(Fig. 4)**. The main extrapulmonary involvement is gastrointestinal with a high prevalence of diarrhea, abdominal pain, and vomiting.[31] Cardiac, neurologic, and renal involvement is seen in a significant percentage of children.[43] Renal involvement is more common in severe COVID-19 infection and in multisystem inflammatory syndrome in children (MIS-C).

Renal Involvement in COVID-19 Infection

The most common renal manifestation in children with COVID-19 is AKI even though early studies from China reported very rare occurrence of renal dysfunction in children.[44] Over the next few months, reports of renal involvement in children appeared in the literature. AKI was most commonly noted in children who were admitted in the pediatric ICU or had clinical features of MIS-C. Many of these children presented with diarrhea and vomiting suggesting a prerenal component in the development of AKI.[45] In a multicentric study conducted to look at the epidemiology of AKI in critically ill children, higher rates of prevalence of AKI were noted.[46] A prevalence of 44% almost compares

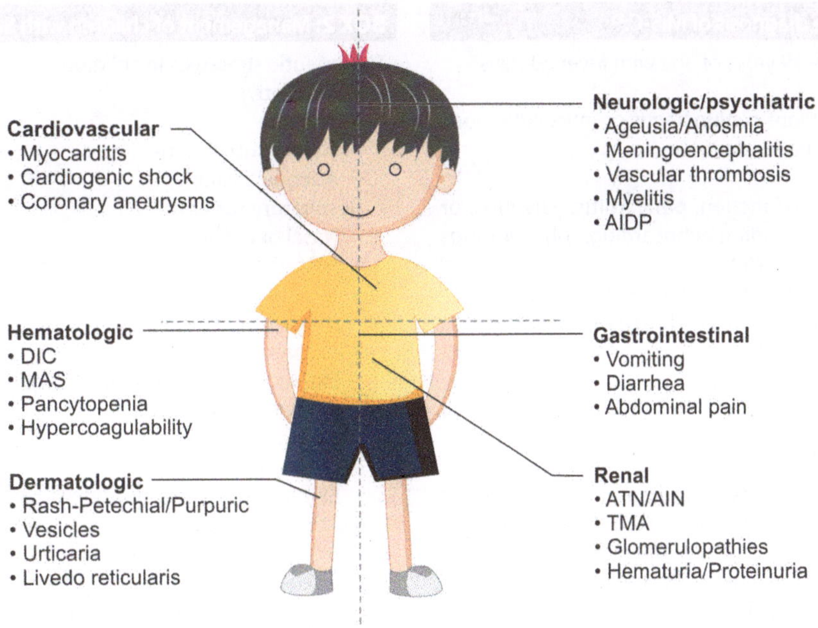

Fig. 4: Extrapulmonary involvement in children with COVID-19. (AIDP: acute inflammatory demyelinating polyneuropathy; AIN: acute interstitial nephritis; ATN: acute tubular necrosis; DIC; disseminated intravascular coagulation; MAS: macrophage activation syndrome; TMA: thrombotic microangiopathy)

to that seen in adults; however, the degree of severity was milder. No child in this cohort needed dialysis. Despite less severity of AKI, 6% of the affected children died. Most studies report AKI in one-fifth of pediatric COVID-19. One-third of these children usually require pediatric intensive care unit (PICU) admission. Not only AKI is associated with increasing morbidity and mortality, but in some children, there is evidence of persistent renal dysfunction following recovery.[47] Some children also develop renal failure secondary to rhabdomyolysis. AKI secondary to rhabdomyolysis is often severe requiring dialysis.[48] Rhabdomyolysis often occurs in the setting of acute COVID-19 infection.

Glomerular disease is reported in association with COVID-19 infection. There are case reports of nephrotic syndrome following COVID-19 infection.[36,37] Treatment is usually with antivirals and steroids. Hematologic abnormalities suggestive of TMA are seen in children, but severe renal failure is rare.[49] TMA resulting in AKI progressing to chronic renal failure is seen in children with MIS-C.[41]

MULTISYSTEM INFLAMMATORY SYNDROME: CHILDREN

Early in the pandemic, it was realized that previously healthy children presented with shock, fever, and hyperinflammation after 4–6 weeks of COVID-19 infection. The first report came from the South Thames Retrieval Service, London, UK, where eight severely ill children presented with shock. This presentation was preceded weeks before by relatively mild/asymptomatic COVID-19 infection.[50] The Royal College of Pediatrics and Child Health (RCPCH) considered this as a pediatric multisystem inflammatory syndrome (PMIS).[51] As more and more cases were recognized worldwide, the WHO and Centers for Disease Control and Prevention (CDC) labeled this syndrome as MIS-C.[52]

The characteristics of this entity are based on six elements:
1. Pediatric age
2. Persistence of fever
3. Presence of markers of inflammation
4. Signs and symptoms of organ dysfunction
5. Lacking an alternate diagnosis
6. Temporal association of COVID-19 infection and exposure

The WHO and Centers for Disease Control and Prevention (CDC) require proof of COVID-19 infection or exposure.[53] The WHO criteria for diagnosis of MIS-C are given in **Box 1**.

The data from India show that MIS-C is seen only in 0.6% of children with COVID-19 infection. Neutrophilia, lymphopenia, and elevated pro-brain natriuretic peptide (BNP) were poor prognostic parameters. The mortality was 4.3%, comparable to that of international reports.[54]

Consistent with the presence of hyperinflammation, the procalcitonin and IL-6 were markedly elevated.[55] The predominance of cardiac manifestations was striking in these children. Majority of them presented with reduced ejection fraction and elevated troponin I.

The involvement of children of all ethnicities, older age, and a higher percentage of cardiovascular collapse differentiates MIS-C from Kawasaki disease.[56]

Acute Kidney Injury and MIS-C

Acute kidney injury is a common finding in children with MIS-C. The cardiovascular instability and systolic dysfunction predispose to AKI. Though common (46% in a study), it is

BOX 1: WHO criteria for the diagnosis of MIS-C.[53]

Children and adolescents 0–19 years of age with fever ≥3 days
AND *two* of the following:
- Rash or bilateral nonpurulent conjunctivitis or mucocutaneous inflammation signs (oral, hands, feet)
- Hypotension or shock
- Features of myocardial dysfunction, pericarditis, valvulitis, or coronary abnormalities (including echocardiographic findings or elevated troponin/NT-pro BNP)
- Evidence of coagulopathy (by PT, PTT, elevated d-dimers)
- Acute gastrointestinal problems (diarrhea, vomiting, or abdominal pain)

AND
Elevated markers of inflammation such as ESR, C-reactive protein, or procalcitonin
AND
No other obvious microbial cause of inflammation, including bacterial sepsis, staphylococcal or streptococcal shock syndromes.
AND
Evidence of COVID-19 (RT-PCR, antigen test, or serology positive) or likely contact with patients with COVID-19

(ESR: erythrocyte sedimentation rate; NT pro-BNP: N terminal pro-brain natriuretic peptide; MIS-C: multisystem inflammatory syndrome in children; PT: prothrombin time; PTT: partial thromboplastin time; RT-PCR: real-time-polymerase chain reaction)

often mild and resolves quickly.[57] Low serum albumin, higher neutrophil counts, and greater degree of systolic dysfunction are predictors of the development of AKI. These children have a prolonged hospital stay.[58]

COVID-19 IN CHILDREN WITH CHRONIC KIDNEY DISEASE

Chronic kidney disease (CKD) is a risk factor for severe and critical illness in adults. This may have a lesser impact on children as the underlying comorbidities that lead to CKD in adults are not common in children. Children who are on immunosuppression for their kidney diseases (transplantation, vasculitis, nephrotic syndrome) have mild symptoms of COVID-19 infection but have a high risk of deterioration. In a study of 1,572 children vulnerable to COVID-19 infection, only three had confirmed infection and none had severe disease.[59]

In transplant recipients, the overall incidence of COVID-19 infection was 0.87% in a multicentric study. There was no incidence of respiratory failure, allograft failure, or death in this cohort.[60]

MANAGEMENT

The overall management of children with COVID-19 infection is depicted in **Box 2** and the reader is directed to refer to the guidelines issued by the Indian Ministry of Health and Family Welfare for further details.[61] Most of the therapeutic interventions are similar to those of adults.

In children with nephrotic syndrome, scant data exists about the impact of immunosuppression on the natural history of COVID-19 infection. Whether to start immunosuppressive therapy depends on the severity of the illness and the risk of immunosuppression. The guidelines suggest initiating immunosuppression except in children with low-grade proteinuria and normal renal function.[62] It may be advisable to defer the use of rituximab until more information is available. Children on immunosuppression also tend to have milder COVID-related disease and there is no evidence to suggest

BOX 2: Management of children with SARS-CoV-2 infection.

Therapeutic strategies in children:
- Conservative:
  - Bed rest
  - Fluid resuscitation
  - Adequate calories
- Respiratory support:
  - Nasal oxygen
  - High-flow oxygen
  - Noninvasive ventilation
  - Invasive ventilation
  - Prone ventilation
  - Extracorporeal membrane oxygenation
  - Inhalation nitric oxide
- Cardiovascular support:
  - Inotropes
  - Extracorporeal membrane oxygenation
- Nutritional support:
  - Adequate calories and fluids
  - Adequate micronutrients, vitamin supplementation
  - Oral and parenteral nutrition
- Drug therapy:
  - Repurposed agents:
    - Chloroquine phosphate
    - Hydroxychloroquine sulfate
    - Ivermectin
    - Lopinavir/Ritonavir
    - Umifenovir
  - Investigational agents:
    - Remdesivir
    - Favipiravir
    - Monulparivir
  - Adjunctive therapies:
    - Tocilizumab
    - Infliximab
    - Baricitinib
- Immunotherapy
  - Steroids
  - Plasma exchange
  - Convalescent plasma
  - Monoclonal antibodies—Casirivimab and Imdevimab
- Dialytic therapies:
  - Continuous kidney replacement therapy, slow low efficiency dialysis, peritoneal dialysis
- Cytokine adsorption treatments:
  - Treatment of MIS-C:
    - Methylprednisolone
    - Intravenous immunoglobulin
- Treatment of comorbidities:
  - Diabetic ketoacidosis
  - Seizures
- Vaccination:
  - Pfizer-BioNTech, Sinovac, Corbevax

BOX 3: Pediatric continuous kidney replacement therapy (CKRT) guidelines.[62]

- Suggested modality of treatment—continuous venovenous hemodiafiltration
- Preemptive CKRT is advised if the child is developing progressive respiratory insufficiency
- Normocarb bicarbonate-based solutions are preferable
- As the COVID-19 infection is a procoagulant state, one-third of the replacement fluid is to be infused prefilter, another third postfilter, and the remaining to be used as dialysate to dilute the circuit
- A high blood flow rate of 4–5 mL/kg/min is advised to enhance cytokine clearance
- Electrolyte monitoring is better every 2 hourly if high-flow CVVHDF is considered
- Nutritional supplementation is required in all children
- Early replacement therapy is advisable to improve hemodynamic stability and cytokine clearance

an association between the number of immunosuppressive medications and severity of COVID disease.[63]

The principles of therapy of AKI are similar to those of treatment in non-COVID-19 situations. Preemptive and early kidney replacement therapy should be considered in a child who is developing respiratory insufficiency. In critically ill pediatric patients, use of high-flow (HF) continuous venovenous hemodiafiltration (CVVHDF) may be better as it may enhance the nonspecific removal of cytokines.[64] The HF-CVVHDF can be started at a flow rate 50 mL/kg/h for the first 12 hours and can be reduced to 25–30 mL/kg/h. The circuit can also connect an adsorption filter if required. The suggestions for kidney replacement therapy are given in **Box 3.**[64,65] In resource-constrained settings, peritoneal dialysis can be considered.

Children on maintenance hemodialysis (HD) have a higher risk of contracting the infection because of their frequent exposure to medical personnel. The guidelines for prevention of infection in children on dialysis are similar to those of CDC guidelines for adult HD patients. UV light disinfection for more than 30 minutes is recommended in pediatric dialysis units.[65] Peritoneal dialysis (PD) effluent should be disinfected with bleach before it is flushed through the toilet drain.

Transplanted children are supposed to continue the same immunosuppression while maintaining utmost precautions. In case the transplanted child is infected, the reduction of immunosuppression should be considered on a case-to-case basis. Systemic corticosteroids can be considered based on the severity of the COVID-19 infection. Antiviral therapy is likely to be beneficial if started early and immunomodulatory therapy can be considered if the child has evidence of a hyperinflammatory state.[66]

VACCINATION

Children who are part of high-risk group (CKD, immunosuppressed, have underlying respiratory ailments) should be considered for vaccination. Trials in children over 12 years of age have been completed or are underway and the CDC has approved vaccination (Pfizer BioNtech) of children more than 12 years of age. There have been reports of cardiac inflammation (myocarditis, pericarditis) in adolescents which have resolved with early clinical intervention. In India, trials are underway with Covaxin in children. There is a report of postvaccination-related hematuria in two children.[67,68]

CONCLUSION

Kidneys have a profound expression of ACE-2 to which SARS-CoV-2 virus has high affinity. Children have milder disease due to potential protective factors such as a strong innate immunity and lack of immunosenescence. With a high probability of further waves of COVID occurring in the near future, we await more evidence and understanding of the aftermath of the disease especially relevant to children.

KEY POINTS

- Renal involvement is increasingly recognized in children as in adults.
- Immunosuppression has not been observed to be a risk for COVID.
- AKI is the most common renal manifestation, especially in children who develop MIS-C.
- ATN, acute interstitial nephritis, collapsing glomerulopathy, and TMA are common renal histopathological entities associated with COVID-19.
- Management of renal injury is mostly supportive and rarely do children need kidney replacement therapy (KRT).

REFERENCES

1. Zhu N, Zhang D, Wang W, Li X, Yang B, Song J, et al. A novel coronavirus from patients with pneumonia in China. N Engl J Med. 2019;382:727-33.
2. WHO. Report of the WHO-China Joint Mission on Coronavirus Disease 2019 (COVID-19). World Health Organization. [online] Available from https://www.who.int/docs/default-source/coronaviruse/who-china-joint-mission-on-covid-19-final-report.pdf [Last accessed May, 2022].
3. CDC COVID-19 Response Team. Coronavirus disease 2019 in children - United States, February 12–April 2, 2020. Morb Mortal Wkly Rep. 2020;69:422-6.
4. Feldstein LR, Rose EB, Horwitz SM, Collins JP, Newhams MM, Son MBF, et al for the Overcoming COVID-19 Investigators and the CDC COVID-19 Response Team. Multisystem inflammatory syndrome in US children and adolescents. N Engl J Med. 2020;383:334-46.
5. Drosten C, Gunther S, Preiser W, van der Werf S, Brodt HR, Becker S, et al. Identification of a novel coronavirus in patients with severe acute respiratory syndrome. N Engl J Med. 2003;348:1967-76.
6. Masters PS. The molecular biology of coronaviruses. Adv Virus Res. 2006;65:193-292.
7. Cyranoski D. Profile of a killer virus. Nature. 2020;581:22-6.
8. Gembrandt F, Sterner-Kock A, Imboden H, Spalteholz M, Reibitz F, Schultheiss HP, et al. Organ-specific distribution

of ACE2 mRNA and correlating peptidase activity in rodents. Peptides. 2005;26:1270-7.

9. Zhou X, Chen K, Zou J, Han P, Hao J, Han Z. Single-cell RNA-seq data analysis on receptor ACE2 expression reveals the potential risk of different organs vulnerable to 2019-nCov infection. Front Med. 2020;14:185-92.
10. Farkash EA, Wilson AM, Jentzen JM. Ultrastructural evidence for direct renal infection with SARS-CoV-2. J Am Soc Nephrol. 2020;31:1683-1687.
11. Martinez-Rojas MA, Vega-Vega O, Bobadilla NA. Is the kidney a target of SARS COV-2? Am J Physiol Renal Physiol. 2020;318:F1454-62.
12. Su H, Yang M, Wan C, Yi LX, Tang F, Zhu HY, et al. Renal histopathological analysis of 26 post-mortem findings of patients with COVID-19 in China. Kidney Int. 2020;98:219-27.
13. Freith M, Erman A, Wechtersbach K, Plesko J, Avsic-Zupanc T, Kojc N. SARS-Cov-2 virions or ubiquitous cell structures? Actual dilemma in COVID-19 era. Kidney Int Rep. 2020;5:1608-10.
14. Anandh U, Gowrishankar S, Sharma A, Salama A, Dasgupta I. Kidney transplant dysfunction in a patient with COVID-19 infection: role of concurrent Sars-Cov 2 nephropathy, chronic rejection and vitamin C-mediated hyperoxalosis: case report. BMC Nephrol. 2021;22:91.
15. Braun F, Lutgehetmann M, Pfefferle S, Wong MN, Carsten A, Lindemeyer MT, et al. SARS-COV-2 renal tropism associates with acute kidney injury. Lancet. 2020;396:597-8.
16. Puelles VG, Lutgehetmann M, Lindenmeyer MT, Sperhake JP, Wong MN, Allweiss L, et al. Multiorgan and renal tropism of SARS-CoV-2. N Engl J Med. 2020;383:590-2.
17. Huang C, Wang Y, Li X, Ren L, Zhao J, Fan G, et al. Clinical Features of patients infected with 2019 novel coronavirus in Wuhan, China. Lancet. 2020;395:497-506.
18. Fu Y, Cheng Y, Wu Y. Understanding SARS-CoV-2 mediated inflammatory responses: from mechanisms to potential therapeutic tools. Virol Sin. 2020;35(3):266-71.
19. Gomez H, Ince C, De Becker D. A unified theory of sepsis-induced acute kidney injury: inflammation, microcirculatory dysfunction, bioenergetics and the tubular cell adaptation to injury. Shock. 2014;41:3-11.
20. Catanzaro M, Fagiani F, Racchi M, Corsinin E, Govoni S, Lanni C. Immune response in COVID-19: addressing a pharmacological challenge by targeting pathways triggered by SARS-CoV-2. Signal Transduct Target Ther. 2020;5:84-90.
21. Iannacone G, Scacciavillani R, Del Buono MG, Camilli M, Ronco C, Lavie CJ, et al. Weathering the cytokine storm in COVID-19: Therapeutic implications. Cardiorenal Med. 2020;10:277-87.
22. Otsuka R, Seino K-I. Macrophage activation syndrome and COVID-19. Inflamm Regen. 2020;40:19.
23. Briet M, Schiffrin EL. Aldosterone effects on the kidney and cardiovascular system. Nat Rev Nephrol. 2010;6:261-73.
24. Cheng Y, Luo R, Wang K, Zhang M, Wang Z, Dong L, et al. Kidney disease is associated with in-hospital death of patients with COVID-19. Kidney Int. 2020;97:829-38.
25. Chan L, Chaudhury K, Saha A, Chauhan K, Vaid A, Zhao S, et al. AKI in hospitalised patients with COVID 19. J Am Soc Nephrol. 2021;32:151-60.
26. Mohammed MMB, Lukitsch I, Torres-Ortiz AE, Walker JB, Varghese V, Hernandez-Arroyo CF, et al. Acute kidney injury associated with coronavirus disease 2019 in urban New Orleans. Kidney 360. 2020;1:614-22.
27. Wang M, Xiong H, Chen H, Li Q, Ruan XZ. Renal injury by SARS-CoV-2 infection: a systemic review. Kidney Dis. 2021;7:100-10.
28. Akilesh S, Nast CC, Yamashita K, Henriksen K, Charu V, Troxell ML, et al. Multicenter clinicopathologic correlation of kidney biopsies presenting with acute kidney injury or proteinuria. Am J Kidney Dis. 2021;77:82-93.e1.
29. Sharma P, Uppal NN, Wancho R, Shah HH, Parikh R, Khanin Y, et al; on behalf of Northwell Nephrology COVID-19 Research Consortium. COVID-19-associated kidney injury: a case series of kidney biopsy findings. J Am Soc Nephrol. 2020;31:1948-58.
30. Fontana F, Cazzato S, Giovanella S, Ballestri M, Leonelli M, Mori G, et al. Oxalate nephropathy caused by excessive vitamin C administration in 2 patients with COVID-19. Kidney Int Rep. 2020;10:1815-22.
31. Stewart DJ, Hartley JC, Johnson M, Marks SD, du Pre P, Stojanovic J. Renal dysfunction in hospitalised children with COVID-19. Lancet Child Adolesc Health. 2020;4:e28-9.
32. Kudose S, Batal I, Santoriello D, Xu K, Barasch J, Peleg Y. Kidney biopsy findings in patients with COVID-19. J Am Soc Nephrol. 2020;31:1959-68.
33. Larsen CP, Bourne TD, Wilson JD, Saqqa O, Sharshir MA. Collapsing glomerulopathy in a patient with COVID-19. Kidney Int Rep. 2020;5(6):935-9.
34. Magoon S, Bichu P, Malhotra V, Alhashimi F, Hu Y, Khanna S, et al. COVID-19-related glomerulopathy: a report of 2 cases of collapsing focal segmental glomerulosclerosis. Kidney Med. 2020;2:488-92.
35. Ng JH, Bijol V, Sparks MA, Sise ME, Izzedine H, Jhaveri KD. Pathophysiology and pathology of acute kidney injury in patients with COVID-19. Adv Chronic Kidney Dis. 2020;27:365-76.
36. Shah SA, Carter HP. New-onset nephrotic syndrome in a child associated with COVID-19 infection. Front Pediatr. 2020;8:471.
37. Alvarado A, Franceschi, Resplandor E, Sumba J, Orta N. COVID-19 associated with onset nephrotic syndrome in a pediatric patient: coincidence or related conditions? Pediatr Nephrol. 2020;36(1):205-7.
38. Noris M, Benigni A, Remuzzi G. The case of complement activation in COVID-19 multi-organ impact. Kidney Int. 2020;98:314-22.
39. Sharma P, Ng JH, Bijol V, Jhaveri KD, Wanchoo R. Pathology of COVID-19 acute kidney injury. Clin Kidney J. 2021;14(Suppl 1):i30-9.
40. Jhaveri KD, Meir LR, Flores Chang BS, Parikh R, Wanchoo R, Barilla-LaBarca ML, et al. Thrombotic microangiopathy in a patient with COVID-19. Kidney Int. 2020;98:509-12.
41. Oi SSP, Muniz MPR, Faria IM, Filho NS, de Brito DJA, Lages JS, et al. Multisystemic inflammatory syndrome and thrombotic microangiopathy as complications of COVID-19 in a child: a case report. Front Pediatr. 2021;9:659069.
42. Lu X, Zhang L, Du H, Zhang Z, Li YY, Qu J, et al. SARS-CoV-2 infection in children. N Engl J Med. 2020;382:1663-5.
43. Brambilla I, Tosca M, De Filippo M, Licari A, Piccotti E, Marseglia G, et al. Special issues for coronavirus disease 2019 in children and adolescents. Obesity. 2020;28:1369-72.
44. Qiu H, Wu J, Hong, Luo Y, Song Q, Chen D. Clinical and epidemiological features of 36 children with coronavirus disease 2019 (COVID-19) in Zhejiang, China: an observational cohort study. Lancet Infect Dis. 2020;20:689-96.
45. Tullie L, Ford K, Bisharat M, Watson T, Thakkar H, Mullassery D, et al. Gastrointestinal features in children with COVID-19: an observation of varied presentation in eight children. Lancet Child Adolesc Health. 2020;4(7):E19-20.
46. Bjornstad EC, Krallman KA, Askenazi D, Zappitelli M, Goldstein SL, Basu RK; on behalf of the SPARC Investigators. Preliminary assessment of acute kidney injury in critically ill children associate with SARS-CoV-2 infection. A multicenter cross sectional analysis. Clin J Am Soc Nephrol. 2021;16:446-8.

47. Kari JA, Shalaby MA, Albanna AS, Alahmadi TS, Alherbish A,Alhasan KA. Acute kidney injury in children with COVID-19: a retrospective study. BMC Nephrol. 2021;22:202.
48. Samies NL, Pinninti S, James SH. Rhabdomyolysis and acute renal failure in an adolescent with coronavirus disease 2019. J Pediatr Infect Dis Soc. 2020;9:507-9.
49. Diorio C, McNerney KO, Lambert M, Paessler M, Anderson EM, Henrickson SE, et al. Evidence of thrombotic microangiopathy in children with SARS-CoV-2 across the spectrum of clinical presentations. Blood Adv. 2020;23:6051-63.
50. Riphagen S, Gomez X, Gonzalez-Martinwz C, Wilkinson N, Theocharis P. Hyperinflammatory shock in children during COVID-19 pandemic. Lancet. 2020:395:1607-8.
51. Royal College of Paediatrics and Child Health. Guidance: paediatric multisystem inflammatory syndrome temporally associated with COVID-19. [online] Available from www.rcpch.ac.uk/resources/guidance-paediatric-multisystem-inflammatory-syndrome-temporally-associated-covid-19. [Last accessed May, 2022].
52. Centers for Disease Control and Prevention. Emergency preparedness and response: multisystem inflammatory syndrome in children (MIS-C) associated with coronavirus disease 2019 (COVID-19).Health advisory. [online] Available from https://emergency.cdc.gov/han/2020/han00432.asp [Last accessed May, 2022].
53. WHO. (2020). Multisystem inflammatory syndrome in children and adolescents with COVID-19. Scientific brief. [online] Available from www.who.int/publications-detail/multisystem-inflammatory-syndrome-in-children-and adolescents-with-covid-19 [Last accessed May, 2022].
54. Jain S, Sen S, Lakshmivenkateshiah S, Bobhate P, Venkatesh S, Udani S, et al. Multisystem inflammatory syndrome in children in children with COVID-19 in Mumbai, India. Indian Pediatrics. 2020;57:1015-9.
55. Grifoni E, Veloriani A, Cei F, Lian J, Gu J, Zhang S, et al. Interleukin-6 as prognosticator in patients with COVID-19. J Infect Dis. 2020;81:452-82.
56. Pouletty M, Borocco C, Ouldali N, Caseris M, Basmaci R, Lachaume N, et al. Paediatric multisystem inflammatory syndrome temporally associated with SARS-CoV-2 mimicking Kawasaki disease (Kawa-COVID-19): a multicentre cohort. Ann Rheum Dis. 2020;79:999-1006.
57. Lipton M, Mahajan R, Kavanagh C, Shen C, Batal I, Dogra S, et al. AKI in COVID-19-associated multisystem inflammatory syndrome in children (MIS-C). Kidney 360. 2021;2:611-8.
58. Basalely A, Gurusinghe S, Schneider J, Shah SS, Siegel LB, Pollack G, et al. Acute kidney injury in pediatric patients hospitalized with acute COVID-19 and multisystem inflammatory syndrome in children associated with COVID-19. Kidney Int. 2021;100:138-45.
59. Mastranglo A, Morello W, Vidal E, Guzzo I, Petruzzelli LA, Bennetti E, et al. Impact of COVID-19 pandemic in children with CKD or immunosuppression. CJASN. 2021;16:449-51.
60. Varnell Jr C, Harshman LA, Smith L, Liu C, Chen S, Al-Akash S, et al. COVID-19 in pediatric kidney transplantation: the Improving Renal Outcomes Collaborative. Sm J Transplant. 2021;21:2740-8.
61. MoHFW. Guidelines for management of COVID-19 in children. [online] Available from https://www.mohfw.gov.in [Last accessed May, 2022].
62. Vasudevan A, Mantan M, Krishnamurthy S, Pais P, Mathew G, Hari P, et al.; for the Indian Society of Pediatric Nephrology. Managing children with renal diseases during COVID-19 pandemic. Indian Pediatr. 2020;57:641-52.
63. Marlais M, Wlodkowski T, Al-Akash S, Ananin P, Bandi VK, Baudouin V, et al. COVID-19 in children treated with immunosuppressive medication for kidney diseases. Arch Dis Child. 2020;106(8):798-801.
64. Raina R, Chakraborty R, Sethi SK, Bunchman T. Kidney replacement therapy in COVID-19 induced kidney failure and septic shock: a pediatric continuous renal replacement therapy (PCRRT) position on emergency preparedness with resource allocation. Front Pediatr. 2020;8; 413.
65. Deep A, Bansal M, Ricci Z. Acute kidney injury and special considerations during renal replacement therapy in children with Coronavirus Disease-19: Perspective from the Critical care nephrology section of the European Society of Paediatric and Neonatal Intensive Care. Blood Purif. 2021;50(2):150-60.
66. Shen Q, Wang M, Che R, Li Q, Zhou J, Wang F, et al. Consensus recommendations for the care of children receiving chronic dialysis in association with the COVID-19 epidemic. Pediatr Nephrol. 2020;35:1351-7.
67. Teoh CW, Gaudreault-Tremblay M-M, Blydt-H TD, Goldberg A, Arora S, Feber J, et al; on behalf of the CST Pediatric Group. Management of pediatric kidney transplant patients during the COVID-19 pandemic: guidance from the Canadian Society of Transplantation Pediatric Group. Canadian J Kidney Health Dis. 2020;7:1-18.
68. Hanan C, Herrera Hernandez LP, Bu L, Kizilbash S, Najera L, Rheault M, et al. IgA nephropathy presenting as macroscopic hematuria in 2 pediatric patients after receiving the Pfizer COVID-19 vaccine. Kidney Int. 2021;100(3):P705-6.

CHAPTER

14.5

Ethics and Pediatric Nephrology: Basic Insights

Priya Pais

INTRODUCTION

The practice of medicine is considered a profession (as opposed to a business enterprise) because physicians have a calling to *care* for and not just *treat* the patient.

In 1996, the Hastings Center, a key bioethics forum, listed these four key "Goals of Medicine":

1. Prevention of disease and promotion of health[1]
2. Relief of pain and suffering from disease
3. Care and cure of those with disease and care for those who cannot be cured
4. Avoidance of premature death and pursuit of peaceful death

These goals define the importance of the doctor-patient relationship in the medical profession. The physician has an obligation to do what is ethically (morally) right for the patient.[2]

PRINCIPLES OF MEDICAL ETHICS

Medical ethics is a set of principles governing the moral conduct of healthcare professionals. In order to guide physicians to make moral decisions, Beauchamp and Childress in 1979 outlined four principles to follow in medical practice.[3] These are nonhierarchical, meaning that all are equally important and one principle is not more important than others.

1. *Principle of beneficence:* The physician is expected to "do good" and act in the best interest of the patient. The health of the patient is of primary consideration.
2. *Principle of nonmaleficence:* It refers to the principle of "Do no harm." The physician must be competent to provide care and ensure the patient's safety while minimizing risk.
3. *Principle of autonomy:* The patient has the right to decide regarding his own treatment. The physician must help the patient make an informed decision, take consent for procedures, and maintain the confidentiality of the patient.
4. *Principle of justice:* The physician must provide an equal standard of care to all the patients without discrimination based on age, religion, or social standing.

Pediatric Bioethics

While caring for children, the pediatrician and the parent are co-fiduciaries (acting in the best interest) of the child who is a patient. Parents have the authority to make decisions on behalf of their child, but they should not refuse medically reasonable alternatives. When parents and pediatricians do not agree on a treatment choice, conflict can arise. In India and most low-resource settings, parental authority is almost absolute. Parents may be within their legal rights to refuse a life-saving treatment and leave against medical advice. This leads to significant distress among pediatric healthcare providers. Therefore, when such conflicts of opinion regarding the treatment arise, it is important to recognize them as *ethical dilemmas*, which may open the door to further counseling and joint decision-making.

ETHICAL DILEMMAS FOR THE PEDIATRIC NEPHROLOGIST

While caring for children with kidney disease, pediatric nephrologists are faced with several unique ethical challenges, arising from not only financial hardship but also broader systemic societal issues.

Common Ethical Dilemmas in Routine Practice

- *Parental refusal of common but invasive procedures:*
  Example: Refusal of micturating cystourethrogram (MCU) in a child with recurrent UTIs.
  The pediatric nephrologist may recommend an MCU guided by the principle of beneficence, to do what is best for the child. The discomfort associated with an MCU is viewed as a minor in comparison to the clinical benefits of this procedure. However, the parents may view this invasive procedure as "harmful" to the child and refuse.
- *Nonadherence to treatment based on family beliefs:*
  Example: Discontinuation of steroids and use of native medications in a child with nephrotic syndrome
  While parents may express their autonomy based on their own cultural beliefs, children have a right to be protected from such medically harmful decisions.

- *Presymptomatic genetic screening for adult-onset disease: Example: A parent with autosomal-dominant polycystic kidney disease (ADPKD) demands genetic testing for his asymptomatic 5-year-old child.*

In such a scenario, there is no clinical indication for testing. The parent may feel that he is within his rights to decide on behalf of the child. However, a positive result may lead to significant stress and anxiety when the child is older, even if he remains asymptomatic. Presymptomatic genetic testing should be performed only when the patient is old enough to participate in decision-making and provide assent (permission).

Dealing with Ethical Dilemmas

Acknowledging that pediatric nephrologists may face frequent ethical dilemmas in patient care, it is important to remember that conflict resolution is best achieved by keeping the best interests of the patient as the primary goal of treatment. Most often, repeated counseling by the physician and an attitude of patience will achieve the required result. Involving the family in each step of decision-making, providing explanations for why a course of action is advised, is critical.

Although time-consuming, these measures will most often resolve the dilemma. However, a "hospital/clinical ethics committee" should be consulted if conflicts are not resolved. A hospital ethics committee should ideally be available in most large hospitals and consists of a group of individuals (doctors, nurses, social workers, and bioethicists). The committee begins by understanding the problem and all points of view, facilitates the discussion, and provides an ethical analysis using bioethical principles, literature review of similar cases, and legal policies. A course of action is then advised, but final decision-making remains with the physician and the family.

SPECIAL ETHICAL CHALLENGES IN PEDIATRIC CHRONIC KIDNEY DISEASE IN LOW-RESOURCE SETTINGS

Refusal of Life-saving Treatment

When advised for the need for dialysis, parents sometimes refuse, for reasons that are unclear, but not solely due to financial difficulties.[4-6] In these circumstances, continuing to care for the child becomes increasingly difficult for the pediatric nephrologist. When a life-saving treatment is clearly indicated, it is morally distressing for the physician to withhold dialysis, due to lack of parental consent. In high-income countries, when parents refuse dialysis, pediatric nephrologists can request social services to intervene. In the absence of social services in countries such as India, removal of the child from the home is not feasible. Are we obligated to continue treating the child, providing only conservative therapy when dialysis is available? Traditionally, conservative care for kidney failure is reserved for those whom dialysis is considered medically futile (the elderly, those with limited life expectancy).

Conservative Care for End-stage Kidney Disease

Families of children with end-stage kidney disease (ESKD) are unable to access dialysis services, either due to the lack of pediatric chronic kidney disease (CKD) care in the vicinity or because they are unable to afford to pay for dialysis. Even if the dialysis is initiated, the high out-of-pocket costs often prove burdensome and drive the entire family into debt. Typically, in low-resource settings, decision-making is deferred to the healthcare team. Should pragmatic consideration of the family's circumstances influence our family counseling? Pediatric nephrologists are often faced with the dilemma of advising harsh pragmatism versus pursuing solely what is in the best interest of the child. However, in our low-resource settings, we are obligated to provide care to patients (and families) even if they choose to withhold dialysis.

Ethical Dilemmas in Kidney Transplantation

Children have inequitable access to kidney transplantation. In low-resource countries, there are few pediatric transplant centers. Finally, there is no national organ-sharing network, and children are not prioritized in the organ-allocation policies. This leads to long wait times, accumulating costs, and the unrelenting burden of care. Children are at a disadvantage when the approach to allocation is based on a "first-come-first-serve" or a utilitarian approach [in a society where the value of an earning adult (often male) is placed above a child's rights].[7]

In settings where ideal treatment is not possible, pediatric nephrologists may be required to care for their patient in the best possible way, offering conservative care, palliation, and end-of-life comfort measures.

CONCLUSION

Pediatric nephrologists often face challenges in determining the "correct" course of treatment, in the context of a particular child and his/her family circumstances. Relying on the principles of medical ethics and not just one's "feelings" is the best way to promote the best interests of patients and avoid moral distress. Recognizing that we are faced with an ethical dilemma is the first step toward conflict resolution. This should open the door to mutual discussion of all points of view and shared decision-making.

KEY POINTS

- The principles of biomedical ethics should guide medical decision-making.
- Four common principles of biomedical ethics are "beneficence," "nonmaleficence," "autonomy," and "justice."

- Pediatric nephrologists frequently face ethical challenges in their daily practice, especially when dealing with pediatric CKD, dialysis, and transplant.
- Resolving ethical dilemmas require mutual discussion, repeated counseling of parents, and openness to shared decision-making.
- A hospital ethics committee is a valuable resource to utilize when are difficulties in resolving conflicts remain despite the efforts mentioned in the above point.

REFERENCES

1. The Hastings Center. The goals of medicine: setting new priorities. Hastings Cent Rep. 1996;26(6):1-6.
2. Timms O. Biomedical Ethics, 2nd edition. Bengaluru: St John's National Academy of Health Sciences; 2019.
3. Ross LF. Theory and practice of pediatric bioethics. Perspect Biol Med. 2016;58(3):267-80.
4. Lantos JD, Saleem S, Raza F, Syltern J, Khoo EJ, Iyengar A, et al. Clinical ethics in pediatrics: an international perspective. J Clin Ethics. 2019;30(1):35-45.
5. Wightman AG, Freeman MA. Update on ethical issues in pediatric dialysis: has pediatric dialysis become morally obligatory? Clin J Am Soc Nephrol. 2016;11(8):1456-62.
6. Pais P, Iyengar A, Wightman A. POS-681 ethical challenges in providing kidney replacement therapy (KRT) for pediatric end stage kidney disease: case series from a referral centre in India. Kidney Int Rep. 2021;6(4):S297-8.
7. Pais P, Blydt-Hansen TD, Michael Raj JA, Dello Strologo L, Iyengar A. Low renal transplantation rates in children with end-stage kidney disease: a study of barriers in a low-resource setting. Pediatr Transplant. 2021;25(2):e13867.

CHAPTER

14.6 Transition to Adult Nephrology: The Handoff

Edwin Fernando M

INTRODUCTION

The transition from pediatric to adult medical services is an important time in the life of an adolescent or young adult with a renal disorder. Transitioning medical care during a time that is filled with social and emotional challenges is a complex process. There are a lot of questions that need to be answered.

- Are they ready?
- Are they going to cope well?
- Will they be able to fulfill their dreams and life goals?
- Are these feelings similar to what one encounters when dropping their child off at college?

Failure of proper transition can lead to medical non-adherence and subsequent loss of follow-up, which could be detrimental to the patient's health **(Flowchart 1)**.

BARRIERS IN TRANSITION OF CARE

There is a growing body of research on transitioning patients with chronic conditions from pediatric to adult care.[1-3] Young adult patients face many challenges throughout this transition process. Some challenges include:[4]

- Difficulty navigating to adult healthcare systems
- Gaps in insurance coverage
- Patient's developmental age
- Lack of health self-efficacy
- Limited experience in self-management
- Patient or family being hesitant to change the care provider
- Lack of financial support for the transition of services

Transition programs have been developed to support the transfer to adult care and to reduce patient vulnerabilities and

Flowchart 1: Algorithm for transition of care.

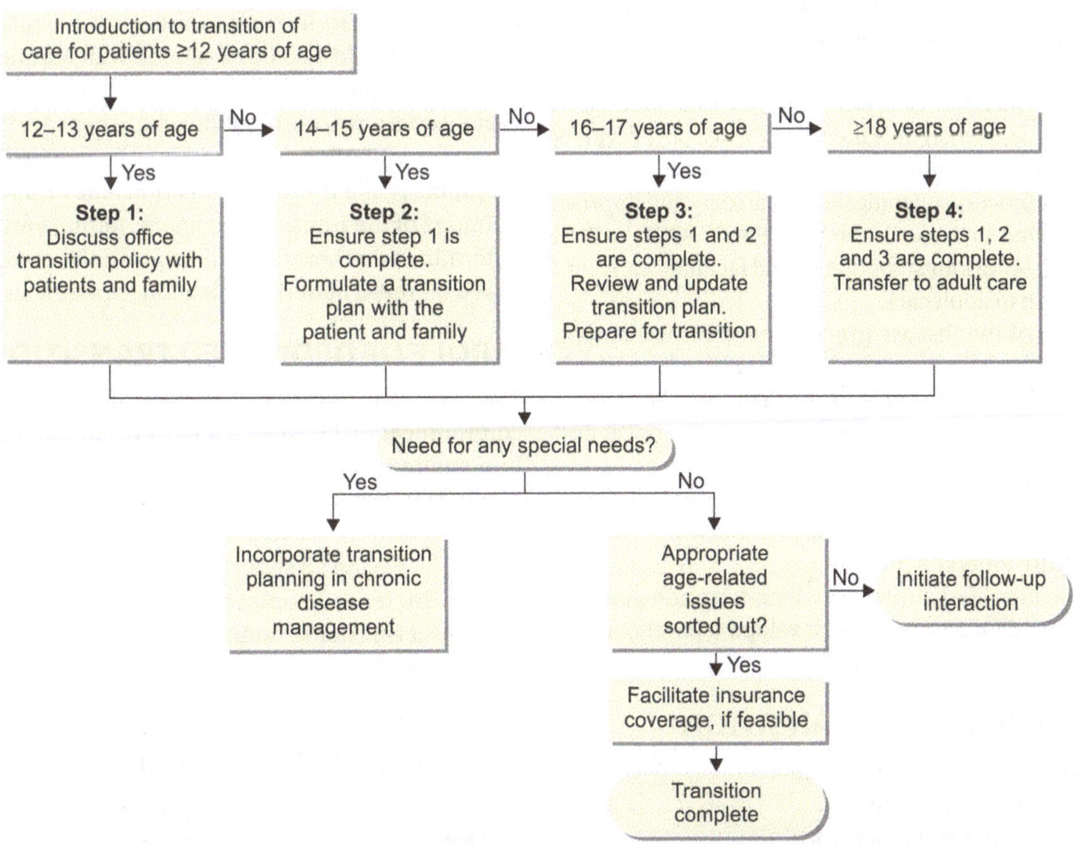

Source: Adapted from McPherson M, et al. A new definition of children with special health care needs. Pediatrics. 1998;102:137-140. doi: 10.1542/peds.102.1.137

interruptions in care. The International Society of Nephrology and the International Pediatric Nephrology Association released a consensus statement which considered 15 components of transition and transfer essential, outlining the ideal clinical management of young adult patients.[5] Since the release of these guidelines in 2011, there has been a growing interest in evaluating transition programs. Several studies highlight the effect of different transition procedures and specialized care (e.g., young adult clinics).[6,7] However, clinical implementation of guidance provided by the consensus statements can be difficult and may, in addition, be hampered by economic and human resource shortages. While most research has focused on clinical outcomes to determine the effectiveness of transition programs, little work has been done to evaluate patients' viewpoints of a transition program.

RECOMMENDED WAYS FOR TRANSITION

The potential (or real) communication barrier could make the process of healthcare transition more challenging. And the only sure way to address this is to have a conversation with the patient and the family. Learn the patients' and their families' language. The process of healthcare transition involves patients, families, healthcare providers, healthcare systems, and the community. The process of transition of care should begin early, at around 12–14 years,[8] continuing until 24–26 years. This might seem very early and a long daunting process. But once patients reach adolescence, they get busier with their personal lives and education, not to mention peer pressure. Starting the process by helping them to understand their disease and the need for compliance to medications can be the first step. Once the fear of the unknown disappears, it can lead to the emergence of more responsible and independent behaviors. Encouraging patients to ask questions will allow us to know them as individuals and could also help them when they meet their new care providers during and after the transition. Involving patients and families in every step of this process can mitigate their anxiety and improve accountability. One such tool is the RISE PROTOCOL,[9] which includes the following four steps that would facilitate early and smooth transition to adult care:

1. Recognition of the disease process, need for transplant, and the healthcare system
2. Insight into the short- and long-term impact of their illness, treatment, consequences of nonadherence, and emotional needs
3. Self-reliance in seeking medical care, making appointments, and self-identifying changes in health status that would require emergency care
4. Establish healthy lifestyle practices, long-term adherence to medicines, and follow-up visits, developing psychosocial, educational, and vocational skills.

CORE ELEMENTS OF TRANSITION

There are six core elements of transition:[9]

1. Developing a transition policy
2. Transition tracking and monitoring
3. Assessing readiness for transition
4. Transition planning
5. Transfer of care
6. Transition completion

Research indicates that successful transition to adult care requires a structured, individualized transition clinic where pediatric and adult providers collaborate on the plan of care. Despite this, many chronically ill young adults do not participate in established transition programs and/or are not educated about their transition process. The adult specialists, whenever encountering newly transitioned patients, have to understand that these are survivors of complex health conditions, who may have cognitive impairment and must deal with the challenges associated with a difficult age in life. A major difference between pediatric and adult care centers is multidisciplinary team support, usually more plenteous in pediatrics and limited in adult settings. Patients transitioning to adult care would benefit from a more comprehensive description of various care providers and referrals in the adult care environment. Patience is the key.

Patients' perceptions of their transition to adult care are instrumental in improving the quality of transition clinic programs. Transition programs will benefit from communicating with patients, clarifying their perception of transition timing. The pediatric team should initiate discussion earlier regarding the opportunity to transition to adult care. Similarly, conversations about the roles of all adult care providers and how to navigate between them should be clear. The adult care providers should incorporate a discussion about the roles of providers and acknowledge that treatment may change with moving to the adult hospital. Transition programs should also be expanded with additional activities that nurture patients' independence during early adult care visits. Additional coordination with other specialty transition programs is another planned improvement to this transition program. While these modifications may improve patients' opinions of the transition program, future work is needed to determine whether they will improve the clinical outcomes based on these patients' transition experiences.

ROLE OF DEDICATED TRANSITION CLINICS

The use of a dedicated transition clinic can improve communication between teams by having all parties involved in a single clinic.[9] Joint appointments with pediatric and adult teams would help foster bidirectional communication. This will also increase patient contact with the healthcare system by having all services delivered in a single day in one facility. Increased contact has been shown to be part of a successful transfer to adult services. Patients' perceptions of their transition timing should be considered by physicians, especially in the severely ill.

KEY GROUPS INVOLVED IN TRANSITION

The seamless efforts of the key teams in transition optimize and facilitate the process completion. These include:[10]

- The patient and family

- Pediatric care providers
- Transition team (adult nephrologist, pediatric nephrologist, allied health professional, social worker, transition coordinator, and community resource provider)
- Adult care providers
- Primary care providers

CHALLENGES FACED BY THE PATIENT AND FAMILY

For the patients, the foremost challenge is that this transition process coincides with a stage filled with major life changes.[10] During adolescence, there is greater opportunity in risk-seeking behavior, added to a poor understanding regarding the underlying condition. The disease condition may limit the overall neurological development which may impair decision-making during further treatment visits. Meanwhile, the family may face difficulties in promoting the patient's autonomy over their caregiving attitude. It may be complicated further by legal aspects of the doctor–patient relationship, due to which the family may no longer be included while discussing certain treatment options. This shall be overcome by educating the patient about their medical condition, and the limitations that the family members shall face in further phases of transit.

CHALLENGES FACED BY THE TREATING TEAM

Of these groups, the pediatric and adult care providers also have their individual barriers that are needed to be overcome.[10] For instance, the long relationship of the pediatrician with the patient may lead to a parental approach finding it difficult to "let go" off the patient. The pediatric care provider is required to hold the responsibility of safe transit while training the young individual to self-report, identifying signs of deterioration in health, and seek their needs and help them understand terms of privacy and confidentiality, because lack of self-management in these growing individuals may translate into poor overall care. Adequate steps need to be taken by the pediatric care provider to familiarize with the community resources and to establish unlimited contact with the adult care provider.

With respect to the adult care provider, the challenges of catering to the needs of smaller adolescent population, in a scenario of preexisting overwhelming patient load, are plentiful. He may not have access to all previous relevant clinical information. He may have minimal expertise in managing childhood disorders in adulthood and may be unfamiliar with psychological issues associated with the disease complex. To overcome these difficulties, the adult care provider needs focused training on adolescent healthcare and develop tolerance toward health risk behavior and immaturity in the young while establishing a rapport with the patient along with his previous care provider.

PRACTICE TOOLS DURING TRANSITION

Some of the practice measures, if followed meticulously, shall help a great deal in the smooth transition to adult care.[11] These measures include:

- Dedicated transition clinics
- Written transition plan
- Checklist of achievement of age-appropriate milestones
- Assuming responsibilities in healthcare, education, financial, and social matters
- Assessment of readiness to transit through questionnaires
- Exchange of treatment guidelines, protocols between an adult and pediatric nephrologist
- Collaboration with adult end-stage kidney disease (ESKD) team

TRANSITION IN CHILDREN WITH CHRONIC KIDNEY DISEASE AND AFTER KIDNEY TRANSPLANTATION

The impact of chronic kidney disease (CKD) on adolescents and young adults can be challenging. Transplanted patients are at very high risk for severe and irreversible complications, resulting from an unsuccessful transition. For adolescents and young adults with pediatric-onset CKD, risk factors associated with the high cardiovascular mortality rate begin early, with calcium–phosphate imbalance, chronic inflammation interspersed with acute illnesses, hypertension, fluid overload, and anemia. Minimizing complications frequently requires close adherence to complex and restrictive, medical regimens, particularly for those on dialysis. However, in addition, frequent visits in the outpatient clinics and many long-term stays in the hospital with possible interventions necessary can minimize the adherence of these patients. Skipping medications and forgetting appointments and poor adherence to fluid restriction before transplantation by such noncompliant patients will lead to severe and irreversible damage. The complicated lives of adolescents on dialysis are often made more challenging by the need for transition. This has also been reported for treatments of other severe chronic health conditions such as diabetes, cystic fibrosis, or organ transplant, possibly resulting in life-threatening complications. Low adherence in teenage years leads to various consequences for patients themselves, their families, and the healthcare system. For chronic conditions, low adherence increases morbidity and medical complications (hospitalization) and contributes to poorer quality of life (fatigue and absenteeism in school) and an overuse of the healthcare system (unnecessary medical consults and investigations). Low adherence increases healthcare costs and may lead a healthcare team to withhold treatment. Among transplant recipients, especially graft loss is most frequently encountered at the age of 16–24 years, primarily due to nonadherence to treatment and difficulty in obtaining insurance services for medical care once adolescence gets over.[11] Among these patients aged 15–19 years, cardiovascular event rates are nearly 1,000-fold higher than those of their age-matched peers, and the mortality rate for those aged 25–34 years is similar to that of 75-year-olds in the general population. In the case of organ transplantation, low adherence is a leading cause of graft rejection and may cause death.[12-14]

CONCLUSION

With the growing need to deliver care for adolescent individuals, a structured transition process becomes mandatory to facilitate the same. The key investment in this process remains detailed communication among both the provider and the recipient of the medical services. Thus, an optimized transition from pediatric to adult renal services would go a long way in preventing poor medical outcomes and decreased hospitalization rates, which shall render the affected youth productive to self and the community.

KEY POINTS

- Healthcare transition from pediatric- to adult-focused care defines transition of care.
- Transition of care demands a multidisciplinary team framework and is a critical need in the kidney care of adolescents.
- Steps in transition care need to be implemented in children from the age of 12 years up to 18 years and include the following steps:
    1. Explain transition policy to parents.
    2. Share the transition plan with parents.
    3. Prepare for transition.
    4. Complete transfer of patient.
- Specific issues of the child and consideration of insurance facilities need focus during transfer of care.

REFERENCES

1. Staa AV, Sattoe JN. Young adults' experiences and satisfaction with the transfer of care. J Adolesc Health. 2014;55:796-803.
2. Yee J. Pediatric-to-adult nephrology: the handoff. Adv Chronic Kidney Dis. 2011;18(5):313-4.
3. Rapley P, Davidson PM. Enough of the problem: a review of time for health care transition solutions for young adults with a chronic illness. J Clin Nurs. 2010;19(3-4):313-23.
4. Watson AR. Problems and pitfalls of transition from paediatric to adult renal care. Pediatr Nephrol. 2005;20:113-7.
5. Watson AR, Harden P, Ferris M, Kerr PG, Mahan J, Ramzy MF. Transition from pediatric to adult renal services: a consensus statement by the International Society of Nephrology (ISN) and the International Pediatric Nephrology Association (IPNA). Pediatr Nephrol. 2011;26:1753-7.
6. Kennedy A, Sawyer S. Transition from pediatric to adult services: are we getting it right? Curr Opin Pediatr. 2008;20:403-9.
7. Hattori M, Iwano M, Sako M, Honda M, Okada H, Akioka Y, et al. Transition of adolescent and young adult patients with childhood-onset chronic kidney disease from pediatric to adult renal services: a nationwide survey in Japan. Clin Exp Nephrol. 2016;20:918-25.
8. West NE, Mogayzel Jr PJ. Transitions in health care: what can we learn from our experience with cystic fibrosis? Pediatr Clin North Am. 2016;63:88797.
9. Raina R, Wang J, Krishnappa V, Ferris M. Pediatric renal transplantation: focus on current transition care and proposal of the "RISE to transition" protocol. Ann Transplant. 2018;23:45-60.
10. Bower WF, Christie D, DeGennaro M, Latthe P, Raes A, Romao RLP, et al. The transition of young adults with lifelong urological needs from pediatric to adult services: an International Children's Continence Society position statement. Neurourol Urodyn. 2017;36(3):811-9.
11. Lam WY, Fresco P. Medication adherence measures: an overview. BioMed Res Int. 2015;2015:217047.
12. Foster BJ. Heightened graft failure risk during emerging adulthood and transition to adult care. Pediatr Nephrol. 2015;30:567-76.
13. Akchurin OM, Melamed ML, Hashim BL, Kaskel FJ, Del Rio M. Medication adherence in the transition of adolescent kidney transplant recipients to the adult care. Pediatr Transplant. 2014;18:538-48.
14. Dobbels F, Ruppar T, De Geest S, Decorte A, Van Damme-Lombaerts R, Fine RN. Adherence to the immunosuppressive regimen in pediatric kidney transplant recipients: a systematic review. Pediatr Transplant. 2010;14:603-13.

SECTION

15

Clinical Practice Resources

CHAPTER

15.1 Nomograms in Pediatric Nephrology

Kiran Sathe, Amish Udani

GROWTH CHARTS BY INDIAN ACADEMY OF PEDIATRICS (IAP) FOR INDIAN CHILDREN

- Girls height and weight charts 0–18 years **(Fig. 1)**[1]
- Boys height and weight charts 0–18 years **(Fig. 2)**[1]
- Girls 5–18 years IAP body mass index charts **(Fig. 3)**[2]
- Boys 5–18 years IAP body mass index charts **(Fig. 4)**[2]
- *World Health Organization (WHO) charts:* 0–5 years girls length/height, weight and head circumference charts **(Fig. 5)**[3]
- WHO charts; 0–5 years boys length/height, weight, and head circumference charts **(Fig. 6)**[3]
- WHO girls weight for height/length charts **(Fig. 7)**[3]
- WHO boys weight for length/height charts **(Fig. 8)**[3]

WEST NOMOGRAM: ESTIMATING BODY SURFACE AREA OF INFANTS AND YOUNG CHILDREN

To determine the BSA of a child, draw a straight line between the child's height and weight. The body surface area (BSA) in square meters is the point where this line crosses the surface area scale **(Fig. 9)**.[4]

BLOOD PRESSURE CENTILE CHARTS FOR CHILDREN

- Blood pressure (BP) levels for boys by age and height percentile **(Table 1)**[5]
- BP levels for girls by age and height percentile **(Table 2)**[5]

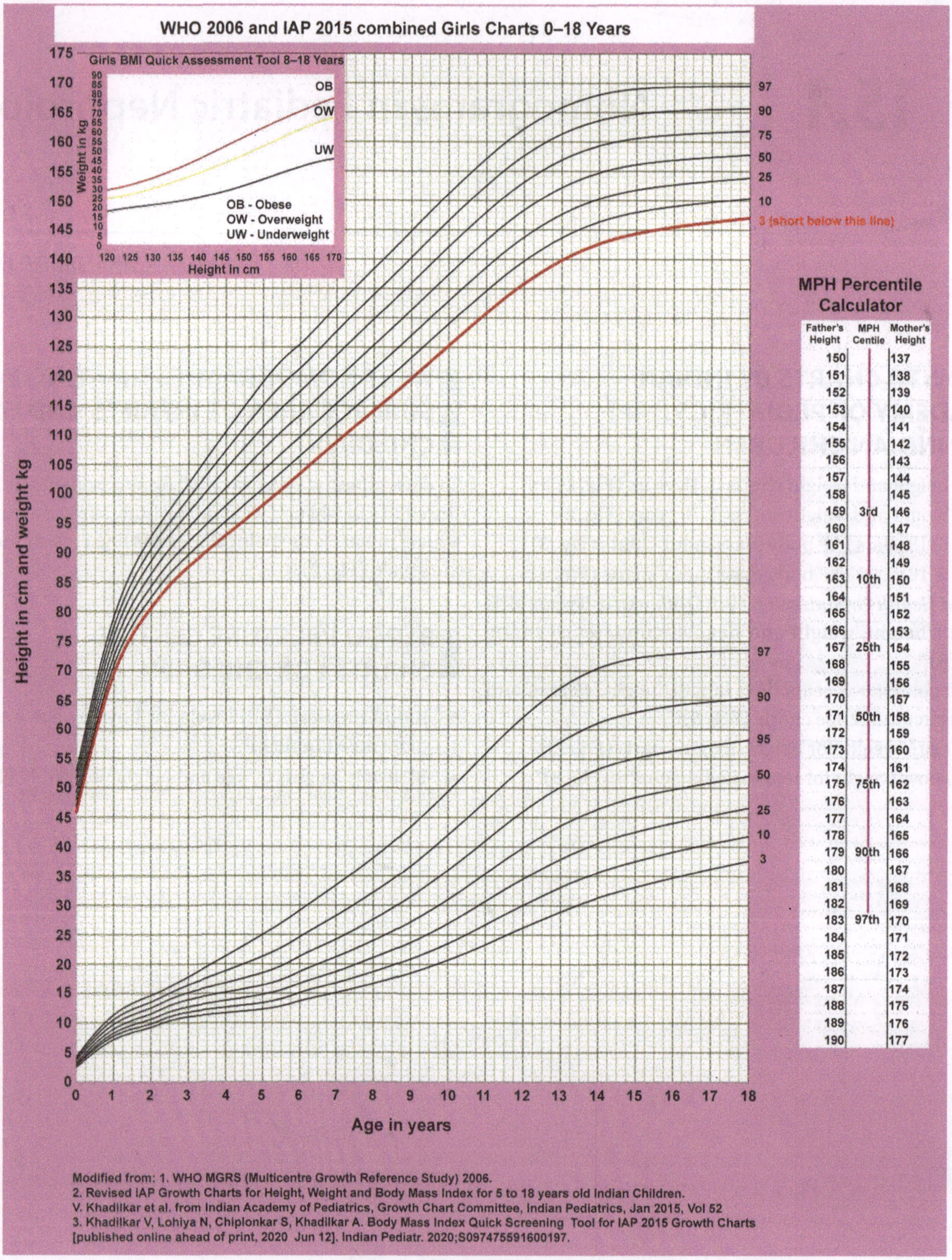

Fig. 1: Girls height and weight charts 0–18 years.

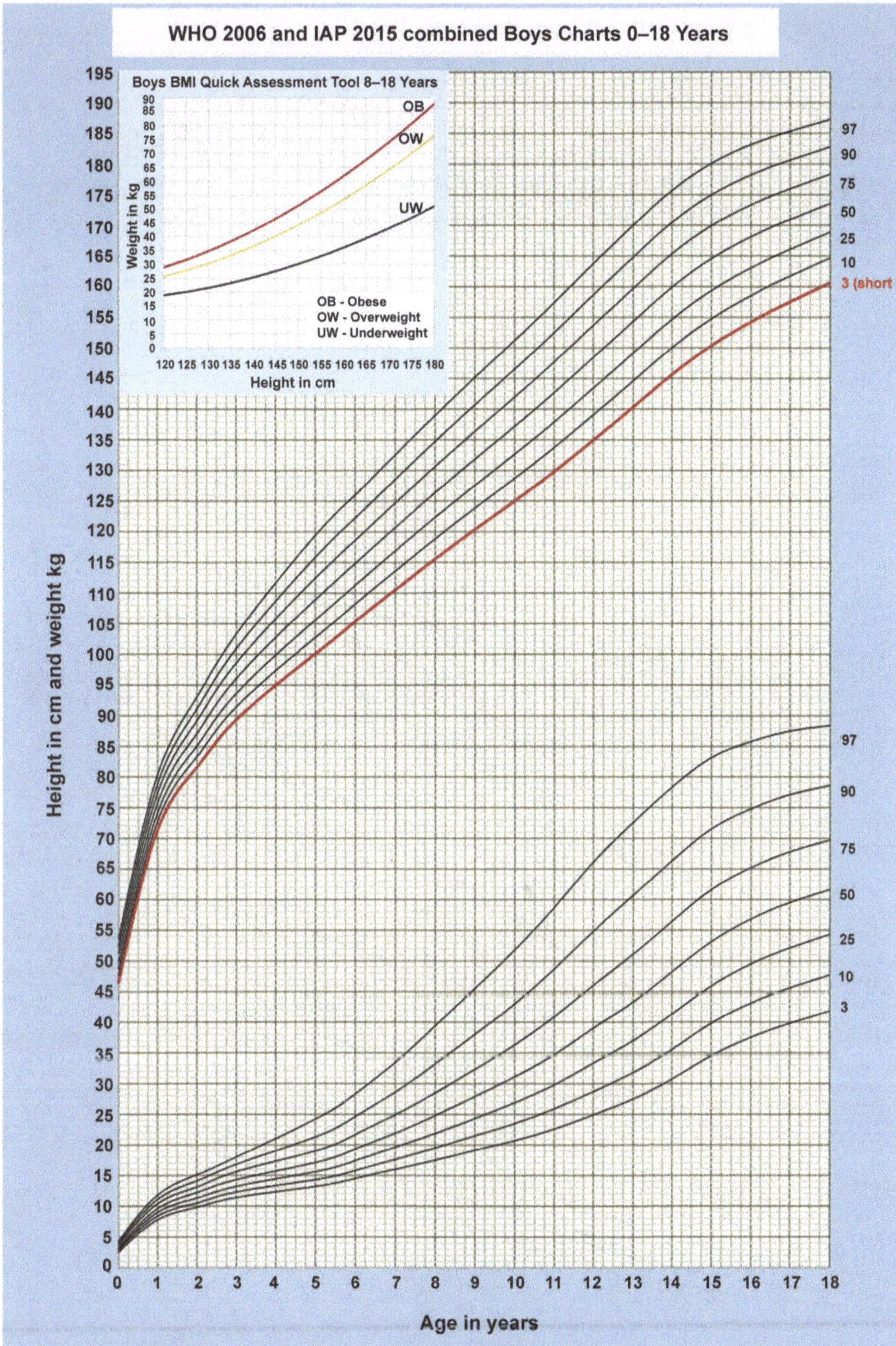

MPH Percentile Calculator

Father's Height	MPH Centile	Mother's Height
150		137
151		138
152		139
153		140
154		141
155		142
156		143
157		144
158	3rd	145
159		146
160		147
161		148
162		149
163	10th	150
164		151
165		152
166		153
167		154
168	25th	155
169		156
170		157
171		158
172		159
173	50th	160
174		161
175		162
176		163
177		164
178	75th	165
179		166
180		167
181		168
182	90th	169
183		170
184		171
185		172
186		173
187	97th	174
188		175
189		176
190		177

Modified from: 1. WHO MGRS (Multicentre Growth Reference Study) 2006.
2. Revised IAP Growth Charts for Height, Weight and Body Mass Index for 5 to 18 years old Indian Children. V. Khadilkar et al. from Indian Academy of Pediatrics, Growth Chart Committee, Indian Pediatrics, Jan 2015, Vol 52
3. Khadilkar V, Lohiya N, Chiplonkar S, Khadilkar A. Body Mass Index Quick Screening Tool for IAP 2015 Growth Charts [published online ahead of print, 2020 Jun 12]. Indian Pediatr. 2020;S097475591600197.

Fig. 2: Boys height and weight charts 0–18 years.

5 to 18 Years : IAP Girls Body Mass Index Charts

Name ______________________

DOB ______________________

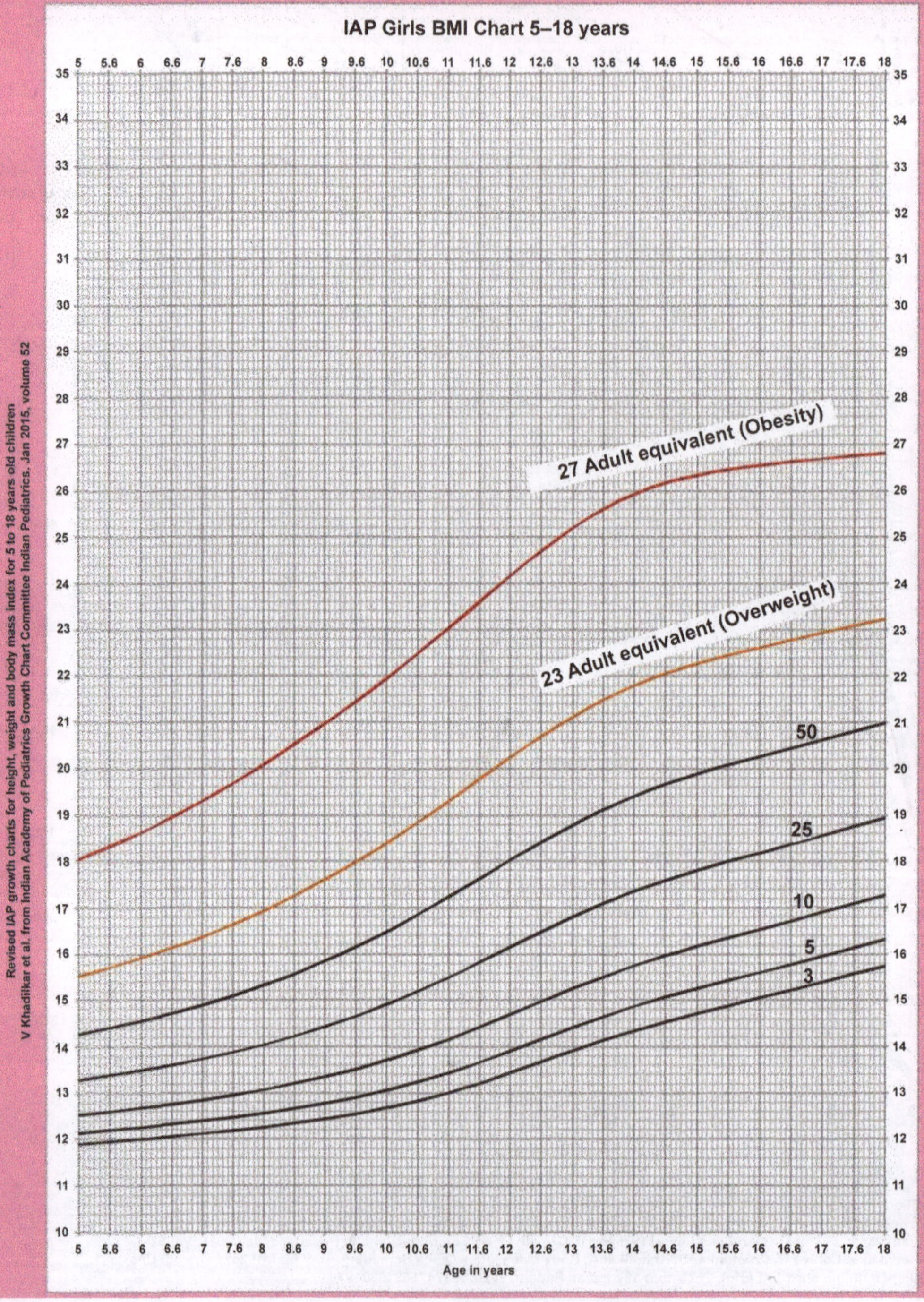

Fig. 3: Girls 5–18 years IAP body mass index charts.

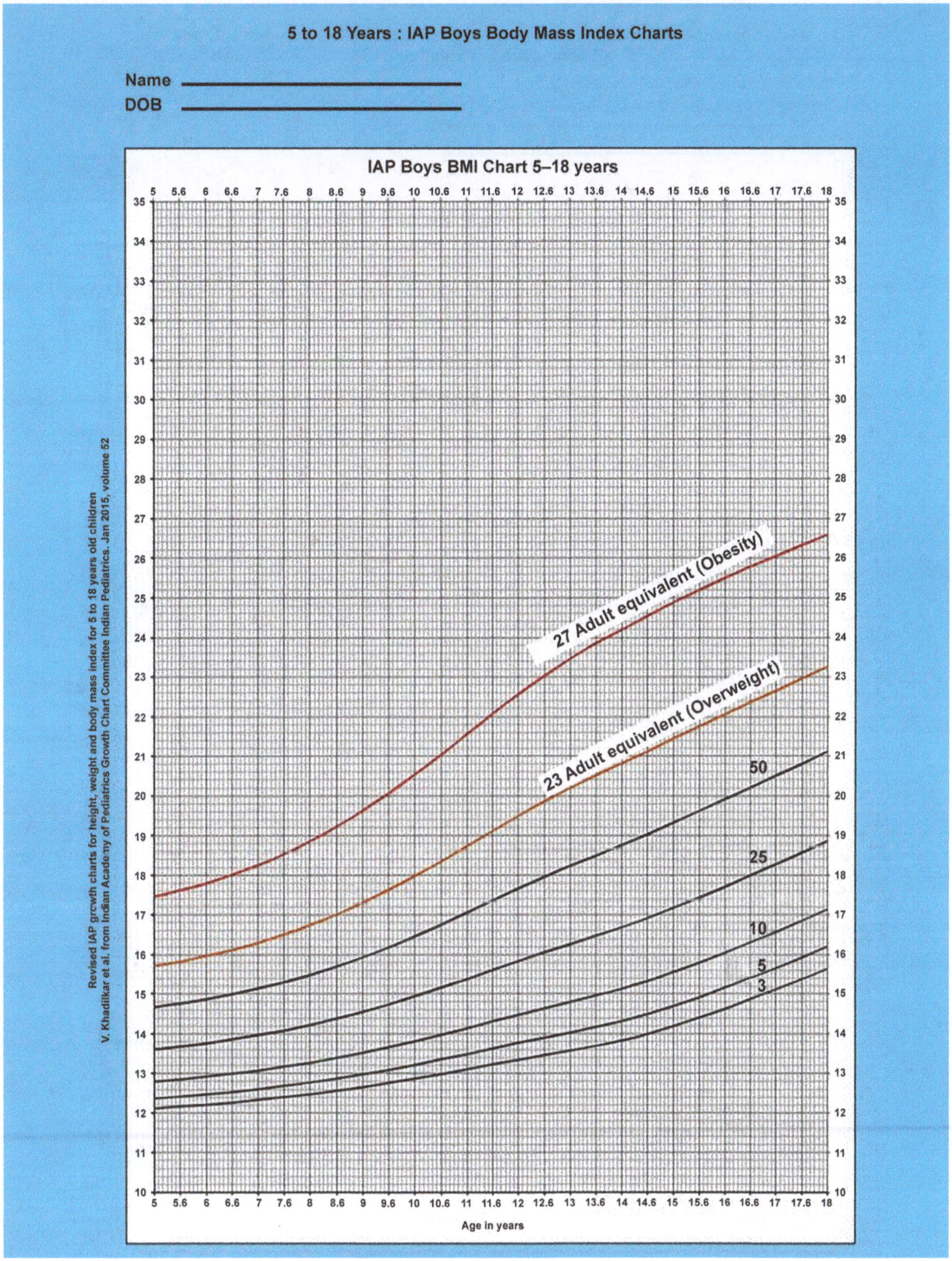

Fig. 4: Boys 5–18 years IAP body mass index charts.

0 to 5 Years: WHO Girls Length/Height, Weight and Head Circumference Charts
(Z Scores are in Parenthesis)

Name : ____________________

DOB : ____________________

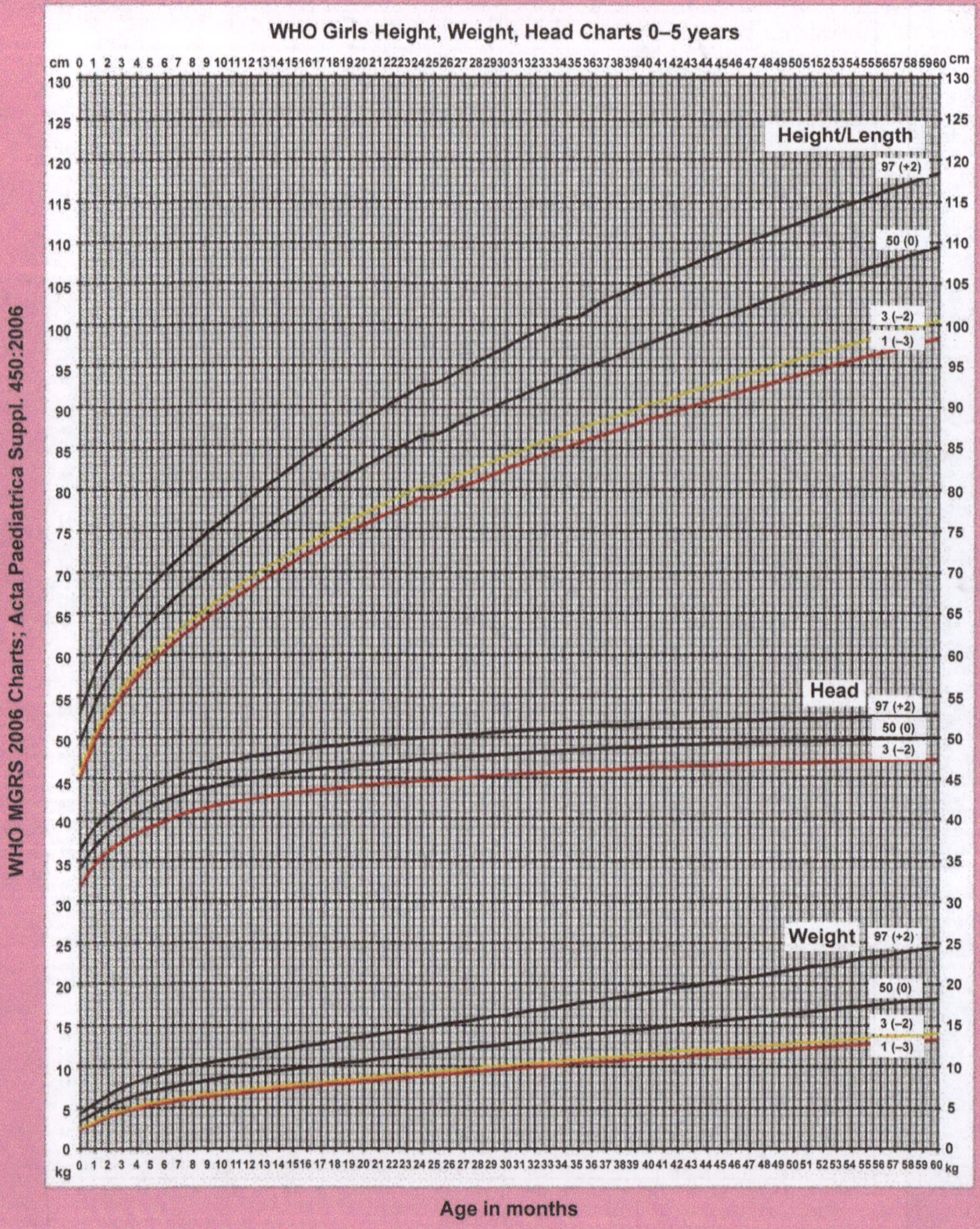

Fig. 5: World Health Organization (WHO) charts: 0–5 years girls length/height, weight and head circumference charts.

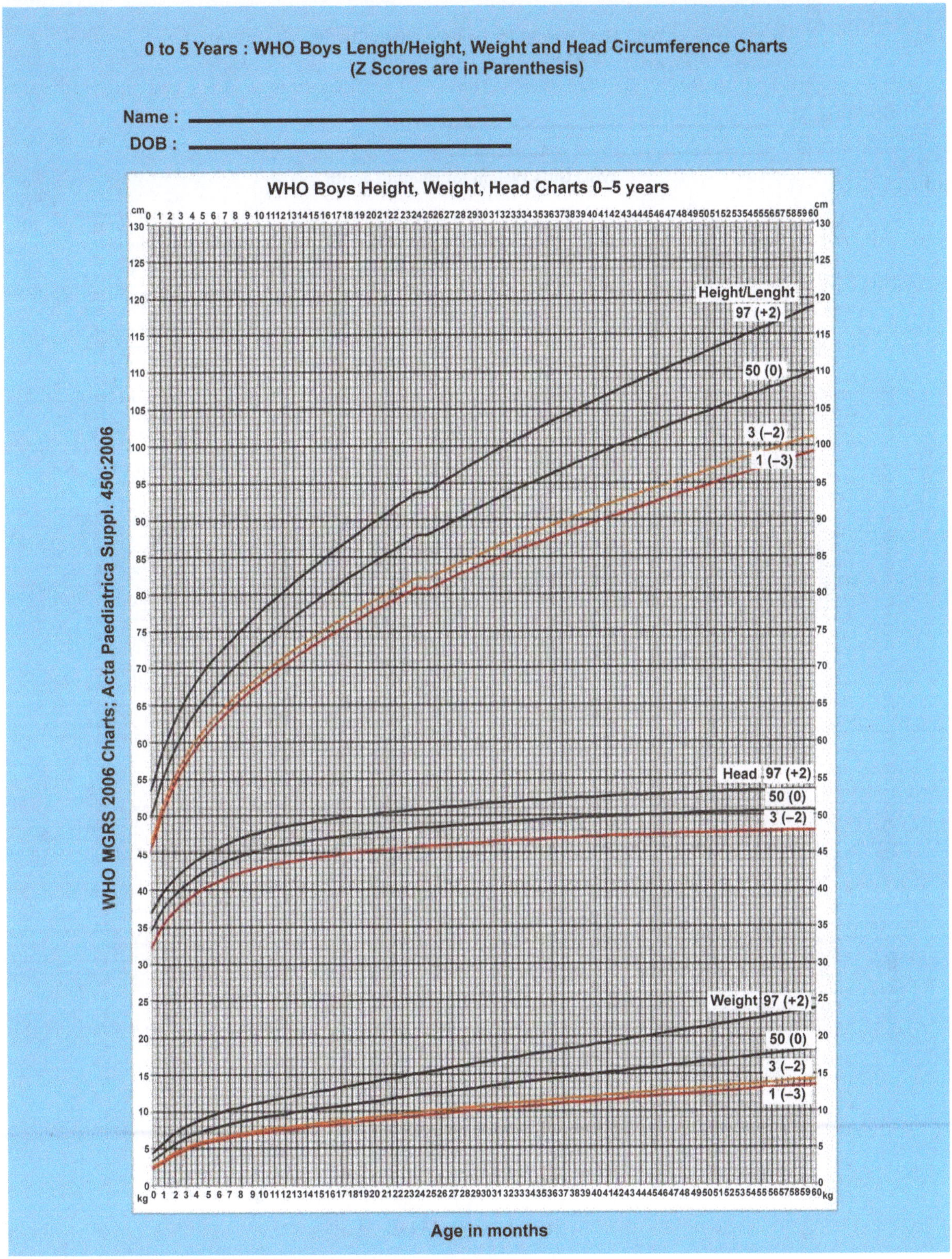

Fig. 6: WHO charts; 0–5 years boys length/height, weight, and head circumference charts.

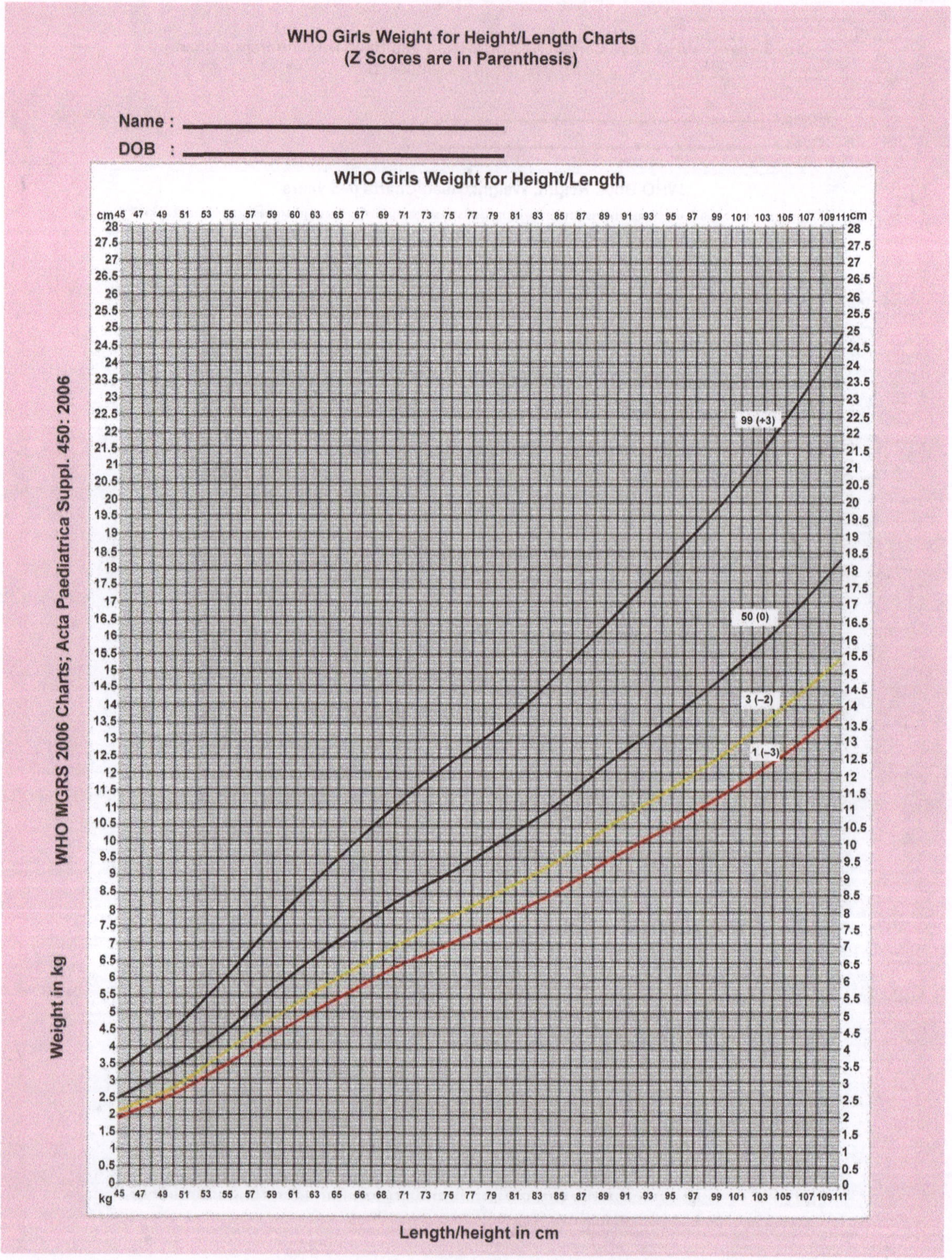

Fig. 7: WHO girls weight for height/length charts.

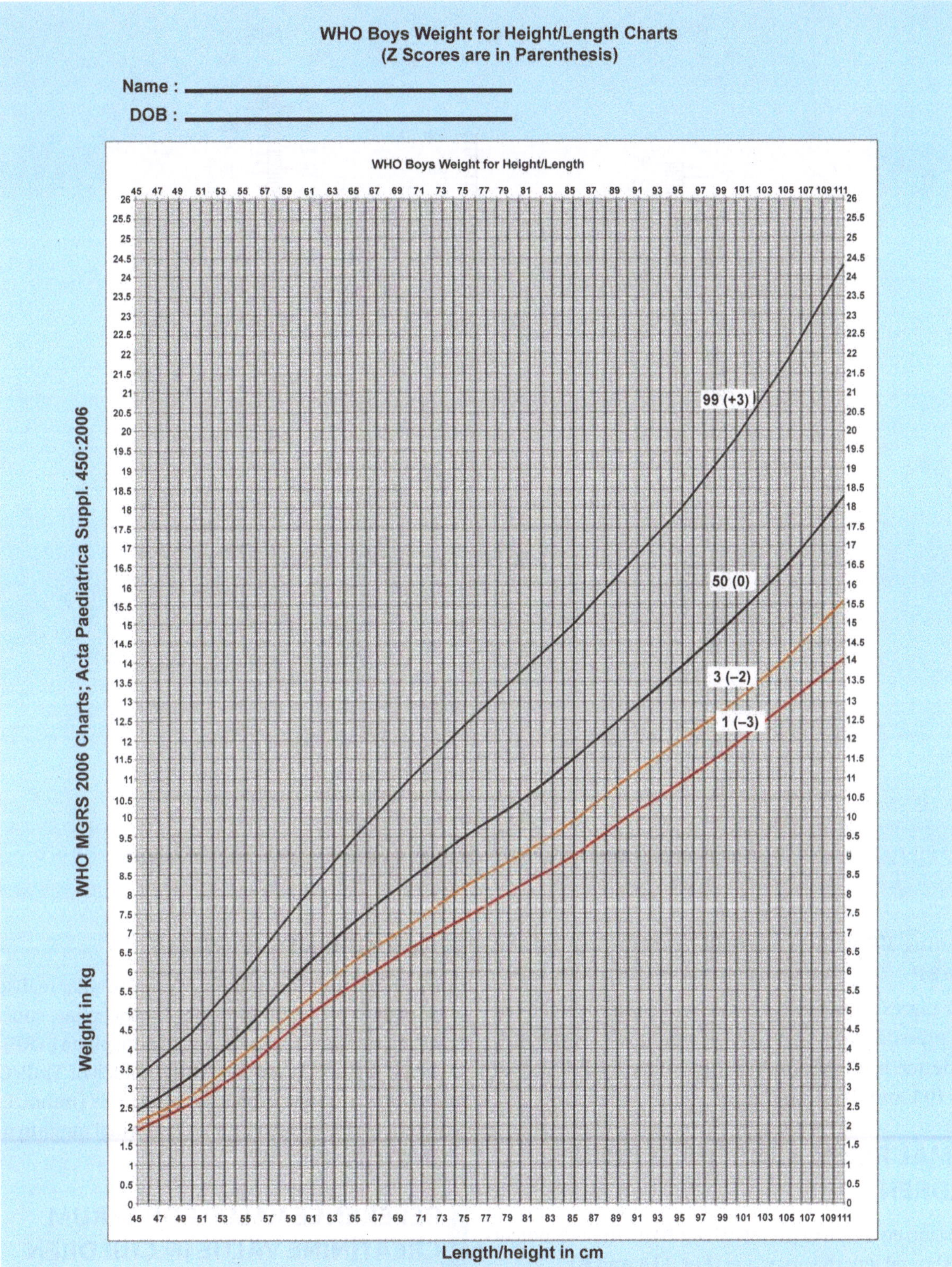

Fig. 8: WHO boys weight for length/height charts.

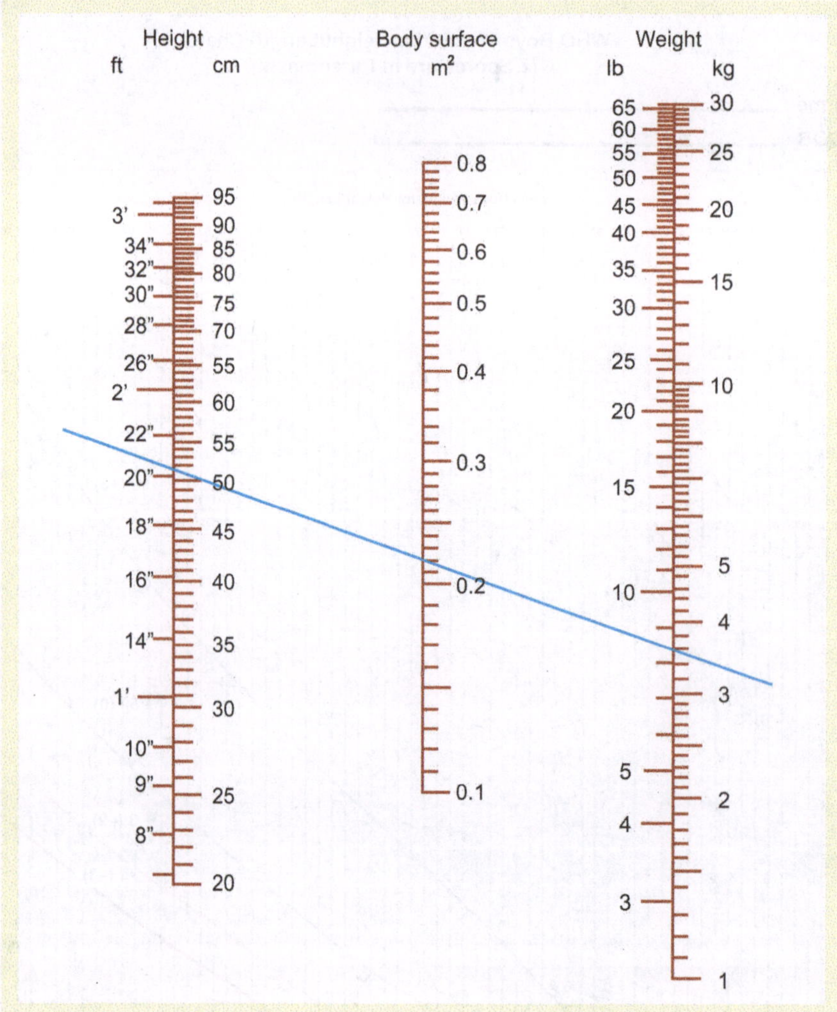

Fig. 9: West nomogram: estimating body surface area (BSA) of infants and young children.

- Screening BP values requiring further evaluation **(Table 3)**[5]
- Linear regression of mean systolic (A) and diastolic (B) blood pressures by postmenstrual age in weeks with 95% confidence intervals (upper and lower dashed lines) **(Figs. 10A and B)**[6]

NORMAL RENAL LENGTHS IN INDIAN CHILDREN

- Regression equation of (A) renal length versus body height and (B) renal length versus age **(Fig. 11A and B)**
- Mean renal length and volume of healthy Indian study children **(Table 4)**[7]

ACID–BASE NOMOGRAM

Shaded areas represent 95% confidence limits of normal respiratory and metabolic compensations for primary disturbances. Points outside the shaded areas represent mixed disorder, assuming absence of laboratory error **(Fig. 12)**.[8]

TmP/GFR NOMOGRAM

Nomogram for the calculation of renal tubular reabsorption of phosphate (TmP/GFR) from plasma phosphate concentration and the fractional reabsorption of phosphate (TRP). The 0.0-2.0 scale is suitable for estimating values of TmP/GFR close to the normal range expressed in SI units (mmol/L) and the 0.0–5.0 scale for values close to the normal range in mass units (mg/100 mL) **(Fig. 13)**.[9]

REFERENCE VALUE FOR SERUM CREATININE VALUE IN CHILDREN YOUNGER THAN 1 YEAR AGE

The reference value for serum creatinine in children younger than 1 year of age is shown in **Figure 14**.[10]

NORMAL UROFLOW CURVES FOR HEALTHY INDIAN CHILDREN 5–15 YEARS

- Uroflowmetry nomogram for maximum flow rates in boys 5–15 years age **(Fig. 15A)**

TABLE 1: BP levels for boys by age and height percentile.

Age (years)	BP percentile	SBP (mm Hg)							DBP (mm Hg)						
		Height percentile or measured height							Height percentile or measured height						
		5%	10%	25%	50%	75%	90%	95%	5%	10%	25%	50%	75%	90%	95%
1	Height (in)	30.4	30.8	31.6	32.4	33.3	34.1	34.6	30.4	30.8	31.6	32.4	33.3	34.1	34.6
	Height (cm)	77.2	78.3	80.2	82.4	84.6	86.7	87.9	77.2	78.3	80.2	82.4	84.6	86.7	87.9
	50th	85	85	86	86	87	88	88	40	40	40	41	41	42	42
	90th	98	99	99	100	100	101	101	52	52	53	53	54	54	54
	95th	102	102	103	103	104	105	105	54	54	55	55	56	57	57
	95th + 12 mm Hg	114	114	115	115	116	117	117	66	66	67	67	68	69	69
2	Height (in)	33.9	34.4	35.3	36.3	37.3	38.2	38.8	33.9	34.4	35.3	36.3	37.3	38.2	38.8
	Height (cm)	86.1	87.4	89.6	92.1	94.7	97.1	98.5	86.1	87.4	89.6	92.1	94.7	97.1	98.5
	50th	87	87	88	89	89	90	91	43	43	44	44	45	46	46
	90th	100	100	101	102	103	103	104	55	55	56	56	57	58	58
	95th	104	105	105	106	107	107	108	57	58	58	59	60	61	61
	95th + 12 mm Hg	116	117	117	118	119	119	120	69	70	70	71	72	73	73
3	Height (in)	36.4	37	37.9	39	40.1	41.1	41.7	36.4	37	37.9	39	40.1	41.1	41.7
	Height (cm)	92.5	93.9	96.3	99	101.8	104.3	105.8	92.5	93.9	96.3	99	101.8	104.3	105.8
	50th	88	89	89	90	91	92	92	45	46	46	47	48	49	49
	90th	101	102	102	103	104	105	105	58	58	59	59	60	61	61
	95th	106	106	107	107	108	109	109	60	61	61	62	63	64	64
	95th + 12 mm Hg	118	118	119	119	120	121	121	72	73	73	74	75	76	76
4	Height (in)	38.8	39.4	40.5	41.7	42.9	43.9	44.5	38.8	39.4	40.5	41.7	42.9	43.9	44.5
	Height (cm)	98.5	100.2	102.9	105.9	108.9	111.5	113.2	98.5	100.2	102.9	105.9	108.9	111.5	113.2
	50th	90	90	91	92	93	94	94	48	49	49	50	51	52	52
	90th	102	103	104	105	105	106	107	60	61	62	62	63	64	64
	95th	107	107	108	108	109	110	110	63	64	65	66	67	67	68
	95th + 12 mm Hg	119	119	120	120	121	122	122	75	76	77	78	79	79	80
5	Height (in)	41.1	41.8	43.0	44.3	45.5	46.7	47.4	41.1	41.8	43.0	44.3	45.5	46.7	47.4
	Height (cm)	104.4	106.2	109.1	112.4	115.7	118.6	120.3	104.4	106.2	109.1	112.4	115.7	118.6	120.3
	50th	91	92	93	94	95	96	96	51	51	52	53	54	55	55
	90th	103	104	105	106	107	108	108	63	64	65	65	66	67	67
	95th	107	108	109	109	110	111	112	66	67	68	69	70	70	71
	95th + 12 mm Hg	119	120	121	121	122	123	124	78	79	80	81	82	82	83
6	Height (in)	43.4	44.2	45.4	46.8	48.2	49.4	50.2	43.4	44.2	45.4	46.8	48.2	49.4	50.2
	Height (cm)	110.3	112.2	115.3	118.9	122.4	125.6	127.5	110.3	112.2	115.3	118.9	122.4	125.6	127.5
	50th	93	93	94	95	96	97	98	54	54	55	56	57	57	58
	90th	105	105	106	107	109	110	110	66	66	67	68	68	69	69
	95th	108	109	110	111	112	113	114	69	70	70	71	72	72	73
	95th + 12 mm Hg	120	121	122	123	124	125	126	81	82	82	83	84	84	85
7	Height (in)	45.7	46.5	47.8	49.3	50.8	52.1	52.9	45.7	46.5	47.8	49.3	50.8	52.1	52.9
	Height (cm)	116.1	118	121.4	125.1	128.9	132.4	134.5	116.1	118	121.4	125.1	128.9	132.4	134.5
	50th	94	94	95	97	98	98	99	56	56	57	58	58	59	59
	90th	106	107	108	109	110	111	111	68	68	69	70	70	71	71
	95th	110	110	111	112	114	115	116	71	71	72	73	73	74	74
	95th + 12 mm Hg	122	122	123	124	126	127	128	83	83	84	85	85	86	86

Contd...

Contd...

Age (years)	BP percentile	SBP (mm Hg)							DBP (mm Hg)						
		Height percentile or measured height							Height percentile or measured height						
		5%	10%	25%	50%	75%	90%	95%	5%	10%	25%	50%	75%	90%	95%
8	Height (in)	47.8	48.6	50	51.6	53.2	54.6	55.5	47.8	48.6	50	51.6	53.2	54.6	55.5
	Height (cm)	121.4	123.5	127	131	135.1	138.8	141	121.4	123.5	127	131	135.1	138.8	141
	50th	95	96	97	98	99	99	100	57	57	58	59	59	60	60
	90th	107	108	109	110	111	112	112	69	70	70	71	72	72	73
	95th	111	112	112	114	115	116	117	72	73	73	74	75	75	75
	95th + 12 mm Hg	123	124	124	126	127	128	129	84	85	85	86	87	87	87
9	Height (in)	49.6	50.5	52	53.7	55.4	56.9	57.9	49.6	50.5	52	53.7	55.4	56.9	57.9
	Height (cm)	126	128.3	132.1	136.3	140.7	144.7	147.1	126	128.3	132.1	136.3	140.7	144.7	147.1
	50th	96	97	98	99	100	101	101	57	58	59	60	61	62	62
	90th	107	108	109	110	112	113	114	70	71	72	73	74	74	74
	95th	112	112	113	115	116	118	119	74	74	75	76	76	77	77
	95th + 12 mm Hg	124	124	125	127	128	130	131	86	86	87	88	88	89	89
10	Height (in)	51.3	52.2	53.8	55.6	57.4	59.1	60.1	51.3	52.2	53.8	55.6	57.4	59.1	60.1
	Height (cm)	130.2	132.7	136.7	141.3	145.9	150.1	152.7	130.2	132.7	136.7	141.3	145.9	150.1	152.7
	50th	97	98	99	100	101	102	103	59	60	61	62	63	63	64
	90th	108	109	111	112	113	115	116	72	73	74	74	75	75	76
	95th	112	113	114	116	118	120	121	76	76	77	77	78	78	78
	95th + 12 mm Hg	124	125	126	128	130	132	133	88	88	89	89	90	90	90
11	Height (in)	53	54	55.7	57.6	59.6	61.3	62.4	53	54	55.7	57.6	59.6	61.3	62.4
	Height (cm)	134.7	137.3	141.5	146.4	151.3	155.8	158.6	134.7	137.3	141.5	146.4	151.3	155.8	158.6
	50th	99	99	101	102	103	104	106	61	61	62	63	63	63	63
	90th	110	111	112	114	116	117	118	74	74	75	75	75	76	76
	95th	114	114	116	118	120	123	124	77	78	78	78	78	78	78
	95th + 12 mm Hg	126	126	128	130	132	135	136	89	90	90	90	90	90	90
12	Height (in)	55.2	56.3	58.1	60.1	62.2	64	65.2	55.2	56.3	58.1	60.1	62.2	64	65.2
	Height (cm)	140.3	143	147.5	152.7	157.9	162.6	165.5	140.3	143	147.5	152.7	157.9	162.6	165.5
	50th	101	101	102	104	106	108	109	61	62	62	62	62	63	63
	90th	113	114	115	117	119	121	122	75	75	75	75	75	76	76
	95th	116	117	118	121	124	126	128	78	78	78	78	78	79	79
	95th + 12 mm Hg	128	129	130	133	136	138	140	90	90	90	90	90	91	91
13	Height (in)	57.9	59.1	61	63.1	65.2	67.1	68.3	57.9	59.1	61	63.1	65.2	67.1	68.3
	Height (cm)	147	150	154.9	160.3	165.7	170.5	173.4	147	150	154.9	160.3	165.7	170.5	173.4
	50th	103	104	105	108	110	111	112	61	60	61	62	63	64	65
	90th	115	116	118	121	124	126	126	74	74	74	75	76	77	77
	95th	119	120	122	125	128	130	131	78	78	78	78	80	81	81
	95th + 12 mm Hg	131	132	134	137	140	142	143	90	90	90	90	92	93	93
14	Height (in)	60.6	61.8	63.8	65.9	68.0	69.8	70.9	60.6	61.8	63.8	65.9	68.0	69.8	70.9
	Height (cm)	153.8	156.9	162	167.5	172.7	177.4	180.1	153.8	156.9	162	167.5	172.7	177.4	180.1
	50th	105	106	109	111	112	113	113	60	60	62	64	65	66	67
	90th	119	120	123	126	127	128	129	74	74	75	77	78	79	80
	95th	123	125	127	130	132	133	134	77	78	79	81	82	83	84
	95th + 12 mm Hg	135	137	139	142	144	145	146	89	90	91	93	94	95	96

Contd...

Contd...

Age (years)	BP percentile	SBP (mm Hg)							DBP (mm Hg)						
		Height percentile or measured height							Height percentile or measured height						
		5%	10%	25%	50%	75%	90%	95%	5%	10%	25%	50%	75%	90%	95%
15	Height (in)	62.6	63.8	65.7	67.8	69.8	71.5	72.5	62.6	63.8	65.7	67.8	69.8	71.5	72.5
	Height (cm)	159	162	166.9	172.2	177.2	181.6	184.2	159	162	166.9	172.2	177.2	181.6	184.2
	50th	108	110	112	113	114	114	114	61	62	64	65	66	67	68
	90th	123	124	126	128	129	130	130	75	76	78	79	80	81	81
	95th	127	129	131	132	134	135	135	78	79	81	83	84	85	85
	95th + 12 mm Hg	139	141	143	144	146	147	147	90	91	93	95	96	97	97
16	Height (in)	63.8	64.9	66.8	68.8	70.7	72.4	73.4	63.8	64.9	66.8	68.8	70.7	72.4	73.4
	Height (cm)	162.1	165	169.6	174.6	179.5	183.8	186.4	162.1	165	169.6	174.6	179.5	183.8	186.4
	50th	111	112	114	115	115	116	116	63	64	66	67	68	69	69
	90th	126	127	128	129	131	131	132	77	78	79	80	81	82	82
	95th	130	131	133	134	135	136	137	80	81	83	84	85	86	86
	95th + 12 mm Hg	142	143	145	146	147	148	149	92	93	95	96	97	98	98
17	Height (in)	64.5	65.5	67.3	69.2	71.1	72.8	73.8	64.5	65.5	67.3	69.2	71.1	72.8	73.8
	Height (cm)	163.8	166.5	170.9	175.8	180.7	184.9	187.5	163.8	166.5	170.9	175.8	180.7	184.9	187.5
	50th	114	115	116	117	117	118	118	65	66	67	68	69	70	70
	90th	128	129	130	131	132	133	134	78	79	80	81	82	82	83
	95th	132	133	134	135	137	138	138	81	82	84	85	86	86	87
	95th + 12 mm Hg	144	145	146	147	149	150	150	93	94	96	97	98	98	99

TABLE 2: BP levels for girls by age and height percentile.

Age (years)	BP percentile	SBP (mm Hg)							DBP (mm Hg)						
		Height percentile or measured height							Height percentile or measured height						
		5%	10%	25%	50%	75%	90%	95%	5%	10%	25%	50%	75%	90%	95%
1	Height (in)	29.7	30.2	30.9	31.8	32.7	33.4	33.9	29.7	30.2	30.9	31.8	32.7	33.4	33.9
	Height (cm)	75.4	76.6	78.6	80.8	83	84.9	86.1	75.4	76.6	78.6	80.8	83	84.9	86.1
	50th	84	85	86	86	87	88	88	41	42	42	43	44	45	46
	90th	98	99	99	100	101	102	102	54	55	56	56	57	58	58
	95th	101	102	102	103	104	105	105	59	59	60	60	61	62	62
	95th + 12 mm Hg	113	114	114	115	116	117	117	71	71	72	72	73	74	74
2	Height (in)	33.4	34	34.9	35.9	36.9	37.8	38.4	33.4	34	34.9	35.9	36.9	37.8	38.4
	Height (cm)	84.9	.86.3	88.6	91.1	93.7	96	97.4	84.9	86.3	88.6	91.1	93.7	96	97.4
	50th	87	87	88	89	90	91	91	45	46	47	48	49	50	51
	90th	101	101	102	103	104	105	106	58	58	59	60	61	62	62
	95th	104	105	106	106	107	108	109	62	63	63	64	65	66	66
	95th + 12 mm Hg	116	117	118	118	119	120	121	74	75	75	76	77	78	78
3	Height (in)	35.8	36.4	37.3	38.4	39.6	40.6	41.2	35.8	36.4	37.3	38.4	39.6	40.6	41.2
	Height (cm)	91	92.4	94.9	97.6	100.5	103.1	104.6	91	92.4	94.9	97.6	100.5	103.1	104.6
	50th	88	89	89	90	91	92	93	48	48	49	50	51	53	53
	90th	102	103	104	104	105	106	107	60	61	61	62	63	64	65
	95th	106	106	107	108	109	110	110	64	65	65	66	67	68	69
	95th + 12 mm Hg	118	118	119	120	121	122	122	76	77	77	78	79	80	81
4	Height (in)	38.3	38.9	39.9	41.1	42.4	43.5	44.2	38.3	38.9	39.9	41.1	42.4	43.5	44.2
	Height (cm)	97.2	98.8	101.4	104.5	107.6	110.5	112.2	97.2	98.8	101.4	104.5	107.6	110.5	112.2
	50th	89	90	91	92	93	94	94	50	51	51	53	54	55	55
	90th	103	104	105	106	107	108	108	62	63	64	65	66	67	67
	95th	107	108	109	109	110	111	112	66	67	68	69	70	70	71
	95th + 12 mm Hg	119	120	121	121	122	123	124	78	79	80	81	82	82	83

Contd...

Contd...

Age (years)	BP percentile	SBP (mm Hg) Height percentile or measured height							DBP (mm Hg) Height percentile or measured height						
		5%	10%	25%	50%	75%	90%	95%	5%	10%	25%	50%	75%	90%	95%
5	Height (in)	40.8	41.5	42.6	43.9	45.2	46.5	47.3	40.8	41.5	42.6	43.9	45.2	46.5	47.3
	Height (cm)	103.6	105.3	108.2	111.5	114.9	118.1	120	103.6	105.3	108.2	111.5	114.9	118.1	120
	50th	90	91	92	93	94	95	96	52	52	53	55	56	57	57
	90th	104	105	106	107	108	109	110	64	65	66	67	68	69	70
	95th	108	109	109	110	111	112	113	68	69	70	71	72	73	73
	95th + 12 mm Hg	120	121	121	122	123	124	125	80	81	82	83	84	85	85
6	Height (in)	43.3	44	45.2	46.6	48.1	49.4	50.3	43.3	44	45.2	46.6	48.1	49.4	50.3
	Height (cm)	110	111.8	114.9	118.4	122.1	125.6	127.7	110	111.8	114.9	118.4	122.1	125.6	127.7
	50th	92	92	93	94	96	97	97	54	54	55	56	57	58	59
	90th	105	106	107	108	109	110	111	67	67	68	69	70	71	71
	95th	109	109	110	111	112	113	114	70	71	72	72	73	74	74
	95th + 12 mm Hg	121	121	122	123	124	125	126	82	83	84	84	85	86	86
7	Height (in)	45.6	46.4	47.7	49.2	50.7	52.1	53	45.6	46.4	47.7	49.2	50.7	52.1	53
	Height (cm)	115.9	117.8	121.1	124.9	128.8	132.5	134.7	115.9	117.8	121.1	124.9	128.8	132.5	134.7
	50th	92	93	94	95	97	98	99	55	55	56	57	58	59	60
	90th	106	106	107	109	110	111	112	68	68	69	70	71	72	72
	95th	109	110	111	112	113	114	115	72	72	73	73	74	74	75
	95th + 12 mm Hg	121	122	123	124	125	126	127	84	84	85	85	86	86	87
8	Height (in)	47.6	48.4	49.8	51.4	53	54.5	55.5	47.6	48.4	49.8	51.4	53	54.5	55.5
	Height (cm)	121	123	126.5	130.6	134.7	138.5	140.9	121	123	126.5	130.6	134.7	138.5	140.9
	50th	93	94	95	97	98	99	100	56	56	57	59	60	61	61
	90th	107	107	108	110	111	112	113	69	70	71	72	72	73	73
	95th	110	111	112	113	115	116	117	72	73	74	74	75	75	75
	95th + 12 mm Hg	122	123	124	125	127	128	129	84	85	86	86	87	87	87
9	Height (in)	49.3	50.2	51.7	53.4	55.1	56.7	57.7	49.3	50.2	51.7	53.4	55.1	56.7	57.7
	Height (cm)	125.3	127.6	131.3	135.6	140.1	144.1	146.6	125.3	127.6	131.3	135.6	140.1	144.1	146.6
	50th	95	95	97	98	99	100	101	57	58	59	60	60	61	61
	90th	108	108	109	111	112	113	114	71	71	72	73	73	73	73
	95th	112	112	113	114	116	117	118	74	74	75	75	75	75	75
	95th + 12 mm Hg	124	124	125	126	128	129	130	86	86	87	87	87	87	87
10	Height (in)	51.1	52	53.7	55.5	57.4	59.1	60.2	51.1	52	53.7	55.5	57.4	59.1	60.2
	Height (cm)	129.7	132.2	136.3	141	145.8	150.2	152.8	129.7	132.2	136.3	141	145.8	150.2	152.8
	50th	96	97	98	99	101	102	103	58	59	59	60	61	61	62
	90th	109	110	111	112	113	115	116	72	73	73	73	73	73	73
	95th	113	114	114	116	117	119	120	75	75	76	76	76	76	76
	95th + 12 mm Hg	125	126	126	128	129	131	132	87	87	88	88	88	88	88
11	Height (in)	53.4	54.5	56.2	58.2	60.2	61.9	63	53.4	54.5	56.2	58.2	60.2	61.9	63
	Height (cm)	135.6	138.3	142.8	147.8	152.8	157.3	160	135.6	138.3	142.8	147.8	152.8	157.3	160
	50th	98	99	101	102	104	105	106	60	60	60	61	62	63	64
	90th	111	112	113	114	116	118	120	74	74	74	74	74	75	75
	95th	115	116	117	118	120	123	124	76	77	77	77	77	77	77
	95th + 12 mm Hg	127	128	129	130	132	135	136	88	89	89	89	89	89	89
12	Height (in)	56.2	57.3	59	60.9	62.8	64.5	65.5	56.2	57.3	59	60.9	62.8	64.5	65.5
	Height (cm)	142.8	145.5	149.9	154.8	159.6	163.8	166.4	142.8	145.5	149.9	154.8	159.6	163.8	166.4
	50th	102	102	104	105	107	108	108	61	61	61	62	64	65	65
	90th	114	115	116	118	120	122	122	75	75	75	75	76	76	76
	95th	118	119	120	122	124	125	126	78	78	78	78	79	79	79
	95th + 12 mm Hg	130	131	132	134	136	137	138	90	90	90	90	91	91	91

Contd...

Contd...

Age (years)	BP percentile	SBP (mm Hg)							DBP (mm Hg)						
		Height percentile or measured height							Height percentile or measured height						
		5%	10%	25%	50%	75%	90%	95%	5%	10%	25%	50%	75%	90%	95%
13	Height (in)	58.3	59.3	60.9	62.7	64.5	66.1	67	58.3	59.3	60.9	62.7	64.5	66.1	67
	Height (cm)	148.1	150.6	154.7	159.2	163.7	167.8	170.2	148.1	150.6	154.7	159.2	163.7	167.8	170.2
	50th	104	105	106	107	108	108	109	62	62	63	64	65	65	66
	90th	116	117	119	121	122	123	123	75	75	75	76	76	76	76
	95th	121	122	123	124	126	126	127	79	79	79	79	80	80	81
	95th + 12 mm Hg	133	134	135	136	138	138	139	91	91	91	91	92	92	93
14	Height (in)	59.3	60.2	61.8	63.5	65.2	66.8	67.7	59.3	60.2	61.8	63.5	65.2	66.8	67.7
	Height (cm)	150.6	153	156.9	161.3	165.7	169.7	172.1	150.6	153	156.9	161.3	165.7	169.7	172.1
	50th	105	106	107	108	109	109	109	63	63	64	65	66	66	66
	90th	118	118	120	122	123	123	123	76	76	76	76	77	77	77
	95th	123	123	124	125	126	127	127	80	80	80	80	81	81	82
	95th + 12 mm Hg	135	135	136	137	138	139	139	92	92	92	92	93	93	94
15	Height (in)	59.7	60.6	62.2	63.9	65.6	67.2	68.1	59.7	60.6	62.2	63.9	65.6	67.2	68.1
	Height (cm)	151.7	154	157.9	162.3	166.7	170.6	173	151.7	154	157.9	162.3	166.7	170.6	173
	50th	105	106	107	108	109	109	109	64	64	64	65	66	67	67
	90th	118	119	121	122	123	123	124	76	76	76	77	77	78	78
	95th	124	124	125	126	127	127	128	80	80	80	81	82	82	82
	95th + 12 mm Hg	136	136	137	138	139	139	140	92	92	92	93	94	94	94
16	Height (in)	59.9	60.8	62.4	64.1	65.8	67.3	68.3	59.9	60.8	62.4	64.1	65.8	67.3	68.3
	Height (cm)	152.1	154.5	158.4	162.8	167.1	171.1	173.4	152.1	154.5	158.4	162.8	167.1	171.1	173.4
	50th	106	107	108	109	109	110	110	64	64	65	66	66	67	67
	90th	119	120	122	123	124	124	124	76	76	76	77	78	78	78
	95th	124	125	125	127	127	128	128	80	80	80	81	82	82	82
	95th + 12 mm Hg	136	137	137	139	139	140	140	92	92	92	93	94	94	94
17	Height (in)	60.0	60.9	62.5	64.2	65.9	67.4	68.4	60.0	60.9	62.5	64.2	65.9	67.4	68.4
	Height (cm)	152.4	154.7	158.7	163.0	167.4	171.3	173.7	152.4	154.7	158.7	163.0	167.4	171.3	173.7
	50th	107	108	109	110	110	110	111	64	64	65	66	66	66	67
	90th	120	121	123	124	124	125	125	76	76	77	77	78	78	78
	95th	125	125	126	127	128	128	128	80	80	80	81	82	82	82
	95th + 12 mm Hg	137	137	138	139	140	140	140	92	92	92	93	94	94	94

TABLE 3: Screening BP values requiring further evaluation.

Age (years)	BP (mm Hg)			
	Boys		Girls	
	Systolic	DBP	Systolic	DBP
1	98	52	98	54
2	100	55	101	58
3	101	58	102	60
4	102	60	103	62
5	103	63	104	64
6	105	66	105	67
7	106	68	106	68
8	107	69	107	69
9	107	70	108	71
10	108	72	109	72
11	110	74	111	74
12	113	75	114	75
≥13	120	80	120	80

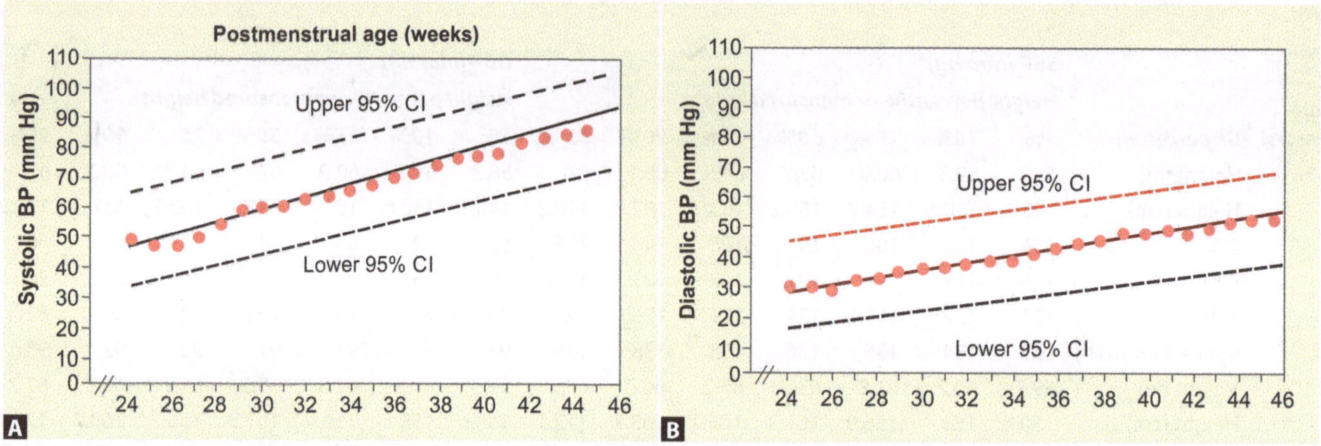

Figs. 10A and B: Linear regression of mean systolic (A) and diastolic (B) blood pressures by postmenstrual age in weeks with 95% confidence intervals (upper and lower dashed lines).

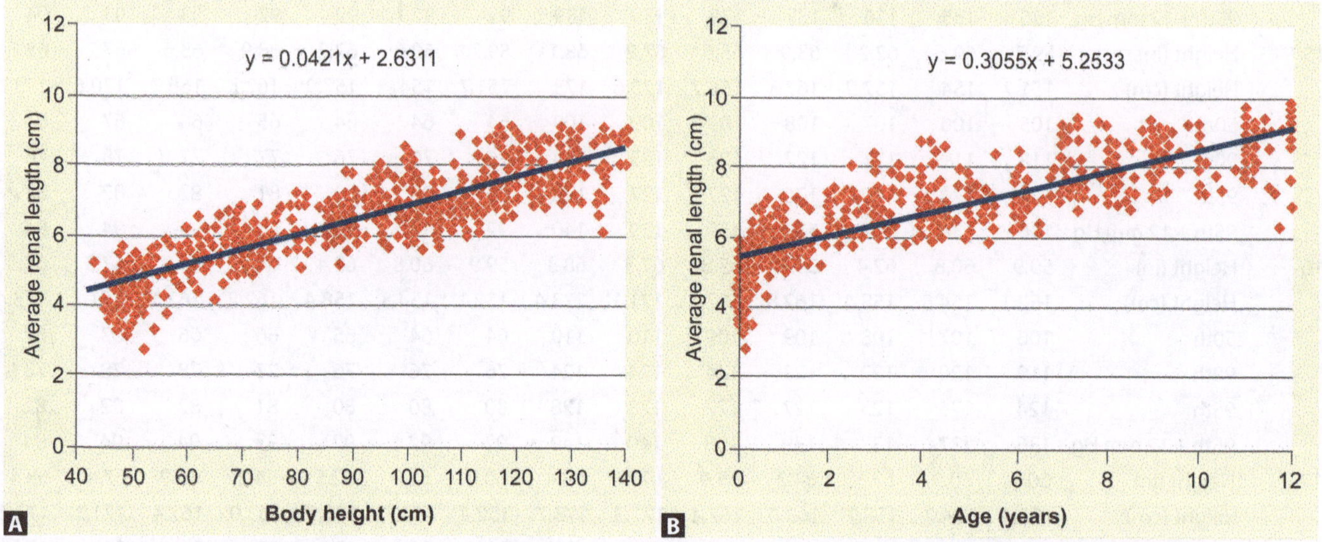

Figs. 11A and B: Regression equation of (A) Average renal length vs body height; (B) Average renal length vs age.

TABLE 4: Mean renal length and volume of healthy Indian study children (*N* = 1000).

Age	*Weight (kg) Mean (SD)*	*Height (cm) Mean (SD)*	*Body surface area (m²) (SD)*	*Renal length (cm) Mean (SD)*	*Renal volume (mL) Mean (SD)*
1 mo (n = 71)	2.5 (0.4)	48.5 (2.1)	0.18 (0.02)	4.3 (0.6)	9.7 (4.7)
3 mo (n = 49)	3.7 (0.9)	53.8 (4.2)	0.23 (0.05)	4.7 (0.7)	12.1 (6.0)
6 mo (n = 61)	5.6 (1.1)	61.8 (4.4)	0.32 (0.05)	5.5 (0.7)	18.3 (7.0)
9 mo (n = 81)	7.3 (0.9)	68.5 (3.7)	0.39 (0.03)	5.6 (0.6)	19.6 (6.8)
1 y (n = 122)	8.5 (1.1)	72.0 (2.8)	0.44 (0.04)	5.7 (0.4)	21.3 (5.5)
2 y (n = 75)	9.7 (1.4)	79.0 (7.6)	0.48 (0.05)	6.1 (0.7)	25.3 (8.2)
3 y (n = 58)	11.2 (1.5)	89.2 (5.0)	0.54 (0.05)	6.7 (0.6)	31.3 (10.0)
4 y (n = 63)	12.9 (1.0)	95.7 (4.2)	0.59 (0.03)	6.8 (0.60)	32.9 (9.1)
5 y (n = 66)	14.0 (1.7)	101.1 (4.3)	0.62 (0.05)	6.7 (0.6)	33.0 (8.9)
6 y (n = 54)	16.5 (2.2)	107.5 (5.2)	0.69 (0.06)	6.7 (0.4)	34.2 (9.4)
7 y (n = 48)	18.0 (2.1)	112.5 (5.5)	0.74 (0.06)	7.2 (0.6)	44.6 (12.7)
8 y (n = 57)	20.6 (2.2)	116.8 (6.0)	0.81 (0.05)	7.6 (0.7)	49.8 (14.8)
9 y (n = 58)	24.0 (2.7)	125.8 (4.1)	0.88 (0.06)	8.0 (0.6)	56.2 (16.7)
10 y (n = 43)	25.9 (3.9)	130.4 (5.8)	0.92 (0.08)	8.0 (0.7)	58.0 (16.2)
11 y (n = 32)	30.9 (4.3)	138.9 (5.3)	1.02 (0.09)	8.5 (0.8)	59.8 (17.3)
12 y (n = 62)	31.9 (4.5)	141.7 (5.8)	1.04 (0.09)	8.6 (0.8)	61.4 (16.5)

(SD: standard deviation; mo = months; y = years).

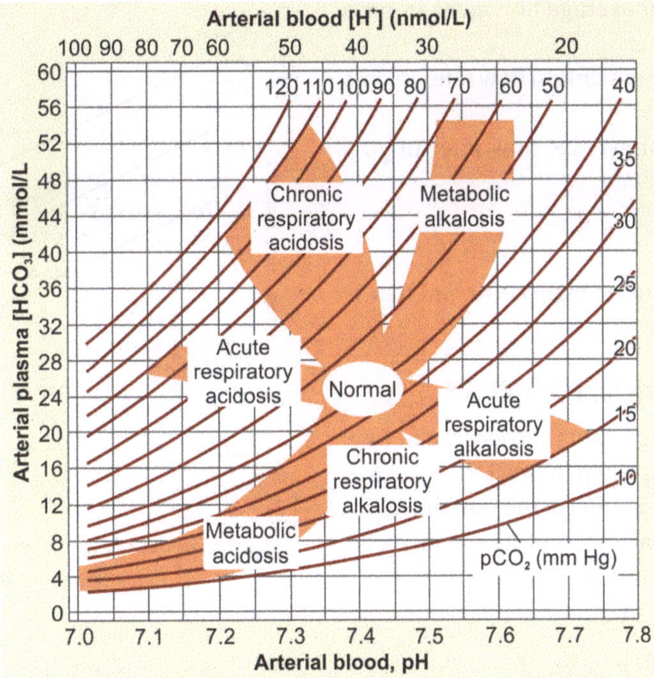

Fig. 12: Acid-base nomogram. Shaded areas represent 95% confidence limits of normal respiratory and metabolic compensations for primary disturbances. Points outside the shaded areas represent mixed disorder, assuming absence of lab error.

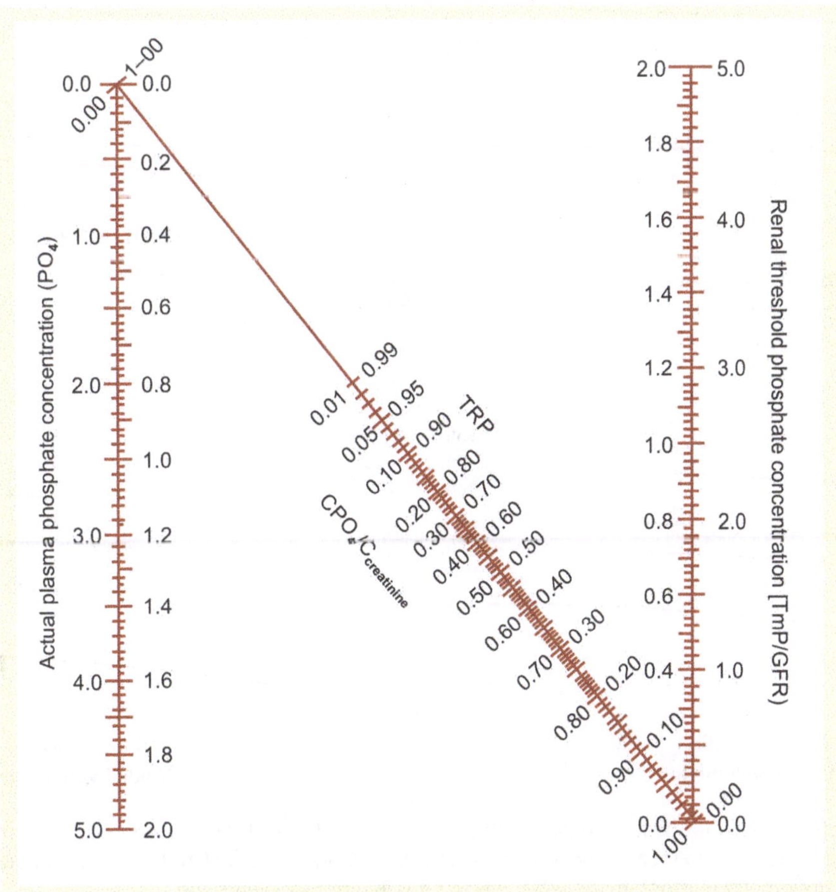

Fig. 13: TmP/GFR nomogram.

- Uroflowmetry nomogram for average flow rates in boys 5–15 years age **(Fig. 15B)**
- Uroflowmetry nomogram for maximum flow rates in girls 5–15 years age **(Fig. 15C)**
- Uroflowmetry nomogram for average flow rates in girls 5–15 years age **(Fig. 15D)**[11]

STONE CHART

A stone chart showing 24-hour urine analysis of children is showing in **Figure 16.**[12]

PERITONEAL EQUILIBRATION TEST

The various peritoneal transporter status categorized as low, low average, high average, and high depending D/Do glucose and D/P creatinine ratios. The numbers at the borders of the four categories represent maximal, mean +1SD, mean, mean -1 SD and minimal values at 4 hours dwell **(Fig. 17).**[13]

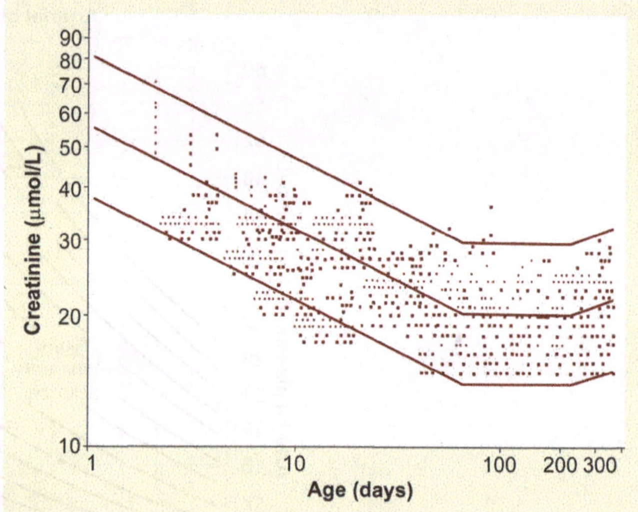

Fig. 14: Reference value for serum creatinine value in children younger than 1 year age.

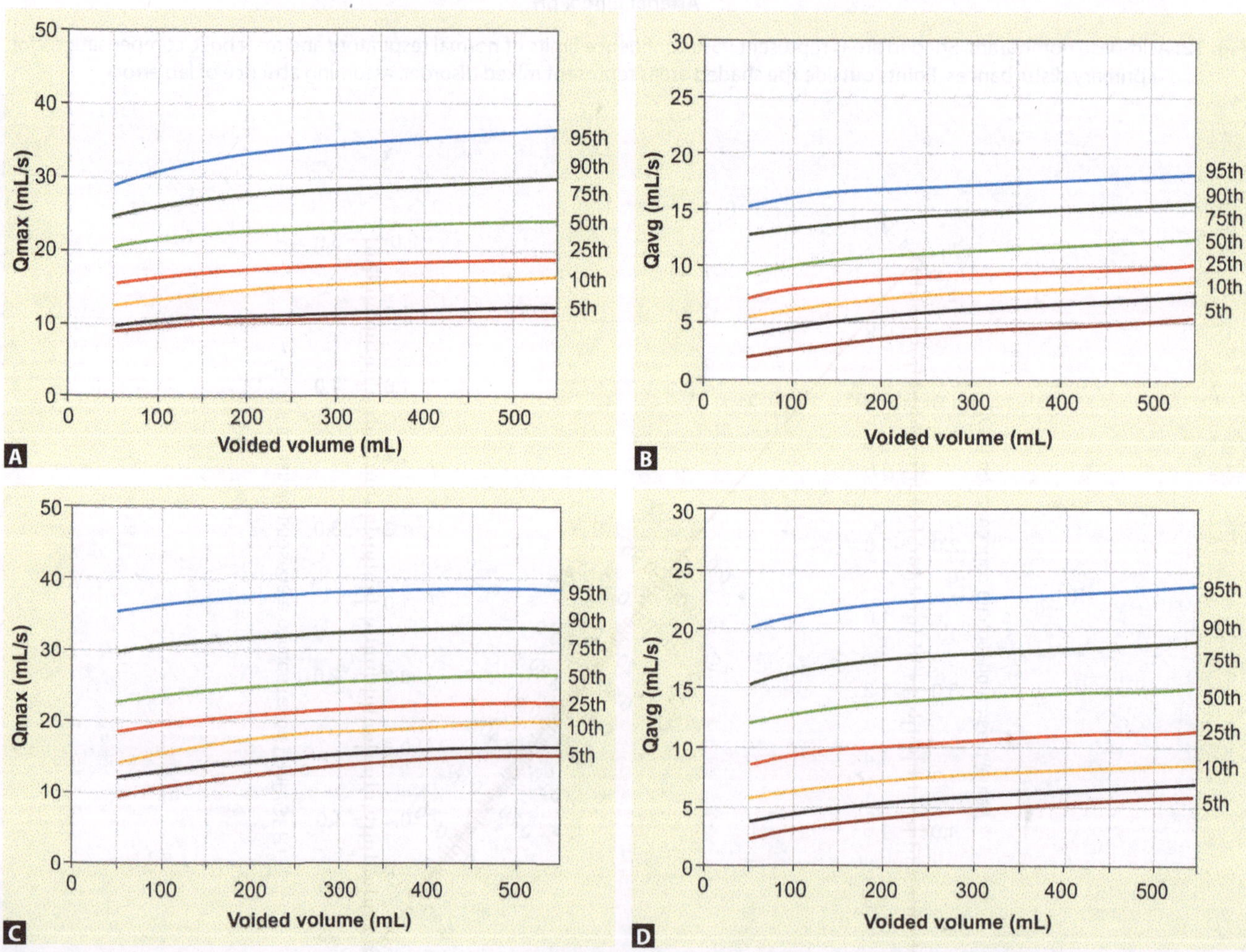

Figs. 15A to D: Normal uroflow curves for healthy Indian children 5–15 years. (A) Uroflometry nomogram for maximum flow rates in boys 5–15 years age; (B) Uroflometry nomogram for average flow rates in boys 5–15 years age; (C) Uroflometry nomogram for maximum flow rates in girls 5–15 years age; (D) Uroflometry nomogram for average flow rates in girls 5–15 years age.

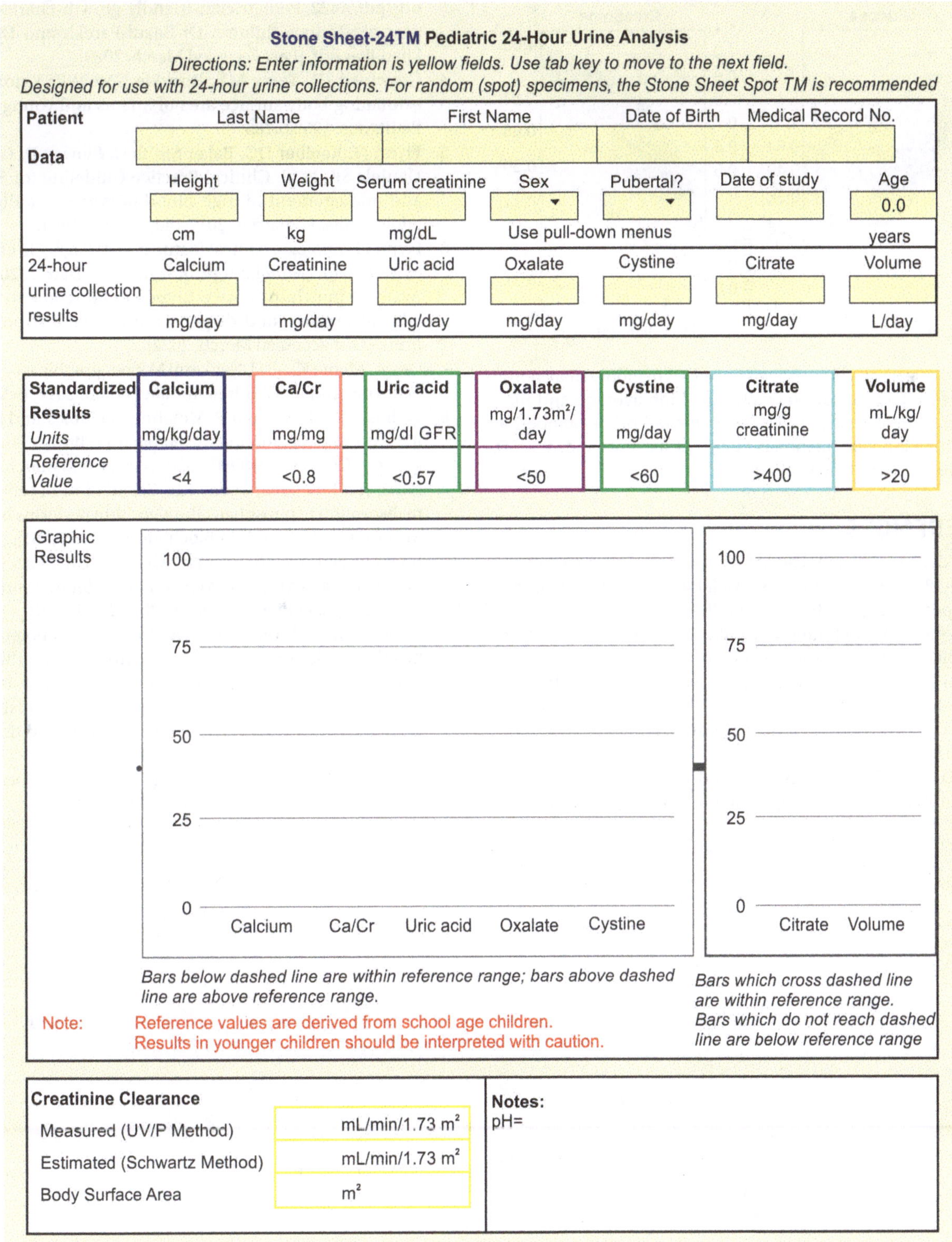

Stone Sheet-24TM Pediatric 24-Hour Urine Analysis

Directions: Enter information is yellow fields. Use tab key to move to the next field.

Designed for use with 24-hour urine collections. For random (spot) specimens, the Stone Sheet Spot TM is recommended

Patient Data	Last Name	First Name	Date of Birth	Medical Record No.		
Height	Weight	Serum creatinine	Sex	Pubertal?	Date of study	Age
						0.0
cm	kg	mg/dL	Use pull-down menus			years

24-hour urine collection results	Calcium	Creatinine	Uric acid	Oxalate	Cystine	Citrate	Volume
	mg/day	mg/day	mg/day	mg/day	mg/day	mg/day	L/day

Standardized Results	**Calcium**	**Ca/Cr**	**Uric acid**	**Oxalate**	**Cystine**	**Citrate**	**Volume**
Units	mg/kg/day	mg/mg	mg/dl GFR	mg/1.73m²/ day	mg/day	mg/g creatinine	mL/kg/ day
Reference Value	<4	<0.8	<0.57	<50	<60	>400	>20

Bars below dashed line are within reference range; bars above dashed line are above reference range.

Bars which cross dashed line are within reference range. Bars which do not reach dashed line are below reference range

Note: Reference values are derived from school age children. Results in younger children should be interpreted with caution.

Creatinine Clearance		**Notes:**
Measured (UV/P Method)	mL/min/1.73 m²	pH=
Estimated (Schwartz Method)	mL/min/1.73 m²	
Body Surface Area	m²	

Fig. 16: Stone chart.

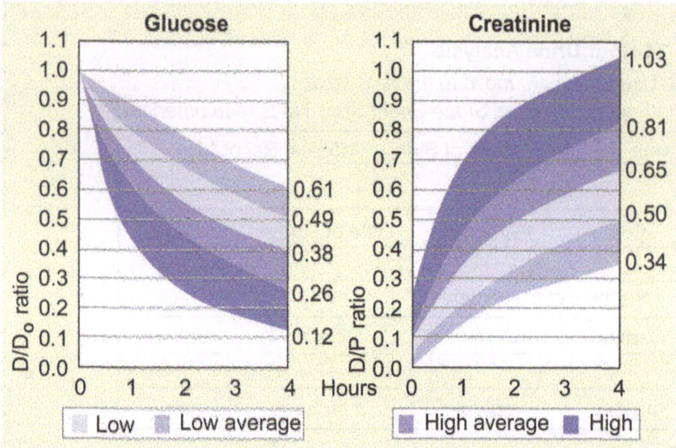

Fig. 17: Peritoneal equilibration test. The various peritoneal transporter status categorized as: Low, low average, high average and high depending D/Do glucose and D/P creatinine ratios. The numbers at the borders of the four categories represent maximal, mean +1SD, mean, mean –1 SD and minimal values at 4 hours dwell.

REFERENCES

1. Parekh BJ, Khadilkar V. Paediatrician friendly IAP growth charts for 0-18 years; 2015. [online] Available from https://iapindia.org/pdf/4422_Pediatrician-friendly-growth-charts-for-0-18-year-old-Indian-children-Dr-Bakul-Parekh-and-Dr-Vaman-khadilkar.pdf. [Last accessed March, 2022].
2. Khadilkar VV, Khadilkar AV. Revised Indian Academy of Pediatrics 2015 growth charts for height, weight and body mass index for 5-18-year-old Indian Children. Indian J Endocr Met. 2015;19:470-6.
3. WHO Growth charts as provided by Indian Academy of Pediatrics (IAP). [online] Available from: https://iapindia.org/pdf/4422_Pediatrician-friendly-growth-charts-for-0-18-year-old-Indian-children-Dr-Bakul-Parekh-and-Dr-Vaman-khadilkar.pdf. [Last accessed March, 2022].
4. Crawford JD, Terry ME, Rourkie GM. WEST nomogram: estimating body surface area of infants and young children. Pediatrics. 1950;5:785.
5. Flynn JT, Kaelber DC, Baker-Smith C, Blowey D, Carroll AE, Daniels SR, et al. Clinical Practice Guideline for Screening and management of high blood pressure in children and adolescents. Pediatrics. 2017;140(3):e20171904.
6. Flynn JT. Etiology, clinical features and diagnosis of neonatal hypertension. Official reprint from UpToDate 2020. [online] Available from https://www.uptodate.com/contents/etiology-clinical-features-and-diagnosis-of-neonatal-hypertension/print. [Last accessed March, 2022].
7. Otiv A, Mehta K, Ali U, Nadkarni M. Sonographic measurement of normal Indian Children. Indian Pediatr. 2012;49:533-6.
8. Dubose TD, Daeihagh P. Metabolic acidosis and alkalosis. Anaesthesia Key. [online] Available from https://images.app.goo.gl/siLZ9RFycDPyDvCw5. [Last accessed March, 2022].
9. Barth JH, Jones RG, Payne RB. Calculation of renal tubular reabsorption of phosphate: the algorithm performs better than the nomogram. Ann Clin Biochem. 2000;37:79-81.
10. Boer DP, de Rijke YB, Hop WC. Cransberg K, Dorresteijn EM. Reference values for serum creatinine in children younger than 1 year of age. Pediatric Nephrol. 2010;25:2107-13.
11. Gupta DK, Sankhwar SN, Goel A. Uroflowmetry nomograms for healthy children 5 to 15 years old. J Urol. 2013;190(3):1008-13.
12. StoneSheet-24TM. Pediatric 24-hour urine analysis. [online] Available from https://docs.google.com/spreadsheets/d/1Uts5I9JxkhXMLHbzrV8nVGPZJG5TdOMdqrSwQLAmYMA/edit?usp=sharing [Last accessed May, 2022].
13. Twardowski ZJ. Clinical values of standard equilibration tests in CAPD patients. Blood Purif. 1989;7:95-108.

CHAPTER

15.2 Drug Preparations and Dosages

Vaishali More, Soumya Reddy, Hamsa V Reddy

INTRODUCTION

Acute kidney injury (AKI) and chronic kidney disease (CKD) are associated with significant alterations in the pharmacokinetics (PK) and the pharmacodynamics (PD) of many drugs. Clinicians must consider the changes in the excretion of these drugs and their active/toxic metabolites while giving the prescription. Despite the advances in the treatment of AKI and CKD, many of them develop decreased kidney function over time. The introduction of many novel kidney replacement therapies (KRTs) for treating AKI and CKD mandates an understanding of their influence on drug disposition and response.

RENAL HANDLING OF DRUGS

The decrease in the renal excretion of drugs is the most evident consequence of abnormal renal functions in handling of drugs resulting in increased plasma drug concentration and a prolonged elimination half-life. Dosage adjustments are required for drugs that are predominantly excreted through renal pathways, which typically rely on an accurate estimation of glomerular filtration rate (GFR).

Patients with reduced GFR also have significantly altered PK of nonrenally eliminated drugs. This altered nonrenal clearance is primarily attributed to decreases in both hepatic drug metabolism and transporter-mediated biliary drug clearance. Ontogeny-mediated changes in essential drug-metabolizing enzymes and transporters in pediatric population further complicate drug dosing in this population.

Another important aspect of drug disposition in patients with reduced GFR is the impact of the dialysis process. Clearance of drugs during dialysis is important for drugs with a narrow therapeutic window, which can lead to subtherapeutic plasma drug concentrations. The physicochemical properties of a drug such as molecular size, protein binding, and volume of distribution and the dialysis prescription such as type of dialyzer membrane, rates of blood/dialysate flow, and type of KRT modality largely determine the dialyzability of drugs.

DRUG DOSING IN KIDNEY REPLACEMENT THERAPY

The drug removal during KRT is dependent on the mode of KRT, frequency, flow rates, filters used, and the pharmacological properties of the drug. It also varies in acute and chronic KRT. The slower flow rate among the blood flow and dialysate flow rate determine the solute clearance and thus the drug removal. For example, in intermittent hemodialysis (IHD), the blood flow rate is half the dialysate flow rate, so it is the blood flow rate that shall determine the dialytic clearance.[1]

In a critically ill child with AKI, volume overload and increased capillary permeability lead to increased volume of distribution of drugs. Acutely ill patients are likely to receive fluid resuscitation causing fluid overload, edema, effusion, and ascites. In addition, the water excretion is decreased in AKI. The increased volume of distribution in turn leads to a decreased serum concentration, especially for hydrophilic drugs such as aminoglycosides and cephalosporins.[1]

Hypoalbuminemia, which is commonly seen in critically ill children, affects the protein-bound fraction of the drug and can either increase drug availability or increase drug elimination. Only the free fraction or the unbound fraction of the drug can easily move across cell membranes. It is known that the protein binding of drugs such as penicillin, aminoglycosides, furosemide, and phenytoin is reduced in AKI and CKD. This leads to a greater distribution of these drugs in the interstitium and hence they are increasingly cleared by the liver, residual function of kidneys, and dialysis. Some studies have shown that the hepatic drug metabolism and transport are affected in AKI. So, it is likely that some drug accumulation may occur due to hepatic dysfunction.[2] Other factors in addition to KRT are increased cardiac output which also increases drug elimination and decreased gastric motility which decreases gastrointestinal absorption, respectively.[1]

The physiology differs in patients with CKD. Though the renal excretion is affected, the acute problems encountered in AKI are not seen in CKD. These patients visit the hospital on an outpatient basis. More vigilant care should be taken as drug dosing adjustment is found to be inadequate in 50–75% of all CKD patients which in turn affects the treatment goals.[3]

Intermittent hemodialysis provides higher clearance than other modes of KRT.[3] Some drug packages have inserts which provide dose adjustments in hemodialysis (HD); these are based on chronic HD and do not apply in acute HD for sick patients with AKI. In these patients, a supplementary dose is recommended after dialysis, which is to be administered postdialysis in addition to the predialysis adjusted dose. This dose should be increased at least by 50% if the available guideline is derived from data where a high-flux dialyzer was used.[2]

Peritoneal dialysis (PD) has two modalities—continuous ambulatory peritoneal dialysis (CAPD) and automated peritoneal dialysis (APD). The factors affecting drug removal in PD are composition of the dialysate, pathology of the peritoneum, volume and exchange rate of dialysate, molecular weight of the molecule, and the osmotic gradient. Most of the studies performed on patients on PD suggest that as most drugs are larger than urea, and the urea clearance is <10 mL/min, there is no enhanced drug removal during PD. Therefore, the recommendations for GFR < 15 mL/min should be used.[4,5] Acute PD which is regularly carried out for children with AKI in our country has frequent continuous cycles without long dwells. There are no recommendations available for dosing in such cases. Common drugs with their dialyzable properties are listed in **Table 1**.[6,7]

Prolonged intermittent kidney replacement therapy (PIKRT) or sustained low-efficiency dialysis (SLED) which is a hybrid therapy prescribed for 6–10 hours also does not have standardization for dose adjustment and is complex due to the variability in prescription. Hence, the PK and PD of drug clearance in SLED are different from other modalities. Clearance is the volume of reference fluid cleared of the drug per unit time. The drug clearance of patients on SLED is higher than continuous kidney replacement therapy (CKRT) and lower than IHD. The patient on SLED is on dialysis for a shorter duration than patients on CKRT and, hence, the overall clearance is lower than CKRT but higher than IHD. Also, the elimination of the drug is faster when the patient is on dialysis and slower when off dialysis. The starting time, duration of SLED, and total hours of treatment should be considered while adjusting the drug doses. Medications given as infusions should be readjusted when the SLED is stopped. Thus, a frequent drug dose review is needed in patients on SLED, and the improvement or decline of residual renal function should also be considered.[5] A stepwise approach is preferred to drug dose modification and is illustrated in **Table 2**.

In CKRT, in addition to the mode of dialysis, other factors which affect the drug removal are the blood and effluent flow rates, surface area, type of dialyzer, and interruptions due to clotting. Usually, high-flux dialyzers are used for CKRT. Also, factors mentioned before such as sepsis and nonrenal clearance of the drug play an important role.

Continuous kidney replacement therapy runs for 24 hours with some interruptions. The dose of prescribed CKRT

TABLE 1: Common drugs and their dialyzable properties.

Drug	*Hemodialysis*	*High permeability dialysis*	*Peritoneal dialysis*
Azathioprine	Yes	L	ND
Basiliximab	U	ND	U
Calcitriol	No	No	U
Carbamazepine	No	ND	No
Cetirizine	No	ND	No
Cyclophosphamide	Yes	L	ND
Cyclosporine	No	L	ND
Dexamethasone	No	ND	No
Enoxaparin	No	ND	U
Epoetin alpha	No	ND	No
Ethambutol	No	No	No
Fosphenytoin	U	ND	U
Furosemide	ND	ND	U
Hydrocortisone	U	ND	U
Isoniazid	No	No	U
IVIg	U	ND	U
Levothyroxine	U	ND	U
Lorazepam	ND	ND	U
Mannitol	Yes	L	Yes
Methotrexate	Yes	Yes	No
Methylprednisolone	Yes	L	Yes
Mycophenolate mofetil	No	ND	No
Phenobarbitone	Yes	L	ND
Pyrazinamide	Yes	Yes	No
Phenytoin	No	Yes	No
Rifampicin	No	No	No
Sevelamer	U	U	U
Valproate	No	ND	No
Warfarin	No	ND	No

(Yes: dialysable; No: nondialysable; L: likely dialyzable but no sufficient data; U: unlikely dialyzable but no sufficient data; ND: no data)

and the actual delivery should be considered as sometimes the actual dose is lower and will affect the drug levels. The sieving coefficients (SC) and saturation coefficients (SA) are used in continuous venovenous hemofiltration (CVVH) and continuous venovenous hemodialysis (CVVHD)/continuous venovenous hemodiafiltration (CVVHDF), respectively. The SC is calculated by measuring the solute/drug concentration in the blood and the dialysate and dividing the later by the former. In case the solute concentration cannot be measured, the normal protein-binding rate can be used (SC = 1 – protein binding). The removal of the drug also depends on the replacement fluid. If the replacement fluid is given prefilter, as dilution of the drug takes place, the drug removal is less. As the effluent rate (dialysate + ultrafiltrate) is higher than the

TABLE 2: Stepwise approach to adjust drug dose.		
Step 1	Obtain history and relevant demographic/clinical information	Assess demographic information, past medical history, current clinical, and laboratory data
Step 2	Estimate GFR	Use most appropriate tools based on age, body size, ethnicity, and concomitant disease status
Step 3	Review current medications	Is it really necessary or not?
Step 4	Calculate individualized treatment regimen	Calculate dosage regimen based on pharmacokinetic characteristics of the drug and the patient's volume status and eGFR or ClCr
Step 5	Monitor	Monitor parameters of drug response and toxicity; monitor levels if available/applicable
Step 6	Revise regimen	Adjust regimen based on step 5

(ClCr: creatinine clearance; eGFR: estimated glomerular filtration rate; GFR: glomerular filtration rate)

TABLE 3: Equations for calculating continuous kidney replacement therapy (CKRT) drug clearance.

CKRT type	Clearance equation
CVVH predilution	$CL_{CVVH(pre)} = Q_{eff} \times SC \times (Q_b/Q_b + Q_{rep})$
CVVH postdilution	$CL_{CVVH(post)} = Q_{eff} \times SC$
CVVHD	$CL_{CVVHD} = Q_d \times SA$
CVVHDF	$CL_{CVVHDF} = (Q_{uf} + Q_d) \times SA$

[CVVH (post): postdilution continuous venovenous hemofiltration; CVVH (pre): predilution continuous venovenous hemofiltration; CVVHD: continuous venovenous hemodialysis; CVVHDF: continuous venovenous hemodiafiltration; Q_b: blood flow rate; Q_d: dialysate flow rate; Q_{eff}: effluent flow rate; Q_{rep}: replacement fluid rate; Q_{uf}: ultrafiltration rate; SA: saturation coefficient; SC: sieving coefficient]

blood flow rate in CKRT, the drug removal is dependent on the effluent rate. **Table 3** lists the equations for calculating drug clearance in CKRT. **Table 4** lists the dose adjustments and supplementary dose for commonly used drugs antimicrobials and non-antimicrobial drugs.

Drugs with high protein binding and predominantly nonrenal elimination do not require adjustment during CKRT, e.g., ceftriaxone, moxifloxacin, clindamycin, azithromycin, tigecycline, polymyxin B, linezolid, voriconazole, posaconazole, caspofungin, micafungin, and AMB. CVVHDF is the most effective in removing drugs followed by CVVHD and CVVHF followed by the intermittent therapies.[8]

For those drugs with no guidelines for renal dosing, the theoretical GFR in various types of CKRT can be used. The GFR for patients on CVVHF is 0–15 mL/min and on CVVHDF is 30–40 mL/min. CAPD four exchanges 5–10 mL/min, IHD 150–200 mL/min during dialysis, and 0–10 mL/min in-between dialysis. Similarly, if the guidelines are not available, it is advisable to use GFR < 10 mL/min.[8] When applying any guidelines, it should be understood that dosing recommendations for one form of KRT usually cannot be applied to other forms of KRT. The clinical judgment is crucial in deciding the drug dose in addition to guidelines as the rate of change of renal function and volume status remain uncertain and variable.[9,10] To conclude, the details on the protocol for preparation and use of common drug infusions in routine clinical practice are mentioned here.[11-15]

PROTOCOLS FOR INFUSION

Immunosuppressive Medications

Methylprednisolone

Pretreatment screening:
- Rule out active infection
- Physical examination to exclude active infections
- Routine blood tests [complete blood count (CBC), renal function test (RFT), serum electrolytes, and liver function test (LFT)].

Contraindications:
- Systemic fungal infection
- Known hypersensitivity to the product or its constituents.

Dose:
10–30 mg/kg/dose (maximum 1,000 mg/dose)—three doses over 3–5 days

Available concentration (mg)	*Reconstitution with bacteriostatic water (mL)*
40	1
125	2
500	8
1,000	16
2,000 mg	30

Reconstituted solution is stale for 48 hours in room temperature. Protect from light.

Infusion protocol:
- No premedication necessary.
- Dilute the reconstituted solution in 100–250 mL normal saline (NS) or 5% dextrose.
- Infuse the solution over 4 hours.
- Strict monitoring of blood pressures (q30 min) and general random blood sugar (q60 min) during the infusion.

TABLE 4: Dose adjustments and supplementary dose for commonly used drugs antimicrobials and nonantimicrobials.

Drug	*Dose for normal renal function*	*GFR < 10*	*GFR 10–29*	*GFR 30–50*	*PD/ CAPD*	*IHD*	*Supplement for patients on PIKRT/SLED*	*Supplement in patients on CVVH/CVVHD*
Antimicrobials:								
Acyclovir	30–80 mg/kg/day q8h	5 mg/kg dose q48h	10 mg/kg dose q24h	10 mg/kg dose q12h	5 mg/kg dose q24h	5 mg/kg dose q24h after dialysis		10 mg/kg dose q12h
Amikacin	15 mg/kg/day q24h or q12h	2 mg/kg dose q24-48h	3–4 mg/kg q24h	5–6 mg/kg q12h	2 mg/kg or IP 25 mg/L, maint 12 mg/L	5 mg/kg after HD	7.5 mg/kg	7.5 mg/kg
Amoxicillin	25–50 mg/kg/day q8h High dose 80–90 mg/kg/ day q12h	8–20 mg/kg/ dose q24h	8–20 mg/kg/ dose q12h	100%	8–20 mg/kg/ dose q24h	8–20 mg/kg/ dose q24h after dialysis		NA
Amoxicillin/clavulanate	25–45 mg/kg/day q12h	8–20 mg/kg/ dose q24h	8–20 mg/kg/ dose q12h	100%	8–20 mg/kg/ dose q24h	8–20 mg/kg/ dose q24h after dialysis		NA
Aztreonam	30–40 mg/kg/dose q8h IV	7.5–10 mg/kg/ dose q12 h	15–20 mg/kg/ dose q8h	100%	7.5–10 mg/kg/ dose q12h	7.5–10 mg/kg/ dose q12h	100%	
Ampicillin sulbactam	Moderate: inf. 100–150 mg/kg/day q6h IM, IV, severe inf. 200–400 mg/ kg/day q6h IM, IV	35–50 mg/kg/ dose q24h	35–50 mg/kg/ dose q12	35–50 mg/kg/ dose q8h	35–50 mg/kg/ dose q24h	35–50 mg/kg/ dose q24h	2 g BD with one dose after dialysis	
Amphotericin B Lipid complex	3–5 mg/kg/day q24h	100%	100%	100%	100%	100%		100%
Ampicillin	100–200 mg/kg/day q6h	35–50 mg/kg/ dose q12h	35–50 mg/kg/ dose q8–12 h	35–50 mg/kg/ dose q6h	35–50 mg/kg/ dose q12h	35–50 mg/kg/ dose q12h	35–50 mg/kg/ dose q6h	35–50 mg/kg/ dose q6h
Azithromycin	10 mg/kg once followed by 5 mg/kg/day q24h	100%	100%	100%	100%	100%		100%
Cefaclor	20–40 mg/kg/day q8–12h	50%	100%	100%	50%	50%		NA
Cefadroxil	30 mg/kg/day q12h	15 mg/kg q36h	15 mg/kg q24h	100%	15 mg/kg q36h	15 mg/kg q24h		NA
Cefazolin	50–100 mg/kg/day q8h	25 mg/kg/dose q24h	25 mg/kg/dose q12h	100%	25 mg/kg/dose q24h IP: LD 500 mg/L, maint: 125 mg/L	25 mg/kg/dose q24h		25 mg/kg/dose q8h
Cefepime	50 mg/kg/dose q8–12h	50 mg/kg/dose q48h	50 mg/kg/dose q24h	50 mg/kg/dose q24h	50 mg/kg/dose q24h	50 mg/kg/dose q24h		50 mg/kg/dose q12h
Cefotaxime	100–200 mg/kg/day	35–70 mg/kg/ dose q24 h	35–70 mg/kg/ dose q12h	35–70 mg/kg/ dose q8–12h	35–70 mg/kg/ dose q24h IP:LD 500 mg/L, maint: 125 mg/L	35–70 mg/kg/ dose q24h		35–70 mg/kg/ dose q12h

Contd...

Contd...

Drug	***Dose for normal renal function***	***GFR < 10***	***GFR 10–29***	***GFR 30–50***	***PD/ CAPD***	***IHD***	***Supplement for patients on PIKRT/SLED***	***Supplement in patients on CVVH/CVVHD***
Ceftazidime	75–150 mg/kg/day q8h	50 mg/kg/dose q48h	50 mg/kg/dose q24h	50 mg/kg/dose q12h	50 mg/kg/dose q48h IP:LD 250 mg/L, maint: 125 mg/L	50 mg/kg/ dose q48h after dialysis	1 g q8h or 2 g q12h	50 mg/kg q12h
Ceftriaxone	50–100 mg/kg/day q12–24h	full dose q24h	100%	100%	50 mg/kg/dose q24h	50 mg/kg/dose q24h		50 mg/kg/dose q24h
Cefuroxime axetil	30 mg/kg/day q12h	15 mg/kg dose q24h	15 mg/kg dose q12h	100%	15 mg/kg dose q24h	15 mg/kg dose q24h		NA
Cephalexin	25–50 mg/kg/day q6h	5–10 mg/kg dose q24h	5–10 mg/kg dose q12h	5–10 mg/kg dose q8h	5–10 mg/kg dose q24h	5–10 mg/kg dose q24h after HD		NA
Ciprofloxacin	20–30 mg/kg/day q12h	10–15 mg/kg dose q24h	10–15 mg/kg dose q18h	100%	10–15 mg/kg dose q24h IP:LD 50 mg/L, maint: 25 mg/L	10–15 mg/kg dose q24h After HD		10–15 mg/kg dose q12h
Clindamycin	*Oral*: 10–30 mg/kg/day q6–8h IV:25–40 mg/kg/day q6h	100%	100%	100%	IP:LD 300 mg/L, maint: 150 mg/L	100%		100%
Caspofungin	70 mg/m² on day 1, then 50 mg/m² q24h	100%	100%	100%	100%	100%		100% Adjust for hepatic dysfunction
Colistin	12.5 mg/kg q12h	50% q12h	75% q12h	No adjustment	50 mg q12h	50 mg q12h	9 million units/ day in three divided doses	
Cefoxitin	80–160 mg/kg/24h q4–8 h IM/IV	20–40 mg/kg/ dose 24h	20–40 mg/kg/ dose q12h	20–40 mg/k/ dose q8h	Same as HD	20–40 mg/kg/ dose q24h		
Cefuroxime sodium (IV)	75–150 mg/kg/24h ÷ q8h	25–50 mg /kg/ dose q24h	25–50 mg/kg/ dose q12 h	100%	25–50 mg /kg/ dose q24h	25–50 mg /kg/ dose q24h after HD	25–50 mg/kg/ dose q8h	
Ceftizoxime	Infant 1–6 months: 100–200 mg/kg/24 h q6–8h IV, IM >6 months: 150–200 mg/kg/day q6–8h IV, IM	50 mg/kg/dose q24h	50 mg/kg/dose q12h	50 mg/kg/dose q8h	50 mg/kg/dose q24h	50 mg/kg/dose q24h after HD	50 mg/kg/dose q8 hourly	
Cefixime	8 mg/kg/24 h q12–24h PO	4 mg/kg/dose q12 h	6 mg/kg/dose q12 h	100%	Not required	Supplemental dose required		
Clarithromycin	7.5–15 mg /kg/dose q12h PO	4 mg/kg/dose q24h	4 mg/kg/dose q12h	100%	4 mg/kg/dose q24h	4 mg/kg/dose q24h		

Contd...

Contd...

Drug	*Dose for normal renal function*	*GFR < 10*	*GFR 10–29*	*GFR 30–50*	*PD/ CAPD*	*IHD*	*Supplement for patients on PIKRT/SLED*	*Supplement in patients on CVVH/CVVHD*
Doxycycline	PO/IV Initial: <45 kg: 2.2 mg/kg/dose BID × 1 day to maximum dose of 200 mg/24 h, >45 kg 100 mg/dose BID × 1 day Maintenance: PO/IV <45 kg: 2.2–4.4 mg/kg/ dose QD–BID >45 kg: 100–200 mg/24 h QD–BID	1 mg /kg/dose q12h	100%	100%	1 mg /kg/dose q12h	1 mg /kg/dose q12h	100%	
Erythromycin	Oral: 30–50 mg/kg/day q6–8 h IV: 15–50 mg/kg/day q6h	10–17 mg/kg/ dose q8h	100%	100%	10–17 mg/kg/ dose q8h	10–17 mg/kg/ dose q8h		100%
Ethambutol	15–25 mg/kg/day q24h	15–25 mg/kg dose q48h	15–25 mg/kg dose q36h	100%	15–25 mg/kg dose q48h	15–25 mg/kg dose q48h		100%
Flucytosine	400–1,200 mg/m²/dose q6 h IV, IM	25–37.5 mg/kg/ dose q24h	25–37.5 mg/kg/ dose q12h	25–37.5 mg/kg/ dose q8h	25–37.5 mg/kg/ dose q24h	25–37.5 mg/kg/ dose q24h	25–37.5 mg/ kg/dose q8 h, monitor serum concentration	
Fluconazole	3–12 mg/kg/day q24h	1.5–6 mg/kg/ day q48h	1.5–6 mg/kg/ day q24h	1.5–6 mg/kg/ day q24h	1.5–6 mg/kg/ day q48h	1.5–6 mg/kg/ day q48h after dialysis		6 mg/kg dose q24h
Foscarnet	90–120 mg/kg/day q24h	Not recommended	50–65 mg/kg q48h	60–80 mg/kg q48h	Not recommended	Not recommended		60–80 mg/kg q48h
Ganciclovir	IV 10 mg/kg/day q12h then 5 mg/kg/day q24h; Oral 30 mg/kg dose q8h	IV 1.25 mg/ kg dose 3/wk, maint: 0.625 mg/kg dose 3/ wk Oral: 30 mg/kg dose q24h	IV 1.25 mg/ kg dose q24h maint: 0.625 mg/kg dose q24 h Oral: 30 mg/kg dose q12h	IV 2.5 mg/kg dose q24h, maint: 1.25 mg/ kg dose q24 h Oral: 100%	IV 1.25 mg/kg dose q3/wk, maint: 0.625 mg/kg dose 3/ wk Oral: 30 mg/kg dose 3/wk	IV 1.25 mg/kg dose q3/wk, maint: 0.625 mg/kg dose 3/wk Oral: 30 mg/kg dose 3/wk After dialysis		IV 2.5 mg/kg dose q24h, maint: 1.25 mg/kg dose q24h Oral: 100%
Gentamicin	2.5 mg/kg dose q8h	2 mg/kg q48–72h, based on serum levels	2–3 mg/kg q24h, monitor serum levels	3–5 mg/kg q24h, monitor serum levels	2 mg/kg	2 mg/kg or IP LD 8 mg/L, maint 12 mg/L	2–2.5 mg/kg post-dialysis	

Contd...

Contd...

Drug	***Dose for normal renal function***	***GFR < 10***	***GFR 10–29***	***GFR 30–50***	***PD/ CAPD***	***IHD***	***Supplement for patients on PIKRT/SLED***	***Supplement in patients on CVVH/CVVHD***
Imipenem	60–100 mg/kg/day q6h	7.5–12.5 mg/kg/ dose q24h	7.5–12.5 mg/kg/ dose q12h	7–13 mg/kg/ dose q8h	7.5–12.5 mg/kg/ dose q24h	7.5–12.5 mg/kg/ dose q24h after dialysis		7–13 mg/kg/dose q8h
Isoniazid	10–15 mg/kg/day q12–24h	100%	100%	100%	100%	100%		100%
Ketoconazole	3.3–6.6 mg/kg/day q24h	100%	100%	100%	100%	100%	100%	100%
Linezolid	10 mg/kg/dose q8h IV/PO	100%	100%	100%	10 mg/kg/dose 12 h	10 mg/kg/dose 12 h	100%	
Levofloxacin	<5 years: 5–10 mg/kg dose q12h >5 years: 5–10 mg/kg dose q24h	All ages: 5–10 mg/kg dose q48h	All ages: 5–10 mg/kg dose q24h	100%	All ages: 5–10 mg/kg dose q48h	All ages: 5–10 mg/kg dose q48h	500 mg q24h	10 mg/kg dose q24h
Lamivudine	4 mg/kg/dose q12 h	1 mg/kg/dose 24 h	2 mg/kg/dose 24 h	4 mg/kg/kg/ dose q24 h	1 mg/kg/dose q24h	1 mg/kg/dose q24h	4 mg/kg/dose q24h	
Meropenem	60–120 mg/kg/day q8h	10–20 mg/kg/ dose q24h	10–20 mg/kg/ dose q12h	20–40 mg/kg/ dose q12h	10–20 mg/kg/ dose q24h	10–20 mg/kg/ dose q24 h after dialysis	1 g q12h	20–40 mg/kg/ dose q12h
Netilmicin	2.25 mg/kg/dose q8h IV	10–20%	20–60%	20–60%	2–4 mg/L/d	Give ½ dose after dialysis	Dose for GFR 10–50, measure plasma serum levels	
Nalidixic acid	15 mg/kg/dose q6h PO	Avoid use						
Metronidazole	15–30 mg/kg/day q6–8h	4 mg/kg/dose q6h	No adjustment	100%		4 mg/kg/dose q6h	4 mg/kg/dose q6h	100%
Ofloxacin	15 mg/kg/day q12h	7.5 mg/kg dose q48h	7.5 mg/kg dose q24h	7.5 mg/kg dose q48h	7.5 mg/kg dose q48h	7.5 mg/kg dose q48h		10 mg/kg dose q24h
Piperacillin + Tazobactam	200–300 mg/kg/day q6h	35–50 mg/kg dose q8h	35–50 mg/kg dose q8h	35–50 mg/kg dose q6h	50–75 mg/kg dose q12h	50–75 mg/kg dose q12h		35–50 mg/kg dose q8h
Pyrazinamide	20–40 mg/kg/day q12–24h	50%	100%	100%	50%	50%		Avoid
Penicillin G/K and Na	450,000–500,000 U/ kg/24 h q4–6h	25–50%	75%	75%	25–50%	Dose after dialysis		
Rifampicin	10–20 mg/kg/day q12–24h	100%	100%	100%	100%	100%	100%	100%
Streptomycin	20–40 mg/kg/day q24h	7.5 mg/kg q72–96h	7.5 mg/kg q48h	7.5 mg/kg q24h	7.5 mg/kg q72–96h	7.5 mg/kg q72–96h		7.5 mg/kg q24h

Contd...

Contd...

Drug	Dose for normal renal function	GFR < 10	GFR 10–29	GFR 30–50	PD/ CAPD	IHD	Supplement for patients on PIKRT/SLED	Supplement in patients on CVVH/CVVHD
Teicoplanin	20/kg divided q12h, maint 6–10 mg/kg/day q24 h	1 mg/kg/dose q24h	1–4 mg/kg/dose q24h	1–4 mg/kg/dose q24h	1 mg/kg/dose q24h IP: LD 400 mg/L, maint 20 mg/L	1 mg/kg/dose q24 h after dialysis		5 mg/kg dose q8h
Tobramycin	2.5 mg/k/ dose q8h	1 mg/kg/dose, then based on serum levels	1 mg/kg/dose, then based on serum levels	1–2 mg/kg/ dose, then based on serum levels	2 mg/kg adjust as per serum concentration IP: LD 8 mg/L, maint: 4 mg/L	2 mg/kg adjust as per serum concentration		2–2.5 mg/kg q12–24 h adjust as per serum concentration
Trimethoprim sulfamethoxazole	5–20 mg/kg/day q6–12h	Not recommended but if used 5–10 mg/kg dose q24h	5–10 mg/kg/ dose q12h	5–7.5 mg/kg/ dose q8h	Not recommended but if used 5–10 mg/kg dose q24 h	Not recommended but if used 5–10 mg/kg dose q24h Or IP LD 320/1600 mg/L, maint 80–400 mg/L	Not enough evidence	5 mg/kg dose q8h
Ticarcillin	200–300 mg/kg/day q 4–6h, Maximum dose 18–24 mg/day	50–70 mg/kg dose q12h	50–70 mg/kg dose q8h	100%	50–70 mg/kg/ dose q12 h	50–70 mg/kg/ dose q12 h	50–70 mg/kg/ dose q8h	
Vancomycin	10 mg/kg/dose q6h or 15 mg/kg/dose q8h	10 mg/kg/dose as needed as per drug level	10 mg/kg/dose q18–24h	10 mg/kg/dose q12h		10 mg/kg/dose as needed as per drug level IP: LD 500 mg/L, maint 30 mg/L	20–25 mg/kg/ dose as needed as per drug level	10 mg/kg/dose every q12–24h
Valganciclovir	Induction 15–18 mg/ kg 12 h, maint: 15–18 mg/kg 24 h	Not recommended	50% dose 48 h followed by 50% dose twice a week	eGFR 40–59: induction: 50% dose 12 h, maint: 50% dose q24 h eGFR 20–40: induction: 50% dose 24 h, maint: 50% dose 48 h	No recommen- dation	50% dose 3/wk AD		Induction 50% dose 24 h, maint: 50% 48 h
Valacyclovir	20 mg/kg/dose q8 hourly PO	10 mg/kg/dose q24h	20 mg/kg/dose q24h	20 mg/kg/dose q12h	10 mg /kg/dose OD	10 mg /kg/dose OD give after dialysis	N/A	

Contd...

Contd...

Drug	*Dose for normal renal function*	*GFR < 10*	*GFR 10–29*	*GFR 30–50*	*PD/ CAPD*	*IHD*	*Supplement for patients on PIKRT/SLED*	*Supplement in patients on CVVH/CVVHD*
Zidovudine	120 mg/m²/dose IV q6 h cont. IV infusion, 20 mg/m²/h or 160 mg/m²/dose PO q8h	50% q8h	100%	100%	50% q8h, unless cont.	50% q8h, unless cont.	100%	
Nonantimicrobials:								
Acetaminophen	10–15 mg/kg/dose q4–6h	100% q8h	100%	100%	100% q8h	100% q8h		100%
Amlodipine	0.05–0.17 mg/kg/day	100%	100%	100%	100%	100%	100%	100%
Atenolol Maximum dose 1/kg	0.8–1.5 mg/kg/day q12–24h	100%	100%	100%	100%	After HD		100%
Allopurinol	Individual protocol	30%	50%	50%	30%	30%		50%
Azathioprine	2–5 mg/kg/day q24 h; then 1–3 mg/kg/day q2h	50% q24h	75% q24h	75% q24h	50% q24h	75% q24h		75% q24h
Acetazolamide	5–10 mg/kg/ dose q6–8h PO	Avoid use	50%	50%				
Aminophylline	Loading dose: 6 mg/kg IV Maintenance dose 1–12 years: 0.8 mg/kg/h IV 12–16 years: 0.7 mg/kg/h IV	100%	100%	100%				
Carbamazepine	5–10 mg/kg/dose q8h PO	75%	100%	100%	75%	75%	Monitor levels	
Captopril	0.1–0.5 mg/kg dose q6–8h, maximum 6 mg/kg/day	50%	75%	75%	50%	50%		75%
Cetirizine	0.25–10 mg/kg/day depending on age group check pediatric dosing	Not recommended	50%	100%	50%	50%		NA
Clonidine	5–10 µg/kg/day q8–12h maximum 0.9 mg/kg/day	100%	100%	100%	100%	100%	100%	100%

Contd...

Contd...

Drug	Dose for normal renal function	GFR < 10	GFR 10–29	GFR 30–50	PD/ CAPD	IHD	Supplement for patients on PIKRT/SLED	Supplement in patients on CVVH/CVVHD
Codeine	0.5–1 mg/kg dose q4–6h	50%	75%	75%	50%	50%		75%
Cyclosporine	Individual protocol	100%	100%	100%	100%	100%		100%
Cyclophosphamide	Individual protocols	75%	100%	100%	75%	50% after dialysis		100% moderately dialyzable
Chlorothiazide	2–20 mg/kg/dose IV q12–24h	Ineffective in GFR < 50						
Digoxin	Pediatric reference	25%	50%	75%	25%	25%		75%
Diazepam	0.1–0.4 mg/kg/dose IV, PR	100% for any GFR						
Diclofenac	1 mg/kg/dose q8–12h PO	25%	25–50%	25–50%				
Enalapril	0.1 mg/kg dose q12–24h	50%	75%	75%	50%	50%		75%
Fexofenadine	>12 years 120–180 mg/ day	30 mg q24h	60 mg q24h	60 mg q24h	30 mg q24h	30 mg q24h		NA
Fentanyl	0.5–2 μg/kg dose or 1–5 μg/kg/h continuous	50%	75%	75%	50%	50%		75% titrate to effect
Gabapentin	10–35 mg/kg/day q8h	75% q48h	75% q24h	75% q12h	75% q48h	75% q48h Additional dose after each 4 h HD		75% q12h Dosing not studied below 12 years
Hydralazine	0.4 mg/kg/dose 12h PO	100% q8–12h	100% q8h	100% q8h	100% q8h	100% q8h	100% q8h	
Hydrochlorothiazide	1–1.5 mg/kg/dose q12–24h PO	Not recommended	Not recommended	100%	Not recommended	Not recommended	100%	
Indomethacin	0.5–1 mg/kg/dose q8h PO	100% for any eGFR						
Labetalol	3–20 mg/kg/day q12h	100%	100%	100%	100%	100%		100%
Lamotrigine	As per pediatric reference	50%	100%	100%	50%	50%		NA
Levetiracetam	5–10 mg/kg/day divided 2–3 times per day, up to 60 mg/kg/day divided 2 times per day	50%	50%	50%	50%	50%		50%
Lisinopril	0.1–1 mg/kg/24 h PO	25%	50%	50%	25%	50% after dialysis	50%	
Metoprolol	1–2 mg/kg/day q12–24h	100%	100%	100%	100%	100% after dialysis		100%

Contd...

Contd...

Drug	*Dose for normal renal function*	*GFR < 10*	*GFR 10–29*	*GFR 30–50*	*PD/ CAPD*	*IHD*	*Supplement for patients on PIKRT/SLED*	*Supplement in patients on CVVH/CVVHD*
Milrinone	Load 50 µg/kg, then 0.25–75 µg/kg/min	0.2 µg/kg/min	0.23–0.33 µg/kg/min	0.33–0.43 µg/kg/min	0.2 µg/kg/min	0.2 µg/kg/min		0.33–0.43 µg/kg/min
Minoxidil	0.25–0.1 mg/kg/day q12–24h	100%	100%	100%	100%	100%		100%
Mycophenolate	600 mg/m² dose 12 h	No more than 600 mg/m²/day	No more than 600 mg/m²/day	100%	No more than 600 mg/m²/day	No more than 600 mg/m²/day		100% Not dialyzable
Methyldopa	3 mg/kg/dose q8h PO	q12–24h	q8–12h	q8h	None	Dose after dialysis	Dose for GFR 10–50	
Nifedipine	0.25–0.5 mg/kg dose q6–8h, maximum 1–2 mg/kg/day	100%	100%	100%	100%	100%		100%
Oxcarbazepine	10–20 mg/kg/day q8–12h	75%	100%	100%	75%	75%		75%
Phenobarbital	3–7 mg/kg/day q12–24h	50% q24h	100%	100%	40–50% removed by PD dependent on number of cycles	100% supplemental dose during and after dependent on patient threshold for seizure		10 mg/kg dose q8h or q6h, monitor serum concentration
Phenytoin	6–9 mg/kg/day depending on age	100%	100%	100%	100%	100%		100%
Prednisolone	Variable	100%	100%	100%	100%	100%		100%
Propranolol	0.5–4 mg/kg/day q6–8h, maximum 16 mg/kg/day	100%	100%	100%	100%	100%		100%
Ranitidine	2–4 mg/kg/dose q8–12h PO	1 mg/kg dose 24 h, IV 0.5 mg/kg/dose q24 h	PO: 1 mg/kg dose q12h IV: 0.5 mg/kg dose q12h	PO: 2 mg/kg/dose q12h IV: 1 mg /kg/dose q12h	PO, 1 mg/kg dose q24h; IV, 0.5 mg/kg dose q24h	PO, 1 mg/kg dose q24h; IV, 0.5 mg/kg dose q24h	PO, 2 mg/kg dose q12 h; IV, 1 mg/kg dose q12h	
Spironolactone	6.25–25 mg/dose q12h PO	Avoid use	q6–12h	q6–12h	Not applicable	Not applicable	Avoid use	
Ramipril	6 mg/m² q24h	25% of dose	50% of dose	No change				
Valproic acid	20–60 mg/kg/day q8–12h if IV use q6h	100%	100%	100%	100%	100%		100%
Sirolimus	3 mg/m² first day; maint: 1 mg/m²/day	100%	100%	100%	100%	100%		100%

Contd...

Contd...

Drug	Dose for normal renal function	GFR < 10	GFR 10–29	GFR 30–50	PD/ CAPD	IHD	Supplement for patients on PIKRT/SLED	Supplement in patients on CVVH/CVVHD
Tacrolimus	0.15–0.4 mg/kg/day divided q12h	Renal and hepatic impairment: Use lowest dose and monitor serum concentration						
Ibuprofen	5–10 mg/kg dose q6h	100%	100%	100%	100%	100%	100%	100%
Lansoprazole								
Meperidine	0.5–2 mg/kg dose q3–4h	50%	75%	75%	Avoid	Avoid		
Methadone	0.05–0.2 mg/kg dose q4–6h for 3–4 doses, then 3–4 doses q8–12h IV: 0.03–0.1 mg/kg dose q4–6h for 3–4 doses then q8–12h	50–75% q12–24h	100%	100%	50–75% q12–24h	50–75% q12–24h		q8–12h
Midazolam	As per pediatric reference	50%	75%	100%	50%	50%		100%
Montelukast								
Morphine	Oral 0.2–0.5 mg/kg dose q4–6h IV 0.05–0.2 mg/kg dose q2–4h	50%	75%	75%	50%	50%		
Omeprazole	0.7–3.5 mg/kg/day q12–24h	100%	100%	100%	100%	100%		100%
Pantoprazole	0.5–1 mg/kg/day	100%	100%	100%	100%	100%		100%
Warfarin	0.1–0.3 mg/kg/day	100%	100%	100%	100%	100%		100%
Enoxaparin	<2 months: prophylaxis 0.75 mg/kg dose q12h Treatment: 1.5 mg/kg dose q12h; >2 months: prophylaxis: 0.5 mg/kg dose q12h, 1 mg/kg q12h	50% q24h	70%	100%	50%	50%		70%
Heparin	50–100 units bolus then 20 U/kg/h	50%	100%	100%	50%	50%		Monitor ACT and PTT

(ACT: activated clotting time; CAPD: continuous ambulatory peritoneal dialysis; CVVH: continuous venovenous hemofiltration; CVVHD: continuous venovenous hemodialysis; eGFR: estimated glomerular filtration rate; GFR: glomerular filtration rate; HD: hemodialysis; IHD: intermittent hemodialysis; IM: intramuscular; IP: intraperitoneal; IV: intravenous; LD: loading dose; NA: not applicable; PD: pharmacodynamics; PIKRT: prolonged intermittent kidney replacement therapy; PO: per oral; PR: per rectal; PTT: partial thromboplastin time; SLED: sustained low-efficiency dialysis)

Side effects:

- Hypertension, hyperglycemia, and fluid retention.

Example: For a 30-kg child
Intravenous (IV) methylprednisolone 500 mg in 250 mL NS over 4 hours daily or alternate day for 3 days.

Rituximab

Pretreatment screening:

- Detailed history regarding active infection, recent hospitalization in the past 2 weeks, comorbidities, and allergies
- Physical examination to exclude active infections
- Routine blood tests (CBC, RFT, SE, and LFT), hepatitis B, and hepatitis C screen if LFT is abnormal
- CD19/CD20 absolute counts
- Confirm present status of remission [if steroid-sensitive nephrotic syndrome (SSNS)]
- *Others:*
  - Chest X-ray (CXR; if indicated especially for suspected tuberculosis)
  - Immunoglobulin levels (if indicated)
- Vaccination should have been given 1 month prior to immunization or 6 months after last dose of rituximab.

Contraindications:

- Hypersensitivity to rituximab or other murine proteins
- Active acute or chronic infection.

Treatment dose and duration:
Initial course:

- Dosing—IV rituximab 375 mg/m²/dose (maximum 500 mg; in those with difficult to treat nephrotic syndrome—may consider dosing based on actual per m² dose)
- Frequency—two doses at weekly intervals; subsequent doses based on CD19 absolute counts (maximum four doses)
- *Monitoring:*
  - To repeat CD19/CD20 after two doses (at least 72 hours following last dose)
  - Target suppression < 5 cells/μL or <1%
  - If >5 cells/μL or >1% → additional doses may be given (maximum two doses, 1 week apart) till target suppression reached.

Subsequent course:

- Indication—relapse despite maintenance immunosuppression within 1 year of first course of rituximab
- Immunoglobulin profile to be considered
- Dosing—375 mg/m² single dose
- Subsequent doses to be based on CD19/CD20 counts
- If >5 cells/μL or >1%—one additional dose can be given (1 week apart from the 1st dose)

Long-term monitoring:

Test	Timing (after second dose of rituximab)		
	3 months	6 months	1 year
CD19/CD20 counts	✓	✓	✓
Complete blood count	✓	✓	✓
Urine albumin	✓	✓	✓
Liver function tests	✓	✓	✓
Follow-up for monitoring of microscopic polyangiitis (MPA) side effects as per the clinician's discretion.			

Maintenance therapy:
Mycophenolate (MMF) is preferred as maintenance immunosuppression.
Dose—600–800 mg/m² (in those with difficult to treat nephrotic syndrome/frequent relapses—can consider 1,000–1,200 mg/m²/day

Rituximab infusion:
Available concentration:

- 500 mg/50 mL
- *Concentration*: 2 mg/mL (make up total volume in NS based on total dose).

Administration:

- Premedication drugs (to be given 30–60 minutes before starting infusion):
  - Injection hydrocortisone (5 mg/kg)
  - Injection chlorpheniramine maleate (0.5 mg/kg)
  - Oral paracetamol (15 mg/kg)
- Start the infusion at 2 mL/h and double the rate every 30 minutes maximum up to 64 mL/h. In case of reactions to previous dose, do not exceed 16 mL/h.

Rituximab reaction management protocol:
Reactions generally occur within 30 minutes to 2 hours of beginning the first infusion. Keep epinephrine (1 mg/mL) intramuscular (IM), diphenhydramine 50 mg IV, and hydrocortisone 100 mg IV available for reaction management.

Common reactions: Fever, headache, rigors, flushing, nausea, rash, and upper respiratory tract infection (URTI) symptoms. Transient hypotension and bronchospasm are usually related to the infusion rate.

Mild-to-moderate reactions: For example, low-grade fever; hypotension <30 mm Hg from baseline

- Halve the infusion rate
- Symptomatic medications if needed
- Once stable, restart IV at one-half previous infusion rate and proceed as ordered.

Moderate-to-severe reactions: E.g., fever >38.5°C, chills, mucosal swelling, shortness of breath, hypotension by >30 mm Hg from baseline

- Stop the infusion and treat the symptoms.

- Administer diphenhydramine 25 mg IV and hydrocortisone 5 mg/kg IV; in an emergent situation, give epinephrine 0.3 mg/0.3 mL IM.
- If hypotensive—IV fluid bolus 10–20 mL/kg.
- The infusion should be restarted at half the previous rate only when the symptoms have resolved.

Late side effects are sepsis, granulocytopenia, and liver failure.

Example: For a 20-kg child [body surface area (BSA) —0.7 m²] Premedicate with hydrocortisone (100 mg), chlorpheniramine maleate (1 mg) and paracetamol (300 mg) 60 minutes prior to rituximab infusion.

Rituximab 250 mg in 250 mL NS:
- 2 mL/h for 30 minutes
- 4 mL/h for 30 minutes
- 8 mL/h for 30 minutes
- 16 mL/h for 60 minutes (if no reactions, then proceed to increase rate)
- 32 mL/h for 120 minutes
- 64 mL/h till infusion ends.

Cyclophosphamide

Pretreatment screening:
- History—ask for active infection, allergies
- Physical examination—to rule out active infection
- Laboratory investigations—complete blood count with differential, serum creatinine, blood urea nitrogen (BUN), serum electrolytes, liver function tests, and urine albumin.

Contraindications:
- Active infection
- Anaphylaxis to previous dose
- Urinary outflow tract obstruction.

Cyclophosphamide infusion:

Dose—500–1,000 mg/m² (maximum—1.2 g/dose)

Renal dose correction:

eGFR (mL/min/1.73 m²)	Dose
>50	100%
25–50	80%
10–25	70%
<10	50%, use with cation

In hemodialysis patients—50% of dose to be given after HD

Available strengths—500 mg, 1 g, 2 g (available as lyophilized powder)

Reconstitution—using 0.9% NaCl or sterile water

Reconstitution of cyclophosphamide:

Strength	Volume of diluent	Cyclophosphamide concentration
500 mg	25 mL	20 mg/mL
1 g	50 mL	
2 g	100 mL	

Dilution of reconstituted cyclophosphamide:

5% dextrose, 5% dextrose + 0.9% sodium chloride injection, 0.45% sodium chloride injection

Dilute the reconstituted cyclophosphamide solution to a minimum concentration of 2 mg/mL with any of the above diluents.

Infusion protocol:
- Commence infusion in the morning to facilitate frequent voiding and prevent accumulation of cyclophosphamide metabolites in the bladder
- Preinfusion hydration—NS (0.9% NaCl) 20 mL/kg (max 1 L) 60–90 minutes prior to infusion
- Premedication—antiemetic—Ondansetron 0.1 mg/kg (IV) 30 minutes prior to infusion
- Cyclophosphamide infusion—over 4 hours
- *Mesna:*
  - Dose—total dose (mg) = 60% of the calculated dose of cyclophosphamide
  - Available doses—100 mg/2 mL, 200 mg/2 mL
  - Administration—in three divided doses at 0 hour, 1 hour, and 4 hours of infusion
- Monitoring—vitals to be checked at baseline and every hour during infusion
- Postinfusion hydration—NS (0.9% NaCl) 20 mL/kg (maximum 1 L) over 60 minutes
- *Advise postinfusion:*
  - Frequent voiding
  - Plenty of oral fluids—1.5–2 L over 24–48 hours.

Monitoring during subsequent doses—complete blood counts, serum creatinine, and disease activity.

To assess response after three doses—if <50% reduction in proteinuria or failure of serum creatinine to return to 25% of baseline (if abnormal)—to consider alternate immunosuppression.

Side effects:

Hemorrhagic cystitis, neutropenia, less commonly myocarditis, and pericardial effusion,

If WBC < 4,000—reduce next dose by 25%.

Example: For a 30-kg child
- 500 mg/m² cyclophosphamide
- Preinfusion—600 mL NS over 1 hour, 60–90 minutes prior
- Premedication—Ondansetron (3 mg IV) 30 minutes prior to infusion
- Cyclophosphamide infusion—500 mg in 50 mL NS over 4 hours
- Mesna 60% of 500 mg = 300 mg—100 mg at 0 hour,1 hour, and 4 hours of infusion
- Postinfusion—600 mL NS over 1 hour.

Antihypertensives

Sodium Nitroprusside

Preparation for infusion:
- 1 vial (5 mL) = 100 mg

- Dilute 100 mg in 5% dextrose to form a total infusion volume of 100 mL
- Concentration 1 mL = 1 mg
- Rate of infusion to start at 0.5 μg per minute and increase by 0.5 μg till desired BP levels are reached.
- Rate of infusion = $\frac{\mu g \times \text{body weight} \times 60 \times 100}{1{,}000 \times \text{drug concentration (100 mg)}}$

Example: For a 10-kg child rate, start at 0.5 μg/kg

$$\text{Rate of infusion} = \frac{0.5 \times 10 \times 60 \times 100 = 0.3\ \text{mL/h}}{1000 \times 100}$$

To increase infusion by 0.5 μg/kg/min, subsequently double the rate of infusion.

Labetalol

Preparation for infusion:

- 1 Ampule (20 mL) = 100 mg
- Preparation: 20 mL + 30 mL NS
- Drug concentration: 1 mL = 2 mg
- Rate of infusion: $\frac{\text{Desired dose (mg)} \times \text{quantity (mL)}}{\text{Total drug content in infusion (mg)}}$

Example: For a weight of 10 kg, start infusion at 0.4 mg/kg/h hence rate of infusion

$$\frac{4\ \text{mg} \times 50\ \text{mL}}{100\ \text{mg}} = 2\ \text{mL/h}$$

Parenteral Iron Therapy

Indications:

Diagnosis of iron-deplete state: Transferrin saturation (TSAT) < 20% and ferritin <100 μg/L

- Poor response to oral iron (6 mg/kg/day for at least 1 month)
- Intolerance to oral iron
- Need to rapidly increase iron levels while on erythropoiesis-stimulating agent (ESA).

Contraindications for parenteral iron therapy:

- Known hypersensitivity to iron
- Clinical/biochemical evidence of acute or chronic infection
- Clinical or biochemical evidence of liver damage
- TSAT > 50%, serum ferritin >500.

Dose of IV iron:

(Ganzoni formula)

Total dose = [Body weight (kg) × (Target Hb - Actual Hb) × 0.24) + Iron stores (Target Hb—12.0)

Iron stores—15 mg/kg if the body weight is <35 kg and 500 if body weight is >35 kg

Iron Preparations

Iron sucrose: Available as 20 mg/mL solution. Each vial contains 100 mg (5 mL).

Dose: Total dose—as per Ganzoni formula

Maximum dose aliquot for the IV iron therapy is 100 mg/day.

Infusion:

- Strict monitoring for anaphylaxis. Ensure that resuscitatory materials are arranged.
- Dilute the required dose of iron sucrose in NS to achieve a concentration of 1 mg/mL.
- Initiate as a slow infusion. The first 25% of the dose is given over 15 minutes.
- If no adverse reactions occur, the remaining dose can be given over the next 45 minutes.
- For patients on hemodialysis: Infuse during the last hour of hemodialysis through the venous limb of the HD circuit.
- For patients on PD: Start with the initiation of.

  Monthly monitoring of ferritin, TSAT, and hemoglobin level to decide the further dosage schedule.

Ferric carboxymaltose: Available as 500 mg/10 mL

Dose—as per Ganzoni formula

Maximum dose of 500 mg/day

Infusion:

- Dilute the dose in NS to a maximum concentration of 2 mg/mL.
- No test dose is required.
- Administer as infusion over 30–60 minutes.
- If total dose >500 mg: Administer as two doses, 1 week apart.
- Watch for hypersensitivity reactions during infusion and for 1-2 hours postinfusion.

Oral iron supplements[15,16]

Iron compound	Preparation	Elemental iron (per tablet/5 mL)
Ferrous sulfate (FS)	FS tablets—100 mg	20 mg
	Fesovit—150 mg	46.8 mg
Colloidal iron	Tonoferon syrup	250 mg
	Tonoferon pediatric syrup	80 mg
	Tonoferon drops (per mL)	25 mg
Ferrous ammonium citrate	Dexorange syrup (each 15 mL)	30 mg
Ferrous fumarate	Livogen capsules	50 mg
	Vitcofol syrup	30 mg

Dose equivalence for conversion from erythropoietin to darbepoetin alpha in a given patient[17]

Previous epoetin alfa dose	OW Aransep° starting dose	
(Units/week)	Adult (μg/week)	Child (μg/week)
<1,500	6.25	–
1,500–2,499	6.25	6.25
2,500–4,999	12.5	10
5,000–10,999	25	20
11,000–17,999	40	40
18,000–33,999	60	60
34,000–89,999	100	100
>90,000	200	200

ANTICOAGULATION (TABLES 5 TO 8)

TABLE 5: Protocol for systemic heparin administration and adjustment for pediatric patients.[18]

I. Loading does: heparin 75 units/kg IV over 10 min

II. Initial maintenance dose: 28 units/kg/h for infants aged < 1 year, 20 units/kg/h for children aged >1 year

III. Adjust hepartin to maintain aPTT of 60–85 second (assuming this reflects an anti-Xa level of 0.35–0.70):

aPTT,s	Bolus, units/kg	Hold, min	% Rate change	Repeat aPTT
< 50	50	0	+10	4 h
50–59	0	0	+10	4 h
60–85	0	0	0	Next day
86–95	0	0	–10	4 h
96–120	0	30	–10	4 h
>120	0	60	–15	4 h

IV. Obtain blood for aPTT 4 h after administration of the heparin loading dose and 4 h after very change in the infusion rate

V. When aPTT values are therapeutic, a daily CBC and aPTT

(aPTT: activated partial thromboplastin time; h: hours)

TABLE 6: Reversal of heparin therapy by protamine. Maximum dose of 50 mg; infusion rate of 10 mg/mL; solution should not exceed 5 mg/min. Hypersensitivity reactions may occur in patients with known hypersensitivity to fish or previous protamine therapy or protamine containing insulin.[18]

Time since last heparin dose, min	Protamine dose
<30	1.0 mg/100 units heparin received
30–60	0.5–0.75 mg/100 units heparin received
60–120	0.375–0.5 mg/100 units heparin received
>120	0.25–0.375 mg/100 units heparin received

TABLE 7: Dose of low-molecular weight (LMW) heparin used in pediatric patients (enoxaparin has 110 antifactor Xa units/mg; dalteparin has 100 antifactor Xa units/mg).[18]

Drug	Weight	Age	Initial treatment dose	Initial prophylactic dose
Weight-dependent dosage of reviparin	<5 kg	na	150 μ/kg/ dose q12h	50 μ/kg/dose q12h
	>5 kg	na	100 μ/kg/ dose q12h	30 μ/kg/dose q12h
Age-dependent dosage of enoxaparin	na	<2 months	1.5 mg/kg/ dose q12h	0.75 mg/kg/ dose q12h
	na	>2 months	1.0 mg/kg/ dose q12h	0.5 mg/kg/ dose q12h
Pediatric (all ages) dose of dalteparin	na	All	129 ± 43 u/kg/dose q2h	92 ± 52 u/kg/dose q24h
Age-dependent dose of tinzaparin	na	0–2	275 μ/kg	—
	na	2–12 months	250 μ/kg	—
	na	1–5 years	240 μ/kg	—
	na	5–10 years	200 μ/kg	—
	na	10–16 years	175 μ/kg	—

TABLE 8: Protocol for oral anticoagulation therapy to maintain INR between 2 and 3 for pediatric patients.[18]

I	Day 1: if the baseline INR is 1.0 to 1.3: Dose = 0.2 mg/kg orally	
II	Loading days 2–4: if the INR is	
	INR	*Action*
	1.1–1.3	Repeat initial loading dose
	1.4–1.9	50% of initial loading dose
	2.0–3.0	50% of initial loading dose
	3.1–3.5	25% of initial loading dose
	>3.5	Hold until INR <3.5 then restart at 50% decreased dose
III	Maintenance oral anticoagulation dose guidelines:	
	1.1–1.4	Increase by 20% of dose
	1.15–1.9	Increase by 10% of dose
	2.0–3.0	No change
	3.1–3.5	Decrease by 10% of dose
	>3.5	Hold until INR <3.5, then restart at 20% decreased dose

(INR: international normalized ratio)

PHOSPHATE BINDERS

Calcium Based

Compound	Calcium content	Calcium absorbed when taken with food	Phosphate bound[19,20]	Advantages	Disadvantages
Calcium carbonate Shelcal (250 mg, 500 mg, 1.25 g, 2.5 g)	40% elemental Ca (200 mg elemental Ca^{2+}/500 mg)	20–30%	39 mg/g	Effective, inexpensive, few GI side effects	Hypercalcemia associated side effects
Calcium acetate Phostat (475 mg, 900 mg)	25% elemental Ca (169 mg elemental Ca^{2+}/667 mg)	22%	45 mg/g Soluble in acidic and alkaline solution	Effective, less GI side effects Less calcium load	Hypercalcemia-associated side effects
Mg + Ca carbonate	28% Mg, 25% Ca	20–30%	1 mg/2.3 mg	Less calcium load Protective effect of Mg	GI side effects

(GI: gastrointestinal)

Noncalcium Based

Compound[19,20]	Phosphate bound (per tablet)	Advantages	Disadvantages
Sevelamer: Hydrochloride Carbonate (400 mg, 800 mg)	65 mg	Useful in those with hypercalcemia or extraskeletal calcifications	GI side effects, metabolic acidosis (HCl form) Lowers fat-soluble vitamins
Lanthanum 500 mg	130 mg	High-binding affinity, Minimal GI side effects	Tissue deposition—long-term effects on bone
Sucroferric oxyhydroxide 500 mg iron	130 mg	Lower pill burden	GI side effects, dysgeusia, stool discoloration
Ferric citrate 210 mg elemental iron/1 g	20 mg	Reduces ESA requirement	GI side effects, stool discoloration, iron toxicity

(ESA: erythropoiesis-stimulating agent; GI: gastrointestinal)

Phosphate: Protein Ratio of Common Foods

Food	Phosphate	Phosphate: protein ratio[21,22]	GI absorption
Egg	86 mg/1 egg	14:1	40–60%
Egg white		1.4:1	
Milk	245 mg/250 mL	29:1	40–60%
Fish	250 mg/100 g	11:1	40–60%
Chicken	150 mg/100 g	8:1	40–60%
Lentils	180 mg/½ cup	20:1	10–30%
Potato	35 mg/100 g	18:1	
Aerated drinks	29 mg/250 mL	–	80–100%

(GI: gastrointestinal)

Potassium Content of Vegetables

Low (<100 mg)[21,22]	Medium (100–200 mg)[21,22]	High (>200 mg)[21,22]
Beetroot	Bitter gourd	Drumstick
Gourds—bottle, ridge, and snake	Brinjal	Potato
Cucumber	Cabbage	Sweet potato
Radish	Carrot	Yam
Peas	Onion	Tapioca
Fenugreek (*methi*)	Ladies finger	Coriander
Lettuce	Beans	Spinach

Potassium Content of Fruits

Low (30–100 mg)[21,22]	Medium (100–200 mg)[21,22]	High (>200 mg)[21,22]
Apple	Watermelon	Amla
Guava	Orange	Banana
Papaya	Pomegranate	Sapota
Blueberry	Jack fruit	Mango
Pears		Custard apple
Pineapple		Apricots, plums, peaches

SUPPLEMENTS

Bicarbonate supplements[21,22]	
Sodamint/nodosis tablet: • 325 mg • 500 mg • 650 mg	 3.8 mEq bicarbonate/tablet 5.6 mEq bicarbonate/tablet 8 mEq bicarbonate/tablet
Nodosis syrup	0.8 mEq bicarbonate/mL
Sodium bicarbonate 7.5% injection (IV)	0.9 mEq bicarbonate/mL
Shohl solution 1,000 mL = 140 g citric acid, 90 g sodium citrate	1 mEq bicarbonate/mL
Potassium and bicarbonate	
Potrate (potassium citrate) syrup	2 mEq bicarbonate/mL 2 mEq potassium/mL
Potassium citrate tablet	25 mEq bicarbonate/tablet 25 mEq potassium/tablet
Potassium supplements	
Potchlor	20 mEq potassium/15 mL
Potassium chloride 15% injection (IV)	2 mEq potassium/mL
Phosphate supplements	
Phosphate sachet	500 mg elemental phosphate/sachet
Joulie solution 1,000 mL = 136 g dibasic sodium phosphate, 58.8 g phosphoric acid	30 mg phosphate/mL

Multivitamin Supplements

	Vitamin B_1	***Vitamin B_2***	***Vitamin B_3***	***Vitamin B_6***	***Folate***	***Vitamin B_{12}***	***Vitamin A***	***Vitamin D***	***Zinc***
Zincovit syrup	0.75 mg	0.75 mg	7.5 mg	0.5 mg		0.5 µg	375 µg	2.5 µg	5 mg
Zincovit tablet	1.4 mg	1.6 mg	18 mg	1 mg	100 µg	1 µg	600 µg	5 µg	10 mg
Becosules syrup	2 mg	2.5 mg	20 mg	2 µg	–	–			
Becosules tablet	10 mg	10 mg	100 mg	3 µg	1,500 µg	100 µg			

Nutritional Supplements

	Serving size (scoop)	***Energy (kcal)***	***Protein (g)***	***Calcium (mg)***	***Phosphorus (mg)***	***Sodium (mg)***	***Potassium (mg)***
Renopro	25 g	117	2.25	57.5	30	28	35
Resource dialysis	7 g	34	1.23	14	18.6	10.4	27.2

REFERENCES

1. Brown P, Battistella M. Principles of drug dosing in sustained low efficiency dialysis (SLED) and review of antimicrobial dosing literature. Pharmacy. 2020;8:33.
2. Aronoff GR, Bennett WM, Berns JS, Brier ME, Kasbekar N, Mueller BA, et al. Drug Prescribing in Renal Failure: Dosing Guidelines for Adults and Children, 5th edition. Philadelphia: American College of Physicians; 2007.
3. Sethi SK, Krishnappa V, Nangethu N, Nemer P, Frazee LA, Raina R. Antibiotic dosing in sustained low-efficiency dialysis in critically ill patients. Can J Kidney Health Dis. 2018;5:1-12.
4. Scoville BA, Mueller BA. Medication dosing in critically ill patients with acute kidney injury treated with renal replacement therapy. Am J Kidney Dis. 2013;61(3):490-500.
5. Saad R, Hallit S, Chahine B. Evaluation of renal drug dosing adjustment in chronic kidney disease patients at two university hospitals in Lebanon. Pharm Pract. 2019;17(1):1304.
6. Sefer S, Degoricija V. About drug dialyzability. Acta Clin Croat. 2003;42:257-67.
7. Harriet Lane Service (Johns Hopkins Hospital), Hughes H, Kahl L. The Harriet Lane Handbook: A Manual for Pediatric House Officers, 22nd edition. Philadelphia, PA: Elsevier; 2020.
8. Millsop A. Drug dosing in patients with renal impairment and during renal replacement therapy. In: Ashley C, Morlidge C (Eds). Introduction to Renal Therapeutics. London: Pharmaceutical Press; 2008. pp. 127-36.
9. Matzke GR, Aronoff GR, Atkinson Jr AJ, Bennett WM, Decker BS, Eckardt KU, et al. Drug dosing consideration in patients with acute and chronic kidney disease—a clinical update from

Kidney Disease: Improving Global Outcomes (KDIGO). Kidney Int. 2011;80:1122-37.

10. Ashley C, Dunleavy A. The Renal Drug Handbook: The Ultimate Prescribing Guide for Renal Practitioners, 5th edition. London: CRC Press; 2019.
11. Food and Drug Administration. (2012). Rituximab Label. [online] Available from: https://www.accessdata.fda.gov/drugsatfda_docs/label/2012/103705s5367s5388lbl.pdf. [Last accessed March, 2022]
12. BCRenal. (2019). Cyclophosphamide infusion protocol for glomerulonephritis. [online] Available from: http://www.bcrenal.ca/resource-gallery/Documents/Cyclophosphamide%20Infusion%20Protocol%20For%20GN.pdf. [Last accessed April, 2022]
13. American Academy of Pediatrics. AAP recommendations for clinical measurement of blood pressures in children and adolescents. 2017.
14. Lurbe E, Agabiti-Rosei E, Cruickshank JK, Dominiczak A, Erdine S, Hirth A, et al. 2016 European Society of Hypertension guidelines for the management of high blood pressure in children and adolescents. J Hypertens. 2016;34(10):1887-920.
15. International Society of Nephrology. (2012). Kidney Disease: Improving Global Outcomes (KDIGO) Clinical Practice Guideline for Anemia in Chronic Kidney Disease. [online] Available from: https://kdigo.org/wp-content/uploads/2016/10/KDIGO-2012-Anemia-Guideline-English.pdf. [Last accessed March, 2022].
16. Naithani R, Saxena R. Hematinics in children. Indian J Pract Paediatr. 2008;10(2):96-105.
17. Food and Drug Administration. Aranesp (Darbepoeitin alpha) Label-FDA. [online] Available from: https://www.accessdata.fda.gov/drugsatfda_docs/label/2011/103951Orig1s5173_103951Orig1s5258lbl.pdf. [Last accessed March, 2022]
18. Monagle P, Chan AKC, Goldenberg NA, Ichord RN, Journeycake JM, Nowak-Göttl U, et al. Antithrombotic therapy in neonates and children: Antithrombotic therapy and prevention of thrombosis, 9th edition. American College of Chest Physicians Evidence-Based Clinical Practice Guidelines. Chest. 2012;141(2 Suppl):e737S-801S.
19. International Society of Nephrology. (2017). KDIGO 2017 Clinical Practice Guideline Update for the Diagnosis, Evaluation, Prevention, and Treatment of Chronic Kidney Disease-Mineral and Bone Disorder (CKD-MBD). [online] Available from: https://kdigo.org/wp-content/uploads/2017/02/2017-KDIGO-CKD-MBD-GL-Update.pdf. [Last accessed March, 2022].
20. Isakova T, Nickolas TL, Denburg M, Yarlagadda S, Weiner DE, Gutiérrez OM, et al. KDOQI US commentary on the 2017 KDIGO Clinical Practice Guideline update for the diagnosis, evaluation, prevention, and treatment of chronic kidney disease-mineral and bone disorder (CKD-MBD). Am J Kidney Dis. 2017;70(6):737-51.
21. Ikizler TA, Burrowes JD, Byham-Gray LD, Campbell KL, Carrero JJ, Chan W, et al. KDOQI Clinical Practice Guideline for nutrition in CKD. AJKD. 2020;3(1):S1-S107.
22. Paediatric Renal Nutrition Taskforce. (2020). Clinical practice recommendations. [online] Available from: https://www.vitaflo-via.com/disorder-resources/paediatric-kidney-disease/paediatric-renal-nutrition-taskforce-clinical-practice. [Last accessed March, 2022].

CHAPTER

15.3 Procedures in Pediatric Nephrology

Neha Bandari, Suprita Kalra, Soumya Reddy

HEMODIALYSIS CATHETER INSERTION

Introduction

Vascular access is necessary for taking up the patients with acute kidney injury (AKI) or chronic kidney disease (CKD) for hemodialysis (HD). Central venous catheters (CVCs) are the most commonly used vascular access in the pediatric age group for initiation of dialysis.

Both temporary and permanent cuffed tunneled catheters can be used in patients requiring HD. Tunneled catheters have lower rates of malfunction, infection, and thrombosis and should be preferred if the patient is expected to need dialysis for more than 1 month.

The recommended ideal initial vascular access point is the internal jugular vein (IJV), and the femoral vein provides the next best alternative site. Use of subclavian vein is generally not recommended due to higher risk of central venous stenosis. Femoral vein is preferred in presence of thrombocytopenia and in critically ill patients with pulmonary edema and/or hyperkalemia and also sometimes if expected dialysis requirement is shorter than 1 week.

Appropriate vascular access should be selected according to the child's age and size. **Table 1** summarizes the recommended catheter size as per the weight of the child. Anatomy of the veins in relation to the large arteries has been found to be variable in almost one-third of the children and, therefore, ultrasound (US) guidance is recommended during CVCs' insertion to increase the success rate of placement and reduce insertion-related complications **(Figs. 1A and B)**.

Indications

For acute or chronic HD.

TABLE 1: Vascular access for hemodialysis.

Patient size	*Catheter size*	*Insertion site*
	Temporary catheter	
<3 kg	4–6 Fr single-lumen or double-lumen 7 Fr	Femoral vein
3–6 kg	Double- or triple-lumen 7 Fr	Internal jugular or femoral
6–15 kg	Double-lumen 8 Fr	Internal jugular or femoral
15–30 kg	Double-lumen 9/10 Fr	Internal jugular or femoral
>30 kg	Double-lumen 10 F or 11.5 F	Internal jugular or femoral
	Permanent (tunneled) catheter	
Pediatric	24 cm, 28 cm	Internal jugular

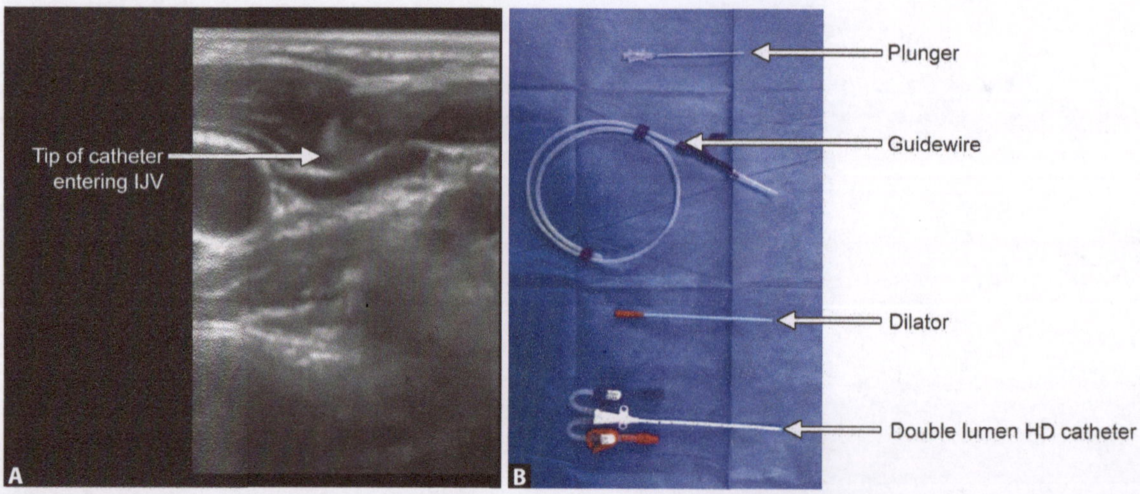

Figs. 1A and B: (A) Ultrasound-guided catheterization of the internal jugular vein (IJV); (B) Double-lumen curved hemodialysis catheter.

Personnel Required

Ideally, two physicians are trained in the procedure of line placement, one physician for administrating sedation and monitoring the child during the procedure and minimum one trained assistant should be present during the procedure.

Steps of the Procedure

1. Take written informed consent.
2. Prepare, ready, and check the equipment, the HD catheter, medications for sedation, and multipara monitor for monitoring the child during the procedure.
3. Keep child nil per orally (NPO) for minimum 4 hours prior to the procedure.
4. Sedate the child with an appropriate dose of midazolam or ketamine or as per institutional policy.
5. Flush the catheter to be used with heparin saline (1 unit heparin/mL of saline).
6. Clean and drape the child maintaining strict asepsis.
7. Visualize the vein and artery carefully using the vascular probe of the US.

For femoral vein:

1. Place the patient in supine position with slight elevation of the ipsilateral hip and in abduction and external rotation.
2. Under direct US visualization, cannulate the femoral vein using the needle and plunger provided or a 16-gauge venous cannula.
3. Insert the guidewire through this. Remember that guidewire should go in freely if the vein has been cannulated correctly and there should be no resistance in the guidewire.
4. Once the guidewire has been inserted and distal end secured by the person assisting the procedure, gently remove the needle/cannula and thread over the dilator, in ascending order of size.
5. Using the Seldinger technique, thread the catheter over the guidewire and remove the guidewire.
6. Check flow in both ends of the catheter and flush with heparin saline and close the ends.
7. Suture the catheter and secure with sterile transparent dressing.

For internal jugular vein:

1. Place the patient in supine position with slight extension and external rotation of the neck toward the opposite side.
2. Under direct US visualization, cannulate the IJV using the needle and plunger provided or a 16-gauge venous cannula.
3. Remove the plunger as soon as free flow blood is observed.
4. Insert the guidewire through the cannula/needle toward the ipsilateral nipple. Remember that guidewire should go in freely if the vein has been cannulated correctly and there should be no resistance in the guidewire.
5. Once the guidewire has been inserted and distal end secured by the person assisting the procedure, gently remove the needle/cannula and thread over the dilators, in ascending order of size to dilate the vein.
6. Using the Seldinger technique, thread the catheter over the guidewire and remove the guidewire.
7. Check flow in both ends of the catheter and flush with heparin saline and close the ends.
8. Suture the catheter and secure with sterile transparent dressing.

For tunneled catheter—IJV ***(Fig. 2)****:*

1. Place the patient in supine position with slight extension and external rotation of the neck toward the opposite side.
2. Under direct US visualization, cannulate the IJV using the needle and plunger provided or a 16-gauge venous cannula.
3. Remove the plunger as soon as free flow blood is observed.
4. Insert the guidewire through the cannula/needle toward the ipsilateral nipple.
5. Confirm the position with fluoroscopy.
6. Gently remove the needle/cannula and thread over the dilator.
7. Make a small skin incision from the dilator exit site laterally.
8. Measure the catheter length and mark the exit site laterally (near the anterior axillary fold) so that the catheter is kink-free.
9. Expose the subcutaneous tissue with blunt dissection and create a subcutaneous pocket. Ensure that the length of the tunnel is such that the cuff is within the tunnel and 1–2 cm from the exit site.
10. Infiltrate the area around the exit site with local anesthesia (use a long needle to infiltrate the tract extending from the exit site to the venotomy insertion site) and make a small skin incision at the exit site.
11. Mount the catheter on the end of the tunneling device and pull the tunneling device from the exit site subcutaneously to the insertion site.
12. Pull the cuff of the catheter into the tunnel and remove the tunnelling device from the catheter.
13. Use dilators (ascending order of size) to dilate the venous tract.
14. After the final dilatation, insert the dilator with the peel-away sheath. Resistance is felt during insertion through the soft tissue and on entering the vein.
15. Remove the dilator and sheath and thread the catheter over the guidewire into the final position.

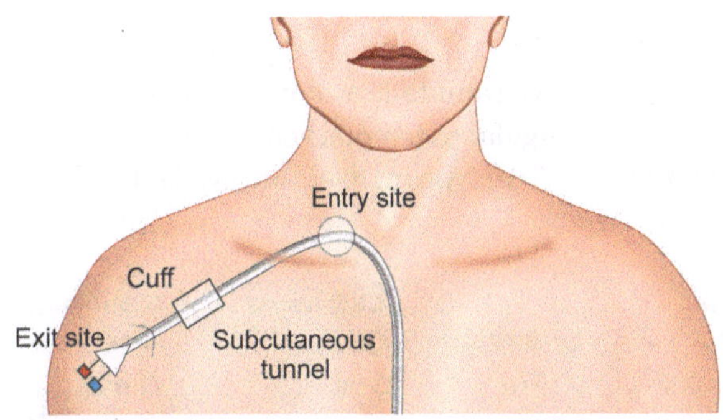

Fig. 2: Pictorial representation of tunneled catheter placement.

16. Pull the catheter back into the tunnel so that the cuff is 1–2 cm from the exit site. Use fluoroscopy to confirm the position of the catheter. Check for good flows in the catheter.
17. Place sutures at the insertion site and to secure the catheter. Avoid exit site suture.

Contraindications

Coagulopathy with deranged prothrombin time (PT), international normalized ratio (INR), and thrombocytopenia (platelet count <1 lakh/mm³) are contraindications for CVC placement. If venous access is required urgently, femoral vein cannulation after appropriate blood component therapy can be done as a high-risk procedure.

Complications

- *Acute*: Arterial puncture, hematoma formation, and pneumothorax/hemothorax in IJV cannulation.
- *Subacute (specific for tunneled catheters):* Suboptimal flow—malposition/kink, clots, and fibrin sheath
- *Chronic:* Thrombosis and line infections causing central line-associated bloodstream infection (CLABSI) and sepsis.

PLASMA EXCHANGE

Plasma exchange is performed for various immune-mediated diseases. It essentially involves separating plasma from rest of the blood which is replaced with fresh frozen plasma (FFP) or albumin. This can be done by apheresis using the HD machine or centrifugation method. A single volume plasma exchange removes approximately 65% of disease mediator when there is no new synthesis or redistribution of the factor. When there is new synthesis or redistribution, however, the volume of circulating disease mediator will rise following treatment. Because of this, a course of consecutive plasma exchanges is performed, the number of which depends on the underlying disease. The American Society for Apheresis (ASFA) has laid down evidence-based recommendations for therapeutic apheresis in a wide range of diseases. **Box 1** lists the conditions in which plasmapheresis is considered first-line therapy, either as standalone treatment or with other modes of treatment. There are numerous other conditions where therapeutic plasmapheresis is performed as second-line or third-line treatment modality.

BOX 1: Diseases where plasmapheresis is the standard first-line therapy.

- Acute inflammatory demyelinating polyradiculoneuropathy
- Chronic inflammatory demyelinating polyradiculoneuropathy
- Antineutrophil cytoplasmic antibody (ANCA)-associated rapidly progressive glomerulonephritis
- Antiglomerular basement membrane disease
- Recurrent focal segmental glomerulosclerosis in transplanted kidney
- Hyperviscosity in monoclonal gammopathies
- Moderate–severe myasthenia gravis
- N-methyl D-aspartate receptor antibody encephalitis
- For desensitization prior to ABO incompatible renal or liver transplantation
- Complement-mediated hemolytic uremic syndrome (HUS): Anti-factor H antibody disease
- Thrombotic thrombocytopenic purpura (TTP)
- Fulminant Wilson's disease

Prerequisites

- *Vascular access:* Double-lumen hemodialysis catheter in the internal jugular or femoral vein
- *Plasma filter:* Two types of filters are available—TPE 1000 and TPE 2000.

Plasma filters	Surface area	ECV (plasma filter)	ECV (blood lines)
TPE 1000	0.15 m²	23 mL	71 mL
TPE 2000	0.35 m²	41 mL	125 mL

- *Replacement solution:* FFP/colloids or crystalloids are used as replacement solution. FFP provides coagulation factors and immunoglobulins. It is cross-matched with recipient blood group. Specific indications for the use of FFP are hemolytic uremic syndrome (HUS)/thrombotic thrombocytopenic purpura (TTP), liver failure, and coagulopathy with inhibitors. 5% albumin lacks coagulation factors and can be used an alternative. An alternative is to infuse one-third replacement with crystalloid such as isotonic saline (NS) or Ringer's lactate (RL) and the remaining two-thirds with 5% albumin.

Procedure

1. *Exchange volume:* Mostly 1–1.5 times plasma volume exchanged. First plasma exchange removes 55% fraction and second plasma exchange removes 70%. Exchanging more than two volumes in 24 hours is not recommended.
2. Estimated plasma volume in mL is:
   Total blood volume (70 or 80 mL/kg) × (1 – hematocrit)
   Or [0.065 × weight (kg)] × [1 – hematocrit] × 1,000
3. *Blood flow rate:* 5 mL/kg/min (minimum 50 mL/min and maximum 250 mL/min); rate of plasma removal should be <50 mL/kg/h.
4. Duration of therapy (min) can be calculated as follows: Plasma volume × Exchange (1–1.5)/Plasma filtration rate.
5. *Anticoagulation with heparin:* Loading dose of 50 IU/kg (maximum 1,000 IU) followed by infusion rate of 15–20 IU/kg/h (maximum 500 IU/h)
6. Prime the circuit with 2 L of normal saline. Watch for hypocalcemia. Replacement fluid and calcium chloride infusion should always be given postfilter.
7. When using albumin as a replacement fluid, monitor PT/PTT before third and subsequent procedures. If it is >1.5 times greater than normal, FP should be used as a replacement fluid.

8. Potassium can be added to prevent hypokalemia (4 mmol K = 2 mL KCl for each liter of albumin).
9. Baseline full blood count, PT/aPTT, ionized calcium, potassium before starting.
10. Premedication to prevent hypersensitivity to replacement fluids:
    - Diphenhydramine 1.25 mg/kg (25–50 mg oral or IV)
    - IV hydrocortisone 10 mg/kg (max 500 mg)
    - Syrup paracetamol 10–15 mg/kg

Complications

- Hypotension
- Hypocalcemia
- Thrombocytopenia
- Hypokalemia
- Allergic reaction to replacement fluid
- Bleeding complications due to anticoagulation with heparin
- Complications secondary to vascular access

Figure 3 shows a child undergoing plasmapheresis through the HD catheter in IJV using hemodialysis machine.

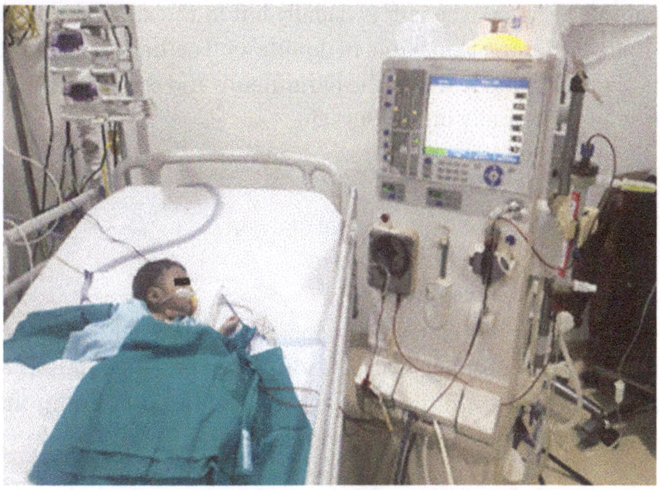

Fig. 3: A child undergoing plasmapheresis.

CYTOSORB THERAPY

The use of extracorporeal blood purification techniques for immunomodulation in acute inflammatory states such as sepsis is being used increasingly in recent years. Cytosorb is made up of biocompatible, highly porous, polyvinylpyrrolidone-coated polystyrene-divinyl-benzene polymer bead. Its estimated size is 300–800 μm with a total surface area of >40,000 m^2 which makes it effective for removal of middle- and low-molecular-weight uremic and other toxins including interleukin-6 (IL-6) and IL-8 and monocyte chemotactic proteins. Endotoxins and IL-10 are however not cleared as adsorption is dependent on the pore size. Therefore, it is used as an adjuvant therapy in patients with septic shock and multiorgan dysfunction including cytokine storm post-COVID infection **(Fig. 4)**. It can be used along with continuous kidney replacement therapy (CKRT) or with SLED therapy or as standalone therapy using the hemodialysis machine in children who do not require dialysis. The therapy is usually offered for up to 24 hours per session, daily for 2–7 consecutive days, and at present the available filter can only be used in children >25 kg.

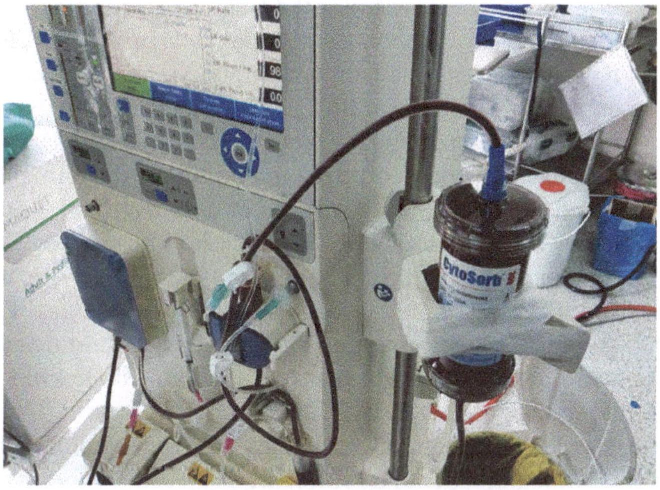

Fig. 4: Cytosorb being done in post-COVID multisystem inflammatory syndrome in children (MIS-C).

PERITONEAL DIALYSIS CATHETER INSERTION

Introduction

Peritoneal dialysis (PD) provides a nonvascular route using the patient's peritoneum as a membrane for kidney replacement therapy in both AKI and CKD. In children with AKI, bedside PD is the most commonly used modality chiefly due to ease of securing the access and providing dialysis, especially in critically ill children who may not tolerate hemodialysis. This is especially true in centers where CKRT is not available or feasible due to financial constraints. Also, vascular access in neonates and infants is difficult to secure and appropriate size catheters and dialyzers are not readily available making PD the most resorted to modality in this subset of patients. Placing children with CKD V on PD gives the advantage of continuing dialysis without having to visit the hospital for the same, ensuring better quality of life. This has made automated PD (APD) a popular alternative to hemodialysis in the management of pediatric dialysis-dependent CKD.

Peritoneal dialysis in AKI can be done using a stiff or a soft cuffed PD catheter, both of which can be placed bedside by trained personnel.

The soft Tenchkoff PD catheters are available as peel-away catheters with an introducer kit for insertion at the patient's bedside under local anesthesia and sedation using the Seldinger technique. These catheters are available both as single and as double cuffs made of Dacron which help to anchor the catheter to the peritoneum and the skin, thereby preventing displacement and infection. When a single-cuff catheter is used, the cuff is usually left in the subcutaneous tissue under the skin while in double-cuff catheters, one cuff is placed deeper just over the peritoneum and the second one is left superficially under the skin.

Indications

For acute or chronic peritoneal dialysis.

Personnel Required

Ideally, two physicians are trained in the procedure of line placement, one physician for administrating sedation and monitoring the child during the procedure and minimum one trained assistant should be present during the procedure.

Steps of the Procedure

1. Take written informed consent.
2. Prior to procedure examine the child to exclude massive hepatomegaly, splenomegaly, or palpable bladder.
3. If presence of coagulopathy or thrombocytopenia is noted, appropriate blood products must be transfused to reduce risk of bleeding during the procedure.
4. Prepare a PD prescription depending on the clinical condition of the child, severity of fluid overload, and biochemical abnormalities. Rapid cycles with short dwell time of 20–30 minutes are preferred in the presence of hyperkalemia or severe acidosis. Similarly, increasing the dextrose concentration of PD fluid with short dwell times helps to pull out more ultrafiltrates per cycle which is required in children with fluid overload.
5. Also, keep PD monitoring chart ready to record inputs and outflow and ultrafiltrate correctly.
6. Prepare, ready and check the PD fluid, the PD catheter, inflow and outflow lines, medications for sedation and multipara monitor for monitoring the child during the procedure.
7. Under strict asepsis, hang two PD fluid bottles on an IV stand and keep them ready for connection to PD catheter inflow track using tubings with Y connector. Hang a Urobag with Urometer for connection to the outflow tract of the PD catheter. Ensure that the circuit is air-free.
8. Mark the insertion point. Midline (1–1.5 cm infraumbilical) insertion is preferred as it is the most avascular plane. Left paramedian (point midway between umbilicus and anterosuperior iliac spine) insertion can be considered in neonates and infants.
9. Keep child nil per orally (NPO) for minimum 4 hours prior to the procedure.
10. Sedate the child with appropriate dose of midazolam (0.1 mg/kg) or ketamine (0.5–1 mg/kg) or as per institutional policy.
11. Clean and drape the child maintaining strict asepsis.

For stiff peritoneal dialysis catheter insertion:

1. Place the patient in supine position.
2. Clean and drape the child's abdomen.
3. Insert a 16G cannula 1–1.5 cm below the umbilicus in the midline to create ascites using 20–30 mL/kg of 1.5 or 1.7% PD fluid such that the flanks are full on palpation. This can be avoided if the patient already has ascites.
4. Put a small stab wound using a sterile blade at the same puncture site and push a stiff PD catheter perpendicularly with the trocar through it till a feeling of give-way is palpable.
5. Once the give is felt, remove the trocar and advance the catheter into the right iliac fossa enough to insert all the side holes intraperitoneally.
6. Connect the catheter through a connector provided using a three way to the inflow and outflow tract kept ready.
7. Open the inflow to fill the abdomen with 30 mL/kg or 1,000–1,200 mL/m^2 of PD fluid. Critically ill children, especially those on ventilator, may have worsening respiratory distress when PD fluid is put in the peritoneum so PD can be started with smaller volumes and the fill volume can be increased gradually.
8. Check outflow and then create a reservoir with 20–30 mL/kg or 1,000–1,200 mL/m^2 of PD fluid and start the first cycle of PD.
9. Suture the catheter (necessary only if there is pericatheter leak) and secure with sterile dressing.

Bedside placement of soft PD catheter by the Seldinger technique:

1. Place the patient in supine position.
2. Clean and drape the child's abdomen.
3. Create ascites as described for stiff PD catheter placement. This is not required in children who already have ascites with full flanks.
4. Make a small stab wound using a sterile blade 1–2 cm below the umbilicus at the same point where a cannula was inserted to create ascites.
5. Insert the guidewire of the introducer kit through the sheath of the cannula used to create ascites.
6. Slowly push the pull-apart sheath and dilator as a single unit along the guidewire into the abdominal cavity.
7. Then insert the Tenchkoff catheter through the sheath, pulling the sheath apart slowly as the catheter is advanced over the guidewire such that the first cuff is placed just above the rectus sheath **(Figs. 5 and 6)**.
8. Make an incision 2–3 cm lateral to the exit site for the subcutaneous tunnel.
9. Attach the tunneling device to the catheter and pull the catheter out through this small incision placing the 2nd cuff in under the skin. An artery forceps may be used for blunt dissection for creating the subcutaneous tunnel.
10. Then connect the titanium connector and lock it by rotating and attach the transfer set to the titanium connector.
11. Flush the catheter two to three times by connecting a bag of PD fluid.
12. The catheter is then ready and can be used for dialysis immediately.

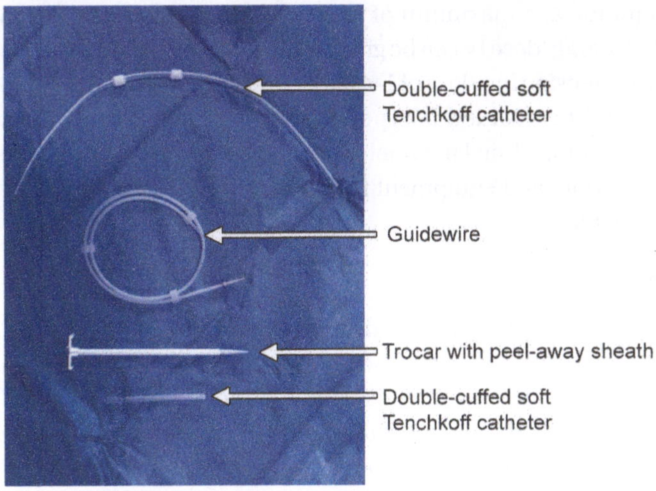

Fig. 5: A double-cuffed soft Tenchkoff catheter.

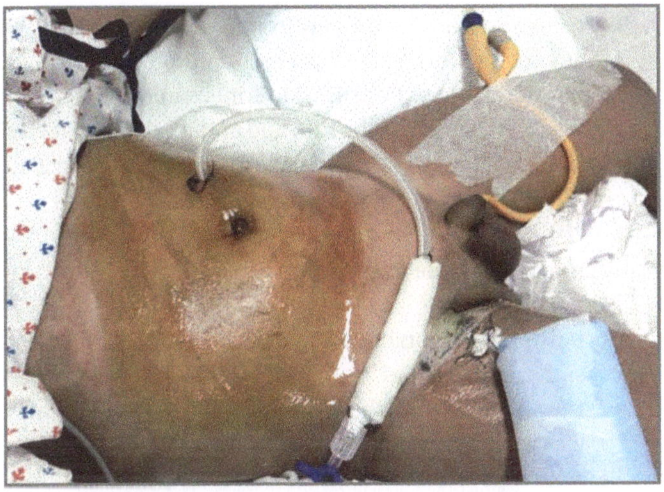

Fig. 6: A child with soft Tenchkoff catheter in situ.

Table 2 summarizes the components of acute PD prescription.

Complications of Peritoneal Dialysis

- *During catheter placement*:
  - Injury to the abdominal viscera
  - Bleeding due to vascular injury
- *Chronic complications*:
  - *Infectious*:
    - Peritonitis
    - Exit-site infection
    - Tunnel infection
  - *Noninfectious*:
    - Peritoneal adhesions and catheter dysfunction
    - Fluid leaks
    - Encapsulating peritoneal sclerosis
    - Hernia
    - Pleural leak (hydrothorax)
- *Metabolic complications*:
  - Hyperglycemia and hyperinsulinemia
  - Inadequate dialysis
  - Hypokalemia
  - Hypophosphatemia

TABLE 2: Components of acute peritoneal dialysis (PD) prescription.

Components	*Comments*
Length of the dialysis session	Length of dialysis session determined by fluid balance, biochemical abnormalities, and urine output
Composition of dialysate (% dextrose)	• Ultrafiltration rate of 1.5% dextrose and 2.5% dextrose (40 mL/kg dwell) is 50–150 and 200–400 mL/h, respectively. A higher concentration of dextrose solution may be used for initial cycles in children with severe fluid overload. • To make 2.5% PD fluid—add 50 mL of 25% dextrose to 1 L of 1.5% PD fluid
Exchange volume	Initial fill volume: 10–20 mL/kg; maximum fill volume: 45 or 1,200 mL/m². <800 mL/m² if age <2 years. Higher the fill volume, greater the clearance and ultrafiltration
Exchange time: Inflow, dwell, and outflow time	• Exchange time is 1 hour—inflow 10 minutes, dwell 30 minutes, outflow 20 minutes for acute intermittent PD using rigid catheter. Dwell time 1–4 hours in continuous PD using flexible catheter. Shorter dwell time (e.g., 15–20 minutes) for rapid fluid, urea and potassium clearance (e.g., severe hyperkalemia or pulmonary edema) and neonates • If hypernatremia develops, extend dwell time if feasible or lower glucose concentration in dialysis solution
Additives to dialysate	• Potassium 4 mEq/L (if K^+ < 3.5 mEq/L) • Heparin 250–1,000 U/L • If blood sugars persistently >250 mg/dL—can add 2–4 IU insulin to 1 L fluid • In hypernatremia to prevent sudden drop in serum sodium—sodium content of dialysate fluid can be increased by adding 3% NaCl (to maintain sodium 10–15 mm Hg below serum levels)
Bicarbonate-based PD fluid	• 250 mL solution A + 500 mL solution B (sodium—140 mEq/L, bicarbonate—40 mEq/L, dextrose—1.5%) • Solution A—440 mL 5% dextrose = 60 mL sodium bicarbonate solution B—500 mL NS
Monitoring	• Fluid balance q4–6 hours • Serum electrolytes q6–12 hours • Blood sugar q6–12 hours (more frequently if using 2.5 or 4.25% dextrose-based dialysis fluid) • Blood urea and serum creatinine q24 hours

RENAL BIOPSY

The renal tissue is biopsied to see histopathology of kidney for confirming diagnosis, for prognostication, and for planning the treatment of primary and secondary renal diseases. The percutaneous renal biopsy (PRB) performed under ultrasound guidance is the standard of care and is performed usually by the nephrologists or radiologists. PRB is done under sedation and local anesthesia with disposable, automated, spring-loaded biopsy guns using 16- or 18-gauge needles. 18-gauge is generally used in infants and for post-transplant biopsies and 16-gauge needles for older children and adults.

Three cores of kidney are recommended to be taken in the biopsy, one for light microscopy which is put in formalin, second for immunofluorescence to be put in normal saline or Michel's solution, and the third core for electron microscopy in glutaraldehyde for transport to the laboratory. The histopathological report correlates the findings of all three and is imperative for accurate diagnosis. A biopsy sample is considered adequate if it contains 20 or more glomeruli.

Indications

- Steroid-resistant nephrotic syndrome
- Nephrotic syndrome with nephritic features
- Prior to starting calcineurin inhibitors
- Rapidly progressive glomerulonephritis
- Nonresolving postinfectious glomerulonephritis
- Recurrent gross or microscopic hematuria with no cause found
- Acute kidney injury >4 weeks without cause
- Tubulointerstitial nephritis

Prerequisites

- Parents need to be explained the procedure and informed consent taken for both kidney biopsy and intravenous sedation.
- Blood pressure (BP) should be checked and antihypertensives started if BP elevated.
- Prior to biopsy, there is a need to check hemoglobin (>8 g/dL), platelet count (>100,000/mm³), and normal coagulation profile (PT/APTT/INR).
- Renal function test to be done and if serum urea elevated, then intranasal desmopressin 2–4 μg/kg/dose 2 hours before the procedure or intravenously and 0.2–0.4 μg/kg/dose over 20 minutes should be given.
- Check history of allergies, especially latex, povidone iodine, and drug history such as aspirin warfarin and heparin use in dialysis.
- Patient should be kept NPO 4–6 hours prior to procedure and IV access secured.
- Single kidney is not an absolute contraindication to a kidney biopsy though biopsy is usually avoided in such children.
- Severe hydronephrosis is a contraindication to the procedure.

Materials Required

Biopsy gun (automatic spring-loaded biopsy device), 18G or 16G (>8 years); dissecting microscope to confirm kidney sample adequate or not; three containers containing isotonic saline/Michel's solution, 20% formaldehyde, glutaraldehyde for transport of biopsy sample to the laboratory.

Sedation

Midazolam injection 0.05–0.1 mg/kg IV slowly over 2–3 minutes (maximum total dose of 10 mg) followed by fentanyl injection 1.0 μg/kg/dose over 2–3 minutes can be repeated every 5 minutes; a maximum of four doses or ketamine injection 1–2 mg/kg/dose IV can be given. Propofol can be used if there is hypertension in a dose of 1–4 μg/kg over 2–3 minutes. Ketamine should be avoided if hypertension is not well controlled. Monitoring of vital parameters should be done throughout the procedure and equipment for resuscitation should be readily available.

Procedure

1. The renal biopsy is done under sedation and local anesthesia in prone position for native kidneys and in supine position for transplanted kidneys. A sandbag/rolled sheet or blanket is used under the abdomen to decrease the mobility of the kidney.
2. Kidney biopsy under real-time ultrasound guidance is recommended **(Figs. 7A and B)**.
3. Biopsies should be obtained from the lower pole of the kidney (or the most easily accessible pole in transplant kidney) and distance from the skin is measured and the point for biopsy is marked on the skin and automated biopsy gun, either 16 or 18-gauge, is used to take three cores as described.

Complications

- Complications due to sedation
- *Hemorrhage:*
  - Perirenal hemorrhage—loin pain, palpable mass, and signs of blood loss
  - Intrapelvic hemorrhage—persistent gross hematuria, clot retention
- Pain at biopsy site
- Infection
- Arteriovenous (AV) fistula

Postbiopsy Care

The child should stay in supine position for 4–6 hours and complete bed rest for 24 hours. Paracetamol should be given 6 hourly for pain relief. Vitals to be monitored every 30 minutes

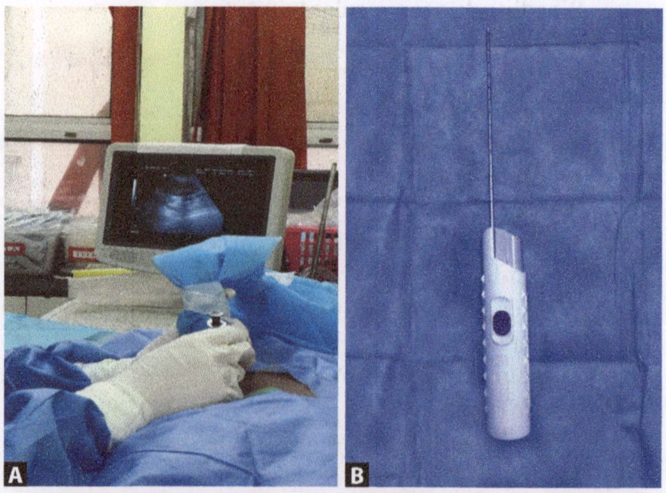

Figs. 7A and B: (A) Kidney biopsy being performed under ultrasound guidance; (B) An automated spring-loaded biopsy gun.

for the first 2 hours followed by hourly monitoring for the next 6 hours. The patient can be discharged 24 hours after biopsy but instructed to avoid climbing stairs, strenuous activity, and playing including running and jumping for 1 week postbiopsy. Collection of urine for three successive samples and naked eye examination to rule out gross hematuria should be done.

Complication management:

- *Gross hematuria*: Postbiopsy ultrasound to see for any perinephric hematoma should be performed. If gross hematuria present or hemoglobin falls by 10–15%, then USG should be repeated to see for any hematoma, fistula, and bladder clots. Mild hematuria gets cleared with IV fluids. Blood transfusion may be needed.
- Rarely embolization by an intervention radiologist or surgical intervention may be needed if gross hematuria continues with circulatory compromise.
- Sedation-related complications such as respiratory depression, laryngospasm, and vomiting can also occur and may require airways suctioning and oxygen therapy.

Adequacy of Biopsy Sample

The minimum number of abnormal glomeruli necessary in a biopsy to assume at least a given percent involvement in the kidney are depicted in **Table 3**.

TABLE 3: Minimum number of abnormal glomeruli to assume at least a given percent involvement in the kidney.

Biopsy size	*Number of abnormal glomeruli in a biopsy*		
	80%†	*50%†*	*20%†*
8	8(100)	7(88)	3(38)
10	10(100)	8(80)	4(40)
12	12(100)	9(75)	5(42)
15	14(93)	11(73)	6(40)
20	19(95)	14(70)	7(35)
25	23(92)	17(68)	9(36)
30	28(93)	20(66)	10(33)
35	32(91)	23(66)	11(31)
40	36(90)	26(65)	12(30)

Note: Figures in parenthesis are the abnormal number of glomeruli in a biopsy.

†Percent involvement in the kidney sought.

PROCEDURES FOR ASSESSMENT OF TUBULAR FUNCTION

Ammonium Chloride Loading Test

This test is used for assessment of urinary acidification.

Protocol

- Ensure that child is not on any bicarbonate supplements.
- Measure blood pH, serum HCO_3, and urine pH at the beginning of the test (if pH < 7.2 and HCO_3 < 15 mEq/L → no need to perform the test).
- Administer 150 mg/kg of NH_4Cl (can be mixed with fruit juice).
- Check urine pH hourly for 4 hours using pH meter.
- Child can be allowed to drink good amount of fluid during this time.
- At 4 hours, check serum HCO_3 and urine pH.

Interpretation

- Urine pH < 5.5 indicates normal urine acidification and the test can be stopped.
- Failure to achieve urine pH < 5.5 indicates distal tubular acidification defect.
- If pH remains >7.2 and HCO_3 > 15 mEq/L at the end of 4 hours, then the test is inconclusive and the test has to be repeated with a higher dose of ammonium chloride.

Furosemide–fludrocortisone Test

It is used for assessment of urinary acidification. Frusemide increases the distal sodium delivery, which in turn enhances distal H^+ secretion. Fludrocortisone also increases H^+ secretion.

Protocol

- Ensure that child is not on any bicarbonate supplements.
- Fast from midnight (not required in infants).
- Check urine Na, K, pH, creatinine, plasma Na, K, TCO_2, urea, and creatinine before starting the test.
- Give an oral or IV dose of 1 mg/kg furosemide and fludrocortisone 0.025 mg/kg.
- Collect urine every 30 minutes for 3 hours and measure the pH.
- After 3 hours, recheck plasma Na, K, TCO_2, urea, and creatinine.
- Prior to discharge, ensure that the child is not clinically dehydrated.

Interpretation

- Urine pH < 5.5 indicates normal urine acidification and the test can be stopped.
- Failure to achieve urine pH < 5.5 indicates distal tubular acidification defect.

Bicarbonate Loading Test

This is used for assessment of urinary acidification and to differentiate impaired HCO_3 reabsorption from impaired H^+ secretion.

Protocol

- Measure serum electrolytes, calcium, and blood gas.
- Administer $NaHCO_3$ 1 mEq/kg by IV infusion.
- Measure urine pH, pCO_2 and plasma HCO_3, pCO_2 concentration every 30 minutes.
- For urine pH, pCO_2 measurement sample has to be collected anaerobically.

Interpretation

Step 1: Calculate fractional excretion of HCO_3

$FE_{HCO_3} = (Urine_{HCO_3} \times Plasma_{Cr}) \div (Plasma_{HCO_3} \times Urine_{Cr})$

Normal FE_{HCO_3} is <5%

>15% suggests proximal RTA.

Usually <5% in distal RTA and occasionally increased to 5–10.

Step 2: Calculate (U – B) P_{CO_2} gradient

Urine to blood P_{CO_2} gradient is used as an index of distal H^+ ion excretion

Normal U – B P_{CO_2} gradient ≥30 mm Hg

In distal RTA, U – B P_{CO_2} gradient ≤10 mm Hg

Water Deprivation and Vasopressin Test (Fig. 8)

Protocol

- This should be done in the morning hours.
- 8 hours test is enough for children.
- Restrict fluid intake; dry food is allowed.
- Weigh the child after emptying bladder.

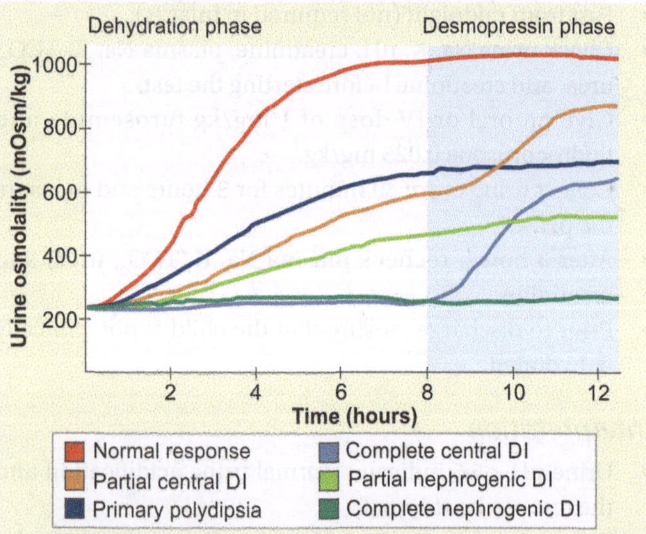

Fig. 8: Response of serum osmolality to water deprivation and desmopressin challenge test. (DI: diabetes insipidus).

- Insert an indwelling catheter if the urine output cannot be measured reliably.
- Measure baseline plasma and urine osmolality.
- Check hourly body weight.
- Measure urine amount and osmolality, serum sodium, and plasma osmolality every 2 hours for a maximum of 8 hours.
- Stop the trial if serum sodium is >150 mEq/L, body weight drops >3%, serum osmolality >300 mOsm/kg, and specific gravity and osmolality differ <30 mOsm/L in two consecutive tests
- At the end of the test, AVP is given if urinary osmolality remains low (**Table 4**). Administer 20 mg (10 IU) DDAVP intranasal or 5 IU S/C vasopressin and repeat the parameters after 2 hours.

Interpretation (Table 4)

- In normal subjects, plasma osmolality remains stable below 300 but the urine output is reduced and its osmolality rises (800–1,200).
- A patient with primary polydipsia, plasma osmolality is low normal (280 mOsm) to start with. The urine/plasma osmolality ratio rises to >2 after water deprivation.
- In patients with DI, the plasma osmolality rises but not the urine osmolality and urine to plasma osmolality ratio remains <1.5.
- Concentration of the dilute urine following DDAVP confirms central DI and no change suggests nephrogenic DI.

MICTURATING CYSTOURETHROGRAM

Micturating cystourethrogram or voiding cystourethrogram (MCU/VCUG) is an essential tool for the diagnosis and evaluation of lower urinary tract in children. It is used to obtain specific diagnostic information not already available from other modalities as it provides a visualization of the lower urinary tract. Anatomy of the lower urinary tract is well delineated with MCU. It also gives information regarding function and coordination of bladder and sphincter. Presence or absence of vesicoureteral reflux can also be determined with MCU.

A low iodine contrast is used for the procedure. There are two phases—filling and voiding phase, which provide

TABLE 4: Water deprivation and vasopressin test—interpretation.

Diagnosis	Thirst at 4 hours	Urine volume at 4 hours	Urine osmolality at 4 hours	Plasma osmolality	Urine osmolality: Plasma osmolality at 4 hours	ADH test after thirst test if urine osmolality low
Normal	±	Decrease	Increase 800–1,400	Stable <300	>2	
Primary polydipsia	Increase	Decrease	Increase	Low normal	>2	
Central DI	Increase	Same	Same Low	High	<1.5	Urine osmolality rises by >50%
Nephrogenic DI	Increase	Same	Same Low	High	<1.5	No increase

(ADH: antidiuretic hormone; DI: diabetes insipidus)

information regarding the anatomical and functional abnormalities of the urinary tract. During the filling phase, the bladder contour and early vesicourethral reflux (VUR) can be appreciated while during the voiding phase urethral anomalies and VUR can be identified. Vertebral and pelvic anomalies can be seen in the scout film.

Indications

- Evaluation of antenatally detected hydronephrosis
- Evaluation of urinary tract infection
- Diagnosis of vesicoureteral reflux
- Evaluation of neurogenic bladder
- Evaluation of urinary tract anatomical anomalies—posterior urethral valve, ureterocele, ureteral duplication, and congenital renal anomalies

Prerequisites

- Counseling parents and the child regarding the procedure with educational aids helps alleviate anxiety, stress, and apprehension.
- Written informed consent must be obtained.
- Timing of MCU—avoid during active UTI. To wait for at least 1–2 weeks after treatment of UTI
- Consumables must be arranged—infant feeding tube of appropriate size, low osmolar iodine contrast medium (150 mg/mL), isotonic saline, fluoroscopy
- Ensure that the procedure room is warm and the contrast medium is maintained at body temperature.
- Preprocedure antibiotic has to be administered—gentamicin (IM)/amikacin (IV).
- Sedation to be avoided for procedure as it interferes with voiding phase.

Calculate bladder capacity:

- *<2 years of age:* Weight (kg) × 7 = Capacity (mL)
- *>2 years of age:* [Age (years) + 2] × 30 = Capacity (mL)

Technique

1. Position the child supine on the fluoroscopy table.
2. Using sterile aseptic precautions, perform per-urethral catheterization with infant feeding tube (smaller size than for age).
3. Obtain a scout film prior to filling of the bladder.
4. Instill the contrast medium (at body temperature, 1:1 dilution with isotonic saline) gradually to fill the bladder to calculated capacity or till periurethral leak is noted.
5. Obtain anteroposterior and oblique films during early filling and full bladder phase.
6. Remove the catheter just prior to voiding (in older children) or when a periurethral leak (younger children) is noted.
7. Obtain anteroposterior and oblique films during voiding and postvoid phase.

Imaging

Intermittent fluoroscopic screening should be done and 4–6 films should be obtained:

1. Scout/control film
2. Early filling film
3. Full bladder film
4. Voiding film (anteroposterior and oblique film must be taken)
5. Full-length film postvoiding

Complications

- Catheter trauma—dysuria, increased frequency, retention, and occasionally hematuria
- Acute urinary tract infection
- Inappropriate placement of catheter in vagina
- Reactions to contrast medium
- Bladder perforation—rare

CLEAN INTERMITTENT CATHETERIZATION

Clean intermittent catheterization (CIC) involves periodic insertion of a catheter into the bladder to evacuate urine. It is an accepted method of management for individuals with voiding disorders and neurogenic bladder.

Prerequisites

- Counseling the patient and family regarding the need for the procedure and importance of compliance to technique and frequency of procedure.
- A clean environment with use of clean material is essential for performing the procedure.
- Consumables required—catheter (infant feeding tube; **Table 5**) or metal catheter), water-soluble lubricant, and hand wipes or cloth soaked with soap and water, collecting container, and four to five clean storage containers
- Maintain voiding diary.

Technique

1. Follow handwashing protocol.
2. Cleanse the perineum or penis with mild soap and water, or with a hand wipe. For girls, spread labia and clean front

TABLE 5: Infant feeding tube size (according to age and weight).

Age	*Weight (kg)*	*Catheter size (French)*
0–6 months	3.5–7	6
1 year	10	6–8
2 years	12	8
3 years	14	8–10
5 years	18	10
6 years	21	10
8 years	27	10–12
12+ years	30+	12–14

to back. For boys, if uncircumcised, pull back foreskin and clean head of penis

3. Lubricate catheter tip, hold the catheter near the tip and gently insert it into the urethra with appropriate angulation until urine flows. Do not use force; if slight resistance is felt, it may help to twist the catheter.
4. Place the other end of the catheter in the collection container before urine flows out of the catheter; hold the catheter in place until urine flow stops. Keep a record of volume of urine drained.
5. Withdraw the catheter gently and slowly; there is often an additional gush of urine.
6. Clean the catheter under running water. The catheter is then left hung to dry or placed on a clean, dry towel in a clean area. Once dried, store in a clean container. The catheter can be reused multiple times till it becomes cloudy or too soft to pass.
7. Repeat procedure of CIC once every 2–3 hours (cycle between four and five catheters in a day. Once a catheter is used, washed, and dried, place in a dry numbered container. Use this catheter again after the other four catheters have been used).
8. Connect catheter to drain bag overnight.

Complications

- Urinary tract infections—can be reduced by strict hand hygiene
- Urethral trauma
- Hematuria
- Urinary leaks

KEY POINTS

- There are many procedures in pediatric nephrology which are essential to accurate diagnosis of underlying etiopathology and those required therapeutically for initiation of kidney replacement therapy.
- Following standard protocols make these procedures effective and safe for the patients.

SUGGESTED READING

1. Al-Imam OA, Al-Nosur NM, Al-Khulaifat. Which is the best way of performing a micturating cystourethrogram in children? Saudi J Kidney Dis Transpl. 2008;19(1):20-5.
2. Bagga A, Sinha A. Renal tubular acidosis. Indian J Pediatr. 2020;87(9):733-44.
3. Daugirdas JT, Blake PG, Ing TS. Handbook of Dialysis, 5th edition. New Delhi: Wolters Kluwer; 2015.
4. de Galasso L, Picca S, Guzzo I. Dialysis modalities for the management of pediatric acute kidney injury. Pediatr Nephrol. 2020;35(5):753-65.
5. Hogan JJ, Mocanu M, Berns JS. The Native Kidney Biopsy: Update and Evidence for Best Practice. Clin J Am Soc Nephrol. 2016;11:354-62.
6. Mantan M, Batra V. Renal biopsy in children. Indian Pediatr. 2020;57:452-58.
7. Phadke K, Goodyer P, Bitzan M. Manual of Pediatric Nephrology, 1st edition. Berlin, Germany: Springer; 2014.
8. Raina R, Vijayaraghavan P, Kapur G, Sethi SK, Krishnappa V, Kumar D, et al. Hemodialysis in neonates and infants: A systematic review. Semin Dial. 2018;31:289-99.
9. Saran R, Robinson B, Abbott KC, Agodoa LYC, Bragg-Gresham J, Balkrishnan R, et al. US Renal Data System 2018 Annual Data Report: epidemiology of kidney disease in the United States. Am J Kidney Dis. 2019;73(3)(Suppl 1):SVII.

CHAPTER

15.4 Links to Key Guidelines and Registries

Soumya Reddy

Nephrotic syndrome	
PodoNet (Europe)	*http://www.podonet.org/index.php?id=home*
NURTuRE (UK)	*https://www.nurturebiobank.org/*
INSIGHT (Canada)	*https://clinicaltrials.gov/ct2/show/NCT01605266*
NEPTUNE (US)	*https://www.neptune-study.org/*
FOrME (Germany)	*https://www.clinicaltrials.gov/ct2/show/NCT03949972*
SUCCESS (China)	*https://clinicaltrials.gov/ct2/show/NCT03001934*
Lupus nephritis	
RELESSER-TRANS	*https://pubmed.ncbi.nlm.nih.gov/26945378/*
Lupus Clinical Trials Consortium	*https://lupustrials.org*
CARRA (US)	*https://carragroup.org/research-reglstry*
Multicentre Registry (China)	*https://clinicaltrials.gov/ct2/show/NCT03791827*
CKD and transplant	
NAPRTCS	*https://naprtcs.org/*
CKiD	*https://clinicaltrials.gov/ct2/show/NCT00327860*
ESPN/ERA-EDTA	*https://espn-reg.org/index.jsp*
IPNA Global KRT	*https://theipna.org/programs/registry/*
USRDS	*https://www.usrds.org/*
OPTN	*https://optn.transplant.hrsa.gov/*
ANZDATA	*https://www.anzdata.org.au/*
Others	
Rare Kidney Stone Consortium Registry • Primary hyperoxaluria • Dent's disease	*https://www.mayo.edu/research/departments-divisions/department-internal-medicine/division-nephrology-hypertension/rare-kidney-stone-consortium-registry/rare-kidney-stone-consortium-registry*
Primary hyperoxaluria	*https://www.ohf.org/patient-registry/*
Polycystic kidney disease	*https://connect.pkdcure.org/*
Cystinosis	*https://www.cystinosisresearch.org/cure-cystinosis-international-registry/*
ASTOR (Alport syndrome)	*https://astor.umn.edu/*
Global aHUS	*https://clinicaltrials.gov/ct2/show/NCT01522183?term=eculizumab*
RaDaR	*https://renal.org/rare-renal/radar*
International Registry of COVID infection in glomerulonephritis (IRoc-GN)	*https://pubmed.ncbi.nlm.nih.gov/33181156/*

(CKD: chronic kidney disease; COVID: coronavirus disease)

GUIDELINES AND RECOMMENDATIONS

Nephrotic Syndrome

- KDIGO Clinical Practice Guideline On Glomerular Diseases, 2020.
  https://kdigo.org/guidelines/gd/
- IPNA clinical practice recommendations for the diagnosis and management of children with steroid-resistant nephrotic syndrome, 2020
  https://pubmed.ncbi.nlm.nih.gov/32382828/
  DOI: 10.1007/s00467-020-04519-1
- ISPN Consensus Guidelines on Management of Steroid-resistant Nephrotic Syndrome, 2020
  https://www.indianpediatrics.net/epub012021/RECOMM-00278.pdf
- ISPN Steroid Sensitive Nephrotic Syndrome: Revised Guidelines, 2021
  https://europepmc.org/article/MED/33742610
- ERKNet-ESPN Consensus Statement on Genetic Aspects of Congenital Nephrotic Syndrome
  https://doi.org/10.1038/s41431-020-0642-8
- *Management of congenital nephrotic syndrome:* Consensus recommendations of the ERKNet-ESPN Working Group
  https://doi.org/10.1038/s41581-020-00384-1

Other Glomerular Disorders

- KDIGO Clinical Practice Guideline on Glomerular Diseases, 2020
  https://kdigo.org/guidelines/gd/
- *Consensus statement on standards and guidelines for the molecular diagnostics of Alport syndrome:* Refining the ACMG criteria, 2021
  https://www.nature.com/articles/s41431-021-00858-1
  DOI: 10.1038/s41431-021-00858-1
- Expert consensus guidelines for the genetic diagnosis of Alport syndrome, 2019.
  https://doi.org/10.1007/s00467-018-3985-4
- Expert guidelines for the management of Alport syndrome and thin basement membrane nephropathy, 2013.
  https://pubmed.ncbi.nlm.nih.gov/23349312/
  DOI: 10.1681/ASN.2012020148
- Clinical practice recommendations for the treatment of Alport syndrome: a statement of the Alport Syndrome Research Collaborative, 2013.
  https://pubmed.ncbi.nlm.nih.gov/22461141/
  DOI: 10.1007/s00467-012-2138-4

Hemolytic Uremic Syndrome

- Hemolytic uremic syndrome in a developing country: Consensus guidelines, 2019.
  https://doi.org/10.1007/s00467-019-04233-7
- An international consensus approach to the management of atypical hemolytic uremic syndrome in children, 2015.
  https://www.researchgate.net/publication/281838127_An_international_consensus_approach_to_the_management_of_atypical_hemolytic_uremic_syndrome_in_children.
  DOI: 10.1007/s00467-015-3076-8

Acute Kidney Injury

- *Kidney Disease:* Improving Global Outcomes (KDIGO) 2012 Clinical Practice Guideline for Acute Kidney Injury (AKI).
  https://kdigo.org/guidelines/acute-kidney-injury/
- ISPD guidelines for peritoneal dialysis in acute kidney injury: 2020 update.
  https://doi.org/10.1177%2F0896860820970834

Tubular Disorders

- Diagnosis and management of Bartter syndrome: Executive summary of the consensus and recommendations from the European Rare Kidney Disease Reference Network Working Group for Tubular Disorders, 2021.
  https://doi.org/10.1016/j.kint.2020.10.035
- Distal Renal Tubular Acidosis: ERKNet/ESPN Clinical Practice Points 2021.
  https://pubmed.ncbi.nlm.nih.gov/33914889/
  DOI: 10.1093/ndt/gfab171
- *Cystinuria:* Clinical Practice Recommendations, 2020.
  https://doi.org/10.1016/j.kint.2020.06.035
- Clinical practice recommendations for the diagnosis and management of X-linked hypophosphataemia, 2019.
  https://doi.org/10.1038/s41581-019-0152-5
- International consensus statement on the diagnosis and management of autosomal dominant polycystic kidney disease in children and young people, 2019.
  https://doi.org/10.1038/s41581-019-0155-2
- *Gitelman syndrome:* Consensus and guidance from a Kidney Disease: Improving Global Outcomes (KDIGO) Controversies Conference, 2017.
  https://doi.org/10.1016/j.kint.2016.09.046
- *Cystinosis in adult and adolescent patients:* Recommendations for the comprehensive care of cystinosis, 2015.
  https://pubmed.ncbi.nlm.nih.gov/26523297/
  DOI: 10.1016/j.nefroe.2015.06.010
- Consensus Expert Recommendations for the Diagnosis and Management of Autosomal Recessive Polycystic Kidney Disease: Report of an International Conference, 2014.
  https://doi.org/10.1016/j.jpeds.2014.06.015
- *Primary hyperoxaluria Type 1:* Indications for screening and guidance for diagnosis and treatment. ERA-EDTA Position Statement, 2012.
  https://doi.org/10.1093/ndt/gfs078

Urinary Tract Infections

- Brazilian consensus on vesicoureteral reflux-recommendations for clinical practice, 2020.
  https://www.scielo.br/j/ibju/a/k74v7s3c8GYZBh5DWRYFRbL/?lang=en.
  DOI: 10.1590/S1677-5538.IBJU.2019.0401
- European Association of Urology Guidelines on Urological Infections, 2019.
  https://uroweb.org/guideline/urological-infections/
- Summary of the UAA-AAUS guidelines for urinary tract infections, 2018.
  https://pubmed.ncbi.nlm.nih.gov/29193372/
  DOI: 10.1111/iju.13493
- *Executive summary of the diagnosis and treatment of urinary tract infection:* Guidelines of the Spanish Society of Clinical Microbiology and Infectious Diseases (SEIMC), 2017.
  https://pubmed.ncbi.nlm.nih.gov/28017477/
  DOI: 10.1016/j.eimc.2016.11.005
- Polish Society of Pediatric Nephrology recommendations for the management of children with urinary tract infection, 2015.
  http://ptnfd.org/
- *Canadian Paediatric Society Urinary Tract Infection in Infants and Children:* Diagnosis and Management, 2014
  https://doi.org/10.1093/pch/19.6.315

- Australian Clinical Practice Guidelines: Diagnosis and Treatment of Urinary Tract Infection in Children, 2014. *https://www.clinicalguidelines.gov.au/portal/2413/* diagnosis-and-treatment-urinary-tract-infection-children
- Indian Society of Pediatric Nephrology. Revised statement on management of urinary tract infections, 2011. *https://www.indianpediatrics.net/sep2011/sep-709-717.htm*
- Clinical practice guideline for the diagnosis and management of the initial UTI in febrile infants and children 2-24 months 2011 (Reaffirmation 2016). *https://doi.org/10.1542/peds.2011-1330*
- *Urinary tract infection in under 16s:* Diagnosis and management NICE, 2007 (Updated 2018). *https://www.nice.org.uk/guidance/cg54*

Chronic Kidney Disease

- *Kidney Disease:* Improving Global Outcomes (KDIGO). 2012 Clinical Practice Guideline for the Evaluation and Management of Chronic Kidney Disease (CKD). *https://kdigo.org/guidelines/ckd-evaluation-and-management/*
- *Anemia:*
  - *Kidney Disease:* Improving Global Outcomes (KDIGO) 2012 Clinical Practice Guideline for Anemia in Chronic Kidney Disease. *https://kdigo.org/guidelines/anemia-in-ckd/*
  - KDOQI US Commentary on the 2012 KDIGO Clinical Practice Guideline for Anemia in CKD. *http://www.ajkd.org/article/S0272-6386(13)00978-5/fulltext*
- *Mineral bone disease:*
  - *Kidney Disease:* Improving Global Outcomes (KDIGO) 2017 Clinical Practice Guideline Update for the Diagnosis, Evaluation, Prevention, and Treatment of chronic kidney disease–mineral and bone disorder (CKD-MBD). *https://kdigo.org/guidelines/ckd-mbd/*
  - KDOQI US Commentary on the 2017 KDIGO Clinical Practice Guideline Update for the Diagnosis, Evaluation, Prevention, and Treatment of Chronic Kidney Disease-Mineral and Bone Disorder (CKD-MBD). *http://www.ajkd.org/article/S0272-6386(17)30898-3/fulltext*
- *Nutrition in CKD (PRNT recommendations):*
  - Energy and protein requirements for children with CKD stages 2–5 and on dialysis—Clinical Practice Recommendations from the Pediatric Renal Nutrition Taskforce, 2019. *https://link.springer.com/article/10.1007%2Fs00467-019-04426-0*
  - The dietary management of calcium and phosphate in children with CKD stages 2–5 and on dialysis—clinical practice recommendation from the Pediatric Renal Nutrition Taskforce 2019. *https://link.springer.com/article/10.1007/s00467-019-04370-z*
  - Assessment of nutritional status in children with kidney diseases—clinical practice recommendations from the Pediatric Renal Nutrition Taskforce, 2020. *https://link.springer.com/article/10.1007/s00467-020-04852-5*
  - Delivery of a nutritional prescription by enteral tube feeding in children with chronic kidney disease stages 2–5 and on dialysis—clinical practice recommendations from the Pediatric Renal Nutrition Taskforce, 2021. *https://link.springer.com/article/10.1007/s00467-020-04623-2*
  - The dietary management of potassium in children with CKD stages 2-5 and on dialysis—clinical practice recommendations from the Pediatric Renal Nutrition Taskforce, 2021. *https://link.springer.com/article/10.1007/s00467-021-04923-1*
  - KDOQI Clinical Practice Guideline for Nutrition in CKD: 2020 Update. *https://www.ajkd.org/issue/S0272-6386(20)X0010-2*
- *Hypertension:*
  - KDIGO 2021 Clinical Practice Guideline for the Management of Blood Pressure in Chronic Kidney Disease. *https://kdigo.org/guidelines/blood-pressure-in-ckd/*
- *Kidney Disease:* Improving Global Outcomes (KDIGO) 2020 Clinical Practice Guideline for Diabetes Management in Chronic Kidney Disease (CKD). *https://kdigo.org/guidelines/diabetes-ckd/*
- *Kidney Disease:* Improving Global Outcomes (KDIGO) 2018 Clinical Practice Guideline for the Prevention, Diagnosis, Evaluation, and Treatment of Hepatitis C in Chronic Kidney Disease. *https://kdigo.org/guidelines/hepatitis-c-in-ckd/*
- *Kidney Disease:* Improving Global Outcomes (KDIGO) 2013 Clinical Practice Guideline for Lipid Management in Chronic Kidney Disease (CKD). *https://kdigo.org/guidelines/lipids-in-ckd/*

Dialysis

- KDOQI Clinical Practice Guideline for Hemodialysis: 2015 Update. *http://www.ajkd.org/article/S0272-6386(15)01019-7/fulltext*
- KDOQI Clinical Practice Guideline for Vascular Access: 2019 Update. *https://www.ajkd.org/article/S0272-6386(19)31137-0/fulltext*

- ISPD recommendations for the evaluation of peritoneal membrane dysfunction in adults: Classification, measurement, interpretation and rationale for intervention, 2021.
  https://doi.org/10.1177/0896860820982218
- *ISPD practice recommendations:* Prescribing high-quality goal-directed peritoneal dialysis, 2020.
  https://journals.sagepub.com/doi/full/10.1177/0896860819895364
- *ISPD Peritonitis Recommendations:* 2016 Update on Prevention and Treatment.
  https://journals.sagepub.com/doi/pdf/10.3747/pdi.2016.00078
- *ISPD Catheter-related Infection Recommendations:* 2017 Update.
  https://journals.sagepub.com/doi/pdf/10.3747/pdi.2016.00120
- KDOQI Peritoneal Dialysis Adequacy, 2006.
  http://kidneyfoundation.cachefly.net/professionals/KDOQI/guideline_upHD_PD_VA/index.htm

Transplant

- *Kidney Disease:* Improving Global Outcomes (KDIGO) 2020 Clinical Practice Guideline on the Evaluation and Management of Candidates for Kidney Transplantation.
  https://kdigo.org/guidelines/transplant-candidate/
- *Kidney Disease:* Improving Global Outcomes (KDIGO) 2017 Clinical Practice Guideline on the Evaluation and Care of Living Kidney Donors.
  https://kdigo.org/guidelines/living-kidney-donor/

Index

Page numbers followed by *b* refer to box, *f* refer to figure, *fc* refer to flowchart, and *t* refer to table.

A

C

D

E

G

M

N

S

T

U

V

W

X

Y

Z